*Compliments of*

THE
ROXANE
INSTITUTE
AND
ROXANE
LABORATORIES,
INC.

# PRINCIPLES AND PRACTICE OF
# SUPPORTIVE ONCOLOGY

# PRINCIPLES AND PRACTICE OF
# SUPPORTIVE ONCOLOGY

*Edited by*

**Ann Berger,** R.N., M.S.N., M.D.
*Assistant Professor of Oncology/Anesthesiology*
*Director of Supportive Care Services*
*Cooper Cancer Institute*
*Cooper Hospital University Medical Center*
*Camden, New Jersey*
*and*
*Medical Director,*
*Lighthouse Hospice/Alternative Hospice Solutions, Inc.*
*Atlanta, Georgia*


**Russell K. Portenoy,** M.D.
*Chairman*
*Department of Pain Medicine and Palliative Care*
*Beth Israel Medical Center*
*New York, New York*


**David E. Weissman,** M.D.
*Professor of Medicine*
*Department of Medicine, Division of Hematology/Oncology*
*Medical College Of Wisconsin*
*Milwaukee, Wisconsin*

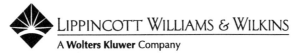

LIPPINCOTT WILLIAMS & WILKINS
A **Wolters Kluwer** Company
Philadelphia · Baltimore · New York · London
Buenos Aires · Hong Kong · Sydney · Tokyo

Manufacturing Manager: Dennis Teston
Production Manager: Larry Bernstein
Production Editor: Pamela Blamey
Cover Designer: Karen Quigley
Indexer: Dorothy Hoffman
Compositor: Lippincott Williams & Wilkins Desktop Division
Printer: Maple Press

Printed in the United States of America

9  8  7  6  5  4  3  2

**Library of Congress Cataloging-in-Publication Data**
Principles and practice of supportive oncology / edited by Ann Berger,
    Russell K. Portenoy, David E. Weissman.
        p.   cm.
    Includes bibliographical references and index.
    ISBN 0-397-51559-6
    1. Cancer—Palliative treatment.   2. Cancer—Complications—Treatment.   3. Cancer pain—Treatment.   I. Berger, Ann.   II. Portenoy, Russell K.   III. Weissman, David E. (David Edward),
1955–
    [DNLM:   1. Neoplasms—therapy.   2. Neoplasms—complications.
3. Pain, Intractable—therapy.   4. Palliative Care. QZ 266 P957 1997]
    RC271.P33P75   1997
    616.99′406—dc21
    DNLM/DLC
    For Library of Congress                                    97-41365
    CIP

To our spouses and children whose love and support make our work possible

Carl, Stephen, Rebecca
Susan, Matthew, Jason, Allison
Mimi, Dan, Aaron

# Contents

# Contributors

**Caroline M. Apovian, M.D.**
*Spence Center for Women's Health*
*300 Granite Street*
*Braintree, Massachusetts 02184*

**Sally S. Bailey, M.P.S.**
*35 North Forest Circle*
*West Haven, Connecticut 06515*

**David Barnard, Ph.D.**
*University Professor of Humanities and Chair*
*Department of Humanities, MC H134*
*The Pennsylvania State University*
*  College of Medicine*
*P.O. Box 850*
*Hershey, Pennsylvania 17033-0850*

**Linda M. Bartoshuk, M.D.**
*Department of Surgery, Section of*
*  Otolaryngology, 248 BML*
*Yale University School of Medicine*
*333 Cedar Street*
*New Haven, Connecticut 06520-8041*

**Ann M. Berger, R.N., M.S.N., M.D.**
*Director of Supportive Care Services*
*Department of Oncology and Anesthesiology*
*Cooper Hospital/University Medical Center*
*Three Cooper Plaza*
*Camden, New Jersey 08103*
*Medical Director of Lighthouse Hospice/*
*  Alternative Hospice Solutions, Inc.*
*3620 DeKalb Technology Parkway, Suite 2120*
*Atlanta, Georgia 30340*

**Julie A. Biller, M.D.**
*Assistant Professor*
*Medicine and Pediatrics*
*Medical College of Wisconsin*
*9200 West Wisconsin Ave., Box 194*
*Milwaukee, Wisconsin 53226*

**J. Andrew Billings, M.D.**
*Assistant Clinical Professor*
*Director, Palliative Care Service*
*Massachusetts General Hospital*
*55 Fruit Street, Founders 604*
*Boston, Massachusetts 02114*

**George L. Blackburn, M.D., Ph.D.**
*Associate Professor of Surgery*
*Department of Surgery*
*Nutrition Support Service*
*Harvard Medical School/*
*  Beth Israel Deaconess Medical Center*
*One Deaconess Road*
*Boston, Massachusetts 02215*

**Howard Brody, M.D., Ph.D.**
*Professor, Family Practice and Philosophy*
*Director, Center for Ethics and Humanities in*
*  the Life Sciences*
*Michigan State University*
*B-100 Clinical Center*
*East Lansing, Michigan 48824*

**Eduardo Bruera, M.D.**
*Professor of Oncology*
*Palliative Care Program*
*University of Alberta*
*Grey Nuns Community Hospital & Health Centre*
*1100 Youville Drive West, Rm. 4324*
*Edmonton, Alberta T6L 5X8*
*Canada*

**Augusto T. Caraceni, M.D.**
*Attending Neurologist*
*Pain Therapy and Palliative Care Division*
*National Cancer Institute of Milano*
*Via Venezia 1*
*20133 Milano*
*Italy*

**Nathan I. Cherny, M.B.B.S., F.R.A.C.P.**
*Department of Medical Oncology*
*Shaare Zedek Medical Center*
*Jerusalem 91031, Israel*

**Elizabeth J. Clark, Ph.D., M.P.H.**
*President*
*National Coalition for Cancer Survivorship*
*1010 Wayne Ave.*
*Silver Spring, Maryland 20910*

**James F. Cleary, M.B., B.S., F.R.A.C.P.**
*Assistant Professor of Medicine*
*Department of Medicine*
*University of Wisconsin*
*K6/518, 600 Highland Avenue*
*Madison, Wisconsin 53792*

**Lawrence R. Coia, M.D.**
*Chairman, Department of Radiation Oncology*
*Community Medical Center*
*99 Highway 37 West*
*Toms River, New Jersey 08755*

**Kevin C. Conlon, M.D., F.A.C.S., F.R.C.S.I., M.B.A.**
*Assistant Professor of Surgery*
*Department of Surgery*
*Memorial Sloan-Kettering Cancer Center*
*1275 York Avenue*
*New York, New York 10021*

**Jeffrey Crawford, M.D.**
*Associate Professor of Medicine*
*Duke University Medical Center*
*P.O. Box 3198*
*Durham, North Carolina 27710*

**Edward T. Creagan, M.D.**
*Consultant, Division of Medical Oncology*
*Professor, Mayo Medical School*
*Department of Medical Oncology*
*The Mayo Clinic*
*200 First Street, SW*
*Rochester, Minnesota 55905*

**David L. Crosby, M.D.**
*Associate Professor of Dermatology*
*Department of Dermatology*
*Medical College of Wisconsin*
*9200 West Wisconsin Avenue*
*Milwaukee, Wisconsin 53226*

**Dorothy Doughty, R.N., M.N., C.E.T.N.**
*Program Director, Wound Ostomy Continence*
*Nursing Education Program*
*Emory University*
*1365 Clifton Road NE, Room M-213*
*Atlanta, Georgia 30322*

**Valerie B. Duffy, Ph.D., R.D.**
*School of Allied Health*
*University of Connecticut*
*Storrs, Connecticut 06269-2101*

**Neil M. Ellison, M.D.**
*Clinical Professor of Medicine*
*Geisinger Medical Center*
*100 North Academy Avenue*
*Danville, Pennsylvania 17822*

**Linda L. Emanuel, M.D., Ph.D.**
*Vice President for Ethics Standards*
*Ethics Standards Division*
*American Medical Association*
*515 N. State Street*
*Chicago, Illinois 60610*

**Barbara G. Fallon, M.D.**
*Assistant Professor of Medicine*
*University of Connecticut School of Medicine*
*Hematology/Oncology Department*
*New Britain General Hospital*
*100 Grand Street*
*New Britain, Connecticut 06050*

**Margaret L. Farncombe, M.D.**
*Palliative Care*
*Queensway-Carleton*
*1455 Woodroffe*
*Nepean, Ontario*
*KZG 1W1, Canada*

**John T. Farrar, M.D.**
*Department of Neurology*
*University of Pennsylvania*
*3400 Spruce Street, 3 West Gates Building*
*Philadelphia, Pennsylvania 19104-4283*

**Katharine Fast**
*Department of Surgery*
*Section of Otolaryngology*
*Yale University School of Medicine*
*333 Cedar Street*
*New Haven, Connecticut 06520-8041*

**Betty R. Ferrell, R.N., Ph.D., F.A.A.N.**
*Associate Research Scientist*
*Department of Nursing Research and Education*
*City of Hope National Medical Center*
*1500 East Duarte Road*
*Duarte, California 91010*

**Bruce A. Ferrell, M.D.**
*Associate Professor of Medicine*
*Department of Geriatric Medicine*
*UCLA School of Medicine and Sepulveda VA*
   *Medical Center*
*16111 Plummer Street*
*Sepulveda, California 91343*

**Alan B. Fleischer, Jr., M.D.**
*Department of Dermatology*
*Wake Forest University Medical Center*
*Medical Center Boulevard*
*Winston-Salem, North Carolina 27157-1071*

**Walter B. Forman, M.D.**
*Professor of Medicine*
*Department of Internal Medicine*
*University of New Mexico*
   *Health Sciences Center*
*2211 Lomas NE*
*Alburquerque, New Mexico 87108*

**Margaret T. Goldberg, R.N., M.S.N., C.E.T.N.**
*118 Hedgerow Drive*
*Cherry Hill, New Jersey 08002*

**Richard M. Goldberg, M.D.**
*Associate Professor of Oncology*
*Department of Medical Oncology*
*The Mayo Clinic*
*200 First Street SW*
*Rochester, Minnesota 55905-0001*

**Richard E. Greenberg, M.D.**
*Clinical Professor of Urology*
*Department of Surgical Oncology*
*Fox Chase Cancer Center*
*7701 Burholme Avenue*
*Philadelphia, Pennsylvania 19111*

**Neil A. Hagen, M.D.**
*Associate Professor of Neurology*
*Department of Clinical Neurosciences*
*University of Calgary*
*1331 29th Street NW*
*Calgary, Alberta T2N 4N2*
*Canada*

**Wendy S. Harpham, M.D.**
*Attending Physician*
*Department of Internal Medicine*
*Presbyterian Hospital of Dallas*
*8200 Walnut Hill Lane*
*Dallas, Texas 75231*

**Steven J. Hirshberg, M.D.**
*Clinical Instructor of Urology*
*Temple University School of Medicine*
*Philadelphia, Pennsylvania 19140*

**Jane M. Ingham, M.B.B.S., F.R.A.C.P.**
*Lombardi Cancer Center*
*Georgetown University Medical Center*
*3800 Resevoir Road*
*Washington, D.C. 20007*

**Nora A. Janjan, M.D.**
*Associate Professor of Radiation Oncology*
*Department of Radiation Oncology*
*The University of Texas,*
   *M.D. Anderson Cancer Center*
*1515 Holcombe Boulevard, Box 97*
*Houston, Texas 77030*

**Albert L. Jochen, M.D.**
*Associate Professor of Medicine*
*Department of Medicine*
*Medical College of Wisconsin*
*9200 West Wisconsin Avenue*
*Milwaukee, Wisconsin 53226*

**Eileen M. Johnston, M.D.**
*Fellow in Hematology and Oncology*
*Duke University Medical Center*
*P.O. Box 3841*
*25125 Morris Building*
*Durham, North Carolina 27710*

**Thomas J. Kilroy, D.D.S.**
*5400 West Jewell*
*Denver, Colorado 80230*

**Michael L. Kochman, M.D.**
*Assistant Professor of Medicine*
*Department of Medicine,*
   *Gastroenterology Division*
*University of Pennsylvania*
*3 Raudin, 3400 Spruce Street*
*Philadelphia, Pennsylvania 19104*

**Mark G. Kris, M.D.**
*Chief, Thoracic Oncology Service*
*Memorial Sloan-Kettering Cancer Center*
*Professor of Medicine*
*Cornell University Medical College*
*1275 York Avenue*
*New York, New York 10021*

**Elisabeth A. Lachmann, M.D.**
*Assistant Professor of Rehabilitation
   Medicine in Surgery*
*Cornell University Medical College*
*Associate Attending Physiatrist*
*Department of Rehabilitation Medicine*
*The New York Hospital*
*525 East 68th Street, Box 142*
*New York, New York 10021*

**Steven B. Leder, Ph.D.**
*Associate Professor of Surgery*
*Department of Surgery, Section of Otolaryngology*
*Yale University School of Medicine*
*P.O. Box 208041*
*New Haven, Connecticut 06520-8041*

**Susan A. Leigh, R.N., B.S.N.**
*Cancer Survivorship Consultant*
*5050 East Golder Ranch Road*
*Tucson, Arizona 85739*

**Randolph J. Lipchik, M.D.**
*Associate Professor of Medicine*
*Department of Pulmonary and Critical Care
   Medicine*
*Medical College of Wisconsin*
*9200 West Wisconsin Avenue*
*Milwaukee, Wisconsin 53226*

**W. Scott Long, M.D.**
*Connecticut Hospice*
*61 Burban Drive*
*Branford, Connecticut 06405*

**Charles L. Loprinzi, M.D.**
*Professor and Chair*
*Department of Medical Oncology*
*The Mayo Clinic*
*200 First Street SW*
*Rochester, Minnesota 55905-0001*

**Matthew J. Loscalzo, M.S.W.**
*Research Associate*
*Department of Oncology*
*The Johns Hopkins University School
   of Medicine*
*600 North Wolfe Street*
*Baltimore, Maryland 21287-8931*

**Laurie A. Lucchina**
*Department of Surgery*
*Section of Otolaryngology*
*Yale University School of Medicine*
*333 Cedar Street*
*New Haven, Connecticut 06520-8041*

**Mary Jane Massie, M.D.**
*Director, Barbara White Fishman Center for
   Psychological Counseling*
*Memorial Sloan-Kettering Cancer Center*
*Department of Psychiatry*
*Cornell University Medical College*
*1275 York Avenue*
*New York, New York 10021*

**Sebastiano Mercadante, M.D.**
*Chief, Pain Relief and Palliative Care*
*S.A.M.O.T.*
*Via Liberta, 191*
*90143 Palermo*
*Italy*

**Christine Miaskowski, R.N., Ph.D.,
   F.A.A.N.**
*Professor and Chair*
*Department of Physiological Nursing*
*University of California, San Francisco*
*School of Nursing*
*Third and Parnassus Avenues*
*Room N-6114, Box 0610*
*San Francisco, California 94143*

**Jason R. Michaels, M.D.**
*Resident, Dermatology*
*Texas Tech University
   Health Sciences Center*
*Lubbock, Texas 79430*

**A. Ross Morton, M.D., M.R.C.P. (UK),
   F.R.C.P.C.**
*Associate Professor of Medicine*
*Department of Medicine*
*Queen's University/Kingston General Hospital*
*76 Stuart Street*
*Kingston, Ontario K7L 2V7*
*Canada*

**John R. Murren, M.D.**
*Associate Professor of Medicine*
*Department of Medicine*
*Yale University School of Medicine*
*333 Cedar Street, NSB 287*
*New Haven, Connecticut 06520*

**Ursula S. Ofman, Psy.D.**
*Private Practice*
*155 East 29th Street*
*New York, New York 10016-6306*

**Karen S. Ogle, M.D.**
*Professor, Family Practice*
*Director, Palliative Care Educational*
*    Research Program*
*College of Human Medicine,*
*    Michigan State University*
*B110 Clinical Center*
*East Lansing, Michigan 48824*

**Irene M. O'Shaughnessy, M.D.**
*Medical College of Wisconsin*
*Department of Endocrinology*
*9200 West Wisconsin Avenue, MCW-CF*
*Milwaukee, Wisconsin 53226*

**Steven D. Passik, Ph.D.**
*Community Cancer Care, Inc.*
*115 West 19th Street*
*Indianapolis, Indiana 46202*

**David K. Payne, Ph.D.**
*Psychiatry Service*
*Memorial Sloan-Kettering Cancer Center*
*1275 York Avenue*
*New York, New York 10021*

**Richard Payne, M.D.**
*Professor of Medicine (Neurology)*
*Department of Neuro-oncology*
*M.D. Anderson Cancer Center*
*1515 Holcombe Boulevard, Box 008*
*Houston, Texas 77030-4095*

**Prema P. Peethambaram, M.B., B.S., D.C.H.**
*Senior Associate Consultant*
*Department of Medical Oncology*
*The Mayo Clinic*
*200 First Street SW, East 12B*
*Rochester, Minnesota 55905-0001*

**Wayne H. Pinover, D.O.**
*Associate Member*
*Department of Radiation Oncology*
*Fox Chase Cancer Center*
*7701 Burholme Avenue*
*Philadelphia, Pennsylvania 19111*

**Katherine M.W. Pisters, M.D.**
*Assistant Professor of Medicine*
*Thoracic/Head and Neck Medical Oncology*
*University of Texas, M.D. Anderson Cancer*
*    Center*
*1515 Holcombe Boulevard, Box 80*
*Houston, Texas 77030*

**Rosemary C. Polomano, Ph.D., R.N., F.A.A.N.**
*Pain Clinical Nurse Specialist*
*Department of Surgical Nursing*
*University of Pennsylvania Medical Center*
*3400 Spruce Street*
*Philadelphia, Pennsylvania 19465*

**Russell K. Portenoy, M.D.**
*Chairman*
*Department of Pain Medicine and*
*    Palliative Care*
*Beth Israel Medical Center*
*First Avenue at 16th Street*
*New York, New York 10003*

**Carla Ripamonti, M.D.**
*Adjunct Clinical Professor of Oncology*
*Department of Oncology*
*University of Alberta*
*Edmonton, Canada*
*Deputy Director, Pain Therapy and*
*    Palliative Care Division*
*National Cancer Institute*
*Via Venezian, 1*
*20133 Milano, Italy*

**Paul S. Ritch, M.D.**
*Professor of Medicine*
*Department of Medicine, Division of*
*    Hematology/Oncology*
*Medical College of Wisconsin*
*9200 W. Wisconsin Avenue*
*Milwaukee, Wisconsin 53226*

**Lary A. Robinson, M.D.**
*Associate Professor of Surgery*
*Director, Division of Cardiovascular and*
*    Thoracic Surgery*
*Department of Cardiothroacic Surgery*
*H. Lee Moffitt Cancer Center and Research*
*    Institute*
*University of South Florida*
*12902 Magnolia Drive*
*Tampa, Florida 33612-9497*

**Sari L. Roth-Roemer, Ph.D.**
*Assistant Professor*
*Department of Psychiatry and Behavioral*
*    Sciences*
*University of Washington School of Medicine*
*Fred Hutchinson Cancer Research Center*
*1100 Fairview Avenue North, FM815*
*Seattle, Washington 98109-1024*

**John C. Ruckdeschel, M.D.**
*Professor of Medicine*
*H. Lee Moffitt Cancer Center and Research*
  *Institute*
*University of South Florida*
*12902 Magnolia Drive*
*Tampa, Florida 33612-9497*

**Lloyd R. Saberski, M.D.**
*Director, Yale Center for Pain Management*
*Associate Clinical Professor*
*Department of Anesthesiology*
*Yale-New Haven Hospital*
*40 Temple Street*
*New Haven, Connecticut 06510*

**Richard G. Schmidt, M.D.**
*Director*
*The Musculoskeletal Tumor and Limb*
  *Reconstruction Center*
*15 North Presidential Blvd. #300*
*Bala Cynwyd, Pennsylvania 19004*

**Michelle Z. Schultz, M.D.**
*Assistant Professor of Medicine*
*Division of Hematology/Oncology*
*Washington University/St. Louis Veterans Affairs*
  *Medical Center*
*915 North Grand Boulevard*
*St. Louis, Missouri 63106*

**Robyn S. Shapiro, J.D.**
*Director and Professor*
*Center for the Study of Bioethics*
*Medical College of Wisconsin*
*8701 Watertown Plank Road*
*Milwaukee, Wisconsin 53226*

**Roland T. Skeel, M.D.**
*Professor, Chief*
*Division of Hematology/Oncology*
*Department of Medicine*
*Medical College of Ohio*
*Richard D. Ruppert Health Center*
*3120 Glendale Avenue*
*Toledo, Ohio 43614-5809*

**Michael C. Soulen, M.D.**
*Associate Professor of Radiology and Surgery*
*Department of Interventional Radiology*
*University of Pennsylvania*
*3400 Spruce Street*
*Philadelphia, Pennsylvania 19104*

**Christopher D. Still, M.S., Ph.D.**
*Associate Physician*
*Department of Internal Medicine*
*Geisinger Medical Center*
*Danville, Pennsylvania 17822*

**Porter Storey, M.D.**
*The Hospice at the Texas*
  *Medical Center*
*1515 Holcombe Boulevard*
*Houston, Texas 77030-4123*

**Barbara A. Supanich, R.S.M., M.D.**
*Assistant Professor of Family Practice*
*Department of Family Practice*
*Michigan State University*
*B100 Clinical Center*
*East Lansing, Michigan 48824*

**Karen L. Syrjala, Ph.D.**
*Associate Professor*
*Department of Biobehavioral Sciences*
*University of Washington School of Medicine*
*Fred Hutchinson Cancer*
  *Research Center*
*1100 Fairview Avenue North, FM815*
*Seattle, Washington 98104-1024*

**James W. Teener, M.D.**
*Assistant Professor, Neurology*
*Department of Neurology*
*University of Pennsylvania*
*3400 Spruce Street,*
  *3 West Gates Bldg.*
*Philadelphia, Pennsylvania 19104-4283*

**Richard S. Tunkel, M.D.**
*Assistant Attending Physiatrist*
*Department of Neurology-Rehabilitation*
  *Service*
*Memorial Sloan-Kettering*
  *Cancer Center*
*1275 York Avenue*
*New York, New York 10021*

**Martha L. Twaddle, M.D.**
*Instructor in Medicine*
*Department of Medicine*
*Northwestern University/*
  *Evanston Hospital*
*2650 Ridge Avenue*
*Evanston, Illinois 60201*

**Mary L.S. Vachon, R.N., Ph.D.**
*Associate Professor*
*Department of Psychiatry and Behavioural*
*  Science*
*University of Toronto, Toronto Sunnybrook*
*  Regional Cancer Centre/*
*  Sunnybrook Health Science Centre*
*2075 Bayview Avenue*
*Toronto, Ontario M4N 3M5*
*Canada*

**Charles F. von Gunten, M.D., Ph.D.**
*Assistant Professor of Medicine*
*Division of Hematology/Oncology*
*Department of Medicine*
*Northwestern University Medical School*
*303 East Chicago Avenue*
*Chicago, Illinois 60611*

**Jamie H. Von Roenn, M.D.**
*Associate Professor of Medicine*
*Division of Hematology/Oncology*
*Department of Medicine*
*Northwestern University*
*303 East Chicago Avenue*
*Chicago, Illinois 60611*

**Sharon M. Weinstein, M.D.**
*Assistant Professor of Medicine (Neurology)*
*Department of Neuro-oncology*
*The University of Texas, M.D. Anderson Cancer*
*  Center*
*1515 Holcombe Boulevard, Box 8*
*Houston, Texas 77030-4095*

**Steven J. Weisman, M.D.**
*Associate Professor of Anesthesiology and*
*  Pediatrics*
*Departments of Anesthesiology and Pediatrics*
*Yale University School of Medicine*
*333 Cedar Street*
*New Haven, Connecticut 06520-8051*

**David E. Weissman, M.D.**
*Professor of Medicine*
*Department of Medicine, Division of*
*  Hematology/Oncology*
*Medical College of Wisconsin, Froedert*
*  Hospital East*
*9200 West Wisconsin Avenue*
*Milwaukee, Wisconsin 53226*

**Brian P. Whooley, M.D.**
*Department of Surgery*
*Memorial Sloan-Kettering Cancer Center*
*1275 York Avenue*
*New York, New York 10021*

**Gabor A. Winkler, M.D.**
*The Musculoskeletal Tumor and Limb*
*  Reconstruction Center*
*15 North Presidential Blvd, #300*
*Bala Cynwyd, Pennsylvania 19004*

**J. William Worden, Ph.D.**
*2 Woodhaven Dr.*
*Laguna Niguel, California 92677*

**James R. Zabora, M.S.W.**
*Research Associate*
*The Johns Hopkins Oncology Center*
*The Johns Hopkins University*
*  School of Medicine*
*600 North Wolfe Street*
*Baltimore, Maryland 21287-8931*

**Wendy Ziai, M.D.**
*Department of Clinical Neurosciences*
*University of Calgary*
*1331 29th Street NW*
*Calgary, Alberta T2N 4N2*
*Canada*

**Ian M. Zlotolow, D.M.D.**
*Chief, Dental Service*
*Department of Surgery*
*Memorial Sloan-Kettering Cancer Center*
*1275 York Avenue*
*New York, New York 10021*

# Preface

The term *supportive oncology* refers to those aspects of medical care concerned with the physical, psychosocial, and spiritual issues faced by persons with cancer, their families, their communities, and their health care providers. In this context, supportive oncology describes both those interventions used to support patients who experience adverse effects caused by antineoplastic therapies and those interventions now considered under the broad rubric of palliative care. The term *palliative* is derived from the Latin *pallium*: to cloak or cover. At its core, palliative care is concerned with providing the maximum quality of life to the patient-family unit at a time when the underlying disease is no longer curable.

In 1990, the World Health Organization (WHO) published a landmark document, *Cancer Pain Relief and Palliative Care,* which clearly defined the international barriers and needs for improved pain and symptom control in the cancer patient.

The WHO definition of palliative care is (1):

> The active total care of patients whose disease is not responsive to curative treatment. Control of pain, of other symptoms, and of psychological, social, and spiritual problems is paramount. The goal of palliative care is achievement of the best quality of life for patients and their families. Many aspects of palliative care are also applicable earlier in the course of the illness in conjunction with anti-cancer treatment.

In 1995, the Canadian Palliative Care Association chose a somewhat broader definition that emphasizes a more expanded role of palliative care (2):

> Palliative care, as a philosophy of care, is the combination of active and compassionate therapies intended to comfort and support individuals and families who are living with a life-threatening illness. During periods of illness and bereavement, palliative care strives to meet physical, psychological, social, and spiritual expectations and needs, while remaining sensitive to personal, cultural, and religious values, beliefs, and practices. Palliative care may be combined with therapies aimed at reducing or curing the illness, or it may be the total focus of care.

In developing this textbook, the editors have brought together those elements of palliative care that are most applicable to the health care professional caring for cancer patients, and have combined this perspective with a detailed description of related therapies used to support patients in active treatment. The editors view these interventions as a necessary and vital aspect of medical care for all cancer patients, from the time of diagnosis until death. Indeed, most patients will have a significant physical symptom requiring treatment at the time of their cancer diagnosis.

Even when cancer can be effectively treated and a cure or life prolongation is achieved, there are always physical, psychosocial, or spiritual concerns that must be addressed to maintain function and optimize the quality of life. For patients whose cancer cannot be effectively treated, palliative care must be the dominant mode and one must focus intensively on the control of distressing symptoms. Planning for the end of life and ensuring that death occurs with a minimum of suffering and in a manner consistent with the values and desires of the patient and family are fundamental elements of this care. Palliative care, as a desired approach to comprehensive cancer care, is appropriate for all health care settings, including the clinic, acute care hospital, long-term care facility, or home hospice.

Palliative care and the broader concept of supportive care involve the collaborative efforts of an interdisciplinary team. This team must include the cancer patient and his or her family, care givers, and involved health care providers. Integral to effective palliative care is the opportunity and support necessary for both care givers and health care providers to work through their own emotions related to the care they are providing.

In organizing this textbook, the editors have recognized the important contributions of medical research and clinical care that have emerged from the disciplines of hospice and palliative medicine;

medical, radiation, and surgical oncology; nursing; neurology and neuro-oncology; anesthesiology; psychiatry and psychology; pharmacology; and many others. The text includes chapters focusing on the common physical symptoms experienced by the cancer patient; a review of specific supportive treatment modalities, such as blood products, nutritional support, hydration, palliative chemotherapy, radiotherapy, and surgery; and, finally, a review of more specialized topics, including survivorship issues, medical ethics, spiritual care, quality of life, and supportive care in elderly, pediatric, and AIDS patients.

As we move toward the year 2000, there are many promising new cancer treatments on the horizon. No matter what these new treatments will offer in terms of curing the disease or prolonging life, cancer will remain a devastating illness, not only for the affected patients, but for their families, community, and health care providers. Providing excellent, supportive care will continue to be a goal for all health care providers.

The authors would like to thank our many contributors for their efforts. We are also grateful to our publisher and secretaries, whose oversight and gentle prodding were essential to our success. Finally, we want to express our gratitude to our families and colleagues, who accommodated our needs in bringing the volume to fruition and provided the support we needed throughout the process.

*Ann M. Berger, R.N., M.S.N., M.D.*
*Russell K. Portenoy, M.D.*
*David E. Weissman, M.D.*

## REFERENCES

1. World Health Organization. *Cancer pain relief and palliative care.* Technical Report Series 804. Geneva: World Health Organization, 1990.
2. Canadian Palliative Care Association. *Palliative care: Towards a consensus in standardized principles and practice.* Ottowa, Ontario: Canadian Palliative Care Association, 1995.

# Symptoms and Syndromes

*Principles and Practice of Supportive Oncology,*
edited by Ann Berger et al.
Lippincott–Raven Publishers, Philadelphia ©1998

CHAPTER 1

# Cancer Pain: Principles of Assessment and Syndromes

Nathan I. Cherny

Surveys indicate that pain is experienced by 30–60% of cancer patients during active therapy and more than two thirds of those with advanced disease (1). This has been corroborated in a series of recent studies, which identified a pain prevalence of 28% among patients with newly diagnosed cancer (2), 50–70% among patients receiving active anticancer therapy (3–8), and 64–80% among patients with far advanced disease (9–11). Unrelieved pain is incapacitating and precludes a satisfying quality of life; it interferes with physical functioning and social interaction, and is strongly associated with heightened psychological distress. Persistent pain interferes with one's ability to eat, sleep, think, and interact with others (12–14). The relationship between pain and psychological well-being is complex and reciprocal; mood disturbance and beliefs about the meaning of pain in relation to illness can exacerbate perceived pain intensity (15,16), and the presence of pain is a major determinant of function and mood (17). The presence of pain can disturb normal processes of coping and adjustment (18–20) and augment a sense of vulnerability, contributing to a preoccupation with the potential for catastrophic outcomes (18). The relationship between pain and psychological distress among cancer patients has been demonstrated in a range of tumor types (7,21–23). This relationship is further evidenced by the observations that uncontrolled pain is a major risk factor in cancer-related suicide (24–27) and that psychiatric symptoms have commonly been observed to disappear with adequate pain relief (28).

The high prevalence of acute and chronic pain among cancer patients, and the profound psychological and physical burdens engendered by this symptom, oblige all treating clinicians to be skilled in pain management (29–31). Relief of pain in cancer patients is an ethical imperative and it is incumbent on clinicians to maximize the knowledge, skill, and diligence needed to attend to this task (29–31). The undertreatment of cancer pain, which continues to be common (32), has many causes, among the most important of which is inadequate assessment (33,34). In a study to evaluate the correlation between patient and clinician evaluation of pain severity, Grossman et al. (34) found that when patients rated their pain as moderate to severe, oncology fellows failed to appreciate the severity of the problem in 73% of cases. In studies of pain relief among cancer patients in the United States (3) and in France (4), the discrepancy between patient and physician evaluation of the severity of the pain problem was a major predictor of inadequate relief. Surveys indicate that the contribution of suboptimal assessment to the problem of inadequate pain management is widely recognized by oncology clinicians (3,35).

## APPROACH TO CANCER PAIN ASSESSMENT

Assessment is an ongoing and dynamic process that includes evaluation of presenting problems, elucidation of pain syndromes and pathophysiology, and formulation of a comprehensive plan for continuing care (36–39). The objectives of cancer pain assessment include: (1) the accurate characterization of the pain, including the pain syndrome and inferred pathophysiology, and (2) the evaluation of the impact of the pain and the role it plays in the overall suffering of the patient. This assessment is predicated on the establishment of a trusting relationship with the patient, in which the clinician emphasizes the relief of pain and suffering as central to the goal of therapy and encourages open communication about symptoms. Clinicians should

N. I. Cherny: Department of Medical Oncology, Shaare Zedek Medical Center, Jerusalem, 91031, Israel.

not be cavalier about the potential for symptom underreporting; symptoms are frequently described as complaints, and there is a common perception that the "good patient" refrains from complaining (40). The prevalence of pain is so great that an open-ended question about the presence of pain should be included at each patient visit in routine oncological practice. If the patient is unable or unwilling to describe the pain, it may be necessary to question a family member regarding the distress or disability of the patient.

## Pain Syndromes

Cancer pain syndromes are defined by the association of particular pain characteristics and physical signs with specific consequences of the underlying disease or its treatment. Syndromes are associated with distinct etiologies and pathophysiologies, and have important prognostic and therapeutic implications. Pain syndromes associated with cancer can be either acute (Table 1) or chronic (Table 2). Whereas acute pains experienced by cancer patients are usually related to diagnostic and therapeutic interventions, chronic pains are most commonly caused by direct tumor infiltration. Adverse consequences of cancer therapy, including surgery, chemotherapy, and radiation therapy, account for 15–25% of chronic cancer pain problems, and a small proportion of the chronic pains experienced by cancer patients are caused by pathology unrelated to either the cancer or the cancer therapy (41–44).

## Pain Characteristics

The evaluation of pain characteristics provides some of the data essential for syndrome identification. These

**TABLE 1.** *Cancer-related acute pain syndromes*

### Acute pain associated with diagnostic and therapeutic interventions

Acute pain associated with diagnostic interventions
  Lumbar puncture headache
  Transthoracic needle biopsy
  Arterial or venous blood sampling
  Bone marrow biopsy
  Lumbar puncture
  Colonoscopy
  Myelography
  Percutaneous biopsy
  Thoracocentesis
Acute postoperative pain

Acute pain caused by other therapeutic interventions
  Pleurodesis
  Tumor embolization
  Suprapubic catheterization
  Intercostal catheter
  Nephrostomy insertion
Cryosurgery-associated pain and cramping
  Acute pain associated with analgesic techniques
  Local anesthetic infiltration pain
  Opioid injection pain
  Opioid headache
  Spinal opioid hyperalgesia syndrome
  Epidural injection pain

### Acute pain associated with anticancer therapies

Acute pain associated with chemotherapy infusion
techniques
  Intravenous infusion pain
    Venous spasm
    Chemical phlebitis
    Vesicant extravasation
    Anthracycline-associated flare reaction
  Hepatic artery infusion pain
  Intraperitoneal chemotherapy abdominal pain
Acute pain associated with chemotherapy toxicity
  Mucositis
  Corticosteroid-induced perineal discomfort
  Taxol-induced arthralgias
  Steroid pseudorheumatism
  Painful peripheral neuropathy
  Headache
    Intrathecal methotrexate meningitic syndrome
    L-asparaginase-associated dural sinuses thrombosis
    *trans*-Retinoic acid headache
  Diffuse bone pain
    *trans*-Retinoic acid

  Colony-stimulating factors
  5-Fluorouracil-induced anginal chest pain
  Palmar-plantar erythrodysesthesia syndrome
  Postchemotherapy gynecomastia
  Chemotherapy induced acute digital ischemia
Acute pain associated with hormonal therapy
  Leutenizing hormone–releasing factor tumor flare in
prostate cancer
  Hormone-induced pain flare in breast cancer
Acute pain associated with immunotherapy
  Interferon-induced acute pain
Acute pain associated with growth factors
  Colony-stimulating factor–induced musculoskeletal pains
  Erythropoietin injection pain
Acute pain associated with radiotherapy
  Incident pains associated with positioning
  Oropharyngeal mucositis
  Acute radiation enteritis and proctocolitis
  Early onset brachial plexopathy
  Subacute radiation myelopathy
  Strontium-89-induced pain flare

### Acute pain associated with infection

Acute herpetic neuralgia

### Acute pain associated with vascular events

Acute thrombosis pain
  Lower extremity deep venous thrombosis

Upper extremity deep venous thrombosis
  Superior vena cava obstruction

**TABLE 2.** *Cancer-related chronic pain syndromes*

### Tumor-related pain syndromes

Bone pain
  Multifocal or generalized bone pain
    Multiple bony metastases
    Marrow expansion
  Vertebral syndromes
    Atlantoaxial destruction and odontoid fractures
    C7-T1 syndrome
    T12-L1 syndrome
    Sacral syndrome
  Back pain and epidural compression
  Pain syndromes of the bony pelvis and hip
    Hip joint syndrome
  Acrometastases
Arthritides
  Hypertrophic pulmonary osteoarthropathy
  Other polyarthritides
Muscle pain
  Muscle cramps
  Skeletal muscle tumors
Headache and facial pain
  Intracerebral tumor
  Leptomeningeal metastases
  Base of skull metastases
    Orbital syndrome
    Parasellar syndrome
    Middle cranial fossa syndrome
    Jugular foramen syndrome
    Occipital condyle syndrome
    Clivus syndrome
    Sphenoid sinus syndrome

  Painful cranial neuralgias
    Glossopharyngeal neuralgia
    Trigeminal neuralgia
Tumor involvement of the peripheral nervous system
  Tumor-related radiculopathy
    Postherpetic neuralgia
  Cervical plexopathy
  Brachial plexopathy
  Malignant brachial plexopathy
  Idiopathic brachial plexopathy associated with Hodgkin's disease
  Malignant lumbosacral plexopathy
  Tumor-related mononeuropathy
  Paraneoplastic painful peripheral neuropathy
    Subacute sensory neuropathy
    Sensorimotor peripheral neuropathy
Pain syndromes of the viscera and miscellaneous tumor-related syndromes
  Hepatic distention syndrome
  Midline retroperitoneal syndrome
  Chronic intestinal obstruction
  Peritoneal carcinomatosis
  Malignant perineal pain
    Malignant pelvic floor myalgia
  Adrenal pain syndrome
  Ureteric obstruction
  Ovarian cancer pain
  Lung cancer pain
Paraneoplastic nociceptive pain syndromes
  Tumor-related gynecomastia

### Chronic pain syndromes associated with cancer therapy

Postchemotherapy pain syndromes
  Chronic painful peripheral neuropathy
  Avascular necrosis of femoral or humeral head
  Plexopathy associated with intraarterial infusion
  Raynaud's phenomenon
Chronic pain associated with hormonal therapy
  Gynecomastia with hormonal therapy for prostate cancer
Chronic postsurgical pain syndromes
  Postmastectomy pain syndrome
  Postradical neck dissection pain
  Postthoracotomy pain
  Postoperative frozen shoulder
  Phantom pain syndromes
    Phantom limb pain

    Phantom breast pain
    Phantom anus pain
    Phantom bladder pain
  Stump pain
  Postsurgical pelvic floor myalgia
Chronic postradiation pain syndromes
  Plexopathies
  Radiation-induced brachial and lumbosacral plexopathies
    Radiation-induced peripheral nerve tumor
  Chronic radiation myelopathy
  Chronic radiation enteritis and proctitis
  Burning perineum syndrome
  Osteoradionecrosis

---

characteristics include intensity, quality, distribution, and temporal relationships.

### *Intensity*

The evaluation of pain intensity is pivotal to therapeutic decision making (45,46). It indicates the urgency with which relief is needed and influences the selection of analgesic drug, route of administration, and rate of dose titration (47). Furthermore, the assessment of pain intensity may help characterize the pain mechanism and underlying syndrome. For example, the pain associated

with radiation-induced nerve injury is rarely severe; the occurrence of severe pain in a previously irradiated region therefore suggests the existence of recurrent neoplasm or a radiation-induced second primary neoplasm.

### *Quality*

The quality of the pain often suggests its pathophysiology. Somatic nociceptive pains are usually well localized and described as sharp, aching, throbbing, or pressure-like. Visceral nociceptive pains are generally diffuse and may be gnawing or crampy when due to obstruction of a hollow viscus, or aching, sharp, or throbbing when due to involvement of organ capsules or mesentery. Neuropathic pains may be described as burning, tingling, or shock-like (lancinating).

### Distribution

Patients with cancer pain commonly experience pain at more than one site (6). The distinction between focal, multifocal, and generalized pain may be important in the selection of therapy, such as nerve blocks, radiotherapy, or surgical approaches. The term "focal" pain, which is used to denote a single site, has also been used to depict pain that is experienced in the region of the underlying lesion. Focal pains can be distinguished from those that are referred to a site remote from the lesion. Familiarity with pain referral patterns is essential to target appropriate diagnostic and therapeutic maneuvers (48–50) (Table 3). For example, a patient who develops progressive shoulder pain and has no evidence of focal pathology needs to undergo evaluation of the region above and below the diaphragm to exclude the possibility of referred pain from diaphragmatic irritation.

### Temporal Relationships

Cancer-related pain may be acute or chronic. Acute pain is defined by a recent onset and a natural history characterized by transience. The pain is often associated with overt pain behaviors (such as moaning, grimacing, and splinting), anxiety, or signs of generalized sympathetic hyperactivity, including diaphoresis, hypertension, and tachycardia. Chronic pain has been defined by persistence for 3 months or more beyond the usual course of an acute illness or injury, a pattern of recurrence at intervals over months or years, or by association with a chronic pathologic process (1). Chronic tumor-related pain is usually insidious in onset, often increases progressively with tumor growth, and may regress with tumor shrinkage. Overt pain behaviors and sympathetic hyperactivity are often absent, and the pain may be associated with affective disturbances (anxiety and/or depression) and vegetative symptoms, such as asthenia, anorexia, and sleep disturbance (51–54).

Transitory exacerbations of severe pain over a baseline of moderate pain or less may be described as "breakthrough pain" (55). Breakthrough pains are common in both acute or chronic pain states. These exacerbations may be precipitated by volitional actions of the patient (so-called incident pains), such as movement, micturition, cough, or defecation, or by nonvolitional events, such as bowel distention. Spontaneous fluctuations in pain intensity can also occur without an identifiable precipitant.

### Inferred Pain Mechanisms

Inferences about the mechanisms that may be responsible for the pain are helpful in the evaluation of the pain syndrome and in the management of cancer pain. The assessment process usually provides the clinical data necessary to infer a predominant pathophysiology.

### Nociceptive Pain

"Nociceptive pain" describes pain that is perceived to be commensurate with tissue damage associated with an identifiable somatic or visceral lesion. The persistence of pain is thought to be related to ongoing activation of nociceptors, primary afferent neurons that transmit information about noxious stimuli. Nociceptive pain that originates from somatic structures (somatic pain) is usually well localized and described as sharp, aching, burning, or throbbing. Pain that arises from visceral structures (visceral pain) is generally more diffuse, and is often described as gnawing or cramping when due to obstruction of a hollow viscus, and aching, sharp or throbbing when due to involvement of organ capsules or other mesentery. From the clinical perspective, nociceptive pains (particularly somatic pains) usually respond to opioid drugs (56,57) or to interventions that ameliorate or denervate the peripheral lesion.

**TABLE 3.** *Common patterns of pain referral*

| Pain mechanism | Site of lesion | Referral site |
|---|---|---|
| Visceral | Diaphragmatic irritation | Shoulder |
| | Urothelial tract | Inguinal region and genitalia |
| Somatic | C7-T1 vertebrae | Interscapular |
| | L1-2 | Sacroiliac joint and hip |
| | Hip joint | Knee |
| | Pharynx | Ipsilateral ear |
| Neuropathic | Nerve or plexus | Anywhere in the distribution of a peripheral nerve |
| | Nerve root | Anywhere in the corresponding dermatome |
| | Central nervous system | Anywhere in the region of the body innervated by the damaged structure |

## Neuropathic Pain

The term "neuropathic pain" is applied when pain is due to injury to, or diseases of, the peripheral or central neural structures or is perceived to be sustained by aberrant somatosensory processing at these sites (58,59). It is most strongly suggested when a dysesthesia occurs in a region of motor, sensory, or autonomic dysfunction that is attributable to a discrete neurologic lesion. The diagnosis can be challenging, however, and is often inferred solely from the distribution of the pain and identification of a lesion in neural structures that innervate this region.

Although neuropathic pains can be described in terms of the pain characteristics (continuous or lancinating) or site of injury (e.g., neuronopathy or plexopathy), it is useful to distinguish these syndromes according to the presumed site of the aberrant neural activity ("generator") that sustains the pain (59). Peripheral neuropathic pain is caused by injury to a peripheral nerve or nerve root and is presumably sustained by aberrant processes originating in the nerve root, plexus, or nerve. In contrast, neuropathic pains believed to be sustained by a central "generator" include sympathetically maintained pain and a group of syndromes traditionally known as the deafferentation pains (e.g., phantom pain). Sympathetically maintained pain may occur following injury to soft tissue, peripheral nerve, viscera, or central nervous system, and is suggested when pain is accompanied by focal autonomic dysregulation (e.g., vasomotor or pilomotor changes, swelling, or sweating abnormalities) or trophic changes (60). This pattern of findings characterizes the syndromes known as reflex sympathetic dystrophy and causalgia (recently termed complex regional pain syndromes Type I and II, respectively).

The diagnosis of neuropathic pain has important clinical implications. The response of neuropathic pains to opioid drugs is less predictable and generally less dramatic than the response of nociceptive pains (56,57,61, 62). Optimal treatment may depend on the use of so-called adjuvant analgesics (63) or other specific approaches, such as sympathetic nerve block.

## Idiopathic Pain

Pain that is perceived to be excessive for the extent of identifiable organic pathology can be termed idiopathic unless the patient presents with affective and behavioral disturbances that are severe enough to infer a predominating psychological pathogenesis, in which case a specific psychiatric diagnosis (somatoform disorder) can be applied (64). When the inference of a somatoform disorder cannot be made, however, the label "idiopathic" should be retained, and assessments should be repeated at appropriate intervals. Idiopathic pain in gen-

eral, and pain related to a psychiatric disorder specifically, are uncommon in the cancer population, notwithstanding the importance of psychological factors in quality of life.

## A Stepwise Approach to the Evaluation of Cancer Pain

A practical approach to cancer pain assessment incorporates a stepwise approach that begins with data collection and ends with a clinically relevant formulation.

### Data Collection

#### History

A careful review of past medical history and the chronology of the cancer is important to place the pain complaint in context. The pain-related history must elucidate the relevant pain characteristics, as well as the responses of the patient to previous disease-modifying and analgesic therapies. The presence of multiple pain problems is common, and if more than one is reported, each must be assessed independently. The use of validated pain assessment instruments can provide a format for communication between the patient and health care professionals and can also be used to monitor the adequacy of therapy (see below).

The clinician should assess the consequences of the pain, including impairment in activities of daily living; psychological, familial, and professional dysfunction; disturbed sleep, appetite, and vitality; and financial concerns. The patient's psychological status, including current level of anxiety or depression, suicidal ideation, and the perceived meaning of the pain, is similarly relevant. Pervasive dysfunctional attitudes, such as pessimism, idiosyncratic interpretation of pain, self-blame, catastrophizing, and perceived loss of personal control, can usually be detected through careful questioning. It is important to assess the patient–family interaction and to note both the kind and the frequency of pain behaviors and the nature of the family response.

Most patients with cancer pain have multiple other symptoms (8,52,53,65). The clinician must evaluate the severity and distress caused by each of these symptoms. Symptom checklists and quality of life measures may contribute to this comprehensive evaluation (8,66,67).

#### Examination

A physical examination, including a neurologic evaluation, is a necessary part of the initial pain assessment. The need for a thorough neurologic assessment is justified by the high prevalence of painful neurologic conditions in this population (68,69). The physical examination should attempt to identify the underlying etiology of the pain problem, clarify the extent of the underlying disease, and discern the relationship of the pain complaint to the disease.

### Review of Previous Investigations

Careful review of previous laboratory and imaging studies can provide important information about the cause of the pain and the extent of the underlying disease.

### Provisional Assessment

The information derived from these data provides the basis for a provisional pain diagnosis, an understanding of the disease status, and the identification of other concurrent concerns. This provisional diagnosis includes inferences about the pathophysiology of the pain and an assessment of the pain syndrome.

Additional investigations are often required to clarify areas of uncertainty in the provisional assessment (68). The extent of diagnostic investigation must be appropriate to the patient's general status and the overall goals of care. For some patients, comprehensive evaluation may require numerous investigations, some targeted at the specific pain problem and others needed to clarify extent of the disease or concurrent symptoms. In specific situations, algorithms have been developed to facilitate an efficient evaluation. This is well illustrated by established clinical algorithms for the investigation of back pain in the cancer patient (70,71), which provide a straightforward approach for those patients at highest risk for epidural spinal cord compression (see below).

The lack of a definitive finding on an investigation should not be used to override a compelling clinical diagnosis. In the assessment of bone pain, for example, plain radiographs provide only crude assessment of bony lesions and further investigation with bone scintigrams, computerized tomography (CT), or magnetic resonance imaging (MRI) may be indicated. To minimize the risk of error, the physician ordering the diagnostic procedures should personally review them with the radiologist to correlate pathologic changes with the clinical findings.

Pain should be managed during the diagnostic evaluation. Comfort will improve compliance and reduce the distress associated with procedures. No patient should be inadequately evaluated because of poorly controlled pain.

The comprehensive assessment may also require additional evaluation of other physical or psychosocial problems identified during the initial assessment. Expert assistance from other physicians, nurses, social workers, or others may be essential.

### Formulation and Therapeutic Planning

The evaluation should enable the clinician to appreciate the nature of the pain, its impact, and concurrent concerns that further undermine quality of life. The findings of this evaluation should be reviewed with the patient and appropriate others. Through candid discussion, current problems can be prioritized to reflect their importance to the patient.

This evaluation may also identify potential outcomes that would benefit from contingency planning. Examples include evaluation of resources for home care, prebereavement interventions with the family, and the provision of assistive devices in anticipation of compromised ambulation.

## Measurement of Pain and Its Impact on Patient Well-Being

Although pain measurement has generally been used by clinical investigators to determine the impact of analgesic therapies, it has become clear that it also has an important role in the routine monitoring of cancer patients in treatment settings (3,4). Since observer ratings of symptom severity correlate poorly with patient ratings and are generally an inadequate substitute for patient reporting (34), patient self-report is the primary source of information for the measurement of pain.

### Pain Measures in Routine Clinical Management

Recent guidelines from the Agency for Health Care Policy and Research (72,73) and the American Pain Society (74,75) recommend the regular use of pain rating scales to assess pain severity and relief in all patients who commence or change treatments. These recommendations also suggest that clinicians teach patients and families to use assessment tools in the home to promote continuity of pain management in all settings. The two most commonly used scales for adults are a verbal descriptor scale (i.e., "Which word best describes your pain: none, mild moderate, severe, or excruciating?") or a numeric scale (i.e., "On a scale from 0 to 10, where 0 indicates no pain and 10 indicates the worst pain you can imagine, how would you rate your pain?) (73).

A recent study demonstrated that the use of a simple verbal pain assessment tool improved the caregiver's understanding of pain status in hospitalized patients (76). Regular pain measurement, using a pain scale included in the bedside chart (Fig. 1), has been incorporated into a continuous quality improvement strategy at a cancer center (77), and preliminary data suggest that nursing knowledge and attitudes regarding the assessment and management of cancer pain have improved as a result. In addition to focusing staff attention on symptom assessment, such

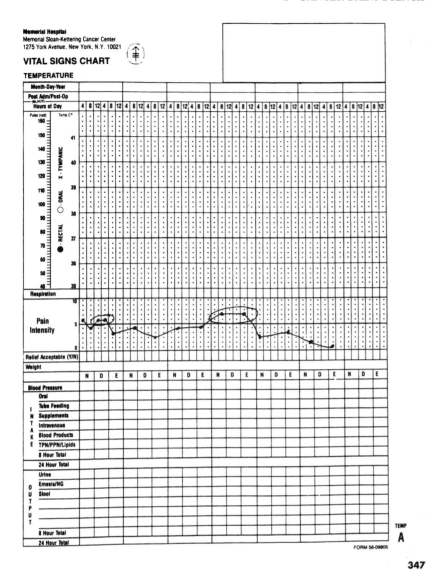

**Memorial Hospital**
Memorial Sloan-Kettering Cancer Center
1275 York Avenue, New York, N.Y. 10021

**VITAL SIGNS CHART**

TEMP
**A**

FORM 56-09805

347

**FIG. 1.** The patient observation chart from Memorial Sloan Kettering Cancer Center. Incorporated into the chart is a 10-point pain scale and an item regarding the adequacy of pain control.

measures may be used as a means of reviewing the quality of patient care and ascertaining situation-specific barriers to symptom control (78,79).

### Instruments for the Measurement of Pain in Research Settings

Pain can be measured using unidimensional or multidimensional scales. Unidimensional scales generally address intensity or relief, using visual analog, numeric, and categorical scales. Multidimensional instruments include the Memorial Pain Assessment Card, the McGill Pain Questionnaire, and the Brief Pain Inventory.

#### Memorial Pain Assessment Card

The Memorial Pain Assessment Card (MPAC) (80) is a brief, validated measure that uses 100 mm visual analog

scales (VASs) to characterize pain intensity, pain relief, and mood, and an 8-point verbal rating scale (VRS) to further characterize pain intensity (Fig. 2). The mood scale, which is correlated with measures of psychological distress, depression, and anxiety, is considered to be a brief measure of global psychological distress (80). Although this instrument does not provide detailed descriptors of pain, its brevity and simplicity may facilitate the collection of useful information while minimizing patient burden and encouraging compliance.

#### Brief Pain Inventory

The Brief Pain Inventory (BPI) (Fig. 3) (81) is a simple and easily administered tool that provides information about pain history, intensity, location, and quality. Numeric scales (range 1–10) indicate the intensity of pain in general, at its worst, at its least, and right now. A

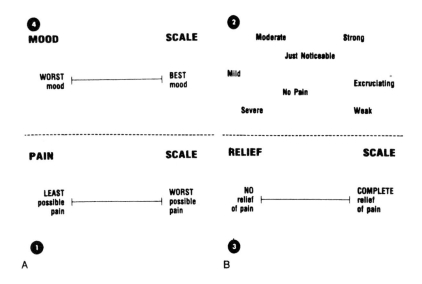

**FIG. 2.** The Memorial Pain Assessment Card (MPAC). Reproduced with permission.

percentage scale quantifies relief from current therapies. A figure representing the body is provided for the patient to shade the area corresponding to his or her pain. Seven questions determine the degree to which pain interferes with function, mood, and enjoyment of life (Fig. 3). The BPI is self-administered and easily understood, and has been translated into several languages.

### The McGill Pain Questionnaire

The McGill Pain Questionnaire (MPQ) (82,83) is a self-administered questionnaire that provides global scores and subscale scores that reflect the sensory, affective, and evaluative dimensions of pain. The scores are derived from ratings of pain descriptors selected by the patient. A 5-point verbal categorical scale characterizes the intensity of pain and a pain drawing localizes the pain. Further information is collected about the impact of medications and other therapies. The impact of pain on function is not assessed. Although the MPQ has been extensively evaluated in chronic pain patients, the utility of the subscale scores has not been demonstrated for cancer pain (84).

### ACUTE PAIN SYNDROMES

Cancer-related acute pain syndromes are most commonly due to diagnostic or therapeutic interventions (Table 1) and they generally pose little diagnostic difficulty. Although some tumor-related pains have an acute onset (such as pain from a pathologic fracture), most of these will persist unless effective treatment for the underlying lesion is provided. A comprehensive pain assessment in such patients is usually valuable, potentially yielding important information about the extent of disease or concurrent issues relevant to therapy.

### Acute Pain Associated with Diagnostic and Therapeutic Interventions

Many investigations and treatments are associated with predictable, transient pain. For those patients with a pre-existing pain syndrome, otherwise innocuous manipulations can also precipitate an incident pain.

### Acute Pain Associated with Diagnostic Interventions

#### Lumbar Puncture Headache

Lumbar puncture (LP) headache is the best characterized acute pain syndrome associated with a diagnostic intervention. This syndrome is characterized by the delayed development of a positional headache, which is precipitated or markedly exacerbated by upright posture. The pain is believed to be related to reduction in cerebrospinal fluid (CSF) volume, due to ongoing leakage through the defect in the dural sheath, and compensatory expansion of the pain-sensitive intracerebral veins (85). The incidence of headache is related to the caliber of the LP needle (0–2% with 27- to 29-gauge, 0.5–7% with 25- to 26-gauge, 5–8% with 22-gauge, 10–15% with 20-gauge, and 20–30% with 18-gauge needles) (86,87). Using a regular beveled needle, the overall incidence can be reduced by the use of a small-gauge needle and by longitudinal insertion of the needle bevel, which presumably induces less trauma to the longitudinal elastic fibers in the dura (85,88,89). Recent evidence suggests that the use of a nontraumatic "Sprotte" needle, which has a conical tip with a lateral opening that spreads the

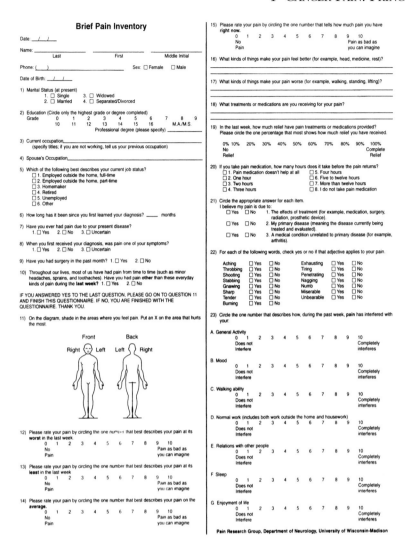

**FIG. 3.** The Brief Pain Inventory. Reproduced with permission.

dural fibers, is associated with a substantially lesser risk of post lumbar puncture headaches compared to regular cannulae (90–94). The evidence that recumbency after LP reduces the incidence of this syndrome is controversial (95–97).

LP headache, which usually develops hours to several days after the procedure, is typically described as a dull occipital discomfort that may radiate to the frontal region or to the shoulders (85,86,89,98). When severe, the pain may be associated with diaphoresis and nausea (98). The duration of the headache is usually brief, hours to days, and routine management relies on bedrest, hydration, and analgesics. Persistent headache may necessitate application of an epidural blood patch (99). Although a recent controlled study suggested that prophylactic administration of a blood patch may reduce this complication (97,100), the incidence and severity of the syndrome do not warrant this treatment. Severe headache has also been reported to respond to treatment with intravenous caffeine (101).

*Transthoracic Needle Biopsy*

Transthoracic fine needle aspiration of intrathoracic mass is generally a non noxious procedure. Severe pain has, however, been associated with this procedure when the underlying diagnosis was a neurogenic tumor (102).

### Acute Pain Associated with Therapeutic Interventions

*Postoperative Pain*

Acute postoperative pain is universal unless adequately treated. Unfortunately, undertreatment is endemic despite the availability of adequate analgesic and anesthetic techniques (72,103,104). Guidelines for management have been reviewed (72,105). Postoperative pain that exceeds the normal duration or severity should prompt a careful evaluation for the possibility of infection or other complications.

*Cryosurgery Associated Pain and Cramping*

Cervical cryosurgery in the treatment of intraepithelial neoplasia commonly produces an acute cramping pain syndrome. The severity of the pain is related to the duration of the freeze period and it is not diminished by the administration of prophylactic nonsteroidal antiinflammatory drugs (NSAIDs) (106).

*Other Interventions*

Invasive interventions other than surgery are commonly used in cancer therapy and may also result in predictable acute pain syndromes. Examples include the pains associated with tumor embolization techniques (107) and chemical pleurodesis.

### Acute Pain Associated with Analgesic Techniques

*Local Anesthetic Infiltration Pain*

Intradermal and subcutaneous infiltration of lidocaine produces a transient burning sensation before the onset of analgesia. Controlled studies demonstrate that this can be attenuated by the coadministration of 0.86% benzyl alcohol without adversely affecting anesthesia (108).

*Opioid Injection Pain*

Intramuscular (IM) and subcutaneous (SC) injections are painful. When repetitive dosing is required, the IM route of administration is not recommended (72,73). The pain associated with SC injection is influenced by the volume injected and the chemical characteristics of the injectant. SC injection of opioids can produce a painful subdermal reaction; this is infrequently observed with morphine or hydromorphone but is common with methadone (109) and fentanyl. For this reason the subcutaneous infusion of methadone (109) and fentanyl is not recommended. There are some data to suggest that the addition of a low concentration of dexamethasone may reduce the likelihood of local irritation (110).

*Opioid Headache*

Rarely, patients develop a reproducible generalized headache after opioid administration. Although its cause is not known, speculation suggests that it may be caused by opioid-induced histamine release.

*Spinal Opioid Hyperalgesia Syndrome*

Intrathecal and epidural injection of high opioid doses is occasionally complicated by pain (typically perineal, buttock, or leg), hyperalgesia, and associated manifestations including segmental myoclonus, piloerection, and priapism. This is an uncommon phenomenon that remits after discontinuation of the drug (111–113).

*Epidural Injection Pain*

Back, pelvic, or leg pain may be precipitated by epidural injection or infusion. The incidence of this problem has been estimated at approximately 20% (113). It is speculated that it may be caused by the compression of an adjacent nerve root by the injected fluid (113).

### Acute Pain Associated with Anticancer Therapies

### Acute Pain Associated with Chemotherapy Infusion Techniques

*Intravenous Infusion Pain*

Pain at the site of cytotoxic infusion is a common problem. Four pain syndromes related to intravenous infusion of chemotherapeutic agents are recognized: venous spasm, chemical phlebitis, vesicant extravasation, and anthracycline-associated flare (114,115). Venous spasm causes pain that is not associated with inflammation or phlebitis, and that may be modified by application of a warm compress or reduction of the rate of infusion (114). Chemical phlebitis can be caused by cytotoxic medications including amasarcine, decarbazine, and carmustine (116,117), as well as the infusion of potassium chloride and hyperosmolar solutions. The pain and linear erythema associated with chemical phlebitis must be distinguished from the more serious complication of a vesicant cytotoxic extravasation (Table 4) (118). Vesicant extravasation may produce intense pain followed by desquamation and ulceration. Finally, a brief venous flare reaction is often associated with intravenous administration of the anthracycline doxorubicin. The flare is typically associ-

**TABLE 4.** *Commonly used tissue vesicant cytotoxic drugs*

Amasarcine
BCNU
Cis-platinum
Decarbazine
Daunorubicin
Doxorubicin
Etoposide
Mitomycin-C
Mitoxantrone
Streptozotocin
Teniposide
Vinblastine
Vincristine
Vindesine

ated with local urticaria and occasional patients report pain or stinging (115).

### Hepatic Artery Infusion Pain

Cytotoxic infusions into the hepatic artery (for patients with hepatic metastases) are often associated with the development of a diffuse abdominal pain (119,120). Continuous infusions can lead to persistent pain. In some patients, the pain is due to the development of gastric ulceration or erosions, or cholangitis (121). If the latter complications do not occur, the pain usually resolves with discontinuation of the infusion. A dose relationship is suggested by the observation that some patients will comfortably tolerate reinitiation of the infusion at a lower dose (119).

### Intraperitoneal Chemotherapy Pain

Abdominal pain is a common complication of intraperitoneal chemotherapy (IPC). A transient mild abdominal pain, associated with sensations of fullness or bloating, is reported by approximately 25% of patients receiving IPC (122). A further 25% of patients reports moderate or severe pain necessitating opioid analgesia or discontinuation of therapy (122). Moderate or severe pain is usually caused by chemical serositis or infection (123). Drug selection may be a factor in the incidence of chemical serositis; it is a common complication of intraperitoneal anthracycline agents, such as mitoxantrone (124–126) and doxorubicin (127,128), but it is relatively uncommon with 5-fluorouracil (129) or cis-platinum (cisplatin). Abdominal pain associated with fever and leukocytosis in blood and peritoneal fluid is suggestive of infectious peritonitis (130).

### Acute Pain Associated with Chemotherapy Toxicity

### Mucositis

Severe mucositis is an almost invariable consequence of the myeloablative chemotherapy and radiotherapy that precedes bone marrow transplantation (131). It is less common with standard intensity therapy. Although the clinical syndrome usually involves the oral cavity and pharynx, the underlying pathology commonly extends to other gastrointestinal mucosal surfaces, and symptoms may occur as a result of involvement of the esophagus, stomach, or intestine (e.g., odynophagia, dyspepsia, or diarrhea). Damaged mucosal surfaces may become superinfected with microorganisms, such as *Candida albicans* and herpes simplex. The latter complication is most likely in neutropenic patients, who are also predisposed to systemic sepsis arising from local invasion by aerobic and anaerobic oral flora. Numerous therapies have been developed to reduce the risk of mucositis, including the use of cryotherapy (132), surface-coating agents (133,134), antibiotics (135), antiviral agents (136), and disinfectant mouthwashes (137). Severe mucositis usually requires both local and systemic analgesic therapies. Studies in bone marrow transplant patients have demonstrated the efficacy of patient-controlled analgesic techniques in this setting (138,139).

### Corticosteroid-Induced Perineal Discomfort

A transient burning sensation in the perineum is described by some patients following rapid infusion of large doses (20–100 mg) of dexamethasone (140). Patients need to be warned that such symptoms may occur. Clinical experience suggests that this syndrome is prevented by slow infusion.

### Steroid Pseudorheumatism

The withdrawal of corticosteroids may produce a pain syndrome that manifests as diffuse myalgias, arthralgias, and tenderness of muscles and joints. These symptoms occur with rapid or slow withdrawal and may occur in patients taking these drugs for long or short periods. The pathogenesis of this syndrome is poorly understood, but it has been speculated that steroid withdrawal may sensitize joint and muscle mechanoreceptors and nociceptors (141). Treatment consists of reinstituting the steroids at a higher dose and withdrawing them more slowly (141).

### Painful Peripheral Neuropathy

Chemotherapy-induced painful peripheral neuropathy, which is usually associated with vinca alkaloids and cisplatin, can have an acute course. The vinca alkaloids (particularly vincristine) are also associated with other, presumably neuropathic acute pain syndromes, including pain in the jaw, legs, arms, or abdomen that may last from hours to days (142,143). Vincristine-induced orofacial pain in the distribution of the trigeminal and glossopharyngeal nerves occurs in approximately 50% of patients at the onset of vincristine treatment (144). The pain, which is severe in about half of those affected, generally begins 2–3 days after vincristine administration and lasts for 1–3 days. It is usually self-limiting and if recurrence occurs it is usually mild (144).

### Headache

Intrathecal methotrexate in the treatment of leukemia or leptomeningeal metastases produces an acute meningitic syndrome in 5–50% of patients (145). Headache is the prominent symptom and may be associated with vomiting, nuchal rigidity, fever, irritability, and lethargy.

Symptoms usually begin hours after intrathecal treatment and persist for several days. CSF examination reveals a pleocytosis that may mimic bacterial meningitis. Patients at increased risk for the development of this syndrome include those who have received multiple intrathecal injections and those undergoing treatment for proven leptomeningeal metastases (145). The syndrome tends not to recur with subsequent injections.

Systemic administration of L-asparaginase for the treatment of acute lymphoblastic leukemia produces thrombosis of cerebral veins or dural sinuses in 1–2% of patients (146). This complication typically occurs after a few weeks of therapy, but its onset may be delayed until after the completion of treatment. It occurs as a result of depletion of asparagine, which in turn leads to the reduction of plasma proteins involved in coagulation and fibrinolysis. Headache is the most common initial symptom, and seizures, hemiparesis, delirium, vomiting, or cranial nerve palsies may also occur. The diagnosis may be established by angiography or by gradient echo sequences on MRI scan (147).

trans-Retinoic acid therapy, which may be used in the treatment of acute promyelocytic leukemia (APML), can cause a transient severe headache (148). The mechanism may be related to pseudotumor cerebri induced by hypervitaminosis A.

### Diffuse Bone Pain

In patients with APMI, trans-retinoic acid therapy often produces a syndrome of diffuse bone pain (149). The pain is generalized, of variable intensity, and closely associated with a transient neutrophilia. The latter observation suggests that the pain may be due to marrow expansion, a phenomenon that may underlie a similar pain syndrome that occurs following the administration of colony stimulating factors (150,151).

### Paclitaxel-Induced Arthralgia

Administration of paclitaxel generates a syndrome of diffuse arthralgias in 10–20% of patients. Joint pains generally appear 1–4 days after drug administration and persist for 3–7 days. The pathophysiology of this phenomenon has not been well evaluated.

### 5-Fluorouracil-Induced Anginal Chest Pain

Patients receiving continuous infusions of 5-fluorouracil (5-FU) may develop ischemic chest pain (152,153). Continuous ambulatory electrocardiographic (ECG) monitoring of patients undergoing 5-FU infusion demonstrated a nearly threefold increase in ischemic episodes over pretreatment recordings (154); these ECG changes were more common among patients with known coronary artery dis-

ease. It is widely speculated that coronary vasospasm may be the underlying mechanism (152–154).

### Palmar-Plantar Erythrodysesthesia Syndrome

Protracted infusion of 5-FU, and potentially treatment with other chemotherapies, can be complicated by the development of a tingling or burning sensation in the palms and soles followed by the development of an erythematous rash. The rash is characterized by a painful, sharply demarcated, intense erythema of the palms and/or soles followed by bulla formation, desquamation, and healing. Continuous low-dose 5-FU infusion (200–300 mg/m²/day) will produce this palmar-plantar erythrodysesthesia syndrome in 40–90% of patients (155–157). It occurs rarely with patients undergoing 96- to 120-hour infusions (158). The pathogenesis is unknown. The eruption is self-limiting in nature and it does not usually require discontinuation of therapy. Symptomatic measures are often required (158) and treatment with pyridoxine has been reported to induce resolution of the lesions (156).

### Postchemotherapy Gynecomastia

Painful gynecomastia can occur as a delayed complication of chemotherapy. Testis cancer is the most common underlying disorder (159,160), but it has been reported after therapy for other cancers as well (159,161,162). Gynecomastia typically develops after a latency of 2–9 months and resolves spontaneously within a few months. Persistent gynecomastia is occasionally observed (159). Cytotoxic-induced disturbance of androgen secretion is the probable cause of this syndrome (159,160,163). In the patient with testicular cancer, this syndrome must be differentiated from tumor-related gynecomastia, which may be associated with early recurrence (see below) (160,164,165).

### Chemotherapy-Induced Acute Digital Ischemia

Raynaud's phenomenon or transient ischemia of the toes is a common complication of bleomycin, vinblastine, and cisplatin (PVB) treatment for testicular cancer (166). Rarely, irreversible digital ischemia leading to gangrene has been reported after bleomycin administration (167, 168).

### Acute Pain Associated with Hormonal Therapy

#### Luteinizing Hormone–Releasing Factor (LHRF) Tumor Flare in Prostate Cancer

Initiation of LHRF hormonal therapy for prostate cancer produces a transient symptom flare in 5–25% of patients (169,170). The flare is presumably caused by an initial stimulation of luteinizing hormone release before suppression is achieved (169,171). The syndrome typically presents as an exacerbation of bone pain or urinary retention; spinal cord compression and sudden death have also been reported (170,172). Symptom flare is usually observed within the first week of therapy and lasts for 1–3 weeks in the absence of androgen antagonist therapy. Coadministration of an androgen antagonist during the initiation of LHRF agonist therapy can prevent this phenomenon (173–175). Among patients with prostate cancer that is refractory to first-line hormonal therapy, transient tumor flares have been observed with androstenedione (176,177) and medroxyprogesterone (178).

### Hormone-Induced Pain Flare in Breast Cancer

Any hormonal therapy for metastatic breast cancer can be complicated by a sudden onset of diffuse musculoskeletal pain commencing within hours to weeks of the initiation of therapy. Other manifestations of this syndrome include erythema around cutaneous metastases, changes in liver function studies, and hypercalcemia. Although the underlying mechanism is not understood, this does not appear to be caused by tumor stimulation, and it is speculated that it may reflect normal tissue response (179).

## Acute Pain Associated with Immunotherapy

### Interferon-Induced Acute Pain

Virtually all patients treated with interferon (IFN) experience an acute syndrome consisting of fever, chills, myalgias, arthralgias, and headache (180). The syndrome usually begins shortly after initial dosing and often improves with continued administration of the drug (180,181). The severity of symptoms is related to type of IFN, route of administration, schedule, and dose. Doses of 1 million to 9 million units of α-interferon are usually well tolerated, but doses greater than or equal to 18 million units usually produce moderate to severe toxicity (180). Acetaminophen pretreatment is often useful in ameliorating these symptoms (181).

## Acute Pain Associated with Growth Factors

### Colony-Stimulating Factor-Induced Musculoskeletal Pains

Colony-stimulating factors (CSFs) are hematopoietic growth hormones that stimulate the production, maturation, and function of white blood cells. Granulocyte-macrophage CSF (GM-CSF), granulocyte CSF (G-CSF), and interleukin-3 commonly produce mild to moderate bone pain and constitutional symptoms such as fever, headache, and myalgias during the period of administration (150,182,183).

### Erythropoietin (r-HuEPO) Injection Pain

Subcutaneous administration of r-HuEPO-α is associated with pain at the injection site in about 40% of cases. Subcutaneous injection of r-HuEPO-α is more painful than r-HuEPO-β (184). α-Erythropoietin injection pain can be reduced by dilution of the vehicle with benzyl alcohol saline or reduction of the volume of the vehicle to 1.0–0.1 ml (185).

## Acute Pain Associated with Radiotherapy

Incident pains can be precipitated by transport and positioning of the patient for radiotherapy. Other pains can be caused by acute radiation toxicity, which is most commonly associated with inflammation and ulceration of skin or mucous membranes within the radiation port. The syndrome produced is dependent on the involved field: head and neck irradiation can cause a stomatitis or pharyngitis (186), treatment of the chest and esophagus can cause an esophagitis (187), and pelvic therapy can cause a proctitis, cystitis-urethritis, or vaginal ulceration. Rare syndromes involve skin or neural tissues.

### Oropharyngeal Mucositis

Radiotherapy-induced mucositis is invariable with doses above 1000 cGy, and ulceration is common at doses above 4000 cGy. Although the severity of the associated pain is variable, it is often severe enough to interfere with oral alimentation. Painful mucositis can persist for several weeks after the completion of the treatment (188).

### Acute Radiation Enteritis and Proctocolitis

Acute radiation enteritis occurs in as many as 50% of patients receiving abdominal or pelvic radiotherapy. Involvement of the small intestine can present with cramping abdominal pain associated with nausea and diarrhea (189,190). Pelvic radiotherapy can cause a painful proctocolitis, with tenesmoid pain associated with diarrhea, mucous discharge, and bleeding (189). These complications typically resolve shortly after completion of therapy but may have a slow resolution over 2–6 months (189,190). Acute enteritis is associated with an increased risk of late onset radiation enteritis (see below) (189).

### Early Onset Brachial Plexopathy

A transient brachial plexopathy has been described in breast cancer patients immediately following radiotherapy to the chest wall and adjacent nodal areas. In retrospective studies, the incidence of this phenomenon has been variably estimated as 1.4–20% (191–193); clinical experience suggests that lower estimates are more accurate. The median latency to the development of symptoms was 4.5 months (3–14 months) in one survey (192). Paresthesias are the most common presenting symptom, and pain and weakness occur less frequently. The syndrome is self-limiting and does not predispose to the subsequent development of delayed onset, progressive plexopathy.

### Subacute Radiation Myelopathy

Subacute radiation myelopathy can occur following radiotherapy of extraspinal tumors (194). It is most frequently observed involving the cervical cord after radiation treatment of head and neck cancers and Hodgkin's disease. In the latter case, patients develop painful, shock-like pains in the neck that are precipitated by neck flexion (Lhermitte's sign); these pains may radiate down the spine and into one or more extremities. The syndrome usually begins weeks to months after the completion of radiotherapy and typically resolves over 3–6 months (194).

### Strontium-89-Induced Pain Flare

Strontium-89 is a systemically administered β-emitting calcium analogue that is taken up by bone in areas of osteoblastic activity (195) and may reduce pain caused by blastic bony metastases. A "flare" response, characterized by transient worsening of pain 1–2 days after administration, occurs in 15–20% of patients (196). This flare is usually resolves after 3–5 days and most affected patients subsequently develop a good analgesic response (196).

## Acute Pain Associated with Infection

### Acute Herpetic Neuralgia

A significantly increased incidence of acute herpetic neuralgia occurs among cancer patients, especially those with hematologic or lymphoproliferative malignancies and those receiving immunosuppressive therapies (197,198). Pain or itch usually precedes the development of the rash by several days and may occasionally occur without the development of skin eruption (198). The pain, which may be continuous or lancinating, usually resolves within 2 months (198). Persistent pain is referred to as postherpetic neuralgia (see below). Patients with active tumor are more likely to disseminate the infection (199). In those predisposed by chemotherapy, the infection usually develops less than 1 month after the completion of treatment. The dermatomal location of the infection is often associated with the site of the malig-

nancy (199): Patients with primary tumors of gynecologic and genitourinary origin have a predilection to lumbar and sacral involvement, and those with breast or lung carcinomas tend to present with thoracic involvement; patients with hematologic tumors appear to be predisposed to cervical lesions. The infection also occurs twice as frequently in previously irradiated dermatomes as nonradiated areas.

## Acute Pain Associated with Vascular Events

### Acute Thrombosis Pain

Thrombosis is the most common complication and the second cause of death in patients with overt malignant disease (200). Thrombotic episodes may precede the diagnosis of cancer by months or years and represent a potential marker for occult malignancy (201). Postoperative deep vein thrombosis (DVT) is more frequent in patients operated for malignant diseases than for other disorders, and both chemotherapy and hormone therapy are associated with an increased thrombotic risk (201).

Possible prothrombic factors in cancer include the capacity of tumor cells and their products to interact with platelets, clotting and fibrinolytic systems, endothelial cells, and tumor-associated macrophages. Cytokine release, acute phase reaction, and neovascularization may contribute to in vivo clotting activation (200). Patients with pelvic tumors (202,203), pancreatic cancer, advanced breast cancer (204), and brain tumors (205) are at greatest risk.

### Lower Extremity Deep Venous Thrombosis

Pain and swelling are the commonest presenting features of lower extremity DVT (206). The pain is variable in severity and is often mild. It is commonly described as a dull cramp or diffuse heaviness. The pain most commonly affects the calf but may involve the sole of the foot, the heel, the thigh, the groin, or the pelvis. Pain usually increases on standing and walking. On examination, suggestive features include swelling, warmth, dilatation of superficial veins, tenderness along venous tracts, and pain induced by stretching (206,207).

The diagnosis can usually be confirmed by noninvasive tests, such as ultrasonography or impedance plethysmography, rather than venography. Ultrasonography is sensitive, effectively defines the anatomic extent of the thrombus; it is the diagnostic standard for symptomatic DVT (208). Impedance plethysmography is a less sensitive alternative (209). When the findings of these noninvasive approaches are at variance with a strong clinical impression, venography should be considered (208).

Among patients with DVT, the development of tissue ischemia or frank gangrene, even without arterial or capillary occlusion, is most commonly seen in patients with underlying neoplasm (210). This condition is characterized by the development of severe pain, extensive edema, and cyanosis of the legs. Gangrene can occur unless the venous obstruction is relieved. When possible, optimal therapy is anticoagulation and thrombectomy. The mortality rate for ischemic venous thrombosis is about 40%, the cause of death usually being the underlying disease or pulmonary emboli (210).

### Upper Extremity Deep Venous Thrombosis

Only 2% of all cases of DVT involve the upper extremity, and the incidence of pulmonary embolism related to thrombosis in this location is approximately 12% (211). The three major clinical features of upper extremity venous thrombosis are edema, dilated collateral circulation, and pain (212). Approximately two thirds of patients have arm pain. Among patents with cancer, the most common causes are central venous catheterization and extrinsic compression by tumor (212). Although thrombosis secondary to intrinsic damage usually responds well to anticoagulation alone and rarely causes persistent symptoms, persistent arm swelling and pain are commonplace when extrinsic obstruction is the cause (213).

### Superior Vena Cava Obstruction

Superior vena cava (SVC) obstruction is most commonly caused by extrinsic compression by enlarged mediastinal lymph nodes (214,215). In contemporary series, lung cancer and lymphomas are the most associated conditions. Patients usually present with facial swelling and dilated neck and chest wall veins. Chest pain, headache, and mastalgia are less common presentations.

## CHRONIC PAIN SYNDROMES

Most chronic cancer-related pains are caused directly by the tumor (Table 2) (17,41,43,216,217). Bone pain and compression of neural structures are the two most common causes (6,17,41,43,216,217).

## Bone Pain

Bone metastases are the most common cause of chronic pain in cancer patients (41,44,216,218,219). Cancers of the lung, breast, and prostate most often metastasize to bone, but any tumor type may be complicated by painful bony lesions. Although bone pain is usually associated with direct tumor invasion of bony structures, more than 25% of patients with bony metastases are pain-free (220), and patients with multiple bony metastases typically report pain in only a few sites. The factors that convert a painless lesion to a painful one are unknown.

Bone metastases could potentially cause pain by any of multiple mechanisms, including endosteal or periosteal nociceptor activation (by mechanical distortion or release of chemical mediators) or tumor growth into adjacent soft tissues and nerves (218).

Bone pain due to metastatic tumor needs to be differentiated from less common causes. Nonneoplastic causes in this population include osteoporotic fractures (including those associated with multiple myeloma); focal osteonecrosis, which may be idiopathic or related to corticosteroids or radiotherapy (see below), and osteomalacia (221).

### Multifocal or Generalized Bone Pain

Bone pain may be focal, multifocal, or generalized. Multifocal bone pains are most commonly experienced by patients with multiple bony metastases. A generalized pain syndrome, which is well recognized in patients with multiple bony metastases, is also rarely produced by replacement of bone marrow (222,223). This bone marrow replacement syndrome has been observed in hematogenous malignancies and, less commonly, solid tumors (222). This syndrome can occur in the absence of abnormalities on bone scintigraphy or radiography, increasing the difficulty of diagnosis. Rarely, a paraneoplastic osteomalacia can mimic multiple metastases (221).

### Vertebral Syndromes

The vertebrae are the most common sites of bony metastases. More than two thirds of vertebral metastases are located in the thoracic spine; lumbosacral and cervical metastases account for approximately 20% and 10%, respectively (224,225). Multiple level involvement is common, occurring in greater than 85% of patients (226). The early recognition of pain syndromes due to tumor invasion of vertebral bodies is essential because pain usually precedes compression of adjacent neural structures and prompt treatment of the lesion may prevent the subsequent development of neurologic deficits. Several factors often confound accurate diagnosis; referral of pain is common, and the associated symptoms and signs can mimic a variety of other disorders, both malignant (e.g., paraspinal masses) and nonmalignant.

### Atlantoaxial Destruction and Odontoid Fracture

Nuchal or occipital pain is the typical presentation of destruction of the atlas or fracture of the odontoid process. Pain often radiates over the posterior aspect of the skull to the vertex and is exacerbated by movement of the neck, particularly flexion (227). Pathologic fracture may result in secondary subluxation with compression of the spinal cord at the cervicomedullary junction. This complication is usually insidious and may begin with symptoms or signs in one or more extremity. Typically, there is early involvement of the upper extremities and the occasional appearance of so-called pseudo-levels suggestive of more caudal spinal lesions; these deficits can slowly progress to involve sensory, motor, and autonomic function in the extremities (228). MRI is probably the best method for imaging this region of the spine (229), but clinical experience suggests that CT is also sensitive. Plain radiography, tomography, and bone scintigraphy should be viewed as ancillary procedures.

### C7–T1 Syndrome

Invasion of the C7 or T1 vertebra can result in pain referred to the interscapular region. These lesions might be missed if radiographic evaluation is mistakenly targeted to the painful area caudal to the site of damage. Additionally, visualization of the appropriate region on routine radiographs might be inadequate due to obscuration by overlying bone and mediastinal shadows. Patients with interscapular pain should therefore undergo radiography of both the cervical and thoracic spines. Bone scintigraphy may assist in targeting additional diagnostic imaging procedures, such as CT or MRI. The latter procedures can be useful in assessing the possibility that pain is referred from an extraspinal site, such as the paraspinal gutter.

### T12–L1 Syndrome

A T12 or L1 vertebral lesion can refer pain to the ipsilateral iliac crest or the sacroiliac joint. Imaging procedures directed at pelvic bones can miss the source of the pain.

### Sacral Syndrome

Severe focal pain radiating to buttocks, perineum, or posterior thighs may accompany destruction of the sacrum (230). The pain is often exacerbated by sitting or lying down and is relieved by standing or walking. The neoplasm can spread laterally to involve muscles that rotate the hip (e.g., the pyriformis muscle). This may produce severe incident pain induced by motion of the hip, or a malignant "pyriformis syndrome," characterized by buttock or posterior leg pain that is exacerbated by internal rotation of the hip. Local extension of the tumor mass may also involve the sacral plexus (see below).

### Back Pain and Epidural Compression

Epidural compression (EC) of the spinal cord or cauda equina is the second most common neurologic complication of cancer, occurring in up to 10% of patients (71). In the community setting, EC is often the first recognized

manifestation of malignancy (231); at a cancer hospital it is the presenting syndrome in only 8% of cases (71). Most EC is caused by posterior extension of vertebral body metastasis to the epidural space (Fig. 4). Occasionally, EC is caused by tumor extension from the posterior arch of the vertebra or infiltration of a paravertebral tumor through the intervertebral foramen (Fig. 5).

Untreated, EC leads inevitably to neurologic compromise, ultimately including paraplegia or quadriplegia. Effective treatment can potentially prevent these complications. The most important determinant of treatment outcome is the degree of neurologic impairment at the time therapy is initiated. Seventy-five percent of patients who begin treatment while ambulatory remain so; the efficacy of treatment declines to 30–50% for those who begin treatment while markedly paretic and is less than 10% for those who are plegic (71,224,232–236). Treatment generally involves the administration of corticosteroids (see below) and radiotherapy (236). Surgical decompression is considered for some patients with radioresistant tumors, those who have previously received maximal radiotherapy to the involved field, those with spinal instability, and those for whom no other tissue is available for histologic diagnosis (71,237). Decompressive laminectomy for posteriorly located lesions and anterior vertebrectomy with spinal stabilization for lesions arising from the vertebral body are the currently recommended procedures (238–241). Decompressive laminectomy in the setting of vertebral body collapse is not recommended because of the risk of neurologic deterioration

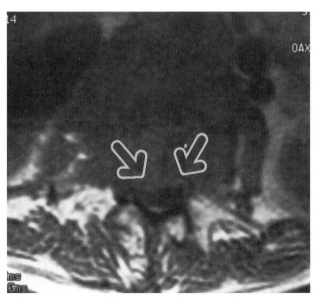

**FIG. 4.** Axial MRI scan of the lumbar spine in a 56-year-old woman with carcinoma of the colon who presented with back pain and L3 radicular pain in the right leg. Performed through L3, the scan demonstrates complete obliteration of the epidural space (*arrows*) and severe compression of the thecal sac.

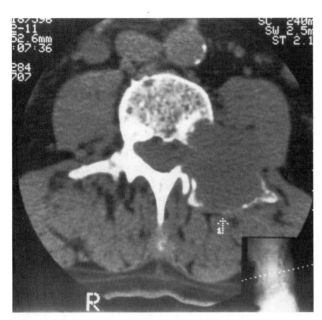

**FIG. 5.** CT scan of lumbar vertebra demonstrating a large metastasis involving the left transverse process, invading into the intervertebral foranen and encroaching into the epidural space.

or spinal instability (22–25%) induced by the procedure (242,243).

Back pain is the initial symptom in almost all patients with EC (71), and in 10% it is the only symptom at the time of diagnosis (244). Because pain usually precedes neurologic signs by a prolonged period, it should be viewed as a potential indicator of EC, which could lead to treatment at a time that a favorable response is most likely. Back pain, however, is a nonspecific symptom that can result from bony or paraspinal metastases without epidural encroachment, from retroperitoneal or leptomeningeal tumor, epidural lipomatosis due to steroid administration (245) or from a large variety of other benign conditions. Because it is infeasible to pursue an extensive evaluation in every cancer patient who develops back pain, the complaint should impel an evaluation that determines the likelihood of EC and thereby selects patients appropriate for definitive imaging of the epidural space. The selection process is based on symptoms and signs and the results of simple imaging techniques.

### Clinical Features of Epidural Extension

Some pain characteristics are particularly suggestive of epidural extension. Rapid progression of back pain in a crescendo pattern is an ominous occurrence (235,246). Radicular pain, which can be constant or lancinating, has similar implications (247). Radicular pain is usually unilateral in the cervical and lumbosacral regions and bilateral in the thorax, where it is often experienced as a tight, belt-like band across the chest or abdomen (246). The likelihood of EC is also greater when back or radicular pain is exacerbated by recumbency, cough, sneeze or strain (233,246). Other types of referred pain are also suggestive, including Lhermitte's sign (248,249) and central pain from spinal cord compression, which usually is perceived some distance below the site of the compression and is typically a poorly localized, nondermatomal dysesthesia (71).

Weakness, sensory loss, autonomic dysfunction, and reflex abnormalities usually occur after a period of progressive pain. Weakness may begin segmentally if related to nerve root damage or in a multisegmental or pyramidal distribution if the cauda equina or spinal cord, respectively, is injured. The rate of progression of weakness is variable; in the absence of treatment, one third of patients will develop paralysis within 7 days following the onset of weakness (250). Patients whose weakness progresses slowly have a better prognosis for neurologic recovery with treatment than those who progress rapidly (251). Without effective treatment, sensory abnormalities, which may also begin segmentally, may ultimately evolve to a sensory level, with complete loss of all sensory modalities below the site of injury. The upper level of sensory findings may correspond to the location of the epidural tumor or be below it by many segments. Ataxia without pain is the initial presentation of epidural compression in 1% of patients; this finding is presumably due to early involvement of the spinocerebellar tracts (224). Bladder and bowel dysfunction occur late, except in patients with a conus medullaris lesion, who may present with acute urinary retention and constipation without preceding motor or sensory symptoms (248).

Other features that may be evident on examination of patients with EC include scoliosis, asymmetric wasting of paravertebral musculature, and a gibbus (palpable step in the spinous processes). Spinal tenderness to percussion, which may be severe, often accompanies the pain.

### Imaging Modalities

Definitive imaging of the epidural space confirms the existence of EC (and thereby indicates the necessity and urgency of treatment), defines the appropriate radiation portals, and determines the extent of epidural encroachment (which influences prognosis and may alter the therapeutic approach) (70). The options for definitive imaging include MRI, myelography, and CT-myelography. MRI, which is noninvasive and offers accurate soft tissue imaging and multiplanar views, is generally preferred. It should be recognized, however, that there are no studies comparing state-of-the-art MRI techniques with myelography in the evaluation of EC, and some data suggest that some techniques, such as a "scanning" midsagittal MRI, are clearly inadequate (252). Myelography remains the investigation of choice for patients who lack access to

MRI and those unable to undergo the procedure. MRI is relatively contraindicated in patients with severe claustrophobia and absolutely contraindicated for patients with metallic implants, cardiac pacemakers, or aneurysm clips. Patients who require total spinal imaging, such as those with multifocal pain or multiple spinal metastases [who have a 10% chance of EC remote from the symptomatic site (231)], can undergo MRI but may need myelography if complete spinal MRI is not feasible for some reason. Those with severe kyphosis or scoliosis, who may not be suitable for MRI scanning due to technical considerations, may also need a different approach. Myelography may also be needed following an MRI scan that is suboptimal or nondiagnostic, particularly in the setting of neurologic deterioration.

### Algorithm for the Investigation of Cancer Patients with Back Pain

Given the prevalence and the potentially dire consequences of EC and the recognition that back pain is a marker of early (and therefore treatable) EC, algorithms have been developed to guide the evaluation of back pain in the cancer patient. The objective of these algorithms is to select a subgroup who should undergo definitive imaging of the epidural space from among the large number of patients who develop back pain (70). Effective treatment of EC before irreversible neurologic compromise occurs is the overriding goal of these approaches.

One such algorithm defines both the urgency and course of the evaluation. Patients with emerging symptoms and signs indicative of spinal cord or cauda equina dysfunction are designated as group 1. The evaluation (and, if appropriate, treatment) of these patients should proceed on an emergency basis. In most cases, these patients should receive an intravenous dose of corticosteroid before epidural imaging is performed. Dexamethasone is used customarily. High doses have been advocated on the basis of animal studies (253), analgesic efficacy (244), and the dose–response relationship that has been observed during treatment of intracranial hypertension from mass lesions. One regimen advocates an initial IV bolus of 100 mg followed by 96 mg/day in divided doses, which is tapered over 3–4 weeks. Although a randomized trial failed to identify any difference in neurologic outcome between a high (100 mg) and low (10 mg) initial dose (254), these findings need to be replicated on a larger sample, and high doses can still be recommended on the basis of a favorable clinical experience.

Patients with symptoms and signs of radiculopathy or stable or mild signs of spinal cord or cauda equina dysfunction are designated as group 2. These patients are also usually treated presumptively with a corticosteroid (typically with a more moderate dose) and are scheduled for definitive imaging of the epidural space as soon as possible.

Group 3 patients have back pain and no symptoms or signs suggesting EC. Unless the back pain has ominous characteristics (e.g., "crescendo" pattern or marked exacerbation with recumbency), these patients should be evaluated in routine fashion starting with plain spine radiographs. The presence at the appropriate level of any abnormality consistent with neoplasm indicates a high probability (60%) of EC (255,256). This likelihood varies, however, with the type of radiologic abnormality; for example, one study noted that EC occurred in 87% of patients with greater than 50% vertebral body collapse, 31% with pedicle erosion, and only 7% with tumor limited to the body of the vertebra without collapse (257). Definitive imaging of the epidural space is thus strongly indicated in patients who have more than 50% vertebral body collapse and is generally recommended for patients with pedicle erosion. Some patients with neoplasm limited to the vertebral body can be followed expectantly; imaging should be performed if pain progresses or changes (e.g., become radicular), or if radiographic evidence of progression is obtained.

Among patients with vertebral collapse it is often difficult to distinguish malignant from nonmalignant pathology. Vertebral metastases are suggested by destruction of the anterolateral or posterior cortical bone of the vertebral body, the cancellous bone or vertebral pedicle; a focal paraspinal soft tissue mass; or an epidural mass. Nonmalignant causes are suggested by cortical fractures of the vertebral body without cortical bone destruction, retropulsion of a fragment of the posterior cortex of the vertebral body into the spinal canal, fracture lines within the cancellous bone of the vertebral body, an intravertebral vacuum phenomenon, and a thin diffuse paraspinal soft tissue mass (258).

Normal spine radiographs alone are not adequate to ensure a low likelihood of epidural tumor in patients with back pain. The bone may not be sufficiently damaged to change the radiograph or the tumor may involve the epidural space with little or no involvement of the adjacent bone (such as may occur when paraspinal tumor grows through the intervertebral foramen). The latter phenomenon has been most strikingly demonstrated in patients with lymphoma, in whom EC presents with normal radiography more than 60% of the time (259). Damage to the vertebra that is not seen on the plain radiograph may potentially be demonstrated by bone scintigraphy. In patients with back pain and normal bone radiography, a positive scintigram at the site of pain is associated with a 12–17% likelihood of epidural disease (232,260). Although such patients can also be followed expectantly, definitive imaging of the epidural space should be considered, particularly if the pain is progressive.

If both radiographs and scintigraphy are normal but the patient has severe or progressive pain, evaluation with CT or, preferably, MRI may still be warranted. If the CT scan demonstrates either a bony lesion abutting the spinal canal, a paraspinal mass, or a paravertebral soft tissue "collar," imaging of the epidural space is still justified (232).

### Pain Syndromes of the Bony Pelvis and Hip

The pelvis and hip are common sites of metastatic involvement. Lesions may involve any of the three anatomic regions of the pelvis (ischiopubic, iliosacral, or periacetabular), the hip joint itself, or the proximal femur (261). The weight bearing function of these structures, essential for normal ambulation, contributes to the propensity of disease at these sites to cause incident pain with ambulation.

### Hip Joint Syndrome

Tumor involvement of the acetabulum or head of femur typically produces localized hip pain that is aggravated by weight bearing and movement of the hip. The pain may radiate to the knee or medial thigh, and occasionally, pain is limited to these structures (261). Medial extension of an acetabular tumor can involve the lumbosacral plexus as it traverses the pelvic sidewall (Fig. 6). Evaluation of this region is best accomplished with CT or MRI, both of which can demonstrate the extent of bony destruction and adjacent soft tissue involvement more sensitively than other imaging techniques (262).

### Acrometastases

Acrometastases are rare and often misdiagnosed or overlooked (263). In the feet, the larger bones contain-

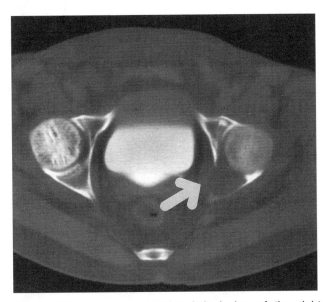

**FIG. 6.** CT scan demonstrating lytic lesion of the right acetabulum with tumor extension into the pelvis (*arrow*).

ing the higher amounts of red marrow, such as the os calcis, are usually involved (264). Symptoms may be vague and can mimic other conditions, such as osteomyelitis, gouty rheumatoid arthritis, Reiter's syndrome, Paget's disease, osteochondral lesions, and ligamentous sprains (265).

### Arthritides

#### Hypertrophic Pulmonary Osteoarthropathy

Hypertrophic pulmonary osteoarthropathy (HPOA) is a paraneoplastic syndrome that includes clubbing of the fingers, periostitis of long bones, and, occasionally, a rheumatoid-like polyarthritis (266,267). Periosteitis and arthritis can produce pain, tenderness, and swelling in the knees, wrists, and ankles. The onset of symptoms is usually subacute, and it may proceed the discovery of the underlying neoplasm by several months. It is most commonly associated with non–small cell lung cancer. Less commonly, it may be associated with benign mesothelioma (268), pulmonary metastases from other sites (269), smooth muscle tumors of the esophagus (270), breast cancer (271), or metastatic nasopharyngeal cancer. Effective anti-tumor therapy is sometimes associated with symptom regression (271,272). HPOA is diagnosed on the basis of physical findings, radiologic appearance, and radionuclide bone scan (267,273).

#### Other Polyarthritides

Rarely, rheumatoid arthritis, systemic lupus erythematosus, and an asymmetric polyarthritis may occur as paraneoplastic phenomena that resolve with effective treatment of the underlying disease (274).

### Muscle Pain

#### Muscle Cramps

Persistent muscle cramps in cancer patients are usually caused by an identifiable neural, muscular, or biochemical abnormality (275). In one series of 50 patients, 22 had peripheral neuropathy, 17 had root or plexus pathology (including 6 with leptomeningeal metastases), 2 had polymyositis, and 1 had hypomagnesemia. In this series, muscle cramps were the presenting symptom of recognizable and previously unsuspected neurologic dysfunction in 64% (27 of 42) of the identified causes (275).

#### Skeletal Muscle Tumors

Soft tissue sarcomas arising from fat, fibrous tissue, or skeletal muscle are the most common tumors involving the skeletal muscles. Skeletal muscle is one of the most unusual sites of metastasis from any malignancy (276). Lesions are usually painless but they may present with persistent ache.

### Headache and Facial Pain

Headache in the cancer patient results from traction, inflammation, or infiltration of pain-sensitive structures in the head or neck (277). Early evaluation with appropriate imaging techniques may identify the lesion and allow prompt treatment, which may reduce pain and prevent the development of neurologic deficits (278).

#### *Intracerebral Tumor*

Among 183 patients with the sole symptom of new-onset chronic headache, investigation revealed underlying tumor in 15 cases (279). The prevalence of headache in patients with brain metastases or primary brain tumors is 60–90% (280,281). The headache is presumably produced by traction on pain-sensitive vascular and dural tissues. Patients with multiple metastases and those with posterior fossa metastases are more likely to report this symptom (280,282,283). The pain may be focal, overlying the site of the lesion, or generalized. Headache has lateralizing value, especially in patients with supratentorial lesions (281). Posterior fossa lesions often cause a bifrontal headache (277). The quality of the headache is usually throbbing or steady, and the intensity is usually mild to moderate (281). The headache is often worse in the morning and is exacerbated by stooping, sudden head movement, or Valsalva maneuvers (cough, sneeze, or strain) (281). In patients with increased intracranial pressure, these maneuvers can also precipitate transient elevations in intracranial pressure, called "plateau waves." These plateau waves, which may also be spontaneous, can be associated with short periods of severe headache, nausea, vomiting, photophobia, lethargy, and transient neurologic deficits (284). Occasionally these plateau waves produce life-threatening herniation syndromes (284).

#### *Leptomeningeal Metastases*

Leptomeningeal metastases, which are characterized by diffuse or multifocal involvement of the subarachnoid space by metastatic tumor, occur in 1–8% of patients with systemic cancer (283). Non-Hodgkin's lymphoma and acute lymphocytic leukemia both demonstrate a predilection for meningeal metastases; the incidence is lower for solid tumors alone. Of solid tumors, adenocarcinomas of the breast and lung predominate.

Leptomeningeal metastases present with focal or multifocal neurologic symptoms or signs that may involve any level of the neuraxis (285,286). More than one-third of patients present with evidence of cranial nerve dam-

age, including double vision, hearing loss, facial numbness, and decreased vision (286). Less common features include seizures, papilledema, hemiparesis, and ataxic gait. Generalized headache and radicular pain in the low back and buttocks are the most common pains associated with leptomeningeal metastases (286,287). The headache is variable and may be associated with changes in mental status (e.g., lethargy, confusion, or loss of memory), nausea, vomiting, tinnitus, or nuchal rigidity. Pains that resemble cluster headache (288) or glossopharyngeal neuralgia with syncope (289) have also been reported.

The diagnosis of leptomeningeal metastases is confirmed through analysis of the CSF. The CSF may reveal elevated pressure, elevated protein, depressed glucose, and/or lymphocytic pleocytosis. Ninety percent of patients ultimately show positive cytology, but multiple evaluations may be required. After a single LP, the false-negative rate may be as high as 55%; this falls to only 10% after three LPs (286,287,290). Tumor markers, such as lactic dehydrogenase (LDH) isoenzymes (291), carcinoembryonic antigen (CEA) (292), and $\beta_2$-microglobulin (293), may help to delineate the diagnosis. Flow cytometry for detection of abnormal DNA content may be a useful adjunct to cytologic examination (294). Imaging studies may also be of value. MRI of the cranium and spinal cord with gadolinium enhancement is the most sensitive imaging modality (Fig. 7) (295,296), but cost and availability may limit its utility at present. Myelography is abnormal in up to 30% of patients, and CT or MRI of the head may demonstrate enhancement of the dural membranes or ventricular enlargement (297,298).

Untreated leptomeningeal metastases cause progressive neurologic dysfunction at multiple sites, followed by

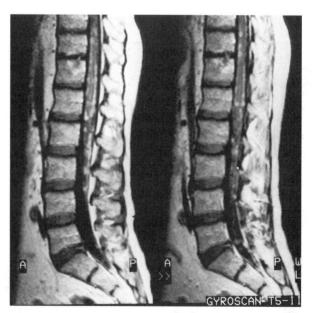

**FIG. 7.** Gadolinium enhanced MRI scan of the thorocolumbar spine demonstrating multifocal meningeal enhancement consistent with leptomeningeal metastases.

death in 4–6 weeks. Treatment, which includes radiation therapy to the area of symptomatic involvement, corticosteroids, and intraventricular or intrathecal chemotherapy, can be salutary; for example, patients with breast carcinoma have a median survival of 7 months following therapy (299).

### Base of Skull Metastases

Base of skull metastases are associated with well-described clinical syndromes (300), which are named according to the site of metastatic involvement: orbital, parasellar, middle fossa, jugular foramen, occipital condyle, clivus, and sphenoid sinus. Cancers of the breast, lung, and prostate are most commonly associated with this complication (300), but any tumor type that metastasizes to bone may be responsible. When base of skull metastases are suspected, axial imaging with CT (including bone window settings) is the usual initial procedure (Fig. 8) (300). MRI is more sensitive for assessing soft tissue extension, and CSF analysis may be needed to exclude leptomeningeal metastases.

### Orbital Syndrome

Orbital metastases usually present with progressive pain in the retroorbital and supraorbital area of the affected eye. Blurred vision and diplopia may be associated complaints. Signs may include proptosis, chemosis

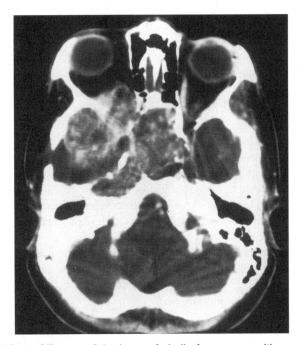

**FIG. 8.** CT scan of the base of skull of a woman with proptosis and right sided facial pain. There is extensive tumor erosion of the orbital wall, clivus, and the floor of the middle cranial fossa.

of the involved eye, external ophthalmoparesis, ipsilateral papilledema, and decreased sensation in the ophthalmic division of the trigeminal nerve. Imaging with MRI or CT scan can delineate the extent of bony damage and orbital infiltration.

### Parasellar Syndrome

The parasellar syndrome typically presents as unilateral supraorbital and frontal headache, which may be associated with diplopia. There may be ophthalmoparesis or papilledema, and formal visual field testing may demonstrate hemianopsia or quadrantinopsia.

### Middle Cranial Fossa Syndrome

The middle cranial fossa syndrome presents with facial numbness, paresthesias, or pain, which is usually referred to the cheek or jaw (in the distribution of second or third divisions of the trigeminal nerve). The pain is typically described as a dull continual ache but may also be paroxysmal or lancinating. On examination, patients may have hypesthesia in the trigeminal nerve distribution and signs of weakness in the ipsilateral muscles of mastication. Occasional patients have other neurologic signs, such as abducens nerve palsy (300, 301).

### Jugular Foramen Syndrome

The jugular foramen syndrome usually presents with hoarseness or dysphagia. Pain is usually referred to the ipsilateral ear or mastoid region and may occasionally present as glossopharyngeal neuralgia, with or without syncope (300). Pain may also be referred to the ipsilateral neck or shoulder. Neurologic signs include ipsilateral Horner's syndrome, and paresis of the palate, vocal cord, sternocleidomastoid, or trapezius. Ipsilateral paresis of the tongue may also occur if the tumor extends to the region of the hypoglossal canal.

### Occipital Condyle Syndrome

The occipital condyle syndrome presents with unilateral occipital pain that is worsened with neck flexion. The patient may complain of neck stiffness. Pain intensity is variable but can be severe. Examination may reveal a head tilt, limited movement of the neck, and tenderness to palpation over the occipitonuchal junction. Neurologic findings may include ipsilateral hypoglossal nerve paralysis and sternocleidomastoid weakness.

### Clivus Syndrome

The clivus syndrome is characterized by vertex headache, which is often exacerbated by neck flexion.

Lower cranial nerve (VI–XII) dysfunction follows and may become bilateral.

### Sphenoid Sinus Syndrome

A sphenoid sinus metastasis often presents with bifrontal and or retroorbital pain, which may radiate to the temporal regions. There may be associated features of nasal congestion and diplopia. Physical examination is often unremarkable, although unilateral or bilateral abducens nerve paresis can be present.

### Painful Cranial Neuralgias

As noted, specific cranial neuralgias can occur from metastases in the base of skull or leptomeninges. They are most commonly observed in patients with prostate and lung cancer (302). Invasion of the soft tissues of the head or neck, or involvement of sinuses, can also eventuate in such lesions. Each of these syndromes has a characteristic presentation. Early diagnosis may allow effective treatment of the underlying lesion before progressive neurologic injury occurs.

### Glossopharyngeal Neuralgia

Glossopharyngeal neuralgia has been reported in patients with leptomeningeal metastases (289), the jugular foramen syndrome (300), or head and neck malignancies (303–305). This syndrome presents as severe pain in the throat or neck, which may radiate to the ear or mastoid region. Pain may be induced by swallowing. In some patients, pain is associated with sudden orthostasis and syncope.

### Trigeminal Neuralgia

Trigeminal pains may be continual, paroxysmal, or lancinating. Pain that mimics classical trigeminal neuralgia can be induced by tumors in the middle or posterior fossa (301,306,307) or leptomeningeal metastases (288). All cancer patients who develop trigeminal neuralgia should be evaluated for the existence of an underlying neoplasm.

### Uncommon Causes of Headache and Facial Pain

Headache and facial pain in cancer patients may have many other causes. Unilateral facial pain can be the initial symptom of an ipsilateral lung tumor (308,309). Presumably, this referred pain is mediated by vagal afferents. Patients with Hodgkin's disease may have transient episodes of neurologic dysfunction that has been likened to migraine (310,311). Headache may occur with cerebral infarction or hemorrhage, which may be due to nonbacterial thrombotic endocarditis, disseminated intravascular coagulation, or other cancer-related phenomena. Headache is also the usual presentation of sagittal sinus occlusion, which may be due to tumor infiltration, hypercoagulable state, or treatment with L-asparaginase therapy (146). Headache due to pseudotumor cerebri has also been reported to be the presentation of superior vena caval obstruction in a patient with lung cancer (312). Tumors of the sinonasal tract may present with deep facial or nasal pain (313).

### Neuropathic Pains Involving the Peripheral Nervous System

Neuropathic pains involving the peripheral nervous system are common and clinically challenging problems in the cancer population. The syndromes include painful radiculopathy, plexopathy, mononeuropathy, and peripheral neuropathy.

### Painful Radiculopathy

Radiculopathy or polyradiculopathy may be caused by any process that compresses, distorts, or inflames nerve roots.

### Tumor-Related Radiculopathy

Painful radiculopathy is an important presentation of epidural tumor and leptomeningeal metastases (see above).

### Postherpetic Neuralgia

Postherpetic neuralgia is defined solely by the persistence of pain in the region of a zoster infection. Although some authors apply this term if pain continues beyond lesion healing, most require a period of weeks to months before this label is used; a criterion of pain persisting for several months beyond lesion healing is recommended (198). One study suggests that postherpetic neuralgia is two to three times more common in the cancer population than in the general population (199). In patients with postherpetic neuralgia and cancer, changes in the intensity or pattern of pain, or the development of new neurologic deficits, may indicate the possibility of local neoplasm and should be investigated.

### Cervical Plexopathy

The ventral rami of the upper four cervical spinal nerves join to form the cervical plexus between the deep anterior and lateral muscles of the neck. Cutaneous branches emerge from the posterior border of the sternocleidomastoid. In the cancer population, plexus injury is frequently due to tumor infiltration or treatment (including surgery or radiotherapy) to neoplasms in this region (314,315).

### Malignant Cervical Plexopathy

Tumor invasion or compression of the cervical plexus can be caused by direct extension of a primary head and neck malignancy or neoplastic (metastatic or lymphomatous) involvement of the cervical lymph nodes (314,315). Pain may be experienced in the preauricular (greater auricular nerve) or postauricular (lesser and greater occipital nerves) regions, or the anterior neck (transverse cutaneous and supraclavicular nerves). Pain may refer to the lateral aspect of the face or head, or to the ipsilateral shoulder. The overlap in the pain referral patterns from the face and neck may relate to the close anatomic relationship between the central connections of cervical afferents and the afferents carried in cranial nerves V, VII, IX, and X (316). The pain may be aching, burning, or lancinating and is often exacerbated by neck movement or swallowing. Associated features can include ipsilateral Horner's syndrome or hemidiaphragmatic paralysis. The diagnosis must be distinguished from epidural compression of the cervical spinal cord and leptomeningeal metastases. MRI or CT imaging of the neck and cervical spine is usually required to evaluate the etiology of the pain.

### Brachial Plexopathy

The two most common causes of brachial plexopathy in cancer patients are tumor infiltration and radiation injury. Less common causes of painful brachial plexopathy include trauma during surgery or anesthesia, radiation-induced second neoplasms, acute brachial plexus ischemia, and paraneoplastic brachial neuritis.

### Malignant Brachial Plexopathy

Plexus infiltration by tumor is the most prevalent cause of brachial plexopathy. Malignant brachial plexopathy is most common in patients with lymphoma, lung cancer, or breast cancer. The invading tumor usually arises from adjacent axillary, cervical, and supraclavicular lymph nodes (lymphoma and breast cancer) or from the lung (superior sulcus tumors or so-called Pancoast tumors) (317). Pain is nearly universal, occurring in 85% of patients, and often precedes neurologic signs or symptoms by months (318,319). Lower plexus involvement (C7, C8, T1 distribution) is typical and is reflected in the pain distribution, which usually involves the elbow, medial forearm, and fourth and fifth fingers. Pain may sometimes localize to the posterior arm or elbow. Severe aching is usually reported, but patients may also experience constant or lancinating dysesthesias along the ulnar aspect of the forearm or hand.

Tumor infiltration of the upper plexus (C5–C6 distribution) is less common. This lesion is characterized by pain in the shoulder girdle, lateral arm, and hand. Seventy-five percent of patients presenting with upper plexopathy subsequently develop a panplexopathy, and 25% of patients present with panplexopathy (317).

Cross-sectional imaging is essential in all patients with symptoms or signs compatible with plexopathy (Fig. 9). In one study, CT scanning had 80–90% sensitivity in detecting tumor infiltration (320); others have demon-

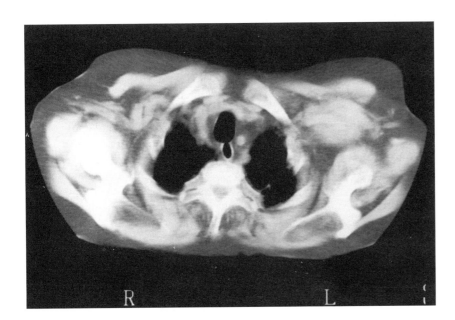

**FIG. 9.** Contrast-enhanced CT scan of the brachial plexus in a 64-year-old woman who has a past history breast cancer and presents with left arm and hand pain. There is a mass in the left brachial plexus.

strated improved diagnostic yield with a multiplanar imaging technique (321). Although there are no comparative data on the sensitivity and specificity of CT and MRI in this setting, MRI does have some theoretical advantages; changes in soft tissue signal intensity on T2-weighted images may help distinguish between tumor and radiation fibrosis, and MRI can reliably assess the integrity of the adjacent epidural space (252).

Electrodiagnostic studies may be helpful in patients with suspected plexopathy, particularly when neurologic examination and imaging studies are normal (319,322). Although not specific for tumor, abnormalities on electromyography (EMG) or somatosensory evoked potentials may establish the diagnosis of plexopathy and thereby confirm the need for additional evaluation. In rare cases, the importance of this diagnosis warrants exploratory surgery (319).

Patients with malignant brachial plexopathy are at high risk for epidural extension of the tumor (232,315). Epidural disease can occur as the neoplasm grows medially and invades vertebrae or tracks along nerve roots through the intervertebral foramina. In the latter case, there may be no evidence of bony erosion on imaging studies. The development of Horner's syndrome, evidence of panplexopathy, or finding of paraspinal tumor or vertebral damage on CT or MRI are highly associated with epidural extension and should lead to definitive imaging of the epidural space (232,315).

### Radiation-Induced Brachial Plexopathy

Two distinct syndromes of radiation-induced brachial plexopathy have been described: (a) early onset transient plexopathy (see above) and (b) delayed onset progressive plexopathy. Delayed onset progressive plexopathy can occur 6 months to 20 years after a course of radiotherapy that included the plexus in the radiation portal. In contrast to tumor infiltration, pain is a relatively uncommon presenting symptom (18%) and when present is usually less severe (317). Weakness and sensory changes predominate in the distribution of the upper plexus (C5, C6 distribution) (317,323,324). Radiation-associated changes in the skin and lymphedema are commonly associated. The CT scan usually demonstrates diffuse infiltration that cannot be distinguished from tumor infiltration. Electromyography may demonstrate myokymia (319,325, 326). Although a careful history combined with these neurologic findings and the results of CT scanning and electrodiagnostic studies, can strongly suggest the diagnosis of radiation-induced injury, repeated assessments over time are needed to confirm the diagnosis. As noted, rare patients require surgical exploration of the plexus to exclude neoplasm and establish the etiology. When due to radiation, plexopathy is usually progressive (315,327), although some patients plateau for a variable period of time.

### Uncommon Causes of Brachial Plexopathy

Malignant peripheral nerve tumor or a second primary tumor in a previously irradiated site can account for pain recurring late in the patient's course (328,329). Pain has been reported to occur as a result of brachial plexus entrapment in a lymphedematous shoulder (323) and as a consequence of acute ischemia many years after axillary radiotherapy (330,331). An idiopathic brachial plexopathy has also been described in patients with Hodgkin's disease (332).

### Lumbosacral Plexopathy

The lumbar plexus, which lies in the paravertebral psoas muscle, is formed primarily by the ventral rami of L1–4. The sacral plexus forms in the sacroiliac notch from the ventral rami of S1–3 and the lumbosacral trunk (L4–5), which courses caudally over the sacral ala to join the plexus (333). Lumbosacral plexopathy may be associated with pain in the lower abdomen, inguinal region, buttock, or leg (334). In the cancer population, lumbosacral plexopathy is usually caused by neoplastic infiltration or compression. Radiation-induced plexopathy also occurs, and occasionally a patient develops the lesion as a result of surgical trauma, infarction, cytotoxic damage, infection in the pelvis or psoas muscle, abdominal aneurysm, or idiopathic lumbosacral neuritis. Polyradiculopathy from leptomeningeal metastases or epidural metastases can mimic lumbosacral plexopathy, and the evaluation of the patient must include consideration of these lesions as well.

### Malignant Lumbosacral Plexopathy

The primary tumors most frequently associated with malignant lumbosacral plexopathy include colorectal, cervical, breast, sarcoma, and lymphoma (315,334). Most tumors involve the plexus by direct extension from intrapelvic neoplasm; metastases account for only one fourth of cases. In one study, two thirds of patients developed plexopathy within 3 years of their primary diagnosis and one third presented within 1 year (334).

Pain is the first symptom reported by most patients with malignant lumbosacral plexopathy. Pain is experienced by almost all patients during the course of the disease, and it is the only symptom in almost 20% of patients. The quality is usually aching, pressure-like, or stabbing; dysesthesias appear to be relatively uncommon. Most patients develop numbness, paresthesias, or weakness weeks to months after the pain has begun. Common signs include leg weakness that involves multiple myotomes, sensory loss that crosses dermatomes, reflex asymmetry, focal tenderness, leg edema, and positive direct or reverse straight leg raising signs.

An upper plexopathy occurs in almost one third of patients with lumbosacral plexopathy (334). This lesion is usually due to direct extension from a low abdominal tumor, most frequently colorectal. Pain may be experienced in the back, lower abdomen, flank or iliac crest, or the anterolateral thigh. Examination may reveal sensory, motor, and reflex changes in an L1–4 distribution. A subgroup of these patients presents with a syndrome characterized by pain and paresthesias limited to the lower abdomen or inguinal region, variable sensory loss, and no motor findings. CT scan may show tumor adjacent to the L1 vertebra (the L1 syndrome) (334) or along the pelvic sidewall, where it presumably damages the ilioinguinal, iliohypogastric, or genitofemoral nerves. Another subgroup has neoplastic involvement of the psoas muscle and presents with a syndrome characterized by upper lumbosacral plexopathy, painful flexion of the ipsilateral hip, and positive psoas muscle stretch test. This has been termed the malignant psoas syndrome (335). Similarly, pain in the distribution of the femoral nerve has been observed in the setting of recurrent retroperitoneal sarcoma (336).

A lower plexopathy occurs in just over 50% of patients with lumbosacral plexopathy (334). This lesion is usually due to direct extension from a pelvic tumor, most frequently rectal cancer, gynecological tumors, or pelvic sarcoma. Pain may be localized in the buttocks and perineum, or referred to the posterolateral thigh and leg. Associated symptoms and signs conform to an L4-S1 distribution. Examination may reveal weakness or sensory changes in the L5 and S1 dermatomes and a depressed ankle jerk. Other findings include leg edema, bladder or bowel dysfunction, sacral or sciatic notch tenderness, and a positive straight leg raising test. A pelvic mass may be palpable.

Sacral plexopathy may occur from direct extension of a sacral lesion or a presacral mass. This may present with predominant involvement of the lumbosacral trunk, characterized by numbness over the dorsal medial foot and sole, and weakness of knee flexion, ankle dorsiflexion, and inversion. Other patients demonstrate particular involvement of the coccygeal plexus, with prominent sphincter dysfunction and perineal sensory loss. The latter syndrome occurs with low pelvic tumors, such as those arising from the rectum or prostate.

A panplexopathy with involvement in an L1-S3 distribution occurs in almost one fifth of patients with lumbosacral plexopathy (334). Local pain may occur in the lower abdomen, back, buttocks, or perineum. Referred pain can be experienced anywhere in the distribution of the plexus. Leg edema is extremely common. Neurologic deficits may be confluent or patchy within the L1-S3 distribution and a positive straight leg raising test is usually present.

Autonomic dysfunction, particularly anhydrosis and vasodilation, has been associated with plexus and peripheral nerve injuries. Focal autonomic neuropathy, which may suggest the anatomic localization of the lesion (337), has been reported as the presenting symptom of metastatic lumbosacral plexopathy (338,339).

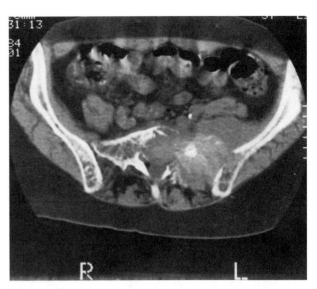

**FIG. 10.** CT scan at the S1 level in a man with low back pain and pain radiating down the posterior aspect of the left leg. The scan shows a large mass invading the left sacrum with extension to the pelvic side wall.

Cross-sectional imaging with either CT or MRI is the usual diagnostic procedure to evaluate lumbosacral plexopathy (Fig. 10). Scanning should be done from the level of the L1 vertebral body through the sciatic notch. When using CT scanning techniques, images should include bone and soft tissue windows. Definitive imaging of the epidural space adjacent to the plexus should be considered in the patient who has features indicative of a relatively high risk of epidural extension, including bilateral symptoms or signs, unexplained incontinence, or a prominent paraspinal mass (232,334).

*Radiation-Induced Lumbosacral Plexopathy*

Radiation fibrosis of the lumbosacral plexus is a rare complication that may occur from 1 to over 30 years following radiation treatment. The use of intracavitary radium implants for carcinoma of the cervix may be an additional risk factor (340,341). Radiation-induced plexopathy typically presents with progressive weakness and leg swelling; pain is not usually a prominent feature (341,342). Weakness typically begins distally in the L5-S1 segments and is slowly progressive. The symptoms and signs may be bilateral (342). If CT scanning demonstrates a lesion, it is usually a non-specific diffuse infiltration of the tissues. Electromyography may show myokymic discharges (342).

*Uncommon Causes of Lumbosacral Plexopathy*

Lumbosacral plexopathy may occur following intraarterial cisplatin infusion (see below) and embolization techniques. This syndrome been observed following attempted embolization of a bleeding rectal lesion. Benign conditions that may produce similar findings include hemorrhage or abscess in the iliopsoas muscle (333), abdominal aortic aneurysms (343), and diabetic radiculoplexopathy (333,344). Vasculitis may also result in lumbosacral plexopathy (333), and an idiopathic lumbosacral plexitis analogous to acute brachial neuritis has been described (345). A subgroup of patients with the latter syndrome have an elevated erythrocyte sedimentation rate and respond to immunosuppressive therapy (346).

### Painful Mononeuropathy

#### Tumor-Related Mononeuropathy

Tumor-related mononeuropathy usually results from compression or infiltration of a nerve from tumor arising in an adjacent bony structure. The most common example of this phenomenon is intercostal nerve injury in a patient with rib metastases. Constant burning pain and other dysesthesias in the area of sensory loss are the typical clinical presentation. Other examples include the cranial neuralgias previously described, sciatica associated with tumor invasion of the sciatic notch, and common peroneal nerve palsy associated with primary bone tumors of the proximal fibula.

#### Other Causes of Mononeuropathy

Cancer patients also develop mononeuropathies from many other causes. Postsurgical syndromes are well described (see below) and radiation injury of a peripheral nerve occurs occasionally. Rarely, cancer patients develop nerve entrapment syndromes (such as carpal tunnel syndrome) related to edema or direct compression by tumor (347).

### Painful Peripheral Neuropathies

Painful peripheral neuropathies have multiple causes, including nutritional deficiencies, other metabolic derangements (e.g., diabetes and renal dysfunction), neurotoxic effects of chemotherapy, and, rarely, paraneoplastic syndromes (285).

#### Toxic Peripheral Neuropathy

Chemotherapy-induced peripheral neuropathy is a common problem, which is typically manifested by painful paresthesias in the feet and hands, and signs consistent with an axonopathy, including "stocking-glove" sensory loss, weakness, hyporeflexia, and autonomic dysfunction (142,348). The pain is usually characterized by continuous burning or lancinating pains, either of which may be increased by contact. The drugs most commonly associated with a peripheral neuropathy are the vinca alkaloids (especially vincristine) (349), cis-platinum (350,351), and paclitaxel. Procarbazine, carboplatinum, misonidazole, and hexamethylmelamine have also been implicated as causes for this syndrome (145,348). One small study has suggested that the neuropathy associated with cisplatin can be prevented by the coadministration of the radioprotective agent S-2-(3-aminopropylamino)ethylphosphorthioic acid (WR 2721) (350).

### Paraneoplastic Painful Peripheral Neuropathy

Paraneoplastic painful peripheral neuropathy can be related to injury to the dorsal root ganglion (also known as subacute sensory neuronopathy or ganglionopathy) or injury to peripheral nerves. These syndromes may be the initial manifestation of an underlying malignancy. Except for the neuropathy associated with myeloma (352,353), their course is usually independent of the primary tumor (354).

Subacute sensory neuronopathy is characterized by pain (usually dysesthetic), paresthesias, and sensory loss in the extremities, and severe sensory ataxia (285,354–356). Although it is usually associated with small cell carcinoma of the lung, other tumor types, including breast cancer, Hodgkin's disease, and varied solid tumors, are rarely associated (285,354–356). Both constant and lancinating dysesthesias occur and typically predate other symptoms. Neuropathic symptoms (pain, paresthesia, sensory loss) are often asymmetric at onset, with a predilection for the upper limbs. The pain usually develops before the tumor is evident and its course is typically independent. The syndrome, which results from an inflammatory process involving the dorsal root ganglia, may be part of a more diffuse autoimmune disorder that can affect the limbic region, brainstem, and spinal cord (285); as a consequence, coexisting autonomic, cerebellar, or cerebral abnormalities are common (356). An antineuronal IgG antibody ("anti-Hu"), which recognizes a low molecular weight protein present in most small cell lung carcinomas, has been associated with the condition (355,357,358).

A sensorimotor peripheral neuropathy, which may be painful, has been observed in association with diverse neoplasms, particularly Hodgkin's disease and paraproteinemias (285,359). The peripheral neuropathies associated with multiple myeloma—Waldenstrom's macroglobulinemia, small-fiber amyloid neuropathy, and osteosclerotic myeloma (359,360)—are thought to be due to antibodies that cross-react with constituents of peripheral nerves (352,353,360). Clinically evident peripheral neuropathy occurs in approximately 15% of patients with multiple myeloma, and electrophysiologic evidence of this lesion can be found in 40% (361). The pathophysiology of the neuropathy that can complicate other neoplasms is unknown.

## Pain Syndromes of the Viscera and Miscellaneous Tumor-Related Syndromes

Pain may be caused by pathology involving the luminal organs of the gastrointestinal or genitourinary tracts, the parenchymal organs, the peritoneum, or the retroperitoneal soft tissues. Obstruction of hollow viscus, including intestine, biliary tract, and ureter, produces visceral nociceptive syndromes that are well described in the surgical literature (362). Pain arising from retroperitoneal and pelvic lesions may involve mixed nociceptive and neuropathic mechanisms if both somatic structures and nerves are involved.

### Hepatic Distention Syndrome

Pain-sensitive structures in the region of the liver include the liver capsule, vessels, and biliary tract (363,364). Nociceptive afferents that innervate these structures travel via the celiac plexus, the phrenic nerve, and the lower right intercostal nerves. Extensive intrahepatic metastases or gross hepatomegaly associated with cholestasis may produce discomfort in the right subcostal region, and less commonly in the right midback or flank (363–365). Referred pain may be experienced in the right neck or shoulder, or in the region of the right scapula (363). The pain, which is usually described as a dull ache, may be exacerbated by movement, pressure in the abdomen, and deep inspiration. Pain is commonly accompanied by symptoms of anorexia and nausea. Physical examination may reveal a hard irregular subcostal mass that descends with respiration and is dull to percussion. Other features of hepatic failure may be present. Imaging of the hepatic parenchyma by either ultrasound or CT will usually identify the presence of space occupying lesions or cholestasis (Fig. 11).

Occasional patients who experience chronic pain due to hepatic distension develop an acute intercurrent subcostal pain that may be exacerbated by respiration. Physical examination may demonstrate a palpable or audible rub. These findings suggest the development of an overlying peritonitis, which can develop in response to some acute event, such as a hemorrhage into a metastasis.

### Midline Retroperitoneal Syndrome

Retroperitoneal pathology involving the upper abdomen may produce pain by injury to deep somatic structures of the posterior abdominal wall, pain-sensitive connective tissue, or vascular and ductal structures; local inflammation; or direct infiltration of the celiac plexus. The most common causes are pancreatic cancer (7) and

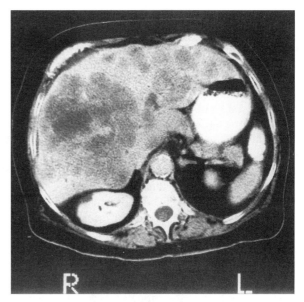

**FIG. 11.** CT scan of the adbdomen of a 72-year-old man with metastatic colon cancer and persistent right upper quadrant abdominal pain. The scan demonstrates extensive liver metastases.

retroperitoneal lymphadenopathy (366). The pain is experienced in the epigastrium, in the low thoracic region of the back, or in both locations. It is often diffuse and poorly localized (7). It is usually dull and boring in character, exacerbated with recumbency, and improved by sitting. The lesion can usually be demonstrated by CT or MRI scanning of the upper abdomen (Fig. 12). If tumor

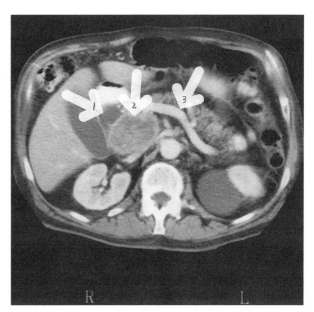

**FIG. 12.** CT scan of the abdomen of a 47-year-old woman with epigastic pain and jaundice. The CT shows a large mass in the head of the pancreas (*arrow 2*), dilatation of the common bile duct (*arrow 1*) and dilatation of the pancreatic duct (*arrow 3*).

is identified in the paravertebral space, or vertebral body destruction is identified, consideration should be given to careful evaluation of the epidural space.

### Chronic Intestinal Obstruction

Abdominal pain is an almost invariable manifestation of chronic intestinal obstruction, which may occur in patients with abdominal or pelvic cancers (367,368). The factors that contribute to this pain include smooth muscle contractions, mesenteric tension, and mural ischemia. Obstructive symptoms may be due primarily to the tumor or, more likely, to a combination of mechanical obstruction and other processes, such as autonomic neuropathy and ileus from metabolic derangements or drugs. Both continuous and colicky pains occur (367,368), which may be referred to the dermatomes represented by the spinal segments supplying the affected viscera. Vomiting, anorexia, and constipation are important associated symptoms. Abdominal radiographs taken in both supine and erect positions may demonstrate the presence of air-fluid levels and intestinal distention. CT or MRI scanning of the abdomen can assess the extent and distribution of intraabdominal neoplasm, which has implication for subsequent treatment options.

### Peritoneal Carcinomatosis

Peritoneal carcinomatosis occurs most often by transcelomic spread of abdominal or pelvic tumor; hematogenous spread of an extra-abdominal neoplasm in this pattern is rare (369,370). Carcinomatosis can cause peritoneal inflammation, mesenteric tethering, malignant adhesions, and ascites (370), all of which can cause pain. Mesenteric tethering and tension appears to cause a diffuse abdominal or low back pain. Tense malignant ascites can produce diffuse abdominal discomfort and a distinct stretching pain in the anterior abdominal wall. Adhesions can also cause obstruction of hollow viscus, with intermittent colicky pain (371). CT scanning may demonstrate evidence of ascites, omental infiltration, and peritoneal nodules (Fig. 13).

### Malignant Perineal Pain

Tumors of the colon or rectum, female reproductive tract, and distal genitourinary system are most commonly responsible for perineal pain (372). Severe perineal pain following antineoplastic therapy may precede evidence of detectable disease and should be viewed as a potential harbinger of progressive or recurrent cancer (372). There is evidence to suggest that this phenomenon is caused by microscopic perineural invasion by recurrent disease (373). The pain, which is typically described as constant

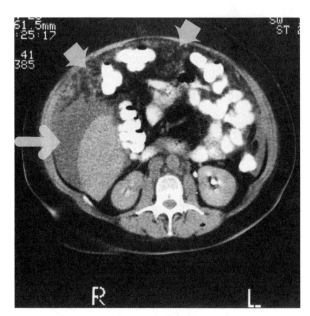

**FIG. 13.** CT scan of the abdomen of a 66-year-old woman with stage IV ovarian cancer. The short arrows indicate areas of peritoneal thickening and infiltration. The large horizontal arrow indicates ascitic fluid interposed lateral to the lower lobe of the liver.

and aching, is often aggravated by sitting or standing, and may be associated with tenesmus or bladder spasms (372).

Tumor invasion of the musculature of the deep pelvis can also result in a syndrome that appears similar to the so-called tension myalgia of the pelvic floor (374). The pain is typically described as a constant ache or heaviness that exacerbates with upright posture. When due to tumor, the pain may be concurrent with other types of perineal pain. Digital examination of the pelvic floor may reveal local tenderness or palpable tumor.

### Adrenal Pain Syndrome

Large adrenal metastases may produce unilateral flank pain and, less commonly, abdominal pain. Pain is of variable severity, and it can be severe (375)

### Ureteric Obstruction

Ureteric obstruction is most frequently caused by tumor compression or infiltration within the true pelvis (376–378). Less commonly, obstruction can be more proximal, associated with retroperitoneal lymphadenopathy, an isolated retroperitoneal metastasis, mural metastases, or intraluminal metastases. Cancers of the cervix, ovary, prostate, and rectum are most commonly associated with this complication. Nonmalignant causes, including retroperitoneal fibrosis resulting from radiotherapy or graft versus host disease, occur rarely (378).

Pain may or may not accompany ureteric obstruction. When present, it is typically a dull chronic discomfort in the flank, which may radiate into the inguinal region or genitalia. If pain does not occur, ureteric obstruction may be discovered when hydronephrosis is discerned on abdominal imaging procedures or renal failure develops. Ureteric obstruction can be complicated by pyelonephritis or pyonephrosis, which often present with features of sepsis, loin pain, and dysuria. Diagnosis of ureteric obstruction can be confirmed by the demonstration of hydronephrosis on renal sonography (378,379). The level of obstruction can be identified by pyelography, and CT scanning techniques will usually demonstrate the cause (377,378).

### Ovarian Cancer Pain

Moderate to severe chronic abdominopelvic pain is the most common symptom of ovarian cancer; it is reported by almost two thirds of patients in the 2 weeks prior to the onset or recurrence of the disease (5). In patients who have been previously treated it is an important symptom of potential recurrence (5).

### Lung Cancer Pain

Even in the absence of involvement of the chest wall or parietal pleura, lung tumors can produce a visceral pain syndrome. In a large case series of lung cancer patients pain was unilateral in 80% of the cases and bilateral in 20%. Among patients with hilar tumors, the pain was referred to the sternum or the scapula. Upper and lower lobe tumors referred to the shoulder and to the lower chest, respectively (380).

### Other Uncommon Visceral Pain Syndromes

Sudden onset severe abdominal or loin pain may be caused by non-traumatic rupture of a visceral tumor. Kidney rupture due to a renal metastasis from an adenocarcinoma of the colon (381) and metastasis-induced perforated appendicitis (382) have been reported. Torsion of pedunculated visceral tumors can produce a cramping abdominal pain (383).

### Paraneoplastic Nociceptive Pain Syndromes

#### Tumor-Related Gynecomastia

Tumors that secrete chorionic gonadotrophin (HCG), including malignant and benign tumors of the testis (164,384–386) and rarely cancers from other sites (163,387–390), may be associated with chronic breast tenderness or gynecomastia. Approximately 10% of patients with testis cancer have gynecomastia or breast tenderness at presentation, and the likelihood of gynecomastia is greater with increasing human chorionic gonadotropin (HCG) level (164). Breast pain can be the first presentation of an occult tumor (384–386).

### Chronic Pain Syndromes Associated with Cancer Therapy

Most treatment-related pains are caused by tissue-damaging procedures. These pains are acute, predictable, and self-limited. Chronic treatment-related pain syndromes are associated with either a persistent nociceptive complication of an invasive treatment (such as a postsurgical abscess) or, more commonly, neural injury. In some cases, these syndromes occur long after the therapy is completed, resulting in a difficult differential diagnosis between recurrent disease and a complication of therapy.

### Postchemotherapy Pain Syndromes

#### Chronic Painful Peripheral Neuropathy

Although most patients who develop painful peripheral neuropathy due to cytotoxic therapy gradually improve, some develop a persistent pain. The characteristics of this pain syndrome were described previously.

#### Avascular (Aseptic) Necrosis of Femoral or Humeral Head

Avascular necrosis of the femoral or humeral head may occur either spontaneously or as a complication of intermittent or continuous corticosteroid therapy. This osteonecrosis may be unilateral or bilateral. Involvement of the femoral head is most common and typically causes pain in the hip, thigh, or knee. Involvement of the humeral head usually presents as pain in the shoulder, upper arm, or elbow. Pain is exacerbated by movement and relieved by rest (217). There may be local tenderness over the joint, but this is not universal. Pain usually precedes radiologic changes by weeks to months; bone scintigraphy and MRI are sensitive and complementary diagnostic procedures. Early treatment consists of analgesics, decrease or discontinuation of steroids, and sometimes surgery. With progressive bone destruction, joint replacement may be necessary.

#### Plexopathy

Lumbosacral or brachial plexopathy may follow cisplatin infusion into the iliac artery (391) or axillary artery (392), respectively. Affected patients develop pain, weakness, and paresthesias within 48 hours of the infusion.

The mechanism for this syndrome is thought to be due to small vessel damage and infarction of the plexus or nerve. The prognosis for neurologic recovery is not known.

*Raynaud's Phenomenon*

Among patients with germ cell tumors treated with cisplatin, vinblastine, and bleomycin, persistent Raynaud's phenomenon is observed in 20–30% of cases (393–395). This effect has also been observed in patients with carcinoma of the head and neck treated with a combination of cisplatin, vincristine, and bleomycin (396). Pathophysiologic studies have demonstrated that a hyperreactivity in the central sympathetic nervous system of resulting in a reduced function of the smooth muscle cells in the terminal arterioles is the responsible mechanism (397).

### Chronic Pain Associated with Hormonal Therapy

*Gynecomastia with Hormonal Therapy for Prostate Cancer*

Chronic gynecomastia and breast tenderness are common complications of antiandrogen therapies for prostate cancer (169). The incidence of this syndrome varies among drugs; it is frequently associated with diethylstilbestrol (398), is less common with flutamide and cyproterone (399–401), and is uncommon among patients receiving LHRF agonist therapy (169). Gynecomastia in the elderly must be distinguished from primary breast cancer or a secondary cancer in the breast (402,403).

### Chronic Postsurgical Pain Syndromes

Surgical incision at virtually any location may result in chronic pain. Although persistent pain is occasionally encountered after nephrectomy, sternotomy, craniotomy, inguinal dissection, and other procedures, these pain syndromes are not well described in the cancer population. In contrast, several syndromes are now clearly recognized as sequelae of specific surgical procedures. The predominant underlying pain mechanism in these syndromes is neuropathic, resulting from injury to peripheral nerves or plexus.

*Postmastectomy Pain Syndrome*

Postmastectomy pain is a chronic and distressing outcome that affects 4–10% of women who undergo breast surgery (404,405). Although it has been reported to occur after almost any surgical procedure on the breast (from lumpectomy to radical mastectomy) (404), it is most common after procedures involving axillary dissection (323,406,407). Pain may begin immediately or begin after many months or, rarely, years. The natural history of this condition appears to be variable, and both subacute and chronic courses are possible (408). The onset of pain later than 18 months following surgery is unusual, and a careful evaluation to exclude recurrent chest wall disease is recommended in this setting.

Postmastectomy pain is usually characterized as a constricting and burning discomfort that is localized to the medial arm, axilla and anterior chest wall (405,407, 409–411). On examination, there is often an area of sensory loss within the region of the pain (411). In some cases a trigger point can be palpated in the axilla or chest wall. The patient may restrict movement of the arm leading to frozen shoulder as a secondary complication.

The etiology of postmastectomy pain is believed to be related to damage to the intercostobrachial nerve, a cutaneous sensory branch of T1, 2, 3 (407,411). There is marked anatomic variation in the size and distribution of the intercostobrachial nerve, and this may account for some of the variability in the distribution of pain observed in patients with this condition (412).

*Postradical Neck Dissection Pain*

Several types of postradical neck dissection pain are recognized. A persistent neuropathic pain can develop weeks to months after surgical injury to the cervical plexus. Tightness, along with burning or lancinating dysesthesias in the area of the sensory loss, are the characteristic symptoms.

A second type of chronic pain can result from musculoskeletal imbalance in the shoulder girdle following surgical removal of neck muscles. Similar to the droopy shoulder syndrome (413), this syndrome can be complicated by development of a thoracic outlet syndrome or suprascapular nerve entrapment, with selective weakness and wasting of the supraspinatus and infraspinatus muscles (414).

Escalating pain in patients who have undergone radical neck dissection may signify recurrent tumor or soft tissue infection. These lesions may be difficult to diagnose in tissues damaged by radiation and surgery. Repeated CT or MRI scanning may be needed to exclude tumor recurrence. Empiric treatment with antibiotics should be considered (415).

*Postthoracotomy Pain*

There have been two major studies of postthoracotomy pain (416,417). In the first (417), three groups were identified: The largest (63%) had prolonged postoperative pain that abated within 2 months after surgery. Recurrent pain, following resolution of the postopera-

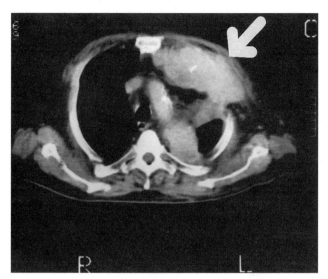

**FIG. 14.** Chest CT scan of a 55-year-old man who had recurrent left-sided chest wall pain 9 months after right upper lobectomy for squamous cell carcinoma of the lung. There is a chest wall recurrence associated with rib destruction and soft tissue mass (*arrow*).

tive pain, was usually due to neoplasm. A second group (16%) experienced pain that persisted following the thoracotomy, then increased in intensity during the follow-up period. Local recurrence of disease and infection were the most common causes of the increasing pain. A final group had a prolonged period of stable or decreasing pain that gradually resolved over a maximum of 8 months. This pain was less associated with tumor recurrence. Overall, the development of late or increasing postthoracotomy pain was due to recurrent or persistent tumor in greater than 95% of patients. This finding was corroborated in the more recent study, which evaluated the records of 238 consecutive patients who underwent thoracotomy; this study identified recurrent pain in 20% of patients, all of whom were found to have tumor regrowth (416).

Patients with recurrent or increasing post-thoracotomy pain should be carefully evaluated, preferably with a CT scan through the chest (Fig. 14). MRI presumably offers a sensitive alternative. Chest radiographs are insufficient to evaluate recurrent chest disease.

*Postoperative Frozen Shoulder*

Patients with postthoracotomy or postmastectomy pain are at risk for the development of a frozen shoulder (418). This lesion may become an independent focus of pain, particularly if complicated by reflex sympathetic dystrophy. Adequate postoperative analgesia and active mobilization of the joint soon after surgery are necessary to prevent these problems.

*Phantom Pain Syndromes*

Phantom limb pain is perceived to arise from an amputated limb, as if the limb were still contiguous with the body. The incidence of phantom pain is significantly higher in patients with a long duration of preamputation pain and those with pain on the day before amputation (419,420). Patients who had pain prior to the amputation may experience phantom pain that replicates the earlier one (420). In a recent study, pain was more prevalent after tumor-related than traumatic amputations, and postoperative chemotherapy was an additional risk factor (421). The pain may be continuous or paroxysmal and is often associated with bothersome paresthesias. The phantom limb may assume painful and unusual postures and may gradually "telescope" and approach the stump. Phantom pain may initially magnify and then slowly fade over time. Two small studies suggested that preoperative or postoperative neural blockade reduces the incidence of phantom limb pain during the first year after amputation (422,423).

Some patients have spontaneous partial remission of phantom pain. The recurrence of pain after such a remission, or the late onset of pain in a previously painless phantom limb, suggests the appearance of a more proximal lesion, including recurrent neoplasm (424).

Phantom pain syndromes have also been described after other surgical procedures. Phantom breast pain after mastectomy, which occurs in 15–30% of patients (425–427), also appears to be related to the presence of preoperative pain (426,427). The pain tends to start in the region of the nipple and then spread to the entire breast (427). The character of the pain is variable and may be lancinating, continuous, or intermittent (427). A phantom anus pain syndrome occurs in approximately 15% of patients who undergo abdominoperineal resection of the rectum (428,429). Phantom anus pain may develop either in the early postoperative period or after a latency of months to years (428,430). Late onset pain is almost always associated with tumor recurrence (430). Rare cases of phantom bladder pain after cystectomy have also been reported (431).

*Stump Pain*

Stump pain occurs at the site of the surgical scar several months to years following amputation. It is usually the result of neuroma development at a site of nerve transection. This pain is characterized by burning or lancinating dysesthesias, which are often exacerbated by movement and blocked by an injection of a local anesthetic (217).

*Postsurgical Pelvic Floor Myalgia*

Surgical trauma to the pelvic floor can cause a residual pelvic floor myalgia, which, like the neoplastic syndrome described previously, mimics so-called tension myalgia (374). The risk of disease recurrence associated with this condition is not known, and its natural history has not been defined. In patients who have undergone anorectal resection, this condition must be differentiated from the phantom anus syndrome (see above).

### Chronic Postradiation Pain Syndromes

Chronic pain complicating radiation therapy tends to occur late in the course of a patient's illness. These syndromes must always be differentiated from recurrent tumor.

#### Radiation-Induced Brachial and Lumbosacral Plexopathies

Radiation-induced brachial and lumbosacral plexopathies were described previously (see above).

#### Chronic Radiation Myelopathy

Chronic radiation myelopathy is a late complication of spinal cord irradiation. The latency is highly variable but is most commonly 12–14 months. The most common presentation is a partial transverse myelopathy at the cervicothoracic level, sometimes in a Brown-Sequard pattern (432). Sensory symptoms, including pain, typically precede the development of progressive motor and autonomic dysfunction (194). The pain is usually characterized as a burning dysesthesia and is localized to the area of spinal cord damage or below. Imaging studies, particularly MRI, are important to exclude an epidural lesion and demonstrate the nature and extent of intrinsic cord pathology, which may include atrophy, swelling, or syrinx (194). The course of chronic radiation myelopathy is usually characterized by steady progression over months, followed by a subsequent phase of slow progression or stabilization.

#### Chronic Radiation Enteritis and Proctitis

Chronic enteritis and proctocolitis occur as a delayed complication in 2–10% of patients who undergo abdominal or pelvic radiation therapy (189,190). The rectum and rectosigmoid are more commonly involved than the small bowel (189), a pattern that may relate to the retroperitoneal fixation of the former structures. The latency is variable (3 months to 30 years) (189,190). Chronic radiation injury to the rectum can present as proctitis (with bloody diarrhea, tenesmus, and cramping pain), obstruction due to stricture formation, or fistulae to the bladder or vagina. Small bowel radiation damage typically causes colicky abdominal pain, which can be associated with chronic nausea or malabsorption (189,190). Barium studies may demonstrate a narrow tubular bowel segment resembling Crohn's disease or ischemic colitis. Endoscopy and biopsy may be necessary to distinguish suspicious lesions from recurrent cancer (189).

#### Burning Perineum Syndrome

Persistent perineal discomfort is an uncommon delayed complication of pelvic radiotherapy. After a latency of 6–18 months, burning pain can develop in the perianal region; the pain may extend anteriorly to involve the vagina or scrotum (433). In patients who have had abdominoperineal resection, phantom anus pain and recurrent tumor are major differential diagnoses.

#### Osteoradionecrosis

Osteoradionecrosis is another late complication of radiotherapy. Bone necrosis, which occurs as a result of endarteritis obliterans, may produce focal pain. Overlying tissue breakdown can occur spontaneously or as a result of trauma, such as dental extraction or denture trauma (188,434). Delayed development of a painful ulcer must be differentiated from tumor recurrence.

### CONCLUSION

Adequate assessment is a necessary precondition for effective pain management. In the cancer population, assessment must recognize the dynamic relationship between the symptom, the illness, and larger concerns related to quality of life. Syndrome identification and inferences about pain pathophysiology are useful elements that may simplify this complex undertaking.

### REFERENCES

1. Bonica JJ, Ventafridda V, Twycross RG. Cancer Pain. In: Bonica JJ, ed. *The management of Pain*, 2nd ed. Philadelphia: Lea & Febiger, 1990: 400–460.
2. Vuorinen E. Pain as an early symptom in cancer. *Clin J Pain* 1993;9: 272–278.
3. Cleeland CS, Gonin R, Hatfield A, et al. Pain and its treatment in outpatients with metastatic cancer. *N Engl J Med* 1994;330:592–596.
4. Larue F, Colleau SM, Brasseur L, et al. Multicentre study of cancer pain and its treatment in France. *Br Med J* 1995;310:1034–1037.
5. Portenoy RK, Kornblith AB, Wong G, et al. Pain in ovarian cancer patients. Prevalence, characteristics, and associated symptoms. *Cancer* 1994;74:907–915.
6. Portenoy RK, Miransky J, Thaler HT, et al. Pain in ambulatory patients with lung or colon cancer: prevalence, characteristics and impact. *Cancer* 1992;70:1616–1624.
7. Kelsen DP, Portenoy RK, Thaler HT, et al. Pain and depression in patients with newly diagnosed pancreas cancer. *J Clin Oncol* 1995;13: 748–755.
8. Portenoy R, Thaler HT, Kornblith AB, et al. The Memorial Symptom Assessment Scale: an instrument for the evaluation of symptom

prevalence, characteristics and distress. *Eur J Clin Oncol* 1994;30: 1326–1336.

9. Tay WK, Shaw RJ, Goh CR. A survey of symptoms in hospice patients in Singapore. *Ann Acad Med Singapore* 1994;23:191–6.

10. Brescia FJ, Portenoy RK, Ryan M, et al. Pain, opioid use, and survival in hospitalized patients with advanced cancer. *J Clin Oncol* 1992;10: 149–155.

11. Donnelly S, Walsh D. The symptoms of advanced cancer. *Semin Oncol* 1995;22(suppl 2):67–72.

12. Feuz A, Rapin CH. An observational study of the role of pain control and food adaptation of elderly patients with terminal cancer. *J Am Diet Assoc* 1994;94:767–770.

13. Thorpe DM. The incidence of sleep disturbance in cancer patients with pain. In: *7th World Congress on Pain: Abstracts*. Seattle: IASP Publications, 1993; abstract 451.

14. Massie MJ, Holland JC. The cancer patient with pain: psychiatric complications and their management. *Med Clin North Am* 1987;71: 243–258.

15. Bond MR, Pearson IB. Psychosocial aspects of pain in women with advanced cancer of the cervix. *J Psychosom Res* 1969;13:13–21.

16. Barkwell DP. Ascribed meaning: a critical factor in coping and pain attenuation in patients with cancer-related pain. *J Palliat Care* 1991; 7:5–14.

17. Daut RL, Cleeland CS. The prevalence and severity of pain in cancer. *Cancer* 1982;50:1913–1918.

18. Fishman B. The treatment of suffering in patients with cancer pain: Cognitive behavioral approaches. In: Foley KM, Bonica JJ, Ventafridda V, ed. *Second international congress on cancer pain*. New York: Raven Press, 1990;301–316. Advances in pain research and therapy; vol 16.

19. Lazarus RS, Folkman C. *Stress, Appraisal and Coping*. New York: Springer, 1984.

20. Syrjala KL. Integrating medical and psychological treatments for cancer pain. In: Chapman CR, Foley KM, ed. *Current and Emerging Isuues in Cancer Pain: Research and Practice*. New York: Raven Press, 1993;393–409.

21. Lancee WJ, Vachon ML, Ghadirian P, et al. The impact of pain and impaired role performance on distress in persons with cancer. *Can J Psychiatry* 1994;39:617–622.

22. Kaasa S, Malt U, Hagen S, et al. Psychological distress in cancer patients with advanced disease. *Radiother Oncol* 1993;27:193–197.

23. Heim HM, Oei TP. Comparison of prostate cancer patients with and without pain. *Pain* 1993;53:159–162.

24. Bolund C. Medical and care factors in suicides by cancer patients in Sweden. *J Psychosoc Oncol* 1985;3:31–52.

25. Breitbart W. Suicide in the cancer patient. *Oncology* 1987;1:49–54.

26. Cleeland CS. The impact of pain on the patient with cancer. *Cancer* 1984;54:2635–2641.

27. Baile WF, Di Maggio JR, Schapira DV, et al. The request for assistance in dying. The need for psychiatric consultation. *Cancer* 1993;72: 2786–2791.

28. Breitbart W. Cancer pain and suicide. In: Foley KM, Bonica JJ, Ventafridda V, ed. *Second International Congress on Cancer Pain*. New York: Raven Press, 1990;399–412. Advances in Pain Research and Therapy; vol 16.

29. Edwards RB. Pain management and the values of health care providers. In: Hill CS, Fields WS, ed. *Drug Treatment of Cancer Pain in a Drug Oriented Society*. New York: Raven Press, 1989;101–112. Advances in Pain Research and Therapy; vol 11.

30. Wanzer SH, Federman DD, Adelstein SJ, et al. The physicians responsibility toward hopelessly ill patients—a second look. *N Engl J Med* 1989;120:844–849.

31. Martin RS. Mortal values: healing, pain and suffering. In: Hill CS, Fields WS, ed. *Drug Treatment of Cancer Pain in a Drug Oriented Society*. New York: Raven Press, 1989;19–26. Advances in Pain Research and Therapy; vol 11.

32. Stjernsward J, Teoh N. The scope of the cancer pain problem. In: Foley KM, Bonica JJ, Ventafridda V, ed. *Second International Congress on Cancer Pain*. New York: Raven Press, 1990;7–12. Advances in Pain Research and Therapy; vol 16.

33. Von Roenn JH, Cleeland CS, Gonin R, et al. Results of a physician attitude toward cancer pain management survey by ECOG. *Proc Am Soc Clin Oncol* 1991;10:abstract 326.

34. Grossman SA, Sheidler VR, Swedeen K, et al. Correlation of patient and caregiver ratings of cancer pain. *J Pain Sympt Manage* 1991;6: 53–57.

35. Cherny NI, Ho MN, Bookbinder M, et al. Cancer pain: knowledge and attitudes of physicians at a cancer cancer. *Proc Am Soc Clin Oncol* 1994;12:abstract 1490.

36. Levy MH. Effective integration of pain management into comprehensive cancer care. *Post Med J* 1991;67(suppl 2):35–43.

37. Ventafridda V. Continuing care: a major issue in cancer pain management. *Pain* 1989;36:137–143.

38. Shegda LM, McCorkle R. Continuing care in the community. *J Pain Sympt Manage* 1990;5:279–286.

39. Coyle N. A model of continuity of care for cancer patients with chronic pain. *Med Clin North Am* 1987;71:259–270.

40. Cleeland CS. Pain control: public and physician's attitudes. In: Hill CS, Fields WS, ed. *Drug Treatment of Cancer Pain in a Drug-Oriented Society*. New York: Raven Press, 1989;81–89. Advances in Pain Research and Therapy; vol 11.

41. Banning A, Sjogren P, Henriksen H. Pain causes in 200 patients referred to a multidisciplinary cancer pain clinic. *Pain* 1991;45(1): 45–48.

42. Foley KM. Clinical assessment of pain. *Acta Anaesth Scand* 1982; 74(suppl):91–96.

43. Twycross RG, Fairfield S. Pain in far-advanced cancer. *Pain* 1982;14: 303–310.

44. Twycross RG, Lack SA. *Symptom Control in Far-Advanced Cancer: Pain Relief*. London: Pitman, 1984.

45. Cherny NI, Portenoy RK. The management of cancer pain. *Ca Cancer J Clin* 1994;44(5):263–303.

46. World Health Organization. *Cancer Pain Relief and Palliative Care*. Geneva: World Health Organization, 1990.

47. Cherny NI, Chang V, Frager G, et al. Opioid pharmacotherapy in the management of cancer pain: A survey of strategies used by pain physicians for the selection of analgesic drugs and routes of administration. *Cancer* 1995;76:1283–1293.

48. Kellgren JG. On distribution of pain arising from deep somatic structures with charts of segmental pain areas. *Clin Sci* 1939;4:35–46.

49. Ness TJ, Gebhart GE. Visceral pain: a review of experimental studies. *Pain* 1990;41:167–234.

50. Torebjork HE, Ochoa JL, Schady W. Referred pain from intraneural stimulation of muscle fascicles in the median nerve. *Pain* 1984;18: 145–156.

51. McCaffery M, Thorpe DM. Differences in perception of pain and the development of adversarial relationships among health care providers. In: Hill CS, Fields WS, ed. *Drug Treatment of Cancer Pain in a Drug Oriented Society*. New York: Raven Press, 1989;19–26. Advances in Pain Research and Therapy; vol 11.

52. Ventafridda V, Ripamonti C, De Conno F, et al. Symptom prevalence and control during cancer patients' last days of life. *J Palliat Care* 1990;6(3):7–11.

53. Coyle N, Adelhardt J, Foley KM, et al. Character of terminal illness in the advanced cancer patient: pain and other symptoms during last four weeks of life. *J Pain Sympt Manage* 1990;5:83–89.

54. Reuben DB, Mor V, Hiris J. Clinical symptoms and length of survival in patients with terminal cancer. *Arch Intern Med* 1988;148(7): 1586–1591.

55. Portenoy RK, Hagen NA. Breakthrough pain: definition, prevalence and characteristics. *Pain* 1990;41(3):273–281.

56. Arner S, Meyerson BA. Lack of analgesic effect of opioids on neuropathic and idiopathic forms of pain. *Pain* 1988;33(1):11–23.

57. Cherny NI, Thaler HT, Friedlander-Klar H, et al. Opioid responsiveness of cancer pain syndromes caused by neuropathic or nociceptive mechanisms: a combined analysis of controlled single dose studies. *Neurology* 1994;44:857–861.

58. Devor M, Basbaum AI, Bennett GJ, et al. Group Report: Mechanisms of neuropathic pain following peripheral injury. In: Basbaum A, Besson J-M, ed. *Towards a New Pharmacotherapy of Pain*. New York: John Wiley and Sons, 1991;417–440.

59. Portenoy RK. Issues in the management of neuropathic pain. In: Basbaum A, Besson J-M, ed. *Towards a New Pharmacotherapy of Pain*. New York: John Wiley and Sons, 1991;393–416.

60. Janig W, Blumberg H, Boas RA, et al. The reflex sympathetic dystrophy syndrome: consensus statement and general recommendations for diagnosis and clinical research. In: Bond MR, Charlton JE, Woolf CJ, ed. *Proceedings of the VIth World Congress on Pain*. Amsterdam:

Elsevier, 1991;373–382. Pain Research and Clinical Management; vol 4.

61. Portenoy RK, Foley KM, Inturrisi CE. The nature of opioid responsiveness and its implications for neuropathic pain: new hypotheses derived from studies of opioid infusions. *Pain* 1990;43(3):273–286.

62. Dubner R. A call for more science, not more rhetoric, regarding opioids and neuropathic pain. *Pain* 1991;47(1):1–2.

63. Portenoy RK. Adjuvant analgesics in pain management. In: Doyle D, Hanks GW, MacDonald N, eds. *Oxford Textbook of Palliative Medicine.* Oxford: Oxford University Press, 1993;187–203.

64. American Psychiatric Association. Somatoform disorders. In: *Diagnostic and Statistical Manual of Mental Disorders (DSM-IV)*, 3rd ed. Washington, DC: American Psychiatric Association, 1994.

65. Portenoy RK, Thaler HT, Kornblith AB, et al. Symptom prevalence, characteristics and distress in a cancer population. *Qual Life Res* 1994;3(3):183–189.

66. Moinpour CM, Feigl P, Metch B, et al. Quality of life endpoints in cancer clinical trials: review and recommendations. *JNCI* 1989;81:485–495.

67. Moinpour CM, Hayden KA, Thomson IM, et al. Quality of life assessment in Southwest Oncology Group trials. In: Tchekmedyian NS, Cella D, ed. *Quality of Life in Oncology Practice and Research.* Williston Park: Dominus Publishing Co., 1991;43–50.

68. Gonzales GR, Elliot KJ, Portenoy RK, et al. The impact of a comprehensive evaluation in the management of cancer pain. *Pain* 1991;47:141–144.

69. Clouston P, De Angelis L, Posner JB. The spectrum of neurologic disease in patients with systemic cancer. *Ann Neurol* 1992;31:268–273.

70. Portenoy RK, Lipton RB, Foley KM. Back pain in the cancer patient: an algorithm for evaluation and management. *Neurology* 1987;37:134–138.

71. Posner JB. Back pain and epidural spinal cord compression. *Med Clin North Am* 1987;71:185–206.

72. Agency for Health Care Policy and Research: Acute Pain Management Panel. *Acute pain management: operative or medical procedures and trauma.* Washington, DC: U.S. Dept. Health and Human Services, 1992; Clinical Practice Guideline.

73. Agency for Health Care Policy and Research: Cancer Pain Management Panel. *Management of Cancer Pain.* Washington, DC: U.S. Dept. Health and Human Services, 1994; Clinical Practice Guideline Number 9.

74. American Pain Society Committee of Quality Assurance Standards. American Pain Society quality assurance standards for the relief of acute pain and cancer pain. In: Bond MR, Charlton JE, Woolf CJ, ed. *Proceedings of the VIth World Congress on Pain.* Amsterdam: Elsevier, 1991;185–190. Pain Research and Clinical Management; vol 4.

75. American Pain Society Quality of Care Committee. Quality improvement guidelines for the treatment of acute pain and cancer pain. *JAMA* 1995;274:1874–1880.

76. Au E, Loprinzi CL, Dhodapkar M, et al. Regular use of a verbal pain scale improves the understanding of oncology inpatient pain intensity. *J Clin Oncol* 1994;12(12):2751–2755.

77. Bookbinder M, Kiss M, Coyle N, et al. Improving Pain Management Practices. In: McGuire DB, Yarbo CH, Ferrell BR, ed. *Cancer Pain Management,* 2nd ed. Boston: Jones and Bartlett Publishers International, 1995.

78. Miaskowski C, Donovan M. Implementation of the American Pain Society quality assurance standards for relief of acute pain and cancer pain in oncology nursing practice. *Oncol Nurs Forum* 1992;19(3):411–415.

79. Miaskowski C. Pain management quality assurance and changing practice. In: Gebhardt GF, Hammond DL, Jensen TS, ed. *Proceedings of the 7th World Congress on Pain.* Seattle: IASP Press, 1994; Progress in Pain Research and Management; vol 2.

80. Fishman B, Pasternak S, Wallenstein SL, et al. The memorial pain assessment card: a valid instrument for the evaluation of cancer pain. *Cancer* 1987;60:1151–1158.

81. Daut RL, Cleeland CS, Flanery RC. Development of the Wisconsin brief pain questionnaire to assess pain in cancer and other diseases. *Pain* 1983;17(2):197–210.

82. Melzack R. The short-form McGill pain questionnaire. *Pain* 1987;30:191–197.

83. Melzack R. The McGill pain questionnaire: major properties and scoring methods. *Pain* 1975;1:277–299.

84. De Conno F, Caraceni A, Gamba A, et al. Pain measurement in cancer patients: a comparison of six methods. *Pain* 1994;57(2):161–166.

85. Morewood GH. A rational approach to the cause, prevention and treatment of postdural puncture headache. *Can Med Assoc J* 1993;149(8):1087–1093.

86. Bonica JJ. Headache and other visceral disorders of the head and neck. In: *The Management of Pain.* Philadelphia: Lea & Febiger, 1953;1263–1309.

87. Tarkkila P, Huhtala J, Salminen U. Difficulties in spinal needle use. Insertion characteristics and failure rates associated with 25-, 27- and 29-gauge Quincke-type spinal needles. *Anaesthesia* 1994;49(8):723–725.

88. Fink BR, Walker S. Orientation of fibers in human dorsal lumbar dura mater in relation to lumbar puncture. *Anesth Analg* 1989;69(6):768–772.

89. Leibold RA, Yealy DM, Coppola M, et al. Post-dural-puncture headache: characteristics, management, and prevention. *Ann Emerg Med* 1993;22(12):1863–1870.

90. Kleyweg RP, Hertzberger LI, Carbaat PA. [Less headache following lumbar puncture with the use of an atraumatic needle; double-blind randomized study]. *Ned Tijdschr Geneeskd* 1995;139(5):232–234.

91. Pittoni G, Toffoletto F, Calcarella G, et al. Spinal anesthesia in outpatient knee surgery: 22-gauge versus 25-gauge Sprotte needle. *Anesth Analg* 1995;81(1):73–79.

92. Harrison DA, Langham BT. Post-dural puncture headache: a comparison of the Sprotte and Yale needles in urological surgery. *Eur J Anaesthesiol* 1994;11(4):325–327.

93. Jones MJ, Selby IR, Gwinnutt CL, et al. Technical note: the influence of using an atraumatic needle on the incidence of post-myelography headache. *Br J Radiol* 1994;67(796):396–398.

94. Muller B, Adelt K, Reichmann H, et al. Atraumatic needle reduces the incidence of post-lumbar puncture syndrome. *J Neurol* 1994;241(6):376–380.

95. Cook PT, Davies MJ, Beavis MJ. Bed rest and post lumbar puncture headache. *Anaesthesia* 1989;44:389–391.

96. De Boer W. Bed rest after lumbar puncture is obsolete. *Anaesthesia* 1989;44(11).

97. Martin R, Jourdain S, Clairoux M, et al. Duration of decubitus position after epidural blood patch. *Can J Anaesth* 1994;41(1):23–25.

98. Raskin NH. Lumbar puncture headache: a review. *Headache* 1990;30(4):197–200.

99. Olsen KS. Epidural blood patch in the treatment of post-lumbar puncture headache. *Pain* 1987;30(3):293–301.

100. Heide W, Diener HC. Epidural blood patch reduces the incidence of post lumbar puncture headache. *Headache* 1990;30(5):280–281.

101. Ford CD, Ford DC, Koenigsberg MD. A simple treatment of post-lumbar-puncture headache. *J Emerg Med* 1989;7(1):29–31.

102. Jones HM, Conces DJ, Tarver RD. Painful transthoracic needle biopsy: a sign of neurogenic tumor. *J Thorac Imag* 1993;8(3):230–232.

103. Marks RM, Sachar EJ. Undertreatment of medical inpatients with narcotic analgesics. *Ann Intern Med* 1973;78:173–181.

104. Edwards WT. Optimizing opioid treatment of postoperative pain. *J Pain Sympt Manage* 1990;5(suppl 1):24–36.

105. Ready LB. The treatment of post operative pain. In: Bond MR, Charlton JE, Woolf CJ, ed. *Proceedings of the VIth World Congress on Pain.* Amsterdam: Elsevier, 1991;53–58. Pain Research and Clinical Management; vol 4.

106. Harper DM. Pain and cramping associated with cryosurgery. *J Fam Pract* 1994;39(6):551–557.

107. Kolmannskog F, Kolbenstvedt AN, Schrumpf E, et al. Side effects and complications after hepatic artery embolization in the carcinoid syndrome. *Scand J Gastroenterol* 1991;26(5):557–562.

108. Williams JM, Howe NR. Benzyl alcohol attenuates the pain of lidocaine injections and prolongs anesthesia. *J Dermatol Surg Oncol* 1994;20(11):730–733.

109. Bruera E, Fainsinger R, Moore M, et al. Local toxicity with subcutaneous methadone. Experience of two centers. *Pain* 1991;45:141–145.

110. Shvartzman P, Bonneh D. Local skin irritation in the course of subcutaneous morphine infusion: a challenge. *J Palliat Care* 1994;10(1):44–45.

111. De Conno F, Caracenti A, Martini C, et al. Hyperalgesia and myoclonus with intrathecal infusion of high-dose morphine. *Pain* 1991;47:337–339.

112. Stillman MJ, Moulin DE, Foley KM. Paradoxical pain following high-dose spinal morphine. *Pain* 1987;(suppl 4):389.

113. De Castro MD, Meynadier MD, Zenz MD. *Regional Opioid Analge-*

*sia*. Dordrecht: Kluwer Academic Publishers, 1991; Developments in Critical Care Medicine and Anesthesiology; vol 20.

114. Molloy HS, Seipp CA, Duffey P. Administration of cancer treatments: practical guide for physicians and oncology nurses. In: De Vita VT, Hellman S, Rosenberg SA, eds. *Cancer: Principles and Practice of Oncology*, 3rd ed. Philadelphia: JB Lippincott, 1989;2369–2402.

115. Curran CF, Luce JK, Page JA. Doxorubicin-associated flare reactions. *Oncol Nurses Forum* 1990;17(3):387–389.

116. Mrozek-Orlowski M, Christie J, Flamme C, et al. Pain associated with peripheral infusion of carmustine. *Oncol Nurses Forum* 1991;18(5):942.

117. Hundrieser J. A non-invasive approach to minimizing vessel pain with DTIC or BCNU. *Oncol Nurses Forum* 1988;15(2):199.

118. Schneider SM, Distelhorst CW. Chemotherapy-induced emergencies. *Semin Oncol* 1989;16(6):572–578.

119. Kemeny N, Cohen A, Bertino J, et al. Continuous intrahepatic infusion of floxuridine and leucovorin through an implantable pump for the treatment of hepatic metastases from colorectal carcinoma. *Cancer* 1990;65:2446–2450.

120. Sugihara K. Continuous hepatic arterial infusion of 5-fluorouracil for unresectable colorectal liver metastases: phase II study. *Surgery* 1995;117:624–628.

121. Botet JF, Watson RC, Kemeny N, et al. Cholangitis complicating intraarterial chemotherapy in liver metastasis. *Radiology* 1985;156:335–337.

122. Almadrones L, Yerys C. Problems associated with the administration of intraperitoneal therapy using the Port-A-Cath system. *Oncol Nurses Forum* 1990;17:75–80.

123. Markman M. Cytotoxic intracavitary chemotherapy. *Am J Med Sci* 1986;291(3):175–179.

124. Dufour P, Maloisel F, Bergerat JP, et al. Intraperitoneal mitoxantrone as consolidation treatment for stage III ovarian carcinoma: a pilot study. *Bull Cancer (Paris)* 1991;78(3):273–280.

125. Gitsch E, Sevelda P, Schmidl S, et al. First experiences with intraperitoneal chemotherapy in ovarian cancer. *Eur J Gynaecol Oncol* 1990;11(1):19–22.

126. Oza AM, ten Bokkel Huinink W, Dubbelman R, et al. Phase I/II study of intraperitoneal mitoxantrone in refractory ovarian cancer. *Ann Oncol* 1994;5(4):343–347.

127. Deppe G, Malviya VK, Boike G, et al. Intraperitoneal doxorubicin in combination with systemic cisplatinum and cyclophosphamide in the treatment of stage III ovarian cancer. *Eur J Gynaecol Oncol* 1991;12(2):93–97.

128. Markman M, Howell SB, Lucas WE, et al. Combination intraperitoneal chemotherapy with cisplatin, cytarabine, and doxorubicin for refractory ovarian carcinoma and other malignancies principally confined to the peritoneal cavity. *J Clin Oncol* 1984;2(12):1321–1326.

129. Schilsky RL, Choi KE, Grayhack J, et al. Phase I clinical and pharmacologic study of intraperitoneal cisplatin and fluorouracil in patients with advanced intraabdominal cancer. *J Clin Oncol* 1990;8(12):2054–2061.

130. Kaplan RA, Markman M, Lucas WE, et al. Infectious peritonitis in patients receiving intraperitoneal chemotherapy. *Am J Med* 1985;78(1):49–53.

131. Chapko MK, Syrjala KL, Schilter L, et al. Chemoradiotherapy toxicity during bone marrow transplantation: time course and variation in pain and nausea. *Bone Marrow Transpl* 1990;4:181–186.

132. Mahood DJ, Dose AM, Loprinzi CL, et al. Inhibition of fluorouracil-induced stomatitis by oral cryotherapy. *J Clin Oncol* 1991;9(3):449–452.

133. Barker G, Loftus L, Cuddy P, et al. The effects of sucralfate suspension and diphenhydramine syrup plus kaolin-pectin on radiotherapy-induced mucositis. *Oral Surg Oral Med Oral Pathol* 1991;71(3):288–293.

134. Pfeiffer P, Madsen EL, Hansen O, et al. Effect of prophylactic sucralfate suspension on stomatitis induced by cancer chemotherapy. A randomized, double-blind cross-over study. *Acta Oncol* 1990;29(2):171–173.

135. Spijkervet FK, Van Saene HK, Van Saene JJ, et al. Effect of selective elimination of the oral flora on mucositis in irradiated head and neck cancer patients. *J Surg Oncol* 1991;46(3):167–173.

136. Redding SW. Role of herpes simplex virus reactivation in chemotherapy-induced oral mucositis. *NCI Monogr* 1990;1990(9):103–105.

137. Ferretti GA, Raybould TP, Brown AT, et al. Chlorhexidine prophylaxis for chemotherapy- and radiotherapy-induced stomatitis: a randomized

138. Hill HF, Chapman CR, Kornell J, et al. Self-administration of morphine in bone marrow transplant patients reduces drug requirement. *Pain* 1990;40:121–129.

139. Hill HF, Mackie AM, Coda BA, et al. Patient-controlled analgesic administration. A comparison of steady-state morphine infusions with bolus doses. *Cancer* 1991;67:873–882.

140. Zaglama NE, Rosenblum SL, Sartiano GP, et al. Single, high-dose intravenous dexamethasone as an antiemetic in cancer chemotherapy. *Oncology* 1986;43:27–32.

141. Rotstein J, Good RA. Steroid pseudorheumatism. *Arch Intern Med* 1957;99:545–555.

142. McDonald DR. Neurological complications of chemotherapy. *Neurol Clin* 1991;9:955–967.

143. Holland JF, Scharlau C, Gailani S, et al. Vincristine treatment of advanced cancer: a cooperative study of 392 cases. *Cancer Res* 1973;33:1258–1264.

144. McCarthy GM, Skillings JR. Jaw and other orofacial pain in patients receiving vincristine for the treatment of cancer. *Oral Surg Oral Med Oral Pathol* 1992;74:299–304.

145. Weiss HD, Walker MD, Wiernik PH, et al. Neurotoxicity of commonly used antineoplastic agents. *N Engl J Med* 1974;291:75–81.

146. Feinberg WM, Swenson MR. Cerebrovascular complications of L-asparaginase therapy. *Neurology* 1988;38:127–133.

147. Moots PL, Walker RW, Sze G, et al. Diagnosis of dural venous sinus thrombosis by magnetic resonance imaging. *Ann Neurol* 1987;2:431–432.

148. Huang ME, Ye YC, Chen SR, et al. Use of all-trans retinoic acid in the treatment of acute promyelocytic leukemia. *Blood* 1988;72:567–572.

149. Castaigne S, Chomienne C, Daniel MT, et al. All-trans retinoic acid as a differentiation therapy for acute promyelocytic leukemia. I. Clinical results. *Blood* 1990;76:1704–1709.

150. Balmer CM. Clinical use of biologic response modifiers in cancer treatment: an overview. Part II. Colony-stimulating factors and interleukin-2. *DICP* 1991;25:490–498.

151. Hollingshead LM, Goa KL. Recombinant granulocyte colony-stimulating factor (rG-CSF). A review of its pharmacological properties and prospective role in neutropenic conditions. *Drugs* 1991;42:300–330.

152. Freeman NJ, Costanza ME. 5-Fluorouracil-associated cardiotoxicity. *Cancer* 1988;61:36–45.

153. Eskilsson J, Albertsson M. Failure of preventing 5-fluorouracil cardiotoxicity by prophylactic treatment with verapamil. *Acta Oncol* 1990;29:1001–1003.

154. Rezkalla S, Kloner RA, Ensley J, et al. Continuous ambulatory ECG monitoring during fluorouracil therapy: a prospective study. *J Clin Oncol* 1989;7:509–514.

155. Lokich JJ, Moore C. Chemotherapy-associated palmar-plantar erythrodysesthesia syndrome. *Ann Intern Med* 1984;101:798–799.

156. Fabian CJ, Molina R, Slavik M, et al. Pyridoxine therapy for palmar-plantar erythrodysesthesia associated with continuous 5-fluorouracil infusion. *Invest New Drugs* 1990;8:57–63.

157. Grem JL, McAtee N, Balis F, et al. A phase II study of continuous infusion 5-fluorouracil and leucovorin with weekly cisplatin in metastatic colorectal carcinoma. *Cancer* 1993;72:663–668.

158. Bellmunt J, Navarro M, Hidalgo R, et al. Palmar-plantar erythrodysesthesia syndrome associated with short-term continuous infusion (5 days) of 5-fluorouracil. *Tumori* 1988;74:329–331.

159. Trump AR, Pavy MD, Staal S. Gynecomastia in men following antineoplastic therapy. *Arch Intern Med* 1982;142:511–513.

160. Saeter G, Fossa SD, Norman N. Gynecomastia following cytotoxic therapy for testicular cancer. *Br J Urol* 1987;59:348–352.

161. Sherins RJ, Olweny CLM, Ziegler JL. Gynecomastia and gonadal dysfunction in adolescent boys treated with combination chemotherapy for Hodgkin's disease. *N Engl J Med* 1978;299:12–16.

162. Schorer AE, Oken MM, Johnson GJ. Gynecomastia with nitrosurea therapy. Cancer Treatment Reports 1978;62:574–576.

163. Hands LJ, Greenall MJ. Gynecomastia. *Br J Surg* 1991;78:907–911.

164. Tseng AJ, Horning SJ, Freiha FS, et al. Gynecomastia in testicular cancer patients. Prognostic and therapeutic implications. *Cancer* 1985;56:2534–2538.

165. Trump DL, Anderson SA. Painful gynecomastia following cytotoxic therapy for testis cancer: a potentially favorable prognostic sign? *J Clin Oncol* 1983;1:416–420.

166. Stefenelli T, Kuzmits R, Ulrich W, et al. Acute vascular toxicity after

combination chemotherapy with cisplatin, vinblastine, and bleomycin for testicular cancer. *Eur Heart J* 1988;9:552–6.

167. Smith E, Harper F, LeRoy E. Raynaud's phenomenon of a single digit following intradermal bleomycin sulphate injection. *Arthritis Rheum* 1985;28:459–461.

168. Elomaa I, Pajunen M, Virkkunen P. Reynaud's syndrome progressing to gangrene aftervincristine and bleomycin. *Arch Dermatol* 1984;216: 323–326.

169. Chrisp P, Sorkin EM. Leuprorelin. A review of its pharmacology and therapeutic use in prostatic disorders. *Drugs Aging* 1991;1:487–509.

170. Thompson IM, Zeidman EJ, Rodriguez FR. Sudden death due to disease flare with luteinizing hormone-releasing hormone agonist therapy for carcinoma of the prostate. *J Urol* 1990;144:1479–1480.

171. Goldspiel BR, Kohler DR. Goserelin acetate implant: a depot luteinizing hormone-releasing hormone analog for advanced prostate cancer. *DICP* 1991;25:796–804.

172. Ahmann FR, Citrin DL, deHaan HA, et al. Zoladex: a sustained-release, monthly luteinizing hormone-releasing hormone analogue for the treatment of advanced prostate cancer. *J Clin Oncol* 1987;5: 912–917.

173. Labrie F, Dupont A, Belanger A, et al. Flutamide eliminates the risk of disease flare in prostatic cancer patients treated with a luteinizing hormone-releasing hormone agonist. *J Urol* 1987;138:804–806.

174. Lunglmayr G. "Zoladex" versus "Zoladex" plus flutamide in the treatment of advanced prostate cancer. First interim analysis of an international trial. International Prostate Cancer Study Group. *Progr Clin Biol Res* 1989;303:145–151.

175. Crawford ED, Nabors W. Hormone therapy of advanced prostate cancer: where we stand today. *Oncology* 1991;5:21–30.

176. Shearer RJ, Davies JH, Dowsett M, et al. Aromatase inhibition in advanced prostatic cancer: preliminary communication. *Br J Cancer* 1990;62:275–276.

177. Davies JH, Dowsett M, Jacobs S, et al. Aromatase inhibition: 4-hydroxyandrostenedione (4-oha, cgp 32349) in advanced prostatic cancer. *Br J Cancer* 1992;66:139–142.

178. Fossa SD, Urnes T. Flare reaction during the initial treatment period with medroxyprogesterone acetate in patients with hormone-resistant prostatic cancer. *Eur Urol* 1986;12:257–259.

179. Henderson IC, Harris JR. Principles in the management of metastatic disease. In: *Breast Diseases,* 2nd ed. Philadelphia: JB Lippincott, 1991;547–678.

180. Quesada JR, Talpaz M, Rios A, et al. Clinical toxicity of interferons in cancer patients: a review. *J Clin Oncol* 1986;4:234–243.

181. Jones GJ, Itri LM. Safety and tolerance of recombinant interferon alfa-2a (Roferon-A) in cancer patients. *Cancer* 1986;8:1709–1715.

182. Chevallier B, Chollet P, Merrouche Y, et al. Lenograstim prevents morbidity from intensive induction chemotherapy in the treatment of inflammatory breast cancer. *J Clin Oncol* 1995;13:1564–1571.

183. Veldhuis GJ, Willemse PH, van GM, et al. Recombinant human interleukin-3 to dose-intensify carboplatin and cyclophosphamide chemotherapy in epithelial ovarian cancer: a phase I trial. *J Clin Oncol* 1995;13:733–740.

184. Morris KP, Hughes C, Hardy SP, et al. Pain after subcutaneous injection of recombinant human erythropoietin: does Emla cream help? *Nephrol Dial Transplant* 1994;9:1299–1301.

185. Frenken LA, van LH, Koene RA. Analysis of the efficacy of measures to reduce pain after subcutaneous administration of epoetin alfa. *Nephrol Dial Transplant* 1994;9:1295–1298.

186. Rider CA. Oral mucositis. A complication of radiotherapy. *NY State Dental J* 1990;56:37–39.

187. Soffer EE, Mitros F, Doornbos JF, et al. Morphology and pathology of radiation-induced esophagitis. Double-blind study of naproxen vs placebo for prevention of radiation injury. *Dig Dis Sci* 1994;39: 655–660.

188. Epstein JB, Schubert MM, Scully C. Evaluation and treatment of pain in patients with orofacial cancer. *Pain Clin* 1991;4:3–20.

189. Earnest DL, Trier JS. Radiation enteritis and colitis. In: Sleisenger MH, Fordtran JS, ed. *Gastrointestinal Disease: Pathophysiology Diagnosis Management,* vol 2. Philadelphia: WB Saunders, 1989; 1369–1382.

190. Buchi K. Radiation proctitis: therapy and prognosis. *JAMA* 1991;265: 1180.

191. Fulton DS. Brachial plexopathy in patients with breast cancer. *Dev Oncol* 1987;51:249–257.

192. Salner AL, Botnick L, Hertzog AG, et al. Reversible transient plexopathy following primary radiation therapy for breast cancer. *Cancer Treat Rep* 1981;65:797–801.

193. Pierce SM, Recht A, Lingos TI, et al. Long-term radiation complications following conservative surgery (CS) and radiation therapy (RT) in patients with early stage breast cancer. *Int J Radiat Oncol Biol Phys* 1992;23:915–923.

194. Cascino TL. Radiation myelopathy. In: Rottenberg DA, ed. *Neurological complications of cancer treatment.* Boston: Butterworth-Heinemann, 1991;69–78.

195. Serafini AN. Current status of systemic intravenous radiopharmaceuticals for the treatment of painful metastatic bone disease. *Int J Radiat Oncol Biol Phys* 1994;30:1187–1194.

196. Robinson RG. Strontium 89: Precursor targeted therapy for relief of blastic metastatic disease. *Cancer* (suppl) 1993;72:3433–3435.

197. Rusthoven JJ, Ahlgren P, Elhakim T, et al. Varicella-zoster infection in adult cancer patients: a population study. *Arch Intern Med* 1988;148: 1561–1566.

198. Portenoy RK, Duma C, Foley KM. Acute herpetic and postherpetic neuralgia: clinical review and current management. *Ann Neurol* 1986; 20:651–664.

199. Rusthoven JJ, Ahlgren P, Elhakim T, et al. Risk factors for varicella zoster disseminated infection among adult cancer patients with localized zoster. *Cancer* 1988;62:1641–1646.

200. Donati MB. Cancer and thrombosis. *Haemostasis* 1994;24:128–131.

201. Rahr HB, Srensen JV. Venous thromboembolism and cancer. *Blood Coagul Fibrinolysis* 1992;3:451–460.

202. Clarke PD, Olt G. Thromboembolism in patients with gyn tumors: risk factors, natural history, and prophylaxis. *Oncology* (Huntingt) 1989;3: 39–45.

203. Bergqvist D, Lindblad B. Thromboembolic problems in colorectal cancer surgery. *Scand J Gastroenterol Suppl* 1988;149:74–81.

204. Levine M, Hirsh J, Gent M, et al. Double-blind randomised trial of a very-low-dose warfarin for prevention of thromboembolism in stage IV breast cancer. *Lancet* 1994;343:886–889.

205. Hamilton MG, Hull RD, Pineo GF. Prophylaxis of venous thromboembolism in brain tumor patients. *J Neurooncol* 1994;22:111–126.

206. Wells PS, Hirsh J, Anderson DR, et al. Accuracy of clinical assessment of deep-vein thrombosis. *Lancet* 1995;345:1326–1330.

207. Henriet JP. Pain in venous thrombosis of the leg. *Phlebologie* 1992;45: 67–76.

208. Wheeler HB, Hirsh J, Wells P, et al. Diagnostic tests for deep vein thrombosis. Clinical usefulness depends on probability of disease. *Arch Intern Med* 1994;154:1921–1928.

209. Anderson DR, Lensing AW, Wells PS, et al. Limitations of impedance plethysmography in the diagnosis of clinically suspected deep-vein thrombosis. *Ann Intern Med* 1993;118:25–30.

210. Hirschmann JV. Ischemic forms of acute venous thrombosis. *Arch Dermatol* 1987;123:933–936.

211. Nemmers DW, Thorpe PE, Knibbe MA, et al. Upper extremity venous thrombosis. case report and literature review. *Orthop Rev* 1990;19: 164–172.

212. Burihan E, de FL, Francisco JJ, et al. Upper-extremity deep venous thrombosis: analysis of 52 cases. *Cardiovasc Surg* 1993;1:19–22.

213. Donayre CE, White GH, Mehringer SM, et al. Pathogenesis determines late morbidity of axillosubclavian vein thrombosis. *Am J Surg* 1986;152:179–84.

214. Escalante CP. Causes and management of superior vena cava syndrome. *Oncology* 1993;7:61–68.

215. Segall M, Shore SA, Miller ME. Superior vena cava syndrome. *RI Med J* 1990;73:109–112.

216. Foley KM. The treatment of cancer pain. *N Engl J Med* 1985;313: 84–95.

217. Foley KM. Pain syndromes in patients with cancer. *Med Clin North Am* 1987;71:169–184.

218. Nielsen OS, Munro AJ, Tannock IF. Bone metastases: pathophysiology and management policy. *J Clin Oncol* 1991;9:509–524.

219. Payne R. Pharmacological management of bone pain in the cancer patient. *Clin J Pain* 1989;5 (suppl 2):43–50.

220. Wagner G. Frequency of pain in patients with cancer. *Rec Results Cancer Res* 1984;89:64–71.

221. Lee HK, Sung WW, Solodnik P, et al. Bone scan in tumor-induced osteomalacia. *J Nucl Med* 1995;36:247–249.

222. Jonsson OG, Sartain P, Ducore JM, et al. Bone pain as an initial symp-

tom of childhood acute lymphoblastic leukemia: association with nearly normal hematologic indexes. *J Pediatrics* 1991;117:233–237.

223. Plezbert JA, Bose M, Carlisle G. Chronic myelogenous leukemia in a 16-yr-old. *J Manip Physiol Ther* 1994;17:610–613.

224. Gilbert RW, Kim JH, Posner JB. Epidural spinal cord compression from metastatic tumor: diagnosis and treatment. *Ann Neurol* 1978;3: 40–51.

225. Sorensen S, Borgesen SE, Rohde K, et al. Metastatic epidural spinal cord compression. Results of treatment and survival. *Cancer* 1990;65: 1502–1508.

226. Constans JP, DeVitis E, Donzelli R, et al. Spinal metastases with neurological manifestations: review of 600 cases. *J Neurosurg* 1983;59: 111–118.

227. Phillips E, Levine AM. Metastatic lesions of the upper cervical spine. *Spine* 1989;14:1071–1077.

228. Sundaresan N, Galicich JH, Lane JM, et al. Treatment of odontoid fractures in cancer patients. *J Neurosurg* 1981;54187–54192, 1981: 187–192.

229. Bosley TM, Cohen DA, Schatz NJ, et al. Comparison of metrimazole computed tomography with magnetic resonance imaging in the evaluation of lesions at the cervicomedullary junction. *Neurology* 1985;35: 485–492.

230. Feldenzer JA, McGauley JL, McGillicuddy JE. Sacral and presacral tumors: problems in diagnosis and management. *Neurosurgery* 1989; 25:884–891.

231. Stark RJ, Henson RA, Evans SJW. Spinal metastases: a retrospective survey from a general hospital. *Brain* 1982;105:189–197.

232. Portenoy RK, Galer BS, Salamon O, et al. Identification of epidural neoplasm. Radiography and bone scintigraphy in the symptomatic and asymptomatic spine. *Cancer* 1989;64:2207–2213.

233. Ruff RL, Lanska DJ. Epidural metastases in prospectively evaluated in veterans with cancer and back pain. *Cancer* 1989;63:2234–2241.

234. Barcena A, Lobato RD, Rivas JJ, et al. Spinal metastatic disease: analysis of factors determining functional prognosis and choice of treatment. *Neurosurgery* 1984;15:820–827.

235. Rosenthal MA, Rosen D, Raghavan D, et al. Spinal cord compression in prostate cancer. A 10-year experience. *Br J Urol* 1992;69:530–533.

236. Maranzano E, Latini P. Effectiveness of radiation therapy without surgery in metastatic spinal cord compression: final results from a prospective trial. *Int J Radiat Oncol Biol Phys* 1995;32:959–967.

237. Grant R, Papadopoulos SM, Greenberg HS. Metastatic epidural spinal cord compression. *Neurol Clin* 1991;9:825–841.

238. Sundaresan N, Galicich JH, Lane JM, et al. Treatment of neoplastic epidural cord compression by vertebral resection and stabilization. *J Neurosurg* 1985;63:676–684.

239. Sundaresan N, Galicich JH, Bains MS, et al. Vertebral body resection in the treatment of cancer involving the spine. *Cancer* 1984; 53:1393–1396.

240. Harrington KD. Anterior cord decompression and spinal stabilization for patients with metastatic lesions of the spine. *J Neurosurg* 1984;61:107–117.

241. Tomita K, Toribatake Y, Kawahara N, et al. Total en bloc spondylectomy and circumspinal decompression for solitary spinal metastasis. *Paraplegia* 1994;32:36–46.

242. Brice J, McKissock W. Surgical treatment of malignant extradural tumors. *Br J Med* 1965;1:1341–1346.

243. Findlay GF. The role of vertebral body collapse in the management of malignant spinal cord compression. *J Neurol Neurosurg Psychiatry* 1987;50:151–154.

244. Greenberg HS, Kim J, Posner JB. Epidural spinal cord compression from metastatic tumor: results with a new treatment protocol. *Ann Neurol* 1980;8:361–366.

245. Stranjalis G, Jamjoom A, Torrens M. Epidural lipomatosis in steroid-treated patients. *Spine* 1992;17:1268.

246. Obbens EAMT, Posner JB. Systemic cancer involving the spinal cord. In: Davidoff RA, ed. *Handbook of the Spinal Cord.* New York: Marcel Dekker, 1987;451–489.

247. Helweg-Larsen S, Srensen PS. Symptoms and signs in metastatic spinal cord compression: a study of progression from first symptom until diagnosis in 153 patients. *Eur J Cancer* 1994;30a:396–398.

248. Stillman M, Foley KM. Breast cancer and epidural spinal cord compression: Diagnostic and therapeutic strategies. In: Harris JR, Hellman S, Henderson IC, Kinne D, eds. *Breast Diseases.* Philadelphia: JB Lippincott, 1991;688–700.

249. Ventafridda V, Caraceni A, Martini C, et al. On the significance of Lhermitte's sign in oncology. *J Neurooncol* 1991;10:133–137.

250. Barron KD, Hirano A, Araki S, et al. Experience with metastatic neoplasms involving the spinal cord. *Neurology* 1959;9:91–100.

251. Helweg-Larsen S, Rasmusson B, Sorensen PS. Recovery of gait after radiotherapy in paralytic patients with metastatic epidural spinal cord compression. *Neurology* 1990;40:1234–1236.

252. Hagen N, Stulman J, Krol G, et al. The role of myelography and magnetic resonance imaging in cancer patients with symptomatic and asymptomatic epidural disease. *Neurology* 1989;39:309.

253. Delattre JY, Arbit E, Thaler HT, et al. A dose response study of dexamethasone in a model of spinal cord compression caused by epidural tumor. *J Neurosurg* 1989;70:920–925.

254. Vecht CJ, Haaxma-Reiche H, van Putten WLJ, et al. Initial bolus of conventional versus high-dose dexamethasone in metastatic spinal cord compression. *Neurology* 1989;39:1255–1257.

255. Rodichok LD, Harper GR, Ruckdeschel JC, et al. Early diagnosis of spinal epidural metastases. *Am J Med* 1981;70:1181–1188.

256. Hill ME, Richards MA, Gregory WM, et al. Spinal cord compression in breast cancer: a review of 70 cases. *Br J Cancer* 1993;68:969–973.

257. Graus F, Krol G, Foley KM. Early diagnosis of spinal epidural metastasis: Correlation with clinical and radiological findings. *Proc Am Soc Clin Oncol* 1986;5:abstract 1047.

258. Laredo JD, Lakhdari K, Bellaiche L, et al. Acute vertebral collapse: CT findings in benign and malignant nontraumatic cases. *Radiology* 1995;194(1):41–48.

259. Haddad P, Thaell JF, Kiely JM, et al. Lymphoma of the spinal epidural space. *Cancer* 1976;38:1862–1866.

260. O'Rourke T, George CB, Redmond J. Spinal computed tomography and computer tomographic metrimazide myelography in the early diagnosis of spinal metastatic disease. *J Clin Oncol* 1986;4:576–581.

261. Sim FH. Metastatic bone disease: lesions of the pelvis and hip. In: Sim FH, ed. *Diagnosis and Management of Metastatic Bone Disease: a Multidisciplinary Approach.* New York: Raven Press, 1988; 183–198.

262. Beatrous TE, Choyke PL, Frank JA. Diagnostic evaluation of cancer patients with pelvic pain: comparison of scintigraphy, CT, and MR imaging. *AJR* 1990;155:85–88.

263. Knapp D, Abdul KF. Fine needle aspiration cytology of acrometastasis. A report of two cases. *Acta Cytol* 1994;38:589–591.

264. Freedman DM, Henderson RC. Metastatic breast carcinoma to the os calcis presenting as heel pain. *South Med J* 1995;88:232–234.

265. Leonheart EE, DiStazio J. Acrometastases. Initial presentation as diffuse ankle pain. *J Am Podiatr Med Assoc* 1994;84:625–627.

266. LeRoux BT. Bronchial cancers with hypertrophic pulmonary osteoarthropathy. *South Afr Med J* 1968;41:1074–1075.

267. Greenfield GB, Schorsch HA, Shkolnik A. The various roentgen appearence of pulmonary hypertrophic osteoarthropathy. *Am J Roentgenol Radium Ther Nucl Med* 1967;101:927–931.

268. Briselli M, Mark EJ, Dickersin GR. Solitary fibrous tumors of the pleura: eight new cases and review of 360 cases in the literature. *Cancer* 1981;47:2678–2689.

269. Margolick J, Bonomi P, Fordham E, et al. Case report. hypertrophic osteoarthropathy associated with endometrial carcinoma. *Gynecol Oncol* 1982;13:399–404.

270. Kaymakcalan H, Sequeria W, Barretta T, et al. Hypertrophic osteoarthropathy with myogenic tumors of the esophagus. *Am J Gastroenterol* 1980;74:17–20.

271. Shapiro JS. Breast cancer presenting as periostitis. *Postgrad Med* 1987;82:139–140.

272. Evans WK. Reversal of hypertrophic osteoarthropathy after chemotherapy for bronchogenic carcinoma. *J Rheumatol* 1980;7: 93–97.

273. Segal AM, Mackenzie AH. Hypertrophic osteoarthropathy: a 10-year retrospective analysis. *Semin Arthritis Rheum* 1982;12:220–232.

274. Bunn PA, Chester-Ridgeway E. Paraneoplastic syndromes. In: DeVita VT, Hellman S, Rosenberg SA, ed. *Cancer: Principles and Practice of Oncology,* 4th ed. Philadelphia: JB Lippincott, 1993; 2026–2071.

275. Steiner I, Siegal T. Muscle cramps in cancer patients. *Cancer* 1989; 63:574–577.

276. Araki K, Kobayashi M, Ogata T, et al. Colorectal carcinoma metastatic to skeletal muscle. *Hepatogastroenterology* 1994;41:405–408.

277. Posner JB. Headache and other head pain. In: Wyngaaden JB, Smith

LH, Claude Bennett J, eds. *Cecil's Textbook of Medicine*, 19th ed. Philadelphia: WB Saunders, 1992;2117–2123.

278. Vecht CJ, Hoff AM, Kansen PJ, et al. Types and causes of pain in cancer of the head and neck. *Cancer* 1992;70:178–184.

279. Vasquez Barquero A, Ibanez FJ, Herrera S, et al. Isolated headache as the presenting clinical manifestation of intracranial tumors: a prospective study. *Cephalgia* 1994;14:270–272.

280. Forsyth PA, Posner JB. Headache associated with intracranial neoplasms. In: Olesen J, Tfelt-Hansen P, Welch KMA, ed. *The Headaches*. New York: Raven Press, 1993;705–714.

281. Suwanwela N, Phanthumchinda K, Kaoropthum S. Headache in brain tumor: a cross-sectional study. *Headache* 1994;34:435–438.

282. Fadul C, Misulis KE, Wiley RG. Cerebellar metastases: Diagnostic and management considerations. *J Clin Oncol* 1987;5:1110–1115.

283. Posner JB, Chernik NL. Intracranial metastases from systemic cancer. *Adv Neurol* 1978;19:575–587.

284. Vick NA, Rottenberg DA. Disorders of intracranial pressure. In: Wyngaaden JB, Smith LH, Claude Bennett J, eds. *Cecil's Textbook of Medicine*, 19th ed. Philadelphia: WB Saunders, 1992;2221–2224.

285. Henson RA, Urich H. *Cancer and the Nervous System*. Boston: Blackwell Scientific, 1982;100–119,368–405.

286. Wasserstrom WR, Glass JP, Posner JB. Diagnosis and treatment of leptomeningeal metastasis from solid tumors: experience with 90 patients. *Cancer* 1982;49:759–772.

287. Kaplan JG, DeSouza TG, Farkash A, et al. Leptomeningeal metastases: comparison of clinical features and laboratory data of solid tumors, lymphomas and leukemias. *J Neurooncol* 1990;9:225–229.

288. DeAngelis LM, Payne R. Lymphomatous meningitis presenting as atypical cluster headache. *Pain* 1987;30:211–216.

289. Sozzi C, Marotta P, Piatti L. Vagoglossopharyngeal neuralgia with syncope in the course of carcinomatous meningitis. *Ital J Neurol Sci* 1987; 8:271–276.

290. Olsen ME, Chernik NL, Posner JB. Infiltration of the leptomeninges by systemic cancer. *Arch Neurol* 1974;30:122–137.

291. Fleisher M, Wasserstrom WR, Schold SC, et al. Lactic dehydrogenase isoenzymes in cerebrospinal fluid in patients with systemic cancer. *Cancer* 1981;47:2654–2659.

292. Twijnstra A, van Zanten AP, Nooyen WJ, et al. Cerebrospinal fluid carcinoembryonic antigen in patients with metastatic and non-metastatic neurological disease. *Arch Neurol* 1986;43:269–272.

293. Twijnstra A, van Zanten AP, Nooyen WJ, et al. Cerebrospinal fluid beta-2-microglobulin: a study in controls and patients with metastatic and non-metastatic neurological disease. *Eur J Cancer Clin Oncol* 1986;22:387–391.

294. Cibas ES, Malkin MG, Posner JB, et al. Detection of DNA abnormalities by flow cytometry in cells from cerebrospinal fluid. *Am J Clin Pathol* 1987;88:570–577.

295. Dillon WP. Imaging of central nervous system tumors. *Curr Opin Radiol* 1991;3:46–50.

296. Manelfe C. Imaging of the spine and spinal cord. *Curr Opin Radiology* 1991;3:5–15.

297. Lee YY, Glass JP, Geoffray A, Wallace S. Cranial computed tomographic abnormalities in leptomeningeal metastasis. *Am J Roentgenol* 1984;143(5):1035–1039.

298. Krol G, Sze G, Malkin M, et al. MR of cranial and spinal meningeal carcinomatosis. *Am J Neuroradiol* 1988;9:709–714.

299. Glass PJ, Foley KM. Carcinomatous meningitis. In: Harris JR, Hellman S, Henderson IC, Kinne D, eds. *Breast diseases*. Philadelphia: JB Lippincott, 1991;700–710.

300. Greenberg HS, Deck MDF, Vikram B, et al. Metastasis to the base of the skull: Clinical findings in 43 patients. *Neurology* 1981;31:530–537.

301. Bullitt E, Tew JM, Boyd J. Intracranial tumors in patients with facial pain. *J Neurosurg* 1986;64:865–871.

302. Gupta SR, Zdonczyk DE, Rubino FA. Cranial neuropathy in systemic malignancy in a va population. *Neurology* 1990;40(6):997–999.

303. MacDonald DR, Strong E, Nielson S, et al. Syncope from head and neck cancer. *J Neurol Oncol* 1983;1:257–267.

304. Weinstein RE, Herec D, Friedman JH. Hypotension due to glossopharyngeal neuralgia. *Arch Neurol* 1986;40:90–92.

305. Dalessio DJ. Diagnosis and treatment of cranial neuralgias. *Med Clin North Am* 1991;75:605–615.

306. Iwasaki K, Kondo A, Otsuka S, et al. Painful tic convulsif caused by a brain tumor: case report and review of the literature. *Neurosurgery* 1992;30:916–919.

307. Ruelle A, Datti R, Andrioli G. Cerebellopontine angle osteoma causing trigeminal neuralgia: case report. *Neurosurgery* 1994;35:1135–1137.

308. Bindoff LA, Heseltine D. Unilateral facial pain in patients with lung cancer: a referred pain via the vagus? *Lancet* 1988;1:812–815.

309. Nestor JJ, Ngo LK. Incidence of facial pain caused by lung cancer. *Otolaryngol Head Neck Surg* 1994;111:155–156.

310. Dulli DA, Levine RL, Chun RW, et al. Migrainous neurological dysfunction in Hodgkin's disease. *Arch Neurol* 1987;44:689–693.

311. Feldmann E, Posner JB. Episodic neurologic dysfunction in patients with Hodgkin's disease. *Arch Neurol* 1986;43:1227–1233.

312. Portenoy RK, Abissi CJ, Robbins B, et al. Increased intracranial pressure with normal ventricular size due to superior vena cava obstruction. *Arch Neurol* 1983;40:598.

313. Abbondanzo SL, Wenig BM. Non-Hodgkin's lymphoma of the sinonasal tract. A clinicopathologic and immunophenotypic study of 120 cases. *Cancer* 1995;75:1281–1291.

314. Hollinshead WH. *Anatomy for Surgeons, Vol 1. The Head and Neck*. Philadelphia: Harper and Row, 1982;472–476.

315. Jaeckle KA. Nerve plexus metastases. *Neurol Clin* 1991;9:857–866.

316. Brodal A. *Neurological Anatomy*. Oxford: Oxford University Press, 1981.

317. Kori SH, Foley KM, Posner JB, et al. Brachial plexus lesions in patients with cancer 100 cases. *Neurology* 1981;31:45–50.

318. iris P, Dyck PJ, Mulder D, et al. Natural history of brachial plexus neuropathy. *Arch Neurol* 1972;27:109–117.

319. Foley K. Brachial plexopathy in patients with breast cancer. In: Harris JR, Hellman S, Henderson IC, Kinne D, ed. *Breast Diseases*. Philadelphia: JB Lippincott, 1991;722–729.

320. Cascino TL, Kori S, Krol G, et al. CT scan of brachial plexus in patients with cancer. *Neurology* 1983;33:1553–1557.

321. Fishman EK, Campbell JN, Kuhlman JE, et al. Multiplanar CT evaluation of brachial plexopathy in breast cancer. *J Comput Assist Tomogr* 1991;15:790–795.

322. Synek VM. Validity of median nerve somatosensory evoked potentials in the diagnosis of supraclavicular brachial plexus lesions. *Electroencephal Clin Neurophysiol* 1986;65:27–35.

323. Vecht CJ. Arm pain in the patient with breast cancer. *J Pain Sympt Manag* 1990;5:109–117.

324. Mondrup K, Olsen NK, Pfeiffer P, et al. Clinical and electrodiagnostic findings in breast cancer patients with radiation–induced brachial plexus neuropathy. *Acta Neurol Scand* 1990;81(2):153–158.

325. Lederman RJ, Wilbourn AJ. Brachial plexopathy: Recurrent cancer or radiation? *Neurology* 1984;34:1331–1335.

326. Harper CM, Thomas JE, Cascino TL, et al. Distinction between neoplastic and radiation-induced brachial plexopathy, with emphasis on EMG. *Neurology* 1989;39:502–506.

327. Killer HE, Hess K. Natural history of radiation-induced brachial plexopathy compared to surgically treated patients. *J Neurol* 1990;237:247–250.

328. Foley KM, Woodruff JM, Ellis FT. Radiation-induced malignant and atypical peripheral nerve sheath tumors. *Arch Neurol* 1980;7:311–318.

329. Aho KA, Sainio K. Late irradiation-induced lesions of the lumbrosacral plexus. *Neurology* 1983;33:953–955.

330. Gerard JM, Franck N, Moussa Z, et al. Acute ischemic brachial plexus neuropathy following radiation therapy. *Neurology* 1989;39:450–451.

331. Mumenthaler M, Narakas A, Billiat RW. Brachial plexus disorders. In: Dyke JP, Thomas PK, Lambert EH, Bune R, ed. *Peripheral Neuropathy*, vol. 2 Philadelphia: WB Saunders, 1987;1384–1424.

332. Lachance DH, O'Neill BP, Harper CJ, et al. Paraneoplastic brachial plexopathy in a patient with Hodgkin's disease. *Mayo Clin Proc* 1991;66:97–101.

333. Chad DA, Bradley WG. Lumbosacral Plexopathy. *Semin Neurol* 1987;7:97–104.

334. Jaeckle KA, Young DF, Foley KM. The natural history of lumbosacral plexopathy in cancer. *Neurology* 1985;35:8–15.

335. Stevens MJ, Gonet YM. Malignant psoas syndrome: recognition of an oncologic entity. *Australas Radiol* 1990;34:150–154.

336. Zografos GC, Karakousis CP. Pain in the distribution of the femoral nerve: early evidence of recurrence of a retroperitoneal sarcoma. *Eur J Surg Oncol* 1994;20:692–693.

337. Evans RJ, Watson CPN. Lumbosacral plexopathy in cancer patients. *Neurology* 1985;35:1392–1393.

338. Dalmau J, Graus F, Marco M. "Hot and dry foot" as initial manifestation of neoplastic lumbosacral plexopathy. *Neurology* 1989;39: 871–872.

339. Gilchrist JM, Moore M. Lumbosacral plexopathy in cancer patients. *Neurology* 1985;35:1392.

340. Glass JP, Pettigrew LC, Maor M. Plexopathy induced by radiation therapy. *Neurology* 1985;35:1261.

341. Stryker JA, Sommerville K, Perez R, et al. Sacral plexus injury after radiotherapy for carcinoma of cervix. *Cancer* 1990;66:1488–1492.

342. Thomas JE, Cascino TL, Earl JD. Differential diagnosis between radiation and tumor plexopathy of the pelvis. *Neurology* 1985;35:1–7.

343. Garcia-Diaz J, Balseiro J, Calandre L, et al. Aortic dissection presenting with neurologic signs. *N Engl J Med* 1988;318:1070.

344. Brown MJ, Asbury AK. Diabetic Neuropathy. *Ann Neurol* 1984;15: 2–12.

345. Evans BA. Lumbosacral plexus neuropathy. *Neurology* 1981;31: 1327–1330.

346. Bradley WG, Chad D, Verghese JP, et al. Painful lumbosacral plexopathy with elevated erythrocyte sedimentation rate: A treatable inflammatory syndrome. *Ann Neurol* 1984;15:457–464.

347. Desta K, O'Shaughnessy M, Milling MA. Non-Hodgkin's lymphoma presenting as median nerve compression in the arm. *J Hand Surg (Br)* 1994;19:289–291.

348. Delattre JY, Posner JB. Neurological complications of chemotherapy and radiation therapy. In: Aminoff MJ, ed. *Neurology and General Medicine.* New York: Churchill Livingstone, 1989;365–387.

349. Casey EB, Jellife AM, LaQuesne PM, et al. Vincristine neuropathy: clinical and electrophysiological observations. *Brain* 1973;96:69–86.

350. Mollman JE, Glover DJ, Hogan WM, et al. Cisplatin neuropathy: risk factors, prognosis and protection by WR-272l. *Cancer* 1988;61: 2192–2195.

351. Mollman JE, Hogan WM, Glover DI, et al. Unusual presentation of cis-platinum neuropathy. *Neurology* 1988;38:488–490.

352. Bardwick BA, Zvaifler NJ, Gill N, et al. Plasma cell dyscrasia with polyneuropathy, organomegaly, endocrinopathy, M protein, and skin changes. *Medicine* 1980;59:311–322.

353. Davis D. Myeloma Neuropathy. *Arch Neurol* 1972;27:507–511.

354. Anderson NE, Cunningham JM, Posner JB. Autoimmune pathogenesis of paraneoplastic neurological syndromes. *Crit Rev Neurobiol* 1987;3:245–299.

355. Posner JB. Paraneoplastic syndromes. *Neurol Clin* 1991;9:919–936.

356. Chalk CH, Windebank AJ, Kimmel DW, et al. The distinctive clinical features of paraneoplastic sensory neuronopathy. *Can J Neurol Sci* 1992;19:346–351.

357. Anderson NE, Rosenblum MK, Graus F, et al. Autoantibodies in paraneoplastic syndromes associated with small-cell lung cancer. *Neurology* 1988;38:1391–1398.

358. Graus F, Elkon KB, Cordon-Cardo C, et al. Sensory neuropathy and small cell lung cancer. Antineuronal antibody that also reacts with the tumor. *Am J Med* 1986;80:45–52.

359. Chad DA, Recht LD. Paraneoplastic syndromes. *Neurol Clin* 1991;9: 901–918.

360. McLeod JG, Walsh JC, Pollard ID, et al. Neuropathies associated with paraproteinemias and dysproteinemias. In: Dyck PJ, Thomas PK, Lambert EH, Bunge R, eds. *Peripheral Neuropathy,* vol 2. Philadelphia: WB Saunders, 1984;1847–1865.

361. Walsh IC. The neuropathy of multiple myeloma: An electrophysiological and histological study. *Arch Neurol* 1971;25:404–414.

362. Silen W. *Cope's Early Diagnosis of the Acute Abdomen,* 16th ed. New York: Oxford, 1983.

363. Mulholland MW, Debas H, Bonica JJ. Diseases of the liver, biliary system and pancreas. In: Bonica JJ, ed. *The Management of Pain,* vol 2. Philadelphia: Lea & Febiger, 1990;1214–1231.

364. Coombs DW. Pain due to liver capsular distention. In: Ferrer-Brechner T, ed. *Common Problems in Pain Management.* Chicago: Year Book, 1990;247–253.

365. Trevisani F, D'Intino PE, Caraceni P, et al. Etiologic factors and clinical presentation of hepatocellular carcinoma. Differences between cirrhotic and noncirrhotic Italian patients. *Cancer* 1995;75:2220–2232.

366. Dieckmann KP, Krain J, Gottschalk W, et al. Atypical symptoms in patients with germinal testicular tumors. *Urologe A* 1994;33:325–330.

367. Ventafridda V, Ripamonti C, Caraceni A, et al. The management of inoperable gastrointestinal obstruction in terminal cancer patients. *Tumori* 1990;76:389–393.

368. Baines MJ. Management of malignant intestinal obstruction in patients with advanced cancer. In: Foley KM, Bonica JJ, Ventafridda V, eds. *Second International Congress on Cancer Pain.* New York: Raven Press, 1990;327–336. Advances in Pain Research and Therapy; vol 16.

369. Walsch D, Williams G. Surgical biopsy studies of omental and peritoneal nodules. *Br J Surg* 1971;58:428–432.

370. Bender MD. Diseases of the peritoneum, mesentery and diaphragm. In: Sleisenger MH, Fordtran JS, ed. *Gastrointestinal Disease: Pathophysiology Diagnosis Management,* 4th ed. Philadelphia: WB Saunders, 1989;1932–1967.

371. Lynch MA, Cho KC, Jeffrey RJ, et al. CT of peritoneal lymphomatosis. *AJR* 1988;151:713–715.

372. Stillman M. Perineal pain: Diagnosis and management, with particular attention to perineal pain of cancer. In: Foley KM, Bonica JJ, Ventafrida V, eds. *Second international congress on cancer pain.* New York: Raven Press, 1990;359–377. Advances in Pain Research and Therapy; vol 16.

373. Seefeld PH, Bargen JA. The spread of carcinoma of the rectum: invasion of lymphatics, veins and nerves. *Ann Surg* 1943;118:76–90.

374. Sinaki M, Merritt JL, Stilwell GK. Tension myalgia of the pelvic floor. *Mayo Clin Proc* 1977;52:717–722.

375. Berger MS, Cooley ME, Abrahm JL. A pain syndrome associated with large adrenal metastases in patients with lung cancer. *J Pain Symp Manag* 1995;10:161–166.

376. Talner LB. Specific causes of obstruction. In: Pollack HM, ed. *Clinical Urography.* vol 2. Philadelphia: WB Saunders, 1990;1629–1751.

377. Greenfield A, Resnick MI. Genitourinary emergencies. *Semin Oncol* 1989;16:516–520.

378. Fair WR. Urologic emergencies. In: DeVita VT, Hellman S, Rosengerg SA, eds. *Cancer: Principles and Practice of Oncology,* 3rd ed. Philadelphia: JB Lippincott, 1989;2016–2028.

379. Frohlich EP, Bex P, Nissenbaum MM, et al. Comparison between renal ultrasonography and excretory urography in cervical cancer. *Int J Gynaecol Obstet* 1991;34:49–54.

380. Marangoni C, Lacerenza M, Formaglio F, et al. Sensory disorder of the chest as presenting symptom of lung cancer. *J Neurol Neurosurg Psychiatry* 1993;56:1033–1034.

381. Wolff JM, Boeckmann W, Jakse G. Spontaneous kidney rupture due to a metastatic renal tumour. Case report. *Scand J Urol Nephrol* 1994;28: 415–417.

382. Ende DA, Robinson G, Moulton J. Metastasis-induced perforated appendicitis: an acute abdomen of rare aetiology. *Aust N Z J Surg* 1995;65:62–63.

383. Reese JA, Blocker SH. Torsion of pedunculated hepatocellular carcinoma. Report of a case in a young woman presenting with abdominal pain. *Mo Med* 1994;91:594–595.

384. Cantwell BM, Richardson PG, Campbell SJ. Gynaecomastia and extragonadal symptoms leading to diagnosis delay of germ cell tumours in young men. *Postgrad Med J* 1991;67:675–677.

385. Mellor SG, McCutchan JD. Gynaecomastia and occult Leydig cell tumour of the testis. *Br J Urol* 1989;63:420–422.

386. Haas GP, Pittaluga S, Gomella L, et al. Clinically occult Leydig cell tumor presenting with gynecomastia. *J Urol* 1989;142:1325–1327.

387. Wurzel RS, Yamase HT, Nieh PT. Ectopic production of human chorionic gonadotropin by poorly differentiated transitional cell tumors of the urinary tract. *J Urol* 1987;137:502–504.

388. Sapone FM, Reyes CV. Unusual faces of lung cancer. *J Surg Oncol* 1985;30:1–5.

389. Herr HW, Hennessy WT, Kantor A. Pelvic sarcoma causing gynecomastia. *J Urol* 1990;143:1008–1009.

390. McCloskey JJ, Germain LE, Perman JA, et al. Gynecomastia as a presenting sign of fibrolamellar carcinoma of the liver. *Pediatrics* 1988;82:379–382.

391. Castellanos AM, Glass JP, Yung WK. Regional nerve injury after intraarterial chemotherapy. *Neurology* 1987;37:834–837.

392. Kahn CE, Messersmith RN, Samuels BL. Brachial plexopathy as a complication of intrarterial cisplatin. *Cardiovasc Intervent Radiol* 1989;12:47–49.

393. Stoter G, Koopman A, Vendrik CP, et al. Ten-year survival and late sequelae in testicular cancer patients treated with cisplatin, vinblastine, and bleomycin. *J Clin Oncol* 1989;7:1099–1104.

394. Bissett D, Kunkeler L, Zwanenburg L, et al. Long-term sequelae of treatment for testicular germ cell tumours. *Br J Cancer* 1990;62: 655–659.

395. Vogelzang N, Bosl G, Johnson K, et al. Raynaud's phenomena: a common toxicity after combination chemotherpy for testicular cancer. *Ann Intern Med* 1980;95:602–608.

396. Kukla LJ, McGuire WP, Lad T, et al. Acute vascular episodes associated with therapy for carcinomas of the upper aerodigestive tract with bleomycin, vincristine, and cisplatin. *Cancer Treat Rep* 1982;66: 369–370.

397. Hansen SW, Olsen N, Rossing N, et al. Vascular toxicity and the mechanism underlying Raynaud's phenomenon in patients treated with cisplatin, vinblastine and bleomycin. *Ann Oncol* 1990;1:289–292.

398. Eberlein TJ. Gynecomastia. In: Harris JR, Hellman S, Henderson IC, Kinne D, eds. *Breast Diseases*. Philadelphia: JB Lippincott, 1991; 46–50.

399. Delaere KP, Van Thillo E. Flutamide monotherapy as primary treatment in advanced prostatic carcinoma. *Semin Oncol* 1991;5:13–18.

400. Neumann F, Kalmus J. Cyproterone acetate in the treatment of sexual disorders: pharmacological base and clinical experience. *Exp Clin Endocrinol* 1991;98:71–80.

401. Goldenberg SL, Bruchovsky N. Use of cyproterone acetate in prostate cancer. *Urol Clin North Am* 1991;18:111–122.

402. Ramamurthy L, Cooper RA. Metastatic carcinoma to the male breast. *Br J Radiol* 1991;64:277–278.

403. Olsson H, Alm P, Kristoffersson U, et al. Hypophyseal tumor and gynecomastia preceding bilateral breast cancer development in a man. *Cancer* 1984;53:1974–1977.

404. Foley KM. Pain syndromes in patients with cancer. In: Bonica JJ, Ventafridda V, eds. New York: Raven Press, 1979:59–75. Advances in Pain Research and Therapy; vol 2.

405. Granek I, Ashikari R, Foley KM. Postmastectomy pain syndrome: clinical and anatomic correlates. *Proc Am Soc Clin Oncol* 1983;3: abstract 122.

406. Watson CPN, Evans RJ, Watt VR. The post-mastectomy pain syndrome and the effect of topical capsaicin. *Pain* 1989;38:177–186.

407. Vecht CJ, Van de Brand HJ, Wajer OJ. Post-axillary dissection pain in breast cancer due to a lesion of the intercostobrachial nerve. *Pain* 1989;38:171–176.

408. International Association for the Study of Pain: Subcommittee on taxonomy. Classification of chronic pain. *Pain* 1986;suppl 3:135–138.

409. Wood IM. Intercostobrachial nerve entrapment syndrome. *South Med J* 1978;76:662–663.

410. Paredes JP, Puente JL, Potel J. Variations in sensitivity after sectioning the intercostobrachial nerve. *Am J Surg* 1990;160:525–528.

411. van Dam MS, Hennipman A, de Kruif JT, et al. Complications following axillary dissection for breast carcinoma. *Ned Tijdschr Geneeskd* 1993;137:2395–2398.

412. Assa J. The intercostobrachial nerve in radical mastectomy. *J Surg Oncol* 1974;6:123–126.

413. Swift TR, Nichols FT. The droopy shoulder syndrome. *Neurology* 1984;34:212–215.

414. Stewart JD. *Focal Peripheral Neuropathies*. New York: Elsevier Science Publishing Co., 1987.

415. Bruera E, McDonald N. Intractable pain in patients with advanced head and neck tumors: A possible role of local infection. *Cancer Treat Rep* 1986;70:691–692.

416. Keller SM, Carp NZ, Levy MN, et al. Chronic post thoracotomy pain. *J Cardiovasc Surg (Torino)* 1994;35(suppl 1):161–164.

417. Kanner R, Martini N, Foley KM. Nature and incidence of postthoracotomy pain. *Proc Am Soc Clin Oncol* 1982;1:abstract 590.

418. Maunsell E, Brisson J, Deschenes L. Arm problems and psychological distress after surgery for breast cancer. *Can J Surg* 1993;36:315–320.

419. Weinstein SM. Phantom pain. *Oncology* (Huntingt) 1994;8:65–70.

420. Katz J, Melzack R. Pain "memories" in phantom limbs: review and clinical observations. *Pain* 1990;43:319–336.

421. Smith J, Thompson JM. Phantom limb pain and chemotherapy in pediatric amputees. *Mayo Clin Proc* 1995;70:357–364.

422. Fisher A, Meller Y. Continuous postoperative regional analgesia by nerve sheath block for amputation surgery—a pilot study. *Anesth Analg* 1991;72:300–303.

423. Bach S, Noreng MF, Tjellden NU. Phantom limb pain in amputees during the first 12 months following limb amputation, after preoperative lumbar epidural blockade. *Pain* 1988;33:297–301.

424. Elliott K, Foley KM. Neurologic pain syndromes in patients with cancer. *Neurol Clin* 1989;7:333–360.

425. Krner K, Knudsen UB, Lundby L, et al. Long-term phantom breast syndrome after mastectomy. *Clin J Pain* 1992;8:346–350.

426. Bressler B, Cohen SI, Magnussen S. The problem of phantom breast and phantom pain. *J Nerv Ment Dis* 1955;123:181–187.

427. Kroner K, Krebs B, Skov J, et al. Immediate and long-term phantom breast syndrome after mastectomy: incidence, clinical characteristic relationship to pre-mastectomy breast pain. *Pain* 1989;36:327–335.

428. Boas RA. Phantom anus syndrome. In: Bonica JJ, Lindblom U, Iggo A, eds. *Proceedings of the Third World Congress on Pain*. New York: Raven Press, 1983;947–951. Advances in Pain Research and Therapy; vol 5.

429. Ovesen P, Kroner K, Ornsholt J, et al. Phantom-related phenomena after rectal amputation: prevalence and characteristics. *Pain* 1991;44: 289–291.

430. Boas RA. Post-surgical perineal pain in cancer: a 5 year follow-up. *Pain* 1990;(suppl 5):376.

431. Brena SF, Sammons EE. Phantom urinary bladder pain-case report. *Pain* 1979;7:197–200.

432. Jellinger K, Strum KW. Delayed radiation in myelopathy in man. *J Neurol Sci* 1971;14:389–408.

433. Minsky B, Cohen A. Minimizing the toxicity of radiation therapy in rectal cancer. *Oncology* 1988;2:21–25.

434. Epstein JB, Wong FLW, Stephenson-Moore P. Osteoradionecrosis: clinical experience and a proposal for classification. *J Oral Maxillofac Surg* 1987;45:104–110.

*Principles and Practice of Supportive Oncology,*
edited by Ann Berger et al.
Lippincott–Raven Publishers, Philadelphia ©1998

# CHAPTER 2

# Primary Cancer Treatment: Antineoplastic

Nora A. Janjan and David E. Weissman

## RADIATION THERAPY

Radiation remains an important modality in palliative care. A number of clinical, prognostic, and therapeutic factors must be considered to determine the optimal treatment regimen in palliative radiotherapy. Adequate management of cancer-related pain is important both during and after completion of palliative irradiation. Efficient and effective palliation is imperative in the treatment of locally advanced and metastatic cancer in order to relieve symptoms, improve function, and minimize morbidity.

Many options exist in the radiotherapeutic management of tumors that cause localized symptoms. Although any site of disease can be effectively palliated, treatment of bone and central nervous system metastases are the most common indications for palliative irradiation with external beam therapy. Spinal cord compression and pathologic fracture represent the two most significant risks for patients with bony metastases. Symptoms related to increased intracranial pressure from brain metastases also can be effectively palliated. Brachytherapy, which delivers localized irradiation using radioactive sources, is an important modality in the treatment of tumors that recur in an area that was previously irradiated. Recurrent endobronchial, esophageal, and cervical cancers and tumors that obstruct the biliary tract are often treated with brachytherapy. Radiopharmaceuticals, like strontium-89, are being used with greater frequency to treat bone metastases both as a primary modality for patients whose symptoms recur in a previously irradiated site and as an adjuvant to external beam irradiation. Because radiation provides treatment only to a localized symptomatic site of disease, it is frequently used in coordination with systemic therapies and surgery. Multidisciplinary evaluation of patients with metastatic disease allows comprehensive management of the associated symptoms and helps coordinate antineoplastic therapy.

### Principles of Radiobiology

Unlike curative therapy, where a sufficient dose of radiation is administered to eradicate the tumor, the radiation dose administered with palliative irradiation is generally intended to result in tumor regression in order to relieve symptoms in patients with limited life expectancies. Therefore, the indications for palliative radiotherapy, the radiation portals, and the doses prescribed are generally indexed to the prognosis. Other factors, like the integration of the radiation schedule with other therapies, are also important considerations in determining the radiation dose prescription.

### Definitions Used in Radiotherapy

Radiotherapy techniques vary considerably based on the involved and adjacent normal structures. The techniques that are applied and the potential side effects of radiotherapy are based on principles of radiobiology and radiation physics (1,2). Radiation therapy is delivered in units designated as the *Gray* (Gy). Relating this to the previously used term *rad*, equivalent doses can be expressed as 1 Gy, 100 centigray (cGy), and 100 rad; 1 rad equals 1 cGy.

Localized radiation may be delivered by either external beam therapy (linear accelerators, cobalt-60 units) or brachytherapy using radioactive isotopes applied directly to the region involved by the tumor. External beam therapy is administered with a prescribed number of daily fractions over several weeks, whereas brachytherapy is a continuous application of radiation to the tumor bed over a number of minutes to days. A variety of radiation energies and biological characteristics

N. A. Janjan: Department of Radiation Oncology, The University of Texas, M.D. Anderson Cancer Center, Houston, TX 77030.

D. E. Weissman: Department of Medicine, Division of Hematology/Oncology, Medical College of Wisconsin, Milwaukee, WI 53226.

are available to help localize treatment to the areas at risk and exclude uninvolved normal tissues.

## Types of External Beam Irradiation

Despite the wide variety of available treatment approaches, external beam irradiation is most commonly used. Included within the classification of external beam radiation are *photons,* which are penetrating forms of radiation, and *electrons,* delivering treatment to superficial areas. External beam irradiation is administered from specialized machines that emit $\tau$ rays from a housed isotope (cobalt-60) or x-rays that are generated in a linear accelerator and are approximately 1000 times as powerful as the x-rays used in diagnostic radiology (1,2).

A wide variety of *photon* energies are available. This allows selective administration of treatment to the tumor and minimizes radiation to uninvolved tissues. Photons derived from cobalt-60 administers 100% of the prescribed dose [defined by the term maximum radiation dose $(D_{max})$] 0.5 cm below the skin surface. The x-rays derived from a 6-MV linear accelerator has a $D_{max}$ of 1.5 cm and the $D_{max}$ of 18-MV photons is 3.5 cm below the skin; tissues 0.5 cm below the skin surface treated with 18-MV photons receive only 30% of the prescribed radiation dose (Table 1). Therefore, high-photon energies deposit radiation in deep structures while sparing superficial structures like skin and subcutaneous tissues. Most commonly, high-energy photons are used to treat tumors in the pelvis and abdomen. Superficial tumors or tumors located in anatomic regions with a small diameter, like the head and neck region or extremities, are best treated with low-energy photons like cobalt-60 or 6-MV photons. The concept of integral dose relates the amount of radiation deposited to uninvolved normal tissues located between the skin surface and tumor; the goal in any radiation plan is to minimize integral dose by selecting the appropriate beam energy (Table 1). To reduce integral dose, parallel opposed radiation portals are routinely used in radiotherapy and each field is treated daily (3).

*Electron beam* irradiation also provides a number of therapeutic options based on the energy selected. The penetration of the beam can roughly be estimated by dividing the energy by different numeric factors. For example, 80% of the radiation dose from a 9-meV electron beam is deposited within 3 cm of the surface (9 divided by 3) whereas essentially all of the radiation is given within 4.5 cm of the skin (9 divided by 2) with no radiation penetrating beyond that depth. A variety of electron beam energies are available to allow precise localization of the radiation to superficial lesions while sparing underlying critical structures.

## Localization of the Radiation Dose/Dosimetry

Treatment often must be initiated emergently in palliative irradiation. Because of the need to rapidly administer therapy, the least complex treatment portals and dose calculations are often used. However, when a large volume of tissue must be included in the radiation portal, such factors as the energy of the radiation beam, angulation of the field, and dose to critical structures such as lung, bowel, eye, and spinal cord must be considered. External beam radiation portals can precisely outline the tissues at risk and exclude uninvolved regions from radiation effects with individualized treatment blocks (3).

## Radiation Doses and Schedules

The intent of palliative irradiation is to relieve suffering and minimize treatment-related morbidity. The treatment should effectively and efficiently eliminate symptoms for the duration of the patient's life. The radiation portals and fractionation should consider the patient's clinical status and prognosis. Hypofractionated irradiation continues to be the most frequently applied treatment schedule in palliative irradiation because large daily doses of radiation are administered over a relatively short period of time. The course of palliative irradiation is abbreviated in order to minimize the commitment of time for therapy and achieve rapid symptomatic relief. Hypofractionated radiation schedules for palliative therapy can range from 2.5 Gy per fraction administered over 3–4 weeks to a single 4-to 8-Gy dose of radiation. Most frequently, 30 Gy is administered in 10 fractions over 2 weeks.

Unlike curative radiotherapy where the cancer is localized and limited in volume, palliative irradiation can involve treatment of large tumors and symptomatic sites in patients who generally have widespread metastases. Radiotherapy that is prescribed with curative intent generally administers daily doses of 1.8–2 Gy over 5–7 weeks. These relatively high doses (50–70 Gy) are

**TABLE 1.** *Concept of integral dose demonstrated by radiation dose distributions (%) for three different energies*[a]

| Skin surface (cm) | Cobalt-60 | 6 MV | 18 MV |
|---|---|---|---|
| 0.5 | 100 | 30 | 25 |
| 1.0 | 98 | 90 | 50 |
| 1.5 | 95 | 100 | 90 |
| 2.0 | 93 | 98 | 96 |
| 2.5 | 90 | 97 | 98 |
| 3.0 | 88 | 95 | 98 |
| 3.5 | 85 | 92 | 100 |
| 5.0 | 80 | 88 | 96 |
| 10 | 55 | 68 | 80 |

[a]$D_{max}$, the maximum dose, refers to the depth at which 100% of the prescribed dose is located below the skin surface. The greater the $D_{max}$, the greater the skin sparing associated with less of an integral dose.

required to achieve local regional control in curative irradiation even though only microscopic residual disease or limited tumor volumes are treated (4–11). As the tumor increases in size, even higher radiation doses are required to kill all of the cancer cells. In most tumors, the potential number of stem cells is directly proportional to the tumor volume (5). The tumor volume is the sum of viable and nonviable cells, and is not always directly proportional to the number of stem cells (6). In some tumors, like soft tissue sarcomas, there is a large necrotic fraction and the rate of cell loss and removal of dead tumor cells from the tumor volume is low (7–9). Necrosis results in tissue hypoxicity, and hypoxic tissues are radioresistant. When treating hypoxic tumors, the radiation dose must be three times higher in order to kill the same number of cells in oxygenated tumors (1,2,12,13). Because of the limited radiation tolerance of the normal tissues adjacent to the tumor, it becomes impossible to administer a large enough dose of radiation to control large tumor volumes in palliative irradiation. The radiation dose required to kill the tumor and the dose tolerated by the normal tissues must be considered in every course of radiotherapy.

Palliative radiation can only administer a radiation dose that is sufficient to reduce the size of the metastatic lesion and relieve symptoms for the remainder of the patient's life. Symptoms that recur after palliative irradiation most commonly result from localized regrowth of tumor. Higher radiation doses may be necessary to kill more tumor cells in order to control symptoms over a longer period of time in patients who have a more extended prognosis. Because the radiation dose may influence the degree and durability of the response to treatment, consideration of the overall prognosis is critical to the radiation schedule selected (14–17).

Radiation tolerance is a function both of the type and the volume of tissue irradiated. Tumor cells and normal tissues vary widely in their tolerance to radiation (18,19).

Relating normal tissue tolerance to a 5% risk of a treatment-related complication at 5 years, the tolerance doses (TD 5/5) for each organ have been determined (18–20). The TD 5/5, when the entire organ is treated, ranges from 10 Gy for the eye, 1.75 Gy for the lung, 45 Gy for the brain, 70 Gy for the larynx. When only one third of the organ is irradiated, the TD 5/5 equals 45 Gy for the lung, 60 Gy for the brain, and 79 Gy for the larynx.

The dose per fraction, total dose, and anatomic distribution of the radiation (dosimetry) are important factors also in determining the efficacy and normal tissue tolerance to radiotherapy. Although the shorter radiation courses administered with palliative irradiation deliver lower total doses, the radiobiological effect of the lower total dose is proportionately greater because palliative radiation schedules use a large dose per fraction. Equivalent normal tissue effects can be achieved with a variety of radiation treatment schedules. For example, the radiation tolerance of the spinal cord is relatively equivalent when 20 Gy is delivered in five fractions, 30 Gy is administered in 10 fractions, 35 Gy in given in 14 fractions, or 40 Gy is prescribed over 20 fractions. The selection of the treatment schedules is indexed to the prognosis and clinical status. Therefore, as the daily radiation dose increases, the total dose must decrease because of the effects on normal tissues (Table 2). The relative equivalence of these radiation schedules is determined by a radiobiological factor known as the $\alpha/\beta$ ratio (3,18–22).

The $\alpha/\beta$ ratio specifically relates to the ability of normal tissues to repair the damage caused by radiation. Because acute radiation reactions do not predict for the development of late radiation sequelae, the $\alpha/\beta$ ratios are different for acute and late- reacting tissues (6,10,11,21–25). Acute reacting tissues, like mucosal surfaces, usually develop an inflammatory radiation reaction during the course of treatment. Late-reacting tissues are slow to or do not regenerate. Examples of late reacting tissues

**TABLE 2.** *Radiation dose schedules*

| Radiation schedule | Dose per fraction | Total dose | Length of treatment |
|---|---|---|---|
| *Curative therapy* | | | |
| Conventional fractionation | 180–200 cGy/day | 5000–7000 cGy | 5–7 weeks |
| Hyperfractionation | 110–120 cGy/fraction; 2 fractions per day separated by 6 hours | 7000–8000 cGy | 6–8 weeks; *longer than* conventional fractionation |
| Accelerated fractionation | 180–200 cGy/day for 5 weeks. Weeks 5–7: 180–200 cGy/day + 150 cGy/fraction given as a 2nd daily boost dose 6 hours later | 6500–7000 cGy | 5–6 weeks; the *same or shorter than* conventional fractionation |
| *Palliative therapy* | | | |
| Hypofractionation | 400–800 cGy given as a single fraction, or 250–400 cGy given as multiple fractions | 400–3500 cGy | 1 day–4 weeks; *shorter than* conventional fractionation |

Dose per fraction is inversely related to total dose: the lower the total dose, the higher the dose per fraction.

include the brain and heart. Scar tissue is the most common form of late radiation effect. The α/β ratio for long-term or late radiation effects is 3, and it is 10 for tumor cell kill and acute radiation reactions. For example, the α/β calculation would indicate that the late radiation effects that occur after the administration of 30 Gy/10 fractions (3 Gy per fraction) would be radiobiologically equivalent to a total dose of 36 Gy given at 2 Gy per fraction. The acute radiation effects, which relate to the number of tumor cells that are killed, would equal 32.4 Gy at 2 Gy per fraction if 30 Gy in 10 fractions were administered (Table 3). In general, the larger the daily dose of radiation, the lower the total dose that can be administered due to normal tissue tolerance.

The total dose of radiation necessary to eradicate a tumor, however, is indexed to the volume of disease and the number of tumor cells killed with each radiation fraction. Proportionately more tumor cells are killed when the daily radiation dose is larger (2,4–6). Obviously, less total dose is required to control microscopic residual disease than bulk disease. The local control rate at 2 years using only radiation to control cervical node metastases in head and neck cancer has been reported to be directly related to the node diameter and total dose (8,10,23,27, 28). Over 85% of patients with lymph node diameters of <2 cm in size are controlled with a median dose of 66 Gy.

Only 69% of nodes measuring between 2.5 cm and 3.0 cm are controlled after 69 Gy and only 59% of nodes >3.5 cm can be controlled after 70 Gy.

Fractionated irradiation allows the normal tissues to repair between each treatment. In contrast to hypofractionated irradiation that is most commonly used in palliative therapy, a variety of radiation schedules have been also been developed that administer high total doses of radiation in an attempt to improve local regional control of the tumor and allow for the repair of normal tissues between radiation doses (23,27–29). These schedules, which are also based on α/β calculations and shown in Table 2, include hyperfractionated radiation that administers two small radiation doses (usually 1.1–1.2 Gy per fraction) each day with a 6-hour separation between doses. Because of the repair of normal tissues between the doses of radiation, radiation doses ranging from 70 to 80 Gy can be administered with hyperfractionated radiotherapy instead of the total doses that range from 50 to 70 Gy with conventional fractionation. Based on α/β calculations, the late normal tissue effects that are observed when total doses of 70–80 Gy are delivered with hyperfractionated irradiation appear equivalent to total doses of 58–68 Gy with conventional radiation given as a daily treatment of 1.8–2.0 Gy per fraction (26). Therefore, higher total doses administered with hyperfractionated irradiation result in more

**TABLE 3.** *α/β calculations*

| Acute radiation effects | Late radiation effects |
|---|---|
| Rapidly proliferating tissues | Slowly proliferating tissues |
| Tumor cells | Nonregenerative tissues |
| Examples: mucositis, diarrhea | Examples: fibrosis, necrosis |
| α/β = 3 | α/β = 10 |

Example 1. The radiobiological equivalent total dose of **30 Gy total dose at 3 Gy per fraction over 10 fractions/ 2 weeks to conventional fractionation of 2 Gy/fraction** is determined with α/β calculations:

$$\alpha/\beta + \text{dose per fraction for total dose (a) divided by } \alpha/\beta + \text{dose per fraction for total dose (b)}$$

| α/β for acute effects | α/β for late effects |
|---|---|
| 3 + 10 divided by 2 + 10 or | 3 + 3 divided by 2 + 3 or |
| 13/12 = α/β ratio of 1.08 | 6/5 = α/β ratio of 1.2 |
| 30 Gy × 1.08 = **32.4 Gy at 2 Gy/fraction** | 30 Gy × 1.2 = **36 Gy at 2 Gy/fraction** |

Example 2. The radiobiological equivalent total dose of **72 Gy total dose at 1.2 Gy per fraction over 60 fractions over 6 weeks to conventional fractionation of 2 Gy/fraction** is determined with α/β calculations:

$$\alpha/\beta + \text{dose per fraction for total dose (a) divided by } \alpha/\beta + \text{dose per fraction for total dose (b)}$$

| α/β for acute effects | α/β for late effects |
|---|---|
| 1.2 + 10 divided by 2 + 10 or | 1.2 + 3 divided by 2 + 3 or |
| 11.2/12 = α/β ratio of 0.93 | 4.2/5 = α/β ratio of 0.84 |
| 72 Gy × 0.93 = **65 Gy at 2 Gy/fraction** | 72 Gy × 0.84 = **60.5 Gy at 2 Gy/fraction** |

*Summary*

| Radiation dose schedule | Dose per fraction | Total dose | α/β | Acute radiation effects/control of tumor relative to conventional fractionation | Late radiation effects relative to conventional fractionation |
|---|---|---|---|---|---|
| Hypofractionation | Increases | Decreases | >1.0 | Decrease | Increase |
| Hyperfractionation | Decreases | Increases | < 1.0 | Increase | Decrease |

tumor cells killed and better rates of local control without excessive late radiation effects. Most commonly, hyperfractionated irradiation is used to treat inoperable, locally advanced cancers, like Pancoast tumors of the lung without associated distant metastases, in order to relieve symptoms and prevent regrowth of the tumor that can result in recurrence of symptoms that often are difficult to manage. This is in contrast to the 30 Gy given at 3 Gy per fraction used in palliative hypofractionated irradiation for patients with disseminated disease and more limited life expectancy; as indicated previously, 30 Gy at 3 Gy per fraction is equivalent to 36 Gy to the tumor at 2 Gy per fraction based on $\alpha/\beta$ calculations (26). Because the effective dose to the tumor with palliative hypofractionated irradiation is essentially half that given with curative therapy, only tumor regression in order to relieve symptoms can be expected. However, it is considered inappropriate to administer an aggressive course of radiotherapy that lasts approximately 2 months and results in significant acute radiation effects to a patient with a limited life expectancy.

### Clinical Application of Radiobiological Principles

These radiobiological concepts can be related to commonly used palliative radiation schedules and the radiation doses used in the Radiation Therapy Oncology Group (RTOG) experience (14,16). A single large radiation fraction has been reported to be as effective in relieving pain as other schedules that have more treatments (30–33). No difference has been reported for either how quickly symptoms resolved or the duration of pain relief when a single fraction of 8 Gy (which is a radiobiologically equivalent dose of 17.6 Gy to normal tissues and only 12 Gy to the tumor if 2-Gy fractions were used) was compared to 30 Gy given in 10 daily fractions (radiobiologically equivalent to 36 Gy at 2 Gy per fraction for normal tissue effects and 32.5 Gy to the tumor) (26,29–31). In each case, symptom relief lasted 3 months in 71%, 6 months in 37%, and 12 months in 21% of cases. Retreatment was necessary in 25% of the 8-Gy treatment arm but all of these patients responded (31). When a single fraction of 4 Gy was compared to a single 8-Gy fraction, the rate of response was essentially equivalent and fewer acute radiation reactions occurred (31). Although large differences exist in the biological dose of radiation administered, reports indicate equivalence in clinical response (29–32). This disparity in dose and clinical response may be accounted for by the limited prognosis in patients with metastatic disease.

The RTOG conducted a prospective trial that included a variety of treatment schedules. In order to account for prognosis, patients were stratified on the basis of whether they had a solitary or multiple sites of bony metastases. The study concluded that low-dose, short-course treatment schedules were as effective as high-dose protracted

treatment programs (14). For solitary bone metastases, there was no difference in the relief of pain when 20 Gy using 4-Gy fractions was compared to 40.5 Gy delivered as 2.7 Gy per fraction. Relapse of pain occurred in 57% of patients at a median of 15 weeks after completion of therapy for each dose level. In patients with multiple bone metastases, the following dose schedules were compared: 30 Gy at 3 Gy per fraction, 15 Gy given as 3 Gy per fraction, 20 Gy using 4 Gy per fraction, and 25 Gy using 5 Gy per fraction. No difference was identified in the rates of pain relief between these treatment schedules. Partial relief of pain was achieved in 83% and complete relief occurred in 53% of the patients studied. Over 50% of these patients developed recurrent pain, the rates of pathologic fracture equaled 8%, and the median duration of pain control was 12 weeks for all of the radiation schedules used in treatment of multiple bony metastases.

In a reanalysis of these data, the definition of a complete response was changed to exclude patients who continued to use any form of analgesics. Using this new definition, the rate of pain relief was significantly related to the number of fractions and the total dose administered (16). Complete relief of pain was achieved in 55% of patients with solitary bone metastases who received 40.5 Gy at 2.7 Gy per fraction as compared to 37% of patients who received a total dose of 20 Gy given at 4 Gy per fraction. A similar relationship was observed in the reanalysis of patients who had multiple bone metastases. Complete relief of pain was achieved in 46% of patients who received 30 Gy at 3 Gy per fraction versus 28% of patients treated to 25 Gy using 5 Gy fractions. In most cases, the interval to response was 4 weeks for both complete and minimal relief of symptoms. The results of the reanalysis demonstrates the importance of defining the parameters of outcome in order to determine a dose–response relationship (16).

These studies suggest that more protracted fractionation (not less than 10 treatments) should be used to relieve symptoms of a solitary metastasis in a patient with a life expectancy of >6 months (15–17,33–35). Often more protracted fractionation will also be used to treat the spine if a significant number of vertebral bodies must be included in the radiation portal and to reduce potential acute radiation side effects to adjacent critical structures like the larynx (35). For patients who have a more limited life expectancy, 20 Gy in 5 fractions in 1 week or 30 Gy in 10 fractions in 2 weeks should be considered. With these treatment schedules, palliation is accomplished in 70% of patients at 3 months with limited treatment-related complications.

### PALLIATIVE EXTERNAL BEAM IRRADIATION

The primary goal of palliative irradiation is the treatment of localized sites of symptomatic tumor without causing significant radiation morbidity. The choice of beam energy, field size and shape, and prescribed total dose and fractionation are dependent on clinical status, tumor extent, tumor location and adjacent normal tissues, and overall prognosis. Because of these factors, hypofractionated regimens are generally preferred. Comfort of the patient in the treatment position should be a priority. The treatment should be administered efficiently with simple setup and blocking techniques. Complex plans and computed tomography (CT)–based dosimetry are rarely indicated. However, documentation of therapy with simulation and portal films is critical because many patients will subsequently require further palliative treatment to nearby lesions. This is particularly important in the treatment of vertebral metastases to avoid overlap of treatment portals.

## Bone Metastases

The treatment of bone metastases is one of the most commonly encountered indications for palliative irradiation, resulting in complete or partial symptomatic relief in over 70% of patients with localized radiation (15,17,33, 35,36). However, the effectiveness of pain relief and its durability are to some extent tumor site and type-dependent.

### Localized Therapy

A number of other factors may influence the response to palliative radiotherapy. Response to palliative irradiation may vary based on the location of the metastatic involvement. Complete pain relief occurs in 71% of spine metastases as compared to a 56% response rate in the limbs, 68% in the pelvis, and 61% in other sites (17). The pathology of the primary tumor generally has not been found to be an important factor in predicting relief of pain after palliative irradiation, except in the case of non–small cell carcinoma of the lung and renal cell carcinoma where complete pain relief is achieved less frequently. The level of pain relief achieved at completion of radiotherapy is an important indicator of the predicted duration of response to therapy. Patients who have a partial response to radiotherapy generally experience only a 4-month interval before pain symptoms progress. By comparison, patients who have a complete resolution of symptoms after radiotherapy have a median 25-month pain- free interval (17).

### Pathological Fracture

Persistent pain following palliative radiation should be investigated to rule out progressive disease under treatment, possible extension of disease outside the radiation portal that results in referred pain, and bone fracture. Bone fracture can result because of reduced cortical strength from the disease itself or instability of the bone.

Instability of the bone is most significant during the interval between tumor regression and healing of the bony cortex. Reduced cortical strength is most evident with lytic metastases and can result in compression, stress, or microfracture (Fig. 1).

Plain radiographs often are more useful than bone scans in follow-up evaluation because they more clearly delineate lytic changes and fracture. The concordance rate with plain x-rays is 91% as compared to 57% with posttherapy bone scans (37). Bone scans are also inferior to magnetic resonance imaging (MRI) in evaluating vertebral body involvement pre- or posttherapy (38,39). This was confirmed in a postmortem of examination of 52 cases of which lung cancer was the primary tumor in 19 of the cases and 28 cases had adenocarcinoma as the primary histology. Metastases were pathologically confirmed in 734 of 1194 vertebrae but were detected in only 50% of plain radiographs, 35% of bone scans, and 100% of MRI evaluations. The pathologic pattern of the metastases included osteoblastic, osteolytic, mixed, and intertrabecular lesions, and compression fracture. Plain film radiographs detected >85% of these lesions except for intertrabecular metastases which were detected only 7% of the time. Although bone scans detect approximately 90% of osteoblastic metastases, they only identify compression fractures 66%, mixed lesions 50%, osteolytic lesions 28%, and intertrabecular tumor 5% of the time. The overall sensitivity for plain radiographs was 50% and 35% for bone scans (38). For this reason, evaluation with an MRI is especially important in patients with persistent back pain after spine irradiation. Progressive disease with epidural extension and spinal cord compression must be excluded. Spinal cord compression can also result from spinal instability and compression fracture. In either case, decompression laminectomy may be required.

Metastases considered at high risk for pathologic fracture include lytic lesions in weight-bearing bones where there is more than a 50% loss in cortex or if a lesion measuring 2.5 cm or greater in size is observed (40). Because these cases are prone to pathologic fracture, prophylactic intramedullary fixation is considered to be beneficial (Fig. 2). It is unclear as to what other specific clinical presentations might benefit from prophylactic surgical fixation; however, current practice considers the extent of disease and the patient's functional status in determining the need for surgical intervention (41–44). Surgical intervention is generally warranted to stabilize a pathologic fracture unless the overall prognosis is poor and the patient is unable to undergo surgical intervention.

The role of radiotherapy following surgical intervention in pathologic fractures is unproven given the lack of prospective trials. Postoperative radiation is frequently administered, however, to treat disease at the fracture site and encourage bony union, particularly in patients with favorable prognostic factors like an isolated bone metastasis. In retrospective evaluations, the stability of the

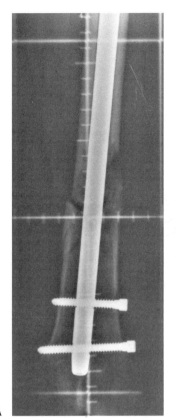
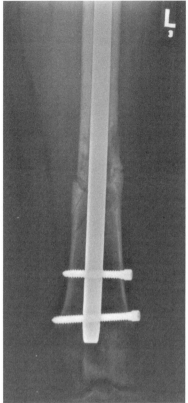
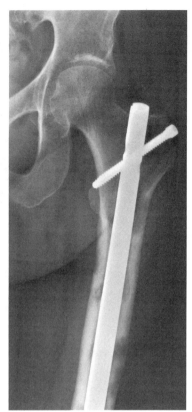

A

B,C

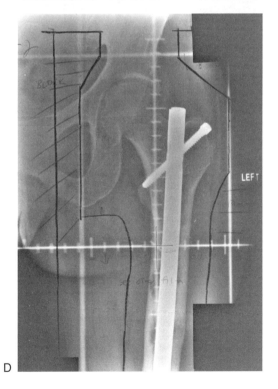

D

**FIG. 1. (A)** Persistent pain was reported in a patient with renal cell carcinoma who had undergone internal fixation of a pathologic fracture involving the distal femur and postoperative irradiation to a localized field (30 Gy/10 fractions). The initial radiation portal only treated the region of the pathologic fracture with a 5-cm margin. **(B)** Subsequent diagnostic x-rays showed stabilization of disease within the radiation portal. **(C)** The patient's persistent pain was explained by the development of lytic metastases in the proximal femur and resulted in instability of the rod. **(D)** Three months after the proximal femur received 30 Gy/10 fractions, the patient experienced near-complete relief of pain and the position of the rod remained stable. Postoperative irradiation following internal fixation should encompass the entire rod whenever possible and reduces the need for subsequent surgical intervention because of progressive disease in the bone resulting in instability of the rod.

bone was improved and there were fewer cases that required reoperation when postoperative radiation was given after surgical stabilization of a pathologic fracture (41–43). Effective rehabilitation can be accomplished in patients with pathologic fracture. About one third of

oncology patients regain the ability to ambulate at discharge from a hospital stay, which on average is only 3 days longer than that required for patients with nonmalignant fractures (43). Outcome was poor in patients who had hypercalcemia or who continued to require parenteral

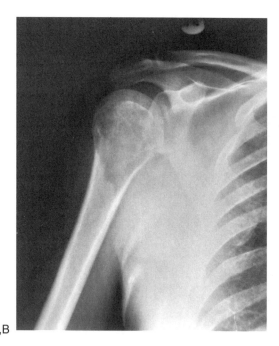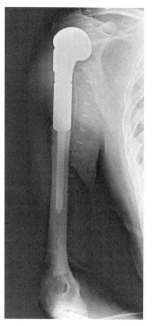

A,B

FIG. 2. (A) The patient had severe pain that did not respond to analgesics due to near-complete replacement of the humeral head and articular surface by metastaic adenocarcinoma. (B) The patient was discharged from the hospital within a week of surgery, had functional improvement, and required only mild analgesics intermittently for postoperative pain. Within two weeks of surgery, postoperative irradiation (30 Gy/10 fractions) was administered.

analgesics to treat the symptoms of diffuse metastatic disease.

Reirradiation can be considered for recurrent or persistent pain. The response rate for retreatment is reported to be 85% (30,33,45). Most frequently, a single 8-Gy or 10-Gy fraction is administered, although other fractionation regimens like 26 Gy per 6 fractions, 28 Gy per 7 fractions, and 30 Gy per 10 fractions also have been used in retreatment. Response to retreatment has been correlated to the initial radiation dose and level of response.

*Summary*

On the basis of the available studies, a moderately protracted course (not less than 30 Gy in 10 treatments) is recommended in treatment of bone metastases. This is particularly important to prevent pathologic fracture in a weight-bearing bone or in the treatment of a solitary metastasis occurring in a patient with a life expectancy of greater than 6 months. In some cases, 40 Gy in 20 fractions over 4 weeks may be delivered based on prognosis and consideration of acute radiation toxicity. A more abbreviated course of radiation is indicated for patients with a more limited life expectancy. Depending on clinical status and the normal tissues in the treatment portal, doses ranging from a single dose of 8–10 Gy to 20 Gy in 5 fractions over 1 week, to 30 Gy in 10 fractions in 2 weeks, to 35 Gy in 14 fractions over 3 weeks are generally administered. These treatment regimens result in effective palliation in 70% of patients at 3 months with essentially no treatment-related complications.

*Wide-Field Irradiation*

After the diagnosis of bone metastases, median survival rates are 1 year with breast cancer, 6 months with prostate cancer, and 3 months with lung cancer resulting in the need for continued management of pain (44). During this time, most patients develop multiple bone metastases. In patients with breast cancer, only 50% will continue to have relief of painful bony metastases 1 year after localized palliative irradiation (17,29,33,34–36). This is because of the development of symptomatic lesions both in and outside of the localized portals of radiation.

Hemibody irradiation has been used to treat multiple sites of asymptomatic bone metastases to delay or prevent their becoming a source of pain. An improvement in the parameters of time to disease progression at 1 year, development of new disease within the treatment volume, and median time to the appearance of new disease was reported in a randomized RTOG study that compared hemibody irradiation to local field irradiation alone (46). Like other studies, palliation of symptoms was accomplished in over 85% of patients, and over 50% experienced stabilization of disease 1 year after hemibody irradiation (47–50). Up to half of patients experience relief from pain relief within 48 hours of treatment.

Hemibody irradiation is used in patients with disseminated bone metastases and has been used to treat a variety of primary histologies including prostate and breast cancer. This technique can be used either alone or as an adjuvant to localized external beam irradiation. Sequential treatment of the upper, middle, or lower body can be delivered in single fraction of 600 cGy. Other approaches have included fractionated regimens of hemibody radiation that total 24–30 Gy in 9–10 fractions (51–54). Acute toxicities of hemibody irradiation, observed in <10% of patients with current practice patterns, can be controlled with premedication and partial shielding to reduce lung dose (46). Hematologic depression is the major dose-limiting toxicity (53). Fractionation of the dose, giving two 4-Gy single doses separated by 2 weeks or five 3-Gy fractions or a 17.5-Gy total dose at 2.5 Gy per fraction, eliminates the need for premedication or postradiation monitoring. In addition to better tolerance of the regimen and administration of a higher total dose, fractionation results in an improved response to therapy that was defined as more complete and durable relief of pain.

Systemic radioisotopes provide an alternative to hemibody irradiation for the treatment of widely disseminated bone metastases (55–57). Advantages include the simplicity and convenience of a single injection of the radioisotope and limited systemic effects.

### Radiopharmaceuticals

Systemic radioisotopes provide an alternative to hemibody irradiation in the treatment of widely disseminated bone metastases. Characterized by the ease of outpatient administration with a single intravenous injection, and limited toxicities, radiopharmaceuticals are being used with greater frequency. Strontium-89 is an approved agent that is commonly used to treat bone metastases due to breast and prostate cancers. Over 80% of patients respond to strontium-89; most responses last 6 months or longer (55–58). Improvements in functional status and quality of life have been observed, and 10–20% of patients have complete resolution of pain following administration of strontium-89 (55,56). Pain control has been reported to be superior in patients with disseminated prostate cancer treated with both strontium-89 and local radiotherapy as compared to localized irradiation alone (57). Myelotoxicity, resulting in a 25% decline of the initial blood cell counts, is usually transient and represents the only significant toxicity associated with strontium-89 (55–58). Patients may receive additional doses of strontium-89 should symptoms recur.

The half-life of strontium-89 is 50 days in diseased bone and about 14 days in normal bone. Strontium-89, a β emitter that has a limited range of radiation, localizes in diseased bone and combines with the calcium component of hydroxyapatite in osteoblastic lesions (56). Therefore little dose is administered to normal bone and essentially no dose is administered to adjacent visceral structures. The only symptomatic side effect is the occasional development of a flare effect in which the pain worsens before it resolves. Because the activity of strontium-89 is limited to bone, use of radiopharmaceuticals is contraindicated when epidural disease is associated with vertebral metastases.

Other radiopharmaceuticals are in development for the treatment of bony metastases. These include tin-117m and samarium-153, which have a more limited uptake in normal bone (59,60). The response rates and relative lack of toxicity are similar to that of strontium-89 and myelotoxicity is even more limited.

### Summary

Many radiotherapeutic options exist in the treatment of bony metastases. Optimization of dose administered and the indications and sequencing of modalities requires further investigation. In order to optimize outcome, prognostic factors and factors that potentially influence response to therapy, like the location of disease, must be considered.

## Treatment of Other Sites

Palliative radiation frequently involves treatment of metastatic lesions other than bone. Visceral metastases that result in symptoms due to tumor mass effect, bleeding, or obstruction of lymphovascular structures can be effectively palliated with radiation. Indications and techniques exist in the treatment of metastases involving the brain and spinal cord, eye, lymphatics, soft tissues, and hollow viscera.

### Central Nervous System

#### Brain Metastases

Metastatic disease that involves the brain or impinges on the spinal cord is the second most common indication for palliative irradiation. A consensus panel recently developed treatment recommendations based on the extent of metastatic disease in the brain (61). Resection of solitary brain lesions should be considered in patients with a good performance status who have achieved local/regional control of the primary lesion, have no other evidence of metastatic disease, and have a lesion that is anatomically accessible. In this selected subpopulation postoperative whole-brain radiation totaling 40–50 Gy has been recommended (62–64). Prognosis remains poor even after resection of a solitary intracerebral metastasis with only 16% of patients surviving more than 1 year after diagnosis (63,64). Median survival rates are 42 weeks with surgery and radiotherapy, 45 weeks with surgery alone, 16 weeks with radiotherapy alone, and 8 weeks with only supportive care (63). Surgical intervention has not been shown to influence survival in cases with multiple intracranial metastases (64). Retrospective evaluations, however, include the bias that therapeutic recommendations are based on the extent of disease.

Recommendations for the treatment of solitary brain metastases in patients who do not fit the criteria for resection or in patients with multiple intracranial lesions depend on clinical status (61–66). Patients with a good to excellent functional status, control of the primary tumor, age <60 years, and limited extent of metastatic disease may be candidates for stereotactic radiosurgery either alone or in combination with whole-brain irradiation. Criteria for stereotactic radiosurgery include limited metastases that are surgically inaccessible and <3 cm in size. Used either alone or as a boost in combination with whole-brain irradiation, stereotactic irradiation delivers a focused single high dose of irradiation, and the integral dose is limited to <10% of the prescribed dose. This dosimetric profile results in little treatment-related morbidity and allows retreatment of metastases that progress after whole-brain irradiation. Disadvantages include the amount of time devoted to the one treatment session, headache, and risk of radiation necrosis. Local control rates with stereotactic radiation are reported to be >80%, representing a twofold improvement when compared to whole-brain irradiation without radiosurgical intervention.

Outside of this setting, a short course of radiation, delivered as either 20 Gy in 5 fractions or 30 Gy in 10 fractions, is recommended (Fig. 3). The use of steroids is controversial in asymptomatic patients. In symptomatic patients, dexamethasone (4 mg q.i.d.) is generally administered during the course of radiotherapy; doses are tapered after completion of irradiation.

*Spinal Cord Metastases*

The dose schedule used in treatment of spinal cord metastases is similar to that used for brain metastases. Other schedules that have been reported deliver 5-Gy fractions daily for 3 days followed by 4 days rest, then an additional five daily fractions of 3 Gy based on experimental evidence suggesting improved initial response with higher daily doses.

The most important predictor of response to radiotherapy in spinal cord compression is the patient's neurologic status at the time of diagnosis. While 66% of ambulatory patients maintain the ability to walk, only 30% of nonambulatory patients and 16% of paraplegic patients regain function (67,68). Prompt initiation of radiotherapy and accurate field placement are critical in the effective palliative treatment of spinal cord compression (Fig. 4). MRI has superseded all other diagnostic tests for suspected spinal cord metastases and should be performed whenever possible to document the extent of disease. This is often multicentric, and not adequately treated by localized fields covering the level of clinical neurologic deficit. Median overall survival is 10 months and patients who were ambulatory prior to surgery, maintained continence, had breast cancer or involvement of only one vertebral body survived longer (68).

Follow-up is important after completion of radiation to monitor for in-field progression of disease and spinal instability and to assess new sites of symptomatology. The risk for progression of disease and spinal cord compression is 9% after a single 6-Gy dose of radiation is

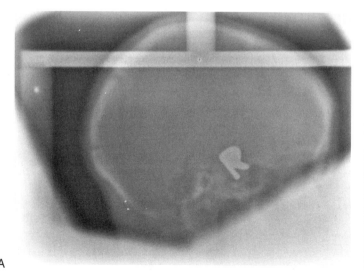
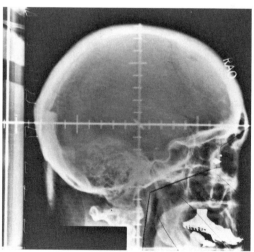

A
B

**FIG. 3. (A)** Trimmer fields are frequently used when radiotherapy is initiated emergently to treat symptomatic intracranial metastases. The borders generally follow a line from the superior orbital ridge to the bottom of the tragus and occiput. **(B)** However, if there is evidence of base of skull or leptomeningeal involvement, blocks are used with posterior angulation of the beam to avoid divergence of the beam to the contralateral eye.

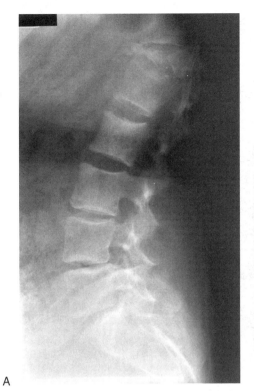
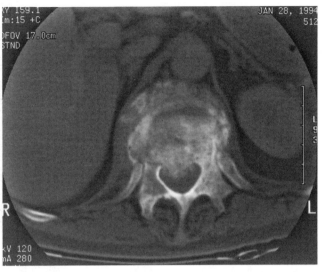

A                                                                                                        B

**FIG. 4. (A)** A compression fracture of T12 is shown on a lateral x-ray of the spine in a lung cancer patient with severe back pain. **(B)** Magnetic resonance imaging demonstrates epidural extension of disease from the vertebral metastases and spinal cord compromise.

used to palliate vertebral metastases (69). Patients who fail to respond to radiotherapy may require surgical intervention to maintain neurologic integrity.

### Eye

Metastatic ocular tumors can include a range of histologies with breast cancer being the most frequent primary. Up to 30% of women with metastatic breast cancer will have retinal metastases that are not often diagnosed due to the dominant clinical manifestations of other sites of disease involvement. The goal of treatment is to preserve vision for the remainder of the patient's life. An MRI of the brain should be considered in patients with ocular metastases to exclude associated central nervous system extension. Palliative irradiation can be administered with either a lateral appositional field or with a wedge pair technique using photons delivering 30 Gy in 10 fractions (Fig. 5). The choice of therapy is dependent on the extent of tumor. The entire retrobulbar orbit should be included in the radiation portal shielding the lacrimal gland whenever possible. Treatment techniques are similar for ocular lymphoma although a dose of 20–30 Gy administered at 1.5–2.0 Gy per fraction is prescribed. Local control is achieved in 85% of patients, with improvement in visual acuity.

### Nodal and Soft Tissues

Both lymphatic and soft tissue tumors can occur in any location. Soft tissue involvement by locally advanced recurrent or metastatic tumors can include skin, subcutaneous tissues, and muscle. Extensive lymphatic or soft tissue metastases can result in compression of vascular and lymphatic channels, and cause edema distal to the obstruction. Symptomatic compression of adjacent nerves by mass lesions can cause symptoms of plexopathy. An example of this is in recurrent breast cancer, which can present with an ulcerative lesion in the skin, multiple subcutaneous nodules, and extensive axillary adenopathy resulting in arm edema and brachial plexopathy.

The fractionation schedule used to treat metastatic lymph node involvement is dependent on the location of the tumor, radiation tolerance of the adjacent normal tissues, and clinical presentation. Factors considered in the clinical presentation include the extent of the local and metastatic disease, intercurrent medical problems, and performance status, all of which relate to overall prognosis. For example, 30 Gy in 10 fractions may be administered to palliate a recurrent rectal tumor that involves pelvic lymph nodes and the sacral plexus in a patient with lower extremity edema, pain, and liver metastases. Treatment of celiac axis involvement by locally advanced pan-

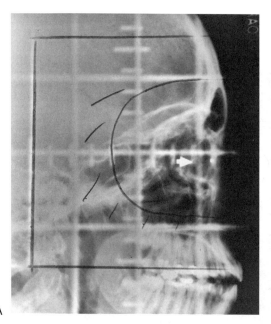
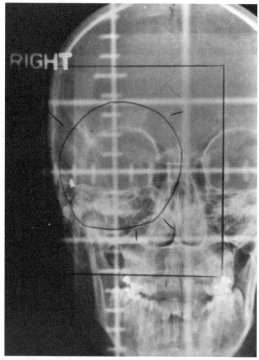

**FIG. 5.** The radiation portals used to treat retinal metastases are demonstrated. The circular areas demarcate the radiation field; anatomic regions outside the circular field are blocked from the radiation beam so that only the eye is treated. Both lateral (**A**) and anterior (**B**) fields are treated each day to deliver a homogeneous dose of radiation to the eye and minimize dose to other structures as the penetrating radiation beam exits.

creatic cancer may be better tolerated using 2.5-Gy fractions to a total dose of 35–40 Gy due to the proximity of the stomach and duodenum. Axillary node involvement with recurrent breast cancer often is treated with high-dose conventional or accelerated fractionation to achieve a more durable regression of the local regional disease, with the understanding that the median survival of these patients is greater than a year.

Metastatic tumors that involve subcutaneous tissues most commonly involve the trunk and can occur with any tumor histology. Tumors most frequently associated with subcutaneous metastases include cancers of the breast, colon, lung, and malignant melanoma. Symptomatic metastatic subcutaneous tumors are generally associated with widely disseminated disease and should be treated with a hypofractionated schedule. Because subcutaneous metastases often are extensive, radiation portals should be limited to symptomatic lesions. Treatment techniques should include tangential portals or electron beam to minimize potential toxicities from radiation of uninvolved deep structures. Recommended doses are 20 Gy in 5 fractions or 30 Gy in 10 fractions, except for melanoma metastases which are usually treated with 5–6 fractions of 6 Gy.

Locally advanced lymphomas and soft tissue sarcomas are often treated with more protracted courses because of the chance for long-term survival. Accounting for the large tissue volumes that are frequently involved, conventional fractionation is frequently preferred for advanced soft tissue sarcoma, even when associated with limited metastatic disease, because palliation of symptoms and limb preservation represents an important aspect of quality of life in these patients with a median survival of over a year. As an alternative to the 5–6 weeks of external beam radiotherapy, an interstitial implant placed at the time of wide local excision can also provide an efficient and effective means of local control in soft tissue sarcoma, delivering 50 Gy to the bed of resection from the fifth to the tenth postoperative day (70–73). This approach is particularly useful in patients with metastases documented at presentation, allowing the prompt relief of tumor-related symptoms and administration of systemic therapy.

### Pelvis and Abdomen

Locally advanced or metastatic disease in the abdomen and/or pelvis often represents a difficult problem for palliative radiotherapy due to the limited radiation tolerance of the bowel. The most common indications for palliative irradiation include pain and bleeding. Colorectal and cervical carcinomas represent the most common tumors requiring palliative therapy. Locally advanced or recurrent pelvic tumors may invade the sacral plexus and cause lymphatic, urinary, or rectal obstruction. A variety of treatment schedules for external irradiation have been used to provide tumor regression sufficient to relieve symptoms due to the mass effect from intraabdominal and pelvic tumors. Bleeding from cervical cancer can often be palliated with localized therapy including intracavitary irradiation or vaginal cone irradiation using orthovoltage irradiation. A tandem placed in the endocervix giving 10–15 Gy in 24 hours is an effective means of controlling hemorrhage. Alternatively, orthovoltage irradiation directed by a vaginal cone that delivers 7.5–10.0 Gy in one to three fractions also is an effective means of palliation.

Hematuria can usually be controlled with 30 Gy in 10 fractions to the pelvis or a single dose of 8–10 Gy. Based on patient assessment of symptoms due to advanced bladder cancer, however, long-term palliation of pain is not generally achieved with hypofractionated irradiation, supporting the use of conventional fractionation in locally advanced tumors, particularly in the absence of other metastases (74).

Liver metastases are treated most frequently by systemic therapy due to the intrinsic radiosensitivity of the liver. Palliative radiation is primarily used for the relief of capsular pain that requires radiation of the entire liver. Treatment regimens of 20–24 Gy in 10–12 fractions or 30 Gy in 12–15 fractions have yielded variable response; higher total doses are not possible due to radiation hepatitis. In rare circumstances where localized radiation fields can be used, such as in the treatment of portal obstruction due to adenopathy, 40–45 Gy using conventional fractionation may be administered with acceptable treatment-related morbidity. Other therapeutic strategies to palliate pain due to hepatic metastases and pancreatic cancer include celiac nerve blocks, which accomplishes pain relief in over 50% of patients at 3 months follow-up. In selected patients, intraluminal brachytherapy may provide palliation to relieve obstruction involving the bile ducts.

## Lung

Palliation is a significant aspect of lung cancer management because the majority of patients are symptomatic at diagnosis. Symptoms associated with lung cancer that frequently require palliation include dyspnea, cough, hemoptysis, postobstructive pneumonia, pain, and superior vena cava obstruction. Definitive radiation, using conventional or other aggressive fractionation schedules, is usually administered in an attempt to achieve local regional control in cases where distant metastases have been excluded. In one study, the response to hypofractionated irradiation evaluated at postmortem examination was reported to be inferior to more aggressive fractionation schedules (75). Conventional fractionation totaling 50 Gy

has been reported to result in a 48% improvement in symptoms and a 74% rate of response.

A similar aggressive treatment approach is advocated for patients with superior vena cava syndrome. An initial dose of 400 cGy followed by conventional fractionation to a total dose of 60 Gy is often administered in patients who have significant symptoms such as cardiopulmonary compromise and edema (Fig. 6). Radiotherapeutic management of a malignant pleural effusion requires hemithoracic irradiation, limited by tolerance of the lung to a total dose of 20–25 Gy with conventional fractionation. Symptom management with evacuation of the pleural fluid and sclerosing agents is also generally performed.

Locally advanced, untreated lung cancer that is associated either with distant metastases or with a poor clinical status is usually treated with hypofractionated irradiation administered as 30 Gy in 10 fractions or 37.5 Gy in 15 fractions. Endobronchial radiation has been used with greater frequency to palliate obstructive symptoms in locally recurrent endobronchial lesions particularly in patients having received prior external beam irradiation. The reported incidence of bronchial obstruction resulting from recurrent tumor ranges from 17% to 28%. Palliation of symptoms is accomplished with endobronchial brachytherapy in >70% of patients for more than 6 months duration, which is superior to the results reported with the use of laser beam therapy alone (76). The prescribed dose is usually 30–50 Gy at 1 cm from the source center. Response rates of >70% with radiographic and bronchoscopic documentation have been reported. Complications, occurring in approximately 10% of patients, can include bronchoesophageal or bronchovascular fistulae. If left untreated, however, many of these patients would develop fistulae related to disease progression. Endobronchial brachytherapy represents an effective and well-tolerated technique to achieve durable palliation of symptoms from malignant airway obstruction in patients who have failed other therapeutic modalities.

## Head and Neck

In general, the best palliation of advanced head and neck tumors is obtained by surgical resection and postoperative radiotherapy. Palliative irradiation can be used to relieve symptoms of respiratory compromise with a protective tracheostomy, functional difficulties in speech and swallowing, bleeding or discharge from exophytic tumors, cranial nerve involvement, and massive lymphadenopathy in locally advanced head and neck cancer. Because most patients present with local regional disease and no evidence of distant metastases, aggressive radiation therapy is often administered using conventional, accelerated, or hyperfractionated dose schedules. In patients with a poor performance status, we have developed a useful palliative regimen of four fractions of 3.5

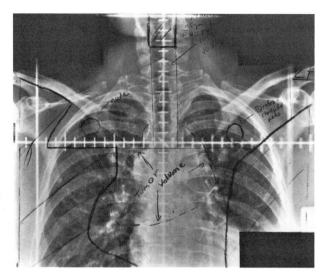

**FIG. 6.** Radiotherapy portal encompassing mediastinal and supraclavicular adenopathy in the patient with superior vena cava syndrome from lung cancer.

Gy given twice a day over two consecutive days, and repeated as necessary at monthly intervals for up to three cycles. This regimen has the advantage of securing worthwhile responses without inducing significant mucositis.

Tumors recurring within an area of previous external beam irradiation that are not associated with distant metastases are primarily approached with surgical salvage. Symptomatic recurrent disease associated with distant metastases that is unresponsive to systemic therapy may be palliated with either brachytherapy or further limited external beam irradiation if any treatment is pursued.

### Brachytherapy

Brachytherapy involves placement of radioactive sources within a tumor bed and represents another means of administering well-localized radiotherapy to limit dose to adjacent uninvolved structures. *Temporary implants* deliver uninterrupted radiation precisely to the tumor bed over a determined length of time. Brachytherapy can be administered with isotopes of relatively low activity and the implant remains in place from 2 to 5 days delivering radiation doses of 20–50 Gy. High-dose-rate radiation uses a high-intensity radiation source to deliver radiation totaling 10–20 Gy over a few minutes. High-dose-rate brachytherapy is commonly used to treat recurrent endobronchial tumors, bile duct tumors, and esophageal cancers by placing a radioactive source adjacent to the tumor. Iridium-192 and cesium are the isotopes used most frequently in temporary implants.

*Permanent implants* insert radioactive sources directly within unresectable tumors that involving deep structures. The radioactive sources most often used in perma-

nent implants include iodine-125, which delivers high total doses (e.g., 150 Gy) of low-energy radioactivity with a long half-life, and gold-198, which administers more intense radiation over a shorter period of time to deliver high doses of radiation that can total over 100 Gy at the center of the tumor. Advantages of brachytherapy include reduced overall treatment time, sparing of uninvolved surrounding structures, and enhanced repair of radiation injury to adjacent normal tissues. Brachytherapy has been used as definitive treatment of localized disease, as a boost in conjunction with external beam irradiation, and for the treatment of disease recurring in an area that was previously irradiated (70,73,77).

### Summary

Antineoplastic therapy can induce tumor regression, provide relief of cancer-related symptoms, and maintain functional integrity. Radiation therapy is an important means of treating localized symptoms related to tumor involvement by providing a wide range of therapeutic options. Radiobiological principles and prognostic factors influence the selection of palliative therapy. The selection of the radiation technique, dose, and fraction size are dependent on normal tissue tolerance and the clinical condition. The optimal dose and radiation schedule, however, are not fully defined. Further study is necessary to integrate validated pain scores, analgesic use, prognostic factors, and radiobiological principles in order to better define the most efficient and efficacious treatment schedule.

Accounting for normal tissue tolerance, additional palliative irradiation can be given to a previously treated area with specific dose fractionation schedules, radiation energies, and orientation of the beam. Other specialized techniques, like brachytherapy, that provide relatively high radiation doses directly to the tumor also are available to provide further treatment to sites of recurrent disease. Because the radiation activity of radiopharmaceuticals is limited to bone, they too provide an important means of treating progressive disease in a previously irradiated area and widespread metastases. Radiopharmaceuticals can also act as an adjuvant to localized external beam irradiation and reduce the development of other symptomatic sites of disease.

Palliative irradiation should be integrated in a multidisciplinary therapeutic approach because of the need to treat associated symptoms and other underlying medical problems. Control of cancer-related pain with the use of analgesics is imperative to allow comfort during and while awaiting response to radiotherapy. Pain represents a sensitive measure of disease activity. Close follow-up should be performed to ensure control of cancer- and treatment-related pain, and assess for progressive disease or recurrent disease.

## SYSTEMIC ANTINEOPLASTIC TREATMENTS

Systemic antineoplastic treatments include chemotherapy, hormonal therapy, and biological therapy. These modalities are used to treat all sites of cancer rather than focal metastatic deposits. Since cancer pain is most often caused by direct tumor involvement, resulting in local pressure and/or invasion of adjacent structures, reducing tumor burden by effective systemic treatments will often result in pain relief.

Analgesic effects are most likely to be seen when systemic treatments are used against cancers that are inherently sensitive to antineoplastic treatments in patients who have had little previous exposure to such treatments. In adults, the most responsive tumors to systemic treatments (response rates to first-line treatment of at least 40%) include both acute and chronic leukemias, germ cell tumors, lymphomas, multiple myeloma, small cell lung cancer, and breast, prostate, and ovarian cancer. Patients with tumors in which there are infrequent responses to systemic treatments (melanoma, hypernephroma, hepatoma) rarely obtain significant analgesic benefit.

The time to onset of analgesia typically mirrors the time course of tumor reduction. This can be as rapid as a few days in a patient with a newly diagnosed large cell lymphoma or germ cell tumor following combination chemotherapy. Alternatively, hormonal therapy for breast or prostate cancer causes a much slower antitumor effect with gradual improvement in pain occurring over 3–6 weeks. For most solid tumors (e.g., lung, colon, head and neck), if there is a substantial antineoplastic effect, it will begin 1–3 weeks following the first course of systemic therapy. Continued antineoplastic therapy will result in

analgesic benefit as long as there is tumor regression or stabilization.

Rarely, patients will report a rapid analgesic benefit that cannot be explained solely by tumor shrinkage, particularly following regional intraarterial chemotherapy (78–84). One theory to explain this phenomenon is that chemotherapy may alter the function of sensory nerves so that pain impulse transmission is modified (85). Although it is well known that certain cytotoxic agents (e.g., vinca alkaloids, cisplatin) will effect peripheral nerve function, it is unknown if these or other cytotoxic agents produce effects on pain transmission. A more likely explanation is that cytotoxic drugs effect the local production of tumor cytokines, nociceptive chemicals, and immune effector cells within and surrounding the tumor (85).

Analgesic improvement is most commonly represented by a decreased need for analgesic drug therapy. Patients will often be able to reduce, if not totally eliminate, their need for analgesics when there has been a good analgesic response. In addition, patients will report improvement in movement, eating, sleeping, and mood. Conversely, a complaint of new or worsening pain, together with new impairment in daily activities, most often represents tumor progression rather than drug tolerance (86).

The decision to administer a systemic antineoplastic treatment is made after careful consideration of multiple tumor and patient factors. These include tumor histology; stage and prognosis; degree of major organ involvement; response to prior antineoplastic treatments; coexisting medical problems such as heart, lung, liver, or kidney disease; and the patient's performance status. The performance status, a measure of functional ability, is the single best predictor of whether or not a patient will respond to chemotherapy, especially for the common solid tumors. Since pain control is rarely the primary goal of systemic therapy, the patient and his or her physician must have an honest and thorough discussion of the expected goals and potential side effects of systemic therapy.

## REFERENCES

1. Khan FM. Interaction of X and photon radiations. In: *The Physics of Radiation Therapy*. Baltimore: Williams & Wilkins, 1984;67–86.
2. Hall EJ. The Janeway Lecture 1992. Nine decades of radiobiology: is radiation therapy any the better for it? *Cancer* 1993; 71:3753–3766.
3. Suit H, duBois W. The importance of optimal treatment planning in radiation therapy. *Int J Radiat Oncol Biol Phys* 1991;21:1471–1478.
4. Taylor JMG, Menenhall WM, Lavey RS. Time-dose factors in positive neck nodes treated with irradiation alone. *Int J Radiat Oncol Biol Phys* 1991;22:167–173.
5. Brenner DJ. Dose, volume and tumor control predictions in radiotherapy. *Int J Radiat Oncol Biol Phys* 1993;26:171–179.
6. Withers HR, Peters LJ. Biologic aspects of radiation therapy. In: Fletcher GH, ed. *Textbook of radiotherapy*. Philadelphia: Lea and Febiger, 1980;103–180.
7. Hermes AF, Barendsen GW. Changes in cell proliferation-characteristics in a rat rhabdomyosarcoma before and after x-irradiation. *Eur J Cancer* 1969;5:173–189.
8. Denekamp J. The relationship between the "cell loss factor" and the

immediate response to radiation in animal tumours. *Eur J Cancer* 1972;8:335–340.

9. Steel GG. *Growth kinetics of tumours.* Oxford: Clarendon Press; 1977.

10. Peters LJ. Biology of modern radiotherapy for head and neck cancer. *Head Neck Cancer* 1985;1:37–47.

11. Thames HD, Bentzen SM, Turesson I, Overgaard M, van den Bogaert W. Time-dose factors in radiotherapy: a review of the human data. *Radiother Oncol* 1990;19:219–23.

12. Young SD, Hill RP. Effects of reoxygenation on cells from hypoxic regions of solid tumors. Anticancer drug sensitivity and metastatic potential. *JNCI* 1990;82(5):371–380.

13. Kallman RF. The phenomenon of reoxygenation and its implications for fractionated radiotherapy. *Radiology* 1972;105:135–142.

14. Tong D, Gillick L, Hendrickson FR. The palliation of symptomatic osseous metastases-final results of the study by the Radiation Therapy Oncology Group. *Cancer* 1982;50:893–899.

15. Bates T. A review of local radiotherapy in the treatment of bone metastases and cord compression. *Int J Radiat Oncol Biol Phys* 1992; 23:217–221.

16. Blitzer PH. Reanalysis of the RTOG study of the palliation of symptomatic osseous metastasis. *Cancer* 1985;55:1468–1472.

17. Arcangeli G, Micheli A, Arcangeli G, Giannarelli D, La Pasta O, Tollis A, Vitullo A, Ghera S, Benassi M. The responsiveness of bone metastases to radiotherapy: the effect of site, histology and radiation dose on pain relief. *Radiother Oncol* 1989;14:95–101.

18. Emami B, Lyman J, Brown A, Coia L, Goiten M, Munzenrider JE, Shank B, Solin LJ, Wesson M. Tolerance of normal tissue to therapeutic irradiation. *Int J Radiat Oncol Biol Phys* 1991;21:109–122.

19. Rubin P, ed. Radiation pathology of other subcritical organs and tissues. In: *Radiation Biology and Radiation Pathology Syllabus.* Chicago: American College of Radiology, 1975;207–217.

20. Stuschke M, Budah V, Klaes W, Sack H. Radiosensitivity, repair capacity, and stem cell fraction in human soft tissue tumors: an in vitro study using multicellular spheroids and the colony assay. *Int J Radiat Oncol Biol Phys* 1992;23:69–80.

21. Geara FB, Peters LJ, Ang KK, Wike JL, Simon FS, Guttenberger R, Callender DL, Malaise EB, Brock WA. Intrinsic radiosensitivity of normal human fibroblasts and lymphocytes after high and low dose rate irradiation. *Cancer Res* 1992;52:6348–6352.

22. Geara FB, Peters LJ, Ang KK, Wike JL, Brock WA. Radiosensitivity measurement of keratinocytes and fibroblasts from radiotherapy patients. *Int J Radiat Oncol Biol Phys* 1992;24:287–293.

23. Sanchiz F, Milla A, Torner J, Bonet F, Artola N, Carreno L, Moya LM, Riera D, Ripol S, Cirera L. Single fraction per day versus two fractions per day versus radiochemotherapy in the treatment of head and neck cancer. *Int J Radiat Oncol Biol Phys* 1990;19:1347–1350.

24. Withers HR. Predicting late normal tissue responses. *Int J Radiat Oncol Biol Phys* 1986;12:693–698.

25. Parsons, JT. The effect of radiation on normal tissues of the head and neck. In: Million RR, Cassisi NJ, eds. *Management of Head and Neck Cancer—a Multidisciplinary Approach.* Philadelphia: JB Lippincott, 1984;173–177.

26. Barton M. Tables of equivalent dose in 2 Gy fractions: a simple application of the linear quadratic formula. *Int J Radiat Oncol Biol Phys* 1995;31:371–378.

27. Horiot JC, Nabid A, Chaplain G, Jampolis S, van den Bogaert W, van der Schueren E, Arcangeli G, Gonzalez D, Svoboda V, Hamers HP. Clinical experience with multiple daily fractionation in the radiotherapy of head and neck carcinoma. *Cancer Bull* 1982;34:230–233.

28. Gardner KE, Parsons JT, Mendenhall WM, Million RR, Cassisi NJ. Time-dose relationships for local tumor control and complications following irradiation of squamous cell carcinoma of the base of tongue. *Int J Radiat Oncol Biol Phys* 1987;13:507–510.

29. Barak F, Werner A, Walach N, Horn Y. The palliative efficacy of a single high dose of radiation in treatment of symptomatic osseous metastases. *Int J Radiat Oncol Biol Phys* 1987;13:1233–1235.

30. Cole DJ. A randomised trial of a single treatment versus conventional fractionation in the palliative radiotherapy of painful bone metastases. *Clin Oncol* 1989;1:56–62.

31. Price P, Hoskin PJ, Easton D, Austin A, Palmer SG, Yarnold JR. Prospective randomised trial of single and multifraction radiotherapy schedules in the treatment of painful bone metastases. *Radiother Oncol* 1986;6:247–255.

32. Hoskin PJ, Price P, Easton D, Regan J, Austin D, Palmer S, Yarnold JR. A prospective randomised trial of 4 Gy or 8 Gy single doses in the treatment of metastatic bone pain. *Radiother Oncol* 1992;23:7478–7482.

33. Bates T, Yarnold JR, Blitzer P, Nelson OS, Rubin P, Maher J. Bone metastases consensus statement. *Int J Radiat Oncol Biol Phys* 1992;23: 215–216.

34. Schocker JD, Brady LW. Radiation therapy for bone metastases. *Clin Orthop Rel Res* 1982;169:38–43.

35. Needham PR, Mithal NP, Hoskin PJ. Radiotherapy for bone pain. *J R Soc Med* 1994;87:503–505.

36. Richter MP, Coia LR. Palliative radiation therapy. *Semin Oncol* 1985; 12 (4): 375–383.

37. Hortobagyi, GN, Libshitz HI, Seabold JE. Osseous metastases of breast cancer-clinical, biochemical, radiographic, and scintigraphic evaluation of response to therapy. *Cancer* 1984;53:577–582.

38. Yamaguchi T, Tamai K, Yamato M, Honma K, Ueda Y, Saotome K. Intertrabecular pattern of tumors metastatic to bone. *Cancer* 1996;78: 1388–1394.

39. Algra PR, Bloem JL, Tissing H, Falke THM, Arndt JW, Verboom LJ. Detection of vertebral metastases: comparison between MR imaging and bone scintigraphy. *RadioGraphics* 1991:11:219–232.

40. Fidler M.: Incidence of fracture through metastasis in long bones. *Acta Orthop Scand* 1981;52:623–627.

41. Weikert, DR, Schwartz, HS: Intramedullary nailing for impending pathological subtrochanteric fractures. *J Bone Joint Surg* 1991;73B: 668–670.

42. Townsend PW, Smalley SR, Cozed SC, Rosenthal HG Hassanein RES. Is radiation therapy beneficial after orthopedic stabilization of impending or pathologic fracture due to metastatic disease? *Int J Radiat Oncol Biol Phys* 1993;27(suppl 1):159.

43. Bunting RW, Boublik M, Blevins FT, Dame CC, Ford LA, Lavine LS. Functional outcome of pathologic fracture secondary to malignant disease in a rehabilitation hospital. *Cancer* 1992;69:98–102.

44. Knudson G, Grinis G, Lopez-Majano V, Sansi P, Targonski P, Rubenstein M, Sharifi R, Gruinan P. Bone scan as a stratification variable in advanced prostate cancer. *Cancer* 1991;68:316–320.

45. Mithal NP, Needham PR, Hoskin PJ. Retreatment with radiotherapy for painful bone metastases. *Int J Radiat Oncol Biol Phys* 1994;29: 1011–1014.

46. Poulter CA, Cosmatos D, Rubin P, Urtasun R, Cooper JS, Kuske RR, Hornback N, Coughlin C, Weigensberg I, Rotman M. A report of RTOG 8206: a phase III study of whether the addition of single dose hemibody irradiation to standard fractionated local field irradiation is more effective than local field irradiation alone in the treatment of symptomatic osseous metastases. *Int J Radiat Oncol Biol Phys* 1992; 23:207–214.

47. Salazar OM, Rubin P, Hendrickson FR, Komaki R, Poulter C, Newall J, Asbell SO, Mohiuddin M, van Ess J. Single dose half-body irradiation for palliation of multiple bone metastases from solid tumors—final Radiation Therapy Oncology Group Report. *Cancer* 1986;58:29–36.

48. Kuban DA, Schellhammer PF, El-Mahdi AM. Hemibody irradiation in advanced prostatic carcinoma. *Urol Clin North Am* 1991;18(1): 131–137.

49. Jones PW, Bogardus CR, Anderson DW. Significance of initial "performance status" in patients receiving halfbody radiation. *Int J Radiat Oncol Biol Phys* 1984;10:1947–1950.

50. Zelefsky MJ, Scher HI, Forman JD, Linares LA, Curley T, Fuks Z. Palliative hemiskeletal irradiation for widespread metastatic prostate cancer: a comparison of single dose and fractionated regimens. *Int J Radiat Oncol Biol Phys* 1989;17:1281–1285.

51. Price P, Hoskin PJ, Easton D, Austin A, et. al.: Prospective randomised trial of single and multifraction radiotherapy schedules in the treatment of painful bone metastases. *Radiother Oncol* 1986;6:247–255

52. Reed RC, Lowery GS, Nordstrom DG: Single high dose-large field irradiation for palliation of advanced malignancies. *Int J Radiat Oncol Biol Phys* 1988;15:1243–1246.

53. Scarantino CW, Caplan R, Rotman M, Coughlin C, Demas W, Delrowe J. A phase I/II study to evaluate the effect of fractionated hemibody irradiation in the treatment of osseous metastases—RTOG 88-22. *Int J Radiat Oncol Biol Phys* 1996;36:37–48.

54. Salazar OM, Da Motta N, Bridgman SM, Cardiges NM, Slawson RG. Fractionated half-body irradiation for pain palliation in widely metastatic cancers : comparison with a single dose. *Int J Radiat Oncol Biol Phys* 1996;36:49–60.

55. Robinson RG, Preston DF, Baxter KG, Dusing RW, et al: Clinical experience with strontium-89 in prostatic and breast cancer patients. *Semin Oncol* 1993;20:44–48.

56. Robinson RG, Preston DF, Schiefelbein M, Baxter KG. Strontium 89 therapy for the palliation of pain due to osseous metastases. *JAMA* 1995;274:420–424.

57. Porter AT, McEwan AJB, Powe JE, Reid R, McGowan DG, Lukka H, Sathyanarayana JR, Yakemchuk VN, Thomas GM, Erlich LE, Crook J, Gulenchyn KY, Hong KE, Wesolowski C, Yardley J. Results of a randomized phase III trial to evaluate the efficacy of strontium-89 adjuvant to local field external beam irradiation in the management of endocrine resistant metastatic prostate cancer. *Int J Radiat Oncol Biol Phys* 1993;25:805–813.

58. Lee CK, Aeppli DM, Unger J, Boudreau RJ, Levitt SH. Strontium-89 chloride (Metastron) for palliative treatment of bony metastases: the University of Minnesota Experience. *Am J Clin Oncol* 1996;19: 102–107.

59. Atkins HL, Mausner LF, Srivastava SC, Meinken GE, Cabahug CJ, D'Alessandro T. Tin-117m(4-)-DTPA for palliation of pain from osseous metastases: a pilot study. *J Nucl Med* 1995;36:725–729.

60. Bayouth JE, Macey DJ, Kasi LP, Fossella FV. Dosimetry and toxicity of samarium-153-EDTMP administered for bone pain due to skeletal metastases. *J Nucl Med* 1994;35:63–69.

61. Coia LR, Aaronson N, Linggood R, Loeffler J, Priestman TJ. A report of the consensus workshop panel on the treatment of brain metastases. *Int J Radiat Oncol Biol Phys* 1992;23:223–227.

62. Sawaya R, Ligon BL, Bindal RK. Management of metastatic brain tumors. *Ann Surg Oncol* 1994;1:169–178.

63. Farnell GF, Buckner JC, Cascino TL, O'Connell MJ, Schomberg PJ, Suman V. Brain metastases from colorectal carcinoma—the long term survivors. *Cancer* 1996;78:711–716.

64. Nussbaum ES, Djalilian HR, Cho KH, Hall WA. Brain metastases: histology, multiplicity, surgery, and survival. *Cancer* 1996;78: 1781–1788.

65. Auchter RM, Lamond JP, Alexander E, Buatti JM, Chappell R, Friedman WA, Kinsella TJ, Levin AB, Noyes WR, Schultz CJ, Loeffler JS, Mehta MP. A multi-institutional outcome and prognostic factor analysis of radiosurgery for resectable single brain metastases. *Int J Radiat Oncol Biol Phys* 1996;35:27–35.

66. Petrovich Z, Luxton G, Formenti S, Jozsef G, Zee CS, Apuzzo MLJ. Stereotactic radiosurgery for primary and metastatic brain tumors. *Cancer Invest* 1996;14:445–454.

67. Leviov M, Dale J, Stein M, Ben-Shahar M, et al: The management of metastatic spinal cord compression: a radiotherapeutic success ceiling. *Int J Radiat Oncol Biol Phys* 1993;27:231–234.

68. Sioutos PJ, Arbit E, Meshulam CF, Galicich JH. Spinal metastases from solid tumors-analysis of factors affecting survival. *Cancer* 1995; 76:1453–1459.

69. Uppelschoten JM, Wanders SL, de Jong JMA. Single dose radiotherapy (6 Gy): palliation in painful bone metastases. *Radiother Oncol* 1995;36:198–202.

70. Shiu MH, Hilaris BS, Harrison LB, Brennan MF. Brachytherapy and function-saving resection of soft tissue sarcoma arising in the limb. *Int J Radiat Oncol Biol Phys* 1991;21:1485–1492.

71. Schray MF. Gunderson LL, Sim FH, Pritchard DJ, Shives TC, Yeakel PD. Soft tissue sarcoma: integration of brachytherapy, resection and external irradiation. *Cancer* 1990;66:451–456.

72. Herskovic A, Ryan J, Han I, Lattin P, Ahmad K, Canady A, Belenky W, Phillipart A, Binns H, White B. Combined interstitial and external beam radiation therapy in soft-tissue tumors: preliminary report. *Endocuriether/Hypertherm Oncol* 1988;4:213–217.

73. Hilaris BS. Adjuvant brachytherapy in the treatment of soft tissue sarcomas of the extremities. *Endocuriether/Hypertherm Oncol* 1987;3: 220–221.

74. Chan RC, Bracken RB, Johnson DE. Single dose whole pelvis megavoltage irradiation for palliative control of hematuria or ureteral obstruction. *J Urol* 1979;122:750–751,

75. Eichhorn HJ. Different fractionation schemas tested by histological examination of autopsy specimens from lung cancer patients. *Br J Radiol* 1981;54:132–135.

76. Mehta MP, Shahabi S, Jarjour NN, Kinsella TJ. Endobronchial irradiation for malignant airway obstruction. *Int J Radiation Oncol Biol Phys* 1989;17:847–851.

77. Mazeron JJ, Langlois D, Glaubiger D, Huart J, Martin M, Raynal M, Colitchi E, Ganen G, Faraldi M, Feuilhade F, Brun B, Marin L, Le Bourgeois JP, Baillet F, Pierquin B. Salvage irradiation of oropharyngeal cancers using Iridium 192 wire implants : 5 year results of 70 cases. *Int J Radiat Oncol Biol Phys* 1987;13:957–962.

78. Estes NC, Morphis JG, Hornback NB, Jewel R. Intra-arterial chemotherapy and hyperthermia for pain control in patients with recurrent rectal cancer. *Am J Surg* 1986;152:597–601.

79. Woodhall B, Pickrell KL, et at . Effect of hyperthermia upon cancer chemotherapy: application to external cancers of head and face structures. *Ann Surg* 1960;151:730–759.

80. Bateman JR, Hazen JG, Stolinsky DC, Steinfeld J. Advanced carcinoma of the cervix treated with intra-arterial methotrexate. *Am J Obstet Gynecol* 1986;96:181–187.

81. Lathrop JC, Frates RE. Arterial infusion of nitrogen mustard in the treatment of intractable pelvic pain of malignant origin. *Cancer* 1980;45: 432–438.

82. Laufe LE, Blockstein RS, Parisi FZ, Lowy AD Jr. Infusion through inferior gluteal artery for pelvic cancer. *Obstet Gynecol* 1966;28:650–659.

83. Beyer JH, vonHyden HW, et al. Intra-arterial perfusion therapy with 5 fluorouracil in patients with metastatic colo–rectal carcinoma and intractable pelvic pain. *Recent Results Cancer Res* 1983;86:33–36.

84. Heim ME, Eberwein S, Georgi M. Palliative therapy of pelvic tumors by intra-arterial infusion of cytotoxic drugs. *Recent Results Cancer Res* 1983;86:37–40.

85. MacDonald N. The role of medical and surgical oncology in the management of cancer pain. In: *Advances in Pain Research and Therapy,* vol 16. New York: Raven Press, 1990;27–39.

86. Collin E, Poulin P, Piquard-Gauvain A, Petit G, Pichard-Leandri E. Is disease progression the major factor in morphine tolerance in cancer pain treatment? *Pain* 1993;55:319–326.

*Principles and Practice of Supportive Oncology,*
edited by Ann Berger et al.
Lippincott–Raven Publishers, Philadelphia ©1998

CHAPTER 3

# Pharmacologic Management of Pain

Richard Payne

## PHARMACOTHERPAY OF PAIN: BASIC PRINCIPLES

Advances in pain management techniques have made it possible to provide adequate control for the vast majority of patients with cancer, acquired immunodeficiency syndrome (AIDS), and other chronic medical disorders, using relatively simple means. Unfortunately, pain very often remains inadequately treated for cancer and many other illnesses (1). Several factors contribute to the undertreatment of cancer pain, including poor physician assessment, inadequate knowledge of management techniques, including pharmacotherapy measures, and negative physician and patient attitudes toward the use of opioids for pain (2).

In a recent large prospective study, physicians identified inadequate pain assessment as the primary reason for poor pain management (2). Successful management of pain in the cancer patient begins with a thorough assessment of the pain complaint. Adequate pain assessment includes the documentation of pain intensity and quality, the evaluation of exacerbating and relieving factors, and requires knowledge of the common pain syndromes occurring in a specific disease or disorder. Principles of pain assessment are covered elsewhere in this book and by other references (1).

Treating the cause of pain should be a high priority for the clinician. For example, in one recent study, 18% of cancer patients evaluated by a pain service required additional antineoplastic therapies to treat their pain (3). Recently, two chemotherapeutic agents, gemcitabine (4) and mitoxantrone (5), were approved by the Food and Drug Administration (FDA) for the palliative treatment of pancreatic cancer and hormone-refractory prostate cancer, respectively. Similarly, radiotherapy is effective in relieving metastatic bone pain. For localized bone pain, external beam treatment will reduce pain in up to 80% of patients (6). More pertinent to the subject of pharmacotherapy, the administration of systemic radioisotopes such as strontium-89 has also been shown to be effective in treating diffuse pain from bone metastases (7). However, pain relief with strontium-89 may not be seen until the third or fourth week after treatment, although it may be sustained for several months (7).

Pharmacotherapy must be individualized to maximize pain relief and minimize adverse effects. The World Health Organization (WHO) has developed a three-step analgesic ladder for the treatment of cancer pain (8), which serves as a model paradigm for pharmacotherapy approaches to pain management (Fig. 1).

The WHO approach advises clinicians to match the patient's reported pain intensity with the potency of the analgesic to be prescribed. For mild pain, one should administer a nonopioid drug such as acetaminophen or a nonsteroidal antiinflammatory drug (NSAID), unless contraindicated (Table 1). For moderate pain that cannot be controlled by an NSAID alone, a so-called weak opioid such as codeine or hydrocodone should be administered, often in a fixed combination with aspirin, another NSAID, or acetaminophen (Table 2). For severe pain, a so-called strong opioid drug such as morphine, hydromorphone, methadone, or fentanyl should be administered (Table 2). NSAIDs and adjuvant analgesic drugs (see below) can be administered at any stage of the WHO ladder. It is important to note that patients presenting with severe pain should not be walked up the ladder starting from the first step but should be administered a strong opioid immediately. This is a common mistake. For example, Cleeland et al. (9) reported that 46% of ambulatory cancer patients were undertreated for pain as measured be a tool called the "pain management index" (PMI). The PMI is based on the WHO anal-

R. Payne: Department of Neuro-oncology, M.D. Anderson Cancer Center, Houston, TX 77030-4095.

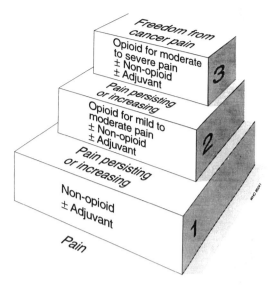

**FIG. 1.** WHO analgesic ladder. Reprinted with permission from WHO (8).

### Acetaminophen and Nonsteroidal Anti-inflammatory Analgesics

The basic principles of pain assessment and management apply when using these agents (Table 3). The NSAIDs constitute a large class of compounds that have analgesic, anti-inflammatory, and antipyretic effects. Of course, aspirin is the prototype drug in this class. Many of these analgesics are available over the counter; a 1995 survey in the *Wall Street Journal* estimated the sales of acetaminophen and NSAIDs to be more than $3 billion in the United States alone, with Tylenol brand of acetaminophen producing almost $800 million in sales alone.

Acetaminophen (APAP) is considered in this class, even though it has only weak antiinflammatory potency (12). Acetaminophen and the NSAIDs constitute the first line of management in the pharmacotherapy of acute and cancer pain, as recommended by the WHO guidelines (8) and the Agency for Health Care Policy and Research (AHCPR) acute pain and cancer pain clinical practice guidelines (13,14). Although widely used by consumers and patients, NSAIDs are seldom the sole agents used to treat pain and are therefore more often part of a multimodal approach to management.

NSAIDs and acetaminophen have a ceiling effect to their analgesic efficacy such that increasing the dose beyond this level will produce no increase in therapeutic effect though it may produce more side effects (15). Therefore their use as sole agents in the management of pain should be restricted to mild or moderate pain because severe pain is often above their ceiling dose for analgesic efficacy.

The minimum effective dose and the ceiling dose of NSAIDs may vary among individuals, however, so that some dose titration may be necessary within a narrow

gesic ladder, and relates the potency of the analgesic regimen prescribed to the patient's reported pain intensity, assigning negative values (indicating undertreatment) when the pain intensity is not matched by an appropriate analgesic class, as often happens when patients with severe pain are inappropriately started on the first or second step of the analgesic ladder. The WHO analgesic ladder approach has been validated (10). However, many of the validation studies have been criticized because they have not included prospective evaluation of individual patient outcomes (11). Nonetheless, the WHO analgesic ladder approach remains the standard method for prescribing pharmacotherapies for pain.

**TABLE 1.** *Partial list of acetaminophen & nonsteroidal anti-inflammatory drugs used for cancer pain*

| Drug type | Name/brands | Typical starting dose |
|---|---|---|
| Acetaminophen | Tylenol and others | 650 mg q 4 h PO |
| Aspirin | Multiple | 650 mg q 4 h PO |
| Ibuprofen | Motrin and others | 200–800 mg q 6 h PO |
| Choline magnesium trisalicylate | Trilisate | 1000–1500 mg tid PO |
| Diclofenac sodium | Voltaren | 50–75 mg q 8–12 h PO |
| Diflunisal | Dolobid | 500 mg q 12 h PO |
| Etodolac | Lodine | 200–400 mg q 8–12 h PO |
| Flurbiprofen | Ansaid | 200–300 mg q 4–8 h PO |
| Naproxen | Naprosyn | 250–750 mg q 12 h PO |
| Naproxen sodium | Anaprox | 275 mg q 12 h PO |
| Oxaprozin | Daypro | 600–1200 mg q daily PO |
| Sulindac | Clinoril | 150–200 mg q 12 h PO |
| Piroxicam | Feldene | 10–20 mg q daily PO |
| Nabumetone | Relafen | 1000–2000 mg q daily PO |
| Ketoprofen | Orudis | 50 mg q 6 h PO |
| Ketorolac | Toradol | 10 mg q 4–6 h PO (not to exceed 10 days??) |
| Ketorolac | Toradol | 30 mg IM or IV × 1 then 15 mg IM or IV q 6 h (not to exceed 5 days) |

**TABLE 2.** *Commonly used opioids for cancer pain*

| WHO Step I/II Opioids | Usual starting dose | Comment |
|---|---|---|
| **Codeine** (with acet or ASA)[a] <br> -Tylenol #2 (15 mg codeine) <br> -Tylenol #3 (30 mg codeine) <br> -Tyleon #4 (60 mg codeine) | 60 mg q 3–4 h PO | Fixed combination with ASA and acet scheduled as DEA III; single entity as DEA II schedule; usually 250 mg acet or ASA/tablet. Take care not to exceed toxic doses of acet and ASA |
| **Hydrocodone** (with APAP or ASA) <br> -Lorcet; Lortab; Vicodan, others | 10 mg q 3–4 h PO | Same as for codeine; <br> Vicodan-ES has 750 mg ASA/tablet |
| **Oxycodone** <br> -Roxicodone (single entity) <br> -Percocet; Percodan; Tylox; others | 10 mg q 3–4 h PO | Available in controlled release formulation (as single entity) |
| **Tramadol** | 50 mg QID PO | Recently approved in the USA. Although a μ opioid agonist, it is not scheduled as an opioid. Also blocks catecholamine reuptake. Nausea common side effect. Seizures may occur in doses >400 mg/day |
| WHO Step II/III Opioids | | |
| **Morphine** <br> -immediate release (MSIR) <br><br> -controlled- and sustained release; (Oramorph; MS Contin; Kadiom) | 30 mg q 3–4 h PO <br> 10 mg q 3-4h IV <br> 30 mg q 12 h PO | Standard by which all other opioids are compared. Some clinicians do not view MS Contin and Oramorph as therapeutically interchangable; MS Contin available in 15-, 30-, 60-, 100-, and 200-mg tablets; Oramorph available in 15-, 30-, 60-, and 100-mg tablets only. Morphine is also available as suppository. MSIR is preferred rescue analgesic for controlled-release preparations |
| **Oxycodone** <br> -immediate release (Roxicodone) <br> -controlled release (Oxycontin) | 10 mg q 4 h PO <br> 20 mg q 12 h PO | Available in 10-, 20-, 40-mg tablets; immediate-release oxycodone also considered step II/III opioid and is recommended as rescue medicine for Oxycontin |
| **Hydromorphone** <br> -Dilaudid; others | 6 mg q 12 h PO | Sustained release formulation in clinical development. Comes in 2-, 4-, and 8-mg tablets. Available as a suppository |
| **Fentanyl** <br> -Duragesic (transdermal) <br><br> -Sublimaze; other | 50 μg/h q 72 h <br><br> 50 μg/h via continuous infusion | The only opioid available for transdermal administration. 100 mcg/hr roughly equianalgesic to morphine 4 mg/hr. Many patients require oral rescue doses. |
| **Methadone** <br> -Dolophine; other | 20 mg q 6–8 h PO <br> 10 mg q 6–8 h IV | Very stigmatized because of use to treat heroin addiction. |
| **Levorphanol** <br> -Levodromoran | 4 mg q 6–8 h PO | Relatively long acting; may have higher incidence of psychotomimetic effects than other opioids |

[a]acet, acetaminophen.

range of doses (15,16). Because patients vary in their response to NSAIDs, a trial of an alternative drug in the same class may be justified if side effects outweigh benefits for a particular drug (16).

The NSAIDs inhibit cyclooxygenase, thereby inhibiting prostaglandin synthesis (17). Prostaglandins are important mediators of the inflammatory process that may serve to activate and sensitize nociceptors; NSAIDs appear to produce analgesia by this peripheral action on prostaglandin inhibition (16). However, recent data also indicate that NSAIDs have a central nervous system (CNS) site of action at the brain or spinal cord level that is important for their analgesic effects (18).

Recently, two isoforms of the enzyme cyclooxygenase (COX-1 and COX-2) have been demonstrated (19). The COX-1 isoenzyme is normally found in blood vessels, stomach, and kidney, whereas COX-2 is induced in peripheral tissues by inflammation. Inhibition of COX-1 is associated with the well-known gastric and renal side effects associated with NSAID use, whereas COX-2 inhibition produces therapeutic effects (Fig. 2).

Most NSAIDs nonselectively inhibit the COX isoenzyme, thereby producing toxic and therapeutic effects. Recently, relatively selective COX-2 inhibitors, such as meloxicam and nabumetone, have been shown to have fewer gastrointestinal (GI) and renal side effects (20).

**TABLE 3.** *Basic principles in use of nonopioid drugs*

1. Perform a comprehensive assessment of the patient.
   Thorough history and physical examination
   Focused neurologic examination
   Assessment of psychosocial complications of the pain and the underlying disorder
2. Use the drugs as part of a multimodal approach to pain treatment
   Physical treatments (e.g., physical therapy, massage, ultrasound for musculoskeletal pain)
   Psychological/behavioral treatments
   Anesthetic treatments
   Neurosurgical treatments
3. Target a specifc pain
4. Use sequential drug trials
   Prepare patient for several drugs and to accept partial analgesia as outcome
   Perform adequate trial (may need several weeks)
   Consider drug combinations (e.g., NSAIDs + opioids)
   Limit side effects (if possible)

Acetaminophen is equipotent to aspirin in terms of analgesic efficacy, and is generally very well tolerated and not associated with the risks of GI hemorrhage associated with NSAID use. Acetaminophen is a weak inhibitor of COX, which presumably explains its poor anti-inflammatory potency. This analgesic is the principle metabolite of phenacetin, which is a known nephrotoxin. Renal failure has been described with long-term use of acetaminophen (21), in addition to its well-known hepatotoxicity. Acute hepatotoxicity occurring during overdose is correlated with acetaminophen plasma concentrations above 200 mg/ml at 4 hours after ingestion, or if plasma concentration persists above 10 mg/ml at 24 hours after ingestion (22). Although not as well correlated with plasma concentrations, it is well known that chronic ingestion of acetaminophen ranging from 2.5 to 4 g/day increases the risk for hepatotoxicity (21). In addition, the odds of chronic renal failure doubled for patients who had a cumulative lifetime intake of more than 1000 pills of acetaminophen (21). NSAID and acetaminophen use is relatively safe, but these data, combined with the well-

known risks of GI bleeding and platelet dysfunction that occur with acute and chronic NSAID use, indicate that these drugs should be used judiciously.

Many NSAIDs are now available. They differ in dosing interval and cost, and to some extent in their analgesic ceiling and safety. The choice of NSAID must be individualized to the patient's needs (see Table 1). Ketorolac is available in an oral and parental formulation; it is currently the only NSAID available in an intramuscular and intravenous formulation. This NSAID is used often in hospitalized patients to manage postoperative pain and other acute pains, including exacerbations of chronic cancer pain and sickle cell pain. Another use of ketorolac occurs for acutely ill patients experiencing side effects such as opioid-induced ileus or delirium, in which the addition of a parenteral NSAID often has an important opioid sparing effect to allow dose reduction and the lessening of GI and CNS side effects of opioids without compromising analgesia.

Several studies have confirmed the effectiveness of the NSAIDs in the treatment of cancer pain (23,24). Of interest, prior studies that documented the additive analgesic effects of NSAIDs when combined with opioids in single-dose postoperative pain studies (27) have not been confirmed in more recent meta-analysis of repeated does studies (24). This is puzzling because NSAIDs and opioids have different mechanisms of action and logically could have additive analgesia. Furthermore, much anecdotal clinical practice suggests that additive analgesic effects do occur when NSAIDs and opioids are coadministered (8), and it is still common clinical practice to use NSAIDs and opioids in combination despite the findings of this recent meta-analysis.

Certain adverse effects are common to most of the drugs in this group. All may be associated with GI toxicity, with the most serious complications being ulceration and bleeding. A recent meta-analysis of the risks of GI toxicity associated with NSAID use compared 12 studies (25). Ibuprofen in doses less than 1600 mg/day was associated with the least risk for serious GI hemorrhage;

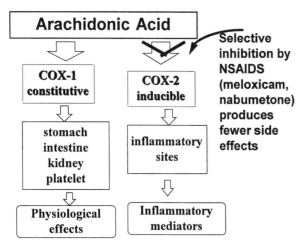

**FIG. 2.** COX inhibitors.

aspirin, indomethacin, naproxen, and sulindac were associated with intermediate risk, and ketoprofen and piroxicam were highest risk (25).

NSAIDs also inhibit platelet function to a variable degree; aspirin is the strongest platelet inhibitor, whereas the non-acetylated salicylates, such as choline magnesium trisalicylate, have minimal effects on platelets (26). However, all NSAIDs must be used with caution in patients with coagulopathies and coexisting GI pathology, and when coadministered with drugs that also have GI toxicity such as with corticosteroids. Another relative contraindication to the use of NSAIDs relates to their antipyretic effects, which may mask fever as an early sign of serious infection in immunocompromised patients.

**Commonly Used Opioids for Pain Management**

Because opioids alter the unpleasant emotional experience associated with nociception and provide pain relief by interacting with specific receptors (28), they are essential components in the pharmacotherapy of pain (8,13,14). Drugs that bind to opioid receptors are classified as agonist (e.g., morphine) if they produce analgesia. Opioids are classified as antagonists (e.g., naloxone) if they block the action of an agonist. Agonist-antagonists (e.g., pentazocine) are opioids that produce analgesia by interacting with a specific receptor (e.g., κ) but they also bind to other receptors and block (e.g., μ) where they can block the action of an agonist. Partial agonist opioids (e.g., buprenorphine) bind to receptors and produce analgesia but unlike morphine they exhibit a ceiling effect: increases in doses do not parallel increases in analgesia (16).

As noted above, the WHO analgesic ladder paradigm classified opioids as "weak" or "strong" depending on their relative efficacy in relieving pain (8), although this concept of distinguishing weak and strong opioids has been challenged, and some have even advocated the elimination of the second step of the WHO analgesic ladder (29). The so-called weak opioids are used for less severe pain because their efficacy is limited by an increased incidence of side effects at higher doses (e.g., nausea and constipation with codeine, CNS excitation with propoxyphene). Furthermore, these weak opioids are usually formulated a fixed oral dose mixture with a nonopioid analgesic so that their efficacy is limited also by the maximum safe daily dose of acetaminophen (4 g/day) or aspirin. By contrast, so-called strong opioids are used for severe pain. Opioids such as morphine, hydromorphone, fentanyl, methadone, and levorphanol have a relatively wide therapeutic window and no ceiling effect for analgesia-increasing doses produce an greater level of analgesia with a lesser likelihood for dose-limiting side effects than the weak opioids. However, as noted below, the management of side effects is critical to achieving optimal results with the administration of opioid in either class.

Codeine, the dimethylated congener of morphine, is the prototype of the weak or step II opioid analgesics. Although a parenteral preparation is available, codeine is nearly always given by mouth, often in a fixed mixture with a nonopioid analgesic. A 200-mg dose is equipotent to 30 mg of morphine (30). The half-life of codeine is 2.5–3 hours; approximately 10% of orally administered codeine is demethylated to morphine: free and conjugated morphine can be found in the urine. The analgesic action is thought to be related to the in vivo conversion to morphine (30). Constipation and nausea are the most common side effects at the usual therapeutic doses of codeine (30–60 mg every 4 hours). Codeine is useful to administer as an alternative to NSAIDs for patients with mild pain in whom the antipyretic, antiplatelet, or GI toxicity of NSAIDs contraindicate their use.

Hydrocodone is a codeine derivative available only in combination with acetaminophen or aspirin. At the usually prescribed doses, its analgesic effect is weak and probably only slightly superior to acetaminophen alone.

Two opioids classified as weak or WHO step II analgesics, meperidine and propoxyphene, although widely used for the treatment of acute and chronic pain, are not generally recommended by pain clinicians for the reasons to be listed below.

Propoxyphene is a synthetic analgesic that is structurally related to methadone. It is approximately equipotent to codeine. Although its analgesic effects lasts only 3–6 hours, the plasma half-life is as long as 6–12 hours. This disparity between the relatively short analgesic duration of effect in comparison to the longer plasma half-life is similar to that of methadone, and patients are at significant risk for sedation and increased toxicity due to drug accumulation when it is dosed according to the analgesic duration of effect. Furthermore, propoxyphene has as its major metabolite norpropoxyphene, which has a long plasma half-life of 30–36 hours and may also be responsible for some of the observed toxicity (31). Norpropoxyphene has local anesthetic effects similar to those of lidocaine and high doses may cause arrhythmias. Seizures occur more often with propoxyphene intoxication than with opiate intoxication. Naloxone antagonizes these toxic effects of propoxyphene (31).

Meperidine is an opioid agonist. The dose equianalgesic to 10 mg of parenteral morphine is 75–100 mg. The reasons for its widespread use in the treatment of pain is unclear. Although often cited as a reason to use meperidine in preference to morphine, the lesser rise in pressure in the common bile duct with meperidine administration has not been shown to be clinically advantageous (32). Furthermore, the CNS excitatory effects that appear after chronic use are well substantiated and occur as a result of the accumulation of the metabolite nor meperidine, which causes multifocal myoclonus and grand mal seizures (33). The nor meperidine toxicity is correlated with plasma concentration and is probably not opioid receptor–mediated because it is not reversed by naloxone. The half-life of meperidine is 3 hours. Normeperidine has a half-life of 15–30 hours and therefore accumulates with repetitive dosing of meperidine, particularly in patients with renal dysfunction. Meperidine also has an important drug interaction with monoamine oxidase (MAO) inhibitors producing two patterns of toxicity: (a) severe respiratory depression or (b) excitation, delirium, hyperpyrexia, and convulsions. This toxicity may lead to fatalities.

Oxycodone is a semisynthetic opioid. Because of its high bioavailability (>50%) after oral dosing, it is a useful opioid analgesic (33). It has a half-life of 2–3 hours and a duration of action of 4–6 hours. It is metabolized in a manner similar to codeine by demethylation and conjugation in the liver and excreted in the urine (34). Part of the analgesic action is mediated by active metabolites. Traditionally, oxycodone has been considered a "weak" or WHO step II analgesic because it is most often used in a fixed combination with acetaminophen and aspirin. These combinations limit its dose to 10 mg every 4 hours. However, oxycodone can also be prescribed as a single-entity compound and as such is often used as a WHO step III or "strong" opioid (35,36), especially now that it is available in a sustained release formulation. Therefore oxycodone straddles the second and third steps of the WHO analgesic ladder, depending on which formulations are used. Oxycodone has been reported to have fewer side effects than morphine (36,37), although these studies have limitations to their interpretation because they were not done in a rigorous study design in which patients were blinded to the specific drugs being administered. Like morphine, the availability of oxycodone in sustained and immediate release formulations provides a means for the clinician to carefully titrate the dose of drug to the patient's response.

Morphine is of course the prototype opioid agonist. The WHO has designated morphine as the "drug of choice" for the treatment of severe pain associated with cancer (8). The half-life of morphine is about 2 hours, and oral immediate release morphine preparations generally provide pain relief for 2–4 hours. Slow release preparations that permit once- or twice-a-day regimens are safe and effective; they are generally best used after dose titration with immediate release morphine sulfate.

Recently, morphine has been shown to have active metabolites. Morphine is metabolized in the liver where it undergoes glucuronidation at the 3 and 6 positions. Morphine-3-glucuronide (M3G) and morphine-6-glucuronide (M6G) accumulate with chronic morphine administration (38). M6G binds to μ receptors with affinity similar to that of morphine (39). M6G appears to be 20 times more potent than morphine when administered directly into the periaqueductal gray (39), indicating that only a fraction of this water-soluble metabolite need cross the blood–brain barrier to produce an analgesic effect (38). In single-dose comparative analgesic trials, the par-

enteral to oral relative potency ratio for morphine was shown to be 1:6 (27). Chronic morphine dosing has been shown to produce a parenteral to oral relative potency ratio of 1:3 (40); this difference is likely due to the presence of the M6G metabolite.

Although the M3G metabolite has a negligible affinity for opioid receptors and does not produce analgesia (39), it may be responsible for some of the toxicity seen with chronic dosing of morphine, especially when relatively large doses are administered. The M3G metabolite has excitatory effects on neurons and can cause myoclonus and possibly a hyperanalgesic state (41,42), paradoxically causing increased pain. Morphine metabolites are eliminated by glomerular filtration; they accumulate in renal failure leading to an increased incidence of side effects (43). Morphine should be used with caution in renal failure, increasing the interval time between doses. Hydromorphone is another semisynthetic opioid agonist commercially available as a highly water-soluble salt. When administered parenterally 1.5 mg of hydromorphone is equipotent to 10 mg of morphine. Its bioavailability is 30–40% when given orally, and the oral to parenteral relative potency ratio is 5:1 (44). Hydromorphone has a half-life of approximately 2 hours. Recently, a 3-0 methyl metabolite of hydromorphone has been measured, which may be responsible for analgesic effects and toxicity such as myoclonus that occurs with continuous high-dose hydromorphone administration (45). Because of its availability in a high-potency formulation (10 mg/ml) and its water solubility, hydromorphone is the drug of choice for the chronic subcutaneous route of administration (44).

Levorphanol is a synthetic potent μ opioid agonist that also binds δ and κ receptors (46). This κ receptor binding may explain its relatively high prevalence of psychotomimetic effects (delirium, hallucinations) in comparison to other opioids when given to patients. When administered parenterally, 2 mg of levorphanol is equianalgesic to 10 mg of morphine (46). This opioid has a half-life of 12–30 hours and a duration of analgesia of 4–6 hours (47). As is the case with other opioids in which the plasma half-life exceeds the duration of analgesia, repeated administration is associated with drug accumulation. Therefore a dose reduction may be required 2–4 days after commencement of the drug in order to avoid side effects from overdose. For the same reason, it is best to avoid this opioid in patients with impaired renal function or encephalopathy. Levorphanol is used as a second- or third-line drug in patients who cannot tolerate morphine, hydromorphone, or fentanyl.

Methadone is a synthetic μ opioid agonist with high oral bioavailability (49). When administered orally, it is rapidly absorbed from the GI tract with measurable plasma concentrations within 30 minutes after oral administration (49). When administered in single parenteral doses it is equipotent to morphine; the duration of analgesia is 4–6 hours (49). The plasma level declines in a biexponential manner with a half-life of 2–3 hours during the initial phase and 15–60 hours during the terminal phase (50). This biexponential decline accounts for the relatively short analgesic action and the tendency for drug accumulation with repeated dosing. A reduction in dose and interval frequency is often needed during the first days of treatment to prevent side effects from overdose (51). Methadone is an effective second-line drug for patients who experience unrelieved pain and intolerable side effects with morphine (54,55).

Because of the large disparity between the plasma half-life and the analgesic duration of effect, dosing recommendations for methadone are complex. For example, it has been recommended to use a tenth of the daily morphine dose as the starting methadone dose, but not to exceed 100 mg, and to give this dose at intervals to be determined by the patient, but not more frequently than every 3 hours (55). The calculated equianalgesic doses of methadone may be as little as 3% of the predicted dose when this opioid is administered chronically (56).

Methadone is an alternative to morphine in several circumstances. Because of its low cost it is an attractive alternative to morphine. It should also be considered for the rare patient who is allergic to morphine because its very different chemical structure makes cross-sensitivity less likely than with other opioids, such as hydromorphone or oxycodone. The pharmacokinetics of methadone can be influenced by impaired renal clearance and decreased plasma protein binding. Methadone is excreted almost exclusively in the feces; it has been proposed as a safe and effective analgesic for patients with chronic renal failure (57).

Fentanyl is a very potent synthetic, lipophilic μ opioid agonist (58). It is 80–100 times more potent than morphine. These properties allow this opioid to be administered by the transdermal route (58). A special rate-controlling membrane provides additional control of drug release although the kinetics of the transdermal fentanyl system can be altered by fever and obesity of the patient. The transdermal absorption of fentanyl is the same from chest, abdomen, and thigh (58). A skin reaction at the application site is found in 4% of patients (58). After application of the transdermal patch the systemic absorption is negligible for the first 4 hours, and then increases steadily from 8 to 24 hours (59). Patients reach steady-state concentrations within 12–24 hours from the application (60,61). Following removal of the transdermal patch the serum fentanyl concentration falls about 50% in approximately 16 hours (61). This apparently long half-life is likely due to the slow washout of fentanyl from cutaneous reservoirs and mobilization of this lipophilic drug from fat stores (61). These pharmacokinetic considerations translate clinically in a several hour delay in the onset of analgesia after an initial application and a persistence of analgesia and eventual side effects long after removal of the transdermal system. In patients with

chronic pain, after a variable period of titration, it is possible to obtain relatively constant serum fentanyl concentrations comparable with continuous intravenous or subcutaneous infusions (61). More recently, the use of oral transmucosal fentanyl has been proposed for the treatment of breakthrough pain (64). Fentanyl can be formulated in a syrup-candy matrix that can be sucked. This fentanyl oral formulation can provide analgesic fentanyl blood concentrations within 5–10 minutes of active sucking, with a peak effect in 20–30 minutes and a duration ranging from 1–4 hours (64). Oral transmucosal fentanyl is being reviewed currently for approval for the treatment of breakthrough pain, defined as acute transient exacerbations of pain on a baseline of otherwise controlled chronic pain (65).

**Intraspinal Administration of Analgesics**

Opioid analgesics can be introduced into the epidural or intrathecal space for the management of pain in selected patients with cancer pain. Small doses of opioids administered by these routes are delivered in close proximity to their receptors in the dorsal horn of the spinal cord, thus achieving high local concentrations. Because the amount of drug administered is reduced, these routes of delivery may produce good analgesia with fewer of the side effects associated with equianalgesic doses of systematically administered opioids (83). Spinally administered opioids should be considered for patients whose pain is at least partially opioid-responsive but who cannot tolerate the side effects of oral or parenteral opioids, especially if attempts at managing these side effects as described above have been unsuccessful.

Adverse effects of spinal opioids are thought to result in part from supraspinal redistribution of drug, and include pruritus, urinary retention, nausea, vomiting, and respiratory depression (83). Respiratory depression may occur early (1–2 hours) or late (6–24 hours), but the risk of respiratory depression in patients who are not opioid-naive is quite low. Tolerance to the analgesic effects of spinal opioids may develop rapidly in some patients, possibly limiting the usefulness of this route of administration in some individuals (83).

When a patient is considered a potential candidate for spinal opioids, an initial trial of opioid administered through a temporary epidural or intrathecal catheter is recommended. If the individual's response to spinal opioids is sufficient to warrant more prolonged therapy, the temporary catheter should be replaced with a permanent implanted catheter to reduce the risks of infection and catheter migration (84). A number of implanted drug delivery systems are available for both epidural and intrathecal administration of opioids. The opioid may be delivered by intermittent bolus or by continuous infusion; the two methods are equally efficacious (85). Catheter placement is associated with a low but definite risk of epidural infection. Nevertheless, long-term epidural analgesia is safe and effective when patients are monitored carefully and receive prompt treatment if signs of infection develop (86). When spinal opioids are considered for the treatment of back pain in the cancer patient, magnetic resonance imaging (MRI) of the spine should ideally precede placement of an epidural catheter. This precaution avoids the potential for unexpected neurologic deterioration from injection in the presence of epidural tumor (83). Co-administration of local anesthetics with opioids into the epidural space such as bupivicaine (0.025% concentration) may also enhance analgesia in selected cases and may be useful when opioid tolerance develops (86).

## Practical Clinical Guidelines for Opioid Use

The onset, peak, and duration of analgesia vary with the opioid drug, the route of administration, and the particular patient. The recognition of this variability allows the appropriate choice of drug, route, and scheduling. When switching from one opioid to another, one half of the calculated equianalgesic dose is recommended as the initial dose for titration (1,8,13,14).

Oral administration is recommended in most patients because it is convenient, well tolerated, and usually the least expensive (8,14). However, transdermal administration of fentanyl has the advantage of convenience and long duration of action, and may improve patient compliance by deemphasizing the need to take something by mouth on a regular basis. However, most patients who take transdermal fentanyl will require an oral or (perhaps in the near future) a transmucosal rescue dose for breakthrough pain. All opioids should be titrated to effect, with intravenous boluses repeated every 15 minutes if necessary, until either analgesia or intolerable side effects develop, and oral doses of an immediate release morphine or oxycodone preparation as often as every 1–2 hours. The concomitant use of NSAIDS, antiemetics, and other coanalgesics is often warranted (8,14).

When pain is continuous, as is often the case, medications should be administered on an around-the-clock basis (8,14,16). Administering medications on an as-needed (prn) basis often results in the patient experiencing multiple episodes of pain during the day, and so is generally undesirable. However, prn administration is highly desirable for the first 24–48 hours following initiation of opioid therapy to determine the 24-hour dose requirement. If patients are started on an around-the-clock regimen and the starting dose is too high, unnecessary sedation and other side effects may occur, thereby reinforcing negative attitudes about taking opioids on the part of the patient. Once the optimum 24-hour dose is determined, the opioid should be prescribed by the clock. Many patients will continue to experience "breakthrough pain," or transitory increases in pain above its baseline level (65). For such pain, prn "rescue dose" of a short-acting opioid should be available that should start at 10–20% of the total scheduled daily dose.

There is enormous interindividual variation in the dose that is necessary to provide adequate analgesia, even among patients with similar pain syndromes. The variability in opioid responsiveness is caused by pharmacokinetic and pharmacodynamic factors (66). Recently, genetic factors such as race and gender have been shown to be important in determining opioid responsiveness (67). For example, 15% of Caucasians lack the oxidative phosphorylative enzyme CYPD211 needed to metabolize codeine to morphine in vivo and thereby require higher doses of codeine than do patients with normal metabolism (67). Kaiko et al. (68) noted that black and Asian patients participating in single-dose clinical trials to determine opioid efficacy reported twice the analgesic effect as whites in a retrospective analysis of the variations in opioid responsiveness. In another important recent study, Levine et al. (69) demonstrated that women achieved greater analgesia than men when administered κ opioid agonist drugs.

Patients on chronic opioid therapy often require relatively large dose increments to control acute exacerbations of pain. An infusion pump with a device for self-administration of extra doses of medication every few minutes (patient-controlled analgesia, PCA) should be used if available (70). The PCA dose can be as high as the hourly rate during the titration phase and when incident pain is a concern. The continuous basal rate should be frequently adjusted based on the patient's report and the PCA usage. When venous access is problematic the subcutaneous route should be used. Once the acute pain exacerbation is controlled the medication should be changed to the oral or transdermal route. Long-term intravenous and subcutaneous opioid administration can be used in patients outside of the hospital; intravenous administration is only possible when long-term access is obtained through a central venous line (71,72).

## Management of Side Effects of Opioid Analgesics

Constipation is the most common adverse effect of opiates. Tolerance to the constipating effects does not usually develop. Opioids cause constipation by a variety of mechanisms: decreased gastric, biliary, pancreatic, and intestinal secretions and a decrease in the propulsive motility of stomach and intestine resulting in delayed passage of increasingly viscous stool. Central and peripheral opioid receptor mechanisms are implicated (73). A prophylactic laxative regimen must be instituted at the same time the opioid is started and maintained for the duration of opioid therapy.

Nausea and vomiting related to opioid administration is thought to be caused by direct stimulation of the chemoreceptor trigger zone for emesis in the area postrema of the medulla (31). Nausea can also be caused by an increased vestibular sensitivity or delayed gastric emptying. A vestibular component is suggested by the fact that nausea is uncommon in recumbent patients and occurs in 40% of ambulatory patients after 15 mg of parenteral morphine (31). It is still unclear whether these effects involve specific opioid receptors because it has not been established as to whether they are reversed by naloxone (31). Tolerance to this effect is the rule and generally the nausea will subside in 2–3 days. Morphine-6-glucuronide may be implicated in some patients with protracted nausea (74). Inadequately treated constipation can be a cause of persistent nausea.

Transient sedation is very common when opioid therapy is initiated (75). Opiate-induced sedation must be differentiated from the predictable deep sleep that follows pain relief in sleep-deprived patients. Excessive sedation is frequently seen when patients are given relatively large doses of opioids to relieve movement-related pain but which have the effect of producing plasma concentrations of opioids that are too high relative to minimal or no pain experienced at rest. Strategies for managing sedation include eliminating of all other (unnecessary) CNS depressant drugs, switching opioid drugs, increasing the caffeine content in the diet, and using potent psychostimulants such as dextroamphetamine or methylphenidate (see below).

Unfounded fears of respiratory depression are often cited as a reason to limit opioid therapy. Respiratory depression is mediated by $\mu_2$ opioid receptors in the brainstem rendering the respiratory centers less responsive to the stimulatory effect of arterial carbon dioxide tension (31). Fortunately, tolerance to the respiratory depressant effect of opioids develops rapidly, and uncontrolled pain is a natural antagonist of opiate-induced respiratory depression. Respiratory depression is always associated with sedation. When a life-threatening opiate overdose is suspected, the patient should be stimulated vigorously to awaken. If this does not reverse sedation and hypoventilation, naloxone, an opiate antagonist, should be given intravenously. Patients on chronic opioids are more sensitive to naloxone than patients relatively naive to opioid administration; therefore it is recommended that a dilute naloxone solution should be used in this setting (14). The 0.4-mg ampule of naloxone can be diluted in 10 ml of normal saline and injected slowly, with titration bringing the dose to effect; this careful titration will prevent the precipitation of severe withdrawal symptoms and return of pain. Naloxone has a half-life of only 1 hour (35) and a short duration of action; therefore, close monitoring and repeated injections might be needed in the event of a morphine overdose. Prolonged monitoring is required with opiates with a longer half-life, like methadone, propoxyphene, and levorphanol. It must be kept in mind that excessive drug intake is a rare cause of encephalopathy and respiratory depression in patients with cancer on a stable dose of opiates. In fact, a recent study indicated that the majority of naloxone administrations in a large cancer center were inappropriate (76) and could have been avoided if more care were taken to determine the true cause of sedation or if the patient were simply physically stimulated.

Other relatively uncommon opioid side effects are listed in Table 4. It should be noted that long-term effects of chronic opiate use on intellectual function have not been demonstrated, although acute transient cognitive effects can be seen when opioid doses are increased (77). Opioids do not mask pain from new or ongoing tissue injury, and fears of masking medical emergencies like "acute abdomen" and myocardial infarction with opioids are unfounded.

## Tolerance, Physical Dependence, and Psychological Dependence

Tolerance implies the need to continuously increase the dose in order to obtain the desired effect, and it is a complex and incompletely understood phenomenon. However, the overwhelming clinical experience with patients on chronic opioids indicates that when the pain is stable, tolerance to the analgesic effects of opiates does not generally develop at the rate that would be predicted by animal studies (78). When rapid escalation of the opioid dose in cancer patients is required, this almost always means that the pain stimulus has increased in relation to progressive disease associated with new or ongoing tissue injury (78). However, because tolerance to the different opioid effects develops at different rates (e.g., rapidly for respiratory depression, slower for analgesic effects, very slow if at all for constipating effects), it is usually possible to titrate the opioid doses to appropriately balance analgesia and side effects. Cross-tolerance among different opiates is incomplete, indicating that analgesia but also side effects might develop when switching to a different strong opiate at an equianalgesic dose (78); a 50% dose reduction of the calculated equianalgesic dose and a gradual upward titration are therefore recommended. It has been observed that true pharmacologic tolerance is seen when, in the setting of an unchanging pain stimulus, the duration of analgesia shortens (78).

Physical dependence is an altered physiologic state, produced by repeated administrations of a drug, which necessitates the continued administration of the drug to

**TABLE 4.** *Side effects of opioid analgesics*

| Common side effects | Uncommon side effects |
|---|---|
| Constipation | Respiratory depression |
| Nausea | Seizures |
| Sedation | Pruritus |
| Mental clouding | Xerostomia |
| | Myoclonus |

prevent the appearance of withdrawal symptoms that are characteristic for the particular drug (31). When opiates are abruptly discontinued, often in error, the withdrawal syndrome consists of lacrimation, rhinorrhea, restlessness, and tremors; these symptoms are usually mild and don't have the dramatic flavor of the withdrawal syndrome seen in the chemically dependent patient. Patients who have received repeated doses of morphine a day for 1 or 2 weeks will have mild and often unrecognized withdrawal symptomatology when the drug is stopped; symptoms are delayed and even less pronounced with opioids with a long half-life like methadone and levorphanol. However, if an opioid antagonist is administered, symptoms of withdrawal may appear after a single dose (31). Appropriate counseling and a gradual taper of the opiate over a few days will effectively prevent the development of a withdrawal syndrome. As discussed above, the inappropriate administration of naloxone may precipitate profound withdrawal in patients taking chronic opioids for pain relief.

Psychological dependence—now the preferred term for addiction— is described as compulsive drug seeking behavior and overwhelming involvement in drug procurement and use (31). The inexperienced clinician may misinterpret the behavior of the patient with severe unrelieved pain for drug seeking behavior because poorly managed pain may produce many of the behaviors that physicians have come to fear in "addicted" individuals. This phenomenon is recognized by the term pseudoaddiction (79). The rarity of psychological dependence following chronic opioid treatment has been clearly documented in several studies and recently reviewed in detail (80). For example, in a study involving 11,882 patients who received at least one opioid prescription, the development of addiction occurred in only four instances (81). The analysis of patterns of drug intake in patients with cancer suggests that chemical dependence does not occur in this population, or occurs only very rarely (82). An exception to this rule is offered by patients with a history of chemical dependence that antedates the cancer. Exaggerated and unfounded fears of addiction should not prevent patients from receiving opioids on a chronic basis for severe pain.

## Adjuvant Analgesics in Cancer Pain Management

The adjuvant analgesics are a heterogeneous group of drugs that were marketed and approved for indications other than pain, but that may be analgesic in certain clinical conditions or counteract adverse effects of conventional opioid and nonopioid analgesics (87). As indicated in Table 5, one can group adjuvant analgesics into three broad categories: (a) general purpose drugs (e.g., tricyclic antidepressants); (b) drugs used in specific pain syndromes such as neuropathic, bone, or visceral pain (e.g., anticonvulsants

for neuropathic pain; radiopharmaceuticals for bone and visceral pain); and (c) drugs used to counteract opioid analgesic side effects (e.g., caffeine, methylphenidate, phenothiazine antiemetics). Adjuvant analgesic drugs usually require several-week trials to determine their utility and often do not provide complete analgesia. Patients should be educated as to these facts so as to make their compliance more likely.

### General Purpose Adjuvant Analgesics

These drugs are utilized for a variety of pains, including those of musculoskeletal, neuropathic, and visceral origin, and chronic headache. The tricyclic antidepressants are the most widely used in this group. They probably produce analgesia by increasing levels of norepinephrine and/or serotonin in the central nervous system and thus may enhance the activity of endogenous pain-modulating pathways (88). Amitriptyline, imipramine, nortriptyline, and desipramine have all been demonstrated to have some analgesic efficacy (89) in chronic pain, especially pain of neuropathic origin. The doses required to produce analgesia are generally lower and the analgesic effect quicker (typical onset within 1 week) in comparison to antidepressant effects.

The new selective serotonin reuptake inhibitors (SSRIs), although attended by fewer side effects than the tricyclic antidepressants, have a mixed picture as analgesics. For example, one randomized controlled trial using fluoxetine in diabetic neuropathy could not demonstrate an analgesic effect in nondepressed patients, although at least some analgesic effect has been demonstrated for paroxetine in the management of painful diabetic neuropathy (90).

In general, one should start with relatively low doses of tricyclic antidepressants (especially in elderly patients) and increase the dose every 3 days. For example, a typical regimen for amitriptyline includes starting at 10 mg at bedtime, and increasing to 25 mg in 3 days, and then increasing by 25 mg every 3–7 days until a dose of 75–150 mg is reached. Sequential trials of different tricyclics should be considered, especially selection of drugs in the secondary amine family (e.g., desipramine or nortriptyline) if the tertiary amine drugs such as amitriptyline are not tolerated because of adverse effects. For this reason, some clinicians prefer initiating tricyclic antidepressant therapy with desipramine or nortriptyline. The SSIs are generally used as second- or third-line agents because the data supporting their efficacy in neuropathic pain are not as strong as those regarding the tricyclic antidepressant family.

Methotrimeprazine is a phenothiazine compound that has analgesic activities. Analgesic studies have confirmed that 15 mg of methotrimeprazine given intramuscularly is equipotent to 10 mg of morphine given intramuscularly (91). This drug is most useful in the setting of hospitalized patients with opioid-induced ileus because it can provide an opioid-sparing analgesic effect. The side

**TABLE 5.** *Adjuvant analgesic drugs used to treat cancer-related pain*

| Drug class and category | Usual dose | Indications |
|---|---|---|
| **1. General purpose, nonspecific** | | |
| Tricyclic antidepressants | Amitriptyline 10–25 mg q HS PO 150 mg/day<br>Nortriptyline 25 mg q HS —> 100–150 mg/day | Neuropathic and musculoskeletal pain |
| Corticosteroids | Dexamethasone 4–16 mg/day PO (2–4 divided doses)<br><br>Prednisone 60–80 mg/day PO (2–4 divided doses) | Essential for spinal cord compression & brain herniation; also useful in malignant bone and nerve pain |
| Phenothiazine | Methotrimeprazine 10–15 mg IM q 6 h | Useful for opioid sparing in very tolerant patients and opioid-induced ileus |
| **2. Neuropathic pain** | | |
| Anticonvulsants | Carbamazepine 200–800 mg/day PO (divided doses)<br>Valproic acid 15–60 mg/kg/day PO (divided doses)<br>Gabepentin 300–900 mg TID PO<br>Clonazapam 0.5–1.0 mg TID PO | Useful for dysesthetic and paroxysmal lancinating pain |
| Antiarrhythmics and local anesthetics | Lidocaine 2–5 mg/kg i.v. continuous infusion in 30 min<br>Mexiletine 450–600 md/day in divided doses PO | Usually reserved for neuropathic pain refractory to anticonvulsants and opioids |
| Topical creams and ointments | Capsaicin 0.075% cream—apply to site of pain at least 4 times a day | Capsaicin most often used for postherpetic neuralgia |
| Baclofen | 5 mg b.i.d. PO–150 mg/day (divided doses) | Useful as second line agent in neuropathic pain in combination with anticonvulsant. Also used in spinal spasticity |
| Eutectic mixture of local anesthetics (EMLA) cream | Apply 60–90 minutes to site prior to procedure | EMLA very useful in children to premedicate for venipunctures and other painful procedures |
| Dissociative "anesthetics" | Ketamine 0.1-0.5 mg/kg/hr IV or SC | Effects on NMDA receptors occur at lower doses than anesthetic effects; psychotomimetic effects may still occur |
| Dextromethorphan | Delsym 15 mg b.i.d. PO–1000 mg/day | Delsym is a single entity slow-release preparation. Dextromethorphan also contained in common cough syrups such as Robitussin-DM® |
| **3. Bone pain** | | |
| Radiopharmaceuticals | Strontium-89 4 µCurie/dose IV | Dose may be repeated if positive analgesic response and adequate marrow reserve |
| Bisphosphonates | Pamidronate 90 mg IV over 2 h, monthly | Inhibits bone resorption and improves bone pain |
| Other osteoclast inhibitors | Calcitonin 25 IU IV b.i.d.–150 IU b.i.d.; 200 IU intranasal g/day | Also used in Paget's disease, phantom pain, and complex regional pain syndromes such as reflex sympathetic dystrophy (RSD) |
| **4. Visceral pain** | | |
| Octreotide | Octreotide 100–600 mg/day via SC bolus or infusion | Useful for secretory diarrhea and malignant bowel obstruction |
| Calcium channel blockers | Diltiazem | |
| Scopolamine | 0.8–2 mg/day SG 1.5–3 mg/g 3 day transdermally | |
| **5. Psychostimulants** | | |
| Over-the-counter preparations | Caffeine 100–200 mg/day PO | One cup of coffee or 12 oz. caffenated beverage contains 65 mg caffeine |
| Controlled substances | Methylphenidate 5–20 mg/day PO<br>Dextroamphetamine sulfate 5–15 mg/day PO | Act additively with opioids for analgesia and improve alertness |
| **6. Marijuana and Cannabinoids** | Dronabinol 2.5–5.0 mg b.i.d. PO | No firm evidence for analgesic effects at usual doses. Effects of smoked marijuana as analgesic reported in anecdotal reports only. Possibly useful as appetite stimulant, antiemetic, and antiglaucoma agent |

effect profile is the same as for other phenothiazines, and orthostatic hypotension and sedation can be dose-limiting effects. Other limitations to its use are caused by its relative expense and the fact that it is not available in an oral formulation in the United States. The parenteral formulation has been used orally by mixing in juice and drinking.

Corticosteroids may enhance analgesia in a variety of situations, including metastatic bone pain, pain related to nerve compression, and pain from epidural spinal cord compression (92). The response to corticosteroids may be rapid and dramatic. Because of the potential for serious adverse effects with prolonged use, corticosteroids are best reserved for patients with advanced disease or for short-term use.

Marijuana has attracted renewed attention as an analgesic, antiemetic, antiglaucoma agent, and appetite stimulant. When smoked, the marijuana delivers over 60 cannabinoid compounds with known or potential pharmacologic activity, although the d-9 tetrahydrocannabinoid ($\Delta$-9 THC) metabolite is the most pharmacologically active (93). This compound, $\Delta$-9 THC, is also available as 2.5-mg dronabinol capsules. A recent controlled trial of dronabinol in doses of 2.5 mg b.i.d. compared to placebo demonstrated effectiveness in increasing appetite, improving mood, and decreasing nausea in patients with AIDS-related anorexia and weight loss (94).

The data regarding the efficacy of $\Delta$-9 THC as an analgesic are less clear. A controlled trial comparing 10- and 20-mg oral doses to placebo and to oral doses of codeine at 30 and 60 mg in patients with cancer pain demonstrated that only the 20-mg dose could be distinguished from placebo, although dysphoria and delirium were quite prominent at this dose (95). There are no studies of the analgesic effect of smoked marijuana, although there are anecdotal reports of the used of inhaled marijuana as an analgesic (96). In summary, the existing data are unclear as to whether inhaled marijuana or $\Delta$-9 THC has any advantage over existing analgesics in terms of analgesic efficacy or side effect profile.

### Adjuvant Analgesic Drugs Used for Bone Pain

A more complete list of drugs useful for metastatic bone pain is given in Table 5. Recently, it has been shown that bisphosphonate compounds inhibit the reabsorption of bone and reduce bone pain in lytic bone metastasis, such as is typical of breast cancer (97). Table 5 lists the usual dosage schedule for pamidronate disodium, perhaps the most widely used bisphosphonate currently. A recent randomized controlled trial in which pamidronate was used in patients with stage IV breast cancer showed that this drug reduced further skeletal complications in this disease and significantly reduced bone pain when compared to placebo controls.

### Adjuvant Analgesics Used in Neuropathic Pain

Many types of pharmacologic agents have been used to manage neuropathic pain including tricyclic antidepressants, anticonvulsants, systemic local anesthetic agents, topical anesthetic creams, and capsaicin, baclofen, and clonidine. Doses of these drugs and their general indications are listed in Table 5. In addition, two old drugs, ketamine and dextromethorphan, are being reevaluated in neuropathic pain because of their ability to inhibit N-methyl-D-aspartate (NMDA) receptors, which have recently been shown to be important in neuropathic pain states (98).

Anticonvulsant drugs are used generally to manage pain refractory to conventional analgesic drugs and as first-line agents to treat lancinating pain of neuropathic origin (99). Current estimates indicate that about 5% of anticonvulsant drug prescriptions are written for neuropathic pain. Generally, these drugs are given in the dose ranges usually administered to treat epilepsy. Gabapentin, a GABA analog, is a relatively new anticonvulsant that has received recent attention for its use in pain, particularly pain associated with neuropathic pain, sympathetically maintained pain, or other complex regional pain syndromes (100). This drug is relatively free of side effects, although drowsiness, dizziness, and ataxia have been associated as dose-related effects.

Systematically administered local anesthetics may have a role in the management of neuropathic pain. Intravenous lidocaine is usually given as a 2–5 mg/kg dose over 20–30 minutes. Most clinicians do the infusion while monitoring blood pressure and heart rate in a monitored environment. Intravenous lidocaine often provides dramatic relief of neuropathic pain (101), but the analgesic effect is usually short-lived although it may persist well beyond the duration of the infusion (101). The efficacy of intravenous lidocaine in the management of cancer-related neuropathic pain has not been established definitively because a placebo-controlled trial could not demonstrate a difference between lidocaine and the inactive treatment (102). Mexiletine, an oral analog of lidocaine, may be administered to patients in doses of 150–600 mg/day (102).

Baclofen is a GABA agonist that has been used many neuropathic pain syndromes, most notably trigeminal neuralgia, in which it is used in combination with carbamazepine when this condition is refractory to carbamazepine alone (103). There is a wide range of effective oral doses, staring at 5 mg b.i.d. up to 150 mg/day.

Epidural clonidine may be effective in selected patients with cancer pain, particularly for neuropathic pain. In a recent study, 85 cancer patients were titrated to pain relief on epidural morphine and then randomized to receive epidural clonidine (30 mg/hour) or placebo, with either group receiving epidural morphine rescue doses as needed. Analgesia was reestablished in 45% of the epidural clonidine group, but only 21% of the placebo group, and was more likely to occur when a neuropathic pain mechanism was the predominant pain (104). Hypotension occurred as a serious complication in only two patients on epidural clonidine.

As mentioned above, activation of the NMDA receptor by endogenous ligands, such as the excitatory amino acids, glutamate, and aspartate, promotes pain and hyperalgesia following experimental peripheral nerve injury, and blockade of this receptor by drugs such as dextromethorphan relieves pain (105). Two old drugs, ketamine and dextromethorphan, are competitive NMDA receptor antagonists and produce analgesia in neuropathic pain (98). Ketamine blocks NMDA receptors and produces analgesia in doses much lower than those needed to produce anesthesia, and is typically given by continuous infusion at 0.1–1.5 mg/kg/hour. The infusion can be repeated as needed. Dextromethorphan is an antitussive and is present in many cough syrup formulations. It also can be given as a single entity in a slow release preparation known as Delsym, in doses ranging from 15 mg to 500 mg BID. Better controlled trials of these agents are required to determine the ultimate usefulness of ketamine and dextromethorphan as NMDA receptor blockers in neuropathic pain. Side effects common to these agents include sedation (ketamine and dextromethorphan) and delirium for ketamine.

### Adjuvant Analgesics Used for Visceral Pain

Several drugs useful for visceral pain are listed in Table 5. Octreotide, a synthetic analog of somatostatin, can be given intrathecally to produce analgesia but has also been administered as a subcutaneous infusion to manage nausea, vomiting, and diarrhea associated with malignant bowel obstruction (106).

### Adjuvant Analgesic Drugs to Counteract Opioid-Induced Side Effects

Psychostimulants such as caffeine (107), methylphenidate, pemoline, and dextroamphetamine also have a place in cancer pain treatment (see Table 5). Methylphenidate has been shown to enhance the analgesic effect of opioid drugs and to decrease the sedation associated with opioid use (108).

### SUMMARY

Currently available pain management techniques make adequate pain control a realistic and achievable goal for virtually all patients with cancer. A thorough evaluation of the pain complaint to establish a pain diagnosis is the key to successful management. Special atten-

tion should be paid to those pain syndromes potentially responsive to primary antineoplastic treatment so that such treatment can be initiated in a timely manner when appropriate.

Individualized pharmacotherapy is the cornerstone of cancer pain management, and most often requires the use of opioid analgesics, often in combination with nonopioid analgesics and adjuvant medications. Opioids should be administered on a scheduled basis with the dose titrated to achieve a balance between pain control and adverse side effects. The risk of addiction in the cancer patient with pain is negligible and should not discourage the appropriate use of this highly effective class of analgesics.

In a minority of patients, cancer pain cannot be adequately controlled by systematically administered analgesics, often because of intractable dose-limiting side effects. For these patients, interventional approaches should be considered, including either anesthetic or neurosurgical procedures. Appropriate patient selection is critical to maximizing the success of these procedures. Optimal pain management in the patient with cancer requires individualization of treatment and the integration of pain management approaches.

Many factors affect the pain experience, including physical, psychosocial, and emotional influences. Conversely, uncontrolled pain may have a disastrous impact on all aspects of patient function and quality of life. Adequate pain management, ideally in a multidisciplinary setting, should therefore be viewed as a high priority for all patients with cancer.

### REFERENCES

1. von Roenn JH, Cleeland CS, Gonin R, Hatfield AK, Pandya KJ. Physician attitudes and practice in cancer pain management: A survey from the Eastern Cooperative Oncology Group. *Ann Int Med* 1993; 119:121–126.
2. Payne R, Weinstein SM, Hill CS. Assessment and management of pain. In: Levin VL, ed. *Cancer in the Nervous System.* New York: Churchill-Livingstone, 1996;411–448.
3. Gonzales GR, Elliott KJ, Portenoy RK, Foley KM. The impact of a comprehensive evaluation in the management of cancer pain. *Pain* 1991;47:141–144.
4. Anderson JS, Burris HA, Casper E et al. Development of a new system for assessing clinical benefit for patients with advanced pancreatic cancer. *Proc Ann Met Am Soc Clin Oncol* 1994;13:A1600.
5. Tannock IF et al. Chemotherapy with mitotoxantrone plus prednisone or prednisone alone for symptomatic hormone-resistant prostate cancer. A Canadian randomized trial with palliative and points. *J Clin Oncol* 1996;14:1754–1764.
6. Hoskin PJ. Scientific and clinical aspects of radiotherapy in the relief of bone pain. *Cancer Surv* 1988;7:69–86.
7. Porter AT, McEwan AJB, Powe JE, et al. Results of a randomized phase III trial to evaluate the efficacy of strontium-89 adjuvant to local field external beam irradiation in the management of endocrine resistant metastatic prostate cancer. *Int J Radiat Oncol Biol Phys* 1993;25:805–813.
8. World Health Organization. *Cancer Pain Relief and Palliative Care: Report of a WHO Expert Committee,* 3rd ed. Geneva, 1996.
9. Cleeland CS, Gonin R, Harfield AK, et al. Pain and its treatment in outpatients with metastatic cancer. *N Engl J Med* 1994;330(9):592–596.

10. Zech DFJ, Grond S, Lynch J, et al. Validation of World Health Organization guidelines for cancer pain relief: a 10-year prospective study. *Pain* 1995;63:65–76.

11. Jadad AR, Browman GP. The WHO analgesic ladder for cancer pain management: stepping up the quality of its evaluation. *JAMA* 1995; 274(23):1870–1873.

12. Hanel AM, Lands WEM. Modification of anti-inflammatory drug effectiveness by ampient lipid peroxides. *Biochem Pharmacol* 1982; 31:3307–3311.

13. Jacox A, Carr DB, Ferrell B et al. Acute pain management: Operative or medical procedures and trauma-clinical practice guidelines. Rockville, MD: U.S. Department of Health and Human Services, 1992, 1–145.

14. Jacox A, Carr DB, Payne R et al. Management of cancer pain, clinical practice guidelines, No. 9, AHCPR Publication No. 94–0592. Rockville, MD: U.S. Department of Health and Human Services, Public Health Service, Agency for Health Care Policy and Research, 1994b.

15. Inturrisi CE. Management of cancer pain: pharmacology and principles of management. *Cancer* 1989;63:2308–2320.

16. Portenoy RK, Kanner RM. Nonopioid and adjuvant analgesics. In: Portenoy RK, Kanner RM, eds. *Pain Management: Theory and Practice.* Philadelphia: FA Davis, 1996;219–276.

17. Vane JR. Inhibition of prostaglandin synthesis as a mechanism of action for aspirin-like drugs. *Nature* 1971;234:231–238.

18. Malmberg AB, Yaksh TL. Hyperalgesia mediated by spinal glutamate or substance P receptor blocked by spinal cyclooxygenase inhibition. *Science* 1992;257:1276–1279.

19. Mitchell JA, Akarasereenomt P, Thiemermann C, Flower RJ, Vane JR. Selectivity of nonsteriodal anti-inflammatory drugs as inhibitors of constitutive and inducible cyclooxygenase. *Proc Natl Acad Sci USA* 1993;90:11593–11597.

20. Laneuville O, Breuer DK, DeWitt DL et al. Differential inhibition of human prostaglandin endoperoxide H synthetase-1 and -2 by nonsteriodal and anti-inflammatory drugs. *J Pharmacol Exper Therap* 1994; 271:927–934.

21. Perneger TV, Whelton PK, Klag MJ. Risk of kidney failure associated with the use of acetaminophen and nonsteroidal anti-inflammatory drugs. *N Engl J Med* 1994;331:1675–1679.

22. Rumack BH, Peterson RC, Koch GG, Amara IA. Acetaminophen overdose. 662 cases with evolution of oral acetycysteine treatment. *Arch Intern Med* 1981;141:380–385.

23. Levick S, Jacobs C, Loukas DF, et al. Naproxen sodium in the treatment of bone pain due to metastatic cancer. *Pain* 1988;35:253–258.

24. Eisenberg E, Berkey CS, Carr DB, et al. Efficacy and safety of nonsteroidal anti-inflammatory drugs for cancer pain: a meta-analysis. *J Clin Oncol* 1994;12:2756–2765.

25. Henry D, Lim LL-Y, Rodriguez LAG, et al. Variability in risk of gastrointestinal complications with individual non-steroid anti-inflammatory drugs: results of a collaborative meta-analysis. *BJM* 1996; 312(7046):1563–1566

26. Ehrlich GE, ed. *The Resurgence of Salicylates in Arthritis Therapy.* Norwalk, CT: Scientific Media Communications, 1983;75–90.

27. Houde RW, Wallenstein SL, Beaver WT. Evaluation of analgesics in patients with cancer pain. In: Lasagna L, ed. *International Encyclopedia of Pharmacology and Therapeutics,* vol 1. New York: Pergamon Press, 1966;59–67.

28. Pert CB, Snyder SH. Opiate receptor: demonstrated in nervous tissue. *Science* 1973;179:1011–1014.

29. Levy M. Drug therapy for cancer pain. *N Engl J Med* 1996;335(15): 1124–1132.

30. Beaver WT, Wallenstein SL, Rogers A, Houde WH. Analgesic studies of codeine and oxycodone in patients with cancer. 1. Comparison of oral with intramuscular codeine and oral with intramuscular oxycodone. *J Pharmacol Exp Ther* 1978;207:92–100.

31. Inturrisi CE, Colburn WN, Verebey K, Dayton KE, Woody GE, O'Brien Cp. Propoxyphene and norpropoxyphene kinetics after single and repeated doses of propoxyphene. *Clin Pharmacol Ther* 1982;31: 157–167.

32. Jaffe JH, Martin WR. Opioid analgesics and antagonists. In: Gillman AG, Rall TW, Nies AS, Taylor P, eds. *Goodman and Gilman's the Pharmacologic Basis of Therapeutics,* 8th ed. New York: Pergamon Press, 1990; 485–521.

33. Kaiko RF, Foley KM, Grabinski PY, Heidrich G, Rogers AG, Inturrisi CE, Reidenberg MM. Central nervous system excitatory effects of meperidine in cancer patients. *Ann Neurol* 1983;13:180–185.

34. Beaver Wt, Wallenstein SL, Rogers A, Houde R. Analgesic Studies of codeine and oxycodone in patients with cancer. 2. Comparison of intramuscular oxycodone with intramuscular morphine and codeine. *J Pharmacol Exp Ther* 1978;207:101–108.

35. Glare PA, Walsh TD. Dose-ranging study of oxycodone for chronic pain in advanced cancer. *J Clin Oncol* 1993;11:973–978.

36. Poyhia R, Vainio A, Kalso E. A review of oxycodone's clinical pharmacokinetics and pharmacodynamics. *J Pain Sympt Manag* 1993;8: 63–67.

37. Kalso E, Vanio A. Morphine and oxycodone for cancer pain. *Clin Pharm Ther* 1990;47:639–646.

38. Portenoy RK, Khan E, Layman M, Lapin J, Malkin MG, Foley KM, Thaler HT, Cerbone DJ, Inturrisi CE. Chronic morphine therapy for cancer pain: plasma and cerebrospinal fluid morphine and morphine-6-glucuronide concentrations. *Neurology* 1991;41:1457–61.

39. Pasternak GW, Bodnar RJ, Clarcke JA, Inturrisi CE. Morphine-6-glucuronide, a potent mu agonist. *Life Sci* 1987;41:2845–49.

40. Twycross R. The use of narcotic analgesics in terminal illness. *J Med Ethics* 1975;1:10–17.

41. Morley JL, Miles JB, Wells JC, Bowsher D. Paradoxical pain. *Lancet* 1992;340(8826):1045(letter).

42. Smith MT, Watt JA, Cramond T. Morphine-3-glucuronide—a potent antagonist of morphine analgesia. *Life Sci* 1990;47:579–585.

43. Osborne RJ, Joel SP, Slevin ML. Morphine intoxication in renal failure: the role of morphine-6-glucuronide. *Br Med J* 1986;292: 1548–1549.

44. Houde RW. Clinical analgesic studies of hydromorphone. *Adv Pain Res Ther* 1986;8:129–135.

45. Babul N, Darke AC, Hagen N. Hydromorphone metabolite accumulation in renal failure (letter). *J Pain Sympt Manag* 1995;10(3):184–186.

46. Tive L, Ginsberg K, Pick CG, Pasternak GW. κ3 receptors and levorphanol analgesia. *Neuropharmacology* 1992;9:851–856.

47. Houde RW, Wallenstein SL, Beaver WT. *Clinical Measurement of Pain: Analgesics.* New York: Academic Press, 1975;75–122.

48. Dixon R. Pharmacokinetics of levorphanol. *Adv Pain Res Ther* 1986; 8:217–224.

49. Faisinger R, Schoeller T, Bruera E. Methadone in the management of chronic pain: a review. *Pain* 1993;52:137–147.

50. Beaver WT, Wallenstein SL, Houde RW, Rogers A. A clinical comparison of the analgesic effects of methadone and morphine administered intramuscularly and of oral and parenterally administered methadone. *Clin Pharmacol Ther* 1967;8:415–426.

51. Sawe J. High dose morphine and methadone in cancer patients. Clinical pharmacokinetic consideration of oral treatment. *Clin Pharmacol* 1986;11:87–106.

52. Inturrisi CE, Colburn WA, Kaiko RF, Houde RW, Foley KM. Pharmacokinetics and pharmacodynamics of methadone in patients with chronic pain. *Clin Pharmacol Ther* 1987;41:392–401.

53. Plummer JL, Gourlay GK, Cherry DA, Cousins MJ. Estimation of methadone clearance: application in the management of cancer pain. *Pain* 1988;33:313–322.

54. Galer BS, Coyle N, Pasternak GW, Portenoy RK. Individual variability in the response to different opioids: report of five cases. *Pain* 1992; 49:87–91.

55. Morley JS, Watt JWG, Wells JC, Miles JB, Finnegan MJ, Leng J. Methadone in pain uncontrolled by morphine. *Lancet* 1993; 342(8881):1243 (letter).

56. Mafredi PL, Borsook D, Chandler S, Payne R. Intravenous methadone for cancer pain unrelieved by morphine and hydromorphone: Clinical observations. *Pain* 1997;70(1):99–101.

57. Kreek MJ, Schecter AJ, Gutjahr CL, Hecht M. Methadone use in patients with chronic renal disease. *Drug Alcohol Depend* 1980;5: 195–205.

58. Roy SD, Flynn GL. Transdermal delivery of narcotic analgesics: Ph, anatomical and subject influences of cutaneous permeability of fentanyl and suffentanil. *Pharm Res* 1990;7:842–847.

59. Hwang SS, Nichols KC, Southam MA. Transdermal permeation: physiological and physiochemical aspects. In: Lehmann KA, Zech D, eds. *Transdermal Fentanyl.* Berlin: Springer-Verlag, 1991;1–7.

60. Varvel Jl, Shafer SL, Hwang SS, Coen PA, Stanski DR. Absorption characteristics of transdermally administered fentanyl. *Anesthesiology* 1989;70:928–934.

61. Portenoy RH et al. Transdermal fontanyl for cancer pain: Repeated dose pharmacokinetics. *Anesthesiology* 1993;78(1):36–43
62. Southam M, Gupta B, Knowles N, Hwang SS. Transdermal fentanyl: an overview of pharmacokinetics, efficacy and safety. In: Lehmann KA, Zech D, eds. *Transdermal Fentanyl.* Berlin: Springer-Verlag, 1991;107–116.
63. Salomaki TE, Laitinen JO, Nuutinen LS. A randomized double-blind comparison of epidural versus intravenous fentanyl infusion for analgesia after thoracotomy. *Anesthesiology* 1991;75:790–795.
64. Fine PG, Marcus M, Just De Boer A, Van der Oord B. An open label study of oral transmucosal fentanyl citrate (OTFC) for the treatment of breakthrough cancer pain. *Pain* 91;45:149–153.
65. Portenoy RK, Hagen NA. Breakthrough pain: definition and manifestations. *Pain* 1990;41:273–281.
66. Portenoy RK, Foley KM, Inturrissi CE. The nature of opioid responsiveness and its implications for neuropathic pain: new hypotheses derived from studies of opioid infusions. *Pain* 1990;43:273–286.
67. Tseng CY, Want SL, Lai MD, Lai ML, Huang JD. Formation of morphine from codeine in Chinese subjects of different CYP2D6 genotypes. *Clin Pharm Therap* 1996;60:177–182.
68. Kaiko RF, Wallenstein SL, Rogers AG, Houde RW. Sources of variation in analgesic responses in cancer patients with chronic pain receiving morphine. *Pain* 1993;15:191–200.
69. Levine and Miaskowski. Gender response in κ opioid agonists. *Nature,* 1996.
70. Citron ML, Johnston-Early A, Boyer M, Krasnow SH, Hood M, Cohen MH. Patient-controlled analgesia for severe cancer pain. *Arch Intern Med* 1986;146:734–736.
71. Portenoy R. Continuous infusion of opioid drugs in the treatment of cancer pain; guidelines for use. *J Pain Sympt Contr* 1986;1: 223–228.
72. Bruera E, Chadwick S, Bacovsky R. Continuous subcutaneous infusion of narcotics using a portable disposable pump. *J Palliat Care* 1985;1:45–47.
73. Paul D, Pasternak GW.Differential blockade by naloxazine of two mu opiate actions: analgesia and inhibition of gastrointestinal transit. *Eur J Pharmacol* 1988;149:403–404.
74. Hagen NA, Foley KM, Cerbone DJ, Portenoy RK, Inturrisi CE. Chronic nausea and morphine-6-glucuronide. *J Pain Sympt Manag* 1991;6:125–128.
75. Bruera E, Roca E, Cedaro L, Carraro S, Chacon R. Action of oral methylprednisolone in terminal cancer patients: a prospective randomized double blind study. *Cancer Treat Rep* 1985;69:751–754.
76. Manfreidi PL, Ribeiro S, Chandler SW, Payne R. Inappropriate use of naloxone in cancer patients with pain. *J Pain Symptom Manag* 1996; 11:131–134.
77. Bruera E, Macmillan K, Hanson J, MacDonald N. The cognitive effects of the administration of narcotic analgesics in patients with cancer pain. *Pain* 1989; 39:13–16.
78. Foley KM. Changing concepts of tolerance to opioids: what the cancer patient has taught us. In: Chapman CR, Foley KM, eds. *Current and Emerging Issues in Cancer Pain: Research and Practice.* New York: Raven Press, 1993;331–350.
79. Weissman DE, Haddox JD. Opioid pseudoaddiction–an iatrogenic syndrome. *Pain* 1989;36(3):363–366.
80. Portenoy RK, Payne R. Acute chronic pain management. In: Lowinson JH, Ruiz P, Millman RB, Langrod JG, eds., *Comprehensive Textbook of Substance Abuse,* 3rd ed. Baltimore, MD: Williams and Wilkins, 1997;563–589.
81. Porter J, Jick, H. Addiction rare in patients treated with narcotics. *N Engl J Med* 1980;302:123 (letter).
82. Kanner RM, Foley KM. Patterns of narcotic use in a cancer pain clinic. In: *Research Developments In Drug and Alcohol Use.* New York: NY Academy of Science, 1981;161–172.
83. Payne R. Role of epidural intrathecal narcotics and peptides in the management of cancer pain. *Med Clin North Am* 1987;71:313–328.
84. Patt RB. Anesthetic procedures for the control of cancer pain. In: Arbit E, ed. *Management of Cancer-Related Pain.* Mount Kisco, NY: Futura Publishing Co., 1993;381–407.
85. Gourlay GK, Plummer JL, Cherry DA, et al. Comparison of intermittent bolus with continuous infusion of epidural morphine in the treatment of severe cancer pain. *Pain* 1991;47:135–140.
86. DuPen SL, Kharasch ED, Williams A, et al. Chronic epidural bupivacaine-opioid infusion in intractable cancer pain. *Pain* 1992;49:293–300.
87. Portenoy RK. Adjuvant analgesics in pain management. In: Doyle D, Hanks GW, MacDonald N, eds. *Oxford Textbook of Palliative Medicine.* Oxford: Oxford University Press, 1993;187–203.
88. Hammond DL. Pharmacology of central pain-modulating networks (biogenic amines and non-opioid analgesics). In: Fields HL, Dubner R, Cervero F, eds. *Advances in Pain Research and Therapy,* vol 9. New York: Raven Press, 1985;499–513.
89. Max MB. Antidepressants as analgesics. In: Fields HL, Lieberkind SC, eds., *Pharmacological Approaches to the Treatment of Chronic Pains: New Concepts and Critical Issues.* Seattle, WA: IASP Press, 1994;229–246.
90. Sindrup SH, Gram LF, Brosen K, et al. The selective serotonin reuptake inhibitor paroxetine is effective in the treatment of diabetic neuropathy symptoms. *Pain* 1990;42:135–144.
91. Lasagna L. Drug interaction in the field of analgesic drugs. *Proc R Soc Med* 1965;58(II, Part 2):978–983.
92. Ettinger AB, Portenoy RK. The use of corticosteroids in the treatment of symptoms associated with cancer. *J Pain Sympt Manag* 1988;3: 99–103.
94. Beal JE, Olson R, Laubenstein L et al. Dronabinol as a treatment for anorexis associated with weight loss in patients with AIDS. *J Pain Sympt Manag* 1995;10:89–97.
95. Noyes et al. The analgesic properties of delta-9-tetrahydrocannabinol and codeine. *Clin Pharmacol Ther* 1975;18(1):84–89.
96. Noyes et al. Cannabinois analgesia. *Compr Psychiatry* 1974;15(6): 531–535.
97. Hortobagyi GN, Theriault RL, Porter L, et al. Efficacy of pamidronate in reducing skeletal complicatons in pateints with breast cancer and lytic bone metastasis. *N Engl J Med* 1996;335:1785–1791.
98. Backjona M, Arndt G, Gombar KA, Check B, Zimmerman M. Response of chronic neuropathic pain syndromes to ketamine: A preliminary study. *Pain* 1994;56(1):51–57.
99. Swerdlow M. Anticonvulsant drugs and chronic pain. *Clin Neuropharmacol* 1984;7:51–82.
101. Kastrup J, Petersen P, Dejgard A, et al. Intravenous lidocaine infusion—a new treatment of chronic painful diabetic neuropathy? *Pain* 1987;28:69–75.
102. Dejgard A, Petersen P, Kastrup J. Mexiletine for treatment of chronic painful diabetic neuropathy. *Lancet* 1988;1:9–11.
103. Fromm GH. Baclofen as an adjuvant analgesic. *J Pain Sympt Manag* 1994;9(8):500–509.
104. Eisenach JC, DuPen SL, Dubois M, et al. Epidural clonidine analgesia for intractable cancer pain. *Pain* 1995;61:391–399.
105. Tal M, Bennett GJ. Dextorphan relieves neuropathic heat-evoked hyperalgesia in the rat. *Neurosci Lett* 1993;151:107–110.
107. Laska EM, Sunshine A, Mueller F et al. Caffeine as an analgesic adjuvant. *JAMA* 1984;251:1711–1718.
108. Bruera E, Brenneis C, Chadwick S, Hanson J, MacDonald RN. Methylphenidate associated with narcotics for the treatment of cancer pain. *Cancer Treat Rep* 1987;71:67–70.

*Principles and Practice of Supportive Oncology,*
edited by Ann Berger et al.
Lippincott–Raven Publishers, Philadelphia ©1998

CHAPTER 4

# Nonpharmacologic Approaches to Pain

Karen L. Syrjala and Sari L. Roth-Roemer

Too many cancer patients do not receive adequate relief for their pain despite the availability of effective medical treatments (1,2). Explanations for this gap between our ability to relieve pain and actual rates of pain relief include almost entirely nonmedical factors: reluctance of patients to take prescribed medications; reluctance of patients to discuss their pain; inadequate assessment; inadequate knowledge of patients about what is appropriate to discuss and what is possible to treat; and myths that disrupt communication between patients, their family members, and health care providers (3–5). While cancer pain experts recognize that barriers to management of pain exist and that nonpharmacologic methods are available, there is little to guide the clinician in how to practically address these issues in the day-to-day workings of a busy medical practice. The basic question becomes not *should* we use nonpharmacological techniques but rather *how can* we use them to our patients' best advantage within the realistic parameters of today's health care.

In this chapter, we review nonpharmacologic methods clinicians will want to integrate into their existing practice of cancer pain management. We focus particularly on simple yet effective communication and educational methods that can be used in any medical practice by any professional treating the cancer patient with pain. We then add information on physical methods of pain relief and provide additional detail on more specialized cognitive-behavioral approaches used by psychologists and other behavioral medicine specialists.

## BACKGROUND

Nonpharmacological approaches are not alternatives to medical treatment; they are valuable adjuncts. One of the most significant roles of nonpharmacologic approaches is to contribute a wider perspective. By providing a broader view of pain management, nonpharmacologic strategies become tools to assist the clinician in identifying stumbling blocks that may be impeding care or suggesting options that may improve patient well-being with no side effects.

All of the methods we discuss are intended to be integrated with medical care. These strategies require the patient to be a participant in this care. They are largely based on verbal methods, which require patients to be interested, willing to be involved, able to maintain adequate attention, and capable of providing some feedback. These requirements are not so different from what is needed of any patient who must be involved in his or her care. Even to take pills as prescribed, a patient must understand the prescription, ask questions when information is unclear, and be willing to follow the treatment recommended. All of these methods work best when they are used early in treatment as part of a comprehensive treatment plan, when patients are motivated, when patients are not excessively fatigued, and when they are not distracted by severe pain. When employed in this way, nonpharmacologic approaches optimize the effectiveness of medical treatment.

These strategies are targeted for use with any patient who is experiencing discomfort. Because we know that psychological factors are influential but not causal in the maintenance of cancer pain symptoms (6,7), we know that any patient can benefit from these strategies—not only those patients in psychological distress or who have a psychiatric diagnosis (8–10). Of course, those patients who do not meet the criteria mentioned above and who are in continuous, severe, disease-related pain will need aggressive medical treatment prior to use of nonpharma-

K. L. Syrjala: Department of Behavioral Sciences, University of Washington School of Medicine, Fred Hutchinson Cancer Research Center, Seattle, WA 98104-1024.

S. L. Roth-Roemer: Department of Psychiatry and Behavioral Sciences, University of Washington School of Medicine, Fred Hutchinson Cancer Research Center, Seattle, WA 98104-1024.

cologic methods. Patients with delirium or severe psychiatric disruption in their functioning will need additional care beyond the methods we will discuss.

Because pain is always a subjective experience with sensory, cognitive, affective, and behavioral components, it is experienced and expressed through how we feel, think, and act. Furthermore, we depend on patients to provide us with these multidimensional cues before we can determine a treatment for pain. Thoughts, feelings, and behaviors are the sources of our information for medical treatment and they are the targets of nonpharmacologic interventions for managing cancer pain. Cognitive-behavioral methods are based on the established fact that how people think and behave affects how they feel. For example, a patient may worriedly complain of leg pain during a follow-up visit with his oncologist. When questioned, the patient may report that the last time he experienced a similar pain it presaged his relapse. As worry about a recurrence escalates, his experience of pain increases accordingly. When the physician asks the patient what activity he did over the past two days, the patient remembers that he walked a much greater distance than usual during his daily walk. This brief conversation suggests another explanation for the leg pain, the meaning of the pain changes, and as the threat from the pain decreases, so does the patient's experience of the pain.

Of course, not all patient discomfort is as simple to ease as in the above example, yet it does help to clarify the relationship between how we think and what we experience. If we can help people to change how they think about their pain, then we can help to change how they feel, behave, and even how they perceive sensations (11). For example, we move people's thoughts from: "This pain is so bad, what if it just keeps getting worse and worse until I'll finally be glad to die," to "I'm hurting, what can I do, I should take another pill before the pain gets too bad. Maybe I'll try some soothing imagery while I'm waiting for the pill to work."

While cognitive strategies were originally developed for treating depression, these methods have been adapted for the treatment of chronic pain and cancer pain (10,12,13). We have found that most cancer patients do not have the maladaptive cognitions and behaviors often found in depression but that some of these methods can still be of benefit to a majority of patients. Thus we have simplified a number of these strategies for use in busy medical practices with generally psychologically healthy people, but the foundation remains the same.

Through the integrated use of nonpharmacologic techniques we can more clearly define the treatment needs of our patients. We help patients understand their symptoms and treatments while also helping them to think about their sensations in more familiar and less frightening ways. As patients understand what is happening to them, their symptoms begin to seem more manageable and their sense of control over their situation increases. They become active participants in their care. For some patients, the introduction of more specialized interventions can offer treatments that patients can learn to do themselves, facilitating even more active participation in their own symptom management.

## ADHERENCE TO MEDICAL TREATMENT

This is a seriously underrecognized problem in the treatment of cancer pain. Most oncologists have told us, "My patients take all of their treatment. They do everything I tell them to because they re so motivated to live." Although this may be true with chemotherapy, when we have gone into patients' homes or they have come to talk to us, we have found a very different picture with regard to symptom-related medications. In this arena, patients act on their own beliefs or their families' beliefs; they are much more likely to adjust doses, to skip doses, and to simply stop taking a medication because they do not like a side effect or are afraid of what they might experience. In part this may be because we need to give people flexible dosing ranges and because we do not spend enough time discussing the value of these medications. Perhaps in giving them less information, but more opportunity for self-control, patients exercise this control by, more often than not, figuring that less is better and none is best.

While extensive discussion has taken place regarding need for increased education of physicians and nurses, far less effort has been directed to understanding patient and family reluctance to take medication as prescribed. The literature on compliance makes it clear as to just how difficult this area is to assess, much less to intervene. Yet the literature is unequivocal that patients in general are shockingly different in their medication usage than their health care providers believe (14). For example, in patients with chronic illness and multiple medications (a description that fits our cancer patients), *80%* of these people do not take their medications as prescribed, and the vast majority of the departures from prescription involve reductions in medications, not increases (14). To solve the problem of inadequate treatment of cancer pain, we must begin to recognize that these descriptions do fit our patients. When patients beliefs do not conform to what we tell them to do, they will not argue with us or even ask questions, but will nod their heads and then proceed to act on their beliefs.

Good evidence of this comes from surveys and taped interviews between physicians and patients. In a survey of ambulatory rehabilitation patients, when asked to indicate how important information was to them, on a possible range from 14 = "not at all important" to 70 = "very important," on all topics the mean score was 65 out of a possible 70 (15). In other words, patients wanted equal information on all topics. They could not select the relative importance of information. Yet these same patients, when tape-recorded with their doctors, initiated an average of three comments, and 28% initiated no comments at all.

When asked why they do not ask more questions, patients say that they don't know what to ask or that there are so many possible questions that they don't know where to start or which questions are important. Furthermore, as with all of us, when we think we know an answer, we don't ask the question. Thus patients have said to us: "I know they save morphine until you're dying" or "I know morphine is addictive." The physician will never hear a question from these patients, will not know that such thoughts are on these patients' minds, but the patients will do anything possible not to take morphine.

For cancer patients the topic of pain is very emotionally laden, and they often believe that pain is inevitable. If pain is inevitable, untreatable, and frightening, what is the use in talking or even thinking about it? The importance of beliefs in influencing pain treatment behavior, the difficulty patients have in knowing what to ask their physicians and nurses, and the strong resistance patients have to taking more pills and especially to taking pills that give them side effects have led us to conclude that we as health care providers must take the initiative in addressing those issues that we know are important to determining whether patients will receive good symptom relief or will be left on their own to suffer unnecessarily.

## INTERVENTIONS FOR PHYSICIANS, NURSES AND OTHER HEALTH CARE PROVIDERS

Communication is the most basic intervention used in patient care. At a time when illness-related concerns become the focus of a patient's and family's thinking, communications with the medical staff are given enormous significance. Words and behaviors are repeated, overinterpreted, and scrutinized for underlying messages. Most often the family uses the medical team as a basis for both their unspoken and spoken rules, beliefs, and behaviors (16). Nurses and physicians routinely convey information; they listen, they reassure patients and family members, and they actively educate patients about both the pain and potential treatments. Each of these interactions can enhance patients' beliefs in their ability to cope with the symptoms, can foster adherence to the medical plan, or, conversely, can escalate patient fear or helplessness often without signaling the health care provider that this is happening.

Patients turn the words of the medical team into internal "cognitions" or thoughts that can either increase fear or provide reassurance when they have pain or other unfamiliar experiences. When the medical team is aware of the types of communication they are providing they can positively influence these cognitions; when they remain unaware of the importance of their words, an opportunity

**TABLE 1.** *Interventions used by all health care providers*

| Interventions | Goals |
| --- | --- |
| Assessment | |
| 0–10 scale for usual and worst pain | Define pain and treatment needs |
| Words to describe pain | Begin use of a shared language |
| Other information about pain | Educate patients in the concepts needed to determine adequate treatment |
| Information | |
| Describe procedure | Make the unknown normal and predictable (we are in control, we know what will happen, what is happening is as expected) |
| Describe sensations with similes | Make familiar ("there is that feeling") |
| "like an insect sting" | Decrease threat |
| "a pull like a strong vacuum cleaner" | Increase tolerance |
| Define time frame | Remember it is not forever |
| Education | |
| How to use treatment prescribed | Improve adherence |
| Myths that disrupt treatment | Reduce fears, counter myths |
| Side effect treatment | Reduce secondary effects of treatment |
| When to call the doctor | Enhance control while improving understanding |
| Easy reframing | |
| What is going well | Increase sense of control |
| What the patient has accomplished | Give a different perspective |
| Quick distraction and imagery | |
| Pleasant place | Evoke pleasure, distract from discomfort |
| Image to counter sensation | Transform sensation |
| Physical methods | |
| Heat and cold | Transform sensation, distract |
| Massage | Relax, evoke pleasure, counter discomfort |
| Expression of thoughts and feelings | Reduce fear and preoccupation; increase feeling can cope |

can be lost or this valuable tool can be unintentionally misused. One of the valuable contributions physicians, nurses, or health care providers can make to the long-term mental health of patients and their families is to model, by example, the acceptability of talking about and planning for pain management, disease progression, and even dying.

## STANDARD PRACTICE TOOLS

In order to provide comprehensive pain management, the following tools should be understood by all practitioners:

1. Assessment
2. Information provision
3. Education
4. Easy reframing
5. Quick distraction and imagery
6. Physical methods
7. Expression of thoughts and feelings

Table 1 lists the communication and physical method tools all health care providers use in regular practice that will either help or hinder patient and family coping efforts. Many of these methods are already part of your practice. They can be used in any communication with patients. Used with insight, these strategies can be strikingly effective in making your work easier while helping patients manage their own pain.

## ASSESSMENT STRATEGIES

Pain assessment is the cornerstone of both pharmacologic and nonpharmacologic techniques. It begins the process of communication that determines medical treatment and begins to teach patients how to think about their pain. By asking the same questions at each assessment and giving the patient some options for answers, the physician and patient begin to develop a common language for communication, e.g., does your pain feel like burning, shooting, electric, or pins and needles, or is it an aching, gnawing, pressing, or throbbing kind of pain? The patient begins to recognize different qualities in pain, and the physician begins to determine whether intervention should be oriented to neuropathic and/or nociceptive treatments. Inadequate assessment will be the first step to inadequate treatment (1,17); adequate assessment may well be the first step to facilitating patient adherence and participation in treatment. In our recent study of an educational intervention for cancer-related pain (9), a patient called to thank us profusely "for teaching me so much about pain. It changed my life and gave me a mission for the time I have left." At first we thanked her but then were quite confused when we realized that she was in the control group that did not receive the pain education. With

further discussion, she told us how she learned so much from our assessment of her pain in the study that it changed the information she gave her doctor and this changed her treatment, bringing her far more pain relief.

If specific questions are not asked during the pain assessment and patients are not given some of the options for how to answer the questions, patients are unlikely to volunteer the information needed by a clinician to adequately determine treatment needs. Cancer patients often do not know what experiences are "normal" or what should be reported. A pain score, rated on a scale from 0 (no pain) to 10 (as much pain as can be), becomes an "objective" tool to determine the need for further evaluation or change in treatment. Pain above a score of 3 or 4 indicates a need to assess more dimensions of the pain experience than just pain severity (18,19).

## INFORMATION PROVISION

Whenever possible, we try to make the unfamiliar more predictable for our patients by informing them of what is going to happen. This can be very reassuring for patients because uncertainty is known to increase distress and threaten one's perceptions of his or her ability to cope (20). Yet the informed consent process used in many hospitals emphasizes provision of medical information that patients often do not fully comprehend (21). The process forces patients to recognize the limits of their own (and the medical staffs') control over the outcome of treatment. Although this process is necessary, it emphasizes the negative and makes it more difficult for patients to believe in their own influence over outcomes.

Some of the effects of this informed consent process and the overall uncertainty about what will happen can be countered by providing other specific information about what is known. Specific information can help patients to "label" their sensations with familiar, less frightening terms. Information can also give patients a way of "reframing," or thinking about their situation from a less threatening or more in-control perspective.

Three kinds of information are helpful to patients:

1. Describing procedures
2. Describing sensations
3. Defining the time frame

*Describing procedures* provides patients with specific information about what will happen or is happening. By giving patients a concrete description of the steps that will occur, patients can remind themselves that what is happening is to be *expected*. It is essential to include the *benign* steps in this description ("you'll sit on the bed and bend your back, we'll clean your back with antiseptic"), not only the invasive steps ("we'll stick a needle into your spine"). This helps patients balance events in a way that reminds them that most of what is happening is nonthreatening. When patients know what to expect, their uncertainty is reduced, which in turn increases confidence that the situation is under control.

*Describing sensations* helps patients because it tells them exactly *how* they will feel. Using specific descriptions of sensations helps patients to label what they feel with familiar, comprehensible terms. Vague terms such as "pain" or "hurt" leave patients worrying about what to expect and whether they will be able to tolerate it. Even something unpleasant can be made less threatening by associating it with something familiar. Describing a sensation as "like an insect sting" or "hot" or "pressure" does not deny discomfort; rather, it allows patients to prepare themselves for specific sensations. When the sensations occur, patients are then able to reassure themselves that these feelings are *expected and familiar*. Use of a simile can be very helpful when describing a sensation and reminding the patient that the experience is tolerable (e.g., "When I pull the marrow, you may feel a pull all the way down your legs as if a strong vacuum cleaner is pulling on your back"). While the feelings are not pleasant, they can be more tolerable and less threatening.

*Time frame* information may be the most important, particularly with pain resulting from procedures or treatment, or when it is brief but recurrent. Telling patients when something is likely to happen and approximately how long it will last is the most useful information we can provide (22). For most people, just knowing there will be an end makes an unpleasant event considerably more tolerable than thinking it might last forever. It is particularly helpful to break the timing of events into the smallest time frames possible. So, for instance, we do not talk about a bone marrow aspiration as taking "only 20 minutes." We break the aspiration down into sections. The local anesthetic might take 30 seconds; the pressure of the needle going into the bone marrow might take 5 seconds; feeling of the pull might take another 10 seconds. Although the overall procedure might take 20 minutes including preparation, we help patients to recognize that the painful section lasts for less than 2 minutes and that most of the procedure is not painful at all. For any of us, our belief in our ability to tolerate 2 minutes of intense discomfort is much greater than our belief that we can withstand 20 minutes of intense physical pain.

In general, procedural information is the most frequently provided form of information; however, it is typically less useful in reducing distress than temporal or sensory information (23,24). The exception to this guideline is the extremely anxious patient who needs a great deal of control. For these patients, procedural information is equally important with temporal and sensory information. At its extreme, these patients may be terrified to the point of phobia or refusal to continue care. For the small number of patients who are phobic of a procedure or cannot tolerate distraction away from the procedure, we recommend systematic desensitization and/or light sedation

(25). If awake, these patients need to receive constant feedback from the person doing the procedure and need opportunities to be in control of the timing of the procedure whenever possible. With these highly anxious, control-oriented patients, there is a tendency for physicians and nurses to want to get the procedure over with as quickly as possible to reduce the patient's distress. Thus we see them pushing ahead as fast as possible while the patient fights all the way. It does initially take longer to slow down and give patients time to gather their control, and to let them say when it is okay to go on to the next step. However, if this extra time is taken with these uncommon patients, the long-term distress and the resistance to further treatment will be far less. For repeat procedures, a psychologist can assist by providing systematic desensitization.

Ideally, patients will receive all three types of information for the greatest effect on pain and distress. Procedure and sensation information work best when provided prior to beginning any new process to familiarize and normalize the experience. During the procedure, the focus can shift onto time frame information and active distraction so that thoughts may be focused away from discomforts that cannot be alleviated. Sensation and procedure information provided in combination have been shown to be superior to sensory information alone in the reduction of patient pain and distress (26).

## EDUCATION

Whereas information provides facts, education requires an interactive process in which patients must acquire and then use knowledge to direct their own behavior. Education does more than label an experience; it allows patients to take the information presented to them, adapt it to their situation, and adjust their coping accordingly. Education involves both the telling of facts and a discussion of patients' questions and concerns. For example, the patient who is underusing prescribed opioids for fear of becoming addicted may be more likely to use the appropriate amount of drug after having had a chance to discuss those concerns with the physician, has learned that addiction is not a concern in cancer patients, and has asked questions about this information.

Clinicians are often frustrated by patients who are given information but seem not to hear it. Anxiety, unfamiliarity, and the medications we use in cancer treatment may impact our patients' ability to retain educational information. Benzodiazepines used for sleep, anxiety, or as antiemetics impair memory (27–29). Data also indicate that opioids, while having minimal effects on most areas of function, do restrict learning and retention of new information (30–32). So while patients may appear to comprehend information immediately during their office visit, they may not be able to retain this information for later recall at home. In addition to these medical aspects of learning interference, the anxiety and helplessness brought about by a cancer diagnosis, and compounded by the experience of unremitting pain, can also make retaining information a difficult task. Recognizing these limitations can help us to consider ways to overcome them.

Concerns about negative effects of educating patients sometimes arise from fears that discussing possible side effects will over-sensitize patients to symptoms. Available research indicates that informing patients about possible side effects of therapy does not increase the occurrence of side effects or have other adverse effects (33,34).

Education can be particularly helpful in addressing patient fears. Mounting evidence supports the observation that patients and their families not only fear cancer pain but believe that pain cannot be effectively controlled without unacceptable consequences. A survey in Wisconsin (35) found 72% of the respondents agreeing that cancer pain can get so bad that a person might consider suicide; 39% agreed that strong pain killers are an indication that a patient is close to death. In relation to effects of opioids, 70% expressed concerns about tolerance; 70% expressed concerns about mental confusion; 63% identified addiction as a concern. In research on cancer patients' beliefs about cancer pain, Ward and colleagues (3,5) reported that a majority of cancer patients and their family members have concerns that pain will not be controlled during the course of the disease. Furthermore, the majority have misperceptions about tolerance, side effects, and addiction. These concerns can interfere with adequate pain treatment. When patients who return home to treat themselves believe that opioids are dangerous, they will not adhere to their physicians' prescriptions of oral medications no matter how effective such treatment might be.

Several educational intervention studies have demonstrated the effectiveness of education as a pain management tool. Rimer and colleagues (36) found that cancer patients who received medication-related education had higher compliance with analgesic medications and had fewer concerns about taking opioids. Furthermore, patients who received training tended to report lower pain levels when compared to the untrained control group. In a study targeted to elderly patients with cancer and their family caregivers, Ferrell and colleagues (37) evaluated a three-part structured pain education program during home care visits. The 66 patients, some with caregivers, received general information about pain, education on pharmacologic interventions, and education about nonpharmacologic interventions such as heat, cold, massage, relaxation, distraction, and imagery. Patients showed increases in knowledge and attitudes toward pain, as well as increases in compliance with pharmacologic and nonpharmacologic treatment. In a recently completed randomized controlled clinical trial we conducted (9), adult cancer patients received either a pain videotape with a handbook and brief nursing intervention or a nutrition videotape with written materials and brief nursing nutrition intervention. Patients who received the pain education demonstrated significant increases in understanding about pain management and decreases in pain report when compared to the nutrition group. These changes remained in three follow-up evaluations out to 6 months following the intervention.

What is the best way to provide educational information to patients? Messerli and colleagues (38) surveyed postmastectomy patients and their surgeons about what the patients identified as their most important sources of education. Whereas surgeons identified talking with a sensitive, understanding doctor as the most important resource, patients identified written materials as their most important source of information. In addition, patients rated having an opportunity to speak with other patients, information from nurses, and receiving videotaped information as useful. Talking with a sensitive, understanding doctor was ranked eighth as a useful source of information. In essence, patients do not want to bother their doctors and do not think of their physicians as a primary source for learning about their treatment.

**TABLE 2.** *Education needs of patients and family members*

1. What treatments are prescribed.
2. When to use treatment: how often, how much at a time.
3. How to know when more medication is needed (e.g., pain is >3 on a 0–10 scale).
4. What symptoms to be concerned about.
5. What symptoms not to be concerned about.
6. There are many treatment options, if something isn't working, there are many other possible treatment choices.
7. Addiction is not a concern.
8. Tolerance will not be a problem; the medication will not stop working.
9. Report symptoms promptly so pain can be treated. Not treating pain can have serious negative health effects.
10. Side effects can be treated; do not stop taking medication if a side effect occurs; treat the side effect or call the doctor.
11. Things to tell the doctor about pain.
12. How to get in touch:
    Who to call (name and number).
    When to call.
    What to say.

These results suggest that physicians will have to specifically ask about symptoms and offer information if they wish to communicate with and educate patients. With time demands on practice, it is equally important to note that written materials, videos, and communication with nurses can be acceptable substitutes for direct education from the physician *as long as the information is reinforced by the physician's communications.* Numerous booklets, books, and videotapes are available to use as educational tools with patients and should be incorporated into routine oncology practice (39–42). Written materials are particularly valuable because they reduce the burden of having to retain information solely in memory. Specific education needs of patients and their family members are listed in Table 2. These targets for education should be addressed when pain is mild and when opioids are first needed.

## EASY REFRAMING

Reframing means, quite simply, thinking about a threatening situation in a different way that reduces its threat. If physicians remember that their exact words will be retained and repeated over and over by patients and families, and if they use this fact to actively choose words to influence patient and family perception, this will be one of the simplest and most helpful strategies they can use. While most patients and families look for statements that offer hope, they will also hang on to negative information. It can be extremely valuable, when providing day-to-day feedback about the patient's condition, to include statements about what is going well without being misleading. It is always possible to find specific positive accomplishments.

Reframing provides an opportunity to look at the situation from a more neutral or positive perspective. When entering the room, symptoms, problems, and patient concerns can be addressed first. This allows patients to express concerns and helps validate their experiences. Next, patients can be asked about what they have been doing and about symptoms the clinician believes they do *not* have. Finally, to reinforce what has just occurred, the clinician can comment on the many accomplishments of the patient and family and on those areas of functioning that are not problematic. For example: "You have been able to walk a little bit each day. That's wonderful— it will help you keep your strength." For a very ill patient for whom getting out of bed is a huge effort, the acknowledgment may be quite different: "You've been able to get a sponge bath. That's great. I know that must have taken a lot of energy and effort." Although the accomplishment may seem small, the patient knows how much energy the activity took and will appreciate having this recognized. In this way the clinician can acknowledge the problems that are of concern to the patient and family, while also

helping them to recognize that no matter how difficult the situation, there are things that are not problems and they are doing a good job. This simple, positive perspective can do much to contribute to feelings of control, self-efficacy, and overall good feelings for patients and their families.

The essence of reframing is to (a) acknowledge and validate the problems; (b) widen the perspective to include things that are not problems and to include specific accomplishments of the patient; and (c) give the patient credit for the accomplishment so that the patient feels recognized and proud of what he or she is doing.

## QUICK DISTRACTION AND IMAGERY

When pain is of brief duration and/or medical treatment cannot reduce discomforts, rather than focusing on the pain, it can be helpful to assist patients in placing their attention elsewhere. This can be accomplished through using simple strategies such as talking to patients about pleasant experiences they have had, helping them to focus on their breathing, or massaging or applying pressure to an area away from the pain. Having the patient tell you a story can also help to engage him or her away from the discomfort. When using this strategy, it is important to elicit from the patient a story that recalls a place where he or she felt particularly at ease and happy. For example, you can ask patients to tell you about a favorite vacation or a favorite place. Encourage them to share as much detail as possible: what the place looks like, the sounds, the feelings, the temperature, the activities available there. Patients can become so engrossed in the reliving of that experience that they become unaware of their pain in the present moment. Recounting these positive events evokes feelings of pleasure which in turn block perceptions of the painful experience.

Brief imagery also can be used to counteract the sensory qualities of pain. To change the pain itself, one can take the patient's description of sensation and create an image to counter this sensory quality. For burning, stabbing pain we might have the patient focus on deep breathing while imagining blowing freezing Arctic air through the sensation; with extreme pressure in the abdomen, we might use an image of a heavy weight lifting off the painful area, lifting higher with each exhalation.

For quick and easy imagery or distraction, the following components are helpful to keep in mind. Have the patient choose an image or participate in the selection so that it is relevant. For intense pain, an image that includes physical action by the patient will be more engaging of attention than a passive, purely relaxing image. Having the patient talk rather than just listen to you helps to maintain his or her focus. Sound made by the patient, whether talking, breathing out through the mouth with a "whooshing" sound, or any other sound, seems to counter acute pain better than silent imagination. Physical stimulus to the patient will help counter the pain stimulus. This can be squeezing the shoulder, having the patient squeeze your hand, having a family member massage feet or hands, or including physical stimulus in the imagery exercise. The goal is to create as much input into the brain as possible in order to flood the brain with non-pain messages and to prevent the pain message from being received.

## PHYSICAL METHODS

Thus far, we have focused largely on verbal methods of relieving pain. Physical methods, such as heat, cold, and massage, are also nonpharmacologic techniques that allow patients and family members to participate in providing pain relief. While no controlled clinical trials establish the efficacy of these methods (43), in clinical reports these techniques are received well by patients and are reported to provide some relief (37,44). Advantages of these methods are that they provide physical contact for patients, they have few (but can have some) side effects, and they give family members an opportunity to be involved, while at the same time they may directly reduce pain.

Choice of heat, cold, or massage and of the technique depends on trial and error. As a rule, patients are more easily convinced to use heat than cold, but cold can be as effective, or more effective, and relief may last longer (37,45,46). Alternating between heat and cold can also be an effective option.

Massage may be most easily accepted by patients and requires the least preparation. It generally requires another person willing to assist, although mechanical massagers can be used. Massage also does not come with the potential risks of heat and cold; as long as sensory perception is intact, the patient's indication of comfort is adequate to ensure safety. Massage of the back and shoulders, of hands, or of feet have reduced pain in clinical reports (37,47,48). Use of a lotion, massage oil, or powder helps reduce friction on the skin. Movements should almost always be continuous, even, and rhythmic (44).

Applying heat can be done with hot-water bottles, electric heating pads, hot moist compresses, bath, or whirlpool/hot tub. Applying cold can be done with ice and water combined in a waterproof bag, terry cloth filled with ice and wrung out, frozen gel packs, bags of frozen peas or corn hit to gently loosen contents. All options should be sealed to prevent dripping, should be wrapped as needed to prevent skin irritation or burning, and should be flexible to conform to body contours. Location directly on the pain or proximal, distal, or contralateral to the pain is a question of trial and error and patient tolerance (44). Patients should be instructed to stop when the area becomes numb, excessively red, blisters, or when they want to. Time of use to be effective

ranges from 5 to 30 minutes. Patients should not sit or lie on the heat or cold packs. Heat should not be used directly over tumor sites (49). Other contraindications include use over a recent radiation therapy site where skin may be more sensitive, if bleeding is occurring, if patients have impaired sensation, or if skin blanches and turns red after application of cold. Those clinicians wishing to integrate these methods into practice are encouraged to obtain more detailed information (44,50).

## IMPORTANCE OF EXPRESSING THOUGHTS AND FEELINGS

The presence of distress, especially distress specific to the pain or cancer situation, will contribute to the patient's perception of pain (7). For patients who are acutely anxious related to a procedure, or who are generally anxious about their pain or cancer, a chance to express their thoughts, concerns, and feelings is essential prior to continuing with any of the nonpharmacologic methods described above. The fact is that patients who are preoccupied will not hear information, will not learn what they need to about their treatment, will not hear reframes, and will not benefit from the distractions of imagery or massage. Consequently, they will be less likely to adhere to treatment. These are the patients who will require more attention and time in the future and will have poorer pain relief. Ten minutes of expressing feelings and addressing concerns can save numerous future appointments and can in itself contribute significantly to improved outcome (51,52). As we discuss below in the section on structured support, talking and expressing concerns has been nearly as effective as more advanced techniques in relieving cancer pain (8,10).

## SPECIALIZED COGNITIVE-BEHAVIORAL INTERVENTIONS

There are times when brief strategies are not enough to manage a chronic or recurring pain. At such times it can be helpful to consult with a psychologist or other behavioral medicine specialist who can help the patient learn more specialized cognitive-behavioral pain management techniques. Table 3 lists coping strategies used most often by psychologists, social workers, nurses, or psychiatrists after specialized training. Because these are skills that can be taught to the patient for use when a therapist is not present, they can be excellent methods for increasing coping options, self-confidence, and self-control of pain. Most practitioners combine the techniques described below into a package of coping skills. The exception is hypnosis, which is often combined only with support for effective pain reduction (8,53).

Although there has been considerable interest in the use of psychological interventions for cancer pain man-

**TABLE 3.** *Specialized cognitive-behavioral interventions*

| Intervention | Assists with |
|---|---|
| Active coping | Reminds of competence |
|   Gather information | Defines the problem and possible solutions |
|   Seek assistance | Reduces aloneness with the problem |
|   Specify plan | Takes back control |
|   Define actions | Takes charge by doing something |
| Distraction | Stimulation competes with pain sensations |
|   Focus on mental activity | Blocks attention to pain |
|   Focus on physical activity | Addition of pleasure to daily experience |
| Relaxation/imagery/hypnosis | Possible neuroendocrine changes |
|   Relaxation | Reduction of autonomic arousal and tension |
|     Progressive muscle relaxation | Learn to identify and change tension |
|     Deep breathing | Learn control over somatic states |
|   Imagery/hypnosis | Mental activity competes with pain |
|     Pleasant places | Introduces feelings incompatible with pain |
|     Analgesic images | Blocks pain sensations |
| Reframing | Reminds the situation is manageable |
| | Reminds of competence |
| Structured support | Decreases isolation/alienation |
| | Allows expression of feelings |
| | May reduce somatic expression of tension, anxiety, depression |

agement, few controlled clinical trials have examined the utility of these techniques. We have completed two prospective studies testing the efficacy of cognitive-behavioral skills training for pain related to bone marrow transplantation for cancer. In both clinical trials we found that when training was completed before cancer treatment, patients learned the skills with brief (two-session) training and used the methods to reduce severe pain even when opioids were used concurrently. The first study randomly assigned patients to one of four groups: hypnosis training, cognitive-behavioral training without hypnosis or imagery, therapist attention control without psychotherapeutic treatment, and standard medical treatment control (53). The two active intervention groups received two sessions of training pretransplant and had two half-hour "booster" sessions per week in the hospital. The hypnosis group reported significantly less pain than all other groups, without using significantly more opioids. In a second trial, we (10) modified the original four groups. The hypnosis group was renamed "relaxation with imagery"; the cognitive-behavioral group included relaxation and imagery along with cognitive skills of distraction and reframing; the third group was active supportive therapy which included education and reframing by the therapist. The standard medical treatment control group received no specialized psychological intervention. The two intervention groups reported significantly less pain than the untreated group. The supportive therapy group was not significantly different from either the standard medical treatment control group or the two intervention groups. We found that patients who received active therapeutic support had lower mean pain report, but the addition of skills training decreased pain further.

A study by Fawzy and colleagues (54,55) did not look specifically at pain but did randomly assign cancer patients to an untreated control group or a group that received coping skills training consisting of four components: brief education, support, training in problem solving, and relaxation with imagery. The advantage of this study was its short duration, six weekly sessions. These researchers found that the intervention significantly reduced patient reports of fatigue and distress while increasing patient use of active cognitive and behavioral coping methods. Results remained at 6-month follow-up. Although not focused specifically on cancer pain, the methodology indicates that relatively brief, cost-effective interventions can have long-lasting results.

## Active Coping

Active coping strategies essentially teach patients to notice when they have a recurring problem or worry and to focus on finding something to do about the problem, even if they can't entirely make it go away. Once a problem is identified, we suggest three major steps:

1. *Collect information.* Talk to doctors, nurses, social workers, other patients, family. Ask them to explain the situation, ask them what can be done, ask them what else can be done if the first steps don't work, and keep asking until the patient finds useful options. Ask for or look for reading material.
2. *Think about what the patient can do to address the problem.* List these options and check them off as the patient does them.
3. *Talk to people who can offer support.* Express concerns so that the patient is not alone with fears.

Once a patient has accomplished these steps, it is time to use methods to put the problem out of his or her mind. At this point, we encourage the use of distraction, imagery, and reframing to change the thoughts one has about a problem—whether it is worry about addiction, actual pain, or other concerns that affect quality of life.

## Distraction

Similar to the quick clinician-assisted distraction strategy described above, distraction skills teach patients how to focus attention away from their discomfort on their own. Distraction is something many of us do automatically when we have exhausted our abilities to solve problems or simply want a break from problems or preoccupations. Just getting through the day comfortably may be the greatest problem for patients suffering from cancer pain. In this case, focusing attention away from discomforts can be one of the more effective coping strategies. Individuals each have their own preferred distractions. We work with patients to identify which distractions work best for them and to help them to plan when, where, and how they will use specific strategies.

Distraction is not the same as denial, which implies an inability to recognize reality. Nor is it the same as avoidance, which implies an unwillingness or inability to cope with reality. Denial can be beneficial in situations where nothing can be done to change the circumstances and focusing on fears may just increase anxiety (56). Avoidance, on the other hand, seems unhelpful as a coping strategy and is related to greater levels of distress (57). Distraction involves a willingness to accept reality while actively attempting to engage ourselves in a positive portion of it. For example, a boy with phantom limb pain resulting from the loss of his left leg to Ewing's sarcoma described how he coped with his difficulty falling asleep at night: "When I start to worry about how bad it hurts, I start to think about the baseball game I went to last week and pretty soon I don't notice the pain anymore and I fall asleep."

Some distractions involve focusing on thoughts or *mental activity*. This can include self-statements (giving encouraging messages to oneself), prayers, reading, listening to someone read, or listening to music. Focusing on pleasant images is another example. Other distractions focus on *active behaviors* such as working on a hobby, playing a game, or using deep breathing or relaxation. One of the most effective distracters reported by patients involves simply spending time with and talking with family and friends. Often the best way to focus attention away from discomfort is to create more pleasant sensations. Massage and exercise such as walking are commonly used. Regardless of the distraction, these type of activities provide a sense of achievement that reminds patients about their control over their own experience.

## Imagery/Hypnosis

Imagery is one of the most easily accepted and useful noninvasive methods for managing pain. While relaxation is not essential for imagery or hypnosis, these methods often begin with relaxation as a way for patients to "tune in" to their bodies and develop greater awareness of internal sensations as preparation for changing these sensations. Progressive muscle relaxation can be provided either by focusing on deep breathing and relaxing muscles from head to toe or by moving through the body and physically tensing and relaxing each muscle in turn (58,59). Learning to recognize the physical sensations of tension and relaxation in the various parts of the body can be helpful to patients so that they may notice tension when it occurs and relax muscles. Once patients understand relaxation and deep breathing, we explore places and events where they have felt comfortable, healthy, strong, and capable. We then help them to develop images of these "pleasant places." Nearly everyone enjoys and responds to these pleasant place images, which provide patients with an opportunity to turn their focus away from their pain and discomfort for a time. In turn, their enjoyment of the experience enhances the likelihood they will continue to use these methods.

Often we will provide an audiotape of the session for patients and ask them to practice between sessions so that they can learn to use these skills on their own, whenever they need to. We have found, as have others (37), that very few patients benefit from just buying or being given an audiotape with imagery. Most people need the connection with a person who understands their unique circumstances and can help them adapt imagery to their preferences and needs. Tapes alone can bias patients against use of imagery, as we often hear in "I tried that; it didn't work."

When possible, we incorporate suggestions for increased comfort and well-being or for analgesia in the painful area (60). Sensory transformation involving the use of images that transform the pain such as seeing the pain as an object and watching as it changes color and shape, moves to a distant location, or decreases in intensity can be very effective for brief or persistent pain (10,60–62). A very short version of this was described in the brief imagery section above.

To assist patients in applying these skills on their own we teach them the steps for using imagery and provide suggestions for how easy and automatic relaxation and imagery can be (63). It is the intentional use of suggestion that is the primary distinction between imagery and hypnosis (60,64,65). For the purpose of pain management, research does not yet allow us to clearly distinguish effects of hypnosis from those of relaxation and imagery. Because of the negative connotations of hypnosis for some patients, we usually use the term "relaxation with imagery" (66).

When in-depth imagery is not possible because the patient is not interested or does not have the needed attention span, brief imagery, or having the patient tell about a favorite experience or place, can still provide a "time out" from pain and illness. When we begin imagery training, hypnosis or imagery itself may last for 20–30 minutes. As patients become familiar with the experience and as they become more ill, sessions may be as brief as 10 minutes.

## Reframing

Just as the messages we give to patients are powerful, so are the messages patients give to themselves. Using this awareness, along with providing information, education, and active coping skills, we help patients prepare "I can cope" statements to use in the face of major stressors, specifically to address the fears of individual patients. For patients with continuous pain or who are giving themselves negative messages, we teach them to do their own reframing. Reframing involves teaching the patient to change negative, unhelpful self-talk into neutral or more positive self-statements.

We prepare these statements by first exploring the messages a person is naturally giving herself. Many patients initially deny having any helpless or self-defeating thoughts. With an accepting approach, exploration, and some provision of examples from other patients, most people acknowledge specific fears or concerns that sometimes enter their minds about what might go wrong, e.g., "This pain is so bad, I can't stand it. It's never going to end." Patients then develop alternative phrases to remind themselves of areas where they have control. Finally, we work out statements to reinforce that they are doing as well as possible in this exceptional experience. The message provided earlier becomes, "Yes, this pain is really bothering me at this moment. What can I do right now? I know that this pain won't last." It is important to emphasize that this approach is most effective when individualized. Specific self-statements and reframes must be adapted by and developed with each patient.

In discussing any cognitive modifications such as this with patients and families, it is essential to assure them that these messages alone will neither cure or kill them. They need not struggle to maintain only the "right" or only positive thoughts. Fears and helpless thoughts are normal and should be understood and tolerated as normal. At the same time, we encourage patients to use these thoughts to help identify when they need more information or when they need reassurance from someone else whose knowledge or support they value.

In addition to working out reframes with patients, we teach them to reframe for themselves. After teaching them to identify negative self-talk, times when they expect the worst, or situations that really bother them, we teach four forms of reframing:

1. Focus on what they have accomplished rather than on what remains to be done.
2. Find something positive that they will gain from the situation and focus on that: "I'm coming through this. This is hard but, I've learned that I'm stronger than I ever imagined."
3. Focus on what they would do to help someone else in the same situation: "If this were happening to your close friend, what would you do to help him or her?"
4. Focus on the temporary nature of what is difficult: "This is difficult, but I know it will not last forever. In a half hour I'll feel better."

One of our major goals in working with patients is to help them to identify aspects of their lives that they are already in control of (e.g., what they eat, what they wear, what they do for leisure). In doing so, we can then help them learn to gain greater control over their own comfort.

## Structured Support

Support is one of the essential needs of patients and family members. Social support is the most common coping strategy used by cancer patients (67). While women are particularly likely to both seek and provide emotional support, men are often more reluctant to use support and are instead more likely to focus on problem-solving types of support provision. Including education as a part of support efforts can be an effective inducement for men who otherwise might resist support groups or individual support.

The value of support is being increasingly recognized in numerous studies examining the relationship of social support to physical and emotional well-being. Recent research demonstrates that cancer patients who receive active psychological support from groups or individuals, with or without skills training, report less pain and live longer (8,10,68,69). Spiegel and Bloom (64) randomly assigned breast cancer patients to one of three groups: support group, support group plus brief hypnosis training, and no psychological treatment. Patients participated in the support groups for a year. Both support groups reported significantly less pain and suffering than the no-treatment group. The hypnosis group did not report significantly less pain than the support-only group. We have found similar results in our research (10). Lower levels of emotional distress have also been associated with the use of social support (67). The expression of feelings and the sharing of experiences involved in supportive interaction may help patients to participate more fully in medical treatment. Researchers are exploring whether these support interventions have effects on survival and function through adherence to treatment, improve treatment through greater education, improve health-related behaviors, or have neuroendocrine or immunologic effects that enhance survival (68–71).

**Psychological or Psychiatric Referrals**

Pain is among the most significant contributors to emotional distress for cancer patients (72–74). Over time, unrelieved pain can engender feelings of helplessness and hopelessness. Helplessness or hopelessness leads to depression. Worries and fears that one will not be able to cope can also result in anxiety reactions. Having to cope with numerous symptoms along with pain can also contribute to generalized distress (75).

The emotional consequences of uncontrolled pain can be so extreme that cancer patients with severe, unrelieved pain are more likely to commit suicide (76,77). Levin et al. (78) found that 69% of cancer patients would consider suicide if their pains were not adequately controlled. Of physicians who have been asked by cancer patients to assist in their deaths, combined persistent pain and terminal illness was identified as the primary reason for these requests (79).

The seriousness of these emotional responses needs to be recognized and treated. They are not simply emotions that are "to be expected," since most cancer patients are not anxious or depressed (80). Medical explanations for the physical symptoms do not mean that psychopharmacologic or psychotherapeutic treatments will not help. In patients with severe pain, the pain should be treated immediately, with psychiatric symptoms treated concurrently, or treated if they remain after pain is better controlled. In other words, never assume pain has a psychological etiology and never treat the "emotional pain" and wait to see whether the physical pain then resolves. Because of the overlap in somatic symptoms of cancer and depression, in assessing for depression and anxiety, affective and cognitive symptoms should be present in addition to somatic symptoms. Even when medications or disease are causing or contributing to the symptoms, depression can be very successfully treated pharmacologically or psychotherapeutically.

**What Works Best?**

Research indicates that nonpharmacologic interventions, when integrated with standard medical care, do reduce cancer pain. In a meta-analysis of 116 psychoeducational intervention studies conducted during the past two decades, Devine and Westlake (81) concluded that psychoeducational interventions were effective not only in increasing knowledge but also in significantly reducing cancer symptomatology, including pain, anxiety, depression, mood, nausea, and vomiting. However, distinguishing which psychoeducational strategies were more effective than others was difficult. The authors concluded that clinicians should be made aware that effective psychoeducational strategies exist and that researchers should continue to examine the relative effectiveness of different types of psychoeducational interventions.

Similarly, a recent review article (70) on a mix of randomized and nonrandomized psychosocial interventions for cancer patients supports the integrated use of psychological interventions. The authors conclude that a variety of structured interventions including education, relaxation/imagery/hypnosis, active coping training, and psychosocial support are effective in cancer symptom management when integrated into the overall medical care of the cancer patient, but no specific methods were singled out as more effective than others.

While all of the interventions described in this chapter have evidence that they are effective in relieving cancer pain, perhaps the strongest controlled clinical trial data are available for the efficacy of support combined with imagery or hypnosis (8,10,53). In a meta-analysis of cognitive behavioral interventions for pain that was not limited to cancer pain, Fernandez and Turk (82) found that all strategies were effective but that imagery consistently showed the largest effect size.

Studies such as these indicate that psychological intervention from trained clinicians helps cancer patients to manage disease-related pain and treatment-related pain. Specific content may be less important than providing the patient with skills for self-management of symptoms and conveying that the patient has the ability to cope with the pain. Our research and that of Fawzy and colleagues clearly indicates that long-term treatment is not necessary and that brief, focused interventions can be effective (10,53,70).

We are more likely to prevent difficult symptom management problems if we begin using nonpharmacologic strategies early in treatment. When pain is mild or new, patients are most open and able to learn strategies to help increase their control over symptoms. Once pain is moderate or has become chronic, patients may benefit from imagery done by a therapist but are less likely to learn new cognitive-behavioral skills for use on their own. Attention span, concentration, and energy are necessary for learning new coping skills; all of these things can be affected by disease and its treatment. When patients are sedated or confused from medical treatments or the disease, or when patients are exhausted and frustrated because all other attempts to manage the pain have failed, we have a very difficult time teaching cognitive techniques for relieving pain. Information and education are always useful, but again they are best provided when the pain problem is in an early, mild stage. Physical methods such as massage or active distraction can be introduced at any point.

Although we do not yet have strong data concerning which psychological methods of cancer pain control are best for which types of patients, clinical experience with patients experiencing pain is quite similar to reports of cancer patients who have other distressing cancer-related

**TABLE 4.** *Steps in using nonpharmacologic strategies*

| Method | Who will benefit |
|---|---|
| Training assessment for communication about pain<br>  Use of 0–10 scale<br>  Verbal descriptors of pain | All patients, but ideally early to optimize care as treatment progresses |
| Education and/or information about medical treatments and myths | All patients, as early in pain treatment as possible |
| Physical methods<br>  Massage<br>  Heat or cold | Patients with a caregiver able to assist or with adequate health to provide heat or cold on their own |
| Brief cognitive-behavioral methods<br>  Distraction, storytelling, or brief imagery | Patients with painful procedures or relatively brief pains |
|   Reframing or meaningful phrase to repeat<br>  Expression of throughts and feelings | Patients with emotional distress contributing to pain experience |
| Specialized cognitive-behavioral methods<br>  Imagery, hypnosis | Patients able to focus attention, relatively alert, with some motivation |
|   Reframing | Patients with persistent pain or with distress related to painful procedures |
|   Active coping skills<br>  Structured support | Patients with moderate to severe distress |

symptoms such as chemotherapy-related nausea and vomiting. We can use this knowledge to provide some general guidelines (see Table 4). Patients who are most anxious, who are avoidant of unpleasant topics, or who expect the physicians and nurses to be in control have difficulty learning cognitive coping skills. These patients initially need supportive listening and assistance with identification of specific areas where they have some control (51). These patients also may do well with hypnosis. After anxiety has been reduced and patients are feeling more in control of their own symptoms, cognitive-behavioral skills may be introduced.

At the other extreme, for patients who cope actively and manage anxiety well, it may be hard to measure improvement with skills training, but these patients are the most eager for active coping techniques and report them to be very effective. Patients with moderate anxiety and those who have not prepared any coping plans may benefit the most from cognitive-behavioral methods (9). These patients are often motivated to learn skills that help them to feel like participants in their care. They feel more in control of their physical reactions when they learn the skills, and they respond well to the additional support provided by the trainer.

## CONCLUSIONS

The nonpharmacologic interventions that we have described provide the clinician with simple and effective tools to assist with the management of cancer pain. In addition, these interventions give patients more control over their pain and treatment, without making them choose between pharmacologic and nonpharmacologic interventions. Because they are based on communication with the patient, the majority of these strategies can be easily used within the context of routine medical visits with the patient.

All patients need, and all clinicians can provide:

1. Assessment that teaches the patient what the physician needs to know to prescribe the appropriate treatment;
2. Procedural, sensory, and time frame information that normalizes the experience, creates nonthreatening expectations, makes the experience more predictable, and reminds the patient that the current situation is not forever;
3. Education that facilitates patient and family participation by teaching about treating pain, addressing barriers to patients reporting pain or taking medication, and informing why and when to call the doctor's office;
4. Reframes that remind patients of what is going well and help them recognize that they are do a good job of coping with a difficult situation;
5. Brief imagery that reduces focus on pain or reduces intensity of pain;
6. Physical methods of heat, cooling, or massage; and
7. Allowance for expression of worries, concerns, fears, or helpless feelings.

With specialized training, clinicians can help patients to significantly reduce pain with the use of active coping, distraction, advanced imagery or hypnosis, reframing skills, and structured support. Nonpharmacologic strategies can become part of the overall treatment plan, alongside pharmacologic treatments, to assure patients optimal pain relief and optimal quality of life.

## ACKNOWLEDGMENTS

This work was supported by grants from the National Cancer Institute (CA38552, CA57807, CA63030, and CA68139).

## REFERENCES

1. Cleeland CS, Gonin R., Hatfield AK, et al. Pain and its treatment in outpatients with metastatic cancer. *N Engl J Med* 1994;330:592.
2. Zhukovsky DS, Gorowski E, Hausdorff J, Napolitano B, Lesser M. Unmet analgesic needs in cancer patients. *J Pain Sympt Manag* 1995; 10:113.
3. Berry PE, Ward SE. Barriers to pain management in hospice: a study of family caregivers. *Hosp J* 1995;10:19.
4. Cleeland CS, Ryan KM. Pain assessment: global use of the Brief Pain Inventory (review). *Ann Acad Med Singapore* 1994;23:129.
5. Ward SE, Goldberg N, Miller-McCauley V, et al. Patient-related barriers to management of cancer pain. *Pain* 1993;52:319.
6. Elliott BA, Elliott TE, Murray DM, Braun BL, Johnson KM. Patients and family members: the role of knowledge and attitudes in cancer pain. *J Pain Sympt Manag* 1996;12:209.
7. Syrjala KL, Chapko ME. Evidence for a biopsychosocial model of cancer treatment–related pain. *Pain* 1995;61:69.
8. Spiegel D, Bloom JR. Group therapy and hypnosis reduce metastatic breast carcinoma pain. *Psychosom Med* 1983;45:333.
9. Syrjala KL, Abrams JR, Cowan J, et al. Is educating patients and families the route to relieving cancer pain? Eighth World Congress on Pain, Vancouver, BC, Canada, 1996.
10. Syrjala KL, Donaldson GW, Davis MW, Kippes M, Carr JE. Relaxation and imagery and cognitive behavioral training reduce pain during marrow transplantation: a controlled clinical trial. *Pain* 1995;63:189.
11. Beck AT, Rush AJ, Shaw BF, Emery G. *Cognitive Therapy of Depression.* New York: Guilford Press, 1979.
12. Turk DC, Meichenbaum D, Genest M. *Pain and Behavioral Medicine: a Cognitive Behavioral Perspective.* New York: Guilford Press, 1983.
13. Turner JA, Clancy S. Comparison of operant behavioral and cognitive-behavioral group treatment for chronic low back pain. *J Consult Clin Psychol* 1988;56:261.
14. DiMatteo MR, Sherbourne CD, Hays RD, et al. Physicians' characteristics influence patients' adherence to medical treatment: results from the Medical Outcomes Study. *Health Psychol* 1993;12:93.
15. Beisecker AE, Beisecker TD. Patient information-seeking behaviors when communicating with doctors. *Med Care* 1990;28:19.
16. Rait D, Lederberg M. The Family of the Cancer Patient. In: Holland JC, Rowland JH, eds. *Handbook of Psychooncology.* New York: Oxford University Press, 1989;585.
17. Von Roenn JH, Cleeland CS, Gonin R, Hatfield AK, Pandya KJ. Physician attitudes and practice in cancer pain management: a survey from the Eastern Cooperative Oncology Group. *Ann Intern Med* 1993;119: 121.
18. Cleeland CS, Syrjala KL. How to assess cancer pain. In: Turk DC, Melzack R, eds. *Handbook of Pain Assessment.* New York: Guilford Press, 1992;360.
19. Serlin RC, Mendoza TR, Nakamura Y, Edwards KF, Cleeland CS. When is cancer pain mild, moderate or severe? Grading pain severity by its interference with function. *Pain* 1995;61:277.
20. Mishel MH. Perceived uncertainty and stress in illness. *Res Nurs Health* 1984;7:163.
21. Penman PT, Holland JC, Bahna GF, et al. Informed consent for investigational chemotherapy: patients' and physicians' perceptions. *J Clin Oncol* 1984;2:849.
22. Johnson JE, Fuller SS, Endress MP, Rice VH. Altering patients' responses to surgery: an extension and replication. *Res Nurs Health* 1978;1:111.
23. Johnson JE, Rice VH, Fuller SS, Endress MP. Sensory information, instruction in a coping strategy, and recovery from surgery. *Res Nurs Health* 1978;1:4.
24. Thompson SC. Will it hurt less if I can control it? A complex answer to a simple question. *Psychol Bull* 1981;90:89.
25. Fishman B, Loscalzo M. Cognitive-behavioral interventions in management of cancer pain: principles and applications. *Med Clin North Am* 1987;71:271.
26. Suls J, Wan CK. Effects of sensory and procedural information on coping with stressful medical procedures and pain: a meta analysis. *J Consult Clin Psychol* 1989;57:372.
27. Curran HV, Gardiner JM, Java RI, Allen D. Effects of lorazepam upon recollective experience in recognition memory. *Psychopharmacology* 1993;110:374.
28. Danion JM, Peretti S, Grange D, Bilik M, Imbs JL, Singer L. Effects of chlorpromazine and lorazepam on explicit memory, repetition priming, and cognitive skill learning in healthy volunteers. *Psychopharmacology* 1992;108:345.
29. Patat A, Perault MC, Vandel B, Ulliac N, Zieleniuk I, Rosenzweig P. Lack of interaction between a new antihistamine, mizolastine, and lorazepam on psychomotor performance and memory in healthy volunteers. *Br J Clin Pharmacol* 1995;39:31.
30. Cleeland CS, Nakamura Y, Howland EW, Morgan NR, Edwards KR, Backonja M. Effects of oral morphine on cold pressor tolerance time and neuropsychological performance. *Neuropsychopharmacology, in press.*
31. Kerr B, Hill H, Coda B, et al. Concentration-related effects of morphine on cognition and motor control in human subjects. *Neuropsychopharmacology* 1991;5:157.
32. Saha N, Datta H, Sharma PL. Effect of morphine on memory: interactions with naloxone, propranolol and haloperidol. *Pharmacology* 1991;42:10.
33. Howland JS, Baker MG, Poe T. Does patient education cause side effects? A controlled trial. *J Fam Pract* 1984;31:62.
34. Wilson JF. Behavioral preparation for surgery: benefit or harm? *J Behav Med* 1981;4:79.
35. Doyle DM, Cleeland CS, Joranson DE. Wisconsin public attitudes toward cancer pain: changes over a seven year period. 10th Annual Meeting of the American Pain Society, New Orleans, 1991.
36. Rimer B, Levy MH, Keintz MK, Fox L, Engstrom P, MacElwee N. Enhancing cancer pain control regiments through patient education. *Patient Educ Counsel* 1987;10:267.
37. Ferrell BR, Ferrell BA, Ahn C, Tran K. Pain management for elderly patients with cancer at home. *Cancer* 1994;74:2139.
38. Messerli ML, Garamendi BA, Romano J. Breast cancer: information as a technique of crisis intervention. *Am J Orthopsychiatry* 1980;50: 728.
39. Agency for Health Care Policy and Research. Clinical Practice Guideline on Management of Cancer Pain. Number 9, Patient Guide. Rockville: US Dept of Health and Human Services AHCPR Publication No. 94-0595, 1994.
40. Ferrell B, Rhiner M. *Managing Cancer Pain at Home.* Duarte, CA: City of Hope National Medical Center, 1993.
41. Levy MH, Rimer B, Keintz MK, MacElwee N, Kedziera P. *No More Pain.* Philadelphia: Fox Chase Cancer Center, 1991.
42. Syrjala KL, Williams A, Niles R, Rupert J, Abrams J. *Relieving Cancer Pain.* Seattle: Academy Press, 1993.
43. Agency for Health Care Policy and Research. Clinical Practice Guideline on Management of Cancer Pain. Number 9. Rockville: US Dept of Health and Human Services AHCPR Publication No. 94-0592, 1994.
44. McCaffery M, Wolff M. Pain Relief Using Cutaneous Modalities, Positioning, and Movement. In: Turk DC, Feldman CS, eds. *Noninvasive Approaches to Pain Management in the Terminally Ill.* New York: Haworth Press, 1992;121.
45. Michlovitz SL. Cryotherapy: The Use of Cold as a Therapeutic Agent. In: Michlovitz SL, ed. *Thermal Agents in Rehabilitation.* Philadelphia: FA Davis, 1990;63.
46. Ramler D, Roberts J. A comparison of cold and warm sitz baths for relief of postpartum perineal pain. *J Obstet Gynecol Neonatal Nurs* 1986;15:471.
47. Cyriax JH. Clinical Applications of Massage. In: Basmajian JB, ed. *Manipulation, Traction and Massage*, 3rd ed. Baltimore: Williams and Wilkins, 1985;270.
48. Weinrich SP, Weinrich MC. The effect of massage on pain in cancer patients. *Appl Nurs Res* 1990;3:140.
49. Lehmann JF, deLateur BJ. Therapeutic Heat. In: Lehmann JF, ed. *Therapeutic Heat and Cold*, 4th ed. Baltimore: Williams and Wilkins, 1990;417.
50. McCaffery M, Beebe A. *Pain: Clinical Manual for Nursing Practice.* St. Louis: CV Mosby, 1989.
51. Burish TG, Tope DM. Psychological techniques for controlling the adverse side effects of cancer chemotherapy: findings from a decade of research. *J Pain Sympt Manag* 1992;7:287.
52. Hathaway, D. Effect of preoperative instruction on postoperative outcomes: a meta-analysis. *Nurs Res* 1986;35:269.
53. Syrjala KL, Cummings C, Donaldson G. Hypnosis or cognitive-behavioral training for the reduction of pain and nausea during cancer treatment: a controlled clinical trial. *Pain* 1992;48:137.

54. Fawzy FI, Cousins N, Fawzy NW, Kemeny ME, Elashoff R, Morton D. A structured psychiatric intervention for cancer patients. I. Changes over time in methods of coping and affective disturbance. *Arch Gen Psychiatry* 1990;47:720.
55. Fawzy FI, Kemeny ME, Fawzy NW, et al. A structured psychiatric intervention for cancer patients. II. Changes over time in immunological measures. *Arch Gen Psychiatry* 1990;47:729.
56. Lazurus RS, Folkman S. *Stress, Appraisal, and Coping.* New York: Springer, 1984;117.
57. Vitaliano PP, Maiuro RD, Russo J, et al. Coping profiles associated with psychiatric, physical health, work, and family problems. *Health Psychol* 1990;9:348.
58. Bernstein DA, Borkevic TD. *Progressive Relaxation Training.* Champaign, IL: Research Press, 1973.
59. Syrjala KL. Relaxation Technique. In: Bonica JJ, Chapman CR, Fordyce WE, Loeser J, eds. *The Management of Pain*, 2nd ed. Philadelphia: Lea & Febiger, 1990;1742.
60. Syrjala KL, Abrams JA. Hypnosis and Imagery in the Treatment of Pain. In: Gatchel RJ, Turk DC, eds. *Chronic Pain: Psychological Perspectives on Treatment.* New York: Guilford Press, 1996;231.
61. Dahlgren LA, Kurtz RM, Strube MJ, Malone MD. Differential effects of hypnotic suggestion on multiple dimensions of pain. *J Pain Symptom Manage* 1995;10:464.
62. Kiernan BD, Dane JR, Phillips LH, Price DD. Hypnotic analgesia reduces R-III nociceptive reflex: further evidence concerning the multifactorial nature of hypnotic analgesia. *Pain* 1995;60:39.
63. Syrjala KL, Danis B, Abrams JR, Keenan R. *Coping Skills for Bone Marrow Transplantation.* Seattle: Printex Press, 1992.
64. Barber J. Hypnosis. In: Bonica JJ, Chapman CR, Fordyce WE, Loeser J, eds. *The Management of Pain*, 2nd ed. Philadelphia: Lea & Febiger, 1990;733.
65. Hilgard ER, Hilgard JR. *Hypnosis in the Relief of Pain.* Los Altos, CA: William Kaufmann, 1975.
66. Hendler CS, Redd WH. Fear of hypnosis: the role of labeling in patients' acceptance of behavioral interventions. *Behav Ther* 1986;17:2.
67. Dunkel-Shetter C, Feinstein LG, Taylor SE, Falke RL. Patterns of coping with cancer. *Health Psychol* 1992;11:79.
68. Fawzy FI, Fawzy NW, Hyun CS, et al. Malignant melanoma: effects of an early structured psychiatric intervention, coping, and affective state on recurrence and survival 6 years later. *Arch Gen Psychiatry* 1993;50:681.
69. Spiegel D, Kraemer HC, Bloom JR, Gottheil E. Effect of psychosocial treatment on survival of patients with metastatic breast cancer. *Lancet* 1989;2:888.
70. Fawzy FI, Fawzy NW, Arndt LA, Pasnau RO. Critical review of psychosocial interventions in cancer care. *Arch Gen Psychiatry* 1995;52:100.
71. Redd WH, Silberfarb PM, Andersen BL, et al. Physiologic and psychobehavioral research in oncology. *Cancer* 1991;67:813.
72. Heim HM, Oei TP. Comparison of prostate cancer patients with and without pain. *Pain* 1993;53:159.
73. Lancee WJ, Vachon ML, Ghadirian P, Adair W, Conway B, Dryer D. The impact of pain and impaired role performance on distress in persons with cancer. *Can J Psychiatry* 1994;39:617.
74. Massie MJ, Holland JC. Depression and the cancer patient. *J Clin Psychiatry* 1990;51:12.
75. Portenoy RK, Thaler HT, Kornblith A, et al. Symptom prevalence, characteristics and distress in a cancer population. *Qual Life Res* 1994;3:183.
76. Breitbart W. Suicide. In: Holland JC, Rowland JH, eds. *Handbook of Psychooncology.* New York: Oxford University Press, 1989;291.
77. Foley KM. The relationship of pain and symptom management to patient requests for physician-assisted suicide. *J Pain Sympt Manag* 1991;6:289.
78. Levin DN, Cleeland CS, Dar R. Public attitudes towards cancer pain. *Cancer* 1985;56:2337.
79. Helig S. The San Francisco Medical Society euthanasia survey. Results and analysis. *San Francisco Med* 1988;61:24.
80. Derogatis LR, Morrow GR, Fetting J, et al. The prevalence of psychiatric disorders among cancer patients. *JAMA* 1983;249:751.
81. Devine EC, Westlake SK. The effects of psychoeducational care provided to adults with cancer: Meta-analysis of 116 studies. *Oncol Nurs Forum* 1995;22:1369.
82. Fernandez E, Turk DC. The utility of cognitive coping strategies for altering pain perception: a meta-analysis. *Pain* 1989;38:123.

*Principles and Practice of Supportive Oncology,*
edited by Ann Berger et al.
Lippincott–Raven Publishers, Philadelphia ©1998

CHAPTER 5

# Interventional Approaches in Oncologic Pain Management

Lloyd R. Saberski

## THE PHILOSOPHY OF INTERVENTIONAL PAIN MANAGEMENT IN CANCER PAIN

A shortcoming of cancer pain therapy, as it is now practiced, is the lack of anticipation for change. Cancer pain is a dynamic process that can progress to the point at which specialized interventions are required and an ever more vigilant and dedicated team is needed to steer the patient and family through the evolving stages of the disease. The latter stages of disease often take a natural course and the clinician who offers specialized interventions should strive to be a partner with the patient rather than a distant director. For example, provision of information on death and dying is a part of supportive care and should be addressed by those who implement interventional approaches (1).

It is common for cancer pain to require a balanced analgesic program that takes advantage of the potential synergy among approaches. In general, no singular approach is a panacea. Interventional therapies, for example, must be balanced by medical and behavioral therapies and by appropriate psychosocial interventions. The approaches chosen should have enough flexibility to accommodate future change. The use of techniques that lack flexibility can mean more trips to providers, thereby defeating a goal of supportive care: to allow patients to maximally enjoy life with family and friends, and to minimize dependency or attachment to health care providers.

A few principles govern the use of interventional approaches: (a) examine the painful region because review of laboratory and radiographic studies alone is never sufficient; (b) always attempt to establish a diagnosis and/or a mechanism for the symptomatology; (c) try

to optimize the balance between efficacy and side effects of therapy; (d) do not rely on high tech to replace practical solutions; for the vast majority of patients, specialized interventional pain management procedures are unnecessary; (e) in most cases, withhold interventional approaches until an optimal oral analgesic regimen fails.

Approximately 60–80% of patients with advanced cancer develop significant pain before death (2). In general, oral opioid administration is the preferred therapy because of ease of administration and widespread patient and clinician acceptance. However, a large proportion of the patients with advanced cancer will require some form of alternative opioid delivery system or an alternative analgesic intervention, which can either improve the efficacy of the systemic opioid or decrease side effects (3). The techniques chosen should not only prove effective medically but should be affordable and easily applied to the given clinical and social situation. The ideal approach takes advantage of the potential of any given patient and allows for the highest level of independence. Although dependence on others may be unavoidable for the cancer patient, therapeutic programs that promote dependency can be counterproductive. In most cases, patients with progressive medical diseases have months or years before the terminal phase. Thus the clinician must strive to avoid interventions that tether the patient and their families. When planning supportive care, the clinician must not only know pharmacology, opioid delivery systems, and ablative and stimulatory techniques, but have a familiarity with individual patient social needs.

The initial approach to analgesic therapy should follow the guidelines promulgated by the World Health Organization (WHO) (4,5). These guidelines should not be interpreted as discrete steps for the management of symptoms. There is ambiguity as to when progression of symptoms occurs, and it is best to consider that the num-

L. R. Saberski: Yale Center for Pain Management, Department of Anesthesiology, Yale-New Haven Hospital, New Haven, CT 06510.

ber of useful options increases as patients become sicker and more complex. The clinician must constantly shift gears to provide for the ever changing patient needs. Pain therapy should never be limited arbitrarily to opioid administration because alternative approaches, including interventional approaches, may offer a better outcome in an individual case.

## GENERAL PRINCIPLES OF ANESTHETIC PAIN MANAGEMENT TECHNIQUES

Making a specific diagnosis improves the chances for a successful intervention. For example, it is important to determine whether a pain is new or different from the previous pain. If the pain is familiar, further laboratory or radiographic evaluation may not be needed. If the pain changes or a new type of pain occurs, the assessment should include the appropriate tests to identify underlying structural etiology.

For most patients, pain therapy begins with an oral opioid, the dose of which is adjusted to achieve the most favorable balance between analgesia and side effects. If dosing is difficult, it is sometimes advantageous to admit the patient to the hospital or hospice unit for titration of the opioid. The amount required to make the patient comfortable during titration can determine the proper oral, intravenous, or neuraxial opioid dose. Use of a patient-controlled analgesia (PCA) system can assist in determining this requirement because the patient is instructed to press the button as often as necessary to be comfortable.

## ALTERNATIVE ROUTES OF OPIOID ADMINISTRATION

### Intravenous Route of Administration

Intravenous opioid infusion produces stable blood levels and is both safe and effective (6–8). A significant problem for the long-term use of this route is the need for intravenous (IV) access. To preserve peripheral IV access as long as possible, it is recommended that IV cannulas be inserted as distal as possible on the arm. Repetitive needle sticks into antecubital veins should be avoided in the chronically ill patient.

Long-term IV therapy usually requires an indwelling vascular access device. There are a number of options:

1. A peripheral long-line catheter is generally placed above the antecubital fossa, threaded 4–6 inches, and does not enter central venous circulation; these catheters can stay in place for several weeks, although the puncture site requires daily inspection.
2. A peripherally inserted central catheter (PICC) is threaded proximal to the antecubital veins into cen-

tral placement; these devices can remain in position for several months.
3. A Hickman-type catheter is inserted surgically in an operating room, usually into the subclavian vein; these devices can be multichannel to accommodate multiple IV therapies, and usually remain in place for 6 months to a year.
4. A subcutaneous access device (Port-a-Cath type) is placed in the central circulation and is totally implanted, which allows bathing without special precautions; the skin must be pierced to access the port but needles can remain in situ for many days and the device itself can be used for years.

The optimal type of IV opioid delivery depends on the availability of the resources and location of the patient (home versus hospice versus hospital). Intermittent bolus injections can be administered by nurses, family members, or the patient. The boluses can be delivered through a capped intravenous access device using a syringe or a demand infusion device. Continuous infusion can be delivered through a gravity-dependent device or a volumetric or pressure-dependent pump system. PCA systems can provide infusions with on-demand boluses. This technique facilitates patient independence and decreases demands on health care providers. Also, such devices enable the providers to easily quantitate opioid requirements for conversion to oral or any other route of administration because patients are instructed to hit the button until they are comfortable.

### Intramuscular Injection

Intramuscular injection should be avoided whenever possible. There is variable response that depends on technique and tissue perfusion. There is also significant patient discomfort with each injection and a risk of troublesome bolus effects (peak concentration toxicity or pain recurrence at the trough). The injection is often not deposited in muscle but placed into poorly perfused adipose tissue.

### Subcutaneous Delivery of Opioids

The subcutaneous (SC) route of delivery is a well-tolerated and effective alternative to oral opioid (9,10). This route can be implemented in the home or inpatient setting. However, an infrastructure must be in place to readily respond to a patient's changing needs. Adequate teaching of patient and family is required (11). SC injection of opioid can be given in the abdomen, chest wall, thigh, or arm. In general, delivery should be into areas that are well perfused. For long-term continuous therapy, a standard 25- to 27-gauge butterfly needle or a commercially available SC needle that enters the skin perpendicularly can be used. SC needles can be left in place for a week but a daily inspection is necessary. Either intermittent or continuous SC delivery can be used. Continuous infusions are preferred, but in situations of limited resources, the intermittent SC injection of an opioid into a capped butterfly is effective when applied on a time-contingent basis. If larger volumes are needed, the injection must be slow to minimize discomfort.

Nonportable or portable pumps can be used for continuous SC infusion. With such devices, the pressure generated by the pump must exceed the resistive forces of the subcutaneous tissues. The opioid is concentrated in accordance to the patient's requirements and the number of cassette or bag changes planned each week. This, of course, is determined by the size of the bags and the cassettes, the availability of nursing resources and/or family, and the patient's ability to participate in the therapy. Many of the portable pumps have 100-ml cassettes and cost savings can be achieved if changes can be limited to twice per week or less.

SC infusion at high flow rates (more than 2–3 ml/hour) can often be accomplished by adding hyaluronidase (e.g., 0.6 units/ml) to the infusate. The long-term stability of hyaluronidase combined with opioid is unknown and hyaluronidase is generally reserved for patients who require daily changes of an infusion bag or only have access to a gravity infusion device rather than a pump. Using hyaluronidase, SC infusion rates of more than 80 ml/hour can be achieved (12).

SC infusion can also be implemented using a pump with a patient-controlled analgesia option. PCA allows the patient to determine the proper dose and maintain a greater degree of control. This flexibility is usually well received by patients. The concentration of infusate should be adjusted to keep total SC volumes less than 2 ml/hour. Because SC absorption requires time, the interval between demand doses should be set at 20–30 minutes. Thus, the maximum number of demand doses delivered per hour is between two and three.

### Sublingual and Buccal Mucosal Delivery of Opioid

Sublingual and buccal mucosal delivery may be an alternative to oral administration. These routes have the potential for rapid absorption and direct passage into systemic circulation without first-pass hepatic metabolism (13). Unfortunately, there are numerous variables that influence absorption, including the length of time the patient keeps the opioid in the buccal mucosa; the degree of mixing with saliva; the pH of the oral cavity; the $pK_a$, the lipid-water partition coefficient, the molecular weight, and the rate of partition of the un-ionized form of the drug (14). There is limited clinical experience with the sublingual or buccal routes in the treatment of cancer pain. If either of these routes is perceived to be necessary,

the following points should be considered: (a) commercially available tablets can be used and are preferred over liquids because liquids mix with saliva and increase the chances of being swallowed; (b) the patient should not swallow for approximately 5 minutes; (c) the dosing interval is the same as for oral opioid; (d) any opioid can be used, but those that are lipophilic (fentanyl, methadone, buprenorphine), as opposed to hydrophilic (morphine), are better absorbed (15); (e) if adequate clinical effect is not obtained with a standard opioid preparation, then consideration can be given to alkalization of the oral mucosa to a pH of 8.5; this increases the un-ionized fraction of the opioid (15), improves absorption, and increases the likelihood of achieving an adequate plasma level.

### Rectal Delivery of Opioid

Preliminary evidence suggests that morphine can be administered rectally in a variety of forms, including aqueous solutions, suppositories, and commercially available tablets, including both immediate release and slow release formulations. Although there is large interpatient variability, acceptable absorption has been observed for all of these preparations (14). It appears that a portion of the absorbed rectal opioid bypasses first-pass hepatic metabolism. If so, the plasma opioid level may be higher than that achieved by oral dose but less than a parenteral dose. In the case of a slow release opioid, one study indicated that the plasma levels for rectal administration were practically identical to oral administration (16). This result is perhaps secondary to the slower rate of absorption for slow release morphine.

### Transdermal Delivery of Opioid

There is currently one commercially available transdermal opioid system, which delivers fentanyl. After steady-state plasma concentration is achieved, the apparent elimination half-life is typically 15–24 hours (17). This long half-life results from ongoing absorption from a subcutaneous depot of drug after the patch is removed. The fentanyl transdermal systems are available in four sizes: 25, 50, 75, and 100 μg/hour. Cancer patients use the transdermal fentanyl for their basal continuous delivery of opioid. Breakthrough medication is usually provided with a short-acting opioid, such as morphine elixir or tablets.

### Inhalation Route of Opioid Delivery

The pulmonary route of administration can be an alternative way to deliver opioid medication and may also decrease the sensation of dyspnea often associated with chronic lung disease (18). Studies have suggested that approximately 15–30% of the opioid reaches the lung when delivered through standard nebulizers (19). Chrubasik et al. randomized 20 patients with postsurgical pain to a continuous-plus-on-demand infusion of inhaled morphine from the oxygen supply's nebulization reservoir versus morphine administered by IV infusion; no significant differences in pain control were found (20).

**Neuraxial Opioid Therapy**

The neuraxial delivery of opioids evolved from the discovery of opioid receptors in the spinal cord and was first used in humans in 1979 (21).These techniques are now commonplace. In the cancer population, less invasive management usually proves adequate (22) and neuraxial opioid delivery should be used only when pain is refractory to less invasive treatments or there are intolerable and untreatable opioid side effects (23,24). For those who do not benefit from systemic opioids, intraspinal opioids can be a major advance. The current literature documents the efficacy of implanted systems for long-term neuraxial delivery of opioid drugs in the management of malignant (25–34) and nonmalignant pain (35–38).

The selection of an intraspinal delivery system is determined by the patient's clinical circumstances, availability of resources, and patient and family understanding and acceptance of the techniques. Before placement of a permanent opioid delivery device, testing with a temporary catheter is suggested. This cannot be carried out if an intraventricular route of opioid administration is chosen, and on occasion clinical circumstances may mitigate against such a trial for the spinal route as well. Once implanted, trained support personnel must be available 24 hours a day for all of these systems.

The neuraxial systems have been classified into six types by Waldman and Coombs (39):

Type I—Percutaneous epidural or intrathecal catheter taped to the patient's back. This is placed at bedside or with radiographic guidance depending on where the catheter tip location is desired. This is the typical device used for testing purposes. It is generally kept in for periods of less than a week or for a few weeks in patients with impending death. This technique has been used for months in special circumstances, but the associated risk of infection precludes this practice on a general basis.

Type II—Percutaneous intrathecal or epidural catheter placement that is either tunneled a few inches from the insertion site using a Tuohy needle as the tunneler or tunneled around the flank in an operating room. The quick bedside procedure is generally done for patients who have a life expectancy not greater than 4 weeks and have difficulty getting to the operating room. The catheter tunneled in the operating room can have a Dacron cuff for security against pull-outs and an antimicrobial secreting cuff to protect against cutaneous infections (40).

Type III—Implanted epidural or intrathecal catheter, tunneled across the flank and attached to an internal injection port that is accessed with a noncoring needle. Such devices are good for more than a year and provide the flexibility of being attached to external drug delivery systems.

Type IV—Implanted intrathecal or epidural catheter, tunneled across the flank and attached to manually activated pumps. This type is not frequently used.

Type V—Implanted intrathecal or epidural catheter, tunneled across the flank and attached to a totally implanted pump that delivers a continuous infusion of opioid at a set rate. The amount of medication is increased or decreased by adjusting the concentration of opioid in the reservoir of the pump.

Type VI—Totally implanted programmable pumps that can deliver from 0.025 to 0.9 ml/hour. This device can be used only for intrathecal placement because the reservoir volume is small. Various bolusing options can be programmed into the pump. However, there is currently no true PCA element.

***Selection of a Neuraxial Delivery System: Epidural, Intrathecal, or Intraventricular***

An intrathecal catheter is technically the easiest type of system to insert. Back-flow of cerebrospinal fluid at the catheter tip confirms its subarachnoid placement. This catheter is less likely to be obstructed by tumor or fibrosis. Very small doses are effective in providing analgesia and, consequently, there is a lower likelihood of systemically mediated side effects with increasing doses. The risk of meningitis is higher, however, and there is a possibility of dural puncture-related leaks and headaches. The delivery systems must be completely implanted (internalized) to minimize infection. The implanted usually systems usually cannot accommodate additional intraspinal drugs because reservoirs have limited capacity. Long-term intraspinal delivery is via programmable pumps implanted surgically into a subcutaneous pocket (25,28).

The catheter for epidural opioid administration should be placed as close as possible to the segmental spinal level receiving input from the site of pain (41,42). The likelihood of meningitis is less than with a subarachnoid catheter and there is less risk of postdural puncture headache and cerebrospinal fluid leaks. There is the risk of catheter migration to a subdural or subarachnoid location, which may result in a serious adverse event. With an epidural system, there is more flexibility in terms of drug combinations and permissible volumes because the catheter is connected to an external pump. The major disadvantage of this route is the likelihood of clogging after 3–6 months, which may be due to epidural fibrosis or tumor. As dose escalation is required, there may be a relatively greater likelihood of systemic side effects than with intrathecal delivery.

Prior to placement of intrathecal/epidural catheters, magnetic resonance imaging (MRI) or computerized tomography (CT) should be performed to ensure that the needle introducer does not go through tumor. If there are significant epidural metastases cephalad and caudad from anticipated needle placement, it may be advantageous to place an intrathecal device, since transport/diffusion of epidural opioid may not be predictable in such circumstance. If there is significant tumor in the region of catheter insertion, the patient may require a catheter at a more rostral level, which can be directed caudad, or require an intraventricular system.

The intraventricular route is usually considered for refractory craniofacial pain but likely works for pain at most sites (43–46). There is little experience with this modality and the risk of infection is a major concern.

### Choice of Opioid

Any opioid can be used for intraspinal administration, assuming that the drug can reach the appropriate receptors. Receptor delivery of opioid is dependent on catheter placement, concentration and volume of the infused opioid, and the lipid solubility of the opioid. A less lipid-soluble opioid will migrate further cephalad and caudad than a more lipid-soluble opioid. Thus, the catheter should be placed as close to the lesion as possible. In the case of epidural placement, a mixture of two different opioids can sometimes be used to take advantage of their different lipid solubilities. Traditionally, preservative-free morphine has been chosen for spinal opioid administration. This is because of reluctance to use opioids containing preservative. This is a costly practice, however, and there is no clear indication that epidurally administered preservative-containing morphine is unsafe in cancer patients. One survey indicated that the chlorobutanol preservative in morphine was not neurotoxic in more than 57,000 epidural injections (40). In the absence of definitive data, it is still recommended that preservative-free opioid be used for intrathecal and intraventricular administration.

### Dose of Opioid

The dose chosen during neuraxial opioid administration depends on technique selected and patient requirements. There is, however, no substitution for titration. Based on clinical experience, the equianalgesic dose of morphine for various routes is oral/parenteral/epidural/intrathecal 300:100:10:1; i.e., the subarachnoid dose is 10 times less than the epidural dose, the epidural dose is 10 times less than the parenteral dose, and the parenteral dose is 3 times less than the oral dose. Hydromorphone is the common second choice for cancer pain and the comparable doses through various routes for this opioid are oral/parenteral/epidural 20:5:1.

### Choice of Adjuvants

Additive or synergistic effects may be achieved by the neuraxial infusion of an opioid combined with another analgesic. The most widely used agents are dilute local anesthetics. Unfortunately, these drugs are difficult to administer intrathecally for prolonged periods of time because adequate volumes for effective distribution are difficult to achieve in totally implanted pump systems. However, local anesthetics, with or without opioids, have been used intrathecally in patients with pain resistant to opioids alone (47–50). There are numerous other agents that can be coadministered with opioids but have not yet achieved widespread acceptance. For example, droperidol can be added to epidural or intrathecal solutions (51–53), and clonidine has proved effective for some neuropathic pain states (54–58). Similarly, antinociceptive efficacy of neuraxially administered somatostatin (59,60) and its synthetic analog octreotide (61,62), calcitonin (63,64), ketamine (65), midazolam (66), baclofen (67), and various α-adrenergic adenosine analogs (68) has been reported.

## REGIONAL ANALGESIA WITH LOCAL ANESTHETICS

Regional analgesia with local anesthetics can be used for diagnostic and therapeutic purposes. Local anesthetic blocks when properly utilized can help to ascertain the specific nociceptive pathways, to define the mechanisms of cancer pain, and to help define the site of noxious stimuli.

Therapeutic blocks with local anesthetics can be used for a variety of purposes. For example, these procedures can provide prompt relief in patients suffering from excruciating pain, temporizing for hours to days until a more definitive treatment plan can be evolved and implemented. Nerve blocks or plexus blocks can be utilized to relieve severe regional pain; for example, a brachial plexus block can relieve arm pain. Continuous segmental epidural block can also provide a regional block for hours to days, or even longer (71–75) and can also be used to help patients with sympathetically maintained pain. The side effects of segmental epidural block include hypotension and motor weakness. Dilute concentrations of local anesthetics can be used in combination with opioids to overcome some of these side effects. Patient-controlled epidural analgesia (PCEA) using local anesthetics, with or without opioids, has been used successfully in postoperative and obstetric patients (76) and can also be used for cancer patients.

Cervicothoracic sympathetic blocks can be effective in treating burning pain experienced by some patients with head and neck cancer. Repeated sympathetic blocks with local anesthetics have also been shown to be effective in treating the symptomatology of causalgia and other complex regional pain syndromes (CRPS), which occasionally afflict the cancer patients with tumor invasion of brachial or lumbosacral plexus (69,70).

Therapeutic local anesthetic blocks can also be used to supplement pharmacologic therapy in patients with less severe pain. For example, injections of local anesthetic into trigger points can ameliorate the pain of myofascial syndromes, which can develop in cancer patients.

## BASIC TENETS OF NEURODESTRUCTIVE TECHNOLOGY

The effective use of opioids and adjuvant analgesics has made it possible to effectively treat greater than 70% of patients with cancer pain (77). Neurolytic blocks should be considered for localized pain that has not responded to conservative techniques. It should be noted that most cancer patients develop multiple sources of pain (78). Thus neurolytic blocks must be used in conjunction with a pain management strategy individualized for the patient. Neuroablation does not stand alone as a therapeutic intervention but is usually combined with medical, psychological, and other therapies to provide a balanced analgesic program.

In most instances, neurolysis is not considered unless a diagnostic block has been performed with a local anesthetic. Although a negative diagnostic block contraindicates a neurolytic procedure, a positive diagnostic block unfortunately does not guarantee a good outcome. The reasons for this are multifactorial and include block-related phenomena, such as lack of blockade specificity and placebo effects. Additional pathways not initially recognized to be carrying nociceptive information exist and these, along with other factors like the development of central pain in conjunction with peripheral pain, the presence of afferent fibers that enter through the ventral spinal cord, the presence of psychological pathology, and lack of specificity of diagnostic neural blockade, all contribute to failure of neurolytic procedures (79). The clinician has little control over most of these factors, but their recognition should sensitize the physician, improve navigation of the patient through the health care system, and perhaps increase the likelihood of success.

### Diagnostic Nerve Block

Because the decision to carry out a neurolytic procedure depends upon the results of a diagnostic nerve block, the need to carry out each block meticulously cannot be overemphasized. To obtain successful regional anesthesia in the operating room environment, it has become customary for anesthesiologists to use large volumes of local anesthetic to achieve various nerve blocks. Although this approach developed out of convenience and operating room needs, as opposed to utility in chronic pain management, it is often used for diagnostic nerve blocks. For example, the stellate ganglion block, frequently used as an adjunct to surgery in order to improve upper extremity perfusion, has been ritualistically performed with 10-ml volumes. Such volumes have been shown to spill onto other somatic fibers (80) and produce a somatic blockade that is generally partial and usually missed on cursory physical exam; it can be discerned, however, with quantitative sensory testing (81,82).

The use of large volumes for diagnostic nerve blocks can affect the precision of needle placement and may not be the preferred technique. When more precise needle placement is desired, such as when considering neurolysis, imaging should be used. Using CT for needle placement during stellate ganglion block, for example, can reduce the volume required from 10 ml to 1.5–3 ml (83). Nerve stimulators can also be used to enhance the precision of needle placement.

The clinician should be aware of the effects of systemic absorption of local anesthetic during diagnostic block. Small amounts of systemically absorbed local anesthetic can improve the pain of a number of neuropathic conditions (84–86). This effect can yield pain relief that is not directly due to neural blockade. Like the placebo response, it reduces the predictive value of nerve blocks. Over one third of patients are placebo responders (87,88). To reduce the importance of the placebo response, careful execution and interpretation of diagnostic nerve blocks is essential. Blinded cross-over injections, alternating between active and inert ingredients, is one way of proceeding.

### Percutaneous Chemical Neurodestructive Technique

Chemical neurolysis (usually the injection of alcohol or phenol) is an important adjunct to pharmacologic therapy for cancer pain. Rarely does neurolysis totally eliminate all painful sensation. The goal of such therapy is to improve the effectiveness of a balanced analgesia program, with reduction of medication side effects and an enhancement of activities. One must remember that neurolytic techniques have a narrow risk/benefit ratio and careful patient selection is required, in addition to a complete informed consent.

The first reported use of neurolytic blockade is probably by Lutton in 1863, who described the injection of an irritant solution into painful areas (89). Since then, phenol and alcohol have been used extensively for neurolysis (90). The primary effect appears to be the denaturing of protein and nonselective damage to neural tissue, both of which are dose-related (91,92). Despite the permanence of alcohol- and phenol-induced neurotoxicity, pain relief is not permanent. This is often the case because of tumor progression and incomplete afferent fiber destruction.

Thus, there is a wide range in outcome after chemical neurodestructive blockade (range 2–6 months, with a mean of 4 months) (93).

Phenol produces segmental demyelination and Wallerian degeneration. Axonal injuries are apparent only after high concentrations (greater than 5%), or with long or repeated exposures (94). The use of lower concentrations produces less damage, and this possibility of a titratable injury is exploited during epidural phenol neurolysis. The local anesthetic properties of phenol initially led investigators to assume that phenol selectively injured smaller myelinated fibers more so than alcohol. However, this has been shown to be incorrect (93). Phenol does have a greater affinity for vascular tissue than for phospholipids and many clinicians avoid phenol near large vascular structures such as the aorta and the inferior vena cava (celiac plexus block).

Alcohol acts by extraction of cholesterol, phospholipid, and cerebroside from neural tissue, leading to precipitation of lipoproteins and mucoproteins. Thus, alcohol injures the myelin sheath and Wallerian degeneration occurs. Partial preservation of the myelin sheath is thought helpful in preventing formation of painful neuroma.

The varying baricities of alcohol and phenol are important for intrathecal injection. Phenol is hyperbaric and will layer out on the dependent side. Alcohol is hypobaric and floats away from gravity's pull. Thus positioning prior to intrathecal injection is critical. Indeed, the decision to use one of these drugs over the other is often a function of which position is most comfortable or practical for the patient to assume for the procedure. Baricity is not a factor for injection into sites outside of the subarachnoid space.

Complications of chemical neurolysis are secondary to either improper placement of the neurolytic solution or systemic absorption. The incidence of local complications from misplaced alcohol/phenol can be minimized by using appropriate radiographic support and meticulous local anesthetic testing. The chances for systemic absorption increase when injecting near blood vessels. This is of little consequence for alcohol but is significant for phenol. Absorbed alcohol will raise the patient's serum osmolarity and render them inebriated. Doses of phenol exceeding 1000 mg can be excitatory to the central nervous system, precipitate seizures, induce renal failure, and be injurious to vascular structures.

### Chemical Neurolytic Techniques

It is essential that the clinicians who perform neuroablative procedures be fully aware of the regional anatomy required for any given procedure. A thorough knowledge of neuroanatomy and regional anesthesia is required. The detailed descriptions that follow may be supplemented by standard anatomy textbooks (95).

### Subarachnoid Neurolysis

The aim of subarachnoid neurolysis is to produce a chemical posterior rhizotomy and interrupt the pain pathways from the affected area. First used in 1955 (96), the technique has become popular because of its relative ease of use. The procedure can be performed at cervical, thoracic, and lumbar subarachnoid spaces. Thoracic injections are the least risky because efferent outflow to limbs are caudad and cephalad. Subarachnoid neurolysis at the lumbar level, though possible at the bedside without specialized equipment, should preferably be carried out in a radiology suite to confirm subarachnoid placement of the needle with injection of radiopaque contrast. Patient selection is important. This procedure is reserved for terminally ill patients who are prepared to accept the risk of bladder, bowel, or motor compromise. If phenol is chosen as the neurolytic agent, 5–6% in glycerine or 7–10% in ionic contrast is used. Alternatively, absolute (100%) alcohol is used.

To perform the neurolysis, the patient is positioned carefully at an approximate 45° angle to permit movement of the alcohol (painful site nondependent) or phenol (painful site dependent) onto the dorsal afferents. Next, a needle is placed into the subarachnoid space and the neurolytic drug is administered at 0.2 ml per injection. The patient is assessed for the location of dysesthesias and a neurologic examination is repeated carefully. Dysesthesia and developing sensory deficits should correlate with the location of pain. If not, the patient is repositioned or the procedure abandoned. If weakness develops, the procedure should be stopped. The total volume injected ranges from 0.5 to 2.0 ml.

When a patient has multisegmental pain, placement of a needle at each involved interspace avoids a single large-volume injection that has more chance of spillage. After injection, the patient is kept in position for 20 minutes. The block produced by phenol tends to be less dense and of shorter duration when compared to the equivalent blockade with alcohol. Alcohol subarachnoid neurolysis achieves peak effect within 5 days and phenol within 2 days. It is not uncommon to require a second injection in up to 20% of the patients. If a repeat block also turns out to be ineffective, an alternative management technique should be sought (97). The incidence of urinary/bowel difficulties after intrathecal neurolysis is about 25% (98).

### Epidural Neurolysis

Epidural neurolysis has not achieved the level of popularity of the subarachnoid neurolytic technique. In part, this is because epidural injection generally requires repeated exposure. However, the risk of spread to the cranial cavity and meningeal irritation is avoided and the incidence of sphincter dysfunction, weakness, and headache should be less. No controlled studies have been conducted comparing epidural and subarachnoid neurolysis with phenol. The technique popularized by Racz et al. during the 1980s (99) requires placement of a phenol-resistant catheter on one side of the epidural space, with the tip of the catheter placed midway between upper and lower limits of the nerve roots to be lysed. Thus, unilateral lesions can be achieved with proper positioning. The phenol diffuses across the dura at an unpredictable rate and it is necessary to titrate this drug to effect. The patient is positioned such that they are in a lateral decubitus position at approximately 30°. The 6–8% phenol mixed in nonionic contrast is injected, 0.5 ml at a time. Each injection is monitored carefully with real-time fluoroscopy. The patient's position is adjusted to ensure layering of the contrast over the roots of interest. If motor blockade is obtained, no further injection is performed that day. However, if the motor block dissipates and there is return of pain, additional careful titration of epidural phenol can continue. Patients will usually require three to five epidural phenol injections.

### Peripheral Chemical Neurolysis

Peripheral chemical neurolysis has been used extensively for malignant and nonmalignant pain syndromes (100). Most frequently used on branches of the trigeminal, glossopharyngeal, and vagus nerves for head and neck malignancies (101), it has also been used effectively to treat entrapment neuropathy, neuroma, perineal pain, and coccydynia. The largest experience involves muscle motor point and lumbar paravertebral somatic blockade for intractable spasticity. Peripheral neurolysis carries the risk of additional injury to nerve and development of deafferentation pain (anesthesia dolorosa). For these reasons, peripheral chemical neurolysis is seldom a first-choice approach in the management of chronic pain.

### Autonomic Blockade

Autonomic blockade can be beneficial for a variety of nonmalignant and malignant pain syndromes. Autonomic blockade entails blockade of either pure sympathetic fibers, as in the case of stellate ganglion block, lumbar sympathetic block, and blockade of ganglion of Walther, or blockade of visceral afferent fibers along with sympathetic fibers, as in case of celiac plexus block and hypogastric block.

*Sympathetic Blockade.* In general, pain syndromes responsive to sympathetic blockade fall into two categories: (a) ischemia-related pain and (b) sympathetically maintained neuropathic pain. Considerable care should be given to the technique used for the diagnostic sympathetic blockade that often precedes neurolysis. Use of the smallest possible volume of local anesthetic, in conjunction with appropriate imaging, improves the prognostic value of the test sympathetic block. Permanent neurolysis of the sympathetic chain should always be performed with radiographic support. This will decrease the incidence of catastrophic events, such as inadvertent intrathecal injection.

Effective sympathetic chemical neurolysis has been performed at the stellate ganglion, the lumbar paravertebral sympathetic chain, and at the ganglion of Impar (Walther). Stellate ganglion neurolysis is indicated for sympathetically maintained neuropathic pain of the face, upper extremity, and chest wall, as well as ischemic pain syndromes of the same. It has been used effectively for angina pectoris and the pain associated with acute and chronic shingles. The blockade is carried out anterior to the longus colli muscle at the level of C6–C7. Use of CT allows injection of smallest effective volume of phenol (1–3 ml).

Lumbar sympathetic neurolysis is used for sympathetically maintained pain of lower extremities, abdomen, pelvis, and genitalia, as well as ischemic pain syndromes of the same regions (102). The block is carried out at the anterior lateral border of the L2–L4 vertebrae, using C-arm radiography for imaging. Ganglion of Walther neurolysis is carried out for midline rectal and perineal pain (103), just anterior to sacrococcygeal junction.

*Visceral Blockade.* Celiac plexus and hypogastric blocks are the commonest procedures utilized for pain related to abdominal visceral organs. Celiac plexus block is most commonly used for pain associated with malignancy of hepatic, pancreatic, or gastrointestinal origin. These patients typically suffer from upper or midabdominal pain, radiating to spine (104). Various techniques of celiac plexus block have been described. All of these require fluoroscopic or CT imaging (105–107). Neurolytic solution is deposited anterior to the aorta and the superior vena cava, at the level of L1 vertebra. Intraoperative placement has been performed and has been recommended if laparotomy is planned (108). Alcohol is the preferred solution for celiac plexus neurolysis because a large volume (30–50 ml) is required and phenol in such a volume may be toxic when placed next to large vessels.

Hypogastric plexus neurolysis is used for lower abdominal and pelvic pain associated with malignancy (109). The block is carried out just anterior to the body of the S1 vertebra with 4–8 ml of phenol.

## PERCUTANEOUS THERMAL NEURODESTRUCTIVE TECHNIQUES: RADIOFREQUENCY AND CRYOLESIONING

Radiofrequency (Rf) energy for medical application dates back to the time of Cushing (1920s), who was trying to determine if it was suitable for electrical surgery. In the 1950s, Rf lesioning in the central nervous system was utilized for the first time (110). The goal was to perform a localized destructive lesion to decrease or otherwise diminish afferent input, without the risk of neurolytic chemical spillage onto critical structures. Unfortunately, there was difficulty focusing the energy and controlling the tissue temperatures. Thus, initial use of Rf energy was associated with tissue charring and boiling. The modern Rf probes are considerably smaller and allow for accurate measurement of impedance, a wide range of frequencies, accurate recording of tissue temperature, and accurate timing of lesioning.

In Rf lesioning, an insulated needle with an uninsulated tip is placed in the tissue and an electrical current is run through the needle. As the current passes into the tissues, heat is generated. The amount of heat generated is a function of the degree of tissue resistance and the current flow (111). It is interesting to note that the needle is cold at the start of the procedure but is warmed by the tissues; it eventually achieves a thermal equilibrium, which is recorded by a temperature sensor. The size of the lesion is determined by current flow, tissue resistance, and duration of the current flow. In most cases, thermal equilibrium is achieved within 1 minute. A large vascular supply to the tissues slows development of thermal equilibrium and necessitates longer durations of current flow.

The most common Rf lesions for cancer pain include percutaneous cordotomy, sympathectomy, trigeminal ganglionotomy, and dorsal root ganglionotomy (112–119). Rf cordotomy is usually performed at the C2 level. A small thermal lesion is placed within the spinothalamic tract in the spinal cord following precise placement of the needle using imaging, impedance monitoring, and stimulation. Pain relief can be obtained from contralateral C5 dermatomal level to the sacrum. Deafferentation pain can develop in those patients who survive longer than 2 years, and this procedure should be reserved for those patients who have intractable pain and relatively short life expectancies. Rf sympathectomies can be performed at lumbar, thoracic, and cervical locations. This is the preferred technique for percutaneous sympathectomy, because the procedure can be done as an outpatient, does not involve a surgical incision and is less likely to be injurious to other structures. When a patient has a monoradiculopathy secondary to tumor infiltration or other cancer-related lesion, a dorsal root ganglionotomy can be performed. This Rf technique is minimally invasive and is performed under fluoroscopic or CT guidance.

Cryoanalgesia is a technique in which low temperatures are used to interrupt afferent flow and produce pain relief. The analgesic effect of low temperature has been known to man for more than a millennium. Hippocrates (460–377 B.C.) provided the first written record of the use of ice and snow packs as a local pain-relieving technique when applied before surgery (120). Early physicians, such as Avicenna of Persia (980–1070 A.D.) and Severino of Naples (1580–1656) recorded their use of cold for pre-operative analgesia (121,122). In 1812, Napoleon's surgeon general, Baron Dominique Jean Larre, recognized that the limbs of soldiers frozen by the Prussian snow could be amputated relatively painlessly (123). Contemporary management with small hand-held cryoprobes is based on the heat absorption capacity of an expanding gas (124,125). The cryoprobes generally consist of an outer tube and a smaller inner tube that terminates in a fine nozzle. High-pressure gas (650–800 lb/in.$^2$) is passed between two tubes and is released via a small orifice into a chamber at the tip of the probe. Within the chamber, the gas expands with a substantial reduction in pressure (80–100 lb/in.$^2$) resulting in a rapid decrease in temperature, and a cooling of the probe tip. The rapid cooling of the cryoprobe produces a tip surface temperature of approximately $-70°C$ (126).

The application of cold to peripheral nerves, whether by direct cooling of localized segments or by complete immersion of tissue in a cold environment, induces a reversible conduction block. The extent and duration of the effect is dependent on the temperature attained in the tissues and the duration of exposure (127). Larger myelinated fibers cease conduction before unmyelinated fibers at 10°C, but at 0°C, all nerve fibers entrapped in the ice ball stop conducting. Fibers resume conduction upon rewarming. To obtain a prolonged effect from a cryolesion, the intracellular contents must be turned into ice crystals, which occurs when the temperature is below $-20°C$ for 1 minute (127). Prolonging the application of cold increases the size of the ice ball and this in turn increases the likelihood of the nerve being encompassed by the cryolesion. In practice, a freeze of 2–3 minutes duration produces the optimum result. Extreme temperatures, prolonged exposure, and repeated freeze–thaw cycles could, however, be beneficial for percutaneous techniques, especially when nerve localization is poor.

Histologically, the axons and myelin sheaths degenerate after cryolesion (Wallerian degeneration), but the epineurium and perineurium remain intact, thus allowing subsequent nerve regeneration. The duration of the block is a function of the rate of axonal regeneration after cryolesion, which is reported to be between 1 and 3 mm/day. Because axonal regrowth is constant, the return of sensory and motor activity is a function of distance between the cryolesion and end-organ. The absence of external damage to the nerve and the minimal inflammatory reaction following freezing ensures that regeneration is exact. Thus, the regenerating axons are unlikely to form painful neuromas. This differs from surgical and thermal lesions, which interrupt the perineurium and epineurium. Other neurolytic techniques (alcohol, phenol) can also potentially produce painful neuromas because the epineurium and perineurium are disrupted.

A cryolesion provides a temporary anesthetic block, which usually lasts for weeks to months. The result is dependent on a number of confounding variables, including operator technique and clinical circumstances. The duration of the analgesia is often longer than the time it takes for the axons to regenerate (128). The reasons for this are unclear but indicate that there is more to cryoanalgesia than the temporary disruption of axons.

A few reports suggest that cryolesions release sequestered tissue proteins or facilitate a change in protein antigenic properties (129). The result is the creation of an autoimmune response targeted at the cryolesioned tissue. The first report of an antigenic response was made by Gander and Soanes (130), who demonstrated tissue-specific autoantibodies following cryocoagulation of a male rabbit accessory gland and regression of metastatic deposits from prostatic adenocarcinoma after cryocoagulation of the primary tumor. Although the significance of these observations for pain management is unclear, they suggest that immunologic mechanisms may play a role in the analgesic response after cryoablation.

Cryoanalgesic therapy is best suited for localized painful conditions, particularly those that originate from small, well-localized lesions of peripheral nerves, such as neuromas and entrapment neuropathies (131). Prolonged block of peripheral nerves may be useful prior to surgery (preemptive analgesia) (132–135) or as a technique for postoperative pain management. Appropriately placed cryolesions can significantly reduce opioid requirements. Frequently used for postthoracotomy pain (136–141), other pains potentially amenable to cryolesioning include coccydyni; ilioinguinal, iliohypogastric, and genitofemoral neuropathies (142,143); and craniofacial pain syndromes including postherpetic neuropathy and irritative neuropathies of the supraorbital, infraorbital, mandibular, mental, auriculotemporal, posterior-auricular, and glossopharyngeal nerves.

## NEUROSURGICAL APPROACHES TO PAIN MANAGEMENT

Neuroablative surgical techniques are appropriate for less than 5% of cancer pain cases. These techniques include rhizotomy, cordotomy, myelotomy, dorsal root entry zone lesion (DREZ), sympathectomy, and hypophysectomy. Cingulotomy, pontine and mesencephalic tractotomy, and thalamotomy are rarely performed. Most of these procedures attempt to interrupt afferent pathways from the periphery into the central nervous system.

### Cordotomy

Cordotomy works best in patients with unilateral somatic pain from the torso to lower extremities. Results are less satisfactory in neuropathic pain, such as postherpetic neuropathy, and visceral pain syndromes. It is very difficult to gauge the results from the literature because cordotomy has been used for both neuropathic and somatic pain, in the presence of disease progression, and with opioid and adjuvant medication. It does appear that complete pain relief is obtained in 60–80% of the patients immediately after the procedure (144–146). At 12 months, effective pain relief is reduced to 50%. This may be because of disease progression and the development of new painful sites.

As a rule, patients with life expectancies greater than 2 years are excluded because of the potential for late-developing post-cordotomy dysesthesias. Complications of the procedure include difficulties with bowel and bladder control, paresis, and pulmonary compromise. The risk of bowel and bladder dysfunction is higher in patients with sacral pain who require a lesion close to the equator of the cord. Paresis is estimated to occur 10–20% and is secondary to posterior extension of the neuroablative lesion. High bilateral cervical cordotomies have been associated with sleep-induced apnea, which may be fatal in 50% of patients. Cordotomy can impair the function of the ipsilateral diaphragm and should generally be eschewed in patients with poor pulmonary function or those with significant disease in the contralateral lung (147). Depression has been observed in up to a third of the patients after cordotomy.

Unilateral percutaneous cordotomy usually is the preferred procedure. Open cordotomy is considered when bilateral lesions are needed. Open procedures are also an option when the patient cannot lie supine for a percutaneous radiofrequency cordotomy, and when the percutaneous technique is not available.

### Commissurotomy

Commissurotomy is an ablative procedure aimed at interrupting the nonspecific nociceptive fibers that run through the center of the spinal cord (148). Indicated for bilateral lower extremity and midline pain affecting the pelvis and perineum (149), surgical commissurotomy requires a multilevel laminotomy with exposure of the indicated lumbar or sacral elements of the cord. A percutaneous, stereotactically guided commissurotomy can be performed at the cervicomedullary junction using radiofrequency (150,151). This provides pain relief over large segments of the body including midline structures. Complications include temporary dysesthesias and apraxia. Motor function and sphincter control are usually spared with both open and closed procedures.

### Dorsal Root Entry Zone Lesion (DREZ)

The DREZ lesion appears to be highly effective for deafferentation pain caused by root avulsion (152). The procedure has been used for other types of neuropathic pain, including that caused by tumor infiltration of brachial or lumbosacral plexus and herpes virus infection (153). The DREZ lesion requires great surgical skill and is performed through a multilevel laminotomy or hemilaminotomy. Interruption of pathways is done with laser, Rf, or surgical instrumentation at the level of Lissauer's tract. This generally preserves medial motor fibers.

## Hypophysectomy

Hypophysectomy, either surgical or chemical, has been reported to be effective for widespread diffuse pain of malignant origin. The mechanism by which the pain relief is provided is unknown but is independent of pituitary hormone levels (154). It is likely that hypophysectomy results in alteration of central processing of pain. Hypophysectomy can cause life-threatening endocrinopathy such as diabetes insipidus, but this can be medically controlled. Pain relief has been described in approximately 50% of the patients [155].

## Rhizotomy and Neurectomy

Surgical dorsal rhizotomy entails section of one or more spinal dorsal roots to relieve pain in the area innervated by these roots. In contrast to chemical rhizotomy, the procedure is seldom performed. Patient selection must consider the overall health of the patient and availability of alternative techniques. Multilevel rhizotomies are frequently required, and the extensive laminectomies needed to facilitate this may not be tolerated by the debilitated cancer patient. Failure may be due to sprouting of nerves from the adjacent skin into denervated area or sprouting within the spinal cord to change the receptive field of existing neurons (156). Unmyelinated afferent fibers entering through the ventral root, which have their cell bodies in dorsal root ganglia, have also been described (157) and may explain failure of dorsal rhizotomy to relieve pain in some cases (158). Availability of newer techniques such as percutaneous dorsal rhizotomy using Rf or cryoprobe has further decreased the need of open surgical approach. Surgical rhizotomy may have a role in patients with pain in the thoracoabdominal region and in patients with pain associated with head and neck malignancy. In the latter population, upper cervical rhizotomies combined with lower cranial rhizotomies may be useful.

Peripheral neurectomy is the surgical resection of a part of the peripheral branch of a spinal or cranial nerve. It is another rarely performed procedure. Most of the peripheral nerves are mixed nerves and sectioning will compromise motor function. Long-term results are not good and pain usually returns. Complications include anesthesia dolorosa, problems related to complete denervation (such as decubiti and Charcot joints), and loss of proprioception.

## NEUROAUGMENTATION AND CANCER PAIN MANAGEMENT

There are four forms of neuroaugmentation: transcutaneous electrical stimulation (TENS), dorsal column stimulation (DCS), peripheral nerve stimulation (PNS), and deep brain stimulation (DBS). The mechanisms for the pain relief produced by these procedures is unknown but may include inhibition of afferent nociceptive input via a gate control mechanism, stimulation of enkephalin release, activation of opioid receptors, or enhanced regional blood flow. TENS should be considered in cancer patients with localized pain that is not satisfactorily responsive to medical intervention. It is minimally invasive and generally well tolerated. DCS is only considered when intractable dysesthetic pain proves refractory to medical management. Such pains can complicate disease progression or result from antineoplastic therapy. The utility of DCS and DBS is limited in pains with disease-related pain because they are inserted and adjusted to treat symptoms at the time of implantation and may not have sufficient flexibility to accommodate for disease progression. In addition, the devices often require revision of electrode position, as well as other servicing. The costs can be relatively high.

DCS is best indicated for deafferentation pain of the limbs or trunk. A test lead is placed percutaneously with fluoroscopic guidance into the epidural space. The minimally sedated patient reports the location of the electrical paresthesias. The electrode is then adjusted until the patient reports a paresthesia overlapping the area of pain. The device is then tunneled or taped to the patient's back and a period of testing usually days to weeks ensues to determine whether the patient is responsive. Placement of a permanent device is rarely indicated without trial stimulation. If the patient improves, the device can be permanently implanted. PNS is only indicated for cases of deafferentation pain confined to a single peripheral nerve—a rare occurrence in cancer pain.

There is a minimum experience with DBS for cancer pain and the procedure is currently reserved for those centers with neurosurgeons skilled in stereotactic deep brain procedures. Thalamic and hypothalamic stimulation has been used successfully in more than 500 published cases (159,160). Unfortunately, long-term follow-up has not been available. Stimulation of periaqueductal and periventricular gray appears to provide good analgesia in less than half the cancer patients (161).

## THE MANAGEMENT OF COMPLEX REGIONAL PAIN IN CANCER PATIENTS

Complex regional pain sydromes (CRPS) refer to a group of poorly understood disorders that have been recently redefined by the International Association for the Study of Pain (IASP) (162). Formerly labeled reflex sympathetic dystrophy (RSD) and causalgia, CRPS type I and type II, respectively, represent symptom complexes as opposed to true diseases with known etiologies. Some of these syndromes are maintained by sympathetic efferent outflow or circulating catecholamines. In the latter subgroup, the pain is termed sympathetically maintained and pain relief may be possible with sympatholytic therapy.

CRPS type I is a syndrome that develops after injury of any variety, possibly a relatively minor trauma. Symptoms are not limited to the distribution of a single nerve. CRPS type II is a similar pain syndrome that develops after injury to a specific nerve. In both syndromes, the pain is frequently described as burning and is made worse with movement. Allodynia and hyperalgesia may be present and not limited to the territory of the nerve injured. Abnormalities of blood flow occur, including changes in skin temperature and color. Edema is usually present. Increased or decreased sweating and impaired motor function can also be present (162).

CRPS types I or II can occur from malignancy or from its treatment (69,70). Clinicians must be aware of such potential outcomes because such cases raise the possibility of sympathetically maintained pain and suggest the utility of sympathetic blocks or other sympatholytic therapies. Depending on the severity of the symptoms and the medical condition of the patient, initial treatment may be medical or some combination of medical therapy and sympathetic blocks. As a rule, it is preferable to direct therapy at the sympathetic chain to determine if future sympathectomy is warranted. If sympathetic block is not feasible, blockade of the sympathetic efferents may be accomplished by local anesthetic injection/infusion into epidural space or peripheral nerve.

## TRANSPLANTED BIOLOGICAL PUMPS

Over the last few years, transplantation of physiologically intact and functionally active cells into the spinal subarachnoid space has emerged as a potentially viable approach to the treatment of pain. Results of studies in experimental models (163–165) and in cancer patients (166–168) suggest that transplantation of adrenal medullary tissue into the spinal subarachnoid tissue can significantly reduce pain. Adrenal medullary chromaffin cells secrete both catecholamines and opioid peptides, which act at the $\alpha_2$ and opioid receptors, respectively. In the subarachnoid space, the compounds may function independently or synergisticly to reduce pain (169–174).

One limiting factor for this technique is the availability of human donor tissue for allografts. A second problem pertains to the need to administer immunosuppressants to prevent rejection. Recently, a bovine adrenal chromaffin cell preparation encapsulated in a semi-permeable membrane has been developed. It is hoped that immunoisolation provided by encapsulating the transplanted cells will overcome the problem of rejection and the need for immunosuppressants. A multicenter trial with this bovine preparation is currently being conducted.

## CONCLUSIONS

To provide the best supportive care, good lines of communication are necessary and clinicians must be prepared for change and willing to alter therapy. In general, most patients are managed with minimally invasive techniques. The best way to ensure maximum benefit from the minimally invasive procedures is to have an overview of the risks and benefits of all interventions. Routine use of invasive therapy in pain management is unwise and rarely effective. Invasive approaches must be used as a part of a balanced analgesia program.

## REFERENCES

1. Newland SB. *How We Die: Reflections on Life's Final Chapter.* New York: Vintage Books, 1993.
2. Foley K. The treatment of cancer pain. *N Engl J Med* 1984;84:313.
3. Bruera E. Subcutaneous administration of opioids in the management of cancer pain. In: Foley K, Ventafridda V, eds. *Advances in Pain Research and Therapy,* vol 16. New York: Raven Press, 1990;203.
4. World Health Organization. Cancer Pain Relief, 2nd ed. Geneva, 1986.
5. Agency for Health Care Policy and Research, *Cancer Pain Treatment: Clinical Practice Guidelines.* Washington, DC: US. Department of Health and Human Services, 1994.
6. Fraser D. Intravenous morphine infusion for chronic pain. *Ann Intern Med* 1980;93:781.
7. Portenoy RK, Moulin DE, Rogers A, et al. IV infusion of opioids for cancer pain: clinical review and guidelines for use. *Cancer Treat Rep* 1986;70:575.
8. Citron M, Johnston-Early A, Fossieck B, et al. Safety and efficacy of continuous intravenous morphine for severe cancer pain. *Am J Med* 1984;77:199.
9. Russell P. Analgesia in terminal malignant disease *Br Med J* 1979;1: 1561.
10. Bruera E, Brenneis C, MacMillan K, et al. The use of the subcutaneous route for the administration of narcotics. *Cancer* 1988;62:407.
11. Sheehan A, Sauerbier G. Continuous subcutaneous infusion of morphine; *Oncol Nurs Forum* 1986;13:92.
12. Hays H, Hypodermoclysis for symptom control in terminal care. *Can Fam Physician* 1985;31:1253.
13. Bruera E, Ripamonti C, Alternate routes of administration of opioids for the management of cancer pain. In: Patt R, ed. *Cancer Pain.* Philadelphia: JB Lippincott, 1993;161–184.
14. De Boer AG, De Leede LGL, Breimer DD, Drug absorption by sublingual and rectal routes. *Br J Anesthesia* 1984;56:69.
15. Weinberg DS, Inturrisi CE, Reidewberg B, et al. Sublingual absorption of selected opioid analgesics. *Clin Pharmacol Ther* 1988;44:335.
16. Kaiko RF, Healy N, Pav J, et al. The comparative bioavailability of MS Contin tablets (controlled-release oral morphine) following rectal and oral administration, In Doyle D (ed), The Edinburgh Symposium on Pain Control and Medical Education 1989, Royal Society Medical Services International Congress and Symposium Series #149, London.
17. Gourlay GK, Kowalski SR, Plummer JL, et al. The transdermal administration of fentanyl in the treatment of postoperative pain: a double-blind comparison of fentanyl and placebo; *Pain* 1990;40:21.
18. Young IH, Daviskas E, Keena V. Effect of low dose nebulized morphine on exercise endurance in patients with chronic lung disease *Thorax* 1989;44:387.

19. Newman SP, Pavia D, Moren F, et al. Deposition of pressurized aerosols in the human respiratory tract, *Thorax* 1981;36:52.

20. Chrubasik J, Wust H, Griedrich G, et al. Absorption and bioavailability of nebulized morphine. *Br J Anesth* 1988;61:228.

21. Benedetti C. Intraspinal Analgesia: A historical overview. *Acta Anaesthesiol Scand* 1987;85:17.

22. Malone BT, Beye R, Walker J, Management of pain in the terminally ill by the administration of epidural narcotics. *Cancer* 1985;55:438.

23. Krames ES, Intrathecal Infusional therapies for intractable pain: Patient management guidelines. *J Pain Sympt Manag* 1993;8:36.

24. Cousins MJ. Anesthetic approaches in cancer pain. *Adv Pain Res Ther* 1990;16:249.

25. Madrid JL, Fatela LV, Alcorta J, Intermittent intrathecal morphine by means of an implantable reservoir: A survey of 100 cases. *J Pain Sympt Manag* 1988;3:67.

26. Harbaugh RE, Coombs DW, Saunders RL. Implanted continuous epidural morphine infusion system. *J Neurosurg* 1992;56:803.

27. Coombs DW, Saunders RL, Gaylor LM. Relief of continuous chronic pain by intraspinal narcotic infusion via an implanted reservoir. *JAMA* 1983;250:236.

28. Krames ES, Gershow J, Glassberg A, et al. Continuous infusion of spinally administered narcotics for the relief of pain due to malignant disorders. *Cancer* 1985;56:696.

29. Shetter AG, Hadley MN, Wilkinson E. Administration of intraspinal morphine for the treatment of cancer pain. *Neurosurgery* 1986;18:740.

30. Penn RD, Paice JA. Chronic intrathecal morphine for intractable pain. *J Neurosurg* 1986;18:740.

31. Dennis GC, DeWitty RL. Management of intractable pain in cancer patients by implantable morphine infusion systems. *J Natl Med Assoc* 1987;79:939.

32. Brazenor GA. Longterm intrathecal administration of morphine: A comparison of bolus injection via reservoir with continuous infusion by implanted pump. *Neurosurgery* 1987;21:484.

33. Onofrio BM, Yaksh TL. Long-term pain relief produced by intrathecal infusion in 53 patients; *J Neurosurg* 1990;72:200.

34. Zimmerman CG, Burchiel KM. The use of intrathecal opiates for malignant and nonmalignant pain: Management of thirty nine patients (Abstract). *Proceedings of the American Pain Society*, New Orleans, 1991.

35. Lamb SA, Hosobuchi Y. Intrathecal morphine sulphate for chronic benign pain, delivered by implanted pump delivery systems. (Abstract). *Proceedings of the International Association for Study of Pain*, Adelaide, Australia, 1990.

36. Krames ES, Lanning RM. Intrathecal infusion analgesia for nonmalignant pain (Abstract). *Proceedings of the American Pain Society*, New Orleans, 1991.

37. Burchiel KJ, Johans TJ. Management of post-herpetic neuralgia with chronic intrathecal morphine (Abstract). *Proceedings of the American Pain Society*, Los Angeles, 1995.

38. Bedder MD, Olsen KA, Flemming BM, Brown D. Diagnostic indicators for implantable infusion pumps in nonmalignant pain (Abstract). *Proceedings of the American Pain Society*, Los Angeles, 1995.

39. Waldman SD, Coombs DW. Selection of implantable narcotic delivery systems. *Anesth Analg* 1989;68:377.

40. DuPen SL, Peterson D, Bogosian, et al. A new permanent exteriorised epidural catheter for narcotic self-administration to control cancer pain. *Cancer* 1987;66:777.

41. Coombs DW Saunders RL, Gaylor LM. Epidural narcotic infusion reservoir: Implantation techniques and efficacy. *Anesthesiology* 1982;56:469.

42. Hamar O, Csomor S, Kazy Z, et al. Epidural morphine analgesia by means of a subcutaneously tunneled catheter in patients with gynecologic cancer. *Anesth Analg* 1986;65:531.

43. Lobato RD, Madrid JL, Fatela LV, et al. Intraventricular morphine for control of pain of terminal cancer patients. *J Neurosurg* 1983;59:627.

44. Roquefeuil B, Benezech J, Blanchet P, et al. Intraventricular administration of morphine in patients with neoplastic intractable pain. *Surg Neurol* 1984;21:155.

45. Cramond T, Stuart G. Intraventricular morphine for intractable pain of advanced cancer. *J Pain Sympt Manag* 1993;8:465.

46. Lenzi A, Galli G, Gandolfini M, et al. Intraventricular morphine in paraneoplastic painful syndrome of the cervicofacial region: Experience in 38 cases. *Neurosurgery* 1985;17:6.

47. Varga CA. Chronic administration of intraspinal local anesthetics in the treatment of malignant pain. *Proceedings of the American Pain Society,* October 26–29, 1989, Phoenix.

48. Krames ES, Lanning RM. Intrathecal infusional analgesia for nonmalignant pain: Analgesic efficacy of intrathecal opioid with or without bupivacaine. *J Pain Sympt Manag* 1993;8:539.

49. Coombs DW, Pageau MG, Saunders RL. Intraspinal narcotic tolerance: Preliminary experience with continuous bupivacaine HCL infusion via implanted infusion device. *Int J Artif Organs* 1982;5(6);379.

50. Berde CB, Sethna NF, Conrad LS, et al. Subarachnoid bupivacaine analgesia for seven months for a patient with a spinal cord tumor. *Anesthesiology* 1990;72:1094.

51. Bach V, Carl P, Ravlo ME, et al. Potentiation of epidural opioids with epidural droperidol. *Anesthesia* 1986;41:1116.

52. Kim KC, Stoelting RK. Effect of droperidol on the duration of analgesia and development of tolerance to intrathecal morphine. *Anesthesiology* 1980;35(suppl):S219.

53. Naji P, Farschtschian M, Wilder-Smith O, et al. Epidural droperidol and morphine for postoperative pain. *Anesth Analg* 1990;70:583.

54. Eisenach JC, Rauck RL, Buzzanell C, et al. Epidural clonidine analgesia for intractable cancer pain: Phase I. *Anesthesiology* 1989;71:647.

55. Coombs DW, Saunders RL, LaChance D, et al. Intrathecal morphine tolerance: Use of intrathecal clonidine, DADL, and intravenous morphine. *Anesthesiology* 1985;62:358.

56. Glynn CJ, Jamous A, Dawson D, et al. The role of epidural clonidine in the treatment of patients with intractable pain. *Pain* 1987;suppl 4:45.

57. Yaksh TL, Reddy SV. Studies in primate on the analgesic effect associated with intrathecal actions of opiates, alpha-adrenergic agonists and baclofen. *Anesthesiology* 1981;54:451.

58. Coombs DW, Allen C, Meier FA, et al. Chronic intraspinal clonidine in sheep. *Reg Anesth* 1994;9:47.

59. Chrubasik J, Meynadier J, Blode S, et al. Somatostatin, a potent analgesic. *Lancet* 1984;2:1208.

60. Meynadier J, Chrubasik J, Dubar M, Wunsch E. Intrathecal somatostatin in terminally ill patients: A report of two cases; *Pain* 1985;23:9.

61. Penn RD, Paice JA, Kroin JS. Octreotide: a potent new non-opiate analgesic for intrathecal infusion. *Pain* 1992;49:13.

62. Candrina R, Galli G. Intraventricular octreotide for cancer pain. *J Neurosug* 1992;76(2):336–337.

63. Fiore CE, Castorina F, Malatino LS, et al. Antalgic activity of calcitonin: Effectiveness of the epidural and subarachnoid routes in man. *Int J Clin Pharmacol Res* 1983;3:257.

64. Eisenach JC. Demonstrating safety of subarachnoid calcitonin: Patients or animals. *Anesth Analg* 1988;67:298.

65. Naguib M, Adu-Gyamfi Y, Absood GH, et al. Epidural ketamine for post-operative analgesia. *Anesth Analg* 1988;67:798.

66. Cripps TP, Goodchild CS. Intrathecal midazolam and stress response to upper abdominal surgery. *Br J Anesth* 1986;58:1324.

67. Wilson PR, Yaksh TL. Baclofen is anti-nociceptive in the spinal intrathecal space of animals. *Eur J Pharmacol* 1978;51:323.

68. Bruera E. Narcotic induced pulmonary edema. *J Pain Sympt Manag* 1990;5:55.

69. Bonica JJ, Benedetti C. Management of Cancer Pain. In: Moossa AR, Robson MC, Schimpff SC, eds. *Comprehensive Textbook of Oncology*. Baltimore: William and Wilkins, 1986;443–477.

70. Hubert C; Recognition and treatment of causalgic pain occuring in cancer patients. In: Jones L, ed. *Abstracts of the Second World Congress on Pain*. Seattle: International Association for Study of Pain, 1978;47.

71. Hassenbusch SJ, Stanton-Hicks MD, Soukup J, et al. Sufentanil citrate and morphine/bupivacaine as alternative agents in chronic epidural infusions for intractable non-cancer pain. *Neurosurgery* 1990;29:76.

72. Nitescu P, Lennart A, Linder L, et al. Epidural versus intrathecal morphine-bupivacaine: Assessment of consecutive treatments in advanced cancer pain. *J Pain Sympt Manag* 1990;5:18.

73. Du Pen SL, Williams AR. Management of patients receiving combined epidural morphine and bupivacaine for the treatment of cancer pain. *J Pain Sympt Manag* 1992;27:125.

74. Van Dongen RTM, Crul BJP, de Bock M. Longterm intrathecal infusion of morphine and morphine/bupivacaine mixtures in the treatment of cancer pain: a retrospective analysis of 51 cases. *Pain* 1993;55:107.

75. Sjoberg M, Karlsson PA, Nordborg C, et al. Neuropathologic findings

after long-term intrathecal infusion of morphine and bupivacaine for pain treatment in cancer patients. *Anesthesiology* 1992;76:173.

76. Naulty JS, Barnes D, Becker R, et al. Epidural PCA versus continuous infusion of sufentanil-bupivacaine for analgesia during labor and delivery. *Anesthesiology* 1990;73:A963.

77. Foley K. The treatment of cancer pain. In: *Cecil's Textbook of Medicine,* 20th ed. Philadelphia: WB Saunders, 1996;100–107.

78. Twycross RG, Lack SA, *Therapeutics in Terminal Cancer.* Edinburgh: Churchill Livingstone, 1986;9.

79. Thimineur MT, Kondamuri S, Kravitz E, Saberski LR, Kitahata LM. Causalgia, RSD and sympathetically maintained pain: a retrospective study of the diagnosis in the clinical setting. *Reg Anesth* 1995; 20(suppl):46.

80. Hogan QH, Erickson SJ, Haddox JD, Abram SE. The spread of solutions during stellate ganglion block. *Reg Anesth* 1992b;17:78.

81. Wahlren L, Torebjork E, Nystrom B, Quantatative sensory testing before and after regional guanethidine block in patients with neuralgia of the hand. *Pain* 1991;46(1):23–30.

82. Treede RD, Davis KD, Campbell JN, Raja SN. The plasticity of cutaneous hyperalgesia during sympathetic ganglion blockade in patients with neuropathic pain. *Brain* 1992;115:607.

83. Hogan QH, Erickson SJ, Abram SE. Computerized tomography guided stellate ganglion blockade. *Anesthesiology* 1992a;77:596.

84. Boas RA, Covino B, Shahnarian A. Analgesic responses to IV lignocaine. *Br J Anaesth* 1982;54:501.

85. Woolf C, Wiesenfeld-Hallin Z. The systemic administration of local anesthetics produces a selective depression of C-afferent fibre evoked activity in the spinal cord. *Pain* 1985;23:361.

86. Tanelian D, MacIver M. Analgesic concentrations of lidocaine suppress tonic A-delta and C fiber discharges produced by acute injury. *Anesthesiology;* 1991;74(5):934–936.

87. Turner JA, Deyo RA, Loeser JD, Von Korff M, Fordyce WE. The importance of placebo effects in pain treatment and research. *JAMA* 1994;271:1609.

88. Verdugo RJ, Ochoa JL. Sympathetically maintained pain, Phentolamine block questions the concept. *Neurology* 1994;44:1003.

89. Luton A. *Archives Generales de Medicin,* Paris, France, 1863.

90. Wood KM. The use of phenol as a neurolytic agent: A review; *Pain* 1978;5:205.

91. Politis MJ, Schaumburg HH, Spencer PS. Neurotoxicity of selected chemicals. In: Spencer PS, Schaumburg HH, eds. *Experimental and Chemical Neurotoxicity.* Baltimore: Williams & Wilkins, 1980.

92. Schaumburg HH, Byck R, Weller RO. The effect of phenol on the peripheral nerve: A histological and electrophysiological study. *J Neuropathol Exp Neurol* 1970;29:615.

93. Lyness WH. Pharmacology of neurolytic agents. In: Racz GB, ed. *Techniques of Neurolysis.* Boston: Kluwer Academic, 1989;13–25.

94. Myers RR, Katz J. Neuropathology of neurolytic and semidestructive agents. In: Cousins, MJ, Bridenbaugh PO, eds. *Neural Blockade in Clinical Anesthesia and Management of Pain.* Philadelphia: JB Lippincott, 1988.

95. Snell R. *Anatomy for Medical Students.* Boston: Little, Brown, 1973.

96. Maher RM. Pain relief in incurable cancer. *Lancet* 1955;1:18.

97. Gerbershagen HU. Neurolysis: subarachnoid neurolytic block. *Acta Anesth Belg* 1981;34:627.

98. Porges P, Zdrahal F. Die intrathekale alkoholneurolyse der unterensakralen wurzeinbeim inoperablen rectumkarzinom. *Anesthetist* 1985; 34:627.

99. Racz GB, Sabongy M, Gintautas J, Kline WM. Intractable pain therapy using a new epidural catheter. *JAMA* 1982;248:579.

100. Katz J, Knott LW, Feldman DJ. Peripheral nerve injections with phenol in the management of spastic patients. *Arch Phys Med Rehab* 1967;48:97.

101. Gordon RA. Diagnostic and therapeutic nerve blocks for head and neck pain. *Can J Otolaryngol* 1975;4:475.

102. Cousins MJ. Anesthetic approaches in cancer pain. In: Foley KM, Bonica JJ, Ventafridda V, eds. *Advances in Pain Research and Therapy,* vol 16. New York: Raven Press, 1990;249.

103. Plancarte R, Amescua C, Patt, et al. Presacral blockade of the ganglion of Walther (ganglion impar). *Anesthesiology* 1990;73:A751.

104. Bridenbaugh LD, Moore DC, Campbell DD. Management of upper abdominal cancer pain: Treatment with a celiac plexus block with alcohol. *JAMA* 1964;190:877.

105. Thompson GE, Moore DC. Celiac plexus, intercostal and minor peripheral blockade. 2nd ed. In: Cousins MJ, Bridenbaugh PO, eds. Philadelphia: JB Lippincott, 1988;503–530.

106. Ischia S, Luzanni A, Ischia A, et al. A new approach to the neurolytic block of the celiac plexus: The transaortic technique. *Pain* 1983;16: 333.

107. Lee MJ, Mueller PR, VanSonnenberg E, et al. CT guided celiac ganglion block with alcohol. *Am J Radiol* 1993;161:633.

108. Flannigan DP, Kraft RO. Continuing experience with palliative chemical splanchnicectomy during laparotomy. *Arch Surg* 1978;113:509.

109. Plancarte R, Amescua C, Patt, et al. Superior hypogastric plexus block for pelvic cancer pain. *Anesthesiology* 1990;73:236.

110. Cosman BJ, Cosman ER. *Guide to Radiofrequency Lesion Generation in Neurosurgery.* Radionics Procedure Technique Series. Burlington, MA: Radionics Inc, 1974.

111. Kline MT. *Stereotaxic Radiofrequency Lesions as Part of the Management of Pain.* Radionics Procedure Technique Series. Orlando, FL: Paul Deutsch Press Inc., 1992.

112. Kantha KS. Radiofrequency Lumbar Sympathectomy: Technique and Review of Indications. In: Racz GB, ed. *Techniques of Neurolysis.* Boston: Kluwer Academic, 1989.

113. Wilkinson HA. Stereotactic radiofrequency sympathectomy. *Pain Clin* 1995;8(1):107.

114. Wilkinson HA. Radiofrequency percutaneous upper thoracic sympathectomy. *N Engl J Med* 1984;311:34.

115. Haynesworth RF, Noe CE. Percutaneous lumbar sympathectomy: a comparison of radiofrequency denervation versus phenol neurolysis. *Anesthesiology* 1991;74:459.

116. Pernak J. Percutaneous radiofrequency thermal lumbar sympathectomy. *Pain Clin* 1995;(80)1:99.

117. Young RF. Clinical experience with radiofrequency and laser DREZ lesions. *J Neurosurg* 1990;72:715.

118. Nash TP. Clinical note percutaneous radiofrequency lesioning of dorsal root ganglia for intractable pain. *Pain* 1986;24:67.

119. Geurts JWM, Stolker RJ. Percutaneous radiofrequency lesion of the stellate ganglion in the treatment of pain in the upper extremity reflex sympathetic dystrophy. *Pain Clin* 1993;6:17.

120. Hippocrates. *Aphorisms,* vol 4. *Heracleitus on the Universe.* Translated by WHS Jones. London: Heinemann, 1931;5:165;7:201.

121. Gruner O. A treatise on the Canon of Medicine of Avicenna. London: Luzac, 1930.

122. Bartholini T. *De nivis usu medico observationes variae.* Hafniae (Copenhagen): Haubold, 1661.

123. Larre D. *Surgical Memoirs of the Campaigns of Russia, Germany and France.* Translated by JC Mercer. Philadelphia: Carey & Lea, 1832.

124. Holden HB. *Practical Cryosurgery.* Chicago: Yearbook and London: Pitman, 1975;2–3.

125. Cooper IS. *J Neurol Sci* 1965;2:493.

126. Amoils SP. The Joule-Thomson cryoprobe. *Arch Opthalmol* 1967;78: 201.

127. Evans P, Cryoanalgesia: the application of low temperatures to nerves to produce anesthesia or analgesia. *Anaesthesia* 1981;36:1003.

128. Lloyd J, Barnard J, Glynn C. Cryoanalgesia: a new approach to pain relief. *Lancet* 1976;2:932.

129. Gonder MJ, Soanes WA, Smith V. Experimental prostate surgery. *Invest Urol* 1965;610.

130. Soanes WA, Ablin RJ, Gonder MJ. Remission of metastatic lesions following cryosurgery in prostatic cancer: immunologic considerations. *J Urol* 1970;104(1):154–159.

131. Pecina M, Krmpotic-Nemanic J, Markiewitz A. Tunnel Syndromes. Boca Raton, FL: CRC Press, 1991;13–83.

132. Wall PD. The prevention of postoperative pain. *Pain* 1988;33:289.

133. Armitage EN. Postoperative pain: prevention or relief? *Br J Anaesth* 1989;63:136.

134. Cousins MJ. Acute pain and injury response: immediate and prolonged effects. *Reg Anesth* 1989;14:162.

135. McQuay HJ, Carroll D, Moore RA. Postoperative orthopedic pain: The effect of opiate premedication and local anesthetic blocks. *Pain* 1988;33:291.

136. Katz J, Nelson W, Forest R, Bruce D. Cryoanalgesia for post-thoracotomy pain. *Lancet* 1980;1:512.

137. Conacher ID, Locke T, Hilton CC. Neuralgia after cryoanalgesia for thoracotomy. *Lancet* 1986;1:277.

138. Orr I, Keenan D, Dundee J. Improved pain relief after thoracotomy: Use of cryoprobe and morphine infusion. *Br Med J* 1981;283.

139. Gough JD, Williams AB, Vaughan RS. The control of post-thoracotomy pain: A comparative evaluation of thoracic epidural fentanyl infusions and cryo-analgesia. *Anesthesia* 1988;43:780.

140. Nelson K, Vincent R, Bourke R. Interoperative intercostal nerve freezing to prevent post-thoracotomy pain. *Ann Thorac Surg* 1974;18(3):280.

141. Maiwand O, Makey AR. Cryoanalgesia for relief of pain after thoracotomy. *Br Med J* 1981;282:49.

142. Wood G, Lloyd J, Bullingham R, Britton F, Finch D. Post-operative analgesia for day case herniorrhaphy patients: a comparison of cryoanalgesia, paravertebral blockade and oral analgesia. *Anesthesia* 1981;36:603.

143. Wood G, Lloyd J, Evans P, Bullingham R, Britton F, Finch D. Cryoanalgesia and day case herniorrhaphy (letter). *Lancet* 1979;2:479.

144. Lahuerta T, Lipton SA, Wells JD. Percutaneous cervical cordotomy: Results and complications in a recent series of 100 patients. *Ann R Coll Surg Engl* 1985;67:41.

145. Lorenz R. Method of percutaneous spinothalamic tract section. In: Krayenbuhl H, ed. *Advances and Technical Standards in Neurosurgery*, vol 3. Vienna: Springer-Verlag, 1976;123–145.

146. Siegfried J, Kuhner A, Sturm V. Neurosurgical treatment of cancer pain. *Cancer Res* 1984;89:148.

147. Rosomoff HL, Krieger AJ, Kuperman AS. Effects of percutaneous cervical cordotomy on pulmonary function. *J Neurosurg* 1969;31:620.

148. Broager B. Commissural myelotomy. *Surg Neurol* 1974;2:71.

149. Cook AW, Kawakami Y. Commissural myelotomy. *J Neurosurg* 1977;47:1.

150. Van Roost D, Gybels J. Myelotomies for chronic pain. *ACTA Neurochir* 1989;46(suppl):69.

151. Hitchcock E. Stereotactic cervical myelotomy. *J Neurol Neurosurg Psych* 1970b;33:224.

152. Thomas DGT. Dorsal root entry zone thermocoagulation. In: Schmidek HH, Sweet WW, eds. *Operative Neurosurgical Technique, Indications, Methods, and Results.* New York: Grune & Stratton, 1988;1169–1175.

153. Richter HP, Seitz K. Dorsal root entry zone lesions for pain relief. *J Neurosurg* 1979;51:59.

154. Levin AB, Ramirez LF, Katz J. The use of sterotaxic chemical hypophysectomy in the treatment of thalamic pain syndrome. *J Neurosurg* 1983;59:1002.

155. Tindall GT, Payne NS, Noxon DW. Trans-sphenoidal hypophysectomy for disseminated carcinoma of the prostate gland. *J Neurosurg* 1979;50:275.

156. Liu CN, Chambers WW. Ultraspinal sprouting of dorsal root axons. *Arch Neurol* 1958;79:46.

157. Coggeshall RE. Afferent fibers in the ventral root. *Neurosurgery* 1979;4:443.

158. Hosobuchi Y. The majority of unmyelinated afferent axons in human ventral roots probably conduct pain. *Pain* 1980;8:167.

159. Fairman D. Thalamic and hypothalamic stimulation. In: Bonica JJ, ed. *Advances in Pain Research and Therapy*, vol 2. New York: Raven Press, 1979;493–498.

160. Mazars G, Merienne L, Cioloca C. Comparative study of electrical stimulation of posterior thalamic nuclei, periaqueductal gray, and other midline mesencephalic structures in man. In: Bonica JJ, ed. *Advances in Pain Research and Therapy,* vol 3. New York: Raven Press, 1979;541–546.

161. Young RF, Chambi V. Pain relief by electrical stimulation of the periaqedudtal and periventricular gray matter. *J Neurosurg* 1987;66:364.

162. Mersky H, Bogduk N. *Classification of Chronic Pain,* International Association for the Study of Pain, Seattle: IASP Press, 1994.

163. Sagen J, Pappas GD, Perlow MJ. Adrenal medullary tissue transplants in the rat spinal cord reduce pain sensitivity. *Brain Res* 1986;384:189.

164. Sagen J, Pappas GD, Pollard HB. Analgesia obtained by isolated bovine chromaffin cells implanted in rat spinal cord. *Proc Natl Acad Sci USA* 1986;83:7522.

165. Sagen J, Wang H, Pappas GD. Adrenal medullary implants in the rat spinal cord reduce nociception in a chronic pain model. *Pain* 1990;42:69.

166. Winnie AP, Krolick TJ, Sagen J, et al. Subarachnoid adrenal medullary transplantation. *Anesthesiology* 1993;79:637.

167. Sagen J, Pappas GD, Winnie AP. Alleviation of pain in cancer patients by adrenal medullary transplants in the spinal subarachnoid space. *Cell Transplant* 1993;2:259.

168. Lazorthes Y, Bes JC, Sagen J, et al. Transplantation of human chromaffin cells for control of intractable cancer pain. *Acta Neurochir* 1995;64(suppl):97.

169. Livett G, Dean DM, Whelan LG, et al. Co-release of enkephalin and catecholamines from cultured adrenal chromaffin cells. *Nature* 1981;289:317.

170. Wilson SP, Chang KJ, Viveros OH. Proportional secretion of opioid peptides and catecholamines from adrenal chromaffin cells in culture. *Anesthesiology* 1982;54:451.

171. Kondo H. Immunohistochemical analysis of the localisation of neuropeptides in the adrenal gland. *Arch Histol Jpn* 1985;48:453.

172. Nguyen TT, de Lean A. Nonadrenergic modulation by clonidine of the cosecretion of catecholamines and enkephalins in adrenal chromaffin cells. *Can J Physiol Pharmacol* 1986;65:823.

173. Lysaght MJ, Frydel B, Emerich D, Winn S. Recent progress in immunoisolated cell therapy. *J Cell Biochem* 1994;56:1.

174. Yaksh TL, Malmberg AB. Interaction of spinal modulatory receptor systems. In: Fields HL, Liebeskind JC, eds. *Progress in Pain Research and Management,* vol 1. Seattle: IASP Press, 1994;151–171.

*Principles and Practice of Supportive Oncology,*
edited by Ann Berger et al.
Lippincott–Raven Publishers, Philadelphia ©1998

CHAPTER 6

# Assessment and Management of Cancer-Related Fatigue

Russell K. Portenoy and Christine Miaskowski

Fatigue is among the most common symptoms experienced by patients with cancer or other progressive diseases. It is often identified by patients as a major impediment to function and quality of life. For patients undergoing active antineoplastic therapy whose disease is stabilized, fatigue may become the most prominent obstacle to functional restoration.

Although recognized for its clinical salience by practitioners, there is a striking lack of empirical research on fatigue. The epidemiology is poorly defined and the range of clinical presentations remains anecdotal. The possibility of discrete fatigue syndromes linked to specific predisposing factors or potential etiologies, and described by unique phenomenologies and pathophysiologies, has not been explored. Indeed, there are very few data to confirm the importance of any particular etiology, and pathophysiology is entirely conjectural. Perhaps most important, there have been almost no clinical trials of putative therapies for fatigue. Treatment, when offered, is based largely on extrapolation of data from other clinical settings and anecdotal experience.

The obvious complexity of fatigue in the medically ill, combined with the lack of research, complicates efforts to define and characterize the symptom and offer clinical guidelines for assessment and management. Nonetheless, it is important to begin this process and thereby increase both the visibility of fatigue as a clinical problem and the willingness of clinicians to explore therapeutic options. In this regard, an abundant theoretical literature can be heuristic (1–12).

R.K. Portenoy: Department of Pain Medicine and Palliative Care, Beth Israel Medical Center, New York, NY 10003.

C. Miaskowski: Department of Physiological Nursing, University of California, San Francisco School of Nursing, San Francisco, CA 94143.

## DEFINITION OF FATIGUE

Fatigue is a symptom and as such is inherently subjective. There is no clear consensus about the nature or duration of the phenomena that would warrant the diagnosis of a fatigue syndrome, or the utility of functional impact as a defining characteristic. Although clinicians generally appreciate that the differentiation between the "normal" fatigue commonly experienced by the population at large and clinical fatigue associated with a disease or its therapy requires specific criteria related to phenomenology, severity, duration, or impact, none of these potential criteria has been evaluated sufficiently to determine a definition on empirical grounds. Indeed, one definition suggests that fatigue is a feeling of weariness, tiredness, or lack of energy that varies in degree, frequency, and duration (2).

Although the multiple dimensions that can be used to characterize the complaint of fatigue (see below) and the lack of extensive survey data combine to complicate efforts to define one or more clinical syndromes, it is valuable to continue this process, even if the basis is mostly clinical observation. The definition provides a focus for research and may increase the visibility of the problem in the clinical setting.

From this perspective, clinically significant cancer-related fatigue can be defined in terms of specific phenomena that occur over time, produce distress or impair function, and are likely to result from the disease or its treatment (Table 1). The specific phenomena comprise a range of sensations, the most important of which are characterized as fatigue, diminished energy, or an increased need to rest that is disproportionate to any recent change in activity. Other sensations may be characterized by diminished motivation or capacity to attend;

**TABLE 1.** *Proposed criteria for fatigue related to cancer or other progressive medical illnesses*

1. An abnormal condition that persists for at least 2 weeks and occurs on most days.
2. The major characteristics are:
   a. Sensations described as fatigue, diminished energy, or an increased need to rest that is disproportionate to any recent change in activity.
   b. These sensations are described as distressing or are associated with a diminished capacity to perform usual physical or intellectual activities.
   c. There is evidence that the condition is causally related to the disease, a medical complication related to the disease, or a treatment for the disease.
   d. There is no evidence that the condition is primarily related to a comorbid psychiatric disorder, such as major depression, somatization, or delirium.
3. The patient may also characterize the condition using other descriptors:
   a. Diminished motivation, volition, mental acuity, interest in activities, or ability to attend.
   b. A feeling of exhaustion, apathy, or lassitude.
   c. A sense of generalized weakness, without true loss of motor function.
   d. A sense of sleepiness, increased need for daytime sleep, insomnia, or the complaint of nonrestorative sleep.
   e. Mood disturbance described as irritability or sadness.

a feeling of exhaustion or generalized weakness; a desire to sleep more than usual; or a disturbance in mood. The adverse functional outcomes may be characterized as a sustained deterioration in the usual ability to perform either physical or intellectual activities.

## EPIDEMIOLOGY OF CANCER-RELATED FATIGUE

Although there are obvious problems in performing valid surveys of a symptom that is yet poorly defined clinically, an abundance of observations in the cancer population together affirm that fatigue is both extremely prevalent and protean in its presentation. The current data are very limited, however, and there continues to be little known about the factors that may predispose to fatigue or produce it, the comorbidities that may influence its expression, and the impact it has on the quality of life of cancer patients.

Among those with metastatic disease, the overall prevalence rate for the complaints of diminished energy or fatigue has been reported to exceed 75% (13–18). A cross-sectional survey of 151 patients with ovarian cancer that evaluated symptom prevalence and characteristics (11) observed that fatigue during the past week was reported by 69% and that approximately half of those who experienced it described it as highly distressing.

A recent population-based survey of 419 randomly selected cancer patients, 31% of whom had been diagnosed during the past year, revealed that 78% experienced fatigue (defined as debilitating tiredness or loss of energy at least once each week) (19). Two thirds of these patients reported that the symptom "significantly" (31%) or somewhat (39%) affected daily routine.

Some surveys have linked the occurrence of fatigue to specific antineoplastic therapies (2,11,12,20–25). The prevalence rates from these surveys must be viewed as tentative because of methodologic concerns, including

the use of nonvalidated assessment techniques in some and, in most cases, the inability to control for a variety of intercurrent phenomena such as other treatments, changes in the disease, and new-onset medical or psychosocial problems. Nonetheless, these surveys suggest that fatigue can occur after surgery, chemotherapy, radiotherapy, or immunotherapy. Prevalence rates as high as 96% have been reported in association with chemotherapy and radiotherapy (2) and severe fatigue has been described as a nearly constant phenomenon associated with some of the biological response modifiers, such as $\alpha$-interferon and interleukin-2 (11,12,25). A relationship between the timing of treatment and the course of fatigue has been observed in several studies (23,24), providing perhaps the strongest evidence of a causative role for the treatment.

Fatigue has been anecdotally associated with many other potential etiologic factors (Table 2), but little is known about the incidence and prevalence of the symptom when these factors exist. Although there is good evidence, for example, that fatigue can be cause by anemia (26), little is known about the relationship between the extent or rate of hemoglobin loss and the development of fatigue. Fatigue has also been associated with many types of major organ dysfunction, including severe cardiac or pulmonary diseases, renal failure, or hepatic failure. Hypothyroidism and adrenal insufficiency, even if relatively mild, may also be etiologically important. Neuromuscular disorders, such as polyneuropathy or Eaton-Lambert syndrome, are also associated with fatigue. More commonly, fatigue is associated with a sleep disorder, systemic infection, or the use of centrally acting drugs such as opioids. It is possible that any of these factors is involved in the pathogenesis of fatigue. Finally, there is a well-recognized association between fatigue and major depression.

Systematic surveys that could confirm the importance of these anecdotal associations have not been performed.

**TABLE 2.** *Possible predisposing factors or etiologies of cancer-related fatigue*

Medical/physical conditions
  Associated with the underlying disease itself
  Associated with treatment for the disease
    Chemotherapy
    Radiotherapy
    Surgery
    Biological response modifiers
  Associated with intercurrent systemic disorders
    Anemia
    Infection
    Pulmonary disorders
    Hepatic failure
    Heart failure
    Renal insufficiency
    Malnutrition
    Neuromuscular disorders
    Dehydration or electrolyte disturbances
  Associated with sleep disorders
  Associated with immobility and lack of exercise
  Associated with chronic pain
  Associated with the use of centrally acting drugs (e.g., opioids)
Psychosocial factors
  Associated with anxiety disorders
  Associated with depressive disorders
    Stress-related
    Related to environmental reinforcers

Consequently, neither the nature of these relationships nor their importance relative to each other is known. Their utility in developing a therapeutic strategy (see below) underscores the need for more research.

The relationships between fatigue and other patient characteristics, including demographics and psychosocial factors, also have been explored very little and there are no reliable conclusions. Older age, more advanced disease, and combined modality therapy were associated with fatigue in one survey (21), and psychological distress was associated in another (23). There continues to be a need for systematic prospective surveys that can confirm and expand these observations.

There are many parallels between cancer and other incurable, progressive diseases, such as acquired immunodeficiency syndrome (AIDS). There is little information about the epidemiology of fatigue in these other disorders. A recent study of 427 ambulatory patients with AIDS (27) suggests the importance of such research. The prevalence of fatigue was 54% and there were strong associations found between the occurrence of fatigue and the number of AIDS-related physical symptoms, current treatment for human immunodeficiency virus (HIV)-related medical disorders, anemia, and pain. In this study, AIDS patients with fatigue were also observed to have relatively poor physical functioning and quality of life, and relatively greater psychological distress, than those who reported no fatigue.

## PATHOGENESIS OF FATIGUE

The mechanisms that precipitate or sustain fatigue in the cancer population are not known. The diversity of factors that may predispose to fatigue, cause it directly, or influence its expression, combined with the equally complex phenomenology of the symptom, suggest that it is not one disorder with a single mechanism. Rather, it is more likely that the fatigue associated with cancer or other medical illnesses actually represents a final common pathway to which many mechanisms may potentially contribute (1,3,5,7–10).

On theoretical grounds, it may be proposed that some fatigue is caused by abnormalities in energy metabolism related to increased need, decreased substrate, or the abnormal production of substances that impair intermediate metabolism or the normal functioning of muscles. Increased need, for example, could be associated with the hypermetabolic state that can accompany tumor growth, infection, fever, or surgery. Decreased substrate may account for the fatigue associated with anemia, hypoxemia of any cause, or poor nutrition.

Based on limited studies of muscle function in cancer patients, it has been suggested that some fatigue could be related to abnormal accumulation of muscle metabolites, such as lactate (28). There is no evidence linking this mechanism to fatigue and, if were to occur, it could still reflect an epiphenomenon related to more fundamental disruption in metabolic activity. The mechanisms that have been most intensively studied involve the production of cytokines, such as tumor necrosis factor and others. There is good evidence that these compounds play a role in the cachexia experienced by some patients with cancer or AIDS (29). The link between cachexia and fatigue observed in the clinical setting, combined with the fatigue that often accompanies the exogenous administration of the biological response modifiers when used as cancer therapy, suggests that similar mechanisms may be primarily involved in the pathogenesis of at least some types of fatigue (30). At the present time, however, there is no direct evidence that any cytokine is causally related to the occurrence of fatigue. Measurement of these and other biochemical factors concurrent with systematic symptom assessment is needed to confirm the relationship.

Other mechanisms for fatigue probably exist as well. Changes in the efficiency of neuromuscular functioning could occur as a direct result of neurologic diseases, such as peripheral neuropathy, and result in fatigue. It is interesting to speculate that the fatigue sometimes reported as associated with immobility and lack of exercise may also be due to reduced efficiency of neuromuscular functioning.

A sleep disorder could possible cause disturbed arousal mechanisms or, equally plausible, be an indicator of a disorder of arousal. These disorders could be primary or related to metabolic disturbances or the use of centrally acting drugs. Again, it is possible to speculate that the pathogenesis of fatigue in some patients relates to these phenomena, but there is no evidence for this at the present time. Studies of the relationships among sleep, daytime arousal, and fatigue would be valuable.

Finally, it may be useful to postulate a mechanism of fatigue that may be specifically related to an affective disorder. The improvement in fatigue often noted by patients who have been successfully treated for a major depression provides some support for this speculation.

Ultimately, it may be possible to assess the fatigue reported by a patient with cancer and infer from this assessment the nature of the underlying pathogenesis. This may, in turn, provide new avenues for therapies targeted to the specific mechanisms involved. A great deal more research is needed before this goal can be attained.

## ASSESSMENT OF FATIGUE

Fatigue is a subjective, multidimensional symptom associated with a broad spectrum of physiologic disorders. Detailed characterization of the symptom, combined with an understanding of the most likely etiologic factors, is needed to fashion a therapeutic strategy that aims to minimize or reverse the likely causes and provide whatever symptomatic therapies are practicable. From this perspective, fatigue is similar to other prevalent symptoms in the cancer population (31). The clinical literature on symptom assessment is most developed for cancer pain, and the guidelines that have been developed for pain assessment offer important lessons for the assessment of fatigue.

### Assessment of Fatigue Characteristics

The comprehensive assessment of fatigue begins with a detailed description of its phenomenology and the elaboration of hypotheses concerning etiology and pathogenesis. This information is acquired through the history, physical examination, and review of laboratory and imaging studies.

As noted, fatigue is multidimensional. Some of the dimensions that could be used to characterize fatigue are like those that could be applied to any other symptom, such as severity or associated distress. Other dimensions, however, are unique to this symptom and reflect the complexity incorporated into the definition of this phenomenon (see Table 1).

As discussed previously, patients may describe fatigue in terms that related to lack of vitality, muscular weakness, dysphoric mood, somnolence, or impaired cognitive functioning. Commonly, the description will focus on several disturbances. The history should clarify the spectrum of complaints and attempt to characterize features associated with each component. In some cases, this information will suggest an approach to therapy. For example, a patient may report a sense of diminished energy throughout the day and somnolence in the morning. If the latter symptom can be related to a nighttime medication, such as an antidepressant, a treatment strategy could be developed that would first address the morning symptoms by changing the drug regimen and then attempt to manage whatever residual fatigue remained.

The distinction between acute fatigue and chronic fatigue is clinically relevant. Acute fatigue has had a recent onset and is anticipated to end in the near future. Chronic fatigue may be defined as fatigue that has persisted for a period of weeks and is not anticipated to remit soon. Although there is obvious imprecision in this distinction, it is important in therapeutic decision making. A patient who is perceived to have chronic fatigue typically warrants a more intensive assessment and an approach to management focused on long-term as well as short-term goals.

Other temporal features, such as onset and course, are also clinically relevant. Fluctuation linked to a discrete event, such as an antineoplastic therapy, is strong evidence of causation.

Information about factors that exacerbate or relieve fatigue should be specifically queried. Like the course over time, this information can suggest an etiology or pathophysiology, or be therapeutically relevant.

In clinical practice, the assessment of fatigue must always include an indication of severity. This can be accomplished simply using a verbal rating scale (none, mild, moderate, severe) or a 11-point numeric scale (where "0" equals no fatigue and "10" equals the worst fatigue imaginable). The clinician should adopt one scale and use it consistently over time. The patient should be given a specific frame of reference when responding. For example, the patient might be asked to indicate the level of fatigue on average during the past week. The clinician can choose a different frame of reference, if this is desired, as long as the same instructions are given whenever the patient is evaluated.

Alternatively, clinicians can make use of a validated fatigue assessment instrument. Although these scales have generally been used in studies, they could easily be scored for clinical use if more precise information were desired.

### Instruments for the Assessment of Fatigue

Fatigue assessment instruments can be unidimensional or multidimensional (4). Unidimensional scales provide an overall measurement fatigue severity (32,33). The same information can be obtained from single items incorporated into symptom checklists (34–36) or the fatigue subscale of the Profile of Mood States (POMS)

(37). Another approach has involved the assessment of specific symptoms associated with fatigue. For example, in a series of studies evaluating psychostimulants in patients receiving opioids, investigators used a visual analog scale (VAS) to assess drowsiness and other scales to evaluate cognitive status (38).

Several multidimensional scales have been validated in the medically ill. The 41-item Piper Fatigue Self-Report Scale addresses the severity, distress, and impact of fatigue and can be administered as either a series of VASs or as numeric scales (39). This scale was developed to assess fatigue in patients receiving radiation therapy and has demonstrated reliability and moderate construct validity in this population.

A 20-item subscale of the Functional Assessment of Cancer Therapy quality-of-life instrument (40) was recently validated to provide information about fatigue and anemia-related concerns (41). Thirteen items of this subscale specifically measure fatigue and can be used alone as a brief, reliable, and valid measure (Table 3). Alternatively, the entire scale can be combined with the larger quality-of-life measure to provide additional information.

Other multidimensional instruments lack the extent of validation in the cancer population of these others. A symptom checklist was used in patients undergoing radiotherapy (42). More recently, a tool that combines a questionnaire with a VAS was developed and tested in a small population of patients with advanced cancer (43). The 18-item Visual Analogue Scale-Fatigue is well validated but has not been tested in cancer patients (44).

## Other Fatigue-Related Evaluation

Identification of factors that may be contributing to fatigue can suggest the use of a specific primary therapy directed to the etiology itself. All patients should undergo a medical and neurologic examination, and an evaluation of psychological status. Most patients should be screened

**TABLE 3.** *Validated fatigue subscale of the functional assessment of cancer therapy measurement system (41)*

I feel fatigued
I feel weak all over
I feel listless ("washed out")
I feel tired
I have trouble starting things because I am tired
I have trouble finishing things because I am tired
I have energy
I am able to do my usual activities
I need to sleep during the day
I am too tired to eat
I need help doing my usual activities
I am frustrated by being too tired to do the things I want to do
I have to limit my social activity because I am tired

for hematologic or metabolic disturbances that may be relevant. The degree to which this and other types of laboratory or radiographic evaluation are pursued must be decided on a case-by-case basis. An extensive and costly evaluation that may be burdensome to the patient is justified only when the etiology is uncertain and the findings of the evaluation could lead to a change in therapy.

### Assessment of Related Constructs

The occurrence of fatigue in the context of a progressive medical illness obligates the clinician to assess the symptom in a broader context. Chronic cancer-related fatigue cannot be addressed clinically without an understanding of the patient's overall quality of life, symptom distress, and the goals of care. These constructs constantly inform decision making.

Quality of life is itself a subjective, multidimensional construct that reflects the overall perception of well-being. It is related to the experience of suffering. The most relevant dimensions that contribute to quality of life or the degree of suffering pertain to physical, psychological, social, and existential or spiritual concerns (45,46). To fully characterize the impact of fatigue, the assessment should attempt to discern the degree to which this symptom contributes to impairment in quality of life and, concurrently, identify other factors that may be equally or more important. These factors may include other symptoms, progressive physical decline, independent psychological disorders, social isolation, financial concerns, spiritual distress, or others. This larger assessment allows the development of a therapeutic strategy that should be more likely to yield improved quality of life, or reduced suffering, than one focused entirely on a single symptom.

In assessing physical and psychological concerns, it is important to recognize that most cancer patients experience multiple symptoms concurrently (14). Studies have generally demonstrated that pain, fatigue, and psychological distress are the most prevalent symptoms across varied cancer populations. The construct of global symptom distress has been useful to characterize overall symptom burden (34–36) and, in some situations, it is useful to consider symptom distress as the critical issue in addressing the impairment in quality of life. Patients who report fatigue should always be queried about the presence of other symptoms.

The issues encountered in the assessment of fatigue may also be clarified by another construct, i.e., the goals of care. At any point during the course of the disease, the patient, the patient's family, and clinicians may emphasize one or more of the major goals in this setting: (a) to cure or prolong life, (b) to maintain function, or (c) to provide comfort. The assessment of the goals of care derives from both the patient's desires and knowledge of the medical realities. Lack of clarity or disagreement about the goals of care can skew the assessment process and undermine the relationship with the patient and family. To avoid these problems, continuing assessment of the goals of care and communication with the patient and family about these goals must be considered to be among the most important and challenging aspects of patient care.

## MANAGEMENT OF FATIGUE

The comprehensive assessment of the patient with cancer-related fatigue allows the development of a strategy that attempts to ameliorate this symptom while addressing the therapeutic requirements posed by the disease itself and the need to provide other elements in the broader approach to palliative care. In some cases, therapy for fatigue should be aggressively pursued, whereas in others, interventions for fatigue can be subordinated to other therapeutic imperatives. These priorities should be developed collaboratively with the patient.

### Establishing Realistic Expectations

Education of the patient about the nature of fatigue, the options for therapy, and the anticipated results is an essential component of any therapeutic approach to fatigue (see below). In some situations, such as fatigue associated with advanced disease and organ failure, there are limited expectations for reversal of the symptom and this should be explained to the patient as part of a plan to improve adaptation. If there is reason to believe that the fatigue will be transitory, this information alone can sometimes suffice as therapy.

### Primary Interventions

Interventions for fatigue can involve primary management of factors that are believed to be causally related, symptomatic interventions, or both. Although the range of factors associated with fatigue (see Table 2) offers many opportunities for primary interventions, the decision to pursue a specific therapy is often difficult. None of these interventions has been studied as a primary treatment for fatigue. The assessment frequently reveals many potential factors, and their relative importance is often unclear. In the medically frail, interventions must be undertaken cautiously. The trial-and-error process of manipulating first one and then another contributing factor can be time consuming and frustrating for the patient. Some of the potential causes, such as the use of centrally acting drugs, are extremely prevalent and it is often difficult to justify efforts to alter these factors when there is risk in doing so and they are so commonly used without the complication of fatigue.

Some primary interventions pose relatively little burden for the patient. The threshold for implementing these interventions is low. For example, all patients who complain of fatigue should undergo review of the drug regimen. Centrally acting drugs that are not essential should be eliminated or reduced. Polypharmacy is extremely common, particularly in the setting of advanced cancer, and there is often a tendency to continue drugs that have questionable benefit due to concern about worsening symptoms if they are stopped. The experience of fatigue shifts the therapeutic index and clearly justifies a trial of dose reduction, at the least. The drugs that are usually considered in this case include antiemetics, hypnotics or anxiolytics, antihistamines (H1 or H2 blockers), and analgesics. If pain is controlled with an opioid, the experience of distressing fatigue often justifies cautious dose reduction (such as 25% of the total daily dose) to determine whether fatigue improves without worsening pain.

The threshold for intervening in an effort to reduce physical inactivity, insomnia, some metabolic abnormalities, or depressed mood is also usually low. The suggestion of exercise, if possible, and nonpharmacologic therapy for a sleep disorder is often accepted enthusiastically by patients (see below). The use of a hypnotic can be useful but clearly requires careful monitoring. If sleep duration increases but the patient perceives it to be nonrestorative, the desired goal has not been achieved. As might be expected, the use of a centrally acting hypnotic can sometimes appear to worsen daytime fatigue.

Fatigue can be associated with varied metabolic disturbances. Some, such as the metabolic derangements associated with renal failure, may not be treatable in the context of the overall disease. Others, such as dehydration, hypercalcemia, hypothyroidism, hypocortisolism, or hypoxia, can be managed at little risk. Interventions to improve these disturbances may be warranted in the overall approach to the fatigued patient.

A trial of an antidepressant in fatigued patient with major depression is strongly indicated. More challenging is the decision to implement antidepressant therapy in the patient who has dysphoric mood but is not anhedonic and lacks other psychological criteria for the diagnosis of major depression. Although there are some risks with this therapy, most clinicians perceive that a treatment trial is warranted with any significant degree of depressed mood, particularly if there are other targets for the drug, such as anxiety or pain. In the setting of fatigue, the use of a relatively less sedating antidepressant, such as one of the serotonin-selective reuptake inhibitors, is appropriate. Buproprion or one of the secondary amine tricyclic antidepressants, such as desipramine, is an alternative to this class.

Recent evidence suggests that anemia may be a major factor in cancer-related fatigue. Anecdotally, transfusion therapy for severe anemia is often associated with substantial improvement in fatigue. Treatment with recombinant human erythropoietin offers another approach to this problem. In three randomized, placebo-controlled trials that enrolled a total of 413 patients, patients who were treated with erythropoietin for 8–12 weeks and experienced an increase in hematocrit of >6% demonstrated significantly improved energy level, daily activities, and overall quality of life (47). The quality of life scores improved approximately 24% from baseline values. A more recent open label study of 2349 patients undergoing cytotoxic chemotherapy at more than 500 community oncology practices demonstrated that erythropoietin treatment for up to 16 weeks was associated with significant increases in energy level, activities, and overall quality of life (26); these changes were correlated with the improvement in hemoglobin and not tumor response.

These data are encouraging, but they do not illuminate the degree of anemia associated with fatigue or the extent of improvement in the hematocrit required to obtain symptomatic benefit. Although erythropoietin is a relatively safe therapy, it is extremely expensive and is difficult to justify if either the fatigue or the anemia is mild, life expectancy is short, or there are other factors that appear to be major contributors to the fatigue. Studies are needed to further clarify the role of anemia in cancer-related fatigue and the cost-benefit of erythropoietin therapy.

**Symptomatic Therapy: Pharmacologic Approaches**

Although pharmacologic therapy for fatigue associated with medical illness has not been evaluated in controlled studies, there is evidence supporting the use of several drug classes for this indication. The utility of the psychostimulants has been suggested in studies of methylphenidate and pemoline (38,48). There is a substantial clinical experience with these drugs in the treatment of opioid-related cognitive impairment (49) and depression in the elderly and medically ill (50–53). Although the evidence suggesting that psychostimulants can improve cancer-related fatigue is not conclusive, there is a favorable enough anecdotal experience to warrant a trial in patients who lack contraindications.

In the cancer population, the largest experience is with methylphenidate. Dextroamphetamine and pemoline have also been used anecdotally. There have been no controlled comparisons of these drugs and clinical experience suggests that the response to one does not necessary predict response to the others. For this reason, sequential trials may be valuable to identify the most useful drug.

Pemoline is a novel psychostimulant with relatively less sympathomimetic activity than the other psychostimulants. This drug has an available chewable formulation that can be absorbed through the buccal mucosa and may be useful in patients who are unable to swallow or absorb oral drugs. There is, however, a very small risk of severe hepatotoxicity from pemoline that has not been

reported with the other psychostimulants (54); this risk may justify the use of methylphenidate as the first-line psychostimulant for most patients.

The potential toxicities associated with the psychostimulants include anorexia; insomnia; anxiety, confusion, and other organic brain syndromes; tremor; and tachycardia. These effects can be particularly problematic in the medically ill, who may be predisposed to the same symptoms for other reasons. Relative contraindications include preexisting anorexia; severe insomnia, anxiety, or agitation (particularly if associated with paranoid ideation); and significant heart disease. To ensure safety, dose escalation of the psychostimulants should be undertaken cautiously, and at intervals long enough to evaluate the full gamut of potential toxicities.

In medically fragile patients, the initial dose of methylphenidate is usually 2.5–5 mg once or twice daily. This dose is then gradually escalated until favorable effects occur or toxicity supervenes. Most patients require low doses; doses above 60 mg/day are very uncommon. Effects sometimes wane over time, a change that could reflect tolerance or progression of the underlying cause of the fatigue, and dose escalation may be needed to maintain effects. The risk of toxicity increases with the dose, however, and the ability to regain lost efficacy may be limited. The starting doses for dextroamphetamine and pemoline are 2.5–5 mg and 18.75 mg, respectively, once or twice daily.

The use of low-dose corticosteroids as a treatment for fatigue has also been supported empirically (55,56). This treatment is usually considered in the population with advanced disease and multiple symptoms. There have been no comparative trials of the different agents in this class. Therapy is usually undertaken with dexamethasone 1–2 mg twice daily or prednisone 5–10 mg twice daily.

Amantadine has been used for the treatment of fatigue due to multiple sclerosis for many years. There is no experience with this drug in populations with other diseases. Nonetheless, amantadine has relatively low toxicity and an empirical trial may be warranted in selected patients with refractory fatigue associated with other diseases.

As noted previously, a therapeutic trial with an antidepressant drug is clearly appropriate if fatigue is related to a clinical depression and an antidepressant that is relatively less likely to be sedating, such as one of the serotonin-specific reuptake inhibitors, secondary amine tricyclics, or buproprion, would be preferred. Some patients appear to experience increased energy disproportionate to any clear effect on mood during treatment with one of these drugs. Theoretically, these "activating" effects could be used to treat fatigue. There have been no clinical trials of these drugs with fatigue as an endpoint, however, and the potential benefit of these drugs in nondepressed patients remains to be studied. In the absence of any data, an empirical trial would only be warranted in cases of severe fatigue refractory to other measures.

## Symptomatic Therapy: Nonpharmacologic Approaches

As noted, all patients with distressing fatigue require education to set realistic expectations. This communication is the simplest of the diverse nonpharmacologic approaches that can be used to manage this symptom. Although there have been empirically evaluations of these nonpharmacologic therapies, anecdotal experience suggests that several types of interventions may be useful (Table 4). Studies are needed to evaluate the effectiveness of these techniques.

Patient preferences must be considered in developing a nonpharmacologic strategy for fatigue. Participation is unlikely unless the patient perceives a substantial chance of benefit and only modest burden. More than one type of nonpharmacologic intervention may be useful depending on the etiology of the fatigue.

### Patient Education

Patient education that contains both procedural and sensory information has been shown to be effective in reducing pain and improving outcomes (57–61). Inadequate information may lead to needless anxiety. As noted previously, the fatigued patient should receive information about the nature of the symptom, the options for therapy, and the expected outcomes. Many patients assume that the problem reflects worsening of the disease and information about alternative explanations, if any are identified, can be very reassuring.

There are large individual differences in patients' preferences for information, and the effort to educate should be provided that is appropriate to the patients' educational level and readiness to learn.

As part of the educational process, patients may find it beneficial to keep a diary of their fatigue. The diary may help clinicians and patients discern a pattern to the fatigue and monitor its severity. This information may be useful in developing a management plan that modifies specific activities and incorporates appropriate periods of rest.

**TABLE 4.** *Nonpharmacologic interventions to manage fatigue*

| |
|---|
| Patient education |
| Exercise |
| Modification of activity and rest patterns |
| Stress management and cognitive therapies |
| Adequate nutrition and hydration |

### Exercise

Exercise may be beneficial in relieving fatigue in cancer patients (61). In one study, a supervised exercise program was effective in reducing the fatigue of women with stage II breast cancer who were receiving chemotherapy (62). Data that would allow the selection of the most appropriate exercise program for patients with various types of cancer or cancer treatments are not available.

Some general principles should be followed when prescribing exercise for a cancer patient. The exercise prescription should be individualized and consider such factors as the patient's age, gender, physical condition, and any intercurrent medical conditions that may affect the individual's ability to exercise. Anecdotally, the type of exercise that appears to be most beneficial in ameliorating fatigue is exercise that involves rhythmic and repetitive movement of large muscle groups. This effect is achieved through walking, cycling, or swimming. An exercise program should be initiated gradually and patients should not exercise to the point of exhaustion. Exercise needs to be done for several days of the week in order for beneficial effects to occur.

Contraindications to low-intensity exercise include cardiac abnormalities, recurrent or unexplained pain, onset of nausea with exercise, extreme fatigability, or cyanosis. A referral to an exercise physiologist may be warranted in order to have a more thorough evaluation and a specific exercise prescription developed for each individual patient.

### Modification of Activity and Rest Patterns

The use of a diary to assess fatigue may identify specific activities that are associated with increased levels of fatigue. This information can facilitate a plan to modify, schedule, or pace these activities throughout the day. Brief, scheduled rest periods may help to reduce fatigue. Naps should be allowed only during the day because a period of sleep in the late afternoon or evening may interfere with the patient's ability to sleep at night.

One of the most important interventions in the area of activity and rest pattern modification is an assessment for sleep disturbances and patient education about basic sleep hygiene principles. Again, education about sleep hygiene principles should be tailored to the individual patient. One of the fundamental principles is the establishment of a specific bedtime and wake time. A specific wake time appears to be particularly important in maintaining a normal sleep–wake rhythm. An additional strategy is the establishment of routine procedures prior to sleep. For example, patients may read a book or watch television prior to falling asleep (63).

Exercise on a consistent basis tends to improve sleep and promote deeper sleep. If exercise is also used, it should be performed at least 6 hours before bedtime. Intense exercise raises the body temperature for at least 6 hours and it appears preferable for this period to pass before sleep.

Additional sleep hygiene measures include reduced environmental stimuli (e.g., loud noises, light) and the use of diversional activities (e.g., music, massage) to promote sleep. Patients also should be instructed to avoid stimulants (e.g., caffeine, nicotine, steroids, methylphenidate) and central nervous system depressants (e.g., alcohol) prior to sleep (63).

### Stress Management and Cognitive Therapies

Anxiety, difficulties in coping with cancer or its treatment, and sleep disturbances are some of the factors that may contribute to the development of fatigue. These factors may be ameliorated using stress reduction techniques or cognitive therapies (e.g., relaxation therapy, hypnosis, guided imagery, distraction). Research has demonstrated that distraction (e.g., gardening, listening to music, taking quiet walks) may be effective in reducing the symptom, particularly for patients with fatigue associated with deficits in attention (64,65). A referral to a psychiatrist or a psychologist for counseling and training in stress management techniques or cognitive therapies may be warranted in some patients.

### Adequate Nutrition and Hydration

Cancer and its treatment can interfere with dietary intake. Fatigued individuals also may underestimate the amount of food and fluid they ingest. To aggressively manage fatigue, patients' weight, hydration status, and electrolyte balance should be monitored and maintained to the extent possible. Regular exercise may improve appetite and increase nutritional intake. Referral to a dietitian for dietary planning and suggestions for nutritional supplements may be beneficial if one of the causes of fatigue is inadequate food or fluid intake.

## CONCLUSION

Despite the high prevalence and distress associated with fatigue, there has been little recognition of this symptom as an important issue for research and clinical guideline development. At the present time, relatively little is known about its epidemiology, etiologies, and management. There is no definitive information about the types of mechanisms that may produce fatigue in discrete populations.

With burgeoning interest in palliative care, it is likely that increasing attention will focus on the problem of fatigue. Extensive research is needed before the symptom will be adequately characterized in terms of phenomenology, pathogenesis, and management.

## REFERENCES

1. Aistars J. Fatigue in the cancer patient: a conceptual approach to a clinical problem. *Oncol Nurs Forum* 1987;14:25–30.
2. Irvine DM, Vincent L, Bubela N, et al. A critical appraisal of the research literature investigating fatigue in the individual with cancer. *Cancer Nurs* 1991;14:188–199.
3. Piper BF, Lindsey AM, Dodd MJ. Fatigue mechanisms in cancer patients: developing nursing theory. *Oncol Nurs Forum* 1987;14:17–23.
4. Varricchio CG. Selecting a tool for measuring fatigue. *Oncol Nurs Forum* 1985;12:122–127.
5. Jacobs LA, Piper BF. The phenomenon of fatigue and the cancer patient. In: McCorkle R, Grant M, Frank-Stromberg M, Baird SB, eds. *Cancer Nursing: A Comprehensive Textbook.* Philadelphia: WB Saunders, 1996; 1193–1210.
6. Glaus A. Assessment of fatigue in cancer and noncancer patients. *Support Care Cancer* 1993;1:305–315.
7. Nail LM, Winningham M. Fatigue. In: Groenwald SL, Frogge MH, Goodman M, Yarbro CH, eds. *Cancer Nursing: Principles and Practice.* Boston: Jones and Bartlett, 1993;608–619.
8. Piper BF. Alterations in comfort: fatigue. In: McNally JC, Somerville E, Miaskowski C, Rostad M, eds. *Guidelines for Oncology Nursing Practice,* 2nd ed. Philadelphia: WB Saunders, 1991;155–162.
9. Smets EMA, Garssen B, Schuster-Uitterhoeve ALJ, de Haes JCJM. Fatigue in cancer patients. *Br J Cancer* 1993;68:220–224.
10. Winningham ML, Nail LM, Burke MB, et al. Fatigue and the cancer experience: the state of the knowledge. *Oncol Nurs Forum* 1994;1:23–35.
11. Piper BF, Rieger PT, Brophy L, et al. Recent advances in the management of biotherapy-related side effects: fatigue. *Oncol Nurs Forum* 1989;16(suppl 6):27–34.
12. Skalla K, Rieger P. Fatigue. In: Rieger PT, ed. *Biotherapy: Comprehensive Review.* Boston: Jones and Bartlett, 1995;221–242.
13. Portenoy RK, Thaler HT, Kornblith AB, Lepore JM, Friedlander-Klar H, Coyle N, Smart-Curley T, Kemeny N, Norton L, Hoskins W, Scher H. Pain in ovarian cancer: prevalence, characteristics, and associated symptoms. *Cancer* 1994;74:907–915.
14. Portenoy RK, Thaler HT, Kornblith AB, et al. Symptom prevalence, characteristics and distress in a cancer population. *Quality Life Res* 1994;3:183–189.
15. Curtis EB, Kretch R, Walsh TD. Common symptoms in patients with advanced cancer. *J Palliat Care* 1991;7:25–29.
16. Dunphy KP, Amesbury BDW. A comparison of hospice and homecare patients: patterns of referral, patient characteristics and predictors of place of death. *Palliat Med* 1990;4:105–111.
17. Dunlop GM. A study of the relative frequency and importance of gastrointestinal symptoms and weakness in patients with far-advanced cancer: student paper. *Palliat Med* 1989;4:37–43.
18. Ventafridda V, DeConno F, Ripamonti C, Gamba A, Tamburini M. Quality of life assessment during a palliative care program. *Ann Oncol* 1990; 1:415–420.
19. Vogelzang N, Breitbart W, Cella D, Portenoy R, Horning S, D Johnson, Scherr S, Parkinson D, Groopman J, Itri L. Patients (Pts), caregivers (CGS), and oncologist (ONCS) perceptions of cancer related fatigue (CF): results of a tripart assessment survey (abstract). *Proc ASCO,* 1997;16:53a.
20. Greenberg DB, Sawicka J, Eisenthal S, Ross D. Fatigue syndrome due to localized radiation. *J Pain Sympt Manag* 1992;7:38–45.
21. Fobair P, Hoppe RT, Bloom J, et al. Psychosocial problems among survivors of Hodgkin's disease. *J Clin Oncol* 1986;4:805–814.
22. Haylock PJ, Hart LK. Fatigue in patients receiving localized radiation therapy. *Cancer Nurs* 1979;2:461–467.
23. Irvine D, Vincent L, Graydon JE, et al. The prevalance and correlates of fatigue in patients receiving treatment with chemotherapy and radiotherapy. *Cancer Nurs* 1994;17:367–378.

24. Pickard-Holley S. Fatigue in the cancer patient. *Cancer Nurs* 1991;14: 13–19.
25. Dean GE, Spears L, Ferrell B, et al. Fatigue in patients with cancer receiving interferon alpha. *Cancer Pract* 1995;3:164–171.
26. Glaspy J, Bukowski R, Steinberg D, et al. The impact of therapy with Epoetin alfa on clinical outcomes in patients with nonmyeloid malignancies during cancer chemotherapy in community oncology practice. *J Clin Oncol.* 1997;15:1218–1234.
27. Breitbart W, McDonald MV, Rosenfeld B, Monkman ND, Passik S. Fatigue in ambulatory AIDS patients. *J Pain Sympt Manag*, in press.
28. Burt ME, Aoki TT, Gorschboth CM, Brennan MR. Peripheral tissue metabolism in cancer-bearing man. *Ann Surg* 1983;198:685–691.
29. Billingsley KG, Alexander HR. The pathophysiology of cachexia in advanced cancer and AIDS. In: Bruera E, Higginson I, eds. *Cachexia-Anorexia in Cancer Patients.* New York: Oxford University Press, 1996; 1–22.
30. Neuenschwander H, Bruera E. Asthenia-cachexia. In: Bruera E, Higginson I, eds. *Cachexia-Anorexia in Cancer Patients.* New York: Oxford University Press, 1996;57–75.
31. Ingham JM, Portenoy RK. Symptom assessment. In: Cherny NI, Foley KM, eds. *Hematology/Oncology Clinics of North America. Pain and Palliative Care.* Philadelphia: WB Saunders, 1996;21–39.
32. Rhoten D. Fatigue and the postsurgical patient. In: Norris CM, ed. *Concept Clarification in Nursing.* Rockville, MD: Aspen Publishers, 1982; 277–300.
33. Pearson PG. Scale analysis of a fatigue checklist. *J Appl Psychol* 1957; 41:186–191.
34. de Haes JCJM, van Kippenberg FCE, Neijt JP. Measuring psychological and physical distress in cancer patients: structure and application of the Rotterdam Symptom Checklist. *Br J Cancer* 1990; 62:1034–38.
35. McCorkle R, Young K. Development of a symptom distress scale. *Cancer Nurs* 1978;1:373–378.
36. Portenoy RK, Thaler HT, Kornblith AB, et al. The Memorial Symptom Assessment Scale: an instrument for the evaluation of symptom prevalence, characteristics, and distress. *Eur J Cancer* 1994;30A(9): 1326–1336.
37. Cella DF, Jacobsen PB, Orav EJ, et al. A brief POMS measure of distress for cancer patients. *J Chronic Dis* 1987;40:939–942.
38. Bruera E, Chadwick S, Brenneis C, MacDonald RN. Methylphenidate associated with narcotics for the treatment of cancer pain. *Cancer Treat Rep* 1987;71:67–70.
39. Piper B F, Lindsey AM, Dodd MJ, Ferketich S, Paul SM, Weller S. The development of an instrument to measure the subjective dimension of fatigue. In: Funk SG, Tornquist EM, Champange MT, Copp LA, Wiese RA, eds. *Key Aspects of Comfort. Management of Pain, Fatigue and Nausea.* New York: Springer Publishing Company, 1989;199–208.
40. Cella DF, Tulsky DS, Gray, G, Sarafian B, Linn E, Bonomi A, et al. The functional assessment of cancer therapy scale: development and validation of the general measure. *J Clin Oncol* 1993;11(3):570–579.
41. Yellen SB, Cella DF, Webster MA, Blendowski C, Kaplan E. Measuring fatigue and other anemia-related symptoms with the Functional Assessment of Cancer Therapy (FACT) measurement system. *J Pain Sympt Manag* 1997;13:63–74.
42. Kobashi-Schoot JAM, Hanewald GJFP, van Dam FSAM, et al. Assessment of malaise in cancer treated with radiotherapy. *Cancer Nurs* 1985; 8:306–314.
43. Morant R, Stiefel F, Berchtold W, Radziwill A, Riesen W. Preliminary results of a study assessing asthenia and related psychological and biological phenomena in patients with advanced cancer. *Support Care Cancer* 1993;1:101–107.
44. Lee KA, Hicks G, Nino-Murcia G. Validity and reliability of a scale to assess fatigue. *Psychiatry Res* 1991;36:291–298.
45. Cherny NI, Coyle N, Foley KM. Suffering in the advanced cancer patient: a definition and taxonomy. *J Palliat Care* 1994;10:57–70.
46. Cella DF. Quality of life: concepts and definition. *J Pain Sympt Manag* 1994;9:186–193.
47. Abels RI, Larholt KM, Drantz KD, Bryant EC. Recombinant human erythropoietin (r-HuEPO) for the treatment of the anemia of cancer. In: Murphy MJ, ed. *Blood Cell Growth Factors: Their Present and Future Use in Hematology and Oncology.* Dayton, OH: AlphaMed Press.
48. Krupp LB, Coyle PK, Doscher C, Miller A, Cross AH, Jandorf L, et al. Fatigue therapy in multiple sclerosis: a double-blind, randomized, parallel trial of amantidine, pemoline and placebo. *Neurology* 1995;45(11): 1956–1961.
49. Bruera E, Brenneis C, Paterson AH, MacDonald RN. Use of methylphenidate as an adjuvant to narcotic analgesics in patients with advanced cancer. *J Pain Sympt Manag* 1989;4:3–6.
50. Breitbart W, Mermelstein H. An alternative psychostimulant for the management of depressive disorders in cancer patients. *Psychosomatics* 1992;33:352–356.
51. Fernandez F, Adams F, Levy JK. Cognitive impairment due to AIDS-related complex and its response to psychostimulants. *Psychosomatics* 1988;29:38–46.
52. Katon W, Raskind M. Treatment of depression in the medically ill elderly with methylphenidate. *Am J Psychiatry* 1980;137:963–965.
53. Kaufmann MW, Murray GB, Cassem NH. Use of psychostimulants in medically ill depressed patients. *Psychosomatics* 1982;23:817–819.
54. Berkovitch M, Pope E, Phillips J, Koren G. Pemoline-associated fulminant liver failure: testing the evidence for causation. *Clin Pharm Ther* 1995;57:696–698.
55. Bruera E, Roca E, Cedaro L, Carraro S, Chacon R. Action of oral methylprednisolone in terminal cancer patients: a prospective randomized double-blind study. *Cancer Treat Rep* 1985;69:751–754.
56. Tannock I, Gospodarowicz M, Meakin W, et al. Treatment of metastatic prostatic cancer with low-dose prednisone. Evaluation of pain and quality of life as pragmatic indices of response. *J Clin Oncol* 1989;7: 590–597.
57. Egbert LD, Battit GE, Welch CE, Bartlett MK. Reduction of postoperative pain by encouragement and instruction of patients. *N Engl J Med* 1964;207:825–827.
58. Fortin F, Kirouac S. A randomized controlled trial of preoperative patient education. *Int J Nurs Studies* 1976;13:11–24.
59. Johnson J, Fuller S, Endress MP, Rice V. Altering patients' responses to surgery: An extension and replication. *Res Nurs Health* 1978;1: 111–121.
60. Johnson J, Rice V, Fuller S, and Endress MP. Sensory information, instruction in a coping strategy, and recovery from surgery. *Res Nurs Health* 1978;1:4–17.
61. Winningham ML. Fatigue. In: Groenwald SL, Frogge MH, Goodman M, Yarbro CH, eds. *Cancer Symptom Management.* Boston: Jones and Bartlett, 1996;42–58.
62. MacVicar SB, Winningham ML. Promoting functional capacity of cancer patients. *Cancer Bull* 1986;38:235–239.
63. Yellen SB and Dyonzak JV. Sleep disturbances. In: Groenwald SL, Frogge MH, Goodman M, Yarbro CH, eds. *Cancer Symptom Management.* Boston: Jones and Bartlett, 1996;151–168.
64. Cimprich B. Attentional fatigue following breast cancer surgery. *Res Nurs Health* 1992;15:199–207.
65. Cimprich B. Developing an intervention to restore attention in cancer patients. *Cancer Nurs* 1993;16:83–92.

*Principles and Practice of Supportive Oncology*,
edited by Ann Berger et al.
Lippincott–Raven Publishers, Philadelphia ©1998

CHAPTER 7

# Fever and Sweats: Including the Immunocompromised Hosts

James F. Cleary

## TEMPERATURE AND ASSOCIATED SYMPTOMS

Temperature has long been used in clinical medicine and was included in the cardinal signs of inflammation described as "tumor, rubor, dolor and fever." The measurement of temperature by thermometer, in the sublingual, subaxillary, or rectal locations, is not a clinical skill practiced regularly by doctors. In most cases, the temperature is recorded by other health workers or the patients themselves. Normal body temperature is considered to be 37°C, the average core temperature for an adult population.

Temperature is tightly controlled within a narrow range in each individual. Fever is defined as any elevation in core body temperature above the normal and results from the upregulation of body temperature. More commonly, a temperature greater that 38°C is considered a clinically significant fever. In oncologic practice and many clinical studies, a significant fever is defined as single temperature reading greater than 38.5°C or three readings (at least an hour apart) of more than 38°C. The term fever (or pyrexia) of unknown origin, or FUO (PUO), is used commonly and often incorrectly in the daily practice of medicine. An FUO is defined as an illness of at least 3 weeks duration with a fever higher than 38°C on more than one occasion and that lacks a definitive diagnosis after 1 week of evaluation in hospital (1).

Fever is often accompanied by other symptoms including sweating and rigors. Sweating, when it accompanies fever, is a cooling response by the body in which heat is released from the body as it evaporates water on the skin's surface. Rigors and shivering also contribute to temperature control and are rapid muscle spasms designed to increase heat production within the body. For adult humans and most large mammals, shivering is the major means of increased heat production in response to a cold environment. Nonshivering thermogenesis, a process involving heat production in brown adipose tissue, is important in the temperature control of infants.

## CONTROL OF TEMPERATURE

It is proposed that core body temperature is controlled by neurologic mechanisms centered at the anterior hypothalamus. The onset of fever in patients results from an elevation of the body's regulated set point temperature through a resetting of the temperature "gauge" in the hypothalamus (2). This may be caused by various drugs or by endogenous pyrogens. As a result of the reset hypothalamic temperature, the body increases the core body temperature to this new level (Fig. 1) through shivering or nonshivering thermogenesis. The continued presence of pyrogen at the hypothalamus results in the maintenance of this higher temperature. Eventually, either as a result of a decrease in the quantity of pyrogen or the administration of an antipyretic, the hypothalamic temperature is reset back to a lower or normal level and the core body temperature is lowered through sweating. This control mechanism may be suppressed in patients administered steroids or antiinflammatory agents. Older patients may not be able to mount the anticipated febrile response.

The endogenous pyrogens that are responsible for the onset of fever are largely derived from monocytes and macrophages. These cells, as a result of challenge by either endotoxin or ineffective sources, release tumor necrosis factor (TNF) and interleukin-1β (IL-1β). Their production is part of the complex cascade that results in the stimulation of other cytokines such as interleukin-6 (IL-6), interleukin-8 (IL-8), and changes in prostaglandin metabolism. Serum levels of IL-6 and IL-8 have been

J. F. Cleary: Department of Medicine, University of Wisconsin, Madison, WI 53792.

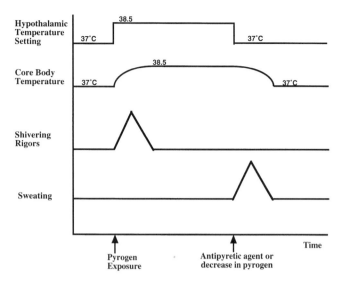

**FIG. 1.** Physiologic mechanisms associated with fever and accompanying symptoms. (Adapted from ref 2.)

**TABLE 1.** *Tumors classically associated with fever*

Hodgkin's disease
Lymphoma
Leukemia
Renal cell carcinoma
Myxoma
Osteogenic sarcoma

found to correlate with core body temperature in febrile neutropenic patients (3). The ultimate endpoint of this cascade is the activation of granulocytes, monocytes, and endothelial cells. While fever appears to be associated with enhanced function of the immune system, it must nonetheless be noted that a direct connection between such phenomena and a beneficial effect of fever on outcome of infections has not been established. Fever, in fact, may be deleterious in the setting of autoimmune disorders or infections (4).

## ETIOLOGY OF FEVER IN CANCER PATIENTS

Fever is commonly seen in cancer patients, both in those with and without infection. The wide range of etiologies of fever in cancer patients will be considered in relation to the pathophysiology of fever in these patients.

### Tumor

Fever associated with tumor is believed to be associated with the release of pyrogens, either directly from a tumor or from stimulation of immunologic mechanisms by the tumor, that cause an elevation in temperature through action on the anterior hypothalamus. The classical association of fever to particular tumor diagnoses relates more to tumors associated with a diagnosis of FUO (Table 1). In the combined results of six studies documenting the etiology of FUO, 23% of adults meeting the defined diagnosis were found to have malignancy as the cause (cf. 8% of children) (5). In another study of 111 elderly (>65 years) patients with FUO, 26 had associated malignancy with 15 patients diagnosed with lymphoma and 4 with renal cell carcinoma (6). Almost 7000 cancer patients with fever were reviewed by Klastersky et al. and

only 47 (0.7%) fit the diagnostic criteria for a FUO (7). Of these 47, 27 had leukemia or lymphoma, with disease rather than infection being the cause of the fever in only 11. Tumor was responsible for fever in 7 patients with widespread metastatic carcinomas and in 6 of these, large liver metastases were present.

Hodgkin's disease has classically been associated with the Pel Epstein fever (Fig. 2), whereby a patient experiences 3- to 10-day cycles of fever alternating with periods of afebrileness (8). While the presence of fever is an important prognostic indicator in patients with Hodgkin's disease, there has been some discussion (9) about the value of Pel Epstein fever as a diagnostic tool, particularly as the original description of the Pel Epstein fever was made in two patients who were subsequently found, on pathologic review, not to have Hodgkin's disease.

Although classical teaching is that particular tumors are associated with fever, fever also occurs in many of the more common cancers (Table 2). Of those who underwent autopsy in this study, 41% had evidence of infection as an explanation of their fever (10). The incidence of infection among the autopsied patients was 50% for acute leukemia, 75% in lymphoma patients, and 80% in those with chronic lymphocytic leukemia. Infection was only found in a third of those with chronic myeloid leukemia, 17% with Hodgkin's disease, and 15% of patients with lung cancer.

### Infection (Including the Neutropenic)

While infection and fever can be a common presentation in cancer patients, it is of particular concern in neutropenic patients. Neutropenia, defined as a peripheral blood neutrophil count of <500/μl, results from either increased destruction or decreased production of white blood cells. Decreased production by the bone marrow may result from either disease involving the marrow or from myelosuppression by chemotherapy. The cause of fever is not identified in some 60–70% of neutropenic patients (11). Risk factors for the development of fever in the setting of neutropenia have been identified and include a rapid decrease in the neutrophil count and a protracted neutropenia of <500 cells/μl for >10 days (12). Of patients with one week of chemotherapy-induced neutropenia, 20% develop a fever and the rate of infection increases with lengthening periods of neutropenia. Other

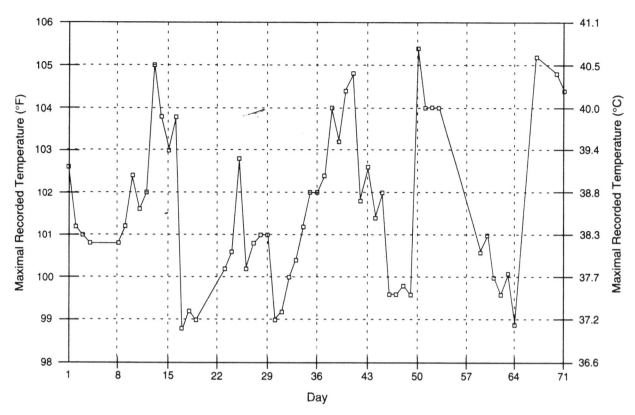

**FIG. 2.** A 50-year-old man had fever, night sweats, and nonproductive cough for 10 weeks. He took antipyretic medications during the febrile periods. His wife recoeded his temperatures, shown above, on 56 of the 71 days. Biopsy of a rapidly enlarging cervical lymph node revealed nodular sclerosing Hodgkin's lymphoma. The patient's fevers and other symptoms promptly disappeared after the first cycle of doxorubicin, bleomycin, vinblastine, and dacarbazine. Reprinted with permission from ref. 8.

factors that may alter the risk of the neutropenic patient include phagocyte function, the status of the patient's immune system, and alterations in the physical defense barriers of the body, e.g., mucositis.

Fever and neutropenia in cancer patients are associated with a high risk of medical complications with a death rate ranging from 4% to 12%. Of patients with febrile neutropenia at the Dana Farber Cancer Center, 21% developed serious medical complications (13), and these investigators identified four risk groups for febrile neutropenic patients. Group 1 were inpatients at the time of onset of fever; group 2, outpatients who developed sig-

**TABLE 2.** *Incidence of fever without evidence of infection at autopsy in patients of different primary tumor types*

| Primary site | No patients observed | Number of patients with fever without associated infection | |
|---|---|---|---|
| | | Number | % |
| Stomach | 1498 | 573 | 41 |
| Kidney | 208 | 39 | 19 |
| Colon and rectum | 113 | 75 | 66 |
| Liver and gallbladder | 98 | 43 | 44 |
| Uterus | 81 | 19 | 36 |
| Squamous ca skin | 41 | 20 | 49 |
| Esophagus | 20 | 7 | 35 |
| Breast | 48 | 16 | 33 |
| Lung | 17 | 8 | 47 |
| Small bowel | 17 | 1 | 6 |
| Prostate | 11 | 7 | 64 |
| Bladder | 10 | 6 | 60 |
| Bone | 10 | 7 | 70 |

From Boggs DR, Frei E. Clinical studies of fever and infection in cancer. *Cancer* 1960; 13:1240–1253.

nificant comorbidity within 24 hours of presentation; group 3, outpatients with uncontrolled cancer but without serious concurrent comorbidity; and group 4, outpatients without serious concurrent comorbidity and whose cancer was well controlled. The model was validated in 444 patients with febrile neutropenia, of whom 36% had a significant comorbidity, 27% had serious medical complications, and 8% died. Group 1 had the greatest risk and group 4 had little risk in relation to medical complications and risk (Table 3).

An important component of this study was the identification of those patients at low risk of medical complication within 24 hours of onset of fever. These low-risk patients were indeed at risk of developing medical complications (5%), but these were either transient and asymptomatic or were heralded by at least 7 days of medical deterioration and were thus readily detectable by appropriate follow-up. Two additional risk factors, a latency period of <10 days from the time of chemotherapy administration to the onset of fever and neutropenia and age >40, correlated with the occurrence of more frequent complications. Mucositis was associated with decreased risk of medical complications, suggesting that infection associated with mucositis may be responsive to antibiotics. The identification of a causative organism or positive blood cultures was not associated with increased risk.

Based on a number of retrospective studies, similar definitions of low risk were applied to pediatric patients with fever and neutropenia (14). Low risk included evidence of bone marrow recovery in culture-negative patients who were afebrile for at least 24 hours and who had no other reason to continue intravenous antibiotics in hospital. The control of any localized infection and the patient's ability to return promptly in the event of fever or other complications were also necessary. In a prospective study of 70 patients who met the above criteria and who were discharged home with neutropenia, none was readmitted with fever. All 7 patients who were inadvertently discharged without evidence of marrow recovery were readmitted with recurrence of fever. Neutropenic children with positive cultures were also assessed to identify risk factors for bacteremia (15). Of cases of bacteremia,

92.5% occurred in those whose cancer was not controlled, were <1 year of age, had <10 days since previous chemotherapy, and had no evidence of marrow recovery.

### Organisms (Bacteriology)

A basic understanding of the classification and sensitivities of the different organisms is essential to the understanding of infection in cancer patients. Over time there have been changes in the underlying organisms associated with febrile neutropenia as evidenced by progressive studies by the EORTC group (16). Gram-negative organisms were the leading cause of infection in febrile neutropenic patient but their incidence has decreased from 71% (1973–1978) of identified causative organisms to 31% (1989–1991). Infection by one of these gram-negative organisms, *Pseudomonas aeruginosa,* has been a driving force in the selection of antibiotics. However, the incidence of *Pseudomonas* infection has also decreased over the last few years as reflected by an incidence of only 0.1% of febrile neutropenic cases at the National Cancer Institute (17). The incidence of gram-positive organisms has increased from 29% (1973–1978) to 69% (1989–1991), requiring a review in treatment regimens used in febrile neutropenic patients. The incidence of both acute and chronic fungal infections has also increased, with up to 33% of febrile neutropenic patients not responding to a week of antibiotic therapy, having a systemic fungal (*Candida* or *Aspergillus)* infection (18).

### Location

Infection can occur throughout the body and needs to be sought carefully with history and examination. Collapse, consolidation, and superimposed infection may develop behind an obstructing bronchial tumor. Aspiration pneumonia may occur in those with esophageal tumor either secondary to an obstruction or as a result of a tracheo-esophageal fistula.

The gastrointestinal system is the most common site of indigent organisms causing infection in neutropenic patients. *Clostridium difficile* infection may present with

**TABLE 3**. *Incidence of multiple medical complications and mortality in febrile neutropenic patients as defined by risk*

| Patient group | No. of patients | Multiple complications (%) | Death (%) |
|---|---|---|---|
| Group I | 268 | 51 (19%) | 25 (9) |
| Group II | 43 | 3 (7) | 5 (12) |
| Group III | 29 | 3 (10) | 4 (14) |
| Group IV | 104 | 0 (0) | 0 (0) |
| All patients | 444 | 57 (13) | 34 (8) |

From Talcott JA, Siegel RD, Finberg R, Goldman L. Risk assessment in cancer patients with fever and neutropenia: a prospective, two center validation of a prediction rule. *J Clin Oncol* 1992;10:316--322.
*Note: Risk groups are defined in text.*

fever and diarrhea and must be considered in those who are already taking antibiotics. Fungal and viral infections of the esophagus need to be suspected in those with dysphagia and odynophagia. Anaerobic infections may be a factor in severe mucositis or gingivitis and in those patients with perianal discomfort. Spontaneous peritonitis may be a cause of fever in patients with ascites. A urinary catheter will increase the risk of urinary tract infection as well as the risk of obstruction but the presence of asymptomatic bacteria in a nonneutropenic cancer patient is not usually an indication for antibiotic treatment.

Central nervous system infections can be difficult to diagnose and usually require lumbar puncture to confirm. Infection is the most common complication of Ommaya reservoirs, used to administer intraventricular chemotherapy, and is more likely to occur in those with previous radiotherapy or in whom repeated surgical procedures have been necessary (19). Most infections are due to *Staphylococcus epidermidis* and usually can be successfully treated with antibiotics (20).

Particular attention to sites of recent surgery is important to exclude them as a source of infection. Surgical collections may include infected hematomas that develop following surgery. The skin is also a common site of infection that may range from infected decubitus ulcers to herpes zoster infections. The use of catheters in oncology has created another portal for the introduction of infection in cancer patients. Of a total of 322 indwelling devices placed in 274 cancer patients by a single surgeon, device-related sepsis occurred in 28 of 209 patients (13%) with catheters and 6 of 113 patients (5%) with subcutaneous ports (21). Triple-lumen catheters were associated with a higher rate of thrombosis but not of infection. The complications of 1630 venous access devices for long-term use in 1431 consecutive patients with cancer were reviewed (22). Three hundred forty-one of 788 (43%) of the catheters inserted had at least one device-related infection compared with 57 of 680 (8%) of the completely implanted ports (p < 0.001). The number of infections per 1000 device days was 2.77 for catheters compared with 0.21 for ports (p < 0.001), and the predominant organisms isolated in catheter-related bacteremia were gram-negative bacilli (55%), compared with gram-positive cocci (65.5%) in port-related bacteremia. Patients with solid tumors were less likely to have device-related infectious morbidity compared with patients with hematologic cancers.

**Transfusion-Related Fever**

Blood products, administered extensively to cancer patients, may be associated with febrile reactions. The incidence of side effects following the administration of over 100,000 units of red blood cells to more than 25,000 cancer patients over a 4-year period was retrospectively reviewed (23). Three-tenths of 1% of all transfused units had a transfusion-associated reaction, of which 51.3% were febrile nonhemolytic and 36.7% allergic urticarial reactions. Only 17 hemolytic reactions (4 immediate, 13 delayed) were documented. The incidence of transfusion-related side effects was significantly lower in this study than that reported in the noncancer population. Infection may also be a source of fever in patients receiving blood products. The Canadian Red Cross (24) estimated that the true positive rate of bacterial contamination of platelet concentrate units was between 4.4 and 10.7 per 10,000 units and recommended screening of all such units. The percentage of those patients developing bacteremia or septicemia from infected units was not discussed.

**Thrombosis**

Trousseau's self-diagnosis of gastric cancer on the basis of venous thrombosis is a reminder that cancer patients are at particular risk of thrombosis. Deep vein thrombosis may present with fever and given the uncertainty of clinical diagnosis, investigation may be necessary in the "at-risk" patient. Pelvic thrombophlebitis may sometimes occur after pelvic surgery and if septic may manifest with either low- or high-grade fever. Pulmonary embolus also needs to be considered in the differential diagnosis of fever in cancer patients. Of 97 patients with confirmed pulmonary embolus in the Urokinase PE Trial, 17 had associated malignancy (25). Of those with confirmed malignancy, 54% had a fever >37.5°C and 19.6% had a fever >38°C. Of the cancer patients, 41% had associated sweating. Pulmonary infarction with the primary signs of tachypnea, tachycardia, and fever may be a presentation of pulmonary thrombi. Other thrombotic syndromes such as cerebral venous thrombosis, while associated with fever, are not common in the setting of malignancy.

**Hemorrhage**

Gastrointestinal bleeding may present with fever and should be considered in the differential diagnosis of a patient with low-grade fever and sweats. However, in a major review of fever in cancer patients (10), serious hemorrhage was followed by fever in a minority of cases; the usual sequence has been that of hemorrhage in an already febrile patient.

**Drugs**

Drug-associated fever is an ill-defined syndrome in which fever is the predominant manifestation of an adverse drug reaction. It is normally a diagnosis of exclusion (26). The drugs commonly associated with fever are antibiotics, cardiovascular drugs, CNS drugs such as phenytoin, cytotoxics, and immune therapy (either as biological response modifiers or growth factors). Antimicrobial agents were responsible for 46 of 148 cases of fever in a review of the experience of two hospitals in Texas and the United Kingdom, with mean lag time from initiation of treatment to onset of fever of 21 days (median 8 days). For 11 cases of cytotoxic-induced fever, the mean lag time was 6.0 days with a median of 0.5 days. Shaking chills were more common with cytotoxic-associated fever than with other drugs (27).

### Cytotoxics

There is a diverse range of cytotoxic drugs whose administration is associated with fever (Table 4). The febrile response to bleomycin was described in the original phase 1 studies (28) and characteristically occurs 3–5 hours after injection and is more common after intravenous than after intramuscular injection. It is seen in about 25% of patients administered the drug, and the fever becomes less frequent with the repeated injections. An anaphylactic reaction manifested by hyperpyrexia, shock, hypotension, urticaria, and asthmatic wheezing can occur in 1% of patients administered bleomycin (29). Fever following the administration of cisplatin was also reported in early clinical trials (30). Streptozocin administration may result in fever associated with chills, as can cytarabine and etoposide. Fever can occur following the administration of 5-fluorouracil (5-FU) and high-dose methotrexate. Confusion concerning the etiology of a fever arises more commonly in the situation of intensive chemotherapy regimens where neutropenic patients may be administered cytotoxic agents that cause fever. Awareness of the symptoms produced by the different agents assists in discerning the etiology of the fever.

### Antibiotics

The antibiotics commonly associated with fever are the penicillins, cephalosporins, and amphotericin. In 50

**TABLE 4.** *Cytotoxic agents associated with fever following administration*

Bleomycin
Cisplatin
Cytarabine
Cyclophosphamide
Etoposide
5-Fluorouracil
Methotrexate
Mustine
Mithramycin
Streptozocin
Thiotepa
Vinblastine
Vincristine

patients administered at least 100 mg of amphotericin B over a minimum of 3 days, fever was experienced by 34% and chills by 56%, with rates of 2.6 and 3.5 mean episodes per patient per treatment course, respectively (31). In patients who had received 20 mg or more of amphotericin B per day for at least 10 consecutive days, shivering was noted to occur first at the test dose, with the percentage of patients who shivered increasing with each successive dose and peaking at the fifth therapeutic dose (32).

### Opioids

The intravenous injection of morphine is often associated with sweating and vasodilatation but is not necessarily associated with fever. Fever may occur as a result of the interaction between pethidine and monoaminoxidase inhibitor, an interaction to be avoided. Drug withdrawal is associated with a syndrome that includes fever and needs to be suspected in febrile cancer patients in whom opioids have been stopped suddenly. Withdrawal from benzodiazepines may also be associated with fever.

### Biological Therapy

Interferons (IFN) are associated with the development of fever (33). Partially purified IFN-$\alpha$, administered at low doses intramuscularly, induces a fever (38–40°C) within 6 hours that persists for some 4–8 hours. More severe side effects are seen when the drug is administered intravenously, intrathecally, or in patients >65 years of age. The use of the highly purified recombinant DNA IFN-$\alpha$ induces similar side effects. IFN-$\alpha$ at doses of 50–120 MU results in a sharp febrile response with severe rigors and associated peripheral cyanosis, vasoconstriction, nausea and vomiting, severe muscle aches, and headaches. In those receiving IFN-$\alpha$ daily, the febrile response and accompanying symptoms usually decrease in intensity and disappear in 7–10 days. Fever, however, persists with intermittent (nondaily) injections and with the daily injection of IFN-$\tau$, which produces a fever that peaks at 6–12 hours and tends to last longer. The administration of other biological factors is associated with the onset of fever, e.g., TNF. The administration of growth factors is associated with the onset of fever although the incidence following G-CSF is very low. Fever occurs much more commonly following GM-CSF administration.

## Graft versus Host Disease

Transplantation in cancer has become much more common and despite the development of autologous transplants the use of nonmatched donors is still common. Death is often caused by infection in acute graft versus host disease. Chronic graft versus host disease is very much like that of a systemic collagen vascular disease and may be associated with infection, with or without the presence of fever.

## Radiation-Induced Fever

Patients receiving radiotherapy alone may present with fever some hours after the initial treatment. Acute radiation pneumonitis may develop 2–3 months after completion of radiation therapy. A high-spiking fever may be part of the syndrome, which consists of dyspnea and an unproductive cough. Lung biopsy may be necessary to establish the diagnosis.

## Other Diseases

Other diseases that may cause fever may coexist in cancer patients, e.g., systemic lupus erythematosis or rheumatoid arthritis. Careful review of past medical history and current symptoms is essential.

## DIAGNOSIS

The classical teaching that history provides 95% of the diagnosis is certainly true when it comes to the symptoms of fever in oncologic patients. Following the physical examination, the use of diagnostic aids is related very much to the relevant history. Although two thirds of neutropenic patients do not have an identifiable cause of their fever, culture of relevant body fluids is still essential in the management of these patients. However, routine surveillance cultures in patients with neutropenia prior to the development of fever are not cost productive (34). While a CXR may not be indicated in symptomatic patients presenting with febrile neutropenia (35), a recent CXR may be an important baseline in a patient without respiratory symptoms or signs who is likely to have a prolonged period of neutropenia.

The diagnosis of fever due to the cancer itself can be confirmed with the use of naproxen (36). The proponents of "the naproxen test" state that it does not result in a decrease in temperature in those with infection. The successful treatment of "neoplastic" fever in 21 cancer patients was demonstrated, with 15 responding to a dose of 250 mg/day, whereas others responded following an increase in the dose of naproxen administered. The true sensitivity and specificity of this test are uncertain but the authors stress that infectious fever and noninfectious fever due to drug toxicity, allergic reaction, and adrenal insufficiency need to be excluded before considering the diagnosis as neoplastic fever.

## TREATMENT

Primary to any treatment of fever in cancer patients is the treatment of the underlying cause of fever. Antibiotics should not be used to control fever in nonneutropenic patients in the absence of evidence of infection, but nonsteroidal antiinflammatory drugs (NSAIDs) may be useful in the treatment of fever associated with infection.

Physical cooling, e.g., through sponging, when used alone is likely to be uncomfortable for febrile patients and should be reserved for those in a hot and humid environment that may impede evaporative heat loss or for those with defective heat-loss mechanisms (37). Sponging, when it does take place, should be with tepid water, as the use of cold water will induce shivering which consequently increases patient discomfort and causes an elevation in temperature (38).

Agents that lower body temperature (antipyretics) primarily comprise three groups: (a) pure antipyretics that do not work in the absence of pyrogen and at usual therapeutic doses do not affect normal temperature, e.g., acetaminophen; (b) agents that cause hypothermia in afebrile subjects by directly impairing thermoregulatory function; and (c) those that are antipyretic in lower doses and cause hypothermia in higher doses, e.g., chlorpromazine.

Only salicylates, acetaminophen, and ibuprofen have been approved for antipyretic use in the United States and none of these agents is likely to cause hypothermia in normothermic patients. Aspirin is not recommended for use in children because of the risk of Reye's syndrome, a disease process that results in liver failure (39). Aspirin has been the standard of reference in nearly two thirds of clinical comparisons of antipyretic activity but only one comparison of aspirin has been performed in cancer patients (40). Patients with low-grade fever received doses of aspirin and placebo in random order. No useful conclusions could be drawn as the mean reduction in temperature for the 600 mg of aspirin was only 0.3°C, not statistically significant from placebo.

In children, acetaminophen has a dose-response effect, with doses of 5, 10, and 20 mg/kg bringing about a reduction in temperature of 0.3, 1.6, and 2.5°C, respectively, after 3 hours (37). Aspirin and acetaminophen appear equally effective at about 10 mg/kg. Ibuprofen 0.5 mg/kg is about as effective as 10 mg/kg aspirin and 12.5 mg/kg acetaminophen and probably lasts longer. Indomethacin has been reported to be more effective than these three compounds in limiting febrile responses to interferon (41) but is not approved for antipyretic use in the United States. Indomethacin (75 mg), naproxen (500 mg), and diclofenac sodium (75 mg) have been found to be equally effective in the management of paraneoplastic fever (42).

## Treatment of Infection

The treatment of fever in a nonneutropenic oncology patient is not in itself a medical emergency. Shock associated with such a patient can make it an emergency. A thorough review of the history and examination and the performance of the appropriate tests should guide both the timing and the type of treatment initiated.

The presence of fever in an immunocompromised patient is a medical emergency and empirical therapy should be initiated as soon as possible. Patients at risk of neutropenia should be instructed to record their temperature and to report the presence of fever to health care staff. An overall schema for the use of antimicrobial agents in neutropenic patients with unexplained fever is presented in Figure 3. A variety of antibiotic treatments were discussed by the Infectious Diseases Society of America Consensus Statement on Febrile Neutropenia (43), and these will be considered together with more recent studies on the choice of antibiotics in febrile neutropenia. The decision as to which antibiotic regimen to use rests with each institution and must take into consideration local experience and infection trends.

The initial choice of antibiotic regimens is most commonly with an aminoglycoside and antipseudomonal β-lactam. These regimes have been extensively used and are particularly recommended for those at high risk of

*Pseudomonas* infection, including cancer patients with severe mucositis and those known to be colonized with the organism. Given the nephro- and ototoxicity associated with aminoglycosides, serum concentrations of these drugs should be monitored regularly. Such a two-drug regimen is considered to be as effective as the combination of a third-generation cephalosporin with an anti-pseudomonal β-lactam such as piperacillin. While safe, these latter regimens are expensive, open to resistance, and may not provide adequate coverage of staphylococcal infections. The addition of vancomycin to either of the above regimens provides additional coverage against staphylococcal infections and if used initially results in fewer incidents of treatment failure. Other studies have shown no difference in mortality and morbidity rates in those patients in whom vancomycin was added at a later date.

The use of monotherapy was not strongly supported by the committee. While initial results of such therapy were good, modification has been required often enough for combination therapy to be preferred as initial therapy. The panel recommended that monotherapy be considered in those at low risk of infection (brief period of neutropenia prior to fever and with counts between 500 and 1000/µl) and that these patients be closely monitored. A meta-analysis has subsequently been performed on 13 studies that compared ceftazadine monotherapy with dif-

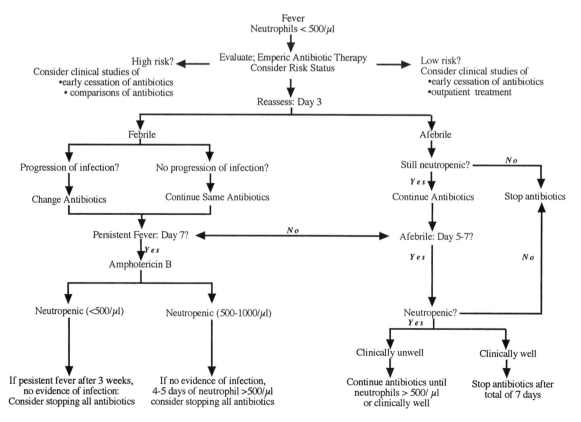

**FIG. 3.** Clinical approach to the treatment of patients with febrile neutropenia.

ferent combination therapies (44). No difference in treatment failure was found and there was no difference in outcome when febrile and bacteremic episodes were considered independently. Similar percentages of modifications for monotherapy and combination therapy were made. In a more recent multicenter, randomized, controlled trial of the treatment of 876 febrile, neutropenic episodes in 696 patients (45), single-agent ceftazidine was found to be safer than piperacillin and tobramycin combined while having similar effectiveness (62.7% versus 61.1%; $p$ - 0.2). Infectious mortality was 6% for ceftazidine and 8% for the combination therapy, and 38 episodes of superinfection developed in each group. An adverse event occurred in 8% of the episodes treated with ceftazidine compared with 20% with combination therapy ($p < 0.001$). Of note, 83% of the patients enrolled in the study were leukemia and transplant patients and often experienced profound and prolonged neutropenia.

The need to continually review a patient's clinical situation and therapy is essential. The Consensus Panel agreed that by day 3, a neutropenic patient who was either afebrile or had continuing fever but with no progression of the infective process could continue on the same antibiotics. Antibiotics should be changed if fever persisted and there was progression of the infective process. Either vancomycin could be added at that stage (if not already in use) or monotherapy, in the form of a third-generation cephalosporin, could be commenced. If the patient remained both neutropenic and febrile after a week and was unlikely to have white cell recovery in the near future, amphotericin should be added (46). Antianaerobic therapy should be considered in those with persistent fever and severe oral mucositis, necrotizing gingivitis, or perianal tenderness.

The current duration of antibiotic treatment where patients with febrile neutropenia have been admitted to hospital for antibiotic treatment until their neutropenia resolved is based on the results of a 1979 study (47). Early stopping of antibiotics at day 7 in 17 patients with resolved fever but persistent neutropenia resulted in the recurrence of fever in 7 patients, of whom 2 died. The consensus committee considered cessation of antibiotics in afebrile patients who were clinically well but with a neutrophil count of <500/μl. While not strongly supported by scientific data, they considered that therapy could be stopped after 7 days provided that the patient was carefully observed, mucus membranes and skin were intact, and no invasive procedure or ablative chemotherapy was imminent.

More recent studies have suggested that in patients at lower risk of complications, outpatient treatment and early stopping of antibiotics may be possible. Thirty febrile neutropenic patients, identified to be of low complication risk after 48 hours of inpatient intravenous treatment, were continued on the same antibiotics at home until neutropenia resolved (48). Four patients were readmitted with medical complications (hypotension, 3; acute renal failure, 1) and five others were readmitted for observation. Overall costs were similar for those treated at home and for those who were medically eligible for home treatment but who were treated in hospital. The higher-than-expected cost of home treatment related to extended periods of neutropenia seen in these patients. Attempts have been made to shorten the hospital stay by discontinuing intravenous antibiotics in blood culture-negative patients who remained clinically stable and afebrile after 48 hours of treatment (49). In a retrospective review of 134 admissions for neutropenic fever, the median duration of intravenous antibiotics decreased significantly from 7 days prior to institution of such a policy to 5 days (4–6) and 4 days (3–5) over the next two consecutive 6-month periods. The median duration of hospital stay decreased from 10 to 7 (5–8) and 6 days (5–7) over the same time periods. The authors concluded that intravenous antibiotics may be discontinued in patients who remain afebrile and clinically stable for 48 hours and who have negative blood cultures, resulting in a shorter duration of hospital stay with the potential for reduction in hospital costs.

Early stopping of antibiotics together with a selective decontamination regimen (neomycin, polymyxin, amphotericin, and pipemidic acid) was prospectively studied in 52 adult patients with hematologic malignancies and a neutrophil count <500/μl (50). Patients experienced 77 febrile episodes while receiving the oral antibiotics and further treatment, either broad-spectrum or disease-specific antibiotics, was initiated only if clinical signs or microbiological culture results indicated an infection. Consequently, antibiotics were adjusted according to culture findings or discontinued if evidence of infection was lacking after 72–96 hours. For the 40 episodes without confirmed infection, the median duration of therapy was 3 days (range 0–13 days) and the survival rate 100% with 15 receiving no additional antibiotics. For the 37 episodes with confirmed infection, the median duration of therapy was 12 days (range 1–49 days, $p < 0.0001$) and the survival rate 85%. Broad-spectrum therapy was only used for the duration of neutropenia in 18% of the treated episodes and none of the six deaths could be attributed to the withholding or stopping of broad-spectrum therapy. It was concluded that in febrile neutropenic patients on this selective decontamination regimen the standard prolonged administration of broad-spectrum antibiotics was not necessary. The authors recommended that systemic antibiotics for this population be discontinued after 3–5 days if infection is unlikely, that a narrower antibiotic spectrum be chosen according to the clinical situation, and that empirical antifungal treatment be considered after 7 days. While very promising, the findings of this study need to be confirmed in randomized clinical trials prior to their widespread implementation.

The place of outpatient treatment of low-risk neutropenic patients was examined at the M.D. Anderson Cancer Center (51). Oral ciprofloxacin combined with clindamycin was as effective in the control of infection as was the combination of intravenous aztreonam and clindamycin. However, the oral regime was associated with increased renal toxicity that resulted in the early termination of the study. The authors recommended the development of better outpatient antibiotic regimens and urged caution, as none of their patients had gram-negative bacteremias or pneumonias, a group that may be difficult to treat. Outpatient treatment was further studied in Pakistan, where 188 low-risk patients with febrile neutropenia were randomized to receive either inpatient or outpatient oral orfloxacin (52). The investigators had previously found oral orfloxacin to be as effective for inpatient care as their standard intravenous regimen (53). The patient group consisted of patients with both solid tumors and leukemias and excluded those in whom the duration of neutropenia was likely to exceed 7 days. Fever control was the same in both groups, with 78% of inpatient and 77% of outpatient fevers resolving without modification of the initial treatment. However, 21% percent of the outpatients required hospitalization. Mortality was 2% in those assigned inpatient treatment and 4% in outpatients, with one death occurring outside of hospital. This approach may be useful but it should be limited to that subset of patients with low-risk factors who are not otherwise on quinolone prophylaxis and in whom close monitoring and surveillance can be performed. Those with an identifiable cause of infection should be treated with the appropriate antibiotics. The issue of limited treatment in low-risk groups needs to be more clearly defined and addressed in further clinical studies (see Fig. 3).

In summary, for patients with fever who continue to have neutropenia for a week or more, broad-spectrum antibiotic therapy for the duration of the neutropenia along with empirical antifungal therapy in those who remain febrile is the current consensus. The use of narrow-spectrum agents or abbreviated courses of antibiotics in these patients is in need of further study, as is their role in those patients at low risk of complications.

Vascular access devices often create a treatment dilemma in patients with febrile neutropenia. Such devices may be left in place in most patients even if bacteremia is detected and managed with antibiotic and local care (54). Catheters should be removed if they are non-patent, are associated with thrombosis, have evidence of septic emboli, or if there is a subcutaneous tunnel infection. Prompt removal of catheters is also done with *Candida* sp. fungemia and bacteremia due to *Bacillus* sp. or a bacteremia that persists for >48 hours after initiation of appropriate antibiotics.

Antiviral medications may be required in neutropenic as well as immunocompromised patients without neu-tropenia. However, the empirical use of antiviral drugs in the management of febrile neutropenia in patients without mucosal lesions or evidence of viral disease is not indicated. The recommended dose of acyclovir for the treatment of established herpes infections in the immunocompromised ranges from 5 mg/kg q8h IV for herpes simplex to 10–12 mg/kg q8h IV in shingles.

While popular throughout the 1970s and 1980s, granulocyte infusion use has faded in recent years despite evidence of efficacy. In a recent review (55) of the use of granulocyte transfusions (GTX), this decline was related to the administration of ineffective doses of granulocytes. The author recommended that physicians assess the outcome of persistent febrile neutropenia in their own institutions and if poor, the addition of GTX, at therapeutic doses ($2–3 \times 10_{10}$ PMN), may be useful along with other changes such as the use of different antibiotics. The use of G-CSF in the collection of white cells was also considered but requires more work before its use is considered standard.

### Treatment of Transfusion Reactions

Transfusion reactions can be prevented by filtering of blood products and also by premedication with an antihistamine. The use of erythropoietin in anemia associated with malignancy may reduce the need for blood transfusions, thus avoiding both transfusion reactions and a source of infection. The cost of such treatment needs to be considered carefully.

### Treatment of Amphotericin-Related Febrile Reaction

A dose of 12.5–25 mg of intravenous meperidine is useful in the prevention of amphotericin-related fever and rigors. However, slowing the rate of amphotericin may reduce toxicity. Amphotericin given over 45 minutes was much more toxic in relation to fever and rigors than the same dose given over 4 hours (56). Less meperidine was required for the control of symptoms in the 4-hour infusion arm. In another study, no difference was found between a 45-minute and a 2-hour infusion (57).

### PROPHYLAXIS

Prophylaxis in the form of antibiotics or other supportive treatment may be useful in the prevention of febrile neutropenia.

### Growth Factors

Hematologic colony-stimulating factors (CSF) reduce treatment-associated myelosuppression by shortening the duration of neutropenia and by reducing the nadir of neutrophil counts. However, much confusion about their appropriate clinical use led to a recent consensus statement from the American Society of Clinical Oncology (58). Two indications for the use of G-CSF administration were addressed: primary CSF use in those receiving their initial chemotherapy and secondary use in those who have previously had chemotherapy-induced neutropenia.

To assess a benefit in primary prevention, the incidence of grade 4 neutropenia following CSF use in different randomized treatment protocols was considered. The incidence of neutropenia ranged from 0% in breast cancer patients receiving the combination of cyclophosphamide, doxorubicin, and 5-FU, to 98% of 102 lung cancer patients administered cyclophosphamide, doxorubicin, and etoposide. G-CSF was found to significantly decrease the incidence of febrile neutropenia, where the placebo group had an incidence of neutropenia greater than 40%. However, in these randomized CSF trials, no difference in infectious mortality, response rates, or survival between CSF- and placebo-treated patients was documented. It was recommended that CSFs only be used with those protocols where the incidence of neutropenia was likely to be >40% without their use. When less myelotoxic chemotherapy is planned, primary administration of CSFs should be reserved for those patients who are at high risk from neutropenic complications due to host- or disease-related factors. Individual cases should also be considered in patients at higher risk of chemotherapy-induced infectious complications, e.g., extensive prior chemotherapy. Elderly patients tolerate chemotherapy as well as younger patients and should not receive CSFs purely on the basis of age.

There were few studies concerning the secondary administration of CSFs available to the ASCO working group. If a patient has already experienced chemotherapy-induced neutropenia, then CSF can be used if there is proven benefit in maintaining the dose. It is important to remember that for primary use of CSF, there was no difference in infectious mortality, tumor response, or survival. In the absence of a reason to maintain the chemotherapy dose, dose reduction should be considered especially if other toxicities not responsive to CSFs are present. No evidence has been found to support the routine use of CSFs in febrile neutropenic patients, although those at particularly high risk may have some benefit. There has been no evidence to recommend the use of CSFs to increase chemotherapy dose intensity outside of clinical trials addressing this issue. CSFs may be useful for mobilizing peripheral blood stem cells (PBSCs) and they have a benefit in reducing the period of neutropenia in autologous and PBSC transplants. However, there was no indication for their use in patients receiving combined chemotherapy and radiotherapy. When used, the group recommended a G-CSF dose of 5 µg/kg/day (GM-CSF, 250 µg/m²/day), without dose escalation, administered 24–72 hours after chemotherapy until the neutrophil

count is >10,000/µl after the neutrophil nadir. However, it may be possible to reduce the cost with the use of a less lengthy treatment period.

The implications, including cost, of the use of G-CSF in the treatment of small cell lung cancer at the University of Indiana were reviewed (59). The overall incidence of neutropenia was 18% in the 137 patients treated with standard chemotherapy and in whom dose reductions were allowed on subsequent courses. The estimated total cost of this treatment was approximately $192,000. There would have been more than a sixfold increase in cost ($1.2 million) if primary treatment of all patients with G-CSF had taken place. The cost of the secondary use of G-CSF in those with a previous episode of fever and neutropenia ($272,000) would have been less than twice that of not using growth factors at all. The authors concluded that the routine use of G-CSF in SCLC patients treated with standard dose chemotherapy was expensive and not associated with obvious therapeutic benefits or cost savings. They suggested that careful analysis of the incidence of infectious complications, rather than granulocyte nadir and duration, be performed.

### Other Prophylactic Measures

Although total protected environments (involving laminar flow, the oral administration of nonabsorbable antibiotic, and cutaneous decontamination) reduce the incidence of infection, using them proved cumbersome and expensive and they have largely been abandoned (17), particularly in those in whom the duration of neutropenia is likely to be short. However, individual components of these regimens continue to be used in many treatment protocols.

There have been mixed results from the oral administration of nonabsorbable drugs such as gentamycin, nystatin, and vancomycin. The consensus panel could make no recommendation as to their use but agreed strongly that the use of aminoglycosides in this situation should be avoided. In a recent review, the use of nonabsorbable antibiotics without concurrent patient isolation was not recommended because of the unpalatability of the antibiotics, their cost, the emergence of resistant organisms, and the lack of constant efficacy (17).

The Infectious Diseases Consensus panel (43) recommended trimethoprim-sulfamethoxazole (TMP-SMZ) prophylaxis for afebrile, uninfected patients with profound neutropenia that was expected to persist for at least a week. This combination has a role in the prevention of *Pneumocystis* infections in transplant patients and has been used in protocols such as MACOP-B. Norfloxacin, an oral quinolone, has been found to reduce gram-negative infection when compared with Bactrim, but the possibility of the development of resistance prevented the consensus group from recommending its routine use. The role of prophylactic ciprofloxacin in reducing the incidence of neutropenic fever in 88 consecutive men receiving intensive chemotherapy for germ cell tumors was reviewed. In total, 88 men received 429 courses of chemotherapy and prophylactic ciprofloxacin was prescribed for 168 courses. The incidence of fever in these patients was significantly reduced from 15% (20/131) to 5% (6/109) ($p = 0.02$) with prophylactic ciprofloxacin. Two patients, one of whom had received prophylactic ciprofloxacin, died of chest infection confirmed on postmortem. The results of this nonrandomized, retrospective study suggest that prophylactic ciprofloxacin 250 mg b.d. is effective in reducing the incidence of fever-complicating neutropenia during chemotherapy for germ cell tumors. To be cost effective, however, it should be given only to neutropenic patients (60). Ciprofloxacin (750 mg b.d.) was found to be as safe and effective as TMP-SMZ (160 mg/800 mg b.d.) in the prevention of bacterial infections in 146 bone marrow transplant patients. However, ciprofloxacin was associated with a lower incidence of *Clostridium difficile* enterocolitis and infections caused by gram-negative bacilli, indicating an advantage for its use in transplant patients (61). Prophylaxis also extends to antiviral medications. Acyclovir use decreases the incidence of herpetic gingivostomatitis in patients with neutropenia, and the administration of acyclovir decreases the incidence of cytomegalovirus pneumonitis in patients who have undergone bone marrow transplant.

## ETHICAL CONSIDERATIONS OF TREATMENT OF INFECTIONS

There is a need for discussion of issues related to nontreatment of infections. There is no doubt that if the intention of treatment is to ensure the prolongation of survival, then treatment of the infective episode needs to be initiated. Dilemmas may arise regarding those patients in whom the intention of treatment is palliation. Antibiotics may make a patient feel more comfortable but they may also prolong the dying process. A balance between the two needs to be assessed in each individual patient, considering in particular factors such as prognosis and treatment goals.

Even if a patient is nearing death, indications for commencement of antibiotics may include convulsions or mental changes attributed to fever, extreme temperature (>40°C), extreme age (very young and very old), and a past history of adverse reaction to fever, marked subjective discomfort pronounced by patient, a prolonged high fever causing significant hypercatabolic state, and a reduced cardiac or pulmonary function to the extent that further tachycardia or tachypnea may be harmful. Further issues pertaining to this will be discussed in other chapters.

## REFERENCES

1. Petersdorf RG, Beeson PB. Fever of unexplained origin: report of 100 cases. *Medicine* 1961;40: 1–29.
2. Boulant JA. Thermoregulation. In: Mackowiak P, ed. *Fever: Basic mechanisms and management.* New York: Raven Press, 1991;1–22
3. Engel A, Kern WV, Murdter G, Kern P. Kinetics and correlation with body temperature of circulating interleukin-6, interleukin-8, tumor necrosis factor alpha and interleukin-1 beta in patients with fever and neutropenia. *Infection* 1994;22:160–4.
4. Ashman RB, Mullbacher A. Host damaging immune responses in virus infections. *Surv Immunol Res* 1984;3: 11–15
5. Greenberg SB, Taber L. Fever of unknown origin. In: Mackowiak P, ed. *Fever: Basic mechanisms and management.* New York: Raven Press, 1991;183–195.
6. Esposito AL, Gleckman RA. Fever of unknown origin in the elderly. *J Am Geriatr Soc* 1978;26:498–505.
7. Klastersky J, Weerts D, Hensgens C, Debusscher L. Fever of unexplained origin in patients with cancer. *Eur J Cancer* 1973;9:649–656.
8. Good GR, Dinubile MJ. Hodgkin's disease. *N Engl J Med* 1995;332: 436.
9. Asher R. *Richard Asher talking sense.* London: Pitman, 1972;21–22.
10. Boggs DR, Frei E. Clinical studies of fever and infection in cancer. *Cancer* 1960;13:1240–1253.
11. Pizzo PA. Evaluation of fever in the patient with cancer. *Eur J Cancer Clin Oncol* 1989;25:S9–S16.
12. Bodey GP, Buckley M, Sathe YS, Friereich EJ. Quantitative relationships between circulating leucocytes and infection in patients with acute leukemia. *Ann Intern Med* 1966;64:328–340.
13. Talcott JA, Siegel RD, Finberg R, Goldman L. Risk assessment in cancer patients with fever and neutropenia: a prospective, two center validation of a prediction rule. *J Clin Oncol* 1992;10;316–322.
14. Buchanan GR. Approach to treatment of the febrile cancer patient with low-risk neutropenia. *Hematol Oncol Clin North Am* 1993;7:919–935.
15. Pappo AS, Buchanan GR. Predictors of bacteremia in febrile neutropenic children with cancer (Abstract). *Proc Am Soc Clin Oncol* 1991;10:331.
16. Klastersky. Therapy of Infections. In: Klastersky J, Schimpff SC, Senn HJ, eds. *Handbook of supportive care in cancer.* New York: Marcel Dekker, 1994;1–44.
17. Pizzo PA. Management of fever in patients with cancer and treatment-induced neutropenia (see comments). *N Engl J Med* 1993;328: 1323–1332.
18. Pizzo PA, Robichaud KJ, Witebsky FG. Emperic antibiotics and antifungal treatment for cancer patients with prolonged fever and neutropenia. *Am J Med* 1982;72:101–111.
19. Machado M, Salcman EM, Kaplan RS. The expanded role of reservoirs in neurooncology. *Neurosurgery* 1985;1:600.
20. Siegal T, Pfeffer MR, Steiner I. Antibiotic therapy for infected Ommaya reservoir systems. *Neurosurgery* 1988;22:97.
21. Eastridge BJ, Lefor AT. Complications of indwelling venous access devices in cancer patients. *J Clin Oncol* 1995;13:233–238.
22. Groeger JS, Lucas AB, Thaler HT, et al. Infectious morbidity associated with long-term use of venous access devices in patients with cancer (see comments). *Ann Intern Med* 1993;119:1168–1174.
23. Huh YO, Lichtiger B. Transfusion reactions in patients with cancer. *Am J Clin Pathol* 1987;87:253–257.
24. Blajchman MA. Bacterial contamination of blood products and the value of pretransfusion testing. *Immunol Invest* 1995;24:163–170.
25. Manganelli D, Palla A, Donnamaria V, Giuntini C. Clinical features of pulmonary embolus. Doubts and certainties. *Chest* 1995;107:S25–S32.
26. Mackowiak PA. Drug fever. In: Mackowiak PA, ed. *Fever: Basic mechanisms and management.* New York: Raven Press, 1991;255–265.
27. Mackowiak PA, LeMaistre CF. Drug fever: a critical appraisal of conventional concepts. An analysis of 51 episodes diagnosed in two Dallas hospitals and 97 episodes reported in the English literature. *Ann Intern Med* 1987;106:728–733.
28. Sonntag RW. Bleomycin (NSC-125066): phase I clinical study. *Cancer Chemother Rep* (Part 1) 1972;56:197–205.
29. Ma DD, Isbister JP. Cytotoxic-induced fulminant hyperpyrexia. *Cancer* 1980;45:2249–2251.
30. Ashford RF, McLachlan A, Nelson I, Mughal T, Pickering D. Pyrexia after cisplatin (letter). *Lancet* 1980;2:691–692.

31. Clements JS Jr, Peacock JE Jr. Amphotericin B revisited: reassessment of toxicity. *Am J Med* 1990;88:22N–27N.
32. Carney-Gersten P, Giuffre M, Levy D. Factors related to amphotericin-B-induced rigors (shivering) (see comments). *Oncol Nursing For* 1991; 18:745–50.
33. Quesada JR, Talpaz M, Rios A, Kurzrock R, Gutterman JU. Clinical toxicity of interferons in cancer patients: a review. *J Clin Oncol* 1986; 4:234–243.
34. Kramer BS, Pizzo PA, Robichaud KJ, Witebsky FG, Wesley R. Role of serial microbiologic surveillance and clinical evaluation in the management of cancer patients with fever and granulocytopenia. *Am J Med* 1982;72:561–568.
35. Feusner J, Cohen R, O'Leary M, Beach B. Use of routine chest radiography in the evaluation of fever in neutropenic pediatric oncology patients. *J Clin Oncol* 1988;6:1699–1702.
36. Chang JC, Gross HM. Neoplastic fever responds to the treatment of an adequate dose of naproxen. *J Clin Oncol* 1985;3:552–558.
37. Clark WG. Antipyretics. In: Mackowiak P, ed. *Fever: Basic mechanics and management.* New York: Raven Press, 1991;297–340.
38. Steele RW, Tanaka PT, Lara RP, Bass JW. Evaluation of sponging and of oral antipyretic therapy to reduce fever. *J Pediatrics* 1970;77: 824–829.
39. Pinsky PF, Hurwitz ES, Schonberger LB, Gunn WJ. Reye's syndrome and aspirin. Evidence for a dose response effect. *JAMA* 1988;260: 657–661.
40. Seed JC. A clinical comparison of the antipyretic potency of aspirin and sodium salicylate. *Clin Pharmacol Ther* 1965;6:354–358.
41. Paolozzi F, Zamkoff K, Doyle M, et al. Phase I trial of recombinant interleukin-2 and recombinant beta-interferon in refractory neoplastic diseases. *J Biol Resp Med* 1989;8:122–139.
42. Tsavaris N, Zinelis A, Karabelis A, et al. A randomized trial of the effect of three non-steroid anti-inflammatory agents in ameliorating cancer-induced fever. *J Intern Med* 1990;228:451–455.
43. Hughes WT, Armstrong D, Bodey GP, et al. Guidelines for the use of antimicrobial agents in neutropenic patients with unexplained fever. *J Infect Dis* 1990;161:381–396.
44. Sanders JW, Powe NR, Moore RD. Ceftazidime monotherapy for empiric treatment of febrile neutropenic patients: a metaanalysis. *J Infect Dis* 1991;164:907–916.
45. De Pauw BE, Deresinski SC, Feld R, Lane-Allman EF, Donnelly JP. Ceftazidime compared with piperacillin and tobramycin for the empiric treatment of fever in neutropenic patients with cancer. A multicenter randomized trial. The Intercontinental Antimicrobial Study Group (see comments). *Ann Intern Med* 1994;120:834–844.
46. Group EIATC. Empiric antifungal therapy in febrile granulocytopenic patients. EORTC International Antimicrobial Therapy Cooperative Group. *Am J Med* 1989;86:668–672.
47. Pizzo PA, Robichaud KJ, Gill FA, et al. Duration of empiric antibiotic therapy in granuloncytopenic patients with cancer. *Am J Med* 1979;67: 194–200.
48. Talcott JA, Whalen A, Clark J, Rieker PP, Finberg R. Home antibiotic therapy for low-risk cancer patients with fever and neutropenia: a pilot study of 30 patients based on a validated prediction rule. *J Clin Oncol* 1994;12:107–114.
49. Tomiak AT, Yau JC, Huan SD, et al. Duration of intravenous antibiotics for patients with neutropenic fever. *Ann Oncol* 1994;5:441–445.
50. de Marie S, van den Broek PJ, Willemze R, van Furth R. Strategy for antibiotic therapy in febrile neutropenic patients on selective antibiotic decontamination. *Eur J Clin Microbiol Infect Dis* 1993;12:897–906.
51. Rubenstein EB, Rolston K, Benjamin RS, et al. Outpatient treatment of febrile episodes in low-risk neutropenic patients with cancer. *Cancer* 1993;71:3640–3646.
52. Malik IA, Khan WA, Karim M, Aziz Z, Khan MA. Feasibility of outpatient management of fever in cancer patients with low-risk neutropenia: results of a prospective randomized trial (see comments). *Am J Med* 1995;98:224–231.
53. Malik IA, Abbas Z, Karim M. Randomised comparison of oral ofloxacin alone with combination of parenteral antibiotics in neutropenic febrile patients (published erratum appears in *Lancet* 1992;Jul 11;340(8811): 128). *Lancet* 1992;339:1092–1096.
54. Newman KA, Reed WP, Schimpff SC, Bustamante CI, Wade JC. Hickman catheters in association with intensive cancer chemotherapy. *Support Care Cancer* 1993;1:92–97.
55. Strauss RG. Granulocyte transfusion therapy. *Hematol Oncol Clin North Am* 1994;8:1159–1166.
56. Ellis ME, al-Hokail AA, Clink HM, et al. Double-blind randomized study of the effect of infusion rates on toxicity of amphotericin B (see comments). *Antimicrob Agents Chemother* 1992;36:172–179.
57. Cleary JD, Weisdorf D, Fletcher CV. Effect of infusion rate on amphotericin B-associated febrile reactions. *Drug Intell Clin Pharmacol* 1988; 22:769–772.
58. ASCO. American Society of Clinical Oncology recommendations for the use of hematopoietic colony-stimulating factors: evidence-based clinical practice guidelines. *J Clin Oncol* 1994;12:2471–2508.
59. Nichols CR, Fox EP, Roth BJ, Williams SD, Loehrer PJ, Einhorn LH. Incidence of neutropenic fever in patients treated with standard-dose combination chemotherapy for small-cell lung cancer and the cost impact of treatment with granulocyte colony-stimulating factor. *J Clin Oncol* 1994;12:1245–1250.
60. Counsell R, Pratt J, Williams MV. Chemotherapy for germ cell tumours: prophylactic ciprofloxacin reduces the incidence of neutropenic fever. *Clin Oncol* (Royal College of Radiologists) 1994;6:232–236.
61. Lew MA, Kohoe K, Ritz J et al. Ciprofloxacin vs. trimethoprim/sulfamethoxazole for prophylaxis of bacterial infections in bone marrow transplant recipients: a randomized, controlled trial. *J Clin Oncol* 1995; 13:239–250.

*Principles and Practice of Supportive Oncology,*
edited by Ann Berger et al.
Lippincott–Raven Publishers, Philadelphia ©1998

CHAPTER 8

# Cancer Anorexia/Cachexia

Charles L. Loprinzi, Richard M. Goldberg, and Prema P. Peethambaram

## DEFINITION, INCIDENCE, AND MAGNITUDE OF THE CLINICAL PROBLEM

Anorexia is defined as an "aversion to food" and cachexia as "a general lack of nutrition and wasting occurring in the course of a chronic disease or emotional disturbance" (1). The anorexia that accompanies malignancy can be characterized by decreased appetite often associated with food aversions and poor food intake. There is evidence that many tumor-bearing individuals who develop cachexia exhibit disordered energy commerce, the metabolic process by which energy is used and stored. These abnormalities commonly culminate in progressive weight loss and wasting.

When present, this collection of symptoms and findings can be both a major cause of physical and psychological morbidity and a determinant of patient survival. In an analysis of 3047 incurable cancer patients treated on 12 cooperative group trials for advanced cancers originating in a variety of primary sites, the loss of more than 6% of premorbid body weight prior to therapy was a more powerful predictor of survival than was any antineoplastic therapy that the patients undertook (2). Patients with such weight loss also did not respond to therapy as often as those with stable or increasing weight.

Patients vary greatly with respect to when in the course of a malignancy, if at all, they manifest cancer-associated anorexia and cachexia and their relative tumor burden when so afflicted. In 15–40% of all cancer patients, anorexia and cachexia are manifest early and may be the presenting complaint (3). During antineoplastic therapy, anorexia and cachexia can be in part related to toxicity of treatment. Near the end of their lives, approximately 85% of 250 consecutive patients with advanced cancer admitted to a palliative care unit reported problematic anorexia

and cachexia (4). This was a greater percentage of patients than indicated that they were troubled by pain. Interestingly, the degree of weight loss does not always correlate with tumor size: i.e., some patients with a small tumor burden will become profoundly wasted whereas others with tumors weighing kilograms will not manifest anorexia or cachexia (2).

## ETIOLOGY

Cancer cachexia is the outcome of a net negative energy balance. The causes of the weight loss associated with cancer are diverse and contribute to the process in different proportions in individual patients. Inadequate intake can be the consequence of changes in the taste or smell of foods; fear of provoking nausea, vomiting, or abdominal cramping; or disinterest in food stemming from depression or uncontrolled pain (5,6). Disordered digestion can lead to inability to convert ingested foods to useful nutrients. Commonly this stems from mechanical effects of the malignancy or its therapy and can include such problems as xerostomia after oropharyngeal radiotherapy, dumping syndrome after upper gastrointestinal surgery, partial bowel obstruction due to tumor encroachment, malabsorption due to pancreatic insufficiency, or mucosal damage caused by chemotherapy. This panoply of contributing factors lead to the same outcome, i.e., the emaciated and weakened state common to patients suffering from cancer-associated anorexia and cachexia.

In many patients with cancer anorexia/cachexia there is a pathologic process at work that cannot be reversed simply by supplying raw materials in usable form. If the process were limited to disordered intake or absorption, then total parenteral nutrition (TPN) would reverse cancer cachexia totally (7). In most cases it does not and in many cases TPN can actually be associated with net harm in the cancer patient. This is effectively illustrated by the finding of a meta-analysis conducted by the American

C.L. Loprinzi, R.M. Goldberg, and P.P. Peethambaram: Department of Medical Oncology, The Mayo Clinic, Rochester, MN 55905-0001.

College of Physicians that found that employment of TPN in some settings, such as during the administration of chemotherapy, was associated with a shortening of survival (8).

The observation that supplying all nutrients necessary to sustain individuals such as those with short gut syndrome could not reverse the cachexia of cancer indicates that the problem is not simply a shortfall of calories on the supply side of the equation. There are many studies in animal models and in humans that document disordered energy utilization on the demand side of the equation in cancer patients with cachexia. These abnormalities have been cataloged in carbohydrate, lipid, and protein metabolism and in one measure of their more global outcome, the basal metabolic rate.

## Abnormal Carbohydrate, Protein, and Lipid Metabolism

Glucose is the body's energy currency. Cachectic cancer patients appear to overproduce glucose despite relative insulin resistance and, in some cases, diminished insulin levels (9,10). Abnormal glucose tolerance often predates cachexia. In cachectic cancer patients the employment of the relatively energy-inefficient pathway of anaerobic gluconeogenesis results in high lactate levels as compared to those found in normal controls or controls during periods of starvation (11). There appears to be a relative imbalance in host energy needs and glucose production through the Cori cycle, a phenomenon labeled "futile cycling."

Generation of glucose via the energy-inefficient breakdown of skeletal muscle protein into its component amino acids contributes to wasting and inanition (12). In the normal control, during starvation, protein turnover is decreased and these stores are mobilized only after depletion of carbohydrate and fat deposits. In the patient with cancer-associated cachexia, protein mobilization is an early source of calories. Increased protein turnover, as measured by the turnover of labeled amino acids and decreased skeletal muscle protein synthesis, has been documented (13–15). The hypoalbuminemia that is often encountered in a cancer patient is due in part to increased breakdown of albumin and in part to hemodilution. The end results of abnormal protein metabolism are a decrease in protein mass, atrophy of skin and skeletal muscle mass, increased risk of infection, poor performance status, decreased serum albumin levels, and diminished wound healing,

In some cases of cancer cachexia there is a depletion of lipid stores (16). This loss of body fat can occur in the absence of anorexia (17). It is unclear to what extent this abnormal state is due to reduced lipogenesis or increased lipolysis or abnormalities in the combination of the two processes. There are conflicting reports as to alterations

in whole-body glycerol turnover, with some studies reporting an increase in turnover and others reporting no change. Decreased lipogenesis, an increased rate of lipid mobilization, and decreased lipoprotein lipase activity have all been described (18–20). Consequently, the cachectic patient often has increased serum triglycerides and glycerol, and decreased high-density lipoproteins and cholesterol (21). A lipolytic factor has been described but not yet been purified that when injected into mice produces weight loss without depressing appetite (22).

More global abnormalities in energy use have been identified as indicated by the presence of abnormal basal metabolic rates in many such patients. Most studies demonstrate that cancer patients have an increased resting energy expenditure compared to controls with similar degrees of weight loss but without cancer. Cohorts of patients with leukemias, sarcomas, and bronchial carcinomas frequently exhibit a hypermetabolic state (23,24). Controversy persists because studies have shown that some severely wasted patients with gastrointestinal tumors exhibit a decreased or normal metabolic rate (25). The mechanism of increased energy expenditure is thought to be due to the alterations discussed above that occur in carbohydrate, fat, and protein metabolism from mediators released by the host or as a part of the host response to the tumor rather than due to the additive effect of the metabolic processes occurring within the tumor plus those of the host.

## Cytokines and Anorexia

In some patients with weight loss related to malignancy a true paraneoplastic syndrome appears to be manifest. These patients exhibit the complex and multifactorial metabolic abnormalities described in the preceding discussion. In order to implicate a paraneoplastic syndrome as the cause, a mediator must be recognized. There is evidence from animal studies that cytokines derived from host macrophages may be causative. Exogenous administration of tumor necrosis factor-$\alpha$ (TNF-$\alpha$) to mice and injection into mice of an ovarian cancer cell line genetically modified to constitutively produce TNF-$\alpha$ causes anorexia associated with weight loss and protein depletion indistinguishable from the syndrome of cancer-associated anorexia and cachexia observed in human cancer patients (26). The administration of an antibody to TNF-$\alpha$ partially abolishes the syndrome (27).

If elevated TNF-$\alpha$ levels could be confirmed in the serum of affected animals, this cytokine would likely be identified as the mediator of this paraneoplastic syndrome. Such confirmatory evidence has proven to be elusive as serum TNF-$\alpha$ levels are not elevated in individuals with the syndrome leading to the postulate that much of the effect of TNF-$\alpha$ is paracrine in nature (28). Because the exogenous administration of interleukin-1, interleukin-6, and γ-interferon also can produce a condition identical to that seen in the cancer anorexia and cachexia syndrome, the causative agent may be an as yet unidentified one (29,30). Alternatively, multiple mediators may be relevant to the process. Although it is clear that administration of these cytokines including TNF-α can reproduce the cancer-associated anorexia and cachexia syndrome, the ultimate proof that these cytokines causes the syndrome in humans remains the subject of ongoing research (31).

The parallel between wasting in cancer and in other disease states such as trauma, sepsis, and in such parasitic infestations as leishmaniasis is striking and harkens back to the definition of cachexia as a condition common to chronic illness (1). The common character of this syndrome among injured, infected, or cancer-bearing hosts suggested the possibility of a host-produced mediator(s) long before the cytokines had been discovered.

## MECHANISMS FOR STUDYING TREATMENTS FOR CANCER ANOREXIA/CACHEXIA

In view of the prominent clinical problem imposed by this condition, a variety of drugs have been studied to assess their impact on cancer anorexia/cachexia. Ideas regarding which drugs to study in this condition have generally come from clinical impressions regarding whether a medication used for an unrelated medical condition causes appetite stimulation and weight gain. At times this has led to pilot or phase II drug trials with appetite and eventual weight gain as study measurements. Although these pilot trials may provide useful information, caution is in order regarding final conclusions as there is clearly a large "placebo effect" regarding potential anti-anorexia agents. This may not truly be a "placebo" interaction. Rather, it might just be a normal waxing and waning of appetite seen with the malignant process or it may be related to other confounding factors (such as radiation therapy or palliative chemotherapy). At any rate, a beneficial effect ascribed to a placebo can occur in 30–40% of patients (32,33). Therefore, randomized controlled clinical trials are important for discerning whether a drug does stimulate appetite in the setting of cancer anorexia/cachexia.

In randomized clinical trials, it is now apparent that, despite its subjective nature, appetite can be reliably measured. One appetite evaluation methodology has undergone some validity testing (34), whereas many others have not. However, even the measurement tools that have not undergone validity testing appear to be useful. Data that lead us to make this statement are elucidated below:

1. Multiple independently developed appetite rating scales have all come to the conclusion that progestational agents do stimulate appetite more so than placebos in prospective clinical trials (33,35–38).

2. There is a strong correlation between patient-reported appetite stimulation and physician-measured nonfluid weight gain in patients receiving megestrol acetate (39).

3. Independent questions within and among these instruments provide similar conclusions (32,33,39).

## PHARMACOLOGIC MANAGEMENT OF CANCER ANOREXIA/CACHEXIA

### Progestational Agents

Over the past several years, progestational agents have been extensively studied as a means of combatting cancer anorexia/cachexia. Most of the data regarding the effects of progestational agents on cancer anorexia/cachexia have been derived from studies utilizing megestrol acetate. The few studies done with the related compound, medroxyprogesterone acetate, suggest that these drugs act in a similar manner.

The initial insight suggesting that progestational agents would be helpful came from observations that patients receiving this drug as hormonal therapy for metastatic breast, endometrial, or prostate cancer reported appetite stimulation and demonstrated nonfluid weight gain (40,41). A pilot trial suggested that increased appetite stimulation and weight gain correlated with higher drug doses (42). This led to the development and subsequent completion of several randomized placebo-controlled clinical trials (33,35–37). The conclusions from these placebo-controlled clinical trials have been remarkably uniform. They have demonstrated that megestrol acetate doses ranging from 240 to 1600 mg/day enhance appetites in patients with non–hormonally responsive, incurable cancers. Similar data have also resulted from trials of megestrol acetate in patients with AIDS anorexia/cachexia (38,43).

Some of the above-noted trials have also reported that this drug has a positive effect on nonfluid weight gain, as measured by clinical examination (33,35,38). More formal body composition trials have demonstrated that the weight gain associated with megestrol acetate is from an increase in true body mass, as opposed to just fluid accumulation (44,45).

Dose-response evaluation trials have demonstrated a positive dose-response effect of megestrol acetate on appetite using doses ranging from 160 to 800 mg/day in patients with anorexia/cachexia associated with cancer (39) or AIDS (38). There is no suggestion of additional benefit for doses greater than 800 mg/day (39).

Two of the early prospective clinical trials provided data that strongly suggested that megestrol acetate had substantial antiemetic properties (33,37). This hypothesis was subsequently confirmed in an additional placebo-controlled randomized clinical trial (46). This antiemetic property can provide incremental value when nausea accompanies anorexia.

In general, megestrol acetate doses up to 800 mg/day are relatively well tolerated. Although not consistent among all trials, there are some data to suggest that megestrol acetate might increase the risk for thromboembolic phenomena to a small degree (33,38,39,43,46,47). This increased incidence of thromboembolic phenomena might be potentiated by concomitant cytotoxic chemotherapy (46). This is similar to what has been reported with another hormone, tamoxifen (48). In some trials, megestrol acetate has been associated with more edema than has a placebo (47,48). This is generally a mild amount of edema that can easily be controlled with a mild diuretic. Reversible impotence has been reported in approximately 10% of patients (38). Megestrol acetate may cause an alteration in menses. The most prominent situation is withdrawal menstrual bleeding, which occurs from 1 to 4 weeks following discontinuation of megestrol acetate therapy (49).

Megestrol acetate appears to cause adrenal suppression from an inhibition of the pituitary-adrenal axis (50). While measurements of adrenal and pituitary functions may be abnormal, these laboratory findings do not appear to cause clinically apparent toxicity in the vast majority of treated patients. Nonetheless, physicians should be aware of this as there are rare reports that progestational agents can cause Cushingoid effects and that they can lead to Addisonian symptoms upon abrupt withdrawal (51). Given this information regarding adrenal suppression in patients who are receiving or have recently discontinued megestrol acetate, such patients should receive stress doses of corticosteroids during medical crisis situations such as significant trauma, infection, or a planned surgical procedure.

Given that progestational agents can improve appetite and cause weight gain in patients with advanced cancer, and that many patients with advanced cancer die of inanition, the question arose as to whether progestational agents might prolong survival and/or quality of life. This question was recently tested in a randomized, placebo-controlled clinical trial utilizing patients with newly diagnosed extensive stage small cell lung cancer (46). This trial was unable to demonstrate any substantive positive or negative effect of megestrol acetate on either quality of life or survival.

## Corticosteroids

Aside from progestational agents, corticosteroids are the most thoroughly studied class of drugs that appear to lead to appetite stimulation in patients with cancer anorexia/cachexia. A number of placebo-controlled, randomized clinical trials, dating back to the 1970s, have been completed (52–55). These trials consistently demonstrated that a variety of corticosteroid drugs can lead to temporary appetite stimulation in patients with advanced cancer. To

date, none of these trials has been able to demonstrate a positive effect on patient weight, suggesting that their effect on appetite is less than what is seen with progestational agents. An advantage of corticosteroid medications over progestational agents is their lower cost. A potential disadvantage is that they are generally associated with considerably more toxicity than is seen with progestational agents. A large prospective clinical trial is in process to compare the corticosteroid dexamethasone to the progestational agent megestrol acetate (see below).

## Dronabinol

Dronabinol is a derivative of marijuana that is clinically available as a tablet. This drug is currently FDA-approved for the treatment of AIDS-associated anorexia/cachexia based on one prospective clinical trial (56). Pilot trials have been done in patients with cancer anorexia/cachexia (57–60). Accepting the uncertainties regarding pilot trials for properly evaluating therapy for cancer anorexia/cachexia, the authors of these pilot trials felt that this was a promising drug. Dronabinol has been tested in cancer patients as an antiemetic. In this situation the drug is frequently associated with side effects (e.g., altered mentation) that are quite bothersome to many patients with cancer. The dronabinol-associated side effects are generally more tolerable for younger patients than for older patients. It is important to note that the dronabinol dose utilized for previous antiemetic trials was 15 mg/day whereas the dose utilized for anorexia/cachexia is 5 mg/day. Currently, efforts are in process to prospectively compare dronabinol to megestrol acetate to the combination of both as means of treating cancer anorexia/cachexia (see below).

## Anabolic Steroids

Anabolic steroids have been utilized by athletes in an illicit manner to augment muscle bulk and strength. Studies have demonstrated that these drugs do increase muscle mass (61). However, the associated side effects from these medications warrant that they be contraindicated in healthy athletes. Some information derived from a pilot study suggests that anabolic steroids may increase appetite and lead to weight gain in patients with cancer (62). A prospective trial is presently in progress to compare the anabolic steroid fluoxymesterone to megestrol acetate and to dexamethasone as a treatment for cancer anorexia/cachexia (see below).

## Cyproheptadine

Cyproheptadine is an antiserotonergic, antihistamine that was first noted to cause appetite stimulation and weight gain approximately three decades ago when it was tested in children for the treatment of asthma (63). Based on multiple trials demonstrating appetite stimulatory properties in patients with anorexia nervosa and other low-weight clinical situations, a large, placebo-controlled, randomized clinical trial was conducted (34). This trial involved 295 patients. The results from this trial demonstrated that cyproheptadine had minimal appetite stimulation properties in patients with advanced cancer anorexia/cachexia. No weight gain was seen in this trial and it was concluded that the appetite stimulatory properties of cyproheptadine were not substantial enough to counteract the prominent clinical process of cancer anorexia/cachexia. An exception to this case might include patients with metastatic carcinoid syndrome. In this situation, the direct blocking of hormonal excess associated with carcinoid syndrome may be responsible for substantial weight gain in these patients (64). Of note, cyproheptadine also appears to decrease carcinoid syndrome-associated diarrhea by approximately 50%.

### Pentoxifylline

Pentoxifylline is a methylxanthine derivative that is FDA-approved for the treatment of intermittent claudication. Based on a report that suggested that pentoxifylline can decrease TNF messenger ribonucleic acid (mRNA) levels in cancer patients (65), a placebo-controlled randomized clinical trial was conducted. Unfortunately, this trial did not demonstrate any suggestion of benefit for the use of this drug in the treatment of cancer anorexia/cachexia (66).

### Metoclopramide

Metoclopramide is a dopamine receptor antagonist that appears to be helpful for treating gastroparesis. It has been utilized in cancer patients as an antiemetic and as a means to help counteract narcotic-induced constipation. A pilot trial suggested that it was helpful for treating anorexia in patients with advanced cancer (67). In addition to improving appetite, this pilot trial suggested that metoclopramide decreased nausea, belching, and bloating. To date, no phase III clinical trial has been performed to evaluate metoclopramide as a treatment for cancer anorexia/cachexia.

### Hydrazine Sulfate

Hydrazine sulfate is an interesting compound that was first developed as a cytotoxic drug. Initial phase I trials were conducted, but they provided little encouragement for further development of this drug (68–70). Proponents of this medication suggested that it did have characteris-

tics that might favorably impact on cancer anorexia/cachexia (71,72). Eventually, a small, prospective, placebo-controlled clinical trial was performed in patients with advanced non–small cell lung cancer (73). Although this trial did not demonstrate evidence of statistically significant benefit overall, a subset analysis suggested that it might have some benefit in patients with favorable performance status. Based on this information, three large, randomized, placebo-controlled clinical trials were initiated. These trials were unable to demonstrate any positive effect from this medication with regard to appetite, weight gain, quality of life, or survival (74–76).

## ONGOING AND PROPOSED CLINICAL TRIALS

As alluded to above, the North Central Cancer Treatment Group is currently nearing completion of a randomized clinical trial that is comparing megestrol acetate (800 mg/day) to dexamethasone (0.75 mg q.i.d) to fluoxymesterone (10 mg b.i.d.) in patients with cancer anorexia/cachexia. The accrual goal of 450 patients (150 patients per arm) was reached in 1996 and should be reported soon thereafter.

Another large, comparative, controlled clinical trial in patients with cancer anorexia/cachexia designed to compare the efficacy of two medications, both of which are FDA-approved for AIDS-associated anorexia/cachexia. This study will compare megestrol acetate to dronabinol to the combination of both of these medications.

## CURRENT RECOMMENDATIONS FOR CLINICAL PRACTICE

Given the information outlined above, what should be done with regard to treatment of cancer anorexia/cachexia in routine clinical practice? Who should be treated? What medications should be utilized? What doses of medication should be utilized?

We believe that it is not clinically appropriate to treat all patients with cancer anorexia/cachexia. In those patients with far advanced disease and a life expectancy of days to a few weeks, there generally are other clinical problems such as pain and organ failure (e.g., kidneys, lungs, and/or liver) that may result in fatigue, confusion, and dyspnea. In this clinical situation, there may be little benefit for trying to treat cancer anorexia/cachexia. However, in a patient in whom anorexia and/or cachexia is a major source of suffering, and when the patient otherwise has a life expectancy measured in months or more, it may be well worthwhile to institute therapy for this clinical problem.

In this situation, we generally recommend the use of megestrol acetate as completed controlled trials suggest that this drug is the most powerful appetite stimulant available and as it is generally quite well tolerated overall. Rational arguments could be made for starting doses ranging from 160 mg up to 800 mg/day. Our current recommendation is to start with 800 mg/day. The most cost-effective form of this medication currently available is a liquid preparation. An 8-ounce bottle of this costs approximately $120.00, and at a dose of 800 mg/day, this will last for approximately 2 weeks. At the 2-week mark, it is worth assessing whether the medication appears to be causing benefit in terms of stimulation of appetite and/or acting as an antiemetic. If there is no evident benefit after 2 weeks, then our recommendation is to stop the megestrol acetate. If there appears to be benefit after the 2-week period, then continuation of the megestrol acetate, either at the same dose or at a lower dose, is recommended. The megestrol acetate can be continued as long as it appears to have beneficial effects. In some situations, patients will gain substantial amounts of weight to the point where further weight gain is undesirable. In these cases, the drug dose should be titrated downward and/or stopped.

Another alternative for treating cancer anorexia/cachexia, either initially or after failure of megestrol acetate, is to utilize a corticosteroid medication such as dexamethasone. Various doses can be defended but a total daily dose of 3 mg/day appears appropriate to try to balance beneficial effects and toxicities. Our clinical bias at this time is that this drug probably does not stimulate appetite as strongly as does megestrol acetate and probably has more clinical toxicity, but it is obtainable at a much lower drug cost.

## SUMMARY

Cancer anorexia/cachexia is an incompletely understood phenomenon that affects a substantial portion of patients with advanced cancer. It is associated with considerable physical and psychological morbidity. Methodology is now available to study new therapeutic endeavors for this prominent clinical problem. Currently, it is reasonable to treat cancer anorexia/cachexia with progestational agents or corticosteroids. It is hoped that ongoing and future trials will provide new helpful information regarding the etiology and treatment of cancer anorexia/cachexia.

## REFERENCES

1. *Stedman's Medical Dictionary,* Baltimore: Williams and Wilkins, 1972.
2. DeWys WD, Begg C, Lavin PT, et al. Prognostic effect of weight loss prior to chemotherapy in cancer patients. *Am J Med* 1980;69:491-497.
3. Shils ME. Principles of nutritional support. *Cancer* 1979;43:2093–2102.
4. Bruera E, MacDonald RN. Asthenia in patients with advanced cancer. *J Pain Sympt Manag* 1988;3:9–14.
5. Brennan MF, Burt ME. Nitrogen metabolism in cancer patients. *Cancer Treat Rep* 1981;65(suppl 5):67–78.
6. Bernstein IL. Etiology of anorexia in cancer. *Cancer* 1986;58:1881–1886.
7. Brennan MF. Total parenteral nutrition and the cancer patient. *N Engl J Med* 1981;305:375–382.
8. American College of Physicians. Parenteral nutrition in patients receiving cancer chemotherapy. *Ann Intern Med* 1989;110:734–736.
9. Rofe AM, Bourgeois CS, Coyle P, Taylor A, Abdi EA. Altered insulin response to glucose in weight-losing cancer patients. *Anticancer Res* 1994;114:647–650.
10. Bennegard K, Lundgren F, Lundholm K. Mechanisms of insulin resistance in cancer associated malnutrition. *Clin Physiol* 1986;6:539–547.
11. Lundholm K, Bylund AC, Schersten T. Glucose tolerance in relation to skeletal muscle enzyme activities in cancer patients. *Scand J Clin Lab Invest* 1977;37:2670–2672.
12. Norton JA, Stein TP, Brennan MF. Whole body protein turnover studies in normal humans and malnourished patients with and without cancer. *Ann Surg* 1980;31:94–96.
13. Carmichael MJ, Clague MB, Kier MJ, Johnston IDA. Whole body protein turnover, synthesis and breakdown in patients with colorectal carcinoma. *Br J Surg* 1980;67:736–769.
14. Shaw JHF, Humberstone DA, Douglas RG, Koea J. Leucine kinetics in patients with benign disease, non-weight-losing cancer, and cancer cachexia: studies at the whole-body and tissue level and the response to nutritional support. *Surgery* 1991;109:37–50.
15. Shaw JHF, Humberstone DM, Wolfe RR. Energy and protein metabolism in sarcoma patients. *Ann Surg* 1988;207:283–289.
16. Axelrod L, Costa G. Contribution of fat loss to weight loss in cancer. *Nutr Cancer* 1980;2:81–83.
17. Groundwater P, Beck SA, Barton C, Adamson C, Ferrier IN, Tisdale MJ. Alterations of serum and urinary lipolytic activity with weight loss in cachectic cancer patients. *Br J Cancer* 1990;62:816–821.
18. Jeevanandam M, Horowitz GD, Lowry SF, and Brennan MF. Cancer cachexia and the rate of whole body lipolysis in man. *Metabolism* 1986;35:304–310.
19. Legaspi A, Jeevanandam M, Starnes Jr HF, and Brennan MF. Whole body lipid and energy metabolism in the cancer patient. *Metabolism* 1987;36:958–963.
20. Mori M, Yamaguchi K, Abe K. Purification of a lipoprotein lipase-inhibiting protein produced by a melanoma cell line associated with cancer cachexia. *Biochem Biophys Res Commun* 1989;160:1085–1092.
21. Klein S, and Wolfe RR. Whole-body lipolysis and triglyceride-fatty acid cycling in cachectic patients with esophageal cancer. *J Clin Invest* 1990;86:1403–1408.
22. Beck SA, Mulligan HD, and Tisdale MJ. Lipolytic factors associated with murine and human cancer cachexia. *JNCI* 1990;82:1922–1926.
23. Dempsey DT, Feurer ID, Knox LS, et al. Energy expenditure in malnourished cancer patients. *Cancer* 1984;53:1265–1273.
24. Fredrix EWHM, Soeters PB, Wouters EFM, Rouflart MJJ, von Meyenfeldt MF, Saris WHM. Effect of different tumor types on resting energy expenditure. *Cancer Res* 1991;51:6138–6141.
25. Fredrix EWHM, Soeters PB, Rouflart MJJ, von Meyerfeldt MF, Saris WHM. Resting energy expenditures in patients with newly detected gastric and colorectal cancers. *Am J Clin Nutr* 1991;53:1318–1322.
26. Oliff A, Defeo-Jones D, Boyer M, et al. Tumors secreting human TNF/cachectin induce cachexia in mice. *Cell* 1987;50:555–563.
27. Feingold KR, Sould M, Stapraus I, et al. Effect of tumor necrosis factor TNF on lipid metabolism in the diabetic rat. Evidence that inhibition of adipose tissue lipoprotein lipase is not required for TNF-induced hyperlipidemia. *J Clin Invest* 1989;83:1116–1121.
28. Strovroff MC, Fraker DI, Norton JA. Cachectin activity in the serum of cachectic, tumor bearing rats. *Arch Surg* 1989;124:94–99.
29. Langstein HN, Doherty GM, Fraker DL, et al. The role of gamma interferon and tumor necrosis factor alpha in an experimental rat model of cancer cachexia. *Cancer Res* 1991;51:415–421.
30. Gelin J, Moldawer LL, Lonnroth C, Sherry R, Chizzonite R, Lundholm. Role of endogenous tumor necrosis factor and interleukin 1 for experimental tumor growth and development of cancer cachexia. *Cancer Res* 1991;51:415–421.
31. Socher SH, Friedman A, Martinez D. Recombinant human tumor necrosis factor induces acute reductions in food intake and body weight in mice. *J Exp Med* 1988;167:1957–1962.
32. Loprinzi CL, Ellison NM, Schaid DJ, et al. Controlled trial of megestrol

acetate for the treatment of cancer anorexia and cachexia. *JNCI* 1990; 82:1127–1132.

33. Kardinal CG, Loprinzi CL, Schaid DJ, et al. A controlled trial of cyproheptadine in cancer patients with anorexia and/or cachexia. *Cancer* 1990;65:2657–2662.

34. Measurement of hunger and food intake in man. In: Silverstone T, ed. *Drugs and Appetite*, New York: Academic Press, 1982;81–92.

35. Bruera E. Macmillan K, Kuehn N, et al. A controlled trial of megestrol acetate on appetite, caloric intake, nutritional status, other symptoms in patients with advanced cancer. *Cancer* 1990;66:1279–1282.

36. Feliu J, Gonzalez-Baron M, Berrocal A, Artal A, Ordonez A, Garrido P, Zamora PO, Garcia de Paredea ML, Montero JM. Usefulness of megestrol acetate in cancer cachexia and anorexia. *Am J Clin Oncol* 1992; 15(5):436–440.

37. Tchekmedyian NS, Hickman M, Siau J, Greco FA, Keller J, Browder H, Aisner J. Megestrol acetate in cancer anorexia and weight loss. *Cancer* 1992;69:1268–1274.

38. Von Roenn JH, Armstrong D, Kotler DP, Cohn DL, Klimas NG, Tchekmedyian NS, et al. Megestrol acetate in patients with AIDS-related cachexia. *Ann Intern Med* 1994;121:393–399.

39. Loprinzi CL, Michalak JC, Schaid DJ, Mailliard JA, Athmann LH, Goldberg RM, Tschetter LK, Hatfield AK, Morton Rf. Phase III evaluatio of four doses of megestrol acetate as therapy for patients with cancer anorexia and/or cachexia. *J Clin Oncol* 1993;11:762–767.

40. Gregory EJ, Cohen SC, Oines DW, et al. Megestrol acetate therapy for advanced breast cancer. *J Clin Oncol* 1985;3:155–160.

41. Bonomi P, Pessis D, Bunting N, et al. Megestrol acetate used as primary hormonal therapy in stage D prostatic cancer. *Semin Oncol* 1985;12: 36–39.

42. Tchekmedyian NS, Tait N, Moody M, et al. High-dose megestrol acetate: a possible treatment for cachexia. *JAMA* 1987;257:1195–1198.

43. Oster MH, Enders SR, Samuels SJ, Cone LA, Hooton TM, Browder HP, et al. Megestrol acetate in patients with AIDS and cachexia. *Ann Intern Med*.

44. Loprinzi CL, Schaid DJ, Dose AM, Burnham NL, Jensen M.D. Body-composition changes in patients who gain weight while receiving megestrol acetate. *J Clin Oncol* 1993;11(1):152–154.

45. Reitmeier M, Hartenstein RC. Megestrol acetate and determination of body composition by bioelectral impedance analysis inc ancer cachexia. *Proc Am Soc Clin Oncol* 1990;9:325(abstr).

46. Rowland KM Jr, Loprinzi CL, Shaw EG, Maksymiuk AW, Kuross SA et al. Randomized double blind placebo controlled trial of cisplatina nd etoposide plus megestrol acetate/placebo in extensive stage small cell lung cancer: A North Central Cancer Treatment Group Study. *J Clin Oncol*, in press.

47. Loprinzi CL, Johnson P, Jensen M. Megestrol acetate for anorexia and cachexia. *Oncology* 1992;49(suppl 2):46–49.

48. Fisher B, Redmond C, Widkerhan DL, et al. Doxorubicin-containing regimens for the treatment of stage II breast cancer: the National Surgical Adjuvant Breast and Bowel Project experience. *J Clin Oncol* 1989;7:572.

49. Loprinzi Cl, Michalak JC, Quella SK, O'Fallon JR, Hatfield AK, Nelimark RA, Dose AM, Fischer T, Johnson C, Klatt NE, Bate W, Rospond RM, Oesterling JE. Megestrol acetate for the prevention of hot flashes. *N Engl J Med* 1994;33(6):347–352.

50. Loprinzi CL. Effect of megestrol acetate on the human pituitary-adrenal axis. *Mayo Clin Proc* 1992;67:1160–1162.

51. Leinung MC, Liporace R, Miller CH. Induction of adrenal suppression by megestrol acetate in patients with AIDS. *Ann Intern Med* 1995;122: 843–845.

52. Moertel CG, Schutt AJ, Reitemeier RJ, Hahn RG. Corticosteroid therapy of preterminal gastrointestinal cancer. *Cancer* 1974;33:1607–1609.

53. Bruera E, Roca E, Cedaro L, et al. Action of oral methylprednisolone in terminal cancer patients: a prospective randomized double–blind study. *Cancer Treat Rep* 1985;69:751–754.

54. Popiela T, Lucchi R, Giongo F. Methylprednisolone as an appetite stimulant in patients with cancer. *Eur J Cancer Clin Oncol* 1989;25: 1823–1829.

55. Wilcox J, Corr J, Shaw J, et al. Prednisolone as an appetite stimulant in patients with cancer. *Br Med J* 1984;288:27.

56. Beal JE, Olson R, Laubenstein L, Morales JO, Bellman P, Yangco B, Lefkowitz L, Plasse TFD, Shepard KV. Dronabinol as a treatment for anorexia associated with weight loss in patients with AIDS. *J Pain Sympt Manag* 1995;10(2):89.

57. Nelson K, Walsh D, Deeter P, Sheehan F. A phase II study of delta-9-tetrahydrocannabinol for appetite stimulation in cancer-associated anorexia. *J Palliat Care* 1994;10(1):14–18.

58. Sacks N, Hutcheson JR, Watts JM, Webb RE. Case report: the effect of tetrahydrocannabinol on food intake during chemotherapy. *J Am Coll Nutr* 1990;9(6):630–632.

59. Plasse TF, Gorter RW, Krasnow SH, Lane M, Shepard KV, Wadleight RG. Recent clinical experience with dronabinol. *Pharm Biochem Behav* 1991;40:695–700.

60. Regelson W, Butler JR, Schulz J, Kirk T, Peek L, Green ML, Zalis MO. q$^9$-Tetrahydrocannabinol as an effective antidepressant and appetite-stimulating agent in advanced cancer patients. In: Brauda MC, Szxara S, eds. *The Pharmacology of Marihuana*. New York: Raven Press, 1976;763–776.

61. Freed DJ, Banks AJ, Longson D, Burley DM. Anabolic steroids in athletics: crossover double-blind trial on weightlifters. *Br Med J* 1975;5: 471–473.

62. Chlebowski RT, Herrold J, Ali I, Ioktay E, Chelbowski JS, et al. Influence of nadrolone decanoate on weight loss in advanced non-small cell lung cancer. *Cancer* 1986;58:183–186.

63. Kardinal CG, Loprinzi CL, Schaid DJ, Hass AC, Dose AM, Athmann LM, Mailliard JA, McCormack GW, Gerstner JB, Schray Marlene Frost, Ph.D., RN. A controlled trial of cyprohepadine in cancer patients with anorexia and/or cachexia. *Cancer* 1990;65(12):2657–2661.

64. Moertel CG, Kvols LK, Rubin J. A study of cyproheptadine in the treatment of metastatic carcinod tumor and the malignant carcinoid syndrome. *Cancer* 1991;67:33–36.

65. Dezube BJ, Fridovbich-Keil JL, Bouvard I, Lange RF, Pardee AB. Pentoxifylline and wellbeing in patients with cancer. *Lancet* 1990;335(1): 662.

66. Goldberg RM, Loprinzi CL, Mailliard JA, O'Fallon JR, Krook JE, Ghosh C, Hestorff RD, Chong SF, Reuter NF, Shanahan TG. Pentoxifylline for treatment of cancer anorexia/cachexia? A randomized, double–blinded, placebo controlled trial. *J Clin Oncol*, 1995;13:2856–2859.

67. Nelson KA, Walsh August 18. Metoclopramide in anorexia caused by cancer-associated dyspepsia syndrome (CADS). *J Palliat Care* 1993; 9(2):14–18.

68. Lerner HJ, Regelson W. Clinical trial of hydrazine sulfate in solid tumors. *Cancer Treat Rep* 1976;60:959–960.

69. Ochua M Jr, Wittes RE, Krakoff LC. Trial of hydrazine sulfate (NSC-150014) in patients with cancer. *Cancer Chemother Rep* 1975;59: 1151–1153.

70. Spremulli E, Wampler GL, Regelson W. Clinical study of hydrazine sulfate in advanced cancer patients. *Cancer Chemother Pharmacol* 1979;3:121–124.

71. Gold J. Use of hydrazine sulfate in temrinal and preterminal cancer patients: results of investigational new drug (IND) study in 84 evaluable patients. *Oncology* 1975;32:1–10.

72. Filov VA, Danova LA, Gershanovich ML, et al. Hydrazine sulfate: experimental and clinical results, mechanism of action. In: Filov VA, Ivin BA, Dementyeva NP, et al, eds. *Medical Therapy of Tumors*. Leningrad: USSR Ministry of Health, 1983;92–139.

73. Chlebowski RT, Bulcavage L, Grosvenor M, et al. Hydrazine sulfate influence on nutritional status and survival in non-small cell lung cancer. *J Clin Oncol* 1990;8:9–15.

74. Loprinzi CL, Goldberg RG, Su JOI, Mailliard J, Maksymiuk A, Kugler J, Jett J, Ghosh C, Pfeifle D, Wender D, Burch P. Placebo-controlled trial of huydrazine sulfate in patients with newly diagnosed non-small cell lung cancer. *J Clin Oncol* 1994;12:1126–1129.

75. Loprinzi CL, Kuross SA, O'Fallon JR, Gesme DH, Gerstner JB, Rospond RM, Cobau CD, Goldberg RM. Randomized placebo-controlled evaluation of hydrazine sulfate in patients with advanced colorectal cancer. *J Clin Oncol* 1994;12:1121–1125.

76. Kosty MPO, Fleishman SB, Herndon JE, Couglin K, Kornblith, AB, Scalzo A, Morris JC, Mortimer J, Green MR. Cisplatin, vinblastine, and hydrazine sulfate in advanced, non small cell lung cancer: a randomized placebo-controlled, double-blind phase III study of the cancer and leukemia group B. *J Clin Oncol* 1994;12(6):1113–1120.

*Principles and Practice of Supportive Oncology,*
edited by Ann Berger et al.
Lippincott–Raven Publishers, Philadelphia ©1998

CHAPTER 9

# Taste and Cancer

Valerie B. Duffy, Laurie A. Lucchina, Katharine Fast, and Linda M. Bartoshuk

Food has an immense impact on our quality of life. Eating, as with the preparation of meals, is often a social activity, and the consistent flavor of packaged cookies or a family recipe subtly reminds us of the few constants in our lives. It stands to reason, then, that changes in the food we know can have a profound effect on us, especially if these changes strike us as unique and arrive at a particularly stressful time, say, after a cancer diagnosis or while undergoing treatment. Changes in a cancer patient's relationship to food can influence response to treatment: diminishing appetite and multiplying aversions to necessary nourishment can compromise a patient's strength, morale, and chances of survival. This chapter aims to familiarize clinicians with the chemosensory mechanisms responsible for the perception of food and the causes of dysfunction in these mechanisms. It will also review reports associated with cancer and its related therapies. This will help the clinician determine whether a patient complaint represents an alteration in sensation per se or an alteration in the pleasure associated with eating food.

## THE CHEMICAL SENSES: A REVIEW OF FUNCTION

Taste buds, clusters of receptor cells containing receptor sites for sweet, sour, salty, and bitter sensations, are present on the tongue itself, between the hard and soft palate, and in the throat. The elongated tips of the receptor cells contain taste receptor sites. These tips project into a space (taste pore) where they come into contact with taste stimuli. On the tongue, taste buds are found in papillae. The fungiform papillae (which resemble small button mushrooms; hence the name) are most densely distributed on the tip and edges of the tongue. The foliate papillae are on the edges at the base of the tongue and the circumvallate papillae are circular structures arranged in an inverted "V" across the base of the tongue. Three cranial nerves innervate taste buds and route taste information to the medulla, then to the ventrobasal thalamus, and finally to the cortex. The facial nerve (VII) innervates taste buds in the fungiform papilla through the chorda tympani branch and innervates taste buds on the palate through the greater superficial petrosal branch; the glossopharyngeal nerve (IX) innervates foliate (these may also be innervated by VII) and vallate papillae on the posterior tongue; and the vagus nerve (X) innervates taste buds in the throat. An individual taste neuron is usually not entirely specific to one quality. This lack of perfect specificity initially led to speculation that taste was not a labeled-line system (1,2), but later work showing that each taste neuron responds best to one quality, e.g., see (3), led to a revision of that view. Each taste neuron is now thought to carry only one quality signal, i.e., taste is a labeled-line system (4). Incidentally, the taste map of our high school textbooks showing sweet perceived on the tip of the tongue, bitter on the back, etc., is incorrect; it stems from the mistranslation of a German thesis. In reality, all four taste qualities can be perceived on all areas of the tongue and palate where there are taste buds (5).

Taste is a remarkably robust sense. Interactions between two of the cranial nerves that mediate taste (VII and IX) are responsible for some of this stability. Although the two nerves do not contact one another in the periphery, the areas they project to in the brain appear to inhibit one another. If one of the nerves is damaged, the inhibition initiated by that nerve stops; thus the taste responses from the other nerve are intensified. This intensification appears to compensate for the taste input lost from the damaged nerve (i.e., release of inhibition). The person whose nerve has been damaged is unaware of this

V. B. Duffy: School of Allied Health, University of Connecticut, Storrs, CT 06269-2101.

L. R. Lucchina, K. Fast, and L.M. Bartoshuk: Department of Surgery, Section of Otolaryngology, Yale University School of Medicine, New Haven, CT 06520-8041.

compensation because the location of taste sensations is controlled by the sense of touch (6).

Smelling through our nostrils can be a passive action that occurs as we breathe or an active action as we concentrate odors by sniffing (i.e., orthonasal olfaction). Air enters the nostrils and moves up past the turbinate bones. A small sample of this air ultimately reaches the top of the nasal cavity and enters a small opening called the olfactory cleft where it contacts the olfactory receptors (located behind the bridge of the nose). The receptors for olfaction are not found on discrete structures (e.g., like the receptor cells for taste) but rather are found on the ciliated dendrites of olfactory neurons. Odors can also reach the olfactory receptors from the mouth where active chewing and swallowing create a pressure gradient and push air from the mouth up behind the palate into the nose (retronasal olfaction). Whether orthonasal or retronasal in origin, once an odor reaches the olfactory receptors, it is carried by the olfactory nerve (I) through the cribriform plate to be distributed to both the cortex and the subcortex.

On the anterior tongue, somatosensory sensations (touch, temperature, and irritation or pain) are mediated by the lingual branch of the trigeminal nerve (V). On the posterior tongue, they are mediated by the glossopharyngeal nerve (IX). Somatosensory stimuli, taste, and smell are so tightly integrated with our experience of eating that we have difficulty teasing them apart. Since retronasal olfactory sensations are accompanied by touch sensations in the mouth (i.e., chewing, swallowing), and as the brain uses touch to localize sensation, the experience is perceptually localized to the mouth. One way to distinguish true taste from olfaction is to ask patients to describe the quality of the experience. If they can identify sweet, salty, sour, and bitter they are describing taste; if they use other descriptors (e.g., chocolate, garlic, smoky) they are describing olfaction.

Our ability to perceive the taste, olfactory, and somatosensory sensations of food varies normally with genetics and hormonal changes. Genetic taste variation was discovered in the early half of this century (7). Some individuals (nontasters) are tasteblind to 6-*n*-propylthiouracil (PROP), whereas others find it bitter (tasters). Family studies, e.g., see (8), showed that nontasters carried two recessive alleles for the trait. More recently, Bartoshuk and colleagues, e.g., see (9,10), have divided tasters into supertasters, individuals who taste PROP as intensely bitter, and medium tasters, individuals who taste PROP as only moderately bitter. Although yet to be proven, Bartoshuk and colleagues suspect that supertasters carry two dominant alleles. Supertasters perceive more intense taste sensations for many bitter and sweet compounds. For example, supertasters perceive more than twice as much sweetness from sugar as nontasters do (9,11). Anatomic studies show supertasters have the most fungiform papillae (and thus the most taste buds); as taste buds are innervated by neurons that carry pain and touch, supertasters also perceive greater pain from oral irritants (e.g., black pepper, chili pepper, alcohol, carbonation) and more intense textural sensations from foods. Greater pain innervation suggests that supertasters would also perceive greater pain from oral lesions, but this has yet to be demonstrated. Since fat in food is perceived as texture (the molecules are too large to be perceived by taste or olfaction), supertasters also perceive more intense sensations from fat in food (12).

Taste appears to vary with the menstrual cycle (13–17) and during pregnancy (14,18,19). The hormone fluctuations of menstruation and pregnancy affect olfaction as well (20).

## SOURCES OF CHEMOSENSORY DISORDERS

Alterations in chemosensory perception can have a devastating effect on an individual. Living with a chronic salty taste in the mouth or an omnipresent foul scent can obviously have tremendous impact on one's day-to-day existence, and while these are extreme (though not uncommon) experiences, less severe dysfunction, such as heightened bitter, diminished sweet, or faded flavors, also reduces the quality of a patient's life.

Though ageusia (the total loss of taste) is rare, hypogeusia (partial losses that can be differential with regard to area or quality) are not. Changes in taste are gauged by applying stimuli to areas innervated by different nerves (21). Through this procedure, pathologies known to damage cranial nerves VII, IX, X (otitis media, influenza, head trauma) have been associated with both the depression and enhancement of localized taste perception (10). The clinical significance of localized taste losses is limited because these losses often go unnoticed by the patient (see discussion of release of inhibition).

One of the most disturbing taste disorders is dysgeusia, the presence of a chronic taste. Sometimes dysgeusia reflects the presence of a real stimulus in the mouth (e.g., reflux, postnasal drip, medications in saliva or gingival fluid), but chronic tastes can also result from abnormal stimulation of a neural structure mediating taste. In the latter case, we call the sensations taste phantoms (akin to phantom limb sensations and tinnitus). To determine whether a persistent taste is indeed a phantom sensation, the mouth can be rinsed with a topical anesthetic preventing nerves VII and IX from receiving taste (21). Since dysgeusia stemming from a tastant present in the mouth is abolished by this anesthesia, if the patient's sensation remains the same or intensifies, it is likely the result of abnormal stimulation in the nervous system.

Olfactory dysfunction may reflect conductive damage, neural damage, or a combination of the two. Conductive damage includes all of those occasions where the delivery of stimuli to the olfactory epithelium is impeded, whether through obstruction or swelling in the paranasal sinuses or interference with the mouth movements necessary to pump odors from the mouth to the nose. Mechanical and chemical damage to the olfactory nerve, most often due to viruses (especially from infection of the upper respiratory tract), results in neural damage (22). A less common but prevalent cause of olfactory loss is repeated exposure to toxins (20). This information, coupled with data demonstrating that older individuals are at high risk for smell loss (23), make it difficult to distinguish olfactory losses associated with the aging process from those due to environmental insult. Parosmia, a distortion of odor perception, and phantosmia, the sensation of odor without a stimulus (24), can be extremely unpleasant for a sufferer. Reports of hypersensitivity to odors do not appear to be associated with altered perception (25).

The peripheral structures for taste and olfaction regenerate. This is the key to recovery from environmental insults. The average life of a taste receptor is 10 days but can extend to a month or more (26); thus, damaged taste buds are likely to regenerate, as are damaged neurons routing sensation to the brain. Olfactory neurons are capable of regeneration at all points between the receptor site and the central nervous system (27,28), though, as demonstrated with head trauma, the degree of regeneration may depend on the severity of damage (29) and perception may be blunted or distorted (30).

## PSYCHOPHYSICAL ISSUES IN THE STUDY OF TASTE AND CANCER

Anecdotal accounts from patients provide convincing evidence that eating can be a very unpleasant experience for many cancer patients. Gilda Radner described her taste problems with chemotherapy in her book, *It's Always Something* (31). She said, "My taste buds were weird. Things tasted weird . . . eating was very unpleasant. I ate what I ordinarily wouldn't eat. I wanted cheeseburgers, cheese, and pickles. Lettuce and vegetables tasted like plastic. The highly salty, tasty things were good, but bland foods tasted like something they weren't and that was too strange. It was too weird when a carrot tasted like a ceramic kitchen magnet." This provides a wonderful example of the difficulty in discerning the source of the alterations. For example, "lettuce and vegetables tasted like plastic" suggests an olfactory loss but Ms. Radner's ability to taste salt remained. "Eating was very unpleasant" could reflect a pure hedonic change or could reflect sensory abnormalities. If we are to provide relief to patients, we must document these changes with careful psychophysical testing. Unfortunately, the psychophysical methods that can reveal real changes in the patient's chemosensory world are deceptive. They often look very simple but in reality require considerable skill

both in execution and in interpretation. We will discuss the problems encountered in any psychophysical evaluation of abnormal sensory experience, review the cancer data with those problems in mind, and suggest appropriate study designs for future research. It should be noted that the best designs to determine whether or not an illness or therapy affects sensory experience is a prospective design where each subject can be his or her own control. With such designs, patients can be tested before and after a given therapy. However, such designs are impractical when studying an illness. Thus, the determination of whether or not cancer per se affects sensory experience is a much harder task than the determination of whether or not a particular therapy affects sensory experience. Obviously, in a clinical setting, an extensive psychophysical evaluation of each cancer patient is impractical. At the end of this chapter we will provide a brief list of suggestions that may help the clinician identify the source of food complaints.

### Threshold versus Suprathreshold Evaluations

The threshold of a particular substance refers to the lowest concentration a subject can either detect or recognize. Threshold measurement seems a simple enough concept but many experimental artifacts exist to plague accurate measurement, and some of the methods that have been used extensively in studies of taste and cancer are open to serious criticism. That aside, even when taste thresholds are measured with appropriate procedures, e.g., see (32–34) for discussions of some of the issues, thresholds provide little information of value for cancer patients. Thresholds merely measure the bottom of the range and cannot demonstrate the actual effect of cancer and/or its therapies on a patient's taste world. As we will show below, the bottom of the range does not predict perceived intensities of foods and beverages because they are at higher concentrations (i.e., suprathreshold).

Figure 1 illustrates some dissociations between threshold and suprathreshold perception for sweet and bitter. We have selected these qualities because they are especially relevant to an explanation of the flaws in one of the most cited cancer papers (35). We will discuss that paper in more detail later in this chapter. The two top panels show psychophysical functions for sucrose (i.e., perceived sweetness intensity plotted against sucrose concentration). In both cases the threshold (i.e., the approximate concentration at which sensation is zero) is elevated. The panel on the left shows taste loss associated with upper respiratory infection across the whole concentration range (36,37); this kind of change involves both a threshold shift and a reduction in perceived intensity. The panel on the right shows an elevated threshold (produced by adapting to sucrose) but no change in the perceived intensity of the highest concentrations (33).

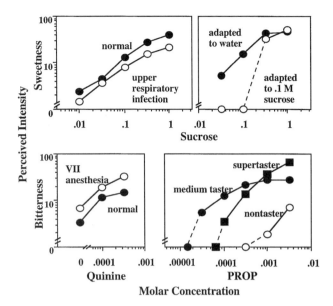

**FIG. 1.** Psychophysical functions for sweet and bitter (see text for explanation). Upper left (36, 37); upper right (33); lower left (38); lower right (10).

The two bottom panels show psychophysical functions for the bitter compounds quinine and PROP. The panel on the left shows the results of a study in which quinine was swabbed onto a circumvallate papilla on one side of the tongue. The "normal" function shows the bitterness before anesthesia and the "anesthesia" function shows the bitterness after the chorda tympani nerve on the contralateral side was anesthetized (38). Note that even water tasted bitter after the anesthesia and the bitterness of the quinine solutions was intensified. The panel on the right shows the thresholds and psychophysical functions for three individuals: a nontaster, a medium taster, and a supertaster of PROP. The thresholds for nontasters are clearly elevated above those for tasters and the suprathreshold intensities for nontasters are reduced below those of tasters. However, among tasters, thresholds do not completely predict how bitter PROP tastes at suprathreshold concentrations. Although on average, individuals who taste PROP to be intensely bitter (i.e., supertasters) have lower PROP thresholds than those who taste PROP to be only moderately bitter (i.e., medium tasters), there are many reversals. The medium taster in the lower right panel actually has a lower threshold than the supertaster. These kinds of dissociations between threshold and suprathreshold intensity have been well documented in taste, e.g., see (33,39,40).

## Cancer and Bitter Thresholds

DeWys and Walters (35) reported that cancer patients had high detection and recognition thresholds for the sweet taste of sucrose and that a subgroup of cancer patients had unusually low recognition thresholds for the bitter taste of urea. The authors stated, "The decreased

taste symptom correlated with an elevated taste threshold for sweet (sucrose), and the symptom of meat aversion correlated with a lowered taste threshold for bitter (urea)." Unfortunately, the conclusions are compromised by a miscalculated $\chi^2$ test (41). Correcting the statistical errors leads to the following corrected conclusions:

1. The sucrose detection and recognition thresholds were significantly elevated (although the $\chi^2$ reported for the recognition threshold, 59.4, should be 5.94).
2. The urea thresholds were *not* significantly lowered ($\chi^2$ was reported to be 10.5 but the correct value is 1.05 which is not significant).
3. Patients with subjective taste loss did have significantly elevated sucrose recognition thresholds.
4. Patients with meat aversions did have significantly lowered urea recognition thresholds.

Gallagher and Tweedle (42) tested cancer patients prior to treatment and reported significantly lower urea thresholds, confirming the DeWys and Walters conclusion that we now know is incorrect. The data were not provided in the paper and therefore their Mann-Whitney U tests cannot be checked; however, since means and standard errors were provided, we can calculate $t$ tests. The $t$ test for cancer patients vs. controls was $t = 0.943$ which is clearly not significant. Thus a second claim that cancer per se lowers urea thresholds does not appear to be correct.

Hall et al (43) studied gastrointestinal (GI) cancer patients before treatment and reported (correctly) that a subgroup had urea thresholds lower than both noncancer GI patients and normal controls. However, their GI noncancer patients had lower urea thresholds than the normal controls, casting doubt on any conclusions about cancer per se. Further, the patients with low urea thresholds did not have meat aversions. Other studies (44–46) found no differences between bitter thresholds in cancer patients who had not received chemotherapy or radiation therapy and control subjects. Bolze and colleagues (47) reported *elevated* thresholds for urea. In this study, cancer patients were significantly older than control subjects and taste thresholds are known to rise with age. For this reason, we reanalyzed the data using only cancer patients and controls under 60 years old. Urea thresholds were still elevated for cancer patients.

These studies do not support the conclusion that cancer lowers bitter recognition thresholds, rendering meat unpalatable because of its bitter components. However, even with the statistical errors, a few patients did have urea thresholds that were very low. These low thresholds raise additional issues regarding bitter thresholds that may be especially relevant to cancer patients. First, bitter dysgeusias have been reported by cancer patients, most often in connection with chemotherapy (more about this below). The presence of a bitter dysgeusia could affect the measurement of bitter thresholds. For example, the Henkin threshold procedure (34,48) presents the patient with three drops: two water and one containing the tastant. The concentration of tastant at which the subject consistently detects the correct drop is the detection threshold; the concentration at which the subject consistently selects the correct drop and provides the correct quality is the recognition threshold. Detection thresholds are generally lower than recognition thresholds. Weiffenbach (personal communication) has noted that if a patient has a chronic bitter taste in her or his mouth, then the recognition threshold will be the detection threshold because all three drops will taste bitter; thus, bitter thresholds will appear reduced.

Another issue relevant to bitter taste and cancer is the suggestion (49,50) that certain types of cancer are not randomly distributed among nontasters, medium tasters, and supertasters of PROP. For example, Milunicová et al. (49) found fewer nontasters than expected among women with malignant tumors of the thyroid gland, breast, uterus, and ovary. If there is association between type of cancer and type of PROP taster (Drewnowski has suggested that this might be mediated by dietary food preferences), then we would expect to find variations in bitter taste thresholds across cancer patients.

Incidentally, food aversions are not explained by lowered bitter thresholds. Food aversions are far more likely to reflect bitter dysgeusia or conditioned aversions.

### Selection of Appropriate Controls for Patient-Control Designs

In order to match controls to patients one must know all of the relevant variables affecting the illness. Any failure to do this renders the conclusions of the study suspect. Obviously, if we knew all of the relevant variables, the investigation at hand would probably be unnecessary; thus we are virtually never certain that a patient-control study is adequate. However, at the very least, variables known to affect the measure under study must be controlled.

Taste and olfactory thresholds rise with age, e.g., see (51) for a review. As we noted above with Bolze et al. (47), the authors report that some taste thresholds were higher among cancer patients (tested prior to radiation therapy) than among controls; however, the patients were significantly older than the controls with which they were compared. A reanalysis of their data using only subjects under 60 diminished the age difference and also diminished the impact of some of the results. Bolze et al. measured detection and recognition thresholds for stimuli representing the four classic taste qualities (sweet, salty, sour, bitter); detection thresholds for NaCl, HCl, and urea (but not sucrose) were elevated and recognition thresholds for HCl and urea were elevated. Our reanalysis showed significant elevations for the HCl recognition threshold and for both the urea detection and recognition thresholds.

The ability to taste varies genetically. To the best of our knowledge, no published paper on taste and cancer has attempted to control for this genetic variation. As we noted above, some authors have suggested the possibility of connections between cancer and PROP tasting. Any such connections are especially important where patient-control studies claim lowered bitter thresholds.

Since the incidence of particular types of cancer is associated with risk factors (e.g., smoking, alcohol abuse), the impact of these risk factors on taste and smell must be considered in the selection of controls. In addition, effects of cancer on incidence of diseases like upper respiratory infections may also produce non-cancer-related differences between patients and controls.

### Limitations on the Suprathreshold Techniques Used to Compare Two Groups (i.e., Patients vs. Controls)

The assessment of chemosensory function most important to an assessment of the patient's everyday taste world is suprathreshold scaling. Suprathreshold scaling produces psychophysical functions that allow us to see how perceived intensity changes across the entire range of sensation from barely detectable (near-threshold) to the most intense sensations possible. This is the most important information but also the most difficult to obtain because we cannot share another person's experiences directly. We have reviewed this dilemma in the context of studies on aging (51) and we briefly summarize that argument in the following section.

### Comparing Sensory Experiences

How do we compare sensory experiences? We do so by finding a standard to which other sensations can be compared. One of the oldest methods is the use of adjectives as standards. For example, with the Natick nine-point category scale we tell subjects to apply numbers to their sensations such that 1 = very weak, 5 = medium, and 9 = very strong. We assume that everyone applies these adjectives to their perceptions of intensity in the same way, so that if two people both call a stimulus very strong, they are perceiving the same absolute intensities. Obviously, we can never know if this assumption is correct but a variety of studies suggest that such adjective scales can be of some value in assessing differences across patients. Their main limitation is that they may fail to detect a difference that is present.

Another way to find a standard is to use another sensory experience. For example, when we explore genetic variation in taste we use a sound standard. We essentially ask subjects to match the intensity of a taste to the intensity of a sound. We know that hearing varies but we have no reason to believe that variations in hearing and taste are related. Thus, on average, we discover that supertasters match saturated PROP to a very loud sound whereas nontasters match the same concentration to a very soft sound. The use of one sensory modality as a standard for variation in another is called magnitude matching (52). This method is usually used with the psychophysical method called magnitude estimation but is applicable to any suprathreshold scaling technique.

We suggest that investigators interested in psychophysical evaluations of cancer patients examine a new scale recently developed by Green and colleagues (53). This line scale is labeled with adjectives spaced such that distances along this scale are essentially equivalent to magnitude estimates (i.e., if two stimuli produce responses of 8 and 4, respectively, the first stimulus is perceived to be twice as intense as the second). This scale is both sensitive to differences across groups and easy for naive subjects to use.

One mistake is particularly devastating when patients are to be compared to controls. Some investigators select a standard, then give it to both patients and controls and tell them what rating the standard represents. This forces patients and controls to give the same ratings even if they are having very different experiences. Needless to say, the results will show no difference between patients and controls for the standard but that result is meaningless. This mistake is easy to make because the practice of providing a standard and assigning it a rating is common when individual differences are not important. Consider the following example that illustrates this problem.

Ames et al. (54) studied the taste of NaCl and sucrose in patients with breast cancer using a method designed for studies related to food (55). The subjects were presented with a 15-cm horizontal line with the endpoints labeled least salty/sweet on the left and most salty/sweet on the right. Subjects were given the most extreme taste concentrations (e.g., 0.04 and 0.756 M NaCl and sucrose) and told that these corresponded to the labels. Subjects were then instructed to mark the line to indicate the perceived intensity of each sample. Note that if the cancer patients had perceived all tastants as weaker than the controls did, this would never have been revealed because cancer patients and controls alike were instructed to rate the top concentration at the most salty/sweet end of the scale. Not surprisingly, there were no differences between cancer patients and controls.

### Distinguishing Hedonic from Sensory Alterations

Taste and smell provide sensory information but also provide affect: pleasure and displeasure. The hedonic attributes of taste and smell serve different functions. The affect of taste is hard-wired; newborns respond to sweet with facial expressions suggesting pleasure and respond to bitter with facial expressions suggesting displeasure (56). On the other hand, the affect of olfaction appears to be largely (if not completely) learned. At 2 years, children do not appear to experience adult-like pleasure and dis-

pleasure from odors (57,58); by 3 years, their responses begin to resemble those of adults (59).

The affect of taste is relatively stable but the affect of olfaction is quite labile. Simple exposure to an odorant can change its pleasantness (60). Pairing an odor with pleasurable experiences like sweet taste (61) or calories (62) can increase the pleasantness and pairing an odor with nausea decreases the pleasantness (63). This latter phenomenon plays an important role in the formation of conditioned food aversions (see below).

When patients say that food does not taste good they may be referring to a genuine sensory alteration but they may also be referring to a hedonic change; the food tastes just as it always did but that taste is no longer pleasant. It is important to question patients to be sure that the nature of the complaint is clear.

## CHEMOSENSORY ALTERATIONS ASSOCIATED WITH CANCER AND ITS RELATED THERAPIES

Most of the literature on chemosensory alterations is focused on taste. For that reason, the discussions in the following sections will also be focused on taste. What is known about cancer-related genuine sensory alterations in olfaction will be summarized later. Conditioned aversions, which reflect hedonic rather than sensory alterations, involve olfaction; these will be discussed toward the end of this chapter.

### Real-World Taste Experience and Cancer

Tumors can obstruct chemoreceptor sites, interfere with neural transmission on the pathway between receptor site and the brain, and affect sensory processing in the brain itself. Several types of intracranial tumors are known to alter both taste and smell. Acoustic neuromas, also called vestibular schwannomas, which grow on the VIIIth cranial nerve, can produce taste loss if the tumor invades the VIIth cranial nerve (21). Chemically, tumor growth may interfere with protein metabolism, leaving patients with diminished immune response and therefore more likely to suffer viral damage to the chemosensory system.

There are two sources of evidence for meaningful taste loss in cancer patients: suprathreshold psychophysical studies and anecdotal reports. We have already discussed the study by Ames et al. (54) on breast cancer patients. Because these patients had only surgery (no chemotherapy or radiation therapy) they would have been an appropriate group to study. However, the results, that there were no effects of cancer per se, were produced by the misuse of the scaling method and have no relevance to cancer per se.

Mossman and Henkin (65) used a different suprathreshold scaling method that can reveal differences between cancer patients and controls. The method used, forced scaling, asks subjects to rate the intensity of taste on a scale from 1 to 100 where 100 equals the most intensely salty, sweet, sour, or bitter solution ever experienced. Patients with head and neck cancer rated taste intensities lower than control subjects did. However, only one of the patients was subjectively aware of any taste loss, which is hard to reconcile with the psychophysical data. This kind of method has one potential flaw. The patients were asked to rate their sensations in comparison to their most intense taste experience. Unfortunately, the most intense taste experience varies with an individual's genetic ability to taste. This means that differences between patients and controls may simply reflect genetic differences. Fortunately, this study also includes within-patient comparisons, which will be discussed in the section on radiation therapy.

Anecdotal descriptions may offer insight into the status of taste function in cancer patients, but the anecdotes must contain sufficient information to ensure that the patient is reporting true taste changes. Bolze et al. (47) reported that 17% of their patients had subjective complaints of loss of taste or abnormal taste when initially interviewed but do not describe how their questions were phrased. Kashima and Kalinowski (65) argue that taste function is frequently disturbed before treatment of laryngeal cancer. The phrasing of their questions is not included in their report; in addition, they were also dealing with patients who may also have experienced damaged taste from some of the risk factors for this cancer (e.g., tobacco and alcohol use). Some reviews of cancer and taste assert that cancer damages taste (66) but the evidence turns out to be the untrustworthy threshold studies (discussed above). Finally, some reports of alterations in taste perception are actually assessments of changes in the palatability of foods (67). In conclusion, there is no good evidence for a general phenomenon of taste loss with cancer per se.

## Chemotherapy and Taste

Cancer therapies suppress tumor growth by destroying cancer cells and can have both direct and indirect impact on the chemical senses. Both chemotherapy and radiation therapy can damage chemosensory structures, disrupt saliva (68) and mucous production, and cause oral mucositis, xerostomia, and dental caries. Antiestrogen drugs such as tamoxifen can alter the body's hormone production, which might affect taste, and also chemotherapy drugs can enter the mouth via gingival fluid (69) and saliva (70,71) and stimulate taste, tactile (72–74), and olfactory (75) sensations. The existence of venous taste was once exploited in the calculation of circulation time; compounds were injected into the bloodstream and the length of time that passed before they were tasted in the mouth was used as a measure of circulation (76,77).

The effect of chemotherapy on a patient's experience with food can often be dramatic. One study demonstrated that over 80% of chemotherapy patients avoided food (78). Many reported taste alterations have been directly linked to drugs such as vinblastine, cisplatin, bleomycin, and methotrexate (26). A study by Soni and Chatterji (79) used electrogustometry (i.e., assessment of thresholds for electric taste) and reported that 10% of the patients treated with bleomycin showed elevated thresholds (compared to control subjects) but that thresholds returned to normal within 10–12 weeks. This paper illustrates a point made above; localized loss often fails to affect real-world perception. Electrogustometry uses a metal probe to stimulate the tongue. The probes are very small and so the stimulation is very localized. Soni and Chatterji reported that only one of five subjects who showed substantially elevated thresholds noticed any loss.

Two suprathreshold psychophysical studies have failed to find impressive effects of chemotherapy. Trant et al. (80) used a 10-cm line labeled no sweetness, sourness, saltiness, or bitterness on the left and extremely sweet, sour, salty, or bitter on the right (subjects were allowed to extend the line if they chose). The intensity scores were not reduced in those patients receiving chemotherapy (compared to other cancer patients). Mulder et al. (81) asked patients to rate taste intensities on a seven-point scale labeled with 0 = no taste and 7 = extremely strong. Patients were tested before chemotherapy and between the seventh and tenth days after the last day of nine courses of chemotherapy. Following chemotherapy, the lowest concentrations were rated stronger than before and the highest concentrations were rated lower than before, the most pronounced effect being on sweet. Note that this is a relatively subtle loss; yet Mulder et al. quote one of their patients as saying, "Everything tastes the same."

The discrepancies between the results of these studies and patient anecdotes suggest several problems. Experimental designs may fail to capture the important events in the effects of chemotherapy on taste. Prospective studies following individual patients may be necessary to identify the critical time at which taste loss occurs, as well as to identify the tumor sites and chemotherapeutic agents most likely to produce damage. New psychophysical methods for suprathreshold scaling are more sensitive than the methods previously in use (52,53). Finally, such patient anecdotes as "Everything tastes the same" actually suggest olfactory losses. The effects of chemotherapy on olfaction have been virtually ignored.

## Radiation Therapy and Taste

The anecdotal accounts of radiotherapy-induced disturbances are compelling. MacCarthy-Leventhal, a physician who underwent radiation for cancer of the pharynx in the 1950s (82), described both a "blindness of the mouth," rendering food tasteless, and a "hallucinatory" taste overwhelming all liquids. More recently, Chencharick and Mossman reported perceived changes in food taste and use of sugar in head and neck cancer patients (83). Before radiation therapy, 25% of these patients reported "changes in taste" and that "foods taste bad," whereas 80% reported such changes after treatment. More than half of patients noticed an abnormal taste with high-protein foods (meat, eggs, dairy) and a quarter reported adding sugar to foods.

The taste losses induced by radiation are not subtle. Radiation therapy may cause dissociation between thresholds and suprathreshold taste as demonstrated in a 52-year-old woman undergoing radiation therapy for a tumor of the neck (33). This patient's taste recognition thresholds initially rose but returned to normal after approximately 60 days. Her suprathreshold functions flattened and did not recover. She lived in a pastel taste world despite her normal thresholds. A study by Mossman and Henkin (64) (discussed above with regard to the effects of cancer) made within-patient comparisons of taste function prior to, 2 weeks after, and 5 weeks after radiation therapy. The psychophysical functions for taste flattened steadily during this time. In a study of the long-term effects of radiotherapy (84), taste losses were still present up to 7 years after therapy. However, taste loss with radiation therapy is by no means universal. Schwartz et al. (85) found only mild impairment in patients tested at varying intervals after therapy (6 months to 19 years).

Of special interest, Bonanni and Perazzi [1965, cited in Rubin and Casarett (86)] followed 50 patients for 1 month to 1 year and reported both suppressed and heightened taste sensations. This is particularly interesting because there are theoretical reasons to expect radiation therapy to be associated with heightened taste. Because radiation is directed to specific areas, one might expect some taste nerves to be affected more than others. Localized damage can lead to intensified taste sensations due to release of inhibition as discussed above.

## CANCER, CANCER THERAPIES, AND OLFACTION

The effects of cancer per se and chemotherapy on the sense of smell have received very little attention. This may reflect the common misunderstanding about the proper distinctions between taste and smell. Anecdotal accounts suggesting that food is flat with no taste actually implies olfactory loss as well as genuine taste loss since a large part of the sensory input from food is olfactory (perceived retronasally).

The effects of radiation therapy on olfaction have been documented by Doty and his colleagues (87,88) and Ophir et al (89). In the study by Ophir et al., patients did not show complete recovery even 6 months after treatment. The influence of cancer and related therapies on olfaction deserves more attention.

## CONDITIONED FOOD AVERSIONS

Garb and Stunkard (90) provided a classic picture of a conditioned aversion: If a person becomes sick after eating a specific food, he may develop an intense dislike, called an *aversion,* for that food, whether or not it was responsible for the illness. Conditioned aversions were used in the treatment of alcoholism as early as 1940 (91). Subsequently, conditioned aversions became of great interest to learning theorists, e.g., see (92,93). Conditioned aversions to foods form in the presence of nausea (63) and they can occur even when an individual recognizes that the nausea was not caused by the food. Nausea is associated with both chemotherapy and radiation therapy but may also be associated with cancer itself. Bernstein (94) was the first to show that conditioned aversions could be produced by therapies for cancer and to suggest that these aversions might play a role in the loss of appetite in cancer patients.

The roles that taste and olfaction play in conditioned aversions are scientifically very interesting. In animals, conditioned aversions are believed to form better to olfactory than to taste stimuli. However, in humans, conditioned aversions are rarely (if ever) specific to sweet, salty, bitter, and sour but rather form to the odors of the food perceived retronasally (95). Part of this apparent difference between the results in animal and human studies may relate to confusion over the proper distinctions between orthonasal olfaction, retronasal olfaction, and taste. Rozin has suggested that the brain may treat olfactory input differently depending on whether its origin is orthonasal or retronasal (96) because orthonasal input provides information about the environment whereas retronasal input provides information about what is in the mouth. To the best of our knowledge, in animal studies the olfactory stimulation is orthonasal. We would expect retronasal olfactory input to condition aversions much more successfully in animals.

Broberg and Bernstein (97) used the properties of conditioned food aversions to provide a behavioral intervention that helps prevent aversions to important dietary items in cancer patients. Children were given either root beer or coconut lifesavers prior to chemotherapy. The lifesavers served as a scapegoat food. Aversions were formed to the scapegoat that prevented the formation of aversions to other foods. Andresen et al. (98) compared novel and familiar scapegoats and found that the novel scapegoat was more effective. Mattes (99) demonstrated the efficacy of this procedure in a large population that included patients receiving radiation therapy (not tested in the previous studies).

One of the interesting features of conditioned food aversions is that some foods become aversive and others do not. Bartoshuk and Wolfe (unpublished data) demonstrated this with aversions formed in college students as the result of illness induced by consumption of alcoholic beverages. Of 61 alcohol-induced aversions, about half occurred when the subject was consuming more than alcohol alone (e.g., vodka and orange juice, beer and buffalo wings). In these cases, about 40% of the time the aversion skipped the alcohol altogether and formed to the accompanying food or beverage. The rest of the time the aversion included the alcoholic beverage. Jacobsen et al. (100) studied the development of aversions to diet items over successive chemotherapy sessions in cancer patients. They found that 46% of the patients developed aversions to at least one food at some time during treatment. They concluded that the number of aversions formed was probably limited by the familiarity of the foods (animal studies indicate that novel foods condition more easily). In addition, the consumption of several foods may have protected individual items.

Although it is clear that nausea produces conditioned aversions (63,101), some aversions appear to form in cancer patients that cannot be closely associated with nausea (100,102–104).

### Phantom Sensations Resulting from Chemotherapy or Radiation Therapy

Some patients report bitter taste sensations during chemotherapy (72–74). Medications tend to taste bitter; thus patients may be tasting their chemotherapeutic drugs. There are two routes by which these drugs might stimulate taste. First, the drugs may gain access to the mouth via saliva, e.g., see (70,71) for examples of medications that enter saliva or (69) for gingival fluid. Second, the drugs may be tasted directly from the bloodstream. The venous taste phenomenon (105) was once used to measure circulation time (106). When a tastant is injected into a vein in the arm, it can be tasted when the blood reaches the taste buds. The speed with which this occurs suggests that the tastant stimulates receptors on the lower portions of taste cells directly from blood without actually entering the mouth. There is a similar venous olfaction phenomenon (75) that might also play a role in producing sensations from chemotherapeutic drugs.

Cancer therapies can produce salivary disorders such as dry mouth, which can abet tissue damage; insufficient saliva leaves tissues unprotected and open to infection, the products of which can be both tasted and smelled.

Nesse et al. (107) reported pseudohallucinations associated with chemotherapy. Some patients described a chemical odor that occurred when they thought about or viewed the clinic. Two patients described being able to taste their chemotherapeutic drugs while under treatment and then tasting them again when thinking about them. Olfactory hallucinations can occur in normal individuals who have been exposed to intensely emotional experiences. Burstein (108) reported two such hallucinations related to posttraumatic stress disorder. A woman who had been in an automobile accident smelled gasoline while riding as a passenger in her husband's car and a man who had been in a fire reported flashbacks in which he smelled smoke as he had in the fire.

## DETERMINING CAUSES OF CHEMOSENSORY COMPLAINTS

Even without extensive psychophysical testing, clinicians can distinguish sensory from hedonic complaints and can obtain information about the source of dysfunctions.

1. Identify genuine losses in taste and/or olfaction:
   - Can the patient recognize the taste of table salt, sugar, lemon, or the bitterness in a sip of coffee?
   - Can the patient identify household odors such as baby powder, coffee, chocolate, cinnamon, and peanut butter?
   - Can the patient identify odors introduced retronasally? This can be easily determined with jellybeans; do not allow the patient to see the jellybean as it is put in the mouth, but ask if the flavor can be identified.
2. Evaluate dysgeusia.
   - Does the patient ever experience a persistent taste in the mouth unrelated to food? If the answer is yes, ask if the patient can identify it as sweet, sour, salty, bitter, or metallic. Can the taste be rinsed away even briefly (this suggests a stimulus actually in the mouth)? If the taste intensifies as the patient chews, the taste may come from saliva or gingival fluid.
   - Topical anesthetics can help identify the source of dysgeusia. If the taste results from a stimulus actually in the mouth, then a topical anesthetic will abolish it. If the taste results from abnormal stimulation of a neural structure mediating taste, a topical anesthesia may intensify it.
3. Evaluate parosmia.
   - Does the patient ever experience a persistent smell and, if so, how would he or she describe it? A taste sensation will have a specific quality (sweet, salty, etc.). An olfactory sensation may evoke a qualitative response (e.g., "like gasoline") or the patient may give a hedonic response (e.g., "unpleasant") and be unable to describe it.

## RECOMMENDATIONS

Strategies designed to improve dietary intake and nutritional status should be individualized. Illness and treatments affect patients differently, making the application of universal recommendations to improve the flavor of food unwise. Patients are likely to benefit from consultation with a registered dietitian. Strategies designed to prevent chemosensory dysfunction secondary to treatment (e.g., minimizing damage to taste and olfactory receptors with shielding during radiation therapy) should be adapted to the needs of the patient, e.g., see (26). The National Cancer Institute has published a booklet, *Eating Hints for Cancer Patients*, that gives recipes that cancer patients and their families have found useful. Finally, reducing the impact of conditioned aversions is especially important. Studies suggest the following:

- Physicians should inform the patient of the possibility of a food aversion occurring with treatment.
- The patient should avoid eating 4 hours prior to and after chemotherapy or bowel irradiation (26).
- The patient may ingest a novel-tasting but nutritionally unimportant food (scapegoat) shortly before irradiation or chemotherapy (97).
- The patient should not consume nutritionally important foods until nausea ends completely (98).

## REFERENCES

1. Pfaffmann C. Gustatory afferent impulses. *J Cell Comp Physiol* 1941; 17:243–258.
2. Pfaffmann C. Gustatory nerve impulses in rat, cat and rabbit. *J Neurophysiol* 1955;18:429–440.
3. Frank ME, Contreras J, Hettinger TP. Nerve fibers sensitive to ionic taste stimuli in chorda tympani of the rat. *J Neurophysiol* 1983;50:941–960.
4. Pfaffmann C, Frank M, Bartoshuk LM, Snell TC. Coding gustatory information in the squirrel monkey chorda tympani. In: Sprague JM, Epstein A, eds. *Progress in physiological psychology.* New York: Academic Press, 1976;1–27.
5. Bartoshuk LM. The biological basis of food perception and acceptance. *Food Qual Pref* 1993;4:21–32.
6. Todrank J, Bartoshuk LM. A taste illusion: taste sensation localized by touch. *Physiol Behav* 1991;50:1027–1031.
7. Fox AL. Six in ten "tasteblind" to bitter chemical. *Sci News Lett* 1931; 9:249.
8. Blakeslee AF. Genetics of sensory thresholds: taste for phenyl thio carbamide. *Proceedings Natl Acad Sci USA* 1932;18:120–130.
9. Bartoshuk LM, Fast K, Karrer TA, Marino S, Price RA, Reed DA. PROP supertasters and the perception of sweetness and bitterness. *Chem Senses* 1992;17:594.
10. Bartoshuk LM, Duffy VB, Reed D, Williams A. Supertasting, earaches, and head injury: genetics and pathology alter our taste worlds. *Neurosci Biobehav Rev* 1996;20:79–87.
11. Lucchina LA, Curtis OF, Putnam P, Drewnowski A, Bartoshuk LM. Psychophysical measurement of 6-n-propylthiouracil (PROP) taste perception, Proceedings of the XII International Symposium on Olfaction and Taste: Annals of the New York Academy of Sciences, in press.
12. Duffy VB, Bartoshuk LM, Lucchina LA, Snyder DJ, Tym A. Supertasters of PROP (6-n-propylthiouracil) rate the highest creaminess to high-fat milk products. *Chem Senses* 1996;21:598.
13. Bhatia S, Sharma KN, Mehta V. Taste responsiveness to phenythiocarbamide and glucose during menstrual cycle. *Curr Sci* 1981;50:980–983.
14. Hoyme LE. Genetics, physiology and phenylthiocarbamide. *J Hered* 1955;46:167–175.
15. Glanville EV, Kaplan AR. Taste perception and the menstrual cycle. *Nature* 1965;206:930–931.
16. Glanville EV, Kaplan AR. The menstrual cycle and sensitivity of taste perception. *Am J Obstet Gynecol* 1965;92:189–194.
17. Than TT, Delay ER, Maier ME. Sucrose threshold variation during the menstrual cycle. *Physiol Behav* 1994;56:237–239.
18. Bhatia S, Puri R. Taste sensitivity in pregnancy. *Ind J Physiol Pharmacol* 1991;35:121–124.
19. Duffy VB, Bartoshuk LM, Striegel–Moore R, Rodin J. Taste changes across pregnancy. Proceedings of the XII International Symposium on Olfaction and Taste: Annals of the New York Academy of Sciences, in press.
20. Corwin J, Loury M, Gilbert AN. Workplace, age, and sex as mediators of olfactory function: data from the National Geographic Smell Survey. *J Gerontol* 1995;50:P179–86.
21. Kveton JF, Bartoshuk LM. The effect of unilateral chorda tympani damage on taste. *Laryngoscope* 1994;104:25–29.
22. Doty R, Bartoshuk L, Snow J. Causes of olfactory and gustatory disorders. In: Getchell TV, Doty RL, Bartoshuk LM, Snow JB, eds. *Smell and taste in health and disease.* New York: Raven Press, 1991; 449–462.
23. Weiffenbach JM. Chemical senses in aging. In: Getchell TV, Doty RL, Bartoshuk LM, Snow JB, eds. *Smell and taste in health and disease.* New York: Raven Press, 1991;369–378.
24. Scott AE. Clinical characteristics of taste and smell disorders. *ENT J* 1989;68:297–315.
25. Doty RL. Olfaction and multiple chemical sensitivity. *Toxicol Indust Health* 1994;10:359–368.
26. Beidler LM, Smith JC. Effects of radiation therapy and drugs on cell turnover and taste. In: Getchell TV, Doty RL, Bartoshuk LM, Snow JB, eds. *Smell and taste in health and disease.* New York: Raven Press, 1991;753–763.
27. Graziadei GAM, Graziadei PPC. Neurogenesis and neuron regeneration in the olfactory system of mammals. II. Degeneration and reconstituion of the olfactory sensory neurons after axotomy. *J Neurocytol* 1979;8:197–213.
28. Graziadei PPC, Graziadei GAM. Neurogenesis and neuron regeneration in the olfactory system of mammals. I. Morphological aspects of differentiation and structural organization of the olfactory sensory neurons. *J Neurocytol* 1979;8:1–18.
29. Esiri MM. Pathology of the olfactory and taste systems. In: Getchell TV, Doty RL, Snow JB, Bartoshuk LM, eds. *Smell and taste in health and disease.* New York: Raven Press, 1991;683–701.
30. Duncan HJ, Seiden AM. Long-term follow-up of olfactory loss secondary to head trauma and upper respiratory tract infection. *Arch Otolaryngol Head Neck Surg* 1995;121:1183–1187.
31. Radner G. *It's always something.* New York: Avon Books, 1989.
32. McBurney DH, Collings VB. *Introduction to sensation/perception*, 2nd ed. Englewood Cliffs, NJ: Prentice-Hall, 1984.
33. Bartoshuk LM. The psychophysics of taste. *Am J Clin Nutr* 1978;31: 1068–1077.
34. Weiffenbach JM, Wolf RO, Benheim AE, Folio CJ. Taste threshold assessment: a note on quality specific differences between methods. *Chem Senses* 1983;8:151–159.
35. DeWys WD, Walters K. Abnormalities of taste sensation in cancer patients. *Cancer* 1975;36:1888–1896.
36. Solomon G. Patterns of taste loss in clinic patients with histories of head trauma, nasal symptoms, or upper respiratory infection. Yale University School of Medicine, 1991.
37. Solomon GM, Catalanotto F, Scott A, Bartoshuk LM. Patterns of taste loss in clinic patients with histories of head trauma, nasal symptoms, or upper respiratory infection. *Yale J Biol Med* 1991;64:280.
38. Lehman CD, Bartoshuk LM, Catalanotto FC, Kveton JF, Lowlicht RA. The effect of anesthesia of the chorda tympani nerve on taste perception in humans. *Physiol Behav* 1995;57:943–951.
39. Lundgren B, Jonsson B, Pangborn RM, et al. Taste discrimination vs hedonic response to sucrose in coffee beverage. An interlaboratory study. *Chem Senses Flavour* 1978;3:249–265.
40. Miller IJ, Bartoshuk LM. Taste perception, taste bud distribution, and spatial relationships. In: Getchell TV, Doty RL, Bartoshuk LM, Snow JB, eds. *Smell and taste in health and disease.* New York: Raven Press, 1991;205–233.
41. Settle RG, Quinn MR, Brand JG, Kare MR, Mullen JL, Brown R. Gustatory evaluation of cancer patients: preliminary results. In: van Eys J, Seelig MS, Nichols BL, eds. *Nutrition and cancer.* New York: SP Medical and Scientific, 1979;171–185.
42. Gallagher P, Tweedle DE. Taste threshold and acceptability of commercial diets in cancer patients. *J Parent Ent Nutr* 1983;7:361–363.
43. Hall JC, Staniland JR, Giles GR. Altered taste thresholds in gastrointestinal cancer. *Clin Oncol* 1980;6:137–142.
44. Barale K, Aker SN, Martinsen CS. Primary taste thresholds in children with leukemia undergoing marrow transplantation. *J Parent Ent Nutr* 1982;6:287–290.
45. Carson JAS, Gormican A. Taste acuity and food attitudes of selected patients with cancer. *J Am Diet Assoc* 1977;70:361–365.

46. Kamath S, Booth P, Lad TE, Kohrs MB, McGuire WP. Taste thresholds of patients with cancer of the esophagus. *Cancer* 1983;52:386–389.

47. Bolze MS, Fosmire GJ, Stryker JA, Chung CK, Flipse BG. Taste acuity, plasma zinc levels, and weight loss during radiotherapy: a study of relationships. *Therapeut Radiol* 1982;144:163–169.

48. Henkin RI, Gill JR, Bartter FC. Studies on taste thresholds in normal man and in patients with adrenal cortical insufficiency: the role of adrenal cortical steroids and of serum sodium concentration. *J Clin Invest* 1963;42:727–735.

49. Milunicova A, Jandova A, Skoda V. Phenylthiocarbamide tasting ability and malignant tumours. *Hum Hered* 1969;19:398–401.

50. Drewnowski A. *Genetic taste markers and dietary choices in cancer patients*. Seattle, Washington: American Association for the Advancement of Science, 1997.

51. Bartoshuk LM, Duffy VB. Taste and smell in aging. In: Masoro EJ, ed. *Handbook of physiology, Section 11: Aging*. New York: Oxford University Press, 1995;363–375.

52. Marks LE, Stevens JC, Bartoshuk LM, Gent JG, Rifkin B, Stone VK. Magnitude matching: the measurement of taste and smell. *Chem Senses* 1988;13:63–87.

53. Green BG, Shaffer GS, Gilmore MM. A semantically-labelled magnitude scale of oral sensation with apparent ratio properties. *Chem Senses* 1993;18:683–702.

54. Ames HG, Gee MI, Hawrysh ZJ. Taste perception and breast cancer: evidence of a role for diet. *J Am Diet Assoc* 1993;93:541–546.

55. Giovanni ME, Pangborn RM. Measurement of taste intensity and degree of liking of beverages by graphic scales and magnitude estimation. *J Food Sci* 1983;48:1175–1182.

56. Steiner JE. Facial expressions of the neonate infant indicating the hedonics of food-related chemical stimuli. In: Weiffenbach JM, ed. *Taste and development: the genesis of sweet preference*. Bethesda, MD: U.S. Department of Health, Education and Welfare, 1977:173–189.

57. Engen T. The origin of preferences in taste and smell. In: Kroeze JHA, ed. *Preference behaviour and chemoreception*. London: IRL, 1979; 263–273.

58. Engen T. *The perception of odors*. New York: Academic Press, 1982.

59. Schmidt HJ, Beauchamp GK. Adult-like odor preferences and aversions in three-year-old children. *Child Dev* 1988;59:1136–1143.

60. Cain WS. Lability of odor pleasantness. In: Kroeze JHA, ed. *Preference behaviour and chemoreception*. London: IRL, 1979:303–315.

61. Zellner DA, Rozin P, Aron M, Kulish C. Conditioned enhancement of human's liking for flavor by pairing with sweetness. *Learn Motiv* 1983;14:338–350.

62. Johnson SL, McPhee L, Birch LL. Conditioned preferences: young children prefer flavors associated with high dietary fat. *Physiol Behav* 1991;50:1245–1251.

63. Pelchat ML, Rozin P. The special role of nausea in the acquisition of food dislikes by humans. *Appetite* 1982;3:341–351.

64. Mossman K, Henkin RI. Radiation-induced changes in taste acuity. *Int J Radiat Oncol Biol Phys* 1978;4:663-670.

65. Kashima HK, Kalinowski B. Taste impairment following laryngectomy. *ENT J* 1979;58:88–92.

66. Strohl RA. Nursing management of the patient with cancer experiencing taste changes. *Cancer Nurs* 1983;6:353–359.

67. Stubbs L. Taste changes in cancer patients. *Nurs Times* 1989;85:49–50.

68. Mossman KL. Frequent short-term oral complications of head and neck radiotherapy. *ENT J* 1994;73:316–320.

69. Alfano M. The origin of gingival fluid. *J Theor Biol* 1974;47:127–136.

70. Juma FD, Rogers HJ, Trounce JR. The kinetics of salivary elimination of cyclophosphamide in man. *Br J Clin Pharmacol* 1979;8: 455–458.

71. Steele WH, Stuart JFB, Whiting B. Serum, tear and salivary concentrations of methotrexate in man. *Br J Clin Pharmacol* 1979;7: 207–211.

72. Greene PG, Seime RJ. Stimulus control of anticipatory nausea. *J Behav Ther Exp Psychiatry* 1987;18:61–64.

73. Fetting JH, Wilcox PM, Sheidler VR, Enterline JP, Donehower RC, Grochow LB. Tastes associated with parenteral chemotherapy for breast cancer. *Cancer Treat Rep* 1985;69:1249–1251.

74. Nerenz PR, Leventhal H, Easterling DV, et al. Anxiety and drug taste as predictors of anticipatory nausea in cancer chemotherapy. *J Clin Oncol* 1986;4:224–233.

75. Maruniak JA, Silver WL, Moulton DG. Olfactory receptors respond to blood-borne odorants. *Brain Res* 1983;265:312–316.

76. Winternitz M, Deutsch J, Brüll Z. Eine klinisch brauchbare Bestim-

mungsmethode der Blutumlaufzeit mettels Decholininjektion. *Medizinische Klinik* 1931;3:986–987.

77. Matsuyama H, Tomita H. Clinical applications and mechanism of intravenous taste tests. *Auris Nasus Larynx* 1986;13:S43–S50.

78. Holmes S. Food avoidance in patients undergoing cancer chemotherapy. *Support Care Cancer* 1993;1:326.

79. Soni NK, Chatterji P. Gustotoxicity of bleomycin. *Otorhino-laryngol Rel Spec* 1985;47:101–104.

80. Trant AS, Serin J, Douglass HO. Is taste related to anorexia in cancer patients? *Am J Clin Nutr* 1982;36:45–58.

81. Mulder NH, Smit JM, Kreumer WM, Bouman J. Effect of chemotherapy on taste sensation in patients with disseminated malignant melanoma. *Oncology* 1983;40:36–38.

82. MacCarthy-Leventhal E. Post radiation mouth blindness. *Lancet* 1959;19:1138–1139.

83. Chencharick JD, Mossman KL. Nutritional consequences of the radiotherapy of head and neck cancer. *Cancer* 1983;51:811–815.

84. Mossman K, Shatzman A, Chencharick J. Long-term effects of radiotherapy on taste and salivary function in man. *Int J Radiat Oncol Biol Phys* 1982;8:991–997.

85. Schwartz LK, Weiffenbach JM, Valdez IH, Fox PC. Taste intensity performance in patients irradiated to the head and neck. *Physiol Behav* 1993;53:671–677.

86. Rubin P, Casarett GW. *Clinical radiation pathology*. Philadelphia: WB Saunders, 1968.

87. Doty RL. A review of olfctory dysfunctions in man. *Am J Otolaryngol* 1979;1:57–59.

88. Carmichael KA, Jennings AS, Doty RL. Reversible anosmia following pituitary irradiation. *Ann Intern Med* 1984;100:532–533.

89. Ophir D, Guterman A, Gross-Isseroff R. Changes in smell acuity induced by radiation exposure of the olfactory mucosa. *Arch Otolaryngol Head Neck Surg* 1988;114:853–855.

90. Garb JL, Stunkard AJ. Taste aversions in man. *Am J Psychiatry* 1974; 131:1204–1207.

91. Voegtlin WL. The treatment of alcoholism by establishing a conditioned reflex. *Amer J Med Sci* 1940;199:802–810.

92. Garcia J, Kimeldorf DJ, Koelling RA. Conditioned aversion to saccharin resulting from exposure to gamma radiation. *Science* 1955; 122:157–158.

93. Smith JC. Radiation: Its detection and its effects on taste preference. In: Stellar E, Sprague JM, eds. *Progress in physiological psychology*, vol 4. New York: Academic Press, 1971;53–118.

94. Bernstein IL. Learned taste aversions in children receiving chemotherapy. *Science* 1978;200:1302–1303.

95. Bartoshuk LM, Wolfe JM. Conditioned taste aversions in humans: are they olfactory aversions? (abstract). *Chem Senses* 1990;15:551.

96. Rozin P. "Taste-smell confusions" and the duality of the olfactory sense. *Perception Psychophys* 1982;31:397–401.

97. Broberg DJ, Bernstein IL. Candy as a scapegoat in the prevention of food aversions in children receiving chemotherapy. *Cancer* 1987;60: 2344–2347.

98. Andresen GV, Birch LL, Johnson PA. The scapegoat effect on food aversions after chemotherapy. *Cancer* 1990;66:1649–1653.

99. Mattes RD. Prevention of food aversions in cancer patients during treatment. *Nutr Cancer* 1994;21:13–24.

100. Jacobsen PB, Bovbjerg DH, Schwartz MD, et al. Formation of food aversions in cancer patients receiving repeated infusions of chemotherapy. *Behav Res Ther* 1993;31:739–48.

101. Carrel LE, Cannon DS, Best MR, Stone MJ. Nausea and radiation-induced taste aversions in cancer patients. *Appetite* 1986;7:203–208.

102. Mattes RD, Arnold C, Boraas M. Learned food aversions among cancer chemotherapy patients. *Cancer* 1987;60:2576–2580.

103. De Silva P, Rachman S. Human food aversions: nature and acquistion. *Behavior Res Ther* 1987;25:457–468.

104. Andrykowski MA, Otis ML. Development of learned food aversions in humans: investigation in a "natural laboratory" of cancer chemotherapy. *Appetite* 1990;14:145–158.

105. Bradley RM. Electrophysiological investigations of intravascular taste using perfused rat tongue. *Am J Physiol* 1973;224:300–304.

106. Fishberg AM, Hitzig WM, King FH. Measurement of the circulation time with saccharin. *Proc Soc Exp Biol Med* 1933;30:651–652.

107. Nesse RM, Carli T, Curtis GC, Kleinman PD. Pseudohallucinations in cancer chemotherapy patients. *Am J Psychiatry* 1983;140:483–485.

108. Burstein A. Olfactory hallucinations. *Hosp Commun Psychiatry* 1987;38:80.

*Principles and Practice of Supportive Oncology,*
edited by Ann Berger et al.
Lippincott–Raven Publishers, Philadelphia ©1998

# CHAPTER 10

# Dysphagia

Steven B. Leder

Eating and life are bound together. Not only is eating one of life's greatest pleasures; it is also necessary to sustain life itself. We eat, however, for many reasons, e.g., for sustenance, for satiety, and to satisfy hedonistic desires (1,2). Just as important, eating is integral to the social network of every society in the world (1,3). Annual feasts, seasonal celebrations, weekly meal planning, and daily treats help to define, order, and enrich a society's, a family's, and an individual's life (3–8). When an attendee at life's celebration cannot participate, the impact is immediate, widespread, and significant (1,4). Inability to eat not only threatens biological survival but represents a barrier to fully sharing life with one's family and society (2).

The impact of the experiential meaning of living with dysphagia on an individual's social, emotional, and psychological life and well-being has seldom been addressed in the professional literature (9). A spousal report (10) discussed the importance of eating, for both the individual and his family, throughout the progression of neurological disease. When eating became impossible for the patients, the family felt that even the smell of favorite foods brought pleasure and a sense of social connection and sharing between the patient and the family.

Only one scientific paper was found that dealt with eating and quality of life (2). It included an extensive discussion of the experiential meaning of eating, a theoretical framework that described dysphagia handicap and adaptiveness, outlined a model for understanding the dysphagic person's concealment of the disorder in the medical encounter, and proposed a strategy for professionals treating the disorder. Dysphagia intervention is intended to increase the patient's feelings of hope, security, and self-respect by focusing on adapting eating to the individual's psychosocial abilities and supporting the individual's feelings of hope for a meaningful life (2,11–13).

The adverse effects on swallowing of both cancer and its treatment are well known (14). Pretreatment dysphagia is caused by the tumor due to mass or neurologic changes, which can lead to malnutrition and, at times, aspiration. Posttreatment dysphagia is caused by the treatment options, with surgery disrupting swallowing ability most significantly, but radiation therapy and chemotherapy, either alone or in conjunction with surgery, also contributing to the severity of dysphagia (14).

The purpose of this chapter is not only to discuss the anatomy and physiology of normal swallowing, etiologies of dysphagia, and diagnostic procedures, but to explore the importance of appropriate rehabilitation and psychosocial intervention with the patient and caregivers in order to foster an optimal supportive environment to either continue or reinstate the act of eating, with all its attendant social importance, into the daily life of the individual.

## ANATOMY AND PHYSIOLOGY

Swallowing is a highly complex, sequential behavior that has a number of interrelated and interdependent motor activity patterns that occur both simultaneously and rapidly in a predetermined order. Successful swallowing is a function critical to a patient's emotional and psychosocial interactions (15), and it impacts directly on medical status due to the potential for aspiration pneumonia and other pulmonary complications (16–18).

It is not the purpose of this chapter to discuss extensively normal swallowing anatomy and physiology. A number of excellent sources are provided for a comprehensive discussion of this area [cf. Miller (19,20), Logemann (21,22), Kennedy and Kent (23), Larson (24), Dodds (25), Gelfand and Richter (26)]. However, a working understanding of normal swallowing anatomy and physiology is required prior to discussing the areas of disordered swallowing and dysphagia diagnostics and rehabilitation.

S. B. Leder: Department of Surgery, Section of Otolaryngolgy, Yale University School of Medicine, New Haven, CT 06520-8041.

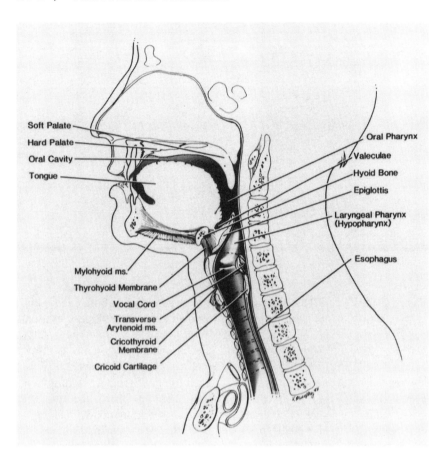

**FIG. 1.** Sagittal view of the head and neck showing relevant musculoskeletal structures involved in swallowing. (From Kahrilas PJ. The anatomy and physiology of dysphagia. In: Gelfand DW, Richter JE, eds. *Dysphagia diagnosis and treatment.* New York: Igaku-Shoin, 1989;11.)

Figure 1 shows the anatomic structures involved in swallowing. Table 1 outlines basic swallowing anatomy and physiology. The swallowing mechanism includes bony and cartilaginous support structures, striated and smooth muscle, and neural substrates. The act of swallowing shapes and moves a bolus from the oral cavity to the stomach by an ordered physiologic chain of events and is commonly divided into four phases: oral preparatory phase, oral phase, pharyngeal phase, and esophageal phase. Dysphagia can occur during one or more of the four phases of swallowing.

Table 2 outlines the sensory and motor nerves and their innervations that are involved in swallowing. The neural control of swallowing involves four main components: efferent motor fibers of the cranial nerves and ansa cervicalis; afferent sensory fibers of the cranial nerves; cerebral and midbrain fibers that synapse with the brainstem swallowing centers; and the paired swallowing centers in the brainstem (25). Input from the cranial and motor nerves and higher cerebral centers send input to the brainstem swallowing centers. The information is processed and, if the afferent neural input is appropriate, a swallow response is activated. The cranial nerves then carry the output signals to the muscles involved in swallowing.

To summarize Table 2, sensory input from the cranial nerves to the brainstem swallowing centers is provided mainly by the glossopharyngeal (C-IX) and vagal (C-X) nerves, with lesser involvement of the maxillary branch of the trigeminal (C-V$_2$) and facial (C-VII) nerves. The facial nerve provides touch sensation from the lips and face and taste from the anterior tongue. The maxillary branch of the trigeminal (C-V$_2$) provides much of the touch sensation from inside the mouth, and the glossopharyngeal (C-IX) completes touch sensation from the posterior tongue and pharynx. The superior laryngeal nerve of the vagus (C-X) provides sensory fibers for the base of tongue and posterior larynx.

Motor innervation of the muscles of mastication and swallowing is continued in Table 2. The facial nerve (C-VII) innervates the muscles of the face and the mandibular branch of the trigeminal (C-V$_3$) nerve innervates the muscles of mastication. The hypoglossal (C-XII) nerve and ansa cervicalis control tongue movement. The vagus (C-X) nerve controls the muscles of the palate and pharynx (except for the tensor veli palitini and stylopharyngeus) and the intrinsic laryngeal muscles. Movement of the hyoid bone and larynx are controlled by multiple nerves (C-V$_3$, C-VII, and C$_1$–C$_2$).

Table 3 outlines basic neural structures and systems involved in swallowing. The exact nature of the neural circuitry that controls the oral, pharyngeal, and esophageal phases of swallowing is not fully known. Two

**TABLE 1.** *Basic swallowing anatomy and physiology*

A. The four phases of swallowing
  1. Oral preparatory phase: manipulation and mastication of bolus; the joy of eating
    a. Lip closure
    b. Facial tone
    c. Rotary and lateral jaw motion
    d. Rotary and lateral tongue motion
    e. Velum contacts pharyngeal aspect of posterior tongue
    f. Variable time period, e.g., dependent on taste, gustatory pleasure, bolus viscosity, mental status
  2. Oral phase: Bolus transport
    a. Lips and buccal muscles contract
    b. Posterior tongue depresses
    c. Tongue stripping action against hard palate and bolus propelled toward anterior faucial arches and oropharynx
    d. Time period: 1 sec
  3. Pharyngeal phase: Bolus transport
    a. Tongue base retracts to posterior pharyngeal wall
    b. Velopharyngeal closure
    c. Glottal closure (airway protection)
      1. Epiglottis flips back, and false and true vocal folds adduct
      2. Laryngeal elevation closes laryngeal vestibule
      3. Cricopharyngeus relaxes for bolus passage
      4. Larynx moves anteriorly and superiorly to open sphincter
      5. Pressure applied to bolus drives it through the cricopharyngeal region
    d. Time Period: 1 sec
  4. Esophageal phase
    a. Peristaltic action
    b. Lower esophageal sphincter opens and bolus enters stomach
    c. Time period: 8–12 sec (dependent on posture and bolus consistency)

theories, with the goal of explaining the neurologic control mechanisms of swallowing, have been reported. They are the reflex chain hypothesis and the central pattern generator hypothesis (19). In the reflex chain hypothesis, a bolus moving in an anterior-to-posterior direction in the oral cavity and pharynx stimulates sensory receptors that sequentially trigger the next phase of swallowing. Swallowing occurs as a result of a chain of reflexes stimulated by and dependent on the previous response, e.g., the late oral phase starts the early pharyngeal phase of swallowing. In the central pattern generator hypothesis, sensory feedback does not influence swallowing behavior once a swallow has been started. The swallowing sequence is preprogrammed by the neurons in the medullary swallowing centers. It is most likely that both theories play a role in the act of swallowing in that swallowing depends on a central pattern generator that is modified by, but not dependent on, feedback from sensory input (25).

**TABLE 2.** *Basic sensory and motor nerves involved in swallowing*

| Sense | Sensory area innervated | Cranial nerve | Motor area innervated |
|---|---|---|---|
| Touch | Soft palate, mouth anterior 2/3 tongue, nasopharynx | V | |
| | | $V_3$ | Mastication muscles |
| | | $V_3$, VII, $C_1$–$C_2$ | Hyoid muscles |
| Taste | Anterior 2/3 tongue | VII | Facial muscles |
| Touch/taste | Posterior 1/3 tongue | IX | Stylopharyngeus, superior constrictor |
| Touch | Oro/hypopharynx | | |
| Touch | Tongue base, interior larynx | X | Palate,[a] pharynx,[b] larynx, esophagus |
| | | XI | With X to larynx, pharynx, pharyngeal constrictors |
| | | XII | Intrinsic and extrinsic tongue muscles[c] |
| | | $C_1$–$C_2$ | Extrinsic tongue muscles[c] |

[a]Except for tensor veli palitini innervated by $V_3$.
[b]Except for stylopharyngeus innervated by IX.
[c]Except for glossopalatinus innervated by X.

**TABLE 3.** *Basic neural structures and systems involved in swallowing*

A. Neural
  1. Cortical
    a. Voluntarily controlled swallowing
  2. Subcortical
    a. Reflexive swallowing
    b. Structures
      1. Basal ganglia
      2. Cerebellum
      3. Thalamus
      4. Limbic system
  3. Brainstem
    a. Motor and sensory nuclei for peripheral muscles
      1. Cranial nerves V (trigeminal), VII (facial), IX (glossopharyngeal), X (vagus), and XII (hypoglossal)
  4. Most swallows triggered by the action of bolus passing against anterior faucial arches and into the pharynx
    a. Not known if the bolus itself or the act of contracting the muscles triggers the swallow reflex
  5. Normal swallow
    a. Cortical signals from lateral motor cortex travel to vicinity of nucleus tractus solitarius (NTS)
    b. Sensory signals sent to rostral part of NTS by C-IX and C-X
    c. The inputs to the NTS activate the brainstem swallowing central pattern generator (SCPG)
    d. The SCPG causes sequential activation of neurons in and near the NTS, nucleus ambiguus, hypoglossal nucleus, and trigeminal nucleus
    e. These neurons are activated in a specific pattern according to the muscles they innervate, i.e., muscles used early in the swallow are innervated before muscles used later in the swallow

Cf. Table 1 for anatomy and physiology involved in swallowing.

## DYSPHAGIA

The term *dysphagia* is derived from the Greek *dys* (with difficulty) and *phagia* (to eat). Passage of a food bolus from the oral cavity through the pharynx without penetration into the trachea constitutes a successful swallow. Dysphagia can occur due to disordered oropharyngeal swallowing and/or following bolus penetration of the vocal folds and aspiration into the trachea and lungs.

When material penetrates the larynx and enters the airway below the level of the true vocal folds aspiration has occurred. Aspiration can occur *before* the swallow, e.g., before triggering of the swallow reflex, *during* the swallow, e.g., due to poor laryngeal closure, or *after* the swallow, e.g., from residual material left supraglottically (21).

Dysphagia results in higher health care costs due to increased length of hospitalization and the more expensive nature of nonoral feeding (27). Just as importantly, dysphagia impacts negatively on both eating and the activities associated with eating by restricting or preventing the normal act of swallowing (1,2,28–31).

## ETIOLOGIES OF DYSPHAGIA

### Head and Neck Cancer Surgery and Reconstruction

The act of swallowing intermixed with respiration and speaking is the most sophisticated coordination of voluntary and involuntary muscle action that exists in the animal kingdom (32). Dysphagia is a very common symptom in patients with head and neck cancer (33). Dysphagia is due to incoordination of the swallowing mechanism, obstruction, neurological changes, or pain caused by the tumor, and the combination of treatment modalities used, e.g., surgery for the resection of the cancer, external beam radiation therapy (EBRT), and chemotherapy. Surgical resection of the oral, pharyngeal, laryngeal, and/or esophageal areas commonly results in varying degrees of dysphagia (21,32,34–37). The limiting factors relative to the type and severity of dysphagia are the number and amount of anatomic structures removed and the reconstructive procedure(s) employed following the resection. In addition, patient motivation and the amount of individualized dysphagia rehabilitation impact on the rate of swallowing recovery (38).

The goal in the treatment of early tumors (stage I–II) is cure with either surgical resection, EBRT, or both. Dysphagia rehabilitation is often not required in these patients, but when it is the success rate for returning to a normal diet is excellent. The goal in the treatment of advanced tumors (stage III–IV) is locoregional control. This is accomplished by either organ preservation therapy, i.e., EBRT and chemotherapy (39–44) with surgical salvage, if necessary, or primary surgery followed by surgical reconstruction to allow for as much preservation of eating and speaking as possible. Organ preservation treatment may cause dysphagia due to mucositis, xerostomia, localized swelling, taste changes, and nausea. Surgical resection, however, often results in dysphagia, which may make eating very difficult (34). The patient's quality of life, dignity, and interpersonal relationships may become severely compromised, resulting in a reclusive behavior pattern and withdrawal from society (32).

## Oropharyngeal Structure Resections and Consequences

Surgical resection(s) involving oral, pharyngeal, laryngeal, and esophageal structures commonly results in dysphagia. The actual functional deficits are dependent on the extent of the specific resection and the reconstructive procedure (36). Although this makes for a heterogeneous population (38), surgical resections nevertheless result in predictable patterns of dysphagia and aspiration risk (37). Common dysphagia symptoms are increased pooling of secretions, drooling, pocketing of food in the lateral and anterior sulci, difficulty with mastication, numbness, decreased temperature and pain sensation, and poor bolus control and transport.

## Oral Cavity

Aspiration is not characteristic in patients with resectons of the anterior tongue and floor of mouth, regardless of the type of closure, i.e., primary or flap. These patients will have problems with the oral preparatory and oral phases of swallowing, but the pharyngeal phase is not disrupted, eliminating significant risk of aspiration (38).

However, resection of the lips, anterior tongue, and floor of mouth has social consequences for the individual. Drooling and bolus loss anteriorly make eating in public difficult and vigilance must be maintained to place the bolus posteriorly in the oral cavity to circumvent an anterior floor of mouth defect or loss of the tongue tip.

More extensive resections of the oral structures require a skin graft, tissue flap, or microvascular free flap. Generally, the larger the resection and subsequent reconstruction, the greater the probability of dysphagia and the higher the aspiration risk. McConnel et al. (45) compared three methods of oral reconstruction and found that the best method of reinstating masticatory and swallowing ability was intraoral skin grafting followed by a myocutaneous flap and, lastly, a tongue flap. Microvascular free flaps have recently shown promise for oral cavity reconstructions that may surpass skin grafting (46).

## Glossectomy

Total glossectomy results in a significant aspiration risk due to the obvious impairment of the oral preparatory and oral phases of swallowing and subsequent failure to trigger the swallowing reflex (47–49). When tumor is extensive and invades the preepiglottic space or the vallecula, it may be necessary to perform a total laryngectomy in conjunction with total glossectomy because of the high risk of life-threatening aspiration, especially in elderly and debilitated patients who are unable to tolerate the risk of recurrent aspiration (49).

Rehabilitation of the total glossectomy patient has focused on prosthetic management, with either a prosthetic tongue or palatal augmentation, to aid in deglutition and articulation (50–52).

## Mandibulectomy

When cancer has invaded bone, a composite resection, i.e., glossectomy, mandibulectomy, and radical neck dissection, is performed for an en bloc resection. Oral preparatory and oral phases of swallowing are affected due to surgical changes in the muscles of the tongue and floor of mouth. Functional deficit is directly proportional to the amount of surgical resection, with the prognosis for prosthetic and functional rehabilitation better when more bone, musculature, and dentition are present postoperatively (53). When the anterior mandibular arch is resected, the genioglossus muscle, which composes the bulk of the tongue and suprahyoid laryngeal support, loses its insertion, resulting in drooling (54). If the mandible is cut the inferior alveolar nerve, a sensory branch of $V_3$, may be severed, resulting in ipsilateral anesthesia of mandibular dentition and alveolar ridge, labial alveolar mucosa and gingiva, and skin and mucus membrane of the lower lip, and skin of the chin; and tactile sensation to the tongue. Bolus loss anteriorly and pocketing of food in the ipsilateral buccal sulcus often occur.

## Palate: Hard and Soft

Palatal defects cause abnormalities in the oral preparatory and oral phases of swallowing. Hard palate defects are successfully handled with an obturator (55) that prevents food from entering the nose via the surgically created oronasal fistula. Soft palate defects are more difficult to solve, as the soft palate is a dynamic muscular structure. Resection often results in velopharyngeal insufficiency due to insufficient length for oronasal separation and neuromuscular deficits due to injury to or severing of C-X. Lateral soft palate defects are more difficult to obturate than midline deficits (53). Both hard and soft palate defects and the obturator itself cause decreased sensation, which may impair oral function resulting in dysphagia. More recent surgical restoration techniques have attempted to preserve sensation along with functional anatomic separation of the oral and nasal cavities by using nerve grafts and scnsate flaps (46).

Objective improvement in swallowing has not yet been demonstrated.

## Pharynx and Esophagus

When the hypopharynx is involved with tumor, resection involves the pharynx and, by necessity, the larynx secondary to life-threatening risk of aspiration. Reconstruction is undertaken by gastric pull-up, jejunal free flap with microvascular anastomisis, regional myocutaneous flap, colon interposition, or radial forearm free flap (37).

Similarly, if the tumor is extensive and involves the esophagus as well, a total pharyngolaryngoesophagectomy with gastric pull-up or jejunal interposition is necessary. Although aspiration cannot occur following these procedures, dysphagia can occur due to a fistula or, more likely, by poor emptying of the gastric segment or jejunal graft because gravity must be relied on to transport material through a low-resistance tube. The patient presents with a "full" feeling at the base of tongue and oral regurgitation occurs if an upright posture is not maintained during and for at least an hour following eating (56).

## Laryngectomy: Total and Partial

There are three distinct types of swallowing problems corresponding to total laryngectomy and partial laryngectomies, i.e., supraglottic and hemilaryngectomy. They are dysphagia secondary to pharyngeal or cricopharyngeal dysmotility (57), recurrent tumor, or benign stricture (58). Partial laryngectomies are performed to save at least one vocal fold for preservation of voice (cf. Chapter XX for additional discussion of the different types of laryngectomies).

The incidence of dysphagia following total laryngectomy is highly variable, i.e., 10% to 58% (58–60). Dysphagia may be underestimated because retrospective analyses may not identify all patients with complaints of dysphagia (59) and because aspiration is eliminated by the surgical separation of the respiratory and digestive tracts. Nonetheless, total laryngectomy alters the swallowing mechanism because there can no longer be laryngeal elevation with the concomitant development of negative pressure in the pharyngoesophageal segment to aid in bolus propulsion. The laryngectomy therefore increases the propulsive pressure generated by the tongue (61). Fistulae may develop secondary to the increased swallowing pressures, especially due to increased mucosal edema in the immediate postoperative period.

It has been recommended that a cricopharyngeal myotomy be performed at the time of total laryngectomy to aid in bolus transit into and through the pharyngoesophageal segment (62). Also, hypopharyngeal stenosis is a relatively common occurrence following total laryngectomy (63) and is most likely due to the nature of the surgery rather than the site of the lesion (61). Dilatation is the most common therapy solution, but microvascular intestinal transfer grafts may be required.

Supraglottic laryngectomy involves resection, in the horizontal plane, of two of the three airway protective mechanisms, i.e., the epiglottis and aryepiglottic folds and false vocal folds (but not the true vocal folds), and often the hyoid bone, which provides skeletal support superiorly for the suspensory mechanism of the larynx (37,64). Supraglottic laryngectomy is organ-sparing surgery that places the patient at high risk for dysphagia and aspiration secondary to poor ability to protect the airway and reduced pharyngeal clearing resulting in aspiration after the swallow (64,65). Recovery of swallowing may take as little as 2 weeks, but some patients never regain functional swallowing. Although an overall failure rate of 8% to 20% was reported (37), the median number of days to resumption of successful oral intake was 106 (65).

Partial laryngectomy involves excision, in the vertical plane, of the aryepiglottic fold, false vocal fold, and true vocal fold unilaterally, sparing the epiglottis (37). Specific oncologic requirements may also necessitate resections involving the hyoid bone, arytenoid cartilage, superior laryngeal nerve, thyroid cartilage, and/or base of tongue, with concomitant increasing swallowing difficulties based on the extent of surgery.

Most patients exhibit some amount of aspiration in the short term following partial laryngectomy, i.e., ranging from 50% to 67% (37). Although life-threatening complications, i.e., pulmonary fibrosis, pneumonia, and lung abscess, can develop, most patients eventually regain the ability to eat by mouth following surgical resection, reconstruction, and dysphagia rehabilitation (66,67).

## Tracheotomy and Tracheotomy Tubes

Dysphagia has been shown to be a problem in both the head and neck cancer and tracheotomized populations. It appears that alterations in oral, pharyngeal, and laryngeal anatomy and physiology secondary to either the cancer and surgical resection and reconstruction or changes secondary to bypassing the upper airway with a tracheotomy place each of these populations at risk for various swallowing difficulties, including aspiration. When the populations overlap, i.e., patients with both head and neck cancer and a tracheotomy, the incidence of aspiration increases (33).

Tracheotomy has become one of the most frequently performed operations in otolaryngology head and neck surgery (68,69) due to the wide variety of conditions for which it is performed, i.e., acute airway obstruction secondary to infection or edema, chronic airway obstruction secondary to a mass or sleep apnea, respiratory difficulties requiring prolonged ventilatory support or to bypass the dead space of the upper airway, and chronic aspiration

(69). Despite such widespread use, the effect of a tracheotomy on the involved anatomic structures and their physiologic relationships is not without consequence.

In humans, the two diverse and mutually exclusive functions of deglutition and respiration share the same anatomic structures in the upper aerodigestive tract. Swallowing is a highly complex activity requiring precise coordination between anatomic structures and the sequencing of physiologic events occurring within a closed aerodigestive system. Tracheotomy inherently violates the closed aerodigestive system and alters the precise interrelated coordination involved in breathing and swallowing (68), i.e., glottic reflexes have been shown to be less sensitive in experimental animals following tracheotomy (70,71).

Although the majority of patients with a tracheotomy swallow successfully, a number of studies reported on aspiration associated with tracheotomy. Explanations as to the cause of aspiration following tracheotomy and placement of a tracheotomy tube include (a) fixation of the larynx causing impaired mechanical ability of the supraglottic larynx to achieve closure and protect the airway by limiting the rostrocaudal excursion of the laryngotracheal complex (68,72–74); (b) esophageal compression caused by a distended trachea secondary to an inflated tracheotomy tube cuff (75,76); (c) desensitization of the larynx secondary to diversion of normal airflow through the tracheotomy (68,73); and (d) neurophysiologic changes, specifically adductor vocal fold dysfunction and a weakened closure response after long-term tracheotomy, and alterations in respiratory abductor function of the larynx secondary to bypassing the upper airway via tracheotomy (68,70,71).

The latter two explanations, i.e., physiologic changes secondary to bypassing the upper airway with a tracheotomy, have been investigated directly by first occluding the tracheotomy tube, thereby reinstating the normal closed aerodigestive tract and allowing expired air to exit via the upper airway, followed by unoccluding the tracheotomy tube and diverting expired air from the tracheotomy tube. Aspiration can then be investigated under these two conditions in the same patient.

A case study (72) reported that the presence of an open tracheotomy tube appeared to have an adverse effect on swallowing; and upon plugging and subsequent removal of the tube the dysphagia resolved. Although tracheotomy caused neurophysiologic changes in both abductor and adductor laryngeal responses, when the tracheotomy cannula was occluded for 3 minutes some motor return was observed (68,71). Muz and colleagues reported on patients with tracheotomy and head and neck cancer. They found that aspiration increased when the tracheotomy tube was unoccluded (77) and that aspiration occurred in all patients with an unoccluded tube but in only half of the same group of patients with an occluded tube (33).

## Organ Preservation

Dysphagia rehabilitation is successful in allowing the patient to resume as near a normal diet as possible, but optimal eating is more likely to be preserved with intact, i.e., non–surgically altered, oral, pharyngeal, and laryngeal anatomy. Recent reports have shown that overall disease-free survival for advanced, i.e., stage III and IV, laryngeal and hypopharyngeal cancers, with laryngeal preservation therapy, i.e., induction chemotherapy combined with definitive radiation, was similar when compared to surgical resection and reconstruction (40–44). However, both EBRT and chemotherapy have side effects that may cause dysphagia. Specifically, an estimated 400,000 cancer patients per year in the United States exhibit oral cavity damage secondary to cancer or its treatment (78), which greatly affects quality of life.

## External Beam Radiation Therapy

Although EBRT does not usually cause physiologically based swallowing problems, as is the case following surgery and reconstruction, a wide variety of oral complications contributing to poor oral intake can occur (78). Complications may become more prevalent when combined treatments are used, e.g., surgery with EBRT, whether given pre- or postoperatively (79). Some problems are temporary, e.g., mucositis, infections, odynophagia, trismus, dysgeusia (80), and will resolve in the months following completion of EBRT. Other problems, e.g., xerostomia, dental caries, osteonecrosis, and tissue necrosis, may be permanent (81).

## Chemotherapy

Similar to EBRT, chemotherapy does not usually cause physiologically based swallowing problems, but it contributes to poor oral intake due to the emergence of taste changes (78). In addition, the cytotoxic effects of chemotherapeutic agents can cause mucositis, xerostomia, increased dental caries, nausea, vomiting, and dysguesia. More severe complications can lead to life-threatening hemorrhage and infections, which are more likely to occur in a chemotherapy patient than in an EBRT patient (82).

## COUNSELING

Preoperative counseling is often quite helpful, not so much to discuss the extent of the upcoming surgery but to prepare the patient for possible swallowing problems and, if they occur, to assure the patient that rehabilitation will be initiated before discharge from the hospital. The use of a nasogastric tube for nutritional maintenance immediately postoperatively and the possibility of a feeding gastrostomy tube if dysphagia persists are discussed. The patient is informed that swallowing diagnostics and rehabilitation will most likely begin before the nasogastric tube is discontinued. The different types of food consistencies, i.e., thin and thick liquid, puree, soft/moist solid, and hard/dry solid, are discussed, and the patient should understand that a diet may be restricted to one or more of the consistencies dependent on swallowing ability postoperatively.

Postoperative counseling deals with long-term issues related to nutritional maintenance, type of food consistency, e.g., restriction to a blenderized diet, and the importance of following swallowing recommendations and therapy exercises following discharge from the hospital. If postoperative EBRT or chemotherapy is to be given, the patient is educated regarding possible consequences, i.e., xerostomia, localized edema, odynophagia with EBRT and mucositis and taste changes with chemotherapy, to decrease anxiety and concern should these side effects occur.

## DIAGNOSTICS

Dysphagia diagnostics has three purposes: (a) to document if dysphagia and aspiration are present; (b) to determine why dysphagia and aspiration occurred; and (c) to make recommendations for rehabilitation strategies, e.g., bolus consistencies, head positions, and swallowing techniques.

The bedside dysphagia evaluation (BDE) follows a standardized protocol, examines the oral preparatory and oral phases of swallowing, and can identify patients at risk for dysphagia (83). The accuracy of such predictions, however, was reported to range from 42% (84) to 66% (85). Despite such variable accuracy, the BDE is widely used in making the initial diagnosis of dysphagia and subsequent recommendations for oral feeding.

The videofluoroscopic swallowing study (VFSS) (86) uses a more extensive test protocol than the original modified barium swallow (21) and is the gold standard for diagnosing dysphagia and recommending rehabilitation. It is performed in a fluoroscopy suite, assesses all four phases of swallowing, and many studies over the past decade have shown it to have excellent sensitivity and specificity (83).

The flexible endoscopic evaluation of swallowing (FEES) (87,88) is a relatively new bedside procedure for assessing the pharyngeal phase of swallowing by using a flexible nasolaryngoscope for visualization of the pharynx and larynx on a video monitor. Objective information can be obtained regarding aspiration, safety of oral feeding, bolus consistency, and optimum positioning in patients for whom a BDE is inadequate or deemed unreliable, and when a VFSS is difficult or impossible to perform.

The relative advantages and disadvantages of the BDE, VFSS, and FEES diagnostic procedures are listed in Table 4.

**TABLE 4.** *Relative advantages and disadvantages of the Bedside Dysphagia Evaluation (BDE), Videofluoroscopic Swallowing Study (VFES), and Fiberoptic Endoscopic Evaluation of Swallowing (FEES) procedures*

| | Advantages | Disadvantages |
|---|---|---|
| (1) BDE | Ease of administration<br>No equipment needed<br>No transport needed<br>Assess oral preparatory and oral phases<br>Use different bolus consistencies<br>Repeat as often as want<br>Cost | Does not assess pharyngeal or esophageal phases<br>Potential to miss "silent" aspirators<br>Adequate mental status to follow directions |
| (2) VFSS | Assess oral preparatory, oral, pharyngeal, and esophageal phases<br>Objective assessment<br>Use different bolus consistencies<br>Team approach, speech-language pathologist and radiologist | X-irradiation exposure<br>Must transport patient to fluoroscopy suite<br>Adequate mental status to follow directions<br>Cost |
| (3) FEES | Direct view of larynx and vocal folds<br>Objective assessment<br>Use different bolus consistencies or saliva<br>Cost<br>Repeat as often as want<br>No transport needed<br>Assess sensitivity in laryngeal region with tip of scope to identify "silent" aspirators | Must tolerate endoscopy<br>Anesthetize one nasal fossa<br>Difficult with agitated patient<br>Trained endoscopist<br>Initial setup cost: nasolaryngoscope, videocamera, videorecorder, TV monitor<br>Only assess pharyngeal phase |

## DIAGNOSTICS WITH SPECIAL POPULATIONS

### Tracheotomy Tubes

As discussed previously, from both a mechanical and a neurophysiologic perspective, a patient with a tracheotomy tube is, *ceteris paribus,* at greater risk for aspiration than one without a tracheotomy tube. When assessing swallowing with a tracheotomized patient, the tracheotomy cuff should always be deflated. The reason for this is that an inflated cuff does not prevent aspiration but only delays its detection. Recent evidence has demonstrated that the occlusion status of the tracheotomy tube does not not influence the prevalence of aspiration, but rather age (>65 years) and overall medical condition predispose the patient for aspiration (89). The deflated cuff allows for immediate identification of aspiration, by either coughing of a food bolus out the tracheotomy tube or evidence of food in the trachea following tracheal suctioning. An inflated tracheotomy cuff does not prevent aspiration (because by definition aspiration has occurred when the bolus is below the true vocal folds) and only delays evidence of aspiration for a short time, i.e., until the aspirated material that has collected just above the cuff migrates between the cuff and tracheal wall and enters the main stem bronchi and lungs.

### Ventilator Dependency

Patients on ventilatory support can eat orally. However, because the tracheotomy cuff cannot be deflated, extra care must be taken during dysphagia diagnostics and subsequent rehabilitation. A careful BDE supplemented by an FEES should be capable of determining the swallowing ability and bolus consistency necessary for successful oral feeding.

## RECOMMENDING ORAL FEEDING

The physician recommends when oral feedings should begin. The dietitian recommends and monitors maintenance of adequate nutritional intake. The speech-language pathologist determines the diet consistency and attempts to reestablish adequate oral feeding as soon as possible.

Once the speech-language pathologist has reviewed the medical history, completed a physical assessment of the swallowing mechanism, and performed a diagnostic dysphagia evaluation, determination of type of oral feeding, if any, can be made. The speech-language pathologist then makes recommendations regarding food consistencies, rehabilitation techniques, aspiration precautions, and criteria for discontinuing oral feedings due to signs of aspiration (Table 5).

**TABLE 5.** *Common aspiration precautions, procedures to decrease risk of aspiration, and features to monitor potential aspiration risk for health care providers*

I. Aspiration precautions
  Instructions to health care provider that patient is at risk to aspirate
  A. Explanation of surgical procedure
  B. Explanation of how swallowing mechanism has been physically altered
  C. Explanation of how edema, pain, fatigue, decreased sensation, and decreased range of motion may impair swallowing skills
  D. Explanation of types of food consistencies necessary for successful swallowing
II. Procedures to decrease risk of aspiration
  A. Health care provider to monitor:
    1. HOB 90° or in chair during eating
    2. Small bolus size
    3. Swallow completely before next bolus
    4. Clear throat or multiple swallows to help clear oropharynx
III. Features to monitor potential risk of aspiration
  A. Direct patient monitoring
    1. Temperature spike
    2. Coughing
    3. Throat clearing
    4. "Wet" sounding (gurgly) vocal quality
    5. Chest x-ray
    6. Weight loss
    7. Fatigue
    8. Poor compliance with recommendations

Individualized aspiration precautions and recommended techniques to improve dysphagia are often placed at the head of the bed on brightly colored paper so that all health care providers are alerted to the fact that a swallowing problem exists and the steps to be followed for successful swallowing. Table 5 lists common aspiration precautions, procedures to decrease aspiration risk, and features of which health care providers should be cognizant of when monitoring the dysphagic individual both during and after eating.

Specific indirect, direct, compensatory, and adaptive rehabilitative strategies are listed in Table 6. Indirect strategies do not use a food bolus and the exercises are focused on improving range of motion and strength of the structures of the swallowing mechanism, from labial closure to airway protection. Direct strategies use a food bolus consistency and quantity that are safe for the patient and direct him or her regarding optimal bolus placement in the oral cavity and specific instructions regarding postures and positioning. Compensatory strategies encompass bolus consistency modifications and steps to be followed for a successful swallow. Adaptive strategies use devices to aid in successful swallowing by optimal bolus placement, manipulation, and transit in the oral cavity [cf. Light (90) for a detailed discussion of oral

**TABLE 6.** *Indirect, direct, compensatory, and adaptive rehabilitation strategies for dysphagia*

A. Indirect: without a bolus
  1. Oromotor exercises to improve bolus manipulation and the voluntary swallow
    a. Lingual range-of-motion exercises
    b. Lingual resistance exercises
    c. Labial range of motion exercises
    d. Labial resistance (closure) exercises
  2. Improved triggering of the swallow reflex
    a. Touch anterior faucial arches with cold laryngeal mirror
  3. Laryngeal closure exercises for improved airway protection
    a. Supraglottic swallow
    b. Hold breath and bear down or pull up on chair arms
    c. Hard glottal attack
B. Direct: with a bolus
  1. Postures and positioning
    a. Head tilted and/or turned to the stronger or unoperated side (left or right)
    b. Head tilted back for gravity-assisted bolus movement
    c. Head tilted forward to open vallecular space and delay bolus slightly in pharynx
    d. Bolus placed in posterior or lateral (left or right) oral cavity
    e. Mendelsohn maneuver (94) (larynx elevated with fingers)
    f. Chin-tuck or chin-up posture
    g. Effortful swallow
C. Compensatory strategies to aid in bolus transport
  1. Bolus consistencies and modifications
    a. Liquid: thin, nectar, honey, custard consistencies
    b. Puree
    c. Soft solid
    d. Solid
    e. When to use food thickener
  2. Bolus volume
  3. Double swallows
  4. Swallow—clear throat—swallow
  5. Alternate solids and liquids to aid in bolus clearing
  6. Supraglottic swallow
D. Adaptive strategies and devices to aid in bolus placement, manipulation, and transit in oral cavity
  1. "Breck" feeder (syringe and catheter)
  2. Long-handled teaspoon
  3. Straw
  4. "Sippy" cup
  5. Cup with cut-out for nose
  6. Intraoral oral prosthesis
  7. Handheld oral prosthesis
E. Tracheotomy tubes
  1. Occlusion status of the tracheotomy tube does not influence prevalence of aspiration.
  2. Age (>65 years) and poor medical status predispose the patient to aspiration.

and oropharyngeal prostheses used to rehabilitate and facilitate swallowing skills].

The following is an example of dysphagia rehabilitation for a patient with decreased lingual range of motion secondary to lingual resection follows. Indirect and direct dysphagia rehabilitation (cf. Table 6) was attempted first but lingual motion remained decreased and food pocketed in the left sulcus. The speech-language pathologist and maxillofacial prosthodontist collaborated on designing a prosthesis to aid in swallowing. The puree bolus consistency was placed on the right side of the oral cavity by a long-handled spoon with the patient's head tilted to the right. The custom-made palatal prosthesis physically lowered the palatal vault to allow for tongue contact.

More normal oral preparatory and oral phases of swallowing were thus achieved. The patient was instructed to swallow twice to clear any residual bolus from the oropharynx. This rehabilitation strategy resulted in a successful swallow.

## THE SUPRAGLOTTIC SWALLOW

The supraglottic swallow is a technique with the goal of adducting the true vocal folds to protect the airway during swallowing. The technique can also be used by patients who have poor vocal fold adduction secondary to tumor involvement or surgical resection of the laryngeal branches of C-X, i.e., the superior laryngeal nerve and right and left recurrent laryngeal nerves, neurologic insult, or partial laryngectomy (65). The supraglottic swallow is composed of the following five steps:

1. Adduct true vocal folds and hold breath (tense neck).
2. Swallow during breath hold.
3. Clear throat or cough vigorously immediately following the swallow; do not inhale at this time.
4. Adduct true vocal folds and hold breath again.
5. Swallow again during breath hold.

## PHARYNGEAL AND ESOPHAGEAL PHASE DYSPHAGIA

There is no direct therapy to improve pharyngeal peristalsis or paralysis, cricopharyngeus dysfunction, or esophageal phase disorders. Pharyngeal phase problems that may indirectly benefit from rehabilitation are stimulation of the swallow reflex, reduced laryngeal closure, and paralysis by compensatory head positions. Other pharyngeal phase disorders, e.g., cervical osteophyte (91), scar tissue, and cricopharyngeus dysfunction (62,92), are treated surgically. Esophageal phase disorders are treated both surgically and medically (92,93).

## CONCLUSION

Successful eating and swallowing are requisites for a normal life. Not only does dysphagia impair the individual's quality of life, but if aspiration occurs the consequence could be life-threatening pneumonia. The patient should be counseled that although the cancer and/or its treatment may cause dysphagia, there are intervention strategies available to make eating as pleasant and successful an experience as possible.

## REFERENCES

1. Gustafsson B, Tibbling L. Dysphagia, an unrecognized handicap. *Dysphgagia* 1991;6:193.
2. Gustaffson B. The experiential meaning of eating, handicap, adaptedness, and confirmation in living with esophageal dysphagia. *Dysphagia* 1995;10:68.
3. Moore, HB. The meaning of food. *Am J Clin Nutr* 1957;5:77.
4. Taylor C. Interpretation and the sciences of man. In: Beehler R, Drengson AR, eds. *The philosophy of society.* London: Methuen, 1978;156.
5. Menzies IEP. Psychosocial aspects of eating. *J Psychosom Res* 1970;14:223.
6. Chappelle ML. The language of food. *Am J Nurs* 1972;72:1294.
7. Murcott A. The cultural significance of food and eating. *Proc Nutr Noc* 1982;41:203.
8. Bayer LM, Bauers CM, Kapp SR. Psychosocial aspects of nutritional support. *Nursing Clin North Am* 1983;1:119.
9. Ekberg O. "I and thou-the lived experience of the dysphagic life". *Dysphagia* 1995;10:67.
10. Schwartz B. Spouse report of Milton S. as I saw it. *Dysphagia* 1987;1:232.
11. Axelsson K, Norberg A, Asplund K. Relearning to eat late after a stroke by systematic nursing intervention: a case report. *J Adv Nursing* 1986;11:553.
12. Norberg A, Sandman PO. Existential dimensions of eating in Alzheimer's patients—An analysis by means of E.H. Erikson's theory of eight stages of man. *Adv Nursing* 1988;21:127.
13. Lundman A, Norberg A. The significance of a sense of coherence for subjective health in persons with insulin-dependent diabetes. *J Adv Nursing* 1993;18:381.
14. Humphreys B, Mathog R, Rosen R, Miller P, Muz J, Nelson R. Videofluoroscopic and scintigraphic analysis of dysphagia in the head and neck cancer patient. *Laryngoscope* 1987;97:25.
15. Hotaling DL. Adapting the mealtime environment: setting the stage for eating. *Dysphagia* 1990;5:77.
16. Johnson ER, McKernzie SW, Sievers A. Aspiration pneumonia in stroke. *Arch Phys Med Rehab* 1993;74:973.
17. Martin BJ, Corlew M. Wood H, et al. The association of swallowing dysfunction and aspiration pneumonia. *Dysphagia* 1994;9:1.
18. Schmidt J, Holas M, Halvorson K, Reding M. Videofluoroscopic evidence of aspiration predicts pneumonia and death but not dehydration following stroke. *Dysphagia* 1994;9:7.
19. Miller AJ. Deglutition. *Physiol Rev* 1982;62:129.
20. Miller AJ. Neurophysiological basis of swallowing. *Dysphagia* 1986;1:91.
21. Logemann JA. *Evaluation and treatment of swallowing disorders.* San Diego: College-Hill Press, 1983.
22. Logemann JA. Upper digestive tract anatomy and physiology. In: Bailey BJ, ed. *Head and neck surgery-otolaryngology.* Philadelphia: JB Lippincott, 1993;485.
23. Kennedy JG, Kent RD. Anatomy and physiology of deglutition and related functions. *Sem Speech Lang* 1985;6(4):257.
24. Larson C. Neurophysiology of speech and swallowing. *Sem Speech Lang* 1985;6(4):275.
25. Dodds WJ. The physiology of swallowing. *Dysphagia* 1989;3:171.
26. Gelfand DW, Richter JE. *Dysphagia diagnosis and treatment.* New York: Igaku-Shoin Medical Publishers, Inc., 1989.
27. Logemann JA. Evaluation and treatment of swallowing disorders. *Am J Speech Lang Pathol* 1994;3(3):41.
28. Tibbling L, Gustafsson B. Dysphagia and its consequences in the elderly. *Dysphagia* 1991;6:200.
29. Gustafsson B, Tibbling L, Theorell T. Do physicians care about patients with dysphagia? A study on confirming communication. *Fam Pract* 1992;9:203.
30. Gustafsson B, Porn I. A motivational approach to confirmation: an interpretation of some dysphagic patients' experiences. *Theor Med* 1994;15:409.
31. Gustafsson B, Theorell T. Adaptedness and coping in dysphagic students. *Dysphagia* 1995;10:86.
32. Dingman DL. Postoperative management of the severe oral cripple. *Plast Reconstr Surg* 1970;45:263.
33. Muz J, Hamlet S, Mathog R, Farris R. Scintigraphic assessment of aspiration in head and neck cancer patients with tracheostomy. *Head Neck* 1994;16:17.
34. Downie PA. The rehabilitation for patients following head and neck surgery. *J Laryngol Otol* 1975;89:1281.
35. Sessions DG, Zill R, Schwartz SL. Deglutition after conservation surgery for cancer of the larynx and hypopharynx. *Otolaryngol Head Neck Surg* 1979;87:779.
36. Baker BM, Fraser AM, Baker CD. Long-term postoperative dysphagia in oral/pharyngeal surgery patients: subjects' perceptions vs. videofluoroscopic observations. *Dysphagia* 1991;6:11.
37. Kronenberg MB, Meyers AD. Dysphagia following head and neck cancer surgery. *Dysphagia* 1994;9:236.
38. Pauloski BR, Logemann JA, Rademaker AW, et al. Speech and swallowing function after anterior tongue and floor of mouth resection with distal flap reconstruction. *J Speech Hear Res* 1993;36:267.
39. McNeil BJ, Weichselbaum R, Pauker SG. Speech and survival, trade-offs between quality and quantity of life in laryngeal cancer. *N Engl J Med* 1981;305:982.
40. Wolf GT, Fisher SG, Hong WK, et al. Induction chemotherapy plus radiation compared with surgery plus radiation in patients with advanced laryngeal cancer. VA laryngeal cancer study group. *N Engl J Med* 1991;324:1685.
41. Kraus DH, Pfister DG, Harrison LB, et al. Larynx preservation with combined chemotherapy and radiation therapy in advanced hypopharynx cancer. *Otolaryngol Head Neck Surg* 1994;111:31.

42. Shirnian MH, Weber RS, Lippman SM, et al. Laryngeal preservation by induction chemotherapy plus radiotherapy in locally advanced head and neck cancer: the M.D. Anderson cancer center experience. *Head Neck* 1994;16:39.

43. Clayman GL, Weber RS, Guillamondegui O, et al. Laryngeal preservation for advanced laryngeal and hypopharyngeal cancers. *Arch Otolaryngol Head Neck Surg* 1995;121:219.

44. de Andres L, Brunet J, Lopez-Pousa A, et al. Function preservation in stage III squamous laryngeal carcinomas: results with an induction chemotherapy protocol. *Laryngoscope* 1995;105:822.

45. McConnel FMS, Teichgraeber JF, Adler RK. A comparison of three methods of oral reconstruction. *Arch Otolaryngol Head Neck Surg* 1987;113:496.

46. Urken ML. The restoration or preservation of sensation in the oral cavity following ablative surgery. *Arch Otolaryngol Head Neck Surg* 1995;121:607.

47. Effron MZ, Johnson JT, Myers EN, Curtin H, Beery Q, Sigler B. Advanced carcinoma of the tongue. *Arch Otolaryngol* 1981;107:694.

48. Biller HF, Lawson W, Baek S. Total glossectomy. *Arch Otolaryngol* 1983;109:69.

49. Pradhan SA, Rajpal RM. Total glossectomy sans laryngectomy—are we justified? *Laryngoscope* 1983;93:813.

50. Light J. Prosthetic functional therapy. *Arch Otolaryngol* 1978;104:442.

51. Leonard R, Gillis R. Effects of a prosthetic tongue on vowel intelligibility and food management in a patient with total glossectomy. *J Speech Hear Dis* 1982;47:25.

52. Robbins KT, Bowman JB, Jacob RF. Postglossectomy deglutitory and articulatory rehabilitation with palatal augmentation prosthesis. *Arch Otolaryngol Head Neck Surg* 1987;113:1214.

53. Hurst PS. The role of the prosthodontist in the correction of swallowing disorders. *Otolaryngol Clin North Am* 1988;21(4):771.

54. Logemann JA, Bytell D. Swallowing disorders in three types of head and neck surgical patients. *Cancer* 1979;44:1095.

55. Meyers EN, Johnson JT, Aramany MA. Reconstruction of the oral cavity. In: English GM, ed. *Otolaryngology*, rev. ed. Philadelphia: JB Lippincott, 1991;4(42);1.

56. McConnel FMS, Hester TR, Mendelsohn MS, Logemann JA. Manofluorography of deglutition after total laryngopharyngectomy. *Plast Reconstr Surg* 1988;81:346.

57. Shobinger R. Spasm of the cricopharyngeal muscle as cause of dysphagia with total laryngectomy. *Arch Otol* 1957;67:271.

58. Balfe DM, Koehler RE, Setzen M, Weyman PJ, Baron RL, Ogura JH. Barium examination of the esophagus after total laryngectomy. *Radiology* 1982;143:501.

59. Jung TK, Adams GL. Dysphagia in laryngectomized patients. *Otolaryngol Head Neck Surg* 1980;88:25.

60. Nayar RC, Sharma VP, Arora MML. A study of the pharynx after laryngectomy. *J Laryngol Otol* 1984;98:807.

61. McConnel FMS, Cerenko D, Mendelsohn MS. Dysphagia after total laryngectomy. *Otolaryngol Clin N Am* 1988;21:721.

62. Horowitz JB, Sasaki CT. Effect of cricopharyngeus mytomy on postlaryngectomy pharyngeal contraction pressures. *Laryngoscope* 1993;103:138.

63. Kaplan JN. The incidence of hypopharyngeal stenosis after surgery for laryngeal cancer. *Otolaryngol Head Neck Surg* 1981;89:656.

64. Logemann JA, Gibbons P, Rademaker AW, et al. Mechanisms of recovery of swallow after supraglottic laryngectomy. *J Speech Hear Res* 1994;37:965.

65. Rademaker AW, Logemann JA, Pauloski BR, et al. Recovery of postoperative swallowing in patients undergoing partial laryngectomy. *Head Neck* 1993;15:325.

66. Schoenrock LD, King AY, Everts EC, Schneider HJ, Shumrick D. Hemilaryngectomy: deglutition evaluation and rehabilitation. *Trans Am Acad Ophth Otolaryngol* 1972;76:752.

67. Weaver AW, Fleming SM. Partial laryngectomy: analysis of associated swallowing disorders. *Am J Surg* 1978;136:486.

68. Buchwalter JA, Sasaki CT. Effect of tracheotomy on laryngeal function. *Otolaryngol Clin North Am* 1984;17:41.

69. Nash M. Swallowing problems in the tracheotomized patient. *Otolaryngol Clin North Am* 1988;21:701.

70. Sasaki CT, Fukuda H, Kirchner JA. Laryngeal abductor activity in response to varying ventilatory resistance. *Trans Am Acad Ophthalmol Otolaryngol* 1973;77:403.

71. Sasaki CT, Suzuki M, Horiuchi M, Kirchner JA. The effect of tracheostomy on the laryngeal closure reflex. *Laryngoscope* 1977;87:1428.

72. Kremen AJ. Cancer of the tongue-a surgical technique for a primary combined en bloc resection of tongue, floor of mouth, and cervical lymphatics. *Surgery* 1951;30:227.

73. Feldman SA, Deal CW, Urquhart W. Disturbance of swallowing after tracheostomy. *Lancet* 1966;1:954.

74. Bonanno PC. Swallowing dysfunction after tracheostomy. *Ann Surg* 1971;174:29.

75. Robbie DS, Feldman SA. Experience with fifty patients treated with artificial ventilation. *Br J Anaesth* 1963;35:771.

76. Betts RH. Post-tracheostomy aspiration. *N Engl J Med* 1965;273:155.

77. Muz J, Mathog RH, Nelson R, Jones LA. Aspiration in patients with head and neck cancer and tracheostomy. *Am J Otolaryngol* 1989;10:282.

78. Beidler LM, Smith JC. Effects of radiation therapy and drugs on cell turnover and taste. In: Getchell TV, Bartoshuk LM, Doty RL, Snow JB, eds. *Smell and taste in health and disease.* New York: Raven Press, 1991;753.

79. Doyle PC. *Foundations of voice and speech rehabilitation following laryngeal cancer.* San Diego: Singular Publishing Group, 1994.

80. Conger AD. Loss and recovery of taste acuity in patients irradiated to the oral cavity. *Radiat Res* 1973;53:338.

81. Kirchner JA. Cancer at the anterior commissure of the larynx. *Arch Otolaryngol* 1970;91:524.

82. Sandow PL, Baughman RA. Dental and oral care for the head and neck cancer patient. In: Million RR, Cassisi NJ, eds. *Management of head and neck cancer,* 2nd ed. Philadelphia: JB Lippincott, 1994;185.

83. Linden P, Siebens AA. Dysphagia: predicting laryngeal penetration. *Arch Phys Med Rehab* 1983;64:281.

84. Splaingard ML, Hutchins B, Sulton LD, Chaudhuri G. Aspiration in rehabilitation patients: videofluoroscopy vs bedside clinical assessment. *Arch Phys Med Rehab* 1988;69:637.

85. Linden P, Kuhlemeier KV, Patterson C. The probability of correctly predicting subglottic penetration from clinical observation. *Dysphagia* 1993;8:170.

86. Palmer JB, Kuhlemeier KV, Tippett DC, Lynch C. A protocol for the videofluorographic swallowing study. *Dysphagia* 1993;8:209.

87. Langmore SE, Schatz K, Olsen N. Fiberoptic endoscopic examination of swallowing safety. a new procedure. *Dysphagia* 1988;2:216.

88. Bastion RW. Videoendoscopic evaluation of patients with dysphagia: an adjunct to the modified barium swallow. *Otolaryngol Head Neck Surg* 1991;104:339.

89. Leder SB, Tarro JM, Burrell MI. Effect of occlusion of a tracheotomy tube on aspiration. *Dysphagia* 1995;11:254–258.

90. Light J. A review of oral and oropharyngeal prostheses to facilitate speech and swallowing. *Am J Speech Lang Pathol* 1995;4(3):15.

91. Kmucha ST, Cravens RB. DISH syndrome and its role in dysphagia. *Otolaryngol Head Neck Surg* 1994;110:431.

92. Attwood, SEA, Eypasch EP, DeMeester TR. Surgical therapies for dysphagia. In: Gelfand DW, Richter JE, eds. *Dysphagia diagnosis and treatment.* New York: Igaku-Shoin, 1989;335.

93. Hewson EG, Richter JE. Gastroesophageal reflux disease. In: Gelfand DW, Richter JE, eds. *Dysphagia diagnosis and treatment.* New York: Igaku-Shoin, 1989;221.

94. Logemnn JA. *Manual for the videofluographic study of swallowing,* 2nd ed. Austin, TX: Pro-Ed, 1993.

*Principles and Practice of Supportive Oncology,*
edited by Ann Berger et al.
Lippincott–Raven Publishers, Philadelphia ©1998

# CHAPTER 11

# Treatment-Related Nausea and Vomiting

Katherine M. W. Pisters and Mark G. Kris

## EMESIS SYNDROMES

Five different syndromes have been identified in patients receiving anticancer chemotherapy. It is important to recognize the various forms of emesis as treatment strategies vary. In addition, cancer patients often experience nausea and/or vomiting for reasons unrelated to chemotherapy. Patients presenting with emesis should undergo a thorough evaluation including a history and physical examination, along with appropriate laboratory and imaging studies. The differential diagnosis of nausea and vomiting in the cancer patient is lengthy. Concomitant medications (such as analgesics, antibiotics, or bronchodilators), tumor-related complications (such as bowel obstruction, hypercalcemia, liver or brain metastases), or peptic ulcer disease are common causes of emesis unrelated to chemotherapy. In these instances, treatment directed at the underlying cause is more important than selection of an antiemetic agent. Therapeutic irradiation, particularly to the abdominal cavity, is another common cause of emesis.

*Acute chemotherapy-induced emesis* has been defined as the nausea and vomiting that occurs in the 24-hour period immediately following chemotherapy administration. Antiemetic research has focused primarily on this type of emesis as it is the most common and severe form of emesis for the patient with cancer. Nausea and vomiting generally begins 1–2 hours following most chemotherapy. Exceptions to this rule are emesis occurring following the administration of cyclophosphamide or carboplatin where 9–18 hours may pass prior to the onset of emesis (2,3) and nitrogen mustard whereby vomiting can start within minutes after the drug is given.

*Delayed emesis* begins 24 or more hours after chemotherapy administration. This type of emesis occurs most commonly in patients treated with high doses of cisplatin or cyclophosphamide and may have a different pathophysiology than acute chemotherapy-induced emesis. This type of emesis tends to be less intense than acute vomiting, but of longer duration. Patients who experience acute emesis are more likely to develop delayed nausea and vomiting; however, delayed emesis can also occur in patients who have no emesis in the 24 hours following chemotherapy.

*Anticipatory emesis* is a Pavlovian conditioned response that occurs *prior* to subsequent chemotherapy. It occurs only in patients who have had poor control of emesis with previous chemotherapy (4,5). As the control of acute chemotherapy-induced emesis has improved, anticipatory emesis has become less common.

*Breakthrough emesis* is a term used to describe vomiting that occurs on the day of chemotherapy despite treatment with appropriate antiemetic prophylaxis.

*Refractory emesis* may develop in patients who have experienced severe vomiting during prior chemotherapy cycles. This emesis is characterized by emesis associated with chemotherapy administration that occurs despite optimal antiemetic prevention and treatment in earlier courses.

## PHYSIOLOGY AND PATHOPHYSIOLOGY OF EMESIS

The mechanism by which anticancer chemotherapy induces emesis is still not completely understood. The studies of Borison and McCarthy (6) established the basis for our current understanding of this complex reflex. Studies performed primarily in cats and dogs led these investigators to propose the existence of two distinct

K. M. W. Pisters: Thoracic/Head and Neck Medical Oncology, University of Texas, M.D. Anderson Cancer Center, Houston, TX 77030.

M. G. Kris: Thoracic Oncology Service, Memorial Sloan-Kettering Cancer Center, and Cornell University Medical College, New York, NY 10021.

areas in the brainstem critical for the control of emesis. One site, termed the "vomiting center," was located in the lateral reticular formation of the medulla near other structures (respiratory, vasomotor, and salivary centers, as well as cranial nerves VIII and X) involved in the vomiting reflex. Electrical stimulation of this area triggered emesis, whereas ablation prevented emesis by a variety of stimuli. Recent studies have suggested that the vomiting center is not an anatomically discrete area but rather a complex system of intertwined neural networks (7,8).

The chemoreceptor trigger zone (CTZ) was the second important area described by Borison and McCarthy (6). The CTZ, located outside the blood–brain barrier at the ventral aspect of the fourth ventricle, is exposed to noxious agents in the blood or cerebrospinal fluid. Stimulation of the chemoreceptor trigger zone cannot produce vomiting independently but only through secondary activation of the vomiting center.

Three other sources of input to the vomiting center have been recognized: the nasopharynx and gastrointestinal (GI) tract, the vestibular system and higher brainstem, and cortical structures. Input from the GI tract occurs primarily through afferent vagal fibers, and an intact CTZ is not essential when vomiting is initiated by this mechanism. The vestibular system is involved primarily in vomiting seen with motion sickness. Higher cortical centers, including the cerebral cortex, hypothalamus, and thalamus, also input to the vomiting center and appear critical in a variety of conditions, including anticipatory emesis.

The elucidation of the neurochemistry of the emetic reflex has been important in the development of effective antiemetic therapy. Initial studies focused on pharmacologic blockade of the many neurotransmitters found in the area postrema and adjacent sites. Serotonin, dopamine, histamine, acetylcholine, and norepinephrine are all found in the vomiting center and area postrema and the development of pharmacologic agents that block specific sets of receptors has resulted in the identification of valuable antiemetic agents. Recent interest has focused on the role of neuroactive substances in the GI tract. Serotonin receptors ($5$-$HT_3$) have been identified on vagal and splanchnic afferents (9). These receptors appear to play a key role in the pathophysiology of chemotherapy-induced emesis. Because antagonists for the $5$-$HT_3$ receptor subtype are so specific, these new compounds have further improved our understanding of the role of serotonin in the vomiting reflex (10). The $5$-$HT_3$ receptor is now recognized as an important mediator of the emetic reflex and is found in both the GI tract (11) and the central nervous system (12). The development of the highly specific $5$-$HT_3$ receptor antagonists has both greatly improved the control of chemotherapy-induced nausea and vomiting and established the role of serotonin in this pathway.

The exact mechanism of chemotherapy-induced nausea and vomiting has not been completely elucidated.

Some recent studies have suggested a peripheral mechanism in cisplatin-induced emesis. Serotonin is released from the mucosa of the small intestine following cisplatin administration in animal models (13,14). A similar event most likely occurs in humans as increased levels of urinary 5-hydroxyindoleacetic acid (5-HIAA) levels have been found following cisplatin administration in patients (15). Serotonin release into the GI tract may induce emesis by binding to afferent vagal and splanchnic $5$-$HT_3$ receptors within the intestinal wall, thereby stimulating vagal input to the vomiting center (16). However, patients who undergo interruption of both vagal trunks and splanchnic nerves as a consequence of esophagogastrectomy for the treatment of esophageal tumors experience vomiting when given cisplatin. As noted above, $5$-$HT_3$ receptor activity has also been demonstrated in the area of the vomiting center (12). In animals, the intracerebroventricular injection of cisplatin alone produces emesis which can be controlled by $5$-$HT_3$ antagonists.

The discovery of the role of $5$-$HT_3$ in emesis has also shed light on the mechanism of action of antiemetic agents, particularly metoclopramide. Whereas low doses of metoclopramide have limited usefulness in controlling emesis, high doses are effective. Metoclopramide is a weak and nonselective inhibitor of the $5$-$HT_3$ receptor and also affects dopamine receptors. When administered in high doses, however, potency issues are overcome and metoclopramide effectively blocks serotonin receptors (17).

Several important questions about the mechanisms of chemotherapy-induced emesis remain unanswered. How much of a role does each of the known receptors play in the physiology of emesis? Are there other receptors that also play a role? Is it the chemotherapeutic agent or some other substance that binds to these receptors to induce emesis? Why is there a difference in the likelihood of causing emesis and in the time of onset of emesis among various chemotherapy drugs? What is the mechanism underlying delayed emesis? Is there a final common pathway leading to the vomiting reflex?

## PATIENT CHARACTERISTICS AND EMESIS

Investigators have identified several patient characteristics that influence emetic outcome. These include incidence and severity of emesis with past courses of chemotherapy; a history of chronic, heavy alcohol intake; age; and gender.

Poor control of emesis with past courses of chemotherapy predisposes a patient to unsatisfactory antiemetic results with any subsequent treatment, regardless of the emetic stimulus or antiemetic employed. Patients with this history can develop anticipatory symptoms and/or become refractory to antiemetic therapy. In one trial in which all patients received the same chemotherapy regimen and the same antiemetic agent, substantial control of emesis was three times more likely to occur in patients who were receiving their initial treatment compared to those who had previously received chemotherapy (18). This finding was confirmed in a prospective, multicenter, double-blind trial in which naive and pretreated patients were randomized to receive the same antiemetic treatment [metoclopramide+methylprednisolone (MM) or metoclopramide+dexamethasone+diphenhydramine (MDD)] for three consecutive cycles of cisplatin chemotherapy (19). Complete protection from vomiting was greater in the chemotherapy-naive patients (62% MM and 74% MDD) versus those with previous chemotherapy (35% MM and 68% MDD). Furthermore, the efficacy of antiemetic treatments studied decreased progressively from the first to the third cycle of chemotherapy, with complete protection from vomiting with the most efficacious antiemetic regimen being 73% in the first cycle to 52% in the third (19).

Emesis is easier to control in patients with a history of chronic, high alcohol intake (>100 g/day or approximately five mixed drinks per day) (20,21). In the one prospective evaluation, of 52 patients receiving high-dose cisplatin and an appropriate combination antiemetic regimen, 93% of those with a history of high alcohol history had no emesis as opposed to 61% of those who did not (20). The mechanism underlying this effect is unknown. It has been postulated that long-term alcohol exposure decreases the sensitivity of the chemoreceptor trigger zone (22). Although vomiting is easier to control, patients with a history of heavy alcohol intake should still receive aggressive antiemetic therapy appropriate for the dose and schedule of chemotherapy administered.

A third important factor is the patient's age. In one large study, complete protection from nausea and vomiting was significantly better in patients ≥65 years than those <50 years (19). This is relevant not only because it may directly affect the control of emesis (22) but because there is a predilection for younger patients to experience acute dystonic reactions when any of the dopamine-blocking antiemetics are administered. In a report summarizing the experience of nearly 500 patients receiving metoclopramide, the incidence of trismus or torticollis was only 2% in those over age 30; by contrast, a 27% occurrence was reported in younger patients (23). In addition, when dopamine-blocking agents are given on consecutive days, as is necessary with the multiple-day chemotherapy regimens used for testicular cancer and various childhood neoplasms, dystonic reactions become more common (24,25). Antiemetic therapy has been greatly improved for younger patients with the advent of the specific 5-HT$_3$ receptor antagonists, which do not cause extrapyramidal symptoms.

It should be emphasized that acute dystonic reactions are not allergic in nature. These reactions can be treated with diphenhydramine, benztropine, or benzodiazepines and should not be viewed as a contraindication to further use of dopamine-blocking drugs if satisfactory antiemetic control was obtained. The specific serotonin antagonists have not been associated with dystonic reactions even when given on consecutive days or at high individual doses (25–28).

Finally, gender has been determined to be an independent predictor for response to antiemetic therapy (22,29). Women consistently experience a greater intensity of nausea, more vomiting episodes, and a longer duration of nausea and vomiting than men given the same chemotherapy and antiemetic regimen. Review of data from a large prospective trial found more women receiving high-dose cisplatin and ondansetron had poorer control of emesis than did men receiving the same chemotherapy regimens (49% versus 29%) (30). It is not known as to whether gender influences emetogenic sensitivity to chemotherapy or the efficacy of antiemetic therapy itself (22). A similar gender difference in the incidence of emesis caused by opiate analgesics has been reported and a possible gender difference in neurotransmitter receptor site distribution or emetic drug binding characteristics has been postulated (31).

Other patient factors such as a history of susceptibility to motion sickness (32) or pregnancy-induced emesis (33) may predict a poor emetic outcome. The type of cancer appears to have little influence (22).

## ACUTE CHEMOTHERAPY-INDUCED EMESIS

### Emetogenic Potential of Chemotherapy Drugs

A recent classification of the acute emetogenicity of antineoplastic chemotherapy agents has been proposed by Hesketh et al. (34). Table 1 groups commonly prescribed chemotherapy agents according to their potential to induce acute (24-hour period after chemotherapy) emesis in the absence of effective antiemetic prophylaxis. The five levels have been defined as follows: level 1, <10% of patients experience emesis; level 2, 10–30%; level 3, 30–60%; level 4, 60–90%; Level 5, >90% experience emesis. In general, agents that frequently cause emesis also induce vomiting of the greatest severity. Differences can occur among patients and even between identical treatment courses in the same patient as noted above.

The dose, route of administration, and infusion schedule of the chemotherapeutic agent can affect the incidence and pattern of nausea and vomiting. In general, the potential for emesis increases with increasing chemotherapy dose (e.g., cisplatin, cyclophosphamide, cytosine arabinoside, doxorubicin, methotrexate). Intravenous chemotherapy is often more emetogenic than oral formulations. Chemotherapy administered as a large intravenous bolus or brief infusion is more likely to cause emesis than smaller divided doses or prolonged

**TABLE 1.** *Emetogenic potential of chemotherapy agents*[a]

| Level | Frequency of emesis | Chemotherapy agent |
|---|---|---|
| 5 | >90% | Carmustine > 250 mg/m$^2$<br>Cisplatin ≥50 mg/m$^2$<br>Cyclophosphamide > 1500 mg/m$^2$<br>Dacarbazine<br>Mechlorethamine<br>Streptozocin |
| 4 | 60–90% | Carboplatin<br>Carmustine ≤ 250 mg/m$^2$<br>Cisplatin < 50 mg/m$^2$<br>Cyclophosphamide >750–1500 mg/m$^2$<br>Cytarabine > 1 g/m$^2$<br>Doxorubicin > 60 mg/m$^2$<br>Methotrexate > 1000 mg/m$^2$<br>Procarbazine (po) |
| 3 | 30–60% | Cyclophosphamide ≤ 750 mg/m$^2$<br>Cyclophosphamide (PO)<br>Doxorubicin 20–60 mg/m$^2$<br>Epirubicin ≤ 90 mg/m$^2$<br>Hexamethylmelamine (PO)<br>Idarubicin<br>Ifosfamide<br>Methotrexate 250–1000 mg/m$^2$<br>Mitoxantrone < 15 mg/m$^2$ |
| 2 | 10–30% | Docetaxel<br>Etoposide<br>5-Fluorouracil < 1000 mg/m$^2$<br>Gemcitabine<br>Methotrexate > 50–250 mg/m$^2$<br>Mitomycin<br>Paclitaxel |
| 1 | <10% | Bleomycin<br>Busulfan<br>Chlorambucil (PO)<br>2-Chlorodeoxyadenosine<br>Fludarabine<br>Hydroxyurea<br>Methotrexate ≤ 50 mg/m$^2$<br>L-Phenylalanine mustard (PO)<br>6-Thioguanine (PO)<br>Vinblastine<br>Vincristine<br>Vinorelbine |

[a]Proportion of patients experiencing emesis in the absence of effective antiemetic prophylaxis.
From Hesketh, *J Clin Oncol*, 1997.

infusions (e.g., cisplatin, doxorubicin). For patients receiving combination chemotherapy, the emetic pattern of each chemotherapeutic agent must be considered when prescribing appropriate antiemetic therapy. The recent classification by Hesketh et al. attempts to address the emetic potential of combinations using information from a large database of patients treated with cyclophosphamide-based combinations. The emetogenic level of a chemotherapy combination is determined by identifying the most emetogenic agent in the combination and then assessing the relative contribution of other agents. When considering other agents, the following rules apply: (a) level 1 agents do not contribute to the emetogenicity of the regimen; (b) adding one or more level 2 agents increases the emetogenicity of the combination by 1 level greater than the most emetogenic agent in the combination; and (c) adding level 3 or 4 agents increases the emetogenicity of the combination by one level per agent (34).

The majority of chemotherapeutic agents typically induce emesis beginning 1–3 hours after chemotherapy. An important exception to this pattern occurs following administration of cyclophosphamide (2) or carboplatin (3). With these agents, the onset of emesis may be delayed until 12 or even 18 hours following chemotherapy administration and continue into the next day.

## Principles of Antiemetic Drug Development

Drugs used to prevent emesis caused by anticancer therapy, like other pharmacologic agents, are developed in a stepwise process. The laboratory animal most commonly used to study acute emesis is the ferret. This animal is given cisplatin, observed for a 4-hour period, and then sacrificed. There is no established laboratory model for delayed emesis. Candidate drugs effective in animal models with acceptable toxicity are then advanced to trials in humans.

In phase I trials, dose, schedule and toxicity are evaluated in the target population of patients. After the treatment regimen and safety are established, phase II efficacy studies are initiated in patients receiving a chemotherapeutic regimen known to cause vomiting. Cisplatin given as a single infusion over 3 hours or less is the standard emetic stimulus because of its widespread use and the certainty and severity of the emesis it produces. Now that several effective antiemetic agents have been identified, the initial testing of new antivomiting drugs is conducted in patients who have vomited despite receiving antiemetic therapy. Once activity has been shown against cisplatin, a phase III randomized trial is necessary to prove that the candidate drug has efficacy and safety at least comparable to that of the current standards. Afterward, most com-

pounds require additional study to define the optimal dose and schedule and to test their utility for additional indications such as delayed emesis or consecutive day chemotherapy.

As control of chemotherapy-induced emesis has improved, criteria for effectiveness have become more stringent and simple. The primary efficacy endpoint for acute emesis is the percentage of patients who have vomiting prevented during the 24 hours following chemotherapy. Additional endpoints are the presence or absence of nausea, the severity of nausea measured by a visual analog scale, or the percentage of patients requiring rescue therapy.

The process described has successfully identified all of the useful antiemetics we have today. The experience gained can rapidly be applied to the testing of new compounds that enter clinical trial.

### Antiemetic Agents

Table 2 lists the classes of antiemetic agents in current use along with recommended doses and schedules. The best studied agents are: ondansetron (Zofran), granisetron (Kytril), dolasetron mesylate (Anzemet), metoclopramide (Reglan), haloperidol (Haldol), dexamethasone

**TABLE 2.** *Antiemetic agents: mechanism of action and recommended dose*

| Antiemetic | Mechanism of action | Dosage |
|---|---|---|
| **5-HT$_3$ antagonist** | | |
| Ondansetron | 5-HT$_3$ Blockade | 8–32 mg IV × 1 dose 2× daily OR 8 mg PO OR continuous infusion (bone marrow transplantation) |
| Granisetron | | 10 µg/kg IV × 1 dose OR 2 mg PO × 1 dose |
| Dolasetron mesylate | | 1.8 mg/kg or 100mg IV × 1 dose or 200 mg PO × 1 dose |
| **Substituted benzamide** | | |
| Metoclopramide | 5-HT$_3$ and dopamine blockade | 1–3 mg/kg IV q2h × 2–5 doses |
| **Corticosteroids** | | |
| Dexamethasone | Unknown | 4–20 mg PO/IV × 1 dose or q4–6h |
| Methylprednisolone | | 250–500 mg IV × 1 dose |
| **Butyrophenones** | | |
| Haloperidol | Dopamine blockade | 1–3 mg IV q2–6h × 3–5 doses |
| **Phenothiazines** | | |
| Prochlorperazine | Dopamine blockade | 10 mg PO/IV q4–6h |
| Promethazine | | 25 mg PO/PR q4–6h |
| Thiethylperazine | | 10 mg PO/PR q4–6h |
| **Cannabinoids** | | |
| Dronabinol | Cannabinoid receptor blockade | 5–10 mg/m² PO q3–4h |
| **Benzodiazepines** | | |
| Lorazepam | Anxiolytic | 1.0–1.5 mg/m² (max 3.0 mg) IV × 1 dose |

5-HT$_3$ = serotonin subtype 3.

(Decadron), lorazepam (Ativan), dronabinol (Marinol), prochlorperazine (Compazine), and chlorpromazine (Thorazine).

### Serotonin Antagonists

#### 5-HT₃ Receptor Antagonists

The specific 5-HT₃ receptor antagonists are the most recently developed class of antiemetic drugs. There are currently three approved selective serotonin antagonists in the United States: ondansetron, granisetron, and dolasetron. An additional 5-HT₃ antagonist, dolasetron, is now in clinical development. Tropisetron is available in many countries. These drugs are the most effective antiemetics currently available for the prevention of chemotherapy-induced emesis. Early studies demonstrated that serotonin antagonists control emesis from a variety of chemotherapeutic agents, including high-dose cisplatin- and cyclophosphamide-containing regimens. These drugs are similar in efficacy and side effects (35), and the choice of one particular agent over another is usually determined by pharmacoeconomic factors.

Phase I studies of the serotonin antagonists have demonstrated excellent safety characteristics over a large dosing range (26,27,36,37a). Initial studies with ondansetron utilized a three-dose schedule, with optimal efficacy seen at doses of 0.1 mg/kg or more (26,27). Further studies have found once daily dosing to be as effective and less cumbersome than multiple or continuous dose regimens (ref. 62b,c). Single-dose studies of granisetron revealed a therapeutic plateau at doses greater than 10 µg/kg (37). A comparative trial by Hesketh et al. found a dose level of 1.8 mg/kg of dolasetron mesylate effective (d). Toxicities have been minor and transient. The most frequently reported side effect of this class of compounds has been headache, which occurs in 10–15% of patients treated. Other effects have included constipation, mild transient elevation in serum levels of hepatic enzymes, and clinically insignificant prolongation of cardiac conduction intervals.

Phase II studies have reported complete control of emesis in 35–68% of patients receiving cisplatin (37–39). Phase III trials have compared these agents to metoclopramide in patients receiving cisplatin. In all of these studies, the 5-HT₃ receptor antagonists yielded superior or equivalent antiemetic efficacy (40–44).

Trials have examined the effectiveness of ondansetron and granisetron given to patients receiving 20–40 mg/m² of cisplatin on consecutive days. In the past, this clinical scenario represented a difficult antiemetic challenge as metoclopramide-based regimens lead to frequent extrapyramidal symptoms, sedation, and required prolonged administration schedules. In studies employing ondansetron, 28–32% of patients experienced no emesis over the entire 5-day study period (25,45,46). The control of emesis declined on days 3 and 4 of these studies, possibly related to the occurrence of delayed emesis. One study administered granisetron to patients receiving cisplatin on consecutive days and 44% of patients were completely protected from emesis (47). Two phase III trials have compared a 5-HT₃ antagonist to metoclopramide-based therapy in the multiple day setting (48,49). The serotonin receptor antagonists yielded improved antiemetic efficacy and were better tolerated in both studies.

The serotonin antagonists have proven effective against a number of different chemotherapy agents (50–54). For patients receiving cyclophosphamide-based regimens, roughly three quarters of patients experience no emesis when pretreated with ondansetron or granisetron as single agents (50,54,55). In most of the cyclophosphamide studies, ondansetron has been successfully administered orally at a dose of 4–8 mg t.i.d. for 3–5 days (50,55,56).

The serotonin antagonists have been compared in several randomized trials for both cisplatin (35,47,57–60d) and non-cisplatin-based chemotherapy (54). The efficacy and toxicity of the agents were remarkably similar. Patient preference was evaluated in several crossover trials (patients received each agent in subsequent chemotherapy cycles), and granisetron was often the preferred agent in the minority of patients who expressed a preference (47,54,57) although no reason was identified for this preference. A review of the preclinical pharmacology and comparative efficacy of the 5-HT₃ receptor antagonists by Perez concluded that although the preclinical pharmacologic profile may differ among the serotonin antagonists in terms of potency, selectivity, dose–response, and duration of action, the comparative clinical trials have shown therapeutic and safety equivalence.

Recent trials of the serotonin antagonists have focused on dosing and schedule. Much of this interest has been spurred by the high cost of these agents. It has now been shown that a single dose of ondansetron is as effective as the original three-dose schedule (61,62b,c). A study by Hesketh et al. (35) reported the antiemetic results of adjusted dose ondansetron—32, 24, or 8 mg—as a single infusion with dexamethasone 20 mg, for highly, moderately high, or moderately emetogenic chemotherapy, respectively. Good control of emesis was achieved in all scenarios. Therefore it seems most appropriate to reserve the 32-mg dose of ondansetron for highly emetogenic chemotherapy regimens and employ a more modest dose for moderately emetogenic chemotherapy. The recommended dose of intravenous granisetron is 10 µg/kg of dolasetron mesylate, 1.8 mg/kg. In a further effort to minimize costs while maximizing convenience, studies are now examining all-oral, single-dose combination antiemetic therapy. A phase II trial in 61 patients receiving high (≥100 mg/m²) or moderate (≥60 mg/m²) dose cisplatin administered dexamethasone plus granisetron 1 mg or 1.5 mg orally (moderate or high-dose cisplatin, respectively). The regimens were given 30 minutes before chemotherapy and 85% of patients had no emesis in the acute period (63). The combination of oral dolasetron 200 mg and oral dexamethasone 20 mg prevented emesis in 75% of patients receiving initial cisplatin (64).

### Metoclopramide

Metoclopramide is most effective when given in high intravenous doses (18). Until recently, metoclopramide was thought to function as an antiemetic through the blockade of dopamine receptors. Research has now shown that high concentrations of this agent effectively block 5-HT$_3$ receptors (17). Maintenance of an adequate level of this antiemetic at the time of emetic vulnerability through the use of an appropriate dosing schedule is required to achieve optimal results. In preventing emesis induced by cisplatin or by cyclophosphamide plus doxorubicin, metoclopramide administration every 2 hours (beginning shortly before chemotherapy) appears to be the most effective schedule. Doses and schedules of metoclopramide are outlined in Table 2. Comparison trials in patients receiving cisplatin have found metoclopramide to be superior, or at least equivalent, to most classes of antiemetic agents other than the specific 5-HT$_3$ antagonists as noted above (18,65–69). Randomized trials comparing metoclopramide to ondansetron for cisplatin-induced emesis have demonstrated antiemetic superiority for patients receiving ondansetron (40,42,70).

The side effects commonly observed with metoclopramide are related to its dopamine receptor antagonism and include mild sedation, dystonic reactions (age-related, as discussed above), and akathisia or restlessness. Diarrhea, often considered an adverse effect of metoclopramide, is often caused by specific chemotherapeutic agents, such as cisplatin (18,23). In general, dystonic reactions and akathisia can be prevented or easily controlled by administering diphenhydramine, benztropine, or a benzodiazepine (23,24,71).

### Corticosteroids

The antiemetic mechanism of action of corticosteroids remains unclear. Several open studies and randomized trials have confirmed their effectiveness (65,66,72–74). Dexamethasone doses have generally been in the range of 4–20 mg per dose. In most studies, adding a corticosteroid to an effective agent of another class has resulted in improved antiemetic efficacy (75,76).

Toxicities associated with short courses of dexamethasone used for antiemetic therapy have been mild and infrequent, generally consisting of insomnia and mild epigastric burning. There has been no evidence for a lessening of chemotherapeutic effect through the use of steroids as antiemetics in controlled trials. The low toxicity of dexamethasone combined with a different mechanism of action makes this agent ideal for use in combination antiemetic regimens and as a single agent for treatment of patients receiving chemotherapy that rarely or infrequently causes emesis.

### Phenothiazines

The phenothiazines were the first family of antiemetic agents and are felt to function through dopaminergic blockade. The results of formal antiemetic trials with this class of agents have been poor. Randomized trials have found prochlorperazine given in oral and intramuscular doses to be less active than metoclopramide (18) or dexamethasone (72), and equivalent or less active than dronabinol (77,78). Side effects include sedation, akathisia, hypotension, and dystonic reactions.

### Butyrophenones

Haloperidol and droperidol are the most frequently used agents of this class and their antiemetic activity is a result of dopaminergic blockade (79,80). These agents have no effect on 5-HT$_3$ receptors (12). A formal study comparing haloperidol with metoclopramide in patients receiving cisplatin found both agents to be effective, although metoclopramide gave better control (68). In that trial demonstrating equivalence, haloperidol was given at doses of 3 mg IV given every 2–6 hours—a regimen rarely used. Toxicities include sedation, dystonic reactions, akathisia, and occasional hypotension.

### Cannabinoids

Interest in the cannabinoids as antiemetics stemmed from anecdotal reports of reduced emesis in patients smoking marijuana during chemotherapy. Most trials have studied dronabinol ($\Delta$9-tetrahydrocannabinol, Marinol), the active ingredient in marijuana. Dronabinol has been tried at many doses with differing schedules. The most useful dosages have been in the range of 5–10 mg/m$^2$, orally, every 3–4 hours (67,81). Dronabinol has been found to be superior to placebo, and equivalent or superior to oral prochlorperazine (77,78). The mechanism of action is not completely understood, but a central mechanism has been postulated. Side effects associated with these agents have limited their usefulness. In middle-aged and older adults, frequent and bothersome dry mouth, sedation, orthostatic hypotension, ataxia, dizziness, disorientation, and euphoria or dysphoria have been observed. Like the butyrophenones, the use of these agents should be reserved for the occasional patient with mild to moderate emesis in whom the safer and more effective agents have failed.

## Adjunctive Agents

### *Benzodiazepines*

Benzodiazepines are potent antianxiety agents that can be useful additions to antiemetic therapy. Lorazepam has been shown to have a high degree of patient acceptance and subjective benefit, but only a small degree of objective antiemetic activity (82). The addition of lorazepam to metoclopramide and dexamethasone resulted in a significant decrease in akathisia and anxiety compared to the same two agents given with diphenhydramine (83). Lorazepam is usually given in doses of 1.0–1.5 mg/m$^2$ (82,83). This dose causes sedation lasting for several hours, limiting its usefulness in some outpatient settings.

### Combination Antiemetic Therapy

The identification of several antiemetic agents and drug classes has not only greatly enhanced emetic outcome for patients receiving anticancer chemotherapy but also made possible the development of combination antiemetic regimens. Similar to combination chemotherapy, antiemetic regimens should ideally be composed of agents with demonstrated single-agent efficacy, differing mechanisms of action, and nonoverlapping toxicities. Current recommendations for antiemetic combination therapy are presented in Table 3.

The corticosteroids have been extensively utilized in combination antiemetic therapy due to their single-agent activity, different mechanism of action, minimal toxicity, and low cost. The addition of a corticosteroid to either metoclopramide or a specific serotonin antagonist has generally resulted in a 20% improvement in complete control of acute emesis. The combination of metoclopramide plus a corticosteroid has proven superior to either agent used alone in controlling cisplatin-induced emesis in several trials (83–86). In addition to improving antiemetic efficacy, dexamethasone also decreased the incidence of diarrhea caused by cisplatin. The optimal dose of dexamethasone has not been determined but most trials have utilized a single 20-mg dose. Additional dosages the night before chemotherapy or hours afterward did not improve results beyond that of a single 20-mg dose of dexamethasone given immediately prior to chemotherapy (83).

The combination of a specific 5-HT$_3$ antagonist and a corticosteroid has also proven more effective than either agent alone (75,76). Complete response rates as high as 90% have been reported when patients receiving moderate dose cisplatin were treated with the combination of a specific serotonin receptor antagonist and dexamethasone (76). A phase III trial comparing ondansetron plus dexamethasone to the combination of metoclopramide, dexamethasone, and diphenhydramine in patients receiving cisplatin ≥50 mg/m$^2$ found the two-drug combination more effective in preventing acute chemotherapy-induced emesis (79% versus 60%, $p < 0.002$). In addition, less sedation and fewer extrapyramidal reactions were seen in the ondansetron arm (75). The authors noted that the metoclopramide regimen provided therapeutic success in many patients (84% with two or fewer vomiting episodes, and 65% with no nausea) and that the cost of the three-drug regimen was much less than that of

**TABLE 3.** *Recommendations for combination antiemetic therapy*

| Corticosteroid | + | Serotonin antagonist | +/– | Antianxiety agent |
|---|---|---|---|---|
| **Dexamethasone** 20 mg IV or PO | | **Granisetron** 10 µg/kg IV × 1 dose -or- | | **Lorazepam** 1.0–1.5 mg/m$^2$ (3 mg maximum) |
| | | 2 mg PO × 1 dose *or* **Ondansetron** 8–32 mg IV × 1 dose *or* 8 mg PO 2× daily Bone marrow transplantation:   8 mg IV, then infusion at 1 mg/h -or-   8 mg PO, 3 × daily *or* **Dolasetron mesylate** 1.8 mg/kg or 100mg IV × 1 dose *or* 200 mg PO × 1 dose | | |

Note: Antiemetic therapy should begin 30 minutes prior to chemotherapy.

ondansetron plus dexamethasone. Extrapyramidal reactions were reported by only 3% of patients and were easily controlled with appropriate therapy.

Adjunctive use of a benzodiazepine, such as lorazepam, in patients receiving high-dose cisplatin with metoclopramide and dexamethasone antiemetic therapy has lessened both treatment-related anxiety and akathisia (71). Despite the fact that lorazepam has added little if any antiemetic effect to these combinations, patients preferred the lorazepam-containing regimens. The addition of lorazepam to a selective 5-HT$_3$ antagonist-containing antiemetic combinations has not been formally studied. The use of lorazepam in this setting should be encouraged because of its proven safety and benefit in completed studies and the high baseline and acute incidence of anxiety in cancer patients about to receive chemotherapy.

As discussed earlier, recent trials have attempted to further simplify antiemetic therapy and allow more convenient, cost-effective therapy. In preliminary trials, the use of single-dose, all-oral antiemetic combination therapy appears to be as efficacious as more cumbersome intravenous regimens and represents a significant cost savings (63,64).

## DELAYED EMESIS

Delayed emesis is defined as vomiting beginning or persisting 24 or more hours after chemotherapy administration (87). The pathophysiology of this problem is unclear. This condition is particularly common after high-dose cisplatin or cyclophosphamide. As the therapy of acute chemotherapy-induced emesis has improved, delayed emesis has emerged as the critical problem in emetic therapy. Progress in the control of delayed emesis has been slow and hindered by the lack of an accepted animal model. In one natural history study, 93% of the studied patients experienced some degree of delayed nausea or vomiting from 24 to 120 hours after high-dose cisplatin, with a peak incidence occurring between 48 and 72 hours (87). The incidence of delayed emesis was lower among patients who had complete protection from acute chemotherapy-induced emesis. Regimens for delayed vomiting have generally utilized drugs of proven efficacy in acute chemotherapy-induced emesis. The combination of oral dexamethasone (8 mg b.i.d. × 2 days, then 4 mg b.i.d. × 2 days) and metoclopramide (0.5 mg/kg q.i.d. × 4 days) has been found to be superior to dexamethasone alone or placebo in a double-blind, randomized trial (88). Fifty-two percent of patients receiving the combination had complete control of delayed vomiting, compared to 35% receiving dexamethasone and 11% placebo. Prochlorperazine spansules (30 mg t.i.d. × 2 days, then 15 mg t.i.d. × 2 days) in combination with dexamethasone (8 mg b.i.d. × 2 days, then 4 mg b.i.d. × 2 days) has also proven efficacious for the treatment of delayed emesis (89).

The majority of trials examining the role of ondansetron as a single agent in the control of delayed emesis have been disappointing (41,90,91). In contrast, one nonrandomized study of oral ondansetron 8 mg t.i.d. × 5 days following treatment with 50–120 mg/m$^2$ of cisplatin did find a complete control rate of 52% (92). In addition, a phase II study with ondansetron (8 mg t.i.d. × 2 days) and dexamethasone (8 mg b.i.d. × 2 days, then 4 mg b.i.d. × 2 days), beginning 16 hours after cisplatin, completely controlled vomiting in the majority of patients treated (63). The Italian Group for Antiemetic Research conducted a randomized delayed emesis trial of ondansetron (8 mg b.i.d. × 3 days) and dexamethasone (8 mg b.i.d. × 2 days, then 4 mg b.i.d. × 1 day) versus metoclopramide (20 mg q.i.d. × 3 days) and dexamethasone (same schedule) in over 300 patients receiving initial cisplatin ≥50 mg/m$^2$. All patients received the same antiemetic treatment for acute emesis, and emetic control for the initial 24 hours was similar between the two arms. Complete protection from delayed vomiting/nausea was 62%/43% for the ondansetron arm and 60%/54% for metoclopramide (no significant difference). For patients who vomited in the first 24 hours, lower complete protection from delayed emesis was seen. However, the ondansetron-treated patients fared better (29% versus 9% complete delayed vomiting protection, $p < 0.05$) (93).

## ANTICIPATORY EMESIS

Anticipatory vomiting is emesis beginning *before* the administration of chemotherapy. It is seen only in patients who experienced vomiting with prior chemotherapy. As this is a conditioned Pavlovian response, the hospital environment, staff, or other treatment-related associations may trigger the onset of emesis unrelated to chemotherapy. Strong emetic stimuli combined with poor

**TABLE 4.** *Management strategy for acute chemotherapy-induced emesis*

| All patients | Education |
|---|---|
| | Reassurance |
| | "PRN" antiemetic prescription: |
| | Metoclopramide 10 PO |
| | Ondansetron 8 mg PO |
| | Granisetron 1 mg PO |
| | Prochlorperazine spansules 15 mg PO |
| Emesis common (>30%) | Combination antiemetics: Serotonin antagonist[a] + Dexamethasone 20 mg + Lorazepam 1–3 mg |
| Emesis uncommon (10–29%) | Dexamethasone 20 mg |

[a]Intravenous dose to be determined by the intensity of emesis expected (see Table 3).

emetic control leads to a greater likelihood of anticipatory emesis (94). As the control of acute emesis has improved, the prevalence and severity of anticipatory nausea and vomiting has decreased (95). For patients who develop anticipatory symptoms, behavioral therapy involving systematic desensitization can be helpful (4). Also, benzodiazepines appear useful (96). The best approach is prevention. The problem of anticipatory emesis again emphasizes the importance of providing the most effective antiemetics with each and every course of emesis-producing chemotherapy.

## BREAKTHROUGH/REFRACTORY EMESIS

Despite the prophylactic use of optimal combination antiemetic therapy, patients may experience breakthrough emesis in the initial 24-hour period following chemotherapy. Treatments for this condition have not been rigorously studied. For patients who received ondansetron or granisetron plus dexamethasone prior to chemotherapy, rescue medications such as metoclopramide, lorazepam, phenothiazines with or without diphenhydramine and dronabinol are used.

Patients who experienced severe nausea and vomiting during previous treatment cycles are often refractory to antiemetic prophylaxis with subsequent chemotherapy. These patients should again receive combination antiemetic therapy and may require inpatient hospitalization to ensure adequate hydration and support during chemotherapy. Further research to establish treatment regimens for breakthrough and refractory emesis are sorely needed.

## RADIATION-INDUCED EMESIS

Therapeutic irradiation to any part of the body has the potential to cause nausea and vomiting. However, symptoms occur most commonly when radiation fields include the GI tract or brain or when total body irradiation is administered. Like chemotherapy-induced emesis, the exact mechanism by which irradiation induces vomiting is not known. Because drugs that block the actions of dopamine and serotonin can attenuate emesis following irradiation, we theorize that irradiation leads to the release of neurotransmitters including dopamine and serotonin somewhere in the body, which in turn initiates the emetic reflex. In general, the same drugs that control chemotherapy-induced emesis are helpful in the control of irradiation-induced emesis. The serotonin antagonists have demonstrated efficacy in patients undergoing abdominal radiotherapy (97), as well as total body irradiation prior to bone marrow transplantation (98). These agents are best used prophylactically, given on each day the patient is scheduled to receive radiotherapy. Oral ondansetron 8 mg, three times daily, has been shown to be efficacious.

## CURRENT MANAGEMENT OF CHEMOTHERAPY-INDUCED EMESIS

Through the appropriate use of antiemetic agents, chemotherapy-related nausea and vomiting can be reduced or eliminated for most patients. To do this requires knowledge of the antiemetic agents, experience in their use in combination, and careful consideration of the individual patient and the chemotherapeutic regimen they are receiving. A management plan to prevent chemotherapy-induced emesis is outlined in Table 4. All individuals receiving chemotherapy should be counseled about the potential for chemotherapy-induced emesis. Each patient should be reassured that optimal antiemetic therapy will be prescribed and that with its use the majority of patients do not experience significant emesis.

The combination of a serotonin antagonist and a corticosteroid is the most efficacious antiemetic prophylaxis tested to date for acute emesis. This combination should be routinely prescribed to patients receiving chemotherapy that causes emesis in 30% or more of the patients receiving it. The adjunctive use of a benzodiazepine may be desirable in anxious patients. Patients receiving emetogenic chemotherapy on consecutive days (such as cisplatin, ifosfamide, or dacarbazine) should receive the same combination of a serotonin antagonist and dexamethasone daily.

A summary of antiemetic treatment recommendations for specific clinical scenarios is presented in Table 4. In some cases, several regimens have proven efficacious.

## RESEARCH

The introduction of the specific serotonin antagonists and our improved understanding of the underlying physiology of vomiting promise better emetic control. Research continues to tackle the remaining vomiting problems by investigating the optimal dose and schedule of available agents, exploring new dosage forms, and identifying new antiemetic agents such as those that block the $NK_1$ receptor, the binding site of substance P.

## REFERENCES

1. Coates A, Abraham S, Kaye SB, et al. On the receiving end—patient perception of the side effects of cancer chemotherapy. *Eur J Cancer Clin Oncol* 1983;19:203.
2. Fetting JH, Grochow LB, Folstein MF, Ettinger DS, Colvin M. The course of nausea and vomiting after high-dose cyclophosphamide. *Cancer Treat Rep* 1982;66(7):1487.
3. Martin M, Diaz-Rubio E, Sanchez A, Almenarez J, Lopez-Vega JM. The natural course of emesis after carboplatin treatment. *Acta Oncol* 1990;29:593.

4. Morrow GR, Morrell C. Behavioral treatment for the anticipatory nausea and vomiting induced by cancer chemotherapy. *N Engl J Med* 1982; 307(24):1474.

5. Wilcox PM, Fetting JH, Nettesheim KM, Abeloff MD. Anticipatory vomiting in women receiving cyclophosphamide, methotrexate, and 5-FU (CMF) adjuvant chemotherapy for breast carcinoma. *Cancer Treat Rep* 1982;66:(8)1601.

6. Borison HL, McCarthy LE. Neuropharmacology of chemotherapy induced emesis. *Drugs* 1983;25:8.

7. Carpenter DO.Neural mechanisms of emesis. *Can J Physiol Pharmacol* 1990;68:230.

8. Miller AD, Wilson VJ. "Vomiting center" reanalyzed: an electrical stimulation study. *Brain Res* 1983;270:154.

9. Fozard JR.Neuronal 5-HT receptors in the periphery. *Neuropharmacology* 1984;23:1473.

10. Bradley PB, Engel G, Feniuk W, et al. Proposals for the classification and nomenclature of functional receptors for 5-hydroxytryptamine. *Neuropharmacology* 1986;25(6):563.

11. Richardson BP, Engel G, Donatsch P, Stadler PA. Identification of serotonin M-receptor subtypes and their specific blockade by a new class of drugs. *Nature* 1985;316(11):126.

12. Kilpatrick GJ, Jones BJ, Tyers MB. Identification and distribution of 5-HT$_3$ receptors in rat brain using radioligand binding. *Nature* 1987;330 (24):746.

13. Gunning SJ, Hagan RM, Tyers MB. Cisplatin induces biochemical and histological changes in the small intestine of the ferret, abstracted. *Br J Pharmacol* 1987;90:135.

14. Endo T, Minami M, Monama Y, et al. Emesis-related biochemical and histopathological changes induced by cisplatin in the ferret. *J Toxicol Sci* 1990;15:235.

15. Cubeddu LX, Hoffmann IS, Fuenmayor NT, Finn AL. Efficacy of ondansetron (GR 38032F) and the role of serotonin in cisplatin-induced nausea and vomiting (see comments). *N Engl J Med* 1990; 322:810.

16. Andrews PLR, Davis CJ, Bingham S, et al. The abdominal visceral innervation and the emetic reflex: Pathways, pharmacology, and plasticity. *Can J Physiol* 1990;68:325.

17. Buchheit KH, Engel G, Mutschler E, Richardson B. Study of the contractile effect of 5-hydroxytryptamine (5-HT) in the isolated longitudinal muscle strip from guinea-pig ileum. *Naunyn-Schmiedeberg's Arch Pharmacol* 1985;329:36.

18. Gralla RJ, Itri LM, Pisko SE, Squillante AE, Kelsen DP, Braun DW. Antiemetic efficacy of high-dose metoclopramide: randomized trials with placebo and prochlorperazine in patients with chemotherapy-induced nausea and vomiting. *N Engl J Med* 1981;305(16):905.

19. Roila F, Tonato M, Basurto C, et al. Protection from nausea and vomiting in cisplatin-treated patients: high-dose metoclopramide combined with methylprednisolone versus metoclopramide combined with dexamethasone and diphenhydramine: a study of the Italian Oncology Group for Clinical Research. *J Clin Oncol* 1989;7:1693.

20. D'Acquisto R, Tyson LB, Gralla RJ, et al. The influence of a chronic high alcohol intake on chemotherapy-induced nausea and vomiting. *Proc Am Soc Clin Oncol* 1986;5:257.

21. Sullivan JR, Leyden MJ, Bell R. Decreased cisplatin-induced nausea and vomiting with chronic alcohol ingestion. *N Engl J Med* 1983;309: 796.

22. Tonato M, Roila F, DelFavero A. Methodolgy of antiemetic trials: a review. *Ann Oncol* 1991;2:107.

23. Kris MG, Tyson LB, Gralla RJ, Clark RA, Allen JC, Reilly LK. Extrapyramidal reactions with high-dose metoclopramide (letter). *N Engl J Med* 1983;309(7):433.

24. Allen JC, Gralla R, Reilly L, Kellick M, Young C. Metoclopramide: dose-related toxicity and preliminary antiemetic studies in children receiving cancer chemotherapy. *J Clin Oncol* 1985;3(8):1136.

25. Einhorn LH, Nagy C, Werner K, Finn AL. Ondansetron: a new antiemetic for patients receiving cisplatin chemotherapy. *J Clin Oncol* 1990;8(4):731.

26. Kris MG, Gralla RJ, Clark RA, Tyson LB. Dose-ranging evaluation of the serotonin antagonist GR-C507/75 (GR38032F) when used as an antiemetic in patients receiving anticancer chemotherapy. *J Clin Oncol* 1988;6:659.

27. Grunberg SM, Stevenson LL, Russell CA, McDermed JE. Dose ranging phase I study of the serotonin antagonist GR38032F for prevention of cisplatin-induced nausea and vomiting. *J Clin Oncol* 1989;7:1137.

28. Carden PA, Mitchell SL, Waters KD, Tiedemann K, Ekert H. Prevention of cyclophosphamide/cytarabine-induced emesis with ondansetron in children with leukemia. *J Clin Oncol* 1990;8(9):1531.

29. Roila F, Tonato M, Basurto C, et al. Antiemetic activity of high doses of metoclopramide combined with methylprednisolone versus metoclopramide alone in cisplatin-treated cancer patients: a randomized double-blind trial of the Italian Oncology Group for Clinical Research. *J Clin Oncol* 1987;5:(1)141.

30. Hesketh PJ, Plagge P, Bryson JC. Single-dose ondasetron for prevention of acute cisplatin-induced emesis: analysis of efficacy and prognostic factors. In: Branch AL, Grelot L, Miller AD, King GL, eds. *Mechanisms and Control of Emesis.* London: INSERM/John Libbey Eurotext, 1992;235.

31. Walsh TD. Antiemetic drug combinations in advanced cancer. *Lancet* 1982;1:1018.

32. Morrow G. Susceptibility to motion sickness and the development of anticipatory nausea and vomiting in cancer patients undergoing chemotherapy. *Cancer Treat Rep* 1984;68:1177.

33. Martin M, Diaz-Rubio E. Emesis during past pregnancy: a new factor in chemotherapy-induced emesis. *Ann Oncol* 1990;1:152.

34. Hesketh PJ, Kris MG, Grunberg SM, et al. Proposal for classifying the acute emetogenicity of cancer chemotherapy. *J Clin Oncol* 1997;15: 103–109.

35. Hesketh P, Beck T, Uhlennhopp M, et al. Adjusting the dose of intravenous ondasetron plus dexmethasone to the emetic potential of the chemotherapy regime. *J Clin Oncol* 1995;13:2117–2122.

36. Addelman M, Erlichman C, Fine S, Warr D, Murray C. Phase I/II trial of granisetron: a novel 5-hydroxytryptamine antagonist for the prevention of chemotherapy-induced nausea and vomiting. *J Clin Oncol* 1990; 8(2):337.

37. Navari RM, Kaplan HG, Gralla RJ, Grunberg SM, Palmer R, Fitts D. Efficacy and safety of granisetron, a selective 5-hydroxytryptamine-3 receptor antagonist, in the prevention of nausea and vomiting induced by high-dose cisplatin. *J Clin Oncol* 1994;12:2204.

38. Kris MG, Gralla RJ, Clark RA, Tyson LB. Phase II trials of the serotonin antagonist GR38032F for the control of vomiting caused by cisplatin. *JNCI* 1989;81:42.

39. Riviere A. Dose finding study of granisetron in patients receiving high-dose cisplatin chemotherapy. *Br J Cancer* 1994;69:967.

40. Marty M, Pouillart P, Scholl S, et al. Comparison of the 5-hydroxytryptamine 3 (serotonin) antagonist ondansetron (GR 38032F) with high-dose metoclopramide in the control of cisplatin-induced emesis. *N Engl J Med* 1990;322:816.

41. DeMulder PH, Seynaeve C, Vermorken JB, et al. Ondansetron compared with high-dose metoclopramide in prophylaxis of acute multicenter, randomized, double-blind, crossover study. *Ann Intern Med* 1990;113(11):834.

42. Hainsworth J, Harvey W, Pendergrass K, et al. A single-blind comparison of intravenous ondansetron, a selective serotonin antagonist, with intravenous metoclopramide in the prevention of nausea and vomiting associated with high-dose cisplatin chemotherapy. *J Clin Oncol* 1991; 9:721.

43. Warr D, Willlan A, Fine S, et al. Superiority of granisetron to dexamethasone plus prochlorperazine in the prevention of chemotherapy-induced emesis. *JNCI* 1991;83(16):1169.

44. Chevallier B, and Granisetron Study Group. The control of cisplatin-induced emesis- A comparative study of granisetron and a combination regimen of high-dose metoclopramide and dexamethasone. *Br J Cancer* 1993;68:176.

45. Hainsworth JD. The use of ondansetron in patients receiving multiple-day cisplatin regimens. *Semin Oncol* 1992;19(suppl 10):48.

46. Fox SM, Einhorn LH, Cox E, Powell N, Abdy A. Ondansetron versus ondansetron, dexamethasone, and chlorpromazine in the prevention of nausea and vomiting associated with multiple-day cisplatin chemotherapy. *J Clin Oncol* 1993;11:2391.

47. Noble A, Bremer K, Goedhals L, Cupissol D, Dilly SG. A double blind, randomized, crossover comparison of granisetron and ondansetron in 5 day fractionated chemotherapy: assessment of efficacy, safety and patient preference. *Eur J Cancer* 1994;30A:1083.

48. Sledge GW, Einhorn L, Nagy C, House K. Phase III double-blind comparison of intravenous ondansetron and metoclopramide as antiemetic therapy for patients receiving multiple-day cisplatin-based chemotherapy. *Cancer* 1992;70(10):2524.

49. The Granisetron Study Group. The antiemetic efficacy and safety of

granisetron compared with metoclopramide and dexamethasone in patients receiving fractional chemotherapy over 5 days. *J Cancer Res Clin Oncol* 1993;119:555.

50. Bonneterre J, Chevallier B, Metz R, et al. A randomized double-blind comparison of ondansetron and metoclopramide in the prophylaxis of emesis induced by cyclophosphamide, fluorouracil, and doxorubicin or epirubicin chemotherapy. *J Clin Oncol* 1990;8(6):1063.

51. Cunningham D, Pople A, Ford HT, et al. Prevention of emesis in patients receiving cytotoxic drugs by GR38032F, a selective 5-HT, receptor antagonist. *Lancet* 1987;1(June 27, 1987):1461.

52. Zulian G, Selby P, Viner C. GR38032F-A safe and effective antiemetic in patients receiving high-dose melphalan (abstract). *Proc Am Soc Clin Oncol* 1988;7:289.

53. Harvey V, Evans B, Mak D. Ondansetron controls carboplatin induced vomiting resistant to standard antiemetics (abstract). *Proc Am Soc Clin Oncol* 1990;9:330.

54. Jantunen IT, Muhonen TT, Kataja VV, Flander MK, Teerenhovi L. 5-HT₃ receptor antagonists in the prophylaxis of acute vomiting induced by moderately emetogenic chemotherapy—A randomized study. *Eur J Cancer* 1993;29A(12):1669.

55. Fraschini G, Ciociola A, Esparza L, et al. Evaluation of three oral dosages of ondansetron in the prevention of nausea chemotherapy. *J Clin Oncol* 1991;9(7):1268.

56. Beck TM, Ciociola AA, Jones SE, et al. Efficacy of oral ondansetron in the prevention of emesis in outpatients receiving cyclophosphamide-based chemotherapy. *Ann Intern Med* 1993;118(6):407.

57. Martoni A, Angelelli B, Guaraldi M, et al. Granisetron versus ondansetron in the prevention of cis-platinum induced emesis: an open randomized cross-over study. *Proc Am Soc Clin Oncol* 1994;13:431.

58. Mantovani A, Maccio L, Curreli L, et al. Comparison of the effectiveness of three 5-HT3 receptor antagonists in the prophylaxis of acute vomiting induced by highly emetogenic chemotherapy (high-dose cisplatin) for the treatment of primary head and neck cancer. *Proc Am Soc Clin Oncol* 1994;13:428.

59. Roila F, De Angelis V, Cognetti F, et al. Ondansetron versus granisetron both combined with dexamethasone in the prevention of cisplatin-induced emesis. *Proc Am Soc Clin Oncol* 1995;14:523.

60. Ritter H, Hall S, Mailliard J, Navari R, Friedman C, and Granesetron Study Group. A comparative clinical trial of granisetron and ondansetron in the prophylaxis of cisplatin-induced emesis. *Proc Am Soc Clin Oncol* 1995;14:528.

61. Beck TM, Madajewicz S, Navari RM, et al. A double blind, stratified, randomized comparison of intravenous (IV) ondansetron administered as a multiple dose regimen versus two single dose regimens in the prevention of cisplatin-induced nausea and vomiting. *Proc Am Soc Clin Oncol* 1992;11:378.

62. Seynaeve C, Schuller J, Buser J, et al. Comparison of the antiemetic efficacy of different doses of ondansetron, given as either a continuous infusion or a single intravenous dose, in acute cisplatin-induced emesis. A multicentre, double-blind, randomized parallel group study. *Br J Cancer* 1992;66:192.

63. Gralla RJ, Rittenberg CN, Lettow L, et al. A unique all-oral, single-dose, combination antiemetic regimen with high efficacy and marked cost saving potential. *Proc Am Soc Clin Oncol* 1995;14:526.

64. Navari RM, Pendergrass KB, Grote TH, et al. All oral regimens of dolasetron and dexamethasone to prevent emesis caused by high-dose cisplatin. *Proc Am Soc Clin Oncol* 1996;15:537.

65. Frustaci S, Tumolo S, Tirell U, et al. High-dose metoclopramide versus dexamethasone in the prevention of cisplatin induced vomiting (abstract). *Proc Am Soc Clin Oncol* 1983;2:87.

66. Aapro MS, Plezia PM, Alberts DS, et al. Double-blind crossover study of the antiemetic efficacy of high-dose dexamethasone versus high-dose metoclopramide. *Proc Am Soc Clin Oncol* 1983;2:93.

67. Gralla RJ, Tyson LB, Bordin LA, et al. Antiemetic therapy: a review of recent studies and a report of a random assignment trial comparing metoclopramide with delta-9-tetrahydrocannabinol. *Cancer Treat Rep* 1984;68(1):163.

68. Grunberg SM, Gala KV, Lampenfeld M, et al. Comparison of the antiemetic effect of high-dose intravenous metoclopramide and high-dose intravenous haloperidol in a randomized double-blind crossover study. *J Clin Oncol* 1984;2:782.

69. Richards PD, Flamm MA, Bateman M, et al. The antiemetic efficacy of secobarbital and chlorpromazine compared to metoclopramide, diphenhydramine, and dexamethasone: a randomized trial. *Cancer* 1986;58:959.

70. De Mulder PHM, Seynaeve C, Vermorken JB, et al. Ondansetron compared with high-dose metoclopramide in prophylaxis of acute and delayed cisplatin-induced nausea and vomiting. *Ann Intern Med* 1990; 113:834.

71. Kris MG, Gralla RJ, Clark RA, Tyson LB, Groshen S. Antiemetic control and prevention of side effects of anti-cancer therapy with lorazepam or diphenhydramine when used in combination with metoclopramide plus dexamethasone. A double-blind, randomized trial. *Cancer* 1987;60:2816.

72. Markman M, Sheidler V, Ettinger DS, Quaskey SA, Mellits ED. Antiemetic efficacy of dexamethasone. Randomized double-blind crossover study with prochlorperazine in patients receiving cancer chemotherapy. *N Engl J Med* 1984;311(9):549.

73. Aapro MS, Alberts DS. High-dose dexamethasone for prevention of cis-platinum-induced vomiting. *Cancer Chemother Pharmacol* 1981;7:11.

74. Cassileth PA, Lusk EJ, Torri S, DiNubile N, Gerson SL. Antiemetic efficacy of dexamethasone therapy in patients receiving cancer chemotherapy. *Arch Intern Med* 1983;143(7):1347.

75. The Italian Group for Antiemetic Research. Dexamethasone, granisetron, or both for the prevention of nausea and vomiting during chemotherapy for cancer. *N Engl J Med* 1995;332:1.

76. Roila F, Tonato M, Cognetti F, et al. Prevention of cisplatin-induced emesis: a double-blind multicenter randomized crossover study comparing ondansetron and ondansetron plus dexamethasone. *J Clin Oncol* 1991;9:675.

77. Frytak S, Moertel CG, O'Fallon JR, et al. Delta-9-Tetrahydrocannabinol as an antiemetic for patients receiving cancer chemotherapy. *Ann Intern Med* 1979;91:825.

78. Sallan SE, Cronin CM, Zelen M, et al. Antiemetics in patients receiving chemotherapy for cancer: a randomized comparison of delta-9-tetrahydrocannabinol and prochlorperazine. *N Engl J Med* 1980;302: 135.

79. Grossman B, Lessin LS, Cohen P. Droperidol prevents nausea and vomiting from cis-platinum. *N Engl J Med* 1979;301:47.

80. Neidhart J, Gayen M, Metz E. Haldol is an effective antiemetic for platinum and mustard induced vomiting when other agents fail (abstract). *Proc Am Soc Clin Oncol* 1980;21:365.

81. Vincent BJ, McQuistion DJ, Einhorn LH, et al. Review of cannabinoids and their antiemetic effectiveness. *Drugs* 1983;25:52.

82. Laszlo J, Clark RA, Hanson DC, Tyson L, Crumpler L, Gralla R. Lorazepam in cancer patients treated with cisplatin: a drug having antiemetic, amnestic, and anxiolytic effects. *J Clin Oncol* 1985;3:864.

83. Kris MG, Gralla RJ, Tyson LB, et al. Improved control of cisplatin-induced emesis with high-dose metoclopramide and with combinations of metoclopramide, dexamethasone, and diphenhydramine. Results of consecutive trials in 255 patients. *Cancer* 1985;55:527.

84. Allan SG, Cornbleet MA, Warrington PS, Golland IM, Leonard RC, Smyth JN. Dexamethasone and high dose metoclopramide: efficacy in controlling cisplatin induced nausea and vomiting. *Br Med J* 1984;289: 878.

85. Strum SB, McDermed JE, Liponi DF. High-dose intravenous metoclopramide versus combination high-dose metoclopramide and intravenous dexamethasone in preventing cisplatin-induced nausea and emesis: a single-blind crossover comparison of antiemetic efficacy. *J Clin Oncol* 1985;3:245.

86. Grunberg SM, Akerley WA, Krailo MD, Johnson KB, Baker CR, Cariffe PA. Comparison of metoclopramide and metoclopramide plus dexamethasone for complete protection from cisplatinum-induced emesis. *Cancer Invest* 1986;4:379.

87. Kris MG, Gralla RJ, Clark RA, et al. Incidence, course, and severity of delayed nausea and vomiting following the administration of high-dose cisplatin. *J Clin Oncol* 1985;3:1379.

88. Kris MG, Gralla RJ, Tyson LB, Clark RA, Cirrincione C, Groshen S. Controlling delayed vomiting: double-blind, randomized trial comparing placebo, dexamethasone alone, and metoclopramide plus dexamethasone in patients receiving cisplatin. *J Clin Oncol* 1989;7:108.

89. Clark R, Kris M, Tyson L, Gralla R, O'Hehir M. Antiemetic trials to control delayed vomiting following high-dose cisplatin. *Proc Am Soc Clin Oncol* 1986;5:257.

90. Kris MG, Tyson LB, Clark RA, Gralla RG. Oral ondansetron for the control of delayed emesis after cisplatin. Report of a phase II study and

a review of completed trials to manage delayed emesis. *Cancer* 1992; 70:1012.

91. Gandara DR, Harvey WH, Monaghan GG, Bryson JC, Finn AL. Efficacy of ondansetron in the prevention of delayed emesis following high dose cisplatin (DDP). *Proc Am Soc Clin Oncol* 1990;9:328.

92. Roila F, Bracarda S, Tonato M, et al. Ondansetron (GR38032) in the prophylaxis of acute and delayed cisplatin-induced emesis. *Clin Oncol* 1990;2(5):268.

93. Roila F, De Angelis V, Contu A, et al. Ondansetron versus metoclopramide both combined with dexamethasone in the prevention of cisplatin-induced delayed emesis. *Proc Am Soc Clin Oncol* 1996;15:528.

94. Morrow GR. Clinical characteristics associated with the development of anticipatory nausea and vomiting in cancer patients undergoing chemotherapy treatment. *J Clin Oncol* 1984;2:1171.

95. Stefanek ME, Sheidler VR, Fetting JH. Anticipatory nausea and vomiting: does it remain a significant clinical problem? *Cancer* 1988;62: 2654.

96. Greenberg DB, Surman OS, Clarke J, Baer L. Alprazolam for phobic nausea and vomiting related to cancer chemotherapy. *Cancer Treat Rep* 1987;71:549.

97. Priestman TJ, Roberts JT, Lucraft H, et al. Results of a randomized, double-blind comparative study of ondansetron and metoclopramide in the prevention of nausea and vomiting following high-dose upper abdominal irradiation. *Clin Oncol* 1990;2:71.

98. Hunter AE, Prentice HG, Pothecary K, et al. Granisetron, a selective 5-HT3 receptor antagonist, for the prevention of radiation induced emesis during total body irradiation. *Bone Marrow Transplant* 1991; 7:439.

*Principles and Practice of Supportive Oncology,*
edited by Ann Berger et al.
Lippincott–Raven Publishers, Philadelphia ©1998

CHAPTER 12

# Nausea and Vomiting Unrelated to Cancer Treatment

Barbara G. Fallon

Scant attention has been paid in the oncology literature to this distressing symptom when it occurs apart from anti-tumor therapy. Several authors have reported that nausea or vomiting occurs in up to half of all patients with advanced cancer across a broad range of tumor diagnoses (1–7); most have shown a female preponderance. These studies have attempted to define the constellation of symptoms that characterize the end of life in patients with cancer and have led to the concept of the terminal cancer syndrome (8). Identifying a common clinical pathway in terminal illness may lead to better palliative care program development and foster clinical research that will ultimately assist the clinician caring for these patients.

This chapter will focus on emesis unrelated to chemotherapy. The mechanisms of emesis will be reviewed as a basis to formulate a differential diagnosis. The evaluation of this symptom is familiar: it is composed of the history, physical examination, and laboratory investigation but the approach must be practical, with a goal toward relief of symptoms as quickly as possible. The choice of therapy for nausea and vomiting may be directed at the cause (e.g., treatment of brain metastases with radiation therapy and dexamethasone) or at the symptom, (e.g., nausea at the initiation of narcotic therapy for pain may be treated by neuroleptic antiemetics rather than by withdrawal of pain medication). Understanding the complex neural pathways that interact to produce this symptom can more accurately target the cause. While successful treatment more often comes from a precise diagnosis, empirical approaches have contributed much to this troubling and common symptom. Two cases will be presented to illustrate common scenarios for the workup and treatment of this symptom. Finally, future directions in the manage-ment of emesis unrelated to anticancer therapy will be discussed.

## PHYSIOLOGY OF EMESIS

A broad range of sensory inputs can lead to nausea and vomiting, a complex motor activity coordinated by the vomiting center (VC), a neuroanatomic region in the lateral reticular formation of the medulla. Vomiting occurs when relaxation of the proximal stomach accompanied by antiperistalsis from the upper jejunum toward the pylorus allows distal gastric contents into the body of the stomach. Esophageal sphincter tone is also relaxed, thereby allowing stomach contents to be expelled. The VC is composed of the nucleus tractus solitarius, the dorsal motor nucleus of the vagus, and the nucleus ambiguous. Stimulation of these motor pathways produces vomiting (9). Because it is a protective reflex designed to rid the body of toxins, complete eradication of this symptom is difficult.

Wang and Borison first proposed that the VC is activated directly by irritation of visceral afferents mediated by the vagus nerve or via the circulation delivering emetic stimuli to the chemoreceptor trigger zone (CTZ) (10). Other pathways with a variety of neuroreceptors have since been elucidated. These signals are integrated in the central nervous system (CNS) and relayed to the VC. Understanding these neural pathways permits a rational approach to pharmacotherapy. Table 1 delineates the causes of emesis unrelated to anticancer treatment, proven or proposed mechanisms, neuroreceptors that have been identified, and antagonists or therapy directed at these neuroreceptors. The list, while extensive, is not all encompassing. It is meant to guide the clinician toward the most common causes of emesis that are persistent or recurrent in advanced cancer patients.

B. G. Fallon: University of Connecticut School of Medicine, Hematology/Oncology Department, New Britain General Hospital, New Britain, CT 06050.

**TABLE 1.** *Nausea and Vomiting Unrelated to Anticancer Treatment: Causes, Mechanisms, Neuroreceptors and Antagonists*

| Causes | Mechanisms | Receptors Identified | Antagonists |
|---|---|---|---|
| Visceral<br>Distension, stasis or obstruction of gastric, bowel, biliary, genitourinary tracts<br>Constipation<br>Cancer of the stomach, pancreas, liver; peritoneal metastases<br>Gastric irritation: drugs, blood<br>External pressure: "squashed stomach syndrome"<br><br>Cardiac pain<br>Paroxysmal or chronic cough | Stimulation of the vomiting center via vagal and sympathetic afferents | Gut: Dopamine $D_2$ & 5 $HT_3$ | Dopamine antagonists: prokinetic agents<br>Serotonergic antagonists |
| Chemical<br>Drugs: narcotics, digitalis, estrogens, alcohol<br><br>Metabolic abnormalities: hypercalcemia, uremia, hyponatremia<br>Toxins: abnormal metabolites or peptides from cancer, infection, radiotherapy | Stimulation of chemoreceptor trigger zone | Dopamine $D_2$ & Serotonin 5 $HT_3$ | Dopamine antagonists: neuroleptic & prokinetic agents<br>Serotonergic antagonists |
| Central Nervous System<br>Primary or metastatic brain tumors<br>Meningitis: carcinomatous, infectious, chemical<br><br>Elevated intracranial pressure<br>Psychological and emotional factors: pain, fear, anxiety | Direct stimulation of the vomiting center: inflammation with increased prostaglandin synthesis, increased intracranial pressure | Histamine $H_1$ (especially from raised intracranial pressure & brain metastases), Muscarinic cholinergic & Serotonin $5HT_3$ | Anti-inflammatory agents: corticosteroids (also may reduce edema)<br>Anxiolytic, anti-histamines |
| Vestibular<br>Drugs: aspirin, narcotics<br>Motion sickness, Meniere's Disease, labyrinthitis<br>Local tumor or metastasis: acoustic neuroma, brain tumor, skull base metastasis | Direct stimulation of the vestibular apparatus | Histamine $H_1$, Muscarinic Cholinergic | Anti-histamines, Belladonna alkaloids |

Nausea and vomiting could represent distinct forms of emetic control (11) or a continuum of responses wherein nausea is triggered from a lower level of stimulation than vomiting (12). Vomiting is easier to suppress than nausea, but the latter may be controlled by a higher dose of antiemetics (13). A phenomenon of chronic nausea in malignancy has been attributed to autonomic dysfunction, which may cause delayed gastric emptying (14).

## Visceral Causes of Vomiting

In patients with advanced cancer the most common mechanism of emesis is stimulation of the VC via the vagal and sympathetic afferents of the viscera, with their vast heterogeneous array of inputs. Distention of the gut can occur from the stomach to the colon and from malignant or benign conditions. Slowed gastric emptying can lead to chronic nausea or may cause vomiting due to overfeeding. Constipation, one of the most prevalent complaints in advanced cancer, can lead to nausea and vomiting via this mechanism. Constipation is often due to multiple causes (15). Typically, a patient with pain becomes progressively immobilized and anorectic, and is prescribed opiates without attention to his bowel status. Such a patient can develop fecal impaction, compounding the problem with pain on defecation. Constipation in less severe forms can result in patient noncompliance with appropriate medications, leading to a downward spiral of unrelieved pain, depression, withdrawal, and worsening of symptoms (16).

Distention of the liver capsule or elsewhere in the biliary tree or along the genitourinary tract may also lead to vomiting via the same mechanism. Pressure on the stomach from a massively enlarged spleen or liver or tumor deposit can produce the squashed stomach syndrome. Other organs are also served by the vagus nerve, e.g., chest pain of cardiac origin and paroxysmal or chronic cough can trigger vomiting (17).

Numerous drugs used in advanced cancer can cause gastric irritation or bleeding that leads to vomiting via these pathways. Non-steroidal antiinflammatory drugs (NSAIDs), mucolytics, expectorants, iron supplements, hormones, and antibiotics are the chief culprits for drug-induced visceral causes of vomiting (17).

## Chemical Causes of Vomiting

In addition to direct stomach irritation, drugs can also produce emesis via stimulation of the CTZ. Common offenders in patients with advanced cancer include narcotics, digitalis, estrogens, and alcohol (1,18). Patients on chronic medication that had been well tolerated may now experience toxic effects because of altered drug metabolism or excretion due to tumor progression in the liver or urinary tract. Anorexia, dehydration, weight loss,

or interactions with other medications can also play a role. Nausea and vomiting may be the first manifestation of paraneoplastic syndromes such as hypercalcemia or hyponatremia. Abnormal metabolites from tumor proliferation, associated infections, or as a result of treatment with radiation therapy may also contribute to nausea and vomiting. All of these chemical causes reach the CTZ via the circulation (1,17).

## CNS Causes of Vomiting

The CNS has direct input into the VC via several types of neuroreceptors (18). Primary or metastatic brain tumors can directly activate histamine receptors in the brain, particularly if they cause increased intracranial pressure. Inflammatory responses to meningitis from carcinoma, chemotherapy, or infection cause vomiting, perhaps due to increased prostaglandin synthesis, and respond to corticosteroids. Psychological or emotional factors can cause or compound symptoms of nausea and vomiting, and addressing these factors can contribute to the successful therapy of emesis.

## Vestibular Causes of Vomiting

Drugs, particularly aspirin and narcotics, directly stimulate the vestibular apparatus, which in turn provides input to the VC. Many of the other causes in this category are incidental to the patient's cancer diagnosis: motion sickness, Meniere's disease, labyrinthitis, acoustic neuroma, or the use of aspirin. Less common causes include bone metastases at the base of skull, brain tumors, or metastases affecting the vestibular apparatus (18).

## FORMULATING A DIFFERENTIAL DIAGNOSIS

It is convenient to categorize the common causes of emesis in advanced cancer according to the mechanisms described above. Visceral causes will be suspected in patients with cancer known to involve the viscera or whose tumors have a natural history consistent with visceral involvement, e.g., ovarian cancer. Central nervous system causes of emesis are usually accompanied by additional abnormalities in neurologic function. Chemical causes will be elucidated by a complete medication list and simple laboratory investigation. Emesis due to vestibular causes is characteristically worsened with head motion and may be accompanied by auditory symptoms; the cause is usually discerned by neurologic exam and tests of vestibular function.

## Workup of Emesis

Rarely, patients will present with nausea and vomiting as a first manifestation of advanced cancer. More often,

**TABLE 2.** *Work-up of Emesis Unrelated to Cancer Treatment: Common Scenarios*

| Suspected Diagnosis | Symptoms | Relevant History | Physical | Laboratories & Radiography | Plan |
|---|---|---|---|---|---|
| Gastric outlet or bowel dilitation or obstruction | (Usually large volume) +/- undigested food +/- fecal odor | Intra-abdominal cancer e.g., stomach, bowel or ovarian. May have colicky abdominal pain. | Non-specific +/-ascites Pattern of distension may suggest level of obstruction. | KUB and CT may support obstruction vs. ileus. Contrast study often helpful. Prior pathology or operative reports may confirm diffuse peritoneal or mesenteric metastasis. | Surgical candidate:consult for bypass or proximal tube drainage and distal alimentation. Non-surgical candidate: Octreotide or gastric tube for elective drainage; consider hyper-alimentation. |
| Constipation, ileus | Variable volume emesis +/-abdominal distension | Often chronic constipation with recent exacerbation by narcotics, immobility dehydration, mental status changes. | Non-specific Should include rectal and neurologic exam. Patient may require disimpaction. | Non-specific, KUB usually helpful. | Vigorous clean-out and prevention of further episodes. |
| Cardiac | Variable volume emesis +/-chest, jaw or arm pain, sweating, SOB, palpitations; occurs after exertion, heavy meal, cold weather activity. | +- cardiac history or meds +/- smoker +/- diabetic | Work-up for cardiac pain or arrhythmias. | Work-up for cardiac cause as appropriate. | Work-up and treat for cardiac pain as appropriate. |
| Cough-induced emesis | Variable volume emesis with known cough; emesis usually occurs at end or during coughing paroxysm. | Lung ca, COPD, pneumonia, esophageal ca or known fistula. CNS metastases with possible or known aspiration. | Lung findings may support pneumonia/ COPD. Neuro may suggest CNS metastases or aspiration. | Confirm diagnosis if not known, e.g., modified barium swallow to confirm aspiration. Chest x-ray to r/o pneumonia | Cough suppressant; NPO if appropriate to reduce aspiration with PEG for nutrition. |
| Chemical-induced emesis | Variable volume emesis, unpredictable, usually recent onset. | Check medication list: any new prescriptions, especially antibiotics and narcotics. Known bone metastases of symptoms; known CNS metastases in symptoms Known squamous cell ca. Tumor lysis: rapidly proliferating tumor or rapid response to treatment. | Non-specific Neuro exam may be helpful. | If not attributable to new medication, check drug toxicity. R/O hyponatremia or hypercalcemia, uremia or liver disfunction. | Remove offending agent and treat metabolic disruption as appropriate. May respond to antiemetic. |
| Central Nervous System mets or primary brain tumor Meningitis Psycho/emotional | Variable volume emesis; may be projectile. Neck stiffness, headaches. Pain, fear, anxiety. | Tumors known to effect CNS. | Careful neurologic exam. Check for meningismus. | CT or MRI of brain. MRI of meninges +/- lumbar puncture. | Dependent upon clinical status of the patient. Emesis and some neuro systems may respond to steroids if infectious meningitis is ruled out. |
| Vestibular | Nausea increases with head motion. +/- tinitis +/- decreased hearing +/- skull or bone tenderness | Aspirin or opiate toxicity Acoustic neuroma History of bone metastases | Unilateral auditory impairment. Tenderness on skeletal exam. | CT or MRI to rule out acoustic neuroma or skull base metastases. Bone scan except in purely lytic disease. | Remove offending agent. Treatment symptomatically. |

patients with advanced cancer who complain of this symptom have the extent of their disease well documented. The diagnosis, prior treatment, and sites of metastases combined with knowledge of the natural history of the tumor suggest a likely etiology and the history can be further tailored to elucidate findings that confirm or refute the suspected diagnosis. The physical examination and, in particular, the neurologic exam are critical to direct the rest of the workup. Emesis of large volumes suggests obstruction of the gastrointestinal tract and attention should be paid to the amount of distention on the abdominal exam. Proximal obstruction may have minimal distention after vomiting, or a large fluid-filled stomach with a succussion splash prior to vomiting. Small bowel obstruction will have moderate to severe distention, whereas distal colon obstruction may present with a peripheral pattern of distention in the presence of a competent ileocecal valve. Laboratory studies will usually include tests of renal and liver function, ionized calcium, electrolytes, as well as a leukocyte count and differential. Serum drug levels may be helpful, e.g., digoxin, if toxicity is suspected. Radiographic studies are most useful when structural causes in the central nervous system or abdomen are suspected. The presence of brain metastases on computed tomography (CT) or magnetic resonance imaging (MRI) scan or the findings of carcinomatous meningitis on MRI are usually diagnostic, although the latter may require examination of cerebrospinal fluid. The abdominal flat plate and upright radiograph, which shows multiple loops of fluid-filled bowel with air-fluid levels and air in the colon, is consistent with an ileus pattern, whereas dilatation of the bowel and lack of distal air suggest a bowel obstruction. Often there is a continuum of findings radiographically and clinically as the situation improves or worsens. A contrast study is usually performed to determine the degree of obstruction and whether more than one site is involved. Care should be exercised in choosing a contrast medium (19). Barium is often preferred technically but should be used with caution, as it can inspissate above the obstruction and convert a partial obstruction to one requiring surgical correction. Water-soluble contrast that is diluted in the sequestered fluid of the bowel may be suboptimal in defining the degree of obstruction and determining whether multiple areas are involved, but it can be used safely in patients who are not surgical candidates. As in other procedures in medicine, the value of radiographs is enhanced when they are chosen on the basis of their positive predictive value. Typical clinical presentations of emesis unrelated to cancer treatment are presented in Table 2.

## TREATMENT OF NAUSEA AND VOMITING IN ADVANCED CANCER PATIENTS

In the past, effective chemotherapy was delivered at a significant price to patient comfort: severe to intractable nausea and vomiting. Compliance in the face of such toxicity was extremely difficult for patients. Thankfully, a much improved understanding of the mechanisms of chemotherapy-induced emesis has spurred successful drug development (9,20). Patients undergoing emetogenic chemotherapy are the beneficiaries of this progress, as are patients with emesis from other causes. Table 1 lists antagonists to the known or proposed neuroreceptors of the pathways believed to be responsible for many of the causes of emesis in patients with advanced cancer. Table 3 lists many useful antiemetics and provides information for oral and alternate routes of administration. Miscellaneous medications that are helpful in visceral causes of nausea and vomiting are described in Table 4.

Not all nausea should prompt suppressive pharmacotherapy. Common sense dictates that if a drug induces a side effect and such drug is not necessary to the patient's well-being, it should be withdrawn or substituted with one better tolerated. Many patients with end-stage cancer should have cardiovascular and diabetic medications reduced or eliminated to reduce side effects and improve comfort. In the case of a patient with bone pain who describes severe nausea and vomiting to morphine, substitution of another opiate or an NSAID can be tried. Nausea that begins with the administration of an NSAID may be due to gastric irritation; in this case, treating the irritation with an acid-blocking agent is preferred to prescribing an antiemetic. Nausea due to constipation will be relieved with a proper bowel regimen (15,21). Malignancy-associated hypercalcemia, hyponatremia, and brain metastases have specific therapies as well (22). Whether to treat the cause or suppress the symptom will depend on the clinical status of the patient and the responsiveness of his tumor.

This section will discuss the treatment of nausea and vomiting in advanced cancer according to the diagnostic categories described previously.

### Treatment of Visceral Causes of Emesis

Nausea and vomiting in advanced cancer is frequently due to mechanical problems in the gut (17,23). Simple distension of viscera not meant to be stretched leads to nausea, and patients may report emesis after simple overfeeding (23). Many patients appear to have slow gastric emptying and autonomic dysfunction has been postulated (14). A cancer-associated dyspepsia syndrome (CADS) has been described in which anorexia is associated with autonomic dysfunction and patients complain of constipation, early satiety, nausea, vomiting, bloating, and belching. These authors believe that it is a precursor to the subsequent development of anorexia and cachexia in advanced cancer. Early satiety, the most common symptom, did not always abate although many patients still responded to metochlopramide. The authors postulate a

**TABLE 3.** *Antiemetic Doses, Routes, and Schedules of Administration*

| Drug | Oral route in MG per 4-8 hr unless otherwise stated | Alternate routes in MG per 4–8 hr unless otherwise stated |
|---|---|---|
| Haloperidol | 1-2 | rectal: 1.3-3 |
| Droperidol | 1-2 | IV or IM: 2.5-10 |
| Metochlopramide | 10-15mg per 6 hr | IV: 10-20mg per 6 hr; higher doses may be effective |
| Ondansetron | 8mg per 8 hr | IV: 24mg per 24 hr in single dose or divided per 8 hr |
| Scopolamine | | transdermal: 0.5mcg per 72 hr |
| Meclizine | 25-50mg per 8-12 hr | |
| Cyclizine | 25-50 | rectal: 25-50 |
| Hydroxyzine | 25-50 | IM: 50-100 |
| Promethazine | 12.5-25 | rectal 25-50 |
| Prochlorperazine | 10-25 | rectal: 10-25; IM: 10-25 |
| Promethazine | 12.5-25 | rectal: 25-50 |
| Chlorpromazine | 10-25 (may be increased) | rectal: 50-100mg per 6-8 hr; IM: 25-50mg |
| Methotrimeprazine | | IM: 10-20mg |
| Lorazepam | 0.5-2 | SL: IM, IV: 1-2 |
| Dronabinol | 5-10mg per 4-6 hr | |
| Dexamethasone | 2-10mg per 4-12 hr | SC, IV: 4-10mg per 6 hr |

possible central appetite-stimulating effect of metochlopromide, as half of these patients had improved appetite (24). Although metochlopramide and cisapride are both prokinetic agents, only metochlopramide has been evaluated in this setting (25–29). Metochlopramide in higher doses has central antiemetic properties, but there is a risk of the side effects associated with dopamine antagonists.

Gastric dilatation can be due to outlet obstruction from tumor infiltration or benign duodenal ulcer. With gastritis or duodenal ulcer, acid blocking agents are recommended. Malignant gastric outlet obstruction is often refractory to medical management (1); prokinetic drugs are usually ineffective and can increase pain. Recently, the percutaneous endoscopically placed gastrostomy (PEG) tube has been used effectively for intractable vomiting due to obstruction of the upper gastrointestinal tract (30–32). Initially developed for enteral feeding, the PEG tube has been adapted for venting the gut. Patients with intraabdominal cancer who have ascites or bowel overlying the stomach were felt to be poor candidates for this procedure; however, ultrasound guidance allows the tube to be placed safely in most patients (33). Patients with discrete obstruction may be candidates for placement of both a venting gastrostomy tube and a feeding jejunos-

tomy tube, effectively bypassing the obstruction externally (34). This method is preferred to surgical placement in that it avoids general anesthesia, is effective, and is less costly.

Bowel obstruction is a common occurrence in advanced cancer and can be due to benign or malignant causes (35,36). It can be partial or complete, with single or multiple areas of involvement. Obstruction can be due to muscle paralysis (paralytic ileus) or luminal occlusion (mechanical ileus) or both, restricting the passage of feces and gas. The distention that results produces vomiting. The optimal management of bowel obstruction in advanced cancer is controversial. When success was measured by surgically correctable causes and survival beyond 60 days from laparotomy, some authors have reported 18–30% of patients with cancer and bowel obstruction were helped by surgery (37–39). For advanced ovarian patients, Krebs and Gopelrud have devised a prognostic index based on age, nutritional status, tumor spread, ascites, prior chemotherapy, and radiation therapy. Only 20% of patients with adverse prognostic scores survived for more than 8 weeks, whereas 84% of those with favorable scores met that measure (40). The combined experience of several investigators in ovarian cancer suggest that

**TABLE 4.** Miscellaneous Agents for Nausea or Vomiting

| Drug | Oral/route in MG 4 times daily unless otherwise stated | Mechanism |
|---|---|---|
| Cisapride | 10–20 | Prokinetic agent to enhance gastric emptying. |
| Misoprostol | 100–200mcg | Inhibits gastric acid secretion; ulcer prophylaxis with NSAID or aspirin. |
| Octreotide | 100–200mcg sc tid | Somatostatin analogue; inhibits gastrointestinal and pancreatic enzymes. |

patients with ascites and diffuse carcinomatosis are poor surgical candidates, especially if they are refractory to chemotherapy (41–45). Moreover, the quantitative measure of success has been criticized for ignoring the quality of that survival (46,47). Surgery did not correct obstruction in all patients and many patients had recurrences or continued to rely on venting apparatus. In this population there are considerable risks, including poor wound healing, infection or dehiscence, enterocutaneous fistulae or anastomotic leaks, venous thrombosis, pulmonary emboli, and gastrointestinal bleeding.

Recently, investigators have sought to apply prognostic factors to retrospective series. Van Ooijen (48) examined the outcome of 59 patients with bowel obstruction and advanced intraabdominal malignancy due to ovarian or other cancers. Twenty-five patients were deemed inoperable at presentation and had placement of gastric drainage tubes. Forty patients underwent laparotomy and two distinct groups emerged. In the first group of 15 patients, the median survival was 154 days and no patients had recurrent obstruction. Five of these patients had newly diagnosed ovarian cancer and the remainder had no palpable abdominal disease or ascites. The second group fared much worse, with only one successful laparotomy and a median survival of 36 days. The authors concluded that surgery should only be offered to patients with bowel obstruction who have no manifest ascites or palpable masses, excepting newly diagnosed ovarian cancer patients for whom effective chemotherapy is available. They advocated placement of a PEG tube for nonsurgical candidates. Surgical palliation in advanced cancer is a complex issue and requires decision making on a case-by-case basis. There seems to be an emerging consensus as to what constitutes poor surgical risk, as shown in Table 5 (41–45,47,48). There is less agreement about how to identify patients who will benefit from surgery (47).

Supportive therapies to enhance comfort in patients with advanced inoperable malignancy have long existed. Moertel et al. (49) showed an improved sense of well-being and appetite in patients with preterminal gastrointestinal cancer given dexamethasone versus placebo; symptomatic improvement did not lead to any objective increase in weight or survival. Specific medical management for intestinal obstruction may be effective, however. Baines et al. (1) reported results in 38 patients treated medically for malignant obstruction. Drugs were administered by the oral, rectal, and/or subcutaneous routes. Colic was treated with loperamide or hyoscine, with atropine reserved for those excessively sedated by hyoscine. Vomiting responded best to phenothiazines or butyrophenones; metochlopramide and domperidone were ineffective and appeared to worsen colic. Diarrhea was treated with loperamide and codeine. Only four patients with enterocutaneous or enterovaginal fistulae had results described as unsatisfactory with this regimen. An excellent review enlarging the experience of Baines and others has been published on the management of bowel obstruction in patients with terminal cancer (47). Regimens recommended for the treatment of pain, colic, and vomiting are included. This experience confirms their prior observation that vomiting unresponsive to medical treatment is usually caused by an obstruction of the upper gastrointestinal tract. In these patients placement of a PEG is preferred to prolonged nasogastric suction. Most authors agree that conventional management of bowel obstruction with nasogastric suction and fluid and electrolyte replacement (what has been referred to as the "drip and suck" method) is at best a temporary measure to reduce symptoms while assessing the patient for surgery or alternate management. Prolonged nasogastric suction is to be avoided because it is painful and can pose risks of nasal erosion, aspiration, and other complications (47,50). Patients rarely welcome the placement of a nasogastric tube.

When symptoms are controlled surgically, oral feeding can resume. In patients requiring a venting PEG the issue of nutrition or hydration usually arises. In hospice settings where relief of symptoms is emphasized, medical therapy often abolishes the need for parenteral nutrition or hydration. Symptoms of thirst are treated with sips of fluid or ice chips, and some patients even tolerate small amounts of their favorite foods. Parenteral nutrition is complex and expensive and has considerable risks (50,51). There is controversy over its role in patients with cancer (52–54). Nonetheless, in a patient with a good performance status in whom nutritional deprivation is the major deterrent to enjoying life, parenteral nutrition ought to be considered. Others have reported acceptable

**TABLE 5.** *Factors Predicitve of Poor Outcome to Surgical Exploration for Bowel Obstruction in Advanced Cancer*

1. End stage disease and poor performance status.
2. Diffuse intraperitoneal carcinomatosis.
3. Palpable abdominal masses or diffuse metastases in liver, lung or pleura.
4. Multiple area of partial bowel obstruction with prolonged evacuation time.
5. Large volume ascites.
6. Small or small and large bowel obstruction is worse than large bowel obstruction alone.
7. Prior chemotherapy especially if refractory.
8. Prior radiation therapy of the abdomen and pelvis.
9. Age greater than 65 years, especially with severe malnutrition.

results and high patient satisfaction in carefully selected patients using this method (55,56). This is discussed further in the first case study below. A new addition to the pharmacologic management of bowel obstruction comes from a somatostatin analog, octreotide. Initially used in cancer patients with malignant diarrhea due to fistulae or after high-dose chemotherapy, it reduced life-threatening diarrhea dramatically (57). Octreotide was then used in patients with copious vomiting due to bowel obstruction (58,59). In a study of 13 patients with refractory ovarian cancer and bowel obstruction, including 5 patients who had more than 10 episodes of vomiting per day, octreotide was administered with excellent results. In doses of 100 to 200 µg subcutaneously three times per day all patients had control of vomiting usually within 3 days of starting therapy. Three patients could resume oral intake (60). Octreotide, a synthetic form of somatostatin, inhibits the release of growth hormone, gastrin, secretin, vasointestinal peptides, insulin, and glucagon. It blocks secretion of pepsin, pancreatic enzymes, bicarbonate, and water (61). By so doing it reduces bowel motility and also reduces gastric acid and bile secretion to relieve the discomfort of obstruction. In these patients it was not necessary to administer additional anticholinergic agents. Octreotide is a local skin irritant and some patients preferred a subcutaneous infusion to multiple daily injections. A long-acting preparation of somatostatin is being studied that could be administered weekly (62). Octreotide and the long-acting analog vapreotide also appear to have analgesic properties, possibly mediated by opioid receptors. Development of these drugs looks promising for the management of painful bowel symptoms in patients with advanced cancer.

As often happens in patients with visceral causes of vomiting, oral medications may be ineffective. Storey et al. (63) recently reviewed subcutaneous infusion as a method of administering medication to patients with advanced cancer who cannot take oral medications. Additional information about alternate routes of antiemetics is provided in Table 3. Medications not classified as antiemetic but helpful in some visceral causes of emesis and referred to in the preceding paragraphs are listed in Table 4.

### Treatment of Chemical, CNS, and Vestibular Causes of Emesis

Because the causes of emesis that are mediated by the chemical, central, and vestibular mechanisms are so varied, clinicians will evaluate the merits of treating the cause of the symptom in individual patients. When the symptoms require medication, the use of antiemetics in appropriate dose and schedule specific to the neuroreceptors will usually yield the best results. Lichter (17,18) has reviewed this topic extensively and has reported

excellent results in patients treated with specific antiemetics rather than an all-purpose antiemetic. In some patients combination antinausea therapy is most effective. Lichter has outlined a procedure for successful treatment with antiemetics: first, to establish the probable cause of emesis; second, to consider the afferent pathways and associated neuroreceptors involved; and finally, to choose the most potent antiemetic with the fewest side effects that acts on those receptors. In a study of 100 consecutive patients with nausea and vomiting, visceral factors including gastric stasis and constipation accounted for more than 50% of the causes of nausea and vomiting; almost one third of patients had drug toxicity or biochemical disturbance. Seventy percent of patients attained control of emesis within 24 hours of administration and 93% of patients came under control on the second day by means of a dose increase or addition of another antiemetic. Lichter emphasized the need to reassess the efficacy of therapy promptly and to be willing to modify the dose of drug or to use combination therapy to attain these results. Vomiting assessed to be due to chemical causes will respond best if those causes can be corrected, but suppression of symptoms can be accomplished with haloperidol, which acts on the CTZ. CNS stimuli not due to edema or increased intracranial pressure will respond to antihistamines, and certain tranquilizers such as lorazepam are also helpful. Cyclizine is the most effective antiemetic in this category. Vestibular causes will respond to antihistamine or muscarinic cholinergic antagonists such as cyclizine or hyoscine.

Two cases that illustrate common presentations for vomiting in patients with advanced cancer are discussed below. The first case describes the difficulty in establishing the diagnosis of partial small bowel obstruction and shows the recurrent nature of this symptom complex. The second case typifies the patient with multiple contributing causes of nausea, vomiting, and pain and illustrates the need for a combined approach to symptom management.

### CASE DISCUSSION: ONE

#### Metastatic Colon Cancer

A 42-year-old man with widespread peritoneal and liver metastases from colon cancer presented to the emergency room after 48 hours of vomiting and severe abdominal pain. Past medical history was significant for enrollment in two prior chemotherapy protocols, each of which produced transient reduction in the size of measurable liver lesions and serum carcinoembryonic antigen (CEA). He was awaiting evaluation for a possible third experimental program when his symptoms progressed. On examination his abdomen was not distended, bowel sounds were active, and there was no focal tenderness. He had modest hepatomegaly and was not jaundiced. A surgical consultant obtained an abdominal radiograph that was negative. The patient was given oral analgesics and antiemetics and discharged home. He was readmitted 24 hours later with continued vomiting, abdominal pain, weakness, and profound dehydration. His abdominal exam remained unchanged. A nasogastric tube was placed for comfort and intravenous rehydration was begun. A transdermal fentanyl patch was applied for pain. Two days later his nausea had subsided and he tolerated clamping of the nasogastric tube. On the following day the tube was removed and he underwent a radiographic contrast evaluation of his upper GI tract. No areas of obstruction were identified. He was discharged on a full liquid diet, transdermal fentanyl patch, and prochlorperazine suppositories as needed. He began palliative chemotherapy and in 4 weeks a brief reduction in his CEA was noted. Two weeks later he developed midabdominal pain and nausea. Liver function tests were mildly abnormal. His fentanyl was increased. He developed vomiting and was unable to maintain enteral hydration. He was admitted for evaluation. His examination had not changed. An abdominal radiograph showed one air-fluid level but no definite signs of obstruction. Liver function tests were slightly worse. CEA had risen to its pretreatment value. The patient understood that further chemotherapy was futile and he elected comfort measures. Intravenous fluids were begun and the patient was given ice chips and sips of liquids for comfort. A trial of metoclopramide produced agitation and increased colicky abdominal pain. Severe abdominal pain occurred sporadically and appeared to be precipitated by oral intake. After a long discussion with the patient and his family he elected total parenteral nutrition via his Port-a-Cath, along with intravenous morphine provided through a patient-controlled pump. His colic subsided and he was able to tolerate an oral bowel regimen with infrequent supplementation by rectal medications or enemas. The clinical diagnosis was intermittent, partial small-bowel obstruction produced by diffuse peritoneal carcinomatosis and was deemed inoperable. A PEG tube was refused by the patient as his vomiting was infrequent (approximately once every 3 or 4 days with minimal oral intake). His pain was well managed with IV morphine, allowing good baseline function and rapid titration for his intermittent painful episodes. His family was pleased with his level of comfort and took him home with assistance from the visiting nurses and a home health care agency supervised by his oncology team. He lived for 6 weeks at home with his family. Terminally, he appeared to suffer an intraabdominal event with sepsis and died 2 days later.

This case typifies the presentation of patients with intraabdominal cancer who complain of intermittent nausea and vomiting. Knowledge of the extent of the patient's disease is very helpful in directing the workup. Review of the operative note at the patient's initial exploratory laparotomy confirmed extensive intraabdomi-

nal disease involving peritoneal surfaces, omentum, and the liver. Often the physical examination and plain radiographs belie the extent of this disease. Contrast studies may show only delayed evacuation. Significant ascites may be present, but it is the insidious progression of metastases along the bowel itself that produces a functional obstruction and intermittent symptoms. Colic was worsened by oral intake and prokinetic medication. Had the colic persisted, scopolamine might have been useful. If vomiting had increased, a PEG tube or octreotide would have been offered. The choice for total parenteral nutrition must be individualized. It is expensive, has risks, and requires cooperation by and training of the patient and family. In this young man it enabled him to participate in his family's activities and settle business until his demise.

## CASE DISCUSSION: TWO

### Metastatic Gastric Cancer

A 70-year-old woman with rapidly progressive metastatic gastric cancer to the liver was referred for hospice care. At diagnosis 6 months prior, the patient had undergone a partial gastrectomy for palliation of bleeding. Recent evaluation had shown diffuse liver metastases and elevated liver function tests. Because of abdominal pain the patient was given long-acting oral morphine, but over the previous 3 days she had developed nausea and vomiting. She described the episodes as unpredictable with large-volume emesis containing undigested food. On evaluation she rated her pain as severe (pain score: 8/10) and constant. Her last bowel movement was 6 days previously. On examination she appeared alert, cachectic, mildly jaundiced with tender hepatomegaly. Her rectal examination showed normal tone and impacted feces. She was assessed to have nausea and vomiting due to liver metastases and constipation. Her unrelieved pain and brief exposure to morphine were contributing causes. No laboratories were obtained.

For immediate pain control the patient was given parenteral hydromorphone 4 mg SC. Long-acting oxycodone 10 mg orally was begun 1 hour later and continued every 12 hours. Parenteral perchlorpromazine 10 mg IM was given. Once comfortable, disimpaction was performed followed by an enema with good results. She was given prescriptions for long-acting oxycodone and oxycodone liquid for breakthrough pain.

On the second day the patient was taking oxycodone 20 mg orally every 12 hours with 10 mg of oxycodone elixir every 4 hours as needed for breakthrough pain. She did not require more than one breakthrough dose. By the end of that day she described her pain control as generally good (pain score: 2/10). She did not require any additional antiemetics. She began a bowel regimen with senna and a stool softener every 12 hours and was instructed to take sorbitol 2 tablespoons every other day if she did not have a bowel movement.

This case illustrates how unrecognized constipation can become a "recipe for therapeutic disaster" (16). A patient develops severe pain and is given an opioid without attention to her baseline bowel function. Vomiting ensues from several possible causes and complicates her oral pain control. During the initial phases of assessment and formulation of a treatment plan the clinician must attend to her comfort: a disimpaction should be performed after her pain and vomiting have been treated. A plan is formulated to address pain and bowel function with oral medications, and antiemetics can be continued if needed. In this case, by the third day the patient's pain relief was described as usually good, and with subsequent regular bowel movements no further emesis was encountered. Initially morphine was discontinued, but it is not clear that morphine caused or contributed to the patient's nausea (64). The patient had little prior opiate experience and no known drug allergies. If indicated, morphine could be tried again in the future.

## SUMMARY

As the creation of this book attests, interest in supportive care for patients with cancer is burgeoning. Newer approaches to nausea and vomiting are likely and may come from technical or pharmaceutical advances. A long-acting preparation of somatostatin is available and is being evaluated in this setting. Further refinements to drug delivery can be expected. For now, in patients with advanced cancer but no preterminal disease, assessment and treatment of the cause of emesis may be appropriate. In preterminal patients or in those who require antiemetics, clinicians should be mindful of the most specific antiemetic directed at the cause of the patient's vomiting and apply the appropriate dose; symptoms that do not respond require reassessment and consideration of combination pharmacotherapy.

## REFERENCES

1. Baines M. Nausea and vomiting in the patient with advanced cancer. *J Pain Sympt Manage* 1988;3:81.
2. Reuben DB, Mor V, Hiris J. Clinical symptoms and length of survival in patients with terminal cancer. *Arch Intern Med* 1988;148:1586.
3. Coyle N, Adelhardt J, Foley KM, Portenoy RK. Character of terminal illness in the advanced cancer patient: pain and other symptoms during the last four weeks of life. J *Pain Sympt Manage* 1990; 5:83.
4. Hoskin PJ, Hanks GW. The management of symptoms in advanced cancer: experience in a hospital-based continuing care unit. *J R Soc Med* 1988;81:341.
5. Curtis EB. Common symptoms in patients with advanced cancer. *J Palliat Care* 1991;7:25.
6. Brescia FJ, Adler D, Gray G, Ryan MA, Cimino J, Mamtani R. Hospitalized advanced cancer patients: a profile. *J Pain Sympt Manage* 1990; 5:221.
7. Donnelly S, Walsh D. The symptoms of advanced cancer. *Semin Oncol* 1995;22:67.
8. Wachtel T, Allen-Masterson S, Reuben D, Goldberg R, Mor V. The end stage cancer patient: terminal common pathway. *Hosp J* 1988;4:43.
9. Bilgrami S, Fallon B. Chemotherapy-induced nausea and vomiting. *Postgrad Med* 1993;94:55.
10. Wang SC, Borison HL. A new concept of organization of the central emetic mechanism: recent studies of the sites of action of apomorphine, copper sulfate and cardiac glycerides. *Gastroenterology* 1952;22:1.
11. Borison HL. Anatomy and physiology of the chemoreceptor trigger zone and area postrema. In: Davis CJ, Lake-Bakaar CV, Grahame-Smith DG, eds. *Nausea and vomiting: mechanisms and treatment.* Berlin: Springer-Verlag, 1986;10.
12. Andrews PLR, Rappeport WG, Sanger GJ. Neuropharmacology of emesis induced by anti-cancer therapy. *Trends Pharmacol Sci* 1988;9: 334.
13. Twycross RG, Lack SA. *Control of alimentary symptoms in far advanced cancer.* London: Churchill Livingstone, 1986;166.
14. Bruera E, Catz Z, Hooper R, Lentle B, MacDonald N. Chronic nausea and anorexia in advanced cancer patients: a possible role for autonomic dysfunction. *J Pain Sympt Manage* 1987;2:19.
15. Levy MH. Constipation and diarrhea in cancer patients. *Cancer Bull* 1991;43:412.
16. Glare P, Lickiss JN. Unrecognized constipation in patients with advanced cancer: a recipe for therapeutic disaster. *J Pain Sympt Manage* 1992;7:369.
17. Lichter I. Results of antiemetic management in terminal illness. *J Palliat Care* 1993;9:19.
18. Lichter I. Which antiemetic? *J Palliat Care* 1993;9:42.
19. Krebs HB, Helmkamp BF. Management of intestinal obstruction in ovarian cancer. *Oncology* 1989;3:25.
20. Grunberg SM, Hesketh PJ. Control of chemotherapy-induced emesis. *N Engl J Med* 1993;329:1790.
21. Lederle FA, Busch DL, Mattox KM, West MJ, Aske DM. Cost-effective treatment of constipation in the elderly: a randomized double-blind comparison of sorbitol and lactulose. *Am J Med* 1990;89:597.
22. Bunn PA Jr, Ridgeway EC. Paraneoplastic syndromes. In: DeVita VT, Hellman S, Rosenberg SA, eds. *Cancer: principles and practice of oncology,* 4th ed. Philadelphia: JB Lippincott, 1993;2026.
23. Storey P. Symptom control in advanced cancer. *Semin Oncol* 1994; 21:748.
24. Nelson KA, Walsh TD, O'Donovan PB, Sheehan FG, Falk GW. Assessment of upper gastrointestinal motility in the cancer-associated dyspepsia syndrome (CADS). *J Palliat Care* 1993;9:27.
25. Shivshanker K, Bennett RW, Haynie TP. Tumor-associated gastroparesis: correction with metoclopramide. *Am J Surg* 1983;145:221.
26. Krasnow S, Vieras F, Smith J, et al. Gastric emptying (GE) in cancer patients. *ASCO Proc* 1990;9:326.
27. Kris MG, Yeh SDJ, Gralla RJ, Young DW. Symptomatic gastroparesis in cancer patients: a possible cause of cancer-associated anorexia that can be improved with oral metoclopramide. *ASCO Proc* 1985;4:267.
28. Nelson KA, Walsh TD. Metoclopramide in anorexia caused by cancer-associated dyspepsia syndrome (CADS). *J Palliat Care* 1993;9:14.
29. Bruera E, Macmillan K, Kuehn N, Hanson J, MacDonald RN. A controlled trial of megestrol acetate on appetite, caloric intake, nutritional status, and other symptoms in patients with advanced cancer. *Cancer* 1990;66:1279.
30. Picus D, Marx MV, Weyman PJ. Chronic intestinal obstruction: value of percutaneous gastrostomy tube placement. *Am J Radiol* 1988;150:295.
31. Marks WH, Perkal MF, Schwartz PE. Percutaneous endoscopic gastrostomy for gastric decompression in metastatic gynecologic malignancies. *Surg Gynecol Obstet* 1993;177:573.
32. Kadish SL, Kochman ML. Endoscopic diagnosis and management of gastrointestinal malignancy. *Oncology* 1995;9:967.
33. Vargo JJ, Germain MM, Swenson JA, Harrison CR. Ultrasound-assisted percutaneous endoscopic gastrostomy in a patient with advanced ovarian carcinoma and recurrent intestinal obstruction. *Am J Gastroenterol* 1993;88:1946.
34. Shike M. Percutaneous endoscopic stomas for enteral feeding and drainage. *Oncology* 1995;9:39.
35. Ventafridda V, Ripamonti C, Caraceni A, Spoldi E, Messina L, De Conno F. The management of inoperable gastrointestinal obstruction in terminal cancer patients. *Tumori* 1990;76:389.
36. Whelan TJ, Dembo AJ, Bush RS, et al. Complications of whole abdom-

inal and pelvic radiotherapy folowing chemotherapy for advanced ovarian cancer. *Int J Radiat Oncol Biol Phys* 1992;22:853.

37. Ketcham AS, Hoye RC, Pilch YH, Morton DL. Intestinal obstruction following treatment for cancer. *Cancer* 1970;25:406.

38. Walsh HPJ, Schofield PF. Is laparotomy for small bowel obstruction justified in patients with previously treated malignancy? *Br J Surg* 1984;71:933.

39. Osteen RT, Guyton S, Steele G, Wilson RE. Malignant intestinal obstruction. *Surgery* 1980;87:611.

40. Krebs HB, Goplerud DR. Mechanical intestinal obstruction in patients with gynecologic disease: a review of 368 patients. *Am J Obstet Gynecol* 1987;157:577.

41. Farias-Eisner R, Kim YB, Berek JS. Surgical management of ovarian cancer. *Semin Surg Oncol* 1994;10:268.

42. Zoetmulder FAN, Helmerhorst ThJM, Coevorden Fv, Wolfs PE, Leyer JPH, Hart AAM. Management of bowel obstruction in patients with advanced ovarian cancer. *Eur J Cancer* 1994;30A:1625.

43. Hogan WM, Boente MP. The role of surgery in the management of recurrent gynecologic cancer. *Semin Oncol* 1993;20:462.

44. Markman M. Is there a role for intraperitoneal therapy in the management of gastrointestinal malignancies? *Cancer Invest* 1995;13:625.

45. Drakes TP. Resolution of bowel obstruction due to newly diagnosed inoperable advanced ovarian cancer with medical therapy. *West J Med* 1991;155:76.

46. Anderson B. Quality of life in progressive ovarian cancer. *Gynecol Oncol* 1994;55:S151.

47. Ripamonti C, De Conno F, Ventafridda V, Rossi B, Baines MJ. Management of bowel obstruction in advanced and terminal cancer patients. *Ann Oncol* 1993;4:15.

48. Van Ooijen B, Van der Burg MEL, Planting ASTh, Siersema PD, Wiggers T. Surgical treatment or gastric drainage only for intestinal obstruction in patients with carcinoma of the ovary or peritoneal carcinomatosis of other origin. *Surg Gynecol Obstet* 1993;176:469.

49. Moertel CG, Schutt AJ, Reitemeier RJ, Hahn RG. Corticosteroid therapy of preterminal gastrointestinal cancer. *Cancer* 1974;33:1607.

50. Collins LS, Daly JM. Nutritional support in the cancer patient. In: MacDonald JS, Haller DG, Mayer RJ, eds. *Manual of oncologic therapeutics*, 3rd ed. Philadelphia: JB Lippincott, 1995;400.

51. Ciocon JO, Silverstone FA, Graver M, Foley CJ. Tube feedings in elderly patients. *Arch Intern Med* 1988;148:429.

52. Terepka AR, Waterhouse C. Metabolic observations during the forced feeding of patients with cancer. *Am J Med* 1956;20:225.

53. Ottery FD. Rethinking nutritional support of the cancer patient: the new field of nutritional oncology. *Semin Oncol* 1994;21:770.

54. McGeer AJ, Detsky AS, O Rourke K. Parenteral nutrition in patients receiving cancer chemotherapy. *Ann Intern Med* 1989;110:734.

55. August DA, Thorn D, Fisher RL, Welchek CM. Home parenteral nutrition for patients with inoperable malignant bowel obstruction. *J Parenter Enter Nutr* 1991;15:323.

56. Chapman C, Bosscher J, Remmenga S, Park R, Barnhill D. A technique for managing terminally ill ovarian carcinoma patients. *Gynecol Oncol* 1991;41:88.

57. Dean A, Bridge D, Lickiss JN. The palliative effects of octreotide in malignant disease. *Ann Acad Med* 1994;23:212.

58. Mercadante S, Maddaloni S. Octreotide in the management of inoperable gastrointestinal obstruction in terminal cancer patients. *J Pain Sympt Manage* 1992;7:496.

59. Mercadante S, Spoldi E, Caraceni A, Maddaloni S, Simonetti MT. Octreotide in relieving gastrointestinal symptoms due to bowel obstruction. *Palliat Med* 1993;7:295.

60. Mangilli G, Franchi M, Mariani A, Zanaboni F, et al. Octreotide in the management of bowel obstruction in terminal ovarian cancer. *Gynecol Oncol* 1996;61:345.

61. Reichlin S. Somatostatin. *N Engl J Med* 1983;24:1495.

62. Stiefel F, Morant R. Vapreotide, a new somatostatin analogue in the palliative management of obstructive ileus in advanced cancer. *Support Care Cancer* 1993;1:57.

63. Storey P, Hill Jr HH, St Louis RH, Tarver EE. Subcutaneous infusions for control of cancer symptoms. *J Pain Sympt Manage* 1990;5:33.

64. Walsh TD. Prevention of opioid side effects. *J Pain Sympt Manage* 1990;5:362.

*Principles and Practice of Supportive Oncology,*
edited by Ann Berger et al.
Lippincott–Raven Publishers, Philadelphia ©1998

# CHAPTER 13

# Diarrhea, Malabsorption, and Constipation

Sebastiano Mercadante

## DIARRHEA

A practical definition of diarrhea is lacking. Normally an average solid stool of 50–200 g/day is passed. It is formed of bacteria, nonabsorbed carbohydrates, water, electrolytes, and short chain fatty acids. The passage of more than 200 g/day of stool may be defined as diarrhea, although this definition is restricted because fecal weight, consistency, and form are correlated with dietary fiber intake. More than 200 g of stool a day may be produced in individuals consuming a diet rich in complex carbohydrates (1–3). Furthermore there are also wide normal variations in stool water content and total solid output. A passage of stool with a water content of more than 75% can be considered as diarrhea. More than an average of two bowel movements per day during a 3-day period is considered abnormal, although the upper limit of normal defecation frequency has not been definitively established. In turn, diarrhea is present when one of the following is present: abnormal increase in daily stool weight, water content, and frequency, whether or not accompanied by urgency, perianal discomfort, or incontinence (3).

Diarrhea is a common complication in the oncologic population; 4–10% of advanced cancer patients have been reported to suffer from this symptom (4–6). Although the influence on therapeutic outcome is not well established, its consequences may be severe. This includes loss of water, electrolytes, albumin, failure to reach nutritional goals, declining immune function, risk of bedsores, or systemic infection. Diarrhea also brings additional work for the nursing staff or family who have to prevent skin maceration and bedsores. Moreover, diarrhea is uncomfortable and adversely affects personal dignity. Diarrhea may lead to dehydration, resulting in asthenia, anorexia, weight loss, and drowsiness, all of which tend to diminish quality of life. Furthermore, dehydration will cause a shift in fluid compartments influencing drug pharmacokinetics, renal blood flow, and acid-base balance, often resulting in hypokalemia and acidosis from potassium and bicarbonate loss (7).

### Absorption and Secretion of Fluids and Electrolytes

Both fluid absorption and secretion are secondary to solute movement. Since diarrhea results from a disturbance in the normal flow and transport of intestinal fluids, the physiology of electrolyte transport and its coupling to fluid movement must be reviewed. The fluid load to the small intestine is large, approximately 7–9 l daily. It includes salivary, gastric, pancreatic, and biliary secretions in addition to the average oral fluid intake of about 2 l/day (1,3,8,9). Most electrolytes and water presented to the gut are absorbed in the small intestine via the enormous intestinal epithelial surface. In contrast to the colon, the small intestine has a limited concentration capacity and the fluid absorbed is isotonic. Absorptive and secretive processes are operative simultaneously. Varying degrees of permeability in different areas of intestinal epithelium may account for passive diffusion. The jejunal mucosa has a higher permeability and a lower resistance than that of the ileum and the colon. Chemical concentration gradients or electrical potential gradients are the forces responsible for generating passive electrolyte movement. A movement against the electrochemical concentration gradient requires an energy-dependent process. An active, carrier-mediated transport process results in sodium extrusion from the cell by Na-K-ATPase, permitting a low intracellular sodium concentration, electronegativity of the cell interior, and, as a consequence, an electrochemical concentration gradient to be maintained (2,3,8,10). Several secretagogues increase lumen negative electrical potential, determining the con-

S. Mercadante: Pain Relief and Palliative Care, SAMOT, 90143 Palermo, Italy.

ditions for sodium secretion. Active chloride secretion has been proposed, although details about the eventual mechanisms are lacking (8).

Only 1.5–2 l/day of fluid is presented to the colon. The colon extracts this amount leaving a mass of colonic bacteria and non-absorbable residue of about 100 g/day. The colon is more efficient in absorbing water and sodium than the small intestine. Moreover, it has a greater absorptive capacity than the small intestine. Diarrhea occurs when the fluid load presented to the colon exceeds 5 l daily (2,8).

The large intestine is characterized by relatively high mucosal resistance and low permeability. The colon differs from the small intestine by the absence of carriers for the transport of sugars and amino acids. Carbohydrates are not absorbed in the colon. On the contrary, these substances are degraded or utilized for protein synthesis by colonic anaerobic bacteria, resulting in short chain fatty acids that are rapidly absorbed across the epithelial membrane by nonionic diffusion or exchanged for bicarbonate. The inward movement of short chain fatty acids enhances sodium and chloride absorption in the colon (11).

A wide variety of chemical substances influence intestinal electrolyte transport (Table 1). Mechanical or chemical factors such as intestinal distention or toxigenic bacteria can directly influence transport tone, stimulating local nervous reflexes (8).

Different diets may mediate hormonal responses and, as a consequence, determine the course of absorption, digestion, or motor mechanisms in the gut. The feeding of rapidly absorbable nutrients causes a release of upper gut hormones including gastrin, insulin, cholecystokinin (CCK) pancreatic polypeptide, and somatostatin, whereas poorly absorbable fibers stimulate the release of distal gut hormones peptide YY (PYY) and enteroglucagon. Starvation causes the release of secretin and vasoactive

intestinal peptide (VIP) which may occur secondary to an increase in gastric acid secretion. Gastrin is capable of increasing absorption of carbohydrate and protein, whereas secretin inhibits jejunal absorption of water, sodium, and glucose. The products of fermentation, short chain fatty acids, stimulate the release of enteroglucagon and PYY (1,3,8,9).

Neural and endocrine factors exert a profound influence on intestinal electrolyte movement. $\alpha_2$-Receptor stimulation reduces secretion, uncoupling sodium–hydrogen exchange, affecting sodium chloride absorption in both the small and large intestine. Angiotensin can promote absorption due to the release of catecholamines.

Somatostatin controls intestinal secretion via a direct effect on enterocytes and an indirect effect on the enteric nerves. It prolongs intestinal transit time and stimulates active sodium chloride absorption. Moreover, somatostatin exerts an inhibitory effect on most neuroendocrine substances. The colon has the highest concentration of VIP, a potent colonic secretagogue and an important inhibitor of smooth muscle contraction (13). Noradrenaline inhibits the release of acetylcholine and VIP from secretomotor nerve fibers (12,14). Cholinergic neurotransmitters modulate both absorptive and secretory processes, probably by influencing intracellular calcium, resulting in inhibition of absorption and stimulating sodium and chloride secretion.

Glucocorticoids and mineralocorticoids regulate electroneural sodium chloride absorption, probably by stimulating Na-K-ATPase. Glucocorticoids increase net sodium and water absorption and potassium secretion (15). In the large intestine mineralocorticoids exert a greater effect than glucocorticoids by stimulating sodium absorption and potassium excretion. Sodium depletion stimulates aldosterone secretion, an important mechanism to compensate for dehydration. Patients with an ileostomy do not have this protective response (8). Moreover, glucocorticoids exert a powerful antiinflammatory effect. They inhibit the synthesis of eicosanoid precursors, known to be potent secretagogues (8,15,16). The arachidonic acid metabolites act as endocrine mediators. Their effects include the stimulation of intestinal secretion, probably acting on transcapillary fluid exchange, resulting in chloride secretion and an inhibition of sodium absorption.

### Intestinal Motility

Intestinal motility is an important factor that influences the absorption/secretion ratio. Intestinal motility allows the propulsion of intestinal contents from the stomach to the rectum. Postprandial intestinal motor activity maximizes absorption before the next meal, assuring the exposure of food to the jejunal epithelium and digestive secretions. Neural, myogenic, and endocrine systems influence propulsion, mediated by complex, repetitive, irregular,

**TABLE 1.** *Agents that stimulate intestinal secretion*

Bacterial toxins
Luminal contents
  Bile acids
  Long chain fatty acids (colon)
Neurotransmitters
  Acetylcholine
  Prostaglandins
  Serotonin
  Histamine
  Vasoactive intestinal peptide
  Neurotensin
  Cholecystokinin
  Secretin
  Bombesin
  Substance P
  Bradykinin
  Glucagon

and propulsive waves over very short distances, originating from the distal stomach, migrating and propelling the chyme slowly down the small intestine. This type of contraction allows for the breakdown of solids, the mixture of food with digestive juices, and increasing contact time with the epithelial surface (17).

During fasting, recurrent propulsive phases alternate with periods of quiescence, associated with changes in transport tone and bursts of intestinal secretion (3). These cyclic phenomenon are regulated by the intrinsic neural plexus but can be modulated by extrinsic nerves, hormones, and drugs. The intrinsic activity of the smooth muscle is modulated by extrinsic innervation from parasympathetic and sympathetic systems, acting either on smooth muscle cells or on the intrinsic neural system. Whereas the parasympathetic nerves increase contractions, the sympathetic nerves have an opposite effect. Cholinergic reflexes have been described in response to feeding and distention. Serotonin, identified in the myenteric plexus, stimulates intestinal contractions. Endogenous opiates act on both the intestinal smooth muscle and the myenteric plexus.

CCK is a physiologic mediator of intestinal and gallbladder motility. This pancreatic polypeptide does not act on intestinal smooth muscle but can modulate the activity of certain enteric neurons which are involved in the regulation of intestinal motility. Somatostatin inhibits intestinal motility, increasing the interval between migrating myoelectric complexes (12,16).

Enteroglucagon appears to act as a growth hormone for small intestine mucosa, but it also inhibits gastric emptying and small bowel transit. Peptide YY is a potent inhibitor of upper gastrointestinal (GI) motility and secretion. Some of its effects are mediated by an inhibition of cholecystokinin. Neurotensin increases the force of nonpropulsive contractions resulting in a substantial delay in intestinal transit. Galanin, a neuropeptide found in the myenteric plexus, exerts a profound inhibitory effect on gastric emptying and small bowel motility (16).

The terminal ileum exerts inhibitory effects on jejunal and gastric motility via a neurohormonal mechanism. Free fatty acids in the terminal ileum will delay intestinal transit by reducing the propagation of contractile activity. This effect is mediated by the release of ileal peptides, such as neurotensin, enteroglucagon, and PYY (16). Ileal peptides are also released after exposure to excessive loads of malabsorbed nutrients. Therefore, the terminal ileum is a fundamental site for the compensatory slowing of small bowel transit that must occur after intestinal resection. This mechanism is interrupted after ileal resection (17).

Colonic motility is mediated by local peristalsis, consisting of ring-like contractions. This motility pattern slows the transit of food, permitting the maximum absorption of water and electrolytes, favoring the activity of fermentative bacteria. Occasionally, a prolonged contraction is propagated toward the rectum. This phenomenon is associated with defecation. Colonic motility is regulated through the interrelationship between myogenic, neurogenic, and humoral factors, although the relative role of each factor has not been well described. The intermittent motor activity, stimulated by colonic distention, is determined by the balance between inherent myogenic activity and inhibitory intrinsic noncholinergic neural tone but can be modulated by activity of extrinsic sympathetic nerves and intrinsic cholinergic neurons. A large degree of inhibitory sympathetic tone mediated by $\alpha_2$-adrenoreceptors is prevalent in the proximal colon (13,18). Prevertebral and paravertebral ganglia may mediate input from the central nervous system or peripheral mechanoreceptors. The lumbar spinal cord seems to provide chronic neural inhibition to the colon. In fact lumbar spinal cord lesions cause an increased colon motility whereas high cord damage results in reduced colonic motility. Chronic neural inhibitory activity of the colon smooth muscle is mediated by the myenteric plexus. Several mediators have been identified to affect smooth muscle and to influence neural release of neurotransmitters. CCK, neurotensin, and substance P have prevalent excitatory effects while VIP appears to be part of the inhibitory limb of autoregulation (17).

In the colon, slow waves are generated by an intrinsic pacemaker. Superimposed spike potentials, similar to those observed in the small intestine, also occur. Moreover, oscillatory potentials initiate spike bursts that migrate distally. The proximal portion of the colon acts as a brake on the forward flow of luminal content allowing a longer mucosal exposure resulting in a more complete absorption of water and electrolytes. The luminal content is moved in a retrograde and anterograde direction by segmental nonpropulsive activity. Thus either increased or decreased colonic contractility may be associated with constipation (13).

After eating, spike activity is superimposed on the slow wave resulting in segmental contractions with an increase in colonic propulsive activity. Fat ingestion stimulates such spike activity, mediated by both the opioid and cholinergic nervous system. Dietary fiber increases the speed of GI transit, especially in the colon, depending on the physical characteristics of the fiber. Bile salts not reabsorbed within the ileum will stimulate colonic motility.

### Defecation

Continence is maintained by a tonically contracted sphincter. Defecation occurs when there is relaxation of the internal anal sphincter in response to rectal distention and relaxation, via voluntary control, of the external anal sphincter. The rectal distention reflex is composed of an afferent limb activated on the rectum, passing through the sacral spinal cord and terminating in the colon wall via an efferent pathway. This sensation of distention warns the person of the presence of material in the anal canal. Impulses to the cortex may initiate the mechanism for voluntary defecation involving increased intraabdominal pressure, relaxation of the pelvic floor, and relaxation of the external anal sphincter. Voluntary contraction of the external sphincter can inhibit defecation. The rectum adapts to its new volume and the stimulus is relieved. Striated musculature, including elevatoris ani, forms an anorectal ring moving forward and upward, providing a sphincter-like mechanism at the anorectal junction. Sensory innervation of the rectum derives from sacral parasympathetic fibers via the pelvic nerves. The external sphincter receives pudendal innervation whereas the internal anal sphincter has autonomic innervation. The sympathetic nerves induce contraction, whereas the parasympathetic nerves provide an inhibitory effect of the internal anal sphincter (17).

## Pathophysiology

All of the circumstances causing diarrhea in the general medical setting can be observed in cancer patients, although some clinical findings are specifically cancer-related (7). The colon absorbs about 1 l of fluid per day, but it is able to increase this capacity up to 4 l/day. After a meal, the intestinal inflow rate may temporarily exceed the absorptive capacity. However, diarrhea does not result because these periods are brief and the colon can hold excessive fluid due to its absorptive and motility properties. This margin of safety is reduced in the presence of small abnormalities in crucial segments of the gut, such as the ileocecal area. Diarrhea may result from many different causes, including the presence in the gut of unusual amounts of poorly absorbable osmotically active solutes, inhibition of ion absorption or stimulation of ion secretion, abnormal intestinal motility as well as exudation from sites of inflammation.

### Osmotic Diarrhea

Any nonabsorbable solute may alter the osmolarity of the luminal content. The osmolality of chyme will tend to move toward that of plasma. The proximal small bowel is highly permeable to sodium but not to solute, secreting water even after the osmolality values between luminal contents and plasma are similar. The ileum and colon have efficient active ion transport mechanisms to compensate for these losses, allowing them to reabsorb sodium and, as a consequence, water even against electrochemical gradients (3).

Carbohydrates and proteins are fermented by colonic bacteria and salvaged as short chain fatty acids and gases. When large amounts of lactulose (a nonabsorbable sugar) are ingested, the protective role of colonic bacteria, favoring the production of absorbable short chain fatty acids,

may be exhausted, resulting in severe diarrhea. An osmotic gap present in the stool, equivalent to the concentration of poorly absorbable solute, confirms the diagnosis. In osmotic diarrhea due to carbohydrate malabsorption, diarrhea is characterized by a low stool pH, due to the presence of short chain fatty acids, a high content of carbohydrates, high stool osmolality, and flatulence. A normal stool pH will be observed in osmotic diarrhea caused by ingestion of magnesium, sulfate, and poorly absorbed salts. Osmotic diarrhea is distinguished by the fact that diarrhea stops when the patient fasts (10).

### Secretory Diarrhea

Secretory diarrhea is caused by stimulation of active secretion that overwhelms the absorptive processes or by inhibition of normal fluid absorption. During changes in active secretion/absorption, other absorptive events such as glucose absorption and sodium pump function may continue normally as will permeability to large molecules. Stools are large in volume and watery, and diarrhea usually persists during periods of fasting.

The substances stimulating the intestine to secrete fluid act mostly via the enteric nervous system or through inflammatory processes, rather than directly on enterocytes. Secretory diarrhea persists in spite of limiting oral intake (3,7).

Endocrine tumors may cause diarrhea via the release of secretagogue transmitters. Small cell lung carcinoma, ganglioneuroma, pheochromocytoma, medullary carcinoma of thyroid, malignant carcinoids, or gastrinomas may cause copious intestinal secretion by liberating a host of substances (VIP, calcitonin, serotonin, bradykinin, substance P, prostaglandins, gastrin). Diarrhea is a common manifestation of the carcinoid syndrome, occurring in up to 70% of patients. Intestinal secretion seems to be mediated by serotonin and substance P. In medullary carcinoma of the thyroid, circulating calcitonin is the major mediator of intestinal secretion. In the Zollinger-Ellison syndrome, secretory diarrhea is the consequence of gastric hypersecretion caused by a high concentration of circulating gastrin, overwhelming the intestinal absorptive capacity. Ileal resection or a postvagotomy state may result in watery diarrhea from the secretory effect of malabsorbed bile acids on colonic mucosa. Malabsorption due to lymphatic obstruction or fibrosis induced by the tumor may contribute to diarrhea (19).

Bacterial enterotoxins induce secretion by a local nervous reflex mediated by enteroendocrine cells. The damage to intestinal epithelium induces an inflammatory response enhancing the cyclooxygenase pathway and the release of prostaglandins, which are potent secretagogues (3,4). This condition is frequently observed in intestinal damage induced by chemotherapy (e.g., 5-fluorouracil) or radiotherapy (20,21). Acute radiation enteritis usually occurs within the initial few weeks of treatment (22,23).

The main mechanism of diarrhea is the interference with absorption due to mucosal damage. Disturbances in motility due to damage of the muscularis propria may also contribute to radiation-induced diarrhea (10).

*Clostridium difficilis,* an anaerobic organism producing an enteric toxin, is a common cause of pseudomembranous enterocolitis, which presents as a severe microbial diarrhea, typically during or following antibiotic administration (3).

Secretory diarrhea is frequently caused by drugs, including diuretics, caffeine, theophylline, antacids, antibiotics, and poorly absorbable osmotically active laxative agents.

### Deranged Motility

Rapid colonic transit is associated with an increased stool weight. Dysmotility can provoke diarrhea even though the epithelial absorptive function remains intact. This is probably due to the reduced exposure time, limiting adequate absorption of chyme into epithelial cells. This can be observed in patients who have a postgastrectomy dumping syndrome or who are postvagotomy, patients who have had an ileocecal valve resection, or those with malignant carcinoid syndrome, medullary carcinoma of the thyroid, or diabetic neuropathy (24).

Diminished colonic motility may also promote bacterial growth, inducing deconjugation of bile acids, resulting in diarrhea. Whereas a complete intestinal obstruction produces irreversible constipation, a partial obstruction often presents as alternating diarrhea and constipation. A rectal or colonic neoplasm may cause a partial intestinal obstruction with an increase in mucus or blood secretion.

An iatrogenic autonomic neuropathy may follow a celiac plexus block, an antalgic procedure used in visceral abdominal cancer pain. Sympathetic denervation of the bowel from this procedure may leave cholinergic innervation unopposed, leading to an increase in intestinal motility and diarrhea. This phenomenon is generally self-limiting (25,26). Diarrhea secondary to dysmotility disorders generally stops after a 1- or 2-day fast.

### Assessment

Stool frequency, quantity, and consistency should be carefully described and recorded along with dietary habits, alcohol consumption, food intolerances, and any history of food allergies. A complete history of antineoplastic treatment, especially any abdominal or pelvic radiation, should be recorded. When the stools are consistently large, light in color, watery or greasy, free of blood or contain undigested food particles, the underlying disorder is likely to be in the small bowel or proximal colon. Diarrhea consisting of small stools that are dark in color, often containing mucus or blood, associated with a sense of urgency, is typical for disorders of the left colon or rectum (3). Tenesmus, the presence of little or no stool despite a sense of rectal urgency, generally indicates a problem in the rectum. A complete physical examination may reveal important clues regarding the origin of the diarrhea, including an abdominal mass, fever, postural hypotension, lymphadenopathy, ascites, abdominal distention, or deteriorated nutritional status (27). When there is sudden diarrhea after a period of constipation, the possibility of a partial obstruction should be raised.

Rectal examination and abdominal palpation should be performed to look for a fecal mass/fecal impaction and intestinal obstruction. Fecal impaction may present as apparent diarrhea because only liquids can bypass a partial obstruction.

Watery diarrhea is often caused by microbial agents. Fever and abdominal tenderness may or may not be present in viral bacterial enteritis. Gram stain and stool culture can help diagnose the presence of *Staphylococcus, Campylobacter,* or *Candida* infection. Multiple stool cultures should be obtained from patients with secretory diarrhea to exclude microorganisms that produce enterotoxins which stimulate intestinal secretion (2,3,11).

An anion gap of more than 50 mmol/l (due to the reduction of stool sodium and potassium) is observed in osmotic diarrhea, whereas a value of <50 mmol/l seems to indicate a secretory diarrhea, a characteristic of endocrine tumors (3). Osmotic diarrhea typically stops or reduces after fasting or stopping the offending drug, whereas secretory diarrhea persists in spite of fasting. In fact, secretory diarrhea usually has nothing to do with food consumption; rather, it is due to abnormal ion transport. A positive stool guaiac test raises the suspicion of an exudative mechanism, such as radiation colitis, colonic neoplasm, or infectious diarrhea.

Secretory diarrhea combined with upper GI symptoms caused by refractory peptic ulcer disease is suggestive of a gastrin-secreting tumor. High circulating serotonin levels in the carcinoid syndrome will cause other symptoms besides diarrhea, including hypotension, sweating, flushing, palpitation, and bronchospasm (3,12). The association of heat intolerance, palpitations, and weight loss suggests possible hyperthyroidism (12).

### Treatment

Current medication should be reviewed, with special attention to the use of laxatives, antacids, theophylline preparations, central nervous system drugs, antiarrhythmics, and antibiotics. Clinical signs of dehydration suggest the need for intensive hydration by the intravenous route, especially in patients suffering from nausea and vomiting (7,28). However, in the majority of cases, oral dietary therapy will provide effective symptom management. Oral hydration solutions containing glucose, electrolytes, and water are the simplest treatments to administer. Adding glucose to electrolyte solutions takes advantage of the presence of the small intestinal sodium-glucose cotransporter to promote increased water and sodium absorption. Addition of complex carbohydrates, rather than monomeric forms, improves water and electrolyte absorption (9).

A gluten-free diet can reduce abdominal cramping and bowel movement frequency in the presence of intestinal fermentation. Binders of osmotically active substances (kaolin-pectin) give a thicker consistency to loose stools, producing a viscous colloidal absorbent solution, but their antidiarrheal effectiveness is disputable. Peeled apples are particularly rich in pectin (27). Other dietary manipulations include avoiding cold meals, milk, vegetables rich in fibers, fatty meat and fish, coffee, and alcohol.

Simethicone, a defoaming antiflatulent, is helpful for gas-related symptoms, reducing intestinal distention due to fermentation. $H_2$-receptor antagonists and bile acid–binding resins may be effective in controlling diarrhea due to ileal surgery (12). Cholestyramine has been effectively used in radiation-induced diarrhea. Aspirin has been reported to be effective in post-radiotherapy diarrhea by reducing prostaglandin synthesis (2,3). Steroids may be effective for radiation enteritis and in reducing edema in intestinal pseudo-obstruction. Furthermore, steroids can reduce hormone secretion in certain endocrine tumors, promoting salt and water absorption (3).

Antibiotic-associated diarrhea (pseudomembranous enterocolitis) requires the discontinuation of antibiotics and the use of either metronidazole or vancomycin. Antibiotic-associated diarrhea often subsides spontaneously after stopping the antibiotics. Bismuth subsalicylate, in doses of 30–60 ml every 30 minutes for eight doses, may bring mild symptomatic relief in patients with acute infectious diarrhea (10).

Clonidine, an $\alpha_2$ agonist, has been reported useful in controlling diarrhea in diabetic patients or in patients with chronic idiopathic secretory diarrhea. The increase in salt and water absorption seen with clonidine is probably due to an interaction with enterocyte receptors and the suppression of secretory transmitter release. However, hypotension and sedation may limit the usefulness of clonidine in advanced cancer patients (7).

### Opioids

Opioids are commonly used for their antidiarrheal properties. The site of action appears to be neuronal rather than muscular. Opioid receptors are represented at different sites, including smooth muscle, myenteric plexus, spinal cord, and brain. Their activation influences intestinal motility and, as a consequence, secretion. Although a central action cannot be excluded, only peripheral mechanisms have been confirmed. Antidiar-

rheal effects can be obtained by both oral and parenteral opioids. Opioids increase ileocecal tone, decrease small intestine and colon peristalsis (increasing electrolyte and water absorption), impair the defecation reflex by inhibiting anorectal sphincteric relaxation, and they diminish anorectal sensitivity to distention. The contact time between intestinal mucosa and luminal contents is enhanced by the reduction of colonic propulsive activity, resulting in a greater fluid absorption (27).

Opioid-like agents, including codeine, morphine, diphenoxylate, and loperamide, represent the best known drugs for the symptomatic treatment of diarrhea. In patients presenting with diarrhea who are already taking codeine or morphine with adequate pain relief, drowsiness and other side effects can result from an increased dosage. Loperamide is able to reduce ileal calcium fluxes, with an activity independent from the opioid effect, and does not cross the blood–brain barrier, whereas diphenoxylate rarely reaches significant opioid effects at a clinical dosage. Loperamide induces a long-lasting stimulation of colonic motility associated with a disorganization of cyclic motor activity, enhancing nonpropulsive contraction in the small intestine and the colon. The effects on the colon are probably mediated by a local mechanism. Loperamide shows the highest antidiarrheal/analgesic ratio among the opioid-like agents. It is the antidiarrheal drug of first choice due to its few adverse effects; the dosage can be titrated to effect (up to 12 mg/day or more). Of note, opiate drugs may cause a paradoxical diarrhea secondary to fecal impaction (5,27).

### Octreotide

Octreotide, an analog of somatostatin with a more favorable pharmacokinetic profile, exerts a wide range of physiologic effects on the GI tract. It suppresses many of the gut peptides implicated in the control of secretory and motor activity. Octreotide induces the appearance of migrating myoelectric complexes characteristic of the fasting state and reduces the duration and vigor of postprandial motility. Data from several clinical trials suggest that this anti-secretory agent may be useful in the symptomatic treatment of diarrhea refractory to other medications. The mechanism is probably multifactorial. Octreotide reduces splanchnic blood flow; inhibits exocrine secretions from the stomach, pancreas, and small intestine; impairs GI motility; and facilitates water and electrolyte absorption. The increased net absorption of water and salts mainly reflects decreased secretion (12,26).

Octreotide has the ability to reduce the plasma concentration of, and the postprandial responses to, many gut peptides. Several cases of a favorable response to octreotide in both early and late dumping syndrome have been reported. The effect of octreotide on both GI transit time and hormone release appears to contribute to the benefits observed in patients with the dumping syndrome (29,30).

Octreotide seems to be an effective agent in the management of chemotherapy-related diarrhea (fluorouracil) and is more effective than loperamide (21). Octreotide has been shown to be an effective and well-tolerated treatment in patients with secretory diarrhea. Its efficacy extends from specific disease control, as in the neuroendocrine tumors, to widespread inhibition of secretion in a range of conditions irrespective of etiology. Octreotide can help control diarrhea due to carcinoid tumors, VIPoma, gastrinoma, and small cell lung cancer, although the hormonal responses to the somatostatin analog do not always parallel clinical responses, probably related to the effects of cosecreted peptides (12). Finally, octreotide has been proved effective in the treatment of diarrhea induced by celiac plexus block, as well as diabetic diarrhea (14,31).

## MALABSORPTION

The term of malabsorption refers to an ineffective absorption of breakdown products in the small intestine. A sound knowledge of normal absorptive processes allows the physician to pursue a logical approach to the diagnosis and treatment of the cancer patient with malabsorption.

Pancreatic secretion of lipase, amylase, and proteases breaks down fat to monoglycerides and fatty acids, carbohydrates to mono and disaccharides, and proteins to peptides and amino acids. Absorption is the passage of these products of digestion from the lumen through the enterocyte to appear in the lymphatics or the portal vein. Several processes are involved in absorption. Active transport requires energy to move nutrients against a gradient, whereas passive diffusion allows nutrients to pass according to gradient differentials. Facilitated diffusion is an intermediate mechanism, similar to passive diffusion, but carrier-mediated and subject to competitive inhibition. Endocytosis is a process in which parts of a cell membrane engulf nutrients.

The simple diffusion of monosaccharides across membranes is slow but important in the presence of high luminal concentrations of glucose. Specific active transport systems, especially via sodium-coupled transporters, mediate efficient transport of these substances when luminal concentrations of glucose are low. Monosaccharides may also enter enterocytes by facilitated diffusion. The uptake of lactose is limited by lactase activity. Xylose is not digested and has a low affinity for carriers.

Carbohydrate absorption occurs predominantly in the proximal small intestine, although not all dietary carbohydrate is absorbed. Some carbohydrates reach the colon and are fermented by bacteria into short chain fatty acids with production of gases, such as hydrogen and methane. Short chain fatty acids are subsequently absorbed by colonic epithelial cells.

Several processes have been recognized to facilitate the absorption of fat from the aqueous luminal environment, including emulsification, enzymatic hydrolysis, dispersion, diffusion, absorption, and intracellular metabolism. Triglycerides are emulsified together with phospholipids, bile salts, and mono- and diglycerides and dispersed into a variety of phases and particles. Lipid digestion by lingual lipase, active at low pH, begins in the mouth and in the stomach promoting emulsion stability and facilitating the action of pancreatic lipases. Gastric and pyloric motility further promote emulsification of lipids. This effect is amplified by bile salts and biliary phospholipids, which also influence the absorption of cholesterol and sterol vitamins. Lipolysis to fatty acids and monoglycerides is mediated by pancreatic lipases.

Fat products rapidly diffuse passively into enterocytes, with the rate of transfer depending on the chain length. Fatty acids and monoglycerides are metabolized into triglycerides and assembled with phospholipids and cholesterol esters into chylomicrons. Short and medium chain fatty acids have a less complex absorptive mechanism. They may be absorbed intact by passive diffusion or completely hydrolyzed, but they are not reesterified inside the enterocytes. Lipid absorption is highly efficient; only small amounts of lipids enter the colon. These may be absorbed by the colonic mucosa or undergo bacterial metabolism.

Bile salts are synthesized from cholesterol in the liver, conjugated with amino acids, secreted into the bile, and recycled back to the liver via the portal system. Minimal daily losses are balanced by hepatic synthesis. Passive diffusion and active transport are involved in bile salt transport in the small intestine to limit fecal loss. A certain amount of bile salt in the colonic lumen is essential for normal colonic function. In the colon, bile salts are not absorbed but they stimulate colonic motility and secretion of NaCl and water. In contrast bile salt deficiency may cause constipation.

Protein digestion begins in the stomach. Acid denaturation prepares proteolysis. Proteolytic enzymes, endopeptidases activated by an acid environment, cleave the internal bonds of large proteins to form nonabsorbable peptides. Pancreatic peptidases convert proteins and polypeptides into amino acids and oligopeptides. After hormonal or neural stimulation, proenzymes are released by the pancreas. Enteropeptidases and trypsin activate a cascade of events that promote the activation of chymotrypsin, elastase, carboxypeptidase A and B, and colipases in the duodenum. Amino acids are absorbed by enterocytes, oligopeptides are digested by the enterocyte, brush border by oligo- or dipeptidases. A specific transport mechanism exists for the intracellular transport of amino acids and dipeptides. Protein absorption is efficient and mainly occurs in the jejunum and ileum (11,19).

## Pathophysiology

Different sequential stages of digestion and absorption may be affected in the cancer patient resulting in malabsorption. The series of events includes the reduction of particle size, the solubilization of hydrophobic lipids and the enzymatic digestion of nutrients to small fragments, the absorption of the products of digestion across the intestinal cells, and the transport via lymphatics.

1. In the *intraluminal stage,* the hydrolysis of fat, protein, and carbohydrate by pancreatic enzymes, as well as solubilization of fat by bile salts, may be altered by several conditions (19). In pancreatic carcinoma or following pancreatic resection, decreased pancreatic enzyme and bicarbonate release may limit the digestion of fat and protein, leading to pancreatic insufficiency. These disorders may also be associated with malabsorption of fat-soluble vitamins. The Zollinger-Ellison syndrome is characterized by an extreme acid hypersecretion causing a low luminal pH, inactivating pancreatic enzymes with consequent fat malabsorption. A decrease in intraluminal bile salts due to disruption of the enterohepatic circulation is also seen in patients with Zollinger-Ellison syndrome. Biliary tract obstruction, terminal ileal resection, or cholestatic liver disease result in decreased bile salts formation or delivery to the duodenum. With limited small bowel resections, malabsorbed bile acids pass into the colon, decreasing water and electrolyte absorption, resulting in diarrhea. In massive small bowel resection, steatorrhea is caused by a diminished bile acid pool from increased intestinal bile salts loss, together with loss of the absorptive intestinal surface and bacterial overgrowth.

Many postsurgical disorders have been associated with a marked proliferation of intraluminal microorganisms including an afferent loop of a Billroth II partial gastrectomy, a surgical blind loop with end-to-side anastomosis, or a recirculating loop with side-to-side anastomosis. Other causes of bacterial overgrowth include obstruction or strictures, autonomic neuropathy, and resection of the ileocecal valve. All of these conditions cause malabsorption by changing the intraluminal environment of the proximal small intestine so that it more closely resembles the colon. Bacterial overgrowth competes with the human host for nutrients causing catabolism of carbohydrates by gram-negative aerobes, deconjugation of bile salts by anaerobes, and the binding of cobalamin by anaerobes (11).

2. The *intestinal stage* includes the hydrolysis of carbohydrates; the epithelial transport of monosaccharides, monoglycerides, and fatty acids, small peptides, and amino acids; as well as the formation of chylomicrons in the epithelial cells. Abnormalities of the small intestinal mucosa or impairment of epithelial cell transport may be seen with radiation enteritis. The pathologic changes from radiation enteritis occur in three phases. During and immediately after irradiation, abnormal epithelial cell proliferation, maturation, and inflammatory cell infiltration occur. An acute vasculopathy coincides in time with the period of maximal epithelial cell damage. Vascular changes may be progressive, even after the resolution of the acute epithelial changes. Subsequently, the intestinal mucosa regenerates to a variable extent depending on the vascular damage. Extensive fibrosis, strictures, and fistulae, with disruption of the mucosal surface, may develop resulting in a chronically inflamed bowel with impairment of mucosal function. Moreover, severe adhesions may develop between loops of intestine leading to the formation of fistulous tracts between adjacent bowel loops. Extensive mucosal damage, lymphatic obstruction, and bacterial overgrowth are the principal mechanisms of radiation-induced malabsorption (23).

Extensive surgical resection of the small intestine also reduces the epithelial surface area available for absorption. The extent and specific level of resection are predictive of severe malabsorption and short bowel syndrome. Most patients with short bowel syndrome either have a high jejunostomy with a residual jejunal length of <100 cm or a jejunocolic anastomosis (32). Resection of more than 50% of the small intestine usually results in significant malabsorption. The inclusion of the distal two thirds of the ileum and ileocecal sphincter in the resected section increases the risk of malabsorption. Enterostomy or intestinal fistulae may also result in a reduced absorption due to the loss of intestinal surface area. Preservation of the ileocecal sphincter is important because it may prevent small bowel contamination from colonic flora and may increase the transit time of the intraluminal content.

Hyperoxaluria may occur in patients with severe steatorrhea after ileal resection. This is attributable to excessive quantities of bowel fatty acids, forming soaps with calcium and reducing the formation of insoluble nonabsorbable calcium oxalate. As a consequence, increased absorption may result in calcium oxalate urinary tract stones. This problem does not exist in patients with enterostomies because the absorption of calcium oxalate occurs in the colon (32). Ileal resection may further lead to malabsorption secondary to loss of ileocolic absorptive capacity for sodium and chloride (33). Large or carbohydrate-rich meals precipitate this motility disturbance, limiting adequate absorption. The recovery from massive small bowel resection depends on the adaptive response of the remaining mucosa.

3. *Lymphatic transport* of chylomicrons and proteins is limited by lymphatic obstruction, leading to dilatation and potential rupture of intestinal lymphatic vessels causing intestinal leakage of proteins, chylomicrons, and

small lymphocytes. Localized ileal tumors, diffuse intestinal lymphomas, metastatic carcinoma, and metastatic carcinoid disease may all lead to lymphatic obstruction, fat malabsorption, and protein-losing enteropathy.

## Assessment

Patients with malabsorption syndrome generally suffer from diarrhea, weight loss, and malnutrition. The stools are bulky, greasy, and malodorous. Documentation of steatorrhea is the cornerstone of the diagnostic evaluation, although quantitative fecal fat is a cumbersome test for many cancer patients. Specific tests of digestion and absorption are usually not necessary in cancer patients.

Certain physical signs are frequently associated with specific deficiency states secondary to malabsorption, such as glossitis in folate or vitamin $B_{12}$ deficiency, hyperkeratosis, ecchymoses, and hematuria due to fat-soluble vitamin deficiency (vitamins A and K). Anemia (chronic blood loss or malabsorption of iron, folate, or vitamin $B_{12}$), leukocytosis with eosinophilia, low serum levels or albumin, iron, cholesterol, and an extension of the prothrombin time are the most common laboratory findings in malabsorption (11,21). Impaired absorption of Ca and Mg may induce weakness, paresthesias, and tetany. Osteopenia and bone pain, spontaneous fractures, and vertebral collapse may develop from vitamin D and calcium deficiency. Peripheral neuropathy may occur after gastric resection due to vitamin $B_{12}$ deficiency. Weakness, severe weight loss, and fatigue result from caloric deprivation. In pancreatic carcinoma, floating, bulky, and malodorous stools and increased gas production are often associated with anorexia. Steatorrhea, peripheral lymphocytopenia, hypoalbuminemia, chylous ascites, and peripheral edema are the hallmarks of abnormalities of lymphatic transport. Symptoms of dumping syndrome after gastrectomy include early nausea, abdominal distention, weakness, and diarrhea after a meal, followed by hypoglycemia, sweating, dizziness, and tachycardia.

Reviewing current drugs is important in the diagnostic evaluation. Colchicine, neomycin, and clindamycin are the most common drugs causing malabsorption, although the pathophysiologic mechanisms are unknown. Dietary phosphate absorption may be limited by use of aluminum-containing antacids, resulting in hypophosphatemia and hypercalciuria.

Small intestinal barium x-rays may define anatomic abnormalities after massive resection. Biochemical examination of the fecal material may give information about the origin of a fistula (pancreatic or enteric). Liver function tests and imaging of the liver or biliary tract may demonstrate parenchymal liver disease as a cause of decreased production of bile salts or a biliary tract obstruction.

## Treatment

After assessing the causes of malabsorption, therapy should be directed to correct the deficiencies including enzyme replacement, bicarbonate supplements, vitamins, calcium, magnesium, and iron. Pancreatic enzyme replacement along with a low-fat, high-protein diet is indicated in the case of malabsorption due to pancreatic insufficiency. The effectiveness of enzyme replacements is variable and, in part, depends on a high enough gastric pH to prevent their degradation in the stomach (4,34). Large doses of pancreatic extract are required with each meal. Sodium and bicarbonate are mainly added to raise the duodenal pH.

Fat intake should be strictly limited, especially in short bowel syndrome. Medium chain triglycerides may be substituted for long chain triglycerides to improve fat absorption after a small intestinal resection, and they are useful in the presence of lymphatic obstruction because they do not require intestinal lymphatic transport (35).

For patients with prominent dumping, dietary modification comprising frequent small, dry meals that are high in protein and low in carbohydrates, along with ingestion of substances that prolong the absorption of carbohydrates such as pectin, may be useful (7).

In the presence of severe malnutrition and dehydration, aggressive measures should be undertaken, especially after surgery. Parenteral nutrition is essential in the immediate postoperative period after massive intestinal resection. The duration of parenteral nutrition that will be necessary is inversely proportional to the length of the remaining intestine. The weaning to oral nutrition depends on several variables including the preoperative nutritional state, the absorptive deficit, and the tolerance to oral intake. Oral feeding should be initiated as soon as possible. Adaptation to resection has been demonstrated by an increase in the mass of the remaining bowel due to enlargement of the remaining villi and an increase in the number of absorptive cells. This absorptive function improves with time and is strictly dependent on the early introduction of oral nutrients (32). There is also evidence that $H_2$-blocking agents favorably influence the rate of adaptation of remaining intestine after massive resection, possibly by a mucosal trophic effect improving nutrient absorption. Moreover, intraluminal nutrients stimulate trophic GI hormones. Nutrients requiring minimal digestion for absorption should be chosen, such as commercial preparations containing simple sugars, amino acids, or oligopeptides, as well as medium chain triglycerides. An excessive osmolar load should be avoided by diluting hypertonic solutions. More complex food should be added gradually.

Vitamin $B_{12}$ replacement is necessary after terminal ileal resection. $H_2$ blockers are used to treat the transient acid hypersecretion after extensive bowel resection. Large doses of $H_2$-receptor antagonists reverse the acid hypersecretion state in patients with gastrinoma (Zollinger-Ellison syndrome) (11). Omeprazole inhibits the hydrogen-potassium proton pump and produces a greater antisecretory effect than that achieved by $H_2$-antagonist drugs alone (34). A low-oxalate diet and a high urinary volume are helpful to prevent the formation of urinary tract stones. The use of cholestyramine should be carefully examined. While it is indicated in limited resections because it binds bile salts and prevents their irritant effects on the colon, in short bowel syndrome after massive resection it may reduce the bile salt pool, increasing fat malabsorption. Cholestyramine has been favorably used in radiation-induced malabsorption (23). The dose suggested is 4 g three times daily before meals. Aluminum hydroxide exerts similar effects.

Antibiotic-associated malnutrition requires discontinuation of any implicated antimicrobial agents. However, if there is stasis with bacterial overgrowth caused by impaired motility or stricture, such as in radiation enteritis or blind loop syndrome, broad-spectrum antibiotics should be administered. A 10-day course of a cephalosporin and metronidazole seems to be effective in suppressing the flora and correcting malabsorption. However, cyclic therapy may be needed (36).

Pharmacological treatment of patients affected by malabsorption with short bowel syndrome aims at reducing intestinal output or transit time. Antidiarrheal agents such as codeine and loperamide may delay the transit time or reduce secretions (37). Somatostatin and, more recently, its derivative octreotide have been used because of their ability to reduce gastric, pancreatic, and biliary secretions. They also reduce intestinal transit time. Somatostatin and octreotide therapy have both been associated with the spontaneous closure of GI fistulae. However, somatostatin has a very short half-life, which makes it essential to give the drug as a continuous intravenous infusion. Octreotide possesses the same spectrum of effects as somatostatin but is more potent, has a long half-life, has less influence on insulin secretion than somatostatin, and, above all, can be administered by the subcutaneous route (26). Dosages from 0.2 to 0.6 mg daily have been advocated. It may reduce or shorten the use of parenteral administration in several postoperative conditions such as enterocutaneous or pancreatic fistulae (37–40). Its use has been favorably reported in terminally ill patients (26,41).

Reversal of a short segment of the bowel or construction of a recirculating loop have been advocated in patients with life-threatening malabsorption and uncontrolled weight loss. However, such operations may lead to stasis and bacterial overgrowth, and may further compromise intestinal absorption. More often than not, these procedures fail to provide significant benefit (42).

## CONSTIPATION

Constipation is an extremely common problem among cancer patients. Understanding the mechanisms of constipation is plagued by the highly variable definition of constipation. The term may have different meanings for different people. Perception of constipation is defined in rank order as straining, hard stools; the desire but inability to defecate; infrequent stools; and abdominal discomfort. Stool weight and consistency are unreliable parameters because of the wide range in normal subjects (43). Stool frequency is typically the most common parameter considered. A frequency of at least three bowel movements per week is viewed as an objective indicator of normalcy. However, frequency per se may not be of much concern to people. Differences in race and gender have been reported; whites and males defecate more frequently than blacks and women, respectively. Depending on the definition, the prevalence of constipation ranges from 5% to 20% in the normal population and occurs in more than 50% of patients referred to a palliative care service (27,44,45).

### Pathophysiology

As a symptom, constipation may be indicative of many diseases. A differential diagnosis should be considered as would be done for any other symptom in the cancer patient (Table 2). In cancer patients, constipation may be secondary to systemic diseases or those solely afflicting the GI tract. It may be directly due to a cancer or to secondary effects of the cancer. Many drugs used by cancer patients may induce constipation. In Table 2 the most frequent causes of constipation are listed.

Constipation is frequently noted by patients with various motor disorders. A visceral neuropathy seems to be present in the majority of patients with severe slow transit constipation. Disturbance in the extrinsic nerve supply to the colon has been found in these patients along with a lack of inhibitory innervation of colonic circular muscle and a diminished release of acetylcholine (13).

Patients with advanced cancer frequently complain of GI symptoms including anorexia, chronic nausea, and early satiety—a symptom complex often associated with physical signs of an autonomic neuropathy. Autonomic neuropathy may also be manifested as severe constipation, including postural hypotension and resting tachycardia. It is a multifactorial syndrome and malnutrition, decreased activity, diabetes, and drugs, such as vinca alkaloids, opioids, and tricyclic antidepressants, are all possible causative factors (46).

**TABLE 2.** *Causes of constipation in cancer patients*

**Neurogenic disorders:**

Periphery: Ganglionopathy
               Autonomic neuropathy

CNS: Spinal cord lesions
               Parkinson's disease

**Metabolic and endocrine diseases:**

Diabetes
Uremia
Hypokalemia
Hypothyroidism
Hypercalcemia
Pheocromocytoma
Enteric glucagon excess

**Malignancy:**

Direct effects:
     Cerebral or spinal cord tumors
     Intestinal obstruction
     Hypercalcemia

Secondary effects:
     Inadequate food intake and low-fiber diet
     Dehydration
     Reduced activity
     Previous bowel surgery
     Autonomic neuropathy
     Radiotherapy

**Drugs:**

Opioids
NSAIDs
Anticholinergics
Anticonvulsants
Antidepressants
Diuretics
Antacids
Anti-Parkinson drugs
Antihypertensive agents
Vinca alkaloids

Diabetic dysmotility has traditionally been thought to reflect a generalized autonomic neuropathy. However, secretions of GI hormones may also be important. Decreased amounts of substance P in the rectal mucosa of constipated diabetic patients has been thought to contribute to the pathogenesis of diabetic constipation (47).

Peripheral neuropathy is a common complication of cancer chemotherapy, particularly after the use of regimens containing the vinca alkaloids vincristine or vindesine. These drugs have been shown to cause symptoms of autonomic polyneuropathy with constipation, bladder atony, and hypotension. Whereas many reports describe the acute neurologic side effects during therapy, little is known about persistent and late damage to the peripheral nervous system. The long-term neurologic side effects in patients with curable malignancies, such as Hodgkin's disease and testicular cancer, may be particularly troublesome. Patients receiving a high cumulative dose of vincristine or cisplatin seem to be at a significantly elevated risk for the development of long-term side effects (48).

The rectosigmoid junction is a key area in the mechanism of constipation. Rectal outlet obstruction and failure of the puborectalis and anal sphincter muscles to relax are frequent findings in patients with neurologic diseases with intractable constipation. Several mechanisms of constipation by outlet obstruction are possible, including a hyperactive rectosigmoid junction, an increased storage capacity of the rectum, spasticity and hypertonicity of the anal canal with incoordination of the reflex between rectum and anus. Anismus is a spastic pelvic floor syndrome, recently termed "rectosphincteric dyssynergia," for its similarity with vesicourethral dyssynergia. Similar extrinsic innervation of the bladder and the rectum has been observed, explaining why patients with severe slow transit constipation often complain of urologic symptoms.

Long-term denervation abolishes the normal pelvic floor muscle activity and may result in the descending perineum syndrome. This neurologic impairment may be produced by nerve damage following chemotherapy, radiotherapy, pelvic surgery, compression, or invasion by neoplastic growth or during prolonged chronic opioid therapy. A loss of the normal rectal muscle tone is also a consequence of prolonged immobility often seen in debilitated cancer patients.

The integrity of the nervous system is essential to maintain normal defecation. Patients with paraplegia often complain of constipation. After spinal cord lesions above the lumbosacral area, incontinence is controlled but defecation is impaired. This is due to interruption of the cortical pathways, demonstrating the importance of supraspinal control of distal colonic function and defecation. Moreover, colonic response to a meal is reduced. However, appropriate stimuli may be sufficient to result in evacuation. In patients with damage to the cauda equina, transit time is prolonged and the rectoanal inhibitory reflex is weaker, offering little protection against fecal incontinence. Impaired modulation of spinal reflexes by cerebral influences or a localized lesion in the conus medullaris or the sacral nervous plexus may influence the capability of defecation. Rectal sensation may be reduced and the rectal capacity to distention increased after lesions of the sacral afferent nerves. This effect has been observed after vincristine treatment, during opioid therapy or as a consequence of neoplastic involvement of the pelvic sacral nerves (49).

Fecal impactions are most commonly encountered in elderly or debilitated patients, in patients treated by chronic opioid therapy or patients taking large doses of sedatives. In cancer patients with Parkinson's disease, constipation is probably caused by the degeneration of the autonomic nervous system, particularly the myenteric plexus (50). Chronic dehydration can also result in dry stools that are difficult to expel. Psychiatric and neurologic diseases are frequently associated with colonic dysmotility. There is a strong link between constipation and personality disorders, such as hypochondria and hysteria (43).

Many drugs induce constipation. Patients treated with carbamazepine may develop severe constipation that is not dose-related but is refractory to the concomitant use of oral laxatives, necessitating drug discontinuation (51). Selective 5-HT$_3$ receptor antagonists cause constipation. They antagonize the ability of 5-HT to evoke cholinergically mediated contractions of the intestinal longitudinal muscle (52).

One of the most striking pharmacologic features of opioids is their ability to cause constipation. Opioids have contradictory effects on the colon. Activation of different receptors at several different levels modulate colonic motility. Opioids activate δ receptors, inhibiting the contraction of colonic longitudinal muscle. Opioids may also suppress the release of VIP, an inhibitory neurotransmitter. VIP is a potent colonic secretagogue and an important inhibitor of smooth muscle contraction. The colon has the highest concentration of VIP of any region of the gut (13). Opioids induce phasic contractions by suppressing VIP release in the colonic circular muscle (53). Opioids increase the frequency and amplitude of segmenting nonpropulsive contractions resulting in an increase in the resistance to flow and a decreased colonic transit time. Typically, gastric emptying is inhibited by opioids and small bowel transit is prolonged, with increased intestinal absorption of fluid and electrolytes.

Postoperative pain relief by both parenteral or intraspinal opioids is often associated with adynamic ileus. Gastric emptying and small bowel transit are inhibited. This is an important consideration for cancer patients undergoing surgical procedures in which the ileus is likely to be a severe problem. Epidural anesthesia with local anesthetics appears to disrupt GI motility less than systemic opioids (54).

Massive colonic dilatation, in the absence of an obstruction or inflammatory process, has been described as pseudo-obstruction or Ogilvie's syndrome. This term describes a variety of states with a similar clinical picture due to intrinsic defects in the intestinal smooth muscle (55). The pseudo-obstruction can be categorized into those with myopathic and those with neuropathic features. Several conditions involving the intestinal smooth muscle are associated with colonic pseudo-obstruction, including endocrine and metabolic disorders, neurologic diseases, nonoperative trauma, surgery, nonintestinal inflammatory processes, infections, malignancy, radiation therapy, drugs, and cardiovascular and respiratory diseases. Extensive damage to the submucosal and myenteric nerve plexus associated with lymphoid infiltrate has been observed as a specific disorder, different from other processes that produce intestinal pseudo-obstruction (56).

## Assessment

Any complaint of constipation should be evaluated. It is of the utmost importance to first establish what the patient means by constipation; are stools too small, too hard, too difficult to expel, too infrequent, or do patients have a feeling of incomplete evacuation after defecation?

A careful history should be taken regarding the onset of constipation, bowel habits, and the use of laxatives. Impaction with overflow should be excluded by performing a rectal examination. The first step is to completely evacuate the bowel. Multiple oil or saline enemas may be needed. Digital fragmentation is unpleasant, but may permit the great majority of fecal impactions in the rectum to be diagnosed. A pseudodiarrhea in the presence of impaired anal sphincter function may be discovered. Gentle digital examination of the rectum may reveal a hard mass, a rectal tumor, rectal ulcers, an anal stenosis, anismus, or a lax anal sphincter. Multiple small fecaliths may cause lower abdominal pain. These stones are usually proximal to a stricture of the intestinal tract, visible on a plain x-ray of the abdomen.

An abdominal radiograph may distinguish between constipation and obstruction. Examination after a barium meal may help to distinguish between paralytic ileus and mechanical obstruction. Barium studies may help reveal a small intestine motility dysfunction in chronic intestinal pseudo-obstruction. In visceral myopathy, intestinal contractions are infrequent, whereas with a visceral neuropathy patients tend to have less distention and faster intestinal transit time due to uncoordinated contractions (55).

When constipation is due to ineffective colonic musculature, measurement of colonic transit time may be a useful tool to detect specific areas of the bowel that are not functioning properly. Pieces of radiopaque nasogastric tube are ingested and the progression of markers along the colon are observed by a daily radiograph until total expulsion. This study may demonstrate delayed transit in the colon, long storage of feces in the rectum, or retrograde movement due to a distal spasm (42,57).

Defecography is a radiologic technique used to investigate anorectal morphology and the dynamics of defecation, the morphology of anorectal structures and the different anorectal angles at rest or during straining. A narrow anorectal angle, not opening during straining to defecate, may help diagnose anismus.

Motor activity of the sigmoid colon may increase to an abnormal degree or decrease after a meal, suggesting two different groups of subjects with delayed transit in the colon: the hypomotor and the hypermotor patients. Recording the electrical activity of the bowel smooth muscle may be diagnostic. Spiking activity consists of rhythmic and stationary bursts of short duration occurring in sequences lasting a few minutes. Sporadic bursts, with more variable duration, correspond to a continuous electrical response. Sporadic bursts are associated with intraluminal pressure waves and significant propulsion of bowel content. Food has the most powerful stimulant effect on the propulsive activity. On the contrary, rest inhibits all types of myoelectric spiking activity. Morphine administration results in the disappearance of propagating spike bursts, whereas bisacodyl increases their number.

Anal sphincter electromyography may demonstrate increased external anal sphincter activity during defecation or demonstrate abnormal activity of the puborectalis muscle, and give information on the integrity of the innervation to and from the spinal cord.

## Treatment

An extensive effort should be made to find a specific cause of constipation and then treatment can be directed at that cause. Etiologic factors, such as physiologic consequences of cancer-associated debility, biochemical abnormalities, including hypercalcemia and hyperkalemia, and drug use, should be identified and reversed wherever possible. An adequate fluid intake is helpful to increase the stool water content.

Fluids, fruit juice, fruit, and bran are all recommended. However, fiber deficiency is unlikely to account for a lower stool weight and there is no justification for the claim that treatment with bran can return stool output and transit time to normal. In far advanced cancer patients, high amounts of fiber, beyond the capacity of most patients, is necessary to minimally increase stool frequency (58,59). Moreover, dietary fiber seems to have no prophylactic value to prevent constipation in hospitalized patients. An unfavorable toilet environment, such as lack of privacy or inappropriate posture, may lead to constipation, and patients should be provided privacy and appropriate facilities in the hospital setting.

Irreversible causes of constipation, such a malignant bowel obstruction or neurologic disorders, cannot be directly treated and symptomatic relief should be provided. Moreover, in spite of prophylaxis, most of these patients will require chronic laxatives, especially in the advanced stage of their disease or when treated with chronic opioid therapy. It is appropriate to begin prophylactic laxative treatment in patients with risk factors for constipation, including the elderly, those who are bedridden, or those requiring drugs known to cause constipation (60).

A low-rectal impaction should be removed manually. Appropriate sedation and analgesics are usually required to make this procedure comfortable. A more proximal mass can be broken by a sigmoidoscope or by delivering a pulsating stream of water against the stool.

### Laxatives

Laxatives will promote active electrolyte secretion, decrease water and electrolyte absorption, increase intraluminal osmolarity, and increase hydrostatic pressure in the gut. Although laxatives can be divided into several groups, no agent acts purely to soften the stool or to stimulate peristalsis (61). Clinical criteria, responsiveness, acceptability, and the patient's preference should guide the selection of the drug.

*Bulk-forming agents* are high-fiber foods containing polysaccharides or cellulose derivatives resistant to bacterial breakdown. Evidence of their effect may take 24 hours or more. They must be taken with water to avoid obstruction. Their effectiveness and feasibility in the advanced cancer patient are doubtful.

*Emollient laxatives* are surfactant substances not adsorbed in the gut, acting as a detergent and facilitating the mixture of water and fat. They also promote water and electrolyte secretion. Docusate alone or in combination with danthron is used at doses of 100–300 mg every 8 hours. It has a latency of action of more than 24 hours. The effectiveness of docusate has been questioned (27).

*Lubricant laxatives* are represented by mineral oil. It lubricates the stool surface. Coated feces may pass more easily and colonic absorption of water is decreased. It may also decrease absorption of fat vitamins. Absorption of small amounts may cause foreign body reactions in bowel lymphoid tissue. Liquid paraffin, 10 cm$^3$/day, may be given orally or rectally with an effect noted in 8–24 hours.

*Saline laxatives* exert an osmotic effect increasing the intraluminal volume. They also appear to directly stimulate peristalsis and increase water secretion. The latency of action is very short (within few hours) and is dose-dependent. The starting dose is 2–4 g daily. Magnesium, sulfate, phosphate, and citrate ions are the ingredients in saline laxatives. Their use may lead to electrolyte imbalances with accumulation of magnesium in patients with renal dysfunction or an excessive load of sodium in hypertensive patients. Moreover, their administration may result in an undesirable strong purgative effect. Administered rectally, they stimulate rectal peristalsis within 15 minutes. Repeated use of a phosphate enema may cause hypocalcemia and hyperphosphatemia or rectal gangrene in patients with hemorrhoids,.

*Stimulant laxatives* are the most commonly used drugs to treat constipation. They are represented by the anthraquinone derivatives, such as senna, cascara, and dantron, and the diphenylmethane derivatives, such as bisacodyl and phenolphthalein. This class of drugs acts at the level of the colon and distal ileum by directly stimulating the myenteric plexus. Senna is converted to an active form by colonic bacteria. As a consequence, its site of action is primarily the colon. Dantron and the polyphenolic agents bisacodyl and sodium picosulfate undergo glucuronidation and are secreted in the bile. The enterohepatic circulation may prolong their effect. An increase in myoelectric colonic activity has been observed after administration of oral senna. Bisacodyl stimulates the mucosal nerve plexus, producing contractions of the entire colon and decreasing water absorption in the small and large intestine. Castor oil is metabolized into ricinoleic acid that has stimulant secretory properties and an effect on glucose absorption. All of these drugs may cause severe cramping. The cathartic action occurs within 8–12 hours. Starting doses proposed are 15 mg daily of senna, 50 mg daily of danthron, or 10 mg daily of bisacodyl. Bisacodyl suppositories promote colonic peristalsis with a short onset due to the rapid conversion to its active metabolite by rectal flora.

*Hyperosmotic agents* are not broken down or absorbed in the small bowel, exerting an osmotic effect in the bowel. Lactulose increases fecal weight and frequency but may result in bloating, colic, flatulence, as well as electrolyte imbalances at high doses. Moreover, it is expensive in comparison to other preparations. The latency of action is 1–2 days. Starting doses are 15–20 ml twice a day. Glycerin can be used rectally as an osmotic and lubricant agent.

*Other drugs.* Cisapride is a prokinetic agent that appears to accelerate orocecal transit and to stimulate the colon. Cisapride enhances the release of acetylcholine from the myenteric nerve endings. Cisapride may alleviate constipation associated with Parkinson's disease (50). It has been shown to correct impaired propulsion in the small bowel of patients with pseudo-obstruction (62). Metoclopramide given by the subcutaneous route, but not by oral route, seems to be effective in narcotic bowel syndrome (63).

### Opioid-Induced Constipation

Opioids cause constipation by binding to specific opioid receptors in the enteric and central nervous system. Opioid use may lead to fecal impaction and spurious diarrhea, bowel pseudobstruction causing abdominal pain, nausea and vomiting, and interference with drug administration and absorption (64).

Although there is no correlation between the dose of opioids and the dose of laxatives, an upward titration of laxatives in parallel to increasing doses of morphine has been observed (44). However, proportionally less laxative is required at a higher opioid dose. Approximate equivalents of laxatives and typical requirements of opioid therapy have been proposed but there is clearly large individual patient variation (4).

Naloxone can reverse the actions of granisetron, morphine, and clonidine on the incidence of defecation (52). Orally administered naloxone has limited systemic bioavailability due to first-pass glucuronidation. Low plasma levels and high enteric wall concentration may explain the desired drug effect (65). For these reasons it has been proposed to reverse opioid-induced constipation (66). Dose titration, beginning with a dose of 4 mg daily, to a maximum of 12 mg, with at least 6 hours between doses, can be safely administered (67).

### Therapeutic Strategy

No data exist to guide the clinician or patient in the optimal choice of laxatives. In general, selection should be made according to the stool consistency. Local measures to soften fecal mass are necessary in case of rectal impaction. The short latency of action of rectal laxatives may be useful to remove hard feces impacted in the rectum. Glycerin suppositories or sorbitol enemas soften the stool by osmosis, also lubricating the rectum wall. Water penetration may be facilitated by a stool softener. Saline enemas cannot be regularly administered and should be used as a last resort. Practical and economic consideration may influence the choice of drug according to the setting (home, hospital, hospice, palliative care unit). While stimulant agents may cause painful colic, softener drugs may be useful in the presence of a hard stool. Peristaltic stimulants are indicated in patients unable to pass soft stool. Senna is the most useful drug in the presence of soft feces in the rectum. The combination of drugs seems to have a synergistic effect with few adverse effects.

In patients suspected of having intestinal obstruction, laxatives with a softening action may be tried (44). However, treatment should be immediately interrupted when transit stops. Patients with colostomies require the same treatment. Before using stimulating agents, an obstruction should be excluded in the absence of feces in a colostomy. Paraplegic patients often require regular manual evacuation. They may also benefit from the use of cisapride. Periodic laxative-free intervals have been advocated for patients with a relatively long prognosis to avoid tolerance (60).

## REFERENCES

1. Dobbins J. Approach to the patient with diarrhea. In: Kelley WN, ed. *Textbook of Internal Medicine.* Philadelphia: JB Lippincott, 1989; 669–680.
2. Field M, Rao MC, Chang EB. Intestinal electrolyte transport and diarrheal disease. *N Engl J Med* 1989;300:800–806.
3. Fine KD, Krejs GJ, Fordtran JS. Diarrhea. In: Sleisenger MH, Fordtran JS, eds. *Gastrointestinal Disease.* Philadelphia: WB Saunders, 1989; 290–313.
4. Regnard CFB, Tempest S. *A Guide to Symptom Relief in Advanced Cancer.* Manchester: Haigh & Hockland LDT, 1992.
5. Walsh TD, O'Shaughnessy C. Diarrhoea. In: Walsh TD, ed. *Symptom Control.* Oxford: Blackwell Scientific, 1989;99–116.
6. Mercadante S, ed. Sintomi gastrointestinali. In: Piccin, ed. *Trattamento del Dolore e dei Sintomi nel Cancro Avanzato.* Padova:Piccin, 1994: 137–154.
7. Mercadante S. Diarrhea in terminally ill patients: pathophysiology and treatment. *J Pain Sympt Manag* 1995;10:298–309.
8. Binder HJ. Absorption and secretion. *Curr Opin Gastroenterol* 1989;5: 63–66
9. Thillainayagam AV, Farthing MJG. Water and electrolyte absorption and secretion. *Curr Opin Gastroenterol* 1990;6:288–197.
10. Krejs GJ. Diarrhea. In: Wyngaarden JB, Smith LH, Bennett JC, eds. *Cecil's Textbook of Medicine,* 19th ed. Philadelphia: WB Saunders, 1992;680–687.
11. Toskes PP. Malabsorption. In: Wyngaarden JB, Smith LH, Bennett JC, eds. *Cecil's Textbook of Medicine,* 19th ed. Philadelphia: WB Saunders, 1992;667–699.

12. Harris AG. Octreotide in the treatment of disorders of the gastrointestinal tract. *Drugs* 1992;4(suppl 3):1–54.
13. Read NW. Colonic motility. *Curr Opin Gastroenterol* 1989;5:57–62
14. Dudl RJ, Anderson DS, Forsythe AB, et al. Treatment of diabetic diarrhea and orthostatic hypotension with somatostatin analogue SMS 201-995. *Am J Med* 1987;83:564–588.
15. Sandle GI, Binder HJ. Corticosteroids and intestinal ion transport. *Gastroenterology* 1987;93:188–196.
16. Buchanan KD. Hormones and the small intestine. *Curr Opin Gastroenterol* 1988;4:222–225.
17. Cohen S, Snape WJ. Movement of the small and large intestine. In: Sleisenger MH, Fordtran JS, eds. *Gastrointestinal Disease*. Philadelphia: WB Saunders, 1989;1088–1102.
18. Maggi CA, Manzini S, Meli A. Contribution of neurogenic and myogenic factors in the response or rat proximal colon to distension. *Am J Physiol* 1987;252:G447–G457.
19. Wright TL, Heyworth MF. Maldigestion and malabsorption. In: Slesinger MH, Fordtran JE, eds. *Gastrointestinal Disease*. Philadelphia: WB Saunders, 1989;263–282.
20. Petrelli NJ, Rodriguez-Bigas M, Rustum Y, et al. Bowel rest, intravenous hydration and continuous high-dose infusion of octreotide acetate for the treatment of chemotherapy-induced diarrhea in patients with colorectal carcinoma. *Cancer* 1993;72:1543–1546.
21. Cascinu S, Fedeli A, Luzi Fedeli S, Catalano G. Octreotide versus loperamide in the treatment of fluorouracil-induced diarrhea: a randomized trial. *J Clin Oncol* 1993;11:148–151.
22. Otterson MF, Sarna SK, Moulder JE. Effects of fractionated doses of ionizing radiation on small intestinal activity. *Gastroenterology* 1988; 95:1249–1257.
23. Earnest DL. Radiation enteritis and colitis. In: Sleisinger MH, Fordtran JS, eds. *Gastrointestinal Disease*. Philadelphia: WB Saunders, 1989; 1369–1382.
24. Boyd K. Diabetes mellitus in hospice patients: some guidelines. *Palliat Med* 1993;7:163–164.
25. Dean AP, Reed WD. Diarrhoea—an unrecognized hazard of coeliac plexus block. *Aust N Z J Med* 1991;21:47–48.
26. Mercadante S. The role of octreotide in palliative care. *J Pain Sympt Manag* 1994;9:406–411.
27. Sykes NP. Constipation and diarrhoea. In: Doyle D, Hanks GW, MacDonald N, eds. *Oxford Textbook of Palliative Medicine*. New York: Oxford Medical, 1993;299–310.
28. Fainsinger R, MacEachern T, Miller M, et al. The use of hypodermoclysis (HDC) for rehydration in terminally ill cancer patients. *J Palliat Care* 1992;8:70–72.
29. Richards WO, Geer R, O'Dorisio TM, et al. Octreotide acetate induces fasting small bowel motility in patients with dumping syndrome. *J Surg Res* 1990;49:483–387.
30. Sawyers JL. Management of postgastrectomy syndromes. *Am J Surg* 1990;159:8–14.
31. Mercadante S. Octreotide in the treatment of diarrhea induced by celiac plexus block. *Pain* 1995;61:345–346.
32. Trier JS, Lipsky M. The short bowel syndrome. In: Sleisenger MH, Fordtran JS, eds. *Gastrointestinal Disease*. Philadelphia: WB Saunders, 1989;1106–1112.
33. Arrambide KA, Santa Ana CA, Achiller LR, et al. Loss of absorptive capacity for sodium chloride as a cause of diarrhea following partial ileal and right colon resection. *Dig Dis Sci* 1989;34:193–201.
34. Nightingale JMD, Walker ER, Farthing MJG, Lennard-Jones JE. Effect of omeprazole on intestinal output in the short bowel syndrome. *Alim Pharmacol Ther* 1991;5:405–412.
35. Jeffries GH. Protein-losing gastroenteropathy. In: Sleisinger MH, Fordtran JS, eds. *Gastrointestinal Disease*. Philadelphia: WB Saunders, 1989;283–290.
36. Toskes PP, Donaldson RM. The blind loop syndrome. In: Sleisenger MH, Fordtran JS, eds. *Gastrointestinal Disease*. Philadelphia: WB Saunders, 1989;1289–1297.
37. Nightingale JMD, Walker ER, Burnham WR, et al. Short bowel syndrome. *Digestion* 1990;45(suppl 1):77–83.
38. Cooper JC, Williams NS, King RFGJ, Barker MCJ. Effects of a long acting somatostatin analogue in patients with severe ileostomy diarrhoea. *Br J Surg* 1986;73:128–131.
39. Ladefoged K, Christensen KC, Hegnhoj J, Jarnum S. Effect of a long

acting somatostatin analogue SMS 201-995 on jejunostomy effluents in patients with severe short bowel syndrome. *Gut* 1989;30:943–949.
40. Nightingale JMD, Lennard-Jones JE, Walker ER, Fathing MJG. Jejunal efflux in short bowel syndrome. *Lancet* 1990;336:765–768.
41. Mercadante S. Treatment of diarrhoea due to enterocolic fistula with octreotide in a terminal cancer patient. *Palliat Med* 1992;6:257–259.
42. Thompson JS. Surgical therapy for the short bowel syndrome. *J Surg Res* 1985;39:81–85.
43. Devroede G. Constipation. In: Sleisenger MH, Fordtran JS, eds. *Gastrointestinal Disease*. Philadelphia: WB Saunders, 1989:331–368.
44. Twycross RG, Harcourt JMV. The use of laxatives at a palliative care centre. *Palliat Med* 1991;5:27–33.
45. Curtis EB, Krech R, Walsh TD. Common symptoms in patients with advanced cancer. *J Palliat Care* 1991;7:25–29.
46. Bruera E, Chadwick S, Fox R, et al. Study of cardiovascular autonomic insufficiency in advanced cancer patients. *Cancer Treat Rep* 1986;70:1383–1387.
47. Lysy J, Karmeli F, Goldin E. Substances-P levels in the rectal mucosa of diabetic patients with normal bowel function and constipation. *Scand J Gastroenterol* 1993;28:49–52.
48. Bokemeyer C, Frank B, Vanrhee J, et al. Peripheral neuropathy following cancer chemotherapy. Long-term results in patients with curable neoplasms. *Tumordiagnostik Therapie* 1993;14:232–237.
49. Menardo G, Bausano G, Corazziari E, et al. Large-bowel transit in paraplegic patients. *Dis Colon Rect* 1987;30:924–928.
50. Jost WH, Schimrigk K. Cisapride treatment of constipation in Parkinson's disease. *Movement Disord* 1993;8:339–343.
51. Ettinger AB, Shinnar S, Sinnett MJ, Moshe SL. Carbamazepine-induced constipation. *J Epilepsy* 1992;5:191–193.
52. Sanger GJ, Wardle KA. Constipation evoked by 5-HT-receptor antagonism. Evidence for heterogeneous efficacy among different antagonists in guinea pigs. *J Pharm Pharmacol* 1994;46:666–670.
53. Bouvier M, Grimaud JC, Naudy B, Salducci J. Effects of morphine on electrical activity of the rectum in man. *J Physiol* 1987;388:153–162.
54. Waitwil M. Postoperative pain relief and gastrointestinal motility. *Acta Chir Scand* 1989(suppl 550):140–145.
55. Scott Jones R, Schirmer BD. Intestinal obstruction, pseudo-obstruction and ileus. In: Sleisenger MH, Fordtran JS, eds. *Gastrointestinal Disease*. Philadelphia: WB Saunders, 1989;369–381.
56. Aristanasr J, Gonzalezromo M, Keirns C, Larrivasahd J. Diffuse lymphoplasmatic infiltration of the small intestine with damage to nerve plexus. A cause of intestinal pseudo-obstruction. *Arch Pathol Lab Med* 1993;117:812–819.
57. Sykes NP. Methods of assessment of bowel function in patients with advanced cancer. *Palliat Med* 1990;4:287–292.
58. Twycross RG, Lack SA. *Control of Alimentary Symptoms in Far Advanced Cancer*. Edinburgh: Churchill Livingstone, 1986.
59. Muller-Lissner SA. Effect of wheat bran on weight of stool and gastrointestinal transit time: a meta-analysis. *Br Med J* 1988;296: 615–617.
60. Portenoy RK, Coyle N. Controversies in the long-term management of analgesic therapy in patients with advanced cancer. *J Palliat Care* 1991;7:13–24.
61. Tedesco FJ, Di Piro JT. American College of Gastroenterology's Committee on FDA-related matters. Laxative use in constipation. *Am J Gastroenterol* 1985;80:303.
62. Heading RC, Wood JD. *Gastrointestinal Dismotility. Focus on Cisapride*. Berlin: Raven Health Care Communications, 1992;269–279.
63. Bruera E, Brenneis C, Michand M, MacDonald N. Continuous subcutaneous infusion of metoclopramide for treatment of narcotic bowel syndrome. *Cancer Treat Rep* 1987;71:1121–1122.
64. Glare P, Lickiss JN. Unrecognized constipation in patients with advanced cancer: a recipe for therapeutic disaster. *J Pain Sympt Manag* 1992;7:369–371.
65. Sykes NP. Oral naloxone in opioid-associated constipation. *Lancet* 1991;337:1475.
66. Kreek MJ, Schaefer RA, Hahn EF, Fishman J. Naloxone, a specific opioid antagonist, reverses chronic idiopathic constipation. *Lancet* 1983;1:261–262.
67. Culpepper-Morgan JA, Inturrisi CE, Portenoy RK, et al. Treatment of opioid-induced constipation with oral naloxone. *Clin Pharmacol Ther* 1992;52:90–95.

*Principles and Practice of Supportive Oncology,*
edited by Ann Berger et al.
Lippincott–Raven Publishers, Philadelphia ©1998

CHAPTER 14

# Bowel Obstruction

Carla Ripamonti

Bowel obstruction is a common complication in patients with abdominal or pelvic cancers, such as those arising from colon, ovary, and stomach. Extraabdominal cancers, such as lung, breast, and melanoma, can also spread to the abdomen and cause secondary bowel obstruction. Although bowel obstruction may develop at any time, it is more common, and may evolve more rapidly, in patients with more advanced disease (1,2). The incidence is 5.5–25% in ovarian carcinoma (1,3–5) and 4.4–24% in colorectal cancer (6–9). In terminal patients with ovarian cancer the incidence can be as high as 42% (2) .

Ovarian carcinoma is the most common cause of bowel obstruction among women with gynecologic disease and bowel obstruction is a major cause of death in this population. Ovarian cancer accounts for 50% of small intestinal obstructions and 37% of large intestinal obstructions treated on a large gynecology service (10). Patients with stage III or IV disease and those with high-grade lesions are at higher risk for treatment failure and therefore develop bowel obstruction more often than patients with stage I or II disease or low-grade tumors. In the population with gynecologic cancer, more than two thirds of patients with bowel obstruction had advanced carcinoma at the time of diagnosis (1,11).

The time interval from diagnosis of cancer to the onset of bowel obstruction varies among tumor types. This interval is significantly longer for intraabdominal neoplasms (mean 22.4 months) then extra-abdominal neoplasms (mean 57.5 months) (1,2,12–15).

## PATHOPHYSIOLOGY

### Structural Factors

Several mechanisms may be involved in the onset of gastrointestinal obstruction (Table 1) and there is variabil-

ity in both presentation and etiology. Bowel obstruction can be partial or complete, single or multiple, and due to benign or malignant factors. In the majority of patients with advanced cancer, there appears to be a slow progression from partial to complete obstruction. However, some patients have intermittent symptoms (8,16).

The site of obstruction varies with tumor type. Pancreatic cancer spreads directly to the duodenum or stomach, whereas cancer of the colon spreads to the jejunum and ileum. Prostate and bladder cancers spread to the rectum (9).

Tumors at the splenic flexure cause obstruction in 49% of cases. Tumors of the right and left colon obstruct in approximately 25% of cases, and tumors of the rectum and rectosigmoid junction cause obstruction in only 6% (6). In patients with ovarian carcinoma, the small bowel is more commonly involved than the large bowel (61% versus 33%), and in 6–22% of cases both are obstructed (12,17).

In cancer patients, the cause of the intestinal blockage is usually recurrent tumor. Less often, adhesions or radiation-associated strictures and fibrosis are causes. Occasionally, the signs and symptoms of an intestinal obstruction can be the first indication of the neoplasm. In patients with gynecologic or colorectal cancers, recurrence is often heralded by obstruction of the large and/or small bowel.

Factors that affect extrinsic neural control to viscera may contribute to obstructive symptoms. These factors may be related to the neoplasms or to intercurrent diseases. Chronic intestinal pseudo-obstruction (CIP), for example, is mainly due to diabetes mellitus, previous gastric surgery, or other neurologic disorders (18). Vagal dysfunction occurs in a majority of patients with CIP associated with diabetes or neurologic disorders.

### Physiologic Factors

Gastrointestinal secretion amounts to 7–8 l/day, and the average fluid intake is about 2 l/day, depending on

C. Ripamonti: Department of Oncology, University of Alberta, Alberta, Canada, and Pain Therapy and Palliative Care Division, National Cancer Institute, 20133 Milano, Italy.

**TABLE 1.** *Pathophysiology of bowel obstruction*

1. **Extrinsic occlusion of the lumen**: enlargement of the primary tumor or recurrence, mesenteric and omental masses, abdominal or pelvic adhesions, postirradiation fibrosis
2. **Intraluminal occlusion of the lumen**: polypoid lesions due to primary cancer or metastases, annular tumoral dissemination
3. **Intramural occlusion of the lumen**: intestinal linitis plastica
4. **Intestinal motility disorders (pseudo-obstruction):** infiltration of the mesentery or bowel muscle and nerves, malignant involvement of the celiac plexus, paraneoplastic neuropathy in patients with lung cancer (75,76)
       Chronic intestinal pseudo-obstruction (CIP) (18)
       Paraneoplastic pseudo-obstruction (18,77)

diet. Most electrolytes and water present in the gut are absorbed in the small intestine owing to its enormous epithelial surface. Although the colon could handle up to 6 l/day, only about 1–1.5 l/day arrives from the small intestine under normal conditions. The colon extracts this amount, leaving a mass of colonic bacteria and unabsorbable residue of about 100 g. A wide variety of chemical substances influence this intestinal transport, including neurotransmitters, hormones, intestinal content, and inflammatory mediators that act on secretomotor receptors. The substances stimulating the intestine to secrete fluid act mostly via the enteric nervous system or inflammatory events.

Occlusion of the lumen prevents or delays the propulsion of the intestinal contents. As a consequence, secretions accumulate and cause abdominal distension and peristaltic motor activity to surmount the obstacle. This motor activity is associated with colicky pain.

Although bowel obstruction limits or prevents through-movement of intestinal contents, the bowel continues to contract with increased uncoordinated peristaltic activity. A vicious circle represented by distension-secretion-motor activity worsens the clinical picture, producing a hypertensive state in the lumen and damage to intestinal epithelium. This, in turn, causes an inflammatory response that induces the release of prostaglandins, which are potent secretagogues, either by a direct effect on enterocytes or by an enteric nervous reflex.

Other disturbances may relate to the release of vasoactive intestinal polypeptide (VIP) into the portal and peripheral circulation. This compound may mediate local intestinal and systemic pathophysiologic alterations accompanying small intestinal obstruction, such as hyperemia and edema of intestinal wall and accumulation of fluid in the lumen. High portal levels of VIP are known to cause hypersecretion and splanchnic vasodilatation. Higher VIP content is present in the duodenal tissue than colonic tissue in an experimental animal bowel obstruction model. These vascular effects may account for the redistribution of blood flow in the obstructed segment and distal to the site of obstruction. A loss of the normal hemodynamic homeostasis may explain the systemic hypotension that can occur during bowel obstruction (19).

## DIAGNOSIS

### Signs and Symptoms

In advanced cancer patients, the onset of obstruction is rarely an acute event because the compression of the lumen is slow, progressive, and passes through a phase of partial obstruction. Symptoms gradually worsen until they become continuous. Initially, vomiting occurs sporadically. Its frequency increases progressively and its prevalence is ultimately in the range of 68–100% (8,20). Vomiting can remain intermittent or become continuous. It develops early and in large amounts in obstruction of the gastric outlet or small intestine, and develops later in large bowel obstruction. Biliary vomiting is almost odorless and indicates an obstruction in the upper part of the abdomen. The presence of foul-smelling fecaloid vomiting can be the first sign of an ileal or colonic obstruction.

The prevalence of colicky pain is 72–76% (8,20), and continuous abdominal pain is present in more than 90% of cancer patients with bowel obstruction (8,20). Pain may be due to abdominal distension, tumor mass, or hepatomegaly, as well as the obstruction itself. The intestine is distended proximal to the obstruction by an accumulation of gas and fluid, most of which is secreted by the gut rather than ingested. Hyperperistaltic pain is of the colicky type and has variable intensity and localization. If it is intense, periumbilical, and occurring at brief intervals, it is often an indication of an obstruction at the jejunoileal level. In large bowel obstruction, the pain is less intense, deeper, and occurs at longer intervals.

An acute pain, which begins intensely and becomes stronger, or pain that is specifically localized suggests a perforation or an ileal or colonic strangulation syndrome. Similarly, a pain that increases with palpation indicates the probability of peritoneal irritation, which may be caused by a new lesion such as an early perforation.

In cases of complete obstruction, there is no evacuation of feces and no flatus. Sometimes overflow diarrhea results from bacterial liquefaction of the fecal material blocked in the sigmoid colon or rectum.

## Clinical Assessment

To diagnose a mechanical obstruction, the presence of constipation and paralytic ileus must first be excluded. Constipation is often the sole cause of obstructive symptoms. It should be considered when patients complain of hard feces and infrequent bowel movements, and when constipating drugs (opioids, belladonna alkaloids, antispasmodics, antidepressants) are being used without laxatives. This situation may be worsened by inactivity, a low-fiber diet, and practical problems such as lack of privacy or the inability to reach a toilet. Physical examination shows a loaded rectum and palpable fecal masses in the abdomen. When the rectum is empty and impaction is high, abdominal radiographs are needed for diagnosis.

Abdominal distension, intermittent borborygmi, anorexia, and "squashed stomach syndrome" (i.e., dyspeptic symptoms associated with the inability of the stomach to distend normally because of hepatomegaly) are also commonly manifested in patients with bowel obstruction. The absence of peristalsis indicates that a paralytic ileus has complicated the mechanical obstruction. This may occur following a period of bowel distension or result from an intercurrent problem, such as perforation.

## Radiologic Assessment

An abdominal radiograph taken in a supine or standing position is the first investigation in patients with suspected small bowel obstruction. This is done to document the dilated loops of bowel, air-fluid interfaces, or both. A radiograph following the ingestion of contrast can distinguish obstruction from metastases, radiation injury, or adhesions (21).

The diagnosis of a motility disorder may also be revealed by the slow passage of barium through undilated bowel, with no demonstrable obstruction.

Abdominal radiographs in different positions are necessary when large bowel obstruction is suspected. This examination can be carried out with a barium enema and colosigmoidoscopy (22–24).

When a complete bowel obstruction is suspected in a patient who is considered to be inoperable, barium must not be used as the contrast medium because it can markedly worsen symptoms. In these cases, the use of a water-soluble medium, such as gastrograffin, is indicated. Retrograde transrectal radiographic contrast studies should be used to rule out or to diagnose isolated or concomitant obstruction of the large bowel.

## THERAPIES

The management of patients with malignant bowel obstruction is one of the greatest challenges for physi-

cians who care for cancer patients. In the face of a clearly incurable situation, significant patient discomfort and suffering must be balanced with the need to simplify the care of those patients with a short time to live.

## SURGERY

Palliative surgery is usually considered when relief from symptoms due to bowel obstruction is not obtained within 48–72 hours of decompression with a nasogastric tube (25–27). In advanced cancer patients, however, guidelines for conservative versus surgical treatment are still unresolved. According to some authors (28,29), surgery should be considered even when multiple episodes have occurred; in contrast, others (30) believe that obstruction due to recurrent cancer has such a small chance of relief that surgery should generally be avoided. This decision to pursue or withhold invasive therapy is further complicated by the fact that the cause of the obstruction may be benign. The rate of bowel obstruction due to benign causes ranges from 6.1% in ovarian and other gynecologic cancers (1,17,31) to 48% in colorectal cancer (13).

The type of obstruction (partial versus complete) and the method of surgical treatment (bypass versus resection and reanastomosis) has no significant effect on the outcome (1,32). In the series of Piver et al. (32), survival was primarily related to the response to postoperative chemotherapy rather than the type of surgery performed. Up to 30% of surgically treated patients can be expected to develop another episode of bowel obstruction.

Not all patients are fit for surgery. The rate of inoperable patients ranges from 6.2% to 50% (1,3,11,12,14,31–34). The most frequent causes are (a) extensive tumor; (b) multiple partial obstructions; and (c) impossibility of surgical correction.

According to van Ooijen et al. (35), intestinal obstruction in patients with chemotherapy-resistant tumors and peritoneal carcinomatosis of the ovary, or of other origin associated with clinically manifest ascitic fluid or palpable masses, should not be treated surgically by laparotomy. Percutaneous gastrostomy should be the method of choice for these patients.

Benefit from surgery is defined as at least 60 days of survival after operation (36). This definition, however, does not take into account the well-being of the patient, the presence or absence of symptoms, postoperative complications, or the length of hospitalization. In the study by Lund and colleagues (3), for example, 56% of patients survived for 60 days after operation, but 43% of these individuals manifested intermittent symptoms of incomplete or complete intestinal obstruction until death.

Thus surgery may not solve the problem of obstruction or control of symptoms in advanced cancer patients. Furthermore, in a large percentage of cases it can lead to fur-

**TABLE 2.** *Complications and survival time after surgery*

| Ref. | No. Pts | Primary cancer | 30-Day mortality (%) | Other operative complications (%) | Survival (months) |
|---|---|---|---|---|---|
| (31) | 64 | Gynecol. | 11 | 15.5 | 2.5 median |
| (3) | 25 | Ovary | 32 | 32.0 | 2.0 median |
| (12) | 43 | Ovary | 9 | 11.5 | 6.8 mean |
| (4) | 23 | Ovary | 13 | 43 | 17% 1 year |
| (17) | 49 | Ovary | 14 | 49 | 4.5 median |
| (11) | 98 | Ovary | 12 | 12 | 3.1 median |
| (1) | 90 | Ovary | 14 | — | 7.0 mean |
| (32) | 60 | Ovary | 16.5 | 31 | 2.5 median |
| (2) | 11 | Ovary | 9 | 9 | 7.0 mean |
| (35) | 20 | Ovary[a] | 30.0 | 90 | 1.0 median |
| (26) | 36 | Various | 19 | — | 11 median |
| (78) | 40 | Various | 27.5 | 22.5 | 7.0 mean |
| (78) | 26 | Various | 46 | 15.0 | 4.5 mean |
| (30) | 32 | Various | — | — | 3 median |
| (15) | 41 | Various | 24.4 | — | 4.5 median |
| (79) | 10 | Various | 40 | 80 | 2 median |
| (33) | 34 | Various | 18 | 44 | 4.0 mean |
| (14) | 89 | Abdominal | 13 | 44 | 4.5 mean |
| (29) | 30 | Colorectal | 37 | 27 | 6.1 median |

—, Not reported.
[a]Presented with clinically manifest ascites and/or palpable masses.

ther complications. Table 2 shows the rate of operative mortality (defined as death from any cause within 30 days of the operation), the morbidity, and the length of survival after surgery for bowel obstruction. The most common complications are wound infections and/or dehiscence, sepsis, enterocutaneous fistulae, further obstruction, peritoneal abscess, anastomosis dehiscence, GI bleeding, and deep venous thrombosis with or without pulmonary embolism.

Several authors have emphasized that prognostic criteria are needed to help doctors select patients who are likely to benefit from surgical intervention. The available data suggest that poor prognostic factors include the following: (a) intestinal motility problems due to diffuse intraperitoneal carcinomatosis (11,15,36–38); (b) patients over 65, particularly if cachectic (11,39); (c) ascites requiring frequent paracentesis (35,37–39), low serum albumin level (39), and low serum prealbumin level (40); (d) nutritional deficits (41); (e) previous radiotherapy of the abdomen or pelvis (4,11); (f) palpable intraabdominal masses (35) and liver involvement or distant metastases, pleural effusion, or pulmonary metastases (1,11,37,38); (g) multiple partial bowel obstructions with prolonged passage time on radiograph examination (39); and (h) elevated blood urea nitrogen levels, elevated alkaline phosphatase levels, advanced tumor stage, and short diagnosis to obstruction interval (39). In contrast to these data, one study (12) could not correlate any of the clinical variables analyzed (patient age, interval after cancer diagnosis, previous radiotherapy, mean number of prior laparotomies, use of perioperative total parenteral nutrition, or site of intestinal

obstruction) with either operability or survival following definitive surgery.

Surgical palliation in advanced cancer patients is a complex issue, and the decision to proceed with surgery must be carefully evaluated for each individual patient. The decision should be made by the physician together with the patient and family members. Surgery must be considered for patients with a life expectancy greater than 2 months (1,11,14).

## NASOGASTRIC SUCTION AND INTRAVENOUS FLUIDS

The usual hospital treatment for symptom control is nasogastric suction and parenteral fluids. This treatment decompresses the stomach and/or intestine, and corrects fluid and electrolyte imbalance before surgery or while a decision is being made. The tube often becomes occluded and requires flushing and/or replacement. The incidence of spontaneous expulsion of the nasogastric tube is about 23% in the first 24 hours (42).

During long-term drainage, a nasogastric tube can interfere with coughing for clearing pulmonary secretions and may be associated with nasal cartilage erosion, otitis media, aspiration pneumonia, esophagitis, and bleeding (43). This treatment can also create discomfort in patients who are already distressed by previous anticancer and surgical therapies. For these reasons, prolonged nasogastric suction and intravenous fluids for symptomatic treatment of inoperable patients is not recommended. Long-term use of nasogastric tube should only be considered when pharmacologic therapy for symptom control is ineffective or when gastrostomy cannot be carried out.

## PHARMACOLOGICAL TREATMENT

The pharmacological management of bowel obstruction due to advanced cancer focuses on the treatment of nausea, vomiting, pain, and other symptoms without the use of a nasogastric tube and intravenous hydration. This approach was first described approximately 10 years ago (8). Other authors were able to verify the efficacy of such a pharmacological approach, and it is now used by palliative care units worldwide. The average survival of inoperable patients treated with drugs differs among studies: 3.7 months (8), 13.4 days with a range of 2–50 (20), 18 days with a range of 2–41 (16), and 29.2 days (44).

### Drug Administration Routes

In patients with bowel obstruction symptoms, the route of drug administration must be individualized. Vomiting is a very frequent symptom, and may eliminate the oral route. Although the rectal and sublingual routes are very safe and easy to use in a home setting (45), only a few drugs are available for these routes of administration. If a central venous catheter has been previously inserted, this can be used to administer drugs. Continuous subcutaneous infusion of drugs using a portable syringe driver allows the parenteral administration of different drug combinations, produces minimal discomfort for the patient, and is easy to use in a home setting (46).

### Drugs Used for Controlling Pain and/or Vomiting

To control continuous abdominal pain, opioids such as morphine, hydromorphone, or diamorphine are usually administered. The dose is gradually increased until symptom control is achieved. The treatment of colicky pain is reported in Table 3.

Table 4 shows the most frequently used drugs to control nausea and vomiting.

Haloperidol is often considered first by palliative care specialists. Parkinsonian side effects may occur with doses higher than 15 mg/day, however, and other adverse effects, such as akinesia, may also compromise therapy. Haloperidol can be combined with scopolamine in the same syringe. Another neuroleptic, methotrimeprazine, is very effective but it causes sedation and subcutaneous irritation.

Metoclopramide is an antiemetic and increases gastric motility. Although most authors (8,9,20,47,48) do not recommend this drug in the presence of complete bowel obstruction because it may increase nausea, vomiting, and

**TABLE 3.** *Colicky pain: pharmacological therapy*

1. Hyoscine butylbromide starting with 40–60 mg/day up to 380 mg/day (16,20,53)
2. Hyoscine hydrobromide 0.8–2.0 mg/day SC (8,9)
3. Hyoscine hydrobromide 0.3–0.6 mg sublingually prn (8,9)
4. Transdermal scopolamine 1.5–3 mg every 3 days (63)
5. Loperamide 2 mg four times daily (8)
6. Opioids increasing the dose until relief is achieved (20,44,53)
7. Celiac plexus block with alcohol

SC, subcutaneously.

colicky pain, Isbister et al. (44) successfully used parenteral metoclopramide (mean dose of 6.9 mg/hour) to control nausea and vomiting in patients who did not have upper GI obstruction. In the latter case, the drug presumably encouraged the stomach to evacuate its contents into the paralyzed reservoir of the bowel. According to Fainsinger et al. (16), metoclopramide used parenterally at a dose of 10 mg every 4 hours can be considered the drug of choice in patients with incomplete bowel obstruction.

Cyclizine is the first choice in some palliative care centers. It can be added to prochlorperazine suppositories and to haloperidol subcutaneously. Crystallization may occur at higher doses or in association with other drugs (9).

Scopolamine (hyoscine) butylbromide is commonly used for both vomiting and colicky pain by some palliative care centers. This drug, which is not available in the United States, differs from both atropine and scopolamine (hyoscine) hydrobromide in having a low lipid solubility. It does not penetrate the blood–brain barrier as well as these other drugs and consequently may produce fewer side effects, such as somnolence and hallucinations, when administered in combination with opioids.

**TABLE 4.** *Nausea and vomiting: pharmacological therapy*

Neuroleptics
Haloperidol 5–15 mg/day SC (8,20)
Methotrimeprazine 50–150 mg/day SC (8)
Prochlorperazine 25 mg 8 hourly rectally (8)
Chlorpromazine 50–100 mg 8 hourly rectally or SC (8,63)
Prokinetic drugs
Metoclopramide 60–240 mg/day SC (16,44)
Cisapride 10 mg A.C. (54)
Antihistamines
Cyclizine 100–150 mg/day SC or 50 mg 8 hourly rectally (8)
Dimenhydrinate 50–100 mg SC prn (16)
Anticholinergics
Hyoscine butyl bromide 40–120 mg/day (SC) (16,53)
Hyoscine hydrobromide 0.8–2 mg/day SC (8)
Somatostatin Analogs
Octreotide 0.2–0.9 mg/day SC (57–60)
Vapreotide 4 mg five times at weekly intervals (61)
Corticosteroids
Dexamethasone 20–40 mg/day (62,63); 8–60 mg/day (16)

SC, subcutaneously.

The anticholinergic activity of scopolamine butylbromide decreases the tonus and peristalsis in smooth muscle. This is due to both a competitive inhibition of muscarinic receptors at the smooth muscle level and impairment of ganglionic neural transmission in the bowel wall (49,50). Muscarinic cholinergic receptors have also been observed on mucosal cells of the intestinal lumen and in human salivary glands (51,52). The distribution of these receptors may explain its analgesic effect on colicky pain, the reduction of intestinal secretions, and its potential side effects.

De Conno et al. (53) described the antiemetic and analgesic role of scopolamine (hyoscine) butylbromide administered subcutaneously by a syringe driver in three patients with inoperable malignant GI obstruction. All patients were treated with total parenteral nutrition through a central venous catheter and all underwent nasogastric drainage. During daily administration of 120, 120, and 80 mg of scopolamine (hyoscine), respectively, the quantities of GI fluids drained through the tube were significantly reduced. After the first week of treatment, it was possible to remove the nasogastric tube in all three cases, and all patients reported good relief of colicky pain. Later, morphine hydrochloride was added to the other drugs to control continuous abdominal pain. Therapy was continued until death and lasted 55, 172, and 54 days, respectively. Dry mouth was reported to be the most significant side effect, but the patients tolerated it by sucking ice cubes and taking small sips of water.

Cisapride is an orally administered prokinetic agent that facilitates or restores motility throughout the length of the GI tract. It is a substituted piperidinyl benzamide that is chemically related to metoclopramide but, unlike metoclopramide, is largely devoid of central depressant or antidopaminergic effects. Cisapride stimulates GI motor activity through an indirect mechanism involving the release of acetylcholine and is mediated by postganglionic nerve endings in the myenteric plexus of the gut. It is an agonist of serotonin at the 5-HT$_4$ receptor as well as an antagonist at the 5-HT$_3$ receptor. Camilleri et al. (54) reported that over a 6-week period cisapride had a beneficial effect on gastric emptying of solids in patients with antral hypomotility (diabetic and idiopathic gastroparesis) and intestinal dysmotility (chronic idiopathic pseudo-obstruction).

Octreotide, a synthetic analog of somatostatin that has a more potent biological activity and a longer half-life, has also been used to manage the symptoms of bowel obstruction. Somatostatin and its analogs have been shown to inhibit the release and activity of GI hormones, modulate GI function by reducing gastric acid secretion, slow intestinal motility, decrease bile flow, increase mucous production, and reduce splanchnic blood flow (55,56). It reduces GI contents and increases the absorption of water and electrolytes at the intracellular level via cAMP and calcium regulation. Submucosal somatostatin-containing neurons activated by octreotide inhibit excitatory nerves, mainly by an inhibition of acetylcholine output. As a result, muscle relaxation can occur, ameliorating the spastic activity responsible for colicky pain.

The inhibitory effect of octreotide on both peristalsis and GI secretions reduces bowel distension and the secretion of water and sodium by the intestinal epithelium, thereby reducing vomiting and pain (57). The drug may therefore break the vicious circle represented by secretion, distension, and contractile hyperactivity. Octreotide may be administered by subcutaneous bolus or continuous subcutaneous infusion. Its half-life is about 1.5 hours after intravenous or subcutaneous administration, and its kinetics are linear.

Octreotide is an expensive drug and its cost–benefit ratio should be carefully considered, especially for prolonged treatment. Mercadante et al. (57) reported the control of vomiting and pain in a patient with bowel obstruction caused by pancreatic cancer through subcutaneous octreotide (0.1 mg/8 hours) and subcutaneous buprenorphine (0.3 mg/8 hours). Symptom control was maintained until death, which occurred 3 weeks later. No side effects were attributable to the drugs. The nasogastric tube was removed, although the occlusion was in the upper bowel. In another patient with bowel obstruction due to colon cancer and diffuse carcinomatosis, vomiting was controlled by subcutaneous administration of octreotide 0.9 mg/day and haloperidol 3 mg/day, both of which were combined in a syringe-driver. There was no further need for analgesics or intravenous fluids. No other episodes of vomiting occurred during the last week of life.

In a recent study, Mercadante et al. (58) treated 14 patients with doses of octreotide ranging from 0.3 to 0.6 mg/day by subcutaneous bolus or by continuous subcutaneous infusion. The drug was employed as an alternative when haloperidol and chlorpromazine were not effective. The administration of octreotide allowed the complete control of vomiting in 12 patients and partial control in 2. In two patients, the nasogastric tube was removed without loss of symptom control. Good effects were observed in the patients with upper bowel obstruction, who are often considered less responsive to medical treatment without a nasogastric tube. Painful injection of octreotide was observed in 7 of the 14 patients and only one patient showed an uncomplicated skin reaction. The vial should be warmed with the hands for a few minutes so as to reduce the pain.

Khoo et al. (59) used octreotide to treat five cancer patients with intractable continual vomiting due to small bowel obstruction that was unresponsive to conventional therapy with prochlorperazine, metoclopramide, cyclizine, and dexamethasone. Octreotide was administered subcutaneously in single doses of 0.1 mg, followed by continuous infusion of 0.3–0.5 mg in 24 hours. Vomiting stopped within one hour of start of treatment in every patient. In a patient with a nasogastric tube, the drainage decreased from 2000 ml/day to <300 ml/day after the start of octreotide treatment. There were no reported side effects.

Riley and Fallon (60) reported 24 patients with obstruction who were treated with octreotide. Fourteen of 24 had a complete response with no further vomiting. Four had a partial response and six had no response. In those responding, relief occurred within 2–4 hours of administration. No side effects were noted. The median daily dose was 0.3 mg/day (range 0.25–0.7 mg/day) given by continuous subcutaneous infusion. The median duration of treatment was 9.4 days. In those patients who did not respond, increasing the dose to 1.2 mg/day did not help.

On the basis of this experience, octreotide can be recommended when symptom control fails with conventional antiemetics. The recommended starting dose is 0.3 mg/day subcutaneously. The dose can be titrated upward until symptom control is achieved.

Vapreotide is a long-acting microencapsulated preparation of a somatostatin analog. Vapreotide has been shown to have similar clinical properties to somatostatin but a longer duration of action. Stiefel et al. (61) used this drug in a patient with obstructive ileus due to pancreatic cancer. Four milligrams of the drug was injected five times at weekly intervals during the last month of the patient's life. Within 2 days after the first injection of vapreotide, the patient no longer complained of nausea and vomiting. The patient vomited only six times in 29 days and reported good symptom control until death.

Several authors recommend the use of corticosteroids for the symptoms of bowel obstruction because it can reduce peritumoral inflammatory edema, thus improving intestinal motility. No controlled clinical trials have been carried out, and administration routes and dosing of these drugs have not been standardized yet. MacDonald et al. (62) suggest either dexamethasone (8 mg/day) or prednisone (25 mg every 12 hours for 5 days), gradually reducing the dose when response is positive. When there was no positive response to dexamethasone with usual doses (5–10 mg/day subcutaneously), Steiner et al. (63) administered single doses of 20, 50, and 100 mg intravenously; in 40% of the treated patients, this dose regimen obtained both temporary symptom control and a reduction in obstruction. Reid (47) reported using dexamethasone in starting doses of 20 mg/day for the temporary relief of GI obstruction and/or nausea.

According to Fainsinger et al. (16), dexamethasone ranging from 8 to 60 mg/day is a very useful agent in managing nausea and vomiting. However, its role in preventing progression to complete bowel obstruction cannot be determined from current experience.

## GASTROSTOMY

If obstruction continues for more then a few days, gastrostomy is a much more acceptable and well-tolerated route for decompression than nasogastric intubation. Intermittent venting of the gastrostomy allows the patient to continue oral intake and maintain an active lifestyle without the inconvenience of a nasogastric tube.

The two options currently available are operative gastrostomy and percutaneous gastrostomy (PG). Tube gastrostomy at the time of surgical exploration is the traditional method of long-term gastric decompression. It adds little time or morbidity to the surgical procedure and should be done whenever the intraoperative impression is that complete bowel obstruction may be prolonged or imminent. Previous surgery or massive carcinomatosis may make placement of the gastrostomy difficult or dangerous, but every effort should be made to place a gastrostomy at the time of exploration if the clinical situation warrants one.

Percutaneous gastrostomy is the insertion of a tube into the stomach through the abdominal wall under fluoroscopic or endoscopic guidance (64,65). It can be done at the bedside. The procedure may be performed under local anesthesia in most patients, and has a lower cost and lower complication rate than operative placement of the gastrostomy tube (66). Percutaneous gastrostomy usually requires a brief hospitalization (an average of 4.6 days).

PG can be performed safely in advanced cancer patients as a venting procedure in patients suffering from nausea and vomiting due to bowel obstruction. According to Malone et al. (64), PG is a superior technique to both nasogastric suction and operative gastrostomy for palliation of small bowel obstruction in terminal ovarian cancer. There are generally no absolute contraindications because of the desperate nature of the clinical situation. PG should be avoided in patients with portal hypertension and ascites, those predisposed to bleeding, and those with active gastric ulceration (67).

The utility of gastrostomy was described by Gemlo et al. (68) who reported the experience of 27 inoperable, terminally ill patients with abdominal cancer and partial or complete bowel obstruction. When the oral and rectal routes were not viable, a central venous catheter was placed for the administration of 2–3 l of standard electrolyte solution per day, and analgesic and antiemetic drugs. In 13 patients, a venting gastrostomy connected to passive drainage was performed to control intractable vomiting due to complete obstruction. All patients were managed at home by nurses after an average stay in the hospital of 11.2 days, during which time the patients and their families underwent extensive training in the use of infusion pumps and gastrostomy tubes. Symptoms were controlled and there were no complications from the gastrostomies. The mean length of survival was 64 days (9–223 days) and home care costs were one sixth those of hospital care. When obstructive symptoms cannot be controlled by drugs, PG is believed to be a more effective and acceptable alternative to the prolonged use of a nasogastric tube.

## FEEDING AND HYDRATION

The need to treat dehydration in terminally ill patients remains a controversial issue. In a prospective evaluation of 32 consecutively admitted terminally ill patients treated in a comfort care unit, thirst was present in only a minority of patients despite water intake inadequate to sustain basal requirements (69). Ice chips, sips of liquid, and mouth care (cleansing, swabbing, and application of lip moisteners) provided relief of dry mouth and thirst for varying periods of time.

Although these data suggest that hydration is not needed, Fainsinger et al. (16) suggest that hydration is indicated in terminal cancer patients to prevent dehydration and prerenal kidney failure. These outcomes may cause agitated delirium directly or through accumulation of drug metabolites, such as morphine-6-glucuronide, that may also result in complications such as myoclonus or seizure.

Hypodermoclysis (HDC) is a technique used to administer fluids into the subcutaneous space. HDC is a simple technique for rehydration that offers many advantages over the intravenous (IV) route, which can be difficult to maintain in this patient group. HDC can be started by any staff member able to give a subcutaneous (SC) injection, without the need for a physician or IV team. It can be stopped and started without concern about thrombosis in the SC needle. In some cases, hospitalization can be avoided or shortened if hydration can be given by this route. Very few local reactions to HDC have been reported. Subcutaneous sites often last for several days (70), and if relief of obstructive symptoms is obtained through palliative treatment, patients are usually able to drink water and other fluids and to eat small amounts of their favorite foods (8,20,44) while continuing some HDC.

The role of total parenteral nutrition (TPN) in the management of patients with inoperable bowel obstruction is controversial (11,35). No data are available on quality of life of advanced cancer patients treated with this modality. Some studies have shown decreased survival in patients given aggressive nutritional support as a result of complications of the therapy and possibly by enhancing tumor growth (71–73).

Clinical experience suggests that the routine use of artificial nutrition should be discouraged. TPN may be useful in rare cases, such as advanced cancer patients who experience hunger but cannot take food orally, patients who will die due to malnutrition long before the cancer attacks vital organs, and patients whose suffering is mainly the result of nutritional deterioration. Any decision regarding the start or the suspension of artificial feeding in advanced cancer patients should be based on a careful assessment of the physical and psychological condition of the patient and his or her wishes and informed consent. Life expectancy must be considered. Artificial feeding should not be used indiscriminately, as it may lead to serious complications and may even prolong the suffering in some patients with severe or terminal illness.

Providing food and fluids only as needed can be an effective means of fulfilling a patient's wishes while alleviating discomfort. As this is accomplished, attention must also be focused on oral hygiene, reduction of dry mouth, and prevention of oral infections and halitosis (74).

## CONCLUSION

The optimal treatment of bowel obstruction in patients with advanced cancer is still an open and widely debated issue. Patients are usually considered suitable candidates for surgery when survival is expected be more than 2 months. Studies of prognostic indicators of survival in advanced cancer patients are necessary to assist doctors in making appropriate therapeutic decisions, together with the patient and family members. Medical treatment by continuous subcutaneous or intravenous administration of opioids, corticosteroids, anticholinergic drugs, octreotide, and antiemetic drugs can be an effective approach for controlling pain, nausea, and vomiting in patients with inoperable GI obstruction. Nasogastric suction or percutaneous gastrostomy may be considered for patients with refractory symptoms and/or upper bowel obstruction who do not respond satisfactorily to pharmacologic measures alone. The efforts of the doctor/nurse team must be aimed at both symptom control and other aspects of the patient's suffering, including psychological distress and spiritual concerns.

## REFERENCES

1. Tunca JC, Buchler DA, Mack EA, et al. The management of ovarian-cancer-caused bowel obstruction. *Gynecol Oncol* 1981;12:186.
2. Beattie GJ, Leonard R, Smyth JF. Bowel obstruction in ovarian carcinoma: a retrospective study and review of the literature. *Palliat Med* 1989;3:275.
3. Lund B, Hansen M, Lundvall F, et al. Intestinal obstruction in patients with advanced carcinoma of the ovaries treated with combination chemotherapy. *Surg Gynecol Obstret* 1989;169:213.
4. Castaldo TW, Petrilli ES, Ballon SC, et al. Intestinal operations in patients with ovarian carcinoma. *Am J Obstet Gynecol* 1981;139:80.
5. Solomon HJ, et al. Bowel complications in the management of ovarian cancer. *Aust N Z J Obstet Gynaecol* 1983;23:65.
6. Phillips RKS, Hittinger R, Fry JS, et al. Malignant large bowel obstruction. *Br J Surg* 1985;72:296.
7. Kyllonen LEJ. Obstruction and perforation complicating colorectal carcinoma. *Acta Chir Scand* 1987;153:607.
8. Baines M, Oliver DJ, Carter RL. Medical management of intestinal obstruction in patients with advanced malignant disease:a clinical and pathological study. *Lancet* 1985;2:990.
9. Baines M. The pathophysiology and management of malignant intestinal obstruction. In: Doyle D, Hanks GWC, MacDonald N, eds. *Oxford Textbook of Palliative Medicine,* 2nd ed. Oxford: Oxford University Press, 1993;311.
10. Krebs HB, Goplerud DR. Mechanical intestinal obstruction in patients with gynecologic disease: a review of 368 patients. *Am J Obstet Gynecol* 1987;157:577.
11. Krebs HB, Goplerud DR. Surgical management of bowel obstruction in advanced ovarian carcinoma. *Obstet Gynecol* 1983;61:327.
12. Rubin SC, Hoskins WJ, Benjamin I, et al. Palliative surgery for intestinal obstruction in advanced ovarian cancer. *Gynecol Oncol* 1989;34:16.
13. Spears H, Petrelli NJ, Herrera L, et al. Treatment of bowel obstruction after operation for colorectal carcinoma. *Am J Surg* 1988;155:383.
14. Turnbull ADM, Guerra J, Starners HF. Results of surgery for obstructing carcinomatosis of gastrointestinal, pancreatic, or biliary origin. *J Clin Oncol* 1989;7:381.

15. Aabo K, Pedersen H, Bach F, et al. Surgical management of intestinal obstruction in the late course of malignant disease. *Acta Chir Scand* 1984;150:173.
16. Fainsinger RL, Spachynski K, Hanson J, et al. Symptom control in terminally ill patients with malignant bowel obstruction. *J Pain Sympt Manag* 1994;9:12.
17. Clarke-Pearson DL, Chin NO, DeLong ER, et al. Surgical Management of intestinal obstruction in ovarian cancer. I. Clinical features, postoperative complications, and survival. *Gynecol Oncol* 1987;26:11.
18. Mathias JR. Pseudo-obstruction syndromes and disorders of the small intestine. In: Fisher RS, Krevsky B, eds. *Motor Disorders of the Gastrointestinal Tract: What's New and What to Do.* New York: Academy Professional Information Services, 1993;121.
19. Mercadante S. International Consensus Conference on Bowel Obstruction. Athens 28–29 October 1994, unpublished data.
20. Ventafridda V, Ripamonti C, Caraceni A, et al. The management of inoperable gastrointestinal obstruction in terminal cancer patients. *Tumori* 1990;76:389.
21. Yuhasz M, Laufer I, Sutton G, et al. Radiography of the small bowel in patients with gynecologic malignancies. *Am J Radiol* 1985;144:303.
22. Ziter FMH. Radiologic diagnosis: small bowel. In: Welch JP, ed. *Bowel Obstruction.* Philadelphia: WB Saunders, 1990;96.
23. Markowitz SK. Radiologic diagnosis: colon. In: Welch JP, ed. *Bowel Obstruction.* Philadelphia: WB Saunders, 1990;108.
24. Maglinte DDT, Peterson LA, Vahey TN, et al. Enteroclysis in partial small bowel obstruction. *Am J Surg* 1984;147:325.
25. Krebs HB, Goplerud DR. The role of intestinal intubation in obstruction of the small intestine due to carcinoma of the ovary. *Surg Gynecol Obstet* 1984;158:467.
26. Walsh HPJ, Schofield PF. Is laparotomy for small bowel obstruction justified in patients with previously treated malignancy? *Br J Surg* 1984;71:933.
27. Editorial: Intubate the bowel and enjoy the sunset. *Lancet* 1985;16:1107.
28. Ketcham AS, Hoye RC, Pilch YH, et al. Delayed intestinal obstruction following treatment for cancer. *Cancer* 1970;25:406.
29. Lau PW, Lorentz TG. Results of surgery for malignant bowel obstruction in advanced, unresectable, recurrent colorectal cancer. *Dis Colon Rect* 1993;36(1):61.
30. Osteen RT, Guyton S, Steele G, et al. Malignant intestinal obstruction. *Surgery* 1980;87(6):611.
31. Soo KC, Davidson T, Parker M, et al. Intestinal obstruction in patients with gynaecological malignancies. *Ann Acad Med* 1988; 17(1):72.
32. Piver MS, Barlow JJ, Lele SB, et al. Survival after ovarian cancer induced intestinal obstruction. *Gynecol Oncol* 1982;13:44.
33. Annest LS, Jolly PC. The results of surgical treatment of bowel obstruction caused by peritoneal carcinomatosis. *Am Surgeon* 1979, 45:718.
34. Taylor RH. Laparotomy for obstruction with recurrent tumor. *Br J Surg* 1985;72:327.
35. van Oojen B, van der Burg MEL, Planting ASTh et al. Surgical treatment or gastric drainage only for intestinal obstruction in patients with carcinoma of the ovary or peritoneal carcinomatosis of other origin. *Surg Gynecol Obstet* 1993;176:469.
36. Larson JE, Podczaski ES, Manetta A, et al. Bowel obstruction in patients with ovarian carcinoma: analysis of prognostic factors. *Gynecol Oncol* 1989;35:61.
37. Gallick HL, Weaver DW, Sachs RJ, et al. Intestinal obstruction in cancer patients. An assessment of risk factors and outcome. *Am Surgeon* 1986;52:434.
38. Glass RL, LeDuc RJ. Small intestinal obstruction from peritoneal carcinomatosis. *Am J Surg* 1973;125:316.
39. Fernandes JR, Seymour RJ, Suissa S. Bowel obstruction in patients with ovarian cancer: a search for prognostic factors. *Am J Obstet Gynecol* 1988;158:244.
40. Rapin ChH, Chatelain C, Weil R, et al. Pour une meilleure qualité de vie en fin de vie: nutrition et hydration. *Age Nutr* 1990;1:22.
41. Clarke-Pearson DL, DeLong ER, Chin EN et al. Surgical management of intestinal obstruction in ovarian cancer II. Analysis of factors associated with complications and survival. *Arch Surg* 1988; 123:42.
42. Rees RGP, Payne-James JJ, King C, et al. Spontaneous transpylorus passage and performance of fine bore polyurethane feeding under a controlled clinical trial. *J Parenter Enter Nutr* 1988;12:469.
43. Pictus D, Marx MV, Weyman PJ. Chronic intestinal obstruction: value of percutaneous gastrostomy tube placement. *Am J Radiol* 1988;150:295.
44. Isbister WH, Elder P, Symons L. Non-operative management of malignant intestinal obstruction. *J R Coll Surg Edinb* 1990;35:369.
45. Ripamonti C, Bruera E. Rectal, buccal, and sublingual narcotics for the management of cancer pain. *J Palliat Care* 1991;7(1):30.
46. Bruera E. Subcutaneous administration of opioids in the management of cancer pain. In: Foley K, Ventafridda V, eds. *Advances in Pain Research and Therapy,* vol 16. New York: Raven Press, 1990;203.
47. Reid DB. Palliative management of bowel obstruction. *Med J Aust* 1988; 148:54.
48. Twycross RG, Lack SA. Gastrointestinal obstruction. In: Twycross RG, Lack SA, eds. *Symptom Control in Advanced Cancer: Alimentary Symptoms,* vol 11. London: Pitman, 1986;239.
49. Bauer VR, Gross E, Scarselli V, et al. Uber Wirkungsunterchiede von Atropin, Scopolamin und einigen ihren quartaren Derivate nach subcutaner und enteralen Gabe unter besonderer Beruchsichtigung des Scopolamin-n-butylbromids. *Arzneimittel Forschung* 1968;18:1132.
50. Weiner N. Atropine, scopolamine and related antimuscarinic drugs. In: Goodman Gilman A, Goodman L, Gilman A, eds. *The Pharmacological Basis of Therapeutics.* New York: Macmillan, 1980;120.
51. Gespach C, Emami S, Chastre E. Membrane receptors in the gastrointestinal tract. *Biosci Rep* 1988;43:199.
52. Giraldo E, Martos F, Gomes A, et al. Characterization of muscarinic receptor subtypes in human tissues. *Life Sci* 1988;43:1507.
53. De Conno F, Caraceni A, Zecca E, et al. Continuous subcutaneous infusion of hyoscine butylbromide reduces secretions in patients with gastrointestinal obstruction. *J Pain Sympt Manag* 1991;6:484.
54. Camilleri M, Malagelada JR, Abele TL, et al. Effect of six weeks of treatment with cisapride in gastroparesis and intestinal pseudo-obstruction. *Gastroenterology* 1989;96:704.
55. Reichlin S. Medical progress. Somatostatin. *N Engl J Med* 1983;309:1495.
56. Arnold R, Lankisch PG. Somatostatin and gastrointestinal tract. *Clin Gastroenterol* 1980;9:733.
57. Mercadante S, Maddaloni S. Octreotide in the management of inoperable gastrointestinal obstruction in terminal cancer patients. *J Pain Symptom Manag* 1992;7(8):496.
58. Mercadante S, Spoldi E, Caraceni A, et al. Octreotide in relieving gastrointestinal symptoms due to bowel obstruction. *Palliat Med* 1993;7:295.
59. Khoo D, Riley J, Waxman J. Control of emesis in bowel obstruction in terminally ill patients. *Lancet* 1992;339:375.
60. Riley J, Fallon MT. Octreotide in terminal malignant obstruction of the gastrointestinal tract. *Eur J Palliat Care* 1994;1:23.
61. Stiefel F, Morant R. Vapreotide, a new somatostatin analogue in the palliative management of obstructive ileus in advanced cancer. *Support Care Cancer* 1993;1:57.
62. MacDonald N. *Palliative Cancer Care: Pain Relief and Management of Other Symptoms.* Geneva: WHO, 1991.
63. Steiner N. Controle des symptomes en soins palliatifs: l'ileus terminal. *Med Hyg* 1991;49:1182.
64. Malone JM, Koonce T, Larson DM, et al. Palliation of small bowel obstructon by percutaneous gastrostomy in patients with progressive ovarian carcinoma. *Obstet Gynecol* 1986;68:431.
65. George J, Crawford D, Lewis T, et al. Percutaneous endoscopic gastrostomy: a two year experience. *Med J Aust* 1990;152:17.
66. Adelson MD, Kazowits MH. Percutaneous endoscopic drainage gastrostomy in treatment of gastrointestinal obstruction from intraperitoneal malignancy. *Obstet Gynecol* 1993;81:467.
67. Forgas I, Macpherson A, Tibbs C. Percutaneous endoscopic gastrostomy. The end of the line for nasogastric feeding? *Br Med J* 1992;304:1395.
68. Gemlo B, Rayner AA, Lewis B. Home support of patients with end-stage malignant bowel obstruction using hydration and venting gastrostomy. *Am J Surg* 1986;152:100.
69. McCann RM, Hall WJ, Groth-Juncker A. Comfort care for terminally ill patients. The appropriate use of nutrition and hydration. *JAMA* 1994; 272(16):1263.
70. Fainsinger RL, MacEachern T, Miller MJ et al. The use of hypodermoclysis for rehydration in terminally ill cancer patients. *J Pain Sympt Manag* 1994;9:298.
71. Torosian M, Daly J. Nutritional support in the cancer-bearing host. *Cancer* 58:1915.
72. Koretz R. Parenteral nutrition: is it oncologically logical? *J Clin Oncol* 1984;2:534.
73. Clamon G, Feld R, Evans W, et al. Effect of adjuvant central IV hyper-

alimentation on the survival and response to treatment of patients with small cell lung cancer: a randomized trial. *Cancer Treat Rep* 1985;69: 167.

74. Ventafridda V, Ripamonti C, Sbanotto A, et al. Mouth Care. In: Doyle D, Hanks GWC, MacDonald N, eds. *Oxford Textbook of Palliative Medicine.* Oxford: Oxford University Press, 1993;434.

75. Addison NV. Pseudo-obstruction of the large bowel. *J R Soc Med* 1983; 76:252.

76. Schuffler MD, Baird HW, Fleming CR. Intestinal pseudo-obstruction as the presenting manifestation of small-cell carcinoma of the lung. *Ann Intern Med* 1983;98:129.

77. Liang BC, Albers JW, Sima AAF, et al. Paraneoplastic pseudo-obstruction, mononeuropathy multiplex, and sensory neuronopathy. *Muscle and Nerve* 1994;17:91.

78. Aranha GV, Folk FA, Greenlee HB. Surgical palliation of small bowel obstruction due to metastatic carcinoma. *Am Surgeon* 1981;47:99.

79. Chan A, Woodruff RK. Intestinal obstruction in patients with widespread intra-abdominal malignancy. *J Pain Sympt Manag* 1992;7:339.

*Principles and Practice of Supportive Oncology,*
edited by Ann Berger et al.
Lippincott–Raven Publishers, Philadelphia ©1998

CHAPTER 15

# Diagnosis and Management of Ascites

Charles F. von Gunten and Martha L. Twaddle

## EPIDEMIOLOGY

Ascites, the accumulation of fluid in the abdomen, is common in patients with certain types of end-stage cancer. Its formation may be a direct result of a malignant process or secondary to unrelated comorbidity. Because the pathophysiology of fluid collection varies, treatment strategies differ. Clinical distinction between malignant and nonmalignant causes is therefore imperative.

Of all patients with ascites, the vast majority have advanced primary liver disease, usually cirrhosis. Secondary liver dysfunction as a result of cardiac or renal failure will also result in the accumulation of ascitic fluid. Rarely, nephrogenic ascites may develop alone (1). Only 10% of patients who have ascites will have a malignancy as the primary cause. In these patients, epithelial malignancies, particularly ovarian, endometrial, breast, colon, gastric, and pancreatic carcinomas, cause over 80% of malignant ascites. The remaining 20% are due to malignancies of unknown origin (2).

In general, the presence of malignant ascites portends a poor prognosis, regardless of the cause. The mean survival in patients with malignant ascites is generally less than 4 months. If it is due to a malignancy that is relatively sensitive to chemotherapy, such as ovarian cancer, the mean survival may be somewhat longer (2).

## PATHOPHYSIOLOGY

### Nonmalignant Ascites

The mechanisms that lead to the development of ascites are many, and controversy exists regarding which

---

C. F. von Gunten: Division of Hematology/Oncology, Department of Medicine, Northwestern University Medical School, Chicago, IL 60611.

M. L. Twaddle: Department of Medicine, Northwestern University/Evanston Hospital, Evanston, IL 60201.

---

factors are most important (3–5). In cirrhosis of the liver, the most common cause of nonmalignant ascites, abnormal sodium retention is mediated by various hormonal and neural mechanisms similar to those responsible for excess fluid retention in congestive heart failure. As the disease progresses, the kidneys are unable to compensate for the increase in the sodium-retaining factors, and the result is an increase in total body sodium and water. Portal hypertension ensues from the restriction of normal blood flow in the venous and lymphatic systems in the liver caused by the cirrhosis. The increase in hepatic venous sinusoidal and portal pressures causes the excess fluid volume to localize to the peritoneal cavity secondary to fluid transudation from the splanchnic capillary bed. Ascites accumulation may be exacerbated by the diminished synthetic capacity of the liver to maintain adequate intravascular oncotic pressure.

Other causes of nonmalignant ascites, which include portal vein thrombosis (Budd-Chiari syndrome), congestive heart failure, pericardial disease, nephrotic syndrome, pancreatitis, and tuberculosis, should be considered in appropriate patients.

### Malignant Ascites

Ascites may result from malignancies in several ways. Most commonly, tumor cells on the peritoneal surface of the abdominal cavity interfere with normal venous and lymphatic drainage, causing fluid to leak into the abdominal cavity. The tumor cell implants may themselves induce fluid secretion into the abdomen. Liver congestion and increased portal pressures may be produced by direct tumor invasion of the liver. This leads to transudation of fluid across the splanchnic bed into the abdominal cavity. If the retroperitoneal space is infiltrated, chylous ascites may result from obstructed lymphatic flow, as from lymphoma.

## DIAGNOSIS

### History

Patients with ascites commonly notice an increase in abdominal girth and a sensation of fullness or bloating. Other useful historical features include recent weight gain or ankle swelling. Patients may describe a vague generalized abdominal discomfort or a feeling of heaviness with ambulation. They may also note indigestion, nausea, and vomiting due to delayed gastric emptying, and esophageal reflux symptoms due to increased intraabdominal pressure. Some may note physical changes in the umbilicus.

### Physical Examination

The physical examination for ascites includes inspection for bulging flanks, percussion for flank dullness, a test for shifting dullness, and a test for a fluid wave.

The abdominal flanks bulge when significant ascites is present because of the weight of abdominal free fluid. The examiner should look for bulging flanks when the patient is supine. However, if less than 2 liters are present, or the patient is significantly obese, this physical finding may be difficult to appreciate or is unreliable. The distinction between excess adipose tissue and ascites may be made by percussing the flanks to assess for dullness (Fig. 1).

The percussion of shifting dullness is a useful maneuver. The flank is tapped, and a mark is made on the skin at the location where the tone changes. The patient is then turned partially toward the side that has been percussed. If the location of the dullness shifts upward toward the umbilicus, this is evidence of intraabdominal ascites (Fig. 2).

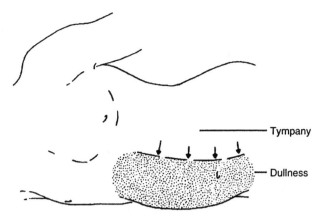

**FIG. 2.** Tympany and dullness.

The elicitation of a fluid wave may also help to confirm the diagnosis. The test is performed by having an assistant place the medial edges of both hands firmly down the midline of the abdomen to block transmission of a wave through subcutaneous fat. The examiner places her hands on the flanks. She taps one flank sharply while simultaneously using the fingertips of the opposite hand to feel for an impulse transmitted through the ascites to the other flank.

Several additional aspects of the physical examination may also be helpful. The liver may be ballottable if it is enlarged and ascites is present. If ascites is severe, the examiner may discern umbilical, abdominal, or inguinal hernias; scrotal or lower extremity edema; or abdominal venous engorgement. The umbilicus may be flattened or slightly protuberant. Two additional maneuvers that have been described for the physical diagnosis of ascites, the puddle sign and auscultatory percussion, are not recommended (6).

Several diagnostic tests may be useful, particularly if the physical examination is equivocal. A plain radiograph of the abdomen may demonstrate a hazy or ground-glass pattern. Ultrasonography or computed tomography of the abdomen will readily identify free fluid. They are most helpful in making the diagnosis when there is a relatively small amount of fluid, or when loculation is present.

### Laboratory Abnormalities

A diagnostic paracentesis of 10 to 20 ml of fluid is useful to confirm the presence of ascites and to help determine its cause. Ultrasonography may be performed if the fluid is difficult to obtain or if loculation is suspected.

We favor using the Z technique to minimize the risk of leaking fluid following the procedure. A location on the abdomen at the midpoint between the umbilicus and the anterior superior iliac crest is identified. After careful cleansing and local anesthetizing, a 2-inch, 20-gauge angiocatheter is attached to a 20-ml syringe. The angio-

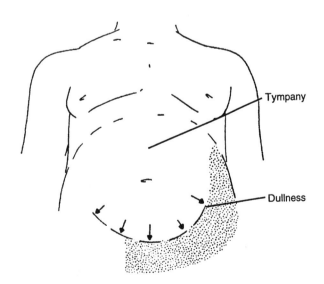

**FIG. 1.** Shifting dullness.

catheter is inserted at a 45° angle to the skin until abdominal fascia is encountered. The needle is then rotated through 90° so that it is now facing in the opposite direction and at 45° from the skin. The needle is slowly advanced while a small amount of negative pressure is applied through the syringe until ascitic fluid is obtained. After the necessary amount of fluid has been obtained, the needle is withdrawn. The fascial planes will overlap to prevent fluid leakage, a common complication with a more direct approach.

The color of the fluid should be noted. A white milky fluid is characteristic of chylous ascites. Bloody fluid is almost always malignant in origin, although it may be due to abdominal tuberculosis. The fluid should undergo cytologic analysis and determinations of cell count with differential and total protein concentrations. A Gram stain with culture should be performed if infection is suspected. Cytology is the most specific test to demonstrate that the ascites is due to malignancy. However, the absence of malignant cells does not exclude malignancy as a cause. The cell count, particularly the absolute neutrophil count, is useful in the presumptive diagnosis of bacterial peritonitis. If the neutrophil count is greater than 250 cells/ml, bacterial peritonitis is presumed. The total protein concentration has been used to classify specimens into the broad categories of exudate (total protein >25 g/l) or transudate (total protein <25 g/l). An exudate is caused by an inflamed, infected, or tumor-laden peritoneal surface. Examples include bacterial or tuberculous peritonitis, pancreatitis, and carcinomatosis. Transudates result from fluid that traverses a normal peritoneal surface because of an imbalance of Starling forces, as in cirrhosis, heart failure, and the nephrotic syndrome.

In some patients, the exudate/transudate concept may not be sufficient to make a clear diagnosis, particularly if serum protein levels are low. A useful measurement in such patients is the serum-ascites albumin gradient, defined as the serum albumin concentration minus the ascitic fluid albumin concentration. The gradient directly correlates with portal pressure. Patients with a gradient of 11 g/l or more have ascites that is due in part to increased portal pressures (7,8). If, for example, a patient is thought to have malignant ascites because cytology has been positive, yet the ascitic fluid is transudative (protein is less than 25 g/l), calculation of the serum-ascites albumin gradient could be used to test for the contribution of portal hypertension to the ascites.

## MANAGEMENT

The overall goals for patient care should be considered before specific choices for managing ascites are made. The prognosis, expected response to antineoplastic therapies, and preferences for treatment should first be established with the patient and family before any treatment plan is instituted. Each ascites treatment modality has associated burdens and benefits, which must be considered and discussed.

The discernment of the ascites as being of either malignant or nonmalignant cause is critical in determining the overall management plan. In general, the intraabdominal fluid is *not* in equilibrium with total body fluid in malignant ascites. Consequently, salt and fluid restriction and diuretics may be of little use. Their injudicious use may result in intravascular volume depletion, diminished renal perfusion, azotemia, hypotension, and fatigue (2). In contrast, nonmalignant ascites *is* in equilibrium with total body fluid, and efforts to affect that balance are often quite useful. Of course, there are patients in whom the causes are mixed, and the judgment of the clinician is required to choose the best management (2).

The intervention for ascites in the supportive or palliative care setting should generally be reserved for patients who are symptomatic. The following symptoms may spur the need for intervention when the ascites seems to be responsible or contributing:

- dyspnea
- fatigue
- anorexia or early satiety
- diminished exercise tolerance

### Dietary Management

The management of ascites, particularly that of nonmalignant origin, begins with sodium and water restriction. Patients with cirrhosis may excrete as little as 5 to 10 mEq of sodium per day in their urine. Because of the tendency to retain water through activation of the renin-angiotensin-aldosterone system, patients are prone to develop dilutional hyponatremia. The management of this condition has typically been fluid restriction, usually on the order of 1 liter per day total. In the patient with advanced disease, when treatment goals are purely palliative, fluid restriction may be quite reasonably perceived as intolerably burdensome. Judicious medical management may be less burdensome.

### Medical Management

*Chemotherapy* may be an effective management strategy for patients with ascites due to a malignancy that is responsive (such as lymphoma, breast, or ovarian cancer). Unfortunately, for the majority of patients, the management of ascites is palliative. That is, the goal of therapy is to minimize the symptoms and optimize the quality of life without the expectation that the underlying cause can be treated.

*Diuretic therapy* is useful in some patients, particularly those whose ascites is due wholly or in part to nonmalignant causes. As with any drug therapy in the supportive care setting, the patient's symptoms should first be ascertained and the benefit versus the burden of therapy considered.

The goal of diuretic therapy is to reduce fluid accumulation. A slow and gradual diuresis that does not exceed the capacity for mobilization of ascitic fluid (approximately 900 ml/day) is the goal of diuretic therapy. In the patient with ascites and edema, the edema will act as a reservoir to buffer the effects of a rapid contraction of plasma volume if the response to the diuretic is brisk. In patients with ascites but without edema, diuresis may be achieved at the expense of the intravascular volume leading to symptomatic orthostatic hypotension. Diuretics should not be administered in order to render the patient edema and ascites free, but rather to remove only enough retained fluid to ensure the patient's comfort (9). Overly aggressive therapy for ascites in a patient with liver disease may lead to the hepatorenal syndrome and death (17).

In patients with ascites for whom diuretics may be helpful, the renin-angiotensin-aldosterone system is activated. Therefore, the initial diuretic for management is usually one that acts at the distal nephron to block the effect of increased aldosterone activity. Spironolactone, beginning with 25 to 50 mg per day (given in the morning), is often a useful agent with which to begin. Spironolactone is sometimes associated with painful gynecomastia. Amiloride, 5 mg per day, is an alternative. The doses may be gradually increased until the desired relief of ascites is achieved. It may take several weeks for a given dose of diuretic to achieve its ultimate effect. As these diuretics are relatively potassium sparing, patients should be advised not to use salt substitutes, as these are usually preparations of potassium chloride. If patients have a suboptimal response despite maximal use of the distal diuretics, a loop diuretic may be added beginning at low doses, such as furosemide, 20 mg orally daily.

In the patient who has limited mobility, urinary tract outflow symptoms such as hesitancy and frequency, poor appetite, and poor oral intake, or who has difficulties related to polypharmacy, diuretic therapy may be excessively burdensome. Injudicious diuretic therapy can result in incontinence with attendant self-esteem and skin care issues, sleep deprivation from frequent urination, fatigue from hyponatremia and/or hypokalemia, and falls from postural hypotension during attempts to get to the bathroom.

### Therapeutic Paracentesis

Large-volume therapeutic paracentesis is a simple procedure and is associated with minimal morbidity or mortality (10–12). Up to 5 liters may be safely removed at a single session, thus assuring rapid amelioration of the symptoms. The symptom response is much faster than when diuretics are used alone. In the patient with malignant ascites, it may be the only therapeutic modality that is effective.

The supplies needed are as follows:

- 16-gauge angiocatheter
- blood collection tubing
- several 1-liter glass vacuum bottles
- antiseptic cleansing solution
- 1% lidocaine
- 20-ml syringe
- Three-way stopcock

The patient is placed in the supine or semirecumbent position. A location on the abdomen either midway between the umbilicus and the symphysis pubis or midway between the umbilicus and the anterior superior iliac crest is identified. The skin is cleansed and infiltrated generously with lidocaine. A large-bore angiocatheter (16 gauge) is inserted by means of the Z technique as described above. A three-way connector may be attached to the angiocatheter to allow both a syringe and heavy-gauge plastic tubing (such as one from a blood collection set) to be attached to the angiocatheter. After the angiocatheter has been appropriately positioned, the distal end of the tubing may be placed in a glass vacuum collection bottle to allow for rapid evacuation of fluid. The collection needle can be moved to successive bottles until the desired amount of fluid has been collected. Repositioning the patient during the procedure may be required if omentum is drawn across the aperture of the angiocatheter. Large-volume paracentesis may be safely performed either in the outpatient clinic setting or in the patient's home.

If the ascites is not due to malignancy, there is a risk that symptomatic hypotension will ensue as the body fluid reequilibrates following large-volume paracentesis. In general, if there is significant peripheral edema, there is adequate body fluid to compensate for the loss of ascitic fluid during paracentesis. However, if there is no edema and the serum albumin is low, some authors have advised the infusion of 40 grams of albumin intravenously both before and 6 to 8 hours after the procedure to increase the intravascular oncotic pressure when large-volume paracentesis (3 to 5 liters) is performed (13). This prevents excessive fluid shifts from the intravascular compartment to the abdominal compartment. Albumin infusion is not necessary if only 1 to 2 liters are removed.

### Surgical Procedures

Peritoneovenous shunts (LeVeen, Denver, and others) are placed surgically during a 30- to 60-minute procedure while the patient is under local anesthesia. Their purpose is to drain ascites fluid from the peritoneal space into the internal jugular vein. Although possibly useful for selected patients with nonmalignant ascites, they are rarely indicated for patients with malignant ascites. Their use in patients with cirrhosis is associated with a significant risk of sepsis and disseminated intravascular coagulation. Malignant ascites characteristically has a high protein content, making flow through the shunts difficult and blockage frequent. As the overall prognosis for such patients is so poor, and the results of paracentesis so good, the need for such a surgical approach is rarely required.

Tenckhoff catheters may be beneficial for selected patients who require repeated large-volume paracenteses for comfort and whose prognosis warrants a surgical procedure. The catheter is surgically placed in the peritoneal cavity with an external drain, which can be accessed intermittently by physicians or nurses or even by trained family members (14).

The transjugular intrahepatic portosystemic shunt (TIPS) has been introduced as a relatively noninvasive approach to the palliation of ascites due to cirrhosis in highly selected patients for whom an interventional radiologic approach would be appropriate. Early reports suggest that patients do not have the same complications as with peritoneovenous shunts (15,16).

## REFERENCES

1. Hammond TC, Takyyuddin MA. Nephrogenic ascites: a poorly understood syndrome. *J Am Soc Nephrol* 1994;5(5):1173–1177.
2. Sharma S, Walsh D. Management of symptomatic malignant ascites with diuretics: two case reports and a review of the literature. *J Pain Symp Manage* 1995;10(3):237–242.
3. Garcia TG. Cirrhotic ascites: pathogenesis and management. *Gastroenterologist* 1995;3(1):41–54.
4. Aiza I, Perez GO, Schiff ER. Management of ascites in patients with chronic liver disease. *Am J Gastroenterol* 1994;89(11):1949–1956.
5. McCormick PA, McIntyre N. Pathogenesis and management of ascites in chronic liver disease. *Br J Hosp Med* 1992;47(10):738–744.
6. Williams JW, Simel DL. Does this patient have ascites? *JAMA* 1992;267(19):2645–2648.
7. Runyon BA, Montano AA, Akriviadis EA, Antillon MR, Irving MA, McHutchison JG. The serum-ascites albumin gradient is superior to the exudate-transudate concept in the differential diagnosis of ascites. *Ann Intern Med* 1992;117:215–220.
8. Runyon BA. Malignancy-related ascites and ascitic fluid humoral tests of malignancy. *J Clin Gastroenterol* 1994;18(2):94–98.
9. Arroyo V, Gines P, Planas R. Treatment of ascites in cirrhosis: diuretics, peritoneovenous shunt, and large-volume paracentesis. *Gastroenterol Clin North Am* 1992;21:237–256.
10. Porayko MK, Wiesner RH. Management of ascites in patients with cirrhosis. What to do when diuretics fail. *Postgrad Med* 1992;92(8):155–158.
11. Gines P, Arroyo V, Vargas B, Plana R, et al. Paracentesis with intravenous infusion of albumin as compared with peritoneovenous shunting in cirrhosis with refractory ascites. *N Engl J Med* 1991;325:829–835.
12. Gines P, Arroyo V. Paracentesis in the management of cirrhotic ascites. *J Hepatol* 1993;17(Suppl 2):S14–18.
13. Salerno F, Badalamenti S, Incerti P, et al. Repeated paracentesis and I.V. albumin infusion to treat tense ascites in cirrhotic patients: a safe alternative therapy. *J Hepatol* 1987;5:102–108.
14. Murphy M, Rossi, M. Managing ascites via the Tenckhoff catheter. *Med Surg Nurs* 1995;4:468–471.
15. Rossle M. The transjugular intrahepatic portosystemic shunt. *J Hepatol* 1996;25:224–231.
16. Arroyo V, Gines P. TIPS and refractory ascites. Lessons from the recent history of ascites therapy. *J Hepatol* 1996;25(2)22–23.
17. Roberts LR, Kamath PS, Ascites and hepatorenal syndrome: pathophysiology and management. *Mayo Clin Proc* 1996;71(9):874–881.

*Principles and Practice of Supportive Oncology,*
edited by Ann Berger et al.
Lippincott–Raven Publishers, Philadelphia ©1998

CHAPTER 16

# Oral Complications of Cancer Therapy

Ann M. Berger and Thomas J. Kilroy

In the discussion of orofacial complications and pain and its management for patients receiving chemotherapy or radiation therapy, we must consider and discuss many factors. In the brief space allocated to oral complications, we shall evaluate dentition, mucosa, and bone to understand the interrelationship of these organ systems and how they interface with orofacial pain.

Orofacial pain that develops during the course of oncology therapy cannot be described simplistically as mucositis. Mucositis is the common definition for the oral symptoms that the oncology patient develops during the course of therapy; however, mucositis is not simply the result of mucosal ulceration from chemotherapy or radiation therapy. We must examine the various causes of orofacial pain, which may arise from different origins (Table 1). The oral environment, when in imbalance, poses a serious threat to the success of both chemotherapy and radiation therapy. There is a complex interrelationship between the oral microflora, occlusal pathology, dental restorations, and mucositis. In chemotherapy, bacteria play a major role in the morbidity associated with mucositis. For patients receiving radiation therpy, both oral microorganisms and restorative dental procedures have a significant impact on both the transient mucositis and the long-term dental mangement.

Oral mucositis is a major problem in patients receiving chemotherapy or radiation therapy. Estimates of oral mucositis in cancer therapy range from 40% of those receiving standard chemotheapy to 76% in bone marrow transplant patients (1). Virtually all patients who receive radiation therapy to the head and neck area develop oral complications. Mucositis is not only painful but also can

limit adequate nutritional intake and decrease the willingness of patients to continue treatment. More severe mucositis with extensive ulceration may require costly hospitalizations with parenteral nutrition and narcotics. Mucositis diminishes the quality of life and may result in serious clinical complications. A healthy oral mucosa serves to clear microorganisms and provides a chemical barrier that limits penetration of many compounds into the epithelium. A mucosal surface that is damaged increases the risk of a secondary infection and may prove to be a nidus for systemic infection. Mucositis may result in the need to reduce dosage in subsequent chemotherapy cycles or to delay radiation therapy, which ultimately may affect patient response to therapy.

It is important to recognize that the dentition, supporting tissue, hard and soft prostheses, and fixed and removable prostheses must be examined thoroughly before the commencement of therapy. Dental caries involving previous restorations or nonrestored teeth will be a source of bacteria that can be implicated in the cause of mucositis. Xerostomia associated with radiation therapy notably increases plaque colonization on the surfaces of the teeth and prostheses. Increases in bacterial volume are related directly to mucositis symptoms and elevated caries activity on the eroded and worn surfaces of the dentition.

## DIRECT STOMATOTOXICITY

Normally, cells of the mouth undergo rapid renewal over a 7- to 14-day cycle. Both chemotherapy and radiation therapy interfere with cellular mitosis and reduce the ability of the oral mucosa to regenerate. Cancer chemotherapeutic drugs that produce direct stomatotoxicity include the alkylating agents, antimetabolites, natural products, and other synthetic agents, such as hydroxyurea and procarbazine hydrochloride (2). Typical sequelae of these cytotoxic agents include epithelial hyperplasia, collagen and glandular degeneration, and epithelial dyspla-

A. M. Berger: Supportive Care Services, Department of Oncology and Anesthesiology, Cooper Hospital/University Medical Center, Camden, NJ 08103, and Lighthouse Hospice/Alternative Hospice Solutions, Inc., Atlanta, GA 30340.

T. J. Kilroy: Private Practice, Denver, CO 80230.

**TABLE 1.** *Etiologic factors contributing to pain in the oncology patient*

Dental
  Root exposure secondary to periodontal
    (gum) attachment loss
  Dental caries
  Dentures
    Denture sores
      Occlusion
      Overextension of borders
      Fractured dentures or denture teeth
    Denture hygiene
  Orthodontic appliances
Soft tissue (mucosa)
  Mucositis
  Pericorinitis
  Gingivitis
  Periodontitis
  Angular cheilosis
  Epulis fissuratum
Bone
  Osteomyelitis
    Osteoradionecrosis
    Denture related dehisence

sia (3). Mucositis is an inevitable side effect of radiation. The severity of the mucositis depends on the type of ionizing radiation, the volume of irradiated tissue, the daily dose, and the cumulative dose. As the mucositis becomes more severe, pseudomembranes and ulcerations develop. Poor nutritional status further interferes with mucosal regeneration by decreasing cellular migration and renewal (4).

Direct stomatotoxicity usually is seen 5 to 7 days after the administration of chemotherapy or radiation therapy. In the nonmyelosuppressed patient, oral lesions heal in 2 to 3 weeks. The mucosa that is most affected is the nonkeratinized mucosa. The most common sites include the labial, buccal, and soft palate mucosa as well as the floor of the mouth and the ventral surface of the tongue. Clinically, mucositis presents with multiple complex symptoms, beginning with asymptomatic redness and erythema and progressing to solitary elevated, desquamative white patches that are slightly painful to contact pressure to large, contiguous, pseudomembranous, acutely painful lesions with associated dysphagia and decreased oral intake. Histopathologically, edema of the retepegs will be noted along with vascular changes that demonstrate a thickening of the tunica intima with concominant reduction in the size of the lumen and destruction of the elastic and muscle fibers of the vessel walls. The loss of epithelial cells to the basement membrane exposes the underlying connective tissue stroma with its associated innervation, which, as the mucosal lesions enlarge, contributes to increasing pain levels. Oral infections that may be the resulting from bacteria, viruses, or fungal organisms can exacerbate mucositis and lead to systemic infec-

tions. If the patient develops both severe mucositis and thrombocytopenia, oral bleeding may occur and be difficult to treat.

A mucositis grading system gives the physician the ability to assess the severity of the mucositis in terms of both pain and the ability of the patient to maintain adequate nutrition so that an appropriate treatment plan can be constructed. There are many different grading systems; however, most are based on two or more clinical parameters, including erythema, pain, and problems with eating. An example of a common grading system is that proposed by the National Cancer Institute, which uses a numbering scale of 0 to 4. Grade 0 means no mucositis; grade 1, the patient has painless ulcers, erythema, or mild soreness; grade 2, the patient has painful erythema, edema, or ulcers but can eat; and grade 4, the patient requires parenteral or enteral support (5).

At the 1989 National Institutes of Health concensus conference on oral complications of cancer therapy, clinicians and researchers agreed that effective prevention of mucositis requires a comprehensive patient examination to identify potentially complicating oral disease before cancer therapy begins. Major problems that must be corrected include poor oral hygiene, periapical pathology, third molar pathology, periodontal disease, dental caries, defective restorations, orthodontic appliances, ill-fitting prostheses, and other potential sources of infection. Bacterial and fungal surveillance cultures are not necessary, but prophylactic use of acyclovir should be considered in patients who are seropositive and at high risk for reactivating herpes simplex virus infection, such as those who undergo bone marrow transplant or who have prolonged and pronounced myelosuppression. If a diagnosis is made of a fungal, viral, or bacterial infection along with the mucosal lesions, prompt treatment is necessary to avoid the risk of systemic infection (6).

## REMEDIES FOR THE PREVENTION AND TREATMENT OF MUCOSITIS

A standardized approach for the prevention and treatment of chemotherapy- and radiation-induced mucositis is essential, although it is unfortunate that the efficacy and safety of most regimens have not been established. The usual prophylactic measures used for the prevention of mucositis include chlorhexidine gluconate (Peridex), saline rinses, sodium bicarbonate rinses, acyclovir, amphotericin, and ice. Regimens commonly used for the treatment of mucositis and the pain associated with the mucositis include a local anesthetic such as lidocaine or Dyclone, Maalox or Mylanta, diphenhydramine (Benadryl), nystatin, or sucralfate. These agents are used either alone or in different combinations consisting of several of these medications made into a mouthwash. Other agents used less commonly include Kaopectate, allopurinol, vitamin E, beta-carotene, Kamillosan liquid, aspirin, anti-prostaglandins, prostaglandins, MGI 209 (marketed as Oratect gel), silver nitrate, and antibiotics. Oral and sometimes parenteral narcotics are used to relieve the pain caused by the mucositis. A new method using capsaicin is currently under study to help relieve the pain associated with mucositis.

## Direct Cyroprotectants

Sucralfate, an aluminum salt of sucrose ocrasulfate, which has been used successfully to treat gastrointestinal ulceration has been tested as a rinse for the prevention and treatment of mucositis. The mechanism of action of sucralfate appears to be by forming an ionic bond to proteins in an ulcer site, thereby creating a protective barrier (7). Additionally, there is evidence that there is an increase in the local production of prostaglandin E2, which results in an increase in mucosal blood flow, mucus production, mitotic activity, and surface migration of cells (8,9).

Anecdotal experience suggests sucralfate might be useful in the prevention and treatment of chemotherapy-induced mucositis; however, data from the studies are conflicting. Solomon (10) reported a 55% objective response rate, which was defined as a decrease of one grade on the cancer and leukemia group B (CALGB) scale of oral toxicity, in 19 patients receiving chemotherapy (10). In 1984 and 1985 Ferraro and Mattern (11,12) reported encouraging results in the use of sucralfate for chemotherapy-induced mucositis. Two randomized, double-blind clinical trials have evaluated sucralfate for the prevention of chemotheapy-induced mucositis. Pfeiffer et al. (13) found a significant reduction in edema, erythema, erosion, and ulceration in 23 evaluable patients of a total of 40 patients receiving cisplatin and continuous infusion with 5-fluorouracil (5-FU) with or without bleomycin (13). Patients favored sucralfate although this preference failed to reach statistical significance. Ten of these patients did not complete the study because the swishing of the sucralfate and the placebo aggravated chemotherapy-induced nausea. To help overcome this problem, the authors suggested that the solution should have a neutral taste and should not be swallowed after swishing. In contrast, results from a similarly designed study, with patients receiving remission-induction chemotherapy for acute nonlymphocytic leukemia, did not support the amelioration of mucositis. The latter study also concluded that chronic administration of the sucralfate suspension had no effect on the incidence of gastrointestinal bleeding and ulceration. The authors did note that some patients reported pain relief from sucralfate (14). Preliminary data from a Phase III randomized trial completed by the Illinois Cancer Council suggest that a topical solution of sucralfate is superior to a solution of Benadryl, Maalox, and Xylocaine. Both treatments provided equal pain

relief and equal use of supplememtal analgesics; however, 5 days after treatment initiation, a greater percentage of patients in the sucralfate group had less severe mucositis than the group receiving Benadryl, Maalox, and Xylocaine combination.

Sucralfate also has been tested in patients receiving radiation therapy. One study compared 21 patients who received standard oral care to the head and neck with 24 patients who received sucralfate suspension four times daily. Results revealed a significant difference in mucosal edema, pain, dysphagia, and weight loss in patients receiving sucralfate (15). In a pilot study done by Pfeiffer et al. (16), sequential patients who received radiation therapy to the head and neck received sucralfate at the onset of mucositis. Most patients had a decrease in pain following the use of sucralfate. A double-blind, placebo-controlled study with sucralfate in 33 patients who received irradiation to the head and neck reported no stastitically significant differences in mucositis; however, the sucralfate group reported less oral pain, and other topical and systemic analgesics were started later in the course of radiation (17). A prospective double-blind study compared the effectiveness of sucralfate suspension versus diphenhydramine syrup plus kaolin-pectin on radiotherapy-induced mucositis. Data were collected daily, including perceived pain, helpfulness of mouth rinses, weekly mucositis grade, weight change, and interruption of therapy. Analysis of the two groups revealed no stastically significant differences between the two groups. In a retrospective review, 15 patients who had not used daily oral rinses were compared with the two groups, and the results suggested that the use of a daily oral rinse with a mouth-coating agent may result in less pain, reduce weight loss, and help prevent interruption of radiation because of severe mucositis (18).

## Prostaglandins, Antiprostaglandins, Nonsteroidal Agents

Prostaglandins are a family of naturally occurring eicosanoids, some of which have known cytoprotective activity. Dinoprostone, or prostaglandin E2 (PGE2), has been reported to be beneficial in healing both gastric ulcers and chronic leg ulcers (19,20). Pilot studies done revealed the need for controlled clinical trials. In a pilot study done by Kuhrer et al. (21), five patients received topical dinoprostone for chemotherapy-induced mucositis. Four of the five patients reported pain relief, with healing of the ulcers within 3 to 7 days. They then tested the prophylactic efficacy of dinoprostone by applying it topically to one patient who was receiving chemotherapy and who had developed previous episodes of mucositis as well as two patients receiving total body irradiation. Only one of the patients who had received the dinoprostone and total body irradiation developed mucositis (21). In a nonblinded study, Porteder treated ten patients receiving 5-FU and mitomycin with concomitant radiation for oral carcinomas with dinoprostone four times daily during treatment. The control group comprised 14 patients who were receiving identical treatments. Eight of the ten patients who received dinoprostone were evaluable, and none developed severe mucositis compared with six episodes in the control arm (22). A third pilot study of 15 patients who received radiotherapy of the head and neck found that an inflammatory reaction in the vicinity of the tumor could only be detected in five patients treated with topically applied $PGE_2$, and none of the patients developed any bullous or desquamating inflammatory lesions (23). A double-blind, placebo-controlled study of $PGE_2$ in 60 patients undergoing bone marrow transplant revealed no significant differences in the incidence, severity, or duration of mucositis. The incidence of herpes simplex virus was higher in those on the $PGE_2$ arm, and in those patients who developed herpes simplex virus, mucositis was more severe (24).

Benzydamine is a nonsteroidal with analgesic, anesthetic, antiinflammatory and antimicrobial properties. Epstein and Stevenson-Moore (25) found in a double-blind, placebo-controlled trial that benzydamine produced stastically significant relief of pain from radiation-induced mucositis (25). Positive responses to benzydamine were reported in at least two other studies (26,27). The study done by Epstein and Stevenson-Moore (25) revealed not only a trend toward reduction in pain but also a stastically significant reduction in the total area and size of ulceration. Another study demonstrated that when indomethacin, an antiprostagalandin, was given orally, it reduced the severity and delayed the onset of mucositis induced by radiation therapy (28).

### Corticosteroids

No placebo-controlled studies on the use of corticosteroids for chemotherapy-induced mucositis have been done; however there have been two reports of pilot work done with patients who received radiation therapy. Abdelaal et al. (29) reported the use of bethamethasone with water mouthwash in five patients receiving radiation therapy. They reported that the mucosa was virtually ulcer free and the patients did not report any pain (29). The proposed mechanism of action of the steroid mouthwash was attributed to inhibition of production of leukotrienes and prostaglandins. Another pilot study done on 21 patients receiving radiation therapy who used an oral rinse consisting of hydrocortisone in combination with nystatin, tetracycline, and diphenhydramine was compared with a placebo rinse. Only 12 of 21 patients were evaluable; however, by the end of radiation treatment, there was a stastically significant difference in mucositis and a trend toward a reduction in pain. No patients in the treatment group needed to interrupt radia-

tion, whereas three patients in the control group needed an interruption in radiation therapy (30).

### Vitamins and Other Antioxidants

Vitamins in pharmacologic doses also have been used to treat mucositis. Vitamin E has been tested in chemotherapy-induced mucositis because it can stabilize cellular membranes and may improve herpetic gingivitis, possibly through antioxidant activity (31–33). The efficacy of vitamin E was demonstrated by Wadleigh et al. (34) in a randomized double-blind, placebo-controlled study. Eighteen patients receiving chemotherapy were randomized to receive a topical application of vitamin E or a placebo. In the vitamin E treated group, six of nine patients had complete resolution of their mucositis in 4 days of initiating therapy, whereas in the placebo group only one of nine had resolution of the lesions during the 5-day study period. This difference was stastically significant (34).

Other antioxidants that have been used clinically include vitamin C and glutathione. Another antioxidant tested in a pilot study is azelastine hyrochloride, which has been used in many allergic diseases and is effective in the treatment of aphthous ulcers in Behcet disease. Osaki et al. (35) reported on a study done with 63 patients who had head and neck tumors and received a combination of radiation therapy with concomitant chemotherapy. Twenty-six patients received regimen 1, which consisted of vitamin C, vitamin E, and glutathione; 37 patients received regimen 2, which consisted of everything in regimen 1 plus azelastine. At the completion of treatment, 21 of the patients in the azelastine arm remained at grade 1 or 2 mucositis, with six patients having grade 3 mucositis and ten having grade 4 mucositis. In the control group, grades 3 and 4 mucositis was induced in six and 15 patients, respectively, with only two cases having grade 1 mucositis and two cases with grade 2 mucositis. The azelastine suppressed neutrophil respiratory burst both in vivo and in vitro as well as cytokine release from lymphocytes. The authors concluded that a regimen including azelastine, which suppresses reactive oxygen production and stabilizes cell membranes, may be useful for the prophylaxis of mucositis due to chemoradiotherapy (35).

Beta-carotene, a vitamin A precursor with known effects on cellular differentiation, has been used on radiation-induced mucositis. B-carotene has been shown to produce regression in oral leukoplakia lesions (36). Mills (37) reported on the use of beta-carotene in treatment-induced mucositis. Ten patients receiving radiation interspersed with two cycles of chemotherapy were given beta-carotene 250 mg/day for the first 3 weeks of therapy and then 75 mg/day for the last 5 weeks of therapy. The control group comprised ten patients with oral cancer who were receiving the identical treatment. At the end of treatment, there was a stastically significant difference in grade 3 to 4 mucositis in the beta-carotene group. There was no difference in the grade 1 and 2 mucositis.

### Silver Nitrate

Silver nitrate, a caustic agent, has been tested in radiation-induced mucositis. Because silver nitrate stimulates cell division when it is applied to normal mucosa, the thought was that if applied before cytotoxic therapy, it might enhance repair and replacement of mucosa that was damaged by cytotoxic therapy. Maciejewski et al. (38) reported on a study of 16 patients who received radiation therapy to bilateral opposing fields; 2% silver nitrate was applied to the left side of the oral mucosa three times per day for 5 days before radiation therapy and during the first 2 days of radiation. The right side of the oral mucosa was unpainted and served as the control. The study revealed significantly less severe mucositis and a decrease in duration of mucositis on the mucosa treated with silver nitrate.

### Miscellaneous Cytoprotectants

An uncontrolled study of 98 patients with different malignancies receiving different medical regimens with either chemotherapy or radiation therapy reported that kamillosan liquid used before and after the development of mucositis helped to prevent and also decreased the duration of mucositis (39). Because this was an uncontrolled study with many different types of patients with different malignancies and different treatments, further well-designed studies need to be done to evaluate the efficacy of kamillason in mucositis. Oshitani et al. (40) reported on the use of sodium alginate topically, an agent thath promotes healing of esophageal and gastric mucosa in radiation-induced mucositis. Thirty-nine patients with mucositis were randomized to receive either sodium alginate or placebo. Those who received sodium alginate had a reduction in both mucosal erosions and in port (40). Other topical agents used clinically for treatment-induced mucositis include Kaopectate, Benadryl, saline, sodium bicarbonate, and gentian violet. Even though the previously mentioned agents are used clinically for treatment-induced mucositis, there are no controlled clinical trials that establish their efficacy.

## Indirect Cytoprotectants

### Hematologic Growth Factors

Hematologic growth factors are currently standard in the treatment of patients receiving high-dose chemotherapy. The effect of the hematologic growth factors on decreasing the depth and duration of chemotherapy-induced neutropenia is well established. Lieschke et al.(41) reported on a study examining the levels of neutrophil count and assessing whether the oral neutrophil count correlated with oral mucositis. It was found that the oral neutrophil count, like that of circulating systemic neutrophils, went to undetectable levels; however, they recovered before the systemic circulating neutrophils. In patients receiving granulocyte colony-stimulating factor (G-CSF), the mean cumulative mucositis score was less than those who did not receive G-CSF (41).

Gabrilove et al. (42) reported on a study done with 27 patients receiving MVAC (methotrexate, vinblastine, doxorubicin, and cisplatin) for bladder carcinoma and escalating doses of G-CSF. The patients received the G-CSF in their first cycle of chemotherapy but not in their second cycle. Significantly less mucositis was seen during the cycle in which patients received G-CSF (42). In this study there may have been a bias in that the patients may have developed less severe mucositis because G-CSF was given only during the first cycle; perhaps there is cumulative toxicity so that with each cycle of chemotheapy, the severity of mucositis increases. Bronchud et al. (43) treated 17 patients with breast or ovarian carcinoma who were receiving escalating doses of doxorubicin with G-CSF support. In this study the G-CSF did not prevent severe mucositis (43). In a fourth study using G-CSF, 41 patients receiving chemotheapy for non-Hodgkins lymphoma received G-CSF, and 39 patients received chemotherapy without G-CSF. In those who did not receive G-CSF, the main cause of treatment delay was neutropenia, whereas in patients who did receive G-CSF, the main cause of treatment delay was mucositis (44).

In a study in which GM-CSF was used in patients undergoing bone marrow transplantation compared with historical controls, recovery of neutrophils was more rapid with the GM-CSF; however, there was no difference in the severity of mucositis or in duration of hospitalization. Patients who received GM-CSF had more severe graft-versus-host disease (45). At this time, most evidence does not support the use of hematologic growth factors to prevent mucositis.

The effect of other biologically active factors on mucositis development is currently under study. In vitro studies have shown that not only is epidermal growth factor (EGF) present in saliva but also that it has the abililty to affect growth, cell differentiation, and cell migration (46,47). It is known that EGF induces chemotaxis of oral epithelial cells, indicating that it may be important in maintaining the integrity of the oral epithelium, especially in wound healing. Patients with peptic ulcers have significantly lower levels of EGF in their saliva, suggesting that EGF may be involved in either protection or repair (48). In an animal study in which the animals received 5-FU with an infusion of EGF for 7 and 14 days versus a placebo, the animals that received the EGF had increased mucosal breakdown. The results of the study indicate that chemotherapy-induced mucositis depends on the rate of epithelial cell growth. The timing of the administration of the EGF in relation to the chemotherapy may determine whether a patient develops increased oral toxicity versus repair of the mucosa (49).

### Antimicrobials

There have been many conflicting studies on the use of chlohexidine mouthwash in both alleviating mucositis and reducing oral colonization by gram-positive, gram-negative, and candida species in patients receiving radiotherapy, chemotherapy, or bone marrow transplantation. In 1990 Ferretti et al. (50), in a randomized controlled trial, demonstrated that prophylactic chlorhexidine mouth rinse reduces oral mucositis and microbial burden in patients with cancer receiving chemotherapy (50). Most studies since that time have not demonstrated a reduction in mucositis in patients receiving intensive chemotherapy (51–53); however, Epstein et al. (52) and Weisdorf et al. (53) did demonstrate a reduction in oral colonization by candida and oral candidiasis. Ferretti et al. (54) found that the use of chlohexidine rinse for the prevention of mucositis was not effective; however, there was a reduction in streptococcal counts. Spijkervet et al., in a placebo-controlled, double-blind study revealed that the colonization index of viridans streptococci was reduced after 5 weeks of chlorhexidine treatment, but it did not decrease the colonization of Candida, *Streptococcus faecalis*, staphlococci, Enterobacteriaceae, Pseudomonadaceae, and Acinetobacter species, and there was no difference in the development and severity of mucositis (55). A recent randomized, double-blind study comparing chlorhexidine mouthwash versus placebo in 25 patients receiving radiation revealed a trend for more mucositis as well as mouthwash-induced discomfort, taste alteration, and teeth staining on the chlorhexidine arm (56). The overall statistical data lead to the conclusion that chlorhexidine may result in improved oral hygiene, but the discomfort from using the rinse negates its minimal benefits.

The endotoxins of aerobic gram-negative bacilli are implicated in the etiology of mucositis. A study by Spijkervet et al. (57) postulated that lozenges containing 2 mg of polymyxin E, 1.8 mg of tobramycin, and 10 mg of amphotericin (PTA) four times daily on the oropharyngeal flora would mediate and control mucositis. They compared the results in 15 irradiated patients using PTA and two other groups of 15 patients using 0.1% chlorhexidine and 15 using placebo. In the selectively decontaminated group, the severity and extent of mucositis were reduced significantly compared with the chlorhexidine and placebo groups (p value less than 0.05). Clinically, all patients in the lozenge group showed erythema only, whereas 80% of both the placebo and chlorhexidine rinse groups suffered severe mucositis with extended pseudomembranes from the third week of irradiation. No nasogastric tube feedings were needed in the PTA group compared with 30% of patients in the other groups (57). The potential role of PTA lozenges remains to be clarified. Another antimicrobial, nystatin suspension, has been studied in the prophylaxis of candidiasis in leukemia and bone marrow transplantation patients. Most publications do not support the use of nystatin (58–65).

### Pharmacolgic Modulation

Another agent that has been evaluated for the prevention and treatment of oral mucositis induced by 5-FU chemotherapy is allopurinol. The rationale for the allopurinol mothwash was based on data that systemic allopurinol was able to decrease 5-FU-induced toxicity by inhibiting the enzme orotidylate decarboxylase and the formation of the metabolites of fluorodeoxyuridine monophosphate (FdUMP) and fluorouridine (FUrd) (66). Two pilot studies support the use of allopurinol for oral mucositis. The study by Clark and Slevin (67) revealed that allopurinol mouthwash substantially decreased the incidence and severity of mucositis in six patients who received bolus 5-FU chemotherapy (67). Another pilot study involving 16 patients receiving 5-day intravenous 5-FU infusions and using allopurinol mouthwashs four to six times per day also found that the allopurinol alleviated the mucositis in all these patients (68). After the success of the pilot studies, the use of allopurinol became routine medical practice in many institutions. The efficacy of allopurinol was tested by the North Central Cancer Treatment Group and the Mayo Clinic in a randomized, double-blind clinical trial. Seventy-five patients were assigned to receive allopurinol mouthwash or placebo while they received their first 5-day course of 5-FU with or without leucovorin. This study demonstrated no protective effect against 5-FU-induced mucositis by the allopurinol regimen (69).

Leucorvin has been used in combination with methotrexate (MTX) to help decrease the oral mucositis that occurs with MTX. In a pilot study with 19 patients who received edatrexate for non-small cell lung carcinoma, there was less mucositis seen than anticipated (70).

Glutamine administration in animal studies led to a reduction in both morbidity and mortality of animals who have received a variety of chemotherapeutic agents, including MTX. The glutamine both preserved the morphological structure of the gut and reduced the incidence of bacteraemia (71,72). In a randomized trial of 28 patients with gastointestinal cancers who received 5-FU and folinic acid and who also received 16 g of glutamine per day for 8 days versus a placebo, there was no effect on oral mucositis in the group who received the glutamine. The authors concluded that perhaps both the dose and duration of exposure to the glutamine were not sufficient to show a decrease in mucositis (73).

Another agent found in laboratory data to protect host tissues selectively from 5-FU toxic effects without loss of antitumor effect is uridine (74). A study of 29 patients with advanced malignancies received PALA and MTX, each at 250 mg/m², followed 24 hours later by increasing doses of 5-FU to 600 to 750 mg/m² per meter with a leucovorin rescue and uridine rescue for a 72-hour infusion. The uridine allowed dose escalation of 5-FU to 750 mg/m² with a decrease in all toxicity of the 5-FU except that mucositis was the only significant chemotherapy-induced toxicity (75). Perhaps additional studies with oral uridine would reveal a reduction of the toxicity from mucositis.

A pilot study using propantheline, an anticholingeric agent that causes xerostomia, was done to test whether the incidence of mucositis could be reduced when patients received etoposide. The hypothesis was that the mucosal toxicity may be related to salivary excretion of etoposide following systemic administration. Propantheline or placebo was given to 12 patients. The results revealed a decrease in the incidence and severity of mucositis in the patients who received propantheline (76).

## Cryotherapy

Cryotherapy, in the form of ice chips and popsicles, have been used for the prevention of mucositis. The North Central Cancer Treatment Group and the Mayo Clinic undertook a controlled randomized trial of oral cryotherapy for preventing 5-FU-induced mucositis. The study found that cryotherapy is helpful in reducing the severity of 5-FU-induced mucositis (77,78). Following this study, another was done in which randomized patients received 30 minutes of cryotherapy versus 60 minutes. A total of 178 evaluable patients were studied. Both cryotherapy groups had similar degrees of mucositis. The conclusion was to continue to recommend the use of 30 minutes of oral cryotherapy for patients receiving bolus intensive courses of 5-FU-based chemotherapy (79). A confirmatory study done following the original study reported by the North Central Cancer Treatment Group and the Mayo Clinic was done and once again confirmed that oral cryotherapy can reduce 5-FU-induced mucositis (80).

## Laser

Laser, as a palliative methodology for mucositis, only recently has begun to be investigated as a potential for lesion and pain control. Laser initially was studied in an animal model. In a study done by Bugai et al. (81), four groups of animals had a mucosal lesion. Three groups received impulse laser exposure from 60 to 600 pulses, and one group was untreated. The only group demonstrating more rapid resolution of the mucosal lesion (14 versus 21–25 days) was the group who received the 600

pulsed exposures (81). A preliminary report revealed that laser may be beneficial in reducing the severity and duration of mucositis. Twenty patients, all with different cancers and chemotherapy protocols, served as controls, and 16 patients constituted a treatment group who received laser treatment. Patients in the treatment arm had a reduced duration of the mucosal lesions from a mean of 19.3 days in the control arm to 8.1 days in those who received laser therapy (82). At this time, double-blind randomized trials are needed to verify these earlier reports.

## Anesthetic Cocktails

Several anesthetic cocktails using agents such as viscous Xylocaine or dyclonine hydrochloride have been used with some success (83). The anesthetic agents relieve the pain, but this relief is temporary and also prevents taste perception, which can further interfere with food intake. Other analgesics and mucosal coating agents that can control pain include Kaopectate, Benadryl, Orabase, and Oratect gel. Even though clinicians use these agents, there is no experimental evidence to establish the efficacy of any of them (84).

## Capsaicin

Capsaicin, the active ingredient in chili peppers, is a remedy that has been used for many different pain syndromes through the years and may prove beneficial for mucositis pain induced by chemotherapy and radiation therapy. Several studies support the medical efficacy of locally applied capsaicin in a cream vehicle in neuropathic pain syndromes. A large multicenter trial comprising 277 patients demonstrated that topically applied capsaicin used for up to 8 weeks significantly reduced pain and improved quality of life in both postherpetic neuralgia and diabetic neuropathy (85–87). Other neuropathic pain syndromes for which capsaicin is effective include postmastectomy pain (88), stump pain (89), trigeminal neuralgia (90), reflex sympathetic dystrophy (91), and Guillain-Barre syndrome (92). Topical capsaicin also decreases the pain associated with rheumatoid arthritis and osteoarthritis (93), and intranasal capsaicin spray reduces the pain associated with cluster headaches (94). Topical capsaicin improves the rate of reepithelialization of wound healing in minipigs and may be efficacious in wound healing in humans (95).

In a pilot project, capsaicin in a candy vehicle (cayenne pepper candy) was given to patients with therapy-induced mucositis. Patients were instructed to allow the candy to dissolve in the mouth without chewing it. After the candy had dissolved, the burn produced by the candy was allowed to fade. The patients rated their pain before and after eating the candy. The reduction in pain was highly

**TABLE 2.** *Formulary of common remedies for oral complications*

Prevention of mucositis
- Povidone iodine rinse 0.5%
  - Rinse 2 to 4 times daily; do not swallow
- Chlorhexidine gluconate 0.12% oral rinse
  - Rinse twice daily for 30 s; do not swallow
- NAHCO$_3$ powder — 3 tbsp or 11.6 g
  - NACl powder — 3 tbsp or 11.6 g
  - Distilled water — 1 gallon
    - Combine all ingredients together; rinse 2 to 4 times per day; do not swallow.

Treatment of mucositis and pain[a]
- Benadryl (diphenhydramine) — 30 ml
  - 12.5 mg/5 ml
  - Viscous lidocaine 2% — 30 ml
  - Maalox — 30 ml
    - Combine all ingredients together; rinse 15 ml 4 to 6 times daily

- Benadryl (diphenhydramine) — 30 ml
  - 12.5 mg/5 ml
  - Tetracycline or penicillin — 60 ml
  - 125 mg/5 ml susp.
  - Nystatin oral suspension — 45 ml
  - 100,000 U/ml
  - Viscous Xylocaine 2% — 30 ml
  - Hydrocortisone suspension — 30 ml
  - 10 mg/5 ml
  - Sterile water for irrigation — 45 ml
    - Combine all ingredients together; rinse with 15 ml 4 to 6 times daily

- Carafate suspension — 1 g 4 times daily
- Viscous Xylocaine 2% solution or — 10–15 ml every
  - Dyclonine hydrochloride 0.5% — 2–3 h
  - or 1% solution
- Benadryl 12.5 mg/5 ml
  - Kaopectate
    - Combine 50% each; swish 10-15 ml 4 to 6 times per day.

- Benadryl 12.5 mg/5 ml — 30 ml
  - Maalox — 30 ml
  - Nystatin 100,000 U/ml — 30 ml
    - Combine all ingredients together; rinse 15 ml 4 to 6 times daily

- Narcotics
  - May use oral or parenteral narcotics (such as patient controlled analgesia. If use oral analgesics, use tablets. Do not use elixir, which contains alcohol and will exacerbate mucositis
- Capsaicin candies
  - One candy every 3–4 h as needed; currently under clinical evaluation

Xerostoma
- Saliva substitutes
  - Xerolube
    - Rinse four to six times daily
  - Salivart synthetic saliva spray
    - Spray four to six times daily
  - Biotene chewing gum
    - Use as needed
- Pilocarpine
  - 5 mg 3 times daily

[a]Many of these medications have been used alone or in combination to treat mucositis.

stastistically significant (96,97). A double-blinded, placebo-controlled study is under way to test the efficacy of oral capsaicin for pain control.

### Narcotics

Many of the agents discussed herein may have some value in preventing mucositis or palliating the pain; however, there, are few controlled clinical trials that have established their efficacy. At present there is no standard treatment for the prevention or treatment of mucositis. When the mucositis is severe and interferes with nutritional intake and quality of life, it is appropriate to use any of the aforementioned treatments as well as oral or, if necessary, parenteral narcotic (Table 2). To discover an efficacious treatment, it is essential to continue studies of available treatments and to develop any promising new approaches.

## ORAL COMPLICATIONS IN RADIATION THERAPY

Before one can discuss orofacial pain, one must understand the nature and necessity of a comprehensive dental examination and how its data interface with the treatment regimen. Therefore, in accordance with the guidelines developed by the National Institute of Health (98), it is of supreme importance to have a team effort for the management of the oncology patient. Therefore, we recommend that a Preventive Dental Oncology Service (PDOS) be established for identification and management of patients receiving head and neck oncological surgery, irradiation, or chemotherapy treatment. The objective of the PDOS program is to evaluate the oncology patient for intraoral problems as related to the specific surgery, radiotherapy, or chemotherapy and to formulate a treatment plan for resolution of the intraoral symptoms associated with therapy.

Radiation therapy for the oncology patient has a significant risk of mucositis; however, the long-term effects of the radiation are of greater concern to the clinical team than the transient mucositis. The decrease in the numbers of osteocytes and the concommitant loss of vascularity in the maxillary or mandibular treatment fields precludes bone healing in the event of osseous surgery after therapy. The impaired, retarded, or nonhealing wound presents as a osteoradionecrosis (ORN), which requires specific management protocols (i.e. hyperbaric oxygen and intravenous antibiotics followed by osseous resection and additional hyperbaric oxygen and intravenous antibiotics). Secondary to the transient mucositis is xerostomia.

### Xerostomia

Xerostomia is a complex phenomenon that cannot be equivocated to radiation damage to the salivary glands alone. To understand xerostomia and the radiotherapy patient more fully, one must review the mechanisms behind saliva production. Secretion of saliva is subject to reflex stimulation not only of a physical but also of a psychic nature (99). Physical stimulation of the salivary gland originates in the taste buds. Psychic stimulation of the salivary glands is via the sensory nerve receptors. Xerostomia presents with a twofold pathogenosis. First, the lack of a wetting medium reduces the ability of the chemoreceptors on the dorsum of the tongue and the palate to accept the stimuli presented with foods or liquids. This loss of physical stimulation (chemical) fails to trigger the neurogenic response to the salivary gland, and the anticipated salivary response never occurs. The minimal thickened, mucinous saliva produced by the affected glands coats the mucosa of the cheeks, tongue, and palate, forming a effective barrier and making the taste buds physically inaccessible to the dietary (chemophores) and physical response to thermal and mechanical stimulation. The cumulative result of not being able to stimulate the taste buds physically has a direct corresponding effect on the psychic component of salivary gland secretions. Histopathologically, the mucosa on the dorsum of the tongue appears atrophied, the end result of which is decreased surface area on the taste buds.

With the xerostomic patient, the clinician notices a significant loss of appetite, which occurrs concomitantly with mucositis. It is important to not discount the role of xerostomia and place the blame of weight loss on stomatitis. When the physical component of salivary stimulation is denegrated by mechanical (mucous) barriers, the anticipated taste sensation associated with specific food groups is altered. When the patient can no longer perceive what should be sour or sweet, he or she will be unable to elicit the correct sensory response through the neurogenic paths; then the second component of salivary stimulation (visual) becomes ineffective and the xerostomia is further exacerbated. When patients can no longer acheive the sensory gratification normally associated with specific food groups, dietary intake decreases and weight loss becomes a significant factor in the continuity of therapy. With the decrease in the salivary enzymes necessary for the initial stages of digestion, a third factor presents itself into the weight loss arena: the inability to assimilate dietary nutrients efficiently. Xerostomia is compounded by other factors, such as antidepressant therapy, diabetes, interstitial nephritis, aging, postmenopausal syndromes, antihypertensives, and diuretics. Vitamin A and nicotinic acid deficiencies also can affect salivary secretions.

The management of xerostomia is complex, requiring attention to the patient's medical history for drug interactions and providing a diet that both physically and psychologically is able to stimulate the salivary responses while maintaining excellent oral hygiene to provide physical access to the taste receptors and monitoring the vitamin A and nicotinic acid levels for deficiencies. Increased intake of nicotinic acid and vitamin A on a specific monitored response to dose program can be effective in increasing saliva flow. Mechanical debridement of the

dorsum of the tongue with a soft toothbrush and the use of a spray mist before and during meals assist in maintaining access to taste buds. Earlier clinical pilot studies by Fox and co-workers (100) and Greenspan and Daniels (101) indicated that low doses of oral pilocarpine reduced radiation-induced xerostomia. Recently, a randomized, double-blind, placebo-controlled trial by Johnson and colleagues (102) found that pilocarpine improved saliva production and relieved symptoms of xerostomia after irradiation for cancer of the head and neck; minor side effects were limited predominantly to sweating.

With effective management of xerostomia, the thickened mucinous film that accumulates on the mucosa of the tongue, floor of mouth, palate, and buccal folds is eliminated. With this simple maintenance step that can be managed by the patient or support staff, a significant reduction in bacterial volume is achieved, and this in turn will reduce the incidence of mucositis significantly. When xerostomia is not controlled, significant plaque and material will accumulate on the surfaces of prosthetic appliances. This bacterial film can contribute to denture irritation that will compound therapy-related mucositis and can lead to fenestration of the supporting mucosa and development of a osteonecrosis in the posttreatment patient. When xerostomia is not monitored and or controlled, the clinical team can anticipate heavy plaque accumulation on the surfaces of the teeth. This plaque film is highly cariogenic and ultimately will cause dental complications involving the teeth (decay) and the supporting tissue (gingivitis and periodontitis). Patients with high plaque indices will not benefit from the anticariogenic treatment using fluoride applicators because plaque is a effective barrier against fluoride absorption. It must be assumed that the elevated plaque matrix resulting from xerostomia poses the greatest risk in the postradiation therapy morbidity of osteoradionecrosis (ORN).

Because of this risk of ORN, it will be necessary for the clinical team to assess not only the pretreatment periodontal health of the patient but also to query the patient about his or her intent to maintain adaquate oral hygiene efforts. If the patient is not psychologically prepared to play a role in his or her own oral hygiene or if the patient is physically or mentally impaired and unable to manage an appropriate personal oral hygiene program, it will be prudent to consider oral surgery to remove all high-risk teeth as a preventative measure. Amputation of a patient's dentition is a serious, irreversible step that must be thoroughly planned by all members of the clinical team before proceeding.

From the dental examination, diagnostic models, and radiographs obtained prior to radiation therapy or chemotherapy, high-risk teeth can be identified and treated restoratively or surgically. The therapy team must recognize and identify teeth and other bone anatomy aberrations that would require posttreatment surgery. Because of the reduction in the vascular network and the permanent alteration of osteocytes in the bone in the treatment ports, it will be necessary to perform all prospective surgeries before the initiation of radiation. This will minimize the potential for osteoradionecrosis in situations where surgery must be performed after radiotherapy has been completed.

High-risk teeth and bone can be summarized as follows: impacted third molars; both bony and soft tissue; teeth diagnosed with periodontal disease that will require mucosal flap surgery for treatment; nonrestored endodontically treated teeth, which have a high risk for traumatic fracture; teeth that have been surgically removed, endodontically treated, and reimplanted; teeth restored with dental implants; teeth with root resorption secondary to orthodontic therapy. Supernumary teeth and ossifications also must be evaluated.

After dentition has been restored and appropriate surgeries have been completed, vacuum-formed vinyl fluoride applicators are made for home-care fluoride application. These applicators provide two functions: The first is to prevent xerostomia-induced dental caries through fluoride induction into the tooth enamel and dentin; secondly, the increased ambient fluroide levels on the tooth surface and the residual fluoride that remains in the oral cavity after each fluoride application reduce the level of oral bacteria and assist in microbial prophylaxis, which aids in the reduction of mucositis. In general, 0.04% stannous fluoride gel appears to be more effective than sodium fluoride 1.1% because it reduces the levels of *Streptococcus mutans*, which causes caries (103). These authors recommend that during the use of fluoride applicators a 0.04% stannous fluoride gel be placed in the applicators before application to the teeth; the applicators should remain for 3 minutes, after which the applicators are removed and the excess fluoride is expectorated. The patient is not allowed to rinse, eat, or drink for 30 minutes. For the week before initiation and weeks 1 and 2 of radiation therapy, we recommend using the fluoride three times daily. This recommendation is in anticipation of discontinuing fluoride therapy during the third, fourth and fifth weeks of radiation. For the first 3 months after radiation therapy, we recommend using fluoride twice daily. After 3 months and a thorough dental assessement, if the plaque indices are below 5%, we will continue the patient on once a day fluoride maintenance for life.

Before beginning radiation therapy, a protective radiation stent is fabricated. These stents are used during radiation therapy for all patients who have natural dentition. The purpose of the stents is to eliminate soft-tissue contact from the surfaces of large dental restorations, thereby eliminating the secondary electron scatter from radiation therapy that will cause significant localized mucositis.

From the diagnostic examination and radiographs, one must determine whether the patient undergoing radiation therapy has had dental implants placed for prosthetic rehabilitation. Oral implantology is rapidly becoming commonplace in the prosthetic rehabilitiation of missing teeth, as support for cleft palate obdurators, and as support for facial muloges and prostheses. If it has been determined that implants are present, the dental oncologist must be prepared to fabricate the appropriate radiation shields and blocks to protect the areas of the bone supporting the implants to minimize increased radiation dosimetry in those portions of the mandible or maxilla.

Keus et al. (104) reported on the effect of customized beam shaping on normal tissue complications in radiation therapy for parotid gland tumors. They evaluated customized beam's eye view as opposed to unblocked portals with field sizes defined by the largest target contour found in any computed tomography (CT) slice. They found the volume of unnecessarily exposed normal tissue that received more than 90% of the prescribed dose was reduced by a factor of 4% to 44% on average when the volume is expressed as a percentage of the target volume in each patient. For a tumor dose of 70 Gy, the average probability of bone necrosis was reduced from 8.4% to 4.1%.

In patients with extensive implanted supported fixed or fixed removable prostheses, a large volume of gold alloy is used in the fixed prostheses and the framework of the fixed removable. For patients with dental implants, removal of the detachable portions of the prosthesis should be completed before radiation therapy, and beam-shaping blocks should be fabricated by the prosthodontist for protection of the mandible containing the titanium implant fixture. These precautions are necessary to reduce the risk of radiation-induced osteoradionecrosis.

## Osteoradionecrosis

Osteoradionecrosis (ORN) carries the greatest morbidity in any radiotherapy program involving osseous tissue. It is not an infection but rather a nonhealing acellular, avascular bone that may have been present for months or years before becoming clinically evident. Continuous monitoring of the radiotherapy patient by the dental oncologist on a 3-month recall is appropriate. This recall schedule will allow evaluation of the plaque indices and monitoring of fluoride compliance and developing dental disease. Even with the best diagnosis, planning, and staging, an ORN can develop spontaneously. Early osteonecrotic changes are subtle and difficult to detect. In many instances ORN presents as asymptomatic dehiscence in the mucosa. As the necrosis progresses, the site can become more erythemotus and painful. At this stage, it is not uncommon for the clinician to misdiagnose the signs as a minor infection and place the patient on a regimen of antibiotics, which will minimize the symptoms but allow the necrosis to continue to progress. If teeth are present, the clinical symptoms are mobility, minimal to moderate pain, and ectopic eruption. In the early stages, routine dental radiographs are insufficient to provide an accurate diagnosis. As the necrosis advances, extraoral fistulas and intraoral antral fistulas will develop. Eventually, occlusion pathology becomes evident, and in many cases pathologic fractures will occur.

Early definitive diagnosis using CT scans, dentiscans, bone density studies, and magnetic resonance imagery will aid in determining the extent of the necrosis so that a surgical template can be made. In very small, isolated solitary lesions of less than 0.5 cm, surgical exposure and cautious debridement along with appropriate prophylactic antibiotics may suffice. Unfortunately, this is seldom the case with ORN, and if remission and healing are not evident within the first 8 weeks, presurgical and postsurgical hyperbaric oxygen, intravenous antibiotics, and radical excision of the necrotic avascular bone will be necessary. Myers and Marx (105) reported on the use of hyperbaric oxygen, which stimulates antiogenesis, with increased neovascularization and optimization of cellular levels of oxygen for osteoblast and fibroblast proliferaton, collagen formation, and support of ingrowing blood vessels. The hypoxic, acellular matrix in the postirradiated field is changed to a hypercellular, hyperoxic or normoxic situation. Oxygen is used as an adjunct to appropriate surgery, but using the two modalities together, the salvage rate for ORN and its complications of orocutaneous fistula, pathologic fractures, and severe bone loss can be increased dramatically (105).

With accurate pretherapy diagnosis, appropriate treatment planning, and therapy staging by all members of the clinical team, the incidence of ORN and other oral complications can be minimized or eliminated. If the pretreatment protocols are not in place, medicolegal accountability is significant and economically devastating. There is no reason for a patient to be denied the availability of a thorough comprehensive examination followed by a well-formulated and staged treatment plan.

## ORAL COMPLICATIONS IN TERMINAL CARE

Comprehensive care of the terminally ill person is as critical as care of patients in any other stage of illness. Untreated oral complications for a terminally ill patient can lead to both physiological and psychological complications. The oral cavity is often the final means by which a patient is able to communicate. It is therefore critical to provide comprehensive oral care to help the patient die with minimal discomfort and maximum dignity.

Infection and inflammation in the oral cavity are common in the terminal phase. Many patients experience significant discomfort from moniliasis, which usually is brought on by the administration of antibiotics or steroids. Treatment with nystatin liquid or troches five times a day quickly ameliorates this problem. Lack of saliva and poor oral care before the terminal phase will lead to rampant caries as well as significant oral inflammation. Orocutaneous fistula, abscesses, and infection are particularly common in patients with head and neck carcinoma. Metronidazole should be used to decrease sepsis as well as pain and discharge (106).

Excessive salivation (*silorrhoea*) is uncommon, but when it occurs it can be extremely uncomfortable as well as a social embarrassment. Silorrhoea can be caused by medications, aphthous ulcers, tumor, and local irritants, such as ill-fitting dentures. Treatment for this problem depends on its cause, that is, whether tumor is present. Training the patient to swallow differently and offering reassurance are sometimes helpful. Suction devices with small catheters can be devised and placed in the floor of the mouth, exiting through the submaxillary area (107).

Patients who are terminally ill may develop unpleasant or bad breath (*halitosis*). The incidence and prevalence of this symptom in patients with cancer are not known. Its causes are many, including diseases of the oral cavity (such as poor oral hygiene and xerostomia), diseases of the respiratory tract secondary to infections or tumor, diseases of the digestive tract (such as dyspepsia or colon stasis), metabolic failure (such as uremia, hepatic failure, or diabetic ketoacidosis), medications (such as antibiotics), and foods (such as garlic and onions). Treatment of halitosis varies with the cause. Gastric stasis may be treated with prokinetic drugs (e.g., metoclopramide or cisapride), and infections sometimes can be treated with systemic antibiotics and or antifungal drugs as well as local antiseptics (e.g., hydrogen peroxide or povidone-iodine mouthwash). General measures that are essential regardless of the cause include dietary advice and good oral hygiene.

Xerostomia is another problem that terminally ill patients may experience. Xerostomia leads to plaque formation around the teeth, which produces caries. The treatment of xerostomia is discussed in a previous section; once again, the most essential element of the treatment plan includes cleaning the teeth and gums at frequent intervals. With the terminally ill patient, this can be done with a soft toothbrush or gauze. At times, near-terminal patients may develop *trismus* (lockjaw), which makes oral care extremely difficult if not impossible. Trismus should be treated with dilators, which may help release the locked muscles (108).

Proper oral care is an integral part of patient care from pretherapy through the terminal phase of illness. In summary, one must conclude that a total team effort is a mandatory requirement for the standard of care necessary to provide the oncology patient with a comprehensive treatment plan that encompasses all the medical and dental health and rehabilitation issues.

# REFERENCES

1. Sonis ST. Oral complications of cancer therapy. In: De Vita VT, Hellman S, Rosenberg SA eds. *Cancer: principles and practice of oncology*, 4th ed. Philadelphia: JB Lippincott; 1993:2385.

2. Sonis ST. Oral complications of cancer therapy. In De Vita VT, Hellman S, Rosenberg SA, eds. *Cancer: principles and practice of oncology*, 4th ed. Philadelphia: JB Lippincott; 1993:2389.

3. Peterson DE, Ambrosio JA. Diagnosis and management of acute and chronic oral complications of nonsurgical cancer therapies. *Dent Clin North Am* 1992;36:945.

4. Sonis ST. Oral complications of cancer therapy. In: De Vita VT, Hellman S, Rosenberg SA, eds. *Cancer: principles and practice of oncology*, 4th ed. Philadelphia: JB Lippincott; 1993:2385–2386.

5. Oken MM, Creech RH, Tormey DC, et al. Toxicity and response criteria of the Eastern Cooperative Oncology Group. *Am J Clin Oncol* 1982;5:649.

6. Conference C. Oral complications of cancer therapies: diagnosis, prevention and treatment. *Conn Med* 1989;53:595.

7. Nagashima R, Hirano T. Selective binding of sucralfate to ulcer lesion. I. Experiments in rats with acetic acid-induced gastric ulcer receiving unlabeled sucralfate. *Arzneimittelforschung* 1980;30:80–83

8. Nagashima R, Yoshida N, Terao N. Sucralfate, a basic aluminum salt of sucrose sulfate II. Inhibition of peptic hydrolysis as it results from sucrose sulfate interaction with protein substrate, serum albumins. *Arzneimittelforschung* 1979;29:73–76.

9. Ferraro JM, Mattern J. Sucralfate suspension for stomatitis. *Drug Intell Clin Pharm* 1984;18:153.

10. Solomon MA. Oral sucralfate suspension for mucositis. *N Engl J Med* 1986;315:459–460.

11. Ferraro JM, Mattern J. Sucralfate suspension for stomatitis (Letter). *Drug Intell Clin Pharm* 1984;18:153.

12. Ferraro JM, Mattern J. Sucralfate suspension for mouth ulcers (Letter). *Drug Intell Clin Pharm* 1985;19:480.

13. Pfeiffer P, Madsen EL, Hansen O, et al. Effect of prophylactic sucralfate suspension on stomatitis induced by cancer chemotherapy. A randomized, double-blind cross-over study. *Acta Oncol* 1990;29:171–173.

14. Shenep JL, Kalwihsky D, Hudson PR, et al. Oral sucralfate in chemotherapy-induced mucositis. *J Pediatr* 1988;113:753.

15. Scherlacher A, Beaufort-Spontin E. Radiotherapy of head-neck neoplasms:prevention of inflammation of the mucosa by sucralfate treatment. *HNO* 1990;38:24–28.

16. Pfeiffer P, Hansen O, Madsen EL, et al. A prospective pilot study on the effect of sucralfate mouth-swishing in reducing stomatitis during radiotherapy of the oral cavity. *Acta Oncol* 1990;29:471–3.

17. Epstein JB, Wong FLW. The efficacy of sucralfate suspension in the prevention of oral mucositis due to radiation therapy. *Int J Radiat Oncol Biol Phys* 1994;28:693–698.

18. Barker G, Loftus L, Cuddy P, et al. The effects of sucralfate suspension and diphenhydramine syrup plus kaolin-pectin on radiotherapy-induced mucositis. *Oral Surg Oral Med Oral Pathol Oral Radiol Endod* 1991;71:288–293.

19. Cohen MM, Clark L. Preventing acetylsalicytic acid damage to human gastric mucosa by the use of prostaglandin $E_2$. *Can J Surg* 1983;26:116–122.

20. Ericksson B, Johansson C, Aly A. Prostaglandin $E_2$ for chronic leg ulcers. *Lancet* 1986;1:905.

21. Kuhrer I, Kuzmits R, Linkesch W, et al. Topical $PGE_2$ enhances healing of chemotherapy-associated mucosal lesions. *Lancet* 1986;1:623.

22. Porteder H, Rausch E, Kment G, et al. Local prostaglandin $E_2$ in patients with oral malignancies undergoing chemo and radiotherapy. *J Craniomaxillofac Surg* 1988;16:371–374.

23. Matejka M, Nell A, Kment G, et al. Local benefit of prostaglandin $E_2$ in radiochemotherapy-induced oral mucositis. *Br J Oral Maxillofac Surg* 1990;28:89–91.

24. Labor B, Mrsic M, Pavleric A, et al. Prostaglandin $E_2$ for prophylaxis of oral mucositis following BMT. *Bone Marrow Transplant* 1993;11:379–382.

25. Epstein JB, Stevenson-Moore P. Benzydamine hydrochloride in prevention and management of pain in mucositis associated with radiation therapy. *Oral Surg Oral Med Oral Pathol Oral Radiol Endod* 1986;62:145.

26. Epstein JB, Stevenson-Moore P, Jackson S, et al. Prevention of oral mucositis in radiation therapy: A controlled study with benzydamine hydrochloride rinse. *Int J Radiat Oncol Biol Phys* 1989;16:1571.

27. Lever SA, Dupuis LL, Chan SL. Comparative evaluation of benzydamine oral rinse in children with antineoplastic-induced stomatitis. *Drug Intell Clin Pharm* 1987;21:359.

28. Pillsbury HC, Webster WP, Rosenman J. Prostaglandin inhibitor and radiotherapy in advanced head and neck cancer. *Arch Otolaryngol Head Neck Surg* 1986;112:552.

29. Abdelaal AS, Barker DS, Fergusson MM. Treatment for irradiation-induced mucositis. *Lancet* 1987;1:97.

30. Rothwell BR, Speltor WS. Palliation of radiation-related mucositis. *Special Care in Dentistry* 1990;10:21–25.

31. Starasoler S, Haber GS. Use of Vitamin E oil in primary herpes gingivostomatitis in an adult. *New York State Dentistry* 1978;44:382.

32. Tampo Y, Yonaha M. Vitamin E and glutathione are required for preservation of microsomal glutathione 5-transferase from oxidative stress in microsomes. *Pharmacology* 1990;66:259.

33. Regan V, Servinova E, Packer L. Antioxidant effects of ubiquinones in microsomes and mitochondria are mediated by tocopherol recycling. *Biochem Biophys Res Commun* 1990;169:851.

34. Wadleigh RG, Redman RS, Graham Ml, et al. Vitamin E in the treatment of chemo-induced mucositis. *Am J Med* 1992;92:481.

35. Osaki T, Ueta E, Yoneda K, et al. Prophylaxis of oral mucositis associated with chemoradiotherapy for oral carcinoma by azelastine hydrochloride with other antioxidants. *Head Neck* 1994;16:331–339.

36. Garewal HS, Meyskens F. Retinoids and carcinoids in the prevention of oral cancer: a critical appraisal. *Cancer Epidemiol Biomarkers Prev* 1992;1:155–159.

37. Mills EE. The modifying effect of beta-carotene on radiation and chemotherapy induced oral mucositis. *Br J Cancer* 1988;57:416–417.

38. Maciejewski B, Zajusz A, Pilecki B, et al. Acute mucositis in the stimulated oral mucosa of patients during radiotherapy for head and neck cancer. *Radiother Oncol* 1991;22:7–11.

39. Carl W, Emrich LS. Management of oral mucositis during local radiation and systemic chemotherapy. A Study of 98 patients. *J Prosthet Dent* 1991;66:361–9.

40. Oshitani T, Okada K, Kushima T, et al. Clinical evaluation of sodium alginate on oral mucositis associated with radiotherapy. *J Jpn Soc Cancer Ther* 1990;25:1129–1137.

41. Lieschke GT, Ramenghi U, O Connor MP, et al. Studies of oral neutrophil levels in patients receiving GCSF after autologous marrow transplantation. *Br J Haematol* 1992;82:589–595.

42. Gabrilove JL, Jakubowski A, Scher H, et al. Effect of granulocyte colony-stimulating factor on neutropenia and associated morbidity due to chemotherapy for transitional-cell carcinoma of the urothelium. *N Engl J Med* 1988;318:1414–1422.

43. Bronchud MH, Howell A, Crowther D, et al. The use of granulocyte colony-stimulating factor to increase the intensity of treatment with doxorubicin in patients with advanced breast and ovarian cancer. *Br J Cancer* 1989;60:121–125.

44. Pettengell R, Gurney H, Radford JA, et al. Granulocyte colony-stimulating factor to prevent dose-limiting neutropenia in non-Hodgkins lymphoma: a randomized controlled trial. *Blood* 1992;80:1430–1436.

45. Atkinson K, Biggs JC, Downs K, et al. GM-CSF after allogenic bone marrow transplantation-accelerated recovery of neutrophil, monocytes and lymphocytes. *Aust N Z J Med* 1991;21:686–692.

46. Game SM, Stone A, Scully C, et al. Tumour progression in experimental oral carcinogenesis is associated with changes in EGF and TGF-beta receptor expression and altered responses to those growth factors. *Carcinogenesis* 1990;11:965–973.

47. Sundqvist K, Liu Y, Arvidson K, et al. Growth regulation of serum free cultures of epithelial cells from normal human buccal mucosa. *In Vitro Cell Dev Biol* 1991;27A:562–568.

48. Maccini DM, Veit BC. Salivary epidermal growth factor in patients with and without acid peptic disease. *Am J Gastoenterol* 1990;85:1102–1104.

49. Sonis ST, Costa JW Jr, Evitts SM, et al. Effect of epidermal growth factor on ulcerative mucositis in hamsters that receive cancer chemotherapy. *Oral Surg Oral Med Oral Pathol Oral Radiol Endod* 1992;74:749–755.

50. Ferretti AG, Raybould TP, Brown AT, et al. Chlorhexidine prophylaxis for chemotherapy and radiotherapy-induced stomatitis:A randomized

double-blind trial. *Oral Surg Oral Med Oral Path Oral Radiol Endod* 1990;69:1331–1338.

51. Wahlin BY. Effects of chlorhexidine mouthrinse on oral health in patients with acute leukemia. *Oral Surg Oral Med Oral Pathol Oral Radiol Endod* 1989;68:279–284.

52. Weisdorf DJ, Bostrom B, Raether D, et al. Oropharyngeal mucositis complicating bone marrow transplantation: prognostic factors and the effect of chlorhexidine mouth rinse. *Bone Marrow Transplant* 1989;4: 89–95.

53. Epstein JB, Vickais L, Spinelli J, et al. Efficacy of chlorhexidine and nystatin rinses in prevention of oral complications in leukemia and bone marrow transplantation. *Oral Surg Oral Med Oral Pathol Oral Radiol Endod* 1992;73:682–689.

54. Ferretti AG, Raybould TP, Brown AT, et al. Chlorhexidine prophylaxis for chemotherapy and radiotherapy-induced stomatitis: a randomized double-blind trial. *Oral Surg Oral Med Oral Pathol Oral Radiol Endod* 1990;69:1331–1338.

55. Spijkervet FKL, Saene HKF, Panders AK, et al. Effect of chlorhexidine rinsing on the oropharyngeal ecology in patients with head and neck cancer who have irradiation mucositis. *Oral Surg Oral Med Oral Pathol Oral Radiol Endod* 1989;67:154–161.

56. Foote RL, Loprinzi CL, Frank AR, et al. Randomized trial of a chlorhexidine mouthwash for alleviation of radiation-induced mucositis. *J Clin Oncol* 1994;12:2630–2633.

57. Spijkervet FK, Saene HK, van Saene JJ, et al. Effect of selective elimination of the oral flora on mucositis in irradiated head and neck cancer patients. *J Surg Oncol* 1991;46:167–173.

58. Epstein JB, Vickais L, Spinelli J, et al. Efficacy of chlorhexidine and nystatin rinses in prevention of oral complications in leukemia and bone marrow transplantation. *Oral Surg Oral Med Oral Pathol Oral Radiol Endod* 1992;73:682–689.

59. Barrett AP. A long-term prospective clinical study of oral complications during conventional chemotherapy for acute leukemia. *Oral Surg Oral Med Oral Pathol Oral Radiol Endod* 1987;63:313–316.

60. DeGregorio MW, Lee WMF, Linker CA, et al. Fungal infections in patients with acute leukemia. *Am J Med* 1982;73:543–548.

61. Bender JF, Schimpff SC, Young VM, et al. A comparative trial of tobramycin vs gentamycin in combination with vancomycin and nystatin for alimentary tract suppression in leukemic patients. *Eur J Cancer* 1979;15:35–44.

62. Barrett AP. Evaluation of nystatin in prevention and elimination of oropharyngeal candida in immunosuppressed patients. *Oral Surg Oral Med Oral Pathol Oral Radiol Endod* 1984;58:148–151.

63. William C, Whitehouse JMA, Lister TA, et al. Oral anti candidal prophylaxis in patients undergoing chemotherapy for acute leukemia. *Med Pediatr Oncol* 1977;3:275–280.

64. Carpentieri V, Haggard ME, Lockhart LH, et al. Clinical experience in prevention of candidiasis by nystatin in children with acute lymphocytic leukemia 1978;92:593–595.

65. Hann IM, Prentice HG, Corringham R, et al. Ketoconazole versus nystatin plus amphotericin B for fungal prophylaxis in severely immunocompromised patients. *Lancet* 1982;1:826–829.

66. Schwartz PM, Dunigan JM, Marsh JC, et al. Allopurinol modification of the toxicity and antitumor activity of 5-fluorouracil. *Cancer Res* 1980;40:1885–1889.

67. Clark PI, Selvin ML. Allopurinol mouthwash and 5-fluorouracil-induced oral toxicity. *Eur J Surg Oncol* 1985;11:267.

68. Tsavaris N, Caraglauris P, Kosmidus P. Reduction of oral toxicity of 5-fluorouracil by allopurinol mouthwashes. *Eur J Surg Oncol* 1988;14: 405–406.

69. Loprinzi CI, Cianflone SG, Dose AM, et al. A controlled evaluation of an allopurinol mouthwash as prophylaxis against 5-fluorouracil induced stomatitis. *Cancer* 1990;65:1879.

70. Lee JS, Murphy WK, Shirinian MH, et al. Alleviation by leucovorin of the dose-limiting toxicity of edatrexate:potential for improved therapeutic efficacy. *Cancer Chemother Pharmacol* 1991;28: 199–204.

71. Fox AD, Kripke SA, Depaula JA, et al. Effect of a glutamine supplemented enteral diet on methotrexate-induced enterocolitis. *J Parent Ent Nutr* 1988;12:325–331.

72. O Dwyer ST, Scott T, Smith RJ, et al. 5-fluorouracil toxicity on small intestinal mucosa but not white blood cells is decreased by glutamine. *Clin Res* 1987;35:367A.

73. Jebb SA, Osborne RJ, Maughan TS, et al. 5-fluorouracil and folinic

acid-induced mucositis: no effect of oral glutamine supplementation. *Br J Cancer* 1994;70:132–135.

74. Martin DS, Stolf RL, Sawyer RC, et al. High dose 5-fluorouracil with delayed uridine rescue in mice. *Cancer Res* 1982;42:3964–3970.

75. Seiter K, Kemeny N, Martin D, et al. Uridine allows dose escalation of 5-fluorouracil when given with N-phosphonacetyl-L-asparatate, methotrexate, and leucovorin. *Cancer* 1993;71:5:1875–1881.

76. Ahmed T, Engelking C, Szalyga J, et al. Propantheline prevention of mucositis from etoposide. *Bone Marrow Transplant* 1993;12:131–132.

77. Dose AM, Mahoud DJ, Loprinzi CL. A controlled trial of oral cryotherapy for preventing stomatitis in patients receiving 5-fluorouracil plus leucovorin. A North Central Cancer Treatment Group and Mayo Clinic Study. *Proc Am Soc Clin Oncol* 1992;9:1242.

78. Mahoud DJ, Dose AM, Loprinzi CL, et al. Inhibition of fluorouracil-induced stomatitis by oral cryotherapy. *J Clin Oncol* 1991;9:449.

79. Rocke LK, Loprinzi CL, Lee JK, et al. A randomized clinical trial of two different durations of oral cryotherapy for prevention of 5-fluorouracil-related stomatitis. *Cancer* 1993;72:7:2234–2238.

80. Cascinu S, Fedeli A, Fedeli SL, et al. Oral Cooling (Cryotherapy), an effective treatment for the prevention of 5-fluorouracil-induced stomatitis. *Oral Oncol Eur J Cancer* 1994;30:4:234–236.

81. Bugai EP, Saprykina VA, Vakhtin VI, et al. The effect of light from a low intensity impulse laser on the processes of experimental inflammation and regeneration in the oral mucosa. *Stomatologica* 1991;2:6–9.

82. Pourreau-Schneider N, Soudry M, Franquin JC, et al. Soft-laser therapy for iatrogenic mucositis in cancer patients receiving high-dose fluorouracil:a preliminary report. *J Natl Cancer Inst* 1992;84:358–359.

83. Poland J. Prevention and treatment of oral complications in the cancer patient. *Oncology* 1991;5.

84. Miaskowski C. Management of mucositis during therapy. *Natl Cancer Inst Monogr* 1990;9:95.

85. Watson CPN, Evans RJ, Watt VR, et al. Post-herpetic neuralgia:208 cases. *Pain* 1988;35:289.

86. Scheffler NM, Sheitel PL, Lipton MN. Treatment of painful diabetic neuropathy with capsaicin 0.075%. *J Am Podiatr Med Assoc* 1991; 81:288.

87. Group CS. Treatment of painful diabetic neuropathy with topical capsaicin: a multicenter, double-blind, vehicle-controlled study. *Arch Intern Med* 1991;151:2225.

88. Watson CPN, Evans RJ, Watt VR. The post-mastectomy pain syndrome and the effect of topical capsaicin. *Pain* 1989;38:177.

89. Weintraub M, Golik A, Rubio A. Capsaicin for treatment of post-traumatic amputation stump pain. *Lancet* 1990;336:1003.

90. Fusco BM, Alessandri M. Analgesic effect of capsaicin in idiopathic trigeminal neuralgia. *Anesth Analg* 1992;74:375.

91. Cheshire WP, Snyder CR. Treatment of reflex sympathetic dystrophy with topical capsaicin: case report. *Pain* 1990;42:307.

92. Morgenlander JC, Hurwitz BJ, Massey EW. Capsaicin for the treatment of pain in Guillian-Barre syndrome. *Ann Neurol* 1990;28:199.

93. Deal CL, Schnitzer JJ, Lipstein E, et al. Treatment of arthritis with topical capsaicin: a double-blind trial. *Clin Ther* 1991;13:383.

94. Sicuteri F, Fusco BM, Marabini S. Beneficial effect of capsaicin application to the nasal mucosa in cluster headache. *Clin J Pain* 1989;5:49.

95. Watcher MA, Wheeland RG. The role of topical agents in the healing of full-thickness wounds. *J Dermatol Surg Oncol* 1989;15:1188.

96. Berger AM, Henderson M, Nadoolman W, et al. Oral capsaicin provides temporary relief for oral mucositis pain secondary to chemotherapy/radiation therapy. *J Pain Symptom Manage* 1995;10:3:243–248.

97. Berger AM, Bartoshuk LM, Duffy VB, et al. Capsaicin for the treatment of oral mucositis pain. *Principles and Practice of Oncology* 1995;9: 1–11.

98. Conference C. Oral complications of cancer therapies: Diagnosis, prevention and treatment. *Conn Med* 1989;53:595.

99. Thoma, Goldman. Oral pathology. St Louis: CV Mosby; 1960;892–893.

100. Fox PC, Atkinson JC, Macynski AA, et al. Pilocarpine treatment of salivary gland hypofunction and dry mouth (xerostomia). *Arch Intern Med* 1991;151:1149–1152.

101. Greenspan D, Daniels TE. Effectiveness of pilocarpine in postradiation xerostomia. *Cancer* 1987;59:1123–1125.

102. Johnson JT, Ferretti GA, Nethery J, et al. Oral pilocarpine for post-irradiation xerostomia in patients with head and neck cancer. *N Engl J Med* 1993;329:390–395.

103. Shenep JL, Kalwihsky D, Hudson PR, et al. Oral sucralfate in chemotherapy-induced mucositis. *J Pediatr* 1988;113:758–753.

104. Keus R, Noach P, de Boer R, Lebesque J. The effect of customized beam shaping on normal tissue complications in radiation therapy of parotid gland tumors. *Radiother Oncol* 1991;21:3:211–217.

105. Myers RA, Marx RE. Uses of hyberbaric oxygen in postradiation head and neck surgery. *Natl Cancer Inst Monogr* 1990;9:151–157.

106. Barret AP.Metronidazole in the management of anerobic neck infections on acute leukemia. *Oral Surg Oral Med Oral Pathol Oral Radiol Endod* 1988;66:287–289.

107. Buckingham RW. Dental care policies for treating the terminal cancer patient. *Dental Hygiene* 1981;55:4:23–26.

*Principles and Practice of Supportive Oncology,*
edited by Ann Berger et al.
Lippincott–Raven Publishers, Philadelphia ©1998

CHAPTER 17

# General Considerations in Prevention and Treatment of Oral Manifestations of Cancer Therapies

Ian M. Zlotolow

## GENERAL STRATEGIES

In 1997, a projected 1.2 million people in the United States will have been diagnosed with cancer (exluding skin cancers). Regardless of therapy (i.e., surgery, radiation therapy, or chemotherapy), recognition of the preexisting dental status is paramount for eliminating or decreasing the sequela of the cancer treatment to the oral cavity. All treatments have an effect on the normal and adjacent hard and soft oral tissues. As the cancer treatment becomes more intensified or complex, the morbidity to the oral cavity must be taken into consideration.

Oral sequelae can have different stages and intensities and will vary from patient to patient, even with the same modality of treatment and stage of disease. Patient compliance and basic understanding of both short- and long-term effects of therapy are essential to alleviating potential problems. It is imperative for the patient's dentist to be familiar with the medical therapy and outcome expectations. Pretreatment dental assessment should be completed and addressed before cancer treatment begins in order to reduce morbidity.

Generally, surgical resections of any anatomical oral or pharyngeal structure will compromise oral function. Many resections (i.e., soft palate, tongue, hard palate, mandible, or combination thereof) can be alleviated by intervention with maxillofacial prosthetics, which can restore function and cosmesis, with some limitations.

Chemotherapeutic toxicity can present with oral manifestations that may include mucosal ulcerations, local infection, and a wide range of oral discomfort.

Radiation therapy for head and neck cancers will have a range of sequela in the oral cavity that may include caries, mucositis, trismus, xerostomia, osteoradionecrosis, and secondary oral and fungal infections, many of which can be minimized or prevented with pretreatment intervention.

Regardless of treatment modality, comprehensive oral evaluation must include clinical and radiographic surveys to identify possible sources of dental infection and elimination of ongoing caries, symptomatic periapical lesions, calculus, plaque, and clinical periodontal disease (including pericoronitis).

It is recommended that any patient anticipating chemotherapy or head and neck radiation therapy undergo dental screening at least 2 weeks before commencement of cancer therapy. This generally allows proper healing of extraction sites (10–14 days), recovery of soft-tissue manipulations, and restoration of teeth, all of which are critical in maintaining overall integral mucosal continuity during treatment (1).

The dental assessment and subsequent treatment rendered should correlate with the overall prognosis. Therefore, consultation with the referring physician is paramount to dental treatment strategies and decision making.

One of the most important problems that will affect the cancer patient, regardless of cancer treatment modality, is lack of or poor oral hygiene. It is advisable to perform a thorough root planning, scaling, and prophylaxis before any cancer treatment is initiated, with the exception of a visible tumor at the site of the anticipated dental manipulation. These procedures can reduce the incidence of oral complications by eliminating bacteria that could lead to local or systemic septicemia. The dentist should note the patient's total white blood cell count, absolute granulo-

I. M. Zlotolow: Department of Surgery, Memorial Sloan-Kettering Cancer Center, New York, NY 10021.

cyte count, and platelet count if the patient has received chemotherapy or is anticipating chemotherapy, especially if the patient requires extractions or periodontal surgery.

It is also important for the dentist, in the pretreatment stage, to establish baseline data for comparison during subsequent examinations and treatment. These pretreatment strategies include eliminating or reducing periodontal disease, dental caries, defective restorations, ill-fitting prostheses, symptomatic third molar pathology, improving oral hygiene, and maintaining an intact, normal condition of all mucous membranes (2).

Patient and family education, counseling, and motivation are all critical to the success of preventive strategies. The dentist has a monumental role and can contribute to an improved quality of life of the patient, especially if the dentist is involved in a pretreatment time frame. Minimization and manifestations of cancer treatment is a major concern for both dentists and physicians.

## HEAD AND NECK SURGICAL RESECTIONS

### Maxillofacial Prosthetic Intervention

Treatment of many head and neck surgical resections may require oral rehabilitation and is an essential component of cancer care (3). Surgical resections often create defects that will cause dysfunction and disfigurement; however, most patients can be rehabilitated and these problems and sequelae reduced. Speech, swallowing, control of saliva, and mastication can be affected. The primary objective of rehabilitation is the restoration of function and appearance. The degree of success in restoration involved multiple factors, including the skill of the maxillofacial prosthodontist, the resultant anatomic physiological makeup of the patient posttreatment, and the psychological makeup of the patient. It is important that the idea of rehabilitation begin immediately after the diagnosis. Consultation between surgeon and maxillofacial prosthodontist can eliminate many unwanted sequelae. In many instance, additional surgery can improve the existing anatomic structures, thus making the maxillofacial prosthesis more successful, and could include creating lingual, buccal, and labial sulcus (vestibuloplasty) to free a tongue or osseoimplants in a microvascular free flap to restore mandibular continuity.

### Maxillary Defects

#### Obturator Prostheses

Tumors that require maxillary resection (maxillectomy or palatectomy) can arise from the antrum or palatal or gingival epithelium. A resection of these tumors will create defects of the maxilla, palate, or adjacent soft tissue

(2). They range from small perforations of the hard or soft palate or extensive resections including the maxilla, soft palate, and adjacent structures such as the orbit and cheek. Defects of these regions can lead to a variety of problems. Hypernasality makes speech unintelligible. Mastication is difficult, particularly for the edentulous patient because dental structures and dental-bearing tissue surfaces are lost; swallowing is awkward because food and liquids are forced up in the nasal cavity and out the nose. The nasal mucous membranes become desiccated by abnormal exposure, nasal and sinus secretions collect in the defect area and may be difficult to control, and facial disfigurement can result from the lack of midface bony support or resection of a branch of the facial nerve. In some cases, tumor invasion requires exenteration of the orbital contents.

Rehabilitation after resection of the hard and soft palate is best accomplished prosthodontically. Traditionally, a temporary or immediate surgical obturator is placed at the time of surgery. During the healing period, this prosthesis can be relined periodically with temporary soft denture liners to compensate for tissue changes secondary to organization and contracture of the wound. When the defect becomes well healed and dimensionally stable (usually 3–4 months after surgery), a definitive obturator prosthesis is made. If, however, the patient receives radiation therapy postoperatively, this healing period can last about 6 months after radiation therapy is completed.

The purpose of a maxillary obturator prosthesis is to restore the physical separation between the oral and nasal cavities, thereby restoring speech and swallowing to normal and providing support for the lip and cheek (4,5).

### Soft Palate Speech Bulb Prosthesis

Defects of the soft palate require different and more complex prosthetic rehabilitation. Palatopharyngeal closure normally occurs when the soft palate elevates and contracts the lateral and posterior pharyngeal walls of the nasopharynx. When a portion of soft palate is excised or when the soft palate is perforated, scarred, or neurologically impaired, complete palatopharyngeal closure cannot occur (6). Speech becomes hypernasal and normal swallowing is compromised. With a pharyngeal speech bulb obturator, the patient may be able to reestablish palatopharyngeal closure. The speech bulb obturator must not interfere with breathing, impinge on soft tissue during postural movements, or interfere with the tongue during swallowing and speech. The soft-palate obturator remains in a fixed position. Prosthetic rehabilitation of the acquired soft palate defect can be one of the most difficult intraoral challenges for a prosthodontist.

## Mandibular Defects

Malignant tumors associated with the tongue, mandible, and adjacent structures also represent a difficult challenge for the prosthodontist in regard to rehabilitation after treatment. These usually include squamous cell carcinoma of the lateral margins of the tongue, base of the tongue, gingiva, buccal cheek, retromolar, trigone, tonsil, and floor of the mouth. The disabilities resulting from such resections would include impaired speech articulation, difficulty in swallowing, deviation of the mandible during functional movements, and poor control of salivary secretions (7). There also can be cosmetic disfigurement. These patients present a far more difficult rehabilitation problem than the patients with maxillary surgical defects, particularly if significant portions of the tongue are involved in the resection. It usually is not possible to restore function to presurgical levels in patients after mandibular resection, and permanent cosmetic disfigurement is inevitable. Recently, advances were made in the reconstruction of such defects by means of microvascular free flaps, which can allow the prosthodontist eventually to rehabilitate these patients more effectively. Before the advent of microvascular reconstruction, conventional and maxillofacial prosthetic rehabilitation offered limited success. With proper multidisciplinary pretreatment planning and postoperative treatment, osseointegrated implants can be placed strategically in patients with reconstructed mandibles to restore occlusal and masticatory functions (8).

The degree to which mastication is affected depends somewhat on the amount of mandible removed, but equally important is the status of the tongue in terms of functioning (9). The tongue must be able to place the food bolus on the occlusal surface of the teeth for mastication to take place. The tongue, which in many instances has limited mobility and strength, is required to balance the position of these removable prostheses. A nonrestored mandible becomes retruded and deviates toward the surgical site. When the mandible opens and closes, previous vertical movements are replaced by an oblique or diagonal motion controlled by the unilateral and temporomandibular joint apparatus. Loss of one temporomandibular joint leads to uncoordinated and less precise movements of the mandible. Loss of muscles of mastication in the resected side also forces the mandible to rotate upward on closure if the coronoid process is present because of the pull of the temporalis musculature. The severity or permanence of this mandibular deviation is unpredictable and depends on numerous complex factors. The loss of the adjacent soft tissue and primary closure of the defect without flap reconstruction contribute to dysfunctional disability. Traditionally, if mandibular continuity is not restored surgically, mandibular guide appliances, hemidentures, or palatal ramps on maxillary prostheses are used to decrease mandibular functional disabilities (10).

The success of mandibular guidance therapy on a nonrestored mandible depends on the amount of bone loss from surgery, radiation fibrosis of the surrounding soft tissues, the cooperation and compliancy of the patient, the patient's dexterity, and the early initiation of therapy. In a few instances, prosthetic teeth can be cantilevered to restore the contour and cosmesis of a lower lip and to decrease pooling of saliva (anteriorly), however tongue dysfunction can limit the usefulness of these prostheses (11).

Microvascular free flap mandibular reconstruction after ablative cancer was described recently, and many series have reported clinical success (12). The advent and success of osseointegrated implants in the edentulous mandible were reported as early as 1977, and their osseointegration and the occurrence of direct contact between titanium bone have been shown to exist on the electron microscopic level. By using fibula free flap mandibular reconstruction with osseointegrated implants on selected cases, occlusal function can be restored (Fig. 1).

### Mandibular Guidance Restorations

If mandibular continuity is not restored surgically, a number of methods can reduce the degree of mandibular deviation. These methods include intermaxillary fixation at the time of surgery, mandibular guide bar restorations, and palatably base guidance restorations.

In the postoperative setting, mandibular guidance appliances usually are delayed until healing (by 2–3 months) has been completed; however, use of a palatal augmentation prosthesis should be considered if portions of the tongue or adjacent soft tissues are involved in the resection. The prognosis of a palatal augmentation prosthesis depends on the location and function of the residual tongue.

The prosthetic prognosis of the mandibular resection patient depends on many factors, including the amount of mandible remaining, the severity of mandibular deviation,

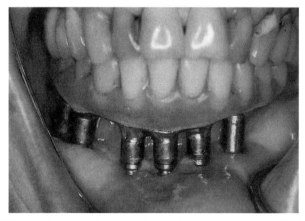

**FIG. 1.** Osseoimplant prosthesis in a microvascular fibula free flap reconstructed mandible.

the character of mandibular movement, postsurgical lip posture and control, tongue control mobility, and previous radiation therapy (13). The status of the remaining tongue is probably the most important prognostic factor. If the patient can move his or her tongue in several directions, it probably will be possible to stabilize a resection denture during function. Obviously, patients who have lost significant volume of tongue in combination with resection of the hypoglossal nerves, accompanied by local paresthesia, have the poorest prosthetic prognosis. Paradoxically, immobility of the tongue creates a minor anatomic advantage and often permits a more aggressive extension of the lingual flange on the nonsurgical side, thus facilitating stability and retention of the prosthesis.

## Facial Defects

Restoration of the facial defect is a difficult challenge for both the surgeon and maxillofacial prosthodontist. Surgical reconstruction and restoration both have distinct limitations. The surgeon is limited by the availability of tissue, the amount of damage to the local tissue beds, and the need for periodic visual inspection of facial defect. The maxillofacial prosthodontist is limited by the materials available for facial restoration, the mobile tissue beds, difficulty in retaining large prostheses, and the patient's willingness to accept the result (14). Whatever the mode of rehabilitation, the patient should be fully informed about limitations and the expected quality of the final result. In patients with extensive facial tumors requiring resection, the method of facial restorations should be considered before surgery. The patient should be involved in this discussion and should participate in the decision-making process.

The choice between surgical reconstruction or prosthetic restoration of large facial defects is difficult and complex and depends on the size and etiology of the defect as well as the wishes of the patient. Surgical reconstruction of small facial defects is possible in most cases and is preferable. Many patients prefer closing a defect with their own tissue rather than a prosthetic restoration. It is safe to say that it is difficult, if not impossible, for the surgeon to fabricate a facial part that is as successful in appearance as a well-made prosthesis. However not everyone will accept an artificial part, and many patients would prefer a permanent, even if less aesthetic, nose or ear. In general, younger patients would rather have a permanent reconstructed facial part rather than an artificial one. The application of osseoimplants in facial deformities has, in part, changed patient perceptions about facial prostheses because of the increased retention that is achievable. Even when surgical reconstruction is deemed possible, significant delay in reconstruction may be necessary to ensure control of the tumor. Surgical reconstruction usually is not considered in patients with larger defects because of the size of defects, previous radiation therapy, or the possibility of recurrence.

A conspicuous prosthesis may produce more anxiety and permit less social readjustment than a simple facial bandage. Successful use of the restoration may depend on the patient's psychological acceptance of it. It is beneficial to have the patient seen by a social worker during the rehabilitation period. The most critical period of acceptance is the first 2 or 3 days after delivery of the prosthesis. The conflicting emotional response of the patient should be anticipated and discussed before delivery. In some cases, the patient will not wear a facial prosthesis because of unrealistic expectations. Because all facial restorations are detectable under close scrutiny, the patient must understand that the prosthesis has two different roles. For family, close friends, or business associates, it can replace the excised tissues only cosmetically. For the public at large, however, it generally provides enough concealment to render the defect inconspicuous.

At present, materials used for facial prostheses exhibit acceptable properties; however, there are frustrating deficiencies, and all materials possess some undesirable characteristics. Most materials are constructed from silicone elastomers (15). Retention can be a problem, especially in silicone materials, but the use of osseointegrated implants for retention can alleviate this concern.

### Midfacial (Combined Oral and Facial) Defects

Large combination defects of the oral cavity and the external face create innumerable problems for the patient. Many of these large orofacial prostheses are required because of the origin of the squamous cell or basal cell carcinoma, which can include the intranasal cavity, premaxilla, gingiva, or lip. Many of the patients who have stage III and IV tumors have had numerous minor surgical removals previously or have had these tumors present a long time. When the integrity of the oral cavity has been resected, food and air escape during swallowing and speech is often unintelligible and saliva control difficult. It is somewhat difficult to adapt the margins of the prosthesis so that tissue contact will be maintained during facial and mandibular movements with the continued orofacial prosthesis.

Facial defects can be reconstructed by using a combination of microvascular free flaps and tissue expanders in conjunction with a maxillofacial prosthesis (Fig. 2). Placement of percutaneous osseointegrated implants in the superior or lateral orbital rim, inferior base of nasal bones, and auricular temporal bone are acceptable treatment modalities. Properly placed osseoimplants, even in irradiated tissue beds, have been successful in many studies with 5-year follow-up (16). Consideration of tumor prognosis is an important factor in this patient population for selection of osseoimplant placement.

Conventional retention of facial prostheses usually relies on skin adhesives placed on the inner surface of the prosthesis and on the skin margins daily. The prostheses

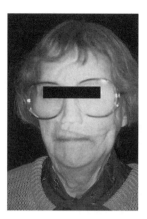

**FIG. 2.** Silicone midfacial prosthesis restoring a large squamous cell carcinoma in conjunction with a rectus abdominus free flap reconstruction (postrhinectomy, orbital exenteration cheek, and upper lip resection).

are removed during sleep, and the skin and adhesives must be removed nightly so as not to have excessive buildup, which will cause deterioration of the prosthetic material. The currently popular silicone materials usually last up to 2 years if maintained properly and if the skin margins are cleansed daily.

Patients requiring facial prostheses are recalled by the maxillofacial prosthodontist approximately every 6 months. Additional tinting can be applied and hygiene instructions re-inforced at this time.

Patients who wear facial appliances are psychologically dependent on the maxillofacial prosthodontist for moral as well as physical support. Availability of these services are an important aspect of total patient care.

## RADIATION THERAPY: PRE-THERAPY DENTAL EVALUATION

Both short- and long-term effects of therapeutic radiation therapy to the head and neck regions will involve the oral cavity. These changes can lead to mucositis, xerostomia, radiation caries, loss of taste, trismus, and possibly osteoradionecrosis (17). The oral sequelae may cause substantial problems during and after radiation therapy. Acute incidents of focal infection, such as periodontal or periapical infection, and severe mucositis occasionally necessitate an adjustment or interruption of the radiation therapy schedule.

Most preventive procedures described in the literature are based on clinical experience. The result is a great diversity in treatment policies and preventive approaches in daily dental practices. Most publications describing patients who have undergone head and neck irradiation are concerned with one sequela. Usually each institution has its own protocol and treatment standards and is extremely concise. The primary issues of patient care before radiation exposure are

screening, consequential treatment, patient motivation, and initiation of preventive measures. Management of the patient during radiation therapy is characterized by prevention and treatment of acute complications and sequelae of radiation exposure, most of which are usually of short duration. Attention also must be addressed at the postradiation situation, as prevention and treatment of chronic dental disease is addressed with close follow-up and continued care of the patient who has had head and neck irradiation.

To maximize the effect of screening patients before radiation therapy, adequate time must be allowed for dental treatment, fabrication of fluoride carriers, radiation protective mouth guards, and wound healing (18). It is suggested that this initial appointment for dental and oral evaluation be made immediately after the diagnosis of oral cancer or within 2 weeks before the onset of radiation therapy, before simulation. At the initial appointment, the patient's dentition should be examined and checked for carious lesions; defective restorations, which are sources of potential irritation of the oral mucosa, should be replaced. The periodontium and vitality of the pulp must be evaluated. Periodontal status is the major dental consideration and should be screened thoroughly by measuring pocket depth and assessment of furcation involvement. Oral hygiene must be evaluated and assessed. Plaque and gingival hemorrhage on dental pocket probing are extremely helpful in deciding the treatment plans regarding dental intervention, such as preradiation extractions. The patient's dental awareness is of utmost importance in this evaluation. The patient must possess motivation to maintain dentition properly and comply completely with the prescribed oral hygiene preventive regimen.

The oral mucosa and alveolar process should be evaluated and considered for possible future prosthetic intervention. Areas evaluated for ulcerations, fibromas, irritation, hyperplasia, bony spicules, and tori should be included in this evaluation. The fit of dentures should be checked because ill-fitting dentures are a potential source of irritation when mucosal surfaces are exposed to radiation, with the possibility of ulceration to underlying bone (19). The maximum mouth opening should be recorded before radiation therapy as a baseline to compare the interarch distance at different times postradiation therapy for evaluating the degree of trismus. Trismus can be anticipated if the temporomandibular joint and other muscles of mastications are included in the field of radiation. Decayed, missing, and filled rates of teeth should be recorded and a generalized periodontal evaluation, including gingival and plaque indices should be noted and recorded. A panoramic radiograph supplemented by intraoral radiographs, when necessary, is most suitable for detection of periodontal disease, periapical infections, cyst, third molar pathology, unerupted or partially erupted teeth, and residual root tips.

As a general rule, any teeth with acute and symptomatic periodontal problems should be considered for extraction before head and neck radiation therapy. In making a decision about extraction before radiation ther-

**TABLE 1.** *Indications for extractions (preradiation therapy)*

Advanced carious lesions with questionable pulpal status or pulpal involvement

Extensive periodontal lesions

Moderate to advanced periodontal disease (pocket depth in excess of 5 mm, especially with advanced bone loss, mobility, or root furcation involvement

Residual root tips not fully covered by alveolar bone or showing radiolucencies.

Incompletely erupted teeth that are not fully covered by alveolar bone or that are in contact with the oral involvement

apy or maintenance of teeth, several factors are important (Table 17-1) and include the patient's motivation to comply with the preventive regimen, with consideration of the tumor prognosis. A lack of motivation on the part of the patient should lead to a decision to extract questionable teeth before radiation therapy. Radiation exposure, type, portal field, fractionization, and total dosage are also part of the decision formula, in addition to the prognosis and expediency of control of the cancer (20).

Deeply impacted teeth that are completely covered by bone and mucosa are usually left without risk of late problems. Teeth that are class II or III mobility, which would serve no benefit as abutment teeth for retention of a prosthesis, also should be considered for extraction before radiation therapy. Extractions of residual root tips, impacted teeth, and other foci that can be potential causes of infection should be performed atraumatically with regard to tissue handling. Alveolectomy and primary wound closure are necessary to speed healing and to eliminate sharp ridges and bone spicules, which could project to the overlying soft tissues. This is particularly important for prosthetic consideration because negligible bone remodeling can be expected after radiation therapy. Generally, dental extraction can be performed in the general dental office.

Nonvital teeth located in the portal fields without periapical radiolucency and not causing symptoms should be treated endodontically. In mandibular molars, endodontics with possible retrograde fillings are preferred because of an increased risk of osteoradionecrosis in this region. Teeth with small, moderate periapical granulomas without periodontal involvement that are important for oral function or rehabilitation should be treated with apicoectomies.

Adequate time for healing of extraction sites before radiation therapy is essential. Healing time of 14 to 21 days generally is considered safe and should be the rule. Routinely, antibiotics are not recommended because there is no evidence that antibiotics influence healing in the absence of infection. Careful examination of extraction sites must be performed before radiation therapy commences. Communication between the dentist, patient, and radiation therapist is the cornerstone for successful maintenance of the oral cavity.

Patients are instructed about effective daily plaque removal. Instructions on the use of soft toothbrushes and a fluoridated tooth paste are essential. The patients are told to brush and floss at least three to four times a day beginning immediately. A neutral 1% sodium fluoride gel, self-applied every night for 5 minutes (21), a brush-on gel, or a fluoride mouth rinse should be prescribed in conjunction with strict oral hygiene measures (Figs. 3 and 4). Acidulated gels usually are not prescribed because they might lead to significant decalcification without sufficient remineralization potential in the presence of xerostomia. In addition, sodium fluoride preparations are preferred to stannous fluoride because the latter has unpleasant side effects, such as bad taste, sensitivity of teeth and gingiva, and staining of arrested lesions. Daily compliancy of fluoride for the rest of the patient's life is more an issue than the modality of fluoride application.

Many topical oral preparations have been reported subjectively to reduce the duration and severity of oral mucositis during radiation treatments. The efficacy of these agents has yet to be established. Agents tested clinically that have produced mixed results include kaolin, magnesium sulfate, antacids, sucralfate, lidocaine (viscous) hydrochloride, and corticosteroids. In modern delivery of radiation therapy to the head and neck, oral mucositis is expected during the last half of treatment (i.e., weeks 4–7) but subsides and diminishes with time (4–8 weeks after completion of therapy). With three-dimensional conformal radiation and cone down techniques, some head and neck patients with base-of-tongue hypopharyngeal or laryngeal carcinoma can have minimal mucositis during their therapeutic treatment.

It is suggested that mucositis be treated palliatively with viscous Xylocaine or Dyclone. The use of equal amounts of 2% viscous xylocaine, Kaopectate, and Benadryl is sometimes beneficial during this period. Patients should avoid spicy or acidic foods and change to a bland diet with frequent intake of water for ease in swallowing.

Oral candidiasis is a common long- and short-term oral sequela of both head and neck chemotherapy and radiation therapy. These lesions may be removable (whitish), chronic

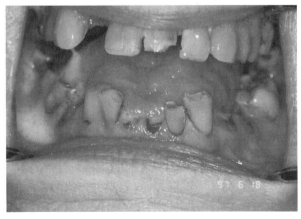

**FIG. 3.** Radiation caries in patient noncompliant with fluoride. (nasopharyngeal carcinoma—post-7200 cGy).

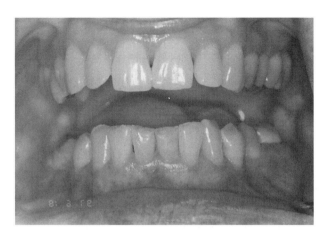

**FIG. 4.** Fluoride compliant patient five years post-6700 cGy for squamous cell carcinoma base of tongue.

or hyperplastic (nonremovable), chronic erythematous (diffused as patchy erythema), and they often appear as angular cheilitis (first signs or symptoms). Treatment of oral candidiasis includes mycostatin (troches), nystatin (oral), or clotrimazole. Pseudomembranous candidiasis is successfully treated topically. Chronic candidiasis usually requires much longer treatment and may require oral keto-conazole, fluconazole, or intraveous amphotericin B.

Xerostomia in head and neck irradiated patients is a major sequela. Its magnitude depends on the radiation dosage, location, and volume of exposed salivary glands; however, significant xerostomia has not been shown to be a sequela in patients treated with chemotherapy alone. The degree of xerostomia usually is reported subjectively by both patients and clinicians. The degree of xerostomia can affect oral comfort, fit of prostheses, and speech and swallowing. Many of the enzymes (mucin) found in xerostomia patients contribute to the growth of caries-producing organisms. This sequela of a decrease in the quantity and quality of saliva can be devastating to the dentition with the formation of caries. Oral hygiene regimens that include the use of water or saline can reduce the colonization and proliferation of oral pathogens.

Sialagogues recently were investigated to stimulate residual salivary parenchyma (pilocarpine, 5- and 10-mg doses). Both doses revealed statistically significant improvement in feelings of mouth comfort, oral dryness, and overall improvement of xerostomia. The major side effect was sweating.

Artificial saliva, usually with carboxymethcellulose as a base, has not been demonstrated to increase oral cavity comfort. Sugarless gum and hard candies frequently are used by patients for comfort with reported subjective improvement. The dental team should encourage the patient to quit or reduce the use of tobacco and alcohol.

The long-term effects of head and neck radiation therapy can include soft-tissue fibrosis and obliterative endoarteritis. These changes become more substantial over time, including trismus and nonhealing or slow healing of mucosal ulcerations. Surgical wounds, (i.e., extraction sites), in the irradiated area usually heal slowly. The muscles of mastication and the temporomandibular joint (if in the field of radiation therapy) can become fibrotic with clinical entities. Early exercises, incluing the use of trismus appliances postradiation, can prevent this sequela. Use of tongue depressors taped together and exercising sets of 10 to 15 times a day for 10-minute sets can be effective.

Osteoradionecrosis (ORN), a relatively uncommon clinical entity, is now described as being related to hypocellularity, hypovascularity, and ischemia of tissues rather than of a bacterial origin (23). This process can be spontaneous but usually is initiated after trauma, such as dental extraction. This process can progress to pathologic fracture, infection of surrounding soft tissues, and severe pain. Most studies have reported ORN following tooth extractions, postradiation, or preradiation if there had not been 10 to 14 days of healing before radiation therapy.

Some authors maintain that traditional treatment of ORN with antibiotics and surgical debridement and curettage is unsuccessful. Recent literature supports hyperbaric oxygen to boost tissue oxygenation in damaged irradiated wounds (24). Further controlled and randomized clinical studies are needed. Dental extractions after radiation therapy require consultation between the dentist and the radiation oncologist to ensure minimizing the risk of ORN. Most studies demonstrate a low incidence of ORN if preradiation dental consultation and treatment are rendered (25–27). Follow-up and recall of the irradiated head and neck patient for dental preventive maintenance and treatment are essential to prevent long-term sequelae in the oral cavity.

## CHEMOTHERAPY

The most common oral complications that arise during chemotherapy or bone marrow transplant treatment are mucosal inflammation, ulceration, hemorrhage and fungal, bacterial, and viral infections (28). These often are painful and difficult to treat and can diminish quality of life. These complications in the oral cavity may interfere and affect the nutritional status of patients. They may become so severe as to cause problems of compliancy and may discourage patients from continuing necessary cancer treatments. The oral cavity may serve as a portal of entry for acute life-threatening or fatal systemic infections. As treatments increase in intensity (often with a concomitant increase in severity of side effects) and as greater numbers of patients survive their cancers for longer periods, these complications can take on an added significance. There is an increased emphasis on developing a means of preventing or minimizing oral complications of chemotherapy. Pretherapy dental intervention may have a great impact on both the incidence and severity of certain oral effects (29).

It has been reported that the oral cavity (mouth) truly reflects the complications of cancer chemotherapy as much as any other part of the body. The infectious, hemorrhagic, cytotoxic, nutritional, and neurologic sides of drug toxicity are reflected in the mouth by changes in the color, character, comfort, and continuity of the mucosa. Similar to the complications from radiation therapy, the oral complications from chemotherapy can vary in pattern, duration, intensity, and time course.

It is recommended that all patients receiving bone marrow or stem cell transplants be seen by a dentist at least 10 days before commencement of therapy. The patient should be informed of possible short-term and long-term side effects of chemotherapy at the initial appointment.

The periodontal condition is assessed and a thorough scaling, root planing, debridement, and prophylaxis are imperative. The hematologic status should be reviewed with the oncologist in regard to platelets, neutrophils, total white blood cell count, protime, and prothrombin time. Home-care hygiene initiatives are commenced. Third molar pathology is evaluated and addressed appropriately. All potential oral sources of bacteremia should be eliminated, including advanced periodontal disease. If symptomatic teeth with periapical lesions are present, pulpotomies or extractions are required.

## SUMMARY

In summary, the availability, accessibility, and visibility of the dental team members and their relationships with medical, surgical, radiation oncologists, and nursing staffs are the keys to preventing oral complications. Preventive dentistry and an ongoing dialogue between physicians, nurses, and dentists, contribute to and are essential for improving quality of life and are standards of care in supportive oncology. Minimizing the oral complications of cancer treatment is a reality.

## REFERENCES

1. Consensus statement: oral complications of cancer therapies. In: *NIH Consensus Development Conference Proceedings, No. 9, Monograph USDH HS*;1990:4–15.
2. Sonis ST, Woods PD, White A. Pre-treatment oral assessment; oral complications of cancer therapies. In: *NIH Consensus Development Conference Proceedings, No. 9, Monograph USDH HS*;1990:29–32.
3. Beumer J, Zlotolow I, Curtis T. Rehabilitation. In: Silverman S, ed. *Oral Cancer*, 3rd edition. New York: American Cancer Society; 1990: 127.
4. Beumer J, Zlotolow I, Curtis T. Rehabilitation. In: Silverman S, ed. *Oral Cancer*, 3rd edition. New York: American Cancer Society; 1990: 128.
5. Beumer J, Curtis J. Restoration of acquired hard palate defects. In:

Beumer J, Curtis T, Marunick M, eds. *Maxillofacial rehabilitation—prosthodontic and surgical considerations.* 2nd ed. St. Louis: Ishiyaku EuroAmerican Inc., 1997.
6. Aram A, Subtelny JD. Velopharyngeal function and cleft palate prosthesis. *J Prosthet Dent* 1959;9:149.
7. Beumer J, Zlotolow I, Curtis T. Rehabilitation. In: Silverman S, ed. *Oral cancer*, 3rd ed. New York: American Cancer Society;1990: 132–142.
8. Zlotolow I, Huryn J, Piro J, Lenchewski E, Hidalgo D. Osseointegrated implants and functional prosthetic rehabilitation in microvascular free flap reconstructed mandibles. *Am J Surg* 1992;165.
9. Cantor R, Curtis T. Prosthetic management of edentulous mandibulectomy patients. Part II. Clinical procedures. *J Prosthet Dent* 1971;25: 546.
10. Curtis T, Taylor RC, Rositano S. Physical problems in obtaining records of the maxillofacial patient. *J Prosthet Dent* 1975;34:539.
11. Beumer J. Marunick M, et al. Acquired defects of the mandible. Beumer J, Curtis T, Marunick M, eds. *Maxillofacial rehabilitation, prosthodontic and surgical considerations*; 2nd ed., St. Louis: Ishiyaku EuroAmerica Inc., 1997;174–180.
12. Hidalgo DA. Fibula free flap: a new method of mandible reconstruction. *Plast Reconst Surg* 1989;84:71–79.
13. Beumer J, Zlotolow I, Curtis T. Rehabilitation. In: Silverman S, ed. *Oral Cancer*, 3rd ed. New York: American Cancer Society;1990: 127–148.
14. Beumer J, Ma T, Marunick, M et al. Restoration of facial defects. In: Beumer J, Curtis T, Marunick M, eds. *Maxillofacial rehabilitation—prosthodontic and surgical considerations;* 2nd ed. St. Louis: Ishiyaku EuroAmerica, Inc., 1997: 385–435.
15. Moore DJ, Glaser ZR, Togacco NJ, Linebaugh MG. Evaluation of Polymeric materials for maxillofacial prosthetics. *J Prosthet Dent* 1977;38: 319.
16. Granstrom G, Tjellstram A, Branemark P-I. Bone-enhanced reconstruction of the irradiated head and neck cancer patient. *Otolaryngology Head Neck Surg* 1993;108:334–343.
17. Beumer J, Curtis T, Nishimura R. Radiation therapy of head and neck tumors. In: Beumer J, Curtis T, Marunick M, eds. *Maxillofacial rehabilitation—prosthodontic and surgical considerations;* 2nd ed., St. Louis: Ishiyaku EuroAmerica, Inc., 1997:43–103.
18. ADA Oral Health Care Guidelines. *Head and neck cancer patients receiving radiation therapy.* American Dental Association Council on Community Health, Hospital, Institutional and Medical Affairs; 1989.
19. Beumer J, et al. Radiation therapy of the oral cavity, sequelae and management. Part I. *Head Neck Surg* 1979;1:303–306.
20. Beumer J, Zlotolow I, Curtis T. Rehabilitation. In: Silverman S, ed. *Oral Cancer.* New York: American Cancer Society; 1990.
21. Dreizen S, Brown LR, Daly TE, et al. Prevention of xerostomia-related dental caries in irradiated cancer patients. *J Dent Res* 1977;56:99–104.
22. Johnson TT, et al. Oral pilocarpine for post irradiation xerostomia in patients with head and neck cancer. *N Engl J Med* 1993;329:390–395.
23. Marx RE. Osteoradionecrosis: a new concept of its pathophysiology. *J Oral Maxillofac Surg* 1983;41:283–288.
24. Marx RE, Johnson RP, Kline SN. Prevention of osteoradionecrosis: a randomized prospective clinical trial of hyperbaric oxygen versus penicillin. *J Am Dent Assoc.*
25. Beumer J, Curtis T, Morris LR. Radiation complications in edentulous patients. *J Prosthet Dent* 1976;36:193.
26. Schweiger JW. Oral complications following radiation therapy: a five year retrospective report. *J Prosthet Dent* 1987;58:78–82.
27. Beumer J, Harrison R, Sanders B, et al. Pre-radiation dental extractions and the incidence of bone necrosis. *Head Neck Surg* 1983;5: 514–521.
28. Toth B, et al. Minimizing oral complications of cancer treatment. *Onocology* 1995;9:851–858.
29. Zlotolow I. Toth et al. Article reviewed. *Onocology* 1995;9:858–864.

*Principles and Practice of Supportive Oncology,*
edited by Ann Berger et al.
Lippincott–Raven Publishers, Philadelphia ©1998

CHAPTER 18

# Pruritus

Alan B. Fleischer, Jr., and Jason R. Michaels

Like the sensation of pain, pruritus can diminish the quality of life in cancer patients. Because of the distress pruritus may cause, the cancer clinician should be aware of its importance and its management. Pruritus in cancer patients may be attributable to a primary skin disease, a coexisting medical condition, a medication, or the cancer itself. The subject of pruritus has been extensively reviewed in articles, chapters, and texts by noted authorities (1–11). This chapter focuses on pruritus and reviews its etiology, diagnosis, and management.

## PRURITUS SENSATIONS

In simplest terms, *pruritus* is the sensation that provokes scratching behavior. Like the sensation of pain, objective analysis cannot easily confirm the presence or severity of pruritus. Scratch marks (*excoriations*), thickening (*lichenification*), and visible cutaneous disease support patients' subjective complaints. To complicate the issue, some patients with typically itchy diseases, such as scabies, deny that they itch. These patients may complain of burning, stinging, tingling, tickling, or a crawling sensation. These symptoms are closely related to pruritus, have similar pathogenic mechanisms, and are treated identically. Bernhard (12) summarized this notion by stating "one man's itch is another man's tickle . . . and one man's stinging itch is another man's pain." For most people, itch is readily distinguished from pain, and many patients with severe pruritus would be happy to have pain instead (8).

Pruritus is a distinct, complex sensation that may be considered a primary sensory modality (9). The itch receptor is a dermal, free, nerve arborization that is diffi-

cult to distinguish from the pain receptor. Unmyelinated C fibers carry these sensations to the thalamus and subthalamus. Experimental injection of histamine into the skin may induce itch or pain. This histamine-induced pruritus may be suppressed by systemic antihistamine administration (13). Because many patients with pruritus show no signs of histamine release, it is likely that other compounds cause most pruritus. The failure of many pruritic conditions to improve with nonsedating antihistamines suggests histamine is a minor pruritus mediator (14,15). Studies have revealed that pruritus may be caused by serotonin and other neuropeptides, prostaglandins, kinins, proteases, and physical stimuli (9). Each of these agents may induce pruritus primarily or act via secondary mediators.

The sensation of pruritus also may arise within the central nervous system. Systemic opioids are known to induce pruritus, and the opioid-antagonist naloxone decreases pruritus (16,17). Exogenous opioids administered in small quantities to spinal levels in spinal anesthesia relieve pain and can stimulate itch (18). Plasma from patients with cholestatic itching cause facial scratching when introduced into the medullary dorsal horn of monkeys, and this scratching is abolished by administering the opioid receptor antagonist naloxone (19). Although opioids may promote histamine release by mast cells (e.g., exacerbating urticarial itch), opioid peptides generally do not cause any release of histamine when injected alone.

Other central nervous system pruritic phenomena include cerebrovascular accident pruritus (20) and phantom limb pruritus (i.e., pruritus in an amputated extremity) (21). Thus, it is clear that pruritus is often not histamine induced and may not arise in the skin.

## DERMATOLOGIC DISEASES AND PRURITUS

Many skin diseases may contribute to the sensation of pruritus. Dry skin, or *xerosis,* is commonly seen in cancer

A. B. Fleischer: Department of Dermatology, Wake Forest University Medical Center, Winston-Salem, NC 27157-1071.

J. R. Michaels: Resident, Dermatology, Texas Tech University Health Sciences Center, Lubbock, TX 79430.

patients who have undergone chemotherapy or radiation therapy. Xerosis makes the skin more susceptible to irritation from environmental assault (22).

Many other diseases may present with pruritus, including scabies, atopic dermatitis, dermatitis herpetiformis, bullous pemphigoid, miliaria, pediculosis, and urticaria (23). These cutaneous diseases often are readily diagnosed by careful clinical examination. Signs of dermatologic diseases may be remarkably subtle or nonspecific in any given patient, particularly in the immunocompromised host. There is no substitute for an excellent physical examination of the skin surface (24–30).

## PRURITUS AND MALIGNANCY

Pruritus may be associated with virtually any malignancy (Table 1) (31–46). Some neoplasms are more frequently associated with pruritus. Primary polycythemia,

**TABLE 1.** *Systemic conditions reported associated with generalized pruritus*

| Organ systems and etiologies | Example |
| --- | --- |
| Autoimmune | Sjögren syndrome |
| Endocrine | Hyperthyroidism |
| | Hypothyroidism |
| | Diabetes mellitus |
| Central nervous system | Cerebrovascular accident |
| | Delusions of parasitosis |
| | Depression |
| | Multiple sclerosis |
| | Neurodermatitis |
| | Psychosis |
| Hematopoietic | Paraproteinemia |
| | Iron deficiency anemia |
| | Mastocytosis |
| Liver | Primary biliary cirrhosis |
| | Extrahepatic biliary obstruction |
| | Hepatitis |
| Malignancy | Breast carcinoma |
| | Carcinoid symdrome |
| | Cutaneous T-cell lymphoma |
| | Hodgkin disease |
| | Gastrointestinal tract cancers: tongue, stomach, and colon |
| | Leukemia |
| | Lung cancer |
| | Multiple myeloma |
| | Non-Hodgkin lymphomas |
| | Polycythemia rubra vera |
| | Prostatic carcinoma |
| | Thyroid carcinoma |
| | Uterine carcinoma |
| Pharmacologic | Drug ingestion |
| Infectious | Human immunodeficiency virus |
| | Parasitic diseases |
| | Syphilis |
| Renal | Chronic renal insufficiency and renal failure |
| | Dialysis dermatosis |

for example, has a pruritus prevalence of 30% to 50% and Hodgkin disease has a prevalence of 15%. Cutaneous T-cell lymphoma, peripheral T-cell lymphoma, and other cutaneous lymphomas are notoriously pruritic. Generally, the etiology of the pruritus in these patients is a poorly understood paraneoplastic phenomenon. The presence of severe pruritus may be more troublesome than from a symptom control perspective alone. Gobbi and colleagues (42) reported that severe pruritus in Hodgkin's disease predicts a poor prognosis.

## PRURITUS AND NONMALIGNANT INTERNAL DISEASES

Cancer patients are not exempt from having concurrent medical conditions. There is no question that other internal diseases may be associated with pruritus. Pruritus has been reported to herald the onset of thyroid disease (47), renal insufficiency (48), liver disease (49), iron deficiency (50), diabetes mellitus (51), paraproteinemia (52), Sjögren syndrome (53), and other conditions. Cancer patients can independently develop other medical conditions, or the cancer itself may cause a systemic condition, such as biliary obstruction, that may cause pruritus. Mechanisms of pruritus induction in most of these diseases are poorly understood. It has been postulated that renal disease may induce a metastatic calcification, hyperphosphatemia, xerosis, mast cell proliferation, and other changes that might be associated with pruritus.

## CANCER THERAPY

Pruritus may be the result of a chemotherapy reaction, radiation therapy, or supportive care. Pruritus has been reported as an adverse reaction to chemotherapeutic agents, including these listed in Table 2 (54–59). New combinations of chemotherapeutic agents in ever increasing dosage regimens undoubtedly will be associated with increased cutaneous toxicity.

Acute radiodermatitis may cause erythema and pruritus. Additionally, chronic radiodermatitis can be associated with severe xerosis, skin thinning, and ease of irritation. Total body electron beam radiation may make the entire skin surface dry and pruritic.

All clinicians managing cancer patients are familiar with the typical morbilliform drug rash from antibiotics and other supportive agents. Appearing similar to this eruption is the engraftment phenomenon in bone marrow transplant recipients; however, many pruritogenic drugs do not induce any rash. As stated, opiates may induce pruritus via central nervous mechanisms. Others, such as estrogens or ketoconazole, may precipitate cholestatis and thus induce pruritus. It is noteworthy that placebo agents may induce may induce pruritus in as many as 5%

**TABLE 2.** *Antitumor agents associated with pruritus*

BCG
Bleomycin
Carmustine
Chlorabmucil
Cisplatin
Cyclophosphamide
Cytosine arabinside and daunomycin
Daunomycin
Doxorubicin
Hydroxyurea
Interleukin-2 with levamisole
L-Asparaginase
Mechlorethamine
Mechlorethamine
Mitomycin
Procarbazine

BCG, Bacille Calmette-Guérin.

of the people treated. More than 100 medications are reported to cause pruritus without a rash (55). Careful review of the medication history and simplification of the drug regimen may aid the patient.

## NEUROPSYCHIATRIC DISEASE AND PRURITUS

Calnan and O'Neill (60) found that in most patients with a chief complaint of generalized pruritus, the itch began at a time of emotional stress. Edwards and colleagues (61) later reported that a high level of psychological stress enhances a person's ability to perceive intense itch stimuli. In cancer patients, psychologic stress, depression, anxiety, and organic brain diseases undoubtedly contribute to cutaneous diseases (62–65). Recognition of neuropsychiatric disease may lead to better control.

## EVALUATION OF THE PRURITIC PATIENT

Obtaining a focused history, a directed review of symptoms, and a focused clinical examination may lead to a clinical diagnosis. The physician first should probe for likely pharmaceutical pruritus exacerbators. A temporal history of therapeutic agent initiation within 2 weeks of the onset of pruritus may be helpful. Other historic points of value include an abnormal or excessive bathing history, others in the family or household with similar problems, and symptoms of neuropsychiatric disease. Complete dermatologic clinical examination will quickly exclude urticaria, scabies, and a host of other dermatologic diagnoses.

Some patients with long-standing, generalized pruritus may require further evaluation. For practicing dermatologic clinicians, further investigation may be warranted. This evaluation should include a careful history, physical examination, and appropriate, limited screening laboratory tests. Extensive, undirected evaluation of these patients rarely leads to a specific attributable cause (66).

There is no single list nor are there specific guidelines for tests that must be performed in any individual patient. Scabies preparations, fungal examinations, and skin biopsies may be needed to diagnose specific dermatologic diseases.

## TOPICAL TREATMENT

Ideally, the physician would choose the single topical medication that corrects the underlying condition. Although this scenario occasionally occurs (e.g., permethrin for scabies infestation), symptomatic treatment is less specific. Therefore, the clinician must use all diagnostic skills to provide the patient with reasonable relief. Table 3 presents the advantages and disadvantages of different topical agents.

**TABLE 3.** *Advantages and disadvantages of topical agents*

| Topical agent | Examples | Advantages | Disadvantages |
|---|---|---|---|
| Emollients and moisturizers | Petrolatum Moisturizing lotions | Inexpensive, reduces irritant dermatitis | May be too greasy, insufficient in inflammatory diseases |
| Corticosteroids | Hydrocortisone Triamcinolone Fluocinonide | Effective for inflammatory dermatoses, mainstay of topical therapy | May cause atrophy, sensitivity, adrenal suppression |
| Anesthetics | Camphor Pramoxine Benzocaine & lidocaine EMLA | Excellent pruritus relief, no atrophy or adrenal suppression | Potentially sensitizing |
| Antihistamines | Diphenhydramine Doxepin | Excellent pruritus relief, no atrophy or adrenal suppression | Potentially sedating and sensitizing |
| Cooling agents | Calamine Menthol Alcohol | May be soothing and cooling | Calamine leaves visible film Alcohol dries the skin |
| Miscellaneous | Coal tar Capsaicin | Coal tar is antiinflammatory Capsaicin works differently than other agents | Tar is not elegant and stains Capsaicin may burn |

One of the most important aspects of skin therapy that must be addressed is hydration of the skin surface (67,68). A simple but sometimes effective therapeutic approach is to apply emollients (lotions, creams and ointments) on the dry skin twice daily. Emollients with camphor and menthol (e.g., Sarna lotion), phenol, pramoxine (PrameGel, Pramosone, or Aveeno antiitch lotion) may provide safe relief from pruritus. Camphor, phenol, and pramoxine have local anesthetic effects, whereas menthol cools the skin acting as a counterirritant (11).

Age-old remedies such as cool compresses (application of a wet washcloth for 20 minutes) and shake lotions (calamine) may prove highly efficacious. Cooling the skin may provide remarkable pruritus relief. Oatmeal baths (Aveeno) or baths in therapeutic salts may also provide short-term symptomatic relief.

Topical corticosteroids may be useful adjunctive agents for pruritus control. When used properly, they should be prescribed in amounts necessary to cover the affected skin. Table 4 provides prescribing quantity information. Although any topical corticosteroid may be useful in a given patient, for widespread pruritus hydrocortisone (1% or 2.5%) or triamcinolone (0.0% to 0.1%), preparations are generally effective. Because of the relatively thin skin of some cancer patients, long-term use of halogenated corticosteroids should be approached with great caution. Overuse of corticosteroids in unsupervised or overzealous patients may be one of the most common causes of dermatologic iatrogenic disease (69). Even when topical corticosteroids are required, the use of emollients remains indicated (70,71).

Capsaicin cream (Zostrix) may be of some benefit in selected patients with a wide range of inflammatory and noninflammatory dermatoses (72,73). Topical capsaicin should be applied thrice daily and may be used indefinately. Its application requires careful patient instruction, as initially it may produce burning or stinging sensations or superficial burns. In many cases, after one or more weeks, the burning sensation diminishes and relief from pruritus follows. Capsaicin may not be appropriate for generalized pruritus because of its significant expense.

Another promising agent now available in the United States is the eutectic mixture of local anesthetics lidocaine, and prilocaine (EMLA); EMLA has already been demonstrated to be helpful in experimentally induced pruritus (74) and may prove useful in recalcitrant pruritic conditions. It can be used twice daily to pruritic areas and may rapidly decrease pruritus symptoms. Analagously, benzocaine (Lanacane), another topical anesthetic, also may provide rapid relief. Topical doxepin (Zonalon), an antidepressant and potent antihistamine, is a useful noncorticosteroid pruritus medication with demonstrated efficacy (75). Clinicians should be aware that all topical agents, including emollients, corticosteroids, antihistamines, and anesthetics have sensitizing potential and may induce allergic contact dermatis.

## ORAL TREATMENT

In patients with pruritus that interferes with sleep or that may have a significant neuropsychiatric component, oral antipruritic agents may prove important in symptomatic relief. Antihistamines, such as hydroxyzine (Atarax) and diphenhydramine (Benadryl), not only are antipruritic but have important central nervous system effects. In a review of the pharmacologic control of pruritus, Winkelmann (16) stated that the most effective antihistamines have central nervous system effects. Moreover, ensuring adequate sedation can be important now that there is good evidence that pruritus disturbs normal sleep (77); however, some patients, especially the elderly, may have increased sensitivity to antihistamines, and memory impairment or impaired psychomotor function may result from their administration (2,3). Cetirizine (Zirtek) is a potent antihistamine that is less sedating than hydroxyzine, but it is more sedating than the nonsedating antihistamines (e.g., loratidine, terfenidine, astemazole).

In conditions other than urticaria, the nonsedating antihistamines may have only marginal therapeutic effect. There are conflicting data on the antipruritic efficacy of terfenadine and acrivastine in atopic dermatitis (15,78). Although they may be outstanding agents in the treatment of urticaria, in nonurticarial conditions, nonsedating antihistamines have limited application. Moreover, in cancer patients the role of histamine in itch mediation is even more questionable. Burtin and colleagues (79) found a decreased skin response to histamine injection in cancer patients. They postulated that the presence of a tumor mimics the effects of general administration of histamine H1 antagonists on the skin response to histamine.

Doxepin, a tricyclic antidepressant with antihistamine activity (80), also may be an effective agent for the treatment of refractory pruritus. Although most antihista-

**TABLE 4.** *Amounts of topical corticosteroid to prescribe*

| Location | One application (g) | BID × 1 wk | BID × 1 mo |
|---|---|---|---|
| Hands, scalp, genitalia, or face | 2 | 30 g (1 ou) | 120 g (4 ou) |
| Upper extremity or one side of trunk | 3 | 45 g (1.5 ou) | 180 g (6 ou) |
| One lower extremity | 4 | 60 g (2 ou) | 240 g (8 ou) |
| Entire body | 30–60 | 540 g (1 lb) | 2,700 g (5 pounds) |

BID, twice daily.

mines have an excellent safety profile compared with other types of drugs, antihistamines may potentiate cardiac dysrhythmias and may exacerbate glaucoma and urinary retention, and these agents also may cause postural hypotension (81). Because of potentially serious cardiac arrhythmias, the nonsedating antihistamines should not be used in patients also taking systemic agents, including azole antifungal agents and erythromycin. Nevertheless, antihistamines are an important class of agents for therapy of pruritus.

Systemic corticosteroids for pruritus are often highly effective, but their use can present certain difficulties. All oncologic practitioners are aware that chronic pathologic states, including hypertension, diabetes, fluid retention, and osteoporosis, all may be exacerbated by intramuscular or oral corticosteroids. Systemic corticosteroids are particularly effective for brief periods for morbilliform drug eruptions and allergic or irritant contact dermatitis. More prolonged use may induce adverse sequelae.

A variety of other systemic agents have been used with some effect in specific disease states. Charcoal (82) and naloxone (17), for instance, have been demonstrated to be effective. Rifampin may be effective for the pruritus of primary biliary cirrhosis (83). Aspirin occasionally exacerbates pruritus but has been reported to be helpful in the treatment of pruritus associated with polycythemia rubra vera (42). Alpha interferon has been used with some success in intractable pruritic conditions (43,44), but its cost and side effects demand careful consideration. Although purely anecdotal, our experience with thalidomide, a teratogenic antiinflammatory agent, suggests that this agent is also extremely useful for intractable pruritus. The reader always should bear in mind that if a patient obtains relief with any given medication, the medication cannot always take credit. In a classic study, Epstein and Pinski (84) found that placebo therapy provides pruritus relief with a surprisingly high success rate.

## PHYSICAL TREATMENT MODALITIES

Ultraviolet A (UVA), ultraviolet B (UVB), and psoralen photochemotherapy (PUVA) have been successfully employed in a wide range of pruritic disorders, from atopic dermatitis to renal disease (85–87). Because of its high degree of efficacy, UVB has become the treatment of choice for uremic pruritus in some centers (87), including our own. We administer UVB, combination UVA-UVB, and PUVA treatments for pruritus. UV doses are usually administered thrice weekly in doses. UV doses are progressively increased until erythema is attained, then the therapy is individually adjusted to accommodate the patients' photosensitivity. To attain symptomatic relief, 20 to 30 treatments may be necessary, and occasionally maintenance weekly therapy is continued.

## CONCLUSIONS

Pruritus in cancer patients is common and provides a diagnostic and therapeutic challenge for the physician. Evaluation may be limited to obtaining an excellent history and physical examination. Alternatively, an exhaustive search for systemic disease occasionally may be indicated. The physician should address the therapeutic intervention to correct the underlying cutaneous disease. Systemic antipruritics are often beneficial and well tolerated but have well-known side effects. Above all, diagnosis and therapy should be individualized for the patient.

## REFERENCES

1. Lober CW. Pruritus and malignancy. *Clins Dermatol* 1993;11:125–128.
2. Higgins EM, du Vivier AW. Cutaneous manifestations of malignant disease. *Br J Hosp Med* 1992;48:552–554.
3. De Conno F, Ventafridda V, Saita I. Skin problems in advanced and terminal cancer patients. *J Pain Symptom Manage* 1991;6:247–256.
4. Rosenberg FW. Cutaneous manifestations of internal malignancy. *Cutis* 1977;20:227–234.
5. Campbell J. Management of pruritus in the cancer patient. *Oncol Nurs Forum* 1981;8:40–41.
6. Bernhard JD. Clinical aspects of pruritus. In: Fitzpatrick TB, Eisen AZ, Wolff K, Freedberg IM, Austen KE, eds. *Dermatology in general medicine*, 3rd ed. New York: McGraw-Hill; 1987:78–90.
7. Jorizzo JI. Generalized pruritus. In: Callen JP, Jorizzo J, eds. *Dermatological signs of internal disease*. Philadelphia: WB Saunders; 1988:80–83.
8. Winkelmann RK. Pruritus. *Semin Dermatol* 1988;7:233–235.
9. Denman ST. A review of pruritus. *J Am Acad Dermatol* 1986;14:375–392.
10. Dangel RB. Pruritus and cancer. *Oncol Nurs Forum* 1986;13:17–21.
11. Gatti S, Serri F. *Pruritus in clinical medicine*. New York: McGraw-Hill, 1991.
12. Bernhard JD. Itches, pains, and other strange sensations. *Current Challenges in Dermatology* 1991;1–10.
13. Arnold AJ, Simpson JG, Jones HE, Ahmed AR. Suppression of histamine-induced pruritus by hydroxyzine and various neuroleptics. *J Am Acad Dermatol* 1979;1:509–512.
14. Krause L, Shuster S. Mechanism of action of antipruritic drugs. *BMJ* 1983;287:1199–1200.
15. Berth-Jones J, Graham-Brown RAC. Failure of terfenidine in relieving the pruritus of atopic dermatitis. *Br J Dermatol* 1989;121:635–637.
16. Bernstein JE, Swift RM, Soltani K et al. Antipruritic effect of the opiate antagonist, naloxone hydrochloride. *J Invest Dermatol* 1982;78:82–83.
17. Bernstein JE, Swift R. Relief of intractable pruritus with naloxone. *Arch Dermatol* 1979;115:1366–1367.
18. Fischer HB, Scott PV. Spinal opiate analgesia and facial pruritus. *Anaesthesia* 1982;37:777–778.
19. Bergasa NV, Thomas DA, Vergalla J, Turner ML, Jones EA. Plasma from patients with the pruritus of cholestasis induces opioid receptor-mediated scratching in monkeys. *Life Sci* 1993;53:1253–1257.
20. King CA, Huff FJ, Jorizzo JL. Unilateral neurogenic pruritus: paroxysmal itching associated with central nervous system lesions. *Ann Intern Med* 1982;97:222–223.
21. Bernhard JD. Phantom itch, pseudophantom itch, and senile pruritus. *Int J Dermatol* 1992;33:856–857.
22. Hunnuksela A, Kinnunen T. Moisturizers prevent irritant dermatitis. *Acta Derm Venereol* 1992;72:42–44.
23. Gilchrest BA. *Skin and aging processes*. Boca Raton, Fl: CRC Press, 1984.
24. Beare JM. Generalized pruritus: a study of 43 cases. *Clin Exp Dermatol* 1976;1:343–352.
25. Botero F. Pruritus as a manifestation of systemic disorders. *Cutis* 1978;21:873–880.
26. Gilchrest BA. Pruritus: pathogenesis, therapy and significance in systemic disease states. *Arch Intern Med* 1982;142:101–105.

27. Camp R. Generalized pruritus and its management. *Clin Exp Dermatol* 1982;7:557–563.
28. Kantor GR, Lookingbill DP. Generalized pruritus and systemic disease. *J Am Acad Dermatol* 1983;9:375–382.
29. Champion RH. Generalized pruritus. *BMJ* 1984;289:751–773.
30. Kantor GR. Evaluation and treatment of generalized pruritus. *Clev Clin J Med* 1990;57:521–526.
31. Cormia FE. Pruritus, an uncommon but important symptom of systemic carcinoma. *Arch Dermatol* 1965;92:36–39.
32. Erskine JG, Rowan RM, Alexander JO, et al. Pruritus as a manifestation of myelomatosis. *BMJ* 1977;1:687–688.
33. Mengel CE. Cutaneous manifestations of the malignant carcinoid syndrome: severe pruritus and orange blotches. *Ann Intern Med* 1963;58:989–993.
34. Beeaff DE. Pruritus as a sign of systemic disease, report of metastatic small cell carcinoma. *Arizona Med* 1980;37:831–833.
35. Thomas S, Harrington CT. Intractable pruritus as the presenting symptom of carcinoma of the bronchus: a case report and review of the literature. *Clin Exp Dermatol* 1983;8:459–461.
36. Shoenfeld Y, Weinburger A, Ben-Bassat M et al. Generalized pruritus in metastatic adenocarcinoma of the stomach. *Dermatologica* 1977;155:122–124.
37. Degos R, Civatte J, Blanchet P, et al. Prurit, seule manifestation pendant 5 ans d'une maladie de Hodgkin. *Ann Med Interne* 3(Paris) 1973;124:235–238.
38. Alexander LL. Pruritus and Hodgkin's disease. *JAMA* 1979;241:2598–2599.
39. Bluefarb SM. *Cutaneous manifestations of malignant lymphomas.* Springfield: Charles C Thomas, 1959.
40. Stock H. Cutaneous paraneoplastic syndromes. *Medizinische Klinik* 1976;71:356–372.
41. Curth HO. A spectrum of organ systems that respond to the presence of cancer: how and why the skin reacts. *Ann NY Acad Sci* 1974;230:435–442.
42. Gobbi PG, Attardo-Parrinello G, Lattanzio G, Rizzo SC, Ascari E. Severe pruritus should be a B-Symptom in Hodgkin's disease. *Cancer* 1983;51:1934–1936.
43. Rosenberg FW. Cutaneous manifestations of internal malignancy. *Cutis* 1977;20:227–234.
44. Fjellner B, Hägermark O. Pruritus in polycythemia: treatment with aspirin and possibility of platelet involvement. *Acta Derm Venereol* 1979;61:505–512.
45. de Wolf JT, Hendriks DW, Egger RC, Esselink MT, Halie MR. Alpha-interferon for intractable pruritus in polycythemia rubra vera. *Lancet* 1991;337:241.
46. Flecknoe-Brown S. Relief of itch associated with myeloproliferative disease by alpha interferon [Letter]. *Aust N Z J Med* 1991;21:81.
47. Barnes HM, Sarkany I, Calnan CD. Pruritus and thyrotoxicosis. Trans St. Johns Hosp *Dermatol Soc* 1974;60:59–62.
48. Gilchrest BA, Rowe JW, Brown RS et al. Ultraviolet phototherapy of uremic pruritus with ultraviolet light therapy: long term results and possible mechanisms of action. *Ann Intern Med* 1979;91:17–21.
49. Sherlock S, Scheyer PJ. The presentation and diagnosis of 100 patients with primary biliary cirrhosis. *N Engl J Med* 1973;289:674–678.
50. Lewiecki EM, Rahman F. Pruritus: a manifestation of iron deficiency. *JAMA* 1976;236:2319–2320.
51. Stawiski MA, Vorhees JJ. Cutaneous signs of diabetes mellitus. *Cutis* 1976;18:415–421.
52. Zelicovici Z, Lahav M, Cahane P, et al. Pruritus as a possible early sign of paraproteinemia. *Isr J Med Sci* 1969;5:1079–1081.
53. Feuerman EJ. Sjögren's syndrome presenting as recalcitrant generalized pruritus. *Dermatologica* 1968;137:74–86.
54. Breathnach SM, Hinter H. *Adverse reactions and the skin.* Oxford: Blackwell Scientific Publications; 1992:281–304.
55. Bork C. *Cutaneous side effects of drugs.* Philadelphia: WB Saunders, 1988.
56. Call TG, Creagan ET, Frytak S, Buckner JC, van Haelst-Pisani C, Homburger HA, Katzmann JA. Phase I trial of combined recombinant interleukin-2 with levamisole in patients with advanced malignant disease. *Am J Clin Oncol* 1994;17:344–347.
57. Hortobagyi GN, Richman SP, Dandridge K, Gutterman JU, Blumenschein GR, Hersh EM. Immunotherapy with BCG administered by scarification: standardization of reactions and management of side effects. *Cancer* 1978;42:2293–2303.
58. Call TG, Creagan ET, Frytak S, Buckner JC, van Haelst-Pisani C, Homburger HA, Katzmann JA. Phase I trial of combined recombinant interleukin-2 with levamisole in patients with advanced malignant disease. *Am J Clin Oncol* 1994;17:344–347.
59. Ogilvie GK, Richardson RC, Curtis CR, Withrow SJ, Reynolds HA, Norris AM, Henderson RA. Klausner JS. Fowler JD. McCaw D. Acute and short-term toxicoses associated with the administration of doxorubicin to dogs with malignant tumors. *J Am Vet Med Assoc* 1989;195:1584–1587.
60. Calnan CD, O'Neill D. Itching in tension states. *Br J Dermatol* 1952;64:274–280.
61. Edwards AE, Shellow WV, Wright ET, Dignam TF. Pruritic skin disease, psychological stress, and the itch sensation. *Arch Dermatol* 1976;112:339–343.
62. Musaph H. Psychodynamics in itching states. *Int J Psychoanal* 1968;49:336–340.
63. Whitlock FA. Pruritus generalized and localised. In: Whitlock FA, ed. *Psychophysiological aspects of skin disease* London: WB Saunders; 1976:110–129.
64. Sheehan-Dare RA, Henderson MJ, Cotterill JA. Anxiety and depression in patients with chronic urticaria and generalized pruritus. *Br J Dermatol* 1990;123:769–774.
65. Fleischer AB Jr. Pruritus in the elderly: management by senior dermatologists. *J Am Acad Dermatol* 1993;28:603–609.
66. Hunnuksela A, Kinnunen T. Moisturizers prevent irritant dermatitis. *Acta Derm Venereol* 1992;72:42–44.
67. Ghiadially R, Halkier-Sorensen L, Elias PM. Effects of petrolatum on stratum corneum structure and function. *J Am Acad Dermatol* 1992;26:387–396.
68. Fransway AF, Winkelmann RK. Treatment of pruritus. *Semin Dermatol* 1988;7:310–325.
69. Watsky KL, Freije L, Leneveu MC, Wenck HA, Leffell DJ. Water-in-oil emollients as steroid sparing adjunctive therapy in the treatment of psoriasis. *Cutis* 1992;50:383–386.
70. Ronayne C, Bray G, Robertson G. The use of aqueous cream to relieve pruritus in patients with liver disease. *Br J Nurs* 1993;2:527–528.
71. Breneman DL, Cardone JS, Blumsack RF et al. Topical capsaicin for hemodialysis-related pruritus. *J Am Acad Dermatol* 1992;26:91–94.
72. Leibsohn E. Treatment of notalgia paresthetica with capsaicin. *Cutis* 1992;49:335–336.
73. Fusco GM, Giacovazzo M. Peppers and pain: The promise of capsaicin. *Drugs* 1997;53(6):909–914.
74. Shuttleworth D, Hill S, Marks R, et al. Relief of experimentally induced pruritus with a novel mixture of local anesthetic agents. *Br J Dermatol* 1988;119:535–540.
75. Drake L, Breneman D, Greene S, et al. Effects of topical doxepin 5% cream on pruritic eczema. *J Invest Dermatol* 1992;98:605.
76. Winkelmann RK. Pharmacologic control of pruritus. *Med Clin North Am* 1982;66:1119–1133.
77. Aoki T, Kushimoto H, Hishikawa Y, Savin JA. Nocturnal scratching and its relationship to the disturbed sleep of itchy subjects. *Clin Exp Dermatol* 1991;16:268–272.
78. Doherty V, Sylvester DGH, Kennedy CTC, et al. Treatment of atopic eczema with antihistamines with a low sedative profile. *BMJ* 1989;298:96.
79. Burtin C, Noirot C, Giroux C, Scheinmann P. Decreased skin response to intradermal histamine in cancer patients. *J Allergy Clin Immunol* 1986;78(1 Pt 1):83–89.
80. Richelson B. Tricyclic antidepressants block $H_1$ receptors of mouse neuroblastoma cells. *Nature* 1978;274:176–177.
81. Monahan BP, Ferguson CL, Killeavy ES, et al. Torsade de pointes occuring in association with terfenadine use. *JAMA* 1990;264:2788–2790.
82. Pederson JA, Matter BJ, Czerwinski AW, Llach F. Relief of idiopathic generalized pruritus in dialysis patients treated with activated oral charcoal. *Ann Intern Med* 1980;93:446–448.
83. Ghent CN, Carruthers SG. Treatment of pruritus in primary biliary cirrhosis with rifampin. Results of a double-blind, crossover, randomized trial. *Gastroenterology* 1988;94:488–493.
84. Epstein E, Pinski JB. A blind study. *Arch Dermatol* 1964;89:548–549.
85. Jekler J, Larko O. UVA solarium versus UVB phototherapy of atopic dermatitis: a paired-comparison study. *Br J Dermatol* 1991;125:569–572.
86. Morison WL, et al. Oral psoralen photochemotherapy of atopic dermatitis. *Br J Dermatol* 1978;98:25–30.
87. Gilchrest BA, Rowe JW, Brown RS, et al. Ultraviolet phototherapy of uremic pruritus with ultraviolet light therapy: long term results and possible mechanisms of action. *Ann Intern Med* 1979;91:17–21.

*Principles and Practice of Supportive Oncology,*
edited by Ann Berger et al.
Lippincott–Raven Publishers, Philadelphia ©1998

CHAPTER 19

# Treatment and Tumor-Related Skin Disorders

David L. Crosby

For trained eyes, the skin can provide a clinical window, at times clear and sometimes foggy, to view significant systemic diseases lying hidden within the patient. Nowhere is this more true than in patients with malignancies. Both the tumor and the therapies used to control the disease may leave indelible marks on the patient's skin. Patients and physicians are both aware of these interactions. All treating physicians have heard the relieved sigh of the patient who thought a benign blemish might be cancer and also have seen the shocked silence of the unfortunate patient who is told that a minor alteration in his or her skin might be a sign of malignancy hiding within. As a completely visible mark (or, as some patients see it, a scarlet letter) of the underlying disease, patients sometimes seem much more concerned and distressed by the signs of the malignancy in the skin than by the malignancy itself.

The study and diagnosis of skin disorders are achieved almost exclusively by visual skills. Nowhere in medicine is physical examination, unsupported by laboratory or other ancillary testing, more important than in dermatology. Although a treatise of words and pictures can provide a primer for those interested in skin diseases, only direct observation of patients suffering from the conditions described in this chapter can fully train the health care provider in the myriad of clinical presentations seen in the diseased skin of oncology patients. Fortunately, all humans are innately careful observers of skin, continuously noting the slight variations signaling the emotions, beauty, and health of those around them. Using this inherent skill to observe the subtle and not so subtle changes in the skin of patients can alert the physician to important changes that then may lead back to this chapter and other works and,

hopefully, to the diagnosis. This chapter provides a systematic approach to the skin conditions frequently encountered in patients with underlying malignancy, starting with treatment-related skin disorders and drug eruptions caused by the therapies used in treating oncology patients, followed by infections and infestations resulting from the immune compromised state of many oncology patients, and ending with paraneoplastic conditions and direct tumor involvement of the skin from the disease itself. I hope readers will use this information wisely to aid in alleviating some of the physical and emotional suffering of their patients.

## CUTANEOUS SEQUELAE OF ANTINEOPLASTIC THERAPY

The skin, mucous membranes, hair, and nails are all rapidly proliferating tissues. It is to be expected that antineoplastic drugs designed to attack rapidly dividing tumor cells will have a variety of adverse sequelae in these epithelial structures (1). Although most of the mucocutaneous complications of antineoplastic therapy are not life threatening, they can produce significant morbidity. This morbidity can be both physical (for example, the mucositis associated with high-dose methotrexate therapy) and psychological (as in the common anagen hair loss associated with many antineoplastic drugs). The cutaneous disfigurement is also a constant, visible reminder to the patient of the cancer and its progressive nature.

It is not always possible to associate definitively a cutaneous finding with a specific antineoplastic drug, as patients undergoing chemotherapy are frequently taking a combination of chemotherapy agents and other medications. Mucocutaneous reactions frequently associated with specific cancer chemotherapy agents are listed in Table 19-1. Some mucocutaneous side effects of antineoplastic agents are dose related and predictable, such as anagen hair loss, whereas others, such as hyperpigmenta-

D. L. Crosby: Department of Dermatology, Medical College of Wisconsin, Milwaukee, WI 53226.

**TABLE 1.** *Adverse mucocutaneous reactions to antineoplastic agents*

| Reaction | Causative agents |
|---|---|
| Stomatitis | Actinomycin-D, amsacrine, bleomycin, cyclophosphamide, daunorubicin, doxorubicin, 5-fluorouracil, interleukin 2, 6-mercaptopurine, methotrexate, mithramycin, mitomycin, nitrosourea, procarbazine, vinblastine, vincristine |
| Alopecia | Amsacrine, bleomycin, cyclophosphamide, cytarabine, dactinomycin, daunorubicin, dacarbazine, doxorubicin, etoposide, 5-fluorouracil, hydroxyurea, interleukin 2 (causes telogen effluvium), methotrexate, nitrosourea, procarbazine, vinblastine, vincristine |
| Hypersensitivity reactions | Amsacrine, L-asparaginase, bleomycin, chlorambucil, cisplatin, cyclophosphamide, daunorubicin, doxorubicin, etoposide, interferons, mechlorethamine, melphalan, methotrexate, procarbazine, triethylenethiophosphoramide |
| Chemical cellulitis | Actinomycin-D, bleomycin, cisplatin, dacarbazine, daunorubicin, doxorubicin, 5-fluorouracil, mechlorethamine, methotrexate, mitoxantrone, mithramycin, mitomycin, streptozocin, vinblastine, vincristine |
| Phlebitis | Actinomycin-D, amsacrine, carmustine, dacarbazine, daunorubicin, doxorubicin, mechlorethamine, mitomycin, mitoxantrone, vinblastine |
| Hyperpigmentation | |
|    Skin: Localized | Bleomycin ("flagellate"; linear), cyclophosphamide, doxorubicin, 5-fluorouracil, mechlorethamine (topical), nitrosourea (topical), triethylenethiophosphoramide |
|    Skin: Diffuse | Busulfan, cyclophosphamide, hydroxyurea, methotrexate |
|    Skin: Nonspecified | Daunorubicin, mithramycin, mitomycin |
|    Mucous membranes | Cyclophosphamide, doxorubicin, 5-fluorouracil, busulfan |
|    Nails | Bleomycin, cyclophosphamide, daunorubicin, doxorubicin, 5-fluorouracil, hydroxyurea |
|    Hair | Methotrexate |
|    Teeth | Cyclophosphamide |
| Inflammation of seborrheic or actinic keratoses | Actinomycin-D, cisplatin, cytarabine, dacarbazine, doxorubicin, 5-fluorouracil, pentostatin, 6-thioguanine, vincristine |
| Radiation enhancement and recall | Actinomycin-D, bleomycin, doxorubicin, etoposide, 5-fluorouracil, hydroxyurea, interferons, methotrexate |
| Photosensitivity | Dacarbazine, 5-fluorouracil, methotrexate, mitomycin, vinblastine |
| Tenderness and/or erythema of palms and soles (acral erythema) | Bleomycin, cytarabine, doxorubicin, 5-fluorouracil, methotrexate |
| Raynaud's phenomenon | Bleomycin with vinblastine |
| Acral sclerosis | Bleomycin |
| Ulceration over pressure areas | Bleomycin, methotrexate |
| Folliculitis | Actinomycin-D, methotrexate |
| Onychodystrophy/onycholysis | Bleomycin, cyclophosphamide, doxorubicin, 5-fluorouracil, hydroxyurea |
| Erythema of face and neck | 5-fluorouracil, mithramycin, procarbazine |
| Exfoliative dermatitis | Chlorambucil/busulfan, methotrexate |
| Atrophy of skin and nails | Hydroxyurea |
| Neutrophilic eccrine hidradenitis | Cytarabine, bleomycin |
| Flag hair | Methotrexate |
| Vasculitis | Cytarabine, hexaethyl-bisacetamide, methotrexate |
| Reaction to UV-light-induced erythema | Methotrexate |
| Erythema/conjunctivitis | Cytarabine |
| Hypertrichosis | Cyclosporine |
| Vesicular eruption with pruritus | Mitomycin |
| Distinctive histopathology | Busulfan, etoposide |
| Mucous erythema with burning erythroderma | Interleukin 2 |
| Exacerbation of psoriasis | Interferons, interleukin 2 |
| Pruritus | Interferons |
| Increased growth of eyelashes | Interferons |

Reprinted with premission from Yokel and Hood, ref 1.

tion and allergic reactions, occur in an idiosyncratic fashion. Table 1 lists mucocutaneous disorders with the causative chemotherapeutic agents. Reactions unique to certain classes and individual chemotherapeutic agents are discussed in detail.

## Alkylating Agents

The antineoplastic effect of the alkylating agents is due to their effect on alteration in the cellular DNA, including strand breaks and chain cross linking. This category of drugs includes cyclophosphamide, mechlorethamine, chlorambucil, melphalan, busulfan, triethylenethiophosphoramide (thio-TEPA), dacarbazine, carmustine, and streptozocin. Mucocutaneous reactions frequently seen with this category of drugs includes IgE-mediated allergic reactions and pigment alteration in the skin, mucosa, hair, and nails.

Cyclophosphamide causes a predictable anagen effluvium at cumulative doses above 5 g (2). Stomatitis is a rare complication of high-dose cyclophosphamide therapy. A more specific, long-term cutaneous complication of cyclophosphamide therapy is hyperpigmentation, which can include generalized hyperpigmentation of the skin and mucous membranes or a localized increase in pigmentation of the hair, nails, palms and soles, or teeth. Nail pigmentation occurs as horizontal bands whose distance from the proximal nail fold corresponds to the time from the last dose of cyclophosphamide (0.1 mm/day or 3 mm/month in fingernails) (Fig. 19-1). Horizontal ridging of the nail surface, or Beau's lines, may overly the pigmentation as a result of interruption of nail growth by chemotherapy. This nail pigmentation will grow out over the life expectancy of the nail, about 3 months in fingernails and 6 months in toenails. Less common hyperpigmented bands of the teeth are permanent enamel stains.

Busulfan also has been reported to cause severe, diffuse hyperpigmentation that can mimic Addison syndrome (3). The busulfan-induced hyperpigmentation can be differentiated from Addison syndrome by its sparing of the palmar crease and mucous membranes.

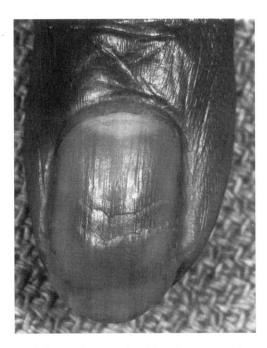

**FIG. 1.** This hyperpigmented nail band measured 6 mm from the proximal nail fold. Its position corresponded to the patient's last cycle of combination chemotherapy that included cyclophosphamide 2 months previously.

Urticaria, angioedema, pruritus, and anaphylactic reactions to cyclophosphamide, mechlorethamine, chlorambucil, and melphalan have been reported. Cross reaction between cyclophosphamide and mechlorethamine has been well documented (1). Topical mechlorethamine, used in the treatment of cutaneous T-cell lymphoma, can cause allergic contact dermatitis and irritant dermatitis in patients or health care workers who injudiciously apply the medication with bare hands (4). Ointment-based preparations, compared with solutions, of mechlorethamine are less likely to sensitize patients. Allergic patients requiring continued topical mechlorethamine can be successfully desensitized (5).

Severe hypersensitivity reactions, and even anaphylaxis, to melphalan have been seen with increased frequency in patients with immunoglobulin A (IgA)-kappa monoclonal gammopathy (6). Thio-TEPA also may cause more severe hypersensitivity reactions, including fever, pruritus, urticaria, and angioedema, which can occur with both systemic and intravesicular (bladder wash) administration of thio-TEPA. Odd pigment alterations also have been reported with thio-TEPA, including hyperpigmentation occurring in sites occluded by adhesive bandages or other devices during administration of the drug.

Dacarbazine may induce severe photosensitivity reactions, with erythema, edema, and blistering after even brief sun exposure (7). Dacarbazine is a prodrug that requires in vivo biotransformation to active metabolites. Photodegradation is one means of activation of this prodrug. The photosensitivity is theorized to be a result of photodegradation of the molecule into a reactivated intermediate in the skin.

## Antimetabolites

The antimetabolites work by inhibiting the biosynthesis of nucleic acids via various mechanisms. This category of drugs includes methotrexate, 5-fluorouracil (5-FU), cytarabine, 6-mercaptopurine, 6-thioguanine, and trimetrexate. Antimetabolites frequently cause mucocutaneous reactions, including mucositis, alopecia, hyperpigmentation, and interactions with ionizing and nonionizing radiation.

The folate antagonist methotrexate predictably causes stomatitis at high doses. This reaction can be severe enough to interfere with oral intake. Severe ulceration is an indication for discontinuing therapy, usually followed by gradual healing of the mucositis over 7 to 14 days. Transient anagen alopecia also has been noted to occur with high-dose methotrexate therapy. Erythema followed by desquamation in areas of pressure, such as the feet, elbows, and intertriginous areas, has been observed in methotrexate-treated patients (8).

Administration of methotrexate within 3 weeks of the completion of radiation therapy can lead to the radiation recall phenomena. Erythema akin to acute radiation toxicity or sunburn erupts in the radiation port 2 to 3 days after administration of the chemotherapeutic agent. Only rarely is severe necrosis of the epidermis and ulceration seen (9). This recall reaction also has been seen with bleomycin, actinomycin-D, doxorubicin, etoposide, 5-FU, hydroxyurea, and interferons (10). A similar phototoxic recall reaction may erupt within the area of a previous sunburn recalled by the administration of methotrexate 2 to 5 days after excessive ultraviolet light exposure.

The administration of 5-FU may cause diffuse cutaneus erythema, scaling, and desquamation, with the most severe reaction manifesting bulla formation (11). Severe photosensitivity with easy sunburning also is frequently associated with systemic 5-FU administration (12). More than half of patients receiving 5-FU develop severe erythema on exposure to doses of sunlight that usually would not cause sunburn. If this reaction is especially severe, it may be followed by permanent alopecia, hyperpigmentation, and atrophy of the skin (13).

Systemic, especially continuous, administration of 5-FU and, less commonly, cytarabine, 6-thioguanine, doxorubicin, or actinomycin-D can lead to an inflammatory reaction in actinic keratoses (cutaneous premalignant lesions found in sun-exposed sites of fair-skinned persons). Two to three weeks after starting the drug infusion, the actinic keratoses develop erythema, crusting, and irritation (Fig. 19-2), followed by sloughing of the crusts and healing over the subsequent 2 to 4 weeks. Ultimately, the actinic keratoses completely resolve. A similar reaction over the same time course is the expected result of topically applied of 5-FU used to treat these premalignant skin lesions.

The antimetabolites 5-FU and 6-mercaptopurine both have the potential to induce pellagra (i.e., niacin deficiency) by inhibition of the conversion of tryptophan to nicotinic acid (14). Patients with poor nutrition from cancer-related cachexia, malabsorption, or alcoholism may develop clinical pellagra on administration of these antimetabolites. The "three D's" of pellagra (diarrhea, photosensitive dermatitis, and dementia) respond rapidly and completely to the systemic administration of nicotinic acid. Those caring for malnourished cancer patients at risk of pellagra should be on alert for the shiny, hyperpigmented eruption on sun-exposed regions of the face, neck, and arms typical of pellagra. Niacin administration will prevent the gradual development of further nutritional deterioration from diarrhea and loss of cognitive abilities as a result of dementia.

Cytarabine may induce an unusual acral erythema. Patients develop tender erythema of the palms and soles, which may be followed by vesiculation and desquamation (Fig. 19-3) that can be especially prominent along the margins of the palms and soles (15). A histologic pattern akin to graft-versus-host reaction is seen in skin biopsy. One possible mechanism of this cutaneous alteration is accumulation of the drug in the eccrine coils of the palmar/plantar skin. Bleomycin, doxorubicin, 5-FU, and methotrexate have been reported to cause a similar palmar/plantar eruption.

Neutrophilic eccrine hydradenitis presents as tender plaques and nodules in a localized distribution on the trunk and extremities, usually during the second week following the first dose of chemotherapy (16). The syndrome most often is seen with cytarabine therapy, although it has also been reported with bleomycin, mitoxantrone, chlorambucil, an even HIV infection (17). Patients typically develop

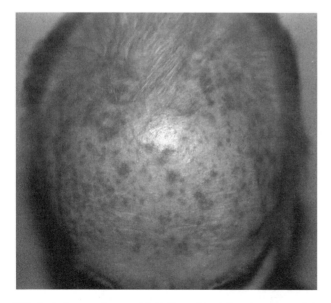

**FIG. 2.** Inflammation and irritation of facial and scalp actinic keratoses 2 weeks after beginning continuous-infusion 5-fluorouracil therapy for colon cancer metastatic to the liver. The infusion continued, and the inflammation and preexisting actinic keratoses resolved over the subsequent 3 weeks.

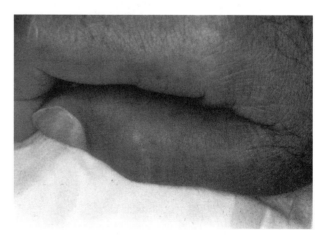

**FIG. 3.** Tender acral erythema developed during cytarabine therapy for lymphoma. The eruption cleared over the next week without residua.

tender, erythematous papules which coalesce over 2 to 3 days into inflamed plaques on the trunk, neck, and extremities. The eruption may occasionally be generalized and is frequently accompanied by fever and malaise. These areas spontaneously resolve over a 2- to 5-day period. Histologic changes within the plaques are distinctive, with neutrophilic infiltration and destruction of the eccrine sweat gland coils. A postulated mechanism is that drug or its metabolites are excreted and concentrated into the eccrine glands.

## Antibiotics

The natural product of Streptomyces which are used as antineoplastic agents include the antibiotics bleomycin, actinomycin-D, doxorubicin, daunorubicin, mithramycin, mitomycin-C, and mitoxantrone. These drugs are all potent cytotoxic agents with common complications including alopecia, mucositis, severe chemical cellulitis if extravasated, pigment alteration, and interaction with ionizing radiation. The antibiotic bleomycin preferentially binds to epithelial cells; therefore, cutaneous reactions are common with this agent due to selective concentration of the drug in the skin. The development of an acute, pruritic, morbilliform eruption is quite common in bleomycin-treated patients (18). Accentuation of this eruption over pressure areas is noted noted. A combination of bleomycin with vincristine has been reported to induce an unusual, Raynaud-like phenomena (19).

Bleomycin is noteworthy for the hyperpigmentation associated with its use. This pigmentation may occur in linear or flagellate hyperpigmented streaks (20) (Fig. 19-4). Similar streaky hyperpigmentation following bleomycin use may be due to pigmentation of striae distensae (stretch marks) (21). Hyperpigmentation may also arise over veins used to administer the bleomycin and, less commonly, 5-FU (22) (Fig. 19-5).

Transient alopecia may occur with the use of actinomycin-D. This hair loss is unique in that the hair may regrow in a different color and texture from the patient's original hair (23). An acneiform drug eruption also has been reported in patients treated with actinomycin-D (24). Unlike usual acne, this eruption generally clears within 1 to 2 weeks after drug administration ends.

Doxorubicin causes severe alopecia in almost all patients. Axillary and pubic hair also may be lost. Using tourniquets or local scalp hypothermia during administration of doxorubicin to reduce the amount of drug reaching the scalp can be helpful in preventing hair loss (25–27). These maneuvers are not always effective, and patients may lose their hair from other agents used in combination chemotherapy regimens. Doxorubicin-induced hyperpigmentation of the nails occurs as longitudinal bands similar to those seen as a result of cyclophosphamide therapy. Hyperpigmentation of the palmar creases, knuckles, buc-

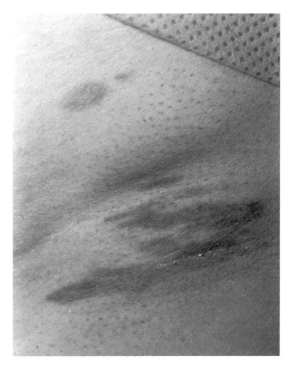

**FIG. 4.** Flagellate hyperpigmentation in a patient treated previously with 5-fluorouracil.

cal mucosa, and tongue also have been reported to occur in doxorubicin-treated patients.

Doxorubicin is noteworthy for the especially severe chemical cellulitis and ulcerations that can develop at the site of drug extravasation (Fig. 19-6). One patient was reported to develop tissue-recall phenomena, in which an earlier, healed site of doxorubicin extravasation followed by cellulitis and ulceration was exacerbated by subsequent administration of doxorubicin at another site (28). Allergic hypersensitivity reactions to doxorubicin are not unusual. One series reported a 3% incidence of urticarial reactions to doxorubicin (29).

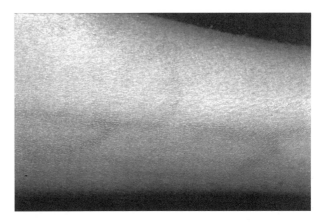

**FIG. 5.** Linear hyperpigmentation overlying the course of veins 1 year after ending bleomycin chemotherapy for head and neck squamous cell carcinoma.

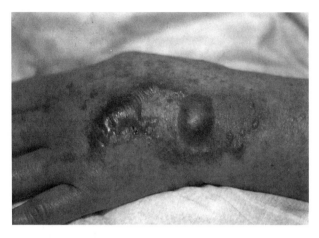

**FIG. 6.** Severe chemical cellulitis with bullae formation and dermal and epidermal necrosis 24 hours after inadvertent infiltration of doxorubicin.

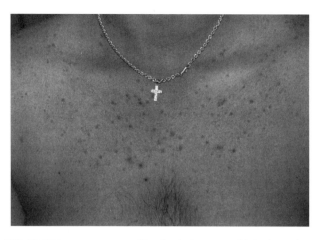

**FIG. 7.** This young man with a brain tumor on high-dose dexamethasone for the previous 4 weeks developed this monomorphic papular eruption of steroid acne. The eruption cleared completely 2 to 3 weeks after the steroids were discontinued. Courtesy of Alan B. Fleischer, Jr., M.D.

Mithramycin causes a unique reaction of macular erythema of the face and neck, seen in 35% of patients in one series (30). This erythema will fade gradually with desquamation and possible residual pigment alteration.

### Vinca Alkaloids

The vinca alkaloids, vincristine and vinblastine, derived from the periwinkle plant, cause reversible alopecia and mucositis. Extravasation of the drugs may lead to vesiculation and ulceration of the epidermis. A photosensitivity reaction similar to but not as severe as seen with dacarbazine has been reported in patients treated with vinblastine (31).

### Miscellaneous Chemotherapeutic Agents

A variety of other agents are used to treat cancer. Reactions of note include severe Ig-E mediated allergic reactions to L-asparaginase. Urticaria and even anaphylaxis has been reported to occur with this drug. Typically, more severe reactions will occur on subsequent rechallenge with the drug. Patients taking oral hydroxyurea for long periods may develop alopecia, hyperpigmentation, scaling dry skin, dystrophy of the fingernails and toenails, and a lichen planus-like skin eruption.

Interleukin 2 can cause a capillary leak syndrome as a result of peripheral vascular dilatation and leaking, with erythema, pruritus, and burning, usually localized to the head and neck region (32). Alpha interferons frequently cause pruritic, transient morbilliform eruptions, and mild alopecia (33). Recrudescence of atopic dermatitis by interferon alpha may occur in atopic patients with a history of childhood eczema.

High-dose therapy can induce steroid acne. Monomorphic papules and pustules usually erupt during the second though fourth week of corticosteroid therapy, peaks in intensity over 2 to 3 weeks, and persists until the medications are discontinued or the dosage decreased (Fig. 19-7). The eruption is limited to the sebaceous gland-rich skin of the chest, back, and face. Usual acne treatments, including topical and oral antibiotics, benzoyl peroxides, and retinoids, are of only limited usefulness.

### DRUG ERUPTIONS

Drug eruptions are a common problem in all drug-treated patients. From 1% to 3% of patients who are treated with a medication will develop a drug eruption of some sort (34). These eruptions usually occur within 2 to 3 weeks of initiation of the medication, and certain medications are more prone to drug eruptions than others (Table 19-2). Listing the drugs started within the prior 2 to 3 weeks before the onset of a drug eruption and using the information in Table 2 as a guide to the drugs most likely to cause a specific type of drug eruption can help to identify the offending agent. It is important to note that patients may become allergic to a medication they have been on for years or be allergic to more than one agent at a time.

The most common type of drug eruption is the macular and papular or exanthematic eruption (Fig. 19-8), usually starting in the trunk. The eruption then spreads distally over 24 to 72 hours, persists for 7 to 14 days, and resolves over a 3- to 7-day period in a proximal to distal manner. Pruritus may be intense, although it is absent in some patients. Rechallenge with the offending agent generally will lead to a similar eruption with an accelerated onset. If the offending drug is continued, one third of patients will persist with the macular and papular eruption, one third will resolve despite the drug being contin-

**TABLE 2.** *Drug eruptions*

| Type of reaction | Drugs commonly associated |
| --- | --- |
| Maculopapular | Penicillins, phenylbutazone, sulfonamides, phenytoin, carbamazepine, gold, gentamicin |
| Erythrodermas | Allopurinol, p-amino salicylic acid, barbiturates, captopril, carbamazepine, cefoxitin, chloroquine, chlorpromazine, cimetidine, diltiazem, gold, griseofulvin, hydantoin derivatives, isoniazid, lithium, nitrofurantoin, D-penicillamine, penicillin, phenylbutazone, quinidine, streptomycin, sulfonamides, sulfonylureas |
| Urticarial | Vaccines, serum, dextrans, penicillins, salicylates, hydralazine, phenylbutazone, hydantoin derivatives, quinidine, radiographic contrast |
| Eczematous | Ethylenediamine antihistamines, mercurials, procaine, p-amino salicylic acid, tolbutamide, chlorpropamide, chlorthiazide |
| Serum sickness | Penicillins, sulfonamides, thiouracils, radiographic contrast, phenytoin, p-amino salicylic acid, streptomycin |
| Lichenoid | Beta-blockers, captopril, thiazides, bold, bismuth, mepacrine, chloroquine, quinine, quinidine, chlorpropamide, penicillamine, carbamazepine, ethambutol, furosemide, isoniazid, methyldopa, p-amino salicylic acid, phenothiazine, phenylbutazone, phenytoin, pyritinol |
| Fixed | Tetracyclines, sulfonamides, barbiturates, oxyphenbutazone, metamizole, acetylsalicylic acid, hyoscine butylbromide, ibuprofen, chlordiazepoxide, dapsone, phenazone, phenolphthalein, quinine, paracetamol, benzodiazepines |
| Erythema multiforme and toxic epidermal necrolysis | Sulfonamides, co-trimoxazole, barbiturates, phenylbutazone, phenolphthalein, rifampicin, penicillins, pyrazolone derivatives, hydantoin derivatives, carbamazepine, phenothiazines, chlorpropamide, thiazide diuretics, sulfones, minoxidil, phenazone, fenbufen, mianserin, sulindac, methaqualone, allopurinol, pentamidine |

Adapted from Breathnach SM. Drug reactions. In: Champion RH, Burton JL, Ebling FJG, eds. *Textbook of dermatology*, 5th ed. London: Blackwell Scientific Publications, 1992:2961.

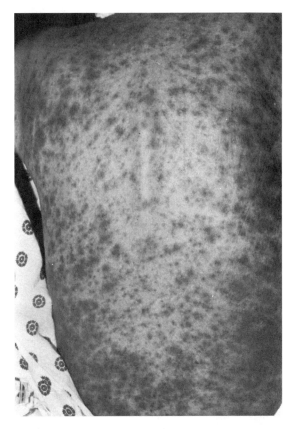

**FIG. 8.** This diabetic patient with an infected foot ulcer developed this maculopapular drug eruption over a 48-hour period on the eighth day of intravenous unasyn therapy. He was diagnosed with ampicillin allergy, and the eruption cleared over a 10-day period after discontinuing the unasyn. Courtesy of Alan B. Fleischer, Jr., M.D.

ued, and the last third will progress into a more severe eruption of generalized exfoliative erythroderma or even toxic epidermal necrolysis.

Other less common clinical types of drug eruptions include exfoliative erythrodermas, urticarial, eczematous (after systemic administration of an agent to which patient is contact allergic), serum sickness, lichenoid (appearing like lichen planus), fixed, and, the most severe of drug eruptions, erythema multiforme and toxic epidermal necrolysis. Fixed drug eruptions are odd drug reactions in which patients treated with a medication break out with an erythematous and vesicular plaque at a specific localized body site each time they are exposed to the medication. The inflammatory reaction will last for 7 to 14 days and then resolve. During periods between dosing of the medication, a hyperpigmented patch may remain at the site of the earlier drug eruption.

## INFECTIONS AND INFESTATIONS DUE TO IMMUNOSUPPRESSION

Patients suffering the latter stages of cancer have numerous insults on their immune systems. Many tumors, especially lymphomas and leukemias, directly impair the immune response. Chemotherapy and radiation therapy used to treat malignancies often weaken the immune system's defenses against infection. The mucositis and frequent breaks in the skin provided by invasive catheters and needles provide ready portals for microbial invasion. For all these reasons, infections of the skin are more common and severe in immunocompromised, debilitated oncology patients. The skin also may be involved as part of a more widespread, multiorgan system (i.e., infection).

Common bacterial infections of the skin include folliculitis, furunculosis, ecthyma, erysipelas, and cellulitis, most commonly resulting from either *Staphylococcus aureus* or *Streptococcus pyogenes*. Gram-negative organism are involved less frequently, usually in infections of intertriginous areas or regions below the patient's waist. Folliculitis is caused by a bacterial invasion of the hair-follicle structures and is especially common in occluded, moist sites, such as the groin, axilla, or anterior thighs. In bedridden patients, the eruption may be most prominent along the back and posterior aspect of the legs and shoulders. If the infection penetrates deeper and wider from the hair follicle, a furuncle, or boil, may develop from a folliculitis lesion. Folliculitis can be treated with either topical (e.g., clindamycin) or oral anti-staphylococcal antibiotics. Furunculosis requires incision and drainage of the infected phlegmon in addition to systemic antibiotics.

Ecthyma arises as a result of excoriation of pruritic folliculitis, with deeper crusted erosions predominating. It is especially prominent on the lower extremities of diabetic or immunocompromised hosts. Ecthyma gangrenosum is a subset of ecthyma that is caused by the Gram-negative organism *Pseudomonas aeruginosa*. The infection presents with a hemorrhagic bulla, which ruptures, leaving a slowly healing, necrotic ulcer as its residua. Intertriginous regions, especially areas of apocrine gland predominance in the groin and axilla, predominate. Traditional teaching was that ecthyma gangrenosum represented the cutaneous manifestation of an underlying Pseudomonas bacteremia; however, a recent report described ecthyma gangrenosum as a primary *P. aeruginosa* infection of the skin in most infected immunocompromised patients (35).

Cellulitis and erysipelas are the sequelae of deeper invasion of bacterial organisms into the dermis and subcutaneous tissue spaces. Although it is most common on the lower extremities, cellulitis can occur on any portion of the skin. Upper extremity cellulitis is common in breast cancer patients with underlying lymphedema. Usually, a preceding break in the cutaneous integrity (e.g., insect bite, abrasion, or tinea) allows penetration of the organism. Bright red, warm, tender, plaques then evolve over a period 2 to 3 days. Cellulitis and erysipelas usually have associated signs of systemic infection, including fever, elevated white blood cell count, and malaise. Erysipelas is distinguished from cellulitis by its more extensive lymphatic involvement, causing well-demarcated, edematous plaques with a peau de orange surface. Treatment of cellulitis or erysipelas requires antibacterial therapy with coverage for *Streptococcus* and *Staphylococcus*.

Viral infections of the skin frequently encountered in immunocompromised oncology patients include recurrent herpes simplex and herpes zoster. Once infected with either the herpes simplex virus during primary orolabial or genital herpes or varicella zoster virus, during chicken pox, the dormant virus is carried in the dorsal sensory root ganglia for the lifetime of the infected host. Immunosuppression facilitates reactivation of herpes simplex virus as cold sores, stomatitis, and anogenital lesions and varicella zoster virus as herpes zoster. Herpes simplex virus type 1 (HSV-1) is a ubiquitous infection of human hosts. More than 95% of urban adults have been previously infected with HSV-1 in orolabial sites (36). Although type 2 HSV infection is less common, 10% to 25% of adults have been infected with HSV-2 in anogenital regions. As the oncology patient's immune system deteriorates, HSV may recur with increased frequency and severity (Fig. 19-9). Primary herpes virus infection is generally more severe than recurrent disease. In the immunocompromised host, a primary eruption may be even more violent. In severely immunocompromised bone marrow transplant patients or other cancer patients undergoing chemotherapy, 20% to 30% per year will develop reactive herpes zoster (shingles). The shingles course may be more prolonged than in immunocompetent persons (usually 2–3 weeks) and may lead to more untoward sequelae, such as acute pain, postherpetic neuralgia (pain persisting 4 weeks after onset of the eruption), and dissemination. Dissemination is arbitrarily defined as more than 10 vesicular lesions outside the primarily affected dermatome.

The primary lesion of both the herpes simplex and varicella zoster viruses is grouped vesicles, papules, or pustules on an erythematous base. In immunocompromised persons, lesions may ulcerate, leaving slow-healing wounds. The lesions of HSV infection tend to localize to one distinct orolabial or genital region, whereas the eruption of shingles is distributed along a single nervous system dermatome.

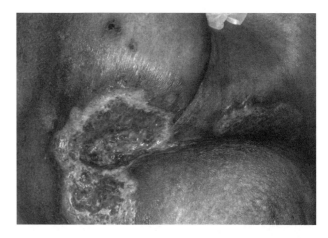

**FIG. 9.** This elderly woman with aplastic anemia developed this slowly growing ulcer over her sacrum 2 months previously. Culture grew herpes simplex virus type 2. Gradual healing occurred over the subsequent month on intravenous acyclovir.

Treatment of herpes viruses is with either acyclovir, famciclovir, or valacyclovir. Acyclovir should be dosed at 400 mg every 4 hours during awake hours (i.e., 5 times daily) for 7 to 10 days for infection and 800 mg every 4 hours while awake for 7 to 10 days for shingles. Intravenous acyclovir is administered at 5 to 10 mg/kg and 10 to 15 mg/kg every 8 hours for HSV and varicella zoster virus infections, respectively. Famciclovir is an alternative in shingles therapy at 500 mg 3 times daily for 7 days. Valacycovir is dosed at 1,000 mg 3 times daily for 7 days. Only famciclovir and valacyclovir decrease the duration of postherpetic neuralgia pain in shingles by a statistically significant amount. Intravenous dosing is required only for patients who are not taking oral medications or in disseminated infection.

Fungal infection of the skin is also more common in immunocompromised patients with tinea caused by dermatophyte fungi and Candida infections of intertriginous areas. Yeast infections of intertriginous areas are especially common in diabetics or in patients on broad-spectrum antibiotics. Diagnosis is established by potassium hydroxide preparation of scale scraped from the margin of the infection. Treatment for tinea includes a topical antifungal imidazole or, if necessary, the oral agent grise-ofulvin, terbinafine, or intraorazole.

Scabies infestation of the skin is not more common in immunocompromised hosts, but the pattern of the infestation can be altered. Patients with limited immunity usually do not itch as profoundly from contact with the scabies mite, limiting the usual removal of the parasite by scratching the insect from the superficial epidermis. Therefore, the mite is able to multiply unrestricted by the host, leading to more extensive infestation. Innumerable, 2- to 6-mm- long burrows may be seen in the areas of scabetic predilection and in the web spaces of the fingers and toes, palms and soles, genitalia, umbilicus, and buttocks. The most severe infestation, called *crusted* or *Norwegian scabies*, is seen in severely immunocompromised patients, typically with some degree of cognitive impairment. These patients have crusted plaques in the groin, axilla, and hands and feet infested with millions of mites. Mites also may live under the fingernails in crusted scabies as hyperkeratotic, subungual plaques. Diagnosis of scabies is established by scraping the mites' burrows off with a scalpel, smearing them onto a glass slide, fixing the specimen under a coverslip with mineral oil, and identifying under low microscopic power the flat, round scabies mite, oval eggs, or clumped, brown mite feces. Treatment of the patient with scabies and all household contacts is with either permethrin or lindane lotion applied from the neck down at bedtime and washed off in the morning. This application is repeated once a week later. All clothing and bed clothing with which the patient has had contact and all household contacts should be washed with laundry detergent the night of the first application. Unlaunderable items, for example, down com-

forters or coats, can be sealed in a plastic bag for 3 days, as the scabies mite will die without a human blood meal for this period. Itching may persist for 3 to 4 weeks after adequate treatment as a result of the residual effects of the infestation.

## PARANEOPLASTIC SYNDROMES

A variety of both common and rare cutaneous disorders have been associated with internal malignancy. Many of these associations are of questionable significance, described in only a limited number of patients or relating common skin disorders with common tumors. A set of criteria were developed by Curth (37) to delineate those conditions that are clearly associated with specific malignancies from those that may be spuriously associated with the cancer. The Curth criteria are (a) a concurrence of onset or recognition of a malignancy when the skin disease is diagnosed; (b) a parallel course, for example, if the tumor is treated, the dermatosis improves or with tumor regrowth the dermatosis recurs; (c) a uniform associated type of neoplasia; (d) a statistically significant association; and (e) a linkage through an inherited syndrome (38). The various skin diseases associated with internal malignancy are listed in Table 19-3. Paraneoplastic conditions of special note are described below. Acanthosis nigricans was the disorder for which Curth originally developed her paraneoplastic criteria. In patients who develop this disorder, after endocrinopathy and obesity are excluded, malignancy within the gastrointestinal tract is frequently found. More than 95% of the tumors associated with acanthosis nigricans are adenocarcinoma, and more than half of all tumors are gastric. Resection or removal of the tumor leads to complete resolution of the eruption, and relapse of the tumor is predictably followed by recurrence of the skin disease.

Patients with acanthosis nigricans develop asymptomatic velvety, hyperpigmented plaques, first in intertriginous areas, then with spread to surrounding nonintertriginous skin, and ultimately a generalized eruption (Fig. 19-10). Disease of the palms and soles usually present as thickening of these regions, but in patients with extensive disease, elsewhere. Velvety, leukokeratotic plaques in the mouth and other mucosal regions represent involvement of these sites.

Erythema gyratum repens is another paraneoplastic condition that fulfills four of five of Curth's criteria (39). Patients, almost exclusively those with lung cancer, develop a scaly, pruritic eruption on the trunk and extremities with a distinctive wood grain appearance (Fig. 19-11). None of the reported cases of erythema gyratum repens have been without an underlying malignancy. In most cases, the eruption was the first sign of malignancy, predating the diagnosis by an average of 9 months. A recent report found immunoreactants directed

**TABLE 3.** *Diseases associated with internal malignancy*

| Disorder | Cutaneous findings | Associated malignancy | Other pertinent findings | Comments |
|---|---|---|---|---|
| *Conditions that fit Curth's criteria* | | | | |
| Acanthosis nigricans | Hyperpigmentation and velvety hyperkeratosis on flexural surfaces | Gastrointestinal adenocarcinoma (often gastric) | Pruritus, weight loss, and mucosal involvement | Lack of endocrinopathy |
| Erythema gyratum repens syndrome | Figurate erythema with wood grain appearance | Lung carcinomas | Weight loss | Rare but striking |
| Sweet's syndrome (acute febrile neutrophilic dermatosis) | Tender erythematous plaques | Myelogenous leukemia | Fever and anemia | Course parallels that of leukemia |
| Necrolytic migratory erythema (glucagonoma syndrome) | Migratory necrolytic erythema or intertriginous and periorificial dermatitis | Alpha cell carcinoma of the pancreas | Glossitis, weight loss, hyperglycemic and decreased plasma amino acids | — |
| Acrokeratosis paraneoplastic (Bazex syndrome) | Three stages: (1) vesicles, periungual hyperkeratosis, nail dystrophy; (2) acral erythema and scaling; (3) dissemination | Squamous cell caner of the upper "aerodigestive" tract | None | Very rare |
| Paraneoplastic pemphigus | Generalized mucocutaneous blistering | Lymphomas and thymomas | Autoantibodies directed at the basement membrane zone and intercellular substance of skin | Newly described |
| Amyloidosis, primary systemic | Pinch purpura, waxy appearance, waxy translucent papules | Multiple myeloma | Macroglossia and organomegaly (spleen, heart, or liver) | Poor prognostic sign, deposition of AL protein |
| Carcinoid syndrome | Flushing and sclerodermoid changes | Carcinoid tumor | Bronchospasm, weight loss, diarrhea, and right-sided cardiac valvular lesions | Intestinal tumor usually metastatic to liver, or bronchial tumor; increased urinary 5-hydroxyindole-acetic acid |
| Hypertrichosis lanuginosa | Excessive growth of lanugo hair | Various cell types and sites | Glossitis and weight loss | Must rule out endocrinopathies |
| *Classic association in questions* | | | | |
| Dermatomyositis | Heliotrope (violaceous rash around the orbits), Gottron's papules (papules and plaques over bony prominences), and poikiloderma in photodistribution | Various cell types and sites; 25% of patients have a cancer; may be concurrent, prior to, or after the diagnosis of diabetes mellitus | Symmetric, proximal muscle weakness | Exhaustive nondirected search not indicated; symptoms or physical findings should direct the search; usual age-appropriate testing is indicated |
| Acquired ichthyosis | Generalized dry, scaling of the skin, with accentuation over the shins | Hodgkin's disease | Occasional pruritus | None |
| Bowen disease | Scaly, erythematous plaque with undulating border | Various cell types and sites | None | Statistics are questionable |
| Exfoliative dermatitis (erythroderma) | Generalized scaly erythroderma | Lymphoproliferative disorders | Weight loss and adenopathy | Only 5–10% association |
| *Hereditary associations* | | | | |
| Gardner's syndrome | Multiple epidermoid cysts, desmoid tumors, fibromas, and lipomas | Colonic adenocarcinoma | Osteomas and polyposis coli (adenomatous polyps) | Autosomal dominant trait; 100% cure with colectomy |
| Multiple hamartoma syndrome (Cowden syndrome) | Periorificial keratotic papules, tricholemmomas, and acral papules | Breast cancer, often bilateral; thyroid or intestinal cancer, rarer | Mucosal papules and intestinal polyposis (hamartomas) | Autosomal dominant trait |
| Neurofibromatosis | Neurofibromas, café-au-lait spots, and axillary freckling (Crowe's sign) | Neurofibrosarcoma, pheochromocytoma leukemia, acoustic neuromas, and Wilms' tumor | Lisch's nodules on the iris, seizures, and mental retardation | Autosomal dominant trait; malignancy is uncommon |
| Peutz-Jeghers syndrome | Mucosal pigmented macules also on acral surfaces | Intestinal neoplasia 5% | Hamartomatous intestinal polyps | Autosomal dominant trait |
| Torres's syndrome | Sebaceous neoplasia, and keratoacanthomas | Multiple colonic carcinomas | None | Autosomal dominant trait |

From Callen JP, Fabré VC. Cutaneous manifestations of systemic diseases. In: Moshella SL, Hurley, eds. *Dermatology*, 3rd ed. Philadelphia: WB Saunders, 1992:1682.

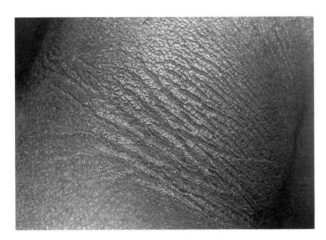

**FIG. 10.** This symmetric, velvety, hyperpigmented plaque of acanthosis nigricans slowly extended outward from the axilla onto the posterior arm in this woman with metastatic gastric adenocarcinoma.

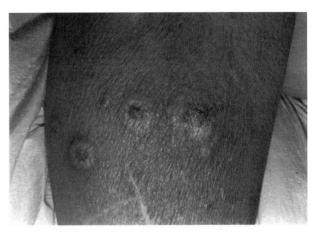

**FIG. 12.** A tender, warm, erythematous plaque surmounted by pseudopustulation due to Sweet syndrome arose suddenly on the leg of a febrile, ill patient with acute myelogenous leukemia. Complete resolution of the eruption occurred over a 72-hour period on prednisone 40 mg per day.

at both the basement membrane zone of the lung carcinoma and skin, suggesting autoimmunity to the patient's tumor with cross reaction to the skin as the etiology of erythema gyratum repens (40).

Paget disease of the breast classically has been included in the paraneoplastic disorders; however, this erosive eruption of the nipple truly represents contiguous tumor spread of an underlying intraductal neoplasia. Paget disease is, unfortunately, a late sign of malignancy, frequently associated with nodal metastases.

In 1964 Sweet (41) described a syndrome he termed *acute febrile neutrophilic dermatosis*. The originally described syndrome consisted of painful, red, raised plaques and nodules appearing anywhere on the skin surface (Fig. 19-12). The tender plaques may be surmounted by lesions that appear to be purulent bullae. Lancing

relieves no pus, revealing their true solid nature. Associated systemic symptoms include arthritis, conjunctivitis, and malaise. Fevers and high white blood cell count are frequently associated signs. Sweet syndrome is associated with an underlying malignancy in about half of the cases, with leukemia, especially acute myelogenous leukemia, the most frequent. The syndrome also occurs in the setting of other carcinomas, including various lymphomas and leukemias and, less commonly, solid tumors. Treatment with systemic steroids (prednisone at 0.5 mg/kg/day) leads to rapid and complete resolution of the eruption and systemic symptoms.

Necrolytic migratory erythema, or glucagonoma syndrome, is a specific marker for glucagon-producing islet cell tumors of the pancreas (42,43). Usually, patients develop scaling, crusted, tender erosions on the face and intertriginous areas, predominantly in a periorificial array. Extensive cases can involve other areas of the skin. Glossitis, stomatitis, dystrophic nails, and alopecia are seen frequently in these patients, with concomitant weight loss, diabetes, and abdominal tumors. Resection of the glucagon-secreting tumor leads to rapid resolution of the eruption.

Acrokeratosis paraneoplastic, or Bazex syndrome, is a rare disorder that presents with violaceous erythema, vesiculation, and scaling on acral areas, for example, the tips of the fingers and toes, nose, and ears (44) (Fig. 19-13). Over time, the eruption will become more hyperkeratotic and generalized. Severe nail dystrophy with paronychia is a hallmark of the condition. Almost all cases of true Bazex syndrome have an associated squamous cell carcinoma of the upper aerodigestive tract, particularly with cervical node metastases. Males are disproportionately affected over females. Bazex syndrome is usually resistant to all therapies except those directed at treating the underlying malignancy.

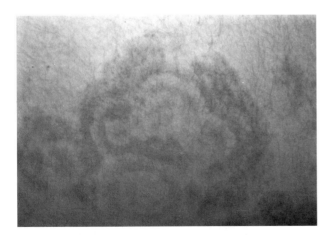

**FIG. 11.** Erythema gyratum repens in a patient diagnosed with lung cancer 3 months after onset of this distinctive eruption of concentric, erythematous rings in a wood grain appearance.

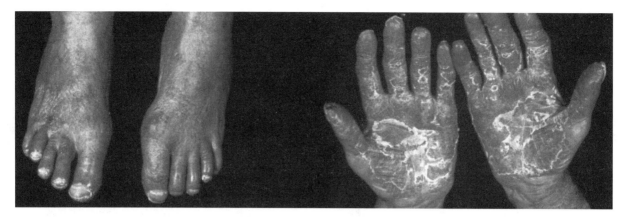

**FIG. 13.** Acrokeratosis paraneoplastica in a man with lung cancer. The violaceous erythema, psoriasiform scaling, and nail dystrophy progressively arose over the past 4 months. Chest radiograph revealed the peripheral tumor nodule and mediastinal metastases of squamous cell carcinoma of the lung. Courtesy of Janet A. Fairley, M.D.

Paraneoplastic pemphigus is a unique form of pemphigus described in association with malignant neoplasms (45). The clinical manifestations of paraneoplastic pemphigus are polymorphous. Patients have sudden eruptions of cutaneous blisters and erosions in association with painful erosions of the oropharynx and lips and pseudomembranous conjunctivitis, all resistant to conventional pemphigus therapy. Immunofluorescence testing in paraneoplastic pemphigus has revealed autoantibodies that bind to desmosome-containing tissues, including squamous, columnar, and transitional cell epithelium; myocardium; skeletal muscle; and thyroid gland. Immunoprecipitation of serum of a patient with paraneoplastic pemphigus reveals a unique antigen complex of four polypeptides with molecular weights of 250, 230, 210, and 190 kD. The pathogenic nature of the paraneoplastic autoantibodies was demonstrated in the mouse model of pemphigus (46). Passive transfer of the autoantibodies to neonatal mice leads to cutaneous blistering within 18 hours of injection. Histological examination of the skin of exposed mice shows intraepidermal acantholytic blistering identical to that found in patients with paraneoplastic pemphigus.

Dermatomyositis has an established but somewhat controversial association with internal neoplasia, frequently predating the diagnosis of the cancer. Bronchogenic is the most frequently associated tumor, with breast, ovary, cervix, and gastrointestinal tract tumors also reported. A cancer is found in about 8% to 10% of all polymyositis/dermatomyositis patients and in 19.2% of male patients aged over 50 years (48). If only dermatomyositis patients are studied, the association is stronger, with 28% to 37% of patients with dermatomyositis having an underlying malignancy (49,50). The clinical manifestations of dermatomyositis with or without malignancy are the same, including periorbital heliotrope; infiltrated erythematous to violaceous scaly plaques on the knuckles, elbows, and knees (Gottron's sign); photodistributed poikiloderma; and atrophic thinning of the skin with telangiectatic vessels and pigment and cutaneous calcinosis. Proximal muscle weakness usually arises concurrently with the skin findings, initially noted as difficulty when arising from a chair or climbing stairs. The activity of paraneoplastic dermatomyositis follows the course of the malignancy, with resolution on treatment and recurrence with relapse of the tumor. The disease may be resistant to other, usual therapies for dermatomyositis, such as systemic steroids and immunosuppressive medications.

Acquired ichthyosis is seen in association with Hodgkin lymphoma. Patients develop dry, scaly areas of skin (*xerosis*), most prominently on the shins and extensor arms and legs. This condition is usually a late manifestation of lymphoma rather than the presenting sign (51).

## DIRECT TUMOR INVOLVEMENT OF THE SKIN

The skin is a common site for discontinuous spread of internal malignancies, found in 5% of 7,316 patients enrolled in the Milton S. Hershey Medical Center tumor registry (52). Cutaneous metastases are usually a late finding in cancer, with skin metastases the presenting sign of internal malignancy in fewer than 5% of patients in most large series. Almost half of all cutaneous metastases are from regional lymphatic spread of breast cancer in women. Patients with melanoma metastases constitute the second largest group in aggregate and are the leading cause of cutaneous metastatic disease in men. Lung and colorectal cancers are responsible for most of the remaining cutaneous metastases in men (Table 19-4).

Cutaneous metastases most commonly occur as dermal or subcutaneous nodules in the skin (Fig. 19-14). Their color varies from flesh toned to red or violaceous. The tumor nodules may be inflammatory, warm, and tender,

**TABLE 4.** *Origin of cutaneous metastases*

| Women | | Men | |
|---|---|---|---|
| Primary site | Incidence | Primary site | Incidence |
| Breast | 71% | Melanoma | 32% |
| Melanoma | 12% | Lung | 12% |
| Ovary | 3% | Colon and rectum | 11% |
| Unknown primary | 3% | Oral cavity | 9% |
| | | Unknown primary | 9% |
| Oral cavity | 2% | | |
| Lung | 2% | Larynx | 6% |

Adapted from Lookingbill et al., ref. 52.

but usually they are asymptomatic and firm to the touch. Cutaneous metastases generally arise as multiple tumor nodules. Metastatic lung carcinoma is a notable exception, with more than half of the patients having a solitary metastases to the skin. Rarer presentations of cutaneous metastases include inflammatory metastases, which clinically mimic plaques of cellulitis or erysipelas. The term *carcinoma erysipeloides* has been used to describe patients with inflammatory, metastatic breast cancer to the skin. Scarring metastases that produce fibrous plaques as a result of stromal reaction to the metastases also have been reported. The term *carcinoma en cuirasse*, likening the metastases to the torso armor of medieval French soldiers, has been used to describe breast carcinoma with extensive scarring metastases to the chest. Rarely, metastases arise in a zosteriform array distributed along one dermatome.

Cutaneous metastases are most common in the regional vicinity of the primary tumor. Metastatic tumors on the chest usually are due to breast or lung metastases, whereas tumors on the abdominal skin are due most frequently to metastases from bowel, ovarian, or bladder carcinoma. A Sister Mary Joseph nodule of the umbilicus, named after Sister Joseph who worked as a nurse at St. Mary's Hospital, Mayo Clinic, has been observed in patients with intraabdominal carcinoma, most often of gastric origin. Metastases also may arise in the scars from the surgical incision used in removal of a carcinoma. Examples include laryngeal carcinoma and tracheostomy site, lung carcinoma and thoracotomy, and abdominal carcinomas and scars. A notable location for distant metastases is the scalp, frequently the site of breast, kidney, lung, or adrenal gland cutaneous metastases.

The primary item in the differential diagnosis of metastatic nodules to the skin is a benign or malignant primary tumors of the dermis or subcutaneous tissues. Usually, metastatic lesions arise suddenly, grow rapidly over 1 to 2 months, and then maintain their size for several months. Primary skin tumors generally demonstrate slower, progressive growth. Metastases are usually harder in consistency than primary tumors of the skin and are asymptomatic. Metastatic tumors of the scalp frequently cause localized loss of hair, causing potential confusion with scarring alopecias.

Cutaneous metastases portend a poor prognosis in cancer patients. The average survival time from the diagnosis of skin metastases to death was documented to be 31 months for breast cancer, 18 months for colorectal cancer, 16 months for melanoma, 9 months for oral cavity cancer, and 5 months for lung cancer (53). Cutaneous metastases may respond to systemic chemotherapy used to control the patient's total tumor burden. If the patient has a limited number of disfiguring or symptomatic metastases, surgical excision or radiation therapy may be used.

## REFERENCES

1. Yokel BK, Hood AF. Mucocutaneous complications of antineoplastic therapy. In: Fitzpatrick TB, Eiser AZ, Wolff R, Freedberg IM, Austen KF, eds. *Dermatology in general medicine.* 4th ed. New York: McGraw-Hill, 1993;1745.
2. Wall RL, Conrad FG. Cyclophosphamide therap: its use in leukemia, lymphoma, and solid tumors. *Arch Intern Med* 1961;108:456.
3. Dahlgren S, Hom G, Svanborg N, Watz R. Clinical and morphological side effects of busulfan (Myleran) treatment. *Acta Med Scand* 1972;192:129.
4. Price NM, Deneau DG, Hoppe RT. The treatment of mycosis fungoides with ointment-based mechlorethamine *Arch Dermatol* 1982;118:234.
5. Constantine VS, Fuks ZY, Farber EM. Mechlorethamine desensitization in therapy for mycosis fungoides. Topical desensitization to mechlorethamine (nitrogen mustard) contact hypersensitivity. *Arch Dermatol* 1975;111:484.
6. Cornwell GG 3d, Pajak TF, McIntyre OR. Hypersensitivity reactions to IV melphalan during treatment of multiple myeloma: cancer and leukemia group B experience. *Cancer Treat Rep* 1979;63:399.
7. Yung CW, Winston EW, Lorincz AL. Dacarbazine-induced photosensitivity reaction. *J Am Acad Dermatol* 1981;4:541.
8. Bell R, Sullivan JR, Burdon JG, Sinclair R. Toxic rash associated with high dose methotrexate therapy. *Clin Exp Pharmacol Physiol* 1979;5:57.
9. Kim YH, Aye MS, Fayos JV. Radiation necrosis of the scalp: A complication of cranial irradiation and methotrexate. *Radiology* 1977;124:813.
10. Stelzer KJ, Griffin TW, Koh W-J. Radiation recall skin toxicity with bleomycin in a patient with Kaposi sarcoma related to acquired immune deficiency syndrome. *Cancer* 1993;71:1322.
11. Kennedy BJ, Theologides A. The role of 5-fluorouracil in malignant disease. *Ann Intern Med* 1961;55:719.
12. Falkson G, Schulz EJ. Skin changes in patients treated with 5-fluorouracil. *Br J Dermatol* 1962;74:229.
13. Vaitkevicius VK, Brennan MJ, Becke HVL, Kelly JE, Talley RW. Clin-

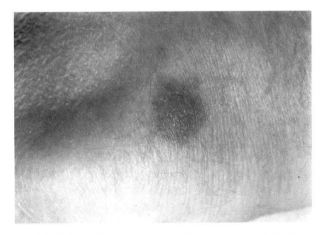

**FIG. 14.** A firm, violaceous, subcutaneous metastatic tumor nodule in an elderly man with adenocarcinoma of the lung.

ical evaluation of cancer chemotherapy with 5-fluorouracil. *Cancer* 1961;14:131.

14. Stevens HP, Ostlere LS, Begent RH, Dooley JS, Rustin MHA. Pellagra secondary to 5-fluorouracil. *Br J Dermatol* 1993;128:578.

15. Burgdorf WHC, Gilmore WA, Ganick RG. Peculiar acral erythema secondary to high-dose chemotherapy for acute myelogenous leukemia. *Ann Intern Med* 1982;97:61.

16. Bernstein EF, Spielvogel RL, Topolsky DL. Recurrent neutrophilic eccrine hidradenitis. *Br J Dermatol* 1992;127:529.

17. Yagoda A, Mukherj B, Young C, et al. Bleomycin, an antitumor antibiotic: clinical experience in 274 patients. *Ann Intern Med* 1972;77:861.

18. Rothberg H. Raynaud's phenomenon after vinblastine-bleomycin chemotherapy. *Cancer Treat Rep* 1978;62:569.

19. Duhra P, Ilchyshyn A, Das RN. Bleomycin-induced flagellate erythema. *Clin Exp Dermatol* 1991;16:216.

20. Tsuji T, Sawabe M. Hyperpigmentation in striae distensae after bleomycin treatment. *J Am Acad Dermatol* 1993;28:503.

21. Hrushesky WJ. Serpentine supravenous 5-fluorouracil (NSC-19893) hyperpigmentation. *Cancer Treat Rep* 1976;60:639.

22. Keidan SE. Actinomycin D in the treatment of cancer in children. *Br J Surg* 1966;53:614.

23. Epstein EH Jr, Lutzner MA. Folliculitis induced by actinomycin D. *N Engl J Med* 1969;281:1094.

24. Lovejoy NC. Preventing hair loss during Adriamycin therapy. *Cancer Nurs* 1979;2:117.

25. Soukop M, Campbell A, Gray MM, Calman KC. Adriamycin, alopecia and the scalp tourniquet. *Cancer Treat Rep* 1978;62:489.

26. Dean JC, Salmon SE, Griffith KS. Prevention of doxorubicin-induced hair loss with scalp hypothermia. *N Engl J Med* 1979;301:1427.

27. Cohen SC, DiBella NJ, Michalak JC. Letter: Recall injury from Adriamycin. *Ann Intern Med* 1975;83:232.

28. Vogelzang NJ. "Adriamycin flare": a skin reaction resembling extravasation. *Cancer Treat Rep* 1979;63:2067.

29. Kennedy BJ. Metabolic and toxic effects of mithramycin during tumor therapy. *Am J Med* 1970;49:494.

30. Breza TS, Hulprin KM, Taylor JR. Photosensitivity reaction to vinblastine. *Arch Dermatol* 1975;111:1168.

31. Gaspari AA, Lotze MT, Rosenberg SA, Stern JB, Kutz SI. Dermatologic changes associated with interleukin 2 administration. *JAMA* 1987;258:1624.

32. Itri LM. The interferons. *Cancer* 1992;70:940.

33. Stern RS, Wintroub BV, Arndt KA. Drug reactions. *J Am Acad Dermatol* 1986;15:1282.

34. El Baze P, Thyss A, Vinti H, Deville A, Dellamonica P, Ortonne JP. A study of nineteen immunocompromised patients with extensive skin lesions caused by *Pseudomonas aeruginosa* with and without bacteremia. *Acta Derm Venereol Suppl (Stockh)* 1991;71:411.

35. Johnson RE, Nahmias AJ, Magder LS, Lee FK, Brooks CA, Snowden CB. A seroepidemiologic survey of the prevalence of herpes simplex virus type 2 infection in the United States. *N Engl J Med* 1989;321:7.

36. Curth HO. Skin lesions and internal carcinoma. In: Adrade R, Gumport SL, Popkin GL, Rees TD, eds. *Cancer of the skin*. Philadelphia: WB Saunders, 1976:1308.

37. Callen JP, Fabré VC. Cutaneous manifestations of systemic diseases. In: Moschella SL, Hurley, eds. *Dermatology*. 3rd ed. Philadelphia: WB Saunders, 1992:1682.

38. Boyd AS, Neldner KH, Menter A: Erythema gyratum repens: a paraneoplastic eruption. *J Am Acad Dermatol* 1992;26:757.

39. Caux F, Lebbe C, Thomine E, et al. Erythema gyratum repens. A case studied with immunofluorescence, immunoelectron microscopy, and immunohistochemistry. *Br J Dermatol* 1994;131:102.

40. Sweet RD. An acute febrile neutrophilic dermatosis. *Br J Dermatol* 1964;76:349.

41. McGavran MH, Unger RH, Recant L, Polk HC, Kilo C, Levin ME. A glucagon-secreting alpha-cell carcinoma of the pancreas. *N Engl J Med* 1966;274:1408

42. Mallinson CN, Bloom SR, Warin AP, Salmon PR, Cox B. A glucagonoma syndrome. *Lancet* 1974;2:1.

43. Bazex A, Griffiths A. Acrokeratosis paraneoplastica: a new cutaneous marker of malignancy. *Br J Dermatol* 1980;103:301.

44. Anhalt GJ, Kim SC, Stanley JR, et al. Paraneoplastic pemphigus: an autoimmune mucocutaneous disease associated with neoplasia. *N Engl J Med* 1990;323:1729.

45. Anhalt GJ, Labib RS, Voorhees JJ, Beals TF, Diaz LA. Induction of pemphigus in neonatal mice by passive transfer of IgG from patients with the disease. *N Engl J Med* 1982;306:1189.

46. Callen JP. Malignancy in polymyositis/dermatomyositis. *Clin Dermatol* 1988;6:55.

47. Bohan A, Peter JB, Bowman RL, Reason CM. A computer assisted analysis of 153 patients with polymyositis-dermatomyositis. *Medicine (Baltimore)* 1977;56:255.

48. Bonnetblanc JM, Bernard P, Fayol J. Dermatomyositis and malignancy. A multicenter cooperative study. *Dermatologica* 1990;180:212.

49. Callen JP, Hyla JF, Bole GG Jr, Kay DR. The relationship of dermatomyositis and polymyositis to internal malignancy. *Arch Dermatol* 1980;116:295.

50. Flint GL, Flam M, Soter NA. Acquired ichthyosis. A sign of nonlymphoproliferative malignant disorders. *Arch Dermatol* 1975;111:1446

51. Lookingbill DP, Spangler N, Sexton FM. Skin involvement as the presenting sign of internal carcinoma: a retrospective study of 7,316 cancer patients. *J Am Acad Dermatol* 1990;22:19.

52. Lookingbill DP, Helm KF. Skin signs of systemic disease. *Clinical dermatology*, 21st revision Philadelphia: JB Lippincott Company, 1994: Unit 32-5.

*Principles and Practice of Supportive Oncology,*
edited by Ann Berger et al.
Lippincott–Raven Publishers, Philadelphia ©1998

CHAPTER 20

# Pressure Ulcers and the Oncology Patient

Margaret T. Goldberg

Pressure ulcers are a common complication in the elderly, immobile patient. These ulcers can be a source of pain and even infection in the seriously compromised person, vastly affecting the patient's quality of life. The prevalence and incidence of pressure ulcers have been difficult to ascertain because of differences in ulcer staging and data collection; however, one acute-care facility reported a 9.2% prevalence (1), and skilled-care facilities and nursing homes have reported prevalences as high as 23% (2). Pressure ulcers also can develop rapidly in the elderly patient with cancer, especially in those experiencing nutritional deficits, incontinence, and immobility. Gallagher (3) related that pressure ulcers pose a threat to the patient when immobility, nutritional deficits, advanced age, incontinence, radiation effects, metabolic abnormalities, pain, and persistent or recurrent disease coexist. Prevention of pressure ulcers is especially important in cancer patients becaise many of these patients may not have the capacity to heal an open ulcer (4).

In view of the problem of pressure ulcers and the costs associated with them, the Agency for Health Care Policy and Research (AHCPR) (5) developed guidelines for the prevention and treatment of pressure ulcers. The AHCPR was created by Congress in 1989 to improve the quality, appropriateness, and effectiveness of health care in the United States. To this end, the AHCPR publishes clinical practice guidelines and systematically developed statements to assist practitioners and patient decisions regarding appropriate health care for specific clinical conditions. These guidelines are developed by independent, multidisciplinary panels of private-sector clinicians and other experts convened by the AHCPR.

The content of the guidelines is derived from extensive literature reviews and expert clinical judgments. In May 1992 *Pressure Ulcers in Adults: Prediction and Preven-*

*tion* was published. This guideline is available in three distinct formats for health care practitioners: The *Clinical Practice Guideline* contains a detailed analysis and discussion of the available research, critical evaluation of the assumptions and knowledge of the field, considerations for patients with special needs, and references. The *Guideline Report* contains a comprehensive discussion of relevant research, including literature reviews and summary evidence tables. The *Quick Reference Guide for Clinicians* contains highlights from the *Clinical Practice Guideline* for easy reference. A fourth publication is available from AHCPR, *A Patient's Guide;* this publication, available in English and Spanish, is prepared for the consumer in easily understood language.

## ETIOLOGY OF PRESSURE ULCERS

A pressure ulcer (also known as decubitus, pressure sore, or bedsore) is any lesion caused by unrelieved pressure resulting in damage of underlying tissue (6). Pressure ulcers develop as a consequence of the occlusion of capillaries from unrelieved external pressure. When pressure is applied from an external surface to a bony prominence (as in the ischial tuberosities when sitting or the coccyx when lying down), the soft tissue is compressed, causing localized ischemia. If the pressure is unrelieved, the capillaries collapse, further disrupting the flow of blood and nutrients. Eventually, hypoxia and edema lead to cellular necrosis (7). Therefore, it is easy to see how pressure ulcers form so readily in the immobile patient.

### Factors that Increase the Risk of Pressure Ulcer Formation

#### Poor Nutrition

Poor nutrition has been identified by numerous studies (8) as a significant factor in the development of pressure

M. T. Goldberg: Cherry Hill, NJ 08002.

ulcers. Severe protein deficiency alters oncotic pressure and causes edema formation, rendering soft tissue susceptible to pressure ulcer formation (9).

### Shearing

Shearing also has been named as a culprit in the creation of pressure ulcers. Shearing occurs when the skin remains stationary and the underlying tissue shifts (i.e., when the head of the bed is raised and the patient slides down toward the foot of the bed). The loosely attached superficial layer of tissue will slide over the well-anchored, deeper tissue through which the blood vessels pass to reach the skin. Vessels may rupture, compress, or become distorted, resulting in deep tissue destruction (10).

### Friction

Friction injuries occur when the skin moves across a coarse surface, such as bed linens (7), and can cause an abrasion of the epidermis and the dermis, resulting in a loss of skin integrity.

### Urinary Incontinence

Urinary incontinence, which allows moisture to remain on the skin, can lead to maceration and excoriation, disrupting the integrity of the skin. Fecal incontinence and diarrhea, positively correlated with the development of pressure ulcer (11).

## PRESSURE ULCER PREVENTION

Prevention of pressure ulcers is vastly preferable to treating pressure ulcers (12); therefore, efforts begin with control or management of pressure ulcer etiology along with contributing factors. A comprehensive plan for pressure ulcer prevention is included in the AHCPR *Guideline Pressure Ulcers in Adults: Prediction and Prevention* (7). To intervene to reduce risk factors, the risk for acquiring a pressure ulcer must be calculated on an ongoing basis and whenever the condition of the patient changes.

### Identification of Patients at Risk

Clinicians are encouraged to select and use a method of risk assessment that ensures systematic evaluation of individual risk factors. Many risk assessment tools exist, but only the Braden Scale (13) and the Norton Scale (14) have been tested extensively. Risk should be reassessed periodically. Care should be modified according to the level of risk. Frequency of reassessment usually depends on patient status and institutional policy.

### Early Interventions

#### Activity or Mobility Deficit: Bedbound Patients

1. Reposition at least every 2 hours.
2. Use pillows or foam wedges to keep bony prominences from direct contact.
3. Use devices that totally relieve pressure on the heels.
4. Decrease skin injury caused by friction and shear forces with proper positioning, transferring, and turning techniques.
5. Use devices that totally relieve pressure on the heels.
6. Avoid positioning directly on the trochanter.
7. Elevate the head of the bed as little and for as short a time as possible.
8. Use lifting devices to move rather than drag patients during transfers and position changes.
9. Place at-risk patients on a pressure-reducing mattress.
10. Do not use a donut-type device.

#### Activity or Mobility Deficit: Chairbound Patients

1. Reposition at least every hour.
2. Have the patient shift weight every 15 minutes if able.
3. Use pressure-reducing devices for seating surfaces. Do not use donut-type devices.
4. Consider postural alignment, distribution of weight, balance and stability, and pressure relief when positioning patients in chairs or wheelchairs.

#### Skin Care and Early Treatment Guidelines

1. Inspect skin at least once a day. Individualize bathing schedule, avoid hot water, and use a mild cleansing agent.
2. Minimize environmental factors, such as low humidity and cold air. Use moisturizers for dry skin.
3. Avoid massage over bony prominences.
4. Use proper positioning, transferring, and turning techniques.
5. Use lubricants to reduce friction injuries.
6. Institute a rehabilitation program.
7. Monitor and document interventions and outcomes.

#### Moisure/Incontence

- Cleanse skin at time of soiling.
- Minimize skin exposure to moisture. Assess and treat urinary incontinence. When moisture cannot be controlled, use underpads or briefs that are absorbent and present a quick-drying surface to the skin.

## Nutritional Deficit

1. Investigate factors that compromise an apparently well-nourished patient's dietary intake (especially protein or calories) and offer support with eating.
2. Plan and implement a nutritional support or supplementation program for nutritionally compromised persons.

Interventions should be monitored and documented. Specific details are needed on who should provide the care, how often, and the supplies and equipment needed. How the care is to be undertaken should be individualized, written, and readily available. Furthermore, results of the interventions and the care being rendered and adjustment in the interventions as indicated by the outcomes should be documented. To ensure continuity, documentation of the plan of care must be clear, concise, and accessible to every caregiver (7).

## MANAGEMENT OF EXISTING ULCERS

### Principles of Wound Management

#### Elimination or Reduction of Causative Factors (15)

The main cause of a pressure ulcer is pressure; however, malnutrition, incontinence, friction, and shearing, if present, must be managed to facilitate wound healing. Assessment for these conditions (Table 1) is necessary and, if present, may lead to interventions such as the following:

1. Implementation of a turning/repositioning schedule if pressure appears to be the main cause.
2. Use of appropriate measures to reduce friction and shearing (e.g., trapeze, turning sheet, socks, use of knee gatch when head of bed is elevated, and so on).
3. Selection of a support surface that can deal with pressure, moisture, friction, or shearing.
4. Management of incontinence with external collection devices, bowel training, prompted voiding.

Doughty (16) maintains that failure to address cause will result in a nonhealing wound despite appropriate systemic and topical therapy.

**TABLE 1.** *Principles of wound management*

| Eliminate/Reduce causative and contributing factors. | 1. Pressure<br>2. Moisture<br>3. Friction<br>4. Shear |
|---|---|
| Provide systemic support<br>Topical therapy—<br>Remove impediments<br>to wound healing | Assess overall patient condition<br>1. Necrosis<br>2. Infection<br>3. Excess exudate<br>4. Retain moisture and heat |

## Systemic Support

Optimizing the overall condition of the patient is necessary to facilitate wound healing. Inadequate oxygen and nutrients will retard or prolong the wound healing process. Interventions are predicated on findings but may include the following:

1. Measures to support tissue oxygenation:
2. Control of diabetes
3. Measures to control insufficient dietary intake
4. Reduction of edema
5. Restoration of blood flow (15)

## Topical Therapy

The purpose of topical therapy is to provide an optimal environment for facilitating wound healing. Principles of topical therapy begin with removal of impediments to healing.

Necrosis in a pressure ulcer provides a medium for bacteria and also prolongs the inflammatory phase of wound healing. Debridement usually is indicated for the necrotic pressure ulcer. Another impediment to wound healing that prolongs the inflammatory phase of wound healing is infection. Pressure ulcers should be assessed for any signs of infection and cultured where appropriate. If the infection invades the surrounding tissue, systemic antibiotics should be considered so that blood and tissue antibiotic levels adequate for infection control can be achieved. Excess exudate can macerate surrounding skin and dilute wound healing factors and nutrients at the wound surface.

Protection of the wound includes maintaining a moist wound surface, thereby preventing desiccation and enhancing epidermal migration. It also promotes angiogenesis and connective tissue synthesis. Thermal insulation of the wound maintains normal tissue temperature, which improves blood flow to the wound bed and enhances epidermal migration (17). Appropriate topical treatment is directed by these principles (15).

## Education

The AHCPR treatment guidelines strongly propose pressure ulcer education not only for health care professionals but also for patients, family, and caregivers. The guidelines themselves can be used to educate colleagues about science-based pressure ulcer treatment. These guidelines are being used by many regulatory agencies to survey health care facilities, and Medicare benefits are being reimbursed according to these guidelines. In addition, the guidelines have been used as the standard of practice in the courtroom (20).

**TABLE 2.** *Assessment of existing ulcers*

| Parameter | Evaluation |
| --- | --- |
| Stage | Ulcer depth |
| Location | Patient positioning |
| Size | Provides baseline |
| Characteristics | Gives direction for wound care |
| Periwound | Identifies drainage, infection |
| Overall condition | Identifies capability of wound healing |
| Nutritional status | Specifies opportunity for improvement |
| Pressure reduction needs | Prevent additional ulcers |

## Assessment

Assessment of the ulcer is the basis for planning treatment as well as evaluating the effects of interventions (Table 2). Establishing a baseline by in-depth assessment also improves communication among caregivers.

### Stage

Staging or grading is a method for classifying wounds according to the tissue damage observed. Staging of a necrotic covered wound cannot be confirmed until the wound base is visible. The Wound Ostomy and Continence Nurses Society (WOCN) in conjunction with the NPUAP has incorporated a four-stage classification system. It should be noted that although progression through the stages may occur, downstaging or reversal of the staging process cannot occur.

#### Stage I

Nonblanchable erythema of intact skin is the heralding lesion of skin ulceration. In patients with darker skin, discoloration of the skin, warmth, edema, induration, or hardness also may be indicators.

#### Stage II

Partial-thickness skin loss involving the epidermis, dermis, or both is seen in stage II.

#### Stage III

Stage II involves full-thickness skin loss involving damage to or necrosis of subcutaneous tissue that may extend down to, but not through, underlying fascia. The ulcer presents clinically as a deep crater with or without undermining adjacent tissue.

#### Stage IV

Full-thickness skin loss with extensive destruction, tissue necrosis, or damage to muscle, bone, or supporting structures (e.g., tendon or joint capsule) occurs in stage IV.

### Location

The location of the pressure ulcer may identify the position in which the patient remained for too long. Pressure ulcers occur only over bony prominences, and the most common sites for pressure ulcers are coccyx/sacral areas and heels(18).

### Size

The length, width, and depth of an ulcer must be measured, and checks should be done for sinus tracks, undermining, and tunneling. Measurements of these areas can be accomplished by using a sterile Q-tip or tongue blade.

### Characteristics

It is important to note the presence of any granulation tissue, epithelialization, necrosis, and slough; measure the percentage present; and document these findings. If drainage is present, the amount, color, and consistency should be documented.

### Periwound

The tissue surrounding the ulcer is inspected, noting any maceration, excoriation, and signs of infection, such as warmth or induration.

### Patient's Overall Physical and Mental Status

Comorbid illnesses (e.g., peripheral vascular disease or diabetes, immune deficiencies, collagen vascular disease, malignancies, and psychosis) may limit an individual patient's capacity to heal.

### Nutritional Status

It must be verified that patient is eating. The health history should be reviewed for recent weight loss and to determine whether the serum albumin level is below 3.5 g/dl. It is important to encourage dietary intake or supplementation. If intake continues to be inadequate, impractical, or impossible, nutritional support (usually tube feeding) should be used to place the patient into positive nitrogen balance with approximately 30 to 35 calories/kg/day and 1.25 to 1.50 g of protein/kg/day according to the goals of care. As much as 2.00 g of protein/kg/day may be needed (19). Vitamin and mineral supplements may be given if deficiencies are confirmed.

### Pressure Reduction Needs

All patients with existing pressure ulcers should be assessed to determine their risk for developing additional pressure ulcers (20). A static support surface can be used if a patient can assume a variety of positions without bearing weight on a pressure ulcer and without "bottoming out." An overlay mattress can be checked at various anatomic sites while the patient assumes various positions an outstretched hand (palm up) under the overlay below the body part. If there is less than an inch of support material, the patient has bottomed out. A dynamic support surface is used when the patient cannot assume a variety of positions without bearing weight on a pressure ulcer, if the patient fully compresses the static support surface, or if the ulcer does not show evidence of healing. If the patient has large stage III or IV pressure ulcers on multiple turning surfaces, a low-air-loss bed or an air-fluidized bed may be indicated (19).

### Local Wound Care Treatments

#### Goals of Treatment

When the initial assessment is completed, patients and family caregivers should be provided with information sufficient to enable them to understand the treatment of pressure ulcers and assist in developing the treatment plan. The treatment plan should reflect the patient's values and explicitly define the goals of therapy. In general, the primary goal is healing of the ulcer, but sometimes the goal of patient comfort may take precedence. A patient who experiences pain or agitation on turning or during administration of tube feedings may simply wish to forgo the sort of intensive management that may be required to heal advanced pressure ulcers (19).

#### Goals of Local Care

After a thorough assessment of the ulcer and the patient, goals are established for the care of the wound. Setting goals for local ulcer care and consistently assessing for progress toward these goals allow new objectives to be set when goals have been met. If debridement is the goal, dressings that encourage debridement are no longer necessary once the necrotic tissue has been removed. In this way, the needs of the dynamic wound are being met constantly.

Topical treatment of wounds usually involves the goals of cleansing, debridement, reduction of bacteria, and pro-

tection. Each of these actions can be accomplished in a variety of ways, however, that in themselves can affect how well the wound heals (17). More than 2,000 wound-care dressings are currently available (21), which leads to much confusion as to when and what to use. To categorize the many products available, Table 3 lists commonly used products and their main overall function according to product inserts. Many of these products may have more than one function; the table lists their main purpose.

### Cleansing

#### Skin

Cleaning the skin involves the removal of wastes and drainage from around the wound. This goal can be accomplished easily by using skin cleansers that emulsify waste materials for ease of removal. Many of these also neutralize odors, which makes them excellent for use on the incontinent patient. Use of these skin cleansers facilitates the removal of surface debris without irritation to the epidermal layers. Some do not require rinsing, and others contain moisturizers that may interfere with adhesion of tapes or dressings. The manufacturer's directions should be followed for each specific product.

#### Wound

There are a number of ways to clean a wound. Absorption of drainage and debris along with preservation of a moist environment or flushing with fluid to remove debris are appropriate methods of wound cleansing.

#### Absorbents

Absorbents are used to absorb exudate and debris from the wound and surrounding tissue. In this way, they reduce drainage and sometimes surrounding tissue edema while cleansing the wound and preserving a moist environment. They vary in the manner in which absorption occurs and the amount of drainage they can absorb. Many absorbents are used to fill in dead space and maintain a moist interface with each wound surface.

#### Irrigants

These fluids are used as mechanical cleansers to clean surface debris. It is the force of the fluid that accomplishes the results rather than the composition of the fluid itself; therefore, irrigants should be chosen with care. Sometimes irrigation fluids are used to wet dressings for packing into wounds to eliminate dead space. Many of these fluids have been found to have some cytotoxic activity and thus may interfere with or delay wound healing

**TABLE 3.** *Wound care products by objective*

| Wound care objective | Product category | Product function | Outcome | Cautions | Example/Manufacturer |
|---|---|---|---|---|---|
| Cleansing: Skin | Liquid/foam skin cleansers | Emulsifies waste materials, neutralizes drainage and odors | Facilitates the removal of surface debris | Use AROUND wounds, not for use IN wounds | Perineal cleans. Foam-Carr. Sproam – Sween Inc. TripleCare – Smith 7 Nephew |
| Cleansing: Wound absorbents | Foam: hydrophilic/hydrophobic K0209–K0215 | Absorption of minimal to heavy adherent, softens necrotic tissue | Moist environment, decreased tissue trauma environment, soothes and protects | Affixed by external dressing to hold in place | Allevyn – Smith & Nephew Epi-Lock – Calgon Vestal Transorb – Brady Medical Vigilon – Bard |
| | Hydrogels: loose K0248–K0249 | Absorb min. – heavy exudate, soften necrotic tissue, non-adherent | Conforms to irregular surface, eliminate dead space, moist environ | Requires cover drsg., replace as needed to keep wound base moist. Not for use in dry wounds | Absorp.Drsg., – Bard Intrasite – Smith & Nephew Hypergel – Scott Wound Care |
| | Non-woven pad: Calcium alginate K0196–0199 | Absorbs heavy exudate, converts to gel for ease of removal. Non-adherent | Exudate absorption, moist environment, one-piece removal | Not for use in dry wounds | Algosteril – Johnson & Johnson Kaltostate – Calgon Vestal Sorbsan – Dow B. Hickam |
| | Powders, beads, granules K0261–K0227 | Applied to wound dry, absorb varying necrosis from wound and surrounding tissue | Cleanses wound, preserves moist environment | Not for dry wounds | Debrisan – Johns. & Johnson Duoderm Granules – ConvaTec |
| | Crystalline sodium Chloride dressing K0222–K0227 | Osmotic action "wicks" exudate, bacteria and necrosis from wound and surrounding tissue | Cleanses reduces edema, retards bacterial growth | Cover with dry dressing to absorb exudate. Not for dry wounds. | Mesalt–Scott Health Care |
| Irrigants | Irrigants: acetic acid, hydrogen peroxide, povidone iodine, Dakin's K0260 | Retard bacterial growth mechanical cleansing action | When used as irrigant, reduces surface debris | Many have been found to be harmful to healthy tissue. Flush wound with saline after irrigating with these products | |
| | Irrigants: Normal saline, sprays | Mechanical cleansing action – sometimes used to 'wet' dressings | Surface debris removal without wound irritation | Do not apply with excessive force | Dermal Wnd Cleanser–S&N Puri Clens–Sween Shur-Clens-Calgon Vestal |
| Debridement: Autolytic | Hydrocolloids K0234–K0241 | Occlusion traps exudate, facilitating WBCs to liquefy and phagocytize necrosis | Selective (specific) debridement, some absorption of exudate | Do not use on any wound suspected of being infected | Duoderm–ConvaTec/Squibb Restore–Hollister Replicare–Smith & Nephew Tegasorb–3M |
| | Hydrogels K0242–K0249 | Moisture helps soften eschar in dry, necrotic wounds | Rehydrates dead tissue for selective debridement | Held in place by external dressing, do not allow to dry out | Aquasorb–DeRoyal Indust. Hypergel–Scott Health Care Nu-gel–Johnson & Johnson SoloSite–Smith & Nephew |
| | MVP films K0257–K0259 | Acts as occlusive, also allows the exchange of gasses, vapors | Selective Debridement | Do not use on infected wounds | Bioclusive–Johnson & Johnson Opsite–Smith&Nephew/United Tegaderm–3M |
| Debridement: Chemical | Enzymes | Chemically digest debris and necrotic tissue | Selective (specific) Debridement | Crosshatch eschar, protect periwound Iodine renders some ineffective | Collagenase–Biozyme C Finbrinolysin–Elase Streptokinase–Varidase Sutilains/Travase–Flint |
| Debridement: Mechanical | Impregnated gauze: Crystalline sodium Chloride dressing | Creates hypertonic environment, "wicks" bacteria, softens necrotic tissue | Selective Debridement | Cover with dry dressings to absorb exudate | Mesalt–Scott Health Care |
| | Surgical | Dissection | Selectivet Debridement | Wound appears to increase in size | |
| | Wet-to-dry | Plain gauze traps wound debris | Non-selective Debridement | Not for patients with bleeding problems. | Nu-Brede–Johnson & Johnson |
| | Whirlpool Irrigations | Mechanical removal of debris, necrosis | Non-selective Debridement | Force rather than solution gives results | |

**TABLE 3.** *Continued*

| Wound care objective | Product category | Product function | Outcome | Cautions | Example/Manufacturer |
|---|---|---|---|---|---|
| Protection: SKIN | Creams, lotions ointments, sprays | Lubricates, softens, some form occlusive barrier | Rehydration and/or protection | Predominantly used on intact skin | Most. Barr. Oint.–Carrington<br>BAZA, Critic Aid–Sween<br>Triple Care–Smith & Nephew<br>Uni-salve–Smith & Nephew |
| | Skin sealants<br>K0250 | Forms layer of plastic polymer over the skin | Protection from corrosive drainage and friction of tape removal | May contain varying amounts of alcohol which "stings" denuded skin | Allkare–Convatec/Squibb<br>Incontinence Barrier Film–Bard<br>No Sting film–3M<br>Skin Gel–Hollister |
| | Gelatin/Pectin wafers | Forms protective impervious skin covering | Protection from corrosive drainage, tape friction | Replace as needed | Skin Prep–Smith & Nephew<br>Premium Barrier–Hollister<br>Stomahesive–ConvaTec/Squibb<br>Sween-A-Peel–Sween |
| | Hydrocolloids<br>K0234–K0239 | As gelatins | As gelatins, conforms to irregular areas | Replace as needed | DuoDerm–ConvaTec/Squibb<br>Replicare–Smith & Nephew<br>Restore–Hollister<br>Tegasorb–3M |
| Protection: Wound | MVP films<br>K0257–K0259 | Forms semi-occlusive seal over wound | Protection, moist wound base | Do not use on infected wounds | Bioclusive–Johnson & Johnson<br>Op-site–Smith & Nephew<br>Tegaderm–3M |
| | Foam dressings<br>K0209–K0215 | Forms semi-occlusive seal over wound, reportedly maintains wound temperature | Protection, moist wound base | Must be affixed by external dressing | Allevyn–Smith & Nephew<br>Epi-Lock–Calgon Vestal<br>Lyofoam–Acme United |
| | Gelatin/pectin wafers | Forms occlusive "seal", absorbs skin moisture prevents maceration | Protection, moist wound base | Do not use on infected wounds | Premium Barrier–Hollister<br>Stomahesive–ConvaTec\Squibb<br>Sween-A-Peel–Sween |
| | Hydrocolloids<br>K0234–K0241 | As gelatins, forms gel over wound bed to decrease removal trauma | Protection, moist wound base, less removal trauma | Do not use on infected wounds | DuoDerm–ConvaTec\Squibb<br>Replicare–Smith & Nephew<br>Restore–Hollister<br>Tegasorb–3M |
| | Ointments, gels, hydrogels | Provides protective, moist environment | Moist wound base | Reapply often to maintain moist environment | Biolex Wound Gel–Catalina<br>Carrington Dermal Wound Gel<br>Dermagram–Dermasciences |

271

(22). Irrigants that have been shown to be nontoxic are preferable, especially for the clean, noninfected wound.

### Hypertonic Dressing

The crystalline sodium-impregnated gauze dressing acts to "wick" exudate, bacteria, and necrotic tissue as it cleanses, reduces edema, and retards bacterial growth. This dressing should be used only on a very wet wound; otherwise, removal can involve mechanical debridement of the wound.

### Debridement

There are three main methods of debridement: autolytic, whereby the body's own fluid breaks down necrotic tissue; chemical, whereby chemicals containing enzymes erode the necrotic tissue; and mechanical, which involves a mechanical force to disrupt the necrotic tissue.

*Autolytic Debridement* Autolytic debridement is also known as self-debridement and includes the following:

1. Occlusive (moisture retentive) dressings: trap exudate, enabling white blood cells to liquefy and phagocytize necrotic tissue. This is selective (specific) debridement in that only necrotic tissue is affected.
2. Film or moisture vapor-permeable dressings: semiocclusive dressings in that they allow the exchange of gasses and vapors but trap exudate under the dressing.
3. Hydrogels/gels: aid in rehydration of necrotic tissue, enabling autolysis to occur. These must be kept moist and not allowed to dry out.

*Chemical Debridement* Enzymes chemically digest debris and necrotic tissue. Eschar must be cross-hatched to facilitate penetration of enzymes. Surrounding skin must be protected from moisture. Iodine renders some chemical debriders ineffective, as does a change in the pH of the wound. Some require a moist environment and multiple dressing changes. As with all dressings, the specific manufacturer's directions must be followed.

### Mechanical Debridement

1. Impregnated gauze: creates a hypertonic environment, which causes wound fluid to soften necrotic tissue. It must be used on wet wounds because it is ineffective on dry wounds.
2. Surgical: most effective selective dissection of necrotic tissue.
3. Wet to dry dressings: Plain gauze, as it dries, traps debris that is removed when dressing is removed. It is nonselective in that all tissue, both necrotic and viable, is removed with the dressing. Gauze with large interstices to trap debris should be used.
4. Whirlpool/Irrigation: the removal of necrosis and debris with fluid as the mechanical force.

In nonselective debridement, the force rather than the solution gives results.

## Protection

### Skin

1. Creams and lotions: lubricate and soften skin to promote rehydration.
2. Ointments: form an occlusive barrier over skin to protect from chemical irritation as in the presence of wound drainage or incontinence.
3. Skin sealants: form a layer of plastic polymer over the skin to protect it from friction of tape removal and irritating drainage. Some contain alcohol and will sting if applied to denuded skin. A new product contains no alcohol and can be applied to excoriated skin.
4. Gelatin/pectin or hydrocolloid wafers: forms seal over skin, excellent dressing to use under tapes.

### Wound

1. Moisture vapor-permeable dressings: semi-occlusive dressings that allow the exchange of gases and vapors; helpful for the protection of superficial wounds.
2. Gelatin/pectin wafers, hydrocolloid wafers (occlusive-moisture retentive dressings: seal off a wound to protect it from the outside world. No fluid or bacteria can penetrate the hydrocolloid dressings. In addition, they provide the wound with an optimal healing environment. Because fluid is formed over the wound bed, trauma from dressing removal is eliminated. These are quite useful with incontinent patients.
3. Ointments, gels: provide protective, moist environment for wounds, prevent desiccation.

Many of these treatments must be reapplied often to maintain moist environment. Always refer to the package inserts and follow manufacturer's directions to achieve optimal outcomes.

## SUMMARY

Pressure ulcers are a pervasive problem among elderly patients. When coupled with cancer and some of its treatments, risk of skin breakdown increases. A review of the literature reflected little information regarding pressure ulcers, specifically in the cancer patient; however, a small British study conducted in 1993 concluded that a protocol for risk assessment and the systematic use of pressure support systems greatly reduced the incidence of pressure sore development in patients in a hospice (23).

Another British hospice with a pressure ulcer prevalence of 43% began using a risk assessment scale, a wound assessment tool. and a wound care protocol. After 3 months, their prevalence rate was 28%. At 6 months and 1 year, that rate has held steady. Use of the pressure sore protocol has encouraged the hospice staff to reconsider wound healing in terminally ill patients. The more it is possible to prevent, heal, or halt deterioration of pressure sores, the more suffering is prevented (24). It would seem that assessment, preventative measures, along with consistent sensible wound care can make a difference to this patient population.

## REFERENCES

1. Meehan M. Multisite pressure ulcer prevalence survey. *Decubitus* 1990;3:14.
2. Langemo Dk, Olson B, Hunter S, Burd C, Hansen D, Cathcart-Silberberg T. Incidence of pressures sores in acute care, rehabilitation, extended care, home health, and hospice in one locale. *Decubitus* 1989;2:42.
3. Gallagher J. Management of cutaneous symptoms. *Seminars in Oncology Nurs* 1995;11:239
4. Goren D. Use of Omiderm in treatment of low-degree pressure sores in terminally ill cancer patients. *Cancer Nurs* 1989;12:165.
5. Panel for the Prediction and Prevention of Pressure Ulcers in Adults. *Pressure Ulcers in Adults: Prediction and Prevention.* Clinical Practice Guideline, No.3. AHCPR Publication No. 92-0047. Rockville MD: Agency for Health Care Policy and Research, Public Health Service, U.S. Department of Health and Human Services. May 1992.
6. National Pressure Ulcer Advisory Panel. Pressure ulcers prevalence, cost and risk assessment:consensus development conference statement. *Decubitus* 1989;2:24.
7. Krasner D. Pressure ulcers: an overview In: Krasner D. ed. *Chronic wound care: A clinical source book for healthcare professionals.* King of Prussia, PA: Health Management Publications; 1990:74.
8. Bryant RA, Shannon ML, Pieper B, Braden BJ, Morris DJ. Pressure Ulcers. In: Bryant RA, ed. *Acute and chronic wounds: nursing management.* St. Louis: Mosby; 1992:105.
9. Mullholland J. Protein metabolism and bed sores. *Ann Surg* 1943;118:1015.
10. Colburn L. Pressure ulcer prevention for the hospice patient. *Am J Hospice Care* 1987;4:22.
11. Allman R. Epidemiology of pressure ulcers in different populations. *Decubitus* 1989;2:30.
12. Low AW. Prevention of pressure sores in patients with cancer. *Oncol Nurs Forum* 1990;17:179.
13. Bergstrom N, Braden BJ, Laguzza A, Holman. The Braden Scale for predicting pressure sore risk. *Nurs Res* 1987;36:205.
14. Norton D. Calculating the risk: reflections on the Norton Scale. *Decubitus* 1989;2:24.
15. Doughty D. Principles of wound healing and wound management. In: Bryant R, ed. *Acute and chronic wounds: nursing management.* St. Louis: Mosby; 1992:31.
16. Doughty D. Topical therapy from concept to results. *Ostomy/Wound Management* 1992;38:16.
17. Granick MS, Solomon MP, Wind S, Goldberg MT. Wound management and wound care. *Adv Plast Surg* 1996;12:99
18. Waltham NL, Bergstrom N, Armstrong N, Norvell K, Braden B. Nutritional status, pressure sores and mortality in elderly patients with cancer. *Oncol Nurs Forum* 1991;18:867.
19. Bergstrom N, Bennett MA, Carlson CE, et al. *Treatment of pressure ulcers.* Clinical Practice Guideline, No. 15. Rockville, MD: U.S. Department of Health and Human Services. Public Health Service, Agency for Health Care Policy and Research. AHCPR Publication No. 95-0652. December 1994.
20. Makelbust J. Pressure ulcers What works. *RN* 1995;Sept:46.
21. Krasner D. Resolving the dressing dilemma:selecting wound dressings by category. *Ostomy/Wound Mangement* 1991;35:62.
22. Doughty D. A rational approach to the use of topical antiseptics. *Journal of Wound Ostomy Continence Nurses Society* 1994;21:224.
23. Bale S, Finlay I, Harding KG. Pressure sore prevention in a hospice. *J Wound Care* 1995;4:465.
24. Walding M. Skin treatment. *Nursing Times* 1994;90:78.

*Principles and Practice of Supportive Oncology,*
edited by Ann Berger et al.
Lippincott–Raven Publishers, Philadelphia ©1998

CHAPTER 21

# Lymphedema

Margaret L. Farncombe

*Lymphedema* is the subcutaneous accumulation of protein-rich fluid caused by damaged or blocked lymphatic vessels. Although lymphedema can be congenital (*primary*) or acquired (*secondary*), only lymphedema secondary to malignant disease is discussed in this text.

Although acquired lymphedema frequently causes patients with progressive cancer (and often also those who have received curative treatment) prolonged and distressing morbidity, the condition is considered benign and not life threatening. Accordingly, lymphedema remains poorly researched and understood, and its true occurrence is probably underdiagnosed. No clearly defined, universally accepted and used diagnostic guidelines have been developed, and, as a consequence, its treatment is often ignored. All too often, comments such as "You will have to live with it" or "There is nothing we can do to help" are the conclusions presented to patients. In other cases, well-intentioned, but inappropriate, treatment may be initiated.

Based on the studies available to date, it is clear that the incidence and prevalence of lymphedema secondary to all types of malignancies make it a common condition and one that instills significant morbidity in patients as well as having far-reaching implications in our health care systems.

## PATHOPHYSIOLOGY

The lymph vascular system's function is to clear the interstitial spaces of macromolecules (proteins too large to reenter the blood vessels directly) and the water that acts as their carrier from the tissues and transport them back to the intravascular circulation (1) (Fig. 21-1). Nor-

mally, this process relies almost entirely on local tissue movement to induce the lymph flow. The flow is therefore a passive process that is dependent on changes in local hydrostatic and osmotic pressures.

Although pure lymphedema remains poorly understood and clinically difficult to induce, it is generally accepted that it occurs when lymphatic production exceeds the lymphatic transport capacity. In most patients with lymphedema secondary to malignant disease or due to treatment of the disease, an obstruction of lymph drainage occurs, resulting in a gradual buildup of the macromolecule proteins within the tissues. The resultant failure of the lymph vascular system to maintain an adequate drainage capability, in combination with an inadequate scavenging of stagnating plasma proteins by macrophages, results in progressive chronic lymphedema.

Chronic edema rarely, however, arises from the failure of one system alone (2). Damage to the vascular system as a result of surgery, radiotherapy, or progression of the disease also frequently causes damage to other vessels. Edema is therefore often secondary to blocked lymphatics plus venous stasis. Recent studies suggested that the pathophysiology of edema in postmastectomy patients also may involve several additional mechanisms, including a possible rise in capillary blood pressure which, in turn, may cause an increase in net capillary filtration, placing an increased load on already damaged lymphatics (3).

## PATIENTS AT RISK

Patients most at risk of developing secondary lymphedema are (4):

1. Breast cancer patients who have had surgery involving nodal dissection. There is an added risk if such patients have undergone postoperative radiotherapy.
2. Patients with malignant melanoma of the arms or legs with nodal dissection or radiotherapy.

M. L. Farncombe: Palliative Care, Queensway-Carleton, Nepean, Ontario, K2G, 1W1 Canada.

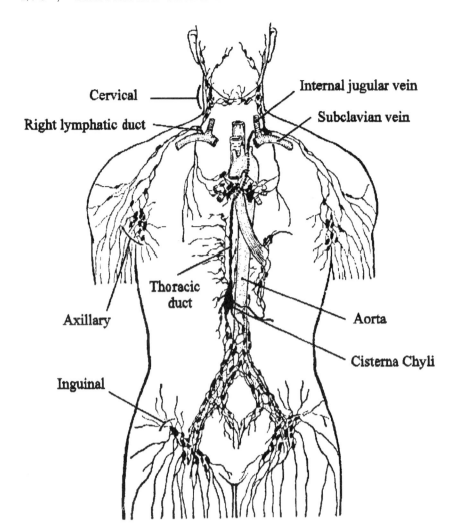

**FIG. 1.** The lymphatic system.

3. Prostate cancer patients who have had surgery or whole pelvic radiation.
4. Patients with gynecologic cancers with advanced disease, surgical procedures, or radiotherapy.
5. Patients with advanced testicular cancer.
6. Patients suffering advanced neoplastic disease in which the metastatic spread is found in the lower quadrants of the abdomen thus impeding venous and lymphatic drainage.

Other factors, such as poor nutritional status and obesity, should be monitored as they may lead to delayed wound healing, which in turn is an important risk factor for the development of lymphedema. Other concomitant diseases, such as diabetes, renal failure, and cardiac disease, also aggravate edema of a limb (5).

## INCIDENCE

The overall incidence of lymphedema is difficult to determine. First, little recent research has been published on its incidence and prevalence. What data do exist tend to be variable and can be misleading because the diagnostic criteria has not yet been standardized, the type and extent of surgery is variable, and the length of the studies undertaken is frequently too short to include patients with late-onset lymphedema.

For most patients, no investigations are currently performed routinely to determine whether the edema is entirely secondary to lymphatic obstruction or also involves damage to other vascular structures. In addition, statistics reported in specific studies tend to refer to lymphedema from one particular malignancy alone, the most widely studied and reported being breast cancer.

Breast cancer is currently the most prevalent malignancy in women in the United States. It is projected that it will affect one in nine women during their lifetime. Surgical and medical therapies based on mastectomy and radiotherapy are increasingly extending patient life spans, but these procedures also may place patients at high risk of developing lymphedema (6). Primarily because of the nonstandard reporting criteria outlined earlier, the available literature suggests that the overall incidence of lymphedema in patients with breast cancer who have had surgical intervention with or without radiotherapy is between 6.7 and 62.5% (7–9). The research, however, does agree that axillary node clearance and postoperative radiotherapy do increase the risk for developing lymphedema, with radiotherapy cited as the most important risk factor (10,11).

Although the reasons for performing either axillary or groin nodal dissections during surgery may have changed from being solely therapeutic to also being important for its staging and diagnostic potential, it still causes profound disability by increasing the risk of lymphedema (12). Early detection and longer survival also have increased the incidence and length of time patients experience this complication.

## STAGES OF LYMPHEDEMA

Edema is generally not detectable clinically until interstitial volume reaches 30% above normal. Symptoms have been reported to occur within days to years of diagnosis and treatment of malignant disease.

Lymphedema frequently occurs in three stages: acute, chronic, and late. During the early stage, edema is pitting and will decrease with elevation of the limb. As the condition progresses untreated, the edema becomes firm and nonpitting, this change being secondary to chronic inflammation, fibrosis, and sclerosis caused by stagnation of the plasma proteins. The late stage results from the overproduction of connective tissue, resulting in hardening of the skin, and the condition is sometimes commonly referred to as *lymphostatic elephantiasis*.

Lymphedema is often graded using the following scale (13):

1. Edema that is barely detectable.
2. A slight indentation is visible when the skin is depressed.
3. A deeper fingerprint returns to normal in 5 to 30 seconds.
4. Edema is the maximal grade; the affected extremity may be 1.5 to 2.0 times its normal size.

This scale has limitations, however, and can be used only during the early stages or when edema is pitting.

## INVESTIGATIONS

Lymphography and lymphangiography previously were considered the "gold standards" for demonstrating lymphatic abnormalities. These techniques are, however, invasive and difficult to perform in the presence of edema. They also are limited in providing information on anatomic detail and frequently visualize only the large subcutaneous collecting lymphatics (14).

Quantitative lymphoscintigraphy (isotope lymphography) (15,16) has been more useful in detecting lymphatic

insufficiency because the dynamics of flow and rate of transit via lymphatic vessels are studied using a gamma camera. It is also a more comfortable procedure for the patient because it is administered by a interstitial injection instead of direct cannulation of peripheral lymphatics.

Magnetic resonance imaging (MRI) also is used sometimes to view soft tissues and lymphatics and is even less invasive. Color Doppler (17) has been used to define or rule out venous abnormalities and can be useful in patients for whom more invasive tests are contraindicated or inappropriate.

In general, for determining the management of lymphedema symptoms, invasive investigations are frequently not necessary in patients with acquired lymphedema secondary to cancer. They may, however, be helpful in determining the management required for patients who do not respond to conservative treatment or in whom a mixed etiology of limb edema is suspected.

## CLINICAL ASSESSMENT

A full clinical assessment for lymphedema (Table 21-1) should address the history of the primary disease, including previous surgery, any nodal dissection, and radiotherapy. It also should include a full history of the duration of the edema, symptoms, complications, and past treatments. The physical examination must include measurements of the affected limb and the contralateral normal limb for comparison. An assessment of motor and sensory function is imperative, and pulses should be checked.

Although pain and other discomforts are common complaints, patients are often even more concerned about the "heaviness" and loss of function in the limb. Many describe the limb as "ugly" and find it impossible to wear their own clothing because of the physical size of the affected limb.

A functional history with specific questions concerning activities of daily living, difficulty with clothing, and other possible limitations secondary to the edema are essential. The patient's sense of self or self-esteem and any

**TABLE 1.** *Clincial assessment.*

| History |
| --- |
|    Primary disease, (including surgery, nodal disection and radiotherapy) |
|    Lymphedema (duration, symptoms, complications, treatment) |
| Functional & social history |
| Changes in activities of daily living, depression, self-esteem |
| Physical examination |
|    Inspection |
|    Pulses |
|    Motor funciton |
|    Sensory function |
|    Measurement of affected and normal limbs |

possible signs and symptoms of depression need to be assessed. Patients frequently feel they have lost their independence and freedom because of both the difficulty experienced in managing the activities of daily living with the often "useless, heavy arm or leg" and the embarrassment of going out and meeting people with "this deformity." For all these reasons, the patient's quality of life is often severely compromised and should be considered to constitute an integral part of the treatment process.

## MONITORING

The size of the limb should be measured before treatment is begun and then at regular intervals during management to permit detailed monitoring of the patient's progress. Several methods of measurement have been used in the past (18). In some centers, the arms are measured at only one location and compared with previous measurements, with a difference of 2.5 cm indicating moderate lymphedema. Other centers use the same basic method but take measurements at two or three levels and compare the results. These methods tend to be unreliable because of the variability of the shape of the limb from point to point and because of differences in shape before and after treatment. Other practitioners advocate submersion of the limb in water and measuring the volume of the displaced liquid. This method, although considered the most accurate, is a complicated and often messy procedure that makes it impractical for home use.

An accurate and more practical method of assessing volume of the limb is shown in Fig. 21-2, which demonstrates measurements for the upper limb. The circumference of the arm is taken at 2-cm intervals using a tape measure with weights at either end, which are allowed to hang freely. Assessment bias can occur if the examiner adjusts the tension on the tape. An adapted formula for the

# LYMPHEDEMA
# UPPER EXTREMITY MEASUREMENT

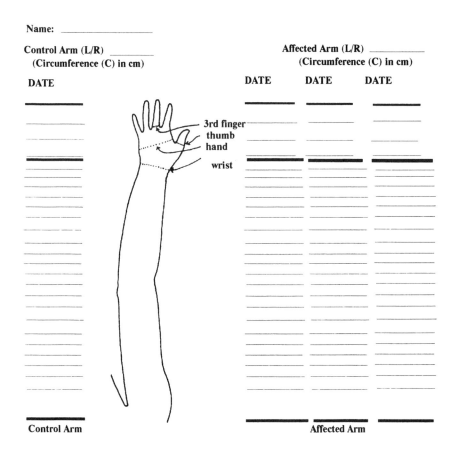

NOTE: Vol = sum of arm circumference measurements from wrist to upper arm value,

each squared and multiplied by 0.159 ie, where Volume for each 2 cm segment

measured = 3.1416 x r squared x h (2 cm)

= c squared x 0.159

**FIG. 2.** Technique for measurement of upper extremity lymphedema.

**TABLE 2.** *Guidelines for limb volume measurements*

At each measuring occasion
  Position the limb at the same height
  Remark the limb
  Record the starting point accurately
  Ensure that tension is not applied to the tape measure
  Ensure that the tape measure is straight
  Use the same number of measurement

volume of a cylinder is used to determine the volume of the arm from wrist to axilla. This methodology is more precise than using only a few comparative points and allows more accurate and detailed comparisons with the other arm and with the same arm over time. It is also much easier and less cumbersome than submersion in water and can be undertaken readily in the patient's home. It does not, however, provide for the volume of the hand, which must be determined and compared separately.

Perhaps more important than the particular method used is the need for consistency in the technique used (Table 21-2) (19). A decrease in limb size indicates that treatment is beneficial and should be maintained; more importantly, such a result also tends to encourage patient compliance because a measurable improvement can be seen readily; this is particularly important at times when visual changes are not obvious. Volumetric measurements provide a quantitative result and are extremely valuable for determining and following the treatment progress.

Several other methods of assessing and monitoring lymphedema are currently being investigated. Studies to assess the elasticity and the viscosity of skin by using a technique involving vertical extensibility by suction may prove useful in assessing functional difficulties in relation to skin infiltration and may be useful in follow-up (20). Subcutaneous interstitial fluid pressure and arm volume also can be measured by the wick-in-needle method (21). Multifrequency bioelectrical impedance analysis may offer a means to an earlier diagnosis and more accurate monitoring of extracelluar fluid changes during and after treatment (22). It is unclear at this time whether any of these techniques will offer any information beyond that provided by a good clinical assessment.

## PREVENTION

Ideally, patients should be assessed preoperatively and taught the appropriate exercises to squeeze soft tissue and encourage proximal lymph flow. These exercises then would be continued postoperatively (23). Patients also should learn to recognize early warning signs, such as tightness, aching, and pain or other sensory changes in the limb. Any signs of infection or cellulitis should be reported and managed appropriately, and delayed wound healing should be regarded as a risk factor for the development of lymphedema.

## TREATMENT

Although the full pathophysiology of lymphedema is still poorly understood, the edema experienced in a limb, whether secondary to the primary diagnosis or resulting from treatment for the disease, such as surgery and radiotherapy, is probably multifactorial with damage, not only to lymphatics but also to the venous circulation system and other tissues as well. For this reason, treatment also must be variable. Lymphedema, however, is a chronic condition, and treatment, therefore, must also be chronic. To be effective and to encourage patient compliance, treatment must be consistent, clearly understood, and convenient.

Management of lymphedema is extremely variable in the medical profession, ranging from aggressive diagnostic procedures to precipitous operations. Scattered between these two extremes are quite a number of various conservative methods (5). Although treatment for lymphedema is usually the same for patients with or without active malignant disease, it is generally perceived that this treatment is more effective if there is no active disease present.

As early as 1855, in the German literature, surgeons Esmarch and Kulenkampff (24) described a treatment modality consisting of hygienic measures, elevation, and compression. Later in 1892, Winiwarter (25), also a surgeon, advocated a similar conservative approach as the first choice of treatment. Excellent results were reported at that time and, with minor alterations, this same treatment plan can still be very effective today. It must be remembered at all times that the single most important factor in management of lymphedema is patient compliance (26).

Treatment is most effective when a multidisciplinary approach involving physicians, nurses, physiotherapists, and occupational therapists is followed. As patient cooperation and compliance is of such great importance in the success or failure of what is often a lengthy course of treatment, an assessment by and continued consultation with a psychiatrist or psychologist is often also valuable in identifying problems and providing appropriate intervention related to the patient's overall psychological adjustment (27). Treatment consists of several basic but important elements (Table 21-3), which should be used in combination for maximum results (28,29).

**TABLE 3.** *Basic treatment for lymphedema*

Education
Massage
Skin care
Containment hosiery
Exercise

## Education

Patients must be aware from the onset that treatment probably will be required for the rest of their lives. It is important for patients to begin management as early as possible and to be consistent and dedicated. To enlist their active cooperation and compliance, they also, however, need to be told about the predicted good results anticipated with treatment (Figs. 21-3 and 21-4). Education includes a thorough discussion about the "do's" and "do not's" of caring for the lymphedematous limb (6). Patients should be instructed to observe skin carefully each day and to report any skin breakdown, weeping, or reddened areas to their doctor immediately. They should not carry heavy objects with the affected arm, avoid having blood pressure or venipuncture in that limb, and avoid excess heat and exposure to detergents and other harmful irritants by wearing gloves while doing housework and gardening.

## Massage

As lymphatics rely almost exclusively on local tissue movement for lymph flow, massage is an important aspect of treatment. Massage is recommended once or twice daily, preferably using a vibrating massager applied directly to the unbandaged limb. Skin-surface massage enhances the movement of lymph through superficial lymphatics in the skin and through the subcutaneous tissue to normal drainage areas. Skin should be free of any lotions when using a battery-operated massager.

The first goal of this treatment is to increase lymphatic activity in the normal lymph vessels. Therefore, gentle pressure is applied to each of the dermal lymphotomes to direct lymph flow to the nonobstructed lymph node area (30). First, this pressure is applied to the contralateral quadrant of the trunk to encourage drainage across the watershed areas and then is continued in the affected

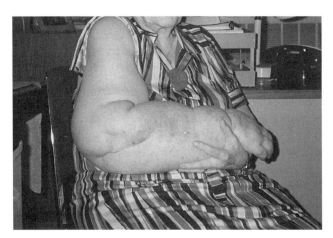

**FIG. 3.** Patient with upper extremity lymphedema prior to treatment.

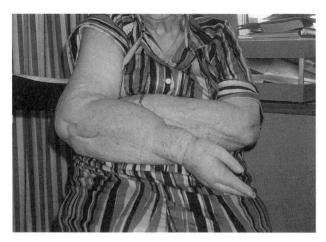

**FIG. 4.** Decrease in lymphedema 1 month after treatment initiated.

limb. The massage is done in segments beginning with the trunk, the upper arm or leg, the forearm or lower leg, and finishing with the hand or foot. Each segment is worked anteriorly and posteriorly, moving from distally to proximally for each segment. Only a gentle pressure is exerted to prevent damage to skin and other tissues. To ensure good results, it is important to teach the patient and a caregiver how to do the massage, including massage of the posterior trunk.

It is imperative that manual lymph drainage (massage) be performed by a qualified physiotherapist or other health care professional with expertise and experience in this treatment modality. In time, patients (and families) can be taught to continue this treatment at home (31).

## Skin Care

Skin care consists of moisturizing the affected limb daily with a water-soluble lotion that is free of perfumes or other irritating additives (26). Skin care is best done after the morning bath and massage. At the same time, routine checking for skin breakdown is advisable. It is important to ensure that the patient visually inspects the limb for any skin changes because sensation in the limb may be impaired and cellulitis or an abrasion, therefore, may not be felt.

## Containment Hosiery

After massage and skin care routines are completed, the affected limb can be bandaged or a compression sleeve or stocking applied. If the limb is large, if it has long-standing nonpitting edema, or if the hand or foot is badly involved, a sleeve or stocking may not be manageable and bandaging may be necessary (2,14). Bandaging must be done by an experienced person who has been appropriately trained. A padding of soft gauze first must be applied to protect the skin, and the limb then is wrapped with an elastic self-adhesive bandaging material, beginning with the fingers or toes and working proximally. Firm pressure must be exerted distally, decreasing the pressure gradually while moving up the arm or leg; this is done to encourage movement of the protein-rich fluid proximally.

If the limb is small enough to fit comfortably into a sleeve or stocking, and if the fingers or toes are not severely affected, a compression sleeve or stocking may be used (32,33); this method is the preferred management because bandaging is costly and time consuming and usually less comfortable for the patient. Sleeves or stockings cover the limb but leave the digits exposed, allowing the patient more freedom in activities of daily living. Sleeves or stockings should be snug but comfortable. If they are too tight, digits will become more edematous, and compliance is likely to be poor. A soft gauze padding should be used at the joints to prevent bunching in these areas, which otherwise could result in constriction. Compression garments may be worn throughout the daytime only or for 24 hours a day except for times of skin care and massage according to the patient's wishes. Some patients are more comfortable wearing the sleeve or stocking and therefore prefer to use it continuously.

## Exercise

The affected limb should be elevated whenever possible and certainly at night if the sleeve is removed. The limb should be exercised when the compression garment or bandaging is worn because these appliances serve to promote improved circulation and fluid return proximally (5). If the edema is mild to moderate and the patient has use of the limb, the usual daily activities may be sufficient exercise. If not, formal exercises within the patient's abilities and range of comfort need to be taught.

## Intermittent Sequential Pneumatic Compression Pumps

These pumps have been used extensively in the treatment of lymphedema, and some reported results have been encouraging, especially over the short term (34); however, for prolonged effects, patients in the studies still wore compression sleeves between sessions with the pump, and it is unclear whether the combination of pump and sleeve or stocking is any better over the long term than the compression garment alone. A study to evaluate the effects of pneumatic massage with uniform pressure, pneumatic massage with differentiated pressure, and manual lymphatic massage showed no difference between uniform-pressure pneumatic massage and man-

ual massage, and both were better than differentiated pneumatic massage. Again, all patients wore compression garments between treatments (35).

Pneumatic pumps necessitate prolonged periods in clinic for treatment or considerable expense to the patient who is buying a pump for home use. Treatment becomes less accessible, more time consuming, and less convenient, all of which affects long-term patient compliance. Pumps may have a more beneficial effect in the early treatment of severe edema to soften the limb, which then would have less negative effects on long-term compliance because most of the treatment still could be done at home with little expense for the patient.

If the pump is used, a compression garment must be applied afterward to prevent recurrence of edema, and care must be taken to ensure that the garment is not too tight if edema recurs. Pumps should never be used in patients with edema involving the trunk.

## Other Treatment Modalities

A variety of other treatments deserve mention:

### Antibiotics

Antibiotics should be used early at any sign of cellulitis. Usually, oral penicillin or erythromycin is sufficient. When weeping edema is present, or for patients experiencing recurrent attacks of cellulitis, antibiotics may be required for a prolonged period (2).

### Steroids

Steroids are often useful when edema is assessed to be secondary to obstruction by tumor or enlarged lymph nodes (2). If there are no contraindications to the use of steroids, a trial of dexamethasone is recommended.

### Diuretics

Diuretics act primarily by limiting capillary filtration and reducing circulating blood volume. They, therefore, may be of benefit in treating limb edema if the swelling is of a mixed origin; however, the function of the lymphatics is to remove protein and other macromolecules from the tissues. With the use of diuretics, fluid can be absorbed back into the vascular compartment, but proteins can return only via lymphatics, or they can be broken down by phagocytosis. Diuretics therefore offer little improvement in true lymphedema and, in fact, may cause complications by mobilizing fluid from everywhere except the lymphedematous limb, resulting in hypotension and electrolyte disturbances (2).

### Benzopyrones

Coumarin, a 5,6-benzo(alpha) pyrone, has been used in Australia to treat lymphedema (36). It is available only in a few centers in North America. It reportedly has provided a therapeutic effect by stimulating macrophages to scavenge plasma proteins. The reduction in lymphedema is reportedly much slower than with decongestive therapy. It would seem reasonable that if coumarin is used, it should be in conjunction with physiotherapy to ensure treatment of both aspects of lymphedema: the decreased lymph flow and the abundance of proteins in the fluid.

Benzopyrones also may cause increased protein catabolism as a result of the continuous degradation of protein molecules. It is unclear at this time whether this could result in troublesome side effects in patients with an inadequate protein intake in their diet.

### Diet

Diet, as a factor in the treatment of lymphedema, has not been widely studied. Two patients with idiopathic unilateral limb lymphedema responded to a diet with restriction of long-chain triglycerides (37). More research is needed to assess any possible benefit of this treatment on patients with lymphedema secondary to malignant disease.

### Surgery

Surgical treatment of chronic limb lymphedema is either *physiologic* (an attempt to improve lymphatic drainage) or *excisional* (removal of edematous subcutaneous tissue with or without overlying skin) (38,39). This intervention is seldom appropriate in patients with malignant disease.

### Intra-arterial Infusion of Autologous Lymphocytes

This still experimental treatment was used recently in a few patients with refractory primary or acquired lymphedema with promising results, including a reduction in size, a decrease in pain, and softening of the limb (40,41).

## COMPLICATIONS

Once treatment for lymphedema is initiated, compliance is of major importance. Factors that can negatively affect compliance include the amount of delay before starting treatment, the size of the limb when treatment is started, the availability of social and financial supports, and the presence of complicating health problems (42).

Untreated lymphedema leads to worsening of the symptoms of fullness, numbness, paraesthesia, weakness, and pain. All too often the weight of the heavy arm in patients with upper-extremity edema can cause shoulder dislocation and further pain and loss of function. Lymphedema also plays an active role in the development of brachial plexus entrapment and carpal tunnel syndrome in patients who have previously had a mastectomy and radiotherapy (43). Recurrent cellulitis or erysipelas also occur more frequently in a lymphadematous limb and can, in turn, lead to further worsening of the edema (44). A more serious but rarer complication is lymphangiosarcoma, which is associated with lymphedema in patients with a previous diagnosis of breast cancer and subsequent radiotherapy treatment. The prognosis for these patients is poor, with metastases to lung, pleura, and chest wall occurring early in the course of the disease.

## CONCLUSION

Lymphedema is not only a prevalent symptom in patients with cancer, but one that causes considerable morbidity and greatly affects the patient's quality of life. It can occur secondary to the disease and subsequent treatment, in particular, surgery including nodal dissection and radiotherapy. Unfortunately, it can appear initially even years after the primary disease diagnosis and also can affect those in whom a cure or remission is achieved.

The treatment of acquired (*secondary*) lymphedema must be chronic and consist of several modalities. Also, however, it must be relatively easy, convenient, inexpensive, and visibly effective to encourage patient compliance over the long term.

## REFERENCES

1. Browse NL, Stewart G. Lymphoedema: pathophysiology and classification. *Cardiovasc Surg* 1985;26:93.
2. Mortimer PS, Badger C, Hall JG. Lymphoedema: *Symptom Management* 4.7:407–415.
3. Bates DO, Levick JR, Mortimer PS. Starling pressures in the human arm and their alteration in postmastectomy oedema. *J Physiol* 1994; 477:355.
4. PDQ supportive care/screening information–lymphedema. *Cancer Fax from the National Cancer Institute* 208/00442. Current as of 09/01/93: 1.
5. Foldi E, Foldi M, Weissleder H. Conservative treatment of lymphoedema of the limbs. *Angiology* 1985;Mar 85:175.
6. Brennan M. Lymphedema following the surgical treatment of breast cancer: a review of pathophysiology and treatment. *J Pain Sympt Manag* 1992;7:110.
7. Markby R, Baldwin E, Kerr P. Incidence of lymphoedema on women with breast cancer. *Professional Nurse* 1991;June 91:502.
8. Kissin MW, Querci della Rovere G, Easton D, Westbury G. Risk of lymphedema following the treatment of breast cancer. *Br J Surg* 1986; 73:580.
9. Hoe AL, Iven D, Ritke GT, Taylor I. Incidence of arm swelling following axillary clearance for breast cancer. *Br J Surg* 1992;79:261.
10. Ryttov N, Holm NV, Qvist N, Blichert-Toft M. Influence of adjuvant irradiation on the development of late arm lymphedema and impaired shoulder mobility after mastectomy for carcinoma of the breast. *Acta Oncol* 1988;27:667
11. Swedborg I, Wallgren A. The effects of pre- and postmastectomy radiotherapy on the degree of edema, shoulder-joint mobility, and gripping force. *Cancer* 1981;47:877–81.

12. Robinson DS, Senofsky GM, Ketcham AS. Role and extent of lymphedenectomy for early breast cancer. *Semin Surg Oncol* 1992;8:78–82.
13. Thiadens S. Eighteen steps to prevention. *National Lymphedema Network*, January 1993:1.
14. Mortimer PS. Investigation and management of lymphoedema. *Vascular Med Rev* 1990;1:1–20.
15. Proby CM, Gane JN, Joseph AEA, Mortimer PS. Investigation of the swollen limb with isotope lymphography. *Br J Dermatol* 1990;123:29–37.
16. Weissleder H, Weissleder R. Lymphedema: evaluation of qualitative and quantitative lymphoscintigraphy in 238 patients. *Radiology* 1988;167:729.
17. Svensson WE, Mortimer PS, Tohno E, Cosgrove DO, Badger C, Al Murrani B. The use of colour Doppler to define venous abnormalities in the swollen arm following therapy for breast carcinoma. *Clin Radiol* 1991;44:249.
18. Badger C. Guidelines for the Calculation of Limb Volume Based on Surface Measurements. *British Lymphology Interest Group Newsletter* Issue 7:1993.
19. Woods M. An audit of swollen limb measurements. *Nursing Standard* 1994;9:24–26.
20. Auriol F, Vaillant L, Pelucio-Lopes C, Machet L, Diridollou S, Berson M. Lorette G. Study of cutaneous extensibility in lymphoedema of the lower limbs. *Br J Dermatol* 1994;131:265.
21. Bates DO, Levick JR, Mortimer PS. Subcutaneous interstitial fluid pressure and arm volume in lymphoedema. *Int J Microcirc Clin Exp* 1992;11:359.
22. Ward LC, Bunce IH, Cornish BH, Mirolo BR, Thomas BJ, Jones LC. Multi-frequency bioelectrical impedance augments the diagnosis and management of lymphoedema in post-mastectomy patients. *Eur J Clin Invest* 1992;22:751.
23. Markowski J, Wilcox JP, Helm PA. Lymphedema incidence after specific postmastectomy therapy. *Arch Phys Med Rehabil* 1981;62:450.
24. Esmarch F, Kulenkampff D. *Elephantiastischen formen.* Hamburg: JF Richter, 1885.
25. Winiwarter A. *Die Chirurgischen Krankheiten der Haut und des Zellgewebes*, Stuttgart: Enke, 1982.
26. Rose KE, Taylor HM, Twycross RG. Long-term compliance with treatment in obstructive arm lymphoedema in cancer. *Palliat Med* 1991:52.
27. Passik S, Newman M, Brennan M, Holland J. Psychiatric consultation for women undergoing rehabilitation for upper-extremity lymphedema following breast cancer treatment. *J Pain Sympt Manag* 1992;8:226.
28. Bunce IH, Mirolo BR, Hennessy JM, Ward LC, Jones LC. Post-mastectomy lymphoedema treatment and measurement. *Med J Aust* 1994;161:125.
29. Farncombe ML, Daniels G, Cross L. Lymphedema: the seemingly forgotten complication. *J Pain Sympt Manag* 1994;9:269.
30. Boris M, Weindorf S, Lasinski PT, Boris G. Lymphedema reduction by noninvasive complex lymphedema therapy. *Oncology* 1994;Sept 94.
31. Földi M, Ed. Treatment of lymphedema [Editorial]. *Lymphology* 1994;27:1.
32. Swedborg I. Effects of treatment with an elastic sleeve and intermittent pneumatic compression in post-mastectomy patients with lymphoedema of the arm. *Scand J Rehabil Med* 1984;16:35–41.
33. Zeissler RH, Rose GB, Nelson PA. Postmastectomy lymphedema: late results of treatment in 385 patients. *Arch Phys Med Rehabil* 1972;Apr 72:162.
34. Richmand DM, O'Donnell TF, Zelikovski A. Sequential pneumatic compression for lymphedema. *Arch Surg* 1985;120:1118.
35. Zanolla R, Monzeglio C, Balzarini A, Martino G. Evaluation of the result of three different methods of postmastectomy lymphedema treatment. *J Surg Oncol* 1984;26:210–213.
36. Casley-Smith JR, Morgan RG, Piller NB. Treatment of lymphedema of the arms and legs with 5,6-benzo-[α]-pyrone. *N Engl J Med* 1993;329:1158.
37. Soria P, Cuesta A, Romero H, Martínez FJ, Sastre A. Dietary treatment of lymphedema by restriction of long-chain triglycerides. *Angiology* 1994;45:703.
38. Mavili ME, Naldoken S, Safak T. Modified Charles operation for primary fibrosclerotic lymphedema. *Lymphology* 1994;27:14.
39. Filippeti M, Santoro E, Graziano F, Petric M. Rinaldi G. Modern therapeutic approaches to postmastectomy brachial lymphedema. *Microsurgery* 1994;15:604.
40. Nagata Y, Murata M, Mitsumori M, Okajima K, Ishigaki T, Ohya N, Fujiwara K, Abe M, Kumada K. Intraarterial infusion of autologous lymphocytes for the treatment of refractory lymphoedema. *Eur J Surg* 1994;160:105.
41. Harada M, Amano Y, Matsuzaki K, Hayashi Y, Nishitani H, Yoshizumi O, Yoshida O, Katoh I. Quantitative evaluation of intraarterial lymphocyte injection therapy for lymph edema using MR imaging. *Acta Radiol* 1994;35:405.
42. Dennis B. Acquired lymphedema: a chart review of nine woman's responses to intervention. *Am J Occup Ther* 1993;47:892.
43. Ganel A, Engel J, Sela M, Brooks M. Nerve entrapments associated with postmastectomy lymphedema. *Cancer* 1979;44:2254.
44. Simon MS, Cody RL. Cellulitis after axillary lymph node dissection for carcinoma of the breast. *Am J Med* 1992;93:543.

*Principles and Practice of Supportive Oncology,*
edited by Ann Berger et al.
Lippincott–Raven Publishers, Philadelphia ©1998

CHAPTER **22**

# Principles of Fistula and Stoma Management

Dorothy Doughty

A significant number of patients with solid tumors involving the abdominal organs will have surgically created stomas or spontaneously occurring fistulas; palliative care for these patients must provide effective containment of the effluent and odor, protection of the peristomal skin, and maintenance of fecal and urinary elimination. This chapter addresses the specific needs of patients with stomas or fistulas involving the intestinal or urinary tracts.

## FISTULA MANAGEMENT

Solid tumors may extend into the bowel or bladder from adjacent organs or may spread from the bowel or bladder to create fistulous openings to the skin, the vagina, or other organs (1–3). Fistulas also may occur as a result of anastomotic breakdown following surgical procedures on the bowel or as a complication of radiation therapy (1,2).

### Classification Systems

Fistulas are commonly classified according to the organs involved, point of drainage, or volume of output (4–7). Fistulas are named according to the organs involved and the pathway followed by the effluent (e.g., enterocutaneous or vesicovaginal). Fistulas also may be classified as internal or external (8). Internal fistulas are abnormal communications between two internal organs (e.g., enteroenteric or enterocolic fistulas); these fistulas may be silent in that they produce no obvious pathology, but they can greatly affect the patient's nutritional status by bypassing absorptive segments of small bowel (3). External fistulas are those communicating with the skin or with organs that drain onto the skin, such as the

vagina; these fistulas produce obvious symptoms and present major challenges in management (3,8). The third mechanism for classifying fistulas is by volume of output; fistulas producing more than 500 ml of output per day have been labeled *high-output fistulas*, and those producing 200 to 500 ml/day are generally classified as *low-* or *moderate-output fistulas* (3–7).

### Fistula Management

Initial interventions for the patient with a fistula involving the intestinal tract include fluid and electrolyte stabilization and infection control (1,4,5,7,9). Specific fluid and electrolyte needs depend on the type and volume of fistula output (5); for example, small bowel fistulas usually produce high volumes of effluent containing significant amounts of sodium, potassium, and bicarbonate (2,5,6). The patient with a high-output fistula requires close monitoring of fluid-electrolyte balance with replacement titrated in response to type and volume of output and laboratory indices (2,5,7). Initial intervention also involves careful evaluation for any intraabdominal infectious process; abscesses are drained via open exploration and irrigation or percutaneous catheter placement (2,5,6).

### *Definitive Management*

Fistula management is typically directed toward fistula closure, either through medical management promoting spontaneous closure or through surgical resection or bypass of the fistulous tract (1,4). Usually, conservative medical management is tried first, assuming there is no intraabdominal infection and that the distal bowel is patent. This approach is based on studies indicating that, in the absence of distal obstruction, about 50% of fistulas will close spontaneously within 4 to 6 weeks and on the fact that surgical closure is frequently ineffective until the underlying factors contributing to fistula development

---

D. Doughty: Wound Ostomy Continence, Nursing Education Program, Emory University, Atlanta, GA 30322.

have been corrected (1,2,4,5,7). The two major principles on which conservative management is based are (a) provision of nutritional support and (b) bowel rest for the involved segment of intestine (1,3). The goal is to ensure adequate intake and absorption of calories and protein to support the healing process while minimizing the volume of drainage through the segment of bowel containing the fistula. These principles are operationalized differently depending on the location of the fistula (3–5). For example, the patient with a fistula in the midportion of the small intestine usually would require NPO (nothing taken orally) status and total parenteral nutrition to promote spontaneous closure. In contrast, the patient with a proximal small bowel fistula usually can be managed via enteral feedings delivered to a site distal to the fistula; of course, it would be necessary to monitor the patient for any significant increase in fistula output following introduction of enteral feedings and to discontinue the feedings should they be associated with a significant increase in output (6). (This patient would also have to be maintained in an NPO status to reduce the volume of drainage through the proximal small bowel.) In establishing a plan to provide both nutritional support and bowel rest, the enteral route for feeding should be selected whenever feasible because enteral feedings are associated with lower cost and fewer complications than parenteral nutrition (1).

Recently, a number of studies demonstrated a significant reduction in fistula output and in time required for spontaneous fistula closure with the administration of somatostatin or its analog, octreotide acetate. Somatostatin is a naturally occurring intestinal hormone that reduces the volume of intestinal secretions (4,6,9).

In some situations, spontaneous fistula closure is not possible; for example, fistulas that undergo mucosal eversion to form pseudostomas do not close spontaneously, nor do fistula tracts lined with epithelium. Malignant involvement also is associated with failure to close, as are distal obstruction and foreign bodies, such as retained sutures (1,3,4,7,9).

When it is recognized that spontaneous closure is unlikely or impossible, a determination must be made regarding further management; the two options are conservative management of the fistula (with no expectation of closure) or surgical intervention. If the decision is made to provide only conservative management, the treatment plan is altered to focus on patient comfort rather than fistula closure. Bowel rest for the involved intestinal segment is no longer a management issue, and patients are allowed oral intake as desired, even if to do so increases the volume of fistula output. Even if surgical intervention is planned, the patient can be allowed oral intake; nutritional status must be maintained via parenteral nutrition (or enteral feedings delivered to a site distal to the fistula), but the principle of bowel rest is no longer relevant (because minimizing output

through the fistula tract has failed to produce spontaneous closure and definitive closure is planned.)

Surgical closure usually is reserved for nonterminal patients whose fistulas fail to close with conservative therapy. Surgical intervention typically involves resection of the fistulous tract with end-to-end anastomosis (1,7). If the involved segment of bowel cannot be isolated because of dense adhesions, it may be necessary to perform a bypass procedure or, occasionally, to divert the fecal stream proximal to the fistula (1,7).

Recently, the literature has contained reports of a procedure for simple fistula closure that is appropriate for patients with advanced cancer; the fistulous tract is closed exteriorly with no intraabdominal access required. The advantage to this procedure is its simplicity and lack of complications; if the closure holds, the patient benefits tremendously and if not, there is no morbidity associated with the attempt (10).

### Conservative Management for the Patient with Cancer

In the patient with advanced malignancy, neither spontaneous closure nor surgical correction of the fistula may be achievable or practical (2). Therapy is directed toward maintenance of patient comfort via containment of drainage and odor and protection of the perifistular skin (1).

A major component of effective fistula management is containment of the effluent and odor and protection of the surrounding skin; these aspects of care have a profound impact on the patient's quality of life (1,11). Today, fistulas usually are treated as spontaneously occurring stomas; management is directed toward effective collection and containment of the drainage and odor.

Many products and techniques are now available for use in containing the drainage and odor and protecting the perifistular skin; selection is determined by the type and volume of drainage, tissue planes and contours in the perifistular area, and perifistular skin integrity (1,3,4,11). Additional factors to be considered include the cost and availability of products, the technical difficulty of the procedures compared to the caregiver's cognitive abilities and technical skills, and availability of professional assistance (e.g., ET nurses and home care nurses).

The volume and characteristics of the effluent dictate the level of skin protection required; drainage that contains proteolytic enzymes or that is highly alkaline or acidic can produce rapid and severe skin breakdown (especially if the fistula is also high output). Thus, gastric, pancreatic, and small bowel fistulas require aggressive protection of all perifistular skin and effective containment of the drainage if at all possible (1,4,5). In contrast, drainage from the colon is usually low volume and nonenzymatic; severe skin breakdown is unlikely, and containment is necessitated more for odor control than for skin protection. Products available for perifistular skin protection include (a) moisture-barrier ointments; (b) copolymer skin sealants; and (c) skin-barrier pastes and barriers (1,4). Moisture-barrier ointments include petrolatum and zinc-oxide based products; these products provide a water-repellent coating on the skin surface but do not provide significant protection against enzymatic drainage; they are incompatible with most pouching systems (because most pouching systems are designed to adhere to the perifistular skin) (4). Therefore, these products are used in combination with absorptive dressings and are appropriate only for low-volume nonenzymatic drainage with minimal odor. Copolymer skin sealants are clear liquid plasticizing agents that provide a protective coating on the skin surface; sealants protect the skin against moisture and against epidermal stripping with tape removal but do not provide adequate protection against enzymatic drainage (4). The most valuable products for perifistular skin protection are the skin-barrier pastes and solid wafers; these products can be used to protect the perifistular skin against enzymatic drainage, to create a smooth pouching surface, and to caulk the perifistular skin between the fistula opening and the pouch (4).

Effective containment of drainage and odor usually involves successful application of an adherent pouching system. Success in pouching depends on adherence to the following principles: (a) the system selected should be compatible with the type of drainage; (b) adhesive pouching systems must be applied to a dry skin surface; and (c) the surface of the pouching system must be compatible with the the perifistular tissue contours (4,11).

There are two primary types of pouching systems: those designed for urinary (or fluid) drainage and those designed for fecal (or particulate) drainage. Urinary systems are equipped with narrow drainage spouts and with antireflux valves that help prevent reflux of drainage onto the perifistular skin, while fecal systems contain no antireflux valves and are equipped with tapered bottom openings to facilitate drainage of thick or solid drainage (4). Several companies now manufacture wound pouches that have both a tapered bottom opening and a spout; these pouches can be used for either fluid or particulate drainage (the spout is cut off for particulate drainage).

Most pouching systems are designed to adhere to the perifistular surface; it is therefore important to create a dry pouching surface. Denuded and weeping perifistular skin will interfere with adhesion; this condition can be treated by application of a skin-barrier powder (e.g., Stomahesive powder by ConvaTec or Premium powder by Hollister) to absorb drainage and create a gummy surface (3,4). (If needed, the area can be blotted with a moist finger or a skin sealant wipe to ensure a dry and nonpowdery surface (3).

Matching the contours of the pouching system to the perifistular planes may be accomplished simply by selecting an appropriate pouching system (i.e., flat flexible versus flat rigid versus convex) or may also require measures to create a flatter pouching surface. A flatter pouching surface can be created by the application of skin barrier paste (e.g., Stomahesive Paste by ConvaTec or Premium Paste by Hollister) to fill surface defects or by use of solid skin barrier strips or wedges to fill uneven perifistular creases (1,4,11).

Most fistulas can be managed via a standard pouching procedure using a standard urinary or fecal pouch or a wound drainage pouch. The standard pouching procedure is outlined in Table 22-1.

In selected patients, the standard approach to pouching is ineffective in providing consistent containment, and leakage occurs frequently. These patients may benefit from the addition of an adhesive to the skin or pouching surface (e.g., Hollister Medical adhesive spray or Skin Bond cement by Smith Nephew United) or from a different approach to pouching. One pouching procedure that is frequently effective when standard pouching fails is the trough procedure (4). It is often effective when the perifistular contours are quite irregular, but its use is limited to fistulas located in open wounds. The basic concept is to protect the perifistular skin with skin-barrier strips and paste and then to place transparent adhesive dressings (such as OpSite by Smith Nephew United) over the wound to seal the wound edges; at the most inferior wound edge, an opening is created in the transparent adhesive dressing, and a pouch is placed over this opening. The wound thus becomes a trough, with drainage funneled to the bottom of the wound where it is collected. The trough procedure is outlined in Table 22-2.

One group of patients with fistulas that cannot be managed by pouching is the patient with a vaginal fistula.

---

**TABLE 1.** *Standard pouching procedure*

Select an appropriate pouch based on type of drainage and abdominal contours.
Size the pouch opening appropriately:
  For fistulas or skin level stomas: size the opening to clear the fistula/stoma margins by 1/4–1/2 in.; this helps prevent tunneling of the drainage under the barrier.
  For protruding stomas: size the opening about 1/8 inch larger than the stoma.
Treat any peristomal skin damage with skin barrier powder and sealant/water.
Use skin barrier paste to fill any surface defects; apply thin layer of paste directly around fecal stoma (Note: Moist finger facilitates paste application).
Press the pouch into place and use gentle pressure to assure adherence.
For fistula: apply thin layer of skin barrier paste to any exposed skin edges and to caulk junction between wound edges and inner edges of pouch.
Change pouch every 5–7 days and as needed for leakage.

**TABLE 2.** *Trough procedure for fistula management*

Treat any damaged perifistular skin with skin barrier powder and sealant or water.

Cut skin barrier strips and apply overlapping strips along periphery of wound. Use skin barrier paste to caulk the junctions between strips and to protect any exposed skin. (Note: The strip placed along the inferior aspect of the wound should be a solid U-shaped strip with no overlapping junctions, since a seam at the inferior aspect of the wound could cause leakage.)

Select transparent adhesive dressing strips that are about 4 in. longer than the widest point of the wound (this assures a 2-in. overlap onto intact skin at each side of the wound bed).

Modify one strip of transparent adhesive dressing as follows:
With paper backing still in place, cut an opening in the adhesive dressing wide enough to encompass the inferior aspect of the wound (if wound diameter is 1½ in. at the inferior aspect, the opening should be cut at least 1¾ in. in diameter).

Select an adhesive-backed ostomy pouch and cut an opening in the pouch that matches the opening in the adhesive dressing—if the opening in the dressing is 1 3/4 in. in diameter, the pouch opening should also be cut 1¾ in. in diameter.

Peel paper backing off the pouch and stick the pouch to the nonadhesive surface of the transparent adhesive dressing strip.

Peel paper backing off transparent adhesive dressing strip with pouch attached and apply to the inferior aspect of the wound.

Apply remaining strips of transparent adhesive dressing in overlapping fashion to cover the remaining area of the wound.

---

**TABLE 3.** *Vaginal fistula management*

Perform a vaginal exam (use a topical anesthetic such as Xylocaine jelly if the patient has significant pain or tenderness) to determine the size of the vaginal vault.

Obtain a soft rubber nipple shield or baby nipple (depending on the size of the vault) and a mushroom catheter.

Cut a small hole in the tip of the nipple shield or nipple, and thread the catheter through so that the mushroom tip is resting within the nipple shield or nipple. Secure the catheter to the nipple shield (or nipple) with waterproof tape.

Fold the nipple shield down around the catheter tubing; lubricate the nipple shield generously with a water-soluble lubricant,[a] and gently push it into the vagina until the entire shield is past the vaginal orifice; gently pull back on the catheter until the nipple shield is seated at the vaginal orifice.

Connect the open end of the catheter to the bedside drainage unit.

---

[a]Consider Xylocaine jelly for patient with significant tenderness.

Patients with rectovaginal fistulas may be managed most effectively by keeping the stool formed (12) to minimize fecal contamination of the vagina. Patients with vesicovaginal fistulas frequently can be managed effectively by placement of an indwelling urethral catheter to decompress the bladder. Patients with enterovaginal fistulas and patients with combined vesicocolovaginal fistulas, however, require containment to prevent significant perineal skin breakdown. An effective approach for these patients is outlined in Table 22-3.

Any patient with a significant fistula can benefit from referral to an ET (wound ostomy continence) nurse specialist; these nurses specialize in management of patients with complex wounds and stomas. Information regarding availability of these specialists can be obtained from the national office of the Wound Ostomy Continence Nurses Society (714-224-9626).

## STOMA MANAGEMENT

Palliative care for patients with gastrointestinal (GI) or genitourinary (GU) stomas must include attention to stoma management and maintenance of GI/GU function.

### Management of Fecal Diversions

#### Descending/Sigmoid Colostomy

A descending or sigmoid colostomy is constructed when the rectum or sigmoid colon or both are removed or bypassed (13,14). The output from a descending/sigmoid colostomy is typically formed stool, and elimination patterns are similar to preoperative bowel patterns for the involved patient (3,15). These patients usually have two options for management (3,14). One option is to wear an odor-proof, drainable pouch and to allow evacuation to occur spontaneously. The other option is to regulate bowel elimination via routine colostomy irrigations; the patient is taught to instill 600 to 1,000 ml of lukewarm tap water into the stoma via a cone tip irrigator that prevents bowel perforation and also prevents backflow of water (3,15). The distention of the bowel stimulates peristalsis, which usually causes evacuation of the left colon within about 30 minutes. Evacuation of this bowel segment typically produces 24 to 48 stool-free hours. Repeated administration of the same stimulus induces some degree of bowel dependence, which over time reduces the potential for fecal spillage between irrigations (3,15). The patient who manages his colostomy with routine irrigation usually can wear a simple stoma cover or a stoma cap between irrigations; the stoma cap provides for absorption of mucus and also deodorizes and vents flatus (15).

Management issues for the patient with a descending or sigmoid colostomy include measures to control odor, reduce gas, and prevent or manage diarrhea and constipation (3,15). Routine measures to control odor include maintenance of an intact pouch seal and a clean pouch opening (the pouch material is odor proof, so odor occurs only if there is a break in the seal or if fecal material is left on the pouch opening); additional measures include the use of pouch deodorants (or the addition of 1 or 2 teaspoons of mouthwash into the pouch each time it is emptied) or administration of oral deodorants (Bismuth subgallate 1 or 2 tablets 3 or 4 × /day or chlorophyllin copper complex 100 mg 1 or 2 × /day) (15,16). Measures to reduce gas include limitation of gas-producing foods, such as broccoli, cabbage, onions, and beans (3,15,16). Diarrhea can occur as a result of a viral illness or in response to some chemotherapeutic agents and is managed similarly to management of diarrhea in the patient with an intact rectum and anus; the patient is counseled to remain on a low-fat, low-fiber diet, to increase fluid intake, and to take over-the-counter antidiarrheal medications if desired (3,15,16). The patient who manages with routine irrigation is instructed to omit irrigations until bowel function and stool consistency return to normal. Constipation is much more common than diarrhea in the patient with advanced malignancy and a descending/sigmoid colostomy because of the antiperistaltic effects of reduced dietary fiber, reduced activity, and increased use of analgesics, a triad common in the setting of advanced disease. Constipation is managed by administration of laxatives (e.g., Milk of Magnesia or bisacodyl tablets) and cleansing irrigations (e.g., 1,000 ml tap water or saline) coupled with initiation of programs to maintain normal bowel function (i.e., administration of bulk laxatives, such as psyllium products or stool softener/stimulant combinations such as docusate and casanthranol (3,15,32).

### Transverse Colostomy

A transverse colostomy most commonly is constructed as a loop stoma to provide fecal diversion in the patient with distal obstruction. Fecal output has a mushy consistency, and the patient typically experiences output following meals and at other unpredictable times (15). Unlike the descending/sigmoid colostomy, a transverse colostomy cannot be regulated by routine irrigation (because of continuous peristalsis in the ascending colon); these patients must wear an odorproof pouch to collect the stool (15). Management issues for these patients include odor and gas control and management of diarrhea (as discussed in the section on descending/sigmoid colostomy) (15). Constipation usually does not occur because the stool in the transverse colon is fairly fluid.

### Ileostomy or Ascending Colostomy

An ileostomy is most commonly done when the entire colon and rectum are removed for disease processes, such as familial polyposis, multiple colon malignancies, or inflammatory bowel disease (14). Cecostomies and ascending colostomies are uncommonly performed but occasionally are required to relieve acute obstruction of the distal ascending or proximal transverse colon (14). Output from these stomas is a thick liquid containing proteolytic enzymes that are extremely damaging to the skin (3,17). Thus, management includes continuous pouching with a well-fitting pouch and meticulous skin care to prevent fecal contact with the peristomal skin. Management issues for the patient with an ascending colostomy include skin protection, maintenance of fluid-electrolyte balance, and medication modifications (15). The patient is taught to size the pouch carefully to fit closely around the stoma and to protect any exposed skin with skin-barrier paste (15). Patients also are taught to maintain a daily fluid intake of about 2 liters to aggressively replace fluids and electrolytes during periods of increased loss (e.g., diarrhea or heavy perspiration) by drinking a glass of replacement fluid each time the pouch is emptied (18) and to report promptly any signs or symptoms of fluid-electrolyte imbalance to the physician (15,16). Medication modifications include avoidance of time-released and enteric-coated medications because these forms are likely to be incompletely and unpredictably absorbed as a result of reduced bowel length and reduced transit time (15). The issues of skin protection, fluid-electrolyte balance, and medication modification are equally critical to the patient with an ileostomy; in addition, the ileostomy patient must be taught how to modify his or her diet to prevent food blockage (3,14,16–19). Food blockage is a complication unique to the patient with an ileostomy and occurs when a bolus of fibrous undigested food obstructs the lumen of the bowel at the point where the bowel is brought through the fascia-muscle layer (a point of potential narrowing) (15). Patients with ileostomies are taught to add high-fiber foods (e.g., raw fruits and vegetables, coconuts, popcorn, and nuts) to their diets one at a time and in small amounts, to chew thoroughly, and to recognize and report signs of partial or complete blockage (high-volume malodorous liquid output or no output coupled with abdominal cramping, distention, and possibly nausea and vomiting) (3,15). Food blockage is managed by ileostomy lavage performed by the physician or ostomy nurse specialist; a catheter is inserted into the stoma until the blockage is reached and 30 to 50 ml of saline is instilled. The catheter then is removed to allow for returns, and the process is repeated until the blockage is removed (3,15,17).

### Continent Fecal Diversions

Most continent fecal diversions are performed for non-malignant conditions affecting the colon, such as familial polyposis and ulcerative colitis (20). These patients, however, are not immune to other malignancies that may progress to an advanced state, and their care must include management of the continent diversion.

A continent ileostomy, such as a Kock Pouch, differs from a standard ileostomy in that an internal reservoir is constructed between the proximal bowel and the abdominal stoma; the diversion is made continent by intussuscepting the segment of bowel between the reservoir and the abdominal stoma, thus creating a one-way valve (14,18,20). The patient drains the reservoir by intubating the stoma and continence mechanism with a large-bore catheter about three or four times daily (19,20); if the stool is too thick to drain readily, the caregiver instills tepid water into the reservoir through a catheter-tipped syringe to fluidize the stool. Management issues include avoidance of foods with peels (because the peels tend to obstruct the drainage catheter) (20) and medication modifications; in addition to avoiding enteric coated and time-released medications, these patients must avoid wax-matrix medications because the wax shells do not dissolve and cannot be drained through the catheter. Patients also are instructed to flush the reservoir until clear one or two times daily to prevent pouchitis (inflammation of the reservoir caused by bacterial overgrowth) (20).

An ileal-anal reservoir is performed in conjunction with a colectomy and proctectomy; the sphincter mechanism is preserved, and a reservoir is constructed from the terminal ileum and anastomosed to the anal canal (3,18,20). Thus, the patient's own sphincter serves as the continence mechanism. The patient with an ileal-anal reservoir has mushy stools with residual enzymes; therefore, meticulous skin care is essential at all times and is even more critical during episodes of diarrhea (3,20). The ileal-anal patient is also at risk for pouchitis; symptoms include burning, itching, bleeding, and fecal urgency, and treatment typically involves clear liquids and metronidazole (3,18,20).

### Management of Retained Nonfunctional Distal Bowel Segment

Patients with a loop or double-barrel colostomy and patients with a Hartmann's pouch have a variable length of distal bowel that is nonfunctional; this segment continues to produce mucus, and some patients require periodic low-volume rectal enemas to cleanse inspissated mucus (3,16). It is also relevant to note that medications can be administered rectally even when the rectum is no longer in continuity with the proximal bowel.

## Management of Urinary Diversions

Urinary diversions are required for patients with pelvic malignancies necessitating removal of the bladder and for patients with ureteral obstruction that cannot be managed with internally placed ureteral stents. Until recently, the standard diversion was the intestinal conduit; currently urinary diversions are more commonly constructed as continent diversions (21).

### Intestinal Conduits

Ileal conduits and other intestinal conduits normally produce clear urine with strands of mucus (as a result of using a bowel segment as the conduit for urine drainage); because there is no reservoir for urine collection, urine drainage is almost continuous, and patients must wear a pouch to contain the output (15,22). The most important management issue is prevention and management of urinary tract infection; patients are taught to maintain adequate fluid intake and to recognize and promptly report signs of urinary tract infection. Confirmation of urinary tract infection and organism identification usually are accomplished via a catheterized specimen for culture and sensitivity; these data provide the basis for organism-specific treatment (15).

### Ureterostomy

Ureterostomies, whether unilateral or bilateral, are rarely constructed because of the numerous problems they cause (i.e., ineffective drainage, stenosis, pouching problems) (22); however, these diversions are done occasionally when it is not feasible to construct an intestinal conduit. Output from a ureterostomy is clear urine without mucus (15); management is the same as for patients with intestinal conduits. In addition, these patients need to be monitored for evidence of stenosis (i.e., reduced output, flank pain, chronic UTI) (22); stomal dilatation or stoma revision may be required for management.

### Continent Urinary Diversions

The trend in urinary diversions is construction of continent reservoirs; a variety of surgical procedures exist, but all involve construction of a low-pressure, high-volume reservoir; an antireflux mechanism between the reservoir and the ureters; and a continent, catheterizable channel between the reservoir and the abdominal surface (20,21). The two most commonly performed are the Kock urostomy and variations of the ileocecal reservoir (e.g., Indiana reservoir, Florida pouch, Miami pouch). Normal output is clear urine with strands of mucus; long-term management involves intermittent intubation of the reservoir (approximately every 3–4 hours and as needed) to drain the urine and daily or bid irrigations of the reservoir (with water or saline) to remove the mucus and prevent pouchitis (20). Adequate fluid intake and close adherence to the catheterization schedule help to prevent urinary tract infections (20). These patients typically need only an absorptive pad over the stoma; significant leakage is uncommon. Patients who develop significant urinary leakage usually are managed by using two-piece pouching systems, which contain the urinary leakage while permitting ready access to the stoma for routine catheterizations. (Routine catheterizations must be continued to prevent urinary retention and resultant infection.)

### Orthotopic Bladder to Urethra

The newest approach to urinary tract reconstruction following cystectomy is construction of a neobladder with anastomosis to the retained urethral sphincter mechanism; this procedure is limited to patients whose malignancy can be resected adequately without compromising the sphincter (20,23,24). Because the neobladder is usually a noncontractile reservoir constructed from detubularized bowel, effective emptying depends on effective relaxation of the voluntary sphincter in combination with abdominal muscle contraction to increase the pressure in the reservoir (20,23,24). Patients must be monitored for urinary retention; patients unable to empty the reservoir completely are taught to augment voluntary voids with clean intermittent catheterization to prevent urinary stasis and resulting infection (20). Another common problem is some degree of urinary leakage, particularly at night (when the sphincter muscle is partially relaxed) (23); depending on the severity of the leakage, absorbent products may be required for containment.

### Principles of and Products for Pouching

As outlined in the section on fistula management, the key principles in stoma management include containment of the drainage and odor and protection of the peristomal skin. The degree of skin protection required is dictated by the characteristics of the drainage; drainage that is proteolytic or highly acidic or alkaline requires meticulous protection of all peristomal skin, whereas nonenzymatic drainage with a pH that is essentially neutral primarily requires protection against pooling of drainage that can macerate the skin (16,25). Thus, ileostomies and ascending colostomies require aggressive skin protection, whereas descending/sigmoid colostomies and urinary diversions primarily require protection against prolonged contact between the drainage and the skin (15).

Products available for protection of peristomal skin include skin sealants and skin barriers; these products are described in the section on fistula management. Table 22-4 lists some of the most widely available products for fistula and stoma management (15).

As discussed earlier, pouching systems are available for both urinary and fecal drainage. Pouching systems are also available as one-piece and two-piece systems. One-piece pouches typically are constructed with a barrier ring and tape border to which the odor-proof pouch is welded; they are available both in precut and cut-to-fit varieties. Two-piece pouches typically consist of a barrier wafer to which a raised flange is attached and a pouch with a matching gasket that is snapped onto the flange

**TABLE 4.** *Commonly available pouching products*

| Company | Pouching systems | Adjunct products |
|---|---|---|
| Convatec Bristol Myers Squibb Princeton, NJ 800-422-8811 | 1-pc. and 2-pc. fecal and urinary pouches, flat and convex Wound pouches (3 sizes) | Skin sealant (Allkare) Stomahesive paste Stomahesive powder Stomahesive barriers |
| Hollister Libertyville, IL 800-323-4060 | 1-pc. and 2-pc. fecal and urinary pouches, flat and convex Wound pouches (3 sizes) | Skin sealant Premium paste Premium powder Premium & Flextend Barriers Medical adhesive |
| Smith Nephew United Largo, FL 800-876-1261 | 1-pc. fecal and urinary pouches, flat only Wound pouches (Bongort): 3 sizes | Skin prep (Sealant) Skin bond cement Transparent adhesive Dressings (OpSite) |
| Colopast Marietta, GA 800-237-4555 | 1-pc. and 2-pc. fecal pouches 2-pc. urinary pouches Wound pouch | Barrier paste |

(15). Application guidelines are the same as those for fistula pouch application and are outlined in Table 1.

### Management of Peristomal Complications

Peristomal complications commonly encountered include epithelial denudation, monilial rash, and allergic reactions to ostomy products. Prompt recognition and appropriate intervention usually result in complete resolution of the problem.

### Denudation

Superficial skin loss typically is caused by a poorly fitting or incorrectly sized pouch that allows the effluent to contact the peristomal skin. The area of damage typically extends from the stoma in the path taken by the effluent; the area is usually red, raw, and painful (15,25). The most important intervention is correction of the underlying problem, that is, modification of the pouching system (15,25). Actual treatment of the denuded areas involves application of a pectin-based skin barrier powder to the denuded areas (3,15,16). The powder can be coated lightly with a skin sealant or with a damp finger to provide a dry or gummy pouching surface. Severely denuded areas may require several layers of powder and sealant/water to provide a thick protective layer. The correctly sized pouching system then can be applied over the treated surface. An alternative approach is to size a hydrocolloid dressing (e.g., DuoDerm by ConvaTec) to fit closely around the stoma and to use this as a primary dressing under the pouch (25).

### Monilial Rash

Peristomal yeast rashes can occur as a result of antibiotic administration with resulting overgrowth of yeast organisms in the bowel or as a result of constant moisture resulting from a leaking pouch or heavy perspiration under a plastic pouch (15,25). The rash has a maculopapular appearance with distinct border (satellite) lesions and is commonly pruritic (15,25). It usually responds promptly to treatment with nystatin powder (15,16,25,26). The powder can be blotted with a sealant or a moist finger to create a dry or sticky pouching surface.

### Allergy

Any product used to protect the peristomal skin or to contain the output can be an allergen. The involved area is typically erythematous and pruritic; vesicles may form in a severe reaction (25). The first step in managment is to identify and eliminate the allergen, which can be a challenge when the patient is using a variety of products on the involved skin (11). Usually the distribution of the reaction helps to identify the offender; patch testing may be required when the identity of the allergen is not clear (15,25,26). Until the specific allergen is identified and the peristomal skin has normalized, product use should be minimized; for example, use of paste, powder, and sealants should be eliminated if possible, and the patient should be managed with a solid barrier and pouch or a nonadhesive silicone ring system, such as the VPI pouch by Cook Products, Spencer, Indiana (because damaged skin is hypersensitive and may react to products that are not true allergens; solid barriers and silicone rings are the products least likely to initiate a further inflammatory response) (26). Patients with severe blistering or pruritis may require topical or systemic antihistamines or corticosteroids in addition to the measures already identified (15,25).

## MANAGEMENT OF STOMAL COMPLICATIONS

Although stomal complications are not common, they can interfere with normal ostomy function or with effective containment of the output; therefore, the clinician needs to be knowledgeable regarding their management.

### Peristomal Hernia

Peristomal hernia involves herniation of the bowel through the muscle defect created by the stoma and into the subcutaneous tissue (26); typically, the hernia reduces spontaneously when the patient is in a reclining position and intraabdominal pressure is reduced. Problems created by peristomal hernias include the potential for strangulation and bowel obstruction, which is uncommon, and difficulty with maintenance of an effective pouch seal, which is more common (26,27). In the patient with advanced cancer, surgical intervention usually is reserved for emergency situations involving strangulation and obstruction (27). Conservative management commonly includes use of a hernia belt, which is an abdominal binder with a cut-out for the stoma and pouch (16,26). The belt is applied while the patient is recumbent and the hernia is reduced, and the resistance provided by the belt helps maintain reduction of the herniated loop of bowel. Colostomy patients who manage their stomas with routine irrigation must be cautioned to irrigate only with a cone-tip irrigator because a catheter could cause perforation of the herniated loop and to try to instill the irrigation fluid while the patient is in a semireclining position (which promotes reduction of the herniated bowel) (17,26).

### Stenosis

Stomal narrowing to a point that interferes with normal function can occur at either the skin level or the fascia level. Stenosis at the skin level may be evidenced by visible narrowing of the stomal lumen, but stenosis at fascia level can be detected only by digital examination. Signs of stenosis include reduced output, cramping pain, and abdominal distention (with fecal diversions) and flank pain or infection (with urinary diversions). Stenosis that interferes with normal function requires surgical revision (16), either local excision of the stenotic area or open laporotomy (26).

### Retraction

Retraction of the stoma to below skin level can occur early postoperatively as a result of tension on the bowel or mesentery or due to breakdown of the mucocutaneous suture line; late retraction can be caused by ascites or intraperitoneal tumor growth causing abdominal distention or traction on the mesentery. Retraction is managed by modification of the pouching system to accommodate the change in the peristomal contours; typically, a convex pouching system is needed (26).

## Prolapse

Factors contributing to stomal prolapse include increased intraabdominal pressure, loop stoma construction, location of the stoma outside of the rectus muscle, and formation of an excessively large aperture in the abdominal wall (28). Prolapse is usually quite upsetting to patients; however, prolapse does not represent a surgical emergency unless there is evidence of incarceration and stomal ischemia (28). Sometimes a prolapsed stoma can be reduced; the patient is placed in a recumbent position to reduce intraabdominal pressure, and manual reduction is attempted. (If the stoma is very edematous, a hypertonic substance, such as salt or sugar, may be applied topically to reduce the edema before reduction is attempted (29). Once the prolapse is reduced, a hernia belt with prolapse overbelt (or a simple abdominal binder) can be used to prevent recurrence (26).

## Bleeding

Slight stomal bleeding during pouch changes is common as a result of the marked vascularity of the stoma (26); however, significant or spontaneous bleeding is not normal and requires investigation and intervention. Bleeding from the stoma itself usually can be managed by direct pressure, application of ice, or AgNO3 cauterization (26). Bleeding originating from the bowel requires further workup, with intervention determined by the causative factors and the patient s overall status (26).

## Specific Issues for Oncology Patients

Some specific ostomy-related issues are relevant only to cancer patients. These issues include management of a stoma in the radiation field, management of stomatitis, and the impact of advancing disease on self-care and management.

## Stoma in Radiation Field

The goal in managing a stoma in the radiation field is to prevent peristomal skin damage. If the radiation oncologist wishes to have the pouch removed for each treatment, the patient should be switched to a nonadhesive pouching system secured with a belt (e.g., Hollister 1-piece Karaya ring pouches or Cook VPI nonadhesive pouches) (30). If the radiation oncologist elects to leave the pouch in place during treatments, the pouching system should be modified to eliminate any metallic agents that could cause scatter of the radiation beam at skin level (e.g., tapes containing zinc oxide) (30). Pectin-based barriers, plastic pouches, and porous paper tape are all safe. Any peristomal damage that does occur can usually be managed by applying a hydrocolloid wafer dressing (e.g., DuoDerm by ConvaTec) to the peristomal skin under the pouch.

## Management of Stomatitis

Stomatitis, a common side effect of both radiation therapy and chemotherapy, is manifested by stomal edema, vasocongestion, and possibly ulceration. The goals of treatment are to prevent secondary infection and to prevent trauma and bleeding. Colostomy patients who manage their stomas with routine irrigation are instructed to omit irrigation during courses of pelvic radiation and during any episodes of stomatitis caused by chemotherapy (30). Patients also are counseled to avoid vigorous cleansing of the stoma and may be advised to add small amounts of mineral oil to lubricate the inside of the pouch if the stoma is friable (30). Patients with continent diversions may need to use smaller catheters, additional lubricant, and extreme caution in intubating the reservoir. Patients who develop stomatitis secondary to chemotherapy usually require treatment with antifungal agents (31) because the entire length of the alimentary canal is likely to be affected.

## Impact of Advancing Disease on Self-Care and Management

One of the most significant issues facing the ostomy patient with advanced disease is self-care and management. It is frequently necessary to modify the patient's management regimen or to teach a family member to change the pouch or intubate the stoma as the patient becomes less able to manage his or her own care. The colostomy patient who has managed with irrigation and who is no longer able to perform this procedure needs to be placed in a drainable pouching system and usually will require administration of a stool softener/peristaltic stimulant combination (e.g., docusate casanthranol) to maintain bowel function (because the bowel has become dependent on the mechanical stimulus of irrigation). As noted earlier in this chapter, constipation is a common problem for the colostomy patient with advanced cancer but usually can be managed with bulk and stimulant laxatives, stool softeners, and irrigations as needed (32). Removal of impacted stool usually can be accomplished by administration of a 1:1 solution of milk and molasses given as irrigation.

The patient with a continent urinary diversion (or orthotopic neobladder) may be managed by insertion of an indwelling catheter into the reservoir if to do so is more feasible for the caregiver than intermittent intubation (24). The home health or hospice nurse can be valuable in assisting the patient and family to modify their care routines in the most effective and manageable way.

## SUMMARY

Effective management of fistulas and stomas requires containment of drainage and odor plus protection of the surrounding skin; these aspects of care have a significant impact on the quality of life for patients with advanced disease.

## REFERENCES

1. Bryant R. Enterocutaneous fistulas: meeting the nursing challenge. *Progressions* 1992;4:3–23.
2. Benson D, Fischer J. Enterocutaneous fistula. In: Fazio V, ed. *Current therapy in colon and rectal surgery*. Philadelphia: BC Decker, 1990; 372–376.
3. Doughty D. *Gastrointestinal disorders*. St. Louis: Mosby Year Book, 1993;245–253; 311–370; 324–337.
4. Bryant R. Management of drain sites and fistulas. In: Bryant R, ed. *Acute and chronic wounds: nursing management*. St. Louis: Mosby Year Book, 1992;248–287.
5. Kimbrough T. Intraabdominal abscesses and fistulas. In: Yamada T. *Textbook of gastroenterology*. Philadelphia: JB Lippincott, 1995; 2289–2298.
6. Pellegrini C, Gordon R. Abdominal abscesses and gastrointestinal fistulas. In: Sleisenger M, Fordtran J, eds. *Gastrointestinal disease: pathophysiology, diagnosis, management*, 5th ed. Philadelphia: WB Saunders, 1993;1962–1976.
7. Wong W, Buie W. Management of intestinal fistulas. In: MacKeigan J, Cataldo P. eds. *Intestinal stomas: principles, techniques, and management*. St. Louis: Quality Medical Publishing, 1993;278–306.
8. Greenstein A. Inflammatory bowel disease: surgical management and ultimate outcome. In: Haubrich W, Schaffner F, Berk J, eds. *Gastroenterology*, 5th ed. Philadelphia: WB Saunders, 1995;1514–1531.
9. Greenstein A. Enterocutaneous fistula. In: Bayless T, ed. *Current therapy in gastroenterology and liver disease*, 4th ed. St. Louis: Mosby Year Book, 1994;341–345.
10. Sarfeh I, Jakowatz J. Surgical treatment of enteric bud fistulas in contaminated wounds: a riskless extraperitoneal method using split-thickness skin grafts. *Arch Surg* 1992;127:1027–1030.
11. Rolstad B, Wong W. Nursing considerations with intestinal fistulas. In: MacKeigan J, Cataldo P, eds. *Intestinal stomas: principles, techniques, and management*. St. Louis: Quality Medical Publishing, 1993;307–328.
12. Hoexter B. Rectovaginal fistula. In: Fazio V, ed. *Current therapy in colon and rectal surgery*. Philadelphia: BC Decker, 1990;28–32.
13. McGarity W. Gastrointestinal surgical procedures. In: Hampton B, Bryant R, eds. *Ostomies and continent diversions: nursing management*. St. Louis: Mosby Year Book, 1992;349–371.
14. Fazio W, Erwin-Toth P. Stomal and pouch function and care. In: Haubrich W, Schaffner F, Berk J, eds. *Gastroenterology*, 5th ed. Philadelphia: WB Saunders, 1995;1547–1560.
15. Erwin-Toth P, Doughty D. Principles and procedures of stomal management. In: Hampton B, Bryant R, eds. *Ostomies and continent diversions: nursing management*. St. Louis: Mosby Year Book, 1992; 29–103.
16. Lavery I, Erwin-Toth P. Stoma therapy. In: MacKeigan J, Cataldo P, eds. *Intestinal stomas: principles, techniques, and management*. St. Louis: Quality Medical Publishing, 19993;60–84.
17. Kodner I. Stoma complications. In: Fazio V, ed. *Current therapy In colon and rectal surgery*. Philadelphia: BC Decker, 1990;420–425.
18. Pemberton J, Phillips S. Ileostomy and its alternatives. In: Sleisenger M, Fordtran J eds. *Gastrointestinal disease*: pathophysiology, diagnosis, management, 5th ed. Philadelphia: WB Saunders, 1993; 1331–1338.
19. Kelly K. Approach to patient with ileostomy and ileal pouch ileostomy. In: Yamada T, ed. *Textbook of gastroenterology*. 2nd ed. Philadelphia: JB Lippincott, 1995;880–892.
20. Rolstad B, Hoyman K. Continent diversions and reservoirs. In: Hampton B, Bryant R, eds. *Ostomies and continent diversions: nursing management*. St. Louis: Mosby Year Book, 1992;129–162.
21. Dalton D. Methods of urinary diversion. In: MacKeigan J, Cataldo P, eds. *Intestinal stomas: principles, techniques, and management*. St. Louis: Quality Medica Publishing, 1993;198–227.
22. Doughty D, Lightner D. Genitourinary surgical procedures. In: Hampton B, Bryant R, eds. *Ostomies and continent diversions: nursing Management*. St. Louis: Mosby Year Book, 1992;249–263.
23. Boyd S, Lieskovsky G, Skiner D. Kock pouch bladder replacement. *Urol Clin North Am* 1991;18:641–648.
24. Marshall F. Ileocolic neobladder after cystectomy. *Urol Clin North Am* 1991;18:631–639.
25. Fry R, Swatske M. Skin problems in stoma management. In: MacKeigan J, Cataldo P, eds. *Intestinal stomas: principles, techniques, and management*. St. Louis: Quality Medical Publishing, 1993;329–338.
26. Hampton B. Peristomal and stomal complications. In: Hampton B, Bryant R, eds. *Ostomies and continent diversions: nursing management*. St. Louis: Mosby Year Book, 1992;105–128.
27. Rubin M, Bailey R. Parastomal hernias. In: MacKeigan J, Cataldo P. *Intestinal stomas: principles, techniques, and management*. St. Louis: Quality Medical Publishing, 1993;245–267.
28. Nogueras J, Wexner S. Stoma prolapse. In: MacKeigan J, Cataldo P. *Intestinal stomas: principles, techniques, and management*. St. Louis: Quality Medical Publishing, 1993;268–277.
29. Myers J, Rothenberger D. Sugar in the reduction of incarcerated prolapsed bowel: report of two cases. *Dis Colon Rectum* 1991;5:416–418.
30. Ratliff C. Principles of cancer therapy. In: Hampton B, Bryant R. *Ostomies and continent diversions: nursing management*. St. Louis: Mosby Year Book, 1992;163–194.
31. Goodman M, Ladd L, Purl S. Integumentary and mucous membrane alterations. In: Groenwald S, Frogge M, Goodman M, Yarbro C, eds. *Cancer nursing: principles and practice*. 3rd ed. Boston: Jones and Bartlett, 1993;737–748.
32. McGuire D, Sheidler V. Pain. In: Groenwald S, Frogge M, Goodman M, Yarbro C, eds. *Cancer nursing: principles and practice*. 3rd ed. Boston: Jones and Bartlett, 1993;530–533.

*Principles and Practice of Supportive Oncology,*
edited by Ann Berger et al.
Lippincott–Raven Publishers, Philadelphia ©1998

CHAPTER 23

# Dyspnea in Patients with Advanced Cancer

Eduardo Bruera and Carla Ripamonti

Dyspnea is a frequent and devastating symptom in patients with advanced cancer (1,2). In addition, there is evidence that good symptom control, even by experienced palliative care teams, is achieved less frequently for dyspnea than for other symptoms, such as pain or nausea (3). Limited research and education are available, however, on the adequate assessment and management of dyspnea in cancer patients.

Dyspnea has been defined as an uncomfortable awareness of breathing (4). Although everybody has experienced the sensation and has an intuitive understanding of this symptom, there is no universal agreement as to its definition. Dyspnea is a subjective sensation and cannot be defined by the physical abnormalities that accompany such unpleasant subjective experience. For the purpose of this chapter, dyspnea is defined as an unpleasant sensation of difficult, labored breathing.

The purpose of this chapter is to review the pathophysiology, clinical presentation, assessment, and treatment of dyspnea in cancer patients. Areas where future research should focus also are discussed.

## PATHOPHYSIOLOGY

Dyspnea is frequently associated with abnormalities in the mechanisms that regulate normal breathing; however, the actual expression of dyspnea by a patient results from a complex interaction between the abnormalities in breathing and the perception of those abnormalities in the central nervous system. Finally, the origins of dyspnea in different clinical settings can be traced to specific abnormalities. These three areas are discussed in the following paragraphs.

E. Bruera: Professor of Oncology, Palliative Care Program, University of Alberta, and Grey Nuns Community Hospital and Health Centre, Edmonton, Alberta T6L 5X8, Canada.

C. Ripamonti: Department of Oncology, University of Alberta, Edmonton, Canada, and Pain Therapy and Palliative Care Division, National Cancer Institute, 20133 Milano, Italy.

## Regulation of Breathing

Figure 23-1 summarizes the regulation of normal breathing and dyspnea. Respiration is integrated as a system with three main components:

### Respiratory Center

The respiratory center is located in the medulla. Its neurons receive information from both central and peripheral chemo receptors and peripheral mechanoreceptors. It also receives information from the cortex of the brain, which regulates voluntary breathing such as occurs during speaking and singing. Its efference stimulates the diaphragm, the intercostal muscles, and the accessory muscles into producing respiration (5,6).

### Receptors

Chemoreceptors located both centrally and peripherally are stimulated by the levels of oxygen and carbon

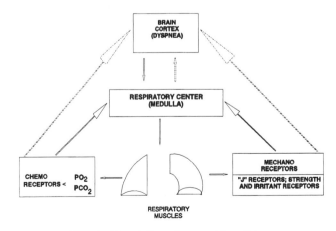

**FIG. 1.** Regulation of normal breathing.

dioxide in the blood. These chemoreceptors are capable of stimulating the respiratory center and increasing respiratory rate (7,8). Although strong debate continues on this subject, recent evidence suggests that chemoreceptors are probably also able to stimulate the brain cortex directly and cause dyspnea. An alternative explanation for the dyspnea caused by increases in PCO₂ and decreases in PO₂ is that these chemoreceptors stimulate the respiratory center. This center increases the respiratory effort, which stimulates mechanoreceptors capable of stimulating the brain cortex.

The mechanoreceptors are located primarily in the respiratory muscles and the lung. These receptors respond to either irritants or, more commonly, pulmonary stretch, including vascular congestion (6). The mechanoreceptors are capable of stimulating the respiratory center and also have a demonstrated effect on causing dyspnea by stimulating the brain cortex.

### *Respiratory Muscles*

The respiratory muscles promote gas exchange. The resulting changes in the PO₂ and PCO₂ are detected by the chemoreceptors. The changes in the tension within the abdominal wall and the lung are detected by the mechanoreceptors. This information is fed back to the respiratory center. Sensory receptors are found inside the respiratory muscles, including the intercostal, sternomastoid, and diaphragm. The balance between the contractual activity and stimulation of the sensory receptors is of great importance in the type of input provided to the respiratory center and the cortex.

Although the three aforementioned factors are the main elements in the regulation of breathing, the actual sensation of dyspnea is a result of cortical stimulation. The production of dyspnea has been demonstrated to be related to the activation of mechanoreceptors both in the respiratory muscles and the lung. Elegant research has shown that both in normal volunteers and patients, different stimuli capable of stimulating mechano receptors are able to produce dyspnea even in absence of increased respiratory activity (6,7). In addition, two more possible mechanisms of dyspnea have been proposed. On one hand, the previously discussed potential role of chemoreceptor stimulation. On the other hand, some authors have proposed a role for efference from the respiratory center as a potential cause of dyspnea by direct ascending stimulation (7–9).

### Production of Dyspnea

Figure 23-2 summarizes the steps in the production of dyspnea. A number of researchers have found great variability in the expression of dyspnea among patients with similar levels of functional abnormalities. Among patients with asthma, about 15% did not express dyspnea

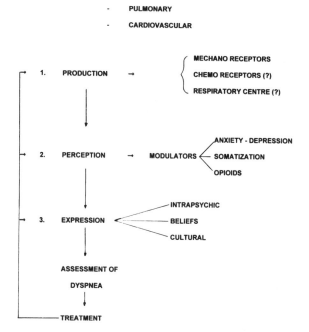

**FIG. 2.** Different stages in the production of dyspnea. No dyspnea worst possible dyspnea 1 2 3: 1. Locally advanced carcinoma—pleural effusion; 2. Major depression episode somatization; 3. Excessive activity poor energy conservation.

despite severe air flow obstruction (forced expiratory volume in 1 second of less than 15% of the predicted) (10). Similarly, among patients with chronic obstructive pulmonary disease (COPD), the complaint of dyspnea was not well correlated with the abnormalities in the pulmonary function tests (11). Among these patients who were defined as having disproportionate dyspnea (complaint of dyspnea in the presence of a mean forced expiratory volume in 1 second of 1.8 L), almost all patients were considered to have a psychiatric diagnosis (mostly anxiety and depression) (11).

These studies suggest that some patients have modulators that either amplify or decrease the intensity of the symptom that is perceived at the cortical level. Patients receiving drugs such as opioids for pain can perceive significantly less dyspnea (1).

Finally, the expression of a certain symptom may be influenced by cultural factors, the belief about the mechanism for the symptom, and other intrapsychic factors (12). Because neither the production or perception of dyspnea can be measured at present, the entire assessment is based on the patient's expression. This issue is discussed in the following section.

### Clinical Situations Associated with Dyspnea

From a pathophysiological point of view, dyspnea can result from three main abnormalities (6):(a) an increase in respiratory effort to overcome a certain load (e.g., obstructive or restrictive lung disease, pleural effusion); (b) an increase in the proportion of respiratory muscle required to maintain a normal workload (e.g, neuromuscular weakness, cancer cachexia, and so on); (c) an increase in ventilatory requirements (hypoxemia, hypercapnia, metabolic acidosis, anemia, etc.).

In many cancer patients, different proportions of the three abnormalities may coexist thereby making the pathophysiological interpretation of the intensity of dyspnea more complex.

## CLINICAL FEATURES

Dyspnea occurs in 21% to 70% of patients with advanced cancer before death. This large variation in reported prevalence is a result of the different natures of patient populations reported by different authors and the lack of a general consensus on the assessment methods for the presence and intensity of dyspnea.

Higginson and McCarthy (3) conducted a prospective study in 86 consecutive patients with advanced cancer referred to a Community Palliative Care Service. Eighteen patients (21%) developed dyspnea as their main symptom before death. The symptom assessment scores for patients with dyspnea showed no change over time as compared with a significant decrease in the intensity of pain reported by this same patient population.

Reuben et al. (13) reported on the prevalence of dyspnea in patients admitted to the National Hospice Study. Dyspnea occurred in 70% of a total of 1,754 patients sometime during the last 6 weeks of life. The frequency of dyspnea increased during the last weeks of life, and more than 28% of patients rated the severity of their symptoms as moderate or worse during the self-report assessment. During the last 6 weeks of life, 27.5% of patients reported dyspnea all the time. Although 33% of patients had the diagnosis of primary or metastatic lung cancer, 24% of patients with dyspnea did not have any known lung or heart disease or evidence of pleural effusion. Grond et al. (14) reported a prevalence of dyspnea of 24% among 1,635 cancer patients referred to a pain clinic. Donnelly et al. (15) found dyspnea in 28% of a total of 1,000 patients referred for consultation to a palliative care service. Of those patients who reported dyspnea, 63% rated this symptom as moderate or severe, that is, of clinical importance.

Twycross and Lack (16) found a prevalence of 51% of dyspnea in 6,677 patients admitted to a palliative care program. Muers (17) found breathlessness to be a presenting complaint for 60% of 289 patients with non-small cell lung cancer, half of whom described their shortness of breath as moderated or severe .

In summary, dyspnea appears to be a common symptom in patients with terminal cancer. It develops more commonly in patients during the last weeks of life. Although it is more common among patients with lung cancer or pulmonary metastases, it is also frequent in patients with no demonstrable tumor involvement in the lung. Most patients who develop dyspnea tend to rate this symptom as one of their main problems.

Table 23-1 summaries the main causes of dyspnea in cancer. It is not uncommon that a patient with advanced cancer and severe dyspnea may have a combination of the different factors reported in the Table 1. Therefore, the pathophysiology in most cancer patients is complex: A given patient may have an increase in respiratory effort necessary to overcome the presence of a large pleural effusion simultaneously with an increase in the proportion of respiratory muscle required for breathing because of cachexia and increased ventilatory requirement resulting from severe anemia.

**TABLE 1.** *Causes of dyspnea in cancer patients[a]*

Direct effect of the tumor
    Primary or metastatic tumor
    Pleural effusion/pericardial effusion
    Superior vena cava syndrome
    Carcinomatous lymphangitis
    Atelectasis
    Phrenic nerve palsy
    Tracheal obstruction
    Trachea-esophageal fistula
    Carcinomatous infiltration of the chest wall
        (carcinoma en cuirasse)
Effect of therapy
    Postactinic fibrosis
    Postpneumectomy
    Mitomycin-vinca alkaloid (acute dyspnea syndrome)
        Bleomycin-induced fibrosis
            Adriamycin- and cyclophosphamide-induced
                cardiomyopathy
Not directly due to the tumor or therapy
    Anemia
    Cachexia
    Ascites
    Metabolic acidosis
    Muscle weakness (i.e., myasthenia gravis,
        Eaten Lambert)
    Rib fracture
    Fever
    Chest wall deformity
    COPD
    Asthma
    Pulmonary embolism
    Pneumonia
    Pneumothorax
    Heart failure
    Neuromuscolar disease (motoneurone disease)
    Obesity
    Thyrotoxicosis
    Psychosocial distress (i.e., anxiety, somatization)

[a]Many different causes may coexist in a patient.

## ASSESSMENT

Although most cancer patients develop dyspnea as a progressive complication over days or weeks, some patients present with sudden onset of dyspnea as an acute medical emergency. The management of the latter group always should be considered a medical emergency. In the following paragraphs, different methods for the assessment of the causes, intensity, and multidimensional assessment of dyspnea are discussed

### Causes of Dyspnea

As discussed above, dyspnea is frequently multicausal in patients with advanced cancer. The cause can be determined easily in most patients by taking an adequate history and physical examination. A chest radiograph, digital oximetry, and simple blood test can rule out another significant number of causes of dyspnea. Pulmonary function tests can be particularly useful in the assessment of obstructive and restrictive pulmonary disorders as well as neuromuscular weakness. These tests can be performed repeatedly at the bedside and are useful in assessing the response to different therapies, mostly bronchodilators.

### Role of Respiratory Muscles

During recent years, a number of authors have found that respiratory muscle weakness has an important role in the dyspnea associated with a number of chronic conditions. Palange et al. (18) found that malnutrition significantly affected the muscle aerobic capacity and exercise tolerance in patients with COPD, and they suggested that high-wasted ventilation might be responsible for the weight loss. Diaphragmatic fatigue has been associated with dyspnea in patients with COPD (19). In chronically malnourished patients without pulmonary disease, malnutrition reduces both respiratory muscle strength and maximal voluntary ventillation; therefore, malnutrition might impair the respiratory muscle capacity to handle increased ventilatory loads in cardiopulmonary disease (20). In normal volunteers, the sensation of dyspnea has been correlated with respiratory muscle fatigue (21).

A recent study in cancer patients determined that the maximal inspiratory pressure, a reliable functional test of the strength of the diaphragm and other respiratory muscles, is impaired severely in cancer patients with dyspnea (D. Dugdeon, personal communication). A number of authors have reported dyspnea in a significant percentage of advanced cancer patients without intrathoraxic malignancy. The National Hospice Study (13) found a prevalence of 24% in patients with no known lung or heart disease. Cachexia occurs in more than 80% of patients with advanced cancer (22). In addition, asthenia and electro-

physiological abnormalities in muscle function are detected in a large proportion of patients with advanced cancer. A recent study in 222 patients with chronic congestive heart failure found that dyspnea was the exercise-limiting symptom in 160 and generalized fatigue in 62 patients. No significant differences were found between any of the cardiovascular parameters of these two groups. The authors concluded that both symptoms are "two sides of the same coin," and they express the same underlying pathophysiological process (23). It is possible that in some patients with advanced cancer, dyspnea may be one clinical expression of the syndrome of overwhelming cachexia and asthenia that is highly prevalent in the comprehensive assessment of these patients, including frequent pulmonary function tests.

### Descriptors of Dyspnea

In the case of pain, specific descriptors are associated with specific pathophysiological syndromes (24). For example, burning or numb sensation traditionally has been associated with neuropathic pain. In many cases, the descriptor alone is enough to make a diagnosis and suggests the need for specific drug therapy. Simon et al. (25) attempted to associate specific descriptors with specific pathophysiology in 53 patients with dyspnea caused by a number of known causes. Patients were asked to choose descriptions of their sensation of breathlessness from a dyspnea questionnaire listing 19 descriptors (Table 23-2). Cluster analysis then was used to identify natural groupings among those descriptors. Although descriptors, such as "rapid" or "heavy," were associated with exercise, "tight" frequently was associated with asthma, and "suffocating" frequently was associated with congestive heart failure.

### Intensity of Dyspnea

As in the case of other symptoms, the expression of dyspnea can be assessed using visual analogue, numerical, and verbal scales (26–30). The intensity of dyspnea is assessed regularly in some of the available supportive care tools, such as the Support Team Assessment Schedule (STASS) (3) or the Edmonton Symptom Assessment System (ESAS) (30). Quality-of-life questionnaires, including the EORTC QL-30, have developed modules such as the lung cancer module, which allows for a more detailed assessment of the intensity of dyspnea (31).

In addition to these more general questionnaires, some specific dyspnea questionnaires have been developed. The chronic respiratory questionnaire (CRQ) was tested against a number of physical parameters in patients with COPD obstructive pulmonary disease (32–34). The Medical Research Council Scale has been tested in patients with dyspnea from a variety of respiratory and cardiovascular

**TABLE 2.** *Descriptor of breathlessness in relation to different cardiopulmonary diseases*

| Questionnaire | Vasc | Neuro | CHF | Inter | Asthma | COPD |
|---|---|---|---|---|---|---|
| My breath does not go in all the way | X | X | | | | |
| My breathing requires effort | | X | X | X | | X |
| I feel that I am smothering | | | X | | X | X |
| I feel a hunger for more air | | | X | | | X |
| My breathing is heavy | | X | X | | X | X |
| I cannot take a deep breath | | | | | X | |
| I feel out of breath | | X | X | X | | X |
| My chest feels tight | | | | X | | |
| My breathing requires more work | | X | | X | | X |
| I feel that I am suffocating | | | X | | | |
| I feel that my breath stops | | | | | | |
| I am gasping for breath | | X | | X | | X |
| My chest is constricted | | | | | X | |
| I feel that my breath is rapid | X | | X | | | |
| My breathing is shallow | | X | | X | | |
| I feel that I am breathing more | | | | | | |
| I cannot get enough air | | | X | | | X |
| My breath does not go out all the way | | | | | X | |
| My breathing requires more concentration | | | | | X | |

Vasc, pulmonary vascular disease; Neuro, neuromuscular and chest wall disease; CHF, chronic heart failure; Inters, interstitial lung disease; COPD, chronic obstructive pulmonary disease.
Modified from Simon et al. (25)

origins (35,36). Mahler et al. (37) compared the MRC scale with a recently developed baseline dyspnea index (BDI) and the oxygen cause diagram (OCD) in 153 patients with various respiratory illnesses who sought medical care because of dyspnea. The authors found correlation between all the dyspnea scores (R = 0.48–0.70, $p<$ 0.001). Agreement between two observers or with repeated use was satisfactory with all three clinical rating methods.

The Borg Category Scale (28,38) originally was developed for rating perceived exertion during exercise. It consists of 15 grades, with numbers ranging from 6 to 20. A more recent modification revised the numbers from 0 to 10, and the verbal descriptors are placed so that doubling the numerical rating corresponds to a twofold increase in sensation intensity.

In addition to these scales, a number of other specific scales have been developed during recent years (39,40). In summary, a large number of scales are available for assessment of the intensity of dyspnea. They range from simple analogue and numerical scales to more complex scales, including multiple items. All these scales were validated adequately and are highly reproducible.

One of the main problems associated with assessment of dyspnea is the variable intensity of this symptom according to the level of activity and even spontaneously during different moments of the day. A similar problem was observed with a subset of patients experiencing pain. This syndrome has been known as *incidental pain* (41,42). The variation in intensity of dyspnea over time makes pharmacological and nonpharmacological symptomatic interventions difficult to assess. In respiratory and cardiovascular populations, one approach to this problem has been the performance of dyspnea-causing activities to be able to compare therapeutic interventions (43,44). Mostly, these interventions consist of progressive exercising on a treadmill or bicycle so that patients or volunteers are subjected to a predictable workload. Dyspnea then is measured at fixed intervals and expressed in relationship to the workload. Unfortunately, most cancer patients are too ill to participate in these stress tests. One potential less invasive approach to the production of dyspnea would be breathholding (45,46), which has been used successfully in volunteers and patients to assess different mechanisms of dyspnea and should be validated prospectively for the assessment of cancer dyspnea.

**Multidimensional Assessment**

Although some researchers have described a good correlation between the abnormality of pulmonary function tests and the intensity of subjective dyspnea (37), other authors found this correlation to be extremely poor (40). In some cases, the authors suggested that the lack of correlation between objective and subjective findings might be due to underlying psychiatric disorders in some of the patients (11).

Figure 2 shows the different stages in the production of dyspnea. Neither the production nor perception of dyspnea can be measured. Expression of the intensity of dyspnea can be influenced by a number of factors described in the figure and should not be interpreted as a direct representation of the intensity of production of dyspnea at the level of mechanoreceptors or chemoreceptors. Whereas the level of glucose in a diabetic patient or the level of blood pressure in a hypertensive patient is generally assumed to be a direct expression of underlying pathophysiological mechanism, dyspnea should be interpreted as a multidimensional construct in which the intensity described by a given patient is a result of the interaction of different factors. Figure 23-3 summarizes the different components in the intensity of dyspnea for a 38-year-old man with advanced carcinoma of the lung. This patient had dyspnea caused by progressive lung disease. The patient's expression of dyspnea (as expressed in a visual analogue scale) summarized the combination of progressive lung cancer plus somatization due to clinical depression and poor use of his energy by trying to be continuously physically active. A unidimensional interpretation of this symptom would have resulted in excessive pharmacological intervention with limited therapeutic success. Instead, a multidimensional assessment identified the need for a combined approach using symptomatic therapy with opioids, antidepressant treatment, and occupational therapy for energy conservation. Determination of the relative contribution of each dimension to the overall symptom expression can be estimated only by disciplined assessment that includes all the relevant dimensions. At this point, it will be possible to plan the therapeutic approach for a given patient in a multidimensional manner.

## TREATMENT

As previously discussed, there are numerous causes of dyspnea in patients with cancer. Many different mechanisms may coexist in a given patient, and adequate planning of treatment can take place only after a comprehensive diagnostic approach, including a number of ancillary

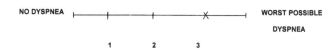

1. **Locally Advanced Carcinoma + Pleural Effusion**
2. **Major Depression Episode → Somatization**
3. **Excessive Activity → Poor Energy Conservation**

**FIG. 3.** Components of the dyspnea compiled in a 38-year-old man with lung cancer.

tests. Treatment dividing the approach between those therapies aimed to modifying a specific pathophysiologic cause and those therapies aimed to provide general symptom control will be discussed in the following section.

### Specific Treatments

Table 1 summarizes the different causes of dyspnea. Several studies have shown that dyspnea is more prevalent among cancer patients with thoracic malignancy, including primary or metastatic cancer in both lungs or the pleural space. Whenever possible, the attempt should be made to treat the underlying malignancy. Unfortunately, most malignancies capable of involving the thoracic space show only a limited response to antineoplastic therapy. Occasionally, treatments or radiation therapy for masses causing bronchial obstruction or a superior vena cava syndrome can bring prompt relief of dyspnea.

#### Superior Vena Cava

The superior vena cava syndrome occurs when there is compression, sometimes accompanied by thrombosis of the large central veins at the upper mediastinum. This syndrome most often is due to lung cancer, although it can also be seen in lymphoma, breast cancer, and other solid tumors. Radiation therapy, usually accompanied by high-dose corticosteroids, can have spectacular symptomatic effects (47,48).

#### Carcinomatous Lymphangitis

Carcinomatous lymphangitis is characterized by the development of severe and continuous dyspnea accompanied by minimal physical findings. This condition most frequently is associated with lung, breast, gastrointestinal, or prostatic carcinoma (49). The radiographic appearance is that of linear infiltrates emerging from the hilar region similar to butterfly wings. These infiltrates may be accompanied by other manifestations of cancer, such as the presence of a large primary tumor, micronodules, or a plural effusion. Although occasionally patients may be candidates for aggressive chemotherapy and show excellent response, most patients with these syndromes present with poorly responsive cancer. High-dose corticosteroids have been suggested to bring prompt, although short-acting, relief.

#### Pleural Effusions

Although most carcinomas have been reported to be capable of metastasizing into the pleural space, lung cancer is the most common cause of malignant pleural effusion, followed by breast, ovarian, and gastric carcinomas.

Lymphomas account for about 10% of all malignant pleural effusions (50). The response to antineoplastic treatments may vary according to the primary tumor, but prompt relief will be achieved in most patients by pleural tapping. Some evidence suggests that thoracentesis can be effective in relieving symptoms even when relatively small volumes are drained (51), probably because this relief results primarily from the reduction in the size of the thoracic cage, thereby allowing the respiratory muscles to operate on a more advantageous portion of their length-dimension curve. In patients in whom repeated pleural effusions are needed, the ideal management is chest tube drainage with installation of a fibrotic agent. Tetracycline hydrocloride appears to be the agent of choice because of its high success rate and minimum toxicity (50).

### Pericardial Effusion

Pericardial effusion is considered a life-threatening emergency. Lung cancer is also the most common cause of severe pericardial effusions. Patients present with decreased cardiac output and severe dyspnea. The specific treatment consists of the creation of a pericardial window. This is a surgical procedure and should be attempted after individualized consideration of the symptomatic advantage of the procedure versus the discomfort of an operation (52–54).

### Cardiovascular Complications

Patients with advanced cancer are at an increased risk for thromboembolic complications, including pulmonary embolism (55). These patients usually respond rapidly to parenteral anticoagulation. Other cardiovascular complications, including congestive heart failure, may occur as a consequence of other risk factors, such as smoking and the toxic effects of certain treatments, including some antineoplastic agents and radiation therapy to the mediastinum, including the heart.

### Chronic Obstructive Pulmonary Disease

Patients with lung cancer and other malignancies, including head and neck tumors, are frequently heavy smokers and have a history of COPD (56). These patients may present with episodes of decompensation of their illness requiring broncodilators, corticosteroids, or antibiotics. Adequate pulmonary function tests and radiological examination should be performed to provide adequate therapy that might result in significant improvement of the symptoms.

### Infections

Infections are responsible for the death of almost half of patients with advanced cancer (57). Lung cancer is the sight of infection in more than half of these patients. When pneumonia is suspected as the cause of sudden onset of dyspnea, adequate antibiotic therapy can bring rapid, definite relief.

### Other Conditions Associated With Dyspnea

In addition to the aforementioned causes, patients may present with severe anaemia, massive ascites, an acute exacerbation of chronic asthma or acute panic attacks as part of a chronic panic disorder, characterized by hyperventilation. Occasionally, metabolic acidosis associated with acute renal failure or lactic acidosis can result in hyperventilation. All these conditions should be considered part of the assessment of a patient with dyspnea and advanced cancer because specific therapy might result in rapid symptom relief.

## Symptomatic Treatment

Symptomatic management of dyspnea is based on three main elements: oxygen therapy, drug therapy, and general measures of support and counselling. Some evidence for the role of these three therapeutic approaches are discussed in subsequent paragraphs. For the purpose of this review, a Medline search of the literature on dyspnea published between 1966 and 1995 was conducted. All studies relating to the symptomatic therapy of dyspnea were reviewed. Studies were classified according to their methodology in three levels of evidence (58).

### Oxygen

Long-term oxygen therapy has beneficial effects on the outcome of patients with chronic obstructive pulmonary disease (59,60); however, the symptomatic effects of this therapy are less clear. Some hospice tests suggest that oxygen has no symptomatic effects in cancer dyspnea (61,62). In addition, the evidence for a symptomatic effect of oxygen in patients with congestive heart failure is also controversial.

Table 23-3 summarizes studies that have addressed the use of oxygen for symptom relief in a number of conditions. Only studies with level 1 evidence (randomized controlled trials) are included in this chapter.

In the case of COPD, most studies suggest that there is a significant symptomatic improvement both at rest and during exercise as a result of the administration of supplemental oxygen (63–66). Liss and Grant (67), however, found that the administration of 0, 2, or 4 liters per minute of oxygen was not superior to air on resting dyspnea of patients with COPD. These authors also found a significant increase in breathlessness after nasal anesthesia with lidocaine. The authors suggested that the reduction in

**TABLE 3.** *The symptomatic effect of oxygen therapy*

| Author (ref) | No. of patients | Dose O2 | Disease | Findings | Level of evidence |
|---|---|---|---|---|---|
| Bruera et al. (70) | 14 | O$_2$ 5 L/min or air | Ca, O$_2$* | + | I |
| Bruera et al. (71) | 1 | O$_2$ 5 L/min or air | Ca, O$_2$* | + | I (no. of one) |
| Swinburn et al. (63) | 10 | O$_2$ 28% 4 L/min or air | ILD | + | I |
| | 12 | | COPD | + | |
| Liss et al. (67) | 8 | O$_2$ 4 L/min or air | COPD | − | I |
| Davidson et al. (64) | 17 | 4 L/min or air | COPD | + | I |
| Woodcock et al. (65) | 10 | O$_2$ 4 L/min or air | COPD | + | I |
| Dean et al. (66) | 12 | O$_2$ 40% or air | COPD | + | I |
| Moore et al. (68) | 12 | O$_2$ of 30% or 50% or air | CHF | + | I |
| Restrick et al. (69) | 12 | O$_2$ 2 L/min or air | CHF | − | I |

*Cancer hypoxemia.
+Effective.
−Not effective.

breathlessness caused by nasal oxygen is a placebo effect caused by wearing the nasal canula and is unrelated to gas flow or the increase of arterial oxygen tension.

In the case of congestive heart failure, one study found that supplemental oxygen could improve subjective scores for fatigue and breathlessness during steady-state exercise (68). Another study, however, found no significant symptomatic benefit from supplemental oxygen on the symptomatic scores of patients subjected to regular walking (69).

Although the balance of evidence suggests that oxygen does have symptomatic effects in COPD and also probably in congestive heart failure, patients with dyspnea due to cancer have most frequently restrictive respiratory failure that might not respond to oxygen in the same way. There are only two randomized controlled trials in which patients with cancer dyspnea were randomized in a crossover design to 5 liters per minute of oxygen or 5 liters per minute of air. In this population of hypoxemic patients, oxygen had a significant symptomatic effect (70,71). Swinburn et al. (63) studied a group of 10 patients with interstitial lung disease in addition to their main sample of 12 patients with COPD (63). Results in their interstitial lung disease patients were as beneficial as those observed in the COPD group.

In summary, although more research is badly needed in this area, there is some compelling evidence for the use of oxygen as a symptomatic treatment of patients with cancer-related dyspnea. Patients who are hypoxemic on room air are quite likely to benefit from this approach. The mechanism of oxygen in these patients is probably a decrease in the chemoreceptor input to the respiratory center and the brain cortex.

It is possible that oxygen would be effective in relieving dyspnea at concentrations higher than those required to maintain optimal saturation of hemoglobin. Anecdotal experience in cancer patients and patients with congestive heart failure suggest that oxygen might give significant symptom relief to patients who are not hypoxemic. This hypothesis could be tested in prospective clinical trials.

When there are doubts about the effectiveness of oxygen for symptom relief in a given patient, particularly when oxygen therapy may be a major problem for a simple and rapid home discharge, an "N of 1" study can be conducted (71). By performing multiple double-blind crossovers between oxygen and air, it is possible to determine with great accuracy in less than an hour whether a specific patient does or does not benefit from the supplemental oxygen.

### Drug Therapy

A number of drugs have been suggested to affect the intensity of dyspnea in patients with cancer and other chronic conditions. The following sections describe those drugs for which more than a single anecdotal report can be found in the literature.

### Opioids

Table 23-4 summarizes studies on the use of opioids in the treatment of dyspnea associated with a number of nonmalignant conditions (72–79). Table 23-5 summarizes studies of systemic opioids in the treatment of cancer-related dyspnea. Most studies found that opioids of different types, doses, and routes of administration are capable of relieving dyspnea (80–83).

In the case of COPD, all the single-dose or short-term studies were positive. Rice et al. (77) reported that four of 11 patients in a 1-month study of codeine dropped out, mostly because of drowsiness. Woodcock et al. (84) attempted long-term therapy with opioids; results were disappointing, mostly as a result of poor patient compliance because of central toxicity and constipation. Problems such as those reported by these authors could be of less relevance in the case of advanced cancer patients, as 80% of these patients already are receiving opioids chronically for the management of cancer pain with minimal side effects.

**TABLE 4.** *Use of opoids in nonmalignant conditions*

| Author (ref) | No. of patients | Opioid | Disease | Study | Level of evidence | Effect on dyspnea | Assessment |
|---|---|---|---|---|---|---|---|
| Browning et al. (72) | 7 | Hydrocodone oral 20 mg m$^2$/day or placebo | COPD | Acute | I | + | VAS |
| Woodcock et al. (73) | 12 | Dihydrocodeine 1 mg/kg (oral) | COPD | Acute | I | + | VAS |
| Johnson et al. (74) | 18 | Dihydrocodeine oral 15 mg 3 times/day or placebo | COPD | 3 weeks | I | + | VAS |
| Robin and Burke (75) | 1 | Hydromorphone suppositories 3 mg 3–4 times/day | COPD | Acute | I n of one | + | Categorical scale |
| Eiser et al. (76) | 4 | Oral diamorphine 2.5 or 5 or 7.5 mg6 hourly or placebo | COPD | 2 weeks | I | − | VAS |
| Rice et al. (77) | 11 | Codeine 30 mg 4 times a day or promethazine 25 mg 4 times/day | COPD | 1 mo | I | + | VAS |
| Light et al. (78) | 13 | 0.8 mg/kg oral morphine or placebo | COPD | Acute | I | + | Borg scale |
| Sackner (79) | 17, 8 | Hydrocodone 5 mg (oral) | COPD | Acute | III | + | Not reported |

VAS,

In the case of cancer-related dyspnea, all the published studies have agreed on the beneficial effect of systemic opioids for cancer dyspnea; however, the optimal type, dose, and modality of administration of opioids has not yet been determined. In addition, the toxicity of systemic opioids for cancer dyspnea is also unclear. Cohen et al. (82) treated eight patients with cancer dyspnea with continuous intravenous morphine. Significant symptomatic relief was observed, but the authors found that in this population of patients with no previous exposure to morphine, the continuous intravenous infusion resulted in a significant increase in the levels of PCO$_2$. On the other hand, Bruera et al. (80,81) conducted two trials using intermittent subcutaneous morphine for the relief of cancer dyspnea. In the first study (81), intermittent doses of up to 2.5 times the regular opioid dose resulted in no significant change in the end-tidal CO$_2$ level in these patients. This result may have been because most of these patients already had been chronically exposed to opioids and therefore had developed tolerance to their respiratory depressant effects.

One of the main methodological problems in the design of clinical trials of opioids in cancer dyspnea is the changing intensity of dyspnea both spontaneously and as a result of definite maneuvers. For these reasons, some groups advocate the use of intermittent opioids as needed when dyspnea occurs or for the anticipation of dyspnea associated with specific maneuvers. This recommendation contrasts with to the commonly recommended approach for the management of cancer-related pain in which regular administration is proposed. It would be consistent, however, with the current approach to incidental pain (pain of minimal intensity while the patient is resting and of moderate or severe intensity

**TABLE 5.** *Use of systemic opioids in the treatment of cancer-related dyspnea*

| Author (ref) | No. of patients | Opioid drug | Daily dose | Disease | Study | Level of evidence | Assessment | Findings |
|---|---|---|---|---|---|---|---|---|
| Bruera et al. (80) | 10 | Morphine SC | 50% higher than regular scheduled dose | Terminal cancer | Acute | I | VAS | + |
| Bruera et al. (81) | 20 | Morphine SC | 5 mg bolus or 2.5 of the regular dose | Terminal cancer | Acute | III | VAS | + |
| Cohen et al. (82) | 8 | Morphine IV bolus, bolus-continuous | 5.6 mg/h (mean dose) | Terminal cancer | Acute | III | Categorical scale | + |
| Ventafridda et al. (83) | 5 | Morphine SC, Chlorpromazine SC | 10 mg 25 mg | Terminal cancer | Acute | III | VAS | + |

when the patient preforms the pain-causing maneuver) (41,42).

*Nebulized Opioids.* During recent years, a number of authors reported symptomatic relief when patients are administered different types and doses of nebulized opioids (summarized in Table 23-6) (85–88). The possibility that opioids might affect receptors in the lung is exciting because of recent evidence suggesting that morphine does have an analgesic effect peripherally (89) and also because a small dose of nebulized morphine might be devoid of the systemic side effects of opioids.

Pharmacokinetic studies suggest that the systemic bioavaliability of nebulized morphine is extremely poor (90). Therefore, the effects reported in most studies would have to be of a local nature. This is further supported by the lack of reports of side effects usually observed when morphine is administered systemically, such as sedation and nausea.

The evidence for a symptomatic effect in patients with COPD is controversial. Two controlled studies suggested a positive effect, in one case for morphine (86) and another case for morphine-6-glucuronide (85). Morphine was ineffective in two different studies (85,87).

The largest uncontrolled study in cancer patients reported beneficial results (88). A recently completed controlled trial in patients with cancer dyspnea currently in preparation showed no symptomic benefit for nebulized morphine compared with placebo (91).

### Benzodiazepines

Benzodiazepines are commonly used in the management of cancer- related dyspnea. Several textbooks on this subject also have been recommended as symptomatic therapy.

Table 23-7 summarizes studies in which benzodaiazepines were used for the management of dyspnea asso-

ciated with both exercise and COPD (92–96). Four of the five studies found no significant difference between benzodiazepines and placebo. Mitchell-Hepp et al. (96) studied four patients with COPD in a controlled, single, blind study comparing diazepam and placebo. The authors reported a sustained benefit for three of four patients after diazepam.

In some patients, benzodiazipines may be used when dyspnea is considered to be a somatic manifestation of a panic disorder or when patients have coexistence severe anxiety; however, both conditions are infrequent in patients with advanced cancer. Therefore, there is no evidence for the regular use of benzodiazepines in the management of dyspnea.

### Corticosteroids

A number of authors have suggested that these drugs are highly effective in the management of dyspnea associated with carcinomatous lymphangitis; however, we are not aware of randomized controlled trials testing their role in this condition. In addition, corticosteroids are used frequently in the management of superior vena cava syndrome, and they are highly effective in treating bronchospasms associated with both asthma and COPD (97,98). On the other hand, evidence exists that corticosteroids induce functional and pathologic alterations in several muscle groups (99). It has been suggested that the effects are more pronounced on the diaphragm than on other muscles. These findings might be important because of the frequent presence of cachexia and muscle weakness in patients with advanced cancer.

### Bronchodilators

Both nebulized and orally administered bronchodilators are useful in the management of bronchospasms

**TABLE 6.** *Nebulized opioids*

| Author (ref) | No. of patients | Drug | Disease | Level of evidence | Findings | Assessment |
|---|---|---|---|---|---|---|
| Davis et al. (85) | 18 | Morphine 12.5 mg or M-6-glucuronide 4 mg or placebo | COPD | I | – + – | Objective measurements |
| Young et al. (86) | 11 | Morphine 5 mg/ 5 ml in 12 min or placebo | COPD | I | + | At end of test each patient was asked about his or her limiting symptoms |
| Beauford et al. (87) | 8 | 1, 4, or 10 mg morphine or placebo | COPD | I | – | VAS & objective measurement |
| Francombe et al. (88) | 40 | 34 patients morphine 5–30 mg/4 h; 17 patients hydromorphone 1–20 mg/4 h; | Cancer, | III | 34 patients + 12 stopped after 1 & 2 doses; | Not described |
| | | 2 patients codeine 15–60 mg/4 h; 1 patient anileridine 25–50 mg/4 h | COPD | | 8 conflicting reports on charts | |

**TABLE 7.** *Effect of psychotropic drugs in the treatment of dyspnea*

| Author (ref) | No. of patients | Opioid drug | Daily dose | Disease | Study | Level of evidence | Effect of dyspnea |
|---|---|---|---|---|---|---|---|
| Stark et al. (92) | 6 | Diazepam | 10 mg | Exercise | Acute | I | − |
| | | Promethazine | 25 mg | | | | − |
| O'Neill et al. (93) | 12 | Promethazine & placebo | 25 mg | Exercise | | | − |
| | | | | | | | − |
| | 6 | Mebhydrolin or placebo (histamine antagonist) | 50 mg | Exercise | Acute | I | − |
| | 6 | Chlorpromazine or placebo | 25 mg | Exercise | | | + |
| Woodcock et al. (94) | 15 | Diazepam | 25 mg | COPD | 2 weeks | I | − |
| | | Promethazine | 125 mg | | | | + |
| Man et al. (95) | 24 | Alprazolam or placebo | 0.5 mg b.i.d. | COPD | 3 weeks | I | − |
| Mitchell-Heggs et al. (96) | 4 | Diazepam | 25 mg | COPD | Acute | I | + |

associated with both asthma and COPD (97). A large proportion of the patients with cancer-related dyspnea have a history of smoking or COPD. Congleton and Muers (56) recently demonstrated that almost half of 57 consecutive patients with lung cancer treated by their group had evidence of airflow obstruction. A strong association was found between airflow obstruction and dyspnea. Only four of the 57 patients were receiving bronchodilators. Of the 17 patients who accepted the offer of a trial of bronchodilator therapy, most experienced significant symptomatic improvement. The authors concluded that untreated airflow obstruction is commonly present in patients with bronchial carcinoma and is strongly associated with breathlessness. These patients may benefit from simple broncodilator treatment. Bronchodilators were underused in this population. In their study, the bronchodilator therapy included a combination of nebulized adrenergic and anticholinergic agents four times a day.

Previous studies suggested that some patients with nonreversible obstructive airway disease can improve from the administration of theophylline (100). Aminophylline, theophylline, and caffeine all improve diaphragmatic contractility both in normal volunteers (100–102) and in patients with COPD (103).

Because of the frequent presence of asthenia and generalized muscle weakness with or without cachexia (22), some cancer patients might benefit from the effect of xanthines on respiratory muscle contractility. This hypothesis should be tested in prospective clinical trials.

### Other Drugs

Several studies suggested that alcohol may be able to decrease the intensity of dyspnea in patients with COPD (73,104). Although there is some consistent evidence for a symptomatic effect for alcohol, the side effects associated with both acute and chronic administration, in addi-

tion to the potentially dangerous interaction with drugs frequently used in cancer patients, including opioid analgesics, suggest that alcohol may be an impractical option for the control of cancer-related dyspnea. A number of drugs, such as indomethocin (105), medroxyprogesterone (106), acetate, and nebulized furosemide (107), are being studied as a potential treatment for dyspnea, but the evidence for a role of these and other agents is very limited, and they could not be recommended for clinical use.

### General Support Measures

A number of measures can be implemented for the support of both the patient and the family. Most of these measures can be implemented in the acute care hospital setting, continuing care hospitals, and at home.

### Activity Level

Dyspnea is a variable symptom. Most of the aggravating factors are related to muscle effort associated with different physical activities. It is important to educate patients and families so that they can recognize the type of manoeuvres associated with episodes of increased dyspnea. Once these manoeuvres are recognized, the two most effective approaches are anticipatory symptom relief and avoidance. Anticipatory relief can include the administration of doses of symptomatic drugs including opioids 30 to 45 minutes before the dyspnea-causing manoeuvre. It may also include phycological support techniques such as relaxation or imaginary in order to decrease the anticipatory components associated with this symptom.

Avoidance implies assisting the patient to the maximum with the manoeuvre in order to minimize the muscle effort and the consequent development of dyspnea. This includes the use of different devices in order to assist the patient with transportation to and from the bathroom and mobilization. This is important for patients and families to understand that they can remain quite active while not necessarily making muscle efforts. With the use of wheelchairs and portable oxygen it is possible for patients to return to the community.

### Ventilatory Support

The role of traditional physiotherapy techniques, including postural drainage and incontinuespirometry, are well established in the management of respiratory complications. This should be established early and maintained during the trajectory of illness (108).

In patients with severe neuromuscular disorders, positive pressure ventilation provides significant relief for respiratory muscle fatigue. The main techniques available are continuous positive pressure ventilation or intermittent positive pressure ventilation. These techniques can be administered by face or nasal masks. By providing respiratory muscle relief, these techniques can decrease the sensation of breathlessness both at rest and during exercise. The recognition of progressive muscle weakness in cancer patients and its possible association with dyspnea suggest that some patients in whom respiratory muscle weakness can be demonstrated possibly could benefit from positive pressure ventilation delivered via a face mask.

### Support of the Patient and Family

Dyspnea can elicit major psychological reactions on both the patient and the family, both of whom may fear choking to death by the patient. It is important to anticipate the possibility of a crisis of respiratory failure. Symptomatic drugs should be made available together with instructions for administration. Telephone numbers of persons to be contacted also should be made available. Even if patients are not requiring oxygen at a given time, it is important that oxygen be available immediately if a respiratory crisis occurs.

Because dyspnea frequently is associated with tachypnea and the use of accesory respiratory muscles, patients may appear to be significantly dyspneic even when they are in good symptom control. It is important for the relatives and members of the staff to remember to assess dyspnea only by asking patients how short of breath they feel rather than by estimating their dyspnea from the degree of tachypnea and use of auxiliary muscles. It is not uncommon that patients who have moderate to severe tachypnea will not complain of respiratory distress. In contrast, patients who are not tachypneic may report severe dyspnea. The goal should be symptomatic therapeutic intervention of the patient's expression of dyspnea rather relief of the objective variables that accompany this symptom.

## REFERENCES

1. Ahmedzai S. Palliation of respiratory symptoms. In: D. Doyle, GWC Hanks, N. MacDonald, eds. *Oxford Textbook of Palliative Medicine.* Oxford: Oxford University Press 1993; 4.4:349–378.
2. Cowcher K, Hanks GW. Long-term management of respiratory symptoms in advanced cancer. *J Pain Sympt Manag* 1990;5:320–330.
3. Higginson I, McCarthy M. Measuring symptoms in terminal cancer: are pain and dyspnoea controlled? *J Royal Society Med* 1989;82:264–267.
4. Baines M. Control of other symptoms. In: CM Saunders, ed.3 *The Management of Terminal Disease.* Chicago: Year Book, 1978.
5. Wasserman K, Casaburi R. Dyspnea: physiological and pathophysiological mechanisms. *Ann Rev Med* 1988;39:503–515.
6. Tobin MJ. Dyspnea: pathophysiologic basis, clinical presentations and management. *Arch Intern Med* 1990;150:1604–1613.
7. Opie LH, Smith AC, Spalding JMK. Conscious appreciation of the effects produced by independent changes of ventilation volume and of end-tidal $pCO_2$ in paralysed patients. *J Physiol (Lond)* 1959;149:494–499.
8. Castele RJ, Connors AF, Altose MD. Effects of changes in $CO_2$ partial pressure on the sensation of respiratory drive. *Appl Physiol J* 1985;59:1747–1757.
9. Altose MA. Dyspnea. In: DH Simmons, ed. *Current Pulmonology,* Chicago: Ill Year Book Medical Publishers Inc 1986;7:199–226.
10. Rubinfeld AR, Pain MCF. Perception of asthma. *Lancet* 1976;882–884.
11. Burns BH, Howell JBL. Disproportionately severe breathlessness in chronic bronchitis. *Quart J Med* 1969;151:277–294.
12. Fainsinger R, Bruera E. Case report: assessment of total pain. *Perspectives in Pain Management* 1991;13–14.
13. Reuben DB, Mor V. Dyspnea in terminally ill cancer patients. *Chest* 1986;89:234–236.
14. Grond S, Zech D, Diefenbach C, et al. Prevalence and pattern of symptoms in patients with cancer pain: a prospective evaluation of 1635 cancer patients referred to a pain clinic. *J Pain Sympt Manag* 1994;9:372–82.
15. Donnelly S, Walsh D. The symptoms of advanced cancer: identification of clinical and research priorities by assessment of prevalence and severity. *J Palliat Care* 1995;11:27–32.
16. Twycross RG, Lack SA. *Control of alimentary symptoms in far advanced cancer.* Edinburgh: Churchill Livingstone 1986.
17. Muers MF. Palliation of symptoms in non-small cell lung cancer: a study by the Yorkshire Regional Cancer Organization Thoraxic Group. *Thorax* 1993;48:339–343.
18. Palange P, Forte S, Felli A, et al. Nutritional state and exercise tolerance in patients with COPD*. *Chest* 1995;107:1206–1212.
19. Kongragunta VR, Druz WS, Sharp JT. Dyspnea and diaphragmatic fatigue in patients with chronic obstructive pulmonary disease. *Am Rev Respir Dis* 1988;137:662–667.
20. Arora NS, Rochester DF. Respiratory muscle strength and maximal voluntary ventilation in undernourished patients. *Am Rev Respir Dis* 1982;126:5–8.
21. Ward ME, Eidelman D, Stubbing DG, et al. Respiratory sensation and pattern of respiratory muscle activation during diaphragm fatigue. *Am Physiol Soc* 1988;2181–2189.
22. Bruera E. Clinical management of cachexia and anorexia in patients with advanced cancer. *Oncology* 1992;49(Suppl 2):35–42.
23. Clark AL, Sparrow JL, Coats AJS. Muscle fatigue and dyspnoea in chronic heart failure: two sides of the same coin? *Eur Heart J* 1995;16:49–52.
24. Foley K. The treatment of cancer pain. *N Engl J Med* 1985;313:84–95.
25. Simon PM, Schwartzstein RM, Weiss JW, et al. Distinguishable types of dyspnea in patients with shortness of breath. *Am Rev Respir Dis* 1990;142:1009–1014.
26. Aitken RCB. Measurement of feelings using viual analogue scales. *Proc R Soc Med* 1969;62:989–993.
27. Mador MJ, Kufel TJ. Reproducibility of visual analogue scale measurements of dyspnea in patients with chronic obstructive pulmonary disease. *Am Rev Respir Dis* 1992;146:82–87.
28. Borg GAV. Psychophysicial bases of perceived exertion. *Med Sci Sports Exerc* 1982;14:377–387.

29. Wilson RC, Jones PW. A comparison of the visual analogue scale and modified Borg scale for the measurement of dyspnea during exercise. *Clin Sci* 1989;76:277–282.

30. Bruera E, Kuehn N, Miller MJ, et al. The Edmonton symptom assessment system (ESAS): a simple method for the assessment of palliative care patients. *J Palliat Care* 1991;7:6–9.

31. Bergman B, Aarouson NK, Ahmedzai S, et al. The EORTC QLQ-LC13: a modular supplement to the EORTC Core Quality of Life Questionnaire (QLQ-C30) for use in lung cancer clinical trials. EORTC Study Group on Quality of Life. *Eur J Cancer* 1994;30A:635–642.

32. Guyatt GH, Townsend M, Keller J, et al. Measuring functional status in chronic lung disease: conclusions from a randomized control trial. *Resp Med* 1991;85(Suppl B):17–21.

33. Wijkstra PJ, Ten Vergert EM, Van Altena R, et al. Reliability and validity of the chronic respiratory questionnaire. *Thorax* 1994;49:465–467.

34. Guyatt GH, Berman LB, Towsend M, et al. A measure of quality of life for clinical trials in chronic lung disease. *Thorax* 1987; 42:773–778.

35. Medical Research Council Committee on research into chronic bronchitis: instruction for use on the questionnaire on respiratory symptoms. Devon: W.J. Holman, 1966.

36. Mahler DA, Wells CK. Evaluation of clinical methods for rating dyspnea. *Chest* 1988;93:580–586.

37. Mahler DA, Rosiello RA, Harver A, et al. Comparison of clinical dyspnea ratings and psychophysical measurements of respiratory sensation in obstructive airway disease. *Am Rev Respir Dis* 1987;135:1229–1233.

38. Mador MJ, Rodis A, Magalang UJ. Reproducibility of Borg scale measurements of dyspnea during exercise in patients with COPD. *Chest* 1995;107:1590–1597.

39. Mahler DA, Weinberg DH, Wells CK, et al. The measurement of dyspnea. Contents, interobserver agreement, and physiologic correlates of two new clinical indexes. *Chest* 1984;85:751–758.

40. Stoller JK, Ferranti R, Feinstein AR. Further specification and evaluation of a new clinical index for dyspnea. *Am Rev Respir Dis* 1986; 134:1129–1134.

41. Portenoy RK, Hagen NA. Breakthrough pain: definition, prevalence and characteristics. *Pain* 1990;41:273–281.

42. Bruera E, Macmillan K, Hanson J, et al. The Edmonton staging system for cancer pain: preliminary report. *Pain* 1989;37:203–209.

43. Morgan A. Simple exercise testing. *Respir Med* 1989;83:383–387.

44. El-Manshawi A, Killian KJ, Summers E, et al. Breathlessness during exercise with and without resistive boading. *J Appl Physiol* 1986;61: 896–905.

45. Taskar V, Clayton N, Atkins M, et al. Breathholding time in normal subjects, snorers, and sleep apnea patients. *Chest* 1995;107:959–962.

46. Nunn JF. Control of breathing: breathholding. In: *Applied respiratory physiology*. 2nd ed. London: Butterworth 1977;95–99.

47. Varricchio C. Clinical management of superior vena cava syndrome. *Heart Lung* 1985;14:411–416.

48. Adelstein DJ, Hines JD, Carter SG, et al. Thromboembolic events in patients with malignant superior vena cava syndrome and the role of anticoagulation. *Cancer* 1988;62:2258–2262.

49. Mestitz H, Pierce RJ, Holmes PW. Intrathoracic manifestation of disseminated prostatic adenocarcinoma. *Respir Med* 1989;83:161–166.

50. Sahn SA. Malignant pleural effusions. *Seminars Respir Med* 1987; 9:43–52.

51. Estenne MC, Vernault JC, De Troyer A. Mechanism of relief of dyspnea after thoracocentesis in patients with pleural effusions. *Am J Med* 1983;74:813–819.

52. Findlay IN. Cardiac complications of malignant disease. In: SB Kay, EM Rankin, eds. *Medical Complications of Malignant Disease*, London: Bailliere Tindall, 1988;283–317.

53. Press OW, Livingston R. Management of malignant pleural effusion and tamponade. *JAMA* 1987;257:1088–1092.

54. Mauch PM, Ullmann JE. Treatment of malignant pericardial effusions. In: VT De Vita, S Hellman, SA Rosenberg, eds. Cancer, *Principles and Practice of Oncology*. Philadelphia: JB Lippincott, 1985; 2141–2144.

55. Kvale PA. Editorial. The cancer patient with dyspnea: unusual cause? *Mayo Clin Proc* 1991;66:215–218.

56. Congleton J, Muers MF. The incidence of airflow obstruction in bronchial carcinoma, its relation to breathlessness, and response to bronchodilator therapy. *Respir Med* 1995;89:291–296.

57. Pizzo PA, Meyers J, Freifeld AG, et al. Infections in the cancer patient. In: VT DeVita, S. Hellman, SA Rosenberg, eds, *Cancer, Principles and Practice of Oncology*, 4th Ed. Philadelphia: JB Lippincott, 1993;2:2292–2337.

58. Cook DJ, Guyatt GH, Laupacis A, et al. Rules of evidence and clinical recommendations on the use of antithrombotic agents. *Chest* 1992; 102:205S–311S.

59. Anthonisen NR. Long-term oxygen therapy. *Ann Intern Med* 1983; 99:519–527.

60. Nocturnal Oxygen Therapy Trial Group. Continuous or nocturnal oxygen therapy in hypoxemic chronic obstructive lung disease. *Ann Int Med* 1980;93:391–398.

61. Billings JA. The managmeent of common symptoms. In JA Billings, ed. *Out-patient management of advanced cancer*. Philadelphia: JB Lippincott, 1985;41:80–87.

62. Twycross RG, Lack SA. *Therapeutics in terminal cancer*, 2nd ed. Edinburgh: Churchill Livingstone 1990:129–132.

63. Swinburn CR, Mould H, Stone TN, et al. Symptomatic benefit of supplemental oxygen in hypoxemic patients with chronic lung disease. *Am Rev Respir Dis* 1991;143:913–915.

64. Davidson AC, Leach R, George RJD, et al. Supplemental oxygen and exercise ability in chronic obstructive airways disease. *Thorax* 1988; 43:965–971.

65. Woodcock AAS, Gross ER, Geddes DM. Oxygen relieves breathlessness in pink puffers. *Lancet* 1981;907–909.

66. Dean NC, Brown JK, Himelman RB, et al. Oxygen may improve dyspnea and endurance in patients with chronic obstructive pulmonary disease and only mild hypoxemia. *Am Rev Respir Dis* 1992; 146:941–945.

67. Liss HP, Grant BJB. The effect of nasal flow on breathlessness in patients with chronic obstructive plumonary disease. *Am Rev Respir Dis* 1988;137:1285–1288.

68. Moore DP, Weston AR, Hughes JMB, et al. Effects of increased inspired oxygen concentrations on exercise performance in chronic heart failure. *Lancet* 1992;339:850–853.

69. Restrick LJ, Davies SW, Noone L, et al. Ambulatory oxygen in chronic heart failure. *Lancet* 1992;334:1192–1193.

70. Bruera E, de Stoutz N, Velasco-Leiva A, et al. The effects of oxygen on the intensity of dyspnea in hypoxemic terminal cancer patients. *Lancet* 1993;342:13–14.

71. Bruera E, Schoeller T, MacEachern T. Symptomatic benefit of supplemental oxygen in hypoxemic patients with terminal cancer: the use of the N of 1 randomized controlled trial. *J Pain Sympt Manag* 1992; 7:365–368.

72. Browning I, D Alonzo GE, Tobin MJ. Effect of hydrocodone on dyspnea, respiratory drive and exercise performance in adult patients with cystic fibrosis. *Am Rev Respir Dis* 1988;137:305 (abst).

73. Woodcock AA, Gross ER, Gellert A, et al. Effects of dihydrocodeine, alcohol, and caffeine on breathlessness and exercise tolerance in patients with chronic obstructive lung disease and normal blood gases. *N Engl J Med* 1981;305:1611–1616.

74. Johnson MA, Woodcock AA, Geddes DM. Dihydrocodeine for breathlessness in pink puffers. *BMJ* 1983;286:675–677.

75. Robin ED, Burke CM. Risk-benefit analysis in chest medicine. Single-patient randomization clinical trial. Opiates for intractable dyspnea. *Chest* 1986;90:889–892.

76. Eiser N, Denman WT, West C, et al. Oral diamorphine: lack of effect on dyspnoea and exercise toelrance in the pink puffer syndrome. *Eur Respir J* 1991;4:926–931.

77. Rice KL, Kronenberg RS, Hedemark LL, et al. Effects of chronic administration of codeine and promethazine on breathlessness and exeercise tolerance in patients with chronic airflow obstruction. *Br J Dis Chest* 1987;81:287–292.

78. Light RW, Muro JR, Sato RI, et al. Effects of oral morphine on breathlessness and exercise tolerance in patients with chronic obstructive pulmonary disease. *Am Rev Respir Dis* 1989;139:126–133.

79. Sackner MA. Effects of hydrocodone bitartrate on breathing pattern of patients with chronic obstructive pulmonary disease and restrictive lung disease. *Mount Sinai J Med* 1984;51:222–226.

80. Bruera E, MacEachern T, Ripamonti C, et al. Subcutaneous morphine for dyspnea in cancer patients. *Ann Intern Med* 1993;119:906–907.

81. Bruera E, Macmillan K, Pither J, et al. The effects of morphine on the dyspnea of terminal cancer patients. *J Pain Sympt Manag* 1990;5:341–344.

82. Cohen MH, Johnston Anderson A, Krasnow SH, et al. Continuous intravenous infusion of moprhine for severe dyspnea. *South Med J* 1991;84:229–234.

83. Ventafridda V, Spoldi E, De Conno F. Control of dyspnea in advanced cancer patients [Letter to the Editor]. *Chest* 1990;98:1544–1545.

84. Woodcock AA, Johnson MA, Geddes DM. Breathlessness, alcohol and opiates. Letter to the Editor, *N Engl J Med* 1982; 306:1363–1364.

85. Davis CL, Hodder C, Love S, et al. Effect of nebulised morphine and morphine-6-glucuronide on exercise endurance in patients with chronic obstructive pulmonary disease. *Thorax* 1994;49:393.

86. Young IH, Daviskas E, Keena VA. Effect of low dose nebulised morphine on exercise endurance in patients with chronic lung disease. *Thorax* 1989;44:387–390.

87. Beauford W, Saylor TT, Stansbury DW, et al. Effects of nebulized morphine sulfate on the exercise tolerance on the ventilatory limited COPD patient. *Chest* 1993;104:175–178.

88. Farncombe M, Chater S, Gillin A. The use of nebulize dopioids for breathlessness: a chart review. *Palliat Med* 1994;8:306–312.

89. Stein C. The control of papin in peripheral tissue by opioids. *N Engl J Med* 1995;332(25):1685–1690.

90. Davis CL, Lam W, Butcher M, et al. Low systemic bioavailability of nebulized morphine: potential therapeutic role for the relieve of dyspnea (meeting abstract). *Proc Annu Meet Am Soc Clin Oncol* 1992;11:A359.

91. Davis C. The role of nebulised drugs in palliating respiratory symptoms of malignant disease. *Eur J Palliat Care* 1995;2:9–15.

92. Stark RD, Gambles SA, Lewis JA. Methods to assess breathlessness in healthy subjects: a critical evaluation and application to analyse the acute effects of diazepam and promethazine on breathlessness induced by exercise or by exposure to raised levels of carbon dioxide. *Clin Sci* 1981;61:429–439.

93. O Neill PA, Morton PB, Stark RD. Chlorpromazine—a specific effect on breathlesslness? *Br J Clin Pharmac* 1985;19:793–797.

94. Woodcock AA, Gross ER, Geddes DM. Drug treatment of breathlessness: contrasting effects of diazepam and promethazine in pink puffers. *BMJ* 1981;283:343–346.

95. Man GCW, Sproule BJ. Effect of alprazolam on exercise and dyspnea in patients with chronic obstructive pulmonary disease. *Chest* 1986;90:832–836.

96. Mitchell-Heggs P, Murphy K, Minty K, et al. Diazepam in the treatment of dyspnoea in the pink puffer syndrome. *Qrtly J Med* 1980; New Series XLIX (193):9–20.

97. Frew AJ, Holgate ST. Clincal pharmaoclogy of asthma. Implications for treatment. *Drugs* 1993;46:847–862.

98. Weir DC, Gove RI, Robertson AS, et al. Corticosteroids trials in non-asthmatic chronic airflow obstruction: a comparison of oral prednisolone and inhaled bechomethasone diproprionate. *Thorax* 1991;45:112–117.

99. Ferguson GT, Irvin CG, Cherniak RM. Effect of corticosteroids on respiratory muscle histopathology. *Am Rev Respir Dis* 1990;142:1047–1052.

100. Mahler DA, Matthay RA, Snyuder PE, et al. Sustained-release theophylline reduced dyspnea in nonreversible obstructive airway disease. *Am Rev Respir Dis* 1985;131:22–25.

101. Aubier M, De Troyer A, Sampson M, et al. Aminophylline improves diaphragmatic contractility. *N Engl J Med* 1981;305:249–254.

102. Wittmann TA, Kelsen SG. The effect of caffeine on diaphragmatic muscle force in normal hamsters. *Am Rev Respir Dis* 1982;126:499–504.

103. Murciano D, Aubier M, Lecocguic Y, et al. Effects of theophylline on diaphragmatic strength and fatigue in patients with chronic obstructive pulmonary disease. *N Engl J Med* 1984;311:349–353.

104. Herxheimer H, Stresemann E. Ethanol and lung function in bronchial asthma. *Arch Int Pharmacodyn Ther* 1963;144:310–314.

105. O Neill PA, Stretton TB, Stark Rd, et al. The effect of indomethacin on breathlessness in patients with diffuse parenchymal disease of the lung. *Br J Dis Ches* 1986;80:72–79.

106. Al-Damluji S. The effect of ventilatory stimulation with medroxyprogesterone on exercise performance and the sensation of dyspnoea in hypercapnic chronic bronchitis. *Br J Dis Chest* 1986;80:273–279.

107. Biancho S, Vaghi A, Robuschi M, et al. Prevention of exercise-induced bronchoconstriction by inhaled frusemide. *Lancet* 1988;July:252–255.

108. Branthwaite MA. Mechanical ventilation at home. *BMJ* 1989;298:1409.

*Principles and Practice of Supportive Oncology,*
edited by Ann Berger et al.
Lippincott–Raven Publishers, Philadelphia ©1998

CHAPTER 24

# Hemoptysis

Randolph J. Lipchik

*Hemoptysis*, the coughing or expectoration of blood that originates in the lung, can be an alarming symptom for both patient and physician. It can range from blood-tinged or streaked sputum to *massive hemoptysis*, the latter defined as blood loss of 400 to 600 ml per day. Massive hemoptysis occurs in fewer than 5% of cases but carries a mortality rate of up to 85% if surgical intervention is not feasible (1,2). The management of hemoptysis, therefore, requires careful consideration of the severity of the process, cause, and functional status of the patient. Management may be more aggressive and invasive early in the course of a malignancy, whereas this could be inappropriate or dangerous for a patient in the terminal stages of an illness.

## PATHOGENESIS

The lung is perfused by two distinct circulations that must be considered when determining the source and planned treatment of hemoptysis. The pulmonary circulation delivers blood under low pressure from the right ventricle to the alveolar capillaries for exchange of oxygen and carbon dioxide. The bronchial circulation, which is about 1% to 2% of the cardiac output, arises from the systemic circulation and provides nutrient flow to the lung parenchyma. A detailed review of the anatomy and physiology of the bronchial circulation has been published (3) and is beyond the scope of this chapter. In brief, two or more arteries arise from the aorta or upper intercostal arteries, enter the lung, and eventually form a plexus, which accompanies the branching airways with small, penetrating arteries, forming another plexus that supplies the bronchial mucosa down to the terminal bronchioles. Farther on, they anastomose with both precapillary pul-

monary arterioles and pulmonary veins. Bronchial venous return is more complex; veins from the proximal airways return blood to the right atrium via the azygos, hemiazygos, or intercostal veins, whereas the intrapulmonary bronchial venous blood returns via the pulmonary veins to the left ventricle. The latter occurs as a result of anastomoses between bronchial and pulmonary veins and carries the bulk of bronchial venous return. Although this circulation is nonessential in the normal adult lung, in the setting of chronic inflammation, neoplasm, or repair after lung injury, bronchial blood flow increases as the result of increases in both the size and number of vessels. Furthermore, elevations of pulmonary vascular pressure can affect the bronchial circulation because of the many anastomoses between the dual circulations. In general, hemoptysis occurs because of disruption of the high-pressure bronchial vessels, which become abnormally enlarged and exposed within diseased airways.

## ETIOLOGY

This discussion concentrates on the malignant causes of hemoptysis, but awareness of other causes is important because many patients will have underlying conditions that may become active problems during treatment of a malignant disease. The differential diagnosis for a patient presenting with hemoptysis is extensive (Table 24-1). Some conditions that are more likely to be associated with massive hemoptysis are shown in Table 24-2. In past years, tuberculosis, bronchiectasis, and lung abscess were the most common causes of massive hemoptysis. The incidence of the latter two has declined in the industrialized nations, but tuberculosis has had a resurgence in parts of the United States and remains a significant problem worldwide. Experience with tuberculosis has helped us to understand the pathophysiology of massive hemop-

R. J. Lipchik: Department of Pulmonary and Critical Care Medicine, Medical College of Wisconsin, Milwaukee, WI 53226.

**TABLE 1.** *Causes of hemoptysis*

**Pulmonary**
  Bronchitis
  Bronchiectasis
  Pulmonary embolism
  Cystic fibrosis
**Infectious**
  Lung abscess
  Mycetoma
  Necrotizing pneumonia
  Viral
  Fungal
  Parasitic
  Septic embolism
**Cardiac**
  Mitral stenosis
  Congestive heart failure
**Neoplastic**
  Bronchogenic carcinoma
  Bronchial adenoma
  Endobronchial hamartoma
  Metastatic disease
  Tracheal tumors
**Hematologic**
  Coagulopathy
  Platelet dysfunction
  Thrombocytopenia
  Disseminated intravascular coagulation
**Vascular**
  Pulmonary hypertension
  Arteriovenous malformation
  Aortic aneurysm
**Traumatic**
  Blunt/penetrating chest injury
  Ruptured bronchus
**Systemic disease**
  Goodpasture's disease
  Vasculitis
  Systemic lupus erythematosus
**Drugs/toxins**
  Aspirin
  Anticoagulation
  Penicillamine
  Solvents
  Crack cocaine
**Miscellaneous**
  Foreign body
  Endometriosis
  Broncholithiasis
  Cryptogenic hemoptysis
**Iatrogenic**
  Lung biopsy
  PA catheterization
  Lymphangiography
  Transtracheal aspirate

(Modified from Cahill BC, Ingbar DH. Massive hemoptysis: assessment and management. *Clin Chest Med* 1994;15:147).

**TABLE 2.** *Causes of massive hemoptysis*

Pulmonary tuberculosis
Bronchiectasis
Lung abscess
Mycetoma
Bronchogenic carcinoma
Pulmonary carcinoid
Pulmonary arteriovenous fistula
Pulmonary vasculitis
Broncholithiasis

walled cavities of chronic tuberculosis, so-called Rasmussen's aneurysms. Rupture occurs secondary to the infection or the associated inflammatory response (4). Healed calcified mediastinal lymph nodes from prior tuberculosis can erode into the bronchial mucosa, also causing significant bleeding. Tuberculosis distorts lung architecture, resulting in bronchiectasis with resulting hypertrophy and proliferation of bronchial vessels. Infection or inflammation in these diseased portions of airway can cause rupture of vessels; the result is massive bleeding caused by the high systemic arterial pressure.

**Nonmalignant Conditions**

Patients with preexisting cavitary lung disease resulting from mycobacterial infections, sarcoidosis, bullous emphysema, lung abscess, lung infarction, and fibrocavitary disease secondary to rheumatoid disease are at risk for mycetoma formation, most often due to Aspergillus. This noninvasive infection results in a thick-walled cavity with vascular granulation tissue and inflammatory cells, the former the result of proliferation of the bronchial circulation. Bleeding is a result of vascular injury from fungal endotoxin, proteolytic activity, or a type III hypersensitivity reaction (5). Bacterial superinfection also can promote hemoptysis in the setting.

Deep venous thrombosis and subsequent thromboembolic disease are a common problem in hospitalized patients, especially those with underlying risk factors. The presence of a malignancy is a major risk factor, and the onset of hemoptysis warrants consideration of the possibility of pulmonary embolism and subsequent infarction. With current standard anticoagulation therapy, pulmonary embolism is a treatable condition with a 2.5% mortality. In a recent prospective study of the clinical course of pulmonary embolism, almost 24% of patients died within one year of diagnosis. Many cases, approximately 35%, had some form of cancer (6). A less well-appreciated and studied source of pulmonary embolism is upper extremity thrombosis resulting from indwelling venous catheters. In some series, the incidence of central line thromboembolism has been as high as 12% (7). Although most commonly seen in the pediatric population, there have been reports of inhaled for-

tysis. Up to 7% of deaths from tuberculosis were attributed to massive hemoptysis, and autopsy examinations revealed ruptured pulmonary artery aneurysms. Rasmussen (4) described localized ruptures of aneurysmal portions of pulmonary arteries passing through thick-

eign bodies in adults that, if unrecognized, have caused hemoptysis (8).

## Malignant Conditions

In a retrospective review of 877 cases of lung cancer, Miller and McGregor (9) reported a 19.3% overall incidence of hemoptysis, with non-life-threatening hemoptysis occurring equally among histologic types (9). Twenty-nine cases (3.3%) were massive and terminal events, due almost exclusively to proximal, cavitary squamous cell carcinomas. In only six of these 29 cases was there no antecedent nonlethal bleeding. The cause of this sudden catastrophic bleeding was tumor hemorrhage or invasion of a pulmonary artery or vein. In another series, Panos et al. (10) also found an association between cavitary squamous cell tumors and fatal hemoptysis. Metastatic endobronchial disease (carcinomas of breast, colon, kidney, and melanoma) is more likely to cause nonfatal hemoptysis rather than a terminal bleeding event. The incidence of hemoptysis in patients with bronchial carcinoid tumors approaches 50% as a result of mucosal ulceration or airway inflammation disrupting the bronchial arteries supplying these tumors. The high incidence of symptomatic bleeding is not surprising, as 85% of carcinoids arise in the proximal airway and are often very vascular (11). Malignant tracheal tumors are uncommon and when present usually result in obstructive symptoms. Hemoptysis does occur from these tumors but less frequently than with bronchogenic carcinoma (12). A Danish series of pulmonary hamartoma cases found that only 39% of patients were symptomatic but that nearly a quarter of those patients suffered from hemoptysis (13).

Patients with a hematological malignancy may develop hemoptysis for many reasons, including thrombocytopenia, coagulation abnormalities, and infections. In one series, fatal hemoptysis was associated strongly with the autopsy findings of vascular invasion, thrombosis, and hemorrhagic infarction secondary to invasive fungal disease (14). Idiopathic alveolar hemorrhage is a rare cause of fatal hemoptysis accounting for only 2 to 3% of leukemia deaths, but it also is associated with nonfatal hemoptysis. This is hypothesized to be attributable to the combination of thrombocytopenia and diffuse alveolar damage, the latter a result of one or more of the following: chemotherapy, radiotherapy, sepsis, or viral infection (14).

Thromboembolic disease already has been discussed in this chapter, but pulmonary embolic disease also may be caused by intravascular tumor metastases, resulting in a clinical presentation indistinguishable from the more common venous thromboembolism. Hemoptysis is unusual, and symptoms of dyspnea and right heart failure predominate. Rarely, massive tumor embolism results in pulmonary infarction with hemoptysis. Pulmonary infarction due to malignant compression of pulmonary veins also has been reported (15).

## DIAGNOSIS

The key element of diagnosis in cases of hemoptysis is the localization of bleeding to the lower respiratory tract. Although blood from the stomach usually has a low pH and blood from the respiratory tract a high pH, bleeding from the nasopharynx, larynx, or gastrointestinal tract may be difficult to distinguish clinically from hemoptysis. Furthermore, bleeding from these sources may result in cough and the appearance of blood misinterpreted as hemoptysis. When there is doubt, a thorough examination of the nasopharynx, larynx, and upper gastrointestinal tract should be performed.

Once the lung has been identified as the source of bleeding, the next step is to localize the site of bleeding. Physical examination alone is not sensitive enough; so a chest radiograph should follow and often is helpful in revealing a tumor or abscess, but it may be misleading because blood may be coughed into uninvolved portions of the lungs. Bronchoscopy is the surest way to visualize the source or at least the segment from which there is active bleeding. Flexible fiberoptic bronchoscopy usually is attempted first because it can be done relatively quickly at the bedside without putting the patient under general anesthesia and can access more distal airways than the rigid bronchoscope. The latter has the advantages of greater suction capability, removal of clots or foreign bodies, and airway control that allows for patient ventilation, which is often necessary in cases of massive hemoptysis. Computed tomography (CT) scan has been compared with bronchoscopy in studies in which hemoptysis is the presenting problem. Patients with preexisting cancer constituted a small proportion of those studied. The CT is superior in identifying bronchiectasis, lung abscess, aspergilloma, and distal parenchymal abnormalities; however, the bronchoscope can obtain material that allows a cytological, histological, and microbiological diagnosis (16,17). In patients with established malignancies, a CT scan may offer important information, as it can delineate peribronchial or mediastinal involvement of tumor that cannot be seen with a bronchoscope. Routine use of CT is not of proven benefit but should be considered in cases in which the chest radiographic findings are inconclusive or to provide a more detailed anatomic localization of an abnormality for the bronchoscopist.

## MANAGEMENT

The severity of hemoptysis determines the pace at which a workup should proceed. In a review of 10 years' experience at Duke University Medical Center, the mortality rate was 9% and 58% percent if blood loss was less than or more than 1000 ml per 24-hour period, respectively (1). A malignant cause for hemoptysis of greater than 1,000 ml per 24 hours increased the mortality rate to 80%. Massive hemoptysis requires rapid intervention to guarantee that the patient has an adequate airway while attempting to control bleeding. If blood loss is minimal and sporadic, a more detailed evaluation can occur without immediate attention to resuscitative efforts. Early consultation with a pulmonary physician and thoracic surgeon is recommended.

Initial diagnostic studies should include chest radiograph, hematocrit, platelet count, blood urea nitrogen and creatinine levels, and coagulation panel, which might include a bleeding time if aspirin or nonsteroidal antiinflammatory agents have recently been used. Oxygenation should be monitored by arterial blood gas determination or pulse oximetry and adequate intravenous access established. Typed and cross-matched blood should be available in cases of significant bleeding. Mild sedation and judicious use of a cough suppressant can be employed, but excessive use will compromise a patient's ability to clear their airway.

If oxygenation is compromised or the patient continues to bleed vigorously, elective intubation should be performed. The endotracheal tube should be large enough to allow passage of a bronchoscope (7.5 or 8.0 mm). If it is known from which side the patient is bleeding, the patient should be placed in a lateral decubitus position with the bleeding side down to help minimize aspiration of blood into the good lung. Placement of a double-lumen endotracheal tube is sometimes necessary to allow separate ventilation of each lung while preventing aspiration of blood throughout the bronchial tree. The two small lumina preclude bronchoscopy with anything but a pediatric bronchoscope, and suctioning is limited because only small-caliber catheters can be passed distally. Newer-generation tubes with larger internal diameters may be less troublesome (18).

### Bronchoscopy

If bronchoscopy identifies the site of bleeding, several maneuvers can be done to stop or slow the bleeding. Bronchial lavage with iced saline (19) application of topical epinephrine (1:20,000) and topical thrombin and fibrinogen-thrombin solutions (20) all have been reported in small series to have varied success; however, they have not been evaluated in large numbers of patients in controlled studies. A 4-French Fogarty balloon catheter can be inflated in the segmental bronchus, leading to the site of bleeding and allowing time for stabilization of the patient and consideration of more definitive therapy (21). Bleeding from visible lesions in the trachea and proximal bronchi can be coagulated with a laser. This is particularly useful when the hemoptysis arises from an obstructing tumor, as both problems can be addressed simultaneously. In a series of 43 patients with advanced bronchogenic carcinoma, 16 with concomitant hemoptysis, 38 were treated successfully (22). One patient died of continued tumor bleeding and aspiration of blood, two required tracheostomy to facilitate management of secretions, there was one pneumothorax, and one transient bronchial obstruction by a tumor fragment mobilized by laser therapy.

### Radiotherapy

High-dose external beam radiation for 6 to 7 weeks usually is employed to attempt cure for inoperable non-small cell carcinoma. In the palliative setting, therapy is delivered in the shortest time possible, with lower doses to achieve symptom relief while minimizing side effects; 8 Gy in 1 fraction up to 20 Gy in 5 fractions in one week or 30 Gy in 10 fractions over 2 weeks have been used with success. Hemoptysis can be stopped in more than 80% of cases by using palliative radiotherapy (23). Although significant symptoms from radiation fibrosis are uncommon, there are reports of massive hemoptysis occurring long after, and attributed to, external beam radiotherapy (24). Such cases are rare, however, probably because most patients succumb to their underlying cancer before significant vascular abnormalities develop.

Endobronchial brachytherapy with iridium[192] is another alternative. A useful summary of this modality was published recently (25). Dose rates can be low (up to 1 Gy per hour), intermediate (2–10 Gy per hour), or high (greater than 10 Gy per hour). The higher dose rates decrease the time of treatment and permit outpatient rather than inpatient therapy. Gollins et al. (25) reported results of high-dose-rate brachytherapy in 406 patients (26). Of 255 patients with hemoptysis, brachytherapy arrested the bleeding in 89% at 1.5 months, 84% at 4 months, and 77% at 12 months after the first treatment. The results were not as favorable for patients who received brachytherapy after failure of external beam radiation; 84%, 56%, and 25% of patients had resolution of hemoptysis 1.5, 4, and 12 months after brachytherapy, respectively. Although most patients died of their cancer during the study (mean survival was 173 days), control of hemoptysis was quite good. Massive hemoptysis as a terminal event occurred in 32 patients (8%). Retrospective palliative results of different brachytherapy dose rates are summarized in Table 3. Brachytherapy has been combined with bronchoscopic laser therapy in some centers (27,28). The Mayo Clinic reported results from 65 patients, 40 of whom had received prior laser therapy. In 24 patients with hemoptysis, bleeding resolved in 19. Response was poorer in patients who had received prior laser therapy, most likely because of more advanced disease (28). Potential complications of brachytherapy include mucositis, fistula forma-

**TABLE 3.** *Endobronchial brachytherapy*

| Study | Year | No. of patients | Dose rate | Palliation[a] (%) | Severe complications[b] (%) |
|---|---|---|---|---|---|
| Seagren et al. (31) | 1985 | 20 | HDR | 100 | 0 |
| Macha et al. (32) | 1987 | 56 | HDR | 74 | 0 |
| Bedwinek et al. (33) | 1992 | 38 | HDR | 76 | 32 |
| Speiser (34) | 1991 | 342 | HDR | 80 | 7 |
| Sutedja et al. (35) | 1992 | 31 | HDR | 71 | 42 |
| Nori et al. (36) | 1993 | 32 | HDR | 91 | 0 |
| Pisch et al. (37) | 1993 | 39 | HDR | 93 | 3 |
| Zajac et al. (38) | 1993 | 82 | HDR | 74 | 2 |
| Chang et al. (39) | 1994 | 76 | HDR | 87 | 4 |
| Speiser and Spratling (40) | 1990 | 45 | IDR | 69 | 0 |
| Allen et al. (41) | 1985 | 15 | LDR | 100 | 0 |
| Schray et al. (28) | 1988 | 65 | LDR | 83 | 11 |
| Mehta et al. (42) | 1990 | 38 | LDR | 70 | 10 |
| Roach et al. (43) | 1990 | 17 | LDR | 60 | 0 |
| Paradelo et al. (44) | 1992 | 32 | LDR | 83 | 0 |
| Suh et al. (45) | 1994 | 37 | LDR | 75 | 30 |

[a] Palliation = Relief of cough, dyspnea, hemoptysis, or radiographic/bronchoscopic improvement.
[b] Severe complications = massive hemoptysis or fistula formation.
HDR, high dose rate; IDR, intermediate dose rate; LDR, low dose rate.
(Modified from Villanueva et al. (25).)

tion, and fatal hemoptysis (29). The latter event has a reported incidence of 6 to 30%.

## Bronchial Artery Embolization

Bronchial artery anatomy is quite variable but generally arises from the ventral surface of the descending aorta or branches from the intercostal arteries at the level of T5 and T6. Intimate knowledge of this vascular anatomy is essential because the anterior spinal artery often arises from the bronchial arteries and inadvertent embolization could result in spinal cord infarction. Bronchiectasis, tuberculosis, and aspergilloma frequently result in hypertrophy of bronchial vessels, but there are often transpleural collaterals from other systemic vessels, such as the subclavian, internal mammary, or intercostal arteries, which must be identified. After angiographic identification of the vessels in question, a variety of agents (e.g., Gelfoam, polyvinyl alcohol particles, and metallic coils) can be injected selectively to stop blood flow. Initial success rates reported in the literature vary between 75% and 90%, with a rebleeding rate of 15% to 30%. Hayakawa and colleagues (30) reported immediate (within 1 month) and long-term results for 63 patients. Of the 12 patients with hemoptysis due to neoplasm, bleeding was controlled in seven patients (58%). Long-term control was documented for four of these seven patients with a median hemoptysis control period of 6 months (range, 0–9 months). All but one of the patients died within the 9-month follow-up period. Patients with bronchiectasis, inflammation, or idiopathic causes had immediate control in 94% of cases with the median period of control lasting 15 months (range, 1–132

months) and a mortality rate of 11%. Recurrent bleeding can be treated with repeat embolization.

## Surgery

The definitive therapy for massive hemoptysis is resection of the diseased portion of the lung; however, this is often precluded by the severity of the underlying lung disease. Similarly, massive hemoptysis from a bronchogenic carcinoma usually results from proximal endobronchial tumor, which is typically not amenable to surgical resection. Therefore, surgery is not an option for the vast majority of palliative care patients.

## REFERENCES

1. Corey R, Hla KM. Major and massive hemoptysis: reassessment of conservative management. *Am J Med Sci* 1987;294:301.
2. Thompson AB, Teschler H, Rennard SI. Pathogenesis, evaluation, and therapy for massive hemoptysis. *Clin Chest Med* 1992;13:69.
3. Deffebach ME, Charan NB, Lakshminarayan S, Butler J. The bronchial circulation: small, but a vital attribute of the lung. *Am Rev Respir Dis* 1987;135:463.
4. Auerbach O. Pathology and pathogenesis of pulmonary arterial aneurysm in tuberculous cavities. *American Review of Tuberculosis* 1939;39:99.
5. Awe RJ, Greenberg SD, Mattox KL. The source of bleeding in pulmonary aspergillomas. *Tex Med* 1984;80:58.
6. Carson JL, Kelley MA, Duff A, et al. The clinical course of pulmonary embolism. *N Engl J Med* 1992;326:1240.
7. Horattas MC, Wright DJ, Fenton AH, et al. Changing concepts of deep venous thrombosis of the upper extremity: report of a series and review of the literature. *Surgery* 1988;104:561.
8. Kane GC, Sloane PJ, McComb B, Chinn B, Gottlieb JE. 'Missed' inhaled foreign body in an adult. *Respir Med* 1994;88:551.
9. Miller RR, McGregor DH. Hemorrhage from carcinoma of the lung. *Cancer* 1980;46:200.
10. Panos RJ, Barr LF, Walsh TJ, Silverman HJ. Factors associated with fatal hemoptysis in cancer patients. *Chest* 1988;94:1008.

11. Davila DG, Dunn WF, Tazelaar HD, Pairolero PC. Bronchial carcinoid tumors. *Mayo Clin Proc* 1993;68:795.
12. Allen MS. Malignant tracheal tumors. *Mayo Clin Proc* 1993;68:680.
13. Hansen CP, Holtveg H, Francis D, Rasch L, Bertelsen S. Pulmonary hamartoma. *J Thorac Cardiovasc Surg* 1992;104:674.
14. Smith LJ, Katzenstein AA. Pathogenesis of massive pulmonary hemorrhage in acute leukemia. *Arch Intern Med* 1982;142:2149.
15. Williamson WA, Tronic BS, Levitan N, Webb-Johnson DC, Shahian DM, Ellis FH. Pulmonary venous infarction secondary to squamous cell carcinoma. *Chest* 1992;102:950.
16. Set PAK, Flower CDR, Smith IE, Cahn AP, Twentyman OP, Shneerson, JM. Hemoptysis: comparative study of the role of CT and fiberoptic bronchoscopy. *Radiology* 1993;189:677.
17. McGuiness G, Beacher JR, Harkin TJ, Garay SM, Rom WN, Naidich DP. Hemoptysis: prospective high-resolution CT/bronchoscopic correlation. *Chest* 1994;105:1155.
18. Shivaram U, Finch P, Nowak P. Plastic endobronchial tubes in the management of life-threatening hemoptysis. *Chest* 1987;92:1108.
19. Conlan AA, Hurwitz SS, Krige L, Nicolaou N, Pool R. Massive hemoptysis: review of 123 cases. *J Thorac Cardiovasc Surg* 1983;85:120.
20. Tsukamoto T, Sasaki H, Nakamura H, et al. Treatment of hemoptysis patients by thrombin and fibrinogen-thrombin infusion therapy using a fiberoptic bronchoscope. *Chest* 1989;96:473.
21. Saw EC, Gottlieb LS, Yokayama T, Lee BC. Flexible fiberoptic bronchoscopy and endobronchial tamponade in the management of massive hemoptysis. *Chest* 1976;70:589.
22. Wolfe WG, Sabiston DC. Management of benign and malignant lesions of the trachea and bronchi with the neodymium-yttrium-aluminum-garnet laser. *J Thorac Cardiovasc Surg* 1986;91:40.
23. Awan AM and Weichselbaum RR. Palliative radiotherapy. *Hematol Oncol Clin North Am* 1990;4:1169.
24. Makker HK, Barnes PC. Fatal hemoptysis from the pulmonary artery as a late complication of pulmonary irradiation. *Thorax* 1991;46:609.
25. Villanueva AG, Lo TCM, Beamis JF. Endobronchial brachytherapy. *Clin Chest Med* 1995;16:445.
26. Gollins SW, Burt PA, Barber PV, Stout R. High dose rate intraluminal radiotherapy for carcinoma of the bronchus: outcome of treatment of 406 patients. *Radiother Oncol* 1994;33:31.
27. Lang N, Maners A, Broadwater J, Shewmake K, Chu D, Westbrook K. Management of airway problems in lung cancer patients using the neodymium-yttrium-aluminum-garnet (Nd-YAG) laser and endobronchial radiotherapy. *Am J Surg* 1988;156:463.
28. Schray MF, McDougall JC, Martinez A, Cortese DA, Brutinel WM. Management of malignant airway compromise with laser and low dose brachytherapy: the Mayo Clinic experience. *Chest* 1988;93:264.
29. Khanavkar B, Stern P, Alberti W, Nakhosteen JA. Complications associated with brachytherapy alone or with laser in lung cancer. *Chest* 1991;99:1062.
30. Hayakawa K, Tanaka F, Torizuka T, et al. Bronchial artery embolization for hemoptysis: immediate and long-term results. *Cardiovasc Intervent Radiol* 1992;15:154.
31. Seagren SL, Harrell JH, Horn RA. High dose rate intraluminal irradiation in recurrent endobronchial carcinoma. *Chest* 1985;88:810.
32. Macha HN, Koch K, Stadler M, Schumacher W, Krumhaar D. New technique for treating occlusive and stenosing tumors of the trachea and main bronchi: endobronchial irradiation by high dose iridium-192 combined with laser canalization. *Thorax* 1987;42:511.
33. Bedwinek J, Petty A, Bruton C, Sofield J, Lee L. The use of high dose rate endobronchial brachytherapy to palliate symptomatic endobronchial recurrence of previously irradiated bronchogenic carcinoma. *Int J Radiat Oncol Biol Phys* 1992;22:23.
34. Speiser B. Advantages of high dose rate remote afterloading systems: physics or biology. *Int J Radiat Oncol Biol Phys* 1991;20:1133.
35. Sutedja G, Baris G, Schaake-Koning C, van Zandwijk N. High dose rates brachytherapy in patients with local recurrences after radiotherapy of non-small cell lung cancer. *Int J Radiat Oncol Biol Phys* 1992;24:551.
36. Nori D, Allison R, Kaplan B, Samala E, Osian A, Karbowitz S. High dose-rate intraluminal irradiation in bronchogenic carcinoma: techniques and results. *Chest* 1993;104:1006.
37. Pisch J, Villamena PC, Harvey JC, Rosenblatt E, Mishra S, Beattie EJ. High dose-rate endobronchial irradiation in malignant airway obstruction. *Chest* 1993;104:721.
38. Zajac AJ, Kohn ML, Heiser D, Peters JW. High-dose-rate intraluminal brachytherapy in the treatment of endobronchial malignancy. *Radiology* 1993;187:571.
39. Chang LF, Horvath J, Peyton W, Ling SS. High dose rate afterloading intraluminal brachytherapy in malignant airway obstruction of lung cancer. *Int J Radiat Oncol Biol Phys* 1994;28:589.
40. Speiser B and Spratling L. Intermediate dose rate remote afterloading brachytherapy for intraluminal control of bronchogenic carcinoma. *Int J Radiat Oncol Biol Phys* 1990;18:1443.
41. Allen MD, Baldwin JC, Fich VJ, Goffinet DR, Cannon WB, Mark JB. Combined laser therapy and endobronchial radiotherapy for unresectable lung carcinoma with bronchial obstruction. *Am J Surg* 1985;150:71.
42. Mehta M, Shahabi S, Jarjour N, Steinmetz M, Kubsad S. Effect of endobronchial radiation therapy on malignant bronchial obstruction. *Chest* 1990;97:662.
43. Roach M 3rd, Lediholdt EM Jr, Tatera BS, Joseph J. Endobronchial radiation therapy (EBRT) in the management of lung cancer. *Int J Radiat Oncol Biol Phys* 1990;18:1449.
44. Paradelo JC, Waxman MJ, Throne BJ, Beller TA, Kopecky WJ. Endobronchial irradiation with 192 Ir in the treatment of malignant endobronchial obstruction. *Chest* 1992;102:1072.
45. Suh J, Dass KK, Pagliaccio L, et al. Endobronchial radiation therapy with or without neodymium yttrium aluminum garnet laser resection for managing malignant airway obstruction. *Cancer* 1994;73:2583.

*Principles and Practice of Supportive Oncology,*
edited by Ann Berger et al.
Lippincott–Raven Publishers, Philadelphia ©1998

CHAPTER 25

# Disorders of the Airways

Julie A. Biller

Disorders of the airways may produce debilitating or life-threatening symptoms in a diverse patient population. Therefore, health care providers, including generalists and those of many subspecialties, may be called on to diagnose and treat these disorders. Often a multidisciplinary approach is needed. Airway obstruction, bronchospasm, stridor, and cough not only may produce symptoms that reduce the quality of life of the patients affected, but they can produce profound distress to those patients' families. In some situations, even our current best therapies will do little to palliate symptoms, and it is my hope that we shall see continued improvement in these areas. In this chapter, the diagnostic and current therapeutic approach to airway disorders are reviewed.

## TRACHEOBRONCHIAL OBSTRUCTION

The tracheobronchial tree quite literally can be "between a rock and a hard place," resulting in airway obstruction. Obstruction may occur on the basis of large exophytic endobronchial tumor causing intrinsic obstruction of the airway. On the other hand, mediastinal pathology can cause obstruction by extrinsic compression of the airways. Etiologies differ somewhat between the two modes of obstruction. *Intrinsic* obstruction usually is caused by primary malignancies arising from the airway epithelium. Two histologic types of tumors, squamous cell carcinoma and adenoid cystic carcinoma, constitute two thirds of the primary tracheal malignancies (1). The remaining third comprises a diverse group of tumors, both benign and malignant, detailed in Table 25-1. More commonly, the trachea can be a site of locally extensive disease, usually from organs in close proximity, such as the lung, larynx, thyroid, and esophagus. Intrinsic obstruction of the bronchial tree most frequently is seen

J. A. Biller: Department of Medicine and Pediatrics, Medical College of Wisconsin, Milwaukee, WI 53226.

in primary cancers of all histologic types. About 5% of metastatic disease to the lungs is predominately endobronchial. Renal cell, colon, rectum, cervical, breast carcinomas, and malignant melanomas are the most common primary malignancies to give rise to endobronchial metastasis (2).

*Extrinsic* obstruction occurs when the airways are surrounded by firm tumor or encased by pathologically enlarged lymph nodes, usually caused by locally advanced disease arising from the lung, esophagus, and thyroid. Lymphoma, which can involve significant lymphadenopathy, is another cause of extrinsic compression. A variety of benign lesions that may imperil airway patency are listed in Table 1.

### Evaluation

Patients with tracheobronchial obstruction usually present with complaints of dyspnea, hemoptysis, wheezing, or stridor and sometimes with pneumonia or atelectasis. The onset of these obstructive symptoms can be insidious, and patients often are treated for other diseases, such as asthma or chronic obstructive pulmonary disease (COPD). Patients occasionally will come to medical attention when pulmonary function tests obtained for other reasons suggest upper airway obstruction.

The evaluation of airway obstruction is primarily through radiographic studies and bronchoscopy. Posteroanterior and lateral chest radiographs should be the first diagnostic study ordered. Grossly abnormal radiographs with a large central parenchymal mass or mediastinal mass/adenopathy causing tracheal narrowing or deviation rapidly raise concern for the patency of the airway. Unfortunately, there can be significant compromise to the airway but only subtle radiographic changes. Therefore, close attention must be paid to the tracheal air column. Often, abnormalities are more obvious on the lateral view.

**TABLE 1.** *Etiologies of airway obstruction*

Intrinsic obstruction
  Malignant
    Primary tumors
    Tracheal
      Squamous carcinoma
      Adenoid cystic carcinoma
    Bronchogenic
      Squamous
      Adenocarcinoma
      Small cell
      Mixed morphology
    Metastatic
      Breast cancer
      Melanoma
      Larynx
      Esophagus
      Renal cell
      Colon
      Rectal
      Cervical
      Kaposi sarcoma (rarely obstructing)
  Benign
    Papillomas
    Chondromas
    Hamartoma
    Lipoma
    Leiomyoma
    Granular cell myoblastoma
    Granuloma 2 retained foreign body
    Hemangiomas
    Postintubation strictures
  Low-grade malignancy
    Carcinoid
Extrinsic obstruction
  Malignancy
    Lung
    Lymphoma
    Esophageal
    Thyroid
  Benign
    Fungal infection
    Reactive lymphadenopathy
    Bronchomalacia
    Mediastinal fibrosis
    Vascular compression
    Goiter

Computed tomography (CT) of the neck and chest are extremely useful for better definition of airway anatomy, allowing accurate measurement of the diameter of the central airways to determine the extent of obstruction. It is important in treatment planning to determine whether the obstruction is primarily intrinsic or extrinsic. This differentiation often can be made by CT scan. In medically stable patients, pulmonary function testing, including spirometry and, most importantly, flow volume loop, may identify upper airway obstruction quickly, inexpensively, and noninvasively. Frequently, it can localize whether the obstruction is extrathoracic or intrathoracic. Figure 25-1A shows the typical flow volume loop in a fixed airway obstruction. The most common causes of this type of lesion are tracheal stenosis, tumor (malignant or benign), goiter, fixation of vocal cords, and a large foreign body. Variable extrathoracic upper airway obstruction (Fig. 1B) affects primarily the inspiratory loop of the flow volume curve. Common causes of this are bilateral vocal cord paralysis, epiglottis, vocal cord adhesions, and foreign body. Variable intrathoracic obstruction (Fig. 1C) affects primarily the expiratory loop of the flow volume curve after the effort-dependent peak expiratory flow, which can be caused by intraluminal polypoid tumors or tracheomalacia.

To complete the evaluation of the patient with upper airway obstruction, more invasive procedures may be necessary, which typically involves fiberoptic evaluation, including laryngoscopy or bronchoscopy. It may necessary to have multiple subspecialists involved in complicated cases, including otolaryngologists, thoracic surgeons, pulmonologists, and anesthesiologists. Bronchoscopy may be performed for several reasons, principally to obtain pathologic material for diagnosis or as a therapeutic maneuver (see below). This is especially important if small-cell lung carcinoma is considered in the differential diagnosis. If there is any question about the adequacy of the airway, bronchoscopy is best performed by a thoracic surgeon in the operating room with an experienced anesthesiologist present. At biopsy, the patient may have complications of airway obstruction or hemorrhage, which may endanger a marginal airway. Frequently, in this patient population, rigid bronchoscopy, with its better suctioning capabilities and ability to ventilate through the bronchoscope, is the procedure of choice.

## Therapy

Patients who have airway obstruction on the basis of primary malignancies of the trachea or larynx, benign strictures (such as postintubation tracheal stenosis or extrinsic compression secondary to goiter or lymphoma) should be referred to the appropriate specialist (surgeon, oncologist, or radiation oncologist) for evaluation of definitive therapy. Palliative therapeutic options for airway management in patients who are not candidates for definitive therapeutic procedures include airway stents, laser therapy, brachytherapy, and tracheostomy. Some patients may be helped by using several of these modalities in combination.

For any palliative therapy to be attempted, the airway must be wide enough to allow passage of a rigid or flexible bronchoscope and still maintain oxygenation and ventilation. In the case of large exophytic tumors that compromise the patency of the central airways, the bronchoscopist still can usually pass a bronchoscope instrument past the tumor. If this is not possible, a rigid bronchoscope may be used to "core out" the obstructing

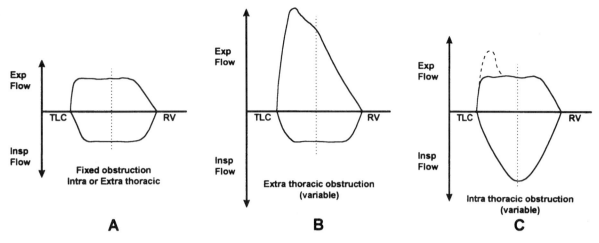

**FIG. 1. A:** Maximal inspiratory and expiratory flow-volume curves in fixed obstruction. **B:** Extrathoracic variable obstruction. **C:** Intrathoracic variable obstruction. **Dashed line** represents a flow transient that occasionally is observed just before the plateau in intrathoracic obstruction. Reprinted, with permission, from Kryger et al. Diagnosis of obstruction of the upper and central airways. *Am J Med* 1976;6185–6193.

tumor, with its tip inserted in corkscrew fashion (1). If significant bleeding occurs, the rigid bronchoscope may be used to exert pressure and tamponade the bleeding. Ventilation can be maintained through the rigid bronchoscope, and it has a large suction channel to clear blood and tissue from the airways. Sometimes it is necessary to pass a fiberoptic bronchoscope through the rigid bronchoscope to clear blood, secretions, or tissue fragments from the more distal airways. Some authors are strong proponents of this technique because although it requires expertise to reduce the risk of complications, such as tracheal perforation, hemorrhage, or rupture of the pulmonary artery, it does not need special equipment and usually requires only one endoscopic procedure. In series from Mathisen and Grillo (3), 51 of 56 patients had significant improvement in airway obstruction after bronchoscopic "core out," and only two patients required a second procedure. The patients who did not improve had distal obstructing disease. Because a rigid bronchoscope is used to perform a "core out," it is best suited for large central airway disease. Distal lesions or those obstructing the upper lobe orifices are less likely to be accessible with a rigid bronchoscope.

The other option for palliative resection of intrinsically obstructing lesions of the large airways is laser endobronchial resection (Figs. 25-2 and 25-3) (3). Lasers transform light energy to heat, which causes tissue coagulation and vaporization. With advances in laser technology, this has become an increasingly popular modality over the past 15 years. Currently, the neodymium:yttrium, alubinum, garnet (ND:YAG)-sourced laser is best suited for endobronchial resection. These lasers can be delivered through both rigid and flexible bronchoscopes. The wavelength of the laser is such that it is poorly absorbed

by hemoglobin and water, resulting in deep tissue penetration. Because of high-power output, it can thermally coagulate blood vessels up to 2 to 3 mm in diameter and vaporize tissue (4). There seems to be a preference toward rigid bronchoscopy because of its ability to ventilate the patient better and its improved suctioning abilities; however, there are many reports of the use of flexible fiberoptic bronchoscopic resections in patients unable to tolerate general anesthesia and rigid bronchoscopy (5,6). In some situations, both types of procedures may be performed in combination. The bronchoscope is passed into the airway, and the base of the tumor is identified. The Nd:Yag laser is aimed at the base of the tumor parallel to the wall of the trachea. Using varying energy levels, pulsations of laser energy are used first to coagulate the tumor mass and then to vaporize the tissue. The tracheal wall is avoided to reduce the risk of perforation or hemorrhage. In addition to these complications, there is also risk of tracheoesophageal fistula formation, combustion and fire within the bronchoscope, and ocular damage to operating personnel if appropriate protective gear is not used. Other drawbacks to laser resection include the need for special equipment and its time-consuming nature. Most patients improve after the first endoscopic resection but may require multiple sessions to complete the excision.

Success rates are quite substantial with most patients having relief of symptoms or reexpansion of obstructed lung. In a series of 100 Nd:YAG laser ablations performed on 40 patients, 22 patients were considered to have an excellent response to therapy and another 10 a fair response (7). Besides improving quality of life, some patients will have prolonged survival from what would otherwise have been a fatal complication of their underlying disease.

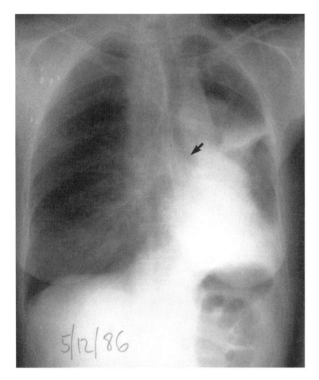

**FIG. 2.** Chest radiograph showing cutoff airway (*arrow*) from obstructing tumor, significant volume loss of the left hemithorax, and postobstructive pneumonia.

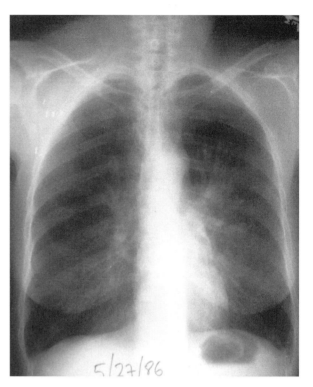

**FIG. 3.** Chest radiograph of the same patient after laser resection of the tumor. Notice the resolution of volume loss and resolving pneumonitis.

Bronchoscopic brachytherapy is the placement of a radiation source in close proximity to an endobronchial tumor. *Brachytherapy*, or short-distance therapy, is in contrast to conventional external beam radiation therapy delivered at a distance from the lesion. Brachytherapy is another modality to palliate locally extensive disease in the airways. Patients first undergo bronchoscopy to evaluate the extent of intraluminal tumor. A catheter then is advanced through a channel in the bronchoscope to the desired level, and the bronchoscope is removed. Correct placement is verified by reinsertion of the bronchoscope. The catheter is secured to the nasal orifice, and a radioactive source, usually iridium-192 or iodine-125, is placed in the catheter. Conventional-dose brachytherapy (50–120 cGy/hour) requires the catheter to remain inserted for 48 to 96 hours with the patient in a shielded hospital room. High-dose brachytherapy (675 cGy/min at 1 cm), delivered by a Gamnaed II™ remote afterloading unit, has a treatment duration of only a few minutes; no special radiation measures are needed for the patient after the afterloading unit is removed. Patients must have sufficient pulmonary reserve to undergo bronchoscopy and catheter placement. Brachytherapy also can be delivered by the insertion of radiation seeds or pellets into endobrachial lesions. Brachytherapy can improve symptoms of dyspnea and hemoptysis in about 90% of patients with stable airway disease (8). Because of the need for a stable airway, several studies combined laser

endobronchial resection with brachytherapy (4,9). High-dose brachytherapy was tolerated better with slightly improved survival compared with conventional dose brachytherapy. Early complications to brachytherapy include airway obstruction secondary to mucus plugs requiring therapeutic bronchoscopy, radiation esophagitis, and laryngospasm. Long-term complications are more ominous, including fatal hemorrhage from fistula formation between airways and major blood vessels as well as airway esophageal fistula formation (9). Long-term survivors are at risk of airway stenosis at the site of laser or radiation therapy (9).

Extrinsic compression of the airway is not amenable to the above-mentioned therapies. Pressure from extraluminal tumor, vasculature, or luminal weakness can cause the airways to narrow or collapse. Intraluminal pressure is needed to counteract these external forces. Over the past two decades, insertion of airway stents to maintain airway patency has gained popularity as an effective palliative treatment for extrinsic compression. Stents can be inserted through both rigid or flexible bronchoscopes. Their most impressive benefit is the immediate palliation of airway obstruction on placement of the stent (Figs. 4 and 5). Several different types of airways stents are available, including silicone stents (Dumon, Montgomery T-tube, Hood) or expandable metallic stents (Gianturco, Wall, William Cook, etc.). Both types of stents are placed in a similar manner. The stents are compressed to an

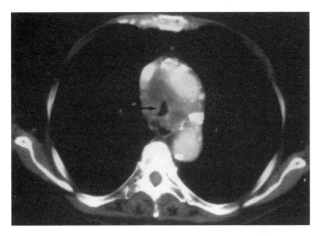

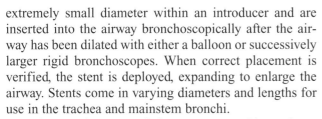

FIG. 4. Tracheal compression causing dyspnea in a 63-year-old woman. Biopsy of the tumor revealed squamous cell carcinoma.

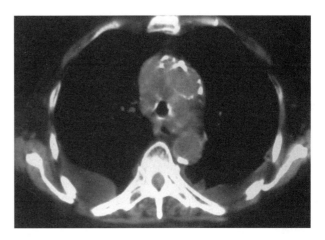

FIG. 5. The same patient after placement of a stent into the trachea which has increased the diameter of the airway and relieved her symptoms.

extremely small diameter within an introducer and are inserted into the airway bronchoscopically after the airway has been dilated with either a balloon or successively larger rigid bronchoscopes. When correct placement is verified, the stent is deployed, expanding to enlarge the airway. Stents come in varying diameters and lengths for use in the trachea and mainstem bronchi.

Unfortunately, none of the stents are without drawbacks. Silicone stents may migrate or even may be coughed completely out of the airway. Therefore, it is extremely important to place the appropriately sized stent, as migration usually is seen with stents that are too small (10). Silicone stents placed in the right mainstem bronchus may obstruct the orifice to the right upper lobe, putting the patient at risk for atelectasis and infectious complications. Silicone stents also are believed to interfere with mucociliary clearance and pulmonary toilet (11). T-tube stents are placed in the trachea and usually require tracheostomy. A rare complication of stent placement is fatal erosion into a central vascular structure. Despite these potential drawbacks, silicone stents are well tolerated and quite successful in the treatment of extrinsic airway obstruction (12,13).

Expandable metallic stents (EMS) are the newest type of stents to be used in the treatment of airway obstruction, but they have many drawbacks. Because these stents are made of loops of wire, they do not obstruct orifices of smaller airways, such as the opening of the right upper lobe, when placed in the right mainstem bronchus. Unfortunately, because of the loops, endobronchial tumor may grow through the stent and compromise the airway. The metallic stents have an irritant effect on the airways; cough and granuloma formation are the most common complications (14). Some patients improve with inhaled corticosteroids and laser resection. Because of the tissue reaction, removal of the stents is difficult, often causing damage to the airways. There have been reports of fatal

hemorrhage, broken suction catheters, stent migration, and stent breakage (15–17).

Lastly, some patients with upper airway obstruction may have relief of symptoms following tracheostomy, which is useful only in patients with laryngeal or very proximal tracheal obstruction. In patients with distal tracheal or small airway obstruction, the tracheostomy tube will not be able to bypass the obstructing lesion. Recent improvements in tracheostomy tube technology can improve patient communication and decrease the risk of complications such as granulation tissue formation and bleeding.

Tracheobronchial obstruction is a devastating complication from both malignant and nonmalignant disease. There are many possible therapies for palliation. These therapies are not mutually exclusive, and their use in combination should be encouraged. Importantly, a multidisciplinary approach with appropriately trained personnel is needed.

## STRIDOR

*Stridor* is loud, harsh breathing, particularly on inspiration. It occurs from obstructed airflow in the upper airway and large intrathoracic central airways. Stridor may indicate a pathologic narrowing of the airway, which is unable to maintain adequate oxygenation and ventilation of the patient. Therefore, evaluation and management of these patients should be done expediently. Treatment for stridor depends on the location of the obstruction and its etiology. When evaluating a patient presenting with stridor, it is useful to consider the airway as three areas or zones (18,19). The first is the *supraglottic zone*, which includes the nose, oral cavity, pharynx, and supraglottic larynx. This area is composed of soft tissues that are only loosely supported and hence more easily obstructed.

Lesions in this area tend to cause stridor only on inspiration. The second is the *extrathoracic tracheal zone*, which is composed primarily of the glottis and subglottis. Because this area has more support, obstruction generally occurs more gradually. Lesions in this area may cause stridor both on inspiration and expiration known as *biphasic stridor*. Last is the *intrathoracic tracheal area*, which also includes the proximal portions of the mainstem bronchi. Stridor from this region may be primarily expiratory and may be confused with wheezing from distal intrathoracic airway obstruction. Of note, patients frequently deviate from these patterns of clinical presentations. The causes of stridor are numerous, some of which are listed in Table 25-2.

## Evaluation

The tempo of evaluation of the patient presenting with stridor is determined by the acuity of the illness. Patients who present in severe respiratory distress with inadequate oxygenation or ventilation need the immediate establishment of an airway. Because they may have lesions that make intubation difficult or impossible, it is necessary to have experienced personnel, including an anesthesiologist and otolaryngologist, available. Fiberoptic-assisted intubation may be necessary and also may be helpful in establishing the etiology of stridor.

In patients who appear stable, a brief history may help in differentiating the causes of stridor. Gradual onset of

**TABLE 2.** *Causes of stridor*

Infection
  Tracheitis: bacterial or viral
  Epiglottitis
  Abscess: peritonsillar or retropharyngeal
  Viral laryngotracheobronchitis
Neoplasm
  See Table 1
Congenital
  Laryngomalacia
  Tracheomalacia/tracheal stenosis
  Vocal Cord cysts/paralysis
  Webs
Trauma
  Facial
  Ingestion
  Inhalation injury
  Postintubation
  Airway fracture
  Postsurgical
Neurologic
  CNS malformation
  Hypoxic encephalopathy
Other
  Foreign bodies (airway, esophageal)
  Psychogenic
  Exercise

symptoms over weeks or months, especially if accompanied by constitutional symptoms, would suggest neoplasm. Stridor that occurs in hours or days, especially if the patient is febrile, is suspicious for an infectious etiology, such as epiglottis croup or abscess. A history of previous intubation is quite important because subglottic stenosis may not appear for months after a traumatic or prolonged intubation. Close questioning regarding episodes of choking or coughing while eating may raise the possibility of aspiration. Foreign body in either the airway or esophagus may cause stridor, especially in younger patients. Pressure exerted from an esophageal foreign body may partially obstruct the airway (20).

Physical examination of a patient with stridor typically begins with the examiner's unaided ear. Loud, noisy breathing is heard. The patient's respiratory rate, depth of respiration, use of accessory muscles of respiration, level of alertness, and evidence of cyanosis should be observed. Inability to handle oral secretions should be noted because it may suggest peritonsillar abscess, retrophargeal hematoma or abscess, epiglottis, or foreign body.

Palpation of the airway should be performed to assess for crepitation suggesting subcutaneous emphysema. A displaced trachea or firm mass could indicate tumor or goiter. Lymphadenopathy could suggest neoplasm. Auscultation of the entire airway may help localize the anatomic location of the lesion; so one should listen especially carefully over the larynx, extrathoracic trachea, and central chest.

Radiologic studies of the chest, as discussed earlier in this chapter, should be obtained to evaluate stridor in stable patients. In addition, anterior-posterior and lateral radiographs of the neck should be obtained. If more detailed imaging of the airway is needed, CT scans should be obtained. Spirometry with flow-volume loops, as discussed in evaluation of tracheobronchial obstruction, may be an important aid in evaluation of stridor.

## Therapy

Stridor secondary to infectious etiologies requires treatment with appropriate antimicrobial therapy. Hemophilus influenza is the most common bacterial cause of epiglottitis, although its incidence has been declining steadily. Respiratory synchial virus infection may cause airway edema resulting in stridor. This infection is typically seen in children, although the virus has been recovered in immunocompromised adults. Treatment with the antiviral drug ribavirin may be considered in the acutely ill patient. Anaerobes, streptococcal species, and a wide assortment of less common agents may cause abscess formation, leading to airway obstruction. While waiting for the culture results, it is appropriate to treat the patient with broad-spectrum antibiotics.

Several therapies are available to stabilize the stridorous patient who is clinically decompensating. Heliox, a mixture of helium and oxygen, has been useful in improving oxygenation, ventilation, and decreasing work of breathing in patients with stridor from a wide variety of causes (21–24). These causes included postextubation edema, extrinsic compression from tumor, and status asthmaticus. Because Heliox has a lower density than ambient nitrogen-oxygen gas mixture, there is decreased airway turbulence and airway resistance. The typical heliox mixture varies from helium 60%-oxygen 40% to maximal concentration helium 80%-oxygen 20%. It can be delivered via a tight-fitting face mask, and relief of respiratory distress is often immediate. Treatment with high-dose intravenous corticosteroids should be started using methyl prednisolone 1 mg/kg every 6 to 8 hours. Racemic epinephrine 2.25%, 0.5 ml in 2.5 ml saline delivered via hand-held nebulizer as often as hourly, but usually every 3 to 4 hours, may be used especially for postextubation stridor (25).

Noninvasive mask ventilation with continuous positive airway pressure (CPAP) or bilevel positive airway pressure (BiPAP) may decrease the work of breathing and overcome large airway obstruction, although currently no studies have evaluated the efficacy of this therapy. Close coordination with a respiratory therapist will be needed if this therapy is initiated. Either a tight-fitting mask over the nose or nasal pillars applied to the nares may be used. Positive pressure of 5 cm $H_2O$ is started and titrated up to a maximum of 20 cm $H_2O$. Most patients are unable to tolerate higher pressures. If needed, supplemental oxygen and humidification can be "bled" into the positive pressure system. Finally, endotracheal intubation or tracheostomy should be considered in appropriate clinical situations for patients severely affected.

## BRONCHOSPASM

*Bronchospasm* is the state of abnormal narrowing of the airways and is usually episodic. Airflow is obstructed and becomes turbulent, resulting in severe dyspnea. Patients complain of dyspnea, chest tightness, or pressure, although occasionally cough is the only symptom. Exacerbation of symptoms frequently occurs in the early hours of the morning, when bronchial tone is normally increased. Wheezing is heard on auscultation of the chest, occasionally needing to be provoked by forced expiration or deep breathing. Expiration time is usually prolonged. Patients may use accessory muscles of respiration and pursed lip breathing.

Bronchospasm is the end result of airway narrowing, which is believed to be a consequence of a state of hyper-responsiveness of the airways to a wide variety of stimuli (26). More recently, airway inflammation is considered of prime importance in the development of airway hyperac-

tivity. The airway epithelium is thickened and friable, and microscopically there is infiltration with inflammatory cells, especially eosinophils and mast cells. Mucus glands are hyperplastic, and goblet cells are more numerous compared with normal persons (27). Bronchial lavage fluid of the lung reveals high concentrations of cytokines, prostagladins, histamine, triptase, and immunoglobulin E (IgE) (26). In severely affected persons, the airways may be plugged with excessive inflammatory secretions and desquamated epithelium (28). Airway muscle is both hyperplastic and hypertrophied, but it has been found to contract normally when stimulated (29). Smooth-muscle mass is increased, probably in response to growth factors, such as histamine, or as a result from increased work (30,31).

### Evaluation

The differential diagnosis for bronchospasm includes asthma, COPD, upper/large airway obstruction (discussed previously), congestive heart failure, bronchiolitis (infectious or inflammatory, medication induced), lymphangitic tumor spread, or rarely pulmonary embolism. Multiple etiologies for bronchospasm are common in an individual patient. The extent of evaluation depends on the complexity of an individual patient's medical condition. In a patient with a significant smoking history, chronic sputum production, and diffuse bronchospasm on examination, it is likely that an exacerbation of COPD explains the clinical situation. Obviously, in a patient who has a similar history but is immunocompromised, the diagnostic possibilities must be widened.

Chest radiographs should be obtained in patients presenting with bronchospasm. Bronchial wall thickening, flattened diaphragm, and increased retrosternal air space are consistent with hyperexpansion and air trapping and would support the diagnosis of asthma or COPD. In addition, the chest radiograph may reveal complications of obstructive lung disease, such as pneumonia, pneumothorax, or atelectasis.

A chest radiograph with no change from the patient's baseline film or with atelectasis or small pleural effusion should alert the clinician to possible pulmonary embolism, and a ventilation/perfusion scan (V/Q) should be obtained to access for pulmonary embolism. The V/Q scan needs to be compared with the chest radiograph for accurate interpretation. A completely normal perfusion scan effectively excludes pulmonary embolism. Segmental perfusion defects in areas of normal ventilation define a high probability V/Q scan, which indicates an 85% to 90% probability of pulmonary embolism, which must be interpreted with care, as one of the few causes of false-positive V/Q scans is bronchospasm. Helical CT scanning of the chest may be more cost effective and more accurate than V/Q scanning in identifying clinically significant pulmonary emboli (32). Again, if the clinical situation warrants further evaluation, noninvasive testing to detect lower extremity deep venous thrombosis or pulmonary angiography may need to be pursued.

Spirometry not only will confirm airway obstruction but can suggest its anatomic location (upper versus intrathoracic) and quantify the extent of airway obstruction. In addition, it also may be helpful in monitoring treatment response. Forced vital capacity (FVC) and forced expiratory volume at one second ($FEV_1$) are reduced in an obstructive lung defect with the reduction in $FEV_1$ greater than that of FVC. In airway obstruction, the ratio of $FEV_1$ to FVC will be less than 70%. The severity of the obstructive defect is graded by the patient's percentage of predicted $FEV_1$ (70% or greater, mild; between 60% and 70%, moderate; between 50% and 60%, moderately severe; between 35% and 50%, severe; and less than 34%, very severe) (33).

The contour of the expiratory portion of a flow volume loop will show concavity, which worsens with the extent of the obstructive lung defect. Patients with chronic obstructive lung disease have fixed airway obstruction but can have some degree of variability in FVC and $FEV_1$ during exacerbations. On the other hand, most patients with asthma should have normal or near normal spirometry between episodes of illness. Spirometry often is obtained before or after use of inhaled bronchodilators. Patients who have at least a 15% improvement in FVC or $FEV_1$ and 200 ml absolute increase in FVC or $FEV_1$ are considered to have a significant immediate response. This group is considered to benefit most from inhaled bronchodilators and corticosteroids, although many studies have reported conflicting results regarding this issue (34). Patients who do not improve immediately after inhaled bronchodilators may have spirometric or clinical improvement with regular use; therefore, these medications should not be withheld.

## Therapy

The goals of therapy in bronchospasm are to dilate the distal airways and reduce inflammation, hence relieving airway obstruction. There are many pharmacologic agents available to treat bronchospasm (Table 25-3). The severity of the patient's symptoms will guide which of these medications and in what order they are used. Beta adrenergic agonists have been, and continue to be, important pharmacologic agents to relieve bronchospasm. They can be administered in many forms: inhaled through metered dose inhalers, inhaled through hand-held nebulizers, taken orally, or injected subcutaneously or intravenously. Over the past decade, there has been a strong

**TABLE 3.** *Medications commonly used to treat bronchospasm*

| Medication | Routes of action | Administration | Typical adult doses |
|---|---|---|---|
| Albuterol (Proventil, Ventalin) | B₂-agonist | Metered-dose inhaler via nebulizer | 2–3 Puffs qid and prn not to exceed 24 puffs/day |
| | | Via nebulizer | 0.5 ml to 0.75 ml in 2.5 ml saline qid may increase frequency for severe symptoms |
| | | Oral | Syrup 2 mg/tsp, 1–2 tsp tid to qid, dose not to exceed 32 mg/day tablets 2 mg and 4 mg |
| Metaproterenol (Alupent) | B₂-agonist | Metered-dose inhaler | 2–3 Puffs qid and prn not to exceed 12 puffs/day |
| | | Via nebulizer | Similar to albuterol |
| | | Oral | Syrup 10 mg/tsp; 1–2 tsp tid to qid tablets 10 mg and 20 mg tid to qid |
| Pirbuterol (Maxair) | B₂-agonist | Metered-dose inhaler | 2–3 Puffs qid and prn, not to exceed 12 puffs/day |
| Ipratropium bromide (Atrovent) | Anticholinergic | Metered-dose inhaler | 2–3 Puffs qid and prn not to exceed 12 puffs/day |
| | | Via nebulizer | 500 mcg in 2.5 ml saline tid to qid compatible with albuterol |
| Cromolyn sodium (Intal) | Antiinflammatory (nonsteroidal) | Metered-dose inhaler | 2 Puffs bid to qid |
| | | Via nebulizer | 1 to 2 ml (10–20 mg) bid to qid |
| Nedocromil sodium (Tilade) | Antiinflammatory (nonsteroidal) | Metered-dose inhaler | 2 Puffs bid to qid |
| Beclomethasone dipropionate (Vanceril, Beclovent) | Antiinflammatory (corticosteroid) | Metered-dose inhaler | 42 mg/puff, 2–4 puffs bid to quid not to exceed 20 puffs/day |
| Flunisolide (Aerobid) | Antiinflammatory (corticosteroid) | Metered-dose inhaler | 250 mg/puff, 2 puffs bid, not to exceed 8 puffs/day |
| Triamcinlone acetonide (Azmacort) | Antiinflammatory (corticosteroid) | Metered-dose inhaler | 100 mg/puff 2–4 puffs bid to qid not to exceed 16 puffs/day |
| Flunisolide propionate (Flovent) | Antiinflammatory (corticosteroid) | Metered-dose inhaler | 44 mcg/puff 110 mcg/puff 220 mcg/puff 1–4 puffs bid |
| Theophylline | unknown | Oral | 400–900 mg/day; monitor serum level 8–12 g/ml |

pid, four times a day; prn, as required; tid, three times a day

movement against using oral beta agonists as their efficacy is similar to the inhaled forms but they have a higher incidence of side effects. Subcutaneous forms are used sparingly for emergency treatments. Intravenous administration of isoproterol is no longer recommended (35).

Beta adrenergic agents promote airway smooth-muscle relaxation by a mechanism that is not completely understood. In addition, they increase mucociliary clearance and increase the secretion of electrolytes by the airways. Side effects include tremor, tachycardia, palpitations, hypokalemia, and hyperglycemia. Usually these side effects are most pronounced when the medications are first initiated and lessen over time. Sustained-release oral beta-adrenergic agonists have a useful role in patients with significant nocturnal symptoms. Patients with mild bronchospasm may be started on beta-adrenergic agonists alone to control symptoms. For patients with more severe presentations, other therapies will be needed. The recent trend has been to have patients use these medications on an as-needed basis for mild symptom control. Recent studies have found equal efficacy between metered dose inhalers and nebulized beta adrenergic agents if proper technique is used and the dose is increased to five or six inhalations. Some patients will benefit by using a spacer device to improve delivery with metered-dose inhalers. The total dose of beta-adrenergic agonist should be 24 or fewer inhalations in a 24-hour period to prevent tachyphylaxis. Patients who do not find relief with use of beta-adrenergic agonists or who must increase their usual dose should be evaluated for additional therapies. The recent spate of literature on safety of beta-adrenergic agonists found that mortality increased when patients were undertreated for asthma (36–39).

Anticholinergic agents act by decreasing parasympathetic bronchoconstriction of the airways. They are most useful in COPD, in which parasympathetic activity is believed to be greater than normal. Ipratropium bromide is the only anticholinergic agent available for inhalational use in the United States. Because of recent reports suggesting inpratropium bromide may be more effective than beta-adrenergic agonists in promoting bronchodilation in patient with COPD, some authors believe it should be the first agent used in maintenance therapy in COPD (40–42).

Corticosteroids are widely used in the treatment of bronchospasm. Patients with mild to moderate symptoms may benefit from inhaled corticosteroids. They are especially attractive because they act locally, with minimal absorption and limited toxicity; however, reports of hypothalamic-pituitary-adrenal axis suppression and cataract formation were recently reported with the use of high-dose inhaled corticosteroids (43). In addition, patients should be cautioned that these medications must be used regularly and may take weeks for therapeutic effect. Therefore, corticosteroids should not be used as monotherapy for acutely symptomatic patients. Inhaled corticosteroids also may allow patients on systemic corticosteroid therapy to have their doses reduced or discontinued altogether. Patients with more serious symptoms or those in respiratory distress require systemic corticosteroids. These medications may take up to 12 hours to have clinical effects. Prednisone 0.5 mg to 1.0 mg/kg per 24 hours may be used for 1 to 2 weeks and then gradually tapered. Seriously ill patients should receive methyl prednisolone 1 mg to 2 mg/kg every 6 to 8 hours IV until improvement is noted. At that time, the intravenous dose may be tapered over several days and the patient switched to oral corticosteroids. Peak flow meters along with physical examination and arterial blood gases will help determine a patient's response to therapy.

Besides corticosteroids, cromolyn sulfate and nedocromial sodium are other antiinflammatory agents. Their exact mode of action is unclear, but likely they act as mast cell stabilizers. These medications are particularly useful in children for symptoms related to exercise or cold air and for patients with a strong allergic component to their bronchospasm. Cromolyn sulfate is available as a metered dose inhaler, two puffs four times a day, or inhalatonal solution 1 to 2 cc four times a day via nebulizer. Nedocromil sodium is used two puffs four times daily via metered-dose inhaler. Again, patients must be educated to use these medications regularly because its maximal effects will not be noted for 4 to 6 weeks.

Theophylline, once a mainstay of therapy, has lost its place as a first-line therapy in the treatment of bronchospasm because of excessive toxicity and potential for serious drug interactions. It is still used in patients with COPD in an effort to augment respiratory muscle function and for its weak bronchodilator effects. In addition, it is used in corticosteroid-dependent asthmatics in hopes of decreasing their daily steroid dose (44). Typically, patients are started on long-acting preparations at a dose of 400 to 900 mg/day to achieve serum levels of 8 to 12 $\mu$/ml. The dose must be individualized depending on concurrent medications, smoking history, and medical history, such as congestive hear failure, as all of these will change drug clearance. Critically ill patients in respiratory failure secondary to bronchospasm who do not respond to maximal therapy including intubation and mechanical ventilation should be considered for bronchial muscle relaxation with inhalational anesthetics.

## COUGH

### Etiology

Cough is a protective, complex reflex that helps clear the airways of foreign material or excessive secretions. It is a common problem that translates into 30 million physician visits per year and millions of dollars spent on over-the-counter medications (45).

The cough reflex is complicated and not fully understood. Suffice it to say that cough results from stimulation of cough receptors, which may be found in the larynx, respiratory epithelium, tympanic membranes, esophagus, pericardium, and sinus mucosa. Afferent impulses travel via the vagus, trigeminal, glossopharyngeal, and phrenic nerves to cough centers in the medulla. Efferent impulses travel via the vagus, phrenic, and spinal nerves to the glottis and respiratory muscles, which produce the high-velocity flow of air that defines a cough (46,47).

## Evaluation

Cough is a common complaint in patients with advanced cancer. In the cancer patient, cough may be secondary to endobronchial tumor, pericardial disease, vocal cord paralysis, or aspiration. Cough also may be due to complications of treatment, such as radiation pneumonitis or chemotherapy-induced interstitial disease (48). In addition, patients with underlying cancer may have all the same causes of cough found in the general population. The most common etiologies of chronic cough include postnasal drip syndrome, asthma, and gastroesophageal reflux (49,50).

A detailed history and physical examination are most helpful in determining the cause of chronic cough (47). Chest radiographs should be obtained early in the evaluation of cough (51). In patients who chronically produce sputum or in whom there is a suspicion of interstitial lung disease, a high-resolution chest CT scan may be helpful. Of patients with interstitial lung disease, 10% to 15% will have a normal chest radiograph; CT scan is very helpful in the evaluation of bronchiectasis.

Sinus imaging, including radiographs and CT scanning, are needed to evaluate for chronic sinus disease. Some authors recommend a trial of antihistamine-decongestants before pursuing sinus radiographic studies (45). Spirometry, before and after inhaled bronchodilators and methacholine challenge, will help to evaluate for asthma or chronic obstructive lung disease. Evaluation for gastroesophageal reflux disease can be undertaken with barium esophagography or 24-hour esophageal pH monitoring. Finally, if no cause has been found for chronic cough, bronchoscopy should be considered to evaluate for occult foreign body aspiration or small endobronchial lesions such as carcinoid tumors or bronchogenic cancer, although studies have found this to be of low yield (49).

## Therapy

Treatment of cough is most successful if it is tailored to a specific etiology. Postnasal drip syndrome may be well controlled with the use of antihistamine-decongestant therapy. Asthma therapy was discussed earlier in this chapter. Gastroesophageal reflux disease is treated with $H_2$ receptor blockers or proton pump inhibitors along with lifestyle changes. In patients for whom no cause is found for their cough or it is due to airway involvement with tumor, empiric medical therapy is reasonable. Some patients will obtain relief with the use of beta$_2$-adrengenic agonists such as Albuterol two or three inhalations every 4 to 6 hours or 0.5 ml Albuterol solution in 2 ml saline via nebulizer every 4 to 6 hours.

For generations, opiates have been used and are variably effective antitussives (46,52). There is no evidence of superior antitussive effect with one preparation over another. Codeine 15 mg to 30 mg every 4 to 6 hours is a reasonable starting dose, with titration upward to control symptoms if the side effects are tolerable. Nonnarcotic cough preparations, such as guaifenesin and dextromethorphan, may be tried, although they have been only weakly effective. Two recent articles review the many conflicting studies evaluating over-the-counter and prescription cough medications (52,53).

Inhaled lidocaine is used to suppress cough during bronchoscopy. Animal studies and a few human studies suggest that lidocaine has an antitussive effect when inhaled via nebulizer, probably acting on afferent C-fibers in the larynx and trachea. The dose is empiric; a starting dose is 5 ml of 2% lidocaine solution every 4 hours via hand-held nebulizer (46,48). Patients should be cautioned regarding anesthesia of the oropharynx and larynx, which puts them at risk for buccal injury or aspiration. The dose may be increased if needed, but there are no studies giving explicit guidelines for this therapy. Generally, during bronchoscopy, doses higher than 300 mg of lidocaine (15 ml of 2% solution) are avoided to decrease the risk of seizures, as there is significant systemic airway absorption of lidocaine.

In patients who have underlying chronic bronchitis, a trial of inhaled ipratropium bromide, two puffs four times a day, may diminish the cough (54). Finally, some patients will respond to corticosteroids. Some of these patients have underlying asthma, whereas others may have other reasons for airway inflammation, such as chronic bronchitis, bronchiectasis, or radiation pneumonitis. Inhaled steroids such as flunisolide two puffs twice daily and triamcinolone 2–4 puffs four times a day may be tried as initial therapy or maintenance therapy after oral agents. Patients not responding to inhaled therapy should be tried on prednisone 0.5 to 1.0 mg/kg per day for 2 to 4 weeks. If the cough subsides, the prednisone should be tapered to the lowest dose to control symptoms, or patients should be switched to inhaled steroids.

## REFERENCES

1. Mathisen DJ. Surgical management of tracheobronchial disease. *Clin Chest Med* 1992;13:151.

2. Braman SS, Whitcomb ME. Endobronchial metastasis. *Arch Intern Med* 1995;135:543.
3. Mathisen DJ, Grillo HC. Endoscopic relief of malignant airway obstruction. *Ann Thorac Surg* 1989;48:469.
4. Lang N, Maners A. Broadwater J, Shewmake K, Chu D, Westbrook K. Management of airway problems in lung cancer patients using the Neodymium-Yhrium-Aluminum-Garnet (Nd:YAG) Laser and endobronchial radiotherapy. *Am J Surg* 1988;156:463.
5. Castro DJ, Saxton RE, Ward PH, Oddie JW, Layfield LJ, Lufkin RB, Calcaterra TC. Flexible Nd:YAG Laser palliation of obstructive tracheal metastatic malignancies. *Laryngoscope* 1990;100:1208.
6. Kao SJ, Shen CY, Hsu K. Nd:YAG Laser application in pulmonary and endobronchial lesions. *Lasers Surg Med* 1986;6:296.
7. Parr GVS, Unger M. Trout RG, Atkinson WG. One hundred Neodymium:YAG Laser ablations of obstructing tracheal neoplasms. *Ann Thorac Surg* 1984;38:374.
8. Marsh BR. Bronchoscopic brachytherapy. *Laryngoscope* 1989;99:1.
9. Schary MF, McDougall JC, Martinez A, Cortese DA, Brutinel WM. Management of malignant airway compromise with laser and low dose rate brachytherapy. *Chest* 1988;93:264.
10. Dumon JF. A dedicated tracheobronchial stent. *Chest* 1990;97:328.
11. Zannini P, Melloni G, Chiesa G, Carretta A. Self-expanding stents in the treatment of tracheobronchial obstruction. *Chest* 1994;106:86.
12 Bolliger CT, Probst R, Tschopp K, Soler M. Perruchoud AP. Silicone stents in the management of inoperable tracheobronchial stenoses. *Chest* 1993;104:1653.
13. Gaer JA, Tsang V, Khaghani A, Gillbe CE, et al. Use of endobronchial silicone stents for relief of tracheobronchial obstruction. *Ann Thorac Surg* 1992;54:512.
14. Nashef SA, Dromer C, Velly JF, Labrousse L, Couraud L. Expanding wire stens in benign tracheobronchial disease: indications and complications. *Ann Thorac Surg* 1992;54:937.
15. Hind CRK, Donnelly RJ. Expandable metal stents for tracheal obstruction: Permanent or temporary? A cautionary tale. *Thorax* 1992;47:757.
16. Sawada S, Tanigawa N, Kobayaski M, Furui S, Ohta Y. Malignant tracheobrachial obstruction lesions: Treatment gianturco expandable metal stents. *Radiology* 1993;188:205.
17. Nomori H, Kobayashi R, Kodera K, Moringa S, Ogawa K. Indications for an expandable metallic stent fpr tracheobronchial stenosis. *Ann Thorac Surg* 1993;56:1324.
18. Santamaria JP, Schafermeyer R. Stridor: a review. *Pediatr Emerg Care* 1992;8:229.
19. Stool SE. Stridor. *Intern Anesth Clin* 1988;26:19.
20. O'Hollaren, MT, Everts EC. Evaluating the patient with stridor. *Ann Allerg* 1991;67:301.
21. Curtis JL, Mahlmeister M, Fink JB, Lampe G, Matthay MA, Stulbarg MS. Helium-oxygen gas therapy use and availablity for the emergency treatment of inoperable airway obstruction. *Chest* 1986;90:455.
22. Orr JB. Helium-oxygen gas mixtures in the management of patients with airway obstruction. *Ear Nose Throat J* 1988;67:866.
23. Skrinskas GJ, Hyland RH, Hutcheon MA. Using helium-oxygen mixtures in the management of acute airway obstruction. *Can Med Assoc J* 1983;R8:555.
24. Gluck E, Onorato DJ, Castriotta R. Helium-oxygen mixtures in intubated patients with status astematicus and respiratory acidosis. *Chest* 1990;98:693.
25. Schmitt G, Hall R, Wood LDH. Management of the ventilated patient. In: Murray JF, Nadel JA, eds. *Textbook of respiratory medicine*, Philadelphia: WB Saunders, 1992.
26. Woolcock AJ. Asthma. In: Murray JF, Nadel JA, eds. *Textbook of respiratory medicine*. 2nd ed. Philadelphia: WB Saunders, 1994:1288.
27. Nadel JA. Regulation of bronchial secretion. In: Newhall HH, ed. *Immunopharmacology of the lung*. New York: Marcel Dekker, 1983:109.
29. Saetta M, Stefano AD, Rosina C, Thiene G. Fabbri LM. Quantitative structural analysis of peripheral airways and arteries in sudden fatal asthma. *Am Rev Respir Dis* 1991;143:138.
28. Hallahan AR, Armour CL, Black JL. Products of neutrophils and eosinophils increase the responsivenes of human isolated bronchial tissue. *Eur Respir J* 1990;3:554.

30. Bai TR. Abnormalities in airway smooth muscle in fatal asthma: A comparison between tracheal and bronchus. *Am Rev Resp Dis* 1991; 143:441.
31. Panathiere RA, Yadish PA, Rubenstein VA, Kelly AM, Kotlikoff MI. Histamine induces proliferation and C-fos transcription in cultured airway smooth muscle. *Am J Physiol* 1990;259:365.
32. Gefter WB, Hatabu H, Holland, GA, Gupta KB, Henschke CI, Palevsky HI. Pulmonary thromboembolism: recent developments in diagnossi with CT and MR imaging. *Radiology* 1995;197:561–574.
33. Crapo RO, Merris, AH, Gardner RM. Reference spisrometric values using techniques and equipment that meed ATS recommendations. *Am Rev Respir Dis* 1981;123:859.
34. Mendella LA, Manfredi J. Warren CPW, et al. Steroid response in stable chronic obstructive pulmonary disease. *Ann Intern Med* 1982;96:17.
35. Stempel DA, Redding GJ. Management of acute asthma. *Pediatr Clin North Am* 1992;(39):1311.
36. Spitzer WO, Suissa S, Ernst p, Horwitz RJ, Habbick B, Cockcroft d, et al. The use of B-agonists and the risk of death and near death from asthma. *N Engl J Med* 1992;326:501.
37. Wong CS, Pavord ID, Williams J, Britton JR, Tattersfield, AE. Bronchodilator, cardiovascular, and hypokatemic effects of fenoterol, salbutamol, and terbutaline in asthma. *Lancet* 1990;336:1396.
38. Burrows B, Lebowitz MD. The B-agonist dilemma. *N Engl J Med* 1992;326:560.
39. Poynter D. Fatal asthma—Is treatment incriminated. *J Allergy Clin Immunol* 1987;80;423.
40. Tashkin DP, Ashutosh K. Bleecker ER, et al. Comparison of the anticholinergic bronchodilator ipratropium bromide with meta proterenol in chronic obstructive pulmonary disease. *Am J Med* 1986;81:81.
41. Marlin GE, Bush DE, Berent N. Comparison of ipratropium bromide and fenoterol in asthma and chronic bronchitis. *Br J Clin Pharmacol* 1978;6:547.
42. Braun SR, Levy SF. Comparison of ipratropium bromide and albuterol in chronic obstructive lung disease a three-center study. *Am J Med* 1991;21:28s.
43. Kamada AK, Szefler SJ, Martin RJ, Boushey HA, et al. Issues in the use of inhaled glucocorticosteroids. *Am J Respir Crit Care Med* 1996;153: 1739–1748.
44. Wrenn K. Slovis CM, Murphy F, Greenberg RS, Aminophylline therapy for acute bronchospastic disease in the emergency room. *Ann Intern Med* 1991;115:241.
45. Pratter MR, Bartter T, Akers S, DuBois J. An Algorithmic approach to chronic cough. *Ann Intern Med* 1993;119:977.
46. Fuller RW, Jackson DM. Physiology and treatment of cough. *Thorax* 1990;45:425.
47. Shuttair MF, Braun SR. Comtemporary management of chronic persistent cough. *Mo Med* 1992;89:795.
48. Cowcher K, Hank GW. Long-term management of respiratory symptoms in advanced cancer. *J Pain Sympt Manag* 1990;5:320.
49. Poe RH, Israwl RH, Utell MJ, Hall WJ. Chronic cough: Bronchoscopy or pulmonary function testing? *Am Rev Respir Dis* 1982;126:160.
50. Irwin RS, Curley FJ, French CL. Chronic cough. *Am Rev Respir Dis* 1990;141:640.
54. Irwin RS, Carley FJ. The treatment of cough: a comprehensive review. *Chest* 1991;99:1477.
52. Irwin RS. Curley FJ, Bennett FM. Approriate use of antitussives and protussives: a practical review. *Drugs* 1993;46:80.
53. Smith MB, Feldman W. Over-the-Counter cold medications. A critical review of clinical trials between 1950 and 1991. *JAMA* 1993;269:2258.
55. Levy MH, Catalano RB. Control of common physical symptoms other than pain in patients with terminal disease. *Semin Oncol* 1985;12:411.
51. Puolijoki H, Lahdensuo A. Causes of prolonged cough in patients referred to a chest clinic. *Ann Med* 1989;21:425.
56. Manthous CA, Hall JB, Malmed A, et al. Heliox improves pulsus paradoxus and peak expiratory flow in non-intubated patients with severe asthma. *Am J Respir Crit Care Med* 1995;151:310.
57. Miller JI, Phillip TW. Neodymium:YAG laser and brachytherapy in the management of inoperable bronchogenic carcinoma. *Am Thorac Surg* 1990;50:190.

*Principles and Practice of Supportive Oncology,*
edited by Ann Berger et al.
Lippincott–Raven Publishers, Philadelphia ©1998

CHAPTER 26

# Management of Pleural and Pericardial Effusions

Lary A. Robinson and John C. Ruckdeschel

One of the most common and troubling problems for the cancer patient is the development of a malignant effusion of any body cavity. When it occurs in the pleural cavity or the pericardium, this abnormal escape of fluid from the blood vessels or lymphatic system may cause severe symptoms or may even be life-threatening. Any type of cancer can metastasize to these serous cavities, and this problem is most common in disseminated malignancies. Although the development of a malignant pleural or pericardial effusion almost always indicates that the patient has an incurable cancer, prompt recognition and diagnosis followed by appropriate treatment can result in excellent palliation and a marked improvement in the patient's quality of life. In addition, it is critical that an accurate diagnosis is made to establish the malignant cause of the effusion, since cancer patients can often develop an effusion from a benign cause such as radiation therapy, infection, chemotherapy, or heart failure. All cancer patients with pleural or pericardial effusions, especially when associated with symptoms, deserve a thorough evaluation and an opportunity for prompt therapy. Their cases should not be just considered terminal and untreatable.

## PLEURAL EFFUSIONS

### Incidence

In a general hospital patient population, 28% to as many as 61% of all pleural effusions are malignant; the highest incidence is in the over-50 age group (1–4). A malignant pleural effusion is the initial manifestation of cancer in 10% to 50% of patients (4,5). In patients with

L. A. Robinson (Division of Cardiovascular and Thoracic Surgery, Department of Cardiothoracic Surgery) and J. C. Ruckdeschel: H. Lee Moffitt Cancer Center and Research Institute, University of South Florida, Tampa, FL 33612-9497.

known breast cancer, almost half will develop a malignant effusion during the course of their illness (3), although this figure may be somewhat lower now with more recent treatment regimens. For lung cancer, 7% to 15% of all patients develop this complication (5). Eventually, about half of all disseminated cancer patients develop a malignant pleural effusion (4). Overall, this is a highly significant clinical problem, since approximately 100,000 malignant pleural effusions occur annually in the United States (6).

The appearance of a symptomatic malignant pleural effusion in a patient with known cancer significantly alters his or her quality of life. Although it is reported that up to 25% of patients with an effusion are asymptomatic, this may prove to be an overestimate if a careful history is elicited (7). In general, a prompt diagnosis accompanied by timely treatment of the effusion can markedly enhance the patient's functional status and should be considered early after the development of this common complication of advanced cancer.

### Etiology

Although about half of pleural effusions in reported hospital series are due to cancer, the most common cause of excess pleural fluid in a general clinical practice is congestive heart failure, which can often be unilateral (3). Once a malignant cause of the effusion has been proved, almost two thirds of the cases are found to be caused by either lung cancer, breast cancer, or lymphoma. However, almost all malignancies are known to metastasize to the pleura to cause an effusion. Table 1 lists the frequency of the various tumor types that are associated with malignant pleural effusions. The tumor origin is not found in 15% of effusions; in such cases the cell type is usually metastatic adenocarcinoma with the primary site unknown.

**TABLE 1.** *Tumor causes of malignant pleural effusions from collected series*

| Tumor type | Incidence (%) |
|---|---|
| Lung | 35 |
| Breast | 23 |
| Lymphoma/Leukemia | 10 |
| Adenocarcinoma, unknown primary | 12 |
| Reproductive tract | 6 |
| Gastrointestinal tract | 5 |
| Genitourinary tract | 3 |
| Primary unknown | 3 |
| Other cancers | 5 |

Reprinted with permission from reference 3.

## Pathophysiology

The pleura is a serous membrane that invests each lung to form a closed sac called the pleural cavity. There is a continuous passage of an almost protein-free fluid (protein content 1.5 g/dl) through the pleural membrane based on hydrostatic and colloid osmotic pressures. The net pressure in the parietal pleura is 9 cm $H_2O$, favoring movement of fluid into the pleural cavity, which is balanced with a net 10 cm $H_2O$ pressure in the visceral pleura, favoring absorption of pleural fluid by the visceral capillaries. Therefore, the overall direction of movement of fluid is from the systemic circulation in the parietal pleura across the pleural cavity back into the pulmonary circulation in the visceral pleura. At any one time, either pleural cavity has only 2 to 5 ml of fluid present, although as much as 5 to 10 liters flow through this space in any 24-hour period (8,9). Any imbalance in these pressures that disturbs the normal equilibrium may lead to a net accumulation of fluid in the pleural cavity.

In the patient with an advanced malignancy, changes occur that may alter the Starling equation governing fluid passage through the pleural space. The normal equilibrium may therefore be interrupted, leading to the accumulation of an effusion. Some of these changes that may occur are (a) increased capillary permeability due to inflammation from infection or tumor cell implantation; (b) increased oncotic pressure of fluid in the pleural space from the inflammatory reaction from tumor cells or infection; (c) decreased systemic oncotic pressure due to hypoalbuminemia from malnutrition; (d) increased negative intrapleural pressure due to atelectasis, possibly from tumor obstructing a bronchus; and (e) increased hydrostatic pressure in the pulmonary circulation, as in congestive heart failure from cardiac or pericardial metastases. In addition, a malignant effusion may result from obstruction of the visceral or parietal lymphatic channels by tumor, resulting in impaired absorption. Most malignant effusions are probably the result of a combination of the factors, with an overall increase in fluid production and a decrease in absorption (3,10).

Pleural effusions caused by a malignancy usually result in an exudate with a high protein content, although rare exceptions have been reported (1,5). However, transudative effusions (low protein) may occur as the indirect result of an advanced cancer, as in the patient with malnutrition and hypoalbuminemia, congestive heart failure due to cardiac or pericardial metastases, malignant ascites, or liver disease secondary to metastases (3).

## Clinical Presentation

The most critical initial step in evaluating the patient with a suspected malignant pleural effusion is to take a complete history and perform a careful physical examination. This simple step will usually exclude other causes of an effusion, such as heart failure or infection.

The clinical presentation of a malignant pleural effusion is almost always related to collapse of lung from the increased pleural fluid and the resulting initial symptom of exertional dyspnea. Later, resting dyspnea and orthopnea develop as the effusion increases in volume. A dry, nonproductive cough, a sense of heaviness in the chest, and occasionally pleuritic chest pain are also experienced. Nevertheless, an occasional patient (<25%) will appear completely asymptomatic in the face of a large effusion (11).

The physical findings of a malignant pleural effusion often include dullness to percussion of the affected hemithorax, decreased vocal fremitus, decreased breath sounds, egophony, and no demonstrable diaphragmatic excursion. Rarely, a very large effusion will result in a mediastinal shift with contralateral tracheal deviation and possibly even plethora or cyanosis from partial caval obstruction (3,7). Other signs and symptoms may be present initially but are usually related to the underlying primary tumor and not the effusion.

## Diagnosis

The approach to the diagnosis and subsequent treatment of a patient with a suspected malignant pleural effusion is shown in Figure 1.

The initial screening exam is the posterior-anterior chest radiograph, including decubitus views, which will confirm the presence of free pleural fluid and will also suggest the presence of any loculated fluid. An upright posterior-anterior chest radiograph that demonstrates blunting of the costophrenic angle will detect 175 to 500 ml of fluid, while a decubitus view will show as little as 100 ml (12).

Computed tomography may play a role in the evaluation of malignant pleural effusion patients. This is especially necessary if the hemithorax is opaque on chest radiograph and the presence of a large effusion (instead of a very large solid tumor filling the chest) must be

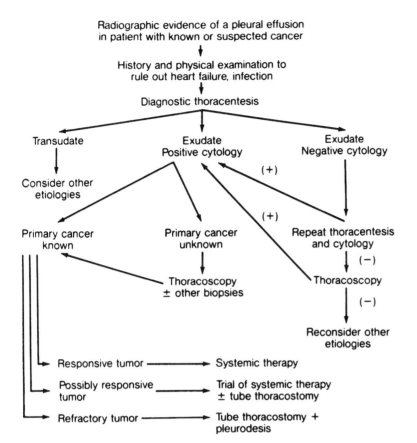

**FIG. 1.** Approach to the diagnosis and treatment of malignant pleural effusions. (+) = study result is positive. (–) = study result is negative. (From reference 7, with permission.)

established before drainage is performed, when a mesothelioma is suspected, or when the underlying primary tumor is unknown. However, a large effusion often obscures an underlying tumor in the lung, and computed tomography may prove more useful after drainage of the effusion and lung reexpansion. Occasionally, chest ultrasonography may prove useful in differentiating between pleural fluid and pleural thickening (13), but its more common application is to localize small effusions as a guide in thoracentesis (14).

After confirmation of a pleural effusion radiographically and after exclusion of any obviously nonmalignant causes, the next step is a diagnostic thoracentesis. In general, when a malignant effusion is suspected, only a small amount of fluid is withdrawn for diagnosis (at least 250 ml is needed for cytology). This leaves a moderate amount behind so that insertion of a chest drainage tube later is easier.

A thoracentesis should be performed by experienced personnel only, using sterile technique. After the chest has been percussed to assure that there is maximal dullness in the targeted area, the procedure is best done with the patient sitting. The approach is usually through the chest wall in the posterior axillary line at the seventh or eight intercostal space. The use of a disposable thoracentesis kit with a specially designed multihole catheter is preferred, since it tends to lessen the chance of complica-

tions such as a pneumothorax. Rapid removal of a large amount of fluid, especially over 1,500 ml, is not advised, since this may result in life-threatening reexpansion pulmonary edema, a real and not infrequent complication of large-volume thoracenteses (15).

The fluid removed should be heparinized and sent to the lab for protein and lactic acid dehydrogenase (LDH) determinations and cytology. Other tests, including pH determination (for which the fluid must be collected in an anaerobic container), glucose level, cell count, and cultures with smears, are usually obtained, although they may not be necessary if the clinical suspicion of cancer is high. With a malignant pleural effusion, the pH and glucose level are often low, but these are nonspecific findings (3). A malignant effusion is frequently hemorrhagic (erythrocyte count >100,000/mm$^3$), but this is also nonspecific and occurs in only one third of cases (5). Very recent or concurrent determinations of serum protein and LDH levels should be obtained to compare with the thoracentesis fluid in order to establish whether the fluid is an exudate or a transudate—an important distinction in planning further evaluation. The Health and Public Policy Committee of the American College of Physicians has reviewed the many published studies of pleural fluid analysis and has developed a set of criteria that reliably determine whether an exudate is present (Table 2) (16). If the fluid is found to be a transudate, then a malignancy is

**TABLE 2.** *Diagnostic tests confirming the presence of an exudate*

| Test | Positive predictive value |
|---|---|
| (1) Fluid LDH >200 International Units | 100% |
| (2) Fluid/blood LDH ratio >0.6 | 99% |
| (3) Fluid protein >3 g/dl | 95% |
| (4) Fluid/blood protein ratio >0.5 | 99% |
| (1), (2), or (4) above | 99% |

Reprinted with permission from reference 16.
LDH = lactic acid dehydrogenase.

essentially excluded. An exudate with a negative cytology result demands a second diagnostic thoracentesis with cytology, which will add approximately 6% to 11% more malignant diagnoses (3).

Cytology is the best method of diagnosing a malignant pleural effusion, although it is somewhat dependent upon tumor type, the experience of the cytopathologist, and the amount of fluid that is sent for cytologic analysis; at least 250 ml is preferred for the best yield (17). In a general hospital patient population, 45% of all effusions will have a positive cytology result (3). But in patients with an effusion eventually proved to be malignant, the first cytology result will be positive in 53% to 59% of cases, rising to 65% when a second thoracentesis is performed (3). In some tumors, such as Hodgkin's disease, the rate of positive cytology results is relatively low at 23%, while with others, such as breast or lung cancer, the diagnosis rate is as high as 73% (3). A variety of immunocytochemical staining techniques and, recently, cytogenetic markers have been added to complement the standard cytologic techniques. These methods have resulted in some increased diagnostic yield, although they often lack sensitivity and specificity, and also the laboratory expense is increased (3,10). We do not recommend using these tests outside of a clinical trial.

If the result of cytologic examination is negative, traditionally a blind pleural biopsy has been attempted, with some expectation of increased diagnostic yield. Although a blind biopsy may be a sensitive test in pleural tuberculosis because of its diffuse involvement, malignancies involving the pleura are commonly patchy in distribution, and a blind pleural biopsy usually adds little to the diagnosis. Although earlier series suggest that the pleural biopsy may be valuable in diagnosing malignancy in a patient with negative cytology results (3), a more recent direct comparison of pleural fluid cytology versus blind pleural biopsy casts doubt on its benefit. In this important series (18), cytology results were diagnostic of cancer in 71% of cases and suggestive in another 8%. Blind biopsy of the pleura gave positive results for malignancy in 45% of cases but provided a diagnosis in only *3%* of cases where the cytology result was nondiagnostic.

Therefore, if two exudative pleural fluid cytology results are negative for malignancy, most clinicians now bypass the blind pleural biopsy and move promptly to video-assisted thoracoscopy (VATS), wherein visually directed pleural biopsies are readily obtained and the diagnostic yield is quite high. In large series, the diagnostic sensitivity of VATS with malignant pleural effusion is 97% (19). Although VATS is a surgical procedure usually requiring general anesthesia, the mortality and morbidity is quite low at 0.5% and 4.7%, respectively (20).

In addition to providing a high diagnostic yield of malignancy by directed biopsies during VATS, this procedure, when the ipsilateral lung is collapsed and the patient is under general anesthesia, permits direct definitive therapeutic intervention with lysis of adhesions, mechanical pleurodesis, pleurectomy, or talc poudrage, with a very low recurrence rate (21). Finally, even when the fluid cytology result is positive but the primary site is unknown, VATS may be employed occasionally to obtain a larger amount of tissue for more definitive studies or to rule out the presence of a mesothelioma, especially when "adenocarcinoma, unknown primary" is the working diagnosis according to cytology. The advent of VATS has virtually eliminated the need for diagnostic open thoracotomy when a malignant effusion is suspected.

## Prognosis

Once the diagnosis of a malignant pleural effusion has been made, the choice of therapy must be put in perspective with the tumor and the condition of the host along with the prognosis. Virtually all of these patients have an incurable disease, so the treatment must be aimed at the most effective palliation for maximal, comfortable time outside of the hospital. For all patients, the overall mean survival time is 3 to 6 months. The mortality is as high as 54% at 1 month and rises to 84% at 6 months (11). Some malignant effusion patients with responsive tumors, such as breast cancer, may have a longer survival averaging 7 to 15 months (11); 20% have a 3-year survival (22). Ovarian cancer patients with a malignant effusion also have a longer expected mean survival of 9 months (23). Conversely, lung cancer patients have a worse prognosis, with a mean survival of 2 months, and 66% will die by 3 months (11).

## Treatment (Table 3)

### Systemic Therapy

When the effusion is small and asymptomatic and the tumor is likely to be sensitive to systemic therapy, as with lymphoma, leukemia, breast cancer, ovarian cancer, small-cell lung cancer, or germ cell tumors, the first line of therapy should be systemic chemotherapy or hormonal therapy, possibly accompanied by thoracentesis or tube

**TABLE 3.** *Methods of controlling malignant pleural effusions*

Systemic chemotherapy
Repeated thoracentesis
External radiotherapy
Tube thoracostomy alone
Tube thoracostomy with drug instillation
Pleurectomy
Pleuroperitoneal shunt
Videothoracoscopy (VATS) with pleurodesis

thoracostomy (7,10). When the tumor is relatively chemoresistant or has been shown to be so in the past, as with non–small-cell lung cancer or pancreatic cancer, the choice then is for prompt tube thoracostomy followed by intrapleural sclerotherapy to create a pleurodesis.

### Thoracentesis

Thoracentesis alone may relieve symptoms briefly, but the fluid usually reaccumulates rapidly. In a study of 94 patients, the mean time to reaccumulation of the pleural effusion after thoracentesis was 4.2 days, and 97% had a recurrence of the fluid by 1 month (24). In addition, repeated thoracenteses carry the risk of empyema, pneumothorax, a trapped lung from inadequate drainage and loculation of fluid, and the real possibility of progressive malnutrition from repeated removal of a large amount of the high-protein effusion fluid.

### Radiation Therapy

Radiation therapy may occasionally be useful as primary therapy, but only when directed at paramalignant effusions caused by mediastinal lymphadenopathy and lymphatic obstruction, usually from lymphoma (25). Improvement is rarely seen before 3 weeks, and therefore radiation has little application in the more acutely symptomatic effusion.

### Tube Thoracostomy

Tube thoracostomy alone has been proposed as effective therapy for malignant effusions (3). But careful review of the results demonstrate that none of these older studies reliably support the conclusion that chest tube drainage alone is efficacious in long-term control (3). However, tube thoracostomy appears quite useful in draining the pleural cavity and maintaining opposition of the pleural surfaces when a therapeutic agent is subsequently instilled into the chest for sclerotherapy. Anderson and associates found that chest tube drainage greatly improved the response to intrapleural nitrogen mustard, compared with instillation of the agent after thoracentesis alone (24). Chest tube drainage on continuous suction is

important in maintaining the pleurae in opposition while the sclerosing agent is causing its inflammatory reaction. The relative direct antitumor effect of any of the sclerosing agents is probably little, or at best some agents are cytostatic (26) and their primary action is mostly local inflammation.

Recently, some enthusiasm has been voiced for the use of small-bore (8 French or 12 French) catheters for gravity drainage or even suction drainage of the pleural cavity followed by intracavitary sclerotherapy. The long-term results of this technique are still undetermined (27), although the selection of patients with free-flowing effusions can enhance the outcome significantly (28). These small-bore catheters rapidly become occluded from debris and fibrin clots, and generally no effective suction can be maintained in the pleural cavity more than a few hours. If, as it is thought, the visceral and parietal pleurae should be kept in direct opposition for a day or two after instillation of the sclerosing agent to obtain a pleurodesis, then it is unlikely that these small catheters will be as successful as larger chest tubes. A national, randomized Intergroup trial of techniques for intrapleural sclerotherapy (ECOG 8592) has recently begun, and one of the therapeutic aspects of this problem that will be studied is a comparison of the effectiveness of larger-bore chest tubes versus small-bore catheters in treating malignant effusions (29).

To achieve the best palliation, the pleural cavity should be drained completely and the lung fully expanded. This is best accomplished by closed tube thoracostomy, with placement of the tube performed by an experienced physician to minimize discomfort and to safely obtain ideal tube position. A No. 24 French or 28 French chest tube is usually inserted in the sixth or seventh interspace in the midaxillary line with the tube directed posterior to the lung to maximize drainage. Generally the patient is given 3 to 6 mg morphine sulfate intravenously just before the procedure for sedation and to ally anxiety. The patient is positioned supine but turned up with the appropriate side of the chest elevated at 45° to 60° and with the surgeon standing behind the patient. After sterile prepping and draping of the skin, 20 to 40 ml 1% lidocaine is infiltrated into the skin, the subcutaneous tissue, and most importantly into the intercostal musculature and pleura of the interspace where the tube will enter. A brief thoracentesis is always performed first at the planned pleural entrance interspace to make sure that there is free aspiration of fluid. If no fluid is obtained, the chest tube entrance site must be altered to a place where fluid is readily obtained by thoracentesis. A small 2- to 3-cm skin incision is made 1 to 1½ interspaces below the target interspace, and a subcutaneous tunnel is created bluntly with a clamp. Likewise, the pleural cavity is initially entered with a blunt clamp, which is spread wide to create a generous opening for the chest tube. A clamp is placed on the introductory end of the chest tube to pass the tube through the subcutaneous tunnel into the pleural space and to direct the tube posterior and cephalad. The opposite end of the tube is also clamped off during the insertion to avoid an open pneumothorax and a gush of fluid from the chest. The surgeon should slowly twirl the tube as he passes it into the chest so he can avoid kinking the tube, since the tube will not twirl easily if the tube bends over inside the chest cavity. As long as the tube remains straight, the tube will twirl easily. Once the tube is inserted to a predetermined depth based on numerical markings on the tube itself, it is firmly sutured into place to the skin with heavy silk suture (0-silk or larger). The tube is then attached to an underwater seal drainage device at approximately 20 cm $H_2O$ suction. If there is a very large effusion, it should not be all drained immediately. Instead, 1,000 to 1,500 ml should be drained initially, and then the tube should be clamped for 30 to 60 minutes, draining approximately 1,000 ml every 60 minutes until the chest is completely empty. More rapid drainage of a large pleural effusion encourages the development of the life-threatening problem of reexpansion pulmonary edema, a real and preventable phenomenon (15). Although some physicians use a trocar chest tube, the risks of laceration of the lung or even the heart or diaphragm are significant, and most thoracic surgeons avoid these devices in favor of blunter, safer instruments.

Chest radiographs are obtained initially and then daily as long as the tube is in place. The chest tube is left on suction for total drainage of the effusion and to encourage reexpansion of all possible lung. When a properly positioned chest tube is completely open and is on suction, essentially all of the fluid that is drainable will have drained within a few hours of insertion and certainly following overnight drainage. Likewise, all lung that is expandable and is not trapped will have expanded following overnight suction. Although some authors suggest waiting an indefinite period of time until the chest tube drainage has decreased to an arbitrary 100 ml per 24 hours (10), waiting this extra time is probably not necessary and may even lessen the chance of success. The prolonged presence of the tube irritating the pleural cavity may encourage loculations and lessen the eventual distribution and effectiveness of the sclerosing agent. Therefore, the decision when to instill the intracavitary agent should rest on the appearance of the chest radiograph and not the daily drainage. Usually, the best time to instill the sclerosing agent is the day following chest tube insertion.

### Lung Expansion

Theoretically, the only time chemical sclerosis and pleurodesis should be effective is when there is complete drainage and complete lung expansion, and the visceral and parietal pleurae are in close contact, as proposed by most authorities in this area (5,20). However, at least one group has had remarkable success with chemical pleurodesis in malignant pleural effusion patients with incompletely reexpanded lungs, noting a successful complete response rate of 90% (9 of 10 patients) in this unfavorable subgroup (30). Nevertheless, if chemical pleurodesis fails in the incompletely reexpanded lung patient, then a more invasive and expensive videothoracoscopic surgery approach can always be employed, provided the patient is a suitable surgical candidate.

### Fibrinolytic Agents

If the chest radiograph the day following chest tube insertion shows apparent residual fluid, and especially if the fluid is thick or gelatinous, it may be worthwhile to try intrapleural instillation of urokinase 100,000 units in 100 ml 0.9% saline, clamping of the tube for 6 hours, and then resumption of suction for another 24 hours (30). This technique has been reported to improve drainage and lung expansion in loculated empyemas as well as with loculated malignant effusions with no side effects or systemic effects on coagulation or fibrinolysis (30,31). Since chest tube drainage alone will rarely control a malignant effusion, the next step is intrapleural sclerotherapy.

### Pleural Sclerotherapy

By far the most common palliative treatment of malignant pleural effusions is drainage of the pleural space with reexpansion of the lung. This is followed by instillation of a chemical agent into the pleural cavity to cause a pleuritis designed to create a symphysis between the visceral and parietal pleurae (also called pleurodesis by sclerotherapy) to prevent reaccumulation of fluid in this space. The most commonly used method to drain the effusion is with a chest tube, as previously described, and at least some nonrandomized studies suggest that this method gives superior results with sclerotherapy compared with drainage and sclerotherapy by needle thoracentesis alone (24).

Another apparent determinant of the success in pleural sclerosis is the glucose level and the pH of the pleural effusion. Several authors have found that a low glucose level (<60 mg/dl) and pH (<7.20) in the malignant effusion result in a higher recurrence rate after attempted chemical pleurodesis as well as an overall shortened patient survival (32,33). Although interesting, the exact significance of these isolated reports is uncertain and probably should not influence the choice of agent or techniques employed.

Controversy abounds as to which is the most effective chemical sclerosing agent for malignant pleural effusions. Comparison of the many published reports about various agents is often difficult because of the difference in reporting response rates, patient criteria, side effects,

**TABLE 4.** *Commonly used guidelines for evaluating the therapeutic efficacy of pleural sclerosis**

Patient must survive one month after the procedure.†
Objective response:
  No major fluid reaccumulation 1 month after pleural sclerosis, as determined by chest radiographs.
  No clinical requirement for thoracentesis within that month.
Failure:
  Reaccumulation of more than 50% of the original effusion volume in comparison with the immediate postpleurodesis chest radiograph.
  Clinical requirement for thoracentesis within 1 month of the pleurodesis.

Table adapted from reference 3. However, we favor a simpler evaluation using time to progression. See text for discussion.
*References 3, 34.
†Reference 35.

methods of evaluating results, and followup. The most widely followed set of guidelines to analyze results in the literature is that published by Hausheer and Yabro (3), which is summarized in Table 4. However, we believe that a simpler and more accurate means of assessing therapeutic efficacy is to follow the time to recurrence compared with the chest radiograph taken after pleurodesis and removal of the chest tube. In many instances, the pleural effusion recurs or progresses, but retreatment is not indicated because the disease has progressed disease elsewhere. For assessment of therapeutic efficacy, these cases still need to be counted as "failures." On the other hand, whether or not the progression is clinically meaningful—that is, needs retreatment—is a significant issue in cost-effectiveness studies.

## Mechanism of Sclerosis

The mechanism of action of sclerosing agents appears to vary somewhat depending on the type of agent and the laboratory model tested. One of the earliest studies (36) employed the rabbit as the test animal and found that the pH of the solution instilled into the pleural cavity appeared to be an important determinant of success. The most acidic solutions tested, including unbuffered tetracycline (the most acid being pH 2.5), were quite effective in creating a small polymorphonuclear-predominant effusion and resulted in complete pleural symphysis on postmortem examination of the animals. Other agents with higher, more neutral pHs, such as nitrogen mustard and quinacrine, had no significant effect on the rabbit pleurae in this study. However, a later study by the same group (37) using the same model but adding bleomycin and sodium hydroxide to the series test agents found that the pleural sclerosing effect was actually independent of pH and was more related to the increasing dosage of tetracy-

cline, the only agent causing a pleural sclerosis in this model.

Another rabbit study explored the effects of various dosages of intracavitary bleomycin versus tetracycline and found similar results of vigorous pleural fibrosis and symphysis with tetracycline, but no effect was seen with bleomycin (38). Minocycline was compared with tetracycline in another study using the rabbit model, and it proved to be as effective as tetracycline in creating a pleurodesis (39). When the mechanical agent talc was instilled by open thoracotomy in a study comparing various methods of pleurodesis using the canine model, this substance was found to cause a very intense pleuritis and a dense pleural symphysis that was even more pronounced than that caused by mechanical abrasion of the pleura or by tetracycline (40).

However, caution must be used in extrapolating the results of these and other laboratory studies to the clinical situation, since the animal models differ significantly in two major respects. The animals did not have a pleural malignancy, and therefore the results may be biased greatly depending on the actual mechanism of action of these agents in humans. In addition, in humans the agents are usually instilled via an indwelling chest tube, which is later returned to suction to keep the pleural surfaces apposed, unlike these animal models, wherein the test agents were instilled by thoracentesis or by thoracotomy. Finally, on a completely pragmatic note, many human clinical studies have shown a significant discrepancy and lack of correlation with animal studies in the efficacy of sclerosing agents such as bleomycin. Bleomycin and even nitrogen mustard have been demonstrated to be highly effective agents in humans (3) despite the complete lack of effect in the rabbit model. For this reason, the results of the animal studies must be viewed as interesting but probably without much clinical relevance.

## Technique of Pleural Sclerotherapy

The most common technique used to instill the sclerosing agent into the pleural cavity has developed primarily from convention and common usage (3,34,41,42) and not on the basis of rigorous studies. Following complete drainage of the pleural cavity with a chest tube and reexpansion of the lung on suction, the tube is clamped and the patient is placed into the lateral decubitus position with the affected hemithorax upward to assure that all of the sclerosing agent initially drains into the chest. Most clinicians will administer a parenteral narcotic such as morphine 3 to 6 mg intravenously 10 minutes before the procedure to minimize the potential and unpredictable pain of the chosen sclerosing agent. Approximately 150 mg lidocaine (15 ml of a 1% solution without epinephrine) are instilled initially into the pleural cavity through the chest tube using a Luer-lock syringe and 22 gauge needle. It is allowed to dwell several minutes for local analgesia. The sclerosing agent dissolved in 50 to 100 ml 0.9% saline is then injected into the chest tube, and the tube is left clamped for 2 hours. The use of talc slurry requires a slightly different technique using a bulb syringe and a saline flush (43).

Usually the patient is then turned and repositioned every 15 minutes for the 2 hours to assure even distribution of the agent throughout the pleural cavity. However, when this patient repositioning maneuver was investigated carefully in a comparative clinical study, rotation of the patient during the time the chest tube was clamped offered no significant benefit to the success of the attempted pleurodesis (42). Despite the results of this small study on position changes, most clinicians still ask the patients to reposition themselves frequently while the tube is clamped, unless there is a reason not to do so, such as a coexisting pathologic fracture. After 2 hours, the chest tube is unclamped and the tube is placed back on suction. The patient is followed with daily chest radiographs to verify continued complete drainage of the pleural cavity. The chest tube is removed when the daily drainage drops to 100 ml or less (41) [or <50 ml/8 hours (29)], and the patient is discharged the same day, once a confirmatory radiograph has been taken after removal of the chest tube. Most surgeons create a moderately long subcutaneous tunnel (1 to 1 1/2 interspaces) through which the chest tube is initially inserted, so that with tube removal the wound seals well without the necessity (and discomfort) of placing sutures to close the skin wound.

With the highly effective agents in common use currently, most patients will be able to have a tube placed the first day with overnight drainage of the pleural cavity and with instillation of the sclerosing agent the second day. The chest tube is then removed on the third or fourth day. Generally, a repeat chest radiograph is performed a month later in the outpatient setting to verify the longer-term success of the pleurodesis. Considering the very limited lifespan of these terminally ill patients, it is important to be as efficient as possible with pleural sclerotherapy to minimize chest tube and hospital time so that the patient can spend the maximal amount of his or her brief remaining time at home.

### Sclerosing Agents

Historically, a wide variety of agents have been instilled into the pleural space in order to create a pleurodesis (3,30,34). Table 5 lists most of the agents that have been described in the literature. These agents have differed greatly as to their effectiveness, side effects, availability, and even cost. Many are of only historical interest, while others such as talc, bleomycin, and doxycycline are in common use. Table 6 summarizes the efficacy of the most widely used sclerosing agents reported in the literature, comparing them with other methods of therapy designed

**TABLE 5.** *Intrapleural sclerosing agents*

Tetracycline
Doxycycline
Minocycline
Bleomycin
Talc
Quinacrine
Nitrogen mustard
Doxorubicin
Radioisotopes ($^{131}$I, $^{90}$Y, $^{32}$P, $^{198}$Au)
Mitoxantrone
*Corynebacterium parvum*
BCG cell wall skeleton
OK432 (streptococcal preparation)
Silver nitrate
Eosinophil colony-stimulating factor
Interleukin-2
Thio-TEPA
5-Fluorouracil
Autologous blood
Cisplatin
Cytarabine
Mechlorethamine
Pirarubicin
Carboplatin
Mustine
Mepacrine
Alpha, beta, or gamma interferon

to prevent the recurrence of malignant pleural effusions. Whenever possible, response rates are compared according to the criteria listed in Table 4.

*Tetracycline.* Since the first description of tetracycline as an agent for intrapleural sclerotherapy in 1972 by Rubinson and Bolooki (52), this agent has gained widespread acceptance and is preferred in the United States (53) and Europe (54). The intrapleural dosage of 500 mg was initially used, but soon as clinical studies began to appear the standard dose became 1 g (20). This agent has demonstrated consistent efficacy, with a mean objective response (using the increased 1-g dose) of 69% to 85%, averaging 72% (3,34). It has been proved to be safe, effective, quite inexpensive, and easily administered, with adverse reactions limited to fever (7% to 33%) and pain (17% to 62%) (3,30). The effect of tetracycline was generally believed to be related to its low pH of 2.0 to 3.5, which caused an extensive pleuritis in the rabbit model. However, a hydrochloric acid solution of the same pH failed to achieve the same sclerosing effect, which suggests that tetracycline had other actions (36).

Over the years, a variety of comparative clinical series, mostly nonrandomized, have been published with disparate methodology, patient selection, and response criteria, as well as retrospective analyses and variable results (3,34). Despite these limitations, most older studies comparing tetracycline with other agents such as nitrogen mustard, quinacrine, mustine, doxorubicin, bleomycin, and *Corynebacterium parvum* consistently demonstrated

**TABLE 6.** *Malignant pleural effusions: response rates of currently available therapy**

| | Response rates (%) | |
|---|---|---|
| Technique | Range | Mean |
| Tube thoracostomy alone | 0–86 | 22 |
| Tube thoracostomy drainage plus | | |
|   Talc | 72–100 | 96 |
|   Bleomycin | 63–85 | 84 |
|   Tetracycline* | 25–100 | 72 |
|   Doxycycline† | 73–95 | 84 |
|   Nitrogen mustard | 27–95 | 44 |
|   Quinacrine | 64–100 | 86 |
|   5-FU/Thio-TEPA | 14–80 | 30 |
|   Doxorubicin‡ | 18–24 | 24 |
| Radioisotopes ($^{198}$Au, $^{32}$P, $^{90}$Y) | 25–89 | 59 |
| External radiation | | |
|   Lymphoma | 88–100 | 94 |
|   Other tumors | 29–43 | 33 |
| Thoracoscopy with talc poudrage§ | 87–95 | 92 |
| Pleurectomy | 88–100 | 98 |

Table adapted from reference 3.

*No longer clinically available after mid-1991; replaced with doxycycline or minocycline.

†References 30, 44–47.

‡Reference 48.

§References 32, 49–51.

that tetracycline gave superior or at least equivalent results with much less toxicity (55). Of the few recent randomized larger trials, the series of Ruckdeschel and associates (56) and Johnson and Curzon (57) comparing intrapleural bleomycin and tetracycline showed a significantly better response to pleurodesis with bleomycin, with similar toxicity profiles. Nevertheless, tetracycline's ready availability and lower cost kept it as the preferred agent for pleurodesis with malignant effusions (53,54). Additionally, tetracycline's popularity was maintained as this agent was also found to be effective as intrapleural therapy for benign spontaneous pneumothoraces from various causes, including opportunistic infections in patients with the human immunodeficiency virus (46).

Despite the widespread use and acceptance of tetracycline, the production of its parenteral form was discontinued by its sole manufacturer in 1991 because it was unable to meet U.S. Food and Drug Administration purity standards (58). In its place, the tetracycline analogs doxycycline and minocycline have been substituted. Of these two, doxycycline has had the widest use and largest number of published studies. Doxycycline may have a mechanism of action similar to that of tetracycline, and it was found in a rabbit study to cause cuboid cellular changes with vacuolated cytoplasm in the pleural mesothelial cells, followed by connective tissue proliferation (59).

Clinical studies with doxycycline have begun to accumulate now, following the demise of parenteral tetracycline, but all thus far have been nonrandomized, noncomparative trials (30,44–47). Despite these limitations, doxycycline has consistently demonstrated effective results: response rates range from 73% to 95%, which is similar to those of bleomycin (see Table 6); yet, its toxicity is also similar, and its pain on administration may actually be less than tetracycline. The 500-mg dosage of doxycycline empirically chosen for these preliminary studies was probably too low, since over one third of patients required repeat dosing to be effective (30). Currently, 1 g doxycycline is considered the standard dose, and this is the dose that is being tested in the randomized, national trial of intrapleural sclerotherapy comparing doxycycline with bleomycin 60 units or talc 5 g in this three-arm study (ECOG 8592). The major problem in using doxycycline, as noted in prior studies, is that it frequently requires several dosings in order to obtain equal efficacy (48), and this seriously reduces its cost effectiveness because of the need for longer hospitalizations (60).

Minocycline has had much less use for pleural sclerotherapy. Rabbit studies (39,48) demonstrate inflammatory changes in the pleura similar to those seen with tetracycline. The only clinical series reported using minocycline (300 mg) was small, with 7 patients, but the complete response rate was 86%, similar to that of doxycycline, and the reported toxicity was likewise low (61). However, little information is currently available on this agent, and its eventual role in pleural sclerotherapy awaits further study.

*Bleomycin.* The most extensively studied cytotoxic chemotherapeutic agent used for intrapleural sclerotherapy is bleomycin. Not only does it play a significant role in the treatment of various solid tumors by parenteral administration, but also it has been shown to be highly effective in the palliative treatment of malignant pleural effusions, with response rates averaging 84% (3). Numerous nonrandomized studies have compared this agent to its primary competitor tetracycline, and most have suggested that there is no significant difference in efficacy or toxicity (55).

A few randomized trials of bleomycin versus tetracycline have been performed, with varying results. Kessinger and Wigton (62), in their study of 41 patients, found no significant difference in the response rates using 89 units bleomycin (67%) versus 500 mg tetracycline (61%), and both agents had similar toxicities. However, Ruckdeschel and associates (56), in their multiinstitutional randomized study of 74 patients receiving either 60 units bleomycin or 1 g tetracycline intrapleurally, found the complete response rate at 1 month to be 64% (18/28) in the bleomycin arm and 33% (9/27) in the tetracycline arm. Unfortunately, not all patients in this trial were restudied at 30 days, although the complete response rates were also significantly different at 90 days with 70% (26/37) and 47% (17/36), respectively. Johnson and Curzon, in their randomized trial of 60 patients, found an 87% complete response rate at 90 days with bleomycin, compared to 56% with tetracycline (57). The acute toxicities of both drugs were similar, although there tended to be a higher incidence of pain in the tetracycline arm in both of the latter studies (56,57).

Although 45% of the intrapleural dose of bleomycin is absorbed (63), myelosuppression is not seen. However, since the plasma half-life of bleomycin increases with renal failure, systemic toxicity with alopecia and mucositis is possible and has rarely been reported in renal failure patients (64). Therefore, caution is advised in using intrapleural bleomycin in patients with renal failure. Some have also recommended using the lower dose of 40 units/m$^2$ body surface area in the elderly because of their potential reduced plasma clearance of the drug (65).

The major disadvantage of bleomycin is its elevated cost in comparison with other agents such as doxycycline and talc, and this has been the major impediment to its widespread use. However, if it proves to be a more effective agent resulting in reduced hospital stays, and if consistently only a single dose is required for sclerotherapy, the cost factor may be overcome and bleomycin may actually be less expensive overall. And it is important to remember that one additional hospital day would pay for any extra cost of this agent, if it is actually more efficient than less expensive agents.

D. K. Fuller (66) and Belani and associates (60) argue that bleomycin is more cost effective overall than talc, tetracycline, and doxycycline on the basis of their questionable post hoc comparative analyses of a variety of disparate clinical studies (often published many years apart)

that commonly used inadequate doses of the test agent in the trials (i.e., 500 mg doxycycline instead of the current 1 g). Actual cost and efficacy comparisons of these agents await the results of the prospective Intergroup trial (ECOG 8592).

### Talc

*Talc Insufflation.* Talc is a generic term referring to a natural product containing the mineral talc (a trilayered magnesium sheet silicate) found in talcose or soapstone, which is usually contaminated with chlorite and trace minerals (quartz, calcite, and dolomite) (50,67) The most important contaminant of talc is asbestos (fibers of actinolyte, amosite, anthophyllite, chrysolite, crocidolite, and tremolite), which has been linked to carcinogenesis. However, for clinical use, USP talc has been purified with particle sizes generally less than 50 μm. Most importantly, USP talc has been asbestos free for many years, although it still requires sterilization prior to use.

Talc is the oldest, cheapest to purchase, and perhaps the most effective agent in causing a pleurodesis. The first description of talc as a pleural sclerosant was in 1935 by a Canadian surgeon, Norman Bethune, who insufflated talc into the pleural cavity of dogs and cats after creating a pneumothorax (51). Two patients were also described receiving an intrapleural dusting of talc just prior to lobectomy in order to create adhesions. Multiple studies with various animal models have followed, with the most recent by Mathlouthi and associates (68) demonstrating that talc insufflated into dogs causes a non–dose-dependent parietal and visceral inflammation followed by a granulomatous pleural reaction. Following talc administration, the resultant intense adhesive pleuritis, possibly accompanied by an adhesion-stimulating factor (50) obliterating the pleural space, is believed to be its primary clinical benefit in preventing the recurrence of malignant pleural effusions (67).

Insufflation of talc into the pleural cavity, or talc poudrage ("powdering"), is highly effective. Many studies demonstrate a response rate with malignant pleural effusions ranging from 87% to 95%, averaging 92% (32,49,50,67). The successful use of talc insufflation has also been described with benign effusions, chylothorax, pneumothorax, and even empyema (50). The primary disadvantage of talc poudrage is the requirement for thoracoscopy to be performed, usually with the patient under general anesthesia, to allow complete collapse of the lung to assure uniform distribution of the talc. An atomizer or bulb syringe is filled with dry talc, usually 2.5–5.0 g, and the talc is blown into the pleural cavity after ensuring that all loculations are removed. In selected patients, the risks of this procedure are small, with low perioperative morbidity and mortality (50). However, many patients with malignant pleural effusions are debilitated and are poor candidates for an operative approach, or they are quite reluctant to have such a procedure because of their short life expectancy. In addition, thoracoscopic talc poudrage usually increases hospitalization time, adds surgical and anesthesia costs, and increases the potential for complications. Fortunately, several studies have suggested that similar results are possible with bedside talc slurry administration through a chest tube, obviating the need for the more invasive operative approach (3,43).

Currently there is an ongoing national cooperative randomized trial of sclerosis of pleural effusions with intrapleural talc comparing delivery by videothoracoscopic insufflation with delivery by chest tube instillation as talc slurry (CALBG 9334). The results of this study should answer the question which is the preferable technique in terms of efficacy and cost effectiveness.

*Talc Slurry.* Twenty-three years after the first described use of talc with an open thoracotomy, J. S. Chambers in 1958 reported the successful use of talc instilled through a tube thoracostomy to control a malignant pleural effusion (69). In subsequent studies (34,43,50,55,70), the administration of talc in a suspension or slurry has proved to be as efficacious as by poudrage (48,67), with response rates ranging from 72% to 100% and averaging 96% (3). The administration of talc slurry is generally performed at the bedside with 2 to 5 g of sterile USP talc suspended in 30 to 50 ml 0.9% saline solution in a bulb syringe instilled into a larger-bore chest tube after complete drainage of the pleural space. Usually, intrapleural lidocaine premedication is used (43,50). The addition of thymol iodine powder to this suspension has been advocated in the hope of increasing the degree of pleuritis (43), but no difference in efficacy has ever been shown with the addition of iodine. At least one allergic reaction to intrapleural iodinated talc has been reported (67).

Although the efficacy of talc is generally well recognized, concerns about its adverse effects and safety have slowed its use. The usual side effects reported are pain on administration in most patients (43), but this is readily manageable, as with other sclerosing agents. Fever also accompanies talc slurry administration 16% to 69% of the time, but it is usually short-lived (67). Talc empyema is reported in 0% to 11% of cases (67) and can be exceedingly difficult to treat effectively, since talc is a foreign body and cannot be removed from the site of infection: the pleural cavity. Nevertheless, in at least one series talc has actually been instilled to obliterate the pleural space following empyema (50).

However, the more worrisome potential adverse effects are rare but definitely can occur, including talc microemboli to the brain (71); pulmonary complications of acute pneumonitis, pulmonary edema, and adult respiratory distress syndrome (72); and death (48,67). The definite mechanism of respiratory complications is unknown, but it is probably related to the suspected uptake of talc by the parietal pleural lymphatic system, with subsequent transport to the mediastinal lymph nodes and thoracic duct and hence to the systemic circulation (72,73). Talc administration has been reported (67) to be associated with a variety of acute cardiovascular complications—arrhythmias, cardiac arrest, chest pain, myocardial infarction, and hypotension—but it is often difficult to attribute these effects to the talc itself versus the other coexisting procedures, such as thoracoscopy in some cases.

The long-term effects of intrapleural talc are also of some concern. The potential decrease in lung compliance or restrictive lung disease was addressed by Lange and associates (74) in a report on 114 patients evaluating their lung function 23 to 35 years after operative talc poudrage treatment of spontaneous pneumothorax. They found mild restriction with a decrease in total lung capacity in patients receiving talc poudrage versus simple drainage, 89% versus 96% of predicted respectively, although the difference might have been related to the operative procedure. McGahren and colleagues (75) studied the pig model and used talc to obliterate the pleural space in young, growing animals, finding only a minimal long-term decrease in pulmonary compliance. Many believe that using the lowest possible dosage of talc, 5 g or less, will minimize the chances for these short- and long-term adverse effects (50,67).

The association of talc with the development of cancer has been described in miners who process talc, but this effect has been attributed to asbestos, which can contaminate unrefined talc in mines (76). When asbestos-free talc is used clinically, there does not appear to be an increased risk of cancer in patients exposed to talc pleurodesis. Lange and associates (74) found no mesothelioma in their series of patients who had undergone talc poudrage 23 to 35 years earlier for benign pneumothoraces. Likewise, Chappell and colleagues (77) found no increase in cancer in their group of talc pleurodesis patients at long-term followup. Generally, there appears to be no increased long-term risk of cancer when asbestos-free talc is used in the pleural cavity.

The last hurdle to the use of talc is the need for sterilization at the point of use, since it has yet to be readily available as a sterile preparation in the United States. Ethylene oxide gas, gamma irradiation, and dry heat sterilization, along with surveillance cultures of each batch of sterilized talc, are methods that have been described, although no one method is considered standard (78). Of these techniques, dry heat sterilization in the least expensive and the most commonly used. A commercially produced disposable spray canister of 4 g asbestos-free talc for use during talc poudrage has recently been described (79), although its availability in the United States has been sporadic and is currently unreliable.

*Quinacrine.* The antimalarial agent quinacrine is effective as a sclerosing agent with malignant pleural effusions; its response rate is as high as 86% on the basis of a variety of uncontrolled studies (3,80). A trial comparing tetracycline with quinacrine pleural sclerosis demonstrated tetracycline to be equally effective, but not associated with such severe adverse reactions (81). The toxicity of quinacrine, including frequent fevers, chest pain, nausea and vomiting, hypotension, hallucinations, and seizures, has made it an unattractive agent that is no longer used (3).

### Other Antineoplastic Agents

One of the first agents used intrapleurally to treat malignant effusions was the cytotoxic agent nitrogen mustard. This alkylating agent is highly reactive and loses its activity within minutes after contact with tissue. The response rates with nitrogen mustard varied greatly in various small series, from 27% to 95%, but averaged only 44% (3). When it was compared with other agents, the response rates were generally lower but the adverse reactions were much higher (3). The toxicity of nitrogen mustard was severe nausea and vomiting, commonly for 24 hours, in addition to local pain and fever (34). The lack of efficacy and its significant toxicity have made this an undesirable agent, of historical interest only (20).

Many other chemotherapeutic agents have been described in various small series, including thio-TEPA, 5-fluorouracil, doxorubicin, combination cisplatin and cytarabine, etoposide, mitoxantrone, and mitomycin-C (3,20,48). Generally, the results have been unimpressive and clearly are no better than those obtained with more common agents, such as tetracycline and its derivatives or bleomycin (3). However, their systemic absorption by intrapleural administration is considerable and often leads to prolonged plasma levels and significant systemic toxicity, including myelosuppression. At present, the use of these agents in this context is investigational and is not generally recommended (10,20,48).

### Biological Agents

#### Corynebacterium parvum

*Corynebacterium parvum* is an anaerobic gram-positive bacterium first described for intrapleural use to cause a pleurodesis in a trial in 6 patients in 1978 (82). Its effect was not found to be from its postulated role as stimulator of cell-mediated immunity. Rather, *C. parvum* recruits neutrophiles to the pleura, causing a subsequent fibrogenic response with fibrotic pleural thickening (83). *C. parvum* averaged response rates of 76% in single-agent studies but consistently demonstrated the same or worse response compared with bleomycin or tetracycline (41,48). *C. parvum* also has moderate toxicity, including fever (5%), pain (43%), cough (6%), and nausea (39%), and furthermore requires multiple instillations over a 2-day period. *C. parvum* offers no advantages as a pleural

sclerosant and is also not available in the United States, resulting in its lack of current clinical usage.

### Interferons and Interleukins

The most recent attempt to use biological therapy for malignant pleural effusions involves the use of interferon-$\alpha$, $\beta$, or $\gamma$ with the intent to stimulate natural killer cells, in addition to their cytotoxic effects (48). The response rates have not been impressive, with only a 41% complete response in a series of 29 patients (84). Intrapleural administration of interferon still remains investigational.

Several recent studies have investigated the use of recombinant interleukin-2 (rIL-2) alone or in combination with lymphokine-activated killer cells in malignant pleural effusions from lung cancer (85,86). These preliminary studies have commonly shown the disappearance of the pleural effusion and occasionally the cancer cells themselves (86), but no serious side effects occurred. These studies are intriguing but require more study in larger patient groups.

### Radioactive Isotopes

Finally, the use of intrapleural radioisotopes, especially radioactive gold ($^{198}$Au) and phosphorus ($^{32}$P), for control of malignant pleural effusions had a period of popularity beginning in 1951 when they were first described (87) until the late 1960s. The overall effectiveness of these agents was less than that of other available agents, with a mean response rate of 59% (3). The isotopes were also expensive and potentially hazardous to hospital personnel, patients needed to be isolated until the radioactive emissions were acceptably low, and special personnel and equipment were needed. Because of their relative ineffectiveness and their many disadvantages, radioisotopes are not currently recommended for pleural sclerotherapy and are of historical interest only (3).

### Surgical Interventions

#### Pleurectomy

A thoracotomy with mechanical pleurodesis, or a pleurectomy to remove most of the parietal pleura, has occasionally been done in the past as a primary procedure for malignant effusions. Martini and associates (88) in 1975 reported the use of pleurectomy in 106 patients with malignant effusion and saw no recurrence in 100%, but there was a 9% mortality and a 23% rate of major complications: bleeding, air leaks, pneumonia, empyema, pulmonary embolus, respiratory insufficiency, and cardiac failure. Currently, this procedure should be considered for application only at the time of thoracotomy when a lung cancer is found to be unresectable with pleural metastases. Occasionally, a well-selected patient of good performance status and a long life expectancy, in whom all other attempts at control of the effusion have failed, might be considered a candidate for open pleurectomy. However, the advent of videothoracoscopy now allows these procedures to be done, if necessary, in a minimally invasive manner, essentially making an open thoracotomy for this purpose rarely necessary.

### Pleuroperitoneal Shunt

Internal drainage of the malignant effusion into the abdomen using an implanted, valved, manually operated pump (Denver shunt, Denver Biomaterials, Denver, CO) was initially described in 1984, with the most recent series reported in 1993 (89). Implantation of this device usually requires general anesthesia (local anesthesia occasionally may be used in selected patients) and the performance of a small thoracotomy and small celiotomy that are needed in order to implant the two limbs; the pump is implanted subcutaneously. Since the shunt must carry fluid from a negative-pressure area (the pleural cavity) to a positive-pressure area (the abdomen), major patient or family participation is necessary. For the shunt to function properly, it requires manual pumping 100 times on five occasions per day. The shunt is occasionally an option in compliant, well-motivated patients with good performance status who have a trapped lung and an intractable effusion (5,10,41). Malfunction of the shunt over time, requiring its replacement, may further limit the usefulness of this device.

### Videothoracoscopy

The minimally invasive approach to intrathoracic disease afforded by videothoracoscopy (VATS) has given us more options in treating malignant effusions, especially refractory effusions in which pleural sclerotherapy by tube thoracostomy has failed. Talc poudrage with VATS, described earlier, is a highly effective technique with a mean 92% success rate. However, since the advent of instillation of talc slurry through a chest tube with its equivalent results, this surgical procedure should generally be reserved for the occasional patient who requires a VATS procedure for diagnosis. Talc poudrage can then be performed at the same time if a frozen section of the pleural tissue definitely verifies the diagnosis of metastatic cancer. If the diagnosis of mesothelioma is suspected at the time of evaluation of the pleura by VATS and the patient may be a candidate for aggressive surgical treatment of this tumor by extrapleural pneumonectomy, or if the diagnosis is in doubt, then a poudrage should not be done.

As experience with VATS grows, some investigators are now reporting series of successful VATS pleurectomy for malignant effusions. Waller and associates (90) performed a VATS parietal pleurectomy on 19 patients (13

mesothelioma and 6 metastatic adenocarcinoma) with no operative deaths or major complications, and the median hospital discharge was on the fifth day. Another approach to VATS pleurectomy was described by Harvey and colleagues (91) in 11 selected patients with malignant pleural effusion in which they performed a parietal pleurectomy assisted by dissection of the pleura with a stream of water (hydrodissection). The effusion did not recur in any patient.

### Another Invasive Technique

An innovative technique for approaching the lung cancer patient with pleural metastasis was described recently by Matsuzaki and associates (92). This approach took advantage of the antineoplastic effect of hyperthermia. The pleural cavity was irrigated using an extracorporeal circuit with a 43°C saline and cis-platinum solution for 2 hours in 12 patients with pleural metastases, who also underwent resection of their primary tumors. The pleural effusion was controlled in all 12 patients, and their median survival was 20 months, compared with 6 months in a cohort of 7 matched control patients with pleural metastases. This report is preliminary but provocative, and the technique bears watching as further work is reported.

### Recommendations

Once the diagnosis of malignant pleural effusion has been made (see Fig. 1), the decision to proceed with therapy requires careful thought. If the cancer is amenable to systemic therapy, then it is most appropriate to begin prompt chemotherapy. However, most malignant effusions occur with tumors that are poorly responsive or nonresponsive to systemic chemotherapy. In this patient population, it is generally best to drain the effusion and reexpand the lung early before it becomes trapped and sclerotherapy is unsuccessful. The preferred treatment is pleural drainage, usually with a large-bore chest tube (a No. 24 to No. 28 French catheter is large enough) and bedside intrapleural sclerotherapy. The optimal agent in terms of efficacy, adverse effects and safety profile, and cost effectiveness for pleural sclerosis is controversial. However, bleomycin, doxycycline, and talc slurry are the best candidates. The recently described technique of ambulatory sclerotherapy (92) using a small-bore catheter and outpatient sclerotherapy is an attractive cost-competitive approach with good preliminary results in a small series, but further study is necessary before this method can be recommended routinely.

Most of the literature in the treatment of malignant pleural effusions contains small retrospective series with loosely defined entrance requirements, variable criteria for assessing response, lack of long-term followup, and a lack of a randomized comparison with other forms of therapy. The few reported prospective trials still have

**TABLE 7.** *Multi-institutional prospective, randomized trial (ECOG 8592) comparing intrapleural bleomycin versus doxycycline versus talc: endpoints to measure (93)*

Time to recurrence of the effusion
Necessity for further treatment of recurrent effusions
Extent of postinstillation complications
Duration of chest catheter following pleurodesis
Duration of hospitalization if retreatment is needed for recurrent effusion
Survival

significant flaws in their study design. For this reason, the Eastern Cooperative Oncology Group designed a three-arm multiinstitutional trial (ECOG 8592) of intrapleural sclerotherapy for malignant pleural effusions (93) employing the most commonly used and effective agents (bleomycin 60 units versus doxycycline 1 g versus talc slurry 5 g). The accrual objective is 480 randomized patients, and the endpoints to be studied are listed in Table 7. It is hoped that this prospective trial will settle some of the controversy surrounding the optimal treatment of malignant effusions. This trial is currently active at the time this chapter is written.

The most perplexing and frustrating problem to deal with is the refractory pleural effusion in which the first attempt at pleural sclerotherapy failed. Generally, a second attempt at tube thoracostomy followed by intrapleural sclerotherapy is recommended, usually employing a different agent. If this second attempt fails, and if the patient has a good performance status and a reasonable estimated life span, then proceeding with VATS talc poudrage or VATS pleurectomy may be an option. Alternatively, such a patient may rarely be a candidate for a pleuroperitoneal shunt.

It is important to remember that the primary goal of therapy of a malignant pleural effusion is entirely palliative. The patient generally has a terminal disease with a very limited life span, usually counted in terms of a few months at best. The choice to treat and the actual treatment chosen must reflect the clinician's realistic understanding of the patient's overall prognosis and a desire to provide these terminally ill patients with the maximum possible comfortable time at home with the best quality of life. The timing of treatment is also critical. Waiting for "significant" symptoms to develop before draining a malignant effusion rarely improves the palliative benefits for the patient.

## PERICARDIAL EFFUSIONS

### Incidence

The appearance of a malignant pericardial effusion in patients with advanced cancer is not uncommon. In col-

lected autopsy studies of patients with disseminated cancer, involvement of the heart and pericardium with metastatic malignancy is seen in up to 21% of cases (41,94–98), with the highest incidence occurring in patients with leukemia (69%), melanoma (64%), and lymphoma (24%) (98). Since a large number of patients with malignant pericardial effusions are asymptomatic, autopsy studies tend to have a higher incidence than in clinical series (99). In terms of the actual clinical impact of symptomatic pericardial effusions, there were 7,000 patients who underwent pericardiectomy for all causes in U.S. hospitals in 1993 (100). Generally, 25% to 50% of all patients requiring surgical pericardial drainage have proven malignant pericardial involvement (101–103). Since not all patients with a malignant pericardial effusion undergo a pericardiectomy, the total number of patients developing this complication of advanced cancer is much higher.

### Etiology

Almost any tumor (except primary tumors of the brain) can metastasize to the pericardium and lead to an effusion (99). However, the most common tumors to involve the pericardium and heart are the same as with malignant pleural effusions: tumors of the lung and breast, lymphoma, and leukemia. These metastatic tumors account for almost 75% of all pericardial malignancies (104). When it metastasizes, melanoma frequently involves the heart, occurring in up to 50% of cases (104). Other malignancies that may spread to the pericardium to cause an effusion include gastrointestinal tumors and sarcomas. Primary tumors of the pericardium can cause effusions, but they are rare and include sarcomas, malignant teratomas, and mesotheliomas. Searching for the cause of a symptomatic pericardial effusion is critically important, since approximately 40% of patients with an underlying cancer have a nonmalignant cause of the effusion (105).

### Pathophysiology

The pericardium, as it is commonly known, is actually the parietal pericardium. The visceral pericardium is a monocellular serosal layer constituting what is also known as the epicardium of the heart. Together, both pericardial layers constitute a serosal sac containing at any one time 15 to 50 ml of low protein fluid. The pericardium is flexible but relatively inelastic. It probably functions to mechanically protect the heart from outside friction, provide a barrier from inflammation, maintain cardiac position against gravitational forces and acceleration, and support the thinner heart chambers such as the atria and the right ventricle (105).

Like the pleurae, the fluid inside the pericardial sac is normally in a balanced steady state of secretion by the serosal surface and reabsorption by the visceral (epicardium) and parietal pericardia. The increase in pericardial fluid that may lead to tamponade generally results from obstruction of the mediastinal lymphatic system, commonly by tumors such as lung and breast cancers that involve the mediastinal lymph nodes. Infiltration of the epicardium by tumor may block subepicardial venous flow, resulting in an outpouring of fluid into the pericardium. The parietal pericardium may also be infiltrated by tumor, resulting in increased fluid secretion. The result of blockage of pericardial fluid reabsorption, as well as often a net increase in secretion, may ultimately result in a symptomatic pericardial effusion (106,107).

When fluid increases slowly, the pericardium will distend greatly, up to as much as 2 liters, before the pericardium becomes tense. However, when the fluid accumulates more rapidly, the pericardium fails to stretch, pericardial pressure rises, and hemodynamic compromise may occur with as little an accumulation as 200 ml (108). The critical effect of this increase in pericardial pressure is impaired diastolic filling of the right side of the heart. The condition termed cardiac tamponade develops when there is "hemodynamically significant cardiac compression due to accumulating pericardial contents that evoke and defeat compensatory mechanisms" (109). On the basis of Starling's law, impaired diastolic filling will result in a depressed stroke volume and cardiac output. A greater volume of pericardial fluid and pressure causes an increase in ventricular diastolic pressure, which further impairs venous return, leading to a declining cardiac output. The autonomic nervous system responds to this decreased stroke volume and initially compensates by a release of catecholamines, resulting in an increased heart rate and arterial and venous vasoconstriction. The kidneys also respond to the decreased cardiac output by increasing sodium and fluid retention, leading to increased intravascular volume and venous pressure. Eventually, these compensatory mechanisms fail as intrapericardial pressure rises (often abruptly), resulting in a further decline in cardiac output with hypotension and circulatory collapse (108).

## Clinical Presentation

### Symptoms

Nearly two thirds of the patients with metastatic tumor involving the heart and pericardium will have no definite cardiovascular signs or symptoms (94), even when a careful history is taken. When the initial symptoms of a malignant pericardial effusion begin, they are often subtle and may be attributed to the underlying primary tumor. The actual development of symptoms depends on the rate at which the effusion accumulates, the actual effusion volume (and how close it is to causing maximal pericardial distension), and the underlying cardiac function, which itself may be impaired because of myocardial metastases or prior chemotherapy, as with doxorubicin (104,108). The actual severity of the symptoms also depends in part upon the rapidity with which the effusion develops. When the intrapericardial pressure increases sufficiently to impair diastolic ventricular filling, then symptoms begin appearing.

The most common and earliest symptom is dyspnea on exertion (93% of symptomatic patients), which may progress to dyspnea at rest as cardiac function is progressively compromised (95,104,108). Dyspnea is also the initial presenting symptom in patients with a malignant pleural effusion, a much more common complication of advanced cancer. A pleural effusion occasionally accompanies a malignant pericardial effusion, and this by itself may draw attention away from the actual pericardial problem and confound the diagnosis. A comparison of the presenting signs and symptoms of pericardial and pleural effusions is found in Table 8 (94,110).Other common symptoms include chest pain or heaviness (63%), cough (30% to 43%), and weakness (26%) (94). Less common symptoms include peripheral edema, low-grade fever, dizziness, nausea, diaphoresis, and peripheral venous constriction. The presence of peripheral edema often

**TABLE 8.** *Comparison of the presenting signs and symptoms of malignant pleural and pericardial effusions*

| Frequency | Pericardial | Pleural |
|---|---|---|
| Common | Dyspnea (exertion) | Dyspnea (exertion) |
| | Dyspnea (rest) | Dyspnea (rest) |
| | Chest pain or heaviness | Orthopnea |
| | | Cough |
| | Cough | Percussion dullness |
| | Jugular venous distension | Egophony |
| | Hypotension | Percussion dullness |
| | Pulsus paradoxus | |
| | Resting tachycardia | |
| Uncommon | Cyanosis | Cyanosis |
| | Peripheral edema | Pleuritic chest pain |
| | Low-grade fever | Anorexia |
| | Distant heart sounds | |
| | Peripheral vasoconstriction | |
| | Narrowed pulse pressure | |
| | Kussmaul's sign | |
| | Low-voltage ECG (limb leads) | |
| | Electrical alternans | |
| | Hepatojugular reflux | |
| | Pleural effusion | |

Adapted from reference 110.

leads unsuspecting clinicians to give diuretics, which significantly worsen the underlying physiologic problem. Cyanosis from decreased venous return and venous hypertension, and agitation and tachypnea from low cardiac output and hypoxia, are late manifestations of pericardial tamponade (104,108).

### Signs

The classic signs associated with cardiac tamponade were described in 1937 by Claude Beck and are often referred to as Beck's triad: quiet heart sounds, hypotension, and venous distension (111). These signs remain the most commonly seen, although the muffled heart sounds may be more difficult to appreciate clinically. Unfortunately, all of these clinical signs appear late in the course of the physiologic deterioration. Therefore, waiting for them to develop before ordering diagnostic tests in inappropriate. Hypotension is found in 41% to 63% of patients, elevated venous pressure is seen in 50% to 63%, and resting tachycardia occurs in 68% to 89% (95). The venous pressure is almost always elevated in cardiac tamponade, although rarely it may be normal or low if the patient is hypovolemic. A central venous pressure greater than 15 mm Hg with hypotension is highly suggestive of tamponade.

The pathophysiologic effects of cardiac tamponade tend to exaggerate the normal fall in systolic blood pressure (usually less than 10 mm Hg) and stroke volume that occur with inspiration. The causes of this normal event are controversial but are thought to involve any or all of the following: (a) inspiratory pooling of blood in the lungs with decreased filling of the left side of the heart, (b) increased right ventricular filling with leftward movement of the interventricular septum to cause reduced left ventricular filling and increased afterload, (c) a fall in left ventricular stroke volume as a result of increased left ventricular transmural pressure, and (d) "reverse thoracic pump" mechanism that is due to a inspiratory decrease of intracavitary left ventricular pressure relative to atmospheric pressure (109). Cardiac tamponade exaggerates this normal physiology and was termed by Kussmaul in 1873 to be a pulsus paradoxus. This term is a misnomer, since it refers to the accentuation of a normal phenomenon, not a reversal of it. Clinically, a patient is considered to have a pulsus paradoxus if the inspiratory drop in the systolic blood pressure is greater than 10 mm Hg. Although strongly associated with tamponade, a pulsus paradoxus may also be detected in other conditions such as pulmonary embolism, chronic obstructive lung disease, obesity, failure of the right side of the heart, and tense ascites.

Other signs, less frequent, that may be present include a narrowed pulse pressure, a visible increase in venous pressure on inspiration (Kussmaul's sign), hepatomegaly, hepatojugular reflux, peripheral edema, cyanosis, pericardial friction rub, arrhythmias, cold clammy extremities, low-grade fever, and ascites.

### Diagnosis

#### Radiographic

In a patient with cancer with or without symptoms, a change in the size and contour of the heart with clear lung fields on a standard chest radiograph should alert the clinician to consider the diagnosis of a pericardial effusion. The cardiac silhouette may resemble the so-called "water-bottle heart" with bulging of the normal contours. Nevertheless, a normal-size heart shadow does not exclude the presence of a pericardial effusion or even a life-threatening tamponade. A coexisting pleural effusion may be present in up to 70% of patients with pericardial effusion (95). Since the accumulation of pericardial fluid and the onset of symptoms may be insidious, re-taking the symptom history carefully may provide useful information when the chest radiograph is changing.

Chest computed tomography (CT) obtained for staging or followup in a cancer patient will occasionally reveal a pericardial effusion with more sensitivity than a standard chest radiograph (95). The chest CT scan may suggest a malignant pericardial process if the effusion has a high density, there is pericardial thickening, masses are contiguous with the pericardium, or there is an obliteration of the tissue planes between the mass and the heart. As a screening tool, however, chest CT has limited usefulness because of the blurring of the pericardial contents on the scan caused by continuous cardiac motion. Magnetic resonance imaging (MRI) provides a more precise view of the myocardium than chest CT, but MRI offers no better evaluation of the pericardium. However, experience with MRI in malignant pericardial effusions is limited, and its use should be limited to clinical investigation only, since it offers no apparent advantages over echocardiography.

Another more invasive diagnostic procedure is catheterization of the right side of the heart, which can easily be done at the bedside in the intensive care unit. The passage of a flow-directed pulmonary artery catheter (Swan-Ganz catheter) is a common critical care procedure that can establish the presence of a cardiac tamponade. The findings from this procedure in true tamponade are depressed cardiac output and the equalization of diastolic pressures in all heart chambers (109). Specifically, the right atrial mean, the right ventricular diastolic, and the pulmonary capillary wedge pressures all tend to equalize in tamponade and can be readily measured with the pulmonary artery catheter. However, if malignant pericardial effusion is suspected, catheterization of the right side of the heart is rarely necessary, since echocardiography is sensitive enough to establish a reliable diagnosis of tamponade noninvasively, thereby allowing for prompt pericardial decompression.

### Electrocardiography

The electrocardiogram often has changes associated with a pericardial effusion, including tachycardia, atrial and ventricular arrhythmias, low-voltage QRS, and diffuse nonspecific ST and T wave abnormalities. Electrical alternans is occasionally seen and consists of alternating large and small P wave and QRS complexes, caused by the increased rotary motion of the heart in the large fluid-filled pericardium. This interesting electrocardiographic abnormality generally resolves immediately with drainage of the effusion (96,109).

### Echocardiography

The most sensitive and precise tool used to evaluate a pericardial effusion is echocardiography, usually in the two-dimensional (2-D) mode (95). Any patient suspected of having an effusion deserves to have an echocardiogram. Not only is this examination rapid and noninvasive, it can be performed quickly at the patient's bedside even with the patient in a sitting position, and this instrument is then available immediately to aid in the performance of a diagnostic or therapeutic pericardiocentesis. Echocardiography is extremely sensitive and may detect as little as 15 ml of fluid, as well as identifying myocardial masses and even loculations of fluid.

Aside from its role in the diagnosis of a pericardial effusion, echocardiography is quite useful in assessing the hemodynamic consequences of the effusion. Cardiac tamponade is suggested by diastolic collapse of the right atrium or ventricle, inspiratory decrease in left ventricular dimensions, inspiratory increase in right ventricular dimensions, or failure of the inferior vena cava to collapse on inspiration (inferior vena cava plethora) (112,113). Prompt performance of an echocardiogram in a patient with a suspected effusion is quite important, since only 69% of patients with echocardiographic signs of tamponade are suspected of having a tamponade clinically prior to the study (114).

The most powerful predictor of the development of subsequent cardiac tamponade is the size of the effusion, since not all effusions will lead to hemodynamic compromise (115). Although the ready availability of echocardiography has allowed the earlier diagnosis of effusions in more patients, it also may have led to some overdiagnoses (116). Small effusions without symptoms are very rarely malignant and almost never require invasive evaluation or treatment. In addition, it is most uncommon for isolated pericardial disease to be the initial manifestation of new malignant disease (116).

### Pericardial Fluid Examination

Percutaneous, ultrasound-guided pericardiocentesis can safely be performed in patients with larger effusions (>1 cm anterior clear space on echocardiogram). It will yield pericardial fluid for examination in approximately 90% of patients and will promptly and temporarily relieve tamponade (95,114). The fluid obtained should be sent to the lab for cytology and for determination of LDH and total protein levels. If the patient has symptoms suggesting an infectious or rheumatologic cause of the effusion, other tests such as glucose, cell count, and culture should be added. This is rarely needed in the patient with an obvious intrathoracic malignancy. In a malignant pericardial effusion, the result of cytology will be positive for malignant cells in 65% to 90% of cases (41,99,109, 117,118). False-negative cytologic results are frequently seen with lymphoma and mesothelioma. However, the lack of malignant cells in the effusion fluid obviously does not exclude the possibility of neoplastic pericarditis, and it is often necessary to obtain pericardial tissue for histology if a malignant diagnosis is still suspected.

Bloody ("crank-case oil" appearance) or serosanguinous fluid is associated with neoplastic pericarditis, but it may also be seen with idiopathic causes. Malignant effusions are bloody or serosanguinous in 76% of cases and serous in the rest (119). This bloody fluid never clots because it is defibrinated by the motion of the heart inside the pericardium in addition to the intrinsic, local fibrinolytic activity of the serosal lining of the pericardium (106). Frankly purulent or milky fluid suggests pyogenic pericarditis. A gold-colored thick fluid may be found in cholesterol or post–myocardial infarction pericarditis. The chemistry values from the effusion fluid may occasionally be useful. Campbell and associates (120), in a study of 25 patients with malignant pericardial effusions, found that an elevated serum LDH and an elevated pericardial fluid LDH, as well as a bloody effusion, were all suggestive of a malignant effusion. However, pericardial fluid protein, glucose, white blood cell count, triglycerides, or cholesterol were not found useful in differentiating between malignant and benign effusions.

### Differential Diagnosis

Since up to 40% of patients with a symptomatic pericardial effusion and an underlying cancer will have a benign cause of the effusion and perhaps require different treatment, it is important to find out the specific cause of the effusion (105). Of particular importance in the differential diagnosis is radiation-related pericardial effusion in patients who have received mediastinal radiation therapy (especially >4,000 cGy) (121). From 7% to 30% of these patients may develop effusive or effusive-constrictive pericardial disease, usually within 24 to 36 months (occasionally within just a few weeks) of the radiotherapy (105,121). Purulent or tuberculous pericarditis is another possibility to consider, especially in the cancer patient who is debilitated and febrile. Drug-induced pericarditis from agents such as procainamide or hydralazine, or even from cancer chemotherapy drugs such as doxorubicin (pericarditis-myocarditis syndrome) (122) may occasionally occur. Idiopathic (viral), uremic, hypothyroid, cholesterol, post–myocardial infarction, or autoimmune pericarditis are other considerations in the differential diagnosis (99). Generally, the pericardial fluid analysis plus the patient's history will exclude most of the potential diagnoses and will pinpoint the actual cause of the effusion.

## Prognosis

Although cancer patients with cardiac tamponade from a malignant pericardial effusion usually are severely ill at presentation, prompt relief of the tamponade will often allow them to return to a surprisingly good functional status for significant time intervals. The quality and quantity of life depends largely on the histology of the malignancy and its extent. After surgical drainage of the pericardial effusion, breast cancer patients have a mean survival of 8 to 18 months (102,116,118,123); lymphoma patients have a mean survival of 10 months (123). Lung cancer patients fare somewhat worse, with a mean 3- to 5-month survival (102,123). However, the extended survival of these advanced cancer patients with malignant pericardial effusions underscores the importance of tailoring treatment of this complication to provide maximal benefit with the least chance of reaccumulation of the effusion.

## Treatment

Patients with obvious end-stage metastatic disease and a pericardial effusion may occasionally be best served by the least invasive intervention, but rarely by none at all. The diagnosis of a malignant pericardial effusion and a life-threatening tamponade should always be considered and investigated in any cancer patient, especially if he or she has had a recent or sudden decline in functional status. Over three decades ago, when interventions for malignant pericardial effusive disease were less common and diagnostic techniques were not as precise, Thurber and associates (97) found that a pericardial tamponade was the direct or contributing cause of death in 85% of their series of 55 advanced cancer patients, and only 30% of patients had a correct antemortem diagnosis. Prompt pericardial decompression can result in prolonging survival and quality of life for many months or longer, depending upon the histologic cell type. Although management decisions involving the treatment of large pericardial effusions in cancer patients must be considered in light of the overall condition, age, symptoms, and prognosis of the patient, an aggressive approach is generally recommended in all cases, even if only minimal symptoms are present.

The optimal therapy for this problem is controversial. The medical literature is filled with reports about various therapeutic options (Table 9) whose results vary as widely as the techniques. When these invasive techniques are compared, it is important to focus on the most recent reports, since the associated morbidity and mortality as well as the results generally improve with further experience. In the discussion that follows, each option in therapy will be discussed, but true comparative data among techniques are not currently available.

### Pericardiocentesis

The earliest described method of nonsurgical drainage of the pericardium, performed by Schuh in 1840, was pericardiocentesis, which he used to relieve a hemorrhagic effusion in 30 patients, of whom 7 subsequently survived (124). As techniques have evolved and safety has improved, pericardiocentesis has remained the most common approach for diagnosis and therapy in patients with malignant pericardial effusions (119). It may be performed quickly under local anesthesia and is the initial procedure of choice in the emergency management of life-threatening tamponade (119).

Pericardiocentesis is best performed from the subxiphoid approach, with the needle inserted between the xiphoid and the left costal arch at a 45° angle directed toward the left shoulder. This is the easiest and safest approach because there is a smaller chance of damaging a coronary artery. The patient is placed in the semi-Fowler's position so that most of the effusion is in the most dependent portion of the pericardium inferiorly (125). In a true emergency, the needle can be advanced blindly or with electrocardiographic monitoring with the needle attached to a V lead. With continuous electrocardiographic monitoring, contact with the epicardium will be seen as an immediate ST segment elevation, often with premature ventricular contractions, warning the clinician to withdraw the needle. If bloody pericardial fluid is

**TABLE 9.** *Treatment options with malignant pericardial effusions*

| |
| --- |
| Pericardiocentesis with or without catheter drainage |
| Intrapericardial sclerosis with chemicals or radioisotopes |
| Chemotherapy |
| Radiotherapy |
| Subxiphoid pericardiectomy ("window") |
| Left anterior thoracotomy with pericardiectomy |
| Median sternotomy with pericardiectomy |
| Videothoracoscopic pericardiectomy |
| Pericardioperitoneal shunt |
| Percutaneous balloon pericardiotomy |

removed, it should not clot and generally has a hematocrit lower than that of intravascular blood. Whenever possible, a thoracic surgeon should be notified that the pericardiocentesis is being performed in case a complication occurs requiring immediate surgical drainage.

Adding echocardiographic guidance to the pericardiocentesis has increased the success rate in obtaining fluid for diagnosis and relieving symptoms to almost 97% and has decreased the complication rate (95,118). Major complications include coronary artery laceration, myocardial puncture, pneumothorax, trauma to abdominal organs (especially the liver), and even death. The complication rate in collected series of pericardiocentesis using echocardiographic guidance is 2.4% with no deaths (118). The hazards of the procedure may be minimized if it is performed only on patients with a significant anterior clear space greater than 1 cm, using echocardiographic guidance, correcting thrombocytopenia prior to the procedure, and avoiding obviously loculated or posterior effusions (95,118,119).

Pericardiocentesis by itself is considered only an initial temporizing procedure to obtain diagnostic fluid and relieve symptoms. It is particularly useful in stabilizing a patient's condition before surgical drainage is performed. However, pericardiocentesis is not considered to be definitive treatment, since most (39% to 56%) malignant effusions will recur even after single or repeated taps (95,118). Insertion of a small No. 7 or No. 8 French multihole pigtail catheter over a guidewire into the pericardial space can be easily accomplished at the time of initial tap, to allow intermittent drainage over several days. Still, a large number of patients treated in this manner will require more definitive surgical drainage for long-term control of the effusion (95).

One word of caution is highlighted by two recent reports of large-volume pericardiocenteses on patients in tamponade. Wolfe and Edelman noted in transient severe symptomatic systolic dysfunction in two women, lasting 1 to 2 weeks after they had undergone pericardiocentesis (650 ml bloody pericardial fluid removed from either patient) to relieve a tamponade for a malignant pericardial effusion from metastatic breast cancer (126). Both patients were treated symptomatically and recovered gradually. Braverman and Sundaresan (127) reported a similar picture in a 27-year-old woman with a pericardial tamponade from benign acute pericarditis who was noted to have global myocardial dysfunction after undergoing pericardiocentesis that removed 500 ml serous fluid. A subxiphoid pericardial window was subsequently made, with removal of 1,000 ml more fluid. Dobutamine was used to treat her low-output syndrome, which resolved completely 3 weeks later. The cause of this phenomenon, which we have also seen, is not known, but it may relate to diminished coronary blood flow during the period of tamponade, leading to a degree of myocardial stunning that was eventually reversible.

## Intrapericardial Sclerosis

The logical extension of pericardiocentesis with catheter drainage is injection a sclerosing agent into the pericardium through the indwelling catheter to prevent a recurrence of the effusion, much like that practiced with malignant pleural effusions. Almost half of the pleural sclerosis agents listed in Table 5 have been used in various small series intrapericardially. Agents were chosen on the basis of their irritating qualities and/or their antitumor activity, but the mechanism of action of the successful agents is unknown.

Nitrogen mustard, thiotepa, and quinicrine were tried in the 1970s in small studies with fair results but with pain and substantial toxicity from bone marrow suppression, leading to abandonment of these agents (41). Intrapericardial tetracycline, the most widely used drug, has had a combined success rate of 85% in the two largest reports (128,129). Tetracycline was instilled in doses of 500 mg to 1 g on several days in all patients (mean 2.9 days), and the pericardial catheters remained in place for a mean 8.8 days in one of the studies (128). Although a fairly effective agent with the expected toxicities of fever (18.7%), pain (9.9%), arrhythmias (12.1%), and catheter plugging (4.4%), tetracycline had the distinct disadvantage of requiring a long hospitalization. Tetracycline is no longer available, and the analog now used, doxycycline, has had a 100% success reported in one small series of 7 patients, but they too required multiple instillations (130). The most recent series using pericardial sclerosis as primary management was larger, involving 85 patients, and had a 73% success rate in controlling the effusion for over 30 days (131). This group used tetracycline early in the series and doxycycline later, but as in prior reports, multiple instillations of drug were also necessary for success.

Bleomycin has also been used in very small series (a total of 15 patients in five series) with fairly good results and minimal toxicity, although these small patient series are difficult to interpret (118). Other anecdotal reports of cisplatin, teniposide, and fluouracil have also appeared, although such small series preclude drawing any conclusions about efficacy and safety.

Immunostimulators interleukin-2 (132) and OK-432 (133) have also been employed by intrapericardial infusion to control malignant effusions. The results from these small series suggest that in two thirds of patients, the effusion can be controlled. However, this novel approach appears to offer no advantage over other agents (118).

One primary concern about the advisability of intrapericardial sclerosis is whether there is an increased risk of pericardial constriction in patients so treated. Lee and associates reported their favorable experience with intrapericardial sclerosis in 20 patients using mitomycin C, and had a 70% success rate (134). Soon afterward, however, the same group reported that in one of their initially successful cases, the patient developed constrictive pericarditis 6 months later. They noted that this complication may occur if the patient survives long enough after pericardial sclerotherapy (135). Despite this concern, late pericardial constriction has not been commonly reported.

Intrapericardial radioisotopes, including gold ($^{198}$Au) and chromic phosphate ($Cr^{32}PO_4$), have been used (95,118). They are only partially effective even in radiosensitive tumors, and the logistical problems associated with them have precluded their use. In a novel approach, radioactive iodine ($^{131}$I) has been tagged to a monoclonal antibody (HMFG2) with intrapericardial administration, and the preliminary excellent results in a small series of four patients suggest that this technique bears further investigation (136).

### Systemic Chemotherapy

Systemic administration of chemotherapy or possibly hormonal therapy (in breast cancer) may be quite appropriate in chemosensitive tumors causing pericardial effusions. Initial pericardiocentesis followed by systemic therapy has been reported to prevent recurrence of the effusion in two thirds of patients and is especially effective in lymphoma (118). Chemotherapy is directed toward long-term control but is not useful when there is hemodynamic compromise from the pericardial effusion (95).

### Radiotherapy

External beam radiotherapy has been advocated for a variety of tumors with cardiac and pericardial involvement (137). In collected series (118), most patients underwent initial pericardiocentesis followed by radiotherapy in the 1,500 to 4,000 cGy dose range, the threshold at which radiation pericarditis and myocarditis can appear (98,138, 139). Approximately 67% of patients so treated will have a positive response, although the best results are found with lymphomas and leukemias (118). Pericardial inflammation is a complication of therapy and may lead to acute pericarditis or possibly late constriction. Generally, radiotherapy is recommended for patients with radiosensitive tumors without hemodynamic compromise, who have not previously received radiotherapy (95).

### Surgical Approaches

Since pericardial tamponade is predominantly a mechanical problem related to compression of the heart by an effusion, it is not surprising that the earliest attempts to treat this problem involved a surgical approach to drainage, and surgery has remained the preferred technique, although it has been considerably refined. In 1649, Jean Riolan first suggested trephination of the sternum to decompress a pericardial effusion compressing the heart, although the technique was not used until several centuries later (140). In 1819, Romero performed the first successful surgical pericardiotomy (141). However, it was Napoléon's famous surgeon, Baron Dominique-Jean Larrey, who first used the subxiphoid approach to drain the pericardial cavity, considering this an easy operation with small risk. He believed, as we do today, that this most dependent portion of the pericardium was best, since the collection of fluid was more prominent and the heart was at the greatest distance away from the pericardium, with the least chance of a rhythm disturbance (142). Techniques have advanced during the intervening 150 years, although Larrey's approach is still favored.

The term *window* in reference to pericardial surgery was described first by Williams and Soutter in 1954 in their description of an anterior thoracotomy through which they created a small opening in the pericardium and held it open by suturing it to the lung (143). The term *subxiphoid pericardial window* was finally used by Fontanelle and associates in 1970, and that term has continued to the present (144).

### Subxiphoid Pericardiectomy ("Window")

The most popular approach to surgical treatment of a malignant pericardial effusion is the subxiphoid pericardiectomy, which offers the distinct advantages of very low mortality (1% or less), 1% major morbidity, 100% immediate efficacy in relieving tamponade, and a long-term recurrence rate of 3% to 7% (41,95,119,145). Diagnostic accuracy is also excellent and approaches 100%, since fluid and pericardial tissue are both removed and are sent for pathologic evaluation. In critically reviewing surgical series, it is important to consider only reports of surgery performed in the last 10 years or so, in the era of the most modern anesthetic techniques, so that the assessment of results reflects current practice with its lower risks. The most recent report involved 82 patients with malignant pericardial effusion who underwent subxiphoid pericardiectomy (146). No postoperative deaths were attributable to the surgical procedure, and there was only a 2.4% recurrence rate in the long term requiring further intervention.

Subxiphoid pericardiectomy may be performed in the operating room in only 30 to 45 minutes on critically ill patients under local anesthesia. Often general endotracheal anesthesia is used if there is no significant hemodynamic compromise or if the pericardium has been decompressed by pericardiocentesis. With general anesthesia, exposure is improved and a larger portion of pericardium may be removed because there is greater muscle relaxation (145). In addition, general anesthesia is necessary if there is extreme obesity or a narrow costal angle, or if there has been a previous upper midline incision. In fact, in these circumstances it may be preferable to divert to a left anterior thoracotomy for the pericardiectomy.

For the subxiphoid approach, a short 4- to 6-cm midline incision is made, extending caudad from the xiphoid with entrance into the preperitoneal space after the linea alba has been opened. The xiphoid may be resected for exposure, if needed, but commonly it is left in place if the procedure is performed with the patient under general anesthesia. The sternum is retracted anterosuperiorly, blunt dissection is carried superiorly directly posterior to the sternum, and the fatty connective tissue from the anterior parietal pericardium is cleared off. The pericardium is sharply incised, and there is commonly a gush of dark bloody fluid, which rapidly reverses any hemodynamic compromise. After fluid has been collected for cytology, the pericardium is explored with the finger to find tumor nodules and to break up loculations. Recurrence of the effusion is best prevented when a large 4x4 cm portion of pericardium is removed for pathologic examination (95). Pericardial tubes can be then inserted anterior and posterior to the heart before the wound is closed. The tubes are left in place 2 to 3 days until the drainage is 50 to 100 ml/day. Commonly, patients are discharged home on the second or third postoperative day.

Occasionally, no obvious tumor nodules are seen on the pericardium when it is visualized directly through the wound. In this situation, the diagnostic yield may be improved with pericardioscopy using a rigid or flexible scope, which can be used to better inspect the rest of the pericardium in order to obtain directed biopsy specimens of suspected lesions (147). Three of 40 patients in the series of Millaire and associates had suspected malignancies confirmed by pericardioscopy alone at the time of surgery, that would have otherwise been missed (147).

Although the term *pericardial window* implies that the communication remains open to drain the pericardium, it is not clear that this is actually the mechanism of action. A subxiphoid pericardiectomy ("window") drains into the preperitoneal space, and probably it seals fairly soon. Sugimoto and associates (148) examined this question in following up their series of 26 patients who had undergone a subxiphoid pericardial window procedure. They found by echocardiography that there was thickening of the pericardium/epicardium and obliteration of the pericardial space. Autopsies of four patients who eventually died of their cancer a mean 120 days after the procedure confirmed the fusion of the visceral and parietal pericardia. These workers concluded that the mechanism allowing success with this procedure is not the maintenance of a "window" draining the effusion continuously, but rather an inflammatory reaction causing fusion of the pericardium to the epicardium, obliterating the former space. They emphasized the necessity of keeping the pericardial space decompressed by suction postoperatively until the fluid drainage is minimal (<50 ml/24 hours) to keep the two pericardial surfaces in opposition to allow fusion.

## Left Anterior Thoracotomy and Pericardiectomy

The first pericardial "window" was made through a thoracotomy incision with creation of a pleuropericardial window that was sutured open (143). The early surgical series using this technique had a fairly respectable success rate of 86%. More recently, the left anterior thoracotomy is performed with resection of 60% to 65% of the parietal pericardium, and this approach is preferred in many centers.

The left anterior thoracotomy for pericardiectomy is quick to perform, has a low morbidity and mortality, and allows examination and biopsy of the contents of the left pleural cavity if desired (125). The procedure is performed through a 10-cm long submammary incision entering the chest through the fifth intercostal space just lateral to the sternum. The pericardium is removed from just anterior to the left phrenic nerve over to the right mediastinal pleural reflection.

Some studies suggest that the amount of pericardium remaining after surgical drainage of the pericardium is directly related to the frequency of development of postoperative complications and recurrent effusion (102). Nevertheless, in collected series of pericardiectomy by left anterior thoracotomy (118), the overall success rate was 83% (freedom from recurrent effusion) and the mortality was 13%—not as favorable as the results with subxiphoid pericardiectomy. The other primary disadvantage of the left anterior thoracotomy is that it is major thoracotomy requiring general anesthesia (118), and it also may be technically difficult to perform because of adhesions in the occasional patient with a lung cancer in the left pleural cavity who has been treated with radiotherapy.

Presently, the left anterior thoracotomy for pericardiectomy is preferred for benign effusive pericarditis, as occurs with purulent pericarditis and viral pericarditis. Benign pericarditis has a propensity to late constriction if most of the pericardium is not removed initially when surgery is performed. Conversely, a subxiphoid pericardial window is generally not recommended for drainage of benign and perhaps some malignant pericardial effusive disease when the patient is expected to have a significant life span (102,118,119).

## Median Sternotomy with Pericardiectomy

The median sternotomy is an even more extensive procedure and gives very wide exposure to most of the pericardium. This approach is preferred only for constrictive pericardial disease, which may occur in the cancer patient as the late result of radiation pericarditis, extensive tumor mass or cake, or possibly as the result of a late failure from a previous approach to pericardial drainage (125). Because of the risk of myocardial laceration and significant bleeding, most surgeons prefer to have cardiopulmonary bypass on standby when dealing with constrictive pericarditis.

One of the most important technical points in the performance of a pericardiectomy for constriction is to remove the pericardium over the left side of the heart first in order to prevent the acute pulmonary edema that may occur if the right side of the heart is decompressed first, which would allow increased blood flow to the constricted left ventricle (125). In addition, it is important to continue the pericardial resection down to include the cavae in order to release them; otherwise, the right-sided failure symptoms may persist postoperatively.

### Videothoracoscopic Pericardiectomy

The recent advent of videothoracoscopic surgery has allowed the surgeon to perform many previously open procedures using this minimally invasive approach (149). Pericardiectomy for effusive disease has proved to be technically feasible with videothoracoscopy, with a recent series of 28 patients by Lui and associates demonstrating 100% long-term success, no significant morbidity, and 0% mortality (150).

Videothoracoscopy has the disadvantages of requiring the lateral decubitus position, minimally increased operating time, and a double-lumen endotracheal tube, and the surgeon must have substantial videothoracoscopic experience in order to perform this procedure effectively and safely. However, this approach is ideal in the patient with simultaneous pulmonary or pleural pathology that needs evaluation and treatment (such as with a pleural abrasion or talc poudrage), a recurrent or loculated pericardial effusion, previous heart surgery or subxiphoid pacemaker insertion, or a previous substernal esophagogastrostomy (150). The videothoracoscopic pericardiectomy may also be performed from either the right side or the left side of the chest. Technically, a large area of pericardium may be removed, as much as 6x8 cm, including pericardium posterior to the phrenic nerve if needed for complete drainage (125).

### Pericardioperitoneal Shunt

An additional alternative drainage method was currently reported by Wang and associates (151) in a small series of four patients. They used the Denver pleuroperitoneal shunt to drain the pericardium into the peritoneal cavity. They performed the procedure with the patients under local anesthesia; the mean hospital stay was 2.8 days in these shunt patients. Further results in larger groups of patients will be needed before any conclusions can be made about the efficacy and safety of this technique.

### Percutaneous Balloon Pericardiotomy

Palacios and associates in 1991 reported a novel approach to drainage of pericardial effusions using a percutaneous balloon pericardiotomy (152). The pericardium is entered by a conventional subxiphoid pericardiocentesis. A guidewire is advanced into the pericardium, over which a Mansfield 20 mm x 3 cm dilating balloon is passed to a point where it straddles the pericardium and is then inflated to create a pericardial window. Usually the pericardial fluid drains into the pleural cavity, as indicated by a new pleural effusion. A catheter is then left in the pericardium until the drainage is minimal.

In their first 50 cases (153), successful long-term decompression of the effusion was accomplished in 92%, with the rest requiring surgery on an urgent or emergent basis. A new left pleural effusion requiring treatment occurred in 16% of patients, and 4% required a chest tube for a pneumothorax. Another 11% developed a fever, but no pericardial infection was found. The current experience by this group includes 88 patients with a success rate of 88% (154). Experience with this new technique thus far is limited to just a few investigative groups. However, the results look promising, especially in patients with recurrent effusions, and this technique bears close observation over the next few years.

### Recommendations

A malignant pericardial effusion is a not uncommon complication of advanced cancers, particularly with cancer of the lung and breast and lymphoma/leukemia. The effusion can rapidly progress to tamponade and if unrecognized may lead to death. Prompt decompression of the effusion has been shown to markedly improve the quality and quantity of life. However, the optimal method of accomplishing this objective is not easily determined because of the difficulty in comparing the large number of nonrandomized disparate series with heterogeneous patient populations employing various techniques and having varying criteria for successful clinical response. No treatment modality clearly emerges as the preferred technique. In addition, therapy to some extent must be individualized, depending on the tumor cell type and its sensitivity to chemotherapy or radiotherapy, the performance status of the host and expected length of survival, and whether the patient presents with pericardial tamponade. Our recommendations are as follows:

1. In a patient without hemodynamic compromise and a chemosensitive tumor, such as lymphoma, leukemia, testicular cancer, or small-cell lung carcinoma, systemic chemotherapy should be given. If symptoms or tamponade appear, then a pericardiocentesis should be performed, possibly followed by subxiphoid peri-

cardiectomy. If chemotherapy fails and the tumor is also radiosensitive, then radiotherapy should be considered as the next step.

2. Patients with a symptomatic, suspected, or proven malignant pericardial effusion, a reasonable life expectancy (3 months or more), and no tamponade should be considered for an elective subxiphoid pericardiectomy. If tamponade and hemodynamic compromise are present, a decompressing pericardiocentesis should be performed and a subxiphoid pericardiectomy should be performed the next day. If the institutional resources are such that surgical decompression is unavailable, a suitable approach would be intrapericardial sclerosis with bleomycin or doxycycline, although a higher failure rate should be expected.

3. Very poor candidates for surgery, on the basis of comorbid disease such as severe chronic obstructive pulmonary disease, should be considered primarily for intrapericardial sclerosis. Patients with a very short life expectancy (less than 1 month) should also be considered for intrapericardial sclerosis.

4. In patients with a history of malignancy and who develop a pericardial effusion in which the diagnosis is uncertain, or when pericardial tissue is necessary for a histologic diagnosis, an operative intervention by the subxiphoid, videothoracoscopic, or left anterior thoracotomy approach is indicated.

5. Videothoracoscopic pericardiectomy is indicated in the setting of coexisting pleural disease requiring evaluation and treatment or when a subxiphoid pericardiectomy is technically not advisable.

6. Patients in whom chemotherapy, radiotherapy, or intrapericardial sclerosis has failed should be managed by surgical pericardiectomy.

In general, patients with pericardial involvement by their primary cancer have a incurable disease. Nevertheless, most patients with symptomatic effusions should be offered treatment, since they usually will respond rapidly and often quite remarkably to pericardial decompression and will have a meaningful period of palliation outside of the hospital at home.

# REFERENCES

1. Light RW, MacGregor MI, Luchsinger PC, Ball WC. Pleural effusions: the diagnostic separation of transudates and exudates. *Ann Intern Med* 1972;77:507–513.
2. Tinney WS, Olsen AM. The significance of fluid in the pleural space: a study of 274 cases. *J Thorac Surg* 1945;14:248–252.
3. Hausheer FH, Yarbro JW. Diagnosis and treatment of malignant pleural effusion. *Semin Oncol* 1985;12:54–75.
4. Matthay RA, Coppage L, Shaw C, Filderman AE. Malignancies metastatic to the pleura. *Invest Radiol* 1990;25:601–19.
5. Fenton KN, Richardson JD. Diagnosis and management of malignant pleural effusions. *Am J Surg* 1995;170:69–74.
6. Lynch TE. The management of malignant pleural effusions. *Chest* 1993;103:385S–89S.
7. Ruckdeschel JC. Management of malignant pleural effusion: an overview. *Semin Oncol* 1988;15:24–8.
8. Agostini E. Mechanics of the pleural space. *Physiol Rev* 1972;52:57–128.
9. Black LF. The pleural space and pleural fluid. *Mayo Clin Proc* 1972;47:493–506.
10. Olopade OI, Ultmann JE. Malignant effusions. *CA* 1991;41:166–79.
11. Chernow B, Sahn SA. Carcinomatous envolvement of the pleura. *Am J Med* 1977;63:695–702.
12. Woodring JH. Recognition of a pleural effusion on supine radiographs: how much fluid is required? *Am J Radiol* 1984;142:59–64.
13. Doust BD, Baum JK, Maklad NF, et al. Ultrasonic evaluation of pleural opacities. *Radiology* 1975;114:135–140.
14. Ravin CE. Thoracentesis of loculated pleural effusions using grey scale ultrasonic guidance. *Chest* 1977;71:666–668.
15. Ratliff JL, Chavez CM, Jamchuk A, et al. Re-expansion pulmonary edema. *Chest* 1973;64:654–656.
16. Health and Public Policy Committee, American College of Physicians. Diagnostic thoracentesis and pleural biopsy in pleural effusions. *Ann Intern Med* 1985;103:799–802.
17. Leff A, Hopewell PC, Costello J. Pleural effusion from malignancy. *Ann Intern Med* 1978;88:532–537.
18. Nance KV, Shermer RW, Askin FB. Diagnostic efficacy of pleural biopsy as compared with that of pleural fluid examination. *Mod Pathol* 1991;4:320–324.
19. Boutin C, Astoul P, Seitz B. The role of thoracoscopy in the evaluation and management of pleural effusions. *Lung* 1990;168(Suppl):1113–1121.
20. Miles DW, Knight RK. Diagnosis and management of malignant pleural effusion. *Cancer Treat Rev* 1993;19:151–168.
21. LoCicero J III. Thoracoscopic management of malignant pleural effusion. *Ann Thorac Surg* 1993;56:641–643.
22. Roy RH, Can DT, Payne WS. The problem of chylothorax. *Mayo Clin Proc* 1967;42:457–467.
23. Van de Molengraft FJJM, Vooijs GP. Survival of patients with malignancy-associated effusions. *Acta Cytol* 1989;33:911–916.
24. Anderson CB, Philpott GW, Ferguson TB. The treatment of malignant pleural effusions. *Cancer* 1974;33:916–922.
25. Weick JK, Kiely JM, Harrison EG Jr, et al. Pleural effusion in lymphoma. *Cancer* 1973;31:848–853.
26. Mackman M, Cleary S, King ME, et al. Cisplatin and cytarabine administered intrapleurally as treatment of malignant pleural effusions. *Med Pediatr Oncol* 1985;13:191–193.
27. Parker LA, Charnock GC, Delany DJ. Small bore catheter drainage and sclerotherapy for malignant pleural effusions. *Cancer* 1989;64:1218–1221.
28. Walsh FW, Alberts WM, Solomon DA, Goldman AL. Malignant pleural effusions: pleurodesis using a small-bore percutaneous catheter. *South Med J* 1989;82:963–965.
29. Rusch VW, Feins RH, Thoracic Intergroup. Summary of current cooperative group clinical trials in thoracic malignancies. *Ann Thorac Surg* 1994;57:102–106.
30. Robinson LA, Fleming WH, Galbraith TA. Intrapleural doxycycline control of malignant pleural effusions. *Ann Thorac Surg* 1993;55:1115–1122.
31. Robinson LA, Moulton AL, Fleming WH, Alonso A, Galbraith TA. Intrapleural fibrinolytic treatment of multiloculated thoracic empyemas. *Ann Thorac Surg* 1994;57:803–814.
32. Sanchez-Armengol A, Rodriguez-Panadero F. Survival and talc pleurodesis in metastatic pleural carcinoma, revisited. *Chest* 1993;104:1482–1485.
33. Sahn SA. Pleural effusions in cancer. *Clin Chest Med* 1993;14:189–200.
34. Austin EH, Flye MW. The treatment of malignant pleural effusion. *Ann Thorac Surg* 1979;28:190–203.
35. Miller AB, Hoogstraten MS, Winkler A. Reporting results of cancer treatment. *Cancer* 1981;47:207–214.
36. Sahn SA, Good JT Jr, Potts DE. The pH of sclerosing agents. *Chest* 1979;76:198–200.
37. Sahn SA, Good JT Jr. The effect of common sclerosing agents on the pleural space. *Am Rev Resp Dis* 1981;124:65–67.
38. Vargas FS, Wang N, Lee HM, et al. Effectiveness of bleomycin in comparison to tetracycline as pleural sclerosing agent in rabbits. *Chest* 1993;104:1582–1584.

39. Dryzer SR, Joseph J, Baumann M, et al. Early inflammatory response of minocycline and tetracycline on the rabbit pleura. *Chest* 1993;104: 1585–1588.

40. Bresticker MA, Oba J, LoCicero J III, Greene R. Optimal pleurodesis: a comparison study. *Ann Thorac Surg* 1993;55:364–366.

41. Pass HI. Treatment of malignant pleural and pericardial effusions. In: DeVita VT Jr, Hellman S, Rosenberg SA, eds. *Cancer: principles and practice of oncology.* 4th ed. Philadelphia: JB Lippincott, 1993: 2246–2255.

42. Dryzer SR, Allen ML, Strange C, Sahn SA. A comparison of rotation and nonrotation in tetracycline pleurodesis. *Chest* 1993;104:1763–1766.

43. Webb WR, Ozmen V, Moulder PV, Shabahang B, Breaux J. Iodized talc pleurodesis for the treatment of pleural effusions. *J Cardiovasc Thorac Surg* 1992;103:881–886.

44. Kitamura S, Sugiyana Y, Izumi T, Hayashi R, Kosaka K. Intrapleural doxycycline for control of malignant pleural effusion. *Curr Therap Res* 1981;30:515–521.

45. Månsson T. Treatment of malignant pleural effusion with doxycycline. *Scand J Infect Dis* 1988;53(Suppl):29–34.

46. Heffner JE, Standerfer RJ, Torstveit J, Unruh L. Clinical efficacy of doxycycline for pleurodesis. *Chest* 1994;105:1743–1747.

47. Seaton KG, Patz EF Jr, Goodman PC. Palliative treatment of malignant pleural effusions: value of small-bore catheter thoracostomy and doxycycline sclerotherapy. *Am J Roentgenol* 1995;164:589–591.

48. Walker-Renard PB, Vaughan LM, Sahn SA. Chemical pleurodesis for malignant pleural effusions. *Ann Intern Med* 1994;120:56–64.

49. Ohri SK, Oswal SK, Townsend ER, Fountain SW. Early and late outcome after diagnostic thoracoscopy and talc pleurodesis. *Ann Thorac Surg* 1992;53:1038–1041.

50. Weissberg D, Ben-Zeev I. Talc pleurodesis: experience with 360 patients. *J Thorac Cardiovasc Surg* 1993;106:689–695.

51. Bethune N. A new technic for the deliberate production of pleural adhesions as a preliminary to lobectomy. *J Thorac Surg* 1935;4:251–261.

52. Rubinson RM, Bolooki H: Intrapleural tetracycline for control of malignant pleural effusion: A preliminary report. *South Med J* 1972; 65:847–9.

53. Sahn SA. Malignant pleural effusions. *Clin Chest Med* 1985;6: 113–125.

54. McAlpine LG, Hulks G, Thompson NC. Management of recurrent pleural effusion in the United Kingdom: survey of clinical practice. *Thorax* 1990;45:699–701.

55. Fentiman IS. Diagnosis and treatment of malignant pleural effusions. *Cancer Treat Rev* 1987;14:107–118.

56. Ruckdeschel JC, Moores D, Lee JY, et al. Intrapleural therapy for malignant pleural effusions: a randomized comparison of bleomycin and tetracycline. *Chest* 1991;100:1528–1535.

57. Johnson CE, Curzon PGD. Comparison of intrapleural bleomycin and tetracycline in the treatment of malignant pleural effusion. *Thorax* 1985;40:210 [Abstract].

58. Heffner JE, Unruh LC. Tetracycline pleurodesis: adios, farewell, adieu. *Chest* 1992;101:5–6.

59. Homma T, Yoneda S, Komuro Y, et al. Pharmacokinetics and pleural reaction of doxycycline after intrapleural administration [English abstract]. *Gan To Kagaku Ryoho* 1983;10:1129–1134.

60. Belani CP, Einarson TR, Arikian SR, et al. Cost-effectiveness analysis of pleurodesis in the management of malignant pleural effusions. *J Oncol Manage* 1995;Jan/Feb:1–11.

61. Hatta T, Tsubuota N, Yoshimura, M, Yanagawa M. Effect of intrapleural administration of minocycline on postoperative air leakage and malignant pleural effusion. *Kyobu Geka* 1990;43:283–286.

62. Kessinger A, Wigton RS. Intracavitary bleomycin and tetracycline in the management of malignant pleural effusions: a randomized study. *J Surg Oncol* 1987;36:81–83.

63. Alberts DS, Chen HSG, Mayersohn M, et al. Bleomycin pharmacokinetics in man: 2. Intracavitary administration. *Cancer Chemother Pharmacol* 1979;2:127–132.

64. Siegel RD, Schiffman FJ. Systemic toxicity following intracavitary administration of bleomycin. *Chest* 1990;98:507.

65. Trotter JM, Stuart JFB, McBeth F, McVie JG, Calman KC. The management of malignant effusion with bleomycin. *Br J Cancer* 1979;40:310 [Abstract].

66. Fuller DK. Bleomycin versus doxycycline: a patient-oriented approach to pleurodesis. *Ann Pharmacother* 1993;27:794.

67. Kennedy L, Sahn SA. Talc pleurodesis for the treatment of pneumothorax and pleural effusion. *Chest* 1994;106:1215–1222.

68. Mathlouthi A, Chabchoub A, Labbene N, et al. Etude anatomopathologique experimentale du talcage pleural. (Experimental anatomical and pathological study of pleural talc.) *Rev Mal Resp* 1992;9:617–621.

69. Chambers JS. Palliative treatment of neoplastic pleural effusion with intercostal intubation and talc instillation. *West J Surg* 1958;66:26–28.

70. Adler RH, Sayek I. Treatment of malignant pleural effusion: a method using tube thoracostomy and talc. *Ann Thorac Surg* 1976;22:8–15.

71. Youmans CR, Williams RD, McMinn MR, Derrick JR. Surgical management of spontaneous pneumothorax by bleb ligation and pleural dry sponge abrasion. *Am J Surg* 1970;120:644–648.

72. Rinaldo JE, Owens GR, Rogers RM. Adult respiratory distress syndrome following intrapleural administration of talc. *Thorac Cardiovasc Surg* 1983;85:823–826.

73. Kennedy L, Harley RA, Sahn SA, Strange C. Talc slurry pleurodesis: pleural fluid and histological analysis. *Chest* 1995;107:1707–1712.

74. Lange P, Mortensen J, Groth S. Lung function 23–35 years after treatment of idiopathic spontaneous pneumothorax with talc poudrage or simple drainage. *Thorax* 1988;43:559–561.

75. McGahren ED, Teague WG Jr, Flanagan T, White B, Rogers BM. The effects of talc pleurodesis on growing swine. *J Pediatr Surg* 1990;25: 1147–1151.

76. Kleinfeld M, Messite J, Kooyman O, Zaki MH. Mortality among talc miners and millers in New York state. *Arch Environ Health* 1967;14: 666–667.

77. Chappell AG, Johnson A, Charles JWJ, et al. A survey of the long-term effects of talc and kaolin pleurodesis. *Br J Dis Chest* 1979; 73:285–288.

78. Kennedy L, Vaughan LM, Steed LL, Sahn SA. Sterilization of talc for pleurodesis: available techniques, efficacy, and cost analysis. *Chest* 1995;107:1032–1034.

79. Colt HG, Dumon J. Development of a disposable spray canister for talc pleurodesis: a preliminary report. *Chest* 1994;196:1776–1780.

80. Taylor SA, Hooton NS, MacArthur AM. Quinacrine in the management of malignant pleural effusion. *Br J Surg* 1977;64:52–53.

81. Bayly TC, Kisner DL, Sybert A, et al. Tetracycline and quinacrine in the control of malignant pleural effusions. *Cancer* 1978;41: 1188–1192.

82. Webb HE, Oaten SW, Pike CP. Treatment of malignant ascitic and pleural effusion with *Corynebacterium parvum*. *Br Med J* 1978;1: 388–440.

83. Rossi GA, Felletti R, Balbi B, et al. Symptomatic treatment of recurrent malignant pleural effusions with intrapleurally administered *Corynebacterium parvum*: clinical response is not associated with evidence of enhancement of local cellular-mediated immunity. *Am Rev Resp Dis* 1987;135:885–890.

84. Rosso R, Rimoldi R, Salvati F, et al. Intrapleural natural beta interferon in the treatment of malignant pleural effusions. *Oncol* 1988;45: 253–256.

85. Astoul P, Viallat J-R, Laurent JC, et al. Intrapleural recombinant IL-2 in passive immunotherapy for malignant pleural effusion. *Chest* 1993; 103:209–213.

86. Dianjun L, Yaorong W, Ziaodong Y, et al. Treatment of patients with malignant pleural effusions due to advanced lung cancer by transfer to autologous LAK cells combined with rIL-2 or rIL-2 alone. *Proc Chinese Acad Med Sci Peking Union Med Coll* 1990;5:51–55.

87. Kent EM, Moses C. Radioactive isotopes in the pallative management of carcinomatosis of the pleura. *J Thorac Surg* 1951;22:503–516.

88. Martini N, Bains BS, Beattie EJ. Indications for pleurectomy in malignant pleural effusions. *Cancer* 1975;35:734–738.

89. Reich H, Beattie EJ, Harvey JC. Pleuroperitoneal shunt for malignant pleural effusion: a one-year experience. *Semin Surg Oncol* 1993;9: 160–162.

90. Waller DA, Morritt GN, Forty J. Video-assisted thoracoscopic pleurectomy in the management of malignant pleural effusion. *Chest* 1995;107:1454–1456.

91. Harvey JC, Erdman CB Beattie EJ. Early experience with videothoracoscopic hydrodissection pleurectomy in the treatment of malignant pleural effusion. *J Surg Oncol* 1995;59:243–245.

92. Matsuzaki Y, Shibata K, Yoshioka M, et al. Intrapleural perfusion hyperthermo-chemotherapy for malignant pleural dissemination and effusion. *Ann Thorac Surg* 1995;59:127–131.

93. A prospective, randomized trial of bleomycin versus doxicycline versus talc for the intrapleural treatment of malignant pleural effusions. CCC-94-10. Eastern Cooperative Oncology Group. Trial No. 8592.

94. Belani CP, Aisner J, Patz, E. Ambulatory sclerotherapy for malignant pleural effusions. *Proc ASCO* 1995;14:524. (abstract)
95. Hawkins JW Vacek JL. What constitutes definitive therapy of malignant pericardial effusion? "Medical" versus surgical treatment. *Am Heart J* 1989;118:428–432.
96. Theologides A. Neoplastic cardiac tamponade. *Semin Oncol* 1978;5:181–192.
97. Thurber DL, Edwards JE, Achor RWP. Secondary malignant tumors of the pericardium. *Circulation* 1962;26:228–241.
98. Lokich JJ. The management of malignant pericardial effusions. *JAMA* 1973;224:1401–1404.
99. Buzaid AC, Garewal HS, Greenberg BR. Managing malignant pericardial effusion. *West J Med* 1989;150:174–179.
100. Vital and Health Statistics, National Center for Health Statistics, U.S. Department of Health and Human Services, Hyattsville, MD. *National Hospital Discharge Survey* 1993; Series 13, No. 122:122 (PHS Pub. No. 95-1783).
101. Miller JI, Mansour KA, Hatcher CR Jr. Pericardiectomy: current indications, concepts, and results in a university center. *Ann Thorac Surg* 1982;34:40–45.
102. Piehler JM, Pluth JR, Schaff HV, Danielson GK, Orszulak TA, Puga FJ. Surgical management of effusive pericardial disease: influence of extent of pericardial resection on clinical course. *J Thorac Cardiovasc Surg* 1985;90:506–516.
103. Palatianos GM, Thurer RJ, Pompeo MQ, Kaiser GA. Clinical experience with subxiphoid drainage of pericardial effusions. *Ann Thorac Surg* 1989;48:381–385.
104. Mills SA, Graeber GM, Nelson MG. Therapy of malignant tumors involving the pericardium. In: Roth J, Ruckdeschel JC, Weisenburger T, eds. *Thoracic oncology*, 2nd ed. Philadelphia: WB Saunders, 1995:492–513.
105. Posner MR, Cohen GI, Skarin AT. Pericardial disease in patients with cancer—the differentiation of malignant from idiopathic and radiation-induced pericarditis. *Am J Med* 1981;71:407–413.
106. Spodick DH. Macrophysiology, microphysiology, and anatomy of the pericardium: a synopsis. *Am Heart J* 1992;124:1046–1051.
107. Miller AJ. Some observations concerning pericardial effusions and their relationship to the venous and lymphatic circulation of the heart. *Lymphology* 1970;2:76–78.
108. Pories WJ, Gaudiani VA. Cardiac tamponade. *Surg Clin North Am* 31975;55:573–589.
109. Spodick DH. The normal and diseased pericardium: current concepts of pericardial physiology, diagnosis and treatment. *J Am Coll Cardiol* 1983;1:240–251.
110. Ruckdeschel JC. Malignant effusions in the chest. In: Kirkwood JM, Lotze MT, Yaska JM, eds. *Current cancer therapeutics*, 2nd ed. Philadelphia: Churchill Livingstone,1996:304–308.
111. Beck CS. Acute and chronic compression of the heart. *Am Heart J* 1937;14:515–525.
112. Settle HP, Adolph RJ, Fowler NO, et al. Echocardiographic study of cardiac tamponade. *Circulation* 1977;56:951–959.
113. Himelman RB, Kircher R, Rockey DC, Schiller NB. Inferior vena cava plethora with blunted respiratory response: a sensitive echocardiographic sign of cardiac tamoponade. *J Am Coll Cardiol* 1988;12:470–477.
114. Markiewicz W, Borovik R, Ecker S. Cardiac tamponade in medical patients: treatment and prognosis in the echocardiographic era. *Am Heart J* 1986;111:1138–1142.
115. Eisenberg MJ, Oken NK, Guerrero S, Saniei MA, Schiller NB. Prognostic value of echocardiography in hospitalized patients with pericardial effusion. *Am J Cardiol* 1992;70:934–939.
116. Buck M, Ingle JN, Giuliani ER, Gordon JR, Therneau TM. Pericardial effusion in women with breast cancer. *Cancer* 1987;6:263–269.
117. Reyes VC, Strinden C, Banerji M. The role of cytology in neoplastic cardiac tamponade. *Acta Cytol* 1982;26:299–302.
118. Vaitkus PT, Herrmann HC, LeWinter MM. Treatment of malignant pericardial effusion. *JAMA* 1994;272:59–64.
119. Press OW, Livingston R. Management of malignant pericardial effusion and tamponade. *JAMA* 1987;257:1088–1092.
120. Campbell PT, Van Trigt P, Wall TC, et al. Subxiphoid pericardiotomy in the diagnosis and management of large pericardial effusions associated with malignancy. *Chest* 1992;101:938–943.
121. Ruckdeschel JC, Chang P, Martin RG, et al. Radiation-related pericardial effusions in patients with Hodgkin's disease. *Medicine* 1975;54:245–270.
122. Calabresi P, Chabner BA. Chemotherapy of neoplastic disease. In: Gilman AG, Rall TW, Nies AS, Taylor P, eds. *The pharmacological basis of therapeutics*, 8th ed. New York: Pergamon Press, 1990:1241–1244.
123. Gregory JR, McMurtrey MJ, Mountain CF. A surgical approach to the treatment of pericardial effusion in cancer patients. *Am J Clin Oncol* 1985;8:319–323.
124. Schuh F: Erfahrungen über die paracentere der brust und des herzbeutels. *Med Jahrb dkk, Öster-staates Wien* (Neuste Folge 24) 1841;33:388.
125. Miller JI Jr. Surgical management of pericardial disease. In: Schlant RC, Alexander RW, O'Roiurke RA, Roberts R, Sonnenblick EH, eds. *The heart, arteries and veins*, 8th ed. New York: McGraw-Hill, 1994:1675–1680.
126. Wolfe MW, Edelman ER. Transient systolic dysfunction after relief of cardiac tamponade. *Ann Intern Med* 1993;119:42–44.
127. Braverman AC, Sundaresan S. Cardiac tamponade and severe ventricular dysfunction. *Ann Intern Med* 1994;120:442.
128. Davis S, Rambotti P, Grignani F. Intrapericardial tetracycline sclerosis in the treatment of malignant pericardial effusion. *J Clin Oncol* 1984;2:631–636.
129. Shepherd FA, Morgan C, Evans WK, Ginsberg JF, Watt D, Murphy K. Medical management of malignant pericardial effusion by tetracycline sclerosis. *Am J Cardiol* 1987;60:1161–1166.
130. Kitamura S, Wagai F, Izumi T, Sugiyama Y, Kosaka K. Treatment of carcinomatous pericarditis with doxycycline: intrapericardial doxycycline for control of malignant pericardial effusion. *Curr Therap Res* 1981;30:589–596.
131. Maher EA, Shepherd FA, Todd JRT. Pericardial sclerosis as the primary management of malignant pericardial effusion and cardiac tamponade. *J Thorac Cardiovasc Surg* 1996;112:637–643.
132. Lissoni P, Barni S, Ardizzoia A. Intracavitary administration of interleukin-2 as palliative therapy for neoplastic effusions. *Tumori* 1992;78:118–120.
133. Imamura T, Tamura K, Takenaga M, et al. Intrapericardial OK-432 instillation for the management of malignant pericardial effusion. *Cancer* 1991;68:259–263.
134. Lee LN, Yang PC, Chang DB. Ultrasound guided pericardial drainage and intrapericardial instillation of mitomycin C for malignant pericardial effusion. *Thorax* 1994;49:594–595.
135. Lin MT, Yang PC, Luh KT. Constrictive pericarditis after sclerosing therapy with mitomycin C for malignant pericardial effusion: report of a case. *J Formosan Med Assoc* 1994;93:250–252.
136. Pectasides D, Stewart S, Courtney-Luck N, et al. Antibody-guided irradiation of malignant pleural and pericardial effusions. *Br J Cancer* 1986;53:727–732.
137. Cham WC, Freiman AH, Carstens HB, Chu FCH. Radiation therapy of cardiac and pericardial metastases. *Radiology* 1975;114:701–704.
138. Terry LN, Kligerman MM. Pericardial and myocardial involvement by lymphomas and leukemias: the role of radiotherapy. *Cancer* 1970;25:1003–1008.
139. Stewart JR, Cohen KE, Fajardo LF, et al. Radiation-induced heart disease: a study of 25 patients. *Radiology* 1967;89:302–310.
140. Riolan J. *Encheiridium anatomicum et pathologicum*. Lugdunum, Batavorum, Ex Officini Adriani, Wyngaarden. 1649:206–212.
141. Baizeau J. Mémorire sur le ponction du péricarde au point de vue chirurgical. *Gaz Med Chir* 1868;1:565–566.
142. Larrey D-J. *Clinique chirurgicale*, vol 2. Paris: Gabon, 1829:303–5, 315–321.
143. William C, Soutter L. Pericardial tamponade: diagnosis and treatment. *Arch Intern Med* 1954;94:571–584.
144. Fontanelle LJ, Cuello L, Dooley BN. Subxiphoid pericardial window. *Am J Surg* 1970;120:679–680.
145. Zwischenberger JB, Bradford DW. Management of malignant pericardial effusion. In: Pass HI, Mitchell JB, Johnson DH, Turrisi AT, eds. *Lung cancer: principles and practice*, 1st ed. Philadelphia: Lippincott-Raven, 1996:655–662.
146. Moores DWO, Allen KB, Faber LP, et al. Subxiphoid pericardial drainage for pericardial tamponade. *J Thorac Cardiovasc Surg* 1995;109:546–52.
147. Milaire A, Wurtz A, de Groote P, Saudemont A, Chambon A, Ducloux G. Malignant pericardial effusions: usefulness of pericardioscopy. *Am Heart J* 1992;124:10304.
148. Sugimoto JT, Little AG, Ferguson MK, et al. Pericardial window: mechanisms of efficacy. *Ann Thorac Surg* 1990;50:442–445.

149. Mack MJ, Aronoff RJ, Acuff TE, Douthit MB, Bowman RT, Ryan WH. Present role of thoracoscopy in the diagnosis and treatment of diseases of the chest. *Ann Thorac Surg* 1992;54:403–409.

150. Liu H-P, Chang C-H, Lin PJ, Hsieh H-C, Chang J-P, Hsieh M-J. Thoracoscopic management of effusive pericardial disease: indications and technique. *Ann Thorac Surg* 1994;58:1695–1697.

151. Wang N, Feikes JR, Mogensen T, Vyhmeister EE, Bailey LL. Pericardioperitoneal shunt: an alternative treatment for malignant pericardial effusion. *Ann Thorac Surg* 1994;57:289–292.

152. Palacios IF, Tuzcu EM, Ziskind AA, Younger J, Block PC. Percutaneous balloon pericardial window for patients with malignant pericardial effusion and tamponade. *Cath Cardiovasc Diag* 1991;22:244–249.

153. Ziskind AA, Pearce AC, Lemmon CC, et al. Percutaneous balloon pericardiotomy for the treatment of cardiac tamoponade and large pericardial effusions: description of techniques and report of first 50 cases. *J Am Coll Cardiol* 1993;21:1–5.

154. Ziskind AA, Rodriguez S, Lemmon CC, et al. Percutaneous balloon pericardiotomy for the treatment of malignant pericardial effusion: long term followup. *Proc Ann Meeting Am Soc Clin Oncol* 1994;13: A1494 [Abstract].

*Principles and Practice of Supportive Oncology,*
edited by Ann Berger et al.
Lippincott–Raven Publishers, Philadelphia ©1998

CHAPTER 27

# Cardiopulmonary Toxicity of Cancer Therapy

Michelle Z. Schultz and John R. Murren

Advances in cancer therapy have produced increasingly complex combinations of chemotherapeutic agents, radiation therapy, and biological-response modifiers. New methods of providing hematopoetic support with growth factors and marrow products have minimized myelosuppression as a barrier to the dose intensification of chemotherapy. As a result, many patients are now at increased risk for cardiopulmonary toxicity. Some of these side effects develop rapidly after exposure to the inciting agent, whereas others may take years before becoming evident. Consequently, the need for vigilant supportive care has intensified. Fortunately, progress also has been made in both the prevention and management of treatment-related toxicity. Optimal management depends on the early recognition of treatment-related toxicity so that the inciting agent can be withdrawn and the appropriate therapy instituted. In addition, patients successfully treated for a malignant disease need to be informed that they remain at risk for potential late cardiopulmonary toxicity and strongly counseled to avoid smoking. With appropriate supportive measures, cardiopulmonary risks to patients undergoing intensive cancer therapy can be minimized despite the narrow therapeutic index of such treatment.

## PULMONARY TOXICITY

Pulmonary complications of cancer therapy include both direct toxicity to the lungs from drugs and radiation as well as indirect effects via immunosuppression and cardiovascular complications. The management of cancer patients with respiratory insufficiency caused by diffuse interstitial infiltrates poses a common challenge. Interstitial pulmonary infiltrates are the hallmark of pulmonary drug toxicity and also may be the presenting feature of a wide variety of other noninfectious and infectious complications of malignancy as listed in Table 1. The lung is the most frequent site of serious infection in cancer patients, and infection is the most common specific diagnosis confirmed when diffuse infiltrates are manifest (1–3).

In addition, congestive heart failure (CHF), pulmonary emboli, the adult respiratory distress syndrome (ARDS), and tumor infiltration can present as diffuse interstitial infiltrates. Dyspnea, dry cough, tachycardia, diffuse rales, and hypoxemia are clinical features common to most of these processes, and there are no unequivocal distinguishing features. Although most toxic reactions have a subacute presentation, some cases exhibit fulminant onset of high fever, chills, and respiratory failure (4). In a series of leukemic patients with diffuse infiltrates, fever was present in 94% and was not helpful in differentiating infectious from noninfectious etiologies (5).

Thus, in the immunocompromised cancer patient, this common nonspecific complex poses a diagnostic and therapeutic challenge. Because of its diverse nature, the optimal therapy of interstitial pneumonitis varies significantly. Nonetheless, noninvasive testing has been of limited use in this setting, and the value of aggressive diagnostic procedures remains controversial. For example, with an open lung biopsy, a specific diagnosis is not always possible, and even if a diagnosis is made, a change in therapy may not be indicated. In a randomized trial comparing immediate open-lung biopsy with empiric antibiotic therapy followed by open-lung biopsy if deterioration occurred after 4 days, no significant difference in survival or complication rate was found. Establishment of a diagnosis rarely resulted in a change of the therapeutic regimen (6).

In contrast, other, nonrandomized series have found lung biopsy helpful in the management of unexplained pulmonary infiltrates in cancer patients. Therapy was modified based on biopsy results in 29% to 78% of cases, but complications rates were as high as 39% (1,2,7). Furthermore, empiric therapy for *Pneumocystis carinii* pneumonia was not necessarily administered. Tenholder and

M. Z. Schultz: Division of Hematology/Oncology, Washington University/St. Louis Veterans Affairs Medical Center, St. Louis, MO 63106.
J. R. Murren: Department of Medicine, Yale University School of Medicine, New Haven, CT 06520.

**TABLE 1.** *Differential diagnosis of diffuse interstitial infiltrates in cancer and bone marrow transplant patients*

Infection
Drug reaction
Radiation toxicity
Lymphangitic tumor spread
Leukemic infiltration
Pulmonary edema
Adult respiration distress syndrome
Pulmonary emboli
Leukoagglutinin reaction
Diffuse alveolar hemorrhage
Idiopathic pneumonia syndrome

Hooper (5) reported that invasive biopsy procedures were most helpful in leukemic patients, who frequently develop diffuse infiltrates during or after induction therapy, because of a high incidence of fungal disease, viral infections, and noninfectious etiologies, including pulmonary hemorrhage and leukemic infiltration. Decisions regarding the use of invasive procedures should therefore be individualized. Patients who are neutropenic and patients who have received prolonged corticosteroid therapy have a high risk of infection with bacteria and *P. carinii*, respectively and may be candidates for empiric therapy. Recently treated leukemia patients and bone marrow transplant patients, on the other hand, may benefit from a more accurate diagnosis (7,8).

Increasingly invasive diagnostic procedures available include bronchoalveolar lavage (BAL), transbronchial biopsy, thoracoscopic biopsy, and open-lung biopsy. For both infectious agents and malignant lesions, BAL has a high diagnostic yield, although false-positive results have been seen with fungi and cytometalovirus (CMV) (9,10). Protected nonbronchoscopic BAL can be used effectively for intubated patients, and for severely myelosuppressed patients it poses less risk of bleeding compared with transbronchial biopsy (3,11,12). Nonetheless, transbronchial forceps biopsy yields more tissue for histopathologic evaluation, which may increase the diagnostic yield in noninfectious processes.

If a diagnosis cannot be established by bronchoscopy, a thoracoscopic or open-lung biopsy may be required. A thoracoscopic procedure requires collapse of the lung being evaluated, although this may not be feasible in some critically ill patients with limited pulmonary reserve. A trial comparing the relative usefulness of thoracoscopic and open-lung biopsies in noncritically ill patients found that equivalent amounts of tissue could be obtained with either method, producing the same diagnostic accuracy but less morbidity with thoracoscopy, and is the preferred procedure in patients who can tolerate single lung ventilation (13).

## Infection

The list of potential pathogens causing interstitial infiltrates is extensive. The most likely infectious etiologies differ somewhat depending on whether the patient has been taking corticosteroids and whether and for how long the patient has been neutropenic (absolute neutrophil count $\leq 500/mm^3$). Patients undergoing bone marrow transplantation are at even higher risk as a result of prolonged marrow aplasia, chronic immunosuppression, and graft versus host disease. The choice of empiric therapy is dictated by the clinical setting (Table 2). For example, neutropenic patients with diffuse infiltrates require broad-spectrum antibacterial agents because of the high risk of both gram-positive and gram-negative bacterial infections. Invasive fungal infections are predominantly a problem in patients with prolonged neutropenia but occasionally occur in nonneutropenic patients who are highly immunosuppressed. In addition, bone marrow transplant patients are at particularly high risk for CMV and other herpes viral infections. *P. carinii* is the most common cause of diffuse interstitial infiltrates in nonneutropenic patients, particularly those on corticosteroids (3,9,14).

An empiric approach to presumed infection should be taken until a definitive diagnosis can be made. In addition

**TABLE 2.** *Predominant infectious causes of interstitial lung disease in cancer patients*

Neutropenia
   Any gram(+) or gram(–) bacteria
   Mycobacteria
   Legionella
   Mycoplasma
   Nocardia
   Fungi (prolnged neutropenia)
   *Pneumocystis carinii*
   Cytomegalovirus
Chronic immunosuppression
   *Pneumocystis carinii*
   Cytomegalovirus
   Herpes simplex virus
   Varicella zoster virus
   Respiratory syncytial virus
   Influenza
   Parainfluenza
   Adenovirus
   Measles
Allogeneic bone marrow transplant
   Early (≤6 wk)
      Bacteria
      Fungi
      Herpes simplex virus
      *Pneumocystis carinii*
   Late
      Cytomegalovirus (2–6 mo)
      Varicella zoster virus (4–12 mo)
      *Streptococcus pneumoniae* (>6 mo; with chronic graft-versus-host disease

to broad-spectrum antibiotics for neutropenic patients, empiric antimicrobial therapy should include erythromycin and trimethoprim-sulfamethoxazole at doses designed to treat atypical bacterial infections (such as legionella, mycoplasma, chlamydia, and nocardia) and *P. carinii*, respectively. If fever persists for more than 5 to 7 days, amphotericin B should be added to cover fungal infection. The decision to proceed with an invasive diagnostic procedure is dictated by the patient's clinical status and response to empiric antibiotics.

## Direct Treatment-related Toxicity

Severe pulmonary injury can result from radiation therapy or chemotherapy alone or in combination (Table 3). The incidence of treatment-related pulmonary toxicity is variable and difficult to establish precisely (15). A small number of agents predictably cause toxicity, whereas most do so exceedingly rarely. The combination of multiple chemotherapeutic agents may produce additive or synergistic toxicity. For example, Bauer et al. (16) reported an 18% incidence of pulmonary toxicity with the M-BACOD regimen consisting of methotrexate, bleomycin, doxorubicin, cyclophosphamide, vincristine, and dexamethasone.

The histopathology of treatment-related interstitial pneumonitis incorporates nonspecific features common to both drug- and radiation-induced lung injury. There is capillary damage characterized by endothelial swelling with fibrinous alveolar exudate in the interstitium and alveolar spaces. Type I pneumocytes are destroyed and thus type II pneumocytes proliferate, sometimes with atypia. There is characteristically a paucity of mononuclear inflammatory cell infiltration, which culminates in thickening of alveolar septae by fibroblasts and collagen (17–20). In addition, hypersensitivity reactions may show eosinophilic infiltrates or granuloma formation (18–21).

### Clinical Features

The severity of toxic reactions varies widely from patient to patient, ranging from incidental asymptomatic cases to life-threatening respiratory insufficiency. Most patients develop subacute onset of progressive dyspnea, nonproductive cough, anorexia, and low-grade fever 1 to 3 months after treatment (17). High fever (>40°C), purulent sputum, and hemoptysis are rarely seen and suggest an infectious etiology (22). Physical findings may include tachypnea, tachycardia, diffuse rales, and occasionally cyanosis. Hypoxemia with respiratory alkalosis may ensue. Chest radiographs typically reveal diffuse interstitial or alveolar infiltrates, particularly prominent at the bases. Pulmonary function tests (PFTs) may display a restrictive pattern and decreased diffusing capacity (18).

There are three predominant patterns of pulmonary injury attributed to drug toxicity: interstitial pneumonitis with pulmonary fibrosis, acute hypersensitivity reactions, and noncardiogenic pulmonary edema. In addition, anaphylactoid reactions have been reported following the administration of several agents (23). In most cases, along with withdrawal of the agent in question, a trial of corticosteroid therapy is warranted, although results and prognosis have been variable (Table 3). Although dosage has not been standardized, 1 mg/kg of prednisone is a common starting dose, followed by a slow, cautious taper.

### Specific Agents

#### Radiation

Irradiating the lung parenchyma results in both acute and chronic lung toxicity consisting of interstitial pneumonitis followed by pulmonary fibrosis (20). The incidence of symptomatic pneumonitis is 5% to 15% in patients irradiated for mediastinal lymphoma, lung can-

**TABLE 3.** *Pulmonary toxicity of commonly used cytotoxic agents and role of corticosteroids*

| Agent | Type of Rxn | | | | | Benefit of corticosteroids* | References |
|---|---|---|---|---|---|---|---|
| | AP | HP | NE | PF | VOD | | |
| Radiation | X | | | X | X | ++ | 20,25,58 |
| Bleomycin | X | X | X | X | X | + | 18,21,57,59 |
| BCNU | X | | | X | X | +/− | 18,21,30,31,57 |
| Mitomycin C | X | | | X | X | ++ | 4,19,32,33,37,57 |
| Cyclophosphamide | | X | X | X | ? | + | 18,19,57,59 |
| Methotrexate | X | X | X | X | | +++ | 18,19 |
| Vinca alkaloids (+MMC) | X | | | | | + | 36,37 |
| Procarbazine | X | | | | | ++ | 18,19,44,45 |
| Cytosine arabinoside | | | X | | | ? | 19,21,47 |
| ATRA for APL | | | X | | | ++ | 54–56 |

Rxn, reaction; AP, acute pneumonitis; HP, hypersensitivity pneumonitis; NE, noncardiogenic pulmonary edema; PF, pulmonary fibrosis; VOD, venoocclusive disease; BCNU, carmastine; MMC, mitomycin C; ATRA, all-*trans*-retinoic acid; APL, acute promyelocytic leukemia.
*Excluding VOD.

cer, or breast cancer(17). The risk of injury is dose and volume related. The acute changes occur 1 to 3 months after completion of radiotherapy. The concomitant use of chemotherapeutic agents or oxygen therapy with radiation may produce synergistic toxicity (17,24,25).

The cardinal feature of acute injury is dyspnea, with or without dry cough and fever. Pleuritic chest pain and blood-tinged sputum sometimes are present (17). Diagnosis usually can be made by chest radiographs revealing a sharply demarcated infiltrate involving the irradiated area (Fig. 1). Diffuse lung injury rarely ensues, making diagnosis more difficult (25). Computerized tomography (CT) is a more sensitive diagnostic technique (17). Pulmonary function tests reveal decreased diffusing capacity and decreased lung volumes. Treatment with corticosteroids most often results in dramatic symptomatic improvement (17,20,25). Moreover, the sudden withdrawal of corticosteroids as in certain chemotherapy regimens may precipitate acute pneumonitis in some irradiated patients and may be avoided by tapering the corticosteroid dose after each cycle (25).

Chronic radiation toxicity is manifested by irreversible pulmonary fibrosis occurring 6 to 24 months after radiotherapy. Most cases of acute pneumonitis eventually evolve into permanent fibrosis (25). Chest radiographs reveal a dense infiltrate with volume loss; however, symptoms are usually minimal if less than 50% of one lung is involved (17). Exertional dyspnea, cyanosis, clubbing, and cor pulmonale may ensue. There is no role for corticosteroid therapy in the chronic phase (25).

Several groups have attempted to develop methods to predict the long-term effect of radiation on a patient's pulmonary function. In patients with lung cancer treated with definitive radiotherapy ($\geq$45 Gy), Choi and Kanarek (26) demonstrated that the loss of pulmonary function after definitive radiotherapy for lung cancer can be predicted by function prior to treatment. Although patients with relatively good function ($FEV_1$ >50% predicted) had a significant decrease in lung function 12 months after treatment, 87% of patients with $FEV_1$ <50% predicted had either no significant change or improvement in pulmonary function after irradiation of their cancers (presumably due to tumor response) (26).

### Chemotherapy

*Bleomycin.* Although it is one of the few cytotoxic agents that is not myelosuppressive, serious toxicity from bleomycin occurs in the form of dose-related pulmonary fibrosis as well as hypersensitivity reactions unrelated to dose (18,21). At therapeutic doses, the incidence of bleomycin-related pulmonary fibrosis appears to be in the range of 3% to 5% (18,19,21). At cumulative doses above 400 to 500 units, the incidence of pulmonary abnormalities rises sharply to above 10% (17–19). Risk factors for the development of toxicity include age over 70 years; radiation therapy concurrent with, preceding, or subsequent to bleomycin administration; and the use of high inspired concentrations of oxygen (18,21). For example,

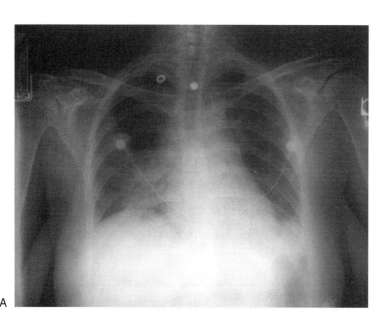
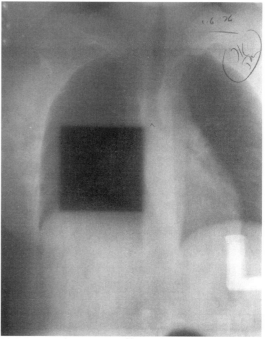

A                                                                                                                            B

**FIG. 1.** Radiation pneumonitis. Unilateral alveolar infiltrate in a woman following radiation treatment for recurrent Hodgkin disease **(A)**. This opacity corresponds with the radiation port **(B)**.

the concurrent use of bleomycin, doxorubicin, cyclophosphamide, vincristine, and chest irradiation for small cell lung cancer (SCLC) resulted in a 23% mortality rate from pulmonary toxicity and virtually eliminated bleomycin from future SCLC regimens (27).

Signs and symptoms of bleomycin-induced pulmonary fibrosis include progressive dyspnea, dry cough, fine basilar rales, and occasionally a pleural friction rub. Fever and peripheral blood eosinophilia may also be present in acute hypersensitivity reactions (18). Chest radiographic findings range from a fine reticular infiltrate early on to nodular alveolar infiltrates and lobar consolidation (Fig. 2). Before to the onset of symptoms or radiographic changes, a decrease in diffusing capacity and forced vital capacity (FVC) can be detected. Most patients with early or mild abnormalities stabilize or improve with discontinuation of the drug, but patients with severe toxicity have a high mortality rate. Corticosteroid therapy is probably beneficial for patients with bleomycin-induced pulmonary toxicity, particularly for hypersensitivity reactions (18,19,21). Extremely high doses of corticosteroids (methylprednisolone 1 $g/m^2$/day) along with azathioprine improved bleomycin lung toxicity refractory to standard corticosteroid doses in one patient (28).

*BCNU.* The pulmonary toxicity of BCNU (carmustine) has been firmly documented as a result of its use as a single agent in the treatment of malignant brain tumors, which spare the lungs and often present in young, otherwise healthy patients. At conventional doses, the incidence of toxicity has been estimated in the range of 20% to 30%, with a clear dose-response effect (18,19,29). Up to 50% of patients develop pulmonary toxicity at cumulative doses exceeding 1,500 $mg/m^2$ (19). Typical BCNU

pulmonary toxicity has an insidious onset similar to that of other subacute chemotherapy drug reactions. Radiographic abnormalities occur late, if at all. In contrast to bleomycin-induced lung damage, there is little evidence that corticosteroid therapy is beneficial. In fact, most reported cases occurred in patients with gliomas who were concurrently receiving corticosteroids (18,19).

More recently, high-dose BCNU has been used in conditioning regimens for bone marrow transplantation. At single doses above 450 $mg/m^2$, there is a precipitous increase in the risk of acute interstitial pneumonitis which, in distinction to the subacute pulmonary fibrosis described above, appears to respond more favorably to corticosteroids (30,31).

*Mitomycin C.* Several authors have documented life-threatening mitomycin C pulmonary toxicity, ranging in incidence from 3% to 12% (4,19,32,33). Signs and symptoms are similar to bleomycin- and BCNU-induced toxicity: insidious onset of dyspnea, decreased diffusing capacity, and a restrictive ventilatory defect. No correlation between total dose received and frequency of toxicity has been demonstrated. Enhancement of toxicity has been associated with oxygen therapy and chest irradiation (4,18). The cumulative mortality rate approaches 50% (18,19). The early institution of corticosteroid therapy and discontinuation of the drug produces dramatic improvement in some patients (33).

*Vinca Alkaloids.* Treatment with vinca alkaloids alone has not been reported to cause lung toxicity; however, in combination with mitomycin C, vinblastine, vindesine, and vinorelbine have been associated with symptoms of acute airway obstruction (34–38). Rivera et al. (37) described a syndrome consisting of severe acute respira-

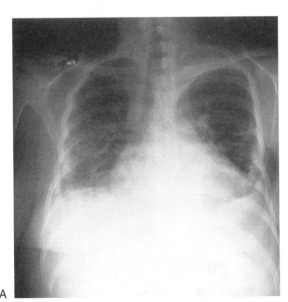
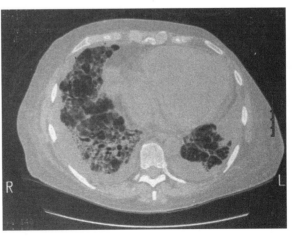

**FIG. 2.** Bleomycin lung. The chest radiograph shows bilateral reticulonodular infiltrates and pleural thickening **(A)**. Computed tomography findings include bibasilar air cysts, bronchiectasis, and reticular opacities associated with extensive bilateral pleural thickening **(B)**.

tory distress within 4 hours of receiving a dose of vinca alkaloid in 4% of 378 patients treated for advanced non-small cell lung cancer. Mitomycin C was administered on the same day in only 32% of cases. Most patients had wheezing, rales or rhonchi, and new diffuse interstitial infiltrates on chest radiograph. Significant improvement occurred within 24 hours in 21 of 25 patients after supportive care with supplemental oxygen and bronchodilators. Eight patients who received corticosteroids for persistent dyspnea all improved; however, residual chronic dyspnea was worse than that before treatment in 63% of patients, and one patient died (37). Rechallenge with vinca alkaloids has resulted in recurrence of symptoms (36,37).

*Cyclophosphamide and Other Alkylating Agents.* Cyclophosphamide is one of the most frequently prescribed chemotherapeutic drugs, but the incidence of pulmonary toxicity remains low (<1%) (18); however, the treatment of small cell lung cancer with very high doses of cyclophosphamide followed by radiation led to symptomatic pulmonary fibrosis 74% of the time in one study (39). No definite dose-response relationship was demonstrated. Clinical features are similar to those of other drugs, although fever is often a prominent feature (18). Corticosteroids may hasten improvement in some cases, with an overall recovery rate of about 60% (18,19,25). A closely related agent, ifosfamide, has very rarely been associated with interstitial pneumonitis to date (40).

Although the therapeutic applications of other alkylating agents, such as chlorambucil, busulfan, and melphalan are not as broad, each also has been reported to cause pulmonary toxicity. All have been associated with the insidious onset of dyspnea and reticular infiltrates months to a few years after therapy. Unlike cyclophosphamide, both chlorambucil and busulfan toxicity appear to be dose related (17,18). The role of corticosteroids for pulmonary toxicity from these agents is equivocal (18,19).

*Doxorubicin.* When administered alone, doxorubicin is not associated with pulmonary injury. It may, however, reduce the tolerance of the lung to radiation. Enhanced toxicity has been identified in patients with Hodgkin disease, breast cancer, and small cell lung carcinoma treated with both doxorubicin-containing chemotherapy and with irradiation (14,41). When administered after chest irradiation, severe pneumonitis can occur, even outside of the radiation port (42). This phenomenon, termed *radiation recall*, was described in a report of 71 patients receiving combined radiation therapy and chemotherapy with cyclophosphamide, doxorubicin, and vincristine. Pneumonitis was the primary toxicity, with a 15% incidence of ARDS and a mortality rate of 10% (41). A 7% incidence and 4% mortality rate from ARDS was reported in a 1992 Cancer and Leukemia Group B (CALGB) study in which a doxorubicin-containing combination was resumed after a course of radiation (43).

Corticosteroids have been reported to be effective treatment for radiation recall pneumonitis (42).

*Methotrexate.* Methotrexate has been associated with hypersensitivity reactions, pulmonary fibrosis, noncardiogenic pulmonary edema, and pleuritis. These reactions may occur after oral, intravenous, or intrathecal administration (18). The presentation of methotrexate pulmonary toxicity may be fulminant with fever, blood eosinophilia, rash, and rapid onset of respiratory failure (Fig. 3). Histopathology often reveals a marked inflammatory infiltrate with granulomas and pulmonary eosinophilia. Nonetheless, the prognosis is favorable, with dramatic responses to corticosteroids reported (18,19).

*Procarbazine.* A hypersensitivity reaction characterized by the abrupt onset of respiratory distress along with fever, rash, arthralgias, and peripheral blood eosinophilia has been described in association with procarbazine therapy (18,19). The subacute onset of dyspnea over 1 to 2 weeks without other signs of hypersensitivity has been reported as well (44,45). Corticosteroids appear to be beneficial in most cases (18,19,44,45).

*Cytosine Arabinoside.* Noncardiogenic pulmonary edema and ARDS have been associated with cytosine arabinoside (Ara-C) (17,19,21,46,47). Pleural and pericardial effusions are present in the minority of cases. There appears to be a dose-response effect, with a 20% to 30% incidence after cumulative doses above 24 g/m². Management consists primarily of aggressive supportive care, and the role of corticosteroids is unclear (21).

*Miscellaneous.* Rare reports of life-threatening pulmonary toxicity have appeared for fludarabine (48,49), irinotecan (CPT-11) (50), and oral etoposide (51). Paclitaxel, or its cremophor vehicle, has been associated with anaphylactoid reactions characterized by hypotension, dyspnea, bronchospasm, and urticaria in up to 10% of patients (23); however, premedication with corticosteroids and H₁- and H₂-antagonists has markedly reduced the incidence of this reaction to below 2% (52). High-dose interleukin-2 was reported to cause severe respiratory distress with diffuse interstitial infiltrates in nine of 199 consecutive patients treated for metastatic melanoma or renal cell carcinoma (53).

## Retinoic Acid Syndrome

A syndrome resembling capillary leak syndrome occurred in up to 25% of patients with acute promyelocytic leukemia (APL) treated with all-*trans*-retinoic acid (ATRA). This entity is characterized by fever, respiratory distress, and interstitial pulmonary infiltrates, often accompanied by weight gain, peripheral edema, pleural or pericardial effusions, and hypotension (Fig. 4). Onset has varied from 2 to 21 days after the start of therapy. Although most patients had increases in white blood cell

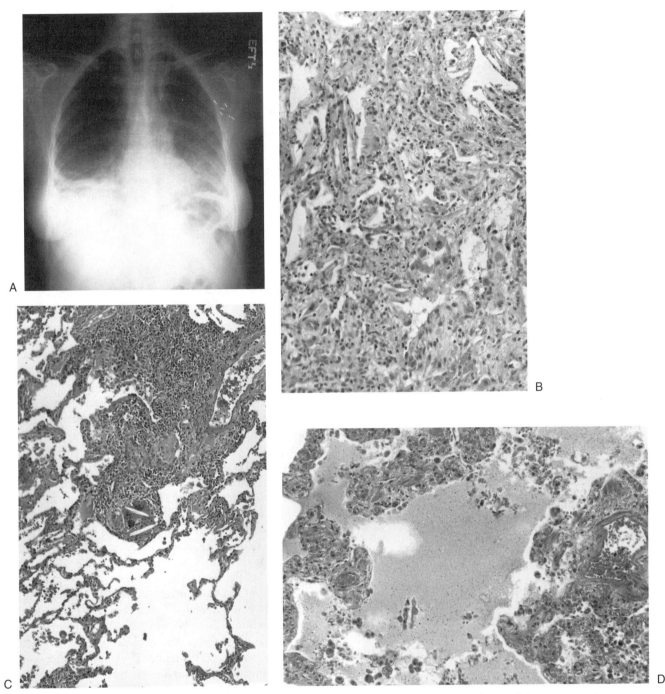

**FIG. 3.** Methotrexate pulmonary toxicity. Alveolar infiltrates, primarily in the bases and bilateral pleural effusions characterize this disease **(A)**. These radiographic findings are consistent with either acute pneumonitis, hypersensitivity pneumonitis, or noncardiogenic pulmonary edema. These entities can be distinguished only by the clinicopathologic findings **(B–D)**. Acute pneumonitis produces expansion of the alveolar walls by a polymorphous inflammatory cell infiltrate. In this section the pneumocytes exhibit moderate atypia **(B)**. With hypersensitivity pneumonitis, there may be patchy interstitial lymphocytic infiltrates and associated bronchiolitis and granuloma formation **(C)**. The pathologic findings of pulmonary edema include expansion of the alveolar spaces by proteinaceous fluid **(D)**.

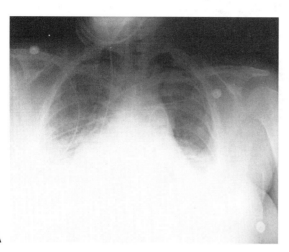 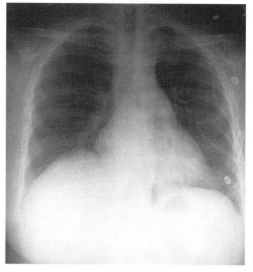

**FIG. 4.** Retinoic acid syndrome. Rapid onset of bilateral pleural effusions and diffuse parenchymal infiltrates **(A)** which resolved with supportive measures **(B)**.

count to ≥20,000, a significant percentage did not have leukocytosis. In early reports, the mortality rate was about 35%. Once respiratory distress had been established, there was no benefit to leukapheresis, chemotherapy, or cessation of ATRA, but early institution of high-dose steroids (dexamethasone 10 mg intravenously every 12 hours for at least 3 days) resulted in prompt recovery in most patients (54–56).

### Pulmonary Venoocclusive Disease (PVOD)

Pulmonary venoocclusive disease (PVOD) is a rare disorder characterized by intimal fibrosis of pulmonary veins and venules, resulting in pulmonary hypertension. Clinical presentation includes progressive dyspnea, hypoxia, and signs and symptoms of cor pulmonale. Diagnosis typically requires open-lung biopsy with special stains for elastic tissue. Although several etiologic factors have been associated with this syndrome, a handful of cases have been attributed to radiation and chemotherapeutic agents, including bleomycin, BCNU, mitomycin C, and possibly cyclophosphamide (57–59).

### Leukoagglutinin Reactions

The leukoagglutinin or pulmonary transfusion reaction is noncardiogenic pulmonary edema caused by activation of the recipient's neutrophils by donor leukocyte antibodies. The clinical presentation is respiratory distress, tachycardia, fever, chills, and often cyanosis and hypotension developing during or after administration of blood products. After discontinuation of the transfusion, treatment is supportive, and in most cases recovery is complete within a few days (60).

### Bone Marrow Transplantation

Pulmonary complications affect 40% to 60% of bone marrow transplant (BMT) recipients and are responsible for more than 30% of transplant-related deaths (61,62). In addition to the multiple infectious and noninfectious pulmonary complications discussed already, there are further complications unique to BMT patients.

In the early phase of bone marrow recovery, diffuse alveolar hemorrhage (DAH) may occur in up to 20% of patients and is associated with mortality rates as high as 80%. Symptoms and signs include progressive dyspnea, hypoxia, and diffuse patchy infiltrates but rarely hemoptysis. The diagnosis is confirmed when BAL yields recovery of progressively bloodier aliquots demonstrating hemosiderin-laden macrophage (63). Diffuse alveolar hemorrhage is associated with white blood cell recovery with or without thrombocytopenia. Risk factors include advanced age, underlying solid tumors, irradiation, severe mucositis, and renal insufficiency. Prompt diagnosis and institution of high-dose corticosteroids may be beneficial (63,64).

Interstitial pneumonitis is the most common pulmonary complication of BMT, occurring in 40% of allogeneic, 17% of syngeneic, and 10% of autologous transplant recipients (62); CMV accounts for most infectious cases. In 30% to 50% of patients, no infectious cause is identified. This noninfectious pneumonitis, termed *idiopathic pneumonia syndrome* (IPS), generally occurs after engraftment and is thought to be related to immunologic reactions coupled with toxicity from the conditioning regimens. Corticosteroids have no proven benefit, and the mortality rate remains close to 80% (62,65).

Acute graft-versus-host disease (GVHD) principally affects the skin, liver, gastrointestinal tract, and immune system; however, respiratory tract involvement may occur as well. Lymphocytic bronchitis is a controversial entity described in up to 25% of patients with acute GVHD (61). Whether it is a specific manifestation of GVHD, however, remains unresolved. Lymphocytic bronchitis presents with dyspnea and nonproductive cough, with a normal chest radiograph and without evidence of airflow obstruction. Bronchoscopy reveals diffuse inflammation of the airways, and pathological evaluation demonstrates small lymphocytes infiltrating the proximal bronchial mucosa, with loss of cilia and damage to the submucosal glands and goblet cells, predisposing to bacterial tracheobronchitis and pneumonia. Increased immunosuppressive therapy for the associated acute GVHD generally improves this syndrome (61,66).

Bronchiolitis obliterans has been described in 10% to 20% of BMT patients, associated with chronic GVHD in most cases (61,62,66). This complication usually occurs 4 to 12 months after BMT and is manifested by exertional dyspnea, nonproductive cough and wheezing. Because of airflow obstruction with gas trapping, physical examination may demonstrate late inspiratory rales, and pulmonary function tests may show obstruction in addition to restriction. BAL demonstrates lymphocytosis and excludes infection. Pathology resembles that of lung allograft rejection. Although mortality rates are as high as 65%, treatment with increased immunosuppressive therapy appears to be beneficial if administered early in the course of disease (62,66,67).

Interstitial pulmonary fibrosis occurs in 20% to 30% of patients within 12 months of allogeneic BMT (61,66). Factors contributing to diffuse lung injury and leading to fibrosis may include conditioning regimens (e.g., BCNU, busulfan, cyclophosphamide, and total body irradiation),

immunosuppressive therapy (methotrexate), transfusion reactions, pulmonary hemorrhage, and hyperleukocytosis. Treatment is supportive, and the mortality rate remains high (61). In severe cases, successful lung transplant has been performed (68,69).

## CARDIAC TOXICITY

Although most anticancer therapies have been reported to cause cardiac arrhythmias during or immediately after administration, few do so predictably or to a clinically meaningful degree (70). Among the chemotherapeutic agents, the anthracyclines are most commonly associated with cardiotoxicity. Combinations of anthracyclines with other cytotoxic agents, including radiation, cyclophosphamide, etoposide, vincristine, bleomycin, busulfan, mitomycin C, methotrexate, and cisplatin all have been reported to potentiate anthracycline-related cardiotoxicity (71–74). In addition, numerous antineoplastic agents have been associated with cardiac complications in patients not exposed to anthracyclines. In some cases, it is difficult to conclude whether toxicity was caused by a single agent or was multifactorial. Cytotoxic therapy may damage the endocardium, myocardium, pericardium, or coronary arteries. Table 4 summarizes the reported cardiotoxicities associated with various agents.

The clinical characteristics of treatment-induced cardiomyopathy are similar to those of other forms of biventricular failure. Risk factors include early and advanced age, underlying cardiac disease, hypertension, poor nutritional status, and mediastinal irradiation (75). Management is similar to that for other causes of cardiac dysfunction. Afterload reduction, inotropic support

**TABLE 4.** *Cardiotoxicity of cancer therapeutic agents*

| Agent | Cardiomyopathy | Ischemia/infarction | Arrhythmia | Pericardial disease |
|---|---|---|---|---|
| Radiation | ++ | ++ | ++ | ++ |
| Doxorubicin | ++ | ++ | ++ | ++ |
| Daunorubicin | ++ | ++ | ++ | ++ |
| Idarubicin | ++ | + | + | − |
| Mitoxantrone | + | + | + | − |
| Amsacrine | ++ | + | ++ | − |
| Bleomycin | − | + | − | + |
| Cyclophosphamide | ++ | − | − | ++ |
| Ifosfamide | + | − | + | − |
| 5-FU | ++ | ++ | ++ | − |
| Ara-C | − | − | − | + |
| Vinca alkaloids | − | + | − | − |
| Cisplatin | + | + | + | − |
| Taxol | − | + | ++ | − |
| Etoposide | + | + | − | − |
| Estramustine | − | + | − | − |
| Estrogens | ++ | ++ | − | − |
| Interferon-α | ++ | ++ | ++ | − |
| Interleukin-2 | ++ | ++ | ++ | ++ |

(++) Strong association; (+) few case reports; (−) no association; 5-FU, 5-fluorouracil; Ara-C, cytosine arabinoside

and correction of any exacerbating factors such as infection or anemia will stabilize or improve the symptoms of CHF in most patients (76). Discontinuation of the causative agent may result in stabilization, progression, or occasionally improvement. Heart transplantation has been performed for patients with end-stage disease (77,78).

## Radiation

The risk of damage to the heart from radiation therapy is related to the volume of heart irradiated and the total dose received (79). Although radiation therapy potentially can damage the pericardium, myocardium, coronary arteries, and conducting system, the incidence of all these toxicities is declining with modern cardiac-shielding techniques that minimize exposure. The cardiotoxic effects of irradiation may be manifested relatively early after completion of therapy, as with acute pericarditis, or delayed for years, as with coronary artery disease. Much of the published data on this subject involve patients treated with mediastinal radiation for Hodgkin disease. In one such series, 46 of 48 patients irradiated before 1977 displayed overt or occult cardiac disease at a mean of 97 months after radiotherapy. Findings included constrictive pericarditis, abnormal hemodynamic response to fluid challenge, coronary artery disease, and left ventricular dysfunction; however, only nine patients required intervention: Two patients had symptomatic CHF, six patients needed pericardiectomy, and three patients underwent coronary artery bypass grafting (80).

Although pericardial disease is the most common cardiotoxicity of mediastinal radiation, this complication has become less common with the modern techniques of the last decade (72,76,81). During the course of treatment of a radiosensitive mediastinal mass, an acute pericarditis may occur, which is believed to be directly related to tumor response rather than to pericardial damage, as it resolves despite continued treatment, and there is no correlation with late cardiac complications (82). In general, however, the onset of symptomatic pericarditis, pericardial effusion, or constriction is delayed for months to decades. Pericardial effusion most commonly develops 4 to 6 months after therapy (72). Of patients who become symptomatic, 10% to 30% develop tamponade, usually within 2 years of treatment. Up to 20% progress to constrictive pericarditis within 5 to 10 years, although a 45-year latency period has been described (72).

A few patients may develop effusive-constrictive pericarditis. This entity presents with signs and symptoms of pericardial tamponade, with persistent elevations in right atrial pressure after pericardiocentesis resulting from fibrosis of the visceral pericardium. Pericardiectomy is required in most symptomatic patients with effusive-constrictive pericarditis (81); however, most cases of radia-

tion pericarditis resolve spontaneously, with or without nonsteroidal antiinflammatory drugs for relief of symptoms (72,76).

Myocardial damage may become evident when pericardiectomy does not improve the signs and symptoms of constrictive pericarditis (82). In historic reports, myocardial dysfunction was reported after high doses of radiation to the heart using techniques that are suboptimal by current standards. With the use of modern techniques, no significant deterioration in left ventricular function has been documented. The concurrent or sequential use of anthracyclines may precipitate severe cardiomyopathy without accompanying pericardial disease (82).

There is substantial evidence demonstrating an increased risk of coronary artery disease in patients who have received mediastinal irradiation. Again, most series have involved patients treated before the cardiac-sparing techniques used over the last decade (76,83). In an autopsy series involving patients under the age of 35, 25% of irradiated patients versus 2.5% of age- and sex-matched nonirradiated controls had significant coronary artery stenosis (84). Large studies demonstrated a 2.6- to 8.8-fold relative risk of mortality from myocardial infarction after mediastinal radiation for Hodgkin disease (76,85). Rutqvist et al. (86) found a threefold relative risk of death of ischemic heart disease in women with cancer of the left breast who received a high-dose volume of radiation before mastectomy compared with surgical controls. There was no increased risk for patients who received radiation to the right breast or whose left chest were treated with electrons postoperatively (i.e., lower doses to the myocardium) (86). More modern techniques have not been demonstrated to confer such a risk, although clearly the duration of follow-up is not as prolonged (83). Nonetheless, monitoring and early intervention for signs of coronary artery disease are warranted for patients who have received radiation therapy to the chest. Both coronary artery bypass surgery and balloon angioplasty have been successful in patients with radiation-induced coronary artery disease (70).

## Chemotherapy

### Doxorubicin

As doxorubicin has the widest spectrum of anticancer activity of the anthracyclines, most information regarding anthracycline cardiotoxicity was derived from its use. Doxorubicn is associated with acute, subacute, chronic, and late cardiotoxicity. The acute effects occur during or immediately after administration and include transient arrhythmias, nonspecific electrocardiographic (ECG) changes, and occasional conduction abnormalities (70, 87). Rare life-threatening ventricular arrhythmias have been reported (88,89). Patients experiencing sympto-

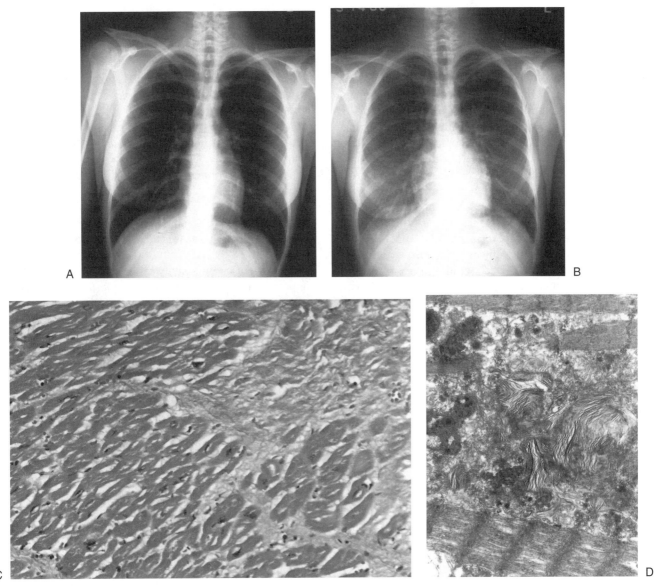

**FIG. 5.** Doxorubicin cardiomyopathy. Films taken three weeks apart show the development of cardiomegaly and the ground glass infiltrates of pulmonary edema secondary to doxorubicin cardiomyopathy **(A,B)**. Biopsy **(C)** depicts myocytes with enlarged and atypical nuclei associated with interstitial fibrosis. Electron micoroscopy **(D)** shows myofibril fragmentation, mitochondrial degeneration, and the accumulation of whorls of membrane proteins (×15,300) **(C)**.

matic atrial or ventricular arrhythmias should receive antiarrhythmic therapy (70).

The subacute form consists of myopericarditis occurring within days of administration, characterized by pericardial effusion and myocardial dysfunction (Fig. 5). Symptoms usually resolve spontaneously with supportive care but are occasionally life threatening (75,87).

The chronic form of doxorubicin cardiotoxicity consists of a congestive cardiomyopathy of insidious onset occurring at a median of 1 month after treatment is discontinued (90). Symptoms range from exercise intolerance to severe dyspnea at rest. The mortality rate for symptomatic patients is 30% to 60% (75,90); however,

with aggressive medical management, the cardiomyopathy may improve over months to a few years (87,91).

There is a well-documented dose-response relationship between cumulative doxorubicin exposure and cardiotoxicity. When administered as an intravenous bolus dose approximately every 3 weeks, doxorubicin induces a 0.1% to 1.2% risk of developing clinically significant cardiomyopathy after doses of less than 500 mg/m$^2$. Beyond a cumulative dose of 550 mg/m$^2$, the risk of CHF rises rapidly, to the range of 10% to 25% (71,90). There is considerable individual variability, however, and CHF has been reported after total doses of only 40 mg/m$^2$, whereas other patients have tolerated more than 1,000 mg/m$^2$ (90). In a retrospective review of 4,018 patients by von Hoff et al. (90), the median cumulative dose of doxorubicin received by patients who developed symptomatic CHF was 390 mg/m$^2$ (90). Rates of cardiotoxicity appear to be lower when doxorubicin is administered as a continuous infusion rather than as a bolus injection and on a weekly schedule rather than every 3 weeks (90). Other risk factors include increasing age, mediastinal irradiation, combination chemotherapy regimens, and history of cardiac disease or hypertension (71,75,90).

Endomyocardial biopsy reveals loss of myofibrils, swelling of the sarcoplasmic reticulum, and cytoplasmic vacuolization involving progressively more myocytes as damage worsens. Diffuse myonecrosis may ensue (92). Endomyocardial biopsy reveals changes much earlier than can be detected clinically or by noninvasive testing. Billingham et al. (92) defined a grading system for progressive pathological changes that correlates well with the degree of heart failure. Because of the biological variability in individual tolerance of doxorubicin therapy, endomyocardial biopsy can be a useful tool in determining the risk-to-benefit ratio of continued anthracycline therapy on an individual basis (92).

Noninvasive testing with radionuclide angiocardiography (RNA) is most often used to monitor patients receiving anthracycline therapy. A fall in ejection fraction has been shown to precede clinical cardiomyopathy. Schwartz et al. (93) demonstrated that, for patients with a normal baseline RNA, a fourfold reduction in the incidence of CHF could be achieved by following serial measurements of ejection fraction, with discontinuation of therapy after an absolute decrease of ≥10% or a decline to <50%. Furthermore, measurement of the ejection fraction in response to exercise may identify patients at risk for cardiotoxicity by uncovering occult preexisting heart disease (94).

Late toxicity is defined as that occurring 5 or more years after treatment. Symptoms may redevelop in patients who recovered from subacute toxicity or may occur de novo. Atrial and ventricular arrhythmias and sudden death have been described as well. In one series, the combination of CHF and arrhythmias developed in previously asymptomatic patients 12 to 18 years after completion of therapy. Pathology at this stage reveals myocardial fibrosis and hypertrophy of myocytes without vacuolization. The degree of cardiac compromise documented within a year of completion of therapy predicts the likelihood of late toxicity (91).

### Other Anthracyclines

Daunorubicin is associated with the same clinical and pathological cardiotoxicity as doxorubicin. The cumulative dose at which the risk of cardiotoxicity increases appears to be greater than 600 mg/m$^2$ (95). Idarubicin initially was reported to cause minimal cardiotoxicity (96); however, later reports indicate a similar risk for CHF with idarubicin and daunorubicin (97–100). Anderlini et al. (101) reported a 5% probability of idarubicin-related cardiomyopathy at cumulative doses ≥150 mg/m$^2$ (102). Epirubicin is associated with a precipitously increased risk of cardiotoxicity at cumulative doses of 900 to 1,000 mg/m$^2$ (102).

Mitoxantrone is an anthracenedione with antitumor activity similar to that of doxorubicin. Although mitoxantrone has been touted to be less cardiotoxic than doxorubicin, the nonhematologic dose-limiting toxicity is cardiac (103,104). Similar to the anthracyclines, cardiotoxicity appears to be cumulative, with a rapid increase in risk above a total dose of 160 mg/m$^2$. Prior anthracycline exposure increases the risk, with toxicity at about 100 mg/m$^2$ (87).

The risk of cardiotoxicity resulting from anthracyclines appears to be related in part to peak plasma concentrations of the drug. Accordingly, treatment schedules in which anthracycline is administered as a continuous infusion over 96 hours, rather than as a bolus injection (71,105) or on a weekly schedule rather than every 3 weeks (90) are associated with a lower risk. Other strategies that ameliorate anthracycline cardiotoxicity include encapsulation within liposomes and the concurrent administration of cardioprotective agents such as dexrazoxane.

Compared with the bolus administration of free drug, liposomal encapsulation results in an improved pharmokinetic profile with a longer plasma life and better drug delivery (106,107). Like the free drug, liposomal doxorubicin produces myelosuppression and stomatitis. Liposomal doxorubicin also can produce acute allergic reactions, and with prolonged therapy, a hand-foot syndrome may ensue (106–109). Liposomal encapsulation appears to reduce the cardiotoxicity of doxorubicin and permit administration of higher cumulative doses more safely (107,109).

Although the precise mechanism of cardioprotection is uncertain, it appears that dexrazoxane is converted intracellularly into a chelating agent that interferes with the formation of iron-mediated free radicals (110). In several randomized trials, dexrazoxane has demonstrated a cardioprotective effect against high cumulative doses of doxorubicin and epirubicin in patients with metastatic breast cancer, small-cell lung cancer, and advanced soft-tissue sarcomas (111–114). In previously untreated patients, differences in cardiac function can be detected by radionuclide scans after cumulative doses of doxorubicin of 150 mg/m$^2$. In heavily pretreated patients (i.e., those who have received more than six cycles of doxorubicin-based chemotherapy), the inclusion of dexrazoxane into subsequent chemotherapy cycles reduces the incidence of clinically evident CHF from 22% to 3% compared with historic controls (115). Dexrazoxane appears to have no clinically significant effect on noncardiac toxicity (102, 112–114,116,117). Whether dexrazoxane impairs the antitumor activity of anthracyclines is unsettled. Two of three randomized trials involving patients with metastatic breast cancer found no effect, whereas a third larger study identified a significantly lower response rate (48% versus 63%) and progression-free survival in patients receiving dexrazoxane (110,115). Accordingly, dexrazoxane currently is indicated only for patients who have received a total dose of doxorubicin of more than 300 mg/m$^2$ in whom continued treatment is warranted.

### Cyclphosphamide

There is a noncumulative dose-response relationship between cyclophosphamide and cardiac damage. When used as a single agent, cyclophosphamide is associated with cardiac complications almost exclusively at high doses such as those used for bone marrow transplantation. Cyclophosphamide toxicity results in myopericarditis characterized by severe CHF, elevated cardiac enzymes, and hemorrhagic pericarditis with pericardial effusion. Pathological evaluation reveals capillary endothelial damage, myocardial hemorrhage, and necrosis with mural edema and serosanguinous pericardial effusion (118). Onset is fulminant within 1 week of beginning treatment, and the mortality rate is 20% to 40% (70,118, 119). With aggressive supportive care with diuretics, inotropic agents, and afterload reduction, patients who recover have no long-term sequelae (70,76). Pericardiocentesis for cardiac tamponade has not been shown to alter outcome (76).

Factors influencing the development of cardiotoxicity include dose, rate of delivery, previous exposure to anthracyclines, and underlying cardiac dysfunction (76). Gottdiener et al. (118) evaluated 32 patients with hematologic malignancies who were treated with 180 mg/kg of cyclophosphamide over 4 days as part of a conditioning regimen for allogeneic bone marrow transplantation. Cardiotoxicity was common, with a 28% incidence of CHF, 19% incidence of pericardial tamponade, and 19% mortality rate. Furthermore, for patients who had received prior anthracycline therapy, the incidence of CHF was 50%. Goldberg et al. (119) reported on a series of 80 young patients undergoing allogeneic bone marrow transplantation for aplastic anemia or immunodeficiency syndromes, none of whom had prior anthracycline therapy or mediastinal irradiation. Twenty-five percent of the patients who received more than 1.55 g/m$^2$/day of cyclophosphamide for 4 days developed CHF compared with 3% in patients who received less than 1.55 g/m$^2$/day. Nearly half of the cases were fatal.

### Ifosfamide

Although ifosfamide is an alkylating agent closely related to cyclophosphamide, similar cardiotoxicity has not been reported; however, a case of cardiomyopathy was reported in a patient treated with ifosfamide in combination with etoposide and cisplatin for testicular cancer (120). In addition, supraventricular arrhythmias have been reported with ifosfamide therapy, and in one case rechallenge with the drug resulted in a refractory arrhythmia (121,122).

### 5-Fluorouracil

The most common cardiotoxic effect of 5-fluorouracil (5-FU) is ischemia, usually manifesting as angina, but rarely progressing to fatal myocardial infarction or cardiogenic shock. Arrhythmias, CHF, and sudden death have been reported as well. Although the overall incidence of cardiotoxicity is low, it appears to be significantly higher in patients with underlying coronary artery disease than in patients without such a history (about 5% versus 1%). Nonetheless, life-threatening ischemia has occurred in patients with normal coronary arteries demonstrated by cardiac catheterization (76,123). The addition of leucovorin to 5-FU has increased cardiotoxicity (124).

Most patients have reported typical precordial pain, sometimes radiating to the arms or jaw, associated with nausea, vomiting, and diaphoresis; ECG abnormalities may include diffuse ST segment depression or elevation, peaked T-waves or T-wave inversions, prolongation of the QT interval, and atrial or ventricular arrhythmias. Symptoms usually start within hours of exposure to the drug and resolve spontaneously or with the administration of nitrates after discontinuation of the drug. Aggressive supportive care with intravenous inotropic agents, diuretics, and vasodilators may be necessary. Although the ECG returns to normal in most patients, continued administration of 5-FU has been associated with the development of Q-waves indicative of completed myocardial infarction. Reversible regional or global left ventricular wall motion abnormalities have been demonstrated. Neither nitrates nor calcium channel blockers have reliably demonstrated efficacy in preventing 5-FU-related ischemia. Relapses on reinstitution of therapy are frequent, and thus the risks and benefits of further treatment with 5-FU should be weighed carefully (76,123).

### Paclitaxel

Cardiotoxicity in the form of arrhythmias, conduction disturbances, and ischemia has been attributed to paclitaxel administration. By far the most common finding is asymptomatic sinus bradycardia, noted in about 30% of patients (125,126). This complication requires no treatment and does not preclude further use of the drug; however, ventricular tachycardia, bundle branch blocks, and second- and third-degree atrioventricular blocks have been reported in about 2% of patients, most of whom also received cisplatin. Complete heart block requiring pacemaker insertion was described in one patient with no history of cardiac disease. In a patient with hypertension and hypercholesterolemia who had received prior mediastinal irradiation for non-small cell lung cancer, a fatal acute inferior-wall myocardial infarction accompanied by complete heart block occurred during paclitaxel infusion (126).

Nevertheless, the likelihood of significant cardiotoxicity in patients without cardiac risk factors appears to be minimal. In a retrospective review of more than 3,400 patients treated with paclitaxel, the incidences of advanced heart block, atrial or ventricular arrhythmias, and myocardial infarction or ischemia were all below 1% (125). Therefore, routine cardiac monitoring has not been recommended. For patients who have or are at high risk for cardiac disease, there is insufficient information regarding the cardiotoxicity of paclitaxel administration. Patients who have developed symptomatic arrhythmias or heart block have been rechallenged safely under controlled conditions, including the use of continuous cardiac monitoring and temporary pacemakers (125,126).

### Etoposide

There are a few reports of myocardial infarction and congestive heart failure during etoposide infusions. Some patients had preexisting coronary artery disease, and others received doxorubicin, cisplatin, bleomycin, or mediastinal irradiation (67,127,128). Hypotension occurs frequently when etoposide is administered by rapid intravenous infusion lasting less than 30 minutes but is reversible with intravenous fluids and slowing of the infusion rate (129).

### Amsacrine

Myocardial infarction, arrhythmias, and CHF all have been reported after administration of amsacrine. The incidence of arrhythmias is below 1%, but ventricular arrhythmias and sudden death have been reported (70, 130). Hypokalemia may be a risk factor for the development of arrhythmias, but most affected patients had normal serum potassium levels (130). Previous anthracycline exposure is a predisposing factor to amsacrine-related cardiomyopathy. In one series, when the combination of anthracycline and amsacrine dose exceeded 900 mg/m$^2$, most patients developed abnormalities in cardiac function (131). Symptoms are often reversible but have been fatal in a number of cases (87,130,131).

### Vinca Alkaloids, Cisplatin, and Bleomycin

Several cases of myocardial ischemia or infarction have been reported in association with combinations of vinblastine or vincristine, with cisplatin and bleomycin (132–134). In some cases, cisplatin was felt to be the causative agent (133). In other reports, vincristine alone was associated with myocardial infarction (135,136).

In addition to myocardial ischemia, vinca alkaloids have been associated with cardiac autonomic neuropathies resulting in orthostatic hypotension and an abnormal heart rate response (137,138). These abnormalities were found more often in patients receiving high cumulative doses (138) or inadvertent overdose (139).

### Estrogens and Estramustine

Estrogen therapy has been effective in the treatment of metastatic breast cancer and metastatic prostate cancer but has largely been replaced by other hormonal agents because of significant cardiovascular toxicity. Diethylstilbestrol (DES) at doses ≥3 mg per day is associated with CHF, myocardial ischemia, myocardial infarction, and thromboembolic episodes in up to 10% of patients (140–142); however, at a dose of 1 mg/day, DES is not associated with an excess incidence of cardiovascular events (141). Although the antineoplastic properties of estramustine are thought be exerted through inhibition of microtubule assembly, its cardiovascular toxicities appear to be related to its estrogenic properties. The incidence of myocardial ischemia or infarction and cardiomyopathy are in the range of 10% to 30%, with the highest incidence in patients with prior cardiac disease (142–144).

### Biologic Response Modifiers

Cardiotoxicity has been described in patients receiving interferons (alpha and gamma) and interleukin-2 (IL-2), both alone and in combination (53,145–149). Interferon has been associated with supraventricular and ventricular arrhythmias, myocardial infarction, and cardiomyopathy. No correlation has been made with either the dose or duration of interferon therapy. Although most patients who have experienced atrial arrhythmias or myocardial ischemia have had underlying heart disease, those developing ventricular arrhythmias or cardiomyopathy have had no such history (145). Although most cases have been reversible on discontinuation of the drug, one case of severe irreversible cardiomyopathy was reported in a patient previously treated with doxorubicin (146).

High doses of IL-2 predictably cause a myriad of adverse effects. The most serious event is the immediate onset of a combination of decreased systemic vascular resistance and capillary leak syndrome. Similar to bacterial sepsis, this reaction to IL-2 is characterized by hypotension, tachycardia, decreased left ventricular function, pulmonary and peripheral edema, oliguria, and renal failure (150). Cardiac effects also have included atrial and ventricular tachyarrhythmias, bradycardia, complete heart block, myocardial ischemia and infarction, myopericarditis, and rarely sudden death (53,147,149–152). Pressor support, mechanical ventilation, or antiarrhythmic therapy often will be required during the course of treatment, but symptoms generally resolve rapidly after discontinuation of the drug (53,150).

# REFERENCES

1. Canham EM, Kennedy TC, Merrick TA. Unexplained pulmonary infiltrates in the compromised patient: an invasive investigation in consecutive series. *Cancer* 1983;52:325.
2. Cheson BD, Samlowski WE, Tang TT, Spruance SL. Value of open-lung biopsy in 87 immunocompromised patients with pulmonary infiltrates. *Cancer* 1985;55:453.
3. Pizzo P, Myers J, Freifeld A, Walsh T. Infections in the cancer patient. In: DeVita VT Jr, Hellman S , Rosenberg SA, eds. *Cancer: principles and practice of oncology.* 4th ed. Philadelphia: JB Lippincott, 1993:2292.
4. Doll DC, Weiss RB, Issell BF. Mitomycin: ten years after approval for marketing. *J Clin Oncol* 1985;3:276.
5. Tenholder M, Hooper R. Pulmonary infiltrates in leukemia. *Chest* 1980;78:468.
6. Browne MJ, Potter D, Gress J, et al. A randomized trial of open lung biopsy versus empiric antimicrobial therapy in cancer patients with diffuse pulmonary infiltrates. *J Clin Oncol* 1990;8:222.
7. Gururangan S, Lawson R, Jones P, Stevens R, Campbell R. Evaluation of the usefulness of open lung biopsies. *Pediatr Hematol Oncol* 1992;9:107.
8. Bustamante CI, Wade JC. Treatment of interstitial pneumonia in cancer patients: Is empiric antibiotic therapy the answer? *J Clin Oncol* 1990;8:200.
9. Pisani R, Wright A. Clinical utility of bronchoalveolar lavage in immunocompromised hosts. *Mayo Clin Proc* 1992;67:221.
10. Crawford S, Bowden R, Hackman R, Gleaves C, Meyers J, Clark J. Rapid detection of cytomegalovirus pulmonary infection by bronchoalveolar lavage and centrifugation culture. *Ann Intern Med* 1988; 18:180.
11. Gaussorgues P, Piperno D, Bachman P, et al. Comparison of nonbronchoscopic bronchoalveolar lavage to open lung biopsy for the bacteriologic diagnosis of pulmonary infections in mechanically ventilated patiets. *Intensive Care Med* 1989;15:94.
12. Rouby J, Rossignon M, Nicholas M, et al. A prospective study of protected bronchoalveolar lavage in the diagnosis of nosocomial pneumonia. *Anesthesiology* 1989;71:679.
13. Bensard D, McIntyre R, Waring B, Simon J. Comparison of video thoracoscopic lung biopsy to open lung biopsy in the diagnosis of interstitial lung disease. *Chest* 1993;103:765.
14. McLoud T, Naidich D. Thoracic disease in the immunocompromised patient. *Radiol Clin North Am* 1992;30:525.
15. Pietra GG. Pathologic mechanisms of drug-induced lung disorders. *J Thorac Imaging* 1991;6:1.
16. Bauer KA, Skarin AT, Balikian JP, Garnick MB, Rosenthal DS, Canellos GP. Pulmonary complications associated with combination chemotherapy programs containing bleomycin. *Am J Med* 1983;74:557.
17. McDonald S, Rubin P, Phillips TL, Marks LB. Injury to the lung from cancer therapy: clinical syndromes, measurable end points and potential scoring systems. *Int J Radiat Oncol Biol Phys* 1995;31:1187.
18. Cooper AD, White DA, Matthay RA. Drug-induced pulmonary disease, Part I: Cytotoxic drugs. *Am Rev Respir Dis* 1986;133:321.
19. Ginsberg SJ, Comis RL. The pulmonary toxicity of antineoplastic agents. *Semin Oncol* 1982;9:34.
20. Gross NJ. Pulmonary effects of radiation therapy. *Ann Int Med* 1977; 86:81.
21. Kreisman H, Wolkove N. Pulmonary toxicity of antineoplastic therapy. In: Perry MC, ed. *The Chemotherapy Sourcebook.* Baltimore: Williams and Wilkins, 1992:598.
22. Patz EFJ. Pulmonary drug toxicity following high-dose chemotherapy with autologous bone marrow transplantation: CT findings in 20 cases. *J Thorac Imaging* 1994;9:129.
23. Weiss RB, Donehower RC, Wiernik PH, et al. Hypersensitivity reactions from taxol. *J Clin Oncol* 1990;8:1263.
24. Mah K, Keane TJ, Van Dyk J, Braban LE, Poon PY, Hao Y. Quantitative effect of combined chemotherapy and fractionated radiotherapy on the incidence of radiation-induced lung damage: a prospective clinical study. *Int J Radiat Oncol Biol Phys* 1995;28:563.
25. Stover DE. Pulmonary toxicity. In: DeVita VT Jr., Hellman S , Rosenberg SA, eds. *Cancer: principles and practice of oncology.* 4th ed. Philadelphia: JB Lipincott, 1993;2362.
26. Choi NC, Kanarek DJ. Toxicity of thoracic radiotherapy on pulmonary function in lung cancer. *Lung Cancer* 1994;10(Suppl 1):S219.
27. Einhorn L, Krause M, Hornback N, Furnas B. Enhanced pulmonary toxicity with bleomycin and radiotherapy in oat cell lung cancer. *Cancer* 1976;37:2414.
28. Maher J, Daly PA. Severe bleomycin lung toxicity: reversal with high dose corticosteroids. *Thorax* 1993;48:92.
29. Weiss RB, Poster DS, Penta JS. The nitrosoureas and pulmonary toxicity. *Cancer Treat Rev* 1981;8:111.
30. Klingemann HG, Shepherd JD, Reece DE, et al. Regimen-related acute toxicities: pathophysiology, risk factors, clinical evaluation and preventive strategies. *Bone Marrow Transplant* 1994;14(Suppl 4): S14.
31. Wheeler C, Antin JH, Churchill WH, et al. Cyclophosphamide, carmustine, and etoposide with autologous bone marrow transplantation in refractory Hodgkin's disease and non-Hodgkin's lymphoma: a dose-finding study. *J Clin Oncol* 1990;8:648.
32. Budzar AU, Legha SS, Luna MA, Tashima CK, Hortobagyi GN, Blumenschein GR. Pulmonary toxicity of mitomycin. *Cancer* 1980; 45:236.
33. Chang AY, Kuebler P, Pandya KJ, Israel RH, Marshall BC, Tormey DC. Pulmonary toxicity induced by mitomycin C is highly responsive to glucocorticoids. *Cancer* 1986;57:2285.
34. Burkes RL, Ginsberg RJ, Shepherd FA, et al. Induction chemotherapy with mitomycin, vindesine and cisplatin for stage III unresectable non-small-cell lung cancer: results of the Toronto phase III trial. *J Clin Oncol* 1992;10:580.
35. Ozols RF, Hogan WM, Ostchega Y, Young RC. MVP (mitomycin, vinblastine and progesterone): a second-line regimen in ovarian cancer with a high incidence of pulmonary toxicity. *Cancer Treat Rep* 1983; 67:721.
36. Luedke D, McLaughlin TT, Daughaday C, et al. Mitomycin C and vindesine associated pulmonary toxicity with variable clinical expression. *Cancer* 1985;55:542.
37. Rivera MP, Kris MG, Gralla RJ, White DA. Syndrome of acute dyspnea related to combined mitomycin plus vinca alkaloid chemotherapy. *Am J Clin Oncol* 1995;18:245.
38. Gralla RJ, Kardinal CG, Clark RA, Otten MC, Hanson DS. Enhancing the safety, efficacy and dose intensity of vinorelbine (navelbine) in combination chemotherapy regimens. *Proc Am Soc Clin Oncol* 1993; 12:336 (abst).
39. Trask CW, Joannides T, Harper PG, et al. Radiation-induced lung fibrosis after treatment of small cell carcinoma of the lung with very high-dose cyclophosphamide. *Cancer* 1985;55:57.
40. Baker W, Fistel SJ, Jones RV, Weiss RB. Interstitial pneumonitis associated with ifosfamide therapy. *Cancer* 1990;65:2217.
41. Johnson RE, Brereton HD, Kent CH. "Total" therapy for small cell carcinoma of the lung. *Ann Thorac Surg* 1978;25:510.
42. McInerney DP, Bullimore J. Reactivation of radiation pneumonitis by adriamycin. *Br J Radiol* 1977;50:224.
43. Aisner J, Goutsou M, Maurer LH, et al. Intensive combination chemotherapy, concurrent chest irradiation and warfarin for the treatment of limited-disease small-cell lung cancer: a Cancer and Leukemia Group B Pilot Study. *J Clin Oncol* 1992;10:1230.
44. Brooks BJ, Hendler NB, Alvarez S, Ancalmo N, Grinton SF. Delayed life-threatening pneumonitis secondary to procarbazine. *Am J Clin Oncol* 1990;13:244.
45. Millward MJ, Cohney SJ, Byrne MJ, Ryan GF. Pulmonary toxicity following MOPP chemotherapy. *Aust NZ J Med* 1990;20:245.
46. Aronchik JM, Gefter WB. Drug-induced pulmonary disease: an update. *J Thorac Imaging* 1991;6:19.
47. Shearer P, Katz J, Bozeman P, et al. Pulmonary insufficiency complicating therapy with high dose cytosine arabinoside in five pediatric patients with relapsed acute myelogenous leukemia. *Cancer* 1994; 74:1953.
48. Cervantes F, Salgado C, Montserrat E, Rozman C. Fludarabine for prolymphocytic leukemia and risk of interstitial pneumonitis. *Lancet* 1990;336:1130.
49. Devlin JW, Wass H, Waters CI. Fludarabine associated pulmonary hypersensitivity. *Can J Hosp Pharm* 1994;47:125.
50. Masuda N, Fukuoka M, Kusunoki Y, et al. CPT-11: a new derivative of camptothecin for the treatment of refractory or relapsed small-cell lung cancer. *J Clin Oncol* 1992;10:1225.

51. Dajczman E, Srolovitz H, Kreisman H, Frank H. Fatal pulmonary toxicity following oral etoposide therapy. *Lung Cancer* 1995;12:81.

52. Pazdur R, Kudelka AP, Kavanagh JJ, Cohen PR, Raber MN. The taxoids: paclitaxel (Taxol) and docetaxel (Taxotere). *Cancer Treat Rev* 1993;19:351.

53. White RL, Schwartzentruber DJ, Guleria A, et al. Cardiopulmonary toxicity of treatment with high dose interleukin-2 in 199 consecutive patients with metastatic melanoma or renal cell carcinoma. *Cancer* 1994;74:3212.

54. Warrell RPJ, De The H, Wang Z, Degos L. Acute promyelocytic leukemia. *N Engl J Med* 1993;329:177.

55. Frankel SR, Eardley A, Lauwers G, Weiss M, Warrell RPJ. The retinoic acid syndrome in acute promyelocytic leukemia. *Ann Intern Med* 1992;117:292.

56. Frankel SR, Eardley A, Heller G, et al. All-trans retinoic acid for acute promyelocytic leukemia—Results of the New York study. *Ann Intern Med* 1994;120:278.

57. Doll DC, Yarbro JW. Vascular toxicity associated with antineoplastic agents. *Semin Oncol* 1992;19:580.

58. Kramer MR, Estenne M, Berkman N, et al. Radiation-induced pulmonary veno-occlusive disease. *Chest* 1993;104:1282.

59. Lombard CM, Churg A, Winokur S. Pulmonary veno-occlusive disease following therapy for malignant neoplasms. *Chest* 1987;92:871.

60. Lalezari P. Leukocyte antigens and antibodies. In: Hoffman R, Benz E Jr, Shattil S, Furie B , Cohen H, eds. *Hematology: basic principles and practice.* New York: Churchill Livingstone, 1991;1566.

61. Krowka MJ, Rosenow EC, Hoagland HC. Pulmonary complications of bone marrow transplantation. *Chest* 1985;87:237.

62. Breuer R, Lossos IS, Berkman N, Or R. Pulmonary complications of bone marrow transplantation. *Respir Med* 1993;87:571.

63. Robbins RA, Linder J, Stahl MG, et al. Diffuse alveolar hemorrhage in autologous bone marrow transplant recipients. *Am J Med* 1989;87:511.

64. Chao NJ, Duncan SR, Long GD, et al. Corticosteroid therapy for diffuse alveolar hemorrhage in autologous bone marrow transplant recipients. *Ann Intern Med* 1991;114:145.

65. Quabeck K. The lung as a critical organ in marrow transplantation. *Bone Marrow Transplant* 1994;14(Suppl 4):S19.

66. Chan CK, Hyland RH, Hutcheon M. Pulmonary complications following bone marrow transplantation. *Clin Chest Med* 1990;11:323.

67. Schwarer AP, Hughes JMB, Trotman-Dickenson B, Krausz T, Goldman JM. A chronic pulmonary syndrome associated with graft-versus-host disease after allogeneic marrow transplantation. *Transplant* 1992;54:1002.

68. Calhoon JH, Levine SM, Anzueto A, Bryan CL, Trinkle JK. Lung transplantation in a patient with a prior bone marrow transplant. *Chest* 1992;102:948.

69. Boas SR, Blakeslee EN, Kurland G, Armitage J, Orenstein D. Pediatric lung transplantation for graft-versus-host disease following bone marrow transplantation. *Chest* 1994;105:1584.

70. Ali MK, Ewer MS, Gibbs HR, Swafford J. Cardiovascular emergencies in cancer patients. *Cancer Bull* 1992;44:173.

71. Praga C, Beretta G, Vigo PL, et al. Adriamycin cardiotoxicity: a survey of 1273 patients. *Cancer Treat Rep* 1979;5:827.

72. Arsenian MA. Cardiovascular sequelae of therapeutic thoracic radiation. *Progress Cardiovasc Dis* 1991;33:299.

73. Watts RG. Severe and fatal anthracycline cardiotoxicity at cumulative doses below 400 mg/m$^2$: evidence for enhanced toxicity with multiagent chemotherapy. *Am J Hematol* 1991;36:217.

74. Quintana J, Beresi V, DelPozo H, et al. Intra-arterial cisplatin given prior to surgery in osteosarcoma: grade of necrosis and size of tumor as major prognostic factors. *Am J Pediatr Hematol Oncol* 1990;13:269.

75. Porembka DT, Lowder JN, Orlowski JP, Bastulli J, Lockrem J. Etiology and management of doxorubicin cardiotoxicity. *Crit Care Med* 1989;17:569.

76. Steinherz LJ, Yahalom J. Cardiac complications of anticancer therapy. In: DeVita VT Jr, Hellman S , Rosenberg SA, eds. *Cancer: principles and practice of oncology.* 4th ed. Philadelphia: JB Lippincott, 1993;2370.

77. Ramrakha PS, Marks D, O Brien SG, Yacoub M, Schofeld JB, Goldman JM. Orthotopic cardiac transplantation for dilated cardiomyopathy after allogeneic bone marrow transplantation. *Clin Transplant* 1994;8:23.

78. Rosado LJ, Wild JC, Huston CL, Sethi GK, Copeland JG. Heart transplantation in patients with treated breast carcinoma. *J Heart Lung Transplant* 1994;13:246.

79. Stewart JR, Fajardo LF. Radiation induced heart disease: An update. *Prog Cardiovasc Dis* 1984;27:173.

80. Appelfeld MM, Wiernik PH. Cardiac disease after radiation therapy for Hodgkin s disease: analysis of 48 patients. *Am J Cardiol* 1983;51:1679.

81. Hancock EW. Neoplastic pericardial disease. *Cardiol Clin* 1990;8:673.

82. Stewart JR, Fajardo LF, Gillette SM, Constine LS. Radiation injury to the heart. *Int J Radiat Oncol Biol Phys* 1995;31:1205.

83. Corn BW, Trock BJ, Goodman RL. Irradiation-related ischemic heart disease. *J Clin Oncol* 1990;4:741.

84. Brosius FC, Waller BF, Roberts WC. Radiation heart disease: analysis of 16 young (aged 15 to 33 years) necropsy patients who received over 3,500 rads to the heart. *Am J Med* 1981;70:519.

85. Boivin JA, Hutchinson GB, Lubin JH, Mauch P. Coronary artery disease mortalitiy in patients treated for Hodgkin's disease. *Cancer* 1992;69:1241.

86. Rutqvist LE, Lax I, Fornander T, Johansson H. Cardiovascular mortalitiy in a randomized trial of adjuvant radiation therapy versus surgery alone in primary breast cancer. *Int J Radiat Oncol Biol Phys* 1992;22:887.

87. Allen A. The cardiotoxicity of chemotherapeutic drugs. In: Perry MC, ed. *The chemotherapy sourcebook.* Baltimore: Williams and Wikins, 1992;582.

88. Cosgriff TM. Doxorubicin and ventricular arrhythmia. *Ann Intern Med* 1980;92:434.

89. Wortman JE, Lucas VS, Schuster E, Thiele D, Logue GL. Sudden death during doxorubicin administration. *Cancer* 1979;44:1588.

90. Von Hoff DD, Layard MW, Basa P, et al. Risk factors for doxorubicin-induced congestive heart failure. *Ann Intern Med* 1979;91:710.

91. Steinherz LJ, Steinherz PG, Tan CTC, Heller G, Murphy ML. Cardiac toxicity 4 to 20 years after completing anthracycline therapy. *JAMA* 1991;266:1672.

92. Billingham ME, Mason JW, Bristow MR, Daniels JR. Anthracycline cardiomyopathy monitored by morphologic changes. *Cancer Treat Rep* 1978;62:865.

93. Schwartz RG, McKenzie WB, Alexander J, et al. Congestive heart failure and left ventricular dysfunction complicating doxorubicin therapy: seven-year experience using serial radionuclide angiocardiography. *Am J Med* 1987;82:1109.

94. Palmeri ST, Bonow RO, Myers CE, et al. Prospective evaluation of doxorubicin cardiotoxicity by rest and exercise radionuclide angiography. *Am J Cardiol* 1986;58:607.

95. Von Hoff DD, Rozencweig M, Piccart M. The cardiotoxicity of anticancer agents. *Semin Oncol* 1982;9:23.

96. Villani F, Galimberti M, Comazzi R, Crippa F. Evaluation of cardiac toxicity of idarubicin (4-demethoxydaunorubicin). *Eur J Cancer Clin Oncol* 1989;25:13.

97. Wiernik PH, Case DC, Periman PO, et al. A multicenter trial of cytarabine plus idarubicin or daunorubicin as induction therapy for adult nonlymphocytic leukemia. *Semin Oncol* 1989;16(Suppl 2):25.

98. Berman E, Heller G, Santorsa J, et al. Results of a randomized trial comparing idarubicin and cytosine arabinoside with daunorubicin and cytosine arabinoside in adult patients with newly diagnosed acute myelogenous leukemia. *Blood* 1991;77:1666.

99. Chan-Lam D, Copplestone JA, Prentice A, Price R, Johnson S, Phillips M. Idarubicin cardiotoxicity in acute myeloid leukaemia. *Lancet* 1992;340:185.

100. Muus P, Donnelly P, Schattenberg A, et al. Idarubicin-related side effects in recipients of T-cell-depleted allogeneic bone marrow transplants are schedule dependent. *Semin Oncol* 1993;6(Suppl 8):47.

101. Anderlini P, Benjamin RS, Wong FC, et al. Idarubicin cardiotoxicity: A retrospective study in acute myeloid leukemia and myelodysplasia. *J Clin Oncol* 1995;13:2827.

102. Weiss RB. The anthracyclines: Will we ever find a better doxorubicin? *Semin Oncol* 1992;19:670.

103. Coleman RE, Maisey MN, Knight RK, Rubens RD. Mitoxantrone in advanced breast cancer—a phase II study with special attention to cardiotoxicity. *Eur J Cancer Clin Oncol* 1984;20:771.

104. Bowers C, Adkins D, Dunphy F, Harrison B, LeMaistre CF, Spitzer G. Dose escalation of mitoxantrone given with thiotepa and autologous

bone marrow transplantation for metastatic breast cancer. *Bone Marrow Transplant* 1993;12:525.

105. Casper ES, Gaynor JJ, Hajdu SI, et al. A prospective randomized trial of adjuvant chemotherapy with bolus versus continuous infusion of doxorubicin in patients with high-grade extremity soft tissue sarcoma and an analysis of prognostic factors. *Cancer* 1991;68:1221.

106. Gabizon A, Catane R, Uziely B, et al. Prolonged circulation time and enhanced accumulation in malignant exudates of doxorubicin encapsulated in polyethylene-glycol coated liposomes. *Cancer Res* 1994; 54:987.

107. Gill PS, Espina BM, Muggia F, et al. Phase I/II clinical and pharmacokinetic evaluation of liposomal daunorubicin. *J Clin Oncol* 1995; 13:914.

108. Harrison M, Tomlinson D, Stewart S. Liposomal-entrapped doxorubicin: an active agent in AIDS-related Kaposi sarcoma. *J Clin Oncol* 1995;13:1777.

109. Uziely B, Jeffers S, Isacson R, et al. Liposomal doxorubicin: antitumor activity and unique toxicities during two complementary Phase I studies. *J Clin Oncol* 1995;13:1777.

110. Seifert CF, Nesser ME, Thompson DF. Dexazoxane in the prevention of doxorubicin-induced cardiotoxicity. *Ann Pharmacother* 1994;28: 1063.

111. Speyer JL, Green MD, Zeleniuch-Jacquotte A, et al. ICRF-187 permits longer treatment with doxorubicin in women with breast cancer. *J Clin Oncol* 1992;10:117.

112. Weisberg SR, Rosenfeld CS, York RM, et al. Dexrazoxane, (ADR-529, ICRF-187, zinecard) protects against doxorubicin-induced chronic cardiotoxicity. *Proc Am J Clin Oncol* 1992;11:190 (abst).

113. Maillard JA, Speyer JL, Hanson K, et al. Prevention of chronic adriamycin cardiotoxcity with the bisdioxopiperazine dexrazoxane (ICRF-187, ADR-529, zinecard) in patients with advanced or metastatic breast cancer. *Proc Am Soc Clin Oncol* 1992;11:191 (abst).

114. Feldmann JE, Jones SE, Weisberg SR, et al. Advanced small cell lung cancer treated with CAV (cyclophosphamide-Adriamycin-vincristine) chemotherapy and the cardioprotective agent dexrazoxane (ADR-527, ICRF-187, zinecard). *Proc Am Soc Clin Oncol* 1992;11:993 (abst).

115. *Physician's desk reference.* 50th ed. Montvale, NJ: Medical Economics, 1996;1961.

116. Vici P, Di Lauro L, Ferraironi A, et al. A randomized tiral of dexrazoxane cardioprotection in patients with metastatic breast cancer and advanced soft tissue sarcoma treated with high-dose epirubicin [Abstract]. *Proc Am Soc Clin Oncol* 1994;13:178.

117. Speyer JL, Green MD, Kramer E, et al. Protective effect of the bis-piperazinedione ICRF-187 against doxorubicin-induced cardiac toxicity in women with advanced breast cancer. *N Engl J Med* 1988; 319:745.

118. Gottdiener JS, Appelbaum FR, Ferrans VJ, Deisseroth A, Ziegler J. Cardiotoxicity associated with high-dose cyclophosphamide therapy. *Arch Intern Med* 1981;141:758.

119. Goldberg MA, Antin JH, Guinan EC, Rappeport JM. Cyclophosphamide cardiotoxicity: an analysis of dosing as a risk factor. *Blood* 1986; 68:1114.

120. Einhorn LH. VP-16 plus ifosfamide plus cisplatin as salvage therapy in refractory testicular cancer. *Cancer Chemother Pharmacol* 1986; 18(Suppl 2):S45.

121. Klein HO, Wickramanayake PD, Coerper C, Christian E, Pohl C, Brock N. High-dose ifosfamide and mesna as continuous infusion over five days—a phase I/II trial. *Cancer Treat Rev* 1983;10:167.

122. Kandylis K, Vassilomanolakis M, Tsoussis S, Efremidis AP. Ifosfamide cardiotoxicity in humans. *Cancer Chemother Pharmacol* 1989;24:395.

123. Anand AJ. Fluorouracil cardiotoxicity. *Ann Pharmacother* 1994; 28:374.

124. Schober C, Papageorgiou E, Harstrick A, et al. Cardiotoxicity of 5-fluorouracil in combination with folinic acid in patients with gastrointestinal cancer. *Cancer* 1993;72:2242.

125. Arbuck SG, Strauss H, Rowinsky E, et al. A reassessment of cardiac toxicity associated with taxol. *J Natl Cancer Inst Monographs* 1993; 15:117.

126. Rowinsky EK, McGuire WP, Guarnieri T, Fisherman JS, Christian MC, Donehower RC. Cardiac disturbances during the administration of taxol. *J Clin Oncol* 1991;9:1704.

127. Schecter JP, Jones SE, Jackson RA. Myocardial infarction in a 27-year-old woman: possible complication of treatment with VP-16-213 (NSC-141540), mediastinal radiation or both. *Cancer Chemother Rep* 1975;59:887.

128. Aisner J, Whitacre M, Van Echo DA, Wiernik P. Combination-chemotherapy for small cell carcinoma of the lung: continuous versus alternating non-cross-resistant combinations. *Cancer Treat Rep* 1982;66:221.

129. Phillips NC, Lauper RD. Review of etoposide. *Clinical Pharmacy* 1983;2:112.

130. Weiss RB, Grillo-Lopez AJ, Marsoni S, Posada JGJ, Hess F, Ross B. Amsacrine-associated cardiotoxicity: an analysis of 82 cases. *J Clin Oncol* 1986;4:918.

131. Steinherz LJ, Steinherz PG, Mangiacasale D, Tan C, Miller DR. Cardiac abnormalities after AMSA administration. *Cancer Treat Rep* 1982;66:483.

132. Dixon AC, Nakamura JM, Oishi N, Wachi DH, Fukuyama O. Angina pectoris and therapy with cisplatin, vincristine and bleomycin. *Ann Intern Med* 1989;111:342.

133. Doll DC, List AF, Greco A, Hainsworth JD, Hande KR, Johnson DH. Acute vascular ischemic events after cisplatin-based combination chemotherapy for germ-cell tumors of the testis. *Ann Intern Med* 1986; 105:48.

134. Samuels BL, Vogelzang NJ, Kennedy BJ. Severe vascular toxicity associated with vinblastine, bleomycin, and cisplatin chemotherapy. *Cancer Chemother Pharmacol* 1987;19:253.

135. Mandel EM, Lewinski U, Djaldetti M. Vincristine-induced myocardial infarction. *Cancer* 1975;36:1979.

136. Somers G, Abramow M, Wittek M, Naets JP. Myocardial infarction: a complication of vincristine treatment? *Lancet* 1976;2:690.

137. Hirvonen HE, Salmi TT, Heinonen E, Antila KJ, Alimaki AT. Vincristine treatment of acute lymphoblastic leukemia induces transient autonomic cardioneuropathy. *Cancer* 1989;64:801.

138. Roca E, Bruera E, Politi PM, et al. Vinca alkaloid-induced cardiovascular autonomic neuropathy. *Cancer Treat Rep* 1985;69:149.

139. Kaufman IA, Kung FH, Koenig HM, Giammona ST. Overdosage with vincristine. *J Pediatr* 1976;89:671.

140. Pritchard KI, Sutherland DJA. The use of endocrine therapy. *Hematol/Oncol Clin North Am* 1989;3:765.

141. Shearer RJ, Hendry WF, Sommerville IF, Fergusson JD. Plasma testosterone: an accurate monitor of hormone treatment in prostatic cancer. *Br J Urol* 1973;45:668.

142. Benson RCJ, Gill GM. Estramustine phosphate compared with diethylstilbestrol: A randomized, double-blind, crossover trial for stage D prostate cancer. *Am J Clin Oncol* 1986;9:341.

143. Hudes GR, Greenberg R, Krigel RL, et al. Phase II study of estramustine and vinblastine, two microtubule inhibitors, in hormone-refractory prostate cancer. *J Clin Oncol* 1992;10:1754.

144. Murphy GP, Slack NH, Mittelman A. Use of estramustine phosphate in prostate cancer by the national prostatic cancer project and by Roswell Park Memorial Institute. *Urology* 1984;23:54.

145. Sonnenblick M, Rosin A. Cardiotoxicity of interferon: A review of 44 cases. *Chest* 1991;99:557.

146. Zimmerman S, Adkins D, Graham M, et al. Case report: Irreversible, severe congestive cardiomyopathy occurring in association with interferon alpha therapy. *Cancer Biother* 1994;9:291.

147. Parkinson DR, Abrams JS, Wiernik PH, et al. Interleukin therapy in patients with metastatic malignant melanoma: a Phase II study. *J Clin Oncol* 1990;8:1650.

148. Mattson K, Niiranen A, Pyrhonen S, Farkkila M, Cantell K. Recombinant interferon gamma in non-small cell lung cancer. *Acta Oncol* 1991;30:607.

149. Kruit WH, Punt KJ, Goey H, et al. Cardiotoxicity as a dose-limiting factor in a schedule of high dose bolus therapy with interleukin-2 and alpha-interferon: an unexpectedly frequent complication. *Cancer* 1994;74:2850.

150. Lee RE, Lotze MT, Skibber JM, et al. Cardiorespiratory effects of immunotherapy with interleukin-2. *J Clin Oncol* 1989;7:7.

151. Samlowski WE, Ward JH, Craven CM, Freedman RA. Severe myocarditis following high-dose interleukin-2 administration. *Arch Pathol Lab Med* 1989;113:838.

152. Thompson JA, Shulman KL, Benyunes MC, et al. Prolonged continuous intravenous infusion interleukin-2 and lymphokine-activated killer-cell therapy for metastatic renal cell carcinoma. *J Clin Oncol* 1992;10:960.

Principles and Practice of Supportive Oncology,
edited by Ann Berger et al.
Lippincott–Raven Publishers, Philadelphia ©1998

CHAPTER 28

# Urologic Issues of Palliative Care

Steven J. Hirshberg and Richard E. Greenberg

The management of patients with a progressive medical disease should allow them to live the remainder of their lives to their fullest potential, maximizing both the quality and quantity of life. The development of complications related to the genitourinary system is not uncommon in these patients. Although some of these problems may merely be considered an annoyance, others can be quite serious and potentially undermine the quality of life. The most serious complications may reduce life expectancy.

A common classification of urinary tract problems differentiates the urinary tract into upper and lower systems. The upper urinary tract refers to those organs proximal to the ureterovesical junction. The lower urinary tract pertains to the bladder, prostate, and urethra. This chapter discusses both the diagnosis and management of upper and lower urinary tract pathology.

## OUTLET OBSTRUCTION

One of the most common problems originating from the urinary tract in men is bladder outlet obstruction, which can result from either benign or malignant processes. In men, the most common organ to obstruct the bladder is the prostate. Both men and women can develop bladder outlet obstruction from direct tumor extension or from other pathology originating from the rectum or urethra; a lesion of the ovary, cervix, or uterus may be the cause in women. The ultimate consequence to the patient with obstructive uropathy, without intervention, is renal failure secondary to chronic urinary retention. This condition will progress more rapidly if there is also underlying infection, a situation not uncommon in patients who fail to empty their bladder adequately.

S. J. Hirshberg: Temple University School of Medicine, Philadelphia, PA 19140.

R. E. Greenberg: Department of Surgical Oncology, Fox Chase Cancer Center, Philadelphia, PA 19111.

A careful history may disclose the lesion responsible for urinary retention. Physiologically, failure to empty the bladder indicates failure to generate a detrusor pressure greater than the urethral resistance, either from primary detrusor failure (e.g., associated with diabetes mellitus or from bladder outlet obstruction at or distal to the bladder neck). A detailed urologic history relating symptoms prior to the episode of urinary retention may clarify the underlying problem. Patients who complain of urinary frequency, urgency, nocturia, and a slow urinary stream frequently have obstruction as the underlying etiology of their urinary retention. In contrast, patients who report a slow stream, impaired bladder sensation, increasing intervals between voids, and decreased urgency are more likely to have primary detrusor failure (1). Because management of these two disorders differs significantly, it is obviously critical to make this distinction before initiating therapy.

### Nonsurgical Treatment

Whereas the initial management of urinary retention secondary to benign prostatic hyperplasia (BPH) may warrant a period of catheter drainage and an empiric trial of selective alpha$_1$-blockers (terazosin or doxazosin), bladder outlet obstruction secondary to a malignant disease is unlikely to respond to this approach. Deconditioning and immobility are additional complicating factors in terminally ill patients; debility in many terminally ill patients may decrease the likelihood for recovery of adequate bladder detrusor function. Patients with BPH who fail initial conservative measures (alpha$_1$-blockers and adequate bladder rest) after an adequate period (e.g., 1–2 weeks) may be candidates for alternative measures. These other options, all of which are invasive to an extent, include chronic urethral or suprapubic bladder drainage, intermittent catheterization, and surgical procedures, including urethral stenting or surgical resection of the obstructing prostate tissue. In patients with malignant disease, these approaches can be considered earlier.

### Hormonal Manipulation

A nonsurgical approach to patients with obstruction caused by prostate cancer involves hormonal manipulation. This approach should be considered especially for patients not previously treated in this fashion. Up to 72% of patients with advanced prostate cancer may have symptoms of bladder outlet obstruction (2). In a 1989 review, Surya and Provet (3) suggested that androgen deprivation may be preferable to surgery as the initial mode of therapy. Androgen deprivation can either be in the form of surgical bilateral orchiectomy or medical orchiectomy with luteinizing hormone-releasing hormone (LHRH) analogues (leuprolide or goserelin) or diethylstilbestrol. In patients who are to be initiated on LHRH analogues, a recent bone scan should be available to rule out significant occult bony disease in the vertebral column. After starting therapy with LHRH analogues, a LH and consequent testosterone surge may occur within the first 2 weeks of therapy, and patients with significant vertebral metastases, whether occult or overt, are at significant risk for spinal cord compression. For similar reasons, patients with bone pain may have increased analgesic needs shortly after beginning treatment with LHRH analogues. To reduce the risk of these adverse events, the authors recommend that all patients be started on flutamide (Eulexin) before the initiation of LHRH agonist therapy to avoid the testosterone flare phenomenon. At a minimum, patients with documented bony disease in the cervical, thoracic, or lumbar axial skeleton should be started on flutamide 7 days before initiating therapy with LHRH analogues. Two to 3 weeks after reduction of serum testosterone to castrate levels, patients who fail to void usually will require surgical intervention or prolonged catheter drainage.

### Clean Intermittent Catheterization

For the medically ill patient who does not wish to undergo a surgical procedure or who is deemed medically unable to tolerate surgery, clean intermittent catheterization (CIC) or chronic indwelling catheterization represent the two most feasible options for adequate bladder decompression; CIC has been the nonsurgical treatment of choice to empty the bladder since Lapides introduced the concept in the late 1960s (4). It enables a motivated patient to maintain freedom from a chronic indwelling catheter, thereby decreasing the attendant risks of infection, stricture, epididymitis, and symptoms associated with a defunctionalized bladder. Once a patient is placed on an adequate CIC schedule, bladder residuals must be monitored so that upper tract deterioration from storing urine at high pressures can be avoided. Common findings on routine urinalysis in patients on CIC include pyuria and bacteriuria. In the absence of systemic evidence of infection (i.e., fever, flank pain, and leukocytosis), the use of broad-spectrum antibiotics in an attempt to sterilize the urine should be avoided to forestall the development of resistant bacterial species (5). In patients with recurrent urosepsis, however, chronic antibiotic prophylaxis using low-dose antibiotics or urinary antiseptic drug regimens may be warranted.

### Indwelling Catheters

Although the use of indwelling catheters is usually limited to acute urinary retention, the benefits and risks of chronic catheterization in the medically ill patient must be carefully weighed. Frequently, a permanent urethral catheter is the most appropriate method of management in the patient with a very short life expectancy. Since these catheters can be changed at longer intervals, they may also be the modality of choice for patients who are technically difficult to catheterize or are unable to catheterize themselves due to functional impairments. Urethral catheters are relatively simple devices, but may cause significant discomfort in those patients who experience bladder spasms. These patients may leak urine around the catheter and appear to be incontinent. Other during long-term catheterization include obstruction of urine drainage secondary to calcification of the catheter itself, calcification of the balloon, urethral stricture, urethritis, epididymitis, and urosepsis. Although insertion of a suprapubic catheter avoids urethral trauma and irritation, and decreases the risk of urosepsis, significant complications may still occur.

## Surgical Treatment

### Transurethral Resection of the Prostate

In patients who fail other treatments, transurethral resection of the prostate (TURP) remains the gold standard for the removal of obstructing tissue. Several newer techniques, however, have been developed for resecting, evaporating, or coagulating the obstructing prostatic tissue. These newer techniques, which include laser prostatectomy, electrosurgical vaporization of the prostate, transurethral needle ablation, and high-frequency radiowave ablation, all claim to have individual benefits to the patient beyond the standard TURP. All these techniques are still evolving, however, and no long-term data are available regarding their overall effectiveness (6). The standard against which any new procedure must be compared remains TURP. During TURP, prostate tissue (benign or malignant) is removed (resected) using an electrocautery loop. Although the procedure itself is usually limited to 1 hour, the potential exists for the development of significant complications, especially in patients with underlying cardiac disease. It has the potential to create large fluid shifts by the absorption of irrigation fluid through venous channels during the resection. In a patient with underlying cardiac disease, this may place an otherwise compensated patient into congestive heart failure. Other risks associated with the procedure include bleeding, which has the potential to be significant during resection of a large gland; urinary tract infection; urethral stricture; dilutional hyponatremia; bladder perforation; erectile dysfunction; and urinary incontinence. The risk of urinary incontinence is a great concern when resecting malignant obstructing prostatic tissue, which causes alteration of the normal anatomic landmarks and may invade the external urethral sphincter directly.

### Channel TURP

An alternative to a standard TURP, in which all of the prostatic tissue is removed out to the surgical capsule, is the channel TURP. Channel TURP is defined as a TURP performed to alleviate obstructive voiding symptoms in the patient with advanced or previously treated cancer. It also may refer to a TURP performed to remove the obstructing tissue without necessarily removing all the tissue to the capsule. The advantage of channel TURP over the traditional TURP is that it is a more limited operation with less associated morbidity.

Mazur and Thompson (7) reviewed 41 patients with known prostate cancer who underwent channel TURP. All these patients were able to void after the procedure, but 11 patients eventually required additional procedures at a minimum of 15 months following the initial resection. The only patients who were totally incontinent were those with invasion of the external sphincter who required intentional resection of this tissue to relieve the obstruction. Although not specifically detailed, the authors stated that there were no complications. Certainly, this duration of response represents a more than adequate period for most of our palliative care patients.

### Urethral Stents

Recent advances with novel materials have led to the creation of self-expanding metal stents for placement into multiple organ systems, including the urinary tract. Because the technology is relatively new, follow-up is necessarily short. Several reports, however, have suggested that these devices may be promising, especially for a patient with a limited life expectancy who wishes to remain free of catheters and external urine collection devices. Insertion of the stent itself is a relatively simple procedure and usually can be performed with local anesthesia and a minimal amount of sedation. Morgentaler

and DeWolf (8) reviewed their experience with self-expanding prostatic stents in 25 patients with symptomatic bladder outlet obstruction. Twenty-one of the 25 patients were in urinary retention, and the remaining four patients had either bladder neck contractures or severe symptoms of BPH. All patients underwent insertion of the Gianturco-Z stent. Initially, 95% of the patients were able to void. At longer follow-up, the success rate had declined to 75% as a result of stent migration in several patients. The authors theorized that the high rate of stent migration was the result of improper selection of stent length.

Additional studies (9–11) evaluated different stents (UroLume Wallstent and Titan intraprostatic stent). The patients enrolled in these studies suffered mainly from BPH and not carcinoma. Overall, there was an almost 100% return of voiding function. The patients who failed to void had detrusor failure secondary to chronic urinary retention. Symptoms following stent insertion were similar to those seen initially following TURP, namely, urinary frequency, urgency, and hematuria. Failures in these studies usually were due to either improper stent length or migration of the stent. Complications were minor, and the patients who required stent removal were able to have it performed without extreme difficulty. Thus, with improvement of stent sizing and insertion technique, intraprostatic stents hold significant promise for treating urinary outflow obstruction in the medically ill patient with bladder outlet obstruction.

## IRRITATIVE VOIDING

### Symptoms

The complex of irritative voiding symptoms refers to the symptoms of urinary frequency, urgency, and dysuria. These symptoms are common in patients seeking urologic evaluation. Rarely, they are the first indication of a severe underlying process. In addition to symptomatic relief, management must be aimed at identifying and treating the underlying disorder. Investigations may be warranted based on clinical presentation and patient prognosis.

### Tumor-related Symptoms

Although significantly less common than urinary tract infection, tumor invasion of the bladder can cause irritative bladder symptoms. Tumor invasion can originate from within the bladder, such as a transitional cell carcinoma, or from within the pelvis. A common genitourinary tumor that presents with irritative voiding symptoms is carcinoma in situ of the bladder. Common malignancies originating outside of the bladder include tumors of the ovary, os cervix, uterus, rectum, prostate, and colon.

The distinction between tumor invasion and urinary tract infection usually can be made on the basis of the history and several tests. Although symptoms are often similar, direct tumor invasion is more likely to have an insidious onset and gross hematuria (12). All patients with irritative voiding symptoms should undergo a detailed urinalysis (dipstick and microscopic analysis). If a urinary tract infection is excluded by urinalysis and urine culture (when indicated), other etiologies must be considered. The differential diagnosis for noninfectious causes of bladder irritability includes stones (secondary to irritation created by a stone in the intramural tunnel), foreign bodies, and tumors. Like urinary tract infection, some of these diseases produce pyuria on routine urinalysis. Unless there is a concurrent urinary tract infection, however, the urine should be sterile, except in the case of the sterile pyuria associated with genitourinary tuberculosis.

Any patient with new-onset irritative voiding symptoms and sterile urine should have a voided urinary cytology. Although not necessarily diagnostic of a urothelial tumor, a positive urine cytology is particularly helpful in diagnosing carcinoma in situ of the bladder. A negative cytology is not diagnostic, however, because this test is relatively insensitive for detecting low-grade superficial papillary transitional cell carcinomas of the bladder or upper tracts. These usually insidious tumors rarely cause any change in the normal voiding pattern. Although carcinoma in situ may be completely asymptomatic, it more commonly presents with irritative voiding symptoms

Patients who develop irritative voiding symptoms associated with microscopic or gross hematuria and a negative urine also deserve additional evaluation. The gold standard for evaluating these patients includes an intravenous pyelogram and cystoscopy. In patients with an advanced medical illness, in whom diagnosis of a urothelial cancer may not change the overall management, this algorithm should be modified. Renal and bladder ultrasound, which now can be performed with relative ease, can detect solid tumors of the kidney or large tumors in the bladder; it would be unlikely, however, to diagnose a small tumor of the urothelium. With the development of fiberoptics and flexible cystoscopes, office or bedside cystoscopy can be performed with minimal discomfort and may be another alternative. If radiologic studies are unrevealing, cystoscopy may be required to rule out an irritative focus, such as tumor or stone within the bladder.

### Treatment

The initial treatment of a tumor that directly invades the bladder wall and causes irritative voiding symptoms should be transurethral resection of the bladder tumor (TURBT). Depending on the extent of the tumor, it can be carried out on an outpatient basis, although some form or anesthesia, usually spinal or general, will be required. Transurethral resection entails using a special cystoscope (resectoscope) with a cutting loop. By application of an electric current, the loop actually cuts the bladder tissue. This loop is used to resect the abnormal urothelium and the underlying layers (submucosa and muscularis) of the bladder. The diagnostic value of TURBT further supports its acceptance as the procedure of choice for the initial evaluation of all bladder tumors. If a full-thickness biopsy is taken, the depth of invasion and the degree of differentiation can be determined with a single procedure.

Patients who persist with disabling irritative voiding symptoms after TURBT may be treated symptomatically. The anticholinergic drugs oxybutynin and hyoscyamine (Ditropan, Levsin SL and Levsinex) are commonly used to treat urinary frequency, urgency, and nocturia. These drugs can be started at low doses and then titrated to effect. Caution must be used in patients who also have a component of bladder outlet obstruction or bowel obstruction because their anticholinergic action may exacerbate urinary retention and gastrointestinal dysmotility. These patients require careful observation of voiding and bowel elimination patterns during treatment. At times, a fine balance between irritative voiding symptoms and urinary retention can be obtained. In addition, there is a relative contraindication to the use of anticholinergic therapy in patients with closed-angle glaucoma. If patients maintain routine pharmacologic therapy for this condition, there should be little chance of clinical deterioration (13,14).

Urinary analgesic drugs, the most well known of which is phenazopyridine (Pyridium), may offer some symptomatic benefit to patients with irritative voiding symptoms. Phenazopyridine is converted from its inactive to its active form in the urinary tract. At times, a combination of this drug and an anticholinergic drug may be particularly helpful in relieving symptoms.

In rare cases, irritative voiding symptoms can be refractory to conservative therapies. If suffering from unrelieved symptoms is severe, urinary diversion may be contemplated. The standard form of urinary diversion with the lowest risk of short-term morbidity is the ileal conduit (see below). This procedure requires general anesthesia, major intraabdominal surgery, and a minimum postoperative recovery of 5 to 7 days. Thus, although it is an alternative for those patients who have experienced a marked loss of independence and quality of life, the risks of the procedure itself must be weighed against the possible benefits.

### Infection

Urinary tract infection is one of the most common conditions treated by physicians. Typical signs of lower urinary tract infection (simple cystitis) include urinary frequency, urgency, dysuria, foul-smelling urine, hematuria, and suprapubic tenderness. Many cases of urinary tract infection in hospitalized or hospice patients are iatrogenic, secondary to urinary tract manipulation, most often by urethral catheters. When evaluating a patient who presents with acute onset of new irritative voiding symptoms, urinary tract infection should be first on the list of differential diagnoses. As previously mentioned, a urinalysis, including both dipstick and microscopic analysis, should be performed before starting empiric antibiotic therapy. Patients who are hospitalized or institutionalized, or who were recently discharged from such a facility, also should have a urine culture and sensitivity performed. The potential virulence of the bacterial flora associated with these facilities justifies this early culture. Likewise, a patient with recent urinary tract instrumentation, including urethral catheterization, who develops signs of urinary tract infection also should have a urine culture obtained at the initial evaluation.

When obtaining urine specimens from patients who appear to have failed appropriate antibiotic therapy, it is particularly important to ensure proper collection of the specimen. This especially holds true for debilitated patients and those with significant functional impairments, who may not be able to properly collect a clean-catch specimen. If the patient is unable to properly collect urine for urinalysis and/or urine culture, a catheterized specimen may be required before continuing or modifying treatment. Additionally, when specimens are collected from patients with either an indwelling catheter or condom catheter, one must take care in interpreting the results. Urine from these patients is almost always colonized with bacteria and consequently, the finding of bacteria on urinalysis does not necessarily indicate active urinary tract infection.

Patients who develop recurrent or relapsing symptomatic infections, should undergo further evaluation to rule out a structural abnormality as the fundamental problem. Obstruction and stasis of urine flow at any level of the urinary tract predisposes to urinary infection. Obstruction can either be secondary to an anatomic abnormality, an obstructing stone or neoplasm, or bladder outlet obstruction. Factors contributing to urinary tract infection include diabetes mellitus and immunosuppression caused by cancer or its therapies. Other patients at risk include those on chronic steroid therapy and those infected with the human immunodeficiency virus (HIV).

Initial evaluation of patients with recurrent urinary tract infections should include a measurement of a post-void residual to rule out the presence of a large residual urine. This measurement can be performed by catheterizing a patient once he has voided to completion. As an alternative, the post-void residual may be measured by ultrasound and should include measurements of bladder volume both before and after voiding. Additional studies can include renal or bladder ultrasound to exclude hydronephrosis or intravenous pyelogram (IVP) to image the entire collecting system. Urine culture and sensitivity are mandatory when infections do not resolve with empiric antibiotic therapy.

**Radiation Cystitis**

It is not uncommon for patients to develop irritative voiding symptoms following external beam or interstitial radiation therapy to the pelvis. Radiation therapy is commonly used to treat genitourinary, gynecologic, and gastrointestinal tumors. Acute radiation cystitis following external beam radiation is characterized by dysuria, frequency, nocturia, and rarely hematuria (15). Dean and Lytton (16) evaluated patients following pelvic irradiation and found that 21% reported urologic symptom; however, in only 2.5% were these truly related to the radiation itself. In most cases, the symptoms were attributable to recurrent or persistent tumor.

Symptoms usually begin to develop after exposure to 3,000 cGy, and there is an increased incidence of cystitis in patients receiving greater than 6,000 to 6,500 cGy. Patients who experience persistent symptoms after completion of radiation fall into the category of chronic radiation cystitis. Open bladder surgery, in the subset of patients who receive higher doses of radiation, appears to be an independent risk factor for the development of chronic radiation cystitis.

Measures used to treat acute radiation cystitis are determined by the associated symptom complex. To address symptoms, drugs such as phenazopyridine and anticholinergics, either alone or in combination, are frequently administered. Unfortunately, patients who are refractory to these symptomatic treatments can become debilitated and experience a marked decline in quality of life as a result of severe urinary frequency, urgency, dysuria, nocturia, and at times urge incontinence. Unfortunately, approaches to treating patients with such intense symptoms are limited to procedures that divert the urine stream. Occasionally, diversion of the urine by a Foley catheter will improve symptoms, although frequently the bladder irritation will actually be exacerbated by Foley balloon trauma . Alternatives to catheter drainage, which have been used with limited success, include small suprapubic tubes and bilateral percutaneous nephrostomies.

Invasive approaches aimed at diverting the urine or enlarging the bladder exist but require major abdominal surgery. A potential contraindication to any surgery involving the bladder in patients with radiation cystitis is the effect of the extensive radiation itself. The risk of complications during or after augmentation cystoplasty or urinary diversion is increased in patients with irradiated bowel or bladder due an underlying vasculitis.

Augmentation cystoplasty involves enlarging the bladder by surgically creating a patch of either small bowel, colon, or stomach and attaching this to the dome of the bladder. Urinary diversion requires constructing either a urostomy with external appliance or continent diversion by creating a pouch that can be catheterized. Again, this procedure requires use of segments of small bowel or large bowel, both of which may have been irradiated. If urinary diversion is entertained, the bladder itself does not necessarily need to be removed. In fact, cystectomy probably should be avoided because of the increased surgical risks following radiation therapy. Although surgical diversion is considered in this discussion for completeness, few patients within the palliative care population are actually candidates for this intervention because of the associated surgical risks and the time required for complete recuperation.

### Chemical Cystitis

Several agents that are administered intravesically for the treatment of either superficial or multifocal transitional cell carcinoma of the bladder or carcinoma in situ can be potentially toxic and irritating. To various degrees, all these agents have the potential to cause a chemical cystitis.

The most common and effective medication used for intravesical treatment of bladder carcinoma is bacille Calmette-Guérin (BCG). A standard course of BCG therapy involves weekly bladder instillations for 6 weeks. Depending on the clinical response and physician preference, maintenance therapy may continue after the initial 6-week regimen. Symptoms of urinary frequency, dysuria, and hematuria usually develop after two or three instillations and may last for about 2 days following each treatment. These symptoms are an expected consequence of the immune stimulation and inflammatory reaction that are thought to be essential components of the mechanism of action of BCG (17). Lamm et al. (18) reviewed the complications of BCG therapy in 1,278 patients and found that 91% developed dysuria, 90% had urinary frequency, and 43% had hematuria. These symptoms seemed to increase with both the duration and frequency of treatments. Although BCG is available in several strains, the local irritative symptoms were not limited to any particular strain.

In patients undergoing a 6-week course of therapy, symptoms usually can be well controlled with the combination of phenazopyridine and anticholinergic medications. Although there have not been any randomized or controlled studies of these medications, several investigators with more than 2,600 patients support their routine use for sympomatic relief (19). For patients refractory to this regimen or who will continue with maintenance therapy, treatment with isoniazid, diphenhydramine, acetaminophen, and nonsteroidal antiinflammatory medications can be helpful. Treatment usually is continued for the duration of symptoms and may be given prophylactically for 3 days starting on the morning of BCG administration. Because all of agents have a different mechanism of action, they frequently are used in combinations, and doses are titrated until a maximal effect is obtained. A rare complication of treatment with BCG is development of a nonfunctional contracted bladder, which occurs in about 0.2% of cases. Because contracted bladders did not develop in patients with severe irritative symptoms who were treated with prophylactic isoniazid, early treatment with antituberculous medication may help prevent this disabling complication.

Local irritative side effects are seen somewhat less frequently with the use of other intravesical chemotherapeutic regimens. Agents used for intravesical treatment of bladder cancer include triethylenethiophosphoramide (Thiotepa), etoglucid (Epodyl), mitomycin C, and doxorubicin. Mitomycin C has been associated with chemical cystitis in 10% to 15% of patients and, in rare cases, can lead to a contracted bladder. Doxorubicin also has been associated with chemical cystitis and defunctionalized bladders. Treatment of cystitis for these agents is similar to that of BCG except that antituberculosis medications will have no effect on irritative symptoms from these agents.

Systemic administration of some cytotoxic drugs also can lead to irritative symptoms. These symptoms are commonly associated with cyclophosphamide and ifosfamide (oxazaphosphorine alkylating agents), Busulfan (1,4-dimethanesulfonayoxybutane), and methenamine mandelate (20).

## HEMATURIA

### General Considerations

Gross hematuria refers to blood in the urine that can be seen with the naked eye. It is important to confirm the presence of red blood cells in urine once dark urine is discovered. There are multiple causes of discolored urine other than blood within the specimen. Some of the more common causes of discolored urine include concentrated urine and systemic administration of flutamide, phenazopyridine, sulfasalazine, phenolphthalein (seen with the use of some over-the-counter laxatives), nitrofurantoin, metronidazole, methylene blue, and vitamin B complex.

Two commonly used methods of detecting blood in urine are the microscopic urinalysis and the urine dipstick test (UDT). The UDT works through a peroxidase reaction; that is, the peroxidase-like activity of hemoglobin causes the oxidation of a chemical indicator impregnated within the dipstick and thereby changes its color. Intact red blood cells are not required for oxidation, and false-positive readings may be caused by hemoglobinuria or myoglobinuria. Although the presence of intact red cells usually causes punctate discoloration of the dipstick rather than the uniform discoloration commonly seen with hemoglobinuria, confirmation of red cells is required. Therefore, all patients with a positive UDT require a microscopic urinalysis in order to confirm the presence of red blood cells. The UDT has a sensitivity greater than 90% when properly used (21–23). Although some controversy exists as to whether hematuria should be defined as 0 to 2 or 0 to 4/5 red blood cells per high-power field, clearly more than five red blood cells per high-power field indicates the presence of blood.

Not uncommonly, the location of urinary tract bleeding can be ascertained by careful history alone. The history should identify the presence or absence of pain, the color of the blood (bright red versus tea color versus light pink), the presence or absence of clots, and the timing of the presence of the hematuria in the urine stream. Also, hematuria must be differentiated from urethral bleeding, which usually presents as either blood at the meatus or spotting on the sheets or undergarments. Bright red blood usually implies that bleeding is from either the prostate or bladder, whereas darker blood more commonly originates from the upper urinary tract. Bleeding only on initiation of the urinary stream (initial hematuria), followed by clear urine, implies that the bleeding originates distal to the level of the bladder neck or prostate. The presence of blood throughout the urine stream (*total hematuria*) usually implies that bleeding is from the kidney, ureter, or bladder, whereas *terminal hematuria* (blood mainly at the end of urination) implies a disease process near either the bladder neck or prostatic urethra.

The evaluation of confirmed hematuria may include urine culture (in patients with concurrent pyuria); voided or catheterized urine cytology; an imaging study to evaluate the kidneys, ureters, bladder, and urothelium; and cystoscopy to evaluate the urethra, prostate, and bladder urothelium. In patients with known urinary tract pathology, the assessment of new-onset hematuria may be modified, especially if previously performed studies have been negative. Because of the tendency of urothelial malignancies to recur, onset of hematuria within 6 months of intial evaluation should prompt consideration of repeating the above studies.

When considering which imaging study to obtain, the test that yields the most information and is considered the gold standard for imaging the entire urinary system is the IVP, although the IVP does have some limitations. If the ureters are unable to be visualized completely, additional studies may be warranted. Retrograde pyelography, which is used to identify lesions of the collecting system, may be performed at the time of cystoscopic evaluation to evaluate or possibly localize upper urinary tract pathology.

Ultrasound can be considered an alternative to IVP in patients at increased risk from exposure to contrast material, including those with azotemia, diabetes mellitus, or history of contrast allergy. Ultrasound is unable to visualize the collecting system unless it is significantly dilated and is not sensitive for detecting small, or even large, abnormalities of the urothelium. Real-time ultrasound is relatively sensitive for detecting calcifications within the renal parenchyma and collecting system, but it does not clarify the clinical significance of such calcifications unless there is significant hydronephrosis, which, in turn, may depend in part on the hydrational status of the patient. If ultrasound is used, it should be coupled with a plain abdominal radiograph (a kidney-ureter-bladder, or KUB film) to examine the remainder of the collecting system for calcifications that could lead to obstruction (e.g., ureteral calculus).

Computed tomographic (CT) scans of the abdomen and pelvis are also not ideal screening tools for urologic pathology. Although CT scans are much more sensitive than IVP for detecting certain types of pathology, such as renal masses, they are less likely to detect subtle obstruction. Because the slices of a CT scan are taken in an axial (transverse) plane, it is sometimes difficult to reconstruct the individual images to create an image in the frontal plane. One of the benefits of IVP is that it is a functional and dynamic study and can be tailored to an individual patient when desired. During a CT scan, there is less control over the technique. Also, because most CT scans are performed with 1-cm-thick slices and 1 cm between slices, some areas of the urinary system will not be imaged. Although this is usually of little consequence, it can make a dramatic difference in detecting a small calcification, such as a 4-mm or 5-mm stone.

## LOWER TRACT BLEEDING

### Asymptomatic

Statistically, most microscopic hematuria of a urologic etiology will be clinically asymptomatic and will arise from the lower urinary tract. The most prevalent cause in men is benign prostatic hyperplasia. Asymptomatic microscopic hematuria rarely, if ever, leads to a significant decrease in the hemoglobin or contributes to iron-deficiency anemia. The significance of this microscopic hematuria lies in the fact that it may be a sign of occult urinary tract pathology. Most urologists believe that even a single detection of microscopic hematuria, without the evidence of infection or prior instrumentation, should be evaluated.

If the detection of urinary tract pathology is unlikely to alter the overall management of the patient, the standard algorithm for evaluating hematuria should be individualized. Cystoscopy is an invasive procedure and may be avoided if an obvious cause for the hematuria is detected. For example, if IVP or ultrasound demonstrates a large renal tumor, additional invasive procedures may not be necessary. Although it is possible that a patient could have a second malignancy, or other bladder pathology (e.g., transitional cell carcinoma of the bladder), further evaluation may not necessarily be in the best interest of the patient.

If the source of microscopic hematuria is not detected by imaging studies and cystoscopy is contemplated, the benefits and risks of cystoscopy must be assessed. With newer flexible cystoscopes, cystoscopy now approaches both the risk and discomfort associated with urethral catheterization; However, both flexible and rigid cystoscopy can place a patient with well-compensated bladder outlet obstruction into urinary retention. Additionally, patients with benign prostatic hyperplasia (BPH), who are likely to have delicate dilated veins on the surface of the prostate as the etiology of their hematuria, may be at risk for developing significant bleeding after this invasive procedure.

Asymptomatic gross hematuria can be managed similarly to microscopic hematuria. Patients who experience gross hematuria should be advised to increase their fluid intake and avoid strenuous activity. As long as the patient does not experience significant voiding difficulties, the evaluation of this disorder may proceed electively, in a similar fashion to that already described.

## Symptomatic

Symptomatic hematuria is less common than asymptomatic hematuria, yet obviously more clinically significant. The spectrum of symptoms in patients with gross hematuria ranges from no change in the voiding pattern to acute urinary retention caused by obstruction from clots. Most cases of gross hematuria are alarming, but relatively few patients actually require immediate intervention. As noted, patients with new-onset gross hematuria should be told to avoid strenuous activities and increase fluid intake. Increased urine production may dilute the blood in the bladder and reduce the risk of forming clots. A patient is unlikely to develop significant voiding difficulties without the formation of blood clots. If clots are passed, significant bleeding should be assumed, and the physician should anticipate the need for intervention. As the concentration of blood increases and larger clots form, a patient eventually will develop clot urinary retention.

The first step in treating a patient with clot urinary retention is to place a large catheter in the bladder and evacuate all the clots. Preferably, a 22 or 24 Foley catheter is used. It will be nearly impossible to evacuate blood clots via 16 or 18 Foley catheters, which are commonly available in catheter kits, because it is not uncommon to irrigate 200 to 300 cc or more of clot from the bladder. It is also wise to insert a three-way Foley catheter, if available, so that continuous bladder irrigation (CBI) can be started if needed. Analogous to increasing the urine flow rate, CBI dilutes the concentration of blood in the urine, thereby helping to prevent new clot forma-

tion. After inserting the catheter and irrigating the bladder free of clot, the cause of the hematuria should be assessed, as described previously. In rare cases, when the bladder cannot be cleared of clot via an irrigating catheter, the patient may need operative intervention, with insertion of a resectoscope and manual clot evacuation with syringes or special equipment. In these patients, one should obtain a complete blood count and coagulation studies to exclude an underlying hematologic problem. Unlike microscopic hematuria, gross hematuria frequently leads to anemia, and the hemoglobin must be monitored, especially with patients debilitated by chronic disease or recently completing chemotherapy or radiation therapy who may have a decreased bone marrow reserves.

The management of patients who present with gross hematuria usually can be temporized with catheter drainage. Once imaging studies are performed, a differential diagnosis will be formulated. When studies of the upper tracts are normal, the pathology is likely to reside either in the prostate or bladder. Cystoscopy should be able to establish the diagnosis and aid in the development of a treatment plan for disorders of either the prostate or bladder. If bleeding is discovered in the prostate during cystoscopy, it may be difficult to control with fulguration (electrocoagulation) alone. More commonly, when bleeding is discovered emanating from the prostate or bladder neck, some prostatic tissue will need to be resected and the friable area will require coagulation. Bleeding in this area can be diffuse, and hemostasis may be achieved after completion of the procedure by placing a Foley catheter on traction, which causes compression and tamponade of vessels in the prostate and bladder neck.

Bleeding that originates from within the bladder is termed *hemorrhagic cystitis* and, as discussed previously, most commonly occurs from either radiation therapy or chemotherapeutic agents (14). Unlike radiation therapy, hematuria that results from chemotherapy drugs will not necessarily be associated with irritative voiding symptoms. The chemotherapeutic agents most commonly associated with hemorrhagic cystitis are cyclophosphamide (Cytoxan) and its analogues. The incidence of hemorrhagic cystitis in early series was reported to be as high as 68%. The compound acrolein is the active metabolite that actually causes the bladder damage produced by cyclophosphamide (24,25). Mesna (2-mercaptoethane sulfonate) was developed specifically to bind to acrolein and thereby reduce the harmful effects of this byproduct (26). Mesna is now given routinely when a patient is treated for malignancy with cyclophosphamide.

As described previously, the hematuria caused by radiation is commonly associated with dysuria, frequency, and urgency. Hemorrhagic cystitis can follow external beam or interstitial radiation treatment of primary genitourinary (prostate and bladder) malignancies, cancers of the cervix or rectum, or other pelvic lesions. The spectrum of hematuria secondary to radiation therapy also ranges from microscopic bleeding to bleeding severe enough to require transfusions. The time course of the development of hematuria ranges from months to years following the initiation of radiation therapy.

The damaging effects of radiation therapy on the bladder are similar to those found in other organs. The clinically significant symptoms in all organs are mediated through vascular damage. Radiation therapy induces a obliterative endarteritis, which leads to telangiectasias, submucosal hemorrhage, and fibrosis of smooth muscle and the interstitium. Ischemia of the mucosal surface resulting from endarteritis produces areas of hypoxic tissue, which can break down and cause ulceration and bleeding. If chronic, these changes may eventuate in fibrosis (27). These derangements also cause an irradiated bladder to be extremely susceptible to injury and slow to heal when injured. Unlike treatment with cyclophosphamide, no prophylactic measures are yet available that can be used to prevent bladder damage. Once radiation hemorrhagic cystitis occurs, aggressive symptomatic intervention should be initiated, and all further radiation exposure must be minimized

As with other types of gross hematuria, initial management of radiation- or chemotherapy-induced cystitis involves insertion of a large Foley catheter. Removal of all clots is paramount for success in eventually clearing the urine. All subsequent therapies will work better in a bladder free of clots, because clot evacuation reduces the naturally occurring fibrinolysins, which may act via the clotting cascade to perpetuate bleeding. If initial conservative management with catheter drainage and CBI fails, alternative therapies to control the bleeding must be sought. Several topical agents can be applied intravesically to aid in cessation of bleeding. Before proceeding with these therapies, cystoscopy should be performed to rule out bleeding from the upper tracts and to fulgurate any obvious bleeding sites.

Empiric therapy may be initiated with epsilon-aminocaproic acid (Amicar) given orally, parenterally (28), or intravesically (29), which reduces fibrinolysis by inhibiting plasminogen activator substances. This drug has been used extensively for idiopathic hematuria (30) and hematuria of unknown etiology associated with sickle cell disease (31,32). Although no controlled or randomized studies have been done on its use in treating hematuria, the above studies and clinical experience substantiate its use for severe hemorrhagic cystitis. Initially given either parenterally or orally, a loading dose of 5 g is followed by hourly doses of 1.0 g to 1.25 g. Maximal response is usually achieved in 8 to 12 hours. Patients who initially respond to the parenteral route can be changed to the oral route for maintenance therapy, which includes dividing the total daily dosage (6–8 g) and dividing it into four doses. When given intravesically, 200 mg is added to each liter of 0.9% saline, and this mixture is administered as CBI. A side effect is the formation of thick, tenacious

clots, which can become difficult for the patient to pass spontaneously and extremely difficult to irrigate in patients with catheters. Administering epsilon-aminocaproic acid to patients with bilateral upper tract bleeding is relatively contraindicated because thick clots in the renal pelvis or ureters can lead to upper tract obstruction, clot colic, or even renal failure.

Silver nitrate 0.5% to 1% mixed in sterile water may be administered into the bladder for treatment of acute bleeding. Rather than being run as CBI, this drug is instilled for 10 to 20 minutes, after which the bladder is emptied. In certain refractory cases, multiple instillations may be required (33).

In treating hemorrhagic cystitis, 1% alum also has shown some efficacy. Unlike silver nitrate, the 1% solution usually is given via CBI (34–36). Although somewhat effective, the rates of success are variable. The advantage of alum is that, apart from allergy, the substance is safe and requires no anesthesia.

The most efficacious and probably the most toxic treatment for hemorrhagic cystitis is intravesical formalin. Formalin is the aqueous solution of formaldehyde, and it acts by fixing the bladder mucosa by cross linking proteins and thereby preventing necrosis, sloughing, and blood loss. Studies have shown formalin to be up to 80% effective in arresting bladder hemorrhage (37–39). Formalin is available as 37% or 40% aqueous formaldehyde, which is diluted with sterile water to yield final concentrations of 10% formalin (3.7% formaldehyde) or 1% formalin (0.37% formaldehyde). Formalin administration is painful and requires regional or general anesthesia. It is administered in concentrations ranging from 1% to 10%, starting at the lowest and progressing to the higher concentrations only as clinically indicated. The usually is filled to capacity using gravity drainage and no more than 15 cm/$H_2O$ pressure. Bladder instillation usually lasts from 10 to 14 minutes (40).

Risks of formalin administration include damage to the bladder and upper tracts. Reflux of formalin to the kidneys can lead to fibrosis, obstruction, hydronephrosis, and papillary necrosis. A cystogram should be performed before formalin administration to rule out vesicoureteral reflux. In patients who have reflux, ureteral balloon catheters may be inserted to prevent retrograde flow of formalin. Also, the procedure can be performed in the reverse Trendelenburg position to minimize reflux. Through its ability to cross-link proteins within the wall of the bladder, administration of formalin can lead to a decrease in bladder capacity and, in extreme cases, a nonfunctional, contracted bladder. Patients must be advised of these potential risks, and formalin therapy must be reserved only for cases of hemorrhagic cystitis that are truly refractory to all other medical treatments.

Two other nonsurgical therapies for hemorrhagic cystitis deserve mention. Several reports (41–43) have described the use of hyperbaric oxygen therapy for radiation-induced hemorrhagic cystitis. In the most recent series, Weiss et al. (41) reported that 12 of 13 patients who had failed formalin or alum and fulguration were treated successfully by hyperbaric oxygen therapy. Hyperbaric oxygen induces hyperoxia, in which increased tissue concentrations of oxygen are attained by the increased dissolved oxygen in the serum. This condition results in neovascularization and secondary growth of healthy granulation tissue. Thus, hyperbaric oxygen tends to reverse the ischemic process caused by radiation therapy. Additionally, hyperoxia itself induces vasoconstriction, which may have a direct effect on bleeding from the bladder mucosa.

Finally, some reports have described the use of conjugated estrogens for treatment of hemorrhagic cystitis. Although the mechanism is unknown, there is a suggestion that estrogens may decrease capillary fragility. Liu et al. (44) reported on five consecutive cases in which bleeding from both radiation therapy and cyclophosphamide was treated successfully with conjugated estrogens. A follow-up study by Miller et al. (45) showed that six of seven patients treated with oral estrogens improved sufficiently to avoid further invasive therapy. Although no standard doses or length of therapy have been established, it appears that the usual starting dose of conjugated estrogens is 2.5 mg twice daily. After an adequate response has been achieved, the dose can be tapered. Final doses appear to be in the range of 1.25 mg daily and sometimes can be weaned to 0.625 mg daily. Conjugated estrogens are well known to induce cardiovascular complications at high doses. Although no thromboembolic or cardiovascular complications occurred in the two aforementioned studies, the long-term safety of estrogens at moderate to high doses is unknown; however, in a terminally ill patient, the benefits of estrogen therapy certainly would seem to outweigh the risks if it could control the significant bleeding associated with hemorrhagic cystitis.

For patients who do not respond to intravesical medical therapy, there are more invasive ways of decreasing bleeding from the bladder. Occasionally, selective embolization of branches of the hypogastric arteries is used to control bleeding. This therapy may be preferred in terminally ill patients who cannot undergo a major surgical procedure because embolization can be performed with the patient under local anesthesia. The procedure works best when arteriography demonstrates a particular vessel responsible for the bleeding; unfortunately, this clinical scenario is unusual. If the entire bladder urothelium appears to be involved, the anterior branches of both hypogastric arteries may need to be occluded. Complications of embolization include claudication of the gluteal muscles, temporary lower-extremity paralysis, and necrosis of the bladder (46).

Some patients fail conservative measures and may require surgery to control the bleeding. Unfortunately, many of these patients are poor surgical candidates because of the ongoing hemorrhage and coagulopathy. These patients, who usually undergo urinary diversion and at times cystectomy, universally do poorly.

## UPPER TRACT BLEEDING

### Asymptomatic

As with bleeding from the lower urinary tract, asymptomatic bleeding from the upper tract rarely requires therapy, and the same algorithm (i.e., urinalysis, imaging study, cystoscopy, and possibly culture) should be applied. Unlike asymptomatic bleeding from the lower urinary tract, however, imaging studies may be more useful than cystoscopy to determine the site of bleeding. For most patients with microscopic hematuria originating in the upper tracts, cystoscopy usually will be normal. In patients with gross hematuria and no symptoms (gross painless hematuria), cystoscopy may be able to lateralize the bleeding if the study is performed while the patient is actively bleeding. Once the bladder is filled with irrigation fluid, a jet of blood may be seen emanating from the ureteral orifice on the side of the pathology.

Although bleeding itself does not necessarily warrant therapy, the pathology causing the bleeding may require treatment. Common causes of upper tract bleeding include renal masses, tumors of the renal pelvis and ureter, stones, and papillary necrosis. Once the side of the bleeding is determined either by imaging studies or cystoscopy, further diagnostic techniques, such as retrograde pyelography, selective ureteral catheterization for cytology, or rarely ureteroscopy, can be entertained. The discussion of further therapy for each pathologic condition in an asymptomatic patient is beyond the scope of this discussion.

### Symptomatic

Symptomatic bleeding from the upper urinary tract is usually manifested by *clot colic*, a term that refers to the acute onset of flank pain secondary to acute ureteral obstruction. Clinically, clot colic mimics renal colic secondary to stones. Differentiating the two can sometimes be difficult, especially because clot colic in the presence of complete ureteral obstruction can present without overt hematuria.

The history and selective imaging studies may assist in the diagnosis of acute ureteral obstruction. Acute-onset flank pain in an elderly person who has no history of kidney stones is more likely caused by clot or tumor. Likewise, upper urinary tract obstruction without evidence of calcifications on IVP or ultrasound is more likely secondary to clot or tumor.

Unlike bleeding from the lower urinary tract, there are only a few noninvasive measures that may benefit the patient with symptomatic upper-tract bleeding. As in lower-tract bleeding, forced diuresis by increasing oral and intravenous fluids may help dilute the blood in the urine sufficiently to prevent clot formation. The administration of -aminocaproic acid can be considered, but, as noted previously, upper-tract bleeding is a relative contraindication for the use of this drug, which can convert small clots that can easily pass through the ureter into large tenacious clots that obstruct the ureter. Small clots that previously could pass through the ureter may become large tenacious clots that can obstruct the ureter. Thus, -aminocaproic acid must be used judiciously in upper-tract bleeding.

For patients who continue to develop clot colic from persistent upper urinary tract bleeding, most interventions to stop the bleeding will require invasive interventions to stop the bleeding. If no pathology is seen on imaging studies, including IVP or CT scan, an arteriogram may be warranted to exclude an arteriovenous fistula. This procedure may be able to identify the area of bleeding so that selective embolization can be performed.

If all studies, including the arteriogram, are normal, one may be faced with the difficult question of whether to remove a kidney or ureter. In this situation, cystoscopy may be extremely helpful in lateralizing the pathology. It is a particularly difficult decision to remove a kidney and ureter without a pathologic diagnosis. In this situation, a patient must be very symptomatic and have failed all other more conservative means.

Patients with advanced renal cell carcinoma and metastatic disease also may develop bleeding and clot formation. Palliative measures may include radiation therapy or chemotherapy. Because the prognosis in these patients is quite poor and surgery to remove the primary tumor will not impact positively on survival, it is again crucially important to document the degree of bleeding and the relative morbidity arising from the bleeding. Only when bleeding and clot colic impact negatively on the quality of life should patients be considered for palliative nephrectomy. Statistically, metastatic tumors are much more likely than primary renal cell carcinomas in terminally ill patients.

## UPPER TRACT OBSTRUCTION

Perhaps the most difficult problem in patients with advanced medical diseases is bilateral ureteral obstruction. Without treatment, these patients die of uremia. It is the physician's responsibility to help the patient make the appropriate decision concerning aggressive or conservative therapy. In patients with a limited life expectancy and poor quality of life, conservative therapy may allow a patient to die with dignity. Patients who have exhausted all primary treatments and cannot improve their functional status should not be considered for aggressive ther-

apy. Patients who have received an adequate trial of all known useful therapy and still have rapidly progressive ureteral obstruction despite the administration of optimal therapy probably will benefit little from urinary diversion. Also, patients with severe, unrelenting, and unmanageable pain are seldom better off after diversion.

Because the ultimate endpoint of bilateral ureteral obstruction is renal failure and uremia, both patient and physician must understand that without treatment the condition will be progressive. The progression of renal failure to uremia is marked by fatigue, decreased appetite, nausea, uremic coma, and eventually death. In a patient who has been suffering with an end-stage malignancy, this may be a welcome situation.

### Percutaneous Nephrostomy

Fortunately, with the advent of modern technology, patients who are acceptable candidates for diversion of the urine have a better chance of experiencing significant improvement with minimum morbidity. Before the 1970s, urinary diversion required an open surgical procedure to divert the flow of urine from the kidneys to the bladder. These procedures were troublesome because most patients with malignant ureteral obstruction are poor surgical candidates as a result of their underlying nutritional, hematologic, and immunologic status. Grabstald and McPhee (47) studied 218 patients who underwent open nephrostomy for malignant ureteral obstruction. They discovered a major life-threatening complication rate of 45% and a 3% operative mortality rate; 43% of these patients did not leave the hospital. A later study by Meyer et al. (48) showed that 30% of patients undergoing an open urinary diversion procedure died within 52 days of surgery and the overall median survival was only 3.3 months. Thus, open nephrostomy subjects the patient to significant operative and perioperative risks without durable responses.

As a result of these outcomes, open surgical procedures have been supplanted by newer percutaneous techniques. In patients who will tolerate anesthesia, cystoscopic insertion of ureteral stents is probably the preferred method of ureteral decompression. Relative contraindications to this procedure include hemodynamic instability and sepsis. When retrograde insertion of ureteral stents is unsuccessful, percutaneous nephrostomy is the technique of choice to relieve ureteral obstruction. As with most procedures, the chances of success and durable response depend mainly on the extent of the underlying disease and whether valid treatment options still exist. Some studies have shown a poor response following percutaneous nephrostomy. Keidan et al. (49) showed that although renal function improved in 85% of patients, the median survival was only 13 weeks, and 55% of the patients required additional hospitalizations for urosepsis and additional procedures. A study by

Gasparini et al. (50) revealed much better results, however, albeit in a patient population that included many patients with newly diagnosed disease. They showed that 77% of patients undergoing either percutaneous nephrostomy (68%) or cystoscopic stent insertion (32%) were able to be discharged home. The mean survival time after urinary diversion was 75 weeks, and one patient lived 4.7 years. There appeared to be a survival advantage for patients who had not previously undergone hormonal or chemotherapy. Also, in contrast to previous studies, there were no perioperative deaths or cardiac, pulmonary, or hemorrhagic complications. Thus, in properly selected patients, endoscopic or percutaneous urinary diversion can be relatively safe and efficacious.

A patient who successfully undergoes percutaneous nephrostomy and returns to a normal lifestyle can be considered for internalization of the nephrostomy tube. This procedure requires placing a ureteral stent into the ureter through an anterograde approach. Hepperlen et al. (51) showed that patients with pigtail ureteral stents, whether inserted initially or after conversion of nephrostomy tube to stent, survived an average of 277 days. More importantly, these patients spent only 8.4% of their remaining time in the hospital. Similarly, Gibbons et al. (52) found no operative mortalities and an 88% satisfaction rate after insertion of a ureteral stent. In contrast, a series by Brin et al. (53), which examined patient outcome after nephrostomy, revealed an average survival of 162 days with 63% of the time spent in the hospital. Thus, there appears to be a significant survival and quality of life advantage in patients with indwelling stents compared with nephrostomy tubes.

Finally, as with urethral obstruction secondary to malignancy, there have been reports of self-expanding metal stents for treatment of ureteral obstruction. Lugmayr and Pauer (54) studied 23 patients who underwent insertion of the Wallstent device for malignant ureteral obstruction. They were successful in implanting the device in 97% of patients, and 83% of the stented ureters remained patent after 30 weeks. Because 81% of patients survived at least 6 months, the patency rate appeared comparable to survival rates. Thus, ureteral stenting may offer a viable option for treating the obstructed ureter.

## CONCLUSION

The ultimate goal with all urologic complications in patients with progressive medical diseases is to maximize the quantity of life without jeopardizing or negatively affecting quality of life. Urologic complications in these patients can arise from benign or malignant disease processes or as a consequence of treatments for an underlying malignancy. With the armamentarium of imaging studies, medications, and surgical interventions, the physician treating these patients can strive to allow them to live the remainder of their lives to their fullest capacity.

## REFERENCES

1. Wein AJ. Neuromuscular dysfunction of the lower urinary tract. In: Walsh PC, Retik AB, Stamey TA, Vaughan ED Jr., eds. *Campbell's urology.* Philadelphia: WB Saunders, 1992;611.
2. Forman JD, Order SE, Zinreich ES, Lee DJ, Wharam MD, Mellitis ED. The correlation of pretreatment transurethral resection of prostatic cancer with tumor dissemination and disease-free survival. *Cancer* 1986; 58:1770.
3. Surya BV, Provet JA. Manifestation of advanced prostate cancer: Prognosis and treatment. *J Urol* 1989;142:921.
4. Lapides J, Diokno AC, Silber SJ, Lowe BS. Clean, intermittent self-catheterization in the treatment of urinary tract disease. *J Urol* 1972; 107:458.
5. Diokno AC. Clean itermittent catheterization in children and adults. In: Seidmon EJ, Hanno PM, eds. *Current urologic therapy.* Philadelphia: WB Saunders, 1994;325.
6. Oesterling JE. Benign prostatic hyperplasia—medical and minimally invasive treatment options. *N Engl J Med* 1995;332:99.
7. Mazur AW, Thompson IM. Efficacy and morbidity of "channel" TURP. *Urology* 1991;38:526.
8. Morgentaler A, DeWolf WC. A self-expanding prostatic stent for bladder outlet obstruction in high risk patients. *J Urol* 1993;150:1636.
9. Kaplan SA, Merrill DC, Mosely WG, et al. The titanium intraprostatic stent: the United States experience. *J Urol* 1993;150:1624.
10. Guazzoni GG, Bergamashi F, Montorsi F, et al. Prostatic Urolume Wallstent for benign prostatic hyperplasia patients at poor operative risk: clinical, uroflowmetric and ultrasonographic patterns. *J Urol* 1993;150: 1641.
11. Milroy E, Chapple CR. The Urolome stent in the management of benign prostatic hyperplasia. *J Urol* 1993;150:1630.
12. Kaye KW, Lange PH. Mode of presentation of invasive bladder cancer: reassessment of the problem. *J Urol* 1982;128;31.
13. Frank MG, Park R. The drug-induced glaucomas. *J Med Soc NJ* 1974; 71:470.
14. Berdy GJ, Berdy SS, Odin LS, Hirst LW. Angle closure glaucoma precipitated by aerosolized atropine. *Arch Intern Med* 1991;151:1658.
15. Goldberg ID, Garnick MB, Bloomer WD. Urinary tract toxic effects of cancer therapy. *J Urol* 1984;132:1.
16. Dean RJ, Lytton B. Urologic complications of pelvic irradiation. *J Urol* 1978;119:64.
17. Lamm DL. Complications of bacillus Calmette-Guérin immunotherapy. *Urol Clin North Am* 1992;19:565.
18. Lamm DL, Stogdill BJ, Crispen RG. Complications of bacillus Calmette-Guérin immunotherapy in 1,278 patients with bladder cancer. *J Urol* 1986;135:272.
19. Lamm DL, Van Der Meijden PM, Morales A, Brosman SA, Catalona WJ, Herr HW, Soloway MS, Steg A, Debruyne FMJ. Incidence and treatment of complications of bacillus Calmette-Guérin intravesical therapy in superficial bladder cancer. *J Urol* 1992;147:596.
20. deVries CR, Freiha FS. Hemorrhagic cystitis: a review. *J Urol* 1990; 143:1.
21. Messing EM, Young TB, Hunt VB, Emoto SE, Webbie JM. The significance of asymptomatic microhematuria in men 50 or more years old: findings of a home screening study using urine dipsticks. *J Urol* 1987; 137:919.
22. Mariani AJ, Luangphinith S, Loo S, Scottolini A, Hodges CV. Dipstick chemical urinalysis: an accurate and cost-effective screening test. *J Urol* 1984;132:64.
23. Hearne CR, Donnell MG, Fraser CG. Assessment of new urinalysis dipstick. *Clin Chem* 1980;26:170.
24. Cox PJ. Cyclophosphamide cystitis and bladder cancer: a hypothesis. *Eur J Cancer* 1979;15:1071.
25. Cox PJ. Cyclophosphamide cystitis: identification of acrolein as the causative agent. *Biochem Pharmacol* 1979;28:2045.
26. Brock N, Pohl J, Stekar J. Detoxification of urotoxic oxazaphosphorines by sulfhydryl compounds. *J Cancer Res Clin Oncol* 1981;100: 311.

27. Scheonrock GJ, Ciani P. Treatment of radiation cystitis with hyperbaric oxygen. *Urology* 1986;27:271.

28. Stefanini M, English HA, Taylor AE. Safe and effective, prolonged administration of epsilon aminocaproic acid in bleeding from the urinary tract. *J Urol* 1990;143:559,

29. Singh I, Laungani GB. Intravesical epsilon aminocaproic acid in management of intractable bladder hemorrhage. *Urology* 1992;40:227.

30. Nash DA Jr, Henry AR. Unilateral essential hematuria: therapy with epsilon aminocaproic acid. *Urology* 1984;23:297.

31. Black WD, Hatch FE, Acchiardo S. Aminocaproic acid in prolonged hematuria of patients with sicklemia. *Arch Intern Med* 1976;136:678.

32. Vega R, Shanberg AM, Malloy TR. The use of epsilon aminocaproic acid in sickle cell trait hematuria. *J Urol* 1971;105:552.

33. Kumar APM, Wrenn EL Jr, Jayalakshmamma B, Conrad L, Quinn P, Cox C. Silver nitrate irrigation to control bladder hemorrhage in children receiving cancer therapy. *J Urol* 1976;116:85.

34. Kennedy L, Snell ME, Witherow RO. Use of alum to control intractable vesical haemorrhage. *Br J Urol* 1984;56:673.

35. Mukamel E, Lupu A, deKernion JB. Alum irrigation for severe bladder hemorrhage. *J Urol* 1986;135:784.

36. Goel AK, Rao MS, Bhagwat AG, Vaidyanathan S, GJoswami AK, Sen TK. Intravesical irrigation with alum for the control of massive bladder hemorrhage. *J Urol* 1985;133:956.

37. Kumar S, Rosen P, Grabstald H. Intravesical formalin for the control of intractable bladder hemorrhage secondary to cystitis or cancer. *J Urol* 1975;114:540.

38. Fair WR. Formalin in the treatment of massive bladder hemorrhage: techniques, results, and complications. *Urology* 1974;3:573.

39. Firlit CF. Intractable hemorrhagic cystitis secondary to extensive carcinomatosis: management with formalin solution. *J Urol* 1973:110:57.

40. Donahue LA, Frank IN. Intravesical formalin therapy for hemorrhagic cystitis: analysis of therapy. *J Urol* 1989;141:809.

41. Weiss JP, Maattei DM, Neville EC, Hanno PM. Primary treatment of radiation-induced hemorrhagic cystitis with hyperbaric oxygen: 10-year experience. *J Urol* 1994;151:1514.

42. Norkool DM, Hampson NB, Gibbons RP, Weissman RM. Hyperbaric oxygen therapy for radiation-induced hemorrhagic cystitis. *J Urol* 1993; 150:332.

43. Rijkmans BG, Bakker DJ, Dabhoiwala NF, Kurth KH. Successful treatment of radiation-induced hemorrhagic cystitis with hyperbaric oxygen. *Eur Urol* 1989;16:354.

44. Liu YK, Hart JI, Steinbock GS, Holt HA Jr, Goldstein DH, Amin M. Treatment of radiation of cyclophosphamide induced hemorrhagic cystitis using conjugated estrogen. *J Urol* 1990;144:41.

45. Miller J, Burfield GD, Moretti KL. Oral conjugated estrogen therapy for treatment of hemorrhagic cystitis. *J Urol* 1994;151:1348.

46. Sieber PR. Bladder necrosis secondary to pelvic artery embolization: case report and literature review. *J Urol* 1994;151:422.

47. Grabstald H, McPhee M. Nephrostomy and the cancer patient. *South Med J* 1973;66:217.

48. Meyer JE, Yatsuhashi M, Green TH. Palliative urinary diversion in patients with advanced pelvic malignancy. *Cancer* 1980;45:2698.

49. Keidan RD, Greenberg RE, Hoffman JP. Is percutaneous nephrostomy for hydronephrosis appropriate in patients with advanced cancer? *Am J Surg* 1988;156:206.

50. Gasparini M, Carroll P, Stoller M. Palliative percutaneous and endoscopic urinary diversion for malignant ureteral obstruction. *Urology* 1991;38:408.

51. Hepperlen TW, Mardis HK, Kammandel H. The pigtail ureteral stent in the cancer patient. *J Urol* 1979;121:17.

52. Gibbons RP, Correa RJ Jr, Cummings KB, Mason JT. Experience with indwelling ureteral stent catheters. *J Urol* 1975;115:22.

53. Brin EN, Schiff M Jr, Weiss RM. Palliative urinary diversion for pelvic malignancy. *J Urol* 1975;113:619.

54. Lugmayr H, Pauer W. Self-expanding metal stents for palliative treatment of malignant ureteral obstruction. *AJR Am J Roentgenol* 1992;159:1091.

*Principles and Practice of Supportive Oncology,*
edited by Ann Berger et al.
Lippincott–Raven Publishers, Philadelphia ©1998

CHAPTER 29

# Primary Renal Failure

W. Scott Long

*Primary renal failure* (PRF) in this chapter is defined as renal parenchymal disease characterized by azotemia, metabolic offsets (e.g., hyperkalemia, acidosis), and in some cases volume overload. Most PRF can be attributed to ischemic or nephrotoxic insults (1). By definition, PRF excludes isolated prerenal or postrenal failure, although either may evolve into parenchymal damage. This chapter does not set a single value of azotemia as a defining level for PRF, nor does the literature. Defining creatinine levels may vary from 2 to 2.5 after rehydration (2–5) to 5.7 mg/dl (6,7) or as increases of 25% to 100% baseline creatinine levels (8–11). The broader term, *acute renal failure* (ARF), often includes prerenal, postrenal, and parenchymal renal failure evolving over hours or days. No single definition exists for it; its meaning must be sought in each article.

Elucidation of ARF as a pathophysiologic entity has a long history in this century and was acclerated with experience of trauma-related renal failure in World War II (12). In the subsequent 25 years, ARF and other renal syndromes specifically related to cancer and its therapies were reviewed (13–21) and continue to be the focus of clinical study.

Epidemiology of renal failure changed over the period from 1956 through 1990 (1,6,7,22,23). The average age of patients treated for renal failure is older. Clinical settings associated with malignancy have become more complicated through wider use of nephrotoxic agents and the increased incidence of sepsis, multiorgan failure, and significant comorbidity, especially cardiovascular disease, superimposed on aging kidneys (7,8,22,24,25). In contrast, improved prevention and care have decreased incidence and mortality of renal failure among trauma and obstetric cases. Overall mortality rates of 40% to 60% in the population of patients with ARF have remained relatively unchanged during this period (1,25).

As discussed in following sections, mortality for cancer patients with PRF remains among the highest in patients with renal failure of any etiology.

This chapter discusses the causes and therapy for PRF in its acute presentation. Brief mention is made of prerenal and postrenal failure because both need to be assessed in diagnosing PRF and because either, if protracted, may evolve into PRF. Care of patients with chronic renal failure (CRF) for the most part is not discussed. The chapter ends with selected topics on the care of cancer patients dying of renal failure.

Although much of the material in this chapter is presented in an isolated clinical perspective, the reader is encouraged to remember that the care of patients and families entails education, emotional support, guidance, patience, and responsibility at each step. This undertaking can rarely, if ever, be accomplished by a single clinician any more than a single clinician can deliver single-handedly the complex clinical care for a cancer patient with PRF. Willing collaboration among clinicians in recognition of individual strengths and limitations promotes good care and furthers cooperation between those giving and those receiving care (26,27).

## INCIDENCE AND CAUSES OF PRF IN CANCER PATIENTS

What is the incidence of ARF among cancer patients? Among 109 cancer patients receiving morphine, 13 had serum creatinine levels of 4 mg/dl or greater (28). Among patients with multiple myeloma more than 50% develop renal involvement. In one large study (2), 18% of 494 patients with previously undiagnosed multiple myeloma suffered from renal failure (creatinine >2 mg/dl). In another striking study, 80 of 85 myeloma patients presented with renal insufficiency (serum creatinine >1.5 mg/dl), and the average serum creatinine level for the 80 patients was 7.9 mg/dl (29). Forty-one of 64 bone marrow

W. S. Long: Connecticut Hospice, Branford, CT 06405.

transplant patients had ARF defined as doubling baseline creatinines (9). Of 349 patients with hematologic neoplasms, 149 (43%) had serum creatinines above 1.7 mg/dl and 43 (12%) required dialysis (10). Among 272 bone marrow transplant patients, 64 (24%) required dialysis; 79 other patients doubled their baseline creatinines but did not require dialysis (30).

In cancer patients, PRF may result from actions of tumor on the kidneys before treatment, from diagnostic and therapeutic procedures, and from both. The major pathophysiologic pathways are nephrotoxicity and ischemia. Comorbidity, including important preexistent renal disease (31,32), plays an important role in predisposition to and evolution of renal compromise (3,6,33).

The most direct action of cancer on kidneys is found in renal cell carcinoma (RCC). In one study, ARF occurred in 13% (33/259) of patients undergoing surgery for RCC (34). Parenchymal infiltration by leukemias and lymphomas commonly found at autopsy and occasionally by renal metastases (e.g., melanoma, thymoma, and also breast, stomach, colon, lung) usually is not associated with renal failure but does occur (16,35).

Acting at greater distance, tumors release antigens, leading most commonly to membranous glomerulopathies, especially in bronchogenic and gastrointestinal tumors, and to minimal change glomerulopathy in Hodgkin lymphomas and much less frequently in other malignancies (20,36). Other paraneoplastic glomerulopathies are less common (20). Vascular changes like thromboses of glomerular and other small-caliber renal vessels are associated with disseminated intravascular coagulation (DIC) in mucinous adenocarcinomas and acute promyelocytic leukemia (16) and with vasculitis in lymphomas. Large-caliber vessels also may be involved, as in renal vein thrombosis in renal cell carcinoma. Renal failure, common in multiple myeloma, is due in part to proximal tubular cellular damage by filtered light chains and to intratubular obstruction (2,29) with associated renal tissue destruction.

A single type of tumor may compromise renal function through multiple pathways. Multiple myeloma produces renal damage by toxic effects of light-chain absorption in proximal tubular cells, by obstruction due to intratubular coagulation, by parenchymal precipitation of calcium phosphate crystals (*nephrocalcinosis*), and by deposition of light chains or amyloid. Renal cell carcinoma compromises renal function not only by parenchymal invasion but also in a small minority of cases by glomerulonephritis and amyloidosis (16) as well as by renal vein thrombosis.

Fluid loss through nausea, vomiting, and diarrhea due to chemotherapy, surgical blood loss, "third spacing" (e.g. ascites and edema), diuretic use, and gastrointestinal drainage all contribute to depletion of extracellular fluid (ECF) volume and decreased effective renal perfusion. If prolonged, these changes produce PRF.

Conditions blocking renal drainage also produce RPF, for example, retroperitoneal adenopathy of genitourinary tumors or lymphomas compressing ureters or intraureteral blocks by clots, by "sludge" of phosphate, urates, and other products of cell breakdown in tumor lysis syndrome or by renal stones. More distal bilateral blockade of ureteral orifices by genitourinary or other pelvic tumors can produce the same deleterious effects, as can benign prostatic hypertrophy (BPH) (18).

Some chemotherapeutic agents create renal parenchymal damage, most commonly cisplatinum and methotrexate. Cisplatinum at 50 to 75 mg/M$^2$ is thought to be directly toxic to renal cells and may present both acutely and chronically. Methotrexate creates damage through intratubular obstruction by precipitated crystals and possibly through direct antimitotic effects on renal cells and afferent arteriolar constriction (14,18,21). Other chemotherapeutic agents, such as nitrosoureas (especially streptozotocin), mitomycin, and ifosfamide, may cause PRF (14,18,21). Dehydration as a result of vomiting or diarrhea associated with chemotherapy further increases likelihood of renal damage.

Other agents (31,32,37–40) used alone or in combination in cancer patients may adversely affect renal function, for example, antibiotics (aminoglycosides, some cephalosporins, amphotericin B, acyclovir), analgesic nonsteroidal antiinflammatory drugs (NSAIDs), radiocontrast dyes (41,42), and cyclosporine A (9) by a variety of mechanisms, including direct tubular toxicity, ischemia, and allergic interstitial nephritis.

Renal failure also occurs in therapeutic settings such as surgery (7,31,34,37,43) or bone marrow transplant (9,30,44). The incidence of renal damage from radiation therapy of abdominal tumors (16) has been reduced in recent years by shielding kidneys from unnecessary radiation and by reduction of dosage delivered and tissue volume exposed (45).

Comorbidity in cancer patients, many of whom are elderly and have other serious illnesses, often exacerbates renal insult. Age alone has been identified as an independent risk factor for renal failure in some studies (3,7,24,33,46) but not all (31,32,47). In intensive care units (ICU), the chances of recovering meaningful life, or life at all, decrease rapidly as additional systems fail (8,24,48).

## DIAGNOSIS AND THERAPIES OF RENAL FAILURE

Initially, patients with renal failure may show no symptoms. Rising azotemia in routine testing is often the first indication of renal insufficiency or failure. Once alerted, the physician begins to search for causes and to measure the rate and consequences of evolving failure. Much depends on early detection and effective treatment, as ARF can evolve into death or into worsening renal failure and then CRF.

Therapies for renal failure in cancer patients can be divided into two large groups depending on clinical context. The first group of therapies is based on the consideration that the life at risk is worth great effort to save or prolong significantly. In this first group, therapy aims to correct underlying pathophysiology and its consequences and to optimize patients' health. The second group of therapies occurs in settings of disease for which active curative therapy is no longer sought. These patients receive care for symptom management, understanding that it will not reverse underlying disease but may make it easier to bear.

During the evolution of renal failure or cancer, placement of patients in these groups may change, as may patient choices. Earlier consultations between patient/family and caregivers, one hopes, will make further decisions easier for all concerned (49).

A physiological perspective divides renal failure of various causes into three categories: prerenal, renal (or parenchymal), and postrenal. Most studies of ARF report hospital (especially ICU) experience and tend to focus on failure resulting from renal parenchymal damage. Community-based studies are fewer and show important roles for prerenal (4) and postrenal (50) failure in "community-acquired" ARF. (Comparison of incidences of prerenal and postrenal failure among studies is difficult because of different defining criteria and patient populations.)

In each category, renal failure can be characterized according to the amount of urine excreted per day: anuric if less than 100 ml/day, oliguric if less than 400 ml/day, and nonoliguric at higher rates. In principle, patients with nonoliguric renal failure should fare better than those in oliguric failure because volume overload is less troublesome, a prediction borne out in several studies (3,31,50–52).

## Prerenal and Postrenal Failure

Prerenal failure indicates that one or more precipitating causes of failure are "upstream" from the kidney. History and physical examination are particularly important in diagnosing prerenal failure. Decreases in daily weights and in fluid intake and output suggest prerenal failure. A history of ECF depletion and an examination revealing poor skin turgor, dry oral mucosa, dry axillae, resting tachycardia, orthostatic pulse and pressure are consistent with prerenal failure.

Generally, patients with prerenal failure produce small amounts of concentrated urine with low sodium content. For example, (urine/plasma) creatinine ratios may be greater than 40, urinary osmolality above 500 mOsm/L, and fractional excretion of sodium less than 0.01 in patients without renal insufficiency and no recent diuretic use. These parameters are less reliable among elderly patients in whom the ability to concentrate urine is re-

duced. Overall such urinary indices can be helpful as additional data but are not diagnostic. Once active therapy starts, they can be used to document evolution of renal failure and treatment (54).

Urinary sediments in prerenal failure are generally free of cellular debris other than clear hyaline tubular casts. "Active" or "busy" sediments of epithelial cells, cellular debris, and tubular casts are associated with parenchymal failure; however, urinary sediments may contain no casts in some cases of PRF. Red-cell casts suggest glomerulonephritis, as tubular casts of leukocytes do for allergic interstitial nephritis (e.g., penicillins, cephalosporins, NSAIDs, and allopurinol).

In some patients, treatment with a cautious fluid challenge is diagnostic of prerenal failure. For example, in ICUs small fluid challenges of 200 ml (with or without low-dose dopamine) with concomitant central venous or capillary wedge pressure measurement, are helpful in assessing ECF status (55). On occasion, patients receive diuretics or mannitol in addition to intravenous fluid to favor evolution of nonoliguric over oliguric renal failure, although these maneuvers have not been shown clearly to be helpful (56,57). Obviously, replacement therapy depends on the composition of fluids lost, especially because renal homeostatic ability is compromised. Close monitoring of ECF volume and composition protects against fluid overload and electrolyte abnormalities such as hyponatremia.

Postrenal failure indicates obstruction downstream from the kidney, whether related to cancer (e.g., of bladder, cervix, prostate) or comorbidity (e.g., BPH). Obstruction predisposes to renal dysfunction and failure through effects of accumulating pressure on circulation and on cell and tissue function. Renal vein thrombosis in renal cell carcinoma causes similar problems.

Many presentations of ARF have more than one cause (31,32,37,39); identification of prerenal or postrenal failure does not rule out parenchymal damage. History from the patient and medical records often reveal comorbidity, with recent events and exposures raising the risk for PRF. Physical examination may be nonrevealing but not omitted. In addition to assessment of fluid status and signs of urinary obstruction, signs of cardiovascular, hepatic, allergic, and neoplastic disease must be sought. The skin is examined for rash (allergy), petechiae (DIC), and purpura both palpable (vasculitis) and nonpalpable (amyloid). Loss of hearing may occur with aminoglycoside excess. Lower-extremity edema and varicocele, especially when developing acutely, raise the question of renal vein thrombosis.

Laboratory testing is helpful in identifying or consolidating a diagnosis of parenchymal damage. Hyperuricemia ≥15 mg/dl with elevated $K^+$, phosphate, and lactate dehydrogenase (LDH) suggest tumor lysis syndrome. Hypercalcemia occurs in several tumors (e.g., breast cancer, squamous cell carcinomas of lung, head and neck, bladder, renal cell carcinoma and in some hematologic tumors, especially multiple myeloma). Schistocytes on blood smear in conjunction with cutaneous signs of coagulopathy and rising fibrin split products suggest a vasculitic process. Eosinophilia on complete blood count suggests allergic interstital nephritis.

Imaging studies with ultrasound, computed tomography (CT), and magnetic resonance images (MRI), often used early to rule out postobstructive lesions, also describe size and number of kidneys with estimation of cortical thickness to identify preexistent CRF. Flow studies, such as duplex Doppler ultrasound and digital subtraction angiography, help to rule out vascular causes or contribution to failure (e.g., bilateral cortical ischemia due to microvascular disease or renal vein thrombosis) (55).

Renal biopsy to guide therapy needs consideration if there are no obvious causes for parenchymal damage or if aspects of history, examination, and laboratory data suggest other causes of renal failure for which specific treatments exist (e.g., glomerular, interstitial, or vascular disease) (58,59). In two series of myeloma patients, 38% to 48% of patients underwent biopsy (5,29) to determine a potential role for dialysis (+/– plasmapheresis) and for prognosis. In series of patients with ARF of all causes, biopsy rates vary from 0 to 24% (6–8,60); in subsets of patients with "medical" causes for ARF, the rates are much higher (6,7).

### Preventive Measures

Preventive measures serve patients' interests whenever risks can be foreseen. Even modest degrees of renal failure may increase mortality, independent of comorbidity (11). Iatrogenic causes of renal failure were identified in 40% to 55% of patients with hospital-acquired renal insufficiency (31,37). Many patients have two or more preexistent factors for renal damage, and more than 50% in one study had more than one acute insult (32). Advanced age, dehydration, the concomitant use of nephrotoxins, and significant comorbidity (like preexistent renal insufficiency, cardiovascular disease, and diabetes mellitus) increase the probability of renal damage. Evaluation of baseline renal function identifies patients already at risk, signals the need for careful preventive measures, and allows quantitation of evolving renal compromise if it arises.

Some cancer patients have forseeable risks for PRF: significant comorbidity, ECF depletion, bulky tumors associated with tumor lysis syndrome, multiple myeloma with hypercalcemia and isosthenuria, planned exposure to chemotherapeutic agents of known nephrotoxicity, continued or potential exposure to other nephrotoxins singly or in combination (e.g., aminoglycosides, NSAIDs, radiocontrast dyes, and cyclosporine A; known drug allergies associated with allergic interstitial nephritis (e.g., cepha-

losporins, penicillins, rifampin, sulfonamides, NSAIDs, some diuretics, captopril). In some cases, hydration and diuresis (urinary alkalinization) minimize risk, such as in protocols to prepare patients for administration of methotrexate or cisplatinum (18) or for radiocontrast dyes (42). Many patients at risk for PRF can be protected by choice among alternative agents, for example, radiocontrast agents (41), antibiotics, anithypertensives, antineoplastics (14,40), diuretics. Furthermore, adjustment of medication dosage or schedule may reduce renal risk in patients requiring potentially nephrotoxic drugs (18,61,62). Drug levels should be monitored, although maintenance of therapeutic levels does not always prevent renal damage, for example, with aminoglycosides (64). Once therapy begins, close monitoring reveals patients with declining renal function, allows correction of metabolic offsets and guides modification of treatment regimen and therapies to limit further renal damage.

### Treatment

Treatment of some problems caused by renal failure may be required soon after detection to protect the patient's status during further workup and therapy and to prevent evolution of renal damage into long-lasting compromise or death. Treatments chosen depend on the severity of signs and symptoms, comorbidity, desired effects, side effects of each agent or intervention, and overall goals of patient and family.

Volume overload most often occurs in patients with oliguric failure unresponsive to cautious fluid challenge. The effectiveness of diuretics like mannitol or furosemide and vasodilators like low-dose dopamine to promote urine flow and to convert oliguric to nonoliguric failure in the early phase of ARF remains unsettled (57,65,66). Medications to correct other aspects of ARF (e.g., sodium bicarbonate for acidosis or urinary alkalinization) may promote volume overload and pulmonary edema. Oxygen should be used to counteract the hypoxia of pulmonary edema. Increasing venous capacitance with morphine sulfate and some other vasodilators may gain time in the most urgent cases of volume overload. Pulmonary edema requires correction with dialysis or hemofiltration unless rapidly resolved by more conservative measures.

In less urgent cases, restriction of salt (<2 g/day) and water (<1 L/day) intake as well as loop diuretics in nonoliguric failure protect patients from fluid overload. The gut also may be used to excrete fluid through the promotion of diarrhea with poorly reabsorbed carbohydrates like sorbitol or lactulose; as much as 4 to 5 L/day can be lost by these means, and [Na$^+$] is followed closely to help guide therapy.

Metabolic acidosis due to decreased acid excretion in PRF and rising acid production in hypercatabolism exerts multiple deleterious effects, e.g. changes in protein structure and function, such as hyperkalemia. Progressively acidotic patients may proceed through confusion to lethargy to coma and death. Cardiovascular effects include decreased cardiac contractility and vasodilation, which may lead to heart failure or hypotension (66a).

Acidosis can be controlled by oral or intravenous bicarbonate replacement to bring its concentration above 15 mEq/L. Monitoring protects patients from adverse consequences of bicarbonate loads, such as hypocalcemia, hypokalemia, alkalosis, and volume overload. In urgent cases, usually in conjunction with other metabolic offsets, acidosis requires dialysis (e.g., for $HCO_3$ less than 10 mEq/L or pH below 7.20) (67). In less severe acidosis, diets low in protein (~0.5 g/kg body weight/day) and high in carbohydrate (~100 g/day) diminish acid production (68).

Hyperkalemia is frequent in PRF of all causes, but its rapid accumulation in the ECF is especially threatening with tissue destruction (e.g., tumor lysis syndrome). Hyperkalemia and its treatment are best monitored with plasma levels and electrocardiographic (ECG) changes. At $[K^+]$ ~7 mEq/L high T-waves and depressed S-T segments occur, followed at $[K^+]$ ~8 mEq/L by intraventricular blocks and loss of P-waves (auricular standstill), which may lead to ventricular fibrillation (69).

Emergent correction of hyperkalemia involves intravenous infusion of calcium gluconate (10 ml of 10% solution over 2–5 minutes) to block life-threatening effects of $K^+$ on cardiac and neuromuscular systems. If ECG changes persist, another dose of calcium gluconate can be administered. Protection occurs within minutes but is not of long duration. Patients not responding rapidly to conservative treatment need hemodialysis. During preparation for dialysis, the following measures for immediate protection are carried out.

Treatment with calcium needs to be followed by longer-acting measures to decrease $K^+$ in ECF and then by removing excess $K^+$ from the body. $K^+$ movement from ECF to intracellular fluid (ICF) is promoted within 30 to 60 minutes by glucose (50 ml of 50% solution) with 10 units of regular insulin added. Bicarbonate (~45 mEq/ampule) can be given over 5 minutes intravenously and repeated in 15 minutes if needed. These maneuvers produce a decrease in $K^+$ of 1 to 2 mEq/L that lasts for hours.

For $[K^+]$ 5.5 to 6.5 mEq/L, less emergent and invasive procedures are effective in removing $K^+$. $K^+$-binding resins like Na-polystyrene sulfonate (15–30 g orally every 4–6 hours) promote intraluminal binding in the gut; resin is given with sorbitol (50–100 ml of 20% solution) to remove the slurry from the gastrointestinal tract. This procedure may be repeated every 4 to 6 hours. If patients cannot take or tolerate resin orally, 50 g of resin in 100 to 200 ml of water can be given as retention enemas. Once again, the use of resin may pose a threat to ECF volume as 1 to 2 mEq sodium replaces each mEq $K^+$. At $K^+$<5.5

mEq/L low $K^+$ diets, discontinuation of $K^+$-sparing diuretics, $K^+$-rich medications (e.g., $K^+$-penicillin, salt substitutes) and $K^+$ supplements usually suffice to protect patients.

Hypercalcemia (>14 mg/dl or 3.5 mM/L, corrected for albumin) is a common metabolic emergency in cancer patients (70–72); its incidence is as high as a third of myeloma patients with PRF (5). Of 50 patients seen for hypercalcemia in hospital setting, cancer was the cause in 41, half of these due to lung cancer (73). Myeloma patients with corrected serum $[Ca^{++}]$ >11.5 mg/dl had a significantly higher incidence of renal failure (49%) than those with lower $Ca^{++}$ levels (10%) (2).

Early presentation of hypercalcemia is often seen with a constellation of nonspecific complaints common in cancer patients: fatigue, lethargy, confusion, pain, anorexia, nausea, constipation. As many as 35% of hypercalcemic patients have more specific findings of polyuria and thirst. Patients with uncorrected progressive hypercalcemia become dehydrated and proceed to stupor, coma, and death. In the most severe cases of hypercalcemia associated with ARF, the ensemble of metabolic abnormalities usually requires dialysis.

When clinical status permits, hydration is the first step in treating hypercalcemia. Rehydration alone may reduce $[Ca^{++}]$ by 2.5 mg/dl. In patients tolerating hydration, 2 to 4 L/day of normal saline can be given intravenously or in some cases by hypodermoclysis for subcutaneous infusion of fluids (74). Adding a loop diuretic like furosemide promotes natriuresis and calciuresis. In milder cases, hydration loop diuretics suffice to correct the problem. (Thiazide diuretics promote $Ca^{++}$ reabsorption and are not used.)

In life-threatening hypercalcemia (>16 mg/dl), hydration must be supplemented by other agents. In addition to osteoclast inhibition, salmon calcitonin (4 U/kg every 12 hours up to 8 units/kg every 6 hours) promotes calciuresis more rapidly than other agents but its effect is relatively weak (~ 2 mg/dl) and not long lasting (nadir in 12–24 hours). Bisphosphonates (e.g., etidronate, clodronate, and pamidronate) block $Ca^{++}$ release from bone and are effective in 60% to 100% patients in a dose-dependent fashion. The most rapid protocol involves a single dose of 60 to 90 mg of pamidronate infused intravenously over a day. More than 95% patients receiving 90 mg of pamidronate administered intravenously regain eucalcemia. Intravenous biphosphonates are followed by oral doses (etidronate) to control $Ca^{++}$ levels often for weeks. Intraveous biphosphonates can be repeated if hypercalcemia recurs. For $[Ca^{++}]$ >3.5 mM/L, a combination of subcutaneous calcitonin and intravenous pamidronate is particularly effective. If objections are raised to intravenous medications, subcutaneous calcitonin and oral biphosphonates may be helpful although not as effective (71).

Successful treatment of underlying disease is the best approach to normocalcemia. In cancer patients, hypercalcemia is often a late manifestation of disease, and this ideal often is not reached (72). In multiple myeloma, hypercalcemia often presents early and is an exception to this generality. Its correction and treatment of the underlying malignancy with chemotherapy±plasmapheresis are associated with improved quality of life and survival.

Hyperuricemia above 15 mg/dl in cancer patients is primarily the result of tumor lysis syndrome. In one series of 43 patients with hematologic tumors, 26% were dialyzed for tumor lysis syndrome (10). Tumor lysis syndrome can occur and should be sought in patients before therapy.

Diagnosis of acute uric acid nephropathy in tumor lysis syndrome is suggested by appropriate history, plasma (uric acid) levels above 15 mg/dl (usually <12 mg/dl in other forms of uncomplicated renal failure), hypocalcemia, and elevation of $K^+$, phosphates, and LDH. Urinary amorphous or crystalline urates are not diagnostic (75). At uric acid levels above 20 mg/dl, crystals form in the acidic and concentrated medullary tissue. Resultant obstruction and inflammation promote renal failure. Sludge of uric acid crystals and amorphous material in the pelvis and ureters may add a postrenal component.

Treatment consists of vigorous intravenous hydration and, in patients not already hyperphosphatemic, urinary alkalinization. Alkalinization must be avoided in hyperphosphatemic patients because alkaline urine favors nephrocalcinosis and creates or worsens failure. Even without sodium bicarbonate or acetazolamide, hydration may produce fluid overload, especially in oliguric renal failure. In such cases, hemodialysis is necessary, sometimes on a daily basis. Peritoneal dialysis clears urate too slowly.

Prevention of hyperuricemia and other metabolic problems in tumor lysis syndrome is preferable to treatment whenever possible. Prevention includes allopurinol (600–900 mg/day) and brisk diuresis (2.5–3 L/day if possible) with bicarbonate-enriched fluids and loop diuretics a day or more (in patients not hyperphosphatemic) before starting chemotherapy and the same period after finishing therapy. Thiazide diuretics promote urate reabsorption and are not used.

Hyperphosphatemia (>5 mg/dl or >1.67 mM/L), like hyperuricemia, is particularly threatening in tumor lysis syndrome. Not only is it associated with nephrocalcinosis, but concomitantly lowered [$Ca^{++}$] may present problems in neuromuscular, cardiac, and central nervous system function. In severe cases, usually associated with other metabolic problems, hyperphosphatemia requires dialysis.

Mild to moderate elevations of serum phosphate concentrations are commonly found in PRF as a result of decreased renal phosphate clearance and increased release of cellular phosphates in acidosis. In these conditions, hyperphosphatemia usually is controlled by phosphate-binding antacids [e.g., aluminum hydroxide ($Al(OH)_3$)], by dietary reduction (including parenteral phosphate) and by avoidance of phosphate-rich enemas (e.g., Fleet enemas).

Infection in many patients precipitates PRF (47,60), exacerbates established RF (39), and disfavors recovery of renal function (47). Sepsis in patients with ARF is associated with increased mortality in some studies (5–7, 10,43,51,60) but not all (3,46). In one study, two thirds of deaths with sepsis and ARF occurred in patients already infected at first detection of ARF (76). Insults to body integrity are superimposed on the compromised immune system in renal failure by urinary catheters, intravascular devices, and intubation. Aseptic conditions must be used in the placement, maintenance, and replacement of these devices. During workup of a serious suspicion of infection, one should begin treatment with antibiotics, chosen to minimize further renal damage and adjusted for ARF and its concurrent therapies (e.g., dialysis).

Some antibiotics can complicate PRF. For example, penicillin G promotes seizure activity, whereas $K^+$ penicillin contributes to hyperkalemia (3 mEq/million units). Trimethoprim, cefoxitin, and cefotetan may cause spuriously high creatinine levels. Tetracyclines may promote uremia through their effects on protein metabolism. Antibiotics dependent on glomerular filtration and tubular secretion (e.g., penicillins, cephalosporins, trimethoprim, and sulfonamides) achieve higher tissue and urine concentrations than those dependent on glomerular filtration alone (e.g., aminoglycosides) (77). Some antibiotics, such as penicillins, cephalosporins, and sulfonadmides, often are associated with allergic interstitial nephritis.

Nutritional support is provided to patients with PRF in partial compensation for protein catabolism, decreased intake, and nutrient loss. Despite the many reasons aggressive nutritional supplementation should promote greater well-being and quicker healing in these patients, clinical studies have not consistently shown better return of renal function and longer patient survival (57,78–81).

Caloric supplementation, protein sparing, and control of ketosis are managed primarily with glucose (~100 g/day) and lipids. To minimize azotemia and to optimize needed protein synthesis, protein supplementation is limited (~0.5 g/kg body weight/day) and uses proteins with a high ratio of essential amino acids/total amino acids. Nitrogen balance studies guide amino acid and protein supplementation. Nutritional needs can vary greatly according to the degree of hypercatabolism, which may be as high as 40% above basal rates in cancer patients with sepsis and multiple organ failure (68,80,82,83).

For complicated patients in ICUs, nutritional supplements should start within 48 to 72 hours. All patients not expected to receive adequate calories by usual means within 5 to 6 days of PRF should start nutritional supplements. Enteral routes are preferred for physiological reasons, immune support, quality of life, decreased infection, and economy. In many cases, dialysis may facilitate nutritional supplementation but at the same time imposes an additional route for nutrient loss needing replacement. Nutritional supplementation entails additional risks, such as electrolyte and acid-base imbalances, and may require more intensive dialysis for control of volume and of increased uremia.

For optimal nutritional support, the managing physician needs collaboration with a nephrologist, a nutritionist, pharmacists, and nurses.

Hematologic problems in PRF include anemia and coagulation problems. Anemia, which is common even in early PRF (12), often has several causes, such as bleeding, blood loss through dialysis or surgery, and diminished erythropoietin synthesis in damaged kidneys. Repletion occurs through hemostasis and transfusions.

Gastrointestinal bleeding occurs in up to a third of patients, usually due to stress ulcers, and it is usually mild. Its role in mortality has decreased with improved prophylaxis and therapy, specifically $H_2$ blockers, sucralfate, and antacids like $Al(OH)_3$ and $CaCO_3$ (48). (Antacids containing magnesium should be avoided because of its accumulation in renal failure). One complication of antacid use is that a more alkaline gastric mucosa favors bacterial growth. Sucralfate suppresses gastric acidity less than the other agents and in one study of ventilated ICU patients was associated with fewer late-developing pneumonias than ranitidine or antacid (84).

Coagulation problems in uremic patients result primarily from platelet dysfunction but also from coagulation factor abnormalities (e.g., von Willebrand factor) and thrombocytopenia (56,85). Dialysis corrects the problem in some but not all patients, but anticoagulation during dialysis may cause additional problems in some patients. Coagulation is usually measured as bleeding time (normally 6–9 minutes); risk of hemorrhage occurs at higher values, especially beyond 10 to 15 minutes. Temporary or partical correction of coagulopathy in preparation for invasive procedures like renal biopsy can be effected by several means, including infusion of cryoprecipitate (86), synthetic vasopressin DDAVP (1-deamino-8-D-arginine vasopressin) (87,88), and infused or oral estrogens (89).

Uremic encephalopathy, as with many clinical consequences of uremia, shows great variations among patients but is generally worse when developing rapidly. Anorexia, insomnia, and restlessness characterize the first phase along with decreased attention and mentation. In untreated encephalopathy, emotional lability, further decreased ability to think, vomiting, and lethargy follow. The most severe consequences are agitated confusion, dysarthria, and bizarre behavior proceeding to stupor, coma, and death (90). Convulsions appear in this phase; in two early studies (12,91), the incidence of seizures varied from 5% to 38%.

The differential diagnosis of such neurologic changes includes other metabolic disorders, such as liver dysfunction and medication-induced changes in neurologic function (e.g., confusion associated with some benzodiazepines or NSAIDs). Meperidine metabolites, penicillins, and theophylline all have been associated with seizures.

Quiet surroundings, reassurance, and reorientation by a small number of familiar caregivers help patients in the early stages of uremic encephalopathy; however, medication is often needed. Many psychotropic medications (see below) can be given relatively safely to patients with renal failure; however, dosing regimens must be monitored and individualized to effect (61,92,93). Advancing neurologic symptoms argue strongly for initiation of dialysis in appropriate patients.

Many drugs and their administration, including antineoplastic medications (94,95), are seriously affected by PRF and its therapies. Manuals and reviews exist to guide dose and schedule modification (40,62,63) in patients in renal failure, treated without or with various forms of hemofiltration or dialysis. Use of analgesics and psychotropics in endstage PRF is discussed below.

Because serum creatinine levels lag behind renal function in developing ARF, Golper and Bennett (77) recommend dosage guidelines with assumed creatinine clearance <10 ml/h) in patients with declining renal function. During the recovery phase, underdosing may occur as a result of similar offset between serum creatinine and renal function. An additional pitfall in recovery is that rising urine flow rates may incorrectly be assumed to correspond with increasing creatinine clearance, which should continue to be measured (77).

### Dialysis

With progressive uncontrolled PRF, dialysis in cancer patients is used (a) urgently to correct signs and symptoms of uremia and (b) prophylactically to protect patients from development or exacerbation of uremia. In patients with or at risk of fluid overload, dialysis can "make room" for other therapies, such as fluid loads of nutrition and intravenous medications.

Although the criteria for urgent dialysis are individualized and vary among nephrologists, the following figures are in keeping with frequently used criteria (3,10,43,46, 67,96): (a) progressive hyperkalemia, e.g., $[K^+]$ 6 to 6.5 mEq/L with ECG changes if not responding rapidly to conservative therapy; (b) severe acidosis with $[HCO_3]$ below 10 mEq/L and pH less than 7.20; (c) volume overload with oliguria, pulmonary edema, congestive heart failure, or hypertension resistant to nondialytic therapy; (d) azotemia, generally blood urea nitrogen levels of 80 to 120 mg/dl and creatinine levels of 8 to mg/dl. Dialysis is begun at lower levels in the presence of threatening uremic signs and symptoms like pericarditis, encephalopathy, hemorrhage, or vomiting. Rapid development of uremia favors these signs and symptoms.

In tumor lysis syndrome, hyperuricemia, hyperkalemia, and hyperphosphatemia with symptomatic hypocalcemia, may prompt initiation of dialysis, as hypercalcemia may in multiple myeloma. Once a patient is stabilized, hemodialysis in general practice is used every other day with the same target blood urea nitrogen levels of 100 to 120 mg/dl (69). In some urgent cases, daily dialysis is needed, such as early in a patient's course with volume overload, hypercatabolism, and ongoing tumor lysis syndrome.

### Different Kinds of Dialysis

Techniques for emergent renal replacement in PRF include hemodialysis, peritoneal dialysis, and slow continuous techniques of ultrafiltration, hemofiltration, and hemodialysis (97–100). Different techniques may be used sequentially in a patient, for example, for maintenance therapy after emergent correction.

Hemodialysis is an episodic, efficient means of altering composition and volume of ECF. In acutely catabolic patients or in patients with life-threatening volume overload or changes in ECF composition, it is often the method of choice; however, this technique is associated with rapid shifts in electrolytes and favors cardiac arrhythmias or hypotension. It is poorly tolerated in patients with cardiovascular instability or multiorgan system failure. Such cardiovascular problems are found in 25% to 50% of hemodialysis patients (97).

Techniques to minimize risks of anticoagulation in hemodialysis include regional anticoagulation in the extracorporeal circuit, use of low-molecular-weight heparin, "tight heparinization," and heparin-free dialysis (99,101).

Peritoneal dialysis produces more gradual changes in volume and composition of ECF than hemodialysis does. Some larger-molecular-weight compounds (e.g., uric acid) are poorly cleared in peritoneal dialysis. Others like $K^+$ are cleared easily but more slowly and continuously, with resultant $K^+$ clearances comparable to those in hemodialysis (once emergent hyperkalemia has been controlled by hemodialysis). In less urgent situations or in patients with hemodynamic instability, peritoneal dialysis may be the method of choice. Recent abdominal surgery or the presence of adhesions mitigate against use of peritoneal dialysis, as do abdominal vascular grafts, which can be infected during bouts of peritonitis (97,98).

Slow continuous techniques (100), also called *continuous renal replacement therapies* (99), involve dialysis, filtration, or ultrafiltration. They offer the advantages of hemodynamic stability coupled with control of ECF volume and composition in cancer patients with multiple problems, including cardiovascular instability, hypercatabolism, and the need for large volumes of fluids (e.g., medication and nutrition). These therapies, however, require indwelling intravascular cathers and intensive nursing care for the length of the procedure. Like hemodialysis, anticoagulation also may complicate its use, although approaches to coagulation problems in hemodialysis are being extended to slow, continuous therapies as well (85,100,101).

### Outcomes

Most patients with ARF either respond to dialysis or die within a month or two of its initiation (2,10,24,29,39, 46). What information exists about outcomes in cancer patients undergoing dialysis? As reviewed in the following section, survival is poor in this population, often elderly, often with significant comorbidity and complications. Most reports describe PRF in ICUs, the setting for many cancer patients with PRF, as part of multisystem organ failure. In contrast, patients with isolated ARF have a mortality rate below 10% (1,102).

In studies of cancer patients who underwent dialysis from 1956 through 1993 (5–10,22,29,30,34,43,103,104), mortality among cancer patients ranged from 9% (34) to 100% (22,43); average mortality for these studies (n= 588) was 62%. In series with malignant and nonmalignant causes of renal failure (6,8,22,30,43), overall mortality was 49% among all patients (n=1,676) with ARF but without cancer. Case mix and differing definitions of renal failure make these estimates very "soft" and statistical comparisons inappropriate.

Fewer pediatric studies exist. Among 138 children with ARF, six of 14 with malignancy-related ARF died (105). Among dialyzed pediatric recipients of bone marrow transplants, 23 of 30 patients (77%) died without renal recovery in fewer than 72 days (mean 12 days) after starting dialysis (106). In contrast, of 486 pediatric patients undergoing bone marrow transplant, only three of 70 deaths occurring in the first 100 days posttransplant were due to ARF (107).

Among survivors of ARF, most live without dialysis, although many have renal insufficiency (108). Reports of those requiring chronic dialysis range from none to nearly a third (8,9,31,32,34,39,109). In one survey, nearly 10% of patients starting dialysis for end-stage renal failure had cancer, and they were more likely to withdraw from dialysis than those without cancer (110). In a survey of 1,309 patients referred for dialysis with end-stage renal disease (ESRD) due to malignancy, the median survival for those with multiple myeloma was about a year and for those with renal cell carcinoma or amyloidosis, about 15 to 20 months (111). Among 234,296 patients entering treatment for ESRD from 1989 through 1992, 1.3% had malignant causes for renal failure. (This number includes primarily patients with multiple myeloma and renal cell carcinoma and a few patients with lymphoma; it excludes patients with amyloidosis and urate nephropathy, some of whom may have had underlying malignancy.) Nearly a third of these patients died within the first year of treatment, a rate surpassed only by acquired immunodeficiency syndrome (AIDS) patients with ESRD (112).

Primary renal failure is commonly encountered early in multiple myeloma, and about half of patients in PRF respond to dialysis (2,5,29) with reversal of renal failure.

In one study of 484 patients, of whom only 18% needed treatment for PRF, response to treatment (chemotherapy± plasmapheresis) for underlying myeloma, not renal function, was the major determinant of survival (2). In two other studies of patients with both PRF and multiple myeloma, survival was longer in patients with good reversal of PRF (5,29), although response to therapy for myeloma was the major determinant of survival time (29). Of myeloma patients, 19% (2,29) survived for months on chronic dialysis. In a study of 23 myeloma patients on chronic dialysis, 1-year actuarial survival was 45%, and about 25% survived longer than 2 years (104).

*Making Decisions About Dialysis*

What response can we have when faced with population data on one hand and an individual cancer patient with PRF on the other? For at least one author, a diagnosis of cancer should not automatically exclude possible dialysis (113); and for some no diagnosis should rule out a trial of dialysis (114). Others cite concerns for cost, limited resources, and individual clinical circumstances in hesitating to initiate dialysis (8,103,115,116).

Many authors emphasize physiological limitations and would exclude dialysis for patients with preexistent poor quality of life or short life-expectancy, for example, those with nonuremic dementia or other irreversible neurologic disease, patients with end-stage liver, cardiovascular, or lung disease limiting the activities of daily living, as well as patients with multisystem failure. Some would specifically not treat or continue dialysis for patients with metastatic or nonresectable solid tumor or hematologic tumors refactory to treatment (115), especially with an expected survival of less than 2 years (117). Other authors state clearly that diagnosis of neoplasm is less prejudicial against dialysis (104,113). In myeloma, PRF often occurs early, before response to antineoplastic therapy is known; and many would agree that dialysis in most of these patients is reasonable (104). Sobel et al. (116) favor dialysis for patients with compensated renal disease, a projected survival of longer than 2 months (e.g., based in part on a Karnofsky index of ≥50%) and an acceptable quality of life. In turning down 25% of 73 dialysis candidates with nonmalignant disease for poor quality of life or a prognosis limited by comorbidity, the physicians encountered no requests for second opinions from patients, families, or referring physicians; and no legal actions occurred (115). Acquiescence by patient and family to treatment denial in more acute settings is likely to be less uniform.

In a cancer patient with PRF, concerned physicians must balance factors for and against dialysis: (a) desires of patient and family concerning treatment; (b) the patient's "baseline" state before PRF and likelihood of tolerating and benefiting from dialysis; (c) the probable course of underlying malignancy and its response to ther-apy. Clearly stated clinical goals, including a timetable for reconsidering of dialysis, should be accepted by patient and family before dialysis begins.

This task is difficult. First, a patient's choice is not fixed or immune to education and experience. Estimation of a patient's baseline state involves not only evaluation of tumor, its stage, and its predicted response to planned therapy but also a patient's comorbidities, performance status, and psychosocial issues, all of which are difficult to quantitate or predict. Some objective criteria do exist, such as Karnofsky and East Coast Oncology Group (ECOG) indices, as well as survival data indexed for a various clinical parameters (52,118). Recent studies present prognostic models for survival and functional status for a closely defined population of seriously ill hospitalized patients (118,119).

Finally, if the situation permits, and it often does not, patient and family may need time to consider options and to ask for further guidance from the physician and other caregivers. In any event, timely decisions must be made. The absence of consensus among patient and family and caregivers presents great problems. Empathy, identification of crucial differences in styles and content, and in some cases legal constraints may help resolve these difficult problems (120).

## CARE OF CANCER PATIENTS DYING OF RENAL FAILURE

When decisions have been made to forgo further curative treatment, the focus of care shifts for cancer patients dying of PRF. Care is directed to alleviation of suffering and to a death as dignified as possible, not to cure of underlying disease(s). Support through the terminal phase often intensifies the interdisciplinary quality (26) of care and involves caregivers from nursing, medical, social work, pastoral fields, and volunteers. In this final phase, a realignment of responsibilities and involvement may occur among the different caregivers. Often nurses and members of the allied services play a more dominant role, although this does not mean physicians should no longer participate in the planning and delivery of care. Doctors who disappear at this time may create or intensify a sense of abandonment and despair in the patient and family. Support, including education, continues to be given directly to patients and also to families and friends; but the content often expands to include more frankly spiritual concerns about dying, death, and grief.

Many signs and symptoms and their treatment in cancer patients have been dealt with in other chapters in this book, such as pain, confusion, and other signs and symptoms of uremic encephalopathy, anxiety, myoclonus, hemorrhage, thirst, and hunger, outside the context of ESRD. The remainder of this chapter concerns two issues: adjustment of analgesic and psychotropic medications in ESRD and discussion of a "good" renal death.

Use of medication in cancer patients with renal failure is guided by several considerations:

1. Significant interindividual variations in pharmacologic parameters and subjective response occur for many drugs in patients with normal renal function. In patients with ESRD, the situation is further complicated by changes in fluid compartment size, reduction or loss of renal metaboslism, effects of uremic toxins on other physiologic systems, and changes in plasma binding. In any event, medication regimens must be tailored to each patient's responses.

2. Medication regimens must be kept as simple as possible to optimize the patient's quality of life.

3. Interventions should be used that are as minimally invasive and disturbing to patients as possible. In some cases, this means increased use of transdermal, rectal, or buccal routes to minimize injections to patients who are no longer able to take oral medication. Subcutaneous injections are often used because they are less painful than intramuscular injections and less likely to produce painful intramuscular hematomas. Pump-driven subcutaneous delivery is a comfortable alternative. In patients electing not to continue dialysis, retention of a central line may in fact be helpful in maintaining an intravenous route for medication.

4. Sedation is considered desirable by and for most patients at the end of their lives but not for all patients. One must ask to know.

5. Most terminally ill patients do not want to have blood drawn frequently to check drug levels; medications with wide therapeutic ranges are helpful.

6. Dosage adjustments for patients usually become less important at the very end of life, so long as patients' comfort is not compromised by risks incurred. For obvious reasons, therapeutic preferences and related issues are best discussed with competent patients before discontinuation of dialysis.

Analgesia is needed for most cancer patients at some time in their illnesses, especially in later phases. A recent study shows that it is not achieved in an important fraction of seriously ill patients, even when additional help is available to physicians (121).

Morphine sulfate (MO) is the most frequently used strong opiate, although in many situations other strong opiates may be as effective and offer other advantages. MO is glucuronidated in the liver; of the two resultant glucuronides, morphine-6-glucuronide (M6G) shares with MO analgesic properties, but it depends more on renal excretion than the parent compound. The question has arisen whether accumulation of M6G in renal failure places patients at risk for significant adverse effects of opiates (e.g., respiratory depression, nausea, myoclonus, cognitive deficits, and obtundation). A series of case reports and small series suggest that the answer is yes (122–124). A study of 109 cancer patients with creatinine levels below 0.5 to 8 mg/dl did not show that increased M6G/MO ratios were significantly associated with myoclonus or decreased cognitive function in these patients; however, M6G concentrations above 2,000 ng/ml in the presence of other metabolic abnormalities (elevated LDH and bilirubin) were associated with respiratory depression or obtundation in a small number of patients (28). More studies like this one will help refine the relationship of opiates and unwanted side effects in patients with renal failure.

Information on the effects of metabolite accumulation for other opiates in renal failure is scanty or nonexistent. Some information suggests that metabolites of hydromorphone (Dilaudid) may accumulate in patients with renal failure (125). Normeperidine, a metabolite of meperidine (Demerol), accumulates in renal failure and facilitates seizures; for this reason, meperidine should not be used in patients with PRF. Among weaker opiates, codeine metabolites show some accumulation in patients in renal failure. Even in a single volume, recommendations vary: One author (93) recommends no adjustment in codeine dosing, whereas another (61) recommends the reductions cited below. Obviously, in each patient, clinical assessment of desired and side effects with consequent adjustment is required.

Analgesia must be provided to patients in pain as long as they desire it. It is suggested that patients with creatinine clearances of 10 to 50 ml/min receive a 25% reduction in doses of morphine or codeine and that those with creatinine clearances below 10 ml/min receive 50% reduction in morphine and codeine doses (61,62). These dose reductions are initial estimates; each patient must be titrated individually for optimal combination of good analgesia and tolerable side effects. Trials of alternative opiates with adjustment for partial cross tolerance can be helpful. Risks of "second effect," i.e., of side effects, such as respiratory depression or sedation hastening death, must be understood and accepted by the patient and family.

Analgesia for neuropathic pain may involve tricyclic antidepressants, anticonvulsants, and other agents (e.g., clonidine). Nortriptyline, a tricyclic antidepressant with fewer anticholinergic side effects and a wider therapeutic window than amitriptyline (92), is used for dull, burning dysesthesias. It can be continued without dose adjustment as long as the patient can take oral medication (61,62). Unadjusted dosing is recommended by some authors (61, 126) for carbamazepine, an anticonvulsant used for lancinating neuropathic pain, whereas others recommend as much as a 25% reduction in ESRD (62,127). Phenytoin may be used as coanalgesic for neuropathic pain.

Some cancer patients with intractable pain, especially neuropathic pain, have received relief with epidural clonidine (128). The medication undergoes significant renal metabolism, can cause sedation and hypotension, and interacts with other medications often used for cancer patients (e.g., tricyclic antidepressants, barbiturates, and other sedatives). However, in transdermal form, it also has been effective in a subpopulation of patients with diabetic neuropathy (129). This route makes it attractive for use in dying patients, although studies of its use in patients dying of ESRD are lacking. In patients with neuropathic pain poorly controlled with other medications, cautious use may be undertaken if patient and family accept the risk.

Calcitonin and biphosphonates may be helpful in combating pain due to bony metastases (71,130) and can be administered by either intravenous and oral routes. Data on this use in patients in renal failure are lacking, but intravenous biphosphonates require small fluid loads and, of little importance here, some may worsen azotemia. For bony pain, NSAIDs may become more relevant in the terminal phase; however, exacerbation of uremic gastritis is a risk in patients with increased bleeding times, even with protection of the gastric mucosa. The same risk occurs with the oral or subcutaneous use of corticosteroids for bony pain, although in some orchidectomized patients with prostate carcinoma, small doses (1–2 mg twice a day) of Decadron may offer good analgesia with reduced risk of side effects. The combination of NSAIDs and corticosteroids should be avoided. $H_2$ blockade is given orally or intravenously in reduced doses for patients with renal failure (61,62). Strontium[89] for bony pain is largely excreted by the kidneys and has too long an interval between administration and analgesia to be useful in dying patients (71).

Phenytoin and phenobarbital are the primary anticonvulsants in terminal patients with ESRD (126). Phenobarbital has a wide therapeutic range and can be given by several routes: orally, intravenously, or intramuscularly; in ESRD it should be started at 75% of its usual range and adjusted. Less sedating than phenobarbital, phenytoin can be given either orally or intravenously. In ESRD it has a lower and narrower therapeutic range than in patients with normal renal function as a result of decreased protein binding. Like these two anticonvulsants, carbamazepine is effective for tonic-clonic as well as for the less frequent partial and complex partial seizures; however, it can be given only orally.

Benzodiazepines are used as anxiolytics and in treating myoclonus; in general, they have a high therapeutic/toxic ratio (92). Benzodiazepines with shorter half-lives and no clinically active metabolites (e.g., lorazepam, clonazepam, oxazepam, and temazepam) are preferred to diazepam with its longer half-life and many active metabolites dependent on renal excretion. These medications undergo primarily hepatic excretion, but a two-thirds reduction is appropriate on grounds of clinical experience (131).

Midazolam, a benzodiazepine with a short half-life, administered intravenously or subcutaneously, is particularly helpful in patients with myoclonus (especially common in patients with renal failure), anxiety, and terminal agitation. Recommended doses vary among physicians (132,133); in severe renal failure, 50% normal doses are used (62). For patients with multifocal myoclonus, an initial dose of 5 to 10 mg subcutaneously every hour is recommended until myoclonus is controlled, followed by continuous subcutaneous or intravenous doses. The same approach and initial dose may be used for moribund patients with grand mal seizures (134). These doses are used for patients without ESRD; starting with lower doses (see above) and titration for desired effects seems appropriate in patients with minimal renal function.

Among drugs to treat confusion, haloperidol and other high-potency antipsychotics have a greater propensity to promote seizures. Chlorpromazine and other low potency antipsychotics have sedating side effects and may be associated with hypotension, both side effects in terminally ill patients that are more acceptable than agitated confusion or seizures. These medications undergo extensive hepatic metabolism. Haloperidol can be given without dose adjustment (62). Recommendations for adjusted chlorpromazine dosing in ESRD vary from suggested avoidance (61) to no changes (62).

*A Good Death in Renal Failure*

Many caregivers have clear ideas and strong feelings about what characterizes acceptable or peaceful death, a good death for their patients; but explicit definition of criteria and their application in actual patients dying of renal failure is rarely published. An interdisciplinary team (two psychiatrists, one nephrologist, one geriatrician, and one social worker) recently published such a study of patients with ESRD of nonmalignant cause withdrawing from chronic dialysis (135). They constructed a quantitative scale measuring the quality of death from three components: (a) duration of dying after stopping dialysis; (b) presence of physical suffering; (c) consideration of psychosocial issues (e.g., decision-making process, level of awareness, involvement of family and friends). The category of "good death" included seven of 11 prospectively studied patients. The remaining four patients' courses after discontinuation of dialysis were compromised by "varying degrees of pain, confusion, agitation, social unrest, and a longer than average survival." Of the four "bad" deaths, the decision to discontinue dialysis was due to acute medical or surgical crisis (e.g., diagnosis of metastatic cancer), to lack of overall improvement on dialysis, or to technical or logistic reasons.

Eight of 11 patients had at least some pain in their final days despite use of analgesics in seven. None required ultrafiltration for pulmonary edema. The authors note the important help of the local hospice program in providing psychosocial and technical support to patients and families.

The number of patients in the study was small and evaluation of the three major components inevitably subjective, but this work suggests that further study to characterize the quality of dying in renal patients will provide needed information and insight into ways we can promote peaceful deaths for them. This is turn helps us accomplish the goals of providing support and comfort to terminally ill patients in our care.

## A NOTE ON RESEARCH

Finally, as observed by others, current research in nephrology suggests improved management and, in some cases, better outcomes for patients with renal failure through (a) extension of quantitative scoring of critically ill patients into outcome prediction for patients with ARF (52); (b) further development of continuous filtration techniques in control of ARF (99,136); (c) expanded use of biocompatible dialysis membranes (137,138); (d) improved dialysis prescriptions (139,140); and (e) further development of the application of biotechnology, such as improved reepithelialization of damaged renal tubules with growth factors (108,141).

## REFERENCES

1. Cameron JS. Acute renal failure—the continuing challenge. *QJM* 1986;59:337.
2. Alexanian R, Barlogie B, Dixon D. Renal failure in multiple myeloma: pathogenesis and prognostic implications. *Arch Intern Med* 1990; 150:1693.
3. Bullock ML, Umen AJ, Finkelstein M, Keane WF. The assessment of risk factors in 462 patients with acute renal failure. *Am J Kidney Dis* 1985;5:97.
4. Kaufman J, Dhakal M, Patel B, Hamburger R. Community-acquired acute renal failure. *Am J Kidney Dis* 1991;17:191.
5. Pozzi C, Pasquali S, Donini U, Casanova S, Banfi G, Tiraboschi G, Furci L et al. Prognostic factors and effectiveness of treatment in acute renal failure due to multiple myeloma: a review of 50 cases. *Clin Nephrol* 1988;29:1.
6. Beaman M, Turney JH, Rodger RSC, McGonigle RSJ, Adu D, Michael J. Changing pattern of acute renal failure. *QJM* 1987;62:15.
7. Turney JH, Marshall SH, Brownjohn AM, Ellis CM, Parsons FM. The evolution of acute renal failure. *QJM* 1990;74:83.
8. Chertow GM, Christiansen CL, Clearly PD, et al. Prognostic stratification in critically ill patients with acute renal failure requiring dialysis. *Arch Intern Med* 1995;155:1505.
9. Kone BC, Whelton A, Santos G, Saral R, Watson AJ. Hypertension and renal dysfunction in bone marrow transplant recipients. *QJM* 1988;69:985.
10. Lanore JJ, Brunet F, Pochard F, et al. Hemodialysis for acute renal failure in patients with hematologic malignancies. *Crit Care Med* 1991; 19:346.
11. Levy EM, Viscoli CM, Horwitz RI. The effect of acute renal failure on mortality: a cohort analysis. *JAMA* 1996;275:1489.
12. Swann RC, Merrill JP. The clinical course of acute renal failure. *Medicine* 1953;32:215.
13. Benabe JE, Martinez-Maldonado M. Tubulo-interstitial nephritis associated with systemic disease and electrolyte abnormalities. *Semin Nephrol* 1988;8:29.
14. Cobos E, Hall RR. Effects of chemotherapy on the kidney. *Semin Nephrol* 1993;13:297.
15. Dafnis EK, Laski ME. Fluid and electrolyte abnormalities in the oncology patient. *Semin Nephrol* 1993;13:281.
16. Fer MF, McKinney TD, Richardson RL, Hande KR, Oldham RK, Greco FA. Cancer and the kidney: renal complications of neoplasms. *Am J Med* 1981;71:704.
17. Flombaum CD. Electrolyte and renal abnormalities in the cancer patient. In: Howland WS, Carlon GC, eds. *Critical care of the cancer patient*. Chicago: Yearbook Medical Publishers, 1985;114.
18. Garnick MB. Urologic complications. In: Holland JF, Frei E III, Bart RC Jr, Kufe DW, Morton DL, Weichselbaum RR, eds. *Cancer medicine*. 3rd ed. Philadelphia: Lea & Febiger, 1993;2323.
19. Garnick MB, Mayer RJ, Abelson HT. Acute renal failure associated with cancer treatment. In: Brenner BM, Lazarus JM, eds. *Acute renal failure*. 2nd ed. New York: Churchill Livingstone, 1988;621.
20. Norris SH. Paraneoplastic glomerulopathies. *Semin Nephrol* 1993; 13:258.
21. Ponticelli C. Oncology and the kidney. In: Cameron S, Davison AM, Grunfeld J-P, Ritz E, eds. *Oxford textbook of clinical nephrology*. Oxford: Oxford University Press, 1992;2316.
22. Abreo K, Moorthy V, Osborne M. Changing patterns and outcome of acute renal failure requiring hemodialysis. *Arch Intern Med* 1986; 146:1338.
23. Turney JH. Acute renal failure—a dangerous condition. *JAMA* 1996; 275:1516.
24. Frost L, Pedersen RS, Bentzen S, Bille H, Hansen HE. Short and long term outcome in a consecutive series of 419 patients with acute dialysis-requiring renal failure. *Scand J Urol Nephrol* 1993;27:453.
25. Turney JH. Acute renal failure—some progress? *N Engl J Med* 1994; 331:1372.
26. Kedziera P, Levy MH. Collaborative practice in oncology. *Semin Oncol* 1994;21:705.
27. Levy MH. Supportive oncology: forward. *Semin Oncol* 1994;21:699.
28. Tiseo PJ, Thaler HT, Lapin J, Inturrisi CE, Portenoy RK, Foley KM. Morphine-6-glucuronide concentrations and opioid-related side effects: a survey in cancer patients. *Pain* 1995;61:47.
29. Ganeval D, Rabian C, Guerin V, Pertuiset N, Landais P, Jungeres P. Treatment of multiple myeloma with renal involvement. *Adv Nephrol* 1992;21:347.
30. Zager RA, O'Quigley J, Zager BK et al. Acute renal failure following bone marrow transplantation: a retrospective study of 272 patients. *Am J Kidney Dis* 1989;13:210.
31. Hou SH, Bushinsky DA, Wish JB, Cohen JJ, Harrington JT. Hospital-acquired renal insufficiency: a prospective study. *Am J Med* 1983: 74:243.
32. Rasmussen HH, Ibels LS. Acute renal failure. Multivariate analysis of causes and risk factors. *Am J Med* 1982;73:211.
33. Groeneveld ABJ, Tran DD, van der Meulen J, Nauta JJP, Thijs LG. Acute renal failure in the medical intensive care unit: predisposing, complicating factors and outcome. *Nephron* 1991;59:602.
34. Campbell SC, Novick AC, Streen SB, Klein E, Licht M. Complications of nephron sparing surgery for renal tumors. *J Urol* 1994; 151:1177.
35. Brodsky GL, Garnick MB. Renal tumors in the adult patient. In: Tisher CC, Brenner BM, eds. *Renal pathology with clinical and functional correlations*. 2nd ed. Philadelphia: JP Lippincott, 1994;1540.
36. Martinez-Vea A, Panisello JM, Garcia C et al. Minimal-change glomerulopathy and carcinoma. Report of two cases and review of the literature. *Am J Nephrol* 1993;13:69.
37. Davidman M, Olson P, Koehn J, Leither T, Kjellstrand C. Iatrogenic renal disease. *Arch Intern Med* 1991;151:1809.
38. Shusterman N, Strom BL, Murray TG, Morrison G, West SZ, Maislin G. Risk factors and outcome of hospital-acquired acute renal failure: a clinical epidemiologic study. *Am J Med* 1987;83:65.
39. Spurney RF, Fulkerson WJ, Schwab SJ. Acute renal failure in critically ill patients: prognosis for recovery of kidney function after prolonged dialysis support. *Crit Care Med* 1991;19:8.
40. Swan SK, Bennett WM. Nephrotoxic acute renal failure. In: Lazarus JM, Brenner BM, eds. *Acute renal failure*. 3rd ed. New York: Churchill Livingstone, 1993;357.
41. Barrett BJ, Carlisle EJ. Metaanalysis of the relative nephrotoxicity of high- and low-osmolality iodinated contrast media. *Radiology* 1993; 188:171.
42. Solomon R, Werner C, Mann D, D'Elia J, Silva P. Effects of saline, mannitol, and furosemide on acute decreases in renal function induced by radiocontrast agents. *N Engl J Med* 1994;331:1416.
43. Lohr JW, McFarlane MJ, Grantham JJ. A clinical index to predict survival in acute renal failure patients requiring dialysis. *Am J Kidney Dis* 1988;11:254.
44. Zager RA. Acute renal failure in the setting of bone marrow transplantation. *Kidney Int* 1994;46:1443.
45. Salant DJ, Adler S, Bernard DB, Silmant MM. Acute renal failure associated with renal vascular disease, vasculitis, glomerulonephritis, and nephrotic syndrome. In: Brenner BM, Lazarus JM, eds. *Acute renal failure*. 3rd ed. New York: Churchill Livingstone, 1988;371.

46. Lien J, Chan V. Risk factors influencing survival in acute renal failure treated by hemodialysis. *Arch Intern Med* 1985;145:2067.

47. Spiegel DM, Ullian ME, Zerbe GO, Berl T. Determinants of survival and recovery in acute renal failure patients dialyzed in intensive-care units. *Am J Nephrol* 1991;11:44.

48. Kleinknecht D. Management of acute renal failure. In: Cameron S, Davison AM, Grunfeld J-P, Kerr D, Ritz E, eds. *Oxford textbook of clinical nephrology.* Oxford: Oxford University Press, 1992;1015.

49. Miller RJ. Supporting a cancer patient's decision to limit therapy. *Semin Oncol* 1994: 21, 787.

50. Feest TG, Round A, Hamad S. Incidence of severe acute renal failure in adults: results of a community based study. *BMJ* 1993;306:481.

51. Corwin HL, Teplick RS, Schreiber MJ, Fang LST, Bonventre JV, Coggins CH. Prediction of outcome in acute renal failure. *Nephrology* 1987;7:8.

52. Maher ER, Robinson KN, Scoble JE, Garrimond JG, Browne DRG, Sweny P, Moorhead JF. Prognosis of critically-ill patients with acute renal failure: APACHE II score and other predictive factors. *QJM* 1989;72:857.

53. Rasmussen HH, Pitt EA, Ibels LS, McNeil DR. Prediction of outcome in acute renal failure by discriminant analysis of clinical variables. *Arch Intern Med* 1985;145:2015.

54. Pru C, Kjellstrand C. Urinary indices and chemistries in the differential diagnosis of prerenal failure and acute tubular necrosis. *Semin Nephrol* 1985;5:224.

55. Rainford DJ, Stevens PE. The investigative approach to the patient with acute renal failure. In: Cameron S, Davison AM, Grunfeld J-P, Ritz E, eds. *Oxford textbook of clinical nephrology.* Oxford: Oxford University Press, 1992;969.

56. Brady HR, Singer GG. Acute renal failure. *Lancet* 1995;346:1533.

57. Conger JD. Interventions in clinical acute renal failure: what are the data? *Am J Kid Dis* 1995;26:565.

58. Faber MD, Kupin WL, Kishna GG, Narins RG. The different diagnosis of acute renal failure. In: Lazarus JM, Brenner BM, eds. *Acute renal failure.* 3rd ed. New York: Churchill Livingstone, 1993;133.

59. Tisher CC. Clinical indications for kidney biopsy. In: Tisher CC, Brenner BM, eds. *Renal pathology with clinical and functional correlation.* 2nd ed. Philadelphia: JP Lippoincott Co, 1994;75.

60. Kleinknecht D, Jungers D, Chanard J, Barbanel C, Ganeval D. Uremic and non-uremic complications in acute renal failure: evaluation of early and frequent dialysis on prognosis. *Kidney Int* 1972;1:190.

61. Aweeka F. Drug reference table. In: Schrier RW, Gambertoglio JG, eds. *Handbook of drug therapy in liver and kidney disease.* Boston: Little, Brown, 1991;285.

62. Bennett WM, Aronoff GR, Golper TA, Morrison G, Singer I, Brater DC. *Drug prescribing in renal failure: dosing guidelines for adults.* Philadelphia: American College of Physicians, 1987.

63. Schrier RW, Gambertoglio JG, eds. *Handbook of drug therapy in liver and kidney disease.* Boston: Little, Brown, 1991.

64. Prins JM, Buller HR, Kuijper EJ, Tange RA, Speelman P. Once versus thrice daily gentamicin in patients with serious infections. *Lancet* 1993;341:335.

65. Lieberthal W, Levinsky NG. Treatment of acute tubular necrosis. *Semin Nephrol* 1990; 10:571.

66. Thadvani R, Pascual M, Bonventre JV. Acute renal failure. *N Engl J Med* 1996;334:1448.

66a. Levinsky NG. Acidosis and alkalosis. In: Isselbacher KJ, Braunwald E, Wilson JD, Martin JB, Fauci AS, Kaster DL, eds. *Harrison's principles of internal medicine,* 13th ed. New York:McGraw-Hill, 1994;253.

67. Ahsan N, Cronin RE. Dialysis considerations in the patient with acute renal failure. In: Henrich WL, ed. *Principles and practice of dialysis.* Baltimore: Williams & Wilkins, 1994;426.

68. Finn WF. Conservative, nondialytic management of acute renal failure. In: Glassock RJ, ed. *Current therapy in nephrology and hypertension.* St Louis: BC Decker, Mosby-Year Book, 1992;258.

69. Kjellstrand CM, Solez K. Treatment of acute renal failure. In: Schrier RW, Gottschalk CV, eds. *Diseases of the Kidney.* 4th ed. Boston: Little, Brown, 1993;1371.

70. Bilezikian JP. Review article: Drug therapy—management of acute hypercalcemia. *N Engl J Med* 1991;326:1196.

71. Kovacs CS, MacDonald SM, Chik CS, Bruera E. Hypercalcemia of malignancy in the palliative care patient: a treatment strategy. *J Pain Sympt Manag* 1995;10:224.

72. Ralston SH, Gallacher SJ, Patel U, Campbell J, Boyle IT. Cancer-associated hypercalcemia: morbidity and mortality. *Ann Intern Med* 1990; 112:499.

73. Kim GH, Lim CS, Han JS, Kim S, Lee JS. Clinical characteristics of hypercalcemia. *Kidney Int* 1992; 39:1066 (abst).

74. Bruera E, Legris MA, Kuehr N, Miller MJ. Hypodermoclysis for the administration of fluids and narcotic analgesics in patients with advanced cancer. *J Pain Sympt Manag* 1990;5:218.

75. Arrambide K, Toto RD. Tumor lysis syndrome. *Semin Nephrol* 1993; 13:273.

76. Woodrow G, Turney JH. Cause of death in acute renal failure. *Nephrol Dial Transplant* 1992;7:230 (Medline abst).

77. Golper TA, Bennett WB. Altering drug dose. In: Schrier RW, Gambertoglio JG, eds. *Handbook of drug therapy in liver and kidney disease.* Boston: Little Brown, 1991;1.

78. Ottery FD. Rethinking nutritional support of the cancer patient: the new field of nutritional oncology. *Semin Oncol* 1994;21:770.

79. Seidner DL, Matarese, Steiger E. Nutritional care of the critically ill patient with renal failure. *Semin Nephrol* 1994;14:53.

80. Sponsel H, Conger JG. Is parenteral nutrition therapy of value in acute renal failure patients? *Am J Kidney Dis* 1995;25:96.

81. Wolfson M, Kopple JD. Nutritional management of acute renal failure. In: Lazarus JM, Brenner BM, eds. *Acute renal failure.* 3rd ed. New York: Churchill Livingstone, 1993;467.

82. Brezis M, Rosen S, Epstein FH. Acute renal failure. In: Brenner BM, Rector FC Jr, eds. *The kidney,* 4th ed. Philadelphia: WB Saunders, 1991;993.

83. Mitch WE, Wilmore DW. Nutritional considerations in the treatment of acute renal failure. In: Brenner BM, Lazarus JM, eds. *Acute renal failure.* 2nd ed. New York: Churchill, Livingstone, 1988;743.

84. Prod'hom G, Leuenberger P, Koerfer J et al. Nosocomial pneumonia in mechanically ventilated patients receiving antacid, ranitidine, or sucralfate as prophylaxis for stress ulcer. *Ann Intern Med* 1994;120:653.

85. Paganini EP. Hematologic abnormalities. In: Daugirdas JR, Ing TS, eds. *Handbook of dialysis.* 2nd ed. Boston: Little, Brown, 1994;445.

86. Janson PA, Jubeliver SJ, Weinstein MJ, Deykin D. Treatment of the bleeding tendency in uremia with cryoprecipitate. *N Engl J Med* 1980; 303:1318.

87. Mannucci PM, Remuzzi G, Pusineri F, Lombardi R, Valsecchi C, Mecca G, Zimmerman TS. Deamino-8-D-arginine vasopressin shortens the bleeding time in uremia. *N Engl J Med* 1983;308:8.

88. Shapiro M, Kelleher SP. Intranasal deamino-8-D-arginine shortens the bleeding time in uremia. *Am J Nephrol* 1984;4:260.

89. Livio M, Mannucci M, Vigano G, Mingardi G, Lonbardi R, Mecca G, Remuzzi G. Conjugated estrogens for the management of bleeding associated with renal failure. *N Engl J Med* 1986;315:731.

90. Fraser CL, Arieff AI. Nervous system complications in uremia. *Ann Intern Med* 1988;109:143.

91. Locke S, Merrill JP, Tyler HR. Neurologic complications of acute uremia. *Arch Intern Med* 1961;108:519.

92. Levy NB. Psychopharmacology in patients with renal failure. *Int J Psychiatry Med* 1990;20:325.

93. Lowenthal DT, Kobasa D. Analgesics and sedatives-hypnotics. In: Schrier RW, Gambertoglio JG, eds. *Handbook of drug therapy in liver and kidney disease.* Boston: Little, Brown, 1991;46.

94. Pahl MV, Vaziri ND. Cancer. In: Daugirdas JR, Ing TS, eds. *Handbook of dialysis,* 2nd ed. Boston: Little, Brown, 1994;537.

95. Stewart CL, Fleming RA, Madden T. Chemotherapy drugs. In: Schrier RW, Gambertoglio JG, eds. *Handbook of drug therapy in liver and kidney disease.* Boston: Little, Brown, 1991;156.

96. Lazarus JM, Hakim RM. Medical aspects of hemodialysis. In: Brenner BM, Rector FC Jr, eds. *The kidney.* 4th ed. Philadelphia: WB Saunders, 1991;2223.

97. Mehta RL. Therapeutic alternatives to renal replacement for critically ill patients in acute renal failure. *Semin Nephrol* 1994;14:64.

98. Owen WF Jr, Lazarus JM. Dialytic management of acute renal failure. In: Lazarus JM, Brenner BM, eds. *Acute renal failure.* 3rd ed. New York: Churchill Livingstone, 1993;467.

99. Paganini EP. General application of continuous therapeutic techniques. In: Henrich WL ed. *Principles and practice of dialysis.* Baltimore: Williams & Wilkins, 1994;98.

100. Sigler MH, Teehan BP, Daugirdas JT, Ing TS. Slow continuous therapies. In: Daugirdas JR, Ing TS, eds. *Handbook of dialysis.* 2nd ed. Boston: Little, Brown, 1994;169.

101. Caruana RJ, Keep DM. Anticoagulation. In: Daugirdas JR, Ing TS, eds. *Handbook of dialysis.* Boston: Little, Brown. 2nd ed. 1994;121.

102. Alexopoulos E, Bakianis P, Kokolina E, et al. Acute renal failure in a medical setting: changing pattern and prognostic factors. *Renal Failure* 1994;16:273 (Medline abst).

103. Harris KPG, Hatterlsey JM, Feehally J, Walls J. Acute renal failure associated with haematological malignancies: a review of 10 years experience. *Eur J Haematol* 1991;47:119.

104. Iggo N, Palmer ABD, Severn A, et al. Chronic dialysis in patient with multiple myeloma and renal failure: a worthwhile treatment. *QJM* 1989;73:903.

105. Gallego N, Gallego A, Pascual J, Liano F, Estepa R, Ortuno J. Prognosis of children with acute renal failure. *Nephron* 1993;64:399.

106. Lane PH, Mauer SM, Blazar BR, Ramsay NK, Kashtan CE. Outcome of dialysis for acute renal failure in pediatric bone marrow transplant patients. *Bone Marrow Transplant* 1994;13:613 (Medline abst).

107. Garaventa A, Porta F, Rondelli R, et al. Early deaths in children after BMT. *Bone Marrow Transplant* 1992;10:419 (Medline abst).

108. Finn WF. Recovery from acute renal failure. In: Lazarus JM, Brenner BM, eds. *Acute renal failure,* 3rd ed. New York: Churchill Livingstone, 1993;357.

109. Kjellstrand CM, Ebben J, Davis T. Time of death, recovery of renal function, development of chronic renal failure and need for chronic hemodialysis in patients with acute tubular necrosis. *Trans Am Soc Artif Intern Organs* 1981;27:45.

110. Neu S, Kjellstrand CM. Stopping long-term dialysis. *N Engl J Med* 1986;314:14.

111. Port FK, Nissenson AR. Outcome of end-stage renal disease in patients with rare causes of renal failure. II. Renal or systemic neoplasms. *QJM* 1989;272:1161.

112. US Renal Data System. 1994 annual data report. Bethesda: The National Institute of Health, National Institutes of Diabetes and Digestive amd Kidney Diseases, 1994. Chapter IV. Incidence and causes of treated ESRD. *Am J Kidney Dis* 1994;24(suppl 2):S48.

113. Epstein AC. Should cancer patients be dialyzed? *Semin Nephrol* 1993;13:315.

114. Carpenter CB, Lazarus MJ. Dialysis and transplantation in the treatment of renal failure. In: Isselbacher KJ, Braunwald E, Wilson JD, Martin JB, Fauci AS, Kaster DL, eds. *Harrison's principles of internal medicine*, 13th ed. New York: McGraw-Hill, 1994;1281.

115. Hirsch DJ, West ML, Cohen AD, Jindal KK. Experience with not offering dialysis to patients with a poor prognosis. *Am J Kidney Dis* 1994;23:463.

116. Sobel BJ, Casciato DA, Lowitz BB. Renal complications. In: Casciato DA, Lowitz BB, eds. *Manual of clinical oncology*. 2nd ed. Boston: Little, Brown, 1988;462.

117. Lowance DC. Factors and guidelines to be considered in offering treatment to patients with end-stage renal disease: a personal opinion. *Am J Kidney Dis* 1993;21:679.

118. Knaus WA, Harrell FE Jr, Lynn J, et al. The SUPPORT prognostic model: objective estimates of survival for seriously ill hospitalized adults. *Ann Intern Med* 1995;122:191.

119. Wu A, Damiano AM, Lynn J et al. Predicting future functional status for seriously ill hospitalized patients. *Ann Intern Med* 1995;122:342.

120. Lowance DC, Singer PA, Siegler M. Withdrawl from dialysis: an ethical perspective. *Kidney Int* 1988;34:124.

121. The SUPPORT Principal Investigators for the SUPPORT Project. A controlled trial to improve care for seriously ill hospitalized patients: the Study to Understand Prognoses and Preferences for Outcomes and Risks of Treatments. *JAMA* 1995;274:1591.

122. Hagen N, Foley KM, Cerbone DJ, Portenoy RK, Inturrisi CE. Chronic nause and morphine-6-glucuronide. *J Pain Sympt Manag* 1991;6:125.

123. Hasselstrom J, Berg U, Lofgren A, Sawe J. Long lasting respiratory depression induce by morphine-6-glucuronide? *Br J Clin Pharmacol* 1989;27:515.

124. Osborne RJ, Joel SP, Slevin ML. Morphine intoxication in renal failure: the role of morphine-6-glucuronide. *BMJ* 1986;292:1548.

125. Babul N, Darke AC, Hagen N. Hydromorphone metabolite accumulation in renal failure. *J Pain Sympt Manag* 1995;10:184.

126. Lauer RM, Glaherty, Gambertoglio JG. Neuropsychiatric drugs. In: Schrier RW, Gambertoglio JG, eds. *Handbook of drug therapy in liver and kidney disease*. Boston: Little, Brown and Co, 1991;207.

127. Nicholls AJ. Nervous system. In: Daugirdas JR, Ing TS, eds. *Handbook of dialysis*. 2nd ed. Boston: Little, Brown, 1994;673.

128. Eisenach JC, DuPen S, Dubois M, Miguel R, Allin D. Epidural clonidine analgesia for intractable cancer pain. *Pain* 1995;61:391.

129. Byas-Smith MG, Max MB, Muir J, Kingman A. Transdermal clonidine compared to placebo in painful diabetic neuropathy using a two-stage "enriched enrollment" design. *Pain* 1995;60:267.

130. Ernst DS, MacDonald N, Paterson AHG, Jensen J, Brasher P, Bruera E. A double-blind, cross-over trial of intravenous clodronate in metastatic bone pain. *J Pain Sympt Manag* 1992;7:4.

131. Levy NB. Psychology and rehabilitation. In: Daugirdas JR, Ing TS, eds. *Handbook of dialysis*. 2nd ed. Boston: Little, Brown, 1994;369.

132. Bottomley DM, Hanks GW. Subcutaneous midazolam infusion in palliative care. *J Pain Sympt Manag* 1990;5:259.

133. Johanson GA. Midazolam in terminal care. *Am J Hospice Palliat Care* 1990;1:13.

134. Twycross RC, Lichter I. The terminal phase. In: Doyle D, Hanks GWC, MacDonald N, eds. *Oxford textbook of palliative medicine*. Oxford: Oxford Medical Publications, 1993;649.

135. Cohen LM, McCue JD, Germain M, Kjellstrand CM. Dialysis discontinuation. A good death? *Arch Intern Med* 1995;155:42.

136. Bellomo R, Farmer M, Parkin G, Wright C, Boyce N. Severe acute renal failure: a comparison of acute continuous hemodiafiltration and conventional dialytic therapy. *Nephron* 1995;71:59.

137. Hakim RM, Wingard RL, Parker RA. Effect of the diaysis membrane in the treatment of patients with acute renal failure. *N Engl J Med* 1995;331:1338.

138. Schiffl H, Lang SM, Konig A, Strasser T, Haider MC, Held E. Biocompatible membranes in acute renal failure: prospective case-controlled study. *Lancet* 1994;344:570.

139. Hull AR. Balancing outcomes in dialysis with economic realities. In: Henrich WL, ed. *Principles and practice of dialysis*. Baltimore: Williams & Wilkins, 1994;457.

140. Leblanc M, Tapolyai M, Paganini EP. What dialysis dose should be provided in acute renal failure. *Adv Ren Replace Ther* 1995; 2:255.

141. Humes HD. Acute renal failure: prevailing challenges and prospects of the future. In: Malluche H, Franz HE, eds. Nephrology at the verge of the century. *Kidney Int* 1995;48:S26.

*Principles and Practice of Supportive Oncology,*
edited by Ann Berger et al.
Lippincott–Raven Publishers, Philadelphia ©1998

CHAPTER 30

# Disorders of Sexuality and Reproduction

Ursula S. Ofman

The medical treatment of cancer patients has become increasingly effective during the past decades, extending lives and increasing survival. As a result, the emotional and physical side effects of cancer treatment have gained increasing importance. Although the long-term sexual side effects of cancer treatments have received considerable attention in clinical research during the past decade, potential infertility and its emotional cost have not been documented as thoroughly, perhaps in part because until recently there was no large cohort of long-term cancer survivors concerned with their own reproductive potential. Therefore, this newly emerging area of interest is to some extent a sign of more effective cancer treatments in younger populations.

After active treatment, survivors attempt to return to their previous daily routines. The challenge this represents for many cancer survivors is not trivial. Sexuality is one of the most complicated areas of functioning to regain. A diagnosis of cancer means having to face one's own mortality, possibly for the first time. The treatments are often painful, frightening, and intrusive and have the potential to erode one's sense of body integrity and body image. Memories of the illness and treatment, together with their emotional aftereffects, present a disruptive mix for sexual interest and functioning. These effects may continue long after active treatment is over and are "stirred" again at every routine follow-up visit.

Many cancer treatments interfere physiologically with some aspect of physical functioning, which also may impede an easy return to pretreatment life. These disruptive long-term effects are not only those that directly affect sexual organs or gonads but also include other aspects of functioning that may interfere with the patient's sexual self-image, such as scars, a change in physique as a result of hormone treatment, ostomies, disfiguring surgery, and so on. Any change in appearance or

functioning and any long-term treatment side effect can be a reminder of the illness and its treatment and may interfere with a sensuous, virile, and confident sexual-self image.

Changes in gender-role behavior resulting from the physical and emotional side effects of cancer surgery or treatment not only may impair the patient's sexual interest but also affect the partner's perception of the patient as a sexual object. For both the patient and the patient's partner, it may be difficult to view each other from the same perspective that had previously drawn them to each other sexually. The patient may have become physically and emotionally dependent on the partner, who in return may have had to assume a nurturing, parenting role. After treatment ends, it may be impossible to return to the previous role distribution in the relationship. Both partners also are faced with the varying reactions of extended family, friends, and colleagues to the illness and subsequent difficulties. These reactions may range from affectionate support to angry withdrawal, adding to the psychosocial difficulty of the posttreatment period. Worries about the possibility of a recurrence, together with uncertainty about the future, heightened anxiety and depression, a sense of personal inadequacy, and diminished sense of control in either or both partners also can interfere seriously with the resumption of a sexual life (1–3).

The psychosexual issues regarding the prospect of infertility in this population appear to be undocumented at this time. To face death and at the same time to surrender one's chance of living on in one's offspring must present a depressing, noxious combination for many of the young, childless patients beginning treatment. On a marital level, the issue of possible infertility undoubtedly has a long-term negative effect on the stability of the relationship as well as the need to renegotiate aspects of the implicit relationship contract. Unattached patients may not worry about possible loss of fertility in the early stages of diagnoses and treatment but still may feel dam-

U. S. Ofman, 155 East 29th St., New York, NY 10016-6306.

aged and limited in their capacity as a potential mate. Research in this area is urgently needed to alert the medical community to this issue and to develop strategies for helping these patients cope with this immense psychosocial stressor.

Although psychosocial causes are responsible for much of the sexual and procreative difficulty that survivors experience, physical causes are to some extent more easily researched and identified. Therefore, the vast majority of studies in this area focus on medically caused sexual and reproductive dysfunction. In the following sections, this literature is reviewed by disease site and systemic treatments.

## SEXUAL AND REPRODUCTIVE SIDE EFFECTS OF CANCER TREATMENT IN WOMEN

### Breast Cancer

Breast cancer patients may be the best researched group in terms of the sexual impact of treatment on sexual functioning. Partly because radical mastectomy had been the treatment of choice for all breast cancer patients, the effects of breast loss on women's sexual experience and life were researched early. In recent years, it has been widely accepted that comparable survival rates may be obtained in early breast cancer patients treated either with traditional surgical procedures (modified radical mastectomy) or with breast-conserving techniques combined with radiation and, increasingly, chemotherapy. The psychological and psychosexual outcomes of these two approaches were compared in a number of studies. Although some studies report a tendency toward better preservation of body image and sexual functioning in patients who elect breast-conserving treatment (4–6), there is no conclusive evidence that these women also have better overall adjustment. Schover (7) questioned the frequently assumed connection between mutilating breast surgery and poor sexual adjustment posttreatment. She suggested that a woman's overall psychological health, relationship satisfaction, and premorbid sexual life appear to be far stronger predictors of postcancer sexual satisfaction than the extent of the damage to the breast and that even a less damaged sense of desirability and better preserved body image may have only a subtle impact on actual sexual functioning after surgery.

In an effort to clarify the nature of women's response to lumpectomy, McCormick and co-workers (1989) (8) studied 74 women following lumpectomy and radiation and reported that 39% of the sexually active patients avoided the treated breast, 20% stated that their partner avoided it, and 48% noted breast discomfort during sexual activity; still, 90% indicated a high level of satisfaction with the results of their treatment.

The implications of breast reconstruction for the psychological adjustment of the mastectomy population is also beginning to receive attention. Rowland et al. (1992) (9) studied 83 women who had undergone reconstruction after modified radical mastectomy for early stage breast cancer and reported that patients generally returned to premorbid levels of sexual satisfaction and comfort.

Although there is now a growing body of research dealing with the emotional and sexual consequences of surgery for early stage breast cancer, little is known about the effects of systemic regimens for breast cancer on sexual functioning. A review of research regarding sexual and reproductive side effects of chemotherapeutic agents is provided below. A further concern is the large cohorts of women now receiving hormonal treatment, especially tamoxifen, for long periods. The long-term side effects of these treatments are only now emerging slowly and require more research in the future. Research to date suggests that tamoxifen actually may produce estrogenic changes in the vaginal mucosa of postmenopausal women (10,11); however, its impact on symptomatic vaginal atrophy in these women is unknown (12).

### Cancer of the Female Reproductive Organs

The incidence of sexual problems in women after gynecologic cancer treatment ranges in various reports from 0 to virtually 100% (13). This reflects both the many methodologic difficulties of assessment in this field and the varied treatments for gynecologic malignancies. These treatments range from laser surgery for cervical carcinoma in situ to total pelvic exenteration and vigorous chemotherapies for advanced gynecologic tumors. The gynecologic malignancies, with their obvious significance for sexual function, deserve comprehensive study to help women recover sexually as fully as possible. As Van de Wiel et al. (1988) (14) point out in their review of the literature on sexual function after cervical cancer treatment, many studies use frequency of intercourse as the sole indicator of the quality of sexual relations; this sheds little light on the true sexual status of the gynecologic cancer survivor. Further refinements in research instruments and methodology hopefully will benefit this population. A review of the research in this area is also available in Berek and Andersen (15) and McCartney and Auchincloss (1992) (16).

### Cervical Cancer

Cervical cancer is the fourth most common neoplasm in women, with 13,000 new cases of invasive disease diagnosed annually in the United States. Excluding in situ lesions, treatment consists of radical hysterectomy, radiation therapy, or a combination of both approaches. For almost two decades, researchers explored and compared the relative incidence of sexual dysfunction in women with cervical cancer after surgery versus after radiation treatment (17,18). These studies indicate that at 6 months posttreatment, both surgery and radiation patients reported no significant changes in sexual functioning; at one year posttreatment, however, both populations reported decreased sexual interest, and radiation patients reported significantly diminished sexual functioning with severe dyspareunia, postcoital bleeding, and pain on penetration. These studies highlight the difficulties posed for sexual recovery by pelvic irradiation for gynecologic cancer. The sequelae of fibrosis, vaginal stenosis, and decreased lubrication (19) are likely to interfere with sexual function unless treated appropriately, promptly, and continuously with vaginal dilators, effective vaginal lubricants (e.g., Astroglide and others) and, in some cases, a hormone-free vaginal moisturizer such as Replens.

Total pelvic exenteration is a surgical procedure occasionally performed to excise advanced pelvic tumors en bloc in the absence of distant metastases. The surgery entails removal of the bladder, urethra, vagina, uterus, ovaries, and rectum; two ostomies are created. The treatment is such a serious challenge to both physical and emotional recovery that early clinical reports explored whether postoperative quality of life justified the continued use of so radical an approach (20,21). Some researchers have reported that construction of a neovagina combined with special support and counseling efforts offers an improved chance for sexual rehabilitation after surgery (22–24). At present, however, many questions remain regarding vaginal reconstruction. The long-term advantage to patient adjustment and satisfaction must be weighed against the risk of these procedures. The psychological and practical adjustments required by exenteration, which include body image, ostomy, and mortality concerns, also merit continued further study.

The impact of gynecologic cancer on a woman's sexual self-esteem or sense of worth as a sexual partner remains an intuitively powerful yet little-studied factor in postcancer distress. Van de Wiel et al. (1988) (14) compared 11 women treated for cervical carcinoma with a group of nonpatient controls and found that although the frequency of sexual activity did not differ between the groups, the patients with cervical cancer valued sexual interactions significantly less and had a lower self-appraisal of themselves as sexual partners. Although the small populations studied and the retrospective nature of the work curtail conclusions one may draw, this report marks a valuable effort to illuminate the subtler but far-reaching consequences of gynecologic cancer for sexual well-being.

### Endometrial and Ovarian Cancer

Endometrial cancer presents most commonly in postmenopausal women. Treatment consists of surgery, radiation therapy, or a combination of both modalities. Ovarian cancer presents in premenopausal and postmenopausal women; surgical evaluation and debulking are ordinarily the first step in treatment, followed by a chemotherapy regimen with a combination of agents. Only with the advent of chemotherapy for ovarian cancer has the previously dismal prognosis for this tumor improved markedly. Studies of the long-term implications of this illness for the survivor's sexual function have begun to appear (13,25,26). Compared with healthy controls, women with these cancers report lower frequency of sexual behaviors, lower levels of arousal, increased incidence of dyspareunia, and problems with body image.

The ovarian cancer patient faces the serial traumata of a serious cancer diagnosis, major pelvic surgery with resultant changes to the vagina, a demanding chemotherapy regimen, treatment-related onset of menopause in the premenopausal patient, and complete loss of fertility. The psychological, physical, and hormonal impact on sexual function in this population merits further careful study.

The endometrial cancer patient must often contend with radiation changes to the vagina and pelvis (27). Vaginal changes include fibrosis with resultant shortening and narrowing; reduced elasticity of the vaginal wall; and diminished lubrication, creating high risk of dyspareunia. As mentioned earlier, the consequences of radiation to the vagina may be avoided or alleviated by the regular use of vaginal dilators, and sexual comfort can be improved by the use of appropriate lubricants, vaginal moisturizers, and intercourse positions. An important area for future inquiry is the implementation of patient support and education plans for women facing pelvic radiation, which may increase contact with health care providers and encourage crucial patient compliance with these strategies during the demanding months of treatment, especially during the first year posttreatment, as radiation changes evolve and produce physical and relationship distress.

### Vulvar Cancer

Vulvar carcinoma is a rare tumor arising primarily in older women. In early stage disease, treatment may consist of wide local excision. In more advanced disease, the lesions are often multicentric and radical vulvectomy is performed, which entails removal of clitoris, labia minora and majora, and bilateral inguinal lymph node dissection. Postoperatively, patients may experience a high degree of complications, including wound infections and lymphedema of the lower extremities as well as introital stricture. Research attention has begun to focus on this population in recent years (21,28,29) and reports document that sexual dysfunction posttreatment for vulvar cancer is common and affects all phases of the sexual response cycle.

## Sexual and Reproductive Implications of Systemic Cancer Treatments in Women

Sexual and reproductive consequences of surgery are obvious, occur at the time of treatment, and are usually permanent. In contrast, the side effects of radiation and chemotherapy may accumulate over time and may not be permanent. Premature menopause, which is a frequent long-term side effect of systemic cancer treatments, such as chemotherapy, hormone therapy, and pelvic irradiation, have implications for both sexual and reproductive functioning. Ovarian failure secondary to single-agent and combination chemotherapy has been documented (30). Alkylating agents appear to be the most notorious cause of ovarian failure in older women (aged 40 and older). Resulting symptoms include amenorrhea and menopausal symptoms, such as hot flashes, irritability, vaginal dryness, and atrophy of the vaginal epithelium. The treatment increases the likelihood of vaginitis, dyspareunia, and decreased sexual interest. Although some women recover normal ovarian functioning after treatment, premature menopause is the long-term outcome for many women. Aside from the specific drug regimen used, age is an important variable in this context, with older women more prone to loss of fertility and early menopause, particularly after treatment with larger, cumulative drug doses.

Gonadal dysfunction and infertility after radiation therapy are difficult to predict. The central location of the ovaries within the pelvis, close to major nodal areas, makes damage from radiation scatter and leakage likely. As with chemotherapy, radiation damage is dose related, cumulative, and age dependent. Loescher et al. (31) found that permanent infertility after 25 treatments of 500 Gy occurred in 60% of women aged 15 to 40 years and in 100% in women aged over 40. Because pelvic radiation interferes with the vasocongestive processes of female sexual arousal, vaginal lubrication also may be impaired, and dyspareunia and vaginitis may develop. Therefore, pelvic radiation may result in long-term adverse effects on female sexual functioning (32).

Radiation treatment is often combined with chemotherapy regimens. In such cases it is difficult to differentiate between toxicity incurred from radiation versus that due to the chemotherapeutic agent(s). Data from women who received combined radiation and chemotherapy for Hodgkin disease suggest that these combination treatments result in additive ovarian toxicity (33).

## CANCER OF THE MALE REPRODUCTIVE ORGANS

### Prostate Cancer

Prostate cancer is the most commonly diagnosed cancer in men. It affects mostly older men; 80% of all diag-

noses are made in men aged 65 years and older. Men and their partners in this age group are often at a developmental stage dominated by losses: retirement, death of peers, and separation from adult children who move away. These losses may include diminished sexual activity secondary to sexual dysfunction that precedes the cancer diagnosis. Changes in sexual functioning due to normal aging are often compounded by age-related chronic diseases, such as hypertension, and their treatment. In a prospective study of 22 men with stage B or C prostate cancer, Schover and von Eschenbach (1983) (34) found that 23% reported painful ejaculation prior to therapy, and 40% reported erectile difficulties. More recently, Zinreich et al. (1990) (35) reported that 63% of 43 patients (mean age, 67.7 years) with varying stages of prostate cancer had erectile dysfunction before undergoing any cancer treatment. Of these, 44% were never able to obtain an erection, and 56% reported difficulty maintaining erections during intercourse. For many elderly couples, the man's erectile difficulty results in a complete cessation of sexual activity.

Treatment for early stage disease commonly consists of surgery or radiation therapy. In early stage prostate cancer, the advances in medical technology have meant gains for sexual functioning posttreatment. Quinlan et al. (1991) (36), in a case series of 500 men, reported an incidence of erectile dysfunction of 32% with nerve-sparing surgery techniques compared with 85% after radical prostatectomy. Recovery of erectile functioning is often slow, however, and may exceed 6 months in some patients (37).

Traditional radiation regimens for prostate cancer also may produce erectile dysfunction as a long-term side effect. Schover (38) found in a review of the literature that the generally estimated 50% of erectile dysfunction after definitive radiotherapy may be inflated and actually may lie between 14% and 46% of all cases. The mechanism believed to be responsible for the development of erectile dysfunction in radiation patients is vascular scarring, which may develop 6 months posttreatment or later.

Advanced-stage prostate cancer is commonly treated with testosterone deprivation, accomplished by bilateral orchiectomy or the administration of estrogen, flutamide, or luteinizing hormone-releasing hormone (LH-RH) analogues. All these interventions produce sexual side effects, including loss of desire for sexual activity and impaired erectile functioning. Men undergoing hormone treatments also are confronted with body image issues, reduced energy levels, and hot flashes, which may contribute to the development of sexual problems.

### Testicular Cancer

Unlike prostate cancer, testicular cancer typically affects young men. It is the most common cancer in men aged 17 to 34 in the United States. These men are confronted with a life-threatening disease at a life stage in which they are supposed to separate from their families of origin and find their own identity as an adult. The demands of the illness interfere with the developmental goals of this population and interfere with the young man's concept of himself as an independent, strong, and virile person.

In the past, treatment routinely included unilateral orchiectomy, retroperitoneal lymphadenectomy (RLND), and either chemotherapy for nonseminomatous tumors or radiation for seminomas. Men with metastatic seminomas may receive chemotherapy in addition to radiation. Fertility issues due to retrograde ejaculation as a result of surgical damage to paraaortic sympathetic nervous system pathways are a prominent concern for men after RLND (39).

Whereas fertility concerns relating to retrograde ejaculation and chemotherapy appear to be the most common sexual side effects of testicular cancer, a number of reports document further sexual difficulties posttreatment (40). Rieker et al. (1989) (41) found in a retrospective study of 223 testicular cancer survivors who were more than 1 year postdiagnosis that 30% experienced overall performance distress, 10% had erectile difficulties, and 6% were anorgasmic. These findings point to the continued need for help in patients who appear to be disease free and whose sexual functioning has returned, at least to a significant degree. These patients often remain troubled in their relationships because of persisting low-grade sexual dysfunction, which is treatable (42).

### Sexual and Reproductive Implications of Systemic Cancer Treatments in Men

Testicular function in adult men is particularly susceptible to injury by chemotherapeutic agents. Affected are the germinal epithelium, the Leydig cells responsible for steroidogenesis (43), and the hypothalamic-pituitary-testicular axis (44). Dysfunction of the testis occurs shortly after initiation of treatment and can persist for months or years after function has returned to other tissues. Manifestations of toxicity are reduction in testicular volume, severe oligospermia or azoospermia, and infertility (45). The effects of the alkylating agents have been particularly well documented. For example, doses of chlorambucil below 400 mg cause reversible oligospermia, and cumulative doses in excess of 400 mg result in azoospermia and germinal aplasia (46). Low sperm count and elevated follicle- stimulating hormone (FSH) levels are physiological indicators of germinal aplasia. The Sertoli cells are more resistant to chemotherapeutic agents, and consequently testosterone levels may remain within the normal range during and after treatment.

Combination chemotherapy regimens may have an even more disruptive effect on the germinal epithelium

than treatment with a single agent. MOPP (nitrogen mustard, vincristine, procarbaazine, and prednisone) results in irreversible germinal dysfunction in male lymphoma patients; however, other regimens that are equally efficacious cause germ cell aplasia in fewer patients, many of which experience the return of spermatogenesis with time (30). Chemotherapeutic agents are not known to affect the male sexual response cycle directly.

In contrast to the consequences of chemotherapeutic regimens on male reproductive capacity, which have been established for a number of antineoplastic agents, the effects of radiation therapy on sexual functioning and fertility have received little attention to date (32). The testis and both the the germinal epithelium and the Leydig cells are very radiosensitive. Damage and recovery appear to be dose dependent. Doses as low as 150 cGy may result in a marked, if transient, suppression of sperm production. Disruption of sperm production increases with accelerating doses; at 2,000 to 3,000 cGy, recovery may take 3 years; at 4,000 to 6,000 cGy, approximately 5 years; and above 6,000 cGy, sterility seems permanent (30). By affecting the vasocongestive mechanisms necessary for erectile functioning, pelvic radiation also may cause erectile dysfunction in men.

## CANCER SITES IN BOTH SEXES

### Bladder Cancer

Bladder cancer arises primarily in older men and women, who already may have experienced age-related changes in sexuality. Whereas in the United States treatment previously consisted of cystectomy for lesions of any stage, early bladder carcinoma in situ without infiltration may now be treated with local excision and bacille Calmette-Guérin (BCG).

In patients with invasive bladder cancer, cystectomy is still the treatment of choice. A common sexual side effect for men after radical cystectomy is erectile dysfunction resulting from transection of the nerves governing erection (47) and loss of ejaculation secondary to excision of the prostate at the time of surgery. Changes in the sensation of orgasm may ensue. Patient response to this loss is not well documented.

In women, cystectomy may result in a narrowed or shortened vagina, scarring, and numbness or loss of sensation, all of which may impair the excitement response. Furthermore, removal of both ovaries during surgery causes premature menopause in premenopausal patients, which may lead to reduced vaginal lubrication and desire. The simultaneous creation of a stoma and external diversion of urine generates concerns about body image, odor, leakage, and spills and thus may contribute to sexual avoidance and other difficulties (48).

## Colorectal Cancer

Cancer of the colon and rectum is the second most common cancer in the United States; approximately 140,000 new cases are diagnosed annually, primarily in older men and women. Surgery remains the mainstay of treatment; resection of the tumor with pelvic lymphadenectomy may be followed by radiation, chemotherapy, or both. Pelvic lymphadenectomy may result in damage to the parasympathetic nervous system, causing erectile dysfunction, and to the sympathetic nervous system, causing retrograde or diminished ejaculation. Past studies have reported a varying incidence of these side effects after treatment (49–51). More recently, Havenga and Welvaart (1991) (52) studied 26 men with rectosigmoid carcinoma, nine of whom were treated with abdominoperineal resection and 17 of whom treated with low anterior resection. Only two of the patients with abdominoperineal resection returned to sexual activity, five had erectile dysfunction, and seven were anorgasmic. Patients who had low anterior resection reported less sexual dysfunction after surgery; 12 maintained sexual activity, and four reported either erectile dysfunction or anorgasmia. Further evidence that abdominoperineal resection produces significant sexual dysfunction was reported by Koukouras et al. (1991) (53), who studied 60 sexually active male patients with colorectal cancer who were treated with high anterior resection, low anterior resection, or abdominoperineal resection. Patients with the abdominoperineal resection had the highest incidence of sexual dysfunction; 65% became sexually inactive, 45% lost all erectile ability, and 50% reported absence of ejaculation.

Hojo et al. (1991) (54) described the use of a nerve-sparing approach to pelvic lymphadenectomy in 134 patients with advanced disease. They found that although bladder dysfunction was best prevented with a nerve-sparing procedure, preservation of sexual function in men is more difficult, requires a high degree of nerve preservation, and therefore is not advisable for patients with locally extensive disease.

In patients with early stage rectal cancer who are treated by amputation of the rectum alone, erectile dysfunction appears to be less prevalent, but problems with the orgasm phase persist (55). There is a glaring shortage of studies focusing on the sexual side effects of treatment for colorectal neoplasms in women.

After the creation of a colostomy, both men and women must contend with issues of changed body image and sensitivity about cleanliness, odor, and fear of accidents. Sutherland and co-workers' early studies (1952) (56) have remained clinically on target; they found that the sexual impact of the ostomy far exceeds the extent of physical handicap. Depression, anger, and fear of being repugnant are common emotional reactions postoperatively and may contribute to a pattern of sexual avoidance. The medical staff must anticipate these issues and offer support to patients, whose challenges include self-care of the ostomy, overcoming fears concerning changed appearance, and regaining physical self-esteem. Other patients who are farther along in this process may provide invaluable help to the recovering colorectal patient in this regard. Overall adjustment to the colostomy may take more than a year, as documented by Hurny and Holland (1985) (57).

Sexual response after colorectal surgery remains an insufficiently understood area, particularly in view of the current high prevalence of this tumor. For women particularly, the issues of sexual recovery after colorectal and bladder cancer remain too little explored. Nonetheless, the impact of pelvic surgeries on the female excitement and orgasm responses, as well as the impact of the ostomy issues on desire, may be surmised to be great. The value of treatment interventions for sexual dysfunction in this population, including both penile prosthesis implantation and sexual counseling for the patient or couple, is also an appropriate area of study.

## Other Cancers

Patients with less common tumors and those with common tumors that do not directly affect the organs of sexual response have received little or no research attention with regard to the sexual sequelae of their treatment. The diagnosis and treatment of all cancers have far-reaching psychological implications for the patient and family that lie beyond the scope of this review. These matters are covered comprehensively elsewhere (58). Some cancer treatments pose a particularly severe challenge to the recovery of normal self-esteem and restored body-image; treatments involving limb amputations, marked facial and other appearance changes, or loss of normal phonation are examples.

The simple passage of time does not heal all wounds. In the area of sexuality, it is not uncommon for problems to become more severe with time (59). The adjustment to cancer and its elements of disfigurement is by nature a slow process, and problems with adjustment and recovery, including those in the sexual and relationship arena, may often be more accessible to counseling by oncology mental health professionals during the first and second posttreatment year than at a later stage in cancer survivorship.

Cancers that require systemic treatment with chemotherapy, whole body irradiation, or bone marrow transplantation challenge the patient physically and emotionally more than most surgeries or radiation regimens. Treatments may be lengthy and arduous, depleting the patient of energy and causing severe side effects. Sexual functioning is clearly affected by many of these regimens. In recent years, the sexual concerns of female bone marrow transplant patients have received some research attention. Ovarian failure secondary to conditioning treatment with melphalan or cyclophosphamide and total body irradiation is associated with profound effects on sexual functioning, most commonly vaginal dryness, loss of desire for sexual activity, and difficulties with sexual intercourse (60). Ostroff et al. (61) found that standard regimens of hormone replacement therapy did not alleviate all sexual impairment experienced by women with treatment-related ovarian failure. In a study comparing bone marrow transplant survivors and a matched sample undergoing maintenance chemotherapy, Altmeier et al. (62) found that bone marrow transplant patients reported a higher incidence of sexual difficulties. Ostroff and Lesko (32) confirmed the prevalence of sexual dysfunction in bone marrow transplant survivors. Clearly, this population is at increased risk for sexual dysfunction and would benefit from further research attention.

Patients with Hodgkin disease are now often successfully treated with aggressive chemotherapy. Treatment is associated with a high degree of infertility in both men (80%–90%) and in women (50%) (63). The interrelationship in young cancer survivors between cancer treatment, loss of desire and sexual dysfunction, lost or impaired fertility, and relationship distress remains clinically inescapable but very little studied.

## PREVENTION AND MANAGEMENT OF SEXUAL AND REPRODUCTIVE DYSFUNCTION IN CANCER PATIENTS

### Medical Strategies to Prevent and Manage Sexual and Reproductive Dysfunction

Efforts have been made to reduce sexual and reproductive morbidity by refining surgical and radiation therapies. Examples include the development of nerve-sparing surgical techniques to preserve erectile function after prostatectomy (64) and nerve-sparing retroperitoneal lymph node dissection for men with clinical stage I nonseminomatous testicular cancer to preserve emission and ejaculation. In some cases, the effort to preserve ejaculatory function and avoid other treatment side effects in men with nonseminomatous tumors who do not evidence metastatic spread led to the use of unilateral orchiectomy followed by careful observation. A further example of the attempt of preserving quality of life is the strategy of offering observation as a treatment for nonmetastatic seminomatous testicular cancer instead of immediately proceeding with chemotherapy postretroperitoneal lymph node dissection, thus preserving gonadal functioning. New nerve-sparing techniques that involve preservation of the superior hypogastric plexus also may contribute to the preservation of ejaculatory functioning (65) in these men.

Similar attempts have been made to preserve sexual functioning in some treatments used for cancers in women. For example, wide local excision for vulvar cancer (28) and lumpectomy of breast tumors mark efforts on the part of surgeons to preserve sexual function and body image as much as possible, without compromising treatment efficacy.

In both men and women, efforts to keep pelvic radiation doses to a therapeutically efficacious minimum may reduce the incidence of radiation-induced sterility and allow recovery of gonadal function. Radiation damage to gonads in men now may be reduced drastically by employing a new testicular shield that reduces scatter to about 10% of the patient's prescription dose. In women, oophoropexy (the surgical transposition of the ovaries to a midline position behind the uterus) reduces the ovarian exposure of women receiving pelvic radiation in about 50% of patients (66). These developments reflect the growing willingness of the oncology world to try to preserve and maintain sexual and reproductive function while providing appropriately aggressive cancer therapy.

Medical treatments for iatrogenic sexual dysfunction and infertility also have begun to be developed. Loss of emission and ejaculation is a frequent side effect of retroperitoneal lymph node dissection (RPLND) in men. Because most men undergoing this procedure are young (17 to 34), this loss is a serious concern. For men with adequate sperm production before sterilizing cancer treatment, cryobanking is usually advised; however, many patients present with suboptimal sperm before treatment. To secure a post-thaw sample adequate for spousal insemination, more than 20 million sperm per milliliter with at least 40% progressive motility is generally required (30). Multiple ejaculates, if time permits, can increase the total of viable sperm for storage. For men after RPLND, antegrade ejaculation may return with time and, in some men, sympathomimetic drugs (ephedrine) or anticholinergic drugs, such as diphenhydramine or imipramine, may help to facilitate normal ejaculation. Electroejaculation is possible to harvest sperm in men who do not recover ejaculatory function (67). Recently, there have also been some encouraging medical developments to help patients overcome sexual difficulties. Particularly notable in this context is pharmacologic injection therapy for erectile dysfunction, and ongoing research exploring the use of topical agents to promote erections in men with organic impotence.

Other interventions to help cancer patients overcome iatrogenic gonadal and sexual dysfunction focus on hormonal intervention. Hall and others (68) treated nine women with acquired hypogonadotropic hypogonadism after therapy for cranial tumors using a physiological replacement regimen of exogenous gonadotrophin-releasing hormone (GnRH); this restored ovulation and fertility in 78% of the participants. Although the technology does not yet exist for the safe thawing of frozen ova, cryobanking of fertilized eggs (i.e., embryos) is possible. Several fertility centers now offer this option. Bone marrow transplant patients may be stimulated with hormonal therapy at the end of chemotherapy to stimulate ova for collection. The fertilized ova are frozen until later implantation in the patient or a surrogate mother. This procedure is experimental and controversial (32) and carries the potential burden for the father to decide how to proceed if the spouse's therapy is not successful.

Women who undergo premature menopause after cancer treatment need medical intervention to alleviate menopausal symptoms and prevent atherosclerosis, hypertension, cardiovascular accidents, and osteoporosis. Unless an estrogen-sensitive tumor was involved, hormonal replacement should be considered (69). Wren (70) argued that hormone replacement may be feasible in most women after genital tract cancer. In his view estrogen/progestogen regimens will not affect malignant cell growth in vulvar and vaginal cancer as well as squamous cell carcinoma of the cervix. Although the endometrium and the ovary contain hormone receptors that may respond to estrogen by increased growth factor production, a large number of women with these cancers were cured by the initial treatment and would benefit from hormone replacement without risk of stimulating cancer growth. Women who were not cured may benefit from treatment with progestogens alone or estrogen and progesterone in combination to relieve any discomfort caused by estrogen deficiency.

Aside from estrogen replacement therapy, nonhormonal medications, such as clonidine, methyldopa, and beta-blockers, may be used to control hot flashes (71). Emotional instability may be addressed with serotonin-reuptake inhibitors, such as fluoxetine or sertraline. Topical solutions to counteract reduced lubrication and changes of the vaginal lining include Replens, vitamin E oil, Chaste berry, 1% to 2 % testosterone cream, and limited doses of estrogen cream or Vagifem (72). Androgen treatment may be indicated in women with reduced bioavailable androgen levels after chemotherapy (73) and may improve sexual interest.

## Psychosocial Prevention and Intervention for Sexual Difficulties

Although efforts are under way to prevent and alleviate adverse sexual and reproductive side effects of cancer treatments medically, severe physical and emotional damage can occur nonetheless. Even patients whose treatments did not affect sexual end organs report being impaired in their sexual enjoyment after cancer treatment. Indeed, impaired sexual functioning during or after cancer treatment can occur regardless of the specific physiological changes that have taken place. The sexual response cycle (desire, arousal, and orgasm) is a complex process that may be disrupted by a wide range of factors, both physiological and psychological. Sexual response during and after cancer treatment is vulnerable to the impact of the cancer itself, medical treatment side effects, other medical problems, medications, pain, depression, anxiety, partner response, and subtler psychological effects, such as changed body image and belief in cancer myths. Cancer patients must face their own mortality, undergo uncomfortable, sometimes lengthy or disfiguring treatments and deal with the effect of their illness on spouse, family, and work. An understandable consequence of this process can be loss of sexual desire and impaired sexual response. Von Eschenbach and Schover (74) found that the most frequent sexual side effect reported by men with cancer is erectile dysfunction, whereas women are more likely to lose interest in sex altogether. Loss or impairment of sexual desire may be triggered by the trauma of diagnosis and treatment, which interferes with the patient's perception of himself or herself as a sexual person. There may be concerns about one's attractiveness and the partner's reaction that contribute to an overall withdrawal from sexual activity. Concerns about sexual functioning may contribute to sexual avoidance even if sexual desire per se is not impaired. Although inhibited sexual desire, sexual avoidance, and erectile dysfunction may be the most frequently observed sexual difficulties in this context, any sexual dysfunction may be caused by the patient's and/the partner of the patient's reaction to the trauma of the experience.

The medical team often fails to help prevent development of sexual dysfunction by not addressing the topic with the patient, which may be due to a number of factors such as discomfort with the topic or a concern about appearing intrusive or presumptuous. When the patients are elderly, young, single, widowed, or homosexual, sexual concerns appear to be particularly difficult to address (42). All too often, sexuality is viewed as being a concern only for men and women who are sexually active within a committed relationship. Every patient, regardless of current level of sexual activity, has a perception of himself or herself as a sexual being and is invested in knowing that he or she can function sexually, even if not pursuing any sexual relationships at the moment. Often the medical staff waits for the patient to open the topic and concludes that there is no interest in sexual issues if the patient remains silent. Vincent et al. (17) found that 80% of patients receiving cancer treatment were interested in more information about sex, although 75% said they would not initiate conversation about it with their doctor. Cancer patients often feel they should be glad to be alive. Asking about sexual concerns may seem ungrateful and frivolous. If physicians and nurses initiate communication about sexual side effects of proposed treatments at the time of treatment decisions, they signal to the patient that sexual functioning is a legitimate concern that can be addressed.

Privacy and confidentiality are crucial prerequisites for discussing sexual concerns with patients. Sexual matters cannot be discussed productively during rounds, when several staff members are present, or when a roommate is within earshot. Under such conditions the clinician is likely to encounter vague responses and little enthusiasm for the topic. Assessment of the patient's sexual status and history at the time of treatment decision provides the crucial basis for members of the medical team to give appropriate support and information about the possible impact of treatment options on sexual functioning. It also signals to the patient that sexual concerns are understood to be an integral component of patients' quality of life. The time of diagnosis and treatment decision is a stressful one for the patient and his or her partner, and sexual concerns are not likely to be in the forefront of their minds; however, sexual functioning needs to be addressed from the start to support the patient in the struggle to adjust to the impact of cancer treatment on self-image and functioning. Clear and detailed information enables patients and their partners to anticipate problems and prepare for them. The nursing staff in particular can be instrumental in helping patients and their partners deal with both emotional and physical side effects by explaining the physiology involved, normalizing the experience, and giving pragmatic advice and coping strategies. The timing of these interventions is determined by the situation. Certainly in emotional or medical crisis situations, such as when a relapse of the cancer is discovered, it is not helpful for the patient to be asked about sexual matters. Sexual advice is best received when it specifically addresses the problems with which the patient and his or her partner are currently struggling.

At the time of treatment decision, the patient needs to know about the sexual and reproductive issues that may arise as a result of the treatment. Patients also need reassurance that help is available should sexual difficulties occur. As treatment proceeds and patients are seen for follow-up visits, the sexual status should be assessed by asking open-ended questions like, "How are things going in your relationship?" and "How are things sexually?" As patients express difficulty, it is easy for the caregiver to normalize the experience of the patient and to offer specific advice on how to improve matters sexually.

Because any change in appearance and functioning may have sexual consequences, the medical staff should consider the potential sexual implications of all treatments offered to the patient and address them with all patients. A good resource for both staff and patients is a pair of booklets published by the American Cancer Society that address sexual concerns of male and female patients after cancer treatment; the booklets are lucid, practical, and informative about both sexual side effects and strategies to deal with them (75). If patients continue to experience sexual difficulty after cancer treatment, referral to a sex therapist for careful evaluation and treatment is indicated.

Often a short course of sexual counseling suffices to facilitate better adaptation and functioning, particularly for patients who had a satisfactory sex life before the cancer diagnosis. Sex therapy with cancer patients is geared to address the specific difficulty expressed by the patient and the patient's partner. Sexual attitudes and fears are explored, and frequently physical exercises are prescribed to do at home. These exercises are designed to reintroduce sexual activity slowly. Usually these exercises follow a graded approach, beginning with general physical pleasuring and gradually becoming more sexually focused. This approach is particularly helpful to patients who have a great deal of performance anxiety, who avoid sexual activity for fear of being unable to complete it, whose confidence in their ability to function is shaken, and who feel unattractive and shy about how their bodies were affected by cancer treatment. Similarly, partners can be traumatized by the experiences they had in the course of the treatment and also may benefit from such exercises.

## SUMMARY

The focus of the available literature is primarily on the incidence of sexual and gonadal dysfunction after cancer treatment. New medical strategies aim at prevention and amelioration of sexual side effects and infertility. Sexual side effects, in particular, can be addressed in brief sexual counseling or therapy. Informing the patient of possible side effects before treatment makes early intervention of psychosexual difficulties possible. Psychosocial aspects of fertility concerns of the cancer patient during active treatment and as a survivor have received little attention so far, possibly because of previous experience, when long-term survival of young patients was rare. With advancing technology in cancer treatment, this cohort of long-term survivors is likely to grow and requires an adequate response to these medical and psychosocial needs.

## REFERENCES

1. Cella D, Tross S. Psychological adjustment to survival from Hodgkin's disease. *J Consult Clin Psychol* 1986;54:616.
2. Ostroff J, Smith K, Lesko L. Promotion of mental health among adolescents cancer survivors and their families. *Proceedings of the Mental Health Services for Children and Adolescents in Primary Care Settings: An NIMH Research Conference,* 1989.
3. Rieker P, Edbril S, Garnick M. Curative testis cancer therapy: Psychosocial sequelae. *J Clin Oncol* 1985; 3:1117.
4. Kiebert GM, De Haes JCJM, Van de Velde CJH. The impact of breast-conserving treatment and mastectomy on the quality of life of early-stage breast cancer patients: A review. *J Clin Oncol* 1991;9:1059.
5. Wolberg WH, Tanner MA, Romsaas EP, Trump DL, Malec JF. Factors influencing options in primary breast cancer treatment. *J Clin Oncol* 1987;5:68.
6. Fallowfield LJ, Hall A. Psychosocial and sexual impact of diagnosis and treatment of breast cancer. *Br Med Bull* 1991;47:388.
7. Schover LR. The impact of breast cancer on sexuality, body image, and intimate relationships. *CA Cancer J Clin* 1991;41:112.
8. McCormick B, Yahalom J, Cox L, Shank B, Massie MJ. The patient's perception of her breast following radiation and limited surgery. *Int J Radiat Oncology Biol Phys* 1989;17:1299.

9. Rowland J, Holland JC, Chaglassian T, Kinne D. Psychological response to breast reconstruction; expectation for and impactonpost mastectomy functioning. *Psychosomatics* 1993;34(3):241–250.

10. Jordan, VC. Long-term adjuvant tamoxifen therapy for breast cancer: the prelude to prevention. *Cancer Treat Rev* 1990;17:15.

11. Love RR. Antiestrogen chemoprevention of breast cancer: Critical issues and research. *Prev Med* 1991; 20:64.

12. Schover LR, Montague DK, Schain WS. Sexual problems. In: DeVita VT, Hellman T, Rosenberg S , eds. *Cancer: principles and practice of oncology*, vol 2, 1993;2464.

13. Andersen BL, Jochimsen PR. Sexual functioning among breast cancer, gynecologic cancer, and healthy women. *J Consult Clin Psychol* 1985; 53:25.

14. Van de Wiehl HBM, Weijmar Schultz WCM, Hallensleben A, Thurkow FG, Bouma J. Sexual functioning following treatment of cervical carcinoma. *J Gyneacol Oncol* 1988:275.

15. Berek JS, Andersen BL. Sexual rehabilitation: Surgical and psychological approaches. In: Hoskins WJ, Perez CA, Young RC, eds. *Principles and practice of gynecologic oncology*. Philadelphia: JB Lippincott. 1992;401–416.

16. McCartney CF, Auchincloss SS. Psychosocial aspects of gynecologic cancer care. In: Hoskins WJ, Perez CA, Young RC, eds. *Principles and practice of gynecologic oncology*. Philadelphia: JB Lippincott, 1992; 387–400.

17. Vincent CE, Vincent B, Greiss FC, Linton EB. Some marital-sexual concomitants of carcinoma of the cervix. *South Med J* 1975;68:52.

18. Schover LR, Fife M, Gershenson DM. Sexual dysfunction and treatment for early stage cervical cancer. *Cancer* 1989;63:204.

19. Seibel MM, Freeman MG, Graves WL: Carcinoma of the cervix and sexual function. *Obstet Gynecol* 1980;55:484.

20. Knorr NJ. A depressive syndrome following pelvic exenteration and ileostomy. *Arch Surg* 1967;94:258.

21. Andersen BL, Hacker NF. Psychosexual Adjustment following pelvic exenteration. *Obstet Gynecol* 1983;61:331.

22. Morley GW, Lindenauer SM, Youngs D. Vaginal reconstruction following pelvic exenteration: Surgical and psychological considerations. *Am J Obstet Gynecol* 1973;116:996.

23. Lamont JA, DePetrillo AD, Sargent ES. Psychosexual rehabilitation and exenterative surgery. *Gynecol Oncol* 1978;6:236.

24. Lacey CG, Stern JL, Feigenbaum S, Hill EC, Braga CA. Vaginal reconstruction after exenteration with use of gracilis myocutaneous flaps: the University of California, San Francisco experience. *Am J Obstet Gynecol* 1988;158:1278.

25. Andersen BL, Lachenbruch PA, Anderson B, DeProsse C. Sexual dysfunction and signs of gynecologic cancer. *Cancer* 1986;57:1880.

26. Mitchell MF, Gershenson DM, Soeters RP, Eifel PJ, Delclos L, Wharton, JT. The long-term effects of radiation therapy on patients with ovarian dysgerminoma. *Cancer* 1991;67:1084.

27. Jenkins B. Sexual healing after pelvic irradiation. *Am J Nurs* 1986;86: 920.

28. Stehman FB, Bundy BN, Dvoretsky PM, Creasman WT. Early stage I carcinoma of the vulva treated with ipsilateral superficial inguinal lymphadenectomy and modified radical hemivulvectomy: a prospective study of the gynecologic oncology group. *Obstet Gynecol* 1992; 79:490.

29. Andreasson B, Moth I, Jensen SB, Bock JE. Sexual function and somatopsychic reactions in vulvectomy-operated women and their partners. *Acta Obstet Gynecol Scand* 1986;65:7.

30. Sherins RJ & Mulvihill JJ. Gonadal dysfunction. In DeVita VT Jr., Hellman S, Rosenberg SA, eds. *Cancer: principles and practice of oncology*. Philadelphia: JB Lippincott, 1989;2170.

31. Loescher L. Surviving adult cancers. Part 1: Physilogical effects. *Ann Intern Med* 1989;3:411–432.

32. Stroff J & Lesko LM. Psychosexual adjustment of patients undergoing bone marrow transplantation: Clinical/research issues and intervention programs. In: Whedon M ed. *Bone marrow transplantation: principles, practice and nursing care*. Monterey, CA: Jones and Bartlett Publishers, 1991;312–33.

33. Horning SJ, Hoppe RT, Kaplan HS. Female reproductive potential after treatment for Hodgkin's disease. *N Engl J Med* 1981;304:1377.

34. Schover LR, von Eschenbach AC. Erectile function in bladder and prostate cancer patients before treatment. Presented at Meeting of the American Urologic Association, Las Vegas, 1983 (abst 17).

35. Zinreich ES, Derogatis LR, Herpst J, Auvil G, Piantadosi S, Order SE. Pretreatment evaluation of sexual function in patients with adenocarcinoma of the prostate. *Int J Radiat Oncol Biol Phys* 1990;19:1001–1004.

36. Quinlan DM, Epstein JI, Carter BS, Walsh PC. Sexual function following radical prostatectomy: influence of preservation of neurovascular bundles. *J Urol* 1991;145:998.

37. Schover LR, Von Eschenbach AC, Smith DB, Gonzalez J. Sexual rehabilitation of urologic cancer patients: a practical approach. *CA Cancer J Clin* 1984; 34:66.

38. Schover LR. Sexual rehabilitation after treatment for prostate cancer. *Cancer* 1993;71(Suppl):1024.

39. Bracken RB, Johnson DE. Sexual function and fecundity after treatment for testicular tumors. *Urology* 1976;7:35.

40. Schover LR, Von Eschenbach AC. Sexual and marital relationships after treatment for nonseminomatous testicular cancer. *Urology* 1985; 25:251.

41. Rieker PP, Fitzgerald EM, Kalish LA, Richie JP, Lederman GS, Edbril SD, Garnick MB. Psychosocial factors, curative therapies, and behavioral outcomes: a comparison of testis cancer survivors and a control group of healthy men. *Cancer* 1989;64:2399.

42. Auchincloss SS. Sexual dysfunction in cancer patients: issues in evaluation and treatment.In: Holland JC, Rowland JH eds. *Handbook of psychooncology*. New York: Oxford University Press, 1989:383–413.

43. Constabile RA. The effects of cancer and cancer therapy on male reproductive function. *J Urol* 1993;149:1327.

44. Chapman RM, Sutcliffe SB, Malpas JS. Male gonadal dysfunction in Hodgkin s disease. A prospective study. *JAMA* 1981;245:1323.

45. Cheviakoff J, Calamera JC, Morgenfeld Ml. Recovery of spermatogenesis in patients with lymphoma after treatment with chlorambucil. *J Reprod Fertil* 1973;33:155.

46. Richter P, Calamera JC, Morgenfeld MD. Effect of chlorambucil on spermatogenesis in the human with malignant lymphoma. *Cancer* 1970;25:1026.

47. Schover LR, Evans R, Von Eschenbach AC. Sexual rehabilitation and male radical cystectomy. *J Urol* 1986;136:1015.

48. Schover LR, Von Eschenbach AC. Sexual function and female radical cystectomy: a case series. *J Urol* 1985;134:465.

49. Bernstein WC, Bernstein EF. Sexual dysfunction following radical surgery for cancer of the rectum. *Dis Colon Rectum* 1966;9:328.

50. Bernstein WC. Sexual dysfunction following radical surgery for cancer of rectum and sigmoid colon. *Medical Aspects of Human Sexuality* 1972;6:156.

51. Yeager ES, Van Heerden JA. Sexual dysfunction following proctocolectomy and abdominoperineal resection. *Ann Surg* 1980;191:169.

52. Havenga K, Welvaart K. Sexual dysfunction in men following surgical treatment for rectosigmoid carcinoma. *Ned Tijdschr Geneeskd* 1991; 135:710.

53. Koukouras D, Spiliotis J, Scopa CD, Kalfarentzos F, Tzoracoleftherakis E, Androulakis J. Radical consequence in the sexuality of male patients operated for colorectal carcinoma. *Eur J Surg Oncol* 1991;17:285.

54. Hojo K, Vernava AM 3d., Sugihara K, Katumata K. Preservation of urine voiding and sexual function after rectal cancer surgery. *Dis Colon Rectum* 1991;34:532.

55. Zenico T, Neri W, Zoli M, Tamburini C, Fabri F, Maltoni G. Sexual dysfunction after excision of the rectum. *Acta Urol Belg* 1989;57:213.

56. Sutherland AM, Orbach CE, Dyk RB, Bard M. The psychological impact of cancer and cancer surgery: I. Adaptation to the dry colostomy: preliminary report and summary of findings. *Cancer* 1952; 5:857.

57. Hurny C, Holland JC. Psychosocial sequelae of ostomies in cancer patients. *CA Cancer J Clin* 1985;36:170.

58. Holland JC, Rowland JH, eds. *Handbook of psychooncology. Psychological care of the patient with cancer*. New York: Oxford University Press, 1989.

59. Chang AE, Steinberg SM, Culnane M, Lampert MH, Reggia AJ, Simpson CG, Hicks JE, White DE, Yang JJ, Glatstein E, Rosenberg SA. Functional and psychosocial effects of multimodality limb-sparing therapy in patients with soft tissue sarcomas. *J Clin Oncol* 1989;7:217.

60. Cust MP, Whitehead MI, Powles R, Hunter M, Milliken S. Consequences and treatment of ovarian failure after total body irradiation for leukaemia. *BMJ* 1989;299:1494.

61. Ostroff J, Stern V, Dukoff R, Bajournas D, Lesko LM. The psychosocial adjustment of prematurely menopausal cancer survivors treated with hormone replacement therapy. American Psychosomatic Society Meeting, 1991.

62. Altmaier EM, Gingrich RD, Fyfe MA. Two-year adjustment of bone marrow transplant survivors. *Bone Marrow Transplant* 1991;7:311.

63. Cella DF. Cancer survival: psychosocial and public issues. *Cancer Invest* 1987;5:59.

64. Walsh PC, Lepor H, Eggelston JC. Radical prostatectomy with preservation of sexual function. *Prostate* 1983;4:473.

65. Takasaki N, Okada S, Kawasaki T, Tonami H, Shimizu A, Ueno N, Hirai K, Miyazaki S. Studies on retroperitoneal lymph node dissection concerning postoperative ejaculatory function in patients with testicular cancer. *Hinyokika Kiyo* 1991;37:213.

66. Thomas PRM, Winstantly D, Peckham MJ. Reproductive and endocrine function in patients with Hodgkin s disease: effeects of oophoropexy and irradiation. *Br J Cancer* 1976;33:226.

67. Bennett CJ, Seager SWJ McGuire EJ. Electroejaculation for recovery of semen after retroperitoneal lymph node dissection. *J Urol* 1987;137:513.

68. Hall JE, Martin KA, Whitney HA, Landy H, Crowley WF Jr. Potential for fertility with replacement of hypothalamic gonadotrophin-releasing hormone in long term female survivors of cranial tumors. *J Clin Endocrinonol Metab* 1994;79:1166.

69. Ettinger B. Overview of the efficacy of hormonal replacement therapy. *Am J Obstet Gynecol* 1987;156:1298.

70. Wren BG. Hormonal therapy following female genital tract cancer. *Int J Gynecol Cancer* 1994; 4:217.

71. Laufer LR, Yohanan E, Meldrum DR. Effect of clonidine on hot flashes in postmenopausal women. *Obstet Gynecol* 1982;60:583.

72. Barbach L. *The pause: postitive approaches to menopause.* New York: Plume/Penguin, 1995;xx–xx.

73. Kaplan HS. A neglected issue: The sexual side effects of current treatments for breast cancer. *J Sex Marital Ther* 1992;18:1.

74. von Eschenbach AC, Schover LR. The role of sexual rehabilitation in the treatment of patients with cancer. *Cancer* 1984;54:2662.

75. Schover LR, Randers-Pehrson M. Sexuality and cancer for the woman who has cancer, and her partner AND Sexuality and cancer for the man who has cancer, and his partner. New York: American Cancer Society 1988.

*Principles and Practice of Supportive Oncology,*
edited by Ann Berger et al.
Lippincott–Raven Publishers, Philadelphia ©1998

CHAPTER 31

# Hypercalcemia

A. Ross Morton and Paul S. Ritch

Hypercalcemia may occur in as many as 8% to 10% of patients with malignancy during the course of their disease, making it one of the most common metabolic complications of cancer. Despite this high frequency, the diagnosis of hypercalcemia is often delayed. An awareness of the tumor types most commonly associated with hypercalcemia, the mechanisms giving rise to hypercalcemia, and the symptoms produced will permit earlier diagnosis and amelioration of morbidity by the use of effective therapeutic interventions.

Since it was first reported in 1924 (1), hypercalcemia has become well recognized in association with various malignant diseases. The mechanisms responsible for the production of hypercalcemia have been increasingly well defined. Hypercalcemia is most commonly seen in association with squamous cell carcinoma of the lung, carcinoma of the breast, and multiple myeloma. This distribution of tumor types associated with hypercalcemia has remained relatively constant over the last decade (2,3). Of considerable interest is the fact that some tumors, including small-cell carcinoma of the lung and carcinoma of the prostate, which frequently metastasize to bone, and some other common tumors, such as adenocarcinoma of the colon and stomach, are rarely associated with hypercalcemia, despite biochemical and histomorphometric data indicating enhanced bone resorption, notably in the case of carcinoma of the prostate (4). The relative frequency of other tumor types associated with hypercalcemia seems to vary with the area of special interest of the investigators reporting the complication. Nevertheless, hypercalcemia is well recognized with squamous tumors of the head and neck and genitourinary neoplasms.

Patients with hypercalcemia and malignant disease are usually in the last weeks of their lives unless effective antitumor therapy is available. Therefore, therapeutic interventions must be as innocuous as they are effective. Fortunately, with modern therapeutic agents, it is possible to restore normocalcemia in most patients without inducing serious side effects.

## ETIOLOGY OF HYPERCALCEMIA IN MALIGNANT DISEASE

A brief review of normal bone and calcium metabolism is important in enhancing the understanding of the mechanisms that lead to hypercalcemia and provides a framework for intelligent therapeutic intervention.

Bone is a dynamic structure that undergoes constant remodeling. The remodeling process is a highly integrated interaction between several cell types (5), the two most important of which are the osteoblasts, or bone-forming cells, and the osteoclasts, or bone-resorbing cells. Responding to as yet incompletely understood stimuli, osteoclasts resorb an area of bone that is to be remodeled over a period of approximately 10 days. Osteoclastic resorption involves the enzymatic degradation of bone proteins such as collagen and the release of calcium from the mineral phase of the bone. The resorption phase is followed by a reversal phase, during which the osteoclasts disappear to be replaced by mononuclear cells. Thereafter, a bone-formation phase, lasting several months, occurs when osteoblasts lay down new bone to repair the defect. To maintain the strength and integrity of the bone, the resorption and formation phases are closely coupled. It is easy to see that any process that could increase osteoclastic bone resorption or decrease osteoblastic bone formation would lead to an increased net calcium flux into the extracellular fluid, which would have to be excreted by the kidneys. If the degree of imbalance is small, a disease process such as osteoporosis would result; however, if the degree of imbalance is quite large, widespread bone lysis and hypercalcemia could be expected.

A.R. Morton: Department of Medicine, Queen's University/ Kingston General Hospital, Kingston, Ontario K7L 2V7, Canada.

P.S. Ritch: Department of Medicine, Division of Hematology/ Oncology, Medical College of Wisconsin, Milwaukee, WI 53226.

The adult human body contains about 1 kg of calcium, of which all but 10 g is lodged in bone. Minute intracellular concentrations of calcium ($10^{-8}$ to $10^{-7}$ molar) are vital to normal cellular function, but most of the nonosseous calcium is present in the extracellular fluid. Under normal circumstances, the total body calcium represents a steady state between calcium intake and excretion. Somewhere between 25% and 50% of the dietary calcium intake of approximately 1 to 1.5 g per day is absorbed. Although bone represents an enormous reservoir of calcium, little transfer (of the order of 500 mg, or 12.5 mmol, per day) occurs between bone and the plasma in the state of good health (6). When net calcium balance is zero, the kidneys are required to excrete about 150 mg of calcium daily. Glomerular filtration of nonprotein bound calcium is of the order of 10 g/day, of which 65% is reabsorbed in the proximal convoluted tubule and 25% in the ascending limb of the loop of Henle, where resorption is independent of hormonal control. Proximal nephron calcium reabsorption is closely linked to sodium reabsorption. In situations of volume depletion (such as those induced by hypercalcemia), inappropriate calcium retention may occur as the kidney attempts to conserve sodium and hence extracellular fluid volume. A variable amount of the remaining calcium is reabsorbed from the distal convoluted tubule. Calcium reabsorption in this area is increased in the presence of parathyroid hormone (PTH), and it is at this site that the fine tuning of calcium homeostasis occurs. Renal calcium losses can increase to accommodate an increase in bone turnover of about 150% before hypercalcemia will occur.

The routinely measured total plasma calcium concentration is composed of a combination of physiologically active or ionized calcium, accounting for about 45% of the total protein-bound calcium, the bulk of which is bound to albumin and accounts for approximately 45% of the total, and the remainder (10%), which is complexed with ions such as bicarbonate and citrate. In terms of patient management, the ionized calcium concentration carries the greatest significance. Although ion-specific electrode measurement of ionized calcium is available, most centers routinely measure the total serum calcium. The correlation between total serum calcium and ionized calcium is, at best, only fair. The proportion of the the total calcium in the unbound or physiologically active state varies with, among other things, the albumin concentration. Numerous algorithms have been designed to attempt to "correct" total serum calcium, particularly in the face of reduced albumin concentrations. The algorithms listed here are clinically useful, and it is imperative that clinical decisions are made not on the basis of a total calcium but at the very least a corrected calcium (7,8).

$$Ca \text{ (corrected)} = Ca \text{ (measured)} + [0.8 \times (4 - \text{albumin concentration})] \textit{ Conventional Units}$$

$$CA \text{ (corrected)} = Ca \text{ (measured)} + [0.02 \times (40 - \text{albumin concentration})] \textit{ SI Units}$$

Under normal circumstances, calcium and bone metabolism are tightly regulated by the action of three main hormones.

Parathyroid hormone (PTH) is an 84 amino acid polypeptide secreted by the parathyroid glands in response to low ionized serum calcium. It enhances calcium resorption from bone by an indirect action on osteoclasts. In addition, PTH diminishes distal nephron calcium excretion and by its action on the renal 1-alpha hydroxylase increases circulating $1,25\text{-}(OH_2)D_3$ (di-hydroxyvitamin $D_3$) (the main active metabolite of the vitamin D complex of sterols).

Most of the biological activity of PTH is contained within the first 34 amino acid residues (9). This is of clinical significance because this amino acid sequence is shared in part with a tumor product, PTH-related peptide (PTHrP, discussed later).

The vitamin D complex is a group of steroid hormones with important effects on bone metabolism and calcium homeostasis. The main active metabolite is $1,25\text{-}(OH)_2D_3$ (di-hydroxyvitamin $D_3$). Hydroxylation of vitamin D is a two-step process. The 25-hydroxylation takes place in the liver and is substrate dependent. Conversion to the active dihydroxy metabolite is the rate-limiting step, which takes place in the kidney and is stimulated by PTH (vide supra) and inhibited by $1,25\text{-}(OH_2D_3)$. Vitamin D brings about its effects by increasing calcium absorption from the gastrointestinal tract and enhancing calcium reabsorption in the kidney.

Calcitonin, the physiological antagonist to PTH, is a 32 amino acid polypeptide hormone secreted by the C cells of the thyroid gland. Using time-lapse photography, calcitonin can be seen to have a powerful and rapid suppressive action on osteoclast activity. Downregulation of calcitonin receptors is known to occur, making its clinical effects generally short lived. The true physiologic role for calcitonin is unclear because biochemical disturbances are unusual in patients who have had complete thyroidectomies or in patients with extremely high levels in medullar carcinoma of the thyroid gland. It may be that calcitonin is a physiologic regulator of postprandial hypercalcemia (10).

Two main mechanisms contribute to the development of hypercalcemia in most patients with malignancy. In local osteolytic hypercalcemia, tumor invasion of bone causes release of large amounts of calcium from destroyed areas of bone. In the humoral hypercalcemia of malignancy, the effects of PTH are mimicked by PTHrP. In this situation, renal tubular reabsorption of filtered calcium is increased in addition to the increased generalized osteoclastic activity throughout the skeleton. These mechanisms are not mutually exclusive because some tumor types that metastasize to bone also manufacture

PTHrP. Enhanced gastrointestinal absorption of calcium is a rare mechanism for hypercalcemia of malignancy, limited mainly to hematological disorders.

## Local Osteolytic Hypercalcemia

Metastatic tumor cells are capable of resorbing bone directly (11), although the classic studies of Glasko (12) suggest that most of the resorption is carried out by osteoclasts. The tumor types commonly associated with this form of hypercalcemia are carcinoma of the breast, multiple myeloma, and other hematological malignancies. A large bony burden of tumor is usually required to produce the hypercalcemia.

### Carcinoma of the Breast

Hypercalcemia is an infrequent finding in patients with carcinoma of the breast in the absence of widespread osseous metastases. Histologic evidence demonstrates that bone destruction is mediated by osteoclasts in close proximity to tumor cells. Breast cancer cell growth regulation is thought to occur in part under the influence of a number of closely associated growth factors (13). Epidermal growth factor (EGF) and transforming growth factor alpha (TGF-$\alpha$) are produced in a paracrine fashion at the site of bone metastases. These substances, which share a common receptor, are potent stimulators of osteoclastic bone resorption. Both TGF-$\alpha$ and EGF can be found by immunohistologic techniques in breast cancer cells. The local release, particularly of TGF-$\alpha$, in bone could be predicted both to increase metastasis growth and to enhance osteoclastic activation and bone resorption, thereby making room for the multiplying tumor cells.

In their classic studies, Galasko and Bennett (14) demonstrated that osteoclast recruitment and bone destruction stimulated by implants of the VX$_2$ carcinoma in rabbits could be reduced by the oral administration of the cyclooxygenase inhibitor indomethacin. Confirmatory evidence for a role for prostaglandins in the development of metastases came from Powles and colleagues (15), who showed a reduced incidence of bone metastases in rats bearing the Walker tumor. Unfortunately, the use of prostaglandin synthesis inhibitors has not been effective in influencing the course of metastatic bone disease in patients with breast cancer.

Despite the fact that most hypercalcemic breast cancer patients have a significant bony metastatic burden, it is clear that not all cases are due to local factors. An enhanced tubular reabsorption of calcium in breast cancer patients has been demonstrated (16). In this study, the authors concluded that approximately 40% of the observed hypercalcemia was accounted for by a renal mechanism. It is known that breast cancer cells can produce and secrete PTHrP (indeed, one of the original tumor types from which PTHrP was isolated was breast cancer) (17). In fact, serum elevation and tumor histochemical localization of PTHrP is common in breast cancer patients, even before the development of hypercalcemia (18).

### Multiple Myeloma

In patients with multiple myeloma, there is an intimate association between the malignant plasma cells and the bone marrow. Fracturing osteopenia and hypercalcemia are frequent complications in these patients. Histologic studies have shown a close association between myeloma cells and activated osteoclasts. Over the last 20 years, significant advances have been made in elucidating the mechanisms of the bone resorption in multiple myeloma. In the mid-1970s, Mundy and colleagues (19) demonstrated that supernatants from myeloma cells in tissue culture had osteoclast-activating activity that lead to the mobilization of $^{45}$Ca from fetal rat long bones. These substances were descriptively named *osteoclast activating factors* (OAF). It has become increasingly clear that more than one substance elaborated by multiple myeloma cells has OAF activity. Several groups of investigators have identified potent osteoclast-activating properties associated with various multifunctional cytokines, including lymphotoxin (tumor necrosis factor $\beta$) (20), interleukin-1 (IL-1) (21), and interleukin-6 (IL-6) (22). Many of these same factors are also potent inhibitors of osteoblastic bone formation.

The multifunctional cytokine IL-6 is well recognized as a growth promoter for myeloma cells. It potentiates the actions of other bone-restoring cytokines such as IL-1 and lymphotoxin, although its effect on bone metabolism is not clear. Levels of IL-6 increase in the advanced phases of disease when widespread osteopenia is manifest, although a direct cause and effect phenomenon cannot be inferred.

Patients with multiple myeloma frequently have abnormal renal function. Reductions in glomerular filtration rate caused by myeloma kidney or light-chain nephropathy hamper the ability of the body to excrete the excessive calcium load. Furthermore, the calcium elevation itself is also nephrotoxic and can lead to a vicious cycle of deteriorating renal function and hypercalcemia.

In rare patients with multiple myeloma or monoclonal gammopathy of undetermined significance (MGUS), the phenomenon of pseudohypercalcemia may occur (23). In this situation, calcium becomes bound to nonalbumin plasma proteins, resulting in a spuriously elevated total serum calcium concentration. The ionized calcium concentration is normal under these circumstances, but correction formulae using albumin will give falsely abnormal results.

## Humoral Hypercalcemia of Malignancy

The concept of a humoral factor being responsible for the genesis of hypercalcemia is not a new one. In 1941 Fuller Albright (24) described the case of a patient with a renal cell carcinoma who was significantly hypercalcemic despite a very low bony metastatic burden. This patient also had significant hypophosphatemia, and the clinical features suggestive of primary hyperparathyroidism had been enough to lead the surgeons to perform a neck exploration. Although PTH could not be recovered from biopsy material from the tumor, Albright postulated that a humoral factor secreted by the tumor was responsible for the hypercalcemia. Indeed, the term *pseudohyperparathyroidism* was popularized in the 1960s (25,26).

In their extensive metabolic evaluation of 50 patients with hypercalcemia and malignant disease in 1980, Stewart and colleagues (27) divided the patients into two groups. One group shared the features of primary hyperparathyroidism, including a tendency to hypophosphatemia, a lowered renal phosphate threshold (RPT), and an elevated nephrogenous cyclic adenosine monophosphate (NcAMP) excretion. These patients mostly had squamous carcinomas, renal carcinomas, and urothelial malignancies. The second group, who mostly had metastatic carcinoma of the breast and multiple myeloma, had low levels of NcAMP excretion. The authors concluded that urinary NcAMP was a surrogate marker for a circulating substance that had PTH-like activity. Using assays available at the time, they were unable to detect elevated levels of PTH in the sera of these patients.

Although they continue to be rare, anecdotal reports of ectopic PTH production causing hypercalcemia (28) do occur; but native PTH is not the substance responsible for most cases of humoral hypercalcemia of malignancy. The strongest evidence came from the fact that using complementary DNA techniques Simpson and colleagues (29) failed to demonstrate the production of PTH by tumors commonly associated with hypercalcemia. The development of a sensitive two-site immunoradiometric assay for PTH helped considerably to overcome the problems of measuring this compound, which has a very short plasma half-life but many products of metabolism that interfere with more conventional assays (30).

### Parathyroid Hormone-related Protein

In 1987 three groups independently published descriptions of a novel polypeptide hormone that had been isolated from tumors associated with the hypercalcemia of malignancy (17,31,32). Parathyroid hormone-related protein is a much larger molecule than PTH. Although the predominant circulating form of PTHrP is not yet known with certainty, the original authors describe several isoforms of this hormone, including 139, 141, and 173 amino acid residues that arise by alternative splicing of RNA and differ only in their carboxy termini. The primary structure of these peptides shows considerable N-terminal homology with native PTH, with eight of the first 13 amino acids being identical; PTHrP interacts the PTH receptor with equal affinity to the native hormone, accounting for its ability to mimic both the renal and bony effects of PTH. Many normal fetal and adult tissues produce PTHrP. Its true physiologic role is unclear, although it has been suggested that it may be involved in lactation and in maintaining the maternal-to-fetal calcium gradient generated by the placenta (33).

Definitive evidence for the biological activity of PTHrP having a causal role in hypercalcemia of malignancy came from studies in nude mice bearing a human tumor responsible for hypercalcemia. By causing an antiserum directed against synthetic human PTHrP, Kukreja and colleagues (34) were able to reverse the biochemical abnormalities of hypercalcemia, hypophosphatemia, and increased NcAMP excretion in these animals. These experiments provided strong evidence that PTHrP was directly responsible for the hypercalcemia.

The development of assays for PTHrP has been plagued by similar problems as those for PTH. The levels in normal serum are quite low (below 2.5 pmol/L), and the nature and reactivity of metabolic byproducts is not clear. Two-site immunoradiometric assays have been developed and are more sensitive. Using a midregional assay, Blind and colleagues (35) reported that 81% of hypercalcemic patients who had squamous tumors had an elevated PTHrP level. Studies using two-site assays have detected elevated serum levels of PTHrP in 90% to 95% of patients with squamous carcinomas and hypercalcemia (36,37).

Whereas PTHrP is commonly considered in the context of humoral hypercalcemia, there are interesting reports of its relationship to bone metastases in patients with breast cancer. Powell and colleagues (38) reported that 92% of bony metastases from breast cancer stain positive for PTHrP immunohistochemically compared with only 17% of metastases at other sites (38). The role of PTHrP in bone tropism is unclear but certainly requires further investigation.

### Vitamin D

Levels of $1,25\text{-}(OH)_2D_3$ are low in most cases of hypercalcemia of malignancy; however, there are a group of malignant (and some nonmalignant) disorders in which $1,25\text{-}(OH)_2D_3$ is elevated and acts as a humoral mediator of hypercalcemia. It has been known for more than 10 years that granulomatous conditions, such as sarcoidosis (39), are associated with extrarenal synthesis of $1,25\text{-}(OH)_2D_3$. The site of the ectopic 1-$\alpha$ hydroxylation is presumably in the macrophages associated with the granulomata. Davies and colleagues (40) described a substrate-dependent conversion of 25-hydroxyvitamin $D_3$ to 1,25-dihydroxyvitamin $D_3$ in a hypercalcemic patient with Hodgkin disease exposed to increased levels of sunlight. This response was no longer seen after successful treatment of the malignancy. Although occasional case reports of hypercalcemia and abnormally elevated 1,25-dihydroxyvitamin $D_3$ have appeared in the literature (41,42), hypercalcemia remains an uncommon complication of hematological malignancies other than myeloma. In a large series of 217 patients with advanced lymphoma, only four cases of hypercalcemia were reported (43).

A significant exception to the rare finding of hypercalcemia in lymphomas is adult T-cell lymphoma, an uncommon tumor in North America that appears to be associated with infection with the human T-cell lymphotropic virus type 1 (HTLV-1). More than half of these patients develop hypercalcemia, which is a common cause of death. Although elevated 1,25-$(OH)_2D_3$ levels have been reported in these patients, there is also evidence for elevation in PTHrP levels, suggesting that an interaction of humoral mediators may be responsible (44). The topic of calcitriol-mediated hypercalcemia in lymphomatous disease has been recently reviewed (45).

## Other Hypercalcemia Factors

Case reports and animal studies have added significantly to the number of mediators that may be responsible for hypercalcemia in malignant disease. Squamous carcinomas have been reported to produce IL-1 either in the presence (46) or absence (47) of hypercalcemia. Furthermore, these tumors also secrete colony-stimulating factors, which may enhance osteoclast precursor generation. Indeed, simultaneous tumor production of IL-1 and PTHrP has been demonstrated (48), and these two hypercalcemia factors may interact synergistically in vitro and in vivo (49). Cosecretion of IL-6 and PTHrP also has been described (50). Similarly, tumor production of prostaglandins associated with the development of hypercalcemia is also well recognized (51).

Although PTH is rarely the humoral factor causing hypercalcemia, secreting carcinomas of the parathyroid glands may occur. In the rare group of multiple endocrine neoplasia syndromes, hyperparathyroidism and asymptomatic hypercalcemia due to PTH secretion is common.

It is likely that many of the substances discussed above, both systemically and locally secreted, combine to cause hypercalcemia in malignant disease. Undoubtedly, further compounds will be found as our understanding of this process increases.

## EVALUATION OF THE HYPERCALCEMIC PATIENT

Hypercalcemia usually occurs in the face of overt malignancy, and so the diagnosis as to the cause of the hypercalcemia is rarely in doubt. In spite of this fact, it is worth considering other causes of hypercalcemia (Table 1),

**TABLE 1.** *Nonmalignant causes of hypercalcemia*

| | |
|---|---|
| Endocrine | Hyperparathyroidism |
| | Hyperthyroidism |
| | Addison disease |
| Iatrogenic | Immobilization |
| | Vitamins A and D |
| | Thiazide diuretics |
| | Lithium |
| Other | Paget disease of bone |
| | Granulomatous disease |

which may be readily amenable to therapeutic intervention. Additionally, aggravating factors such as immobilization should be sought and attempts made to rectify these factors.

## Clinical Findings

The symptoms of hypercalcemia are often vague and nonspecific. Furthermore, there is an imperfect correlation between the calcium level and the degree of symptomatology. Indeed, severe hypercalcemia may be an incidental finding on a biochemical screen of a patient with malignant disease. The rate of development of hypercalcemia may influence the occurrence of symptoms.

Gastrointestinal upset occurs in most symptomatic individuals. Nausea, anorexia, and vomiting are common, but they may be ascribed to the side effects of chemotherapy or to symptoms produced by the tumor itself. By inducing dehydration and hence aggravating the hypercalcemia, these complications set up a vicious cycle. Constipation is common, and complete ileus may occur at severely raised calcium levels. Cramping abdominal pains such as those seen in primary hyperparathyroidism are encountered occasionally, but acute pancreatitis or peptic ulceration complicating the hypercalcemia of malignancy is extremely rare. It is likely that the relative acuteness of the disease as compared with, say, primary hyperparathyroidism accounts for the low incidence of these latter adverse effects.

Hypercalcemia per se is toxic to the renal tubules. It causes a reversible impairment in renal concentrating ability, resulting in the production of large volumes of dilute urine. This polyuria serves to aggravate the volume depletion produced by the gastrointestinal effects and results in a fall in the glomerular filtration rate, which, in turn, causes further impairment of the kidney's ability to handle the abnormal calcium load, and the viscious cycle continues. Although the major disturbance in tubular function is related to changes in urinary concentrating ability, another important renal effect is that of an inappropriate natriuresis. The extracellular fluid volume contraction results in attempts by the proximal tubule to conserve sodium, and because of a linkage between renal sodium and calcium handling, calcium is also retained. Despite the fact that the thirst mechanism is intact and polydypsia occurs, the gastrointestinal upset is often so great that severe volume depletion occurs. Impaired mental status may further compromise fluid intake. Solute washout of potassium and magnesium can occur as a result of the polyuria, and some of the neuromuscular effects of hypercalcemia can be aggravated by relative deficiencies of these ions.

Hypercalcemia frequently is overlooked as a cause of neuropsychiatric symptoms in patients with advanced malignant disease. Rather, these are often ascribed to the underlying neoplasm or to medications the patient may be taking, such as narcotic analgesics, antiemetics, or sedatives. Muscle weakness may be profound, confining the patient to bed and aggravating the hypercalcemia because of immobility. As hypercalcemia worsens, confusion and finally coma supervene. Reversible focal neurological symptoms with hypercalcemia have been reported but are rare.

Cardiac muscle appears relatively immune to the effects of hypercalcemia, which has a digitalis-like effect on cardiac contractility. Reduction of the $QT_c$ may be observed occasionally on ECG, but unless the patient is given cardiac glycosides, the cardiac effects are of little clinical significance. Arrhythmias are more likely to occur because of associated hypokalemia or hypomagnesemia during the treatment phase when rapid intravascular volume expansion is occurring.

Bone pain is a frequent symptom of both malignant disease and hypercalcemia. Although this pain may be due in part to the presence of bony metastases, the symptom is also present in the absence of demonstrable metastatic disease. Calcium may act as a neurosensitizer, decreasing the pain threshold, but the precise mechanism of pain generation in hypercalcemia is unclear.

The syndrome of hypercalcemia of malignancy, therefore, presents itself with anorexia, fatigue, apathy and polyuria but may rapidly progress to obtundation and death.

### Laboratory Investigations

The diagnosis and management of hypercalcemia in a patient with malignant disease require little in the way of investigations. A complete blood count and estimation of the platelet count should be performed. Measurement of serum electrolytes, blood urea nitrogen, and creatinine is mandatory. The ionized calcium level is the best clinically relevant measurement to perform; however, it is less readily available and more expensive than a total calcium level. The total serum calcium level is a poor indicator of the biologically active component and should not be used alone to direct initial management without the use of a correction algorithm to take into account the effect of altered albumin concentrations. In asymptomatic patients with hypercalcemia and multiple

myeloma, a serum ionized calcium should be obtained to exclude pseudohypercalcemia.

Renal function and the response of the calcium to therapy should be monitored daily until the calcium concentration normalizes. Close attention should be paid to changes in potassium and magnesium levels, which may drop dramatically during the early treatment phase because of volume expansion and increased glomerular filtration rate as the hypercalcemia is corrected. An underlying potassium deficiency caused by poor dietary intake is frequently unmasked at this time. Serum phosphate levels may fall precipitously in some patients, particularly when potent antiresorptive therapy is used.

Once the calcium level returns to normal, weekly estimation can act as a guide to the need for further antihypercalcemia therapy. Of course, investigations should be individualized depending on the patient's clinical condition and response to therapy.

From the academic viewpoint, greater insight into the mechanism behind the hypercalcemia can be gained from more complex investigations. These have few practical implications given the current therapeutic options but may become more relevant if, say, effective blockade of the parathyroid hormone receptor becomes possible or monoclonal antibodies to PTHrP are developed for clinical use. In the absence of a readily available assay for PTHrP, biochemical clues to its presence include hypophosphatemia, hyperchloremia, and a mild metabolic acidosis, although these could not be considered diagnostic. Urinary excretion of calcium is high in all cases of hypercalcemia (despite inappropriate calcium resorption stimulated by PTHrP). The renal phosphate threshold is low in the presence of PTHrP, indicating a renal phosphate leak, and significant hypophosphatemia may result following the treatment of hypercalcemia.

The serum immunoreactive PTH is low or undetectable unless the primary site of malignancy is the parathyroid gland itself. Vitamin D metabolites are also frequently low in most cases of hypercalcemia, despite the fact that PTHrP is capable of stimulating the renal 1-α hydroxylase in animal models. The reason for this paradox is not clear, although it has been suggested that tumors may secrete an independent inhibitor of 1-α hydroxylase (52). Measures of osteoblastic function, such as alkaline phosphatase and bone gla-protein (osteocalcin), have little to offer in the diagnosis of hypercalcemia. Although plain radiography and isotope bone scans may help with other aspects of management, they are of little use in the diagnosis and management of hypercalcemia in the face of established disease.

### Grading Hypercalcemia in Malignant Disease

The appearance of hypercalcemia in patients with malignant disease is a poor prognostic indicator in most clinical situations. The major exception is in patients recently indicated on tamoxifen therapy for breast cancer. The mechanism by which tamoxifen causes hypercalcemia is unclear. It is likely, however, that prostaglandins play a central role in this phenomenon of tamoxifen-induced "flare," which is frequently associated with bone pain and a response of the tumor to therapy.

From a practical point of view, it is important to note that the development and severity of symptoms do not correlate well with the serum calcium level. Indeed, patients with symptoms readily relatable to hypercalcemia should be classified and treated as severe, independent of the absolute calcium level. An observation that is frequently made, but poorly understood, is that patients with tumor-induced hypercalcemia often have greater symptomatology for any given rise in calcium level compared with patients with primary hyperthyroidism.

Patients with a corrected serum calcium level below 3.0 mmol/L (<12 mg/dl) who are asymptomatic can be considered as having mild hypercalcemia. This condition may have been detected as part of the routine biochemical workup in patients with tumor types known to predispose to hypercalcemia. Often these patients are being monitored in the outpatient clinic. With the new development of hypercalcemia, it is important to reevaluate the current antineoplastic therapy because this complication may be an early indication of a diminishing response. Immediate treatment of the hypercalcemia may not be indicated, but it is important to remember that the natural history will be for the hypercalcemia to worsen unless a tumor response can be initiated or some intercurrent illness that has precipitated the hypercalcemia can be reversed.

In asymptomatic patients with a serum calcium of 3.0 to 3.5 mmol/L (12–14 mg/dl), the situation is more serious. Any event that induces volume depletion or reduces the glomerular filtration rate, including the institution of medication such as nonsteroidal antiinflammatory agents, may be enough to lead to severe hypercalcemia. Patients with a corrected serum calcium concentration of greater than 3.5 mmol/L (>14 mg/dl) require urgent treatment, as do patients with asymptomatic hypercalcemia.

## TREATMENT OF HYPERCALCEMIA

### General Considerations

It is possible to lower the serum calcium concentration in almost all patients with tumor-induced hypercalcemia. The basic principles to be used are relatively simple. Most patients with hypercalcemia are sodium and water deplete and require aggressive rehydration. The best therapeutic strategy is one directed at removing the cause of the hypercalcemia, including the judicious use of surgery, radiotherapy, and chemotherapy. Hypercalcemia is maintained by two main pathways. Enhanced osteoclastic bone resorption is present in virtually all cases of hypercalcemia. Specific antiresorptive therapy is available and should be used early in the management of the complication. Increased renal reabsorption of calcium is present in cases where PTHrP is acting on the kidneys. In an attempt to offset this problem, high urine volume should be maintained, but direct antagonism of the effects of PTHrP on the kidney is not readily available.

Dietary restriction of calcium containing products seems intuitively appropriate; however, it is important to remember that, except where the mechanism of the hypercalcemia is thought to be vitamin D dependent, gastrointestinal absorption of calcium will be very low. Every effort should be made to maintain the mobility of the patient, and medications predisposing to hypercalcemia, such as thiazide diuretics and vitamin D and A supplements, should be avoided. Table 2 summarizes potential options for the management of hypercalcemia in malignant disease.

### Ethical Considerations

When embarking on the treatment of hypercalcemia in malignant disease, it is important to have clear goals in mind. If no therapeutic intervention directed at the underlying malignancy is available or planned, patient survival is short lived. Ralston and colleagues (52) reported a median survival time of 30 days for 100 hypercalcemic patients in whom no antitumor therapy was available; indeed, all patients in this group had died by 120 days. These data are similar to those presented by Nussbaum and colleagues (53), who report a median survival of 1.4 months. If such a patient is relatively asymptomatic or already obtunded, it may be that aggressive attempts to normalize calcium levels are unwarranted. In most patients with symptomatic hypercalcemia, however, the mental status abnormalities and confusion as well as the chronic nausea and constipation are so troublesome as to make palliative antihypercalcemic therapy worthwhile. Indeed, even in cases in which symptoms may be severe, normalization of serum calcium and resolution of symptoms can be achieved with appropriate therapy, which may allow a terminally ill patient less of a chance to see and speak with family members and clergy, attend to legal matters, and complete unfinished business. We find that early consultation with the palliative care team is extremely useful in these circumstances, as long-term antihypercalcemia therapy can be given on an outpatient basis or even in the patient's home.

### Extracellular Fluid (ECF) Volume Expansion

The combined effects of anorexia, vomiting, compromised mental status, and nephrogenic diabetes insipidus

**TABLE 2.** *Therapeutic options for hypercalcemia[a]*

| Treatment | Dose | Response[b] | Comments |
|---|---|---|---|
| Saline diuresis | 3 L/day IV or more | Rarely complete | Important component of therapy for severe hypercalcemia due to accompanying dehydration (see text) |
| Furosemide | 40–80 mg/day PO or IV | See comment | Useful for maintaining diuresis in patients receiving aggressive hydration (especially elderly) to avoid fluid overload |
| Pamidronate | 60–90 mg IV over 4 h | Approximately 90% | Highly effective, well tolerated, convenient for outpatient administration |
| Etidronate | 7.5 mg/kg IV over 2 h for 3–5 days | 25–40% | Historic interest only |
| Gallium nitrate | 200 mg/m²/day for 5 days | 75–80% | Inconvenient schedule, potentially nephrotoxic |
| Plicamycin (Mithramycin) | 25 µg/kg IV (approx. 1.5–2.0 mg) | Approx. 40% | Emetogenic, vessicant; increased response with repeated daily dosing but with increased myelosuppression, hepatic and renal toxicity |
| Calcitonin | 4 MRC U/kg SQ q 12 h to 8 MRC U/kg SQ q 6 h (approx. 300–600 U) | See comment | Rapid effect but seldom complete normalization of serum calcium; tachyphylaxis |
| Glucocorticoids | Prednisone 40–100 mg/day or equivalent | See comment | Effective in hematological malignancies with cytokine or 1,25-(OH)$_2$D$_3$ mediated hypercalcemia and hormone-induced skeletal flare response |
| Antiprostaglandins | Indomethacin 75–100 mg/day or equivalent | Rare | Little value |
| Inorganic phosphorus | 1 g/day in divided doses titrated to 2–3 g/day | Maintenance usage | Dose-limiting diarrhea |

[a]Currently approved in the United States.
[b]Normalization of albumin-adjusted serum calcium.
IV, intravenously; PO, orally; SQ, subcutaneously.

render most patients with hypercalcemia significantly volume depleted, as much as 5 to 10 L. Under these circumstances, the glomerular filtration rate is reduced and inappropriate calcium retention will occur as the kidneys attempt to conserve sodium. Normal saline solution should be infused, initially as rapidly as the patient's cardiac status will tolerate. Thereafter a saline infusion should be continued until normocalcemia is restored by other means. If a state of mild volume overload can be induced, the fractional excretion of calcium can be increased significantly. Hosking and colleagues (54) demonstrated that it was possible to produce a mean drop in calcium concentration of 0.6 mmol/L in their study of 16 hypercalcemic patients. The authors conclude that most of the calcium-lowering effect was based on improving the glomerular filtration rate and increasing the fractional excretion of sodium, permitting appropriate off-loading of calcium by the kidneys. Interestingly, they noted three patients in whom the tubular resorption rate of calcium appeared fixed. Presumably, those patients were reabsorbing calcium under the influence of PTHrP. Although restoration of fluid volume rarely restores the calcium level to the normal range (the mean postrehydration value in Hosking's study was 3.24 mmol/L (12.8 mg/dl), a failure to rehydrate the patients will certainly compromise the efficiency of other therapeutic maneuvers.

## Antiresorptive Therapy

Enhanced osteoclastic bone resorption, either driven hormonally by the effects of PTHrP or in a paracrine fashion by factors released from tumor deposits within bone, is the final common pathway in the genesis of hypercalcemia in malignant disease. It is of little surprise, therefore, that osteoclast inhibitors are effective in the treatment of hypercalcemia. In the last decade, the introduction of newer, more effective, and less toxic antiresponsive medications have replaced more conventional methods for the management of the hypercalcemia of malignancy.

## Bisphosphonates

The bisphosphonates are structural analogs of pyrophosphate (PP$_i$) in which the P-O-P bond is replaced by a P-C-P bond that is resistant to enzymatic cleavage by endogenous pyrophosphatases (Fig. 1). The commonly used bisphosphonates are etidronate (1-hyroxyethylidene-1, 1-bisphosphonate); clodronate (dichloromethylene bisphosphonate); and the aminobisphosphonates, pamidronate (3-amino-1-hydroxypropylidene-1, 1-bisphosphonate) and alendronate (4-amino-1-hyroxybutylidene-1, 1-bisphosphonate).

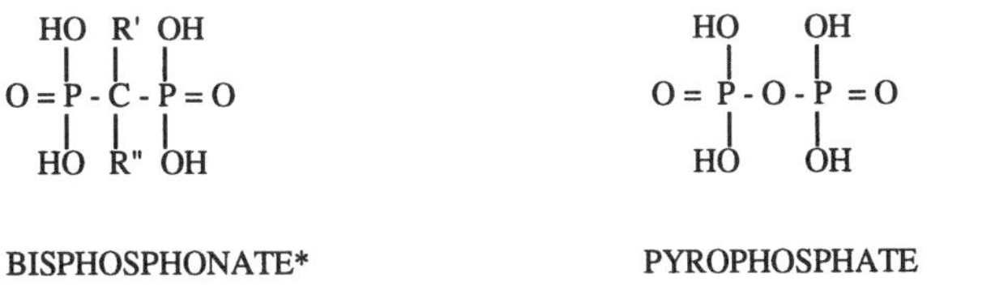

**FIG. 1.** Chemical structure of commonly used bisphosphonates compared with pyrophosphate.

Bisphosphonates share poor and unpredictable oral bioavailability. Furthermore, the bioavailability is reduced almost to zero if they are ingested with food. In the setting of symptomatic hypercalcemia of malignancy, the intravenous route is preferred because nausea and vomiting are such frequent occurrences. Once absorbed, about half of the ingested dose is excreted unchanged in the urine. Bone mineral has a high affinity for bisphosphonates, which are rapidly absorbed onto the bone surface (55). Although the bulk of any absorbed bisphosphonate is rapidly relocated to the bone, this is nonhomogeneous, with most of the bisphosphonate located in areas of highest bone turnover.

The method by which bisphosphonates inhibit osteoclast function is unclear, and it is likely that several mechanisms are involved. The high-affinity adsorption of bisphosphonates to hydroxyapatite crystals suggests that an important physicochemical process may operate. Bisphosphonates affect the ionic composition of the hydration layer that normally surrounds bone crystals (56). The altered concentrations of calcium and phosphate in this microenvironment may be responsible for the relative stability induced by the bisphosphonates.

Osteoclast attachment to bone may be reduced in the presence of bisphosphonates. Carano and colleagues (57) demonstrated a 30% reduction in bone binding by osteoclasts in tissue culture in the presence of etidronate, clodronate, and pamidronate. An inhibition of osteoclast acid hydrolases also has been described (58). Given that these enzymes are so important in bone resorption, this may account in part for some of the effects of the bisphosphonates. Other effects suggested for bisphosphonates include a reduction in osteoclast progenitor maturation, interference with energy-producing enzymes, and a direct cytotoxic effect on osteoclasts.

### *Etidronate*

Etidronate was the first commercially available bisphosphonate. It has been studied extensively in patients with various metabolic bone diseases, including Paget disease of bone and osteoporosis. In a large double-blind multicenter trial of more than 200 patients, etidronate given in a dosage of 7.5 mg/kg/day for 3 consecutive days resulted in normalization of the corrected serum calcium in 24% of patients (59), although the corrected calcium fell into the normal range in only 7% of the control group, who had received saline infusions alone. The effect of the drug is seen after about 48 hours, with the nadir calcium value occurring afer 7 to 10 days. The hypocalcemic effect of etidronate is transient, although it has been suggested that the duration of response can be increased by the use of oral etidronate 20 mg/kg (60).

Comparative studies demonstrated that etidronate is the least effective of the newer antihypercalcemic agents. A European study of the three commonly available bisphosphonates at the time (i.e., etidronate, clodronate, and pamidronate) demonstrated that a single intravenous infusion of 30 mg pamidronate induced a more rapid and more pronounced fall in serum calcium than 600 mg of clodronate as a single intravenous dose or 7.5 mg/kg etidronate intravenously for 3 days (61). A randomized, double-blind multicenter study comparing the hypocalcemic effects of etidronate and pamidronate confirmed the superiority of the latter bisphosphonate. Seventy percent of patients receiving a single dose of 60 mg pamidronate achieved a normal corrected calcium concentration compared with only 41% of patients receiving 7.5 mg/kg/day etidronate for 3 days (62). Furthermore, a randomized, double-blind study comparing etidronate 7.5 mg/kg/day with gallium nitrate 200 mg/m$^2$/day showed that whereas a normal corrected calcium was achieved in 43% of etidronate-treated patients, the success rate was 82% for gallium nitrate-treated patients (63).

### Clodronate

Clodronate is a highly efficacious bisphosphonate. The appearance of three cases of acute leukemia in 664 patients in a multicenter study involving its use in the United States led to the temporary withdrawal of this agent (64). Despite this concern, clodronate has continued to be used both intravenously and orally for the management of hypercalcemia and other neoplastic effects on bone in Europe and Canada. It is an effective agent in restoring normocalcemia, with a reported response rate of 89% (24 of 27 patients) in one study of patients receiving 100 to 300 mg/day for 3 to 10 days (65). Oral clodronate also appears able to induce a normocalcemic response (66). In the clinical situation of the acute management of hypercalcemia, the intravenous route is preferred; however, long-term treatment with oral clodronate may be a useful therapy to maintain normocalcemia.

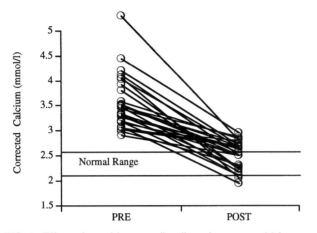

**FIG. 2.** Effect of pamidronate disodium therapy on 30 hypercalcemic patients. From Morton et al. (68).

### Pamidronate

Pamidronate disodium is the first aminobisphosphonate licensed for clinical use. It is effective in restoring normocalcemia (Fig. 2), with expected response rates of the order of 90% (67). Although an early dose-response study suggested little advantage to increasing the dose beyond 0.25 mg/kg, a large multicenter trial in the United States has shown that a single starting dose of 90 mg may be optimum (3). In initial studies, pamidronate was given in divided doses over a period of several days; however, the normocalcemic effect can be achieved with single-dose therapy (68). Dodwell and colleagues (69) recently studied more rapid infusion rates and found that the drug can be given safely and efficaciously over a 2-hour period.

Pamidronate was shown to be the most effective of the bisphosphonates available in 1989 (61). In a comparative randomized, crossover study Thürlimann and colleagues (70) demonstrated that a single intravenous dose of 60 mg pamidronate was more effective than a dose of 20 µg/kg of plicamycin. No primary failures occurred in the pamidronate-treated group, and those primary failures in the plicamycin treated group became normocalcemic when treated with pamidronate. Although one randomized study comparing 30 mg with 90 mg pamidronate failed to show a significant difference in therapeutic efficacy (71), other prospective and retrospective evaluations identified a clear dose-response relationship over this dose range (3,72). This may have important clinical implications, particularly for patients with severely elevated serum calcium levels in whom higher doses may be necessary to achieve normocalcemia. For most patients, 60 mg pamidronate appears adequate to restore the serum calcium to normal. In the United States, initial approval restricted pamidronate administration to a 24-hour intravenous infusion. Subsequently, the approval was liberalized to allow shorter duration infusions over 4 hours, thus facilitating outpatient or home administration.

### Alendronate

Alendronate disodium is an aminobisphosphonate that is undergoing extensive study in the management of osteoporosis. Like other bisphosphonates, it is a powerful antihypercalcemic agent (73). A dose-response and duration of response study demonstrated that normalization of corrected calcium can be expected in about 90% of patients given 10 mg of this agent intravenously over 2 or 24 hours (74). As with pamidronate, the efficacy and safety of a rapid infusion rate lend itself to outpatient management.

### Effect of Tumor Type on Response to Bisphosphonates

Recent evidence has begun to suggest that cases of hypercalcemia that are mediated mainly by PTHrP may be more resistant to antiresorptive therapy. Gurney and colleagues (75) demonstrated that patients with a low renal phosphate threshold (indicative of the effects of PTHrP) responded less well to pamidronate therapy, and Dodwell and colleagues (76) demonstrated a statistically significant relationship between circulating PTHrP concentration and the time to normalization of hypercalcemia. Others (77) similarly noted decreased responsiveness to pamidronate when the hypercalcemia was associated with elevated levels of PTHrP. Relative resistance to the extremely powerful investigational bisphosphonate BM21.0955 (ibandronate) also was reported in patients with elevated serum PTHrP levels (78).

### Duration of Response to Bisphosphonate Therapy

The true duration of response to bisphosphonates is difficult to determine. The mortality rate in this group is high, and many patients die without becoming hypercalcemic again. Furthermore, effective antitumor therapy is introduced whenever possible, confounding the issue of time to recurrence of hypercalcemia. It appears that the duration of response for both etidronate and clodronate is of the order of a few days. For pamidronate the median duration of normocalcemia was found by Thiébaud and colleagues to be 35 days (79), significantly longer than the 9 to 13 days reported by Nussbaum and colleagues (3). The latter appears to be a more accurate estimate of the true response duration measured from the time normocalcemia is actually achieved to the time of the last normal serum calcium before relapse occurs. A prospective randomized study evaluating oral clodronate maintenance therapy is currently under way. Unfortunately, it is not possible to predict the length of time that any specific patient will remain normocalcemic.

### Side Effects of Bisphosphonates

Bisphosphonates have a wide therapeutic index, making them a good choice of agent for patients with advanced malignancy. Oral formulations tend to be associated with gastrointestinal intolerance, which may be dose limiting. This is not usually a problem in the acute setting, when intravenous therapy is indicated, but may limit their role chronically. Rapid intravenous infusions of etidronate and clodronate have been associated with the deterioration of kidney function in patients with myeloma and preexisting renal compromise (80). Low-grade pyrexia is noted in 10% to 15% of patients. Hyperphosphatemia is noted with etidronate therapy, but hypophosphatemia is seen with clodronate and pamidronate treatment. The mechanisms of phosphate imbalance are unclear and are rarely of clinical significance. Ocular adverse reactions occasionally may be observed, including anterior uveitis, scleritis, or episcleritis, and nonspecific conjunctivitis (81).

In addition to the four bisphosphonates described, several newer, more potent bisphosphonates are undergoing clinical trials for the management of various metabolic bone disorders.

### Gallium Nitrate

The antiresponsive mechanism of gallium nitrate is incompletely understood. It appears that this element has a direct action on bone to reduce the solubility of hydroxyapatite crystals (82). Bone resorption is significantly reduced, as indicated by a reduction in urinary calcium excretion in patients receiving this agent. Its hypocalcemic effects were discovered serendipitously as a side effect of antineoplastic therapy (83). Gallium is effective at restoring normocalcemia (84) (Fig. 3). As mentioned, it has been shown to be more potent than etidronate in a randomized, double-blind trial (63). Similarly, it is also more effective than calcitonin, as demonstrated by Warrell and colleagues (85). In this study, the normocalcemic response to gallium was 82% compared with only 43% for calcitonin. Gallium nitrate is well tolerated, although it may cause renal dysfunction if patients are not well hydrated or are receiving concomitant nephrotoxic agents. The most frequently used regimen of administration involves a continuous 5-day infusion at a rate of 200 mg/m². This limits the drug's usefulness with respect to long-term management.

### Plicamycin

Plicamycin, formerly mithramycin, is an antitumor antibiotic that has antiosteoclastic activity. Its mechanism of osteoclast inhibition is incompletely understood, but it appears to interfere with mRNA synthesis within the cells (86). Although highly effective in restoring normocalcemia, much concern has been raised over the potential side effects of marrow, hepatic, and renal toxicity. In fact, an infusion of 25 μg/kg over 4 to 6 hours is approximately one tenth the dose at which those side effects are commonly seen but will restore normocalcemia in about 80% of patients (87), although when albumin-adjusted calcium values are used, the response rate is only about 40% (70). The onset of the hypocalcemic effect is rapid with plicamycin, being evident within the first 24 hours. As with other agents, the individual duration of response is unpredictable, and close monitoring is necessary to avoid serious rebound hypercalcemia.

Plicamycin may be used with success in patients with recalcitrant hypercalcemia, although the weight of evidence favors bisphosphonate therapy (70). When necessary, repeated doses of plicamycin over 2 or 3 days may restore normocalcemia in refractory cases but may be associated with more significant myelosuppression and prolonged thrombocytopenia.

### Calcitonin

The hypocalcemic effects of calcitonin are due in part to a direct inhibition of osteoclast function. Normocalcemia is rarely restored with this agent; however, its actions are rapid, and it can be combined effectively with one of the powerful bisphosphonates (88,89). This may be particularly useful in patients in whom neurological symptoms due to the hypercalcemia are troublesome.

An additional advantage for calcitonin is that it induces a mild degree of renal calcium wasting that begins promptly after administration (90). Unfortunately, tachyphylaxis develops within 2 to 3 days due to downregulation of calcitonin receptors, and although this effect may be reduced by the simultaneous administration of corticosteroids (91), the effects of calcitonin are not long lasting. The suggested dose is 4 MRC U/kg every 12 hours

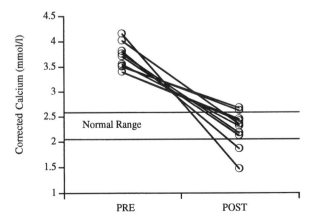

**FIG. 3.** Effect of gallium nitrate therapy on 13 hypercalcemic patients. From Warrell et al. (84).

by injection, although doses as high as 8 MRC U/kg every 6 hours may be used. A test dose of 1 MRC unit intradermally has been recommended to identify allergic individuals. An alternative route of administration is by rectal suppository (92).

### Prostaglandin Synthesis Inhibitors

Given the fact that some tumor types could cause hypercalcemia in association with the high renal excretion of prostaglandin synthetase inhibitors, it was hoped that these agents would be a powerful addition to the oncologist's armamentarium. Unfortunately, responses to these agents are relatively rare.

### Other Therapy

#### Furosemide

The loop diuretic furosemide continues to be used frequently in the management of hypercalcemia. Evidence for its effectiveness comes from a study in 1970 by Suki and colleagues (93), who used high doses of furosemide, in the order of 80 to 100 mg every 2 to 4 hours to achieve their effect. Generally speaking, this regimen is impractical because intensive fluid and electrolyte monitoring with appropriate replacement is required. The use of diuretics before establishing mild hypervolemia may even be counterproductive by enhancing the renal resorption of calcium linked to sodium from the proximal convoluted tubules.

Furosemide should be limited to patients in whom aggressive fluid replacement can potentially induce congestive cardiac failure. It has no place in the chronic management of hypercalcemia.

#### Corticosteroids

Glucocorticoids are another group of agents that are frequently used in the management of hypercalcemia of malignancy despite evidence that their role is very limited (Fig. 4) (94,95). Certain tumor types are inherently responsive to glucocorticoid therapy, including multiple myeloma and lymphoma. Osteolytic cytokines mediating the hypercalcemia may be inhibited by corticosteroids, and these agents also may be useful in managing the flare response occasionally seen after initiating hormonal therapy for breast cancer. In cases in which hypercalcemia is mediated by excessive $1,25\text{-}(OH)_2D_3$, glucocorticoids may have an antagonistic effect on calcium absorption from the gut (96).

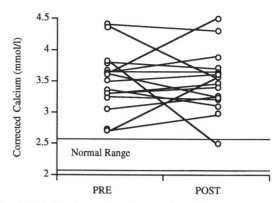

**FIG. 4.** Effect of varying doses of corticosteroids on ten hypercalcemic patients with solid tumors. (From Thalanissos and Joplin (94).

#### Phosphate

Oral phosphate, with its chelating action on intestinal calcium, may be useful as an adjunct for the long-term management of hypercalcemia. The dose-limiting side effect is diarrhea.

### Experimental Agents

Established antitumor agents such as cisplatinum have been used in an attempt to control hypercalcemia. The total dose used by Lad and colleagues (97) in their study of 13 patients with hypercalcemia was 100 mg/m², which the authors reported was nontoxic. Aside from its antineoplastic effects, the mechanism of hypopcalcemia with cisplatinum is unclear. It is recognized that this agent is toxic to the loop of Henle in the kidney, and this may represent the source of calcium wasting.

Ethiofos (WR-2721) is a myeloprotective agent that appears able to suppress parathyroid hormone secretion and bone resorption. Its effects on PTHrP release are currently unknown, but this agent may have great potential if it could suppress the release of this tumor product. It is associated with mild nausea and vomiting as well as potentially troublesome hypotension. Clinical experience in the management of hypercalcemia with this agent is limited.

### SUMMARY

Hypercalcemia of malignancy is a common problem. If promptly recognized, useful palliation may be made available. Strategies aimed at removing or reducing the underlying tumor burden should be sought. Where no effective therapy for the tumor is available, patients are normally in the last few weeks to months of their lives. A thoughtful decision should be made before embarking on antihypercalcemic therapy in terminally ill patients who may be relatively asymptomatic. Volume repletion is the mainstay of therapy, followed by the use of antiresponsive medications. The aminobisphosphonates are effective, safe agents in this regard. They may be given over short infusion times, which can allow therapy to take place in the outpatient or home setting. Individualization of therapy is required because the duration of response to any of the hypercalcemic agents is relatively unpredictable.

# REFERENCES

1. Zondek H, Petow H, Seibert W. Die Bedeutung der Calciumbestimmung im Blute für die Diagnose der Niereninsuffizienz. *Z Klin Med* 1924;99:129.
2. Fisken RA, Heath DA, Bold AM. Hypercalcaemia—a hospital survey. *QJM* 1980;196:405.
3. Nussbaum SR, Younger J, VandePol CJ, et al. Single-dose intravenous therapy with pamidronate for the treatment of hypercalcemia of malignancy: comparison of 30-, 60-, and 90-mg dosages. *Am J Med* 1993;95:297.
4. Percival R, Urwin G, Harris S, et al. Biochemical and histological evidence that carcinoma of the prostate is associated with enhanced bone resorption. *Eur J Surg Oncol* 1987;13:41.
5. Raisz LG, Kream BL. Regulation of bone formation. *N Engl J Med* 1983;309:29,83.
6. Parfitt AM. Equilibrium and disequilibrium hypercalcaemia: new light on an old concept. *Metabolic Bone Disease and Related Research* 1979;1:279.
7. Payne RB, Little AJ, Williams RB, Milner JR. Interpretation of serum calcium in patients with abnormal serum proteins. *BMJ* 1973;4:643.
8. Morton AR, Hercz G. Hypercalcemia in dialysis patients: comparison of diagnostic methods. *Dialysis and Transplantation* 1991;20:661.
9. Potts JT Jr, Kronenberg HM, Rosenblatt M. Parathyroid hormone: chemistry, biosynthesis and mode of action. *Adv Protein Chem* 1982;35:323.
10. VanderWeil CJ, Talmage RV. Ultrastructural and physiological evidence for calcitonin-induced postprandial calcium in bones of rats. *Calcif Tissue Int* 1981;33:417.
11. Eilon G, Mundy GR. Direct resorption of bone by human breast cancer cells in vitro. *Nature* 1978;276:726.
12. Galasko CSB. Mechanisms of bone destruction in the development of skeletal metastases. *Nature* 1976;263:507.
13. Dickson RB, Lippman ME. Growth factors and oncogenes. In: Powles TJ, Smith IE, eds. *Medical management of breast cancer.* London: Martin Dunitz 1991;5.
14. Galasko CSB, Bennett A. Relationship of bone destruction in skeletal metastases to osteoclast activation and prostaglandins. *Nature* 1976;263:508.
15. Powles TJ, Clark A, Easty DM, Easty GC, Neville MA. The inhibition by aspirin and indometacin of osteolytic tumor deposits and hypercalcaemia in rats with walker tumour, and its possible application to human breast cancer. *Br J Cancer* 1973;28:316.
16. Percival RC, Yates AJP, Gray RES, et al. Mechanisms of malignant hypercalcemia in carcinoma of the breast. *BMJ* 1985;291:776.
17. Burtis WJ, Wu T, Bunch C, et al. Identification of a novel 17,000-dalton parathyroid hormone-like adenylate cyclase-stimulating protein from a tumor associated with humoral hypercalcemia of malignancy. *J Biol Chem* 1987;62:7151.
18. Bundred NJ, Ratcliffe WA, Walker RA, Coley S, Morrison JM, Ratcliffe JG. Parathyroid hormone related protein and hypercalcemia in breast cancer. *BMJ* 1991;303:1506.
19. Mundy GR, Raisz LG, Cooper RA, Schechter GP, Salmon SE. Evidence for the secretion of an osteoblast stimulating factor in myeloma. *N Engl J Med* 1974;291:1041.
20. Garrett R, Drurie BGM, Nedwin GE, et al. Production of lymphotoxin, a bone-resorbing cytokine, by cultured human myeloma cells. *N Engl J Med* 1987;317:526.
21. Kawano M, Yamamoto I, Iwato K, et al. Interleukin-1 beta rather than lymphotoxin as the major bone resorbing activity in human multiple myeloma. *Blood* 1989;73:1646–1649.
22. Black K, Garrett IR, Mundy GR. Chinese hamster ovarian cells transfected with murine interleukin-6 gene cause hypercalcemia as well as cahexia, leukocytosis and thrombocytosis in tumor-bearing nude mice. *Endocrinology* 1991;128:2657–2659.
23. Merlini G, Fitzpatrick LA, Siris ES, et al. A human myeloma immunoglobulin G blinding four moles of calcium associated with asymptomatic hypercalcemia. *J Clin Immunol* 1984;4:185.
24. Albright F. Case records of the Massachusetts General Hospital, no. 27461. *N Engl J Med* 1941;225:789.
25. Fry L. Pseudohyperparathyroidism with carcinoma of the bronchus. *BMJ* 1962;1:301.
26. Lafferty FW. Pseudohyperparathyroidism. *Medicine* 1966;45:247.
27. Stewart AF, Horst R, Deftos LJ, Cadman EC, Lang R, Broadus AE. Biochemical evaluation of patients with cancer-associated hypercalcemia. *N Engl J Med* 1980;303:1377.
28. Nussbaum SR, Gaz RD, Arnold A. Hypercalcemia and ectopic secretion of parathyroid hormone by an ovarian carcinoma with rearrangement of the gene for parathyroid hormone. *N Engl J Med* 1990;323:1324.
29. Simpson EL, Mundy GR, D'Souza SM, Ibbotson KJ, Bockman R, Jacobs W. Absence of parathyroid hormone messenger RNA in nonparathyroid tumors associated with hypercalcemia. *N Engl J Med* 1983;309:325.
30. Nussbaum SR, Zahradnik RJ, Lavigne JR, et al. Highly sensitive two-site immunoradiometric assay of parathyrin, and its clinical utility in evaluating patients with hypercalcemia. *Clin Chem* 1988;33:1364.
31. Moseley JM, Kubota M, Diefenbach-Jagger H, et al. Parathyroid hormone-related protein purified from a human lung cancer cell line. *Medical Sciences* 1987;84:5048.
32. Strewler GJ, Stern PH, Jacobs JW, et al. Parathyroid hormone like protein from human renal carcinoma cells. *J Clin Invest* 1987;80:1803.
33. Law F, Ferrari S, Rizzoli R, Bonjour J-P. Parathyroid hormone-related protein: physiology and pathophysiology. In: Grünfeld J-P, Bach JF, Kries H, Maxwell MH, eds. *Advances in nephrology,* vol 23. St Louis: Mosby, 1994;281.
34. Kukreja SC, Shevrin DH, Wimbiscus SA, et al. Antibodies to parathyroid hormone-related protein lower serum calcium in athymic mouse models of malignancy-associated hypercalcemia due to human tumors. *J Clin Invest* 1988;82:1798.
35. Blind E, Raue F, Meinel T, et al. Diagnostiche Bedeutung von parathormone-related-protein bei Tumorpatienten mit Hypercalcämie. *Dtsch Med Wochenschr* 1993;118:330.
36. Ratcliffe WA, Norbury S, Heath DA, Ratcliffe JG. Development and validation of an immunoradiometric assay of parathyrin-related protein in unextracted plasma. *Clin Chem* 1991;37:678.
37. Pandian MR, Morgan CH, Carlton E, Segre GV. Modified immunoradiometric assay of parathyroid hormone-related protein: clinical application in the differential diagnosis of hypercalcemia. *Clin Chem* 1992;38:282.
38. Powell GJ, Southby J, Danks JA, et al. Localization of parathyroid hormone-related protein in breast cancer metastases: increased incidence in bone compared with other sites. *Cancer Res* 1991;51:3059.
39. Barbour GL, Coburn JW, Slatopolsky E, Norman AW, Horst RL. Hypercalcemia in an anephric patient with sarcoidosis: evidence for extrarenal generation of 1,25-dihydroxyvitamin D. *N Engl J Med* 1981;305:440.
40. Davies M, Mawer EB, Hayes ME, Lumb GA. Abnormal vitamin D metabolism in Hodgkin's lymphoma. *Lancet* 1985;1:1186.
41. Breslau NA, McGuire JL, Zerwekh JE, Frenkel EP, Pak CYC. Hypercalcemia associated with increased serum calcitrol levels in three patients with lymphoma. *Ann Intern Med* 1984;100:1.
42. Rosenthal N, Insogna KL, Godsall WJ, Smaldone L, Waldrone JA, Stewart AF. Elevations in circulating 1,25-dihydorxyvitamin D in three patients with lymphoma-associated hypercalcemia. *J Clin Endocrinol Metab* 1985;60:29.
43. Canellos GP. Hypercalcemia in malignant lymphoma and leukemia. *Ann NY Acad Sci* 1974;230:240.
44. Johnston SR, Hammond PJ. Elevated serum parathyroid hormone related protein and 1,25-dihydroxycholecalciferol in hypercalcaemia associated with adult T-cell leukaemia-lymphoma. *Postgrad Med J* 1992;68:753.
45. Seymour JF, Gagel RF. Calcitriol: the major humoral mediator of hypercalcemia in Hodgkin's disease and non-Hodgkin's lymphoma. *Blood* 1993;82:1383.

46. Sato K, Fujii Y, Ono M, Nomura H, Shizume K. Production of interleukin 1α-like factor and colong-stimulating factor by a squamous cell carcinoma of the thyroid (T3M-5) derived from a patient with hypercalcemia and leukocytosis. *Cancer Res* 1987;47:6474.

47. Fried RM, Voelkel EF, Rice RH, Levine L, Gaffney EV. Two squamous cell carcinomas not associated with humoral hypercalcemia produce a potent bone resorption stimulating factor which is interleukin-1α. *Endocrinology* 1989;125:742.

48. Sato K, Fujii Y, Kasono K, Tsushima T, Shizume K. Production of interleukin-1α and a parathyroid hormone-like factor by a squamous cell carcinoma of the esophagus (EC-GI) derived from a patient with hypercalcemia. *J Clin Endocrinol Metab* 1988;67:592–601.

49. Sato K, Fujii Y, Kasono K, et al. Parathyroid hormone-related protein and interleukin-1α synergistically stimulate bone resorption in vitro and increase the serum calcium concentration in vivo. *Endocrinology* 1989;124:2172–2178.

50. Weissglas M, Schamhart D, Löwik C, Papapoulos S, Vos P, Kurth K-H. Hypercalcemia and cosecretion of interleukin-6 and parathyroid hormone related peptide by a human renal cell carcinoma implanted into nude mice. *J Urol* 1995;153:854–857.

51. Seyeberth HW, Segre GV, Morgan JL, Sweetman BJ, Potts Jr JT, Oates JA. Prostaglandins as mediators of hypercalcemia associated with certain types of cancer. *N Engl J Med* 1975;293:1278.

52. Fukumoto S, Matsumoto T, Yamoto H, et al. Suppression of serum 1,25-dihydroxyvitamin D is caused by elaboration of a factor that inhibits renal 1,25-dihydroxyvitamin $D_3$ production. *Endocrinology* 1989;124:2057.

53. Ralston SH, Gallacher SJ, Patel U, Campbell J, Boyle IT. Cancer-associated hypercalcemia: morbidity and mortality. *Ann Intern Med* 1990;112:499.

54. Hosking DJ, Cowley A, Bucknall A. Rehydration in the treatment of severe hypercalcemia. *QJM* 1981;200:473.

55. Jung A, Bisaz S, Fleisch H. The binding of pyrophosphate and two diphosphonates on hydroxyapatite crystals. *Calcif Tissue Res* 1973;11:269.

56. Robertson WG, Morgan DB, Fleisch H, Francis MD. The effects of diphosphonates on the exchangeable and non-exchangeable calcium and phosphate of hydroxyapatitite. *Biochim Biophys Acta* 1972;261:517.

57. Carano A, Teitelbaum SL, Konsek JD, Schlesinger PH, Blair HC. Bisphosphonates directly inhibit the bone resorption activity of isolated avian osteoclasts in vitro. *J Clin Invest* 1990;85:456.

58. Felix R, Russell RGG, Fleisch H. The effects of several diphosphonates on acid phosphohydrolases and other lysosomal enzymes. *Biochim Biophys Acta* 1976;429:429.

59. Singer FR, Ritch PS, Lad TE, et al. Treatment of hypercalcemia of malignancy with intravenous etidronate: a controlled, multicenter study. *Arch Intern Med* 1991;151:471.

60. Ringenberg QS, Ritch PS. Efficacy of oral administration of etidronate disodium in maintaining normal serum calcium levels in previously hypercalcemic cancer patients. *Clin Ther* 1987;9:318.

61. Ralston SH, Gallacher SJ, Patel U, et al. Comparison of three intravenous biphosphonates in cancer-associated hypercalcemia. *Lancet* 1989;2:1180.

62. Gucalp R, Ritch P, Wiernik PH, et al. Comparative study of pamidronate disodium and etidronate disodium in the treatment of cancer-related hypercalcemia. *J Clin Oncol* 1992;10:134.

63. Warnell RP Jr, Murphy WK, Schulman P, O'Dwyer PJ, Heller G. A randomized double-blind study of gallium nitrate compared with etidronate for acute control of cancer-related hypercalcemia. *J Clin Oncol* 1991;9:1467.

64. Witte RS, Koeller J, Davis TE, et al. Clodronate: a randomized study in the treatment of cancer-related hypercalcemia. *Arch Intern Med* 1987;147:937.

65. Urwin GH, Yates AJP, Gray RES, et al. Treatment of hypercalcemia of malignancy with intravenous clodronate. *Bone* 1987;8(suppl1):S43.

66. Chapuy MC, Meunier PJ, Alexandre CM, Vignon EP. Effects of disodium dichloromethylene diphosphonate on hypercalcemia produced by bone metastases. *J Clin Invest* 1980;65:1243.

67. Harinck HIJ, Bijvoet OLM, Plantingh AST, et al. Role of bone and kidney in tumor-induced hypercalcemia and its treatment with bisphosphonate and sodium chloride. *Am J Med* 1987;82:1133.

68. Morton Ar, Cantrill JA, Craig AE, Howell A, Davies M, Anderson DC. Single dose versus daily intravenous aminohydroxypropylidene bisphosphonate (APD) for the hypercalcaemia of malignancy. *BMJ* 1988;296:811.

69. Dodwell DJ, Howell A, Morton AR, Daley-Yates PT, Hoggarth CR. Infusion rate and pharmacokinetics of intravenous pamidronate in the treatment of tumour-induced hypercalcaemia. *Postgrad Med J* 1992;68:434.

70. Thürlimann B, Waldburger R, Senn HJ, Thiébaud D. Plicamycin and pamidronate in symptomatic tumor-related hypercalcemia: a prospective randomized crossover trial. *Ann Oncol* 1992;3:619.

71. Gallacher SJ, Ralston SH, Fraser WD, et al. A comparison of low versus high dose pamidronate in cancer-associated hypercalcaemia. *Bone Min* 1991;15:249–256.

72. Body JJ, Dumon JC. Treatment of tumor-induced hypercalcaemia with the bisphosphonate pamidronate: dose-response relationship and influence of tumour type. *Ann Oncol* 1994;5:359–363.

73. Bickerstaff DR, O'Doherty DPJ, McCloskey EV, et al. Effects of aminobutylidene diphosphonate in hypercalcaemia due to malignancy. *Bone* 1991;12:17.

74. Nussbaum SR, Warrell RP Jr, Rude R, et al. Dose-response study of alendronate sodium for the treatment of cancer-associated hypercalcemia. *J Clin Oncol* 1993;11:1618.

75. Gurney H, Kefford R, Stuart-Harris R. Renal phosphate threshold and response to pamidronate in humoral hypercalcaemia of malignancy. *Lancet* 1989;2:241.

76. Dodwell DJ, Abbas SK, Morton AR, Howell A. Parathyroid hormone-related protein [50-69] and response to pamidronate therapy for tumour-induced hypercalcaemia. *Eur J Cancer* 1991;27:1629.

77. Wimalawansa SJ. Significance of plasma PTH-rp in patients with hypercalcemia of malignancy treated with bisphosphonate. *Cancer* 1994;73:2223–2230.

78. Blind E, Raue F, Meinel T, Wüster C, Ziegler R. Levels of parathyroid hormone-related protein (PTHrP) in hypercalcemia of malignancy are not lowered by treatment with the bisphosphonate BM21.0955. *Horm Metab Res* 1993;25:40.

79. Thiébaud D, Jaeger PH, Jacquet AF, Burckhardt P. Dose-response in the treatment of hypercalcemia of malignancy by a single infusion of the bisphosphonate AHPrBP. *J Clin Oncol* 1988;6:762.

80. Bounameaux HM, Schifferli J, Montani JP, Chatelanat F. Renal failure associated with intravenous diphosphonates. *Lancet* 1983;1:471.

81. Macol V, Fraunfelder FT. Pamidronate disodium and possible ocular adverse drug reactions. *Am J Ophthalmol* 1994;118:220–224.

82. Bockman RS. Studies on the mechanism of action of gallium nitrate. *Semin Oncol* 1991;8(suppl5):21.

83. Krakoff IH, Newman RA, Goldberg RS. Clinical toxicologic and pharmacologic studies of gallium nitrate. *Cancer* 1979;44:1722.

84. Warrell RP, Bockman RS, Coonley CJ, Isaacs M. Staszewski H. Gallium nitrate inhibits calcium resorption from bone and is effective treatment for cancer-related hypercalcemia. *J Clin Invest* 1984;73:1487.

85. Warrell RP, Israel R, Frisone M, Snyder T, Gaynor JJ, Bjockman RS. Gallium nitrate for acute treatment of cancer-related hypercalcemia: a randomized double-blind comparison to calcitonin. *Ann Intern Med* 1988;108:669.

86. Minkin C. Inhibition of parathyroid hormone stimulated bone resorption in vitro by the antibiotic mithramycin. *Calcif Tissue Res* 1973;13:249.

87. Perlia CP, Gubisch NJ, Wolter J, Edelberg D, Dederick MM, Taylor SG. Mithramycin treatment of hypercalcemia. *Cancer* 1970;25:389.

88. Fatemi S, Singer FR, Rude RK. Effect of salmon calcitonin and etidronate on hypercalcemia of malignancy. *Calcif Tissue Int* 1992;50:107.

89. Luce K, O'Donnell DE, Morton AR. A combination of calcitonin and bisphosphonate for the emergency treatment of severe tumor-induced hypercalcemia. *Calcif Tissue Int* 1993;52:70.

90. Cochran M, Peacock M, Sachs G, Nordin BEC. Renal effects of calcitonin. *BMJ* 1970;1:135.

91. Binstock ML, Mundy GR. Effect of calcitonin and glucocorticoids in combination on the hypercalcemia of malignancy. *Ann Int Med* 1980;93:269.

92. Thiébaud D, Burkhardt P, Jaeger P, Azria M. Effectiveness of salmon calcitonin administered as suppositories in tumor-induced hypercalcemia. *Am J Med* 1987;82:745–750.

93. Suki WN, Yium JJ, Von Minden M, Saller-Hebert C, Eknoyan G, Martinez-Maldonado M. Acute treatment of hypercalcemia with furosemide. *N Engl J Med* 1970;283:836.

94. Thalassinos NC, Joplin GF. Failure of corticosteroid therapy to correct the hypercalcemia of malignant disease. *Lancet* 1970;2:537.

95. Pervical RC, Yates AJP, Gray RES, Neal FE, Forrest ARW, Kanis JA. Role of glucocorticoids in management of malignant hypercalcemia. *BMJ* 1984;289:287.

96. Anderson JC, Dent CE, Harper C, Philpot GR. Effect of cortisone on calcium metabolism in sarcoidosis with hypercalcemia: possible antagonistic actions of cortisone and vitamin D. *Lancet* 1954; 2:720.

97. Lad TE, Mishoulam HM, Shevrin DH, Kukla LJ, Abramson EC, Kukreja SC. Treatment of cancer-associated hypercalcemia with cisplatin. Arch Intern Med 1987:147:329.

*Principles and Practice of Supportive Oncology,*
edited by Ann Berger et al.
Lippincott–Raven Publishers, Philadelphia ©1998

# CHAPTER 32

# Metabolic Disorders in the Cancer Patient

Irene M. O'Shaughnessy and Albert L. Jochen

Endocrine disorders occur in persons with advanced malignancy under various circumstances. Cancer may produce effects through the excess production of hormones, cytokines, and growth factors, the so-called paraneoplastic syndromes (Table 32-1). Conversely, the cancer or its metastases may interfere with the normal function of endocrine organs, resulting in hormone-deficiency states. Most commonly, patients have a metabolic disorder such as diabetes, thyroid dysfunction, or hyperparathyroidism that predates the diagnosis of their malignancy or is diagnosed incidentally during the course of their malignancy. This chapter discusses the most common paraneoplastic syndromes and hormone-deficiency states associated with malignancy as well as the management of diabetes and thyroid disease in the cancer patient.

## ENDOCRINE PARANEOPLASTIC SYNDROMES

### Inappropriate Antidiuresis

The differential diagnosis of hyponatremia in the cancer patient is similar to that in the general population and includes hepatic and cardiac failure, renal disease, overdiuresis, factitious hyponatremia associated with hyperglycemia, and other conditions. In the syndrome of inappropriate antidiuretic hormone (SIADH), hyponatremia results from the overproduction of vasopressin (AVP) by the posterior pituitary gland in response to a stimulus by tumor cells, by the actual production of vasopressin or vasopressin-like peptides by tumor cells, or as a side effect of medications able to stimulate vasopressin production.

### *Epidemiology*

The most common malignancies causing SIADH are small-cell lung cancer and carcinoid tumors; SIADH also

I. M. O'Shaughnessy (Department of Endocrinology) and A. L. Jochen (Department of Medicine): Medical College of Wisconsin, Milwaukee, WI 53226.

is seen with cancers of the esophagus, pancreas, duodenum, colon, adrenal cortex, prostate, thymomas, and lymphomas. In one series, the incidence of clinically significant SIADH was 9% among 523 small-cell lung cancer patients. A larger fraction of patients had milder abnormalities in AVP metabolism without hyponatremia. Thus, about half of patients had abnormal renal handling of water loads that were subclinical (1,2). Another study found that 41% of patients with all types of lung cancers and 43% of colon cancer patients had significantly elevated levels of AVP without evidence of clinically significant SIADH (3).

### *Clinical Features*

The clinical features of hyponatremia depend on the degree of hyponatremia and the rate of its development. Most patients with chronic hyponatremia are asymptomatic. Generally, symptoms do not occur until the serum sodium falls below 115 to 120 mmol/L (4). When they occur, the signs and symptoms of SIADH are caused by water intoxication (i.e., hypoosmolality and hyponatremia) and are manifested by confusion, lethargy, seizures, or coma. Occasionally, patients may present with focal neurologic deficits.

### *Diagnosis*

Because most cases of SIADH are asymptomatic, the diagnosis is usually first suspected by noting a low serum sodium on routine chemistries. Other causes of hyponatremia, such as hypovolemia, hypervolemia (occuring in renal or hepatic disease, or cardiac failure), hypothyroidism, and adrenal insufficiency must be excluded before the diagnosis of SIADH can be considered. Urine chemistries show urinary osmolality greater than serum osmolality and a high urinary sodium concentration (>20 mEq/L). Medications commonly used by cancer patients

**TABLE 1.** *Common paraneoplastic syndromes*

| Syndrome | Tumor type |
| --- | --- |
| Inappropriate antidiuresis (SIADH) | Lung cancer, all types |
| Cushing's syndrome | Lung cancer, all types |
| Hypocalcemia | Bone metastases |
| Hypophosphatemia | Mesenchymal tumors |
| Hyperthyroidism | Lung cancer, all types |
| Gynecomastia | Lung cancer, all types |
| Calcitoninemia | Medullary carcinoma of the thyroid, lung cancer, breast cancer |
| Acromegaly | Carcinoids, pheochromocytoma, pancreatic cancer |

associated with SIADH include morphine, vincristine, cyclophosphamide, phenothiazines, and tricyclic antidepressants. Most drugs cause SIADH by stimulating posterior pituitary secretion of AVP (Table 32-2).

### Treatment

The treatment of SIADH is determined by the rate of development of hyponatremia and by the presence of neurologic sequelae. If the patient is symptomatic and has a serum sodium level below 130 mEq/L, fluid restriction to 800 to 1,000 ml per 24 hours is effective in slowly raising serum osmolality over a period of 7 to 10 days. Acute hyponatremia with neurologic symptoms has a mortality rate of 5% to 8% and warrants more aggressive treatment. For patients with more severe hyponatremia, the intravenous administration of hypertonic saline (3% saline at a rate of 0.1 mg/kg per minute) and furosemide may be necessary (5). Careful monitoring of vital signs and urinary losses of sodium and potassium is indicated. Rapid correction of severe hyponatremia has been associated with central pontine myelinosis, which presents with quadriparesis and bulbar palsy 1 to 2 days after correcting hyponatremia. A safe rate of correction is 0.5 to 2.0 mEq/L per hour (6,7).

Fluid restriction is not feasible in some patients who require long-term treatment of SIADH. In these patients, medications, including demeclocycline, lithium carbonate, and urea have been tried. Demeclocyline causes partial nephrogenic diabetes insipidus by inhibiting the formation of AVP-induced cyclic adenosine monophosphate (cAMP) in distal tubules. It is initially administered orally in divided doses of 900 to 1,200 mg/day and then reduced to maintenance doses of 600 to 900 mg/day. Side

effects are mainly gastrointestinal, although hypersensitivity and reversible nephrotoxicity can occur. Similar to demeclocycline, lithium carbonate also causes a reversible, partial form of nephrogenic diabetes insipidus but is less effective. Urea acts as an osmotic diuretic and allows an the patient to maintain a normal fluid intake. Urea can be administered intravenously or orally. When given by mouth, the usual dosing is 30 g of urea dissolved in 100 ml of orange juice or water once daily (8).

### Cushing's Syndrome

Endogenous Cushing's syndrome is due to one of three causes: overproduction of glucocorticoid by a primary adrenal neoplasm, excessive production of adrenocorticotropic hormone (ACTH) by a pituitary adenoma, or a paraneoplastic syndrome in which either ACTH or corticotrophic hormone (CRH) are produced ectopically by the tumor. A number of tumors are capable of producing ACTH, its prohormone "big ACTH," or pro-opiomelanocortin (POMC) (Table 32-3). The POMC gene is located at p23 on the short arm of chromosome 2 near N-myc oncogene at p24. The expression of the POMC gene normally is influenced by glucocorticoids, which suppress transcription, and CRH, which stimulates transcription via cAMP. The activation of alternative steroid-insensitive promoters may result in ectopic ACTH production that is insensitive to glucocorticoid suppression. Pituitary cells and some tumors produce the normal 1,200-base mRNA transcript; however, some nonpituitary tissues produce either a larger or smaller POMC mRNA transcript. Alternative posttranscription processing of POMC gives rise to a large number of biologically active peptides in addition

**TABLE 2.** *Diagnosis of syndrome of inappropriate antidiuresis (SIADH)*

Plasma sodium level below 135 mEq/L
Urine osmolality greater than serum osmolality
Elevated urine sodium (>20 mEq/L)
Normal extracellular fluid volume
Rule out other causes of euvolemic hyponatremia

**TABLE 3.** *Tumors associated with ectopic ACTH/CRH serotonin*

Small-cell lung carcinoma
Thymoma
Pancreatic islet-cell carcinoma
Carcinoid tumors (lung, gut, pancreas, ovary)
Medullary carcinomas of the thyroid
Pheochromocytomas

to ACTH. These include pro-ACTH and a number of different peptides containing melanocyte-stimulating hormone (MSH) (α-MSH, ACTH, pro-ACTH, β-MSH, τ-lipotropin (LPH), β-LPH, τ-MSH, N-POMC, pro-τ-MSH), all of which can lead to generalized hyperpigmentation (9,10). Radioimmunoassays differ in their abilities to detect aberrant ACTH. The immunoradiometric assay (IRMA) for ACTH is able to distinguish between ACTH and its larger precursors, pro-ACTH, and POMC (11).

### Epidemiology

Ectopic ACTH is most frequently secreted by lung carcinomas. A number of other tumor types are also capable of producing this syndrome (Table 3). In the general population, about 65% of patients with Cushing's syndrome have pituitary adenomas producing ACTH (Cushing's disease), 20% have primary adrenal tumors, and 14% have ectopic ACTH. Therefore, ectopic ACTH production is the least common of the three major causes in the general population.

### Clinical Features of Ectopic ACTH Syndrome

Manifestations of the ectopic ACTH syndrome include hypokalemia, hyperglycemia, edema, muscle weakness (especially proximal) and atrophy, hypertension, and weight loss. Features typically seen in long-standing pituitary or adrenal Cushing's syndrome, such as central obesity, plethoric facies, cutaneous striae, buffalo hump, and hyperpigmentation are less common in highly malignant tumors such as small-cell lung carcinoma but occur more frequently in more indolent tumors such as carcinoids, thymomas, and pheochromocytomas.

### Diagnosis

The biochemical diagnosis of Cushing's syndrome is suggested by an elevated 24-hour urinary-free cortisol (>100 μg/24 hours). The other principal screening test is the overnight low-dose dexamethasone suppression test. The test is positive when 1 mg of dexamethasone given at midnight is unable to suppress the following 8:00 a.m. cortisol to less than 5 μg/dl. Failure of cortisol to suppress following high-dose dexamethasone (8 mg at midnight) suggests either ectopic ACTH or a primary adrenal tumor (12). These two are differentiated by measuring plasma ACTH. In primary adrenal tumors, ACTH levels are below 20 pg/ml, whereas in ectopic ACTH levels are generally greater than 100 to 200 pg/ml and frequently are elevated above 1,000 pg/ml. Inferior petrosal sinus sampling of ACTH is useful in confirming the diagnosis of pituitary Cushing's syndrome (13), but it is rarely indicated in the patient with advanced malignancy secreting ectopic ACTH.

Difficulties arise in differentiating those rare tumors producing ectopic CRH from the more common ectopic ACTH production; CRH stimulates release of pituitary ACTH. The clinical presentation and biochemical results are identical for ectopic CRH and ACTH. The prognosis and therapy are identical for the two disorders.

### Treatment of Ectopic ACTH Syndromes

Where possible, the treatment of ectopic ACTH syndrome should be directed primarily at the tumor. Palliative treatment of Cushing's syndrome involves inhibition of steroid synthesis. Drugs successfully used include aminoglutethamide, metyrapone, mitotane, ketoconazole, and octreotide (14). Rarely, bilateral adrenalectomy is considered.

Aminoglutethamide blocks the first step in cortisol biosynthesis. At higher doses, it inhibits production of glucocorticoids, mineralocorticoids, and androgens, whereas at lower doses it primarily inhibits the conversion of androgens to estrogens, contributing to its efficacy in the treatment of postmenopausal breast cancer. At the higher doses required to treat ectopic ACTH syndrome, many patients experience sedation, ataxia, and skin rashes. Metyrapone inhibits 11β-hydroxylase and 18-hydroxylase, resulting in adrenal atrophy and necrosis. It is a toxic drug with significant gastrointestinal side effects, including anorexia, nausea, vomiting, and diarrhea and central nervous system side effects, including lethargy and somnolence. For these reasons, it is used as second-line therapy.

Ketoconazole acts mainly on the first step of cortisol biosynthesis but also inhibits the conversion of 11-deoxycortisol to cortisol. It can cause rare but significant reversible hepatotoxicity and is associated with nausea and vomiting.

Octreotide, a long-acting analog of somatostatin, can reduce ectopic ACTH secretion. It must be injected, is expensive, and is only partially effective in most patients. The efficacy of these treatments can be monitored by 24-hour urine cortisol measurements. As levels return to normal and then fall below normal, replacement with glucocorticoids and mineralocorticoids in physiologic doses similar to patients with Addison's disease is frequently necessary. In cases of stress, these patients require stress doses of glucocorticoids (e.g., hydrocortisone 100 mg intravenously every 8 hours).

## Hypocalcemia

Hypocalcemia is an uncommon paraneoplastic syndrome occurring primarily in patients with bony metastases. It occurs most commonly in association with osteoblastic metastases of the breast, prostate, and lung; its incidence is about 16% (15). Tetany is a rare complication of tumor-associated hypocalcemia. The etiology of the hypocalcemia is not understood. Ectopic calcitonin secretion from the underlying tumor has been rarely implicated.

## Hypophosphatemia

An acquired form of adult-onset, vitamin D-resistant rickets is associated with benign mesenchymal tumors that occur in soft tissues or bone (16). These tumors are also referred to as ossifying mesenchymal tumors, giant cell tumors of bone, sclerosing hemangioma, or cavernous hemangioma. This syndrome has been rarely reported with other cancers, such as lung and prostate. The clinical syndrome can precede the discovery of the tumor by several years. Clinical and laboratory features include bone pain, severe phosphaturia, renal glycosuria, hypophosphatemia, normocalcemia (normal PTH [parathyroid hormone] levels), low 1,25-dihydroxyvitamin D levels, and increased alkaline phosphatase. The proposed mechanisms for this syndrome include inhibition of the conversion of 25-hydroxyvitamin D to 1,25-dihydroxyvitamin D and a substance produced by the tumor with a phosphaturic effect. Treatment is directed at surgical resection of the underlying tumor. When this is not possible, treatment with high doses of vitamin D and phosphate is often required.

## Hyperthyroidism

Human chorionic gonadotrophin (hCG) most commonly is secreted by trophoblastic or germ cell tumors (17). Because of its evolutionary homology with TSH, hCG has intrinsic thyrotropic action. Overt hyperthyroidism usually occurs with large tumors secreting large quantities of hCG, such as gestational trophoblastic disease (e.g., choriocarcinoma, hydatidform mole) and testicular tumors. The hyperthyroidism resolves with surgical resection of the underlying tumor. When necessary, treatment of the hyperthyroidism is achieved by using antithyroid drugs such as prophylthoiuracil or methimazole.

## Gynecomastia

*Gynecomastia* is defined as palpable breast tissue in men (18) and may be caused by drugs that lower testosterone levels (19), including alkylating agents, vinca alkaloids, and nitroureas. Antiemetics, such as metoclopramide and phenothiazines, may produce gynecomastia by stimulating prolactin production. Alternatively, tumor production of gonadotrophins or estrogens may result in gynecomastia; these include adrenal and testicular tumors and hepatomas. Tumors that produce hCG can stimulate estrogen production by interstitial and Sertoli cells of the testes, resulting in gynecomastia. The approach to the treatment of gynecomastia includes treatment of the underlying tumor and, if implicated, cessation of drugs known to cause gynecomastia.

Treatment of gynecomastia with antiestrogens and androgens such as tamoxifen, clomiphene, topical dishydrotestosterone, and danazol is generally unsuccessful. For more severe cases, long-term management with liposuction and subcutaneous mastectomy may be necessary. Low-dose radiation therapy has been used with some success for the treatment of painful gynecomastia.

## Calcitoninemia

Calcitonin is a polypeptide hormone produced by the C cells of the thyroid. It diminishes the release of calcium from bone and increases the excretion of urine calcium, sodium, and phosphate. Interestingly, no clinical syndromes are associated with tumor production of calcitonin except for one reported case of a small-cell carcinoma patient with hypercalcitoninemia and hypocalcemia (20). Calcitonin plays an important role as a tumor marker in monitoring patients with medullary carcinoma of the thyroid and in the diagnosis of multiple endocrine neoplasia type 2 (MEN IIA), a familial disorder characterized by medullary carcinoma of the thyroid, parathyroid adenomas, and pheochromocytoma. In addition to medullary thyroid carcinoma, a number of other cancers have been associated with elevations in calcitonin, including small cell (48%–64%) and other lung cancers, carcinoid, breast cancer, colon cancer (24%), and gastric cancer (38%). With the exception of medullary thyroid carcinoma, the clinical usefulness of serum calcitonin levels as a tumor marker remains undetermined (21).

## Acromegaly

Most cases of acromegaly result from growth hormone overproduction by pituitary tumors. Growth hormone elevations also may result from production of growth hormone releasing hormone (GHRH) by tumors, particulary pancreatic islet-cell tumors and bronchia carcinoids. Treatment of this paraneoplastic syndrome is directed at treatment of the underlying tumor. Occasionally, GHRH secretion responds to administration of long-acting somatostatin anologs (22).

## Carcinoid Syndrome

The classic carcinoid syndrome is characterized by flushing, diarrhea, and bronchospasm. Less frequent signs and symptoms include coronary artery spasm leading to angina pectoris, pellagra, endocardial fibrosis, arthropathy, glucose intolerance, and hypotension. The symptoms are due primarily to the production of 5-hydroxytrytophan (serotonin), although secretion of other hormones, such as bradykinin, hydroxytryptophan, and prostaglandins, also may play a role. Carcinoid tumors are found throughout the gastrointestinal tract, including the esophagus, stomach, duodenum, jejunum, ileum, the Meckel diverticulum, appendix, colon, rectum, bile ducts, pancreas, and liver. They also have been found in the larynx, thymus, lung, breast, ovary, urethra, and testis.

The medical treatment of the carcinoid syndrome is directed at inhibiting serotonin synthesis and at blocking its effects peripherally. Different drugs can be used to accomplish these goals (23,24). Antiserotonin agents such as cyproheptadine and methysergide can ameliorate the diarrhea. For long-term treatment, cyproheptadine is the preferred medication because of the risk of retroperitoneal, cardiac, and pulmonary fibrosis associated with methysergide. Antidiarrheal agents such as loperamide and diphenoxylate also can be quite helpful in controlling the diarrhea.

The flushing appears to be due to the secretion of histamine. The administration of a combination of H1 and H2 histamine receptor antagonists often can control this symptom. Long-acting somatostatin antagonists such as octreotide are effective in controlling the symptoms of flushing and diarrhea in up to 75% of patients. Octreotide is administered subcutaneously every 8 hours. Side effects include hypoglycemia, steatorrhea, and cholelithiasis. Carcinoid syndrome associated with bronchial carcinoid tumors has distinctive features and is treated differented. Many patients experience improvement in symptoms with glucocorticoids or phenothiazines.

## Extrapancreatic Tumor Hypoglycemia

Tumors most likely to cause hypoglycemia are of mesodermal origin, such as fibrosarcomas and mesothemliomas, or of epithelial origin, such as hepatomas, adrenal cortical carcinomas, and gastrointestinal adenocarcinomas. Hypoglycemia usually occurs in the late stages of malignancy. The mechanism by which hypoglycemia occurs involves a combination of impaired hepatic glucose production and increased peripheral glucose utilization. Many patients have a poor nutritional status, with depleted stores of the glycogen and protein needed to sustain hepatic glycogenolysis and gluconeogenesis. Hepatic damage from metastases further limits the ability to sustain gluconeogenesis. In most patients, however, hypoglycemia results predominantly from increased peripheral glucose utilization, raising the possibility of production of hormones with insulin-like properties. Insulin levels, as well as levels of insulin-like growth factor I (IGF-I) and growth hormone, are low, whereas insulin-like growth factor II (IGF-II) levels are usually normal. Recent work has focused on tumor production of an abnormally processed variant of IGF-II, "big IGF-II." This variant is not measured in usual radioimmunoassays for IGF-II but possesses normal biologic activity. It is likely "big IGF-II" accounts for many or most cases of tumor hypoglycemia (25,26).

Symptoms of hypoglycemia result from neuroglycopenia (confusion, seizures, and coma) or from activation of the adrenergic nervous system (sweating, palpitations, hunger, and tremors). The presence of tumor-associated hypoglycemia is established by demonstrating a low serum glucose level (less than 40 to 50 mg%) in a patient with symptoms of hypoglycemia who responds to oral or intravenous glucose. No further diagnostic workup is necessary. The primary treatment is nutritional support, either oral or intravenous. For immediate relief of symptomatic hypoglycemia, glucose is given as an intravenous bolus of 50% dextrose and then continued as a drip of 10% glucose. Refractory hypoglycemia can be treated with the counterregulatory hormones glucagon or cortisone.

## ENDOCRINE DISEASES IN CANCER PATIENTS

Malignancies often occur in patients with preexisting medical conditions such as diabetes mellitus and thyroid disease. Treatment of these conditions must continue during and after treatment of the malignancy and during palliative care. In each condition, goals of treatment must be reevaluated with prognosis of the underlying malignancy in mind.

### Diabetes Mellitus

Standard guidelines for the treatment of both type I and type II diabetes mellitus generally can be followed in the cancer patient; however, the appropriateness of "tight control" needs to be addressed in these patients. Based on results of the Diabetes Control and Complications Trial (DCCT) (27), it is accepted that intensive insulin treatment of type I diabetes results in a decrease in microvascular complications. These results have been extrapolated to type II diabetes mellitus; however, in the cancer patient with a limited life expectancy, intensive insulin therapy to prevent long-term complications is not a reasonable goal. The major complication of intensive insulin therapy is an increased risk of hypoglycemia. In patients with malignancies and poor nutrition, the risk of hypoglycemia is increased further. Additionally, intensive insulin treatment also requires frequent blood sugar monitoring, which may place a further burden on the patient and his or her caregivers. Sulfonylurea agents frequently are included in treatment regimens for type II diabetes. In the cancer population with suboptimal nutrition, recent weight loss, or impaired kidney or liver function, these agents should be used with extreme caution. Severe prolonged hypoglycemia can result from using sulfonyurea drugs. Many type II diabetics previously treated with these agents can have their diabetic medication discontinued because of normalization of blood sugars secondary to weight loss and poor calorie intake.

Diets should be tailored to meet the needs of the individual patient. Patients with poor appetite and decreased oral intake should be allowed to liberalize their diets from the traditional "diabetic diet." Patients may experience early satiety and mechanical problems with chewing and swallowing; nutritional supplementation with commercial products may be necessary. Consultation with a registered dietitian is helpful when devising and appropriate diet for the cancer patient with diabetics.

In summary, when choosing an appropriate treatment for diabetes mellitus in the cancer population, reasonable goals should be chosen. An attempt should be made to avoid symptomatic hyperglycemia, to decrease the risk of hypoglycemia, and to provide the patient with as many dietary choices as possible.

## Euthyroid Sick Syndrome

Severe illness, whether acute or chronic, can cause changes in thyroid physiology, leading to what has been referred to as the *euthyroid sick syndrome* (28). Changes can occur in levels of thyroxine (T4) and, to a lesser extent, thyroid stimulating hormone (TSH) levels. T4 is decreased due to its decreased binding to its serum transport proteins. The decrease in T3 results from inhibition of 5′-deiodinase, the enzyme that converts T4 to T3. Low T4 levels are associated with a higher mortality rate; TSH levels are generally helpful in distinguishing euthyroid sick syndrome from pituitary hypothyroidism.

## Adrenal Insufficiency

Because of the vascular nature of the adrenal cortex, the adrenal glands are common sites of metastatic disease. Typically, adrenal metastases are found incidentally during abdominal computed tomography (CT) and (MRI) scans and are usually of no functional significance. In a minority of cases, bilateral adrenal cortical destruction is sufficiently advanced to impair normal functioning and result in deficient production of cortisol (29). Symptoms of adrenocortical deficiency overlap with typical symptoms of advanced malignancy and include weight loss, fatigue, nausea, anorexia, and hypotension. The presence of hyponatremia or hyperkalemia further suggests the diagnosis.

The ACTH stimulation test is the most direct diagnostic study used to exclude adrenocortical insufficiency. A normal test contains the following three elements: an a.m. basal cortisol of at least 7 to 9 µg/dl, an increase greater than 7 µg/dl 30 minutes after administration of 0.25 mg intravenous ACTH, and a maximum response to intravenous ACTH of 20 µg/dl or greater.

Severely symptomatic adrenal insufficiency (*adrenal crisis*) is treated with intravenous saline and stress doses of hydrocorticone, 100 mg intravenously every 8 hours, tapered to a chronic oral maintenance dose of 20 mg every morning and 10 mg every evening. Patients with concomitant aldosterone deficiency resulting in hyperkalemia also may require the addition of the oral aldosterone analog fludrocortisone acetate (0.05–0.2 mg daily).

## REFERENCES

1. Hansen M, Hammer M, Humer L. Diagnostic and therapeutic implications or ectopic hormone production in small cell lung cancer. *Thorax* 1980;35:101.
2. Comis RL, Miller M, Ginsberg SJ. Abnormalities in water homeostasis in small cell anaplastic lung cancer. *Cancer* 1980;45:2414.
3. Odell WD, Wolfsen AR. Humoral syndromes associated with cancer. *Am Rev Med* 1978;29:379.
4. Sorensen JB, Andersen MK, Hansen HH. Syndrome of inappropriate secretion of antidiuretic hormone (SIADH) in malignant disease. *J Int Med* 1995;238:97.
5. Hantman D, Rossier B, Zohlman R. Rapid correction of hyponatremia in the syndrome of inappropriate secretion of antidiuretic hormone: an alternative treatment to hypertonic saline. *Ann Intern Med* 1973;78:870.
6. Sterns RH. Severe symptomatic hyponatraemia: treatment and outcome. *Ann Intern Med* 1987;107:656.
7. Ayns JC, Olivero JJ, Frommer JP. Rapid correction of severe hyponatraemia with intravenous hypertonic saline solution. *Am J Med* 1982;72:43.
8. Decaux G, Brimioulle S, Genette F. Treatment of the syndrome of inappropriate secretion of antidiuretic hormone by urea. *Am J Med* 1980;69:99.
9. Hale AC, Besser GM, Rees LH. Characterisation of pro-opiomelanocortin derived peptides in pituitary and ectopic adrenocorticotrophin secreting tumors. *J Endocrinol* 1986;108:49.
10. Tanaka K, Nicolson WE, Orth DN. The nature of immunoreactive lipotropins in human plasma and tissue extracts. *J Clin Invest* 1978;62:94.
11. Raff H, Findling JW, Aron DC. A new immunoradiometric assay for corticotropin evaluated in normal subjects and patients with Cushing's syndrome. *Clin Chem* 1989;35:596.
12. Tyrell JB, Findling JW, Aron DC, et al. An overnight high-dose dexamethasone suppression test for rapid differential diagnosis of Cushing's syndrome. *Ann Intern Med* 1986;104:180.
13. Oldfield EH, Chrousos GP, Schulte HM, et al. Preoperative lateralisation of ACTH-secreting pituitary microadenomas by bilateral and simultaneous inferior petrosal venous sinus sampling. *N Engl J Med* 1985;312:100.
14. Pierce ST. Paraendocrine syndromes. *Curr Opin Oncol* 1993;5:639.
15. Raskin P, McClain CJ, Medsger TA. Hypocalcemia associated with metastatic bone disease. *Arch Intern Med* 1973;132:539.
16. Salassa RM, Jowsey J, Arnaud C. Hypophosphatemia osteomalacia associated with "nonendocrine" tumors. *N Engl J Med* 1970;283:65.
17. Caron P, Salandini AM, Plantavid M. Choriocarcinoma and endocrine paraneoplastic syndromes. *Eur J Med* 1993;2:499.
18. Glass AR. Gynecomastia. *Endocrinol Metab Clin North Am* 1994;23:825.
19. Thompson DF, Carter JR. Drug-induced gynecomastia. *Pharmacotherapy* 1993;13:37.
20. Gropp C, Havemann K, Scheuer A. Ectopic hormones in lung cancer patients at diagnosis and during therapy. *Cancer* 1980;46:347.
21. Silva OL, Broder LE, Doppman JL, et al. Calcitonin as a marker for bronchogenic cancer: a prospective study. *Cancer* 1979;44:680.
22. Lamberts SW, van der Lely AJ, de Herder. Octreotide. *N Engl J Med* 1996;334:246.

23. Gregor M. Therapeutic principles in the management of metastasizing carcinoid tumors: drugs for symptomatic treatment. *Digestion* 1994; 55(Suppl3):60.

24. Diaco DS, Hajarizadeh H, Mueller CR. Treatment of metastatic carcinoid tumors using multimodality therapy of octreotide acetate, intra-arterial chemotherapy and hepatic arterial chemoembolization. *Am J Surg* 1995;169:523.

25. Phillips LS, Robertson DG. Insulin-like growth factors and non-islet cell tumor hypoglycemia. *Metabolism* 1993;42:1093.

26. Zapf J. Role of insulin-like growth factor II and IGF binding proteins in extrapancreatic tumor hypoglycemia. *Horm Res* 1994;42:20.

27. DCCT Research Group. Epidemiology of severe hypoglycemia in the Diabetes Control and Complications Trial. *Am J Med* 1991;90:450.

28. Docter R, Krenning EP, de Jong M. The sick euthyroid syndrome: changes in thyroid hormone serum parameters and hormone metabolism. *Clin Endocrinol* 1993;39:499.

29. Redman BG, Pazdur R, Zingas AP. Prospective evaluation of adrenal insufficiency in patients with adrenal metastasis. *Cancer* 1987;60:103.

*Principles and Practice of Supportive Oncology*,
edited by Ann Berger et al.
Lippincott–Raven Publishers, Philadelphia ©1998

CHAPTER 33

# Headache and Other Manifestations of Intracranial Pathology

Wendy Ziai and Neil A. Hagen

Intracranial pathology often results in a variety of distressing symptoms. Fortunately, the underlying cause often can be identified and treated, and the accompanying symptoms commonly respond to supportive measures.

This chapter is divided into two sections. The first deals with headache and other symptoms of intracranial pathology and reviews their pathogenesis and management strategies. Whereas nausea and vomiting are common in patients with intracranial pathology, this topic is covered elsewhere in this volume. The second section reviews cancer-related neurological syndromes, such as brain metastasis, base of skull metastasis, and cerebrovascular disease; oncologic interventions and supportive care strategies are outlined for each.

## SYMPTOMS OF INTRACRANIAL PATHOLOGY

### Headache

#### Assessment

General principles of headache assessment (1) also are applied appropriately for patients with a cancer history, with one important exception: The potential for headache to be the presenting symptom of a serious complication of the disease or its treatment compels an early and thorough assessment for structural disease in any cancer patient who develops this symptom. This assessment begins by confirming the onset, duration, progression, and focality of the headache. Pain characteristics include qualitative descriptors, severity, exacerbating and relieving features, associated symptoms, and the outcome of analgesic drugs or other therapies. Although prior

W. Ziai and N.A. Hagen: Department of Clinical Neurosciences, University of Calgary, Calgary, Alberta T2N 4N2, Canada.

headache history is important, the burden of proof is to rule out a new and serious cause of headache; brain metastasis can present with a headache similar to a previously experienced benign headache (2).

Cancer or its treatment can cause headache in a variety of ways. Some processes are considerably more likely to occur at particular points along the course of the disease. For example, about 90% of patients who die of melanoma have central nervous system metastases at autopsy; disseminated metastases are less likely to occur until regional metastases have developed. Therefore, the cancer history, extent of known disease, and prior treatments should be determined for all cancer patients with a headache.

The physical examination of the cancer patient with headache begins with a general physical examination and screening neurological examination, including examination of the ocular fundi, range of motion of the cervical spine, and assessment for meningismus. Provocation of the pain by the examiner can be informative: an underlying pathologic process is usually not far from the area of tenderness. Sites of pain indicated by the patient should be inspected and palpated. The examiner should palpate over facial sinuses, bony skull prominences, the occipitonuccal junction, and neck arteries. The orbits should be gently palpated and examined for proptosis. If the patient's pain is provoked by any of these maneuvers, the pain referral pattern should be noted.

Although comprehensive investigations can help document the cause of headaches caused by cancer, the extent of investigation should be guided according to the clinical situation. Bone scintigram, computed tomography (CT) of the head with fine bone windows, magnetic resonance imaging (MRI), and spinal fluid examinations are all commonly used in headache assessment. Blood tests can include serum hemoglobin, oxygen and $CO_2$ level, and sedimentation rate.

Head pain usually originates from intracranial or extracranial pain sensitive structures. Nociceptive input from these sites arises by displacement, distention, or inflammation of vascular structures; by sustained contraction of muscles; or by direct pressure on nerves. Alternatively, head pain may arise from nonnociceptive mechanisms arising from damage to peripheral or central pain pathways that subserve the head.

### Physiology of Head Pain

Pain-sensitive structures in the head include the fifth, ninth, and tenth cranial nerves; the upper three cervical nerves; and the great venous sinuses and their tributaries from the surface of the brain; in addition, all the tissues covering the cranium, especially the arteries, are pain sensitive. The cranial bones, diploic and emissary veins, brain parenchyma, parts of the dura, most of the pia mater and arachnoid, and the ependymal lining of the ventricles and choroid plexus are insensitive to pain.

Nociceptive input from supratentorial structures, including the superior surface of the tentorium cerebelli, causes pain to be felt anterior to a line drawn from the ears across the top of the head. Damage to these structures activates branches of the trigeminal nerve. Nociceptive input from infratentorial structures, including the inferior surface of the tentorium cerebelli, causes pain to be experienced posterior to this line and is conveyed by sensory fibers in the fifth, seventh, ninth, and tenth cranial nerves and the upper three cervical nerves (3).

### Primary and Secondary Headaches

Primary headaches encompass migraine, tension-type headaches, cluster headache, and others and are the most frequent headache type in Western society. They are functional disorders which by definition are characterized by the absence of a structural lesion.

In contrast, secondary headaches are symptomatic of an underlying disease, either an intracranial lesion or systemic process. The International Headache Society has provided a comprehensive classification of headache that identifies eight groups of secondary headaches (4) (Table 33-1). Although a temporal relationship between the headache and the underlying disorder is usually apparent, the diagnosis can be challenging because of to the high prevalence and similar features of primary headaches.

The incidence of headache in patients with primary or metastatic brain tumors is about 50% (5). Headache is a presenting symptom in 30% to 60% of adult brain tumor patients, and 60% to 70% of patients will develop headache during the course of this illness (6,7). Primary and metastatic brain tumors have a similar incidence of headache.

**TABLE 1.** *Secondary causes of headache*

| |
|---|
| Head trauma |
| Vascular disorders |
| Nonvascular intracranial disorder |
| Substances or their withdrawal |
| Noncephalic infection |
| Metabolic disorder |
| Disorder of cranium, neck, eyes, ears, nose, sinuses, teeth, mouth or other facial structures, cranial neuralgias, nerve trunk pain and deafferentation pain |
| Headache not classifiable |

Modified with permission after Olesen (4).

Factors reported to influence the incidence of headache in patients with brain tumors are tumor location, rate of growth, increased intracranial pressure, size of the enhancing lesion, amount of midline shift, and a history of previous headache (2). Headache occurs more commonly in infratentorial (64%–84%) than supratentorial (34%–60%) tumors (5–9) and is especially common with midline and basal tumors (95% and 70%, respectively). Slowly growing tumors, such as low-grade supratentorial astrocytomas and neuroepithelial tumors, including ganglogliomas, dysembryoplastic neuroepithelial tumors, and pleomorphic xanthoastrocytomas, have a low headache incidence but frequently are associated with seizures (10–13). Faster growing tumors, particularly malignant gliomas, have been reported to cause headache in about half of patients but have a lower incidence of seizures.

The classic brain-tumor headache is characterized by its progressively increasing severity, frequency, and duration; early morning awakening; disappearance after rising; association with nausea and vomiting; and aggravation by the Valsalva maneuver. This syndrome is actually uncommon, occurring in only 17% to 28% of patients (5,14). In reality, no single headache pattern is typical of a brain tumor. The most common headache profile is bifrontal, often worse ipsilaterally, dull, nonthrobbing, and aching in nature. These characteristics are similar to a tension-type headache. The pain is usually mild to moderate, intermittent, and relieved by simple analgesics in about half of patients. Severe headaches are reported by about 40% of patients, and 45% indicate that headache is the worst symptom. Also, 30% to 70% of patients experience nocturnal headache, and only 18% to 36% report early morning headache. Positional changes, either supine to standing or standing to supine, induce or aggravate headache in 20% to 32%; in 18% to 23% of patients, the headache worsens with Valsalva maneuvers. Nausea and vomiting are associated with headache in 36% to 48% of patients (5,6,7,15).

Brain-tumor headaches may mimic primary headaches. Forsyth and Posner (2) found that tumor headaches were similar to tension-type headaches in 77% of patients; 9% had migraine-like headaches, and 14%

had other types. In one study of cancer patients with a significant history of prior headache, 78% experienced new headaches associated with their brain tumor (5). The brain-tumor headache may be similar to the patient's prior headache but is generally more severe, frequent, or associated with new symptoms or abnormal signs.

The location of the headache in relation to tumor site, the presence of raised intracranial pressure, and the localizing value of focal headache depend on the mechanism by which headache is produced. Two mechanisms commonly account for headache in brain tumor patients: (a) direct traction or distortion of pain-sensitive structures by the tumor mass; and (b) distant traction through extensive displacement of brain tissue, either directly by the mass (e.g., herniation syndromes) or by hydrocephalus caused by obstruction of cerebrospinal fluid (CSF) pathways (15). Direct traction accounts for the localizing value of headaches in patients without raised intracranial pressure (ICP). Supratentorial tumors not associated with raised ICP often produce bilateral headache in the frontal region (85%). Unilateral headache is present in 28% to 53% (5,7), and the headache usually lateralizes to the side of the tumor. With the exception of cerebellopontine-angle tumors, which are more likely to produce symptoms by compression of adjacent cranial nerves, posterior fossa tumors often present with posterior head pain as the first symptom.

The headache of increased ICP tends to be severe, aching, and constant; is unrelieved by simple analgesics; is worse in the morning and with Valsalva maneuvers; and is associated with nausea or vomiting. It is most commonly located in the frontal region, neck, and either bifrontal region or vertex or in the neck alone. Occasionally, increased ICP accounts for the surprising occurrence of occipital headaches in association with a supratentorial tumor or frontal headache in association with a posterior fossa tumor.

Increased ICP is not necessary for the occurrence of headache, nor is it always associated with headache. Headache is commonly associated with "plateau waves," however, which may occur when increased ICP is severe. Plateau waves are transient elevations in ICP, which range from 25 to 60 mm Hg and last 1 to 10 minutes (16). They may be either spontaneous or induced by Valsalva maneuvers or changes in body position. In addition to headache, these episodes may be associated with impaired hearing or vision, nausea, vomiting, photophobia, lethargy, and transient neurological deficits. Severely increased ICP ultimately can result in life-threatening cerebral herniation syndromes and sudden death.

### Relief of Pain Caused by Intracranial Pathology

Management strategies for patients with pain from intracranial pathology derive from the general principles of supportive care and focus on both oncologic interventions and analgesic interventions (Table 33-2). The role of oncologic interventions, including surgery, to treat brain metastases, particularly for patients with single lesions and limited or absent disease elsewhere, is reviewed below. The use of surgery to manage symptoms from intracranial pathology is limited to highly selected patients who may be offered procedures to relieve specific syndromes that are refractory to more conservative treatment. For example, rare patients undergo resection of a large cerebellar metastasis to reduce severe headache, despite the presence of other, less symptomatic metastatic lesions. Others are offered percutaneous aspiration of a tumor cyst through an Ommaya reservoir if relief of mass effect on initial aspiration results in significant relief of symptoms (17).

Radiotherapy is frequently effective to relieve pain or other symptoms from metastatic disease, even if the primary tumor is relatively radiation resistant (18–20). If the goal of treatment is limited to symptom control alone, patients are generally candidates for radiotherapy if life expectancy is greater than 2 months and symptoms are not easily managed with more conservative means.

Chemotherapy can be palliative for metastatic intracranial disease from a small number of tumor primaries, including breast (21), small-cell carcinoma of the lung (22), testes (23), and others. Hormonal therapy can be well tolerated and can be effective to shrink metastatic disease in patients with breast or prostate cancer who have not been exposed to such treatment previously.

The role of corticosteroids to manage symptoms from intracranial pathology requires particular emphasis. An empiric course over a few days can be used to establish efficacy (24). Although dexamethasone is usually preferred, prednisone (25), prednisolone (26), and adrenocortitropic hormone (ACTH) (27) also have been reported to relieve symptoms from intracranial pathology. Dexamethasone is available in both oral and parenteral formulations, generally lacks mineralocorticoid effect, and is historically the corticosteroid of choice for management of symptoms related to brain tumors. Nonfluorinated corticosteroids such as prednisone may have less risk of causing myopathy (25,26). Controlled trials com-

**TABLE 2.** *Management strategies for pain from intracranial pathology*

Oncologic interventions
   Radiation therapy
   Surgery
   Chemotherapy
Analgesic interventions
   Pharmacotherapy
   Physical measures
   Psychological measures
   Neurolytic or anesthetic procedures
   Neurostimulatory procedures

paring the efficacy and side effect profile of different steroids are needed.

In brain tumor patients, cushinoid facies predict the presence of steroid myopathy (25). Other side effects of steroids include hyperglycemia, cataracts, osteoporosis, and neuropsychiatric effects. Side effects can become disabling over time. To reduce the risk of side effects, the lowest effective dose of steroid should be identified by methodical titration upward or downward.

### Neuropathic Pain Due to Central Nervous System Disease

Central pain is defined as pain associated with a lesion of the central nervous system, particularly of the spinothalamic tract or thalamus (28). Central pain must be differentiated from other types of neuropathic pain associated with lesions of the peripheral nervous system and from nociceptive pain associated with ongoing stimulation of nociceptors by a tissue-damaging lesion.

Many types of structural lesions in the brain and spinal cord can cause central pain. Although the type, duration, and size of the lesion can influence the tendency to produce central pain, similar lesions may or may not be painful, or they may produce different types of pain (29). Only a minority of patients with susceptible lesions actually develop central pain. The locations of most painful lesions are in the spinal cord, lower brainstem, and ventral posterior part of the thalamus (30–32). The most common causes of these lesions are spinal cord trauma and cerebrovascular accidents. The prevalence of central pain is highest in syringomyelia; most patients with this lesion develop central pain during the course of the disease. Central pain is less common in traumatic spinal cord injuries (30%) and multiple sclerosis (23%). Interestingly, intracranial and spinal tumors have a low prevalence of central pain. Several patients with central pain due to meningioma have been reported (33). In a series of 49 patients with thalamic tumors, only one had central pain (34).

The diagnosis of central pain depends on a detailed neurological history and examination along with laboratory investigations, including CT or MRI scans, CSF analysis, neurophysiologic testing, and other tests as appropriate. Psychiatric consultation may be indicated, although symptoms characteristic of central pain are rarely psychogenic in origin (29).

The onset of central pain may be immediate or delayed for years after the appearance of the lesion. Although the pain typically has a burning, tingling, or pins and needles quality, it may be superficial, deep, or both; is not always dysesthetic; and can have a variety of descriptors in the same or different regions. The pain may be triggered by physical activity, stress, loud noise, vibrations, weather change, altered muscle or visceral function, or seizures (30). It is usually constant, varies in severity from mild tingling to unbearable and may have more than one element: Commonly, a severe intermittent component is superimposed on constant pain. Central pain is usually permanent, although transient pain in spinal cord injury patients and complete cessation of pain either spontaneously or following the occurrence of new lesions have been reported (29,35,36). Although not necessary for its development, central pain usually is associated with a sensory deficit in the same area as the pain. Hypesthesia to temperature is the most common finding. Sensory deficits are consistent with the site of the known lesion; for example, ventral posterior thalamic lesions may be associated with a hemibody sensory loss, and low brainstem infarcts may produce a crossed, dissociated sensory loss.

The treatment of central pain is based largely on clinical experience. Treatment modalities include pharmacotherapy, sensory stimulation, neurosurgical procedures, and sympathetic blockade (30,37). The first-line drugs are antidepressants, specifically amitriptyline and antiepileptics (AEDS) with carbamazepine being frequently used. The best central pain response to antidepressants is seen in poststroke patients, whereas AEDS seem to be most effective for paroxysmal central pain, especially in multiple sclerosis (29). A range of other therapies are used, including opioid analgesics and other adjuvant drugs.

### Cranial Neuralgias

Cranial neuralgias are of particular significance to the cancer patient because a diagnosis of neuralgia frequently lends to a search for skull base or neck metastases. Also, the frequent response of these pain syndromes to a regimen containing selected adjuvant analgesics (e.g., anticonvulsants) highlights the value of prompt diagnosis. Trigeminal neuralgia and glossopharyngeal neuralgia are characterized by paroxysmal lancinating pain in the face or throat and neck, respectively. Pain lasts from a few seconds to a minute or two, with frequent recurrence. The pain is often spontaneous in onset, but it may be initiated by sensory stimuli such as touch or tickle applied to certain trigger areas; movements such as chewing or talking also can precipitate pains. Other features, such as continuous dull aching, burning, or pressure pain, are not infrequently reported (38). The differential diagnosis includes disorders of the jaw, teeth, sinuses, base of skull, and neck. Although these neuralgias are most commonly idiopathic, the onset of cranial neuralgia in a patient with a cancer history mandates a search for metastatic disease. Radiological studies include CT or MRI with views of the skull base and sinuses. Plain radiographs or tomograms of the skull base may show abnormalities.

## Seizures

A seizure may be defined as an episode of uncontrolled motor, sensory, or psychological activity caused by the sudden excessive discharge of cerebral cortical neurons (39,40), followed by a postictal phase of metabolic cerebral depression lasting a variable period. There are two broad types: primary generalized seizures and partial (also called focal or secondary) seizures. A partial seizure is caused by an epileptogenic lesion. Clinically, a seizure discharge is most effectively identified by electroencephalography (EEG), whereas an epileptogenic lesion may be demonstrated by CT or MRI scanning. The first appearance of any seizure during adulthood, with or without a localizing aura, is sufficiently suspicious to warrant an investigation for neoplasm.

Generalized or focal seizures occur in 20–50% of patients with brain tumors (41). The occurrence of a seizure depends on tumor site, type, and infiltration or expansive properties. In patients with supratentorial tumors, seizures are a presenting symptom in up to half of patients (42,43). In patients with low grade astrocytoma, oligodendroglioma, or meningioma, all relatively slow growing tumors, seizures may predate other symptoms for years. Focal seizures are associated with tumors involving motor cortex, sensory cortex, or the temporal lobe. Temporal lobe gliomas typically produce psychomotor seizures, with or without olfactory hallucinations (uncinate fits), abnormal visual or auditory perception, déja vu phenomenon, or automatic behavior (44). Parietal lobe tumors may cause generalized or focal sensory seizures, and occipital lobe neoplasms have been associated with an aura of flashing lights, but not formed images. Infratentorial tumors and neoplasms involving the white matter only are not commonly associated with seizures.

In patients with intracerebral metastases (ICM), the incidence of seizures as a presenting symptom ranges from 15% to 21% (14,45,46). In one study, late seizures developed in 10% of patients from 1 to 59 weeks after diagnosis of ICM (47). With the exception of malignant melanoma and choriocarcinoma, metastatic brain neoplasms are less likely to cause seizures than primary brain tumors. The presence of multiple metastases or combined brain and leptomeningeal metastases are the conditions most frequently associated with seizures (48).

Seizures also can be an indication of tumor progression or recurrence, often occurring late after initial oncologic therapy. Other etiologies, such as electrolyte disturbances (e.g., hyponatremia), drug interactions, and noncompliance with anticonvulsants, may predispose to the late development of seizures. *Status epilepticus*, which may be defined as a persistent seizure (usually considered to last longer than 5 minutes) or repeated seizures without interictal return of consciousness, is an important neurooncological emergency. All clinicians should be familiar with the treatment of this condition. Acute management begins with assurance of the airway, ventilation, and perfusion. Blood should be sampled for urgent electrolyte screen and other appropriate tests, and a dose of glucose should be given (usually 50 ml of a 50% solution) before any results are known. The typical treatment protocol involves the intravenous administration of a benzodiazepine, such as diazepam or lorazepam followed by intravenous loading with phenytoin. If seizures recur, treatment with either phenobarbital or diazepam by continuous infusion may be started with close monitoring of ventilation. For persistent convulsions, barbiturate anesthesia may be necessary with halothane and neuromuscular blockade. Although focal continuous epilepsy (epilepsy partialis continua) is also treated promptly, this syndrome is less injurious to the patient and usually is treated without the high-dose intravenous drugs administered for generalized status (49). The routine use of prophylactic anticonvulsants in brain tumor patients was recommended in patients who present with seizures and in patients undergoing craniotomy. The most commonly prescribed drug is phenytoin, in doses of 300 to 400 mg/day. Carbamazepine, phenobarbital, and sodium valproate also are used. Initially, monitoring of serum levels is required. Patients with benign brain tumors and no history of seizures do not require prophylaxis.

There is currently conflicting advice regarding the use of prophylactic anticonvulsants in patients with malignant primary or metastatic brain tumors who have never had a seizure. In one study, a 10% incidence of late seizures in patients with brain metastases was noted whether or not prophylactic phenytoin was given (47); serum anticonvulsant levels were subtherapeutic in two thirds of the patients who developed seizures, however, which may explain the therapeutic failure. Preliminary results from a recent randomized, controlled trial of prophylactic anticonvulsants in brain tumor patients who had no prior history of seizures demonstrated no protection against late seizures (50).

Therapeutic levels can be difficult to achieve in brain tumor patients, especially with concomitant use of dexamethasone, which increases the required dose of phenytoin (51). Interaction between phenytoin and dexamethasone also reduces the bioavailability of the dexamethasone (52). Toxic phenytoin levels may occur with frequent dosage adjustments and can produce side effects such as nystagmus and ataxia, which can suggest tumor recurrence. Other potential complications from phenytoin include erythema multiforme and Stevens-Johnson syndrome, which have been associated with the combined administration of whole-brain radiotherapy and phenytoin (53); myopathy (54); and immunosuppressive effects specifically targeted against cell-mediated immunity (55,56).

Discontinuation of seizure prophylaxis in patients with a benign tumor and preoperative seizures has been recommended only for patients with complete excision of a benign tumor who remain seizure-free after 12 months. The risk of relapse remains at least 35% if the patient has had previous seizures (57).

## Singultus (Hiccups)

Singultus (hiccups) is a forceful involuntary inspiration caused by spasmodic contraction of the diaphragm that terminates with sudden closure of the glottis. Closure of the glottis results in the characteristic hiccup sound. Hiccups serve no known physiological function (58) and are usually a transient benign disorder that resolves without medical therapy. Chronic hiccups may reflect underlying pathology, including a lesion that irritates the peripheral vagus or phrenic nerves, drug toxicity, metabolic abnormalities, infection, and intracranial disease. Rarely, chronic hiccups are psychogenic.

The mechanism of hiccup may involve dysfunction of peripheral components or central connections of the reflex arc. The afferent neural pathway is composed of sensory branches of the phrenic and vagus nerves as well as dorsal sympathetic afferent from T6 through T12. The principal efferent limb, which produces the diaphragmatic contraction, includes motor fibers of the phrenic nerve and efferent branches to the glottis and external intercostal muscles (inspiratory). There is reciprocal inhibition of the expiratory intercostal muscles. The separate innervation of right and left hemidiaphragms and the long course of the two phrenic nerves, each of which contacts various organs, account for the large variety of reported mechanisms for hiccup. Hiccups may be bilateral or unilateral; most occur in the left diaphragm. The central control of hiccups, although not yet fully defined, is believed to include a supraspinal center that is integrated with the respiratory center output to respiratory motor neurons in the spinal cord (59). The reported rate of repetitive hiccups is between 4 and 60 per minute; the most frequent rate is 17 to 20 per minute, not surprisingly similar to the respiratory rate (60).

The central nervous system causes of hiccups include parenchymal lesions within the medulla and local pathology causing medullary compression; both of these lesions can produce dysfunction at the level of the vagal nucleus and the nucleus tractus solitarius (61). It also has been suggested that central nervous system conditions causing hiccups may release the normal inhibitory tone on the hiccup reflex arc (58). Specific lesions of the medulla include neoplasms, syringomyelia, infarction (often the territory of the posterior inferior cerebellar artery), and infections, including meningitis, encephalitis, neurosyphilis, and human immunodeficiency virus (HIV) encephalopathy. Compressive lesions causing hiccups include neoplasms, hematomas, and bleeding into the fourth ventricle (62).

Identification of serious underlying causes of hiccups depends on their duration, severity, and associated conditions. Benign hiccup bouts may last up to 48 hours and usually are related to gastric distension, alcohol ingestion, or emotional factors. Persistent hiccups are defined as a hiccup episode lasting longer than 48 hours but less than 1 month, and intractable hiccups are defined as a hiccup episode persisting longer than a month. Both are assumed to have an organic etiology until proven otherwise by extensive medical and laboratory investigations (63).

Neurogenic hiccups may require urgent management. Some patients experience severe fatigue as a result of sleep deprivation. Others develop respiratory irregularity or even respiratory arrest, probably related to a lesion at the medullary respiratory control centers (64). When respiratory difficulties occur, associated brainstem symptoms or signs are usually present. It should be noted that, with the exception of intubated patients or those with a tracheotomy, hiccups alone do not produce any significant ventilatory effect because the glottis closes almost immediately after the onset of diaphragmatic contraction (59).

The management of hiccups includes physical, pharmacological, and surgical interventions. Initial therapy should focus on elimination or treatment of the underlying cause. Physical stimulation of afferent nerve endings or certain end-organs may interrupt the hiccup reflex arc (65) and are the basis of anecdotal folk remedies, such as swallowing granulated sugar, breathing into a bag, and breath-holding. Physiologically, the hiccup reflex is inhibited by high arterial carbon dioxide tension (66).

Pharmacologic measures for hiccough are supported by anecdotal experience. Drugs in the following classes have been used: antipsychotics, tricyclic antidepressants, anticonvulsants, antiarrhythmics, central nervous system stimulants, muscle relaxants, inhalation agents, local anesthetics, and gastric motility agents. The most commonly used and most consistently effective agent is chlorpromazine, a centrally acting major tranquilizer and dopamine antagonist. It is especially effective given as an intravenous bolus (67). The second drug of choice is metoclopramide, a gastric motility agent and dopamine antagonist (68–70). Other valuable agents include the anticonvulsants carbamazepine, phenytoin, and valproic acid and the antispasmodic baclofen. Surgical interventions are reserved for intractable hiccups that fail to respond to physical or pharmacologic therapy. Phrenic nerve transection, crushing, or anesthetic blockade may be complicated by severe respiratory impairment, especially if both phrenic nerves are disrupted. In addition, such a procedure may fail to relieve hiccups (67). Phrenic nerve surgery is therefore a last resort and should be preceded by a local anesthetic block to assess efficacy and the potential respiratory compromise from diaphragmatic paralysis (71).

## Neurologic Impairments
## Caused by Intracranial Pathology

Focal neurological symptoms, such as weakness, numbness, incoordination, and visual impairment, can interfere significantly with function. If correctly diagnosed, treatment of the underlying cause may be possible. In all cases, measures to accommodate the deficit can be helpful. Although the spectrum of manifestations resulting from intracranial disease are protean, two complex neurological syndromes and specific neuropsychiatric conditions deserve emphasis because of the high degree of impairment and the clinical difficulty in making a correct diagnosis.

Patients with bifrontal disease may appear to the family as lacking initiative and sparkle. Speech is sparse or nonexistent (*mutism*), and yet the patient is fully aware of the conversation around him or her. There may be urinary urgency or incontinence (unwitting wetting); a shuffling, wide-based gait; and an apparent slowness of thought processes. Damage to both frontal lobes can be a sequela of radiation therapy, or it can result from multiple bilateral metastases, hydrocephalus, leptomeningeal tumor, cerebrovascular disease, or other causes. Findings on examination that support the diagnosis include bilateral grasp reflexes, a snout reflex, a positive glabellar tap, presence of bilateral palmomental reflexes, and an apraxic gait. Patients' families need to be aware that the patient may be cognitively intact and able to later recall details of events that occurred while sick. Understanding that the lack of motivation is neurologic, rather than psychologic, may help the family cope with the patient's condition.

In the nondominant parietal syndrome, there is denial of illness; the patient may believe he or she should be able to manage alone at home despite severe impairment. Brain metastases and cerebrovascular disease are the most common causes. The diagnosis of a nondominant parietal syndrome is confirmed by identifying focal sensory or motor deficits (usually affecting the left side of the body), hemianopsia, dressing and constructional apraxia, agnosia, and denial of body parts. The overall management and rehabilitation strategies are similar to those used for other neuropsychological impairments. The prognosis for improvement is poor as a result of the patient's lack of insight.

Intracranial pathology also can cause delirium and specific disorders of mood or perception. Delirium is an acute organic disorder of attention and cognition. Thinking, perception, memory, and psychomotor status all may be disturbed in the delirious patient (72). In contrast to dementia, delirium is acute and potentially reversible. Delirium involves a wide differential diagnosis in which toxic and metabolic disorders are prominent. In addition to neoplasm, many other structural disorders may be responsible, including hydrocephalus, stroke, subdural hematoma, cranial arteritis, and trauma (73). Delirium also may be caused by seizures. New onset of delirium requires prompt assessment for treatable causes.

Personality changes, including depression, euphoria, loss of inhibition, and impulsive behaviour, also may reflect intracranial disease, including raised ICP secondary to a space-occupying lesion. Temporal lobe lesions have been noted to produce bizarre thinking and immature emotion behavior (44). The diagnosis of these conditions, particularly the organic mood disorders, may be challenging given the high prevalence of primary psychiatric disorders in the cancer population.

## CANCER-RELATED
## NEUROLOGICAL SYNDROMES

### Brain Metastases

Clinically evident brain metastases occur in 20% to 30% of patients with systemic cancer and are found at autopsy in up to 50% (18,74–78). Metastases are the most common malignant tumor of the brain (75) and have an annual incidence three times that of primary brain tumors (76,77). The three most common cancers that metastasize to the brain are lung, breast, and melanoma (75).

Brain metastases tend to be a late finding, and evidence of other metastatic disease is usually present; only 19% of 201 patients with brain metastases studied at the Memorial Sloan-Kettering Cancer Center lacked evidence of systemic metastases on initial evaluation (18). The interval between diagnosis of the primary malignancy and the discovery of brain metastases depends on the tumor type. Small-cell lung cancer, for example, metastasizes early; there is an 11% incidence of silent metastases at diagnosis (79). Other tumors, such as breast carcinoma, typically develop brain metastases late, once disseminated disease is present (80–82). In addition to the primary cancer, factors that influence brain metastases include age and gender (83). Some tumors, such as colon, pelvic, abdominal, and renal cancers, tend to cause single lesions, whereas others, such as melanoma, lung, and breast cancer, and tumors of unknown origin, are more likely to cause multiple metastases (84,85). In lung cancer and melanoma patients, men have a greater predilection to develop brain metastases than women, perhaps reflecting the more common site of melanoma in men on the head, neck, and trunk; for lung cancer, explanations for this observation are lacking (83).

The distribution of brain metastases is proportional to cerebral blood flow as well as brain weight (86). The cerebral hemispheres receive 85% of cerebral blood flow and are the site of about 80% of brain metastases. The posterior fossa, the recipient of 15% of cerebral flow, is the site in 20% of metastases (16% are in the cerebellum and 3% are in the brainstem) (83,87). The observation that there is a predilection of gastrointestinal and pelvic malignancies to metastasize to the posterior fossa suggests a route of dissemination via Batson's plexus, which may receive venous drainage from the pelvic organs, but the evidence for this is not certain (81,84,88).

Approximately two thirds of patients with brain metastases discovered at autopsy have had clinical findings during life (89). Patients usually have focal findings, which typically exhibit an onset over months, and a progressive course. Although focal signs often suggest the site of metastases, false localizing signs may occur as a a a result of compression of distant structures by shifts caused by increased ICP. These signs may cause a perplexing constellation of symptoms and signs. Generalized neurologic dysfunction caused by raised ICP may present in an acute or gradual manner.

Headache is the most common initial complaint. It occurs in half of patients with a single brain metastasis, and almost all these patients will manifest other signs or symptoms. Patients with multiple or cerebellar metastases have a higher incidence of headache (83,90). Surprisingly, the finding of papilledema occurs in less than one quarter of patients with brain metastases (85,88). Focal weakness, the second most common presenting symptom, is reported in about 40% of patients, although examination reveals weakness in up to two thirds of patients (87,91). Mental or behaviorial changes, an initial finding in 30% of patients, may reflect multiple brain metastases or focal lesions causing raised intracranial pressure or hydrocephalus. One study reported that three quarters of brain metastasis patients failed to score normally on standard mental status tests (92). Seizures, either focal or generalized, are the first sign in 15% to 20% of patients. Occasionally, transient neurological events occur with complete resolution; excluding seizures, an acute onset of symptoms has been reported in fewer than 10% of patients. The complaint of gait ataxia can result from posterior fossa, a large frontal lobe lesion, or hydrocephalus. These patients may lack significant unsteadiness on examination. Other presenting symptoms include sensory disturbance and visual loss, typically hemianopsia. The onset of neurologic dysfunction is usually insidious, over weeks or months. Intratumoral hemorrhage may cause an acute worsening of preexisting, slowly evolving symptoms.

The most sensitive diagnostic test for brain metastases is MRI. This test should be considered for any cancer patient with an unexplained neurologic disturbance and also is indicated for neurologically asymptomatic patients undergoing attempted curative treatment of a primary tumor with high metastatic potential to brain, such as lung cancer or metastatic melanoma (90).

Evaluation of the status of the systemic cancer is important in determining appropriate therapy for an intracranial metastasis. Factors that affect the choice of treatment modality for brain metastases include patient age, size and location of the metastasis, neurologic status, patient performance status, extent of the primary tumor, other sites of metastatic disease, and response to prior therapy (83,89). Therapeutic options range from no treatment, which may be appropriate in patients near death with disseminated disease, to emergency surgery for potentially reversible but otherwise imminently fatal lesions. Most commonly, various combinations of medical, radiation, and surgical therapy are employed.

Without treatment, patients with brain metastases have a median survival of about 1 month (93,94). Corticosteroids double the median survival to 2 months (95,96). About 70% of patients show significant improvement by day 2 of treatment (97). To reduce the risk of side effects, steroid dose is tapered downward from the starting dose, as tolerated.

Whole-brain radiation therapy (WBRT) is reported to increase median survival to 3 to 6 months (92,98,99). Two thirds of patients with serious neurologic dysfunction and one third of patients with moderate dysfunction obtain relief or improvement of symptoms (83,100). The standard dose is 3,000 cGy in 10 fractions (300 cGy per treatment), although regimens vary depending on the center. Protracted radiation therapy regimens (2,000 cGy in 20 fractions) are advised when anticipated survival is greater than one year due to a lesser rate of later neurologic complications associated with this regimen (101). Accelerated radiation therapy may be used to achieve rapid palliation in patients whose condition is deteriorating quickly. Other irradiation modalities include interstitial brachytherapy and radiosurgery, which uses either a stereotactic linear accelerator or a gamma knife to deliver high doses of radiation to a small intracranial target (102).

Although no randomized trial comparing the results of radiosurgery with conventional surgery for metastatic brian tumors has been reported to date, radiosurgery (as an alternative treatment for brain metastases) has undergone an expotential growth and may eventually replace surgery as the primary treatment modality for small brain metastases not producing life-threatening mass effect. One series reported about 88% local control with a single fraction of 1,600 to 3,500 cGy (almost double the local control rate achieved with standard whole-brain radiation) (102). Factors influencing the efficacy of radiosurgery include size and shape of the lesion, number of tumors, and nature of the primary tumor. In general, well-demarcated, spherical tumors of small volume (5 cc) respond best to radiosurgery. All of these characterize cerebral metastases. The risk for distant recurrences increases significantly when more than three metastases are treated in one patient. Radiosurgery treatment for metastases secondary to melanoma and renal cell carcinoma has been associated with high quality of life even in the presence of multiple metastases compared with lung cancer patients, who have a significantly shorter life expectancy. Relative contraindications to stereotactic radiosurgery include large tumors, hemorrhagic tumors, and those producing significant mass effect. Conventional treatment with surgery followed by WBRT is then recommended.

Of patients who exhibit an initial clinical response to radiotherapy, about 80% maintain clinical improvement at 3 months and 60% are stable at 6 months (82). Two thirds of patients who show a major response to radiotherapy die of systemic disease, and only 15% die solely as a result of neurologic deterioration (90). Extent of systemic cancer is, therefore, a strong prognostic indicator in patients with brain metastases. The presence of liver or lung metastases predicts poor survival in patients who develop brain metastases.

Surgical interventions in patients with brain metastases encompass procedures to relieve ICP, biopsy to establish diagnosis (principally in patients with an unknown primary), and resection of metastatic lesions. Surgical resection of brain metastases is most likely to benefit those with a solitary lesion in a surgically accessible location, with either no evidence of systemic disease or controlled systemic disease and with a life expectancy greater than 2 months (82,103–105). Unfortunately, only about 25% of patients with brain metastases fulfill these indications, as only half of brain metastases are single and half of single metastases are excluded based in inaccessibility of the tumor, extensive systemic disease, or other factors. In patients who are surgical candidates, resection followed by adjunctive WBRT has been shown in prospective randomized studies to improve survival and local control compared with whole-brain radiation therapy without surgery. Patchell et al. (103), for example, reported a median survival of 40 weeks in the surgery plus radiotherapy compared with 15 weeks in the radiation group; recurrence at the original site was 20% and 52% in the surgical and radiation groups, respectively (103). Patients treated with surgery remained functionally independent for a median of 38 weeks versus 8 weeks in the radiated group. An additional benefit of surgical intervention is the tissue diagnosis; in one study, 11% of patients did not have metastatic tumors despite radiographic findings (103). The role of radiotherapy following surgery in single brain metastases is currently being evaluated.

For most patients, treatment of multiple brain metastases remains WBRT with corticosteroids. Uncommonly, surgical resection can be considered for easily accessible metastases if other criteria for surgery are met. The contribution of chemotherapy to the management of brain metastases remains uncertain for most types of cancer. Regression of brain metastases has occurred following effective systemically administered cytotoxic chemotherapy (21,22,23).

## Leptomeningeal Metastases

The syndrome of leptomeningeal metastases (or meningeal carcinomatosis) refers to diffuse or multifocal seeding of the leptomeninges by systemic cancer (106). Leptomeningeal metastases are identified at autopsy in up to 8% of patients with systemic cancer. The most frequent cancers to metastasize to the leptomeninges are breast and lung, followed by melanoma. Some cancers have a high affinity for the nervous system, however, and leptomeningeal disease may be clinically evident in almost half of patients (107). The duration from discovery of the primary malignancy to the diagnosis of leptomeningeal involvement is very broad, from 3 months to 6 years in some series (108).

Two characteristic features suggest a diagnosis of leptomeningeal cancer. First, neurologic dysfunction appears at multiple levels of the neuraxis in the absence of brain or spinal epidural metastases on radiographic examination. The patient may present with a variety of complaints and tends to accumulate new symptoms over weeks as the disease progresses. Second, neurological signs tend to be much more prominent than symptoms. Although most patients initially complain of symptoms in one anatomic area, examination reveals signs of neurological abnormality in two or more areas in more than 80% of patients.

Symptoms referable to the brain are the initial complaint in about half of patients, with headache the single most frequent initial symptom; headache is reported by one third of patients at presentation (106). The headache can occur in a variety of locations, including bifrontal, diffuse, or radiating from the occipital region into the neck. Nausea or vomiting, light headedness, and cognitive disturbances are associated features. Changes in mental status alone are a common finding and eventually occur in 80% of patients; these changes are characterized by lethargy, confusion, and memory deficit. Other common symptoms and signs include seizures, cranial nerve palsies, weakness, numbness, pain, ataxia, fecal incontinence, and urinary retention. Occasionally, asymptomatic urinary retention occurs.

The diagnosis of leptomeningeal metastases is based on clinical findings and CSF analysis. The finding of malignant cells in the CSF is the diagnostic gold standard; positive cytology is eventually found in 90% of patients, although three or more examinations of large volumes of CSF may be required (106,108,109). Associated CSF findings include elevated protein, decreased glucose, and lymphocytosis. Other investigations include flow cytometry of CSF content, myelography, CT of the head, and the most sensitive radiologic examination, MRI of the head and spine with gadolinium (107–115).

Treatment of leptomeningeal metastases is aimed at prolonging survival and improving or stabilizing neurologic disability. Untreated, leptomeningeal metastases from a variety of tumor types have a median survival of 4 to 6 weeks (116,117). Meningeal lymphoma and breast cancer have a more favorable prognosis, which is usually measured in many months. Management may include radiation therapy to symptomatic sites of the neuroaxis, intrathecal or intraventricular chemotherapy, and steroids.

### Base of Skull Metastases

The base of the skull includes the temporal, sphenoid, and occipital bones (including the clivus) as well as the bony orbit. Base of skull metastases are most commonly secondary to tumors of the breast, lung, and prostate. Other tumors that may metastasize to the skull base include head and neck tumors, lymphoma, and other tumors that metastasize to bone. The median interval from primary tumor diagnosis to onset of neurologic signs was 23 months in one study; two thirds of patients had metastatic disease elsewhere when the base of skull metastases were diagnosed (118). Several discrete neurological syndromes have been described, characterized by dysfunction of cranial nerves as they pass through bony foramen. Common areas include the bony orbit, parasellar region, middle cranial fossa, jugular foramen, occipital condyle, clivus, and sphenoid sinus.

Base of skull metastases may present with head pain, cranial nerve palsies, or both. Treatment is usually effective and includes pharmacologic analgesic interventions (usually nonsteroidals with opioids) and focal radiation therapy. Recovery of cranial nerve function tends to be slow.

### Cerebrovascular Disease in Cancer Patients

After metastases, cerebrovascular lesions are the next most common neurologic finding at autopsy in cancer patients. In one autopsy series, 14.6% of patients had cerebrovascular lesions (119); of these, about half had clinical symptoms of cerebrovascular disease during life. The usual risk factors in the general population for stroke, including age, hypertension, coronary artery disease, and diabetes, are less important in this population than the pathophysiologic effects of neoplastic disease and its treatment (120).

Cerebral metastases and coagulator disturbances are the usual causes of intracerebral hemorrhage (ICH) in cancer patients. The reported overall incidence of hemorrhage from an intracranial tumor is 1% to 15%. (121). One neurosurgical series demonstrated an overall tumor hemorrhage rate of 14.6%, of which 5.4% were classified as macroscopic and 9.2% as microscopic (122). As a cause of spontaneous ICH, however, tumor-induced ICH is not a common etiology (only 2% of 461 autopsy cases in one study) (123).

The tumors with the highest incidence of bleeding are metastatic melanoma, germ-cell tumors (particularly choriocarcinoma), and bronchogenic carcinoma. The usual presentation mimics an acute vascular event, such as a hypertensive hemorrhage or ruptured berry aneurysm (124). Headache, progressive obtundation, and focal neurologic signs have been reported in two thirds of cancer patients with intracranial hemorrhage. Occasionally, patients present with seizures. Hypertensive hemorrhages may be distinguished from intratumoral bleeding by the presence of a history of high blood pressure and location of the hemorrhage in the basal ganglia in 90% of cases. Neoplastic aneurysms, although uncommon, are another cause of intracranial hemorrhage in cancer patients.

Coagulopathy may be an indirect effect of the tumor or result from iatrogenic causes, including chemotherapy-related thrombocytopenia and treatment with warfarin, which is usually undertaken for deep venous thrombosis. Disease-related coagulopathy may be consumptive, such as disseminated intravascular coagulation. Neurologic complications from the latter disorder may be either hemorrhagic, including intracerebral and subdural hematoma, or ischemic. Hemorrhage may complicate the other disorders. Coagulopathy-induced intraparenchymal hemorrhage is most commonly associated with leukemia, in which case the hemorrhage is often fatal (119). Patients with solid tumors and thrombocytopenia have a low incidence of ICH and coagulopathy-related ICH in this population usually occurs as a terminal event (120). Anticoagulant-induced intracranial hemorrhage is not common.

Clinically, patients with either spontaneous cerebral hemorrhage from a coagulopathy or hemorrhage into a brain tumor present with a combination of headache, vomiting, progressive decline in level of consciousness, and focal neurologic deficits. Disseminated intravascular coagulation can present with encephalopathy, even in the absence of abnormalities in blood clotting parameters or low platelets. Suspected intratumoral hemorrhage should be investigated with CT scan or MRI. Management is primarily medical, and includes elevation of the head, corticosteroids, reversal of hemostatic abnormalities (if possible) and antitumor therapy if appropriate. Spontaneous intracerebral hemorrhage in acute promyelocytic leukemia has been reduced significantly with prophylactic heparin, chemotherapy, and transretinoic acid (125–127).

In patients with leukemia, another cause of intracerebral hemorrhage is hyperleukocytosis (elevation of the peripheral blast count to greater than 100,000 cells per $mm^3$), which causes early death secondary to ICH in a reported 15% of patients (128). Clinically, such patients develop multiple intraparenchymal hemorrhages, occasionally associated with intraventricular or subarachnoid hemorrhage. Chemotherapy and leukophoresis to lower the peripheral blast count reduced but did not eliminate the risk of ICH (119,128).

Causes of cerebral infarction in cancer patients include atherosclerosis, nonbacterial thrombotic endocarditis (NBTE), cerebral disseminated intravascular coagulation, venous sinus thrombosis, infection, tumor embolism, and treatment complications. Atherosclerosis and NBTE are the two most frequent causes of cerebral infarction in cancer patients; NBTE is most commonly associated with adenocarcinoma, especially mucin-producing carcinomas of the lung or gastrointestinal tract. The clinical presentation is usually an acute onset of focal neurologic signs, most frequently aphasia, which either stabilize or progressively worsen. A diffuse encephalopathy also commonly accompanies focal signs. Systemic bleeding, venous thrombosis, and pulmonary embolism are part of the spectrum of coagulopathy that may accompany NBTE. Cerebral infarction from NBTE is diagnosed by CT or MRI findings of infarction (120). In the absence of associated systemic findings, diagnosis can be difficult. Treatment focuses on the underlying cause of the syndrome. Heparin has been shown to improve symptoms from cerebral ischemia but carries the risk of intracerebral and systemic bleeding (120).

Radiation of the head and neck for treatment of Hodgkin disease, head and neck carcinomas, breast cancer, and primary brain tumors can produce accelerated carotid atherosclerosis causing symptomatic carotid occlusive disease from 6 months to decades following radiation therapy. The total dose is usually greater than 50 Gy and accelerated atherosclerotic disease is limited to vessels within the irradiated area. There is no association with generalized atherosclerosis beyond concurrent patient-related factors, such as cigarette smoking. The process is accelerated with concurrent hypercholesterolemia (129). The presentation mimics nonradiation-related atherosclerosis and may include transient ischemic attacks, infarction, amaurosis fugax, or seizures. Cerebral angiography shows occlusion or extensive stenosis disproportionately affecting the common carotid artery (130). This complication has been managed with either carotid endarterectomy or with bypass grafting with favorable results (131). Another complication of neck radiation is acute rupture of the carotid artery, which usually follows resection of head and neck malignancies in which necrosis of the skin flap and surgical wound infection have occurred. Although low-dose heparin may reduce the risk of infarction, the prognosis is poor because of potential exanguination or infarction if the carotid artery is ligated (13–134)

Thrombosis of cerebral venous sinuses or large cortical veins in patients with cancer may be either a metastatic or nonmetastatic complication. In both cases, the superior sagittal sinus is most frequently involved. Metastatic tumor directly causes sagittal sinus thrombosis by either external compression or infiltration of the sinus, which results in stasis or a nidus around which a thrombus may form (135). Nonmetastatic sagittal sinus occlusion may be caused by local injury to the sinus, but is more likely related to a hypercoagulable state of malignancy. Metastatic involvement of the sagittal sinus is seen in lymphoma and some solid tumors, such as neuroblastoma and lung cancer. Nonmetastatic venous thrombosis is less common and occurs in patients with hematologic malignancies; it usually is associated with advanced disease. Clinically, nonmetastatic sagittal sinus thrombosis usually presents as an acute onset of seizures, which may be accompanied by encephalopathy and focal signs if infarction has occurred (120). Metastatic sagittal sinus thrombosis presents with subacute signs of increased ICP, such as headache and vomiting; cerebral infarction can also occur. Diagnosis is best made by MRI, magnetic resonance venography, or coronal views during enhanced CT scan. When patients present early in their disease, prognosis is usually good, often with spontaneous recovery. Patients with advanced disease have a poor prognosis. The benefit of heparin in the cancer population is not certain, given the risk of major hemorrhage. Cranial irradiation is indicated for metastatic sagittal sinus thrombosis.

Cerebral hemorrhage or infarction also can occur as complications of treatment of neoplastic disease. Chemotherapy such as aspariginase, mitomycin, and others have been associated with a variety of cerebral complications, either hemorrhagic or ischemia (120,136).

## CONCLUSION

Symptoms from neurologic complications of malignancy are common and serious and can be difficult to diagnose. Treatment of these disorders may prolong life, improve its quality, or both. Because of their prevalence and potential for effective palliation, intracranial manifestations of malignancy and their treatment deserve the attention of all cancer health care providers.

## REFERENCES

1. Saper JR, Silverstein S, Gordon CD, Hamel RL. *Handbook of headache management: a practical guide to diagnosis and treatment of head, neck and facial pain.* Baltimore: William & Wilkins, 1993;4–15.
2. Forsyth PA, Posner JB. Headaches in patients with brain tumours: a study of ill patients. *Ann Neurol* 1992;32:289.
3. Wolff HG. Headache mechanisms—a summary. In: *Pain research publication association of research and nervous and mental disease,* vol 23. Baltimore: William & Wilkins, 1943.
4. Olesen J. Headache classification committee of the International Headache Society: Classification and diagnostic criteria for headache disorders, cranial neuralgias, and facial pain. *Cephalgia* 1988;7(suppl 8):1.
5. Forsyth PA, Posner JB. Intracranial neoplasms. In: Oleson J, Hansen P, Welch KMA, eds. *The headaches.* New York: Raven Press, 1993;705.
6. Rushton JG, Rooke ED. Brain tumour headache. *Headache* 1962; 2:147.
7. Suwanwela N, Phanthumchinda K, Kaoropthum S. Headache in brain tumour: a cross-sectional study. *Headache* 1994;34:435.
8. Northfield DWC. Some observations on headache. *Brain* 1938; 61:133.
9. Vijayan N. Headache after acoustic neuroma. *Notes of the Acoustic Neuroma Association* 1991;39:3.
10. Daumas-Dupont C, Scheithauer BW, Chodkiewicz JP, Laws ER, Vedrenne C. Dysembryoplastic neuroepithelial tumour: a surgically curable tumour of young patients with intractable partial seizures. *Neurosurgery* 1988;23:545.
11. Kaylan-Raman UP, Olivero WC. Ganglioglioma: a correlative clinicopathological and radiological study of ten surgically treated cases with follow-up. *Neurosurgery* 1987;20:428.

12. Kepes JJ, Rubenstein LJ, Eng LF. Pleomorphic xanthoastrocytoma: a distinctive meningocerebral glioma of young subjects with relatively favourable prognosis. *Cancer* 1979;44:1839.

13. Piepmeier JM. Observations on the current treatment of low grade astrocytic tumours of the cerebral hemispheres. *J Neurosurg* 1987; 67:177.

14. Zimm S, Wampler GL, Stablein D, et al. Intracerebral metastases in solid-tumor patients: natural history and results of treatment. *Cancer* 1981;48:384.

15. Lavyne MH, Patterson RH. Headache associated with brain tumour. In: Dalessio DJ, ed. *Wolff's Headache and other head pain.* New York: Oxford University Press, 1987;343.

16. Ropper AH. Trauma of the head and spinal cord. In: Wilson JD, Braunwald E, Isselbacher KJ, et al., eds. *Harrison's principles of internal medicine.* 12th ed. New York: McGraw-Hill, 1991;2002.

17. Rogers LR, Barnett G. Percutaneous aspiration of brain tumor cysts via the Ommaya reservoir system. *Neurology* 1991;41:279.

18. Cairncross JG, Kim J-H, Posner JB. Radiation therapy for brain metastases. *Ann Neurol* 1980;7:529.

19. Hagen NA, Cirrincione C, Thaler HT, DeAngelis LM. The role of radiation therapy following resection of single brain metastasis from melanoma. *Neurology* 1990;40:158.

20. Coia LR. The role of radiation therapy in the treatment of brain metastases. *Int J Radiat Oncol Biol Phys* 1992;23:229.

21. Rosner D, Nemoto T, Lane WW. Chemotherapy induces regression of brain metastases in breast carcinoma. *Cancer* 1986;58:832.

22. Kristensen CA, Kristjansen PE, Hansen HH. Systemic chemotherapy of brain metastases from small cell lung cancer: a review. *J Clin Oncol* 1992;10:1498.

23. Spears WT, Morphies VGII, Lester SG, et al. Brain metastases and testicular tumors: longterm survival. *Int J Radiat Oncol Biol Phys* 1992;22:17.

24. Posner JB. Blood-nervous system barrier dysfunction: pathophysiology and treatment. In: Posner JB, ed. *Neurologic complications of cancer.* Philadelphia: FA Davis, 1995;37.

25. Dropcho EJ, Soong SJ. Steroid-induced weakness in patients with primary brian tumors. *Neurology* 1991;41:1235.

26. Kofman S, Garvin SJ, Nagamani D, Taylor SG. Treatment of cerebral metastases from breast carcinoma with prednisolone. *JAMA* 1957; 163:1473.

27. Raaf J, Stanisby DL, Larson WLE. The use of ACTH in conjunction with surgery for neoplasms in the parasellar area. *J Neurosurg* 1954; 11:463.

28. Bonica JJ. Definitions and taxonomy of pain. In: Bonica JJ, ed. *The management of pain.* 2nd ed. Philadelphia: Lea and Febiger, 1990; 18.

29. Boivie J. Central pain. In: Wall PD, Melzack R, eds. *Textbook of pain.* 3rd ed. Edinburgh: Churchill Livingstone, 1994;871.

30. Tasker R. Pain resulting from nervous system pathology (central pain). In: Bonica JJ, ed. *The management of pain.* Philadelphia: Lea and Febiger, 1990;264.

31. Bonica JJ. Introduction: somatic, epidemiologic, and educational issues. In: Casey KL, ed. *Pain and central nervous disease: the central pain syndromes.* New York: Raven Press, 1991;13.

32. Boivie J. Hyperalgesia and allodynia in patients with CNS lesions. In: Willis EDJ, ed. *Hyperalgesia and allodynia.* New York: Raven Press, 1992;363.

33. Bender MB, Jaffe R. Pain of central origin. *Med Clin North Am* 1958;42:691.

34. Tovi D, Schisano G, Lilequist B. Primary tumours of the region of the thalamus. *J Neurosurg* 1961;18:730.

35. Beric A, Dimitrijevic MR, Lindblom U. Central dysesthesia syndrome in spinal cord injury patients. *Pain* 1988;34:109.

36. Britell CW, Manano AJ. Chronic pain in spinal cord injury. Physical medicine and rehabilitation: *State of Art Reviews* 1991;5:71.

37. Loh L, Nathan PW, Schott GD. Pain due to lesions of central nervous system removed by sympathetic block. *BMJ* 1981;282:1026.

38. Rushton JG, Stevens JC, Miller RH. Glossopharyngeal (vagoglossopharyngeal) neuralgia. *Arch Neurol* 1981;38:201.

39. Adams RD, Victor M. Epilepsy and other seizure disorders. In: Adams RD, Victor M, eds. *Principles of neurology companion handbook.* 4th ed. New York: McGraw-Hill, 1991;129.

40. Andreoli TE, Carpenter CCJ, Plum F, Smith Jr LH, eds. *Cecil essentials of medicine.* 2nd ed. Philadelphia: WB Saunders, 1990;786.

41. Adams RD, Victor M. *Principles of neurology.* 5th ed. New York: McGraw-Hill, 1993;562.

42. Ketz E. Brain tumors and epilepsy. In: Vinken PJ, Bruyn GW, eds. *Handbook of clinical neurology.* Amsterdam: North Holland Publishing, 1974;16:254.

43. Deutschman CS, Haines SJ. Anticonvulsant prophylaxis in neurological surgery. *Neurosurgery* 1985;17:510.

44. Obbens EAMT, Shapiro WR. Neurological complications of malignant brain tumours. In: Wiley GR, ed. *Neurological complications of cancer.* New York: Marcel Dekker, 1995;103.

45. Galicich JH, Arbit E. Metastatic brain tumors. In: Youmans JR, ed. *Neurological Surgery,* 3rd ed. Philadelphia: WB Saunders, 1990;3209.

46. Paillas JE, Pellet W. Brain metastases. In: Vinhen PJ, Bruyn GW. Eds. *Handbook of clinical neurology.* New York: Elsevier, 1976;201–232.

47. Cohen N, Strauss G, Lew R, Silver D, Recht L. Should prophylactic anticonvulsants be administered to patients with newly diagnosed cerebral metastases? a retrospective analysis. *J Clin Oncol* 1988;6:1621.

48. Jacobs M, Phuphanich S. Seizures in brain metastases and meningeal carcinomatosis. *Proc ASCO* 1990;9:96(abst).

49. Plum F, Posner JB. *The diagnosis of stupor and coma.* 3rd ed. Philadelphia: FA Davis, 1992;352–353.

50. Weaver S, Forsyth P, Fulton D, et al. A prospective randomized trial of prophylactic anticonvulsants in patients with primary or metastatic brain tumors and without prior seizures: a preliminary analysis of 67 patients. *Neurology* 1995;45(suppl 4):A263(abstr 371P).

51. Wong DD, Longenecker RG, Liepman M, et al. Phenytoin-dexamethasone: a potential drug interaction. *JAMA* 1985;254:2062.

52. Chalk JB, Ridgeway K, Brophy TR, Yelland JDN, Eddie MJ. Phenytoin impairs the bioavailability of dexamethasone in neurological and neurosurgical patients. *J Neurol Neurosurg Psychiatry* 1984;47:1087.

53. Delattre J, Safai B, Posner JB. Erythema multiforme and Stevens-Johnson syndrome in patients receiving cranial irradiation and phenytoin. *Neurology* 1988;38:194.

54. Barclay CL, McLean M, Hagen N, Brownell AKW, MacRae ME. Severe phenytoin hypersensivity with myopathy: a case report. *Neurology* 1992;42:4303.

55. Bardana EJ, Gabourel JD, Davis G et al. Effects of phenytoin on man's immunity. Evaluation of changes in serum immunoglobulins, complements, and antinuclear antibody. *Am J Med* 1983;74:289.

56. Kikuchi K, McCormick C, Neuweit EA. Immunosuppression by phenytoin: implication for altered immune competence in brain tumour patients. *J Neurosurg* 1984;61:1085.

57. Agbi CB, Bernstein M. Seizure prophylaxis for brain tumour patients: brief review and guide for family physicians. *Can Fam Physician* 1993;39:1153.

58. Loft LM, Ward RF. Hiccups. A case presentation and etiologic review. *Arch Otolaryngol Head Neck Surg* 1992;118:1115.

59. Davis JN. An experimental study of hiccup. *Brain* 1970;93:851.

60. Mayo CW. Hiccups. *Surg Gynecol Obstet* 1932;55:700.

61. Howard RS. Persistent hiccups [Editorial]. *BMJ* 1992;305 (6864): 1237.

62. Plum F, Posner JB. *The diagnosis of stupor and coma.* 3rd ed. Philadelphia: FA Davis, 1982;39.

63. Kolodzik PW, Eilers MA. Hiccups (singultus): renew and approach to management. *Ann Emerg Med* 1991;20:565.

64. Howard RS, Wiles CM, Hirsch NP, Loh L, Spencer GT, Davis N Jr. Respiratory involvement in multiple sclerosis. *Brain* 1992;115:479.

65. Ashenasy JJ. About the mechanism of hiccup. *Eur Neurol* 1992;32: 159.

66. Bellingham-Smith E. The significance and treatment of obstinate hiccough. *Practitioner* 1938;140:166.

67. Williamson VWA, MacIntyre IMC. Management of intractable hiccups. *BMJ* 1977;2:501.

68. Lipsky MS. Chronic hiccups. *Am Fam Phys* 1986;34:173.

69. Haubrich WS. Hiccup. In: Brockus HL, ed. *Gastroenterology.* 4th ed. Philadelphia: WB Saunders, 1985;1:195.

70. Douthwaife AH. Hiccup. *Lancet* 1968;1:144.

71. Gigot AF, Flynn PD. Treatment of hiccups. *JAMA* 1952;150:760.

72. Plum F, Posner JB. *The diagnosis of stupor and coma.* 3rd ed. Philadelphia: FA Davis, 1982;4.

73. Ramsdell JW, et al. Evaluation of cognitive impairment in the elderly. *J Gen Intern Med* 1990;5:55.

74. Rosenberg SA, ed. *Surgical treatment of metastatic cancer.* Philadelphia: JB Lippincott, 1987;165.

75. Routh A, Khansur T, Hichmann BT, Bass D. Management of brain metastases: past, present and future. *South Med J* 1994;87:1218.

76. Boring CC, Squires TS, Tong T. Cancer statistics. *CA Cancer J Clin* 1993;43:7.

77. Mehta MP, Rozental JM, Levin AB. Defining the role of radiosurgery in the management of brain metastases. *Int J Radiat Oncol Biol Phys* 1992;24:619.

78. Posner J. Management of central nervous system metastases. *Semin Oncol* 1977;4:81.

79. Salbeck R, Graulte HC, Artmann H. Cerebral tumor staging in patients with bronchial carcinoma by computed tomography. *Cancer* 1990;66:2007.

80. Takahura K, Suno K, Hojo S, Hirano A. *Metastatic tumours of the central nervous system.* Tokyo: Igaku-Shoin, 1982;126.

81. Trillet V, Catajur JF, Croisile B, et al. Cerebral metastases as first symptom of bronchogenic carcinoma: a prospective study of 37 cases. *Cancer* 1991;67:2935.

82. O'Neill BP, Ruchner JC, Cotley RJ, Dinapoli RP, Shaw EG. Brain metastatic lesions. *Mayo Clin Proc* 1994;69:1062.

83. Sawaya R, Ligon BL, Bindal RK. Management of metastatic brain tumours. *Annals of Surg Oncol* 1994;1:169.

84. Delattre JY, Krol G, Thaler HT, Posner JB. Distribution of brain metastases. *Arch Neurol* 1988;45:741.

85. Decker DA, Decker VL, Hershovic A, Cummings GD. Brain metastases in patients with renal cell carcinoma: prognosis and treatment. *J Clin Oncol* 1984;2:169.

86. Weiss L, Gilbert HA, Posner JB, eds. *Brain metastasis.* Boston: GK Hall, 1980;11.

87. Galicich JH, Arbit E, Wronski M. Metastatic brain tumors. In: Wilkins RH, Rengachary SS, eds. *Neurosurgery.* New York: McGraw-Hill, 1996;819.

88. Batson OV. Role of vertebral veins in metastatic processes. *Ann Intern Med* 1942;16:38.

89. Cairncross JG, Posner JB. The management of brain metastases. In: Walker MD, Ed. *Oncology of the nervous system.* Boston: Martinus Nijhoff Publishers, 1983;341.

90. Posner JB. Intracranial metastases. In: Posner JB, ed. *Neurologic complications of cancer.* Philadelphia: FA Davis, 1995;77.

91. Paillas JE, Pellet W. Brain metastases. In: Vinken PJ, Bruyn GW, eds. *Handbook of clinical neurology,* vol 18. New York: Elsevier, 1975;201.

92. Young DF, Posner JB, Chu F, et al. Rapid-course radiation therapy of cerebral metastases: Results and complications. *Cancer* 1974;34:1069.

93. Markesbery WR, Brooks WH, Gupta GD, Young AB. Treatment for patients with cerebral metastases. *Arch Neurol* 1978;35:754.

94. Richards P, Makissock W. Intracranial metastases. *BMJ* 1963;1:15.

95. Ruderman NB, Hall TC. Use of glucocorticoids in the palliative treatment of metastatic brain tumours. *Cancer* 1965;18:298.

96. Horton J, Baxter DH, Olson KB. The management of metastases to the brain by irradiation and corticosteroids. *AJR Am J Roentgenol* 1971;3:334.

97. Weissman DE. Glucocorticoid treatment for brain metastases and epidural spinal cord compression: a review. *J Clin Oncol* 1988;6:543.

98. Cairncross JG, Kim JH, Posner JB. Radiation therapy for brain metastases. *Ann Neurol* 1980;7:529.

99. Decley TJ, Edwards JMR. Radiotherapy in the management of cerebral secondaries from bronchial carcinoma. *Lancet* 1968;1:1209.

100. Order SE, Hellman S, Von Essen CF, Kligerman MM. Improvement in quality of survival following whole-brain irradiation for brain metastases. *Radiology* 1968;91:149.

101. DeAngelis LM, Delattre JW, Posner JB. Raiation-induced dementia in patients cured of brain metastases. *Neurology* 1989;39:789.

102. Loehler JS, Alexander E III. Radiosurgery for the treatment of intracranial metastases. In Alexander E III, Loehler JS, Lunsford LD, eds. *Stereotactic radiosurgery.* New York: McGraw-Hill, 1993;197–206.

103. Patchell RA, Tibbs PA, Walsh JW et al. A randomized trial of surgery in the treatment of single metastases to the brain. *N Engl J Med* 1990;322:484.

104. Buckner J. Surgery, radiation therapy and chemotherapy for metastatic tumours to the brain. *Curr Opin Oncol* 1992;4:518.

105. Sause WT, Crowley JJ, Morantz R, et al. Solitary brain metastases: results of an RTOG/SWOG protocol evaluation surgery plus RT versus RT alone. *Am J Clin Oncol* 1990;13:427.

106. Olson ME, Chernik NL, Posner JB. Infiltration of the leptomeninges by systemic cancer: a clinical and pathologic study. *Arch Neurol* 1974;30:122.

107. Posner JB, Chernik NL. Intracranial metastases from systemic cancer. *Adv Neurol* 1978;19:575.

108. Wasserstrom WR, Glass JP, Posner JB. Diagnosis and treatment of leptomeningeal metastases from solid tumours: experience with 90 patients. *Cancer* 1982;49:759.

109. Madow L, Alpers BJ. Encephalitic forms of metastatic carcinoma. *Arch Neurol Psychiatry* 1951;65:161.

110. Cibas ES, Malkin MG, Posner JB, et al. Detection of DNA abnormalities by flow cytometry in cells from cerebrospinal fluid. *Am J Clin Pathol* 1987; 88:570.

111. Dillon WP. Imaging of central nervous system tumours. *Curr Opin Radiol* 1991;3:46.

112. Manelfe C. Imaging of the spine and spinal cord. *Curr Opin Radiol* 1991;3:5.

113. Lee YY, Glass JP, Geoffray A, et al. Cranial computed tomographic abnormalities in leptomeningeal metastasis. *Am J Neurol* 1984;5:559.

114. Krol G, Sze G, Malkin M, Walker R. MR of cranial and spinal meningeal carcinomatosis. *AJNR Am J Neuroradiol* 1988;9:709.

115. Lazlo MH, Levine MA. Low cerebrospinal fluid content in meningeal and intracranial neoplasia. *JAMA* 1965;193:834.

116. Rubenstein MK. Cranial mononeuropathy as the first sign of intracranial metastases. *Ann Intern Med* 1969;70:49.

117. Posner JB. Leptomeningeal metastases. In: Posner JB, ed. *Neurologic complications of cancer.* Philadelphia: FA Davis, 1995;143.

118. Greenberg HS, Deck MDF, Vikram B, et al. Metastases to the base of the skull: clinical findings in 43 patients. *Neurology* 1981; 31:530.

119. Graus F, Rogers LR, Posner JB. Cerebrovascular complications in patients with cancer. *Medicine* 1985;64:16.

120. Rogers LR. Cerebrovascular complication of cancer. In: Wiley RG. *Neurological complications of cancer.* New York: Marcel Dekker, 1995;123.

121. Destian S, Sze G, Krol G, et al. MR imaging of hemorrhagic intracranial neoplasms. *AJNR* 1988;9:115.

122. Kondziolka D, Bernstein M, Resch L, et al. Significance of hemorrhage into brain tumours: clinicopathological study. *J Neurosurg* 1987;67:852.

123. Hirano A, Matsui T. Vascular structures in brain tumours. *Human Pathol* 1975;6:611.

124. Little JR, Dial B, Belanger G, Carpenter S. Brain hemorrhage from intracranial tumour. *Stroke* 1979;10:283.

125. Drapkin RL, Gee TS, Dowling MD, et al. Prophylactic heparin therapy in acute premyelocytic leukemia. *Cancer* 1978;41:2484.

126. Gralnick HR, Bayley J, Abrell E. Heparin treatment for the hemorrhagic diathesis of acute promyelocytic leukemia. *Ann J Med* 1972; 52:167.

127. Castaigne S, Chromienne C, Daniel MT, et al. All-trans retinoic acid as a differentiation therapy for acute promyelocytic leukemia: I, clinical results. *Blood* 1990;76:1704.

128. Wald BR, Heisel MA, Ortega JA. Frequency of early death in children with acute leukemia presenting with hyperleukocytosis. *Cancer* 1982; 50:150.

129. Loftus CM, Biller J, Hart MN, et al. Management of radiation-induced accelerated carotid atherosclerosis. *Arch Neurol* 1987;44:711.

130. Silverberg GD, Britt RH, Goffinet DR. Radiation-induced carotid artery disease. *Cancer* 1978;41:130.

131. Atkinson JLD, Sundt TM, Dale AJD, et al. Radiation-associated atheromatous disease of the cervical carotid artery: report of seven cases and review of the literature. *Neurosurgery* 1989;24:171.

132. McCready RA. Hyde GL, Bivins BA, et al. Radiation-induced arterial injuries. *Surgery* 1983;93:306.

133. Razack MS, Saho K. Carotid artery hemorrhage and ligation in head and neck cancer. *J Surg Oncol* 1982;19:189.

134. Leihensohn J, Milko D, Cotton R. Carotid artery rupture: management and prevention of delayed neurologic sequelae with low dose heparin. *Arch Otolaryngol* 1978;104:307.

135. Sigsbee B, Deck MDF, Posner JB. Non-metastatic superior sagittal sinus thrombosis complicating systemic cancer. *Neurology* 1979;29:139.

136. Wall JG, Weiss RB, Norton L. et al. Arterial thrombosis associated with adjuvant chemotherapy for breast carcinoma: a cancer and leukemia Group B study. *Am J Med* 1984;87:501.

*Principles and Practice of Supportive Oncology,*
edited by Ann Berger et al.
Lippincott–Raven Publishers, Philadelphia ©1998

CHAPTER 34

# Management of Spinal Neoplasm and Its Complications

Sharon M. Weinstein

## EPIDEMIOLOGY

The spine is the most frequent site of bony involvement in patients with metastatic malignancy (1), and complications related to this lesion are commonly encountered in clinical practice. Tumor of the vertebral bodies has been demonstrated in 25% to 70% of patients with metastatic cancer (2), and spinal metastases are present in 40% of patients who die from cancer (3). Metastatic lesions are three to four times as common as primary bony tumors of the spine (4).

Pain and neurologic injury are the major complications caused by metastatic and primary tumors of the spine. Compression of neural structures may be caused directly by tumor mass or by displacement of bony fragments into the spinal canal. Each year in the United States, about 20,000 cancer patients are treated for malignant epidural spinal cord compression or cauda equina compression (MESCC), which affects 5% to 10% of adult solid tumor patients and 5% of pediatric solid tumor patients (5,6). These figures are corroborated by autopsy series (7,8). Half of patients presenting with MESCC are not known to have cancer at the time pain or neurologic deficits begin (9).

The distribution of spinal tumors reflects the prevalence of specific primary malignancies and the physiology of metastasis. Multiple myeloma is the most common primary bone tumor, representing 10% to 15% of malignant epidural spinal disease. Osteogenic sarcoma is the second most common primary spinal tumor, usually affecting children and adolescents. Fifty percent of chordomas affect the sacrococcygeal bones, and 35% affect the base of the skull. Chondrosarcoma and Ewing sar-

coma are other bone tumors that are rarely primary in the vertebrae.

Primary tumors of the breast, lung, and prostate frequently spread to the spinal column (Table 34-1). The spine is also a frequent site of metastasis of an osteogenic sarcoma that originates at a site other than the spine. Spinal metastases are less common in renal carcinoma, melanoma, soft-tissue sarcoma, Ewing sarcoma, germ-cell tumors, neuroblastomas, and carcinomas of the head and neck, thyroid, and bladder. Rarely, malignant neoplasms of the brain affect the bony spinal column. Ten percent of symptomatic spinal metastases originate from unknown primary tumors (3). Some malignancies spread to the intraspinal space without directly affecting bone. Lymphoma and neuroblastoma often invade the spinal canal through the intervertebral foramina; chloroma rarely do the same. Ewing sarcoma may be primary in the epidural space, as may osteosarcoma. In general, primary epidural tumors are rare.

Thoracic metastases occur twice as frequently as lumbar and four times as frequently as cervical metastases (10). In clinical practice, almost two thirds of metastatic spinal lesions present in the thoracic region (11), although in some autopsy series lesions of the lumbar spine were most prevalent (3).

The level of spinal involvement varies with tumor type. Breast and lung tumor metastases are distributed equally throughout the spine. Prostate, renal, and gastrointestinal metastases are found more often in the lower thoracic, lumbar, and sacral levels. Tumors of the uterus and uterine cervix most commonly spread to the lower lumbar and sacral spine. Pancoast tumors of the apex of the lung extend directly into the cervicothoracic spine in 25% of cases (11) often by intraforaminal extension. Multiple noncontiguous levels of spinal tumor are present in 10% to 38% of cases (12). This pat-

S. M. Weinstein: Department of Neuro-oncology, The University of Texas, M.D. Anderson Cancer Center, Houston, TX 77030-4095.

**TABLE 1.** *Distribution of primary neoplasm in 1,432 patients with malignant epidural spinal cord compression (MESCC)*

| Primary site | % of patients |
|---|---|
| Breast | 13–28 |
| Lung | 12–32 |
| Prostate | 4–18 |
| Lymphoma | 6–10 |
| Unknown | 3–14 |
| Renal | 3–10 |
| Sarcoma | 7–8 |
| Myeloma | 4–5 |
| Gastrointestinal | 3–5 |
| Genitourinary | 1–8 |

Data from Grant et al. (5).

tern is relatively less common in patients with lung cancer (9).

In 85% to 90% of cases, MESCC is caused by extension of tumor from the vertebral body (11) and is less likely to arise from tumor in the vertebral laminae and pedicles than the vertebral body; MESCC from tumor in the posterior elements occurs in less than 15% of patients. In pediatric patients, MESCC from tumor of the posterior elements is more likely, and intraforaminal spread of tumor from paraspinal sites also occurs more frequently than in adults (12). Tumor metastases to the epidural space seldom breach the dura (3,13).

The prevalence of MESCC varies according to tumor type. In a series of 103 patients with lung cancer, 26% with squamous histology, 9% with adenocarcinoma, and 14% with small cell tumors had spinal cord compression (14). The prevalence of all neurological complications in this series was about 40%.

Breast cancer accounts for almost a fourth of MESCC cases diagnosed in cancer hospitals. Vertebral metastases are identified in 60% of breast cancer patients, and multiple levels of epidural compression are common. Rarely is MESCC the inital presentation or an early finding in breast cancer, and biopsy usually is not required to establish the diagnosis of metastasis (15).

About 7% of prostate cancer patients develop MESCC; it was noted in 12.2% of patients with poorly differentiated tumors and 2.9% of those with well-differentiated tumors (16). The risk of developing MESCC increases in patients with stage D2 prostate cancer compared with those without bony disease. The average time from initial prostate cancer diagnosis to MESCC is 2 years, shorter in stage D2. In about 30% of prostate cancer patients with MESCC, it is the initial manifestation of the cancer (17).

Renal cell carcinomas infrequently cause MESCC secondary to bony metastasis. Testicular cancer rarely metastasizes to bone but may grow into the spinal canal from the retroperitoneal space. Malignant melanoma may produce MESCC from vertebral disease, but intradural and leptomeningeal involvement are more common.

Head and neck cancers rarely metastasize beyond the cervical lymph nodes, and about 80% of distant metastases are detected within 2 years of initial diagnosis.

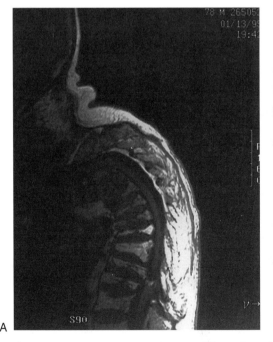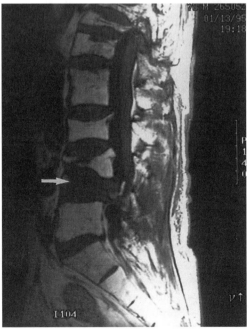

**FIG. 1.** Magnetic resonance image of the spine of advanced multiple myeloma. **A:** Extreme spinal deformity. **B:** Note complete replacement of L4 vertebral body (*arrow*). Clinical presentation of upper and lower back pain, with mild cauda equina syndrome. Over the course of 5 years during progression of disease, the patient's daily oral morphine requirement reached a maximum of over 2 g per day, and subsequently fell to a minimum of 120 mg daily.

Therefore, a head and neck cancer patient presenting with MESCC after 2 years should be evaluated for a second primary malignancy. MESCC occurred at all levels of the spine in one small series of patients with head and neck cancers (18).

Esophageal cancers rarely may cause MESCC by direct invasion to the thoracic spinal column (19). Carcinoid tumors are associated with neurologic complications in fewer than 20% of cases, the most frequent being MESCC due to spinal metastases. Although MESCC generally represents a late complication, it may be the presenting sign of carcinoid tumors.

In plasmacytoma and multiple myeloma, MESCC is usually due to bony collapse and occurs in more than 10% of patients. Epidural extension of tumor and primary epidural tumor are less frequent. There is typically a slow progression of spinal deformity with deterioration of neurologic function, which may be minimal compared to the bony change (Fig. 34-1).

Hodgkin disease and non-Hodgkin lymphomas are associated with 5% incidence of MESCC, usually in the presence of extranodal or extensive nodal disease. The thoracic spine is most often involved, in many cases by intraforaminal spread of tumor rather than by bony extension (20). Patients with MESCC due to lymphoma are at high risk for meningeal disease as well. Cerebrospinal fluid examination should be considered along with spinal imaging as concurrent meningeal lymphoma is common and will affect the antineoplastic treatment regimen. Vertebral compression fracture with radicular pain may be the presenting sign of acute leukemia (21).

In up to 30% of pediatric cases, MESCC is the presenting sign of cancer. The time interval to presentation with MESCC may be twice as long in children without a known cancer compared with those already diagnosed with malignancy (22). Children without a cancer history presenting with MESCC often are initally misdiagnosed (23); MESCC, the most frequent neurologic complication of Ewing sarcoma (24), may occur earlier in the course of Ewing sarcoma compared with rhabdomyosarcoma and osteosarcoma.

## DIFFERENTIAL DIAGNOSIS

The differential diagnosis of back pain and neurologic dysfunction secondary to MESCC includes many benign tumors, such as vertebral hemangiomas, osteochondroma, osteoid osteoma, osteoblastoma, giant cell tumor, eosinophilic granuloma, and hemangioma. Meningiomas occur more frequently in patients with breast cancer (25). Other nonmalignant conditions, including aneurysmal bone cysts, fibrous dysplasia, extramedullary hematopoesis, and lipoma, also occur. Coexisting nonmalignant disease of the spine may affect as many as 30% of patients with MESCC (26). Degenerative, inflammatory, and

infectious processes affect the spinal structures, and soft-tissue injuries causing back pain are quite common (27). In the pediatric population, spine pain is less frequent but more commonly associated with malignant pathology than in adults. Trauma is the most common cause of back pain in children; other nonmalignant conditions, such as Scheuermann disease and scoliosis (28), present in this age group. Numerous nonspinal conditions may refer pain to the back. Back pain in cancer patients also may be caused by vertebral osteoporosis resulting from radiation therapy or corticosteroids.

Spinal cord or cauda equina dysfunction may be related to tumor or treatment without MESCC. Leptomeningeal disease, intradural extramedullary or intramedullary spinal cord disease, paraneoplastic necrotizing myelopathy, and myelopathy induced by radiation or intrathecal chemotherapy should be considered if no epidural compressive lesion is found. Myelopathy is a late complication of radiation, and epidural lipomatosis may be caused by corticosteroid therapy. Vascular events of the spinal cord may occur more often in the presence of tumor.

## PATHOGENESIS OF NEUROLOGIC DYSFUNCTION AND PAIN

The high incidence of metastasis to the vertebrae, despite their poor blood supply, is explained by specific physiologic features. The vertebrae have a large capillary capacity, promoting local stasis of blood. The walls of the vascular sinusoids are discontinuous, and intersinusoidal cords form cul-de-sacs for tumor. Tumor products, such as prostaglandin E2, osteoblast activating factor, parathormone-like factor, tumor growth factor (TGF)-$\alpha$, and the products of bone resorption act to stimulate tumor growth (29). Monocytes producing interleukin-1 may promote resorption of normal bone (30). Metastases may occur more commonly in previously damaged bone (31).

Batson's plexus is a valveless system of epidural veins in which blood may flow rostrally or caudally. On Valsalva maneuver, this system drains the viscera and may be a route of metastatic spread. The neck tends to drain toward the left side, the breasts to the thoracic plexus, and the prostate through pelvic veins to Batson's plexus in the lower spine. Tumor also reaches bone via the arteries and lymphatics and by direct extension.

Epidural tumor produces dysfunction of neural structures by direct compression and by secondary demyelination, ischemia, and tissue edema. Inflammatory process accompanying the tumor also may have several consequences. For example, inflammatory mediators may change vascular permeability and disrupt the blood-spinal cord barrier at the tumor site. This effect was demonstrated in an animal model in which a serotonin antagonist reduced the level of prostaglandin E2, vascular permeability, and cord edema (12). The release of excitatory amino acids by injured neurons may further promote ischemia and injury.

In the initial stage of epidural cord compression, there may be white matter edema and axonal swelling with normal blood flow. These changes are due to direct compression or venous congestion. Over time, progressive compression decreases blood flow and disturbs vascular autoregulation, leading to the development of vasogenic edema. Spinal cord infarction may result from interruption of venous outflow or occlusion of small arteries or from interruption of the major arterial supply to the spinal cord, including the artery of Adamkeiwicz or radicular arteries in the intervertebral foramina.

Pencil-shaped softenings (*infarction*) may extend over several segments of the compressive lesion. A necrotic cavity, usually located in the ventral portion of the posterior columns or dorsal horn, was visualized on magnetic resonance imaging (12). The effects of cord compression also may be due to coup and contrecoup injury, which is not easily predicted on the basis of tumor location in relation to spinal cord. Rat, cat, and monkey models implicate demyelination rather than ischemia as the primary mechanism of gradually worsening neurologic dysfunction (5). This is supported by pathologic examination demonstrating greater demyelination of white matter than grey matter, a pattern that does not conform to arterial supply. Animal experiments indicate that the rate of neural compression partly determines the type of pathology, with more rapid ischemic change producing a greater degree of irreversible neurologic injury (32,33). Similar observations were made in human spinal cord. There is limited experimental work on the cauda equina syndrome.

Pain caused by malignancy of the spine may result from activation of afferent nociceptive neurons by mechanical distortion and inflammatory mediators (*nociceptive pain*) or from neural dysfunction (*neuropathic pain*). Nociceptors innervate the periosteum, soft tissues (i.e., posterior and anterior longitudinal ligament), facet articular cartilage, dura mater, nerve root sheaths, and blood vessels. Vertebral collapse and structural instability can give rise to mechanical pain through injury to these structures, which worsens during spine loading and weight shifting. Neuropathic pain results from altered peripheral and central neural activity that may be induced by injury of the nerve roots, axonal injury, or other processes.

## PATIENT EVALUATION

Although it is widely recognized that pain is the cardinal symptom of spinal neoplasm, accurate assessment of back and neck pain in the cancer patient may present a challenge to even the experienced clinician. A complete history and physical examination, including thorough neurological examination, are essential to localize the underlying pathology and to choose diagnostic and therapeutic interventions correctly. Inadequate evaluation increases the likelihood of mistaken diagnoses, which may eventaute in neurologic compromise. In a retrospective survey of cancer patients presenting with back pain, misdiagnosis was attributed to poor history, inadequate examination, and insufficient diagnostic evaluation (34). In a review of cancer pain consultations performed by a neurology-based pain service, the comprehensive evaluation of pain led to a new diagnosis in 65% of cases (35).

## History

Up to 95% of adult and 80% of pediatric patients with MESCC present with pain (12,36). The difference in the prevalence of pain between adults and children may reflect greater difficulty in pain assessment and underreporting of pain in children. Pain precedes other symptoms by a median of 7 weeks. This interval may vary by tumor type; it is generally shorter for lung cancer than breast cancer (37). In some cases, pain precedes other symptoms and signs by 1 year (12). Overall, patients experience pain for an average of 4 to 5 months before presentation (3).

Pain may be local at the site of pathology, referred in a nonradicular distribution, referred in a radicular (dermatomal) distribution, or have combined features. Radicular or root pain is reported in 90% of lumbosacral MESCC, 79% of cervical MESCC, and 55% of thoracic MESCC (37). Radicular pain may be bilateral in thoracic lesions and is often described as a tight band around the chest or abdomen. It is important to note that radicular pain may be experienced in only one part of a dermatome. For example, pain in the distal lower extremity may be caused by injury of the L5 or S1 root. It may be difficult for the clinician to distinguish nonradicular referred pain from radicular pain and radicular pain from peripheral nerve symptoms. When a nerve root lesion produces chest or abdominal pain, the complaint may be mistakenly identified as referred pain of visceral origin. Radicular lesions usually are associated with segmental findings on examination. Nonradicular referred pain may be associated with vague paraesthesias and tenderness at the painful site.

The character of pain associated with MESCC varies. It may be continuous at rest and markedly aggravated by body movements (*incident pain*). Although local pain from a vertebral lesion will be worsened with loading due to upright posture, pain from MESCC is often greatly increased by lying supine, perhaps because of increased filling of Batson's venous plexus. A lesion confined to the vertebral body also may produce nonradicular referred pain: Disease at C7 may refer pain to the interscapular region, and pain due to disease at L1 may be referred to the iliac crests, hips, or sacroiliac region. Sacral disease often causes midline pain radiating to the buttocks, which is made worse by sitting. Radicular pain in particular may be paroxysmal, spontaneous, or provoked by movement or sensory stimulation. Valsalva maneuver may produce or aggravate both local and radicular pain. Pain on neck flexion or straight leg raising implies dural traction, and Lhermitte's sign indicates a spinal cord lesion. In addition to Lhermitte's sign, compression of the cervical spinal cord rarely produces funicular pain, which is referred to the lower extremities, thorax, or abdomen as a band of paraesthesias. *Pseudoclaudication* of legs may be an isolated lumbar root symptom (38).

The neurologic findings associated with MESCC also vary. Clinicians interpret the pattern of neurologic dysfunction as indicative of the level and severity of the lesion. Upper motor neuron weakness may occur with lesions of the spinal cord (above the L1 vertebral body). This finding, present in 75% of patients with MESCC at diagnosis (11), usually affects the proximal lower extremities initially. Rare patients experience complete and sudden areflexic paralysis. Sensory disturbances occur in about half of patients at presentation; sensory complaint without pain is exceedingly rare. Sensory changes include paraethesias and sensory loss, which can be segmental or below the level of injury. One should remember to inquire about loss of sensation of voiding or evacuation. Bladder and bowel dysfunction are evident in more than half of patients on presentation with spinal cord or cauda equina compression. Constipation usually precedes urinary retention or incontinence (39).

## Examination

The physical examination begins with observation of posture, spinal curvature, symmetry of paraspinal muscles, extremities, and skin. Vital signs should be measured. Latent herpes virus may be activated by tumor, and the dermatomal distribution of skin lesions may correspond to the level of tumor involvement. Lower extremity edema is a late feature of immobility and weakness. Palpation of the back and spine is essential. The practitioner may appreciate tenderness of the spinous processes on palpation or percussion, although this may not correlate with the level of spinal disease. Gibbus deformity and vertebral misalignments are frequently palpable; actual crepitus of the spine is unusual. Tenderness or spasm of the paraspinal muscles also may be noted. Urinary retention may be demonstrated by bladder percussion. Laxity of the anal sphincter may be apparent on digital rectal examination. Specific areas of sacral or coccygeal tenderness may be identified by external palpation or by rectal or pelvic examination.

Spinal maneuvers to elicit pain should be performed carefully. Thoracic and abdominal radicular pain may be provoked on lateral flexion and rotation of the trunk. Increased pain on neck flexion and straight leg raise sign may be "pseudomeningeal" signs of dural traction due to epidural tumor. If neck rigidity is present, the examiner should use extreme caution with range-of-motion maneuvers. Muscle spasm may be triggered by bony instability of the cervical spine, and movements may dislodge bony fragments causing acute spinal cord or brainstem injury.

The neurological examination will reveal positive findings in most patients with MESCC. The examination should include assessment of mental status, cranial nerves, motor function, reflexes, sensation, coordination, and gait. Proximal lower extremity weakness may be initally evident only as difficulty rising from a chair. Weakness may be due to upper or lower motor neuron dysfunction. Although weakness due to upper motor neuron dysfunction usually is associated with increased tone and hyperreflexia, acute "spinal shock" can cause a flaccid areflexic paralysis. In the subacte phase of recovery from spinal shock, "mass reflexes" appear and consist of flexor spasms, hyperhydrosis, and piloerection resulting from autonomic dysfunction. Lower motor neuron weakness may be accompanied by flaccidity, atrophy, muscle fasiculations, and hyporeflexia. A cervical lesion can produce segmental hyporeflexia in the arm or arms and increased reflexes below. Lesions above the pyramidal decussation of the corticospinal tracts in the lower brainstem may be associated with loss of contralateral abdominal reflexes; lesions below the decussation produce loss of ipsilateral abdominal reflexes. Segmental motor dysfunction caused by thoracic nerve-root disease may produce asymmetric abdominal muscle contraction and loss of abdominal reflexes. Beevor's sign (upward movement of the umbilicus on attempted flexion of the trunk) indicates a lesion at or near the T10 level. Lesions of the roots of the upper lumbar plexus produce hip-flexion weakness and a dropped knee-jerk reflex; lesions of the roots to the lower lumbar plexus may produce footdrop and dimished ankle-jerk reflex. Hand atrophy without weakness is considered a false localizing sign when it is the result of upper cervical pathology (40). Loss of bulbocavernosus and anal reflexes may accompany conus and cauda equina lesions (39).

Although the sensory examination may help in determining the level of epidural disease, MESCC results in a broad variation of sensory dysfunction, with incomplete lesions the rule. The level of reduced sensation may be determined to be up to five segemental levels below or one to two segments above the level of cord compression. A sensory level on the trunk sparing the sacral dermatomes may occur in up to 20% of patients with thoracic or high lumbar compression (41). Suspended partial sensory levels or unilateral bands of sensory loss may be seen with spinal cord lesions up to the brainstem. Compression of the conus of the spinal cord may produce sensory loss in the saddle area (buttocks and perineum). A "neck-tongue" syndrome of numbess of the tongue resulting from high cervical lesions has been attributed to a connection between the lingual nerve, hypoglossal nerve, and the C2 root (42); facial numbness also may be due to upper cervical lesions. Lesions of the upper thoracic nerve roots may result in Horner syndrome, with autonomic dysfunction of the face and upper extremity.

Gait ataxia is an uncommon isolated symptom of spinal cord compression. Other unusual features are symptoms or signs of raised intracranial pressure; facial paresis, lower extremity fasciculations or sciatica with cervical tumor; nystagmus with thoracic tumor; spinal myoclonus; an inverted knee jerk reflex; and "painful legs and moving toes" (12).

### Diagnostic Evaluation

Several imaging methods are available to confirm MESCC. It is strongly recommended that clinicoradiographic correlation be made by the examining physician because the correct interpretation of symptomatic and asymptomatic lesions on diagnostic imaging studies requires thorough knowledge of the patient's clinical presentation.

Plain radiographs will confirm tumor and assess structural stability of the spinal elements. In the cancer patient at risk for spinal metastases with neck, shoulder, or upper extremity pain, flexion and extension views of the cervical spine should not be forced. Although plain radiographs are more than 90% sensitive and 86% specific for demonstrating abnormalities in the patient with symptomatic spinal metastases, autopsy series suggest that up to 25% of spinal lesions are invisible on radiography (43). Breast cancer lesions are more likely (94%) to produce abnormal radiographs compared with lung cancer lesions (74%), and perhaps only one third of radiographs are abnormal in lymphoma and pediatric spinal tumors (12). False negatives occur due to a mild degree of pathology or poor visualization (e.g., the first thoracic vertebra) or because the abnormality is missed on interpretation. The false-positive rate for interpreting collapsed vertebrae as malignant may be as high as 20% (44).

It is estimated that a 30% to 50% change in bone mass is needed before plain films are considered abnormal (36). On anterior/posterior view, spinal radiographs may show pedicle erosion (the "winking owl" sign), increased interpeduncular distance, paraspinal widening, or paraspinal soft-tissue shadow. On lateral view, vertebral collapse (wedging of the body), scalloped bodies, discspace destruction, a narrow spinal canal, hypertrophied facets, and disc calcification may be seen. Oblique views are needed to discriminate spondylolytic osteophytic

encroachment from tumor causing foraminal abnormality (5). Greater than 50% vertebral collapse and pedicle erosion are especially predictive of MESCC.

On plain radiography, multiple vertebral involvement is noted in up to 86% of patients with spinal tumor (5) and in greater than 30% of patients with MESCC. The risk of epidural tumor extension based on radiographic findings alone and with symptom correlation is shown in Table 34-2.

Computed tomography (CT) may be useful to better delineate pathology using restricted fields of view (43) and is superior to other imaging techniques for demonstrating cortical bone architecture (45). In one study of 32 cases of malignant spontaneous vertebral collapse, the frequent findings on CT included destruction of anterolateral or posterior cortical bone of the vertebral body, destruction of cancellous bone of the body, destruction of a pedicle, focal paraspinal soft tissue mass, and epidural mass (46).

Before the availability of magnetic resonance imaging (MRI), CT, in combination with myelography, was considered the gold standard for demonstrating the level and extent of epidural disease; CT myelography may be considered if the index of suspicion for epidural disease is high and other imaging studies are normal or if MRI cannot be interpreted or peformed. Lumbar puncture should precede cervical puncture in most cases. Injection of air to supplement contrast medium may better image cerebrospinal fluid (CSF) block. If the upper and lower extent of the block cover a long spinal segment, myelography may be repeated after treatment to determine whether multiple discrete lesions are present and to define radiotherapy portals better. If repeated imaging is anticipated, oil-based contrast medium may be used to allow for follow-up radiographic imaging without repeated punctures. Another advantage of myelography over other diagnostic imaging tests is the collection of CSF for analysis; how-

**TABLE 2.** *Symptoms, radiographic findings, and MESCC*

| Symptoms | Radiograph* | Likelihood of MESCC |
|----------|-------------|---------------------|
| Positive | Positive | 86% |
| Negative | Positive | 43% |
| Positive | Negative | 8% |
| Negative | Negative | 3% |

| *Positive radiograph | Likelihood of MESCC |
|----------------------|---------------------|
| >50% collapse of body | 87% |
| Pedicle erosion | 31% |
| Tumor of multiple bodies | 10% |
| Vertebral body tumor, no collapse | 7% |

Data from Graus F, Krol G, Foley KM. Early diagnosis of epidural metastases (SEM): correlation with clinical and radiological findings. *Proc Am Soc Clin Oncol* 1985;4:269; and Hewitt and Foley (36).

MESCC, malignant epidural spinal cord compression or cauda equina compression.

ever, there is a risk of worsening neurologic function after dural puncture in the patient with partial CSF block as a result of "coning" of the spinal cord as pressure below the block is relieved. This risk may be as high as 15% (12,47). It is therefore recommended that under these conditions, prepuncture corticosteroids be administered.

Radionuclide bone scintigrams will reveal a 5% to 10% change in bone tissue (36). Bone scintigrams are more sensitive than radiographs except in multiple myeloma (12). They are not as specific as radiographs in identifying the level of MESCC. False positives may be the result of nonmalignant skeletal conditions, and false negatives may be due to lytic lesions, for example,

myeloma or solid tumors such as lung and melanoma, and prior radiation therapy. If all the skeleton is involved by tumor, no contrast in the radionuclide uptake can be appreciated. New technology of immunoscintigraphy may prove to be more sensitive (43).

Currently, MRI is considered by many experts to be the imaging procedure of choice for MESCC. Without contrast enhancement MRI may eliminate the need for other imaging studies. Its sensitivity and specificity rival that of CT-myelography and are better with contrast. In the patient with back pain and radicular symptoms but no bony tumor on plain radiograph, gadolinium enhanced MRI is indicated to identify intraforaminal disease such

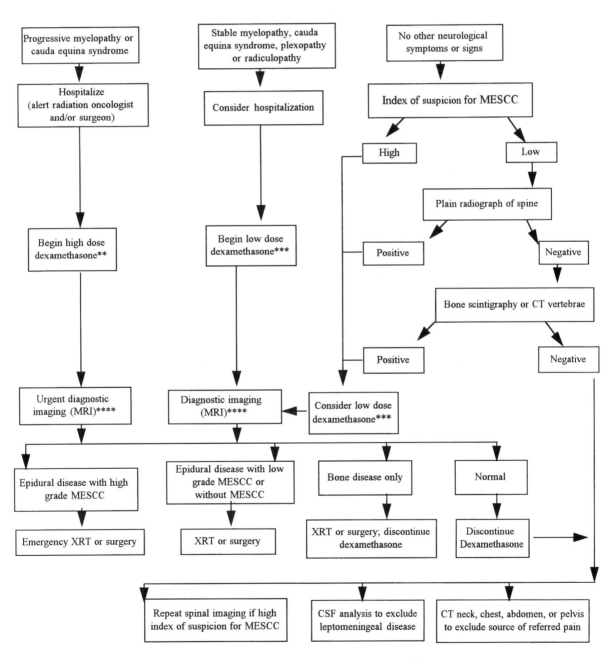

**FIG. 2.** Cancer patient with back or neck pain.

as occurs in lymphoma and sometimes solid tumors (36). Double-dose gadolinium-enhanced MRI may increase accuracy. Both MRI without and with contrast excludes vertebral metastases, paravertebral lesions, MESCC, intramedullary tumor, and many leptomeningeal processes. Fat suppression and T2 weighting, not supplemented by addition of contrast, may improve detection of myeloma lesions (48). In previously irradiated bone, MRI signal intensity is increased, and gadolinium contrast enhancement is decreased. The MRI images are distorted by scoliosis, contraindicated with pacemakers, and obscured by metallic implants. In addition, MRI may cost less than CT myelography.

In the cancer patient with back pain and suspected MESCC, complete spine MRI is indicated when there is a high risk of noncontiguous or skip lesions. A full spine sagittal "screening" image to identify targets for more detailed imaging is suggested (5). Often the cervical spine is not imaged because it adds significantly to sequencing time. Failure to identify multiple levels of MESCC may compromise radiotherapy if untreated lesions become symptomatic and are detected later. The cost/effectiveness ratio of sagittal screening studies for identifying treatable lesions has not yet been determined. In patients with claustrophobia or severe pain in the supine position, conscious sedation or general anesthesia may be required to complete the MRI. The risk of sedation or anesthesia for MRI must be weighed against the risks of alternative imaging procedures, such as CT myelography, for each individual patient.

The selection of specific imaging tests is guided by the clinical presentation. In each individual case, the "neurologic urgency" for further diagnostic tests must be modified according to the potential for treatment, the patient's condition and overall prognosis (Fig. 34-2).

Usually, CSF examination is not required for the diagnosis of epidural tumor, and, as noted above, dural puncture may pose some risk to the patient with MESCC. CSF analysis may show elevated protein with normal glucose and rarely pleiocytosis.

The patient presenting with MESCC and an unknown primary tumor generally will undergo a battery of tests to identify the primary neoplasm. At times biopsy of a vertebral, epidural, or parapsinal lesion is needed to determine the tumor histology, and this may be percutaneous and guided by CT.

## MANAGEMENT OF ACUTE MESCC

### Pharmacologic Interventions

Corticosteroids, the mainstay of pharmacologic therapy for MESCC, facilitate neuronal excitability and transmission, increase spinal blood flow due to beta-receptor activation, and impede vasoconstriction by inhibiting prostaglandin and thromboxane. Administration of these agents also prevents lipid peroxidation of neuronal cell membranes, ischemia, and increased intracellular calcium (49). Vasogenic edema in MESCC was responsive to corticosteroids. Cytotoxic edema also may play a role. Alternative steroids and other agents to treat edema, such as mannitol, may be used.

The timing of administration and dosage of corticosteroids may affect neurologic outcome, and there is some evidence for a therapeutic window (38,49). Better analgesic effect of higher-dose regimens was demonstrated in one study (50). Many authors favor a prolonged course of high-dose corticosteroids, for example, the equivalent of a bolus of 100 mg of dexamethasone, followed by 96 mg per day in divided doses, tapered over a few weeks for high-grade MESCC and the lower dosage (i.e., 20 mg dexamethasone followed by 16 mg per day in divided doses with a taper) for low-grade MESCC (5,50,51).

High-dose therapy may be more analgesic but increases the risk of side effects. Side effects depend on duration of drug administration, cumulative dose, and regimen: neuropsychiatric, musculoskeletal, endocrine, metabolic, gastrointestinal, cardiovascular, ophthalmic, dermatologic, and immunologic complications occur. In one prospective study of MESCC patients treated with high-dose corticosteroids, depressive symptoms and disorders were more common than in similar patients not receiving such treatment (52). Suppression of the hypothalamic-pituitary-adrenal axis occurs with sustained dosing; it is suggested that dosing be readministered after withdrawal in situations of severe physiologic stress. Adrenal failure is actually rare in neurooncology patients treated with high doses of corticosteroids. Steroid-induced osteoporosis may be reversible in young patients (53). Other withdrawal symptoms, including pneumocystis infection, have been reported. Corticosteroids are metabolized by the cytochrome P450 system, which has implications for drug interactions with anticonvulsants and other medications; this potential interaction with anticonvulsants may be least with valproate (49). Clinicians should be aware that rapid administration of steroids causes severe burning pain in the perineum; therefore, it is preferable that doses not be given as intravenous push. Corticosteroids should be held before making the cancer diagnosis if lymhoma is suspected because of the immediate oncolytic effect, which would impede diagnosis.

Virtually all patients presenting with MESCC have severe pain requiring opioid analgesics. During the acute phase, concurrent with bolus high-dose corticosteroid, many patients will require rapid titration of an opioid agonist to achieve analgesia. In some settings, this may be best accomplished with an intravenous patient controlled pump. Patient-controlled analgesia (PCA) facilitates the quick adjustment of dose in both directions according to patient need and allows the patient a rapid bolus for severe incident or movement-related pain. Regardless of the setting and the means used, the practitioner should be prepared to titrate opioid to effect, and this may at least briefly require high doses, especially in patients with neurologic involvement of tumor (54).

## Nonpharmacologic Interventions

### Radiation Therapy

Radiation therapy for MESCC is chosen to inhibit tumor growth, restore and preserve neurologic function, treat pain and improve quality of life. The course of external beam radiotherapy (XRT) for spinal metastases and MESCC depends on the radiosensitivity of the tumor and its extent. Currently, XRT is considered by many clinicians to be the primary treatment for MESCC. The usual treatment schedule is 3000 cGy in 10 fractions. The course may be accelerated for patients in severe pain. A greater total dose may be given in more fractions if there is risk to the viscera (e.g., the stomach). The spinal section treated routinely includes two vertebral segments above and below a single site of neurologic compression. Anterior/posterior portals are set to include the vertebral body, especially in low thoracic and lumbar lesions. A single-port field can be used in very cachectic patients. Lateral portals are used in the cervical region to block the larynx and upper aerodigestive tract. Fields also are designed to accommodate paravertebral tumor. With multiple sites of spinal disease, as there are no known predictive factors for epidural progression, the decision to treat asymptomatic noncontiguous sites depends on clinical judgment. Factors to be considered are the type of tumor, presence of vertebral collapse, and anticipated future difficulty in matching radiation portals. Special techniques are required to reirradiate or give higher doses. When spinal cord tolerance is balanced against the tumoricidal dose needed, the decision usually will weigh against reirradiation. Fortunately, XRT alone is more than 85% effective for MESCC in radiosensitive tumors (3). Motor improvement is seen in 49% and stabilization of function in another 31%. Fewer than 50% of patients will regain lost function (3). In general, patients with slowly progressive deficits respond to XRT, regardless of tumor type. The frequency of MESCC may be reduced by XRT to affected bones; it is uncertain whether the radiation is treating micrometastases or preventing them. The response to XRT may be delayed in some cases; the factors accounting for this observation are not well understood (55). Brachytherapy can be used for adjacent paraspinal masses and may prevent MESCC (56). It is also now recognized that high-dose XRT may not cause spinal cord edema.

### Surgery

Indications for surgery have been established by clinical consensus to be (a) to establish the cancer diagnosis when it is in doubt and tissue is required for histological examination, (b) to achieve surgical cure for the primary neoplasm, (c) to treat prior irradiated tumor with symptomatic progression of MESCC, (d) to decompress neural structures and stabilize the spine, (e) to halt a rapid clinical deterioration, and (f) to treat radioresistant tumor with symptomatic progression of MESCC (3,57,58).

The goals of surgery are to resect pathology, restore load-bearing capacity, decompress neural structures, maintain stability, treat pain, and improve quality of life. In 10% of patients with spinal metastases, pain is due to bony instability. Spinal instability occurs if tumor crosses two or more adjacent bodies, anterior and posterior elements are involved at the same level, there is significant vertebral body collapse, the odontoid is destroyed, there are bone or disk fragments in the spinal canal, or any combination of these factors. Unstable spinal lesions are common in breast cancer and multiple myeloma. Surgery may be considered for stabilization when pain occurs because of bony instability of the spine (similar to an appendicular fracture requiring stabilization) (59) or if instability is associated with greater than 50% collapse of the vertebral body (60).

Many factors affect the choice of surgical technique: tumor location, spinal level, tumor extent, integrity of adjacent segments, and general debility. In vascular tumors, such as renal and thyroid, operative intervention may be preceded by vascular embolization. Tumor decompression and stabilization may be achieved through either an anterior vertebrectomy or laminectomy. The anterior approach usually involves corpectomy and stabilization using bone graft, a plate, or prostheses. Posterior decompression through wide laminectomy is generally followed by stabilization to prevent kyphosis (60–63). Posterior stabilization is accomplished by bone struts, steel rods, and methylmethacrylate. Supplemental posterior stabilization may be required in the cervical region. Titanium prostheses allow MRI to be performed. New posterolateral techniques are being developed for specific MESCC syndromes in advanced cancer patients.

In one thorough retrospective study (64) of 110 patients following aggressive surgical intervention for spinal metastases, 82% of patients showed improvement in pain relief and ambulatory status. The goals of treatment were identified as gross total resection of tumor and spine reconstruction. Half of the patients had prior treatment and were deteriorating clinically. The "traditional" criteria for surgery, such as relapse after radiation therapy, and for determination of histology, were expanded to include gross tumor resection for radioresistant or solitary lesions and for spinal stabilization. In this series, more complex surgical instrumentation was used than previously reported. Most patients received ongoing systemic therapy, partly confounding the analysis of long-term outcomes. The complication rate of 48% correlated in patients aged over 65, who had prior spinal treatment,

**TABLE 3.** *Predictive factors for poor prognosis following surgical intervention*[a]

Leg strength 0/5–3/5
Multiple vertebral body involvement
Lung or colon cancer

[a]Spine surgery considered contraindicated if two or more factors present.
Data from Sioutos PJ, Arbit E, Meshulam BS, Galicich JH. Spinal metastases from solid tumors: analysis of factors affecting survival. *Cancer* 1995;76:8:1453.

and who had paraparesis. These factors also correlated with greater morbidity and poorer survival. In this series, however, nearly half of the patients were alive at 2 years, an improvement over prior studies comparing the posterior surgical laminectomy and radiation therapy to radiation therapy alone. This improvement in survival was noted in patients with more advanced cancer and prior treatment in the tertiary care center. These authors concluded based on prior reports (65,55) and the data from this series that the anterior surgical approach with stabilization may improve outcomes and suggested further

definition of the subset of patients that might benefit from early anterior resection and spinal stabilization.

In a prior report of 26 patients undergoing the anterior surgical approach, 30% mortality was attributed to poor condition of many of the patients, although most did improve in ambulatory status and pain relief (67). Early reviews of surgical outcomes confirmed higher morbidity and mortality in patients with prior spine irradiation, age over 70 years, and those with poor performance status at surgery (65).

In a recently reported series, 109 patients followed after surgical decompression of the spinal cord had a median survival of 10 months. The factors predictive of shorter survival were poorer preoperative neurologic status, anatomic site of the primary carcinoma, and the number of vertebral bodies involved. These authors concluded that patients with two or more poor prognostic indicators have limited life expectancy; therefore, radical surgery is not recommended in this group because benefits are not likely to be realized (Table 34-3). Several authors suggested that a limited posterolateral approach to tumor resection be reserved for patients with expected survival less than 6 months (64,68). Few data are available regarding surgical

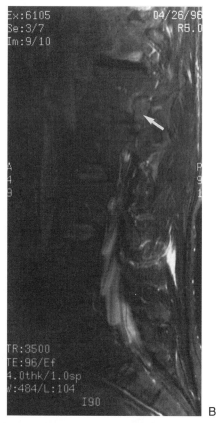

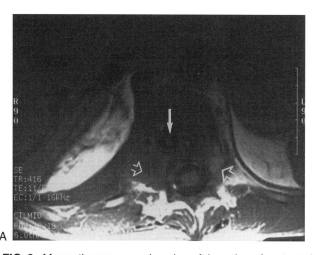

**FIG. 3.** Magnetic resonance imaging of the spine of metastatic colon carcinoma. **A:** Massive recurrence at the site of prior vertebrectomy and placement of stabilization plug (*arrow*). Paravertebral soft-tissue extension involving T11 and T12 nerve roots (open arrows). **B:** Noncontiguous nerve root lesion at L1–2 neural foramen (arrow). Clinical presentation of right L1 radicular pain, and partial suspended sensory level T11–12.

intervention for lateral epidural or intraforaminal disease. In a recent experience, a small group of patients symptomatic from spinal metastases and not considered candidates for major surgical procedures, benefitted from limited resection of lateral epidural tumor. Surgery was preceded by careful correlation of symptoms with tumor mass and good outcomes were recorded in all eight patients (69). This experience supports careful consideration in each case until criteria for primary surgical intervention are more fully delineated.

The complication rate for spinal surgery may be as high as 30% in patients who have undergone prior XRT (3). Coagulopathy and exogenous anticoagulants increase the risk of hematoma at the operative site. Difficult wound healing, infection, bony instability, nonfusion, displacement of implants, and other complications may occur (Figs. 34-3 and 34-4).

The concepts and execution of surgical management for MESCC have evolved steadily (68). In choosing primary surgical versus radiotherapeutic intervention, the prognosis for neurologic improvement and expected impact on functional status must be considered. Clinical outcomes

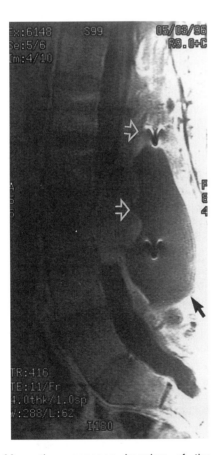

FIG. 4. Magnetic resonance imaging of the spine of metastatic osteosarcoma. Recurrent tumor at the site of prior resection and stabilization. Postoperative pseudomeningocele (*arrow*), and multilocular appearance suggesting infection with abscess formation (*open arrows*). Clinical presentation of back pain with draining sinus.

following laminectomy and radiation therapy may not be better than radiation alone. In some series, radiation therapy has been shown to be equally effective to laminectomy and radiation but with less than 50% neurologic improvement overall (11). De novo anterior-posterior resection with spine stabilization may result in better outcomes than laminectomy and radiation or radiation alone, as surgical complications are generally manageable, survival is improved (although the 2-year survival for lung cancer may be 10% and for colorectal cancer only 17%), and patients may remain ambulatory longer (64). The data are as yet insufficient to draw final conclusions regarding pain and quality of life outcomes. The decision to recommend initial radiation therapy versus surgical intervention depends on many factors; it has been suggested that without bony instability, the speed of progression of neurologic deficit and radiosensitivity of the tumor are the main factors to consider. Severe deficits hold a poor prognosis independent of treatment. Randomized, prospective trials are in progress to compare radiation therapy and surgery for MESCC. It is anticipated that in the future, the indications for primary surgery versus radiotherapy for MESCC will be better defined.

Nonsurgical stabilization of the bony spine can be accomplished with a cervical collar or body bracing (see below). The cancer patient with neck pain and suspected cervical spine disease should be placed in a collar while diagnostic evaluation is being conducted.

**Hormonal and Chemotherapy**

Antineoplastic hormonal and chemotherapeutic agents are considered as treatment for acute MESCC (a) when the patient is asymptomatic or has early symptoms and signs, with mild epidural disease, (b) when no further radiation or surgery is possible, and (c) in conjunction with radiation or surgery (51). Chemotherapy is indicated especially for MESCC in Hodgkin lymphoma, seminoma, and Ewing sarcoma.

**ONGOING CARE**

**Pain Management**

Extended corticosteroid administration (i.e., for the duration of life in patients with MESCC and short prognosis) has not been well studied but is common in clinical practice. Corticosteroids are extremely effective antiinflammatory agents and confer analgesia for bone tumors.

Nonsteroidal antiinflammatory drugs (NSAIDs) are uniquely efficacious for bone pain (70). Bisphosphanates are used to manage hypercalcemia; they inhibit osteoclast activity and may not be as effective in blastic metastases, such as in prostate cancer (71). Second-generation bisphosphanates given with calcium can prevent steroid induced osteoporosis (72). Calcitonin may have analgesic efficacy when given intrapsinally but is not yet approved for this indication.

Guidelines for the use of NSAIDs, opioids, and adjuvant analgesics for neuropathic pain were published in recent years (73–75). Chronic opioid therapy often is required for persistent pain following treatment of MESCC. Cases have been reported in which patients with MESCC required prolonged high-dose intrathecal infusion of opioid and local anesthetic in order to obtain adequate analgesia (76,77).

Strontium-89 is a beta-emitting radionuclide that preferentially localizes in areas of active bone formation, such as osteoblastic tumors. The agent functions as a calcium analog that emits beta particles while decaying to yttrium-89. Clinical studies demonstrated an analgesic effect, especially in prostate cancer. Strontium-89 may relieve pain by blocking release of algesic substances from tumor, or it may suppress tumor blastic activity. Transient worsening of pain within 48 hours of administration has been observed. Dosing for adults is 40 to 60 microCi/kg. Dosing may be repeated at 3-month intervals to a maximum of eight doses. Patients should be monitored for hematologic toxicity (i.e., leukopenia and thrombocytopenia) (78). The overall response rate to Sr-89 may be as high as 80% (4). The analgesic efficacy of strontium-89 has not been studied specifically in verterbal lesions as compared to appendicular metastases.

Neuroablative procedures are considered when the benefit-to-risk ratio favors analgesia over the potential for further neurologic compromise. Destruction of nervous tissue may be accomplished by anesthetic or surgical means. Chemical epidural neurolysis may be chosen to effect single or multiple nerve root interruption. Intrathecal neurolysis would be anticipated to achieve analgesia over a wider territory and may be selected when the epidural space is compromised. Both approaches entail risk of acute neurologic deterioration, which may be irreversible (79). Neurosurgical ablation of nerve roots (rhizotomy) involves major surgery and is indicated less often in very sick patients. Midline myelotomy may be indicated for patients with severe midline sacral pain and bladder or bowel compromise due to tumor of the sacrum. Spinothalamic tractotomy or cordotomy, although more easily performed as a percutaneous procedure, is not generally useful for pain in association with spine disease or MESCC. Hypophysectomy for diffuse painful metastatic bone disease may yield success rates as high as 90% in some endocrine responsive tumors (80). Its efficacy in treating spine disease has not been evaluated thoroughly.

Physical therapy techniques for pain include massage, ultrasound, and transcutaneous electrical nerve stimulation (TENS). Integration of pharmacologic and nonpharmacologic analgesic therapies is needed for the vast majority of patients with MESCC. A multidisciplinary approach to pain management and rehabilitation of patients with resected sacral chordoma has been reported (81).

## Rehabilitation

Each patient's rehabilitation program must be individually tailored and continually reassessed and modified. For some patients, comprehensive care, including patient and family education and training, mobility, activities of daily living training, equipment-needs evaluation, psychosocial support, and discharge planning, may be best accomplished in a formal rehabilitation setting (82). Specific rehabilitation goals are to improve ambulation, achieve weight-bearing and transfers, restore bladder and bowel function, and protect the skin.

Spinal orthotics stabilize the spine and may decrease spinal pain by limiting motion. Orthoses themselves may be uncomfortable to wear, however. The soft cervical or Philadelphia collars do not completely restrict cervical range of motion. Halo devices and sternal-occipital-mandibular immobilizers (SOMI) devices are more effective for immobilization and also are more cumbersome. Custom-fabricated thoracolumbosacral orthoses (TLSO) with a high margin or sternal extension may be used. Standard TLSO braces are available for the lower thoracic and lumbar region. Soft thoracolumbar corsets do not stabilize the spine but may reduce pain by restricting motion somewhat or by cueing the patient to limit their own spinal motion. Bracing is considered when increased mobility is desired.

About 50% of patients require urinary catheterization before and after XRT for MESCC (3). Intermittent urinary catheterization may produce urethral bleeding of friable mucosa. Urethral stricture may follow radiation therapy, making catheterization more difficult. Bladder management may therefore incorporate minor surgical procedures. Sexual dysfunction in women and men may be treatable with specific physical interventions.

A number of medical problems common to the cancer population may limit aggressive rehabilitation efforts. Organ failure due to the disease or its treatment, poor nutrition, and multiple physical and psychological symptoms may complicate rehabilitation. Anemia reduces exercise tolerance. Thrombocytopenia increases the risk of bleeding with more vigorous physical activity. An active exercise program may have to be modified accordingly. Weakness due to spinal cord or nerve root compression may be complicated by peripheral neuropathy or myopathy, common complications of antineoplastic treatment. The skin of many cancer patients is relatively more prone to breakdown and infection due to tumor, radiation, chemotherapy, and poor nutrition. Skin care and protection are essential, especially in the bedridden patient. Caregivers for these patients should remember to observe appropriate infection precautions.

The risk of fracture in osteoporotic or tumor-laden bones should be evaluated carefully before initiating a mobility program. In paraparetic or paraplegic patients, prophylactic fixation of upper extremity lesions may be considered to aid mobility and weight bearing. In bedridden patients with multiple impending fractures, positioning and transfers must be undertaken with great caution. Chronic musculoskeletal problems may occur in children following spine irradiation during growth because of the development of secondary spinal deformities.

The goals of physical medicine and rehabilitation in the patient with MESCC range from active programs to restore independent function, to supportive care (83). Preventive rehabilitation therapy is directed toward achieving maximal functional restoration in patients cured or in stable remission from their cancer. Continued encouragement for the effort required in aggressive rehabilitation is needed for a successful outcome. Supportive rehabilitation therapy attempts to help patients adapt to progressive decline in function due to advancing disease. For patients with limited prognosis, usually considered to be less than 6 months' life expectancy, family participation receives more emphasis and, if indicated, an inpatient rehabilitation stay usually will be short. The needs of the patient will tend more toward dependent care as cancer progresses, and the goals of rehabilitation will be more supportive (i.e., to address problems of bedridden patients). One may consider therapies to prevent complications of immobility, such as prophylactic subcutaneous heparin, antiembolic stockings, venous compression pumps, and frequent position changes. Palliative rehabilitation interventions are intended to provide comfort in the terminal stages of cancer.

## Psychological Interventions

Ongoing psychological support of the patient with metastatic spine disease is essential. Issues of loss of independence, loss of control over bodily functions, and loss of sexual function require sympathetic attention. Families often benefit from emotional support for anticipatory grieving, and professional assistance may be required as the the burden of care increases with the patient's progressing disease.

## OUTCOMES

The potential for recovery of function in patients with tumor involvement of the spine and associated neurologic structures varies by tumor type (primary or metastatic), the number of vertebrae involved, the nature and degree of neurologic involvement, the oncologic status, and general medical condition. In most series, about 50% of patients with metastatic spine tumors are ambulatory at presentation, 35% are paretic, and 15% are plegic (38).

Up to 30% of patients with weakness become plegic within the first week of presentation (5). The prognosis for regaining ambulatory status in MESCC patients who begin therapy while ambulatory is 75%; prognosis declines to 30% to 50% for patients who begin therapy paretic and to 10% for those who begin therapy plegic (36). The duration of neurologic symptoms before treatment also affects prognosis for neurologic recovery: if paraplegia is present for days or urinary retention present for more than 30 hours, the likelihood of recovery is decreased (84). Rapidly progressing symptoms confer a worse prognosis.

Patients who remain unable to ambulate following irradiation for MESCC have a particularly poor prognosis for survival as a result of complications of paresis (infection, decubitus ulcers, venous thrombosis) and other factors relating to more advanced disease. Survival rates for patients with MESCC are 40% at 1 year if ambulatory before and after radiation treatment, 30% at 1 year, 20% at 3 years for patients who are nonambulatory before and ambulatory after treatment, and 7% at 1 year for patients who are nonambulatory after treatment (3).

Response to treatment for MESCC and survival vary with the nature of the malignancy. In patients with prostate cancer, the response to treatment of neurological complications depends on whether the patient has received prior hormonal therapy, and better response to hormonal manipulation correlates with longer survival. The median survival of prostate cancer patients after diagnosis with MESCC is 6 months, and only 34% survive at least 1 year (85). Renal cancer is poorly radioresponsive, and median survival time after diagnosis with MESCC is less than 4 months (86). Hemorrhagic complications of spinal surgery for metastatic renal tumor may be avoided by preoperative embolization (87). In testicular cancer, chemotherapy is effective for untreated lesions or for responsive tumors (88), but radiation and surgery may be considered if the disease is not chemoresponsive (86). Up to 75% of melanoma patients with MESCC will respond to radiation therapy (89–91). Patients with carcinoid tumor and MESCC have a median survival of 6 months. Ambulatory status may be preserved with radiation in up to 90% of patients with carcinoid tumors (19). In myeloma, long-term survival is common. In a series of patients with multiple myeloma, the 1-year survival was 100% and median survival 37 months after MESCC was diagnosed (92). Solitary plasmacytomas will generally be irradiated and surgically removed. Multiple myeloma patients often receive radiation therapy to maximum spinal cord tolerance before surgical intervention is considered. Most lymphomas respond to radiation. In pediatric patients, surgery may be preferred for radioresistant sarcomas and small-cell tumors (Ewing sarcoma, neuroblastoma, lymphoma, and germ-cell tumors) presenting with rapid neurologic deterioration. A trend toward extended survival was shown after surgical decompression in Ewing sarcoma. Many small-cell tumors will respond to chemotherapy or radiation. Younger age may confer greater risk of radiation complications (93). Complete resection of primary spinal extraosseous epidural Ewing sarcoma may be difficult. The 18-month survival was less than 40% in a small series of patients with this unusual malignancy (94).

The survival prognosis for all patients treated for MESCC is less than 50% at 2 months (11). Definitive intervention for MESCC is considered in the context of the patient's overall disease status. Systemic antineoplastic therapy at times may precede or entirely supplant intervention targeted at MESCC. In patients with very advanced cancer, the burden of intervention to reverse MESCC often outweighs minimal potential gains in function. Although few studies of quality of life issues have been conducted in this population, pain control should remain a high priority regardless of prognosis. Given limited available data, the clinician caring for patients with spinal neoplasm and its complications must select medical interventions carefully to achieve therapeutic goals for each individual patient.

# REFERENCES

1. Loeser JD. Neurosurgical approaches in palliative care. In: Doyle D, Hanks GWC, MacDonald N, eds. *Oxford textbook of palliative medicine*. Oxford: Oxford University Press, 1993;221.
2. Posner, JB. *Neurologic complications of cancer*. Contemporary Neurology Series Vol. 45. Philadelphia: FA Davis, 1995;112.
3. Perrin RG, Janjan NA, Langford LA. Spinal axis metastases. In: Levin VA, ed. *Cancer in the nervous system*. New York: Churchill Livingstone, 1996;259.
4. Byrne TN, Waxman SG. *Spinal cord compression: diagnosis and principles of management*. Contemporary Neurology Series Vol. 33. Philadelphia: FA Davis, 1990;xx–xx.
5. Grant R, Papadopoulos SM, Greenberg HS. Metastatic epidural Spinal Cord Compression. In: Patchell RA, ed. *Neurologic complications of Systemic Cancer*. Neurologic Clinics. Philadelphia: WB Saunders, 1991;9:4:825.
6. Klein SL, Sanford RA, Muhlbauer MS. Pediatric spinal epidural metastases. *J Neurosurg* 1991;74:70.
7. Barron KD, Hirano A, Araski S, et al. Experiences with metastatic neoplasms involving the spinal cord. *Neurology* 1959;9:91.
8. Byrne TN, Waxman SG. *Spinal cord compression: diagnosis and principles of management*. Contemporary Neurology Series Vol. 33. Philadelphia: FA Davis, 1990;66.
9. Stark RJ, Henson RA, Evans SJW. Spinal metastases: a retrospective survey from a general hospital. *Brain* 1982;105:189.
10. Posner JB. *Neurologic complications of cancer*. Contemporary Neurology Series Vol. 45. Philadelphia: FA Davis, 1995;113.
11. Obbens EAMT. Neurological problems in palliative medicine. In: Doyle D, Hanks GWC, MacDonald N, eds. *Oxford textbook of palliative medicine*. Oxford: Oxford University Press, 1993;460.
12. Byrne TN. Spinal metastases. In: Wiley RG, ed. *Neurologic complications of cancer*. New York: Marcel Dekker, 1995;23.
13. Harrington KD. Metastatic disease of the spine. In: Harrington KD, ed. *Orthopedic management of metastatic bone disease*. St. Louis: CV Mosby, 1988;309.
14. Misulis KE, Wiley RG. Neurological complications of lung Cancer. In: Wiley RG, ed. *Neurologic complications of cancer*. New York: Marcel Dekker, 1995;295.
15. Anderson NE. Neurological complications of breast cancer. In: Wiley RG, ed. *Neurologic complications of Cancer*. New York: Marcel Dekker, 1995;319.
16. Kuban DA, El-Mahdi AM, Sigfred SV, Schellhammer PF, Babb TJ. Characteristics of spinal cord compression in adenocarcinoma of the prostate. *Urology* 1986;28:364.
17. Flynn DF, Shipley WU. Management of spinal cord compression secondary to metastatic prostatic carcinoma. *Urol Clin North Am* 1991;18:145.
18. Moots PL, Wiley RG. Neurological disorders in head and neck cancers. In: Wiley RG, ed. *Neurologic complications of cancer*. New York: Marcel Dekker, 1995;353.
19. Hagen NA. Neurological complications of gastrointestinal cancers. In: Wiley RG, ed. *Neurologic complications of cancer*. New York: Marcel Dekker, 1995;395.
20. Friedman M, Kim TH, Panahon AM. Spinal cord compression in malignant lymphoma: treatment and results. *Cancer* 1976;37:1485.
21. Ribeiro RC, Pui CH, Schell MJ. Vertebral compression fracture as a presenting feature of acutye lymphoblastic leukemia in children. *Cancer* 1988;61:589.
22. Jennings MT. Neurological complications of childhood cancer. In: Wiley RG, ed. *Neurologic complications of cancer*. New York: Marcel Dekker, 1995;503.
23. Klein SL, Sanford RA, Muhlbauer MS. Pediatric spinal epidural metastases. *J Neurosurg* 1991;74:70.
24. Molloy PT, Phillips PC. Neurological complications of sarcomas. In: Wiley RG, ed. *Neurologic complications of cancer*. New York: Marcel Dekker, 1995;417.
25. Posner JB. *Neurologic complications of cancer*. Contemporary Neurology Series Vol. 45. Philadelphia: FA Davis, 1995;132.
26. Galasko CSB, Sylvester BS. Back pain in patients treated for malignant tumours. *Clin Oncol* 1978;4:273.
27. Kanner RM. Low back pain. In: Portenoy RK, Kanner RM, eds. *Pain management: theory and practice*. Contemporary Neurology Series Vol 48. Philadelphia: FA Davis, 1996;126.
28. Sty JR, Wells RG, Conway JJ. Spine pain in children. *Semin Nucl Med* 1993;23:4:296.
29. Manishen WJ, Sivananthan K, Orr FW. Resorbing bone stimulates tumor cell growth. A role for the host microenvironment in bone metastasis. *Am J Pathol* 1986;123:39.
30. Posner JB. *Neurologic complications of cancer*. Contemporary Neurology Series vol 45. Philadelphia: FA Davis, 1995;30.
31. Powell N. Metastattic carcinoma in association with Paget's disease of bone. *Br J Radiol* 1983;56:582.
32. Tarlov IM, Klinger H. Spinal cord compression studies. II: Time limits for recovery after acute compression in dogs. *Arch Neurol Psychiatry* 1954;71:271.
33. Gledhill RF, Harrison BM, McDonald WI. Demyelination and remyelination after acute spinal cord compression. *Exp Neurol* 1973;38:472.
34. Burger EL, Lindeque BG. Sacral and non-spinal tumors presenting as backache: a retrospective study of 17 patients. *Acta Orthop Scand* 1994;65:93:344.
35. Gonzales GR, Elliott KJ, Portenoy RK, Foley KM. The impact of a comprehenisve evaluation in the management of cancer pain. *Pain* 1991;47:2:141.
36. Hewitt DJ, Foley KM. Neuroimaging of pain. In: Greenberg JO, ed. *Neuroimaging*. New York: McGraw-Hill, 1995;41.
37. Gilbert RW, Kim JH, Posner JB. Epidural spinal cord compression from metastatic tumor: diagnosis and treatment. *Ann Neurol* 1978;3:40.
38. Posner JB. *Neurologic complications of cancer*. Contemporary Neurology Series, vol 45. Philadelphia: FA Davis, 1995;119.
39. Posner JB. *Neurologic complications of cancer*. Contemporary Neurology Series, vol 45. Philadelphia: FA Davis, 1995;192.
40. Smith R. An evaluation of surgical treatment for spinal cord compression due to metastatic carcinoma. *J Neurol Neurosurg Psychiatry* 1965;28:152.
41. Posner JB. *Neurologic complications of cancer*. Contemporary Neurology Series, vol 45. Philadelphia: FA Davis, 1995;122.
42. Posner JB. *Neurologic complications of cancer*. Contemporary Neurology Series, vol 45. Philadelphia: FA Davis, 1995;140.
43. Posner JB. *Neurologic complications of cancer*. Contemporary Neurology Series, vol 45. Philadelphia: FA Davis, 1995;127.
44. Wong DA, Fornasier VL, MacNab I. Spinal metastases: the obvious, the occult, and the imposters. *Spine* 1990;15:1.
45. Byrne TN, Waxman SG. *Spinal cord compression: diagnosis and Principles of management*. Contemporary Neurology Series vol. 33. Philadelphia: FA Davis, 1990;164.
46. Laredo JD, Lakhdari K, Bellaiche L, et al. Acute vertebral collapse: CT

findings in benign and malignant nontraumatic cases. *Radiology* 1995; 194:1:41.

47. Posner JB. *Neurologic complications of cancer*. Contemporary Neurology Series, vol 45. Philadelphia: FA Davis, 1995;129.

48. Rhamouni A, Divine M, Mathieu D, et al. Detection of multiple myeloma involving the spine: efficacy of fat-sppression and contrast-enhanced MR imaging. *AJR Am J Roentgenol* 1993;160:5:1049.

49. Vecht CJ, Verbiest HBC. Use of glucocorticoiuds in neuro-oncology. In: Wiley RG, ed. *Neurologic complications of cancer*. New York: Marcel Dekker, 1995;199.

50. Greenberg HS, Kim JH, Posner JB. Epidural spinal cord compression from metastatic tumor: results with a new treatment protocol. *Ann Neurol* 1980;8:361.

51. Posner JB. *Neurologic complications of cancer*. Contemporary Neurology Series Vol. 45. Philadelphia: F.A. Davis, 1995;134.

52. Breitbart W, Stiefel F, Kornblith AB, Pannullo S. Neuropsychiatric disturbances in cancer patiens wih epidural spinal cord compresion receiving high dose corticosteroids: a prospective comparison study. *Psychooncology* 1993;2:223–245.

53. Pocock NA, Eisman JA, Dunstan CR, et al. Recovery from steroid induced osteoporosis. *Ann Intern Med* 1987;107:319.

54. Yoshioka H, Tsuneto S, Kashiwagi T. Pain control with morphine for vertebral metastases and sciatica in advance cancer patients. *J Palliat Care* 1994;10:1:10.

55. Posner JB. *Neurologic complications of cancer*. Contemporary Neurology Series, vol 45. Philadelphia: FA Davis, 1995;135.

56. Armstrong JG, Fass DE, Bains M, et al. Paraspinal tumors: Techniques and results of brachytherapy. *Int J Radiat Oncol Biol Phys* 1991;20:787.

57. Byrne TN, Waxman SG. *Spinal cord compression: diagnosis and principles of management*. Contemporary Neurology Series, vol 33. Philadelphia: FA Davis, 1990;160.

58. Posner JB. *Neurologic complications of cancer*. Contemporary Neurology Series, vol 45. Philadelphia: FA Davis, 1995;139.

59. Galasko CSB, Sylvester BS. Back pain in patients treated for malignant tumours. *Clin Oncol* 1978;4:273.

60. Posner JB. *Neurologic complications of cancer*. Contemporary Neurology Series, vol 45. Philadelphia: FA Davis, 1995;137.

61. Galasko CSB. Orthopaedic principles and management. In: Doyle D, Hanks GWC, MacDonald N, eds. *Oxford textbook of palliative medicine*. Oxford: Oxford University Press, 1993;274.

62. Findlay GFG. Adverse effects of the management of malignant spinal cord compression. *J Neurol Neurosurg Psychiatry* 1984;47:761.

63. McBroom R. Radiation or surgery for metastatic disease of the spine? Royal Society of Medicine Current Medical Literature. *Orthopedics* 1988;1:97.

64. Sundaresan N, Sachdev VP, Holland JF, et al. Surgical treatment of spinal cord compression from epidural metastasis. *J Clin Oncol* 1995; 13:9:2330.

65. Sundaresan N, Digiacinto GV, Hughes JEO, Cafferty M, Vallejo A. Treatment of neoplastic spinal cord compression: results of a prospective study. *Neurosurgery* 1991;29:645.

66. Siegal T, Siegal TZ. Surgical decompression of anterior and posterior maligant epidural tumors compressing the spinal cord: a prospective study. *Neurosurgery* 1985;17:424–432.

67. Moore AJ, Uttley D. Anterior decompression and stabilization of the spine in malignant disease. *Neurosurgery* 1989;24:713.

68. Perrin RG. Metastatic tumors of the axial spine. *Curr Opin Oncol* 1992;493:525.

69. Weller SJ, Rossitch E Jr. Unilateral posterolateral decompression without stabilization for neurological palliation of symptomatic spinal metastases in debilitated patients. *J Neurosurg* 1995;82:5:739.

70. Portenoy RK. Pharmacologic management of chronic pain. In: Fields HL, ed. *Pain syndromes in neurologic practice*. New York: Butterworth, 1990;257.

71. Payne R, Weinstein SM, Hill CS. Management of cancer pain. In: Levin VL, ed. *Cancer in the nervous system*. New York: Churchill Livingstone, 1996;411.

72. Reid IR, King AR, Alexander CJ, et al. Prevention of steroid-induced osteoporosis with (3-amino-1-hydroxypropylidene)-1,1-bisphosphanate (APD). *Lancet* 1988;1:143.

73. *World Health Organization cancer pain relief and palliative care*. Geneva: World Health Organization, 1990.

74. Jacox A, Carr DB, Payne R, et al. *Management of cancer pain*. Clinical Practice Guideline No. 9. AHCPR Publication No. 94-0592. Rockville, MD: Agency for Health Care Policy and Research, U.S. Department of Health and Human Services, Public Health Services, March 1994.

75. American Pain Society. *Principles of analgesic use in the treatment of acute pain and cancer pain*, 3rd ed. American Pain Society, 1992.

76. Payne R, Cunningham M, Weinstein SM, Ribeiro S, Patt RB, Chiang J. Intractable pain and suffering in a cancer patient. *Clin J Pain* 1995;11: 70.

77. Aguilar JL, Espachs P, Roca G, et al. Difficult management of pain following sacrococcygeal chordoma: thirteen months of subarachnoid infusion. *Pain* 1994;59:2:317.

78. Dana WJ. Therapeutics review: strontium-89. *University of Texas M. D. Anderson Cancer Center Pharmacy Bulletin* 1994;12.

79. Morgan RJ, Steller PH. Acute paraplegisa following intrathecal phenol block in the presence of occult epidural malignancy. *Anesthesia* 1994; 49:2:142.

80. Waldman SD, Feldstein LS, Allen ML. Neuroadenolysis of the pituitary: description of a modified technique. *J Pain Sympt Manag* 1987; 2:45.

81. Watling C, Allen RR. Treatment of neuropathic pain associated witrh sacrectomy. *Proceedings of the 48th Annual Scientific Meeting of the American Academy of Neurology*, 1996.

82. Schlicht LA, Smelz JK. Metastatic spinal cord compression. In: Garden FH, Grabois M, eds. *Cancer rehabilitation: physical medicine and rehabilitation*. State of the Art Reviews. Philadelphia: Hanley and Belfus. 1994;345.

83. Garden FH, Gillis TA. Principles of cancer rehabilitation. In: Braddom RL, ed. *Physical medicine and rehabilitation*. Philadelphia: WB Saunders, 1996;1199.

84. Bach F, Larsen BH, Rohde K, Brgesen SE, Gjerris F, Bge-Rasmussen T, Agerlin N, Rasmusson B, Satjernholm P, Srensen PS. Metastatic spinal cord compression: occurrence, symptoms, clinical presentation and progression in 398 patients with spinal cord compression. *Acta Neurochir (Wien)* 1990;107:37–43.

85. Delattre JY, Krol G, Thaler HT, Posner JB. Distribution of brain metastases. *Arch Neurol* 1988;45:741.

86. Fadul CE. Neurological complications of genitourinary cancer. In: Wiley RG, ed. *Neurologic complications of cancer*. New York: Marcel Dekker, 1995;388.

87. Sundaresan N, Choi IS, Hughes JEO, Sachdev VP, Berenstein A. Treatment of spinal metastases from kidney cancer by presurgical embolization and resection. *J Neurosurg* 1990;73:548.

88. Cooper K, Bajorin D, Shapiro W, Krol G, Sze G, Bosl GJ. Decompression of epidural metatstases from germ cell tumors with chemotherapy. *J Neurooncol* 1990;8:275.

89. Rate WR, Solin LJ, Turrisi AT. Palliative radiotherapy for metastatic malignant melanoma: brain metastases, bone metastases, and spinal cord compression. *Int J Radiat Oncol Biol Phys* 1998;15:859.

90. Herbert SH, Solin LJ, Rate WR, Schultz DJ, Hanks GE. The effect of palliative radiation therapy on epidural compression due to metastatic malignant melanoma. *Cancer* 1991;67:2472.

91. Henson JW. Neurological complications of malignant melanoma and other cutaneous malignancies. In: Wiley RG, ed. *Neurologic complications of cancer*. New York: Marcel Dekker, 1995;333.

92. Spiess JL, Adelstein DJ, Hines DJ. Mutiple myeloma presenting with spinal cord compression. *Oncology* 1988;45;88.

93. Mayfield JK, Riseborough EJ, Jaffe N, et al. Spinal deformities in children treated for neuroblastoma. *J Bone Joint Surg* 1981;63:183.

94. Kaspars GJ, Kamphorst W, et al. Primary spinal epidural extraosseous Ewing's sarcoma. *Cancer* 1991;68:648.

*Principles and Practice of Supportive Oncology,*
edited by Ann Berger et al.
Lippincott–Raven Publishers, Philadelphia ©1998

CHAPTER 35

# Neuromuscular Dysfunction and Supportive Care

James W. Teener and John T. Farrar

The neuromuscular disorders experienced by cancer patients may cause weakness, fatigue, sensory loss, and pain, including cramps and dyesthesias. To determine accurately the etiology of these symptoms and guide treatment, a logical approach to assessment is necessary. First, a careful history and neurologic examination are needed to identify potential neuromuscular dysfunction. Second, a specific diagnosis is sought through confirmatory testing or appropriate consultation. Finally, appropriate therapy is prescribed. In this chapter, such an approach is explored with reference to common cancer-associated neuromuscular diseases.

The term *neuromuscular* refers to the peripheral nervous system, which includes the anterior horn cell, the dorsal root ganglion, the sensory and motor nerve roots, the plexi, the peripheral nerves, the neuromuscular junction and muscle. Patients with cancer can develop neuromuscular dysfunction through direct compression or innvasion by the neoplasm, toxic effects of antineoplastic therapies, or paraneoplastic (remote) effects.

## EXAMINATION

A careful examination of the patient complaining of fatigue, weakness, sensory disturbance, or pain will help the practitioner differentiate a neuromuscular problem from dysfunction caused by central nervous system (CNS) or nonneurologic pathology. For example, weakness of one side of the body suggests a CNS lesion, whereas weakness of distal leg and hand muscles often is caused by a neuropathy. Proximal weakness is more typical of myopathies or defects in neuromuscular transmission. Similarly, a sensory level over the trunk is typical of

spinal cord compression, whereas foot and hand numbness in a stocking/glove pattern is more typical of a neuropathy. Both positive (e.g., tingling) and negative (e.g., numbness) sensory complaints are common with peripheral nerve injury. Reflexes are usually brisk when weakness is caused by a CNS lesion and reduced in cases of neuropathy. Reflexes are often normal in myopathy but may be reduced if the myopathy is severe.

Often, the physical examination is not definitive, and other diagnostic procedures must be used. Figure 35-1 presents diagnostic studies that may be useful in identifying the specific pathologic lesion resulting in neuromuscular dysfunction. Electrodiagnostic studies frequently provide localization, and the additional studies listed may allow a specific diagnosis to be made.

Table 35-1 presents the symptoms that may be caused by neuromuscular dysfunction and the most typical neuromuscular disorders causing those symptoms. Some of the symptoms, such as fatigue and diffuse weakness, have little specific localizing value. Others, such as muscle tenderness or focal pain, may lead to an anatomic localization.

## NEUROMUSCULAR DISORDERS

### Neuropathy

Neuropathy is the most frequently encountered neuromuscular complication of cancer. Although neurotoxic chemotherapy is most commonly implicated, neuropathy also may be caused by direct or metastatic tumor infiltration of nerve or by remote (paraneoplastic) effects of the cancer. Nerve involvement may be focal or widespread, and, consequently, symptoms and signs may be focal or diffuse. Reflexes are generally reduced or absent in the affected areas. Dysesthetic pain, often burning, is a fre-

J. W. Teener and J. T. Farrar: Department of Neurology, University of Pennsylvania, Philadelphia, PA 19104-4283.

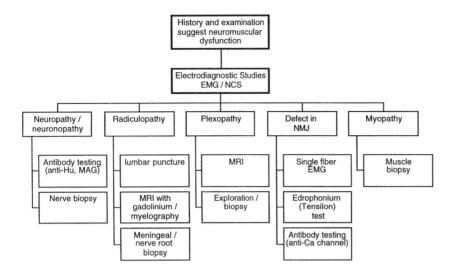

**FIG. 1.** Evaluation of neuromuscular dysfunction in patients with cancer. Electrodiagnostic studies confirm the presence of a suspected neuromuscular disorder. Always consider nonneoplastic causes and screen with appropriate laboratory studies as indicated (glucose, thyroid function, vitamin B12, lyme titer, cyroglobulins, serum protein electrophoresis, and so on). MRI, magnetic resonance imaging; NMJ, neuromuscular junction; EMG/NCS, electomyography/nerve conduction studies.

quent complaint. Fatigue and muscle cramps also may be troublesome.

It is useful to divide neuropathy according to the primary modalities affected: sensory, motor, or sensorimotor. The neuropathy may be further classified according to the predominant pathology: axonal loss, demyelination, or neuron cell body death (Fig. 35-2). Disorders that affect sensation or strength exclusively most often are caused by lesions of the dorsal root ganglion cells or anterior horn cells, respectively, and thus are described most accurately as neuronopathies. In most neuropathies, sensation and strength are both involved to some degree, although one deficit may predominate.

The evaluation of a neuropathy usually involves an electromyogram (EMG) and nerve conduction studies, which help differentiate neuronal or axonal injury from primary injury to myelin and to confirm a focal or diffuse process. Nerve biopsy is rarely indicated but can be helpful in differentiating direct tumor invasion (possibly amenable to chemotherapy or radiation) from a toxic or paraneoplastic process. A lumbar puncture is frequently appropriate if there is a possibility of nerve root involvement. Cerebrospinal fluid (CSF) surrounds nerve roots, and examination of this fluid may clarify pathology at

this level. It may also be important to evaluate some of the nonneoplastic causes of neuropathy. A useful scheme for evaluation of neuropathy was presented by Brown (1).

The primary treatment of a neuropathy, if any, is generally cause specific and is discussed with each syndrome. The treatment of neuropathy-related symptoms depends primarily on the predominant symptom (i.e., weakness, sensory loss, pain, and so on) and is discussed under Symptomatology in the next section.

### Chemotherapy Toxicity

Chemotherapeutic agents are the most frequently encountered cause of clinically important neuropathy in cancer patients. A wide variety of chemotherapeutic agents have been associated with the development of neuropathy. Vincristine, cisplatin, and paclitaxel are most frequently prescribed; other drugs include misonidazole (2), procarbazine (3), suramin (4), cytozine arabinoside (ARA-C)(5), etoposide (6), and ifosfamide (7).

Patients who may have chemotherapy-related neuropathy should undergo a standard neuropathy evaluation, as already described. It is occasionally useful to follow elec-

**TABLE 1.** *Cardinal symptoms of neromuscular dysfunction; most symptoms have a large number of nonneromuscular causes*

| | Focal weakness | Diffuse weakness | Sensory loss/ dysesthesia | Focal pain | Muscle cramps | Myalgias | Fatigue |
|---|---|---|---|---|---|---|---|
| Polyneuropathy | | + | + | | + | + | + |
| Mononeuropathy | + | | + | + | | | |
| Sensory neuropathy | | | + | | | | |
| Motor neuropathy | + | + | | | + | | + |
| Plexopathy | + | | + | + | + | | |
| Radiculopathy | + | + | + | + | + | | |
| Defect in neruomuscular transmission | | + | | | | + | |
| Myopathy | + | + | | + | + | + | + |

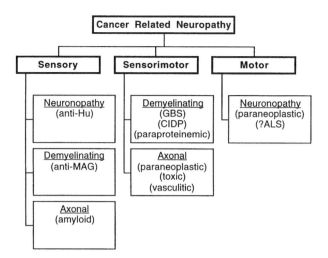

**FIG. 2.** Cancer-related neuropathy subdivided by modality affected and primary pathology. Most common causes are in parentheses. GBS, Guillan-Barre syndrome; CIDP, chronic imflammatory demyelinating neuropathy; ALS, amyotrophic lateral sclerosis; MAG, myelin-associated glycoprotein.

trodiagnostic markers of nerve dysfunction prospectively to identify impending nerve dysfunction early in the course of chemotherapy. Somatosensory-evoked responses are generally affected first, followed later by a reduction in sensory amplitudes on nerve conduction studies (8).

Treatment usually includes attempts to limit the patient's exposure to the offending medication. Symptomatic therapy is detailed below. Chemoprotective agents are under investigation and ultimately may allow prophylactic therapy for neurotoxicity. A compound called WR-2721, for example, has demonstrated protective effects against the development of neuropathy in patients treated with cisplatin (9).

Vincristine uniformly causes a peripheral neuropathy when used at the usual weekly doses of 1.4 mg/m$^2$ or greater (10). The first clinically apparent sign is the loss of ankle reflexes. Parasthesias often develop first in the fingers. Although mild sensory loss does not warrant a reduction in dosage, weakness may develop rapidly and, when severe, is a dose-limiting side effect. Signs of impending motor involvement include cramps and mild clumsiness. Weakness typically reverses when the dose is reduced or the drug is stopped. The parasthesias take longer to disappear, and mild sensory deficits may persist. Occasional patients develop prolonged or permanent dysfunction. Electrodiagnostic studies reveal the neuropathy to be an axonal sensorimotor polyneuropathy.

Cisplatin may begin to cause neurotoxicity or ototoxocity at a cumulative dose of about 300 mg/m$^2$, and more than 50% of patients who receive 600 mg/m$^2$ develop symptoms (9,11). The neuropathy is predominantly sensory. Deep tendon reflexes are progressively lost along with decreases in vibration sensation and perception of

light touch and pinprick. The loss of proprioception may result in a sensory ataxia. On discontinuation of the drug, the neuropathy may appear to progress for weeks before stabilizing. Recovery occurs over months, but is often incomplete (12). Weakness develops rarely and only in the most severely affected patients.

Paclitaxel predominantly causes a large fiber sensory polyneuropathy. Pain, tingling, and numbness may begin within 1 to 3 days after a single high-dose treatment (13). Weakness occasionally develops but invariably improves when the drug is discontinued. Neurotoxicity is generally not dose limiting. Risk factors for the development of neuropathy include a prior neuropathy, high doses (>250 mg/m$^2$), and perhaps older age (14).

### Cancer-related Neuropathies

A large number of acute and chronic sensorimotor neuropathies have been associated with cancer itself. In most cases, the pathologic mechanism or mechanisms are not known. The syndromes are grouped according to the predominant pathologic process.

#### Axonal Sensorimotor Neuropathy

*Polyneuropathy.* Patients with advanced malignancy often develop a mild sensorimotor neuropathy, which is of little clinical importance. Much less frequently, a clinically significant axonal sensorimotor neuropathy accompanies or even precedes the diagnosis of cancer. This neuropathy typically presents with numbness and tingling in the feet. The lesion may progress to cause more widespread sensory disturbance as well as distal leg and hand weakness. Nerve conduction studies confirm an axonal neuropathy; CSF protein may be normal or rarely slightly elevated. The pathogenesis of this neuropathy is unknown in most cases. In some patients with non-Hodgkin's lymphoma, a lymphomatous infiltration of nerve roots and nerves has been detected on nerve biopsy; these patients may respond to antineoplastic treatment (15–18).

*Focal Neuropathy.* Isolated mononeuropathies also may develop in patients with cancer. Peroneal neuropathies at the fibular head typically develop in bed-bound patients with recent weight loss. Loss of the usual fatty cushion predisposes the peroneal nerve to compression at this site. Nutritional, metabolic, and microcirculatory factors also may contribute to this neuropathy. Focal compression neuropathies generally improve with simple measures, such as careful positioning to avoid further compression and padding of vulnerable areas such as the elbow and fibular head (19).

Malignant cells may invade nerves and cause axonal degeneration resulting in a focal neuropathy. Widespread metastatic infiltration of nerves by lymphoma or melanoma may result in a multifocal neuropathy that is indistinguishable from a sensorimotor polyneuropathy (20). If no other cause is found, contrast-enhanced magnetic resonance imaging (MRI) of the affected area may be positive. A nerve biopsy should be considered if further antineoplastic therapy is a possibility.

*Vasculitic Neuropathy.* Peripheral nerves may be damaged by a cancer-associated vasculitis, which typically causes either an acute or chronic sensorimotor neuropathy, usually beginning as a painful asymmetric neuropathy or a pattern consistent with a mononeuritis multiplex. Nerve conduction studies demonstrate evidence of axonal damage. The diagnosis is confirmed by the demonstration of lymphocytic infiltration and necrosis of blood vessels on nerve or muscle biopsy. Treatment with corticosteroids or other immunosuppressants may result in symptomatic improvement (21,22).

### Demyelinating Neuropathy

*Acute Inflammatory Demyelinating Polyneuropathy (Guillain Barré Syndrome).* Guillain Barré syndrome has a higher incidence in patients with Hodgkin's lymphoma and solid tumors, particularly those involving the lung. Patients suspected of having this disorder require immediate hospitalization for careful monitoring of their respiratory vital capacity and cardiac function. The rate of progression of this disease is highly variable, and patients can deteriorate acutely in the first few days. Cancer patients appear to respond to the same therapies used for non-cancer-related Guillain Barré syndrome such as plasmaphoresis or intravenous immunoglobulin (23,24).

*Chronic Inflammatory Demyelinating Neuropathy (CIDP).* Rarely is CIDP associated with cancer (25). The pattern of weakness and sensory loss may be quite asymmetric, and nerve conduction studies reveal classic demyelinating physiology; CSF protein is almost universally elevated. Remissions are reported following removal of the tumor, and the neuropathy also may respond to treatment with corticosteroids or intravenous immunoglobulin (17,26).

### Paraproteinemic Neuropathy

A variety of neuropathies may be associated with paraproteinemia secondary to multiple myeloma, osteosclerotic myeloma, Waldenstrom macroglobulinemia, primary systemic amyloidosis, or monoclonal gammopathy of undetermined significance (MGUS). Axonal or demyelinating subacute or chronic neuropathies occur in up to 13% of patients with multiple myeloma (27). In some patients with Waldenstrom macroglobulinemia or MGUS, an immunoglobulin M (IgM) antibody directed against myelin-associated glycoprotein (MAG) can be detected in serum and in the myelin sheath. These patients have a pre-

dominantly sensory demyelinating neuropathy (28). In most other cases, the pathogenesis of the neuropathy is uncertain, and the paraprotein may not be involved directly in the pathogenesis. A predominantly motor-demyelinating neuropathy can be identified in up to 50% of patients with osteosclerotic myeloma. The neuropathy may occur as part of a syndrome consisting of polyneuropathy, organomegaly, endocrinopathy, monoclonal gammopathy, and skin changes (POEMS). These neuropathies may markedly improve with treatment of the tumor (29).

Patients with primary systemic amyloidosis may develop a neuropathy that is predominantly sensory and typically involves small unmyelinated or thinly myelinated fibers. Autonomic dysfunction is a prominent feature. The diagnosis is made by demonstration of the amyloid material on nerve biopsy. Unfortunately, this disorder has a grim prognosis, and there is no effective primary treatment (30).

## Neuronopathy

Paraneoplastic processes preferentially attack nerve cell bodies. The cell bodies of motor and sensory neurons are found in the anterior horn of the spinal cord and the dorsal root ganglion, respectively. Damage to the cell bodies of these neurons produce a lesion that is most accurately called a *neuronopathy*. Patients presenting with exclusively sensory or motor dysfunction should be evaluated for the presence of neuronopathy, as outlined below. Symptomatic therapy again depends on the predominate symptoms and is discussed in a later section.

### Motor Neuronopathy

Three separate syndromes are currently best understood as motor syndromes and probably are due to a remote effect of cancer. Treatment of the tumor is of uncertain benefit, and there is no effective primary therapy. Physical and occupational therapy can maximize patients' functional capabilities.

### Subacute Motor Neuronopathy

This syndrome, which presents with slowly progressive, painless weakness predominantly in the legs, is a well-established remote effect of non-Hodgkin and Hodgkin lymphoma (31–33). Bulbar involvement and upper motor neuron signs are not seen. The symptoms often develop following radiation or when the lymphoma is in remission. After a period of progression, symptoms may improve slowly over months to years. Electrodiagnostic studies demonstrate widespread denervation. The cause of the subacute motor neuronopathy is uncertain.

## Paraneoplastic Encephalomyelitis (PEM)

Motor neuron involvement is also seen as a feature of PEM, which typically is associated with a sensory neuronopathy, but neurons at any level of the nervous system, including the motor neurons of the anterior horn, may be affected. When PEM is caused by small-cell lung cancer, an antineuronal antibody associated with cancer, which is known as anti-Hu is typically present.

## Amyotrophic Lateral Sclerosis (ALS)

Rarely is ALS related to a neoplasm. Altough large epidemiological studies generally conclude that the incidence of cancer is not increased in patients with ALS (34), case reports have described cancer patients with typical ALS who improved after removal of the tumor (35). Most patients with typical ALS do not need an evaluation for malignancy. Only patients who do not fit the typical age profile or patients with sensory complaints or other evidence of more widespread nervous system involvement should be considered for a search for an underlying occult malignancy.

## Sensory Neuronopathy

So-called subacute sensory neuronopathy, often referred to as a sensory neuropathy, is the most widely recognized neuromuscular paraneoplastic syndrome (36,37). Patients typically present with numbness, dysesthesias, parasthesias, and occasionally aching pain. The findings can be asymmetric. A sensory ataxia due to loss of proprioception is typical and can be severe. Electrodiagnostic studies are consistent, with damage to the dorsal root ganglion with markedly decreased or absent sensory nerve action potentials. Motor nerve conduction studies should be normal.

Patients who develop sensory neuronopathy without a known cancer require a detailed and perhaps repeated search for an underlying malignancy. Small-cell lung cancer is by far the most commonly associated cancer; but breast, ovarian, uterine, and gastrointestinal carcinomas also must be considered. The presence of anti-Hu antibodies is highly suggestive of the presence of a small cell lung cancer. In about 70% of patients with an anti-Hu antibody, there is evidence of CNS or lower motor neuron involvement as well (38). In these patients, an immune mechanism has been supported by the identification of a complement-binding IgG antibody that binds to an antigen found in the tumor and a 35- to 38-kD brain nuclear protein (39,40). Treatment of the underlying tumor may result in stabilization of the sensory neuronopathy or, in rare cases, improvement. Some patients can learn to adapt to the sensory ataxia by using visual cues, but in severe cases function is permanently lost and patients become wheelchair bound. The other neuropathic symptoms are treated as discussed in the later section on symptomatology. Although treatment trials with intravencus immunoglobulin and plasmaphoresis have been reported, the efficacy of these treatments has not been demonstrated.

## Radiculopathies

Radiculopathy implies dysfunction of the nerve roots. Tumors originating from the spinal column commonly compress nerve roots as well as the spinal cord. Pain is usually the first symptom of compressive radiculopathy. Symptoms and signs of sensory or motor dysfunction may follow, depending on the nerve roots involved and the progression of the lesion.

Radiculopathy also may be caused by leptomeningeal spread of tumor, and meningeal carcinomatous or lymphoma also can cause radicular pain, sensory loss, weakness, and areflexia. Signs of meningeal irritation such as meningismus and occasionally headache may be present. Leptomeningeal spread is most common with cancers of the breast, lung, and gastrointestinal tract, melanoma, and lymphoma but is possible with any tumor. With extension lesions, the tumor can invade multiple roots and produce a polyradiculopathy that closely resembles a severe sensorimotor polyneuropathy. Cranial polyneuropathies resulting from invasion of the cranial nerves as they traverse the subarachnoid space occur regularly.

Evaluation of a patient with suspected meningeal carcinomatous or lympha should begin with spinal fluid examination. In nearly all cases, the spinal fluid proves to be abnormal. Spinal fluid cytology may provide a specific diagnosis, but repeated sampling may be required. In one study, 50% of patients had false negative CSF cytology at the initial lumbar puncture, but the CSF almost always had some abnormality (41). Most experts suggest that at least three lumbar punctures separated by several days be performed if cytologies remain negative (42). Electrodiagnostic studies may demonstrate the typical electrodiagnostic findings of radiculopathy. Contrast-enhanced MRI may demonstrate enhancement of thickened nerve roots, particularly when the cauda equina is affected. If an MRI is contraindicated, myelography will sometimes demonstrate multiple nodular defects on nerve roots, again primarily in the cauda equina. Rarely, a meningeal or nerve root biopsy is needed if a high degree of suspicion remains despite an unrevealing noninvasive evaluation.

Meningeal tumors can sometimes be controlled for a time with radiation and intrathecal or intracerebroventricular chemotherapy (43). The long-term prognosis is grim, however.

## Plexopathies

The diagnosis of plexopathy in the cancer patient is perhaps the most challenging neuromuscular complication. Because of the proximity of the brachial and lumbar plexus to frequently used radiation ports, plexopathy may be a complication of radiation therapy. Differentiating between recurrent cancer and radiation-induced plexopathy can be difficult, and has obvious implications for therapy. As with all peripheral nerve injury, plexopathies usually presents with both positive (e.g., tingling) and negative (e.g., numbness) sensory complaints and weakness of the involved limb. In general, malignant plexopathy is more painful than radiation-induced plexopathy. A severely painful plexopathy can be assumed to be tumor related, but radiographic or tissue diagnosis is strongly recommended before proceeding with additional tumor therapy.

Other causes of plexopathy are rare. Idiopathic brachial plexopathy has been reported in patients with Hodgkin disease (44). Brachial plexopathy can complicate a lymphedematous shoulder (45), and lumbosacral plexopathy can occur following psoas muscle hemorrhage or abscess (46). Regional intraarterial infusion of chemotherapeutic agents has produced local neurotoxicity manifesting as brachial or lumbosacral plexopathies (47).

Diagnostic studies are required to confirm the diagnosis. Electromyographic can help localize the lesion and, in some cases, suggest an etiology. Radiation-induced plexopathy tends to be associated with a more diffuse injury on EMG, and myokymia and rhythmic repetitive spontaneous discharges may be found. Myokymia occurs frequently in patients with radiation-induced plexopathy but has not been reported in those with malignant plexopathy (48,49). An MRI may reveal a mass in the region of the plexus or enhancement along the nerve trunks. Occasionally, the etiology of a plexopathy cannot be established noninvasively, and exploration of the plexus with a biopsy is required (50,51).

The treatment of a plexopathy is difficult. In patients with malignant plexopathy, radiotherapy may provide pain relief. Neurologic signs may not improve, however, and pain can persist and become a difficult management problem. Radiation-induced plexopathy is generally less painful but is slowly progressive and eventually causes significant disability. There is no specific primary treatment.

### Brachial Plexopathies

Brachial plexopathies are typically unilateral. Local extension or metastatic spread of breast or lung cancer are the most common causes (52,53). Lymphoma, sarcoma, melanoma, and other types of cancer less commonly invade the brachial plexus. Patients with malignant brachial plexopathy typically experience pain that radiates from the shoulder girdle into the medial arm and hand (52,54). The lower nerve trunk of the brachial plexus is usually most involved, producing hand weakness, atrophy, and sensory disturbance that may mimic an ulnar neuropathy. Horner syndrome is seen in up to 50% of patients. Exacerbation of lymphedema of the arm is seen occasionally.

Radiation may induce a brachial plexopathy when given at a dose greater than 6,000 cGy. Brachial plexopathy is a late manifestation of radiation therapy, and onset has been reported from 3 months to 26 years after treatment. Unlike neoplastic plexopathies, parasthesias and swelling of the arm predominate over pain. Also, the upper nerve trunk or entire brachial plexus is more likely to be involved.

For brachial plexopathy, these clinical features, which usually distinguish malignant from radiation-induced plexopathy, are pain severity (worse with neoplasm), presence or absence of Horner syndrome (present with neoplasm), lymphedema (not common following radiation), and the distribution of the arm weakness (proximal with radiation injury and distributed from neoplastic invasion). A painful lower nerve trunk lesion with Horner syndrome suggests a metastatic plexopathy, whereas a painless upper nerve trunk lesion with a swollen arm is more typically a sign of a radiation plexopathy (52).

### Lumbosacral Plexopathies

Lumbosacral plexopathies are most commonly caused by direct extension of intraabdominal neoplasms, such as colorectal or cervical cancer, or by radiation (55,56). Pain is a frequent early feature, and the upper, lower, or entire nerve plexus can be affected. The plexopathy is frequently slowly progressive, and bilateral symptoms may be seen. Computerized tomography (CT) or MRI scanning of the region of the lumbosacral plexus typically demonstrates the responsible mass. A biopsy is required only if there is no previous tissue diagnosis.

Radiation-induced lumbosacral plexopathy generally presents as slowly progressive weakness. Pain occurs in 50% of patients. Like radiation-induced brachial plexopathy, the plexopathy may follow radiation by months to years. Myokymia is seen on electrodiagnostic studies in 50% of patients.

## Neuromuscular Junction Disorders

Myasthenia gravis and the Lambert-Eaton myasthenic syndrome are the two most frequently encountered disorders of neuromuscular transmission. Myasthenia gravis may be associated with thymoma but probably is not associated with extrathymic tumors.

Although rare, the Lambert-Eaton myasthenic syndrome (LEMS) is associated with cancer in 50% to 70% of people with the syndrome. In patients with cancer-associated LEMS, 80% have a small-cell lung cancer. There have been case reports of association between LEMS and many other types of cancer, but these associations may be incidental. In patients aged under 40 years, the syndrome is more likely to be autoimmune than paraneoplastic; LEMS occurs more frequently in men than in women (about a 2:1 ratio), and cancer is the cause more often in men (70%) than women (25%)(57).

The cause of LEMS is IgG antibodies directed against the voltage-sensitive calcium channels of the motor and autonomic nerve terminals. The antibodies interfere with the voltage-dependent release of neurotransmitter at the neuromuscular junction and in autonomic nerves. Calcium channel antibody titers can be measured in the serum of LEMS patients. The immunologic stimulus is likely the voltage sensitive calcium channel of the carcinoma cells.

Proximal muscle weakness in patients with LEMS is typical, and there may be mild myalgias and tenderness of the muscles. Given these findings, LEMS can be misdiagnosed as polymyositis. Bulbar and ocular muscles are rarely affected and never are affected to the degree seen in myasthenia gravis. The patients may complain of severe fatigue and weakness but on examination often will have only mild demonstrable weakness. Occasionally, strength may improve following exercise but then weaken further as activity is sustained. Deep tendon reflexes tend to be reduced or absent at rest but may increase if tested immediately after a brief strong contraction of the appropriate muscle. Most patients complain of dry mouth, and some patients have other autonomic manifestations, including impotence, hypotension, and constipation.

Confirmation of LEMS is through electrodiagnostic studies. On routine nerve conduction studies, the motor amplitudes are often markedly reduced due to impaired release of acetylcholine. A small decrement is seen with repetitive stimulation at low rates; however, with high rates of stimulation or immediately following a brief contraction of the muscle, the motor amplitudes will markedly increase to at least double their resting size, most likely because of an increase in the concentration of calcium in the nerve terminals, leading to increased acetylcholine release. In questionable situations, the diagnosis can be confirmed with single-fiber EMG (58).

Therapy for LEMS should be tailored to the individual patient and based on clinical severity, the presence of underlying disease, and life expectancy. If the diagnosis of LEMS has been confirmed in a patient without a known malignancy, an extensive search for malignancy must be carried out. Computed tomography scanning of the chest and sometimes bronchoscopy are recommended. If a small-cell lung cancer is identified, initial therapy

should aimed at treating the cancer. Weakness associated with LEMS frequently improves with effective cancer therapy (59,60), and frequently no further treatment is needed. Cholinesterase inhibitors, such as pyridostigmine, usually do not produce significant improvement, but in rare patients there is some benefit. Pyridostigmine can be tried at a dose of 30 to 120 mg every 4 to 6 hours if required. Immunotherapy with plasma exchange, intravenous immunoglobulin, corticosteroids, or azathioprine may be used if the weakness is severe and unresponsive to less aggressive therapy. The orphan drug 3-4 diaminopyridine improves strength and lessons autonomic symptoms in most patients with LEMS (61).

As with myasthenia gravis, drugs that could adversely affect neuromuscular transmission should be avoided. These include the aminoglycosides, beta blockers, calcium channel blockers, and anti-arrhythmics such as quinine, quinidine, or procainamide. Neuromuscular blocking agents typically used during intubation have a exaggerated and prolonged effect in patients with LEMS.

## Myopathy

Except for the local invasion of myofascial structures, primary muscle dysfunction associated with cancer most often arises as a remote effect. The best known example is dermatomyositis. Some cancer therapies, particularly the corticosteroids, also can cause a myopathy. Myopathy should be suspected in the patient with progressive weakness, especially if proximal, and no sensory symptoms. Most myopathies are associated with an elevated creatinine phosphokinase (CK). Myopathy often can be confirmed by EMG, and a muscle biopsy may help to define the syndrome fully. Treatment usually involves primary therapy for the specific underlying disorder. There are few symptomatic therapies.

### Inflammatory Myopathies

Historically, there has been considerable confusion regarding the relationship between cancer and the inflammatory myopathies. Whereas some studies have demonstrated an increased incidence of neoplasm in patients with both polymyositis and dermatomyositis, others failed to find such a relationship. Currently, little evidence exists that either inclusion-body myositis or polymyositis is associated with cancer; however, there does appear to be an increased incidence of malignancy in patients with dermatomyositis, particularly among older patients. In a recent series, about 25% of patients with dermatomyositis had a known malignancy at presentation, or a malignancy was detected soon after the diagnosis of dermatomyositis (62).

The distinction between polymyositis and dermatomyositis is based on the presence or absence of the characteristic skin manifestations of dermatomyositis. These include a purplish (heliotrope) periorbital rash and a more widespread erythematous pruritic scaly rash over extensor surfaces and sun-exposed areas.

Dermatomyositis associated with malignancy usually responds to immunosuppressive therapy with oral corticosteroids, such as prednisone at 40 to 60 mg per day for at least 1 to 2 months, followed by a slow taper. The daily dose can be reduced by 5 mg every week until 30 mg per day, with further tapering at only 2.5 mg per week. Relapse frequently occurs after early or rapid reduction in steroid doses. Other immunosuppressive agents, including methotrexate, cyclophosphamide, chlorambucil, and azathiaprine, have been used, most typically in patients who do not respond to corticosteroids or cannot tolerate their side effects. Intravenous immunoglobulin at a total dose of 2 g/kg divided over several days also was recently demonstrated to be effective (63). Treatment of the underlying tumor also may result in improvement of the myositis (64).

### Cancer-related Muscle Necrosis

A rare rapidly progressive fatal muscle degeneration has been linked to small-cell lung cancer and to gastrointestinal, breast, and bladder cancers (65). This disorder presents with a rapidly progressive weakness that spreads from limbs to involve bulbar and respiratory muscles. Electrodiagnostic studies are typical for a myopathy. On muscle biopsy there is profound muscle-fiber necrosis with little or no inflammation. In general, no treatment has proven helpful.

### Carcinoid Tumor-associated Myopathy

Carcinoid tumors may cause muscle damage and progressive proximal weakness, perhaps related to the secretion of serotonin or other substances by the tumor (66). Most histopathologic changes are nonspecific, with preponderance of type I fiber and type II fiber atrophy. The symptoms sometimes improve with a serotonin antagonist such as cyproheptadine or methysergide.

### Steroid-induced Myopathy

Corticosteroids often produce myopathy, which can be progressive. The weakness typically has an insidious onset but may be sudden. Despite profound weakness, the serum CK is typically normal or only mildly elevated, and EMG may or may not reveal myopathic changes. Muscle biopsy may demonstrate the nonspecific finding of type II muscle-fiber atrophy. Necrosis and regenerating fibers are rarely seen. Susceptibility to steroid myopathy varies widely. Patients who develop significant cushingoid body

habitus seem to be more at risk (67). The fluorinated corticosteroids, such as dexamethasone, betamethasone, or triamsinolone, more often are implicated in the development of steroid myopathy.

Patients often improve with a reduction in the steroid dose. Strength in some patients who are receiving a fluorinated drug improves if therapy is changed to a nonfluorinated steroid, such as prednisone or hydrocortisone. Physical exercise also can help prevent muscle weakness and atrophy.

## SYMPTOMATIC TREATMENTS

If primary treatment of the oncologic or neuromuscular lesion is feasible and appropriate given the medical conditions and goals, it should be provided to halt or reverse neurological deficits and possibly provide some degree of symptom control. Symptomatic therapies are often needed as well and become the major interventions for those who cannot benefit from primary therapy.

### Pharmacologic

Aside from muscular cramps, symptoms involving the peripheral nervous system are predominately neuropathic in origin, specifically sensory loss, paresthesias, dysesthesias, or nondysesthetic pain. Pain is usually the most compelling symptom, and management can be challenging. Opioid drugs combined with nonopioid analgesics and adjuvant analgesic drugs are commonly administered. The adjuvant analgesics are particularly important in the treatment of neuropathic pain, which overall is less responsive to the opioids than other types of pain.

Occasional patients with refractory pain may be candidates for an anesthetic, neurostimulatory, or neurosurgical intervention. The decision to undertake an invasive therapy must carefully consider risk and benefit and relies on a comprehensive assessment of the patient.

Muscle cramps can be particularly troublesome in patients with cancer. Although cramps are often thought of as nonspecific, in reality they typically point to underlying neuromuscular or metabolic dysfunction. In a recent study of 50 cancer patients who complained of muscle cramps, examination and evaluation led to a specific etiology in 82% (68). Peripheral neuropathy was identified in 22 of the patients, nerve root or plexus lesions in 17 patients, and polymyositis in 2 patients. Hypomagnesemia was thought to account for the muscle cramps in one patient. Thus, muscle cramps typically mark the presence of an identifiable and often previously unsuspected neurologic disorder.

Cramps are most effectively eliminated by treating the underlying lesion. Unfortunately, in patients with cancer, this is rarely possible. Cramps occasionally may be successfully treated using muscle membrane stabilizing agents such as quinine, phenytoin, or carbemazepine. Quinine appears to most effective in treating nocturnal cramps, whereas phenytoin or carbemazepine should be used to treat daytime cramping. Strict attention to adequate hydration and electrolyte balance are also critical. Other agents, such as benzodiazepines, baclofen, anti-inflammatory agents, or narcotics, have not been effective, but their sedating effects may help patients sleep more readily.

The mainstay of pharmacologic treatment of neuropathic symptoms (e.g., dysesthesias, paresthesias, radiating pain, and so on) are neuroactive agents. The primary agents are tricyclic antidepressants and anticonvulsants (69,70). Less well studied are baclofen, the benzodiazepines, oral anesthetic agents, and alpha-adrenergic blockers.

The following are important principles for use: (a) to choose each medication carefully, considering both the intended effects and potential side effects; (b) always to start at a very low dose, increasing slowly every 3 to 5 days to allow patients to become tolerant to the side effects; and (c) to push the dose of each medication until the desired effect is achieved, side effects become unmanageable, or high therapeutic drug levels are obtained; (d) that these medications may require several weeks to reach their maximum efficacy.

## Rehabilitation

Rehabilitation should play an important role in the treatment of any neuromuscular complication of cancer. There is increasing evidence that monitored exercise can improve muscle strength and endurance while reducing the complications of joint contractures, disuse atrophy, joint stiffness, osteoporosis, and pain. In a study of 301 terminal cancer patients, an increase in the Barthel mobility index from 12 to 19 was achieved with a supervised program of rehabilitation in the hospice setting. The rehabilitation program was thought to be effective by most patients and their families. In another study, a supervised program of active resistance and endurance exercise was shown to maintain and even increase muscular strength in patients with neuromuscular disease (71). Although the special features of neuromuscular disease in cancer patients were not addressed specifically in these studies, it is reasonable to conclude that supervised rehabilitation efforts, particularly physical therapy, can be effective in maximizing the function of patients suffering from neuromuscular complications of cancer.

Over time, weakness can lead to contractures of the affected joint. Regular stretching exercises may prevent this complication. Splinting in a neutral position also may be needed to prevent contractures in the setting of severe weakness of any type. In addition to exercise, appropriate devises can increase patient function.

Orthotic braces may allow a weak joint to function more normally. For example, molded ankle-foot orthotics, which stabilize the ankle in neutral position and eliminate foot drop, can help a patient maintain ambulation.

Significant loss of proprioception often results in gait instability. A cane or walker can provide additional stability that often helps people to feel more secure. Walking should be encouraged, as gait tends to improve as the brain adapts to a reduced level of proprioceptive input. Use of a cane, walker, or even wheelchair should be encouraged to allow continued independence. Reduced sensation in the hands produces difficulty with fine manipulation, such as buttoning a shirt. Special devices can been created to improve head and finger function and are best evaluated and fitted by a trained occupational therapist.

Other techniques that may be of use for pain or other neuromuscular symptoms include heat (72), cold (73), massage (74), transcutaneous electrical nerve stimulation (TENS) (75), and acupuncture (76). The available literature is generally inconclusive about the efficacy of these therapies. Trials were recommended by a recent expert panel (77).

## Psychologic

Cognitive interventions, such as relaxation and imagery (78,79) distraction and reframing (80,81), hypnosis (82), and biofeedback (78) can be helpful in managing pain or improving function. Because the success of these techniques is highly dependent on the patient's ongoing commitment to use them, the clinician must endeavor to match patients with the technique that is best suited for the specific patient.

## SUMMARY

Through a logical approach guided by the physical examination and selected additional studies, the etiology of most neuromuscular complications of cancer can be determined. In many cases, therapy aimed at the specific etiology is effective, and symptomatic therapies always should be considered to enhance function and improve comfort. Although many of the neuromuscular manifestations of cancer lace effective primary therapy, significant palliation should be possible in most patients.

## REFERENCES

1. Brown MJ. Evaluating the perplexing neuropahthic patient. *Semin Neurol* 1987;7:1.
2. Dische S, Saunders MI, Lee ME, Adams GE, Flockart IR. Clinical testing of the radiosensitizer R0 7-0582: experience with multiple doses. *Br J Cancer* 1977;35:567.
3. Weiss HD, Walker MD, Wiernik PH. Neurotoxicity of commonly used antineoplastic agents. *N Engl J Med* 1974;291:71.

4. La Rocca RV, Meer J, Gilliat RW, et al. Suramin-induced polyneuropathy. *Neurology* 1990;40:954.

5. Baker WJ, Royer GL, Weiss RB. Cytarabine and neurologic toxicity. *J Clin Oncol* 1992;9:679.

6. Falkson G, van Dyk JJ, van Eeden EB, van der Merwe AM, van den Berg JA, Falkson HC. A clinical trial of the oral form of 4-demethyl-epipodophyllotoxin-*d*-ethylidene-glucoside. *Cancer* 1975;35:1141.

7. Patel SR, Forman AD. High-dose ifosfamide-induced exacerbation of peripheral neuropathy. *J Natl Cancer Inst* 1994;86:305.

8. Bird SJ, Kaji R, Mollman J. Sensory evoked potentials are a sensitive indicator of cisplatin neuropathy. *Neurology* 1989;39:263.

9. Mollman JE, Glover DJ, Hogan WM. Cisplatin neuropathy: risk factors, prognosis and protection by SR-2721. *Cancer* 1988;61:2192.

10. Casey EB, Jelliffe AM, LeQuesne PM, Millett YL. Vincristine neuropathy-Clinical and electrophysiological observations. *Brain* 1973;96:69.

11. Roelofs RI, Hrushesky W, Rogin J, Rosenberg L. Peripheral sensory neuropathy and cisplatin chemotherapy. *Neurology* 1984;34:934.

12. Cersosimo RJ. Cisplatin neurotoxicity. *Cancer Treat Rev* 1989;16:195.

13. New P. Neurotoxicity of taxotere. *Proc Am Assoc Cancer Res* 1993;34:233.

14. Donehower RC, Rowinsky EK. An overview of experience with Taxol in the U.S.A. *Cancer Treat Rev* 1993;19(suppl C):63.

15. Prineas J. Polyneuropathies of undetermined cause. *Acta Neurol Scand* 1970;40(suppl):1.

16. Sumi SM, Farrell DF, Knauss TA. Lymphoma and leukemia manifested by steroid responsive polyneuropathy. *Arch Neurol* 1983;40:577.

17. McLeod JG. Paraneoplastic neuropathies. In: Dyck PJ, Thomas PK, eds. *Peripheral neuropathy*. 3rd ed. Philadelphia: WB Saunders, 1993;1583.

18. McLeod JG. Peripheral neuropathy associated with lymphoma, leukemia, and polycythemia vera. In: Dyck PJ, Thomas PK, eds. *Peripheral neuropathy*. 3rd ed. Philadelphia: WB Saunders, 1993;1591.

19. Dawson DM, Hallett M, Millender LH. *Entrapment neuropathies*. 2nd ed. Boston: Little Brown, 1990;156.

20. Barron KD, Rowland LS, Zimmerman HM. Neuropathy with malignant tumor metastases. *J Nerv Ment Dis* 1960;131:10.

21. Oh SJ, Slaughter R, Harrell L. Paraneoplastic vasculitis neuropathy. A treatable neuropathy. *Muscle Nerve* 1991;14:152.

22. Vincent D, Dubas F, Hauw JJ, et al. Nerve and muscle microvasculitis in peripheral neuropathy: a remote effect of cancer? *J Neurol Neurosurg Psychiatry* 1986;49:1007.

23. Lisak RP, Mitchell M, Zweiman B, Orrechio E, Asbury AK. Guillain-Barré syndrome and Hodgkin's disease: three cases with immunological studies. *Ann Neurol* 1977;1:72.

24. Klingon DG. The Guillain-Barré syndrome associated with cancer. *Cancer* 1965;18:157.

25. Croft PB, Urich H, Wilkinson M. Peripheral neuropathy of sensorimotor type associated with malignant disease. *Brain* 1967;90:31.

26. Croft PB, Wilkinson M. The course and prognosis in some types of carcinomatous neuromyopathy. *Brain* 1969;92:1.

27. Kelly JJ, Kyle RA, Miles JM, O'Brien PC, Dyck PJ. The spectrum of peripheral neuropathy in myeloma. *Neurology* 1981;31:24.

28. Kelly JJ. Peripheral neuropathies associated with monoclonal proteins. *Muscle Nerve* 1985;8:138.

29. Kelly JJ, Kyle RA, Miles JM, Dyck PJ. Osteosclerotic myeloma and peripheral neuropathy. *Neurology* 1983;33:202.

30. Kelly JJ, Kyle RA, Obrien PC. The natural history of peripheral neuropathy in primary systemic amyloidosis. *Ann Neurol* 1979;6:1.

31. Walton, JN, Tomlinson BE, Pearce GW. Subacute "poliomyelitis" and Hodgkin's disease. *J Neurol Sci* 1968;6:435.

32. Rowland LP, Schneck SA. Neuromuscular disorders associated with malignant neoplastic diseases. *J Chronic Dis* 1963;16:777.

33. Younger DS, Rowland LP, Latov N, et al. Lymphoma, motor neuron diseases, and amyotrophic lateral sclerosis. *Ann Neurol* 1991;29:78.

34. Rosenfeld MR, Posner JB. Paraneoplastic motor neuron disease. *Adv Neurol* 1991;56:445.

35. Evans BK, Fagan C, Arnold T. Paraneoplastic motor neuron disease and renal cell carcinoma: improvement after nephrectomy. *Neurology* 1990;40:960.

36. Horwich MS, Cho L, Porro S, Posner JB. Subacute sensory neuropathy: a remote effect of carcinoma. *Ann Neurol* 1977;2:7.

37. Schold SC, Cho ES, Somasundaran M, Posner JB. Subacute motor neuronopathy: a remote effect of lymphoma. *Ann Neurol* 1979;5:271.

38. Dalmau J, Graus F, Rosenblum MK. Anti-Hu-associated paraneoplastic encephalomyelitis/sensory neuronopathy: a clinical study of 71 patients. *Medicine (Baltimore)* 1992;71:59.

39. Graus F, Ramon R. Paraneoplastic neuropathies. *Eur Neurol* 1993;33:279.

40. Graus F, Elkon KB, Cordon-Cardo C, Posner JB. Sensory neuronopathy and small cell lung cancer: antineuronal antibody that also reacts with the tumor. *Am J Med* 1986;80:45.

41. Wasserstrom W, Glass JP, Posner JB. Diagnosis and treatment of leptomeningeal metastases from solid tumors: Experience with 90 patients. *Cancer* 1982;49:759.

42. Posner JB. *Neurologic complications of cancer*. Philadelphia: FA Davis, 1995;158. (Contemporary Neurology Series; vol 45).

43. Grant R, Naylor B, Greenberg HS. Clinical outcome in aggressively treated meningeal carcinomatosis. *Arch Neurol* 1994;51:457.

44. Lachance DH, O'Neill BP, Harper CM, Banks PM, Cascino TL. Paraneoplastic brachial plexopathy in a patient with Hodgkin's disease. *Mayo Clin Proc* 1991;66:97.

45. Vecht CJ. Arm pain in the patient with brest cancer. *J Pain Sympt Manag* 1990;5:109.

46. Chad DA, Bradley WG. Lumbosacral plexopathy. *Semin Neurol* 1987;37:97–104.

47. Castellanos AM, Glass JP, Yung WK. Regional nerve injury after intraarterial chemotherapy. *Neurology* 1987;37:834–837.

48. Lederman RJ, Wilbourn AJ. Brachial plexopathy: recurrent cancer or radiation? *Neurology* 1984;34:1331.

49. Roth G, Magistris MR, Le-Fort D, Desjacques P, Della Santa D. Post-radiation brachial plexopathy: persistent conduction block. Myokymic discharges and cramps. *Rev Neurol* 1988;144:173.

50. Payne R, Foley K. Exploration of the brachial plexus in patients with cancer. *Neurology* 1986;36(suppl):329.

51. Kline DG, Kott J, Barnes G, Bryant L. Exploration of selected brachial plexus lesions by the posterior subscapular approach. *J Neurosurg* 1978;49:872.

52. Kori S, Foley KM, Posner JB. Brachial plexus lesions in patients with cancer: 100 cases. *Neurology* 1981;31:45.

53. Thomas JE, Colby MY. Radiation-induced or metastatic brachial plexopathy? A diagnostic dilemma. *JAMA* 1972;222:1392.

54. Bagley FH, Walsh JW, Cady B, Salzman FA, Oberfield RA, Pazianos AG. Carcinomatous versus radiation-induced brachial plexus neuropathy in breast cancer. *Cancer* 1978;41:2154.

55. Jaeckle KA, Young DF, Foley KM. The natural history of lumbosacral plexopathy in cancer. *Neurology* 1985;35:8.

56. Evans RJ, Watson CPN. Lumbosacral plexopathy in cancer patients. *Neurology* 1985;35:1392.

57. O'Neill JH, Murray NMF, Newsom-Davis J. The Lambert-Easton myasthenic syndrome: a review of 50 cases. *Brain* 1988;111:577.

58. Sanders DB. Lambert-Eaton myasthenic sysndrome: Pathogenesis and treatment. *Semin Neurol* 1994;14:111.

59. Jenkyn LR, Brooks PL, Forcier RJ, Maurer LH, Ochoa J. Remission of the Lambert-Eaton myasthenic syndrome and small cell anaplastic carcinoma of the lung induced by chemotherapy and radiotherapy. *Cancer* 1980;46:1123.

60. Chalk CH, Murray NM, Newsom-Davis J, O'Neill JH, Spiro SG. Response of the Lambert-Eaton myasthenic syndrome to treatment of associated small-cell lung carcinoma. *Neurology* 1990;40:1552.

61. Sanders DB, Howard JF, Massey JM. 3,4-Diaminopyridine in Lambert-eaton myasthenic syndrome and myasthenia gravis. *Ann NY Acad Sci* 1993;681:588.

62. Callen JP. Myositis and malignancy. *Curr Opin Rheumatol* 1994;6:590.

63. Dalakas MC, Illa I, Dambrosia JM, et al. A controlled trial of high dose intravenous immune globuline infusions as treatment for dermatomyositis. *N Engl J Med* 1994;329:1993.

64. Cox NH, Lawrence CM, Langtry JAA, Ire FA. Dermatomyositis. *Arch Dermatol* 1990;126:61.

65. Brownell B, Hughes JT. Degeneration of muscle in association with carcinoma of the bronchus. *J Neurol Neurosurg Psychiatry* 1975;38:363.

66. Swash M, Fox KP, Davidson AR. Carcinoid myopathy: Serotonin-induced muscle weakness in man. *Arch Neurol* 1975;32:572.

67. Khaleeli AA, Edwards RHT, Gohil K, et al. Corticosteroid myopathy: a clinical and pathologic study. *Clin Endorinol* 1983;18:155.

68. Steiner I, Siegal T. Muscle cramps in cancer patients. *Cancer* 1989;63:574.

69. Ventafridda V, Bonezzi C, Caraceni A, et al. Antidepressants for cancer

pain and other painful syndromes with deafferation component: comparison of amitriptyline and trazodone. *Ital J Neurol Sci* 1987;8:579.

70. Yajnik S, Singh GP, Singh G, Kumar M. Phenytoin as a coanalgesic in cancer pain. *J Pain Symt Manag* 1992;7:209.

71. Vignos PJ. Physical models of rehabilitation in neuromuscular disease. *Muscle Nerve* 1983;6:323.

72. Lehman JF, de Lateur BJ. Therapeutic heat. In: Lehman JF, ed. *Therapeutic heat and cold.* 4th ed. Baltimore: Williams and Wilkins, 1990; 417.

73. Vasudevan S, Hegmann K, Moore A, Cerletty S. Physical methods of pain management. In: Raj PP, ed. *Practical management of pain.* 2nd ed. Baltimore: Mosby Year Book Medical Publishers, 1992;669.

74. McCaffery M, Wolf M. Pain relief using cutaneous modalities, positioning, and movement. *Hospice J* 1992;8:121.

75. Avellanosa AM, West CR. Experience with transcutaneous electrical nerve stimulation for the relief of intractable pain in cancer patients. *J Med* 1982;13:203.

76. Patel M, Gutzwiller F, Paccaud F, Marazzi A. A meta-analysis of acupuncture for chronic pain. *Int J Epidemiol* 1989;18:900.

77. Jacox A, Carr DB, Payne R. *Management of cancer pain.* Clinical Practice Guideline No. Rockville, MD: Agency for Health Care Policy and Research, U.S. Department of Health and Human Services, Public Health Service, 1994:

78. McCaffery M, Beebe A. *Pain: clinical manual for nursing practice.* St. Louis: CV Mosby, 1989;130.

79. Graffam S, Johnson A. A comparison of two relaxation strategies for the relief of pain and its distress. *J Pain Sympt Manag* 1987;2:229.

80. Beck SL. The therapeutic use of music for cancer-related pain. *Oncol Nurs Forum* 1991;18:1327.

81. McCaul KD, Malott JM. Distraction and coping with pain. *Psychol Bull* 1984;95:516.

82. Spiegel D, Bloom JR, Kraemer HC, Gottheil E. Effect of psychosocial treatment of survival of patients with metastatic breast cancer. *Lancet* 1989;2:888.

*Principles and Practice of Supportive Oncology,*
edited by Ann Berger et al.
Lippincott–Raven Publishers, Philadelphia ©1998

CHAPTER 36

# Delirium

Jane M. Ingham and Augusto T. Caraceni

Delirium has been defined as a transient organic brain syndrome characterized by the acute onset of disordered attention and cognition and accompanied by disturbances of psychomotor behavior and perception (1). It is highly prevalent in the medically ill and has been associated with a wide range of etiologic factors. Given data from studies in other medical populations (2,3), it is likely that delirium is underrecognized by medical and nursing staff in the oncology setting. Unless promptly reversed, this condition can increase family distress and precipitate conflict between staff and families (4). The presence of delirium has been shown to prolong hospital stay and increase mortality (5,6). Those caring for oncology patients must be cognizant of the prevalence and phenomenology of delirium, and be able to initiate and monitor appropriate treatment interventions.

## TERMINOLOGY

The study of mental status changes in patients with cancer and other illnesses has been hampered by a lack of consistency in terminology. A plethora of terms have been used to describe the clinical syndrome consistent with delirium. The *Diagnostic and Statistical Manual of Mental Disorders (DSM-IV)* of the American Psychiatric Association (7) provides the current gold standard for syndrome definition in psychiatry. This document provides the definition that will be utilized throughout this chapter. Delirium is considered to be a single nosologic entity (8), and the *DSM-IV* proposes specific diagnostic criteria for its diagnosis (Table 1). Although the earlier *DSM-III-R* criteria had classified delirium as one of the organic brain syndromes (9), this classification was seen to imply that other psychiatric illnesses had no biologi-

cal correlates. To correct this apparent anomaly, the term "organic brain syndromes" was revised in the *DSM-IV,* which classifies delirium in the category entitled "Delirium, Dementia and Amnestic and Other Cognitive Disorders" (7).

The diagnostic criteria for delirium have evolved over time, yet the term "delirium" is frequently used without adherence to these criteria. In the past, for example, delirium has been used to describe conditions linked to febrile states characterized by agitation and associated with perceptual abnormalities, clouding of consciousness, and disorientation (10). In addition, other terms, particularly "confusion" and "encephalopathy," have been widely utilized in the clinical setting to describe the mental status changes that would fulfill the criteria for delirium. The French literature described the phenomena found in these states as "oneirism" or "oneiric consciousness," with the most striking case of a confused oneiric state being delirium tremens due to alcohol withdrawal.

The terms "encephalopathy" and "acute confusional state" have been used by neurologists to describe acute changes in mental status (11,12). These terms are applied in lieu of the psychiatric classification based on the *DSM* criteria. As a consequence, a dichotomous tendency exists between the psychiatric and neurologic literature. This dualism is usually only semantic. The *DSM* classification criteria are preferred because they have the advantage of defining the essential features of the syndrome (see below) while leaving open the door to further classifying clinical and pathophysiologic subtypes.

In the clinical setting, the imprecise terminology has been compounded by a lack of understanding of the important distinction between symptoms and pathologic processes or diagnoses. Symptom are subjective "physical or mental phenomena . . . accompanying a disorder and constituting evidence for it" (13). When used to describe a subjective experience "confusion" is a symptom. When used by medical and nursing staff to describe a patient's mental state, however, the term is a broad

J. M. Ingham: Lombardi Cancer Center, Georgetown University Medical Center, Washington, DC 20007.

A. T. Caraceni: Pain Therapy and Palliative Care Division, National Cancer Institute of Milano, 20133 Milano, Italy.

**TABLE 1.** *Criteria for diagnosing delirium: DSM-IV*

A. Disturbance of consciousness with reduced ability to focus, sustain or shift attention
B. Change in cognition (such as memory deficit, disorientation, language disturbances, or perception disturbances) that is not better accounted for by preexisting, established, or evolving dementia
C. The disturbance develops over a short period of time (usually hours to days) and tends to fluctuate during the course of the day
D. There is evidence from the history, physical examination, or laboratory findings that the disturbance is caused by the direct physiological consequences of a general medical condition

Adapted from ref 7.

descriptor that is neither a symptom nor a diagnosis. It should never be used synonymously with the diagnosis of delirium. "Confusion" has no diagnostic specificity and may characterize numerous disease states including both delirium and dementia. Given evidence of confusion, a clinician should consider a detailed clinical examination to facilitate a diagnosis for the mental status change and to seek out etiologic factors.

The problems with inconsistent terminology that have characterized both the study of delirium and its diagnosis in the clinical setting may be minimized by the use of *DSM* criteria. Instruments have been developed based on these criteria that facilitate the diagnosis and allow the monitoring of the syndrome (see below). As further research efforts are directed to delirium, it may be that the diagnostic criteria will be further refined. Although the *DSM* criteria for delirium are now considered the gold standard for diagnosis, these criteria and the DSM-IV-classified disorders are reflections of a consensus of the formulations of current knowledge in psychiatry. This is an evolving field, and the classification is likely to evolve further and indeed may, as it exists now, not encompass all conditions that may be legitimate targets for treatment or research.

## PATHOPHYSIOLOGY OF DELIRIUM

Delirium is an altered mental state characterized by altered alertness and impaired cognition that has been described by Engels and Romano as a syndrome of cerebral insufficiency (14). It is considered to be a stereotyped response of the brain to a spectrum of differing insults and has been viewed as a state on the continuum between normal wakefulness and stupor and coma. The number of possible etiologies, including head trauma, metabolic abnormalities, and innumerable drugs, suggests the existence of a final common pathway with diverse inciting pathophysiologies. An alternative interpretation is that each of the clinical subtypes of delirium is a final common pathway for a set of etiologies or pathophysiologies that share characteristics. The current state of knowledge regarding the pathogenesis of delirium has been most comprehensively reviewed by Trzepacz (15).

Anatomically, it is known that both subcortical and cortical structures are important in the development of the syndrome (15). Any pathologic process that, either structurally or functionally, affects most or all of the cortical mantle may modify the level of consciousness (16). This mechanism of diffuse damage or dysfunction is likely to play a part in the pathophysiology of many cases, particularly in delirium triggered by metabolic dysfunction.

Some specific brain structures have also been implicated in the pathogenesis of delirium (15). These include the brainstem nuclei and tracts that subserve normal wakefulness and the regulation of the sleep–wake cycle (17), as well as hypothalamic-cortical pathways (18). Mesulam et al. observed that right-sided cerebral infarcts are more often associated with delirium (19). The prefrontal, orbital, and nondominant parietal regions, and the thalamic and hippocampal structures, are also likely to be important structures (15).

Abnormalities in cerebral blood flow have been described in delirium, although the etiologic implications of these observations are uncertain (15). A reduction in cortical flow has been demonstrated in subclinical hepatic encephalopathy (20) and in posttraumatic delirium (21). Cerebral blood flow has been reported to be globally increased in delirium tremens (22).

Many neurotransmitters have been implicated in the pathogenesis of delirium (15). For example, abnormalities in cholinergic neurotransmission have been implicated in the pathophysiology of many different forms of delirium. It has been postulated that a reduction of acetylcholine synthesis and release may unify many clinical observations in etiologically diverse forms of delirium (15). Other neurotransmitters have also been tentatively implicated in specific types of delirium (15). For example, overstimulation of the $\tau$-aminobutyric acid (GABA) system has been linked to hepatic failure encephalopathy and benzodiazepine intoxication; GABA system understimulation may relate to benzodiazepine and alcohol withdrawal; N-methyl-D-aspartate (NMDA) receptor blockade could be involved in phencyclidine delirium; serotonin antagonism could be a causal factor in *d*-lysergic acid dimethylamide (LSD) hallucinations and delirium; and dopaminergic overactivity has been considered a cause of hyperactive deliria (15).

These diverse associations further suggest the existence of a final common metabolic and cellular pathway for delirium (23). Hypoglycemia, hypoxia, ischemia, and other insults may affect oxidative metabolism and induce profound changes in the cholinergic system. Such insults potentially also impact on the function of other neurotransmitters including dopamine and glutamate. These changes may occur in association with conditions that predispose to delirium, including nutritional cofactor deficiencies (e.g., thiamine), aging processes, and disease states such as Alzheimer's disease. The cellular link between neurotransmitter deficiency, altered brain metabolism, and the clinical manifestations of delirium is postulated to be based on abnormalities of the second messenger systems such as calcium, cyclic GMP, and the phosphatidylinositol cascade (23).

It is clear that there is a need for a greater understanding of the pathophysiology of delirium. As such an understanding evolves, it may in time allow the development of treatment strategies aimed at specific abnormalities in second messenger systems, neurotransmitters, or other abnormalities.

## ELECTROPHYSIOLOGY OF DELIRIUM

The electroencephalogram (EEG) of patients with delirium, regardless of the etiology of the delirium, demonstrates a generalized symmetric slowing of the EEG with reduction of the alpha rhythm and an increase in delta and theta frequencies (14). These changes are not dissimilar to those found in stages of the sleep pattern. In general, the degree of EEG slowing correlates with decrease in arousal. In some conditions, EEG fast wave activity, beta activity, is also present (24). This activity is more prevalent in delirium characterized by hyperactive phenomena, such as delirium tremens.

Recent studies have suggested that EEG techniques may be useful in the study of delirium, clarifying the differential diagnosis and severity, and providing a better method for serial monitoring (25–28). EEG findings, specifically decreased alpha and increased delta and theta frequencies, have been demonstrated to correlate with low Mini-Mental State Examination scores in delirious patients (26,27). In these investigations the reduction of alpha rhythm, demonstrated using quantitative spectral analysis techniques, was particularly useful in diagnosing delirium whereas the pattern of theta and delta waves was more useful in differentiating dementia from delirium. The utility of EEG in the differential diagnosis of delirium has also been demonstrated in the differentiation of nonconvulsive status epilepticus from delirium and several specific diagnostic entities. For example, the EEG associated with delirium produced by high-dose ifosfamide shows rhythmic complexes typical of seizure-like activity, in contrast to generalized symmetric slowing of the EEG considered to be typical of other types of delirium (29).

Evoked potential techniques have seldom been applied to the study of delirium (15). Abnormalities of brainstem acoustic responses and visual evoked potentials have been observed in hepatic encephalopathy (30). Long latency evoked potentials, which are influenced by cognitive processes, can be an interesting tool for exploring the early manifestations of delirium, pattern of recovery, and therapeutic interventions. These potentials have been used in identifying subclinical encephalopathy in liver transplant candidates (30), interleukin administration (31), and in recovery from head trauma (32).

## PREVALENCE AND INCIDENCE OF DELIRIUM

In hospitalized medical and surgical patients, the prevalence of delirium is approximately 10% (5,10,33). In hospitalized cancer patients, the prevalence ranges from 8% to 40% (34–36). A higher prevalence, reaching as high as 50% in some studies, has been demonstrated in specific subpopulations, including the elderly, patients in the postoperative period, patients presenting to the emergency room, and patients in the terminal phase of illness (5,10,36–40). With the exception of several studies in the terminally ill (36,37), studies specifically exploring the prevalence of delirium have not been undertaken in the population with malignant disease.

Although small numbers of patients have been studied in the setting of terminal illness related to cancer, the incidence of delirium has been even less widely investigated than its prevalence, particularly in the oncology setting (36,37,41). In a review of 26 relevant and valid studies on postoperative delirium, Bitondo Dyer et al. concluded that the overall incidence was almost 36.8%, with wide variation (0–73.5%) (38). Similar variability in the incidence of delirium (14–56%) has been reported in hospitalized, medically ill, elderly patients (5,33,42–44).

Clinical experience suggests that the risk of delirium varies during the course of a disease, including cancer. The incidence of delirium is likely to be relatively high during episodes of sepsis; postoperatively; when multiple drugs are administered, including chemotherapeutic agents, opioids, and anticholinergics; and in the terminal phases of illness. In the oncology setting, two studies have reported on delirium and/or cognitive failure and demonstrated that these entities developed in over 80% of cancer patients nearing death (37,41). One study, which did not use strict criteria for diagnosis of delirium, suggested that the incidence of delirium in patients after surgery for head and neck cancer was 9–25% (45).

The reported variation in the prevalence and incidence of delirium reflects differences in the diagnostic criteria and variation in the populations studied. Although the studies cited previously specifically sought to define cases of delirium, delirium may appear to be less prevalent in the clinical setting than the reports would suggest. The most likely factor contributing to this perception is underdiagnosis. It is well documented that the symptoms of delirium are frequently attributed to other disorders or, alternatively, not observed at all (2,3,46,47). In the emergency room setting, for example, one study demonstrated that only 6% of delirium diagnoses were detected by the emergency room physician (47). In a series of elderly medical patients, the physicians' diagnoses correctly identified only 8 of 47 patients as being delirious or acutely confused (3).

## PREDISPOSING, PREDICTIVE, AND ETIOLOGIC FACTORS IN DELIRIUM

The sociodemographic and disease-related factors that may predispose to delirium or predict its occurrence have not been documented in cancer patients. The studies that have investigated delirium in the oncology setting have generally sought to address the spectrum and prevalence of a range of psychiatric diagnoses rather than to address factors involved in specific diagnoses, such as delirium (34–36). As a consequence, the number of delirious cancer patients that has been studied has not been large enough to allow investigators to draw conclusions that relate to predictive factors.

Although there is a paucity of studies in the cancer population and further research is needed in this area, studies that have explored delirium in the hospitalized elderly and in patients prior to surgery may have some application in the cancer population. This is particularly so given that a high proportion of cancer patients are elderly and many undergo surgery. Unfortunately, many of the studies of delirium predictors have significant methodologic limitations. In some studies, for example, standardized validated instruments were not used for delirium diagnosis. Other studies failed to distinguish baseline vulnerability and precipitating factors. Inouye and Charpentier have proposed a multifactorial model for delirium in the hospitalized elderly that may be relevant in the cancer population (33,40). The model involves the interaction between "baseline vulnerability" and "precipitating factors or insults" (Fig. 1) (40). In this model, baseline vulnerability is defined by the predisposing factors present at the time of admission to hospital, and the precipitating factors are the noxious insults that occurred during hospitalization. Patients who have a high baseline vulnerability may develop delirium with any precipitating factor, whereas those with a low baseline vulnerability will be more resistant to the development of delirium, even with noxious insults.

The factors that Inouye et al. specifically demonstrated to be contributory to baseline vulnerability in the elderly include visual impairment, severe illness, cognitive impairment, and an elevated serum urea nitrogen/creatinine ratio of 18 or greater (48). Other studies have implicated risk factors including: each of the aforementioned factors, age, dementia, depression, alcohol abuse, the preoperative use of anticholinergic drugs, poor functional status, and markedly abnormal preoperative serum sodium, potassium, or glucose levels (38,42,49–53). Cer-

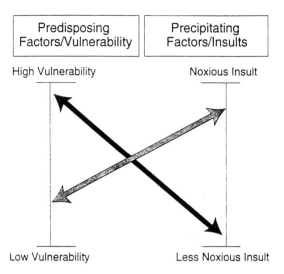

**FIG. 1.** Multifactorial model of delirium. The development of delirium involves a complex interrelationship between baseline patient vulnerability (line to left) and precipitating factors or insults (line to right). For example, a patient with low vulnerability would require noxious insults to develop delirium (gray arrow.) Conversely, a highly vulnerable patient may develop delirium even with relatively trivial insults (black arrow). Reproduced with permission from: Figure 1 in Inouye, S.K. Charpentier, P.A. Precipitating factors for delirium in hospitalized elderly persons: Predictive model and interrelationship with baseline vulnerability. JAMA 275(11): 852-857, 1996.

tain medications have also been implicated as risk factors for delirium, including neuroleptics, opioids, and anticholinergic drugs (42,50,54).

Several authors have suggested predictive models for the stratification of patients at risk for delirium (40,45,48, 51,52). The Inouye et al. predictive model for elderly hospitalized patients is based on the four baseline vulnerability factors (discussed above) and five precipitating factors (the use of physical restraints, malnutrition, more than three medications added, use of a bladder catheter, and any iatrogenic event) (40,48). Although the precipitating factors may not in themselves represent the "cause" of delirium, each may reflect an array of risk factors. Such "risk" may be a consequence of the factor's direct effect on cerebral function; or it may relate to the fact that the presence of the factor increases the likelihood of other delirium precipitants or risks also being present, including immobility or infection. Precipitating factors occurred during hospitalization, whereas baseline factors were present at admission to hospital. The precipitating and baseline vulnerability factors were shown to be highly interrelated and contributory to delirium development in independent, substantive, and cumulative ways (40).

Other authors have attempted to define predictive models in the elderly and in surgical populations based, for the most part, on the admission characteristics of patients rather than on in-hospital events (40,45,48,51, 52). In one of the few studies undertaken in oncology patients, Weed et al. sought to define a method of preoperative identification of patients at risk for delirium after major head and neck cancer surgery (45). In this study, the defined criteria included factors related to age, alcohol abuse, cognitive impairment, biochemical abnormalities, and function. Although these may indeed be valid predictive factors, the study methodology did not use strict criteria for the definition of delirium.

In cancer patients the potential etiologies of delirium, as distinct from "risk factors," may be divided into direct effects related to tumor involvement and indirect effects (Table 2) (55). The latter category includes drugs, electrolyte imbalance, cranial irradiation, organ failure, nutritional deficiencies, vascular complications, paraneoplastic syndromes, and many other factors (55–61). No large prospective survey has assessed the relative contributions of these factors. A survey of cancer patients referred initially for a neurology consultation demonstrated a multifactorial etiology in most of the 94 patients with encephalopathy. The average number of contributing factors in each patient was 4.62. Metabolic causes were found to be contributory in 89% of patients and were the primary cause in 44%. Medications were contributory in 97% of cases, but the primary cause in only 29%. Bacteremia was only documented in 4%, but 50% of patients had fever and evidence of systemic infection. Disseminated intravascular coagulation was a contributing factor in 11%. Central nervous system metastases were found in 32% and were a major cause in all of these patients. Another report establishes delirium as a possible complication of leptomeningeal disease (63).

Drug interactions and metabolic failure (especially renal impairment) can produce unexpected toxicities especially in the patient with advanced disease (64–66). Potentially reversible factors, which are often underestimated in this population, include dehydration (67), borderline renal function, and the accumulation of opioid metabolites (68,69).

## MENTAL STATUS CHANGES AND CLINICAL APPLICATIONS OF DIAGNOSTIC CRITERIA

Investigators have proposed two theoretical models of mental status change to explain the clinical manifestations of delirium. One model suggests a homogeneous deterioration of cognitive functions (10) and the other, based on the studies by Chedru and Geschwind, suggests that the cognitive deficits are secondary to attention failure (70–72). The latter theory suggests that common clinical features—distortion and disorganization of memories, orientation, thinking, and language—occur due to an abnormal attention matrix and that the cognitive performances with the highest attentional demand, including language and writing abilities, are likely to be the most affected. Although in the clinical setting disturbed attention failure is a prominent feature of the syndrome and is considered to be among the essential criteria for diagnosing delirium (see Table 1) (7), the variety and intensity of symptoms suggests that regional areas of the brain are likely to be functioning abnormally and contributing to the clinical picture (15). The common clinical features of delirium are listed in Table 3.

**TABLE 2.** *Causes of delirium in cancer patients*

Primary tumors of the nervous system
Metastases to the central nervous system
    Cerebral tumor
    Leptomeningeal tumor
Nonmetastatic complications of cancer
    Metabolic encephalopathy due to organ failure
    Other metabolic disturbances:
        Electrolyte imbalance including disturbances of sodium, calcium, and others
        Hypo- or hyperglycemia
    Infection
    Hematologic abnormalities
    Nutritional deficiencies
    Paraneoplastic syndromes
    Vasculitic processes
Treatment side effects from:
    chemotherapeutic agents:
    steroids
    radiation
    opioids
    anticholinergics
    antiemetics
    other medications

Adapted from refs 59 and 129.

**TABLE 3.** *Delirium symptoms*

Insomnia and daytime somnolence
Nightmares
Restlessness, agitation
Irritability
Distractibility
Hypersensitivity to light and sound
Anxiety
Difficulty in marshaling our own thoughts
Concentration difficulty
Fleeting illusions, hallucinations, and delusions
Emotional lability
Attention deficits
Memory disturbances

Several of the characteristic clinical features of delirium contribute to the tendency to underdiagnose the condition. For example, the symptoms and signs fluctuate and the diagnosis may be overlooked if careful attention is not given to the changes in mental status examination over time. Additionally, subtle changes frequently precede the onset of delirium. These minor symptoms and behavioral changes may go unnoticed, only to be recalled later in family or staff interviews. Even when the symptoms of delirium are most apparent, the fact that these symptoms are highly prevalent in advanced cancer (73–75) contributes to diagnostic confusion. A patient with cancer may, for example, be restless, anxious, depressed, irritable, angry, or emotionally labile. Clinicians must be cognizant of the fact that these symptoms are not specific for a diagnosis. The spectrum of symptoms must be assessed because in isolation each may be a manifestation of an adjustment disorder, may represent a symptom of delirium, or may be a consequence of any

of a large number of conditions, including dementia (Table 4). Finally, although most patients have disturbances in multiple aspects of cognition and behavior, the highly variable clinical manifestations of the syndrome result in significant interpatient variability.

In the early stages of delirium, some patients experience an isolated disturbance that may be related to an organic cause that alone may not fulfill the criteria for a diagnosis of delirium. Findings frequently include daytime somnolence with nighttime insomnia, and subtle mood and personality changes (see Table 3). For example, a patient may experience hallucinations or a mood disturbance in the absence of any other evidence of cognitive dysfunction. Such problems must be fully assessed and monitored over time. If other disturbances occur later, the criteria for a diagnosis of delirium may then be met.

Although the clinical presentation of delirium is often extremely varied, the diagnosis can be established on the basis of new-onset disturbances involving cognition, affective state, perception, or arousal and responsiveness. Table 1 outlines the specific *DSM-IV* criteria for diagnosis of delirium and each of these criteria must be met for diagnosis.

The first of the *DSM* diagnostic criteria for delirium relates to disturbance of consciousness and impaired attention. This disturbance can be highly variable, characterized by increased or decreased arousal, or merely by distractibility and reduced responsiveness. Three clinical variants of delirium have been described based on the type of arousal disturbance: hypoalert-hypoactive, hyperalert-hyperactive, and mixed type (with fluctuations from hypoalert to hyperalert) (76,77). The hypoactive form is characterized by lethargy and appears to be associated

**TABLE 4.** *Differential features of delirium, dementia, and psychosis*

| Characteristics | Delirium | Dementia | Psychosis |
|---|---|---|---|
| Onset | Sudden | Insidious | Sudden |
| Course over 24 hr | Fluctuating with nocturnal exacerbations | Stable | Stable |
| Consciousness | Reduced | Clear | Clear |
| Attention | Globally disordered | Normal except in severe cases | May be disordered |
| Cognition | Globally disordered | Globally impaired | May be selectively impaired |
| Hallucinations | Visual or visual and auditory | Often absent | Auditory |
| Delusions | Fleeting, poorly systematized | Often absent | Sustained and systematized |
| Orientation | Usually impaired at least for time | Often impaired | May be impaired |
| Psychomotor activity | Increased, reduced or shifting unpredictably | Often normal | Retarded or hyperactive depending on type of psychosis |
| Speech | Often incoherent, slow or rapid | Difficulty in finding words, perseveration | Normal, slow or rapid |
| Involuntary movements | Often asterixis or coarse tremor | Often absent | Usually absent |
| EEG | Abnormal, fast or slow | Often abnormal slow | Normal |

Adapted from ref 77.

with less "positive" clinical phenomena than the hyperactive form, which is often accompanied by hallucinations, delusions, and illusions. In one study, 15% of cases presented hyperactive delirium, 19% had the hypoactive form, 52% had mixed forms, and 14% had neither (76).

Although few studies have explored the variation in arousal, it has been suggested that this aspect of delirium phenomenology may be related to specific etiologic factors. For example, a small study of patients with hepatic encephalopathy found that those patients were more likely to be hypoalert or somnolent than those in whom fever was the main etiologic factor. In the latter group, patients were equally likely to have a somnolent (hypoalert) or a hyperactive (hyperalert) delirium (78). This study demonstrated a trend toward a hyperactive delirium in patients with alcohol withdrawal, an observation that is consistent with clinical experience. Except in cases of alcohol-related delirium, a definite relationship between etiology and clinical subtypes has not been consistently supported by neurodiagnostic studies (15). To date, no study has specifically described the phenomenology of delirium in cancer patients. Nonetheless, the diagnosis of delirium may be overlooked if the existence of differing phenomenologic subtypes, particularly the less apparent hypoactive delirium, is not recognized.

Specific attention disturbances are manifest not only by the level of arousal but also by changes in the patient's ability to concentrate, which can be subtle. Attention disturbances may be evidenced by an inability to maintain a conversation or to attend to its flow. Concentration may be assessed using a variety of assessment instruments for delirium (discussed below). The Mini-Mental State Examination (79), for example, contains a specific question that seeks to define the patient's ability to concentrate by assessing the ability to subtract serial 7's or to spell the word *world* backward. Although specific assessment of concentration is an invaluable tool in the clinical evaluation of mental status, it is important to recognize that apparent abnormalities of attention that may be influenced by language skills, hearing deficits, and other abilities or impairments (80,81).

The second *DSM* criterion for delirium relates to the presence of changed cognition, e.g., disorientation, memory deficits, and disturbances of language, reasoning, and perception. It is important to recognize that a diagnosis of delirium may be established in the presence of any one of these cognitive abnormalities. For example, a patient who is not disoriented may still fulfill the criteria for a diagnosis of delirium if he or she is experiencing memory, language, or perceptual disturbances.

Orientation to time, place, and persons is one of the features most commonly associated with the syndrome. Although other features are also common, the perception that the prevalence of disorientation is high may, in part, be a consequence of the ease with which it is assessed.

Clinical experience suggests that orientation in time is the first to be affected (10). Patients who are disoriented frequently locate themselves in a known space, e.g., in a familiar hospital or house. Recognition of family and self is usually preserved whereas the ability to recognize less well-known people, such as housestaff, is often lost. This hierarchical organization of person, space, and time orientation has also been observed in other conditions, such as the progressive recovery from electroshock (82).

Memory is another aspect of cognition that is often affected. Impairments in short-term memory are most probably due to the presence of attention failure. Remote memory can also be affected and more familiar memories appear to be retained more commonly than others; for example, patients frequently lose the ability to recall presidents' names before the name of their hometown (70). In addition to memory loss, memories may be disrupted and disorganized, with paramnesias and duplications (83).

Language abnormalities are frequently present in delirium and are often compounded by the presence of incoherent reasoning. Language may lack fluency and spontaneity, and conversation may be prolonged and interrupted by long pauses or repetitions. The language may reflect an inability to find the correct word or to name objects (anomia) and may be characterized by "passepartout" words (nonspecific phrases that substitute for specific language, e.g., "you know what I mean"), stereotypes, and cliches. The general meaning of speech may be lost due to incoherence or the patient's inability to sustain attention. Geschwind and Chedru have provided a series of unique observations on the neuropsychology of delirium and demonstrated that writing abilities are affected early and more severely than other language-related skills (84). This aspect of the neurologic dysfunction can be useful in both the diagnosis and study of delirium. For this abnormality to be fully appreciated, it is optimal to have skilled interpretation of a substantial number of written words rather than simply a short written phrase.

Delirium may affect reasoning in complex ways. As the ability to reason and to think in the abstract requires intact attention, this aspect of cognition may be most difficult to evaluate. Nonetheless, patients frequently demonstrate irrelevant or rambling thinking, abnormal conceptualization, and altered insight with anosognosia (85).

Perceptual abnormalities may be more prevalent in particular delirium subtypes, such as delirium tremens. In some cases, these perceptions may be frightening and associated with agitated behavior. In one series of delirious medical and surgical patients, 24% experienced hallucinations, 18% delusions, and 9% illusions (78). Illusions and hallucinations usually involve visual phenomena although auditory and tactile features may also be present.

Delusions may be associated with hallucinations. These delusions are frequently poorly organized and characterized by paranoid features, which may incorporate themes that relate, for example, to homicide, imprisonment, or jealousy. Occupational delusions are among the most common with the patient locating himself or herself in a familiar time and space and attending to usual activities. Lipowski describes "the law of the unfamiliar mistaken for the familiar" (10) and suggests that perceptions are influenced by the emotional color of the situation and the patient's personality characteristics. For example, doctors around the bed may be perceived to be ghosts announcing death. It has been observed that some patients may manifest similar delusional themes in more than one episode of delirium and in episodes triggered by different etiologic factors (10,86).

Although they are not among the diagnostic criteria, affective disturbances may characterize delirium. Such disturbances range from dysphoria to hypomania. The prevailing emotion of patients with delirium is probably anxiety (86). When insight is lost mood often appears to be depressed and apathetic. The patient may suffer from his or her own confusion and may painfully try to keep focused and to understand the disease process and the surrounding world. There may be emotional lability with fluctuating restlessness, irritability, anger, sadness, and anxiety. In the few available reports from patients recovering from delirium, the experience is usually described as a frightening, twilight dreamy state (10). Little is known about the associations that may exist between lack of insight, symptoms, and level of distress during episodes. A recent small study of 14 patients with cancer pain and severe cognitive failure found that during episodes of agitated cognitive failure, pain intensity as assessed by a nurse was significantly higher than the patient's assessment had been before and after the episode (4). Upon complete recovery, none of these patients recalled having had any discomfort during the episode. Although interpretation of these data are difficult, the authors suggest that patients who recover from a severe episode delirium may have no memory of the experience, including the pain, and that medical and nursing staff are likely to overestimate the discomfort of patients with this condition.

The third criterion for diagnosis of delirium relates to the time course of the disturbance. For diagnosis there must be evidence confirming that the disturbance has developed over a short period of time and tends to fluctuate during the course of the day. This pattern of disturbance is characteristic of delirium but, as with the other diagnostic criteria, this pattern is not specific for delirium. The development of mental status changes over a short period may occur in other conditions, including certain types of dementia.

Fluctuation in the clinical manifestations of delirium is usually apparent in disturbance of the sleep–wake cycle. Patients usually experience insomnia and may be agitated at night and somnolent during the day. As noted previously, this change in sleep pattern is often found to be among the prodromal symptoms of the syndrome. The phenomenon known as "sundowning" refers to the worsening of symptoms toward evening and probably has more to do with a sleep–wake abnormalities than with environmental factors (10).

In addition to mental status changes, described above, the neurologic examination may identify findings associated with diffuse brain dysfunction, such as multifocal myoclonus and asterixis. Some findings may be relatively specific for one or more etiologies. For example, tremulousness is typical of alcohol withdrawal states; miosis and mydriasis suggest opioid toxicity and anticholinergic toxicity, respectively; and tachypnea may be a manifestation of a central process, or of sepsis or hypoxemia.

The final *DSM* criterion for diagnosis requires evidence of a general medical condition judged to be etiologically related to the disturbance. The criteria do not state that proof of etiology is necessary. The implication of this criterion is that a medical condition that could feasibly have resulted in delirium must be present. As outlined in Table 2, numerous conditions can fulfill this criterion, including electrolyte disturbances, infection, fever, multisystem failure, and treatment with centrally acting drugs. A detailed history and physical examination may reveal findings that point to the etiology of the delirium and is therefore essential for establishing the diagnosis of delirium in addition to being essential for the assessment of treatment options (see below).

In summary, a comprehensive history, combined with both careful observation and a mental status examination, will frequently provide evidence for the criteria necessary for a *DSM-IV* diagnosis (see Table 1). A physical exam and review of laboratory data will frequently assist in defining the etiology of the syndrome.

## CLINICAL FEATURES OF DELIRIUM IN SPECIFIC SUBPOPULATIONS

It is useful to distinguish several subpopulations in which the prevalence of delirium is high. Syndromes characterized by delirium may complicate withdrawal from alcohol and sedative-hypnotic drugs (87–92). Given that the lifetime prevalence of alcohol disorders in the United States is considered to be approximately 13% (93), alcohol is likely to be an important risk factor for delirium. In the oncology setting, the risk that alcohol withdrawal could be an etiologic factor in delirium is increased in those populations who have tumors associated with alcohol consumption, such as those undergoing surgery for head and neck cancer (90).

The severity of alcohol withdrawal varies from minor symptoms of tremulousness through to the most severe form, delirium tremens (DT) (88,92). DT is usually seen in patients with a long history of alcoholism who are admitted to hospital for an intervening medical problem. Characteristically, these patients become delirious after 2 or 3 days, but symptoms may occur as late as 14 days after alcohol consumption has decreased or stopped (87,88,91). The onset is usually sudden although the delirium may be preceded by tremulousness. It is characterized by agitation, tremors, vivid hallucinations, sleeplessness, and signs of autonomic hyperactivity. When hallucinations are related to withdrawal and DT, visual hallucinations tend to predominate; and auditory and tactile perceptual hallucinations are less common (94). Of note, alcoholic hallucinations may occur in the presence of a clear sensorium, as separate, isolated phenomena unrelated to delirium (89,92). These hallucinations are frequently auditory. Seizures may also occur in DT. In most cases, the withdrawal syndrome continues for less than 72 hours and is associated with spontaneous recovery, frequently followed by a period of deep sleep (92,95). DT can be associated with severe autonomic instability. This disturbance and intercurrent illness account for a mortality for DT between 5% and 15%.

Delirium is common in the postoperative setting. Numerous factors may contribute to a higher likelihood of delirium in this setting (see below) (38). Although this group of patients has been extensively investigated, there have been no studies to suggest that the clinical picture in postoperative delirium is significantly different than delirium from metabolic disturbances or other causes. Those who experience delirium in the postoperative setting have a higher mortality, lesser functional recovery, and longer hospital stays than those who do not develop this complication (5,6,51,96).

Delirium is highly prevalent in patients with advanced terminal illness who are approaching the end of life (36,37,41,52). Accordingly, the assessment and treatment of mental status changes are a very important aspect of palliative care. "Terminal restlessness" is a term that is frequently used to describe the clinical appearance of some patients as they approach death. This condition would be more accurately described as "agitated delirium in a dying patient" (97). Unfortunately, this group of patients has rarely been studied using strict diagnostic criteria for delirium. Although surveys of the last few weeks of life frequently cite "confusion" as a problem, this term does not provide diagnostic specificity. Clinical experience suggests that terminal delirium is prevalent in the hospice setting and may be associated with multifocal myoclonus and convulsions. The etiology of this condition is likely to be multifactorial, with metabolic and drug-related factors in the setting of multisystem failure being contributory.

## APPROACH TO ASSESSMENT

Assessment of the patient with a change in mental status should seek to both clarify the diagnosis and define the etiology of the change. Assessment should also aim to provide the clinician with a view of the patient in the context of the overall medical condition. This view should include an understanding of both the impact of the symptoms and disease, and the goals of treatment. The latter is imperative, as the patient's and family's goals of care, particularly in case of advanced illness, will influence decisions regarding the extent of the diagnostic workup and the options for interventions.

A thorough evaluation should be considered when any change in mental status is observed (see above). This applies not only to the presence of "confusion" and prominent psychiatric symptoms, such as hallucinations and paranoia, but also to other psychological symptoms, including anxiety, fear, sleep disturbance, somnolence, and others (see Table 3). Each of these symptoms may be components of delirium. In assessment it is important to consider symptoms as multidimensional experiences that may be evaluated in terms of their specific characteristics and their impact (73,98–101). The symptoms associated with delirium should be assessed in terms of their frequency, severity, and distress. Psychiatric symptoms must be assessed also in relation to their perceptual characteristics and the patient's interpretation of their meaning (102). The impact of symptoms and the mental status changes associated with the overall syndrome should be explored in relation to the patient's level of distress; family or caregiver distress; behavior patterns, including behavior that may predispose to injury; and spheres of functioning.

A full medical history is a vital component of the workup of delirium. The degree to which the patient can respond cogently is an important part of the evaluation (102). Even when the patient is capable of giving the history, insight may be lacking as a direct consequence of the evolution of the delirium. An interview with those caring for the patient, perhaps family or nursing staff, may be necessary. For example, nighttime symptoms or subtle evidence of cognitive impairment may have been noticed by the caregivers and not by the patient. The interview must also explore the patient's medical and psychiatric history, systems review, social and family history, medications, previous drug reactions, and allergies. Some symptoms, such as fever, may assist in establishing the etiologic factors. All drugs consumed by the patient in the days preceding the episode should be carefully be reviewed with attention to the pattern of administration and dosing in relation to the delirium. Although the extent of the disease may in some cases be known, in others this may need to be defined.

As discussed above in relation to the *DSM* criteria, physical examination, including a mental status and neurologic examination should seek to define the neurologic and psychiatric syndrome (103,104) and should assess for evidence of potential contributory factors, including sepsis, dehydration, or major organ failure. Given the importance of the detection of subtle changes

**TABLE 5.** *Diagnostic tests to consider in a patient with delirium*

Blood glucose
Electrolytes (Na, K, Cl, Ca)
Urea and creatinine
$PO_2$, $PCO_2$, $HCO_3$, pH (arterial blood)
Full blood count
Osmolality
Electrocardiogram
Cerebrospinal fluid examination: blood, glucose, protein, cells, culture
Screen for disseminated intravascular coagulation
Liver function tests
Infection screens: Blood, urine and other cultures
Thyroid and adrenal function tests
Head CT scan or MRI
Electroencephalography

in mental status for detection and diagnosis of delirium, assessment of baseline mental status should be routine in the assessment of patients with acute illness or prior to the administration of therapies that may precipitate delirium. The use of an evaluation instrument may be useful for both baseline and ongoing assessment (see below).

Assessment of laboratory parameters will allow assessment of the possible role of metabolic abnormalities, such as hypercalcemia, and other problems such as hypoxia or disseminated intravascular coagulation (Table 5). Bedside assessments, such as oxygen saturation and blood glucose, may also provide important information. The choice of investigations should be guided by the clinical situation and the goals of care. EEG may supplement the clinical assessment and assist in the clarifying the diagnosis, particularly if there is concern that the differential diagnosis includes epileptiform activity or central nervous system pathology characterized by specific EEG findings. Similarly, brain imaging studies and assessment of the cerebrospinal fluid may be useful when considering the evaluation of etiologic factors.

Studies in patients with advanced cancer have demonstrated the utility of this thorough diagnostic assessment (37,62,105). One study found that 68% of delirious cancer patients improved with treatment, despite a 30-day mortality of 31% (62). Another found that one third of the episodes of cognitive failure improved following an evaluation that yielded a cause for these episodes in 43% (37).

## DIFFERENTIAL DIAGNOSIS OF DELIRIUM

Although the most important diagnoses to be differentiated from delirium are dementia and other psychiatric conditions, the differential diagnosis of delirium encompasses almost the whole spectrum of psychiatric disease as well as an array of neurologic disorders (106,107). As discussed above, it is most important for clinicians to be cognizant of the spectrum of symptoms that may be features of delirium and aware that almost any psychiatric symptom may be a manifestation of delirium. As a consequence, the mental status examination is an important aspect of the assessment of all psychiatric symptoms in the cancer patient, including anxiety, tearfulness, nervousness, depression, irritability, and others. Although these symptoms may be within the normal spectrum of response to serious illness or represent a primary psychiatric disorder, they could indicate a subtle delirium.

When the mental status examination reveals impaired cognition, the potential diagnoses include delirium, dementia of various types, amnestic disorders, and drug-induced disorders. The *DSM-IV* categorizes this group as "cognitive impairment disorders" (7). Table 4 reports some of the features that facilitate the differentiation of these conditions (77).

The dementias are characterized by progressive cognitive impairment. A history of a chronic decline without alteration in level of arousal assists in distinguishing these syndromes from delirium. Nonetheless the assessment can be challenging. Dementia increases the risk of delirium and the two conditions may occur concurrently, particularly in the elderly. Demented patients are particularly sensitive to drug toxicities, especially to drugs with anticholinergic activity, and to metabolic and physical stress, including surgery (49). A history of the patient's baseline mental status, level of cognitive impairment, and behavioral pattern is important in the assessment of the demented patient who may be experiencing delirium.

The acute psychoses also can be difficult to differentiate from delirium. The term *pseudodeliria* has been introduced to describe these episodes, which usually occur in patients with a psychiatric history (77). Vigilance is usually preserved and the EEG is normal. Delusions tend to be more systematized and bizarre in cases of psychosis. A patient with a known history of psychiatric disease who develops an episode of confusion requires careful screening of possible organic causes.

Mood disorders are also common, both in the elderly and in the cancer population, and may contribute to diagnostic uncertainly in the evaluation of cognitive impairment (34,35,46,108–112). Although mood disorders, in particular depression, are common, depressive symptoms are also a common manifestation of delirium. A recent study of elderly patients found that 42% of the patients who were referred for evaluation of depressive symptoms had a diagnosis of delirium (46). This diagnosis had only been considered by the referring health care provider in 3% of cases. The high prevalence of both mood disorders and delirium in the ill population serves to emphasize the need for a comprehensive assessment that incorporates neurologic, psychiatric, and cognitive evaluation.

It is well known that cognitive functions may be affected by brain lesions. When metastases or other structural disease is possible, a full assessment of cognitive impairment must include a comprehensive neurologic examination including aspects of speech and other higher cortical functions (106). An apparent case of delirium manifest by language disturbance may be found, on further examination, to relate to a dysphasic syndrome secondary to a focal cerebral lesion.

Finally, the diagnosis of delirium can be challenging when isolated aspects of the disorder occur without fulfilling the criteria for delirium. Just as depressive symptoms may occur in a patient who does not meet the criteria for a formal psychiatric diagnosis (111–113), drug-induced hallucinations may occur in isolation without cognitive impairment (114). As alluded to above, the presence of isolated symptoms should prompt comprehensive assessment, monitoring, and, if necessary, treatment to minimize distress.

## EVALUATION INSTRUMENTS FOR THE ASSESSMENT OF DELIRIUM

Instruments useful in delirium assessment include those developed for the assessment of cognitive impairment and those specifically developed for the assessment of delirium (Table 6) (115,116). These instruments can be utilized to identify and quantify cognitive impairment, and to determine the likelihood that the impairment can be ascribed to the diagnosis of delirium. As the *DSM-IV* criteria define cognitive impairment as a component of delirium, the abnormalities found on screening tests for cognitive impairment, although not diagnostic of delirium, can be useful in alerting the clinician to the presence of cognitive impairment. Smith et al. have recently comprehensively reviewed the evaluation tools for delirium assessment (116).

Instruments for assessment of cognitive impairment include the Mini-Mental Status Examination (79) and the Blessed Orientation-Memory-Concentration Test (117). Although these tools are sensitive indicators of cognitive impairment (36,37,118), the diagnosis of delirium requires further assessment with either a clinical interview or the administration of another validated instrument.

The clinical psychiatric interview using the *DSM* criteria remains the gold standard for the evaluation and diagnosis of delirium (7,102). Instruments that are available to facilitate the diagnosis (116) include the Confusion Assessment Method (119), the Delirium Symptom Interview (120), and the Delirium Rating Scale (121). These instruments were developed based on the earlier criteria outlined in the *DSM-III* (122) or *DSM-III-R* (9) and use an interview format to characterize the features of the

**TABLE 6.** *Evaluation methods and instruments for delirium assessment and research in cancer patients (115,116)*

Diagnostic Classification Systems
  DSM-III (122), DSM-III-R (9), DSM-IV (7), ICD-9 (195),ICD-10 (195)
Instruments for Assessment and Screening for Cognitive Impairment
  Mini-Mental State Exam (MMSE) (79)
  Short Portable Mental Status Questionnaire (SPMSQ) (196)
  Cognitive Capacity Screening Examination (CCSE) (197)
  Blessed Orientation Memory Concentration Test (BOMC) (117)
Other Screening Instruments, Checklists, and Algorithm Methods
  Confusion Rating Scale (CRS) (198)
  Saskatoon Delirium Checklist (SDC) (199)
  Confusion Assessment Method (CAM) (119)
Diagnostic Interviews
  Delirium Symptom Interview (DSI) (120)
Delirium Rating Scales
  Delirium Rating Scale (DRS) (121)
  The Memorial Delirium Assessment Scale (MDAS) (123)
Laboratory Examinations
  EEG, brain imaging
  Serum anticholinergic activity

Adapted from ref 200.

cognitive impairment. The Memorial Delirium Assessment Scale (MDAS) is a rating scale that has undergone early validation studies in cancer patients and may prove a useful clinical and research tool if further studies confirm its utility (123). Many of these instruments use either a score above a cutoff point or an algorithm to document the presence or absence of delirium. Although none of the currently available instruments has been adequately validated as a measure of delirium severity, instruments may have a useful role in providing a method for the monitoring of patients predisposed to delirium or receiving treatment for this condition. Although this potential exists, many of the instruments utilized to date in screening have lacked adequate validation (115,116).

The instruments for delirium diagnosis have an important role in research, but none have been widely used in routine clinical practice. Their use in this manner could focus staff attention on assessment and be used to review the quality of patient care and situation-specific barriers to symptom control (36,124–126). In considering routine use, simplicity and brevity are important features. For this reason, some clinicians have selected the Mini-Mental State Examination (79) for routine monitoring (36,124–127). If using the instrument for this purpose, clinicians should be aware that it has population- specific limits relating to age, language, and education (80,128). Additionally, as mentioned previously, the instrument does not fully assess the criteria necessary for a diagnosis of delirium.

## TREATMENT

The management of delirium comprises interventions directed at symptom control and interventions directed at underlying causes (62,105,107,118,129,130). The degree to which these treatments are pursued is determined by the goals of care.

### Etiologic Interventions

As discussed previously, the etiology may be related to one factor or many factors (see Table 2). Although in advanced disease the goals of care may dictate a limited workup, the identification and correction of the underlying cause(s) should be pursued, to whatever degree is appropriate and feasible, concurrently with the implementation of symptomatic therapies. In complex cases, it may be possible to address at least one, if not several, of the etiologic factors. For example, a drug-induced delirium may be ameliorated by dose reduction, if feasible, or by switching to an alternative drug. Even those patients in whom the etiology of delirium is multifactorial may be observed to benefit following reversal of one or more factors (36,62,69,131,132).

In many patients, drugs are contributory factors in delirium (62). All nonessential drugs should be stopped.

When opioid-induced delirium is the most likely diagnosis it may be useful to institute a switch from one opioid to another (133–135). Although no opioid has been shown to have a more favorable central nervous system side effect profile than any other, this practice may identify a drug with a more favorable balance between analgesia and side effects in an individual patient. Bruera et al. have suggested that in terminal cancer patients careful monitoring of cognitive function, attention to dehydration, and opioid rotation can reduce the incidence of agitated delirium and the need for neuroleptic medication (134).

### Behavioral and Environmental Management

Treatment measures for delirium, regardless of cause, include the manipulation of the environment to provide a safe, quiet, and reorienting milieu, and support and reassurance through communication with the patient and family. Where possible, measures should be implemented that increase structure and familiarity, and reduce anxiety and disorientation. These measures may include encouraging the family to sit with the patient and placing the patient in a quiet, well-lit room with familiar personnel. The use of orienting devices, such as clocks, calendars, and familiar objects from the patient's home, may be useful.

The safety of the patient with delirium must be ensured. One-to-one nursing observation may be necessary. Occasionally, physical restraint may be needed for a brief time to prevent harm to the patient and others. The use of physical restraints must be minimized, implemented strictly according to national and institutional policies and regulations, and relinquished as soon as behavioral control is attained with drugs.

Patient and family counseling is an important part of delirium treatment. At any time, but especially when the condition is associated with terminal disease, the communication difficulties associated with the condition may cause distress in family members (136). Table 7 highlights some of the issues that should be addressed in family counseling. Although psychological expertise may be helpful in complex cases, a discussion between the physician and family will usually suffice to allay family con-

**TABLE 7.** *Critical issues in counseling for the family of delirious patients*

Communication barrier
Patient's awareness of physical and psychological suffering
Reversibility
Short-term prognosis
Fluctuations of cognitive functions
Role of opioid and other therapies in etiology
Role and goal of sedation
Goals of care

cerns, guide the family's approach to the patient, and assist them in decision making. Importantly, a family member is frequently the proxy for health care decision making for the cognitively impaired patient, and, for this reason as well as many others, family should be kept apprised of the patient's medical condition.

During an episode of delirium, the patient may experience fear related to an awareness of the impairment. In such circumstances, the patient may require repeated reassurance. The importance of patient counseling before the potential onset of postoperative delirium and of systematic reorientation during the episode has been demonstrated in two studies (137,138). These studies confirm the often cited importance of environmental approaches directed to maximizing safety and providing psychosocial support (139,140).

## Pharmacologic Therapy

Symptomatic treatment of delirium is often, but not always, necessary. It is appropriate, while treatment is being instituted for etiologic factors, to alleviate distress in severe cases, to reduce the risk of mortality in delirium tremens, and to manage cases with unknown or untreatable etiologies. Except in the case of delirium tremens, for which a benzodiazepine is the first-line drug, a neuroleptic is generally the most appropriate drug for the initial management of delirium (Table 8). The benefits of treating mild delirium without distress have not been established, nor has the value of neuroleptic therapy been confirmed in hypoactive delirium. Psychostimulants have been suggested for the treatment of the latter condition (125,141,142).

Haloperidol is considered the drug of choice for hallucinations and agitation related to delirium in the medically ill (10,36,140,143–153). Other neuroleptic drugs may also be efficacious, e.g., thioridazine, droperidol, and chlorpromazine. The role of the newer antipsychotic drugs with fewer extrapyramidal side effects, such as risperidone, buspirone, sulpiride, and clozapine, has not to date been clarified (154–158). Although comparative trials are lacking, the preference for haloperidol is based on both clinical experience and anecdotal evidence (10,

118,152). Haloperidol is a potent dopamine blocker with useful sedating effects and a relatively low incidence of cardiovascular and anticholinergic effects.

Haloperidol can be used via the oral, intramuscular, intravenous, or subcutaneous route. The oral route may be appropriate in mild delirium cases; agitation and uncooperative behavior necessitate parenteral administration. Although the intravenous route has not been approved by the U.S. Federal Drug Administration, this route has been reported to be safe and effective (159–161) and is widely used for treatment of delirium in the severely ill (152,160). The subcutaneous route has been frequently used in the palliative care setting (118,162,163). Parenteral doses of haloperidol are roughly twice as potent as oral doses and clinical effects are usually observed within 30 minutes after intravenous administration and may last for 4–8 hours (152). The half-life of haloperidol is between 14 and 20 hours and the drug is widely distributed and may remain in the body for long periods (164,165).

Empirical guidelines have been proposed for the treatment of agitated delirium (152,160). These guidelines recommend the initial administration of intravenous haloperidol in a dose between 2 and 5 mg. The dose can be repeated after 20–30 minutes, with a limit of 5 mg every 15 minutes. Generally, unless agitation is very severe, dosing should be titrated against symptoms at intervals of 45–60 minutes (166). Typical doses are likely to range between 0.5 and 20 mg administered in the first hour. When the patient is calm, haloperidol is continued by either the oral or parenteral route. The usual dose is 0.5–3 mg one to three times daily, which can be given on an as-needed basis or on a fixed schedule. When delirium is mild, treatment can be initiated with haloperidol 1–2 mg orally or 0.5–1 mg parenterally.

Although most guidelines recommend initial treatment with small doses, published series have actually reported varying dose regimens. For example, one study of less severe cases, which included hypoactive delirium, noted that low doses (3 mg) of haloperidol appeared to improve symptoms (167). A survey of the management strategies used for intoxicated or head trauma patients observed that average cumulative doses of 8.2 mg were helpful in

**TABLE 8.** *Common medications used for the management of delirium in adult cancer patients*

| Drug | Commonly used routes |
| --- | --- |
| Neuroleptics | |
|   Haloperidol | Oral intramuscular, intravenous, subcutaneous |
|   Thioridazine | Oral |
|   Chlorpromazine | Oral, intramuscular, intravenous, |
|   Methotrimeprazine | Oral, subcutaneous |
| Benzodiazepines | |
|   Lorazepam | Oral, intramuscular, intravenous |
|   Midazolam | Intravenous, subcutaneous |

Adapted from ref 200.

reducing aggressive behavior (144). A study of AIDS delirium reported symptomatic improvement with combination therapy of haloperidol (average daily dose 42 mg) and lorazepam (average daily dose 7.5 mg) (146) and surveys in intensive care units have reported the use of high doses of intermittently administered or continuously infused haloperidol (48–1155 mg/day) (166,168,169). Despite the high doses administered in the latter studies, clinical experience would suggest that most patients respond to doses of less than 20 mg haloperidol in a 24-hour period.

A drawback to the use of haloperidol and other neuroleptic drugs is the potential for extrapyramidal side effects and movement disorders (36,170). Acute dystonias and other extrapyramidal side effects generally respond to antiparkinsonian medications, including diphenhydramine, benztropine, and trihexyphenidyl. Akathisia may respond to low doses of either propranolol (5 mg two to three times per day) or lorazepam (0.5–1 mg two to three times per day) (171). A trial of benztropine (1–2 mg once or twice per day) may prove to be useful; however, this medication is not generally used as a first-line treatment for akathisia (171). It is important to be vigilant for this latter side effect, which may go unnoticed in a patient with restlessness associated with the delirium itself.

A rare and serious complication of neuroleptic medications is the neuroleptic malignant syndrome (NMS), which may occur as an isolated event or may be triggered by a concurrent illness or fever (170,172). This syndrome may be fatal and must be treated as a potential medical emergency. Although NMS usually occurs after prolonged, high-dose administration of neuroleptics, it may occur spontaneously in patients on lower doses. It is characterized by hyperthermia, increased confusion, leukocytosis, muscular rigidity, myoglobinuria, and high serum creatine phosphokinase. Treatment measures should include discontinuation of the neuroleptic, general supportive measures, treatment of precipitating factors, and the use of dantrolene sodium and bromocriptine mesylate (170,172).

In addition to its neurologic side effects, haloperidol may be associated with cardiac arrhythmias (e.g., torsades de pointes) through prolongation of the QT interval on the electrocardiogram (173–175). Haloperidol should be used with caution in conjunction with other drugs that may prolong the QT interval. Given this risk, consideration should be given to the need for careful monitoring of hypokalemia, hypomagnesemia, and a widening QT interval when administering haloperidol (173–175).

Haloperidol alone may fail to control the symptoms of delirium. In such cases, either a benzodiazepine or another sedative, or a neuroleptic other than haloperidol, can be added. Anecdotal experience is greatest with lorazepam and midazolam. Clinical experience, along with one case series in the cancer population, confirms the need for the use of more than one drug for delirium management in patients with advanced cancer (36). Of the 39 cancer patients reported in the one reported series, 20% were controlled with haloperidol alone, 13% with lorazepam alone, 26% with a combination of lorazepam and haloperidol, and 40% needed another neuroleptic medication (chlorpromazine or methotrimeprazine). Overall, 26% of the patients needed sedation, usually achieved with midazolam, to control delirium.

The choice of a second drug in the management of delirium should be guided by the drug pharmacokinetics and side effects profile, and by the goals of care. For example, propofol, midazolam, or lorazepam have been recommended in the critical care setting because their pharmacokinetics favor rapid dose titration in the initial phases of treatment (152). Chlorpromazine is not recommended in these circumstances because of the likelihood of hypotension and other anticholinergic effects. When sedation would be an acceptable or even favorable outcome, for example, in the terminal setting where the patient has lost the ability to interact, chlorpromazine or a benzodiazepine may be a valuable drug. Other factors may also be considered in some patients: the patient with hypotension should be treated with the medication with the least effect on blood pressure, and the delirious postoperative patient who has an ileus or urinary retention should receive the antipsychotic medication with the fewest anticholinergic effects.

In contrast to neuroleptic drugs like haloperidol, benzodiazepines do not clear a delirious patient's sensorium or improve cognition. In a double-blind, randomized trial comparing haloperidol, chlorpromazine, and lorazepam, Breitbart et al. demonstrated that lorazepam alone, in doses up to 8 mg in a 12-hour period, was ineffective in the treatment of delirium and contributed to worsening cognitive impairment (176). Both of the neuroleptic drugs, in low doses (approximately 2 mg haloperidol equivalent per 24 hours), were highly effective in controlling the symptoms of delirium and in improving cognitive function. Benzodiazepines should not therefore be considered as first-line treatments for delirium but rather as sedatives that may be useful to reduce agitation. In some cases, particularly in the last days of life, clearing the sensorium and improving cognition may not always be attainable goals. The processes causing delirium may, as death nears, be ongoing and irreversible. Ventafridda, Fainsinger, and their respective colleagues have reported that a group (10% to 50%) of terminally ill patients experience delirium that can only be controlled by sedation to the point of a significantly decreased level of consciousness (124,126,177). In such cases, and occasionally in the course of management of reversible delirium, a common strategy in the management of agitated delirium is to supplement the regimen of haloperidol with parenteral benzodiazepine (146,166).

Lorazepam is generally considered to be the drug of first choice when a benzodiazepine is necessary. This drug undergoes glucuronidation and has an intermediate half-life. These characteristics and the observation that lorazepam, unlike other benzodiazepines, has no active metabolites have suggested the superiority of this drug when treating elderly patients or patients with liver disease (178). It can be safely administered even in the critically ill (152,179–181). Dosing usually begins at doses of 1–2 mg orally in mild cases, or 0.5–2 mg (0.044 mg/kg) administered intravenously or intramuscularly in severe cases (152,181). This medication can be administered by the oral, intramuscular, or intravenous route.

Some authors have expressed a preference for the use of midazolam for the management of delirium. It has been reported to be of use in cases of agitated delirium attributed to the excitatory effects of high-dose opioids and for the management of terminal delirium (97,182). Although theoretically any benzodiazepine may be useful for the latter indication, midazolam can be administered via the subcutaneous route, which can be viewed as a significant advantage in the palliative care setting (97,182).

During acute dosing, midazolam is short acting and has a rapid onset of effect (within minutes) (152). Reported doses ranges have been between 20 and 60 mg/day although higher doses (up to 200 mg/day) have been administered without untoward incidents (97,182). The drug is rapidly redistributed and is likely to require continuous infusion to maintain its effects. Long-term administration results in prolongation of the clinical effects of the drug. Active metabolites can accumulate in liver failure. These factors contribute to the observation that midazolam is associated with a less rapid awakening than lorazepam. Consequently, midazolam is considered to be less suitable for use when prolonged treatment is likely to be needed and recovery is expected (152). Aside from its pharmacokinetic profile, the comparative cost of this drug has also been cited as a reason for a preference for lorazepam when prolonged treatment is required (152).

Methotrimeprazine is also commonly used to control confusion and agitation in the setting of terminal disease (183). Dosages range from 12.5 mg to 50 mg every 4–8 hours, up to 300 mg/24 hours. Hypotension and sedation may limit the utility of this drug. However, often the goal of treatment with this medication, as with midazolam, may be to achieve quiet sedation at the end of life.

Alcohol withdrawal and sedative hypnotic withdrawal are special cases of delirium in that their treatment relies on the use of benzodiazepines (88,90,91,94,178,184–188). In alcohol withdrawal benzodiazepines are recommended both to prevent the severe manifestations of DT in patients with minor symptoms of withdrawal and for first-line treatment. This "prophylactic" role in high-risk patients with mild withdrawal has not been explored for delirium related to other etiologic factors and, currently, is unique to the management of the alcohol withdrawal syndrome. The risk of seizures and the high mortality of this condition are

factors that contribute to need for early treatment. Diazepam, chlordiazepoxide, and lorazepam are the most commonly utilized benzodiazepines but, to date, controlled trials have not settled the ongoing debate as to which of these medications is the drug of first choice (178). Haloperidol may be useful, however, in the management of alcohol-related hallucinations.

## PROGNOSTIC ISSUES

The resolution of delirium is likely to depend on many factors and the course may be complicated. Although frequently the clinical perception is that the condition is transient and brief, in a study of elderly delirious patients, the average duration of an episode was found to be longer than 2 weeks (19.5 ± 15.4 days) (6). In this group the most common etiologies for delirium were stroke, infections, and metabolic disorders; coexistent structural brain disease was present in many (81%). Levkoff et al. evaluated a group of acutely hospitalized elderly patients and demonstrated that among those with delirium resolution of symptoms was often incomplete with only 4% experiencing resolution of all new symptoms before hospital discharge, and 20.8% and 17.7% had symptom resolution by 3 and 6 months, respectively (5). To complicate this issue further, many patients experience delirium in the terminal phases of illness and have no resolution of symptoms prior to death (37,41,52). In the Levkoff et al. study, almost one third of the group were found to be experiencing individual symptoms of delirium although they did not meet the full criteria. These data suggest that delirium may be substantially less transient than currently believed and that incomplete manifestations of the syndrome may be frequent.

The mortality associated with delirium has been reported to be between 10% and 65% (5,6,33,189,190). Delirium is more frequent in patients with multiple medical problems and it is likely that these processes, rather than the delirium itself, contribute to the high mortality rate. Nonetheless, delirium has been shown to be an indicator of poor prognosis (2,191). In the elderly, the presence of delirium identified those patients at risk for prolonged hospitalization, loss of independent community living, and future cognitive decline (192–194).

## CONCLUSION

Delirium is a highly prevalent disorder in the medically ill. It is associated with both patient and family distress and frequently presents significant management problems. In many instances, delirium is overlooked in the clinical setting, and a vigilant and thorough approach to detection and assessment is essential. Given that delirium is frequently reversible, the management should align with the overall goals of care for the patient and appropriate treatment strategies should be implemented based on detailed assessment of contributory factors. Further research is needed to assess many aspects of this condition, both in the general medical population and the oncology setting.

# REFERENCES

1. Lipowski ZJ. Delirium (acute confusional states). *JAMA* 1987; 258(13):1789–1792.

2. Trzepacz PT, Teague GB, Lipowski ZJ. Delirium and other organic mental disorders in a general hospital. *Gen Hosp Psychiatry* 1985; 7(2):101–106.

3. Johnson JC, Kerse NM, Gottlieb G, Wanich C, Sullivan E, Chen K. Prospective versus retrospective methods of identifying patients with delirium. *J Am Geriatr Soc* 1992;40(4):316–319.

4. Bruera E, Fainsinger RL, Miller MJ, Kuehn N. The assessment of pain intensity in patients with cognitive failure: a preliminary report. *J Pain Sympt Manage* 1992;7(5):267–270.

5. Levkoff SE, Evans DA, Liptzin B, Cleary PD, Lipsitz LA, Wetle TT, et al. Delirium. The occurrence and persistence of symptoms among elderly hospitalized patients. *Arch Intern Med* 1992;152(2):334–340.

6. Koponen HJ, Riekkinen PJ. A prospective study of delirium in elderly patients admitted to a psychiatric hospital. *Psychol Med* 1993;23(1): 103–109.

7. American Psychiatric Association. *Diagnostic and statistical manual of mental disorders,* 4th ed. Washington, DC, 1994.

8. Lipowski ZJ. Transient cognitive disorders (delirium, acute confusional states) in the elderly. *Am J Psychiatry* 1983;140(11): 1426–1436.

9. American Psychiatric Association. *Diagnostic and Statistical Manual of Mental Disorders,* 3rd ed., Revised. Washington, DC, 1987.

10. Lipowski ZJ. *Delirium: acute confusional states.* New York: Oxford University Press, 1990.

11. Aninoff MJ. *Neurology and general medicine: The neurological aspects of medical disorders.* New York: Churchill Livingstone, 1995.

12. Adams RD, Victor R, Ropper AM. Delirium and other acute confusional states. In: *Principles of neurology,* 6th ed. New York: McGraw-Hill, 1997.

13. *The new shorter Oxford English dictionary.* Oxford: Clarendon Press, 1993.

14. Engel GL, Romano J. Delirium a syndrome of cerebral insufficiency. *J Chronic Dis* 1959;9:260–277.

15. Trzepacz PT. The neuropathogenesis of delirium. A need to focus our research. *Psychosomatics* 1994;35(4):374–91.

16. Plum F, Posner JB. *The diagnosis of stupor and coma.* Philadelphia: FA Davis, 1980.

17. Moruzzi G, Magoun HW. Brain stem reticular formation and activation of the EEG. *Electroenceph Clin Neurophysiol* 1949;1:455–473.

18. Ross CA. Etiological models and their phenomenological variants. CNS arousal systems: possible role in delirium. *Int Psychogeriatrics* 1991;3(2):353–371.

19. Mesulam MM, Waxman SG, Geschwind N, et al. Acute confusional state with right cerebral artery infarction. *J Neurol Neurosurg Psychiatry* 1976;39:84–89.

20. Trzepacz P, Tarter R, Shah A, et al. SPECT scan and cognitive findings in subclinical hepatic encephalopathy. *J Neuropsychiatry Clin Neurosci* 1994;6:170–175.

21. Deutsch G, Eisemberg HM. Frontal blood flow changes in recovery from coma. *J Cereb Blood Flow Metab* 1987;7:29–34.

22. Hemmingsen R, Vostrup S, clemmesen L, et al. Cerebral blood flow during delirium tremens and related clinical states. *Am J Psychiatry* 1988;145:1384–1390.

23. Gibson GE, Blass JP, Huang H, Freeman GB. The cellular basis of delirium and its relevance to age-related disorders including Alzheimer disease. *Int Psychogeriatrics* 1991;3(2):373–395.

24. Itil T, Fink M. EEG and behavioral apects of the interaction of anticholinergic hallucinogens with centrally active compounds. *Prog Brain Res* 1968;28:149–168.

25. Trzepacz PT, Brenner RP, Coffman GC, van Thiel DH. Delirium in liver transplantation candidates: discriminant analysis of multiple test variables. *Biol Psychiatry* 1988;24:3–15.

26. Koponen H, Partanen J, Paakkonen A, Mattila E, Rikkinen PJ. EEG spectral analysis in delirium. *J Neurol Neurosurg Psychiatry* 1989;52: 980–985.

27. Jacobson SA, Leuchter AF, Walter DO, Weiner H. Serial quantitative EEG among elderly subjects with delirium. *Biol Psychiatry* 1993; 34(3):135–140.

28. Jacobson SA, Leuchter AF, Walter DO. Conventional and quantitative EEG in the diagnosis of delirium among the elderly. *J Neurol Neurosurg Psychiatry* 1993;56(2):153–158.

29. Wengs WJ, Talwar D, Bernard J. Ifosfamide-induced nonconvulsive status epilepticus. *Arch Neurol* 1993;50:1104–1105.

30. Basile A, Jones A, Skoenick P. The pathogenesis and treatment of hepatic encephalopathy: evidence for the involvement of benzodiazepine receptor ligands. *Pharmacol Rev* 1991;43(1):27–71.

31. Caraceni A, Martini C, Belli F, Mascheroni L, Rivoltini L, Arienti F, et al. Neuropsychological and neurophysiological assessment of the central effects of interleukin-2 administration. *Eur J Cancer* 1993; 29A(9):1266–1269.

32. Onofrj M, Curatola L, Malatesta G, Bazzano S, Colamartino P, Fulgente T. Reduction of P3 latency during outcome of posttraumatic amnesia. *Acta Neurol Scand* 1991;83:273–279.

33. Inouye SK. The dilemma of delirium: clinical and research controversies regarding diagnosis and evaluation of delirium in hospitalized elderly medical patients. *Am J Med* 1994;97:278–288.

34. Derogatis LR, Morrow GR, Fetting J, Penman D, Piasetsky S, Schmale AM, et al. The prevalence of psychiatric disorders among cancer patients. *JAMA* 1983;249(6):751–757.

35. Levine PM, Silberfarb PM, Lipowski ZJ. Mental disorders in cancer patients: a study of 100 psychiatric referrals. *Cancer* 1978;42(3): 1385–1391.

36. Stiefel F, Fainsinger R, Bruera E. Acute confusional states in patients with advanced cancer. *J Pain Sympt Manage* 1992;7(2):94–98.

37. Bruera E, Miller L, McCallion J, Macmillan K, Krefting L, Hanson J. Cognitive failure in patients with terminal cancer: a prospective study. *J Pain Sympt Manage* 1992;7(4):192–195.

38. Bitondo Dyer C, Ashton CM, Teasdale TA. Postoperative delirium. A review of 80 primary data collection studies. *Arch Intern Med* 1995; 155:461–465.

39. Naughton BJ, Moran MB, Kadah H, Heman-Ackah Y, Longano J. Delirium and other cognitive impairment in older adults in an emergency department. *Ann Emerg Med* 1995;25(6):751–755.

40. Inouye SK, Charpentier PA. Precipitating factors for delirium in hospitalized elderly persons: predictive model and interrelationship with baseline vulnerability. *JAMA* 1996;275(11):852–857.

41. Massie MJ, Holland J, Glass E. Delirium in terminally ill cancer patients. *Am J Psychiatry* 1983;140(8):1048–1050.

42. Schor JD, Levkoff SE, Lipsitz LA, Reilly CH, Cleary PD, Rowe JW, et al. Risk factors for delirium in hospitalized elderly. *JAMA* 1992; 267(6):827–831.

43. Inouye SK, Viscoli CM, Horwitz RI, Hurst LD, Tinetti ME. A predictive model for delirium in hospitalized elderly medical patients based on admission characteristics. *Ann Intern Med* 1993;119(6):474–481.

44. Inouye SK. The dilemma of delirium: clinical and research controversies regarding diagnosis and evaluation of delirium in hospitalized elderly medical patients. *Am J Med* 1994;97(3):278–288.

45. Weed HG, Lutman CV, Young DC, Schuller DE. Preoperative identification of patients at risk for delirium after major head and neck cancer surgery. *Laryngoscope* 1995;105(10):1066–1068.

46. Farrell KR, Ganzini L. Misdiagnosing delirium as depression in medically ill elderly patients. *Arch Intern Med* 1995;155(22):2459–2464.

47. Lewis LM, Miller DK, Morley JE, Nork MJ, Lasater LC. Unrecognized delirium in ED geriatric patients. *Am J Emerg Med* 1995;13(2): 142–145.

48. Inouye SK, Viscoli CM, Horwitz RI, Hurst LD, Tinetti ME. A predictive model for delirium in hospitalized elderly medical patients based on admission characteristics. *Ann Intern Med* 1993;119(6):474–481.

49. Erkinjutti T, Wikstrom J, Palo J, Autio K. Dementia among medical inpatients. Evaluation of 2000 consecutive admission. *Arch Intern Med* 1986;146:1923–1926.

50. Williams-Russo P, Urquhart BL, Sharrock NE, Charlson ME. Postoperative delirium: predictors and prognosis in elderly orthopedic patients. *J Am Geriatr Soc* 1992;40(8):759–767.

51. Marcantonio ER, Goldman L, Mangione CM, Ludwig LE, Muraca B, Haslauer CM, et al. A clinical prediction rule for delirium after elective noncardiac surgery. *JAMA* 1994;271(2):134–139.

52. Pompei P, Foreman M, Rudberg MA, Inouye SK, Braund V, Cassel CK. Delirium in hospitalized older persons: outcomes and predictors. *J Am Geriatr Soc* 1994;42(8):809–815.

53. Parikh SS, Chung F. Post-operative delirium in the elderly. *Anesth Analg* 1995;80:1223–1232.

54. Tune LE, Bylsma FW. Benzodiazepine-induced and anticholinergic-induced delirium in the elderly. *Int Psychogeriatrics* 1991;3(2):397–408.

55. Posner JB. Neurologic complications of systemic cancer. *Disease-a-Month* 1979;25:1–60.

56. Silberfarb PM, Philibert D, Levine PM. Psychosocial aspects of neoplastic disease: II. Affective and cognitive effects of chemotherapy in cancer patients. *Am J Psychiatry* 1980;137(5):597–601.

57. Oxman TE, Silberfarb PM. Serial cognitive testing in cancer patients receiving chemotherapy. *Am J Psychiatry* 1980;137(10):1263–1265.

58. Silberfarb PM. Chemotherapy and cognitive defects in cancer patients. *Annu Rev Med* 1983;34(35):35–46.

59. Patchell RA, Posner JB. Cancer and the nervous system. In: Holland JC, Rowland JH, eds. *Handbook of psychooncology*. New York: Oxford University Press, 1989;327–341.

60. Meyers CA, Abbruzzese JL. Cognitive functioning in cancer patients: effect of previous treatment. *Neurology* 1992;42:434–436.

61. Barbato M. Thiamine deficiency in patients admitted to a palliative care unit. *Palliat Med* 1994;8:320–324.

62. Tuma R, DeAngelis L. Acute encephalopathy in patients with systemic cancer. *Ann Neurol* 1992;32:288.

63. Weitzner MA, Olofsson SM, Forman AD. Patients with malignant meningitis presenting with neuropsychiatric manifestations. *Cancer* 1995;76(10):1804–1808.

64. Stiefel F, Morant R. Morphine intoxication during acute reversible renal insufficiency. *J Palliat Care* 1991;7(4):45–47.

65. Fainsinger R, Schoeller T, Boiskin M, Bruera E. Palliative care round: cognitive failure (CF) and coma after renal failure in a patient receiving captopril and hydromorphone. *J Palliat Care* 1993;9(1):53–55.

66. Bortolussi R, Fabiani F, Savron F, Testa V, Lazzarini R, Sorio R, et al. Acute morphine intoxication during high-dose recombinant interleukin-2 treatment for metastatic renal cell cancer. *Eur J Cancer* 1994;30A(12):1905–1907.

67. Seymour DG, Henschke PJ, Cape RDT, Campbell AJ. Acute confusional states and dementia in the elderly: the role of dehydration volume depletion, physical illness and age. *Age Ageing* 1980;9(3):137–146.

68. Bruera E. Severe organic brain syndrome. *J Palliat Care* 1991;7(1):36–38.

69. de Stoutz ND, Tapper M, Faisinger RL. Reversible delirium in terminally ill patients. *J Pain Sympt Manage* 1995;10:249–253.

70. Chedru F, Geschwind N. Disorders of higher cortical functions in acute confusional states. *Cortex* 1972;8:395–411.

71. Mesulam M-M. Attention, confusional states, and neglect. In: Mesulam MM, eds. *Principles of behavioral neurology*, vol 26. Philadelphia: FA Davis, 1985;125–168.

72. Osmon DC. Luria-Nebraska neuropsychological battery case study: a mild drug related confusional state. *Int J Clin Neuropsychol* 1984;6(4)

73. Portenoy RK, Thaler HT, Kornblith AB, Lepore JM, Friedlander KH, Coyle N, et al. Symptom prevalence, characteristics and distress in a cancer population. *Qual Life Res* 1994;3(3):183–189.

74. Coyle N, Adelhardt J, Foley KM, Portenoy RK. Character of terminal illness in the advanced cancer patient: pain and other symptoms during the last four weeks of life. *J Pain Sympt Manage* 1990;5(2):83–93.

75. Lichter I, Hunt E. The last 48 hours of life. *J Palliat Care* 1990;6(4):7–15.

76. Liptzin B, Levkoff SE. An empirical study of delirium subtypes. *Br J Psychiatry* 1992;161(1):843–845.

77. Lipowski ZJ. Delirium in the elderly patient. *N Engl J Med* 1989;320(9):578–582.

78. Ross CA, Peyser CE, Shapiro I, Folstein MF. Delirium: phenomenologic and etiologic subtypes. *Int Psychogeriatrics* 1991;3(2):135–147.

79. Folstein MF, Folstein SE, McHugh PR. Mini-Mental State. *J Psychiatr Res* 1975;12:189–198.

80. Crum RM, Anthony JC, Basset SS, Folstein MF. Population-based norms for the Mini-Mental State Examination by age and educational level. *JAMA* 1993;269(18):2386–2391.

81. Wallesch CW, Hundsalz A. Language function in delirium: a comparison of single word processing in acute confusional states and probable Alzheimer's disease. *Brain Lang* 1994;46(4):592–606.

82. Daniel WF, Crovitz HF, Weiner RD. Neuropsychological aspects of disorientation. *Cortex* 1987;23:169–187.

83. Geschwind N. Disorders of attention: a frontier in neuropsychology. *Phil Trans R Soc Lond* 1982;B 298:173–185.

84. Chedru F, Geschwind N. Writing disturbances in acute confusional state. *Neuropsychologia* 1972;10:343–353.

85. Weinstein EA, Kahn RL. *Denial of illness*. Springfield, IL: Charles C Thomas, 1955.

86. Wolf HG, Curran D. Nature of delirium and allied states. *Arch Neurol Psychiatry* 1935;33:1175.

87. Lerner WD, Fallom HJ. The alcohol withdrawal syndrome. *N Engl J Med* 1985;313:951–952.

88. Turner RC, Lichstein PR, Peden JG, Busher JT, Waivers LE. Alcohol withdrawal syndromes: a review of pathophysiology, clinical presentation and treatment. *J Gen Intern Med* 1989;4:432–443.

89. McMicken DB. Alcohol withdrawal syndromes. *Emerg Med Clin North Am* 1990;8:805–819.

90. Newman JP, Terris DJ, Moore M. Trends in the management of alcohol withdrawal syndrome. *Laryngoscope* 1995;105(1):1–7.

91. Naranjo CA, Sellers EM. Clinical assessment and pharmacotherapy of the alcohol withdrawal syndrome. In: Galanter M, ed. *Recent developments in alcoholism*, vol 4. New York: Plenum Press, 1986;265–281.

92. Adams RD, Victor R, Ropper AM. Alcohol and alcoholism. In: *Principles of neurology*, 6th ed. New York: McGraw-Hill, 1997;1166–1185.

93. Michels R, Marzuk PM. Progress in psychiatry. *N Engl J Med* 1993;329(8):552–560.

94. Platz WE, Oberlaender FA, Seidel ML. The phenomenology of perceptual hallucinations in alcohol-induced delirium tremens. *Psychopathology* 1995;28(5):247–255.

95. Victor R, Adams RD. Effect of alcohol on the nervous system. *Res Publ Assoc Res Nerv Mental Dis* 1953;32:526–523.

96. Russo P, Urquhart BL, Sharrock NE, Charlson ME. Postoperative delirium: predictors and prognosis in elderly orthopedic patients. *J Am Geriatr Soc* 1992;40:759–767.

97. Burke AL, Diamond PL, Hulbert J, Yeatman J, Farr EA. Terminal restlessness—its management and the role of midazolam. *Med J Aust* 1991;155(7):485–487.

98. Dunlop GM. A study of the relative frequency and importance of gastrointestinal symptoms and weakness in patients with far advanced cancer. *Palliat Med* 1989;4:37–43.

99. Welch JM, Barlow D, Richardson PH. Symptoms of HIV disease. *Palliat Med* 1991;5:46–51.

100. McCorkle R, Young K. Development of a symptom distress scale. *Cancer Nurs* 1978;1(373–78)

101. Ingham JM, Portenoy RK. Symptom assessment. In: Cherny NI, Foley KM, eds. *Hematol Oncol Clin North Am* 1996;10(1):21–40.

102. Othmer E, Othmer SC. *The clinical interview using DSM IV:* fundamentals, 2nd ed, vol 1. Washington DC: American Psychiatric Press; 1994.

103. Seidel HM, Ball JW, Davis JE, Benedict GW. *Mosby's guide to physical examination,* 3rd ed. St. Louis: CV Mosby, 1991.

104. Adams RD, Victor R, Ropper AM. *Principles of neurology*. New York: McGraw-Hill, 1997.

105. Leipzig RM, Goodman H, Gray G, Erle H, Reidenberg MM. Reversible, narcotic-associated mental status impairment in patients with metastatic cancer. *Pharmacology* 1987;35:47–54.

106. Posner JB, Plum F. *Diagnosis of stupor and coma*, 3rd ed. Philadelphia: FA Davis, 1982.

107. Murray GB. Confusion, delirium, and dementia. In: Hackett TP, Cassem NH, eds. *Massachusetts General Hospital handbook of general hospital psychiatry*. Littleton, MA: PSG, 1987;84–115.

108. Holland JC, Massie MJ. Psychosocial aspects of cancer in the elderly. *Clin Geriatr Med* 1987;3(3):533–539.

109. Massie MJ, Holland JC. Depression and the cancer patient. *J Clin Psychiatry* 1990;51(Suppl):12–17.

110. Draper B. Potentially reversible dementia: a review. *Aust N Z J Psychiatry* 1991;25(4):506–518.

111. van Marwijk H, Hoeksema HL, Hermans J, Kaptein AA, Mulder JD. Prevalence of depressive symptoms and depressive disorder in primary care patients over 65 years of age. *Fam Pract* 1994;11(1):80–84.

112. Glasser M, Stearns JA, de Kemp E, van Hout J, Hott D. Dementia and depression symptomatology as assessed through screening tests of older patients in an outpatient clinic. *Fam Pract Res J* 1994;14(3):261–272.

113. Bukberg J, Penman D, Holland JC. Depression in hospitalized cancer patients. *Psychosom Med* 1984;46(3):199–212.

114. Bruera E, Schoeller T, Montejo G. Organic hallucinosis in patients receiving high doses of opiates for cancer pain. *Pain* 1992;48(3):397–399.

115. Trzepacz PT. A review of delirium assessment instruments. *Gen Hosp Psychiatry* 1994;16(6):397–405.

116. Smith MJ, Breitbart WS, Platt MM. A critique of instruments and methods to detect, diagnose, and rate delirium. *J Pain Sympt Manage* 1995;10(1):35–77.

117. Katzman R, Brown T, Fuld P, Peck A, Schechter R, Schimmel H. Validation of a short orientation-memory-concentration test of cognitive impairment. *Am J Psychiatry* 1983;140(6):734–739.

118. Fainsinger RL, Tapper M, Bruera E. A perspective on the management of delirium in terminally ill patients on a palliative care unit. *J Palliat Care* 1993;9(3):4–8.

119. Inouye SK, Van Dyck CH, Alessi CA, Balkin S, Siegal AP, Horwitz RI. Clarifying confusion: the confusion assessment method. *Ann Intern Med* 1990;113:941–948.

120. Albert MS, Levkoff SE, Reilly C, Liptzin B, Pilgrim D, Cleary PD, et al. The delirium symptom interview: an interview for the detection of delirium symptoms in hospitalized patients. *J Geriatr Psychiatry Neurol* 1992;5(1):14–21.

121. Trzepacz PT, Baker RW, Greenhouse J. A symptom rating scale for delirium. *Psychiatr Res* 1988;23:89–97.

122. American Psychiatric Association. *Diagnostic and statistical manual of mental disorders*, 3rd ed. Washington, DC, 1980.

123. Breitbart W, Rosenfeld B, Roth A, Smith MJ, Cohen K, Passik S. The Memonal Delirium Assessment Scale. *J Pain Synptom Manage* 1997;13:128–137.

124. Fainsinger R, Bruera E. Treatment of delirium in a terminally ill patient. *J Pain Sympt Manage* 1992;7(1):54–56.

125. Stiefel F, Bruera E. Psychostimulants for hypoactive-hypoalert delirium? *J Palliat Care* 1991;7(3):25–26.

126. Fainsinger R, Miller MJ, Bruera E, Hanson J, MacEachern T. Symptom control during the last week of life on a palliative care unit. *J Palliat Care* 1991;7(1):5–11.

127. Folstein MF, Fetting JH, Lobo A, Niaz U, Capozzoli KD. Cognitive assessment of cancer patients. *Cancer* 1984;53(May 15 supplement):2250–2257.

128. Anthony JC, Le Resche L, Niaz U, Von Korff MR, Folstein MF. Limits of the "Mini-Mental State" as a screening test for dementia and delirium among hospital patients. *Psychol Med* 1982;12:387–408.

129. Fleishman S, Lesko LM. Delirium and dementia. In: Holland JC, Rowland JH, eds. *Handbook of psychooncology*. New York: Oxford University Press, 1989;342–355.

130. Fleishman SB, Lesko LM, Breitbart W. Treatment of organic mental disorders in cancer patients. In: Breitbart W, Holland JC, eds. *Psychiatric aspects of symptom management in cancer patients*. Washington, DC: American Psychiatric Press, 1993;23–47.

131. Fainsinger RL, Miller MJ, Bruera E. Morphine intoxication during acute reversible renal insufficiency. *J Palliat Care* 1992;8(2):52–53.

132. Caraceni A, Martini C, De Conno F, Ventafridda V. Organic brain syndromes and opioid administration for cancer pain. *J Pain Sympt Manage* 1994;9(8):527–533.

133. MacDonald N, Der L, Allan S, Champion P. Opioid hyperexcitability: the application of alternate opioid therapy. *Pain* 1993;53:353–355.

134. Bruera E, Franco JJ, Maltoni M, Watanabe S, Suarez-Almazor M. Changing pattern of agitated impaired mental status in patients with advanced cancer: association with cognitive monitoring, hydration and opioid rotation. *J Pain Sympt Manage* 1995;10:287–291.

135. Cherny NJ, Chang V, Frager G, Ingham JM, Tiseo PJ, Popp B, et al. Opioid pharmacotherapy in the management of cancer pain: a survey of strategies used by pain physicians for the selection of analgesic drugs and routes of administration. *Cancer* 1995;76(7):1283–1293.

136. Borreani C, Caraceni A, Tamburini M. The role of counselling for the confused patient and the family. In: Portenoy RK, Bruera E, eds. *Topics in palliative care*. New York: Oxford University Press; 45–54. In press.

137. Owens JF, Hutelmyer CM. The effect of preoperative intervention on delirium in cardiac surgical patients. *Nursing Res* 1982;31:60–62.

138. Williams MA, Campbell EB, Raynor WJ, Mylnrazyk SM, Ward SE. Reducing acute confusional states in elderly patients with hip fractures. *Res Nursing Health* 1985;8:329–337.

139. Rabins PV. Psychosocial and management aspects of delirium. *Int Psychogeriatrics* 1991;3(2):319–324.

140. Rummans TA, Evans JM, Krahn LE, Fleming KC. Delirium in elderly patients: evaluation and management. *Mayo Clin Proc* 1995;70(10):989–998.

141. Levenson JA. Should psychostimulants be used to treat delirious patients with depressed mood? *J Clin Psychiatry* 1992;53(2):69.

142. Breitbart W, Bruera E, Chochinov H, Lynch M. Neuropsychiatric syndromes and psychological symptoms in patients with advanced cancer. *J Pain Sympt Manage* 1995;10(2):131–141.

143. Settle EJ, Ayd FJ. Haloperidol: a quarter century of experience. *J Clin Psychiatry* 1983;44(12):440–448.

144. Clinton JE, Sterner S, Stelmachers Z, Ruiz E. Haloperidol for sedation of disruptive emergency patients. *Ann Emerg Med* 1987;16:319–322.

145. Adams F. Neuropsychiatric evaluation and treatment of delirium in cancer patients. *Adv Psychosom Med* 1988;18:26–36.

146. Fernandez F, Levy JK, Mansell PW. Management of delirium in terminally ill AIDS patients. *Int J Psychiatry Med* 1989;19(2):165–172.

147. Breitbart W, Marotta R, Platt MM, Weisman H, Dervenco M, Grav C, Corbera K, Raymond S, Lund S, Jacobsen P. A double-blind trial of Halopendol, Chlorpromazine, and Lorezepam—The treatment of delirium in hospitalized AIDS patients. *Am J Psychiatry* 1996;153:231–237.

148. Stiefel F, Holland J. Delirium in cancer patients. *Int Psychogeriatrics* 1991;3(2):333–336.

149. Fainsinger R, Bruera E. Treatment of delirium in a terminally ill patient. *J Pain Sympt Manage* 1992;7(1):54–56.

150. Lipowski ZJ. Update on delirium. *Psychiatr Clin North Am* 1992;15(2):335–346.

151. Sumner AD, Simons RJ. Delirium in the hospitalized elderly. *Cleve Clin J Med* 1994;61(4):258–262.

152. Shapiro BA, Warren J, Egol AB, Greenbaum DM, Jacobi J, Nasraway SA, et al. Practice parameters for intravenous analgesia and sedation for adult patients in the intensive care unit: an executive summary. Society of Critical Care Medicine. *Crit Care Med* 1995;23(9):1596–1600.

153. Seneff MG, Mathews RA. Use of haloperidol infusions to control delirium in critically ill adults. *Ann Pharmacother* 1995;29(7–8):690–693.

154. Pourcher E, Filteau M, Bouchard RH, Baruch P. Efficacy of the combination of buspirone and carbamazepine in early post-traumatic delirium. *Am J psychiatry* 1994;151(1):150–151.

155. FDA approved new drug bulletin: risperidone (Risperdal). *Rn* 1994;57 6):45–46.

156. Chouinard G, Arnott W. Clinical review of risperidone. *Can J Psychiatry* 1993;38(Supp 3):589–595.

157. Kane JM. Newer antipsychotic drugs. A review of their pharmacology and therapeutic potential. *Drugs* 1993;46(4):585–593.

158. Owens DG. Extrapyramidal side effects and tolerability of risperidone: a review. *J Clin Psychiatry* 1994;55(Supp):29–35.

159. Ayd PJ. Intravenous haloperidol therapy. *Int Drug Ther Newslett* 1987;13:20–23.

160. Gelfand SB, Indelicato J, Benjamin G. Using intravenous haloperidol to control delirium. *Hosp Commun Psychiatry* 1992;43(3):215.

161. Riker RR, Fraser GL, Cox PM. Continuous infusion of haloperidol controls agitation in critically ill patients. *Crit Care Med* 1994;22:433–440.

162. Fainsinger R, Schoeller T, Boiskin M, Bruera E. Palliative care round: cognitive failure and coma after renal failure in a patient receiving captopril and hydromorphone. *J Palliat Care* 1993;9(1):53–55.

163. Breitbart W, Holland JC. Psychiatric complications of cancer. *Curr Ther Hem Oncol* 1988;3:268–274.

164. Anderson BS, Adams F, McCredie KB. High dose of neuroleptics for acute brain failure after intensive chemotherapy for acute leukemia. *Acta Psychiatr Scand* 1984;70:193–197.

165. Volavka J, Cooper T, Czobar P. Haloperidol blood levels and clinical effects. *Arch Gen Psychiatry* 1992;49:354–361.
166. Adams F, Fernandez F, Andersson BS. Emergency pharmacotherapy of delirium in the critically ill cancer patient. *Psychosomatics* 1986;27(Suppl 1):33–37.
167. Platt MM, Breitbart W, Smith M, Marotta R, Weisman H, Jacobsen PB. Efficacy of neuroleptics in hypoactive delirium. *J Neuropsychiatry Clin Neurosci* 1994;6(1):66–65.
168. Dixon D, Craven J. Continuous infusion of haloperidol. *Am J Psychiatry* 1993;150(4):673.
169. Levenson JL. High-dose intravenous haloperidol for agitated delirium following lung transplantation. *Psychosomatics* 1995;36(1):66–68.
170. Rodnitzky RL, Keyser DL. Neurologic complications of drugs. *Psychiatr Clin North Am* 1992;15(2):490–510.
171. Kaplan HI, Benjamin JS, Grebb JA. Biological therapies. In: *Kaplan and Sadocks synopsis of psychiatry,* 7th ed. Baltimore: Williams and Wilkins, 1994;865–1015.
172. Cooper PE. Disorders of the hypothalamus and pituitary gland. In: Joynt RJ, eds. *Clinical neurology*, vol 3. Philadelphia: JB Lippincott, 1994;31–32.
173. Metzger E, Friedman R. Prolongation of the corrected QT and torsades de pointes cardiac arrhythmia associated with intravenous haloperidol in the medically ill. *J Clin Psychopharmacol* 1993;13(2):128–132.
174. Hunt N, Stern TA. The association between intravenous haloperidol and torsades de pointes. *Psychosomatics* 1995;36(6):541–549.
175. DiSalvo TG, O'Gara PT. Torsade de Pointes caused by high-dose intravenous halpoeridol in cardiac patients. *Clin Cardiol* 1995;18(5):285–290.
176. Breitbart W, Marotta R, Platt MM, Weisman H, Derevenco M, Grau C, et al. A double-blind trial of haloperidol, chlorpromazine, and lorazepam in the treatment of delirium in hospitalized AIDS patients. *Am J Psychiatry* 1996;153(2):231–237.
177. Ventafridda V, Ripamonti C, De CF, Tamburini M, Cassileth BR. Symptom prevalence and control during cancer patients' last days of life. *J Palliat Care* 1990;6(3):7–11.
178. Bird RD, Makela EH. Alcohol withdrawal: what is the benzodiazepine of choice? *Ann Pharmacother* 1994;28(1):67–71.
179. Dundee JW, Johnston HM, Gray RC. Lorazepam as a sedative-amnesic in an intensive care unit. *Curr Med Res Opin* 1976;4(4):290–295.
180. Simpson PJ, Eltringham RJ. Lorazepam in intensive care. *Clin Ther* 1981;4(3):150–163.
181. Deppe SA, Sipperly ME, Sargent AI, Kuwik RJ, Thompson DR. Intravenous lorazepam as an amnestic and anxiolytic agent in the intensive care unit: a prospective study. *Crit Care Med* 1994;22(8):1248–1252.
182. Bottomley D, Hanks G. Subcutaneous midazolam infusion in palliative care. *J Pain Sympt Manage* 1990;5(4):259–261.
183. Oliver DJ. The use of methotrimeprazine in terminal care. *Br J Clin Pract* 1985;39:339–340.
184. Adinoff B. Double-blind study of alprazolam, diazepam, clonidine, and placebo in the alcohol withdrawal syndrome: preliminary findings. *Alcohol Clin Exp Res* 1994;18(4):873–878.
185. Lohr RH. Treatment of alcohol withdrawal in hospitalized patients. *Mayo Clin Proc* 1995;70(8):777–782.
186. Miller NS. Pharmacotherapy in alcoholism. *J Addict Dis* 1995;14(1):23–46.
187. Verbanck PM. The pharmacological treatment of alcoholism: from basic science to clinical medicine. *Alcohol Alcoholism* 1995;30(6):757–764.
188. Peppers MP. Benzodiazepines for alcohol withdrawal in the elderly and in patients with liver disease. *Pharmacotherapy* 1996;16(1):49–57.
189. Weddington WW. The mortality of delirium: an underappreciated problem? *Psychosomatics* 1982;23:1232–1235.
190. Rabins PV, Folstein MF. Delirium and dementia: diagnostic criteria and fatality rates. *Br J Psychiatry* 1982;140:149–153.
191. van Hemert AM, van der Mast RC, Hengeveld MW, Vorstenbosch M. Excess mortality in general hospital patients with delirium: a 5-year follow-up of 519 patients seen in psychiatric consultation. *J Psychosom Res* 1994;38(4):339–346.
192. Thomas RI, Cameron DJ, Fahs MC. A prospective study of delirium and prolonged hospital stay. *Arch Gen Psychiatry* 1988;45(10):937–940.
193. Francis J, Kapoor WN. Prognosis after hospital discharge of older medical patients with delirium. *J Am Geriatr Soc* 1992;40(6):601–606.
194. Kolbeinsson H, Jonsson A. Delirium and dementia in acute medical admissions of elderly patients in Iceland. *Acta Psychiatr Scand* 1993;87(2):123–127.
195. World Health Organization. *Mental disorders: glossary and guide to their classification in accordance with the ninth revision of the international classification of diseases.* Geneva, 1978.
196. Pfieffer E. A short portable mental status questionnaire for the assessment of elderly psychiatric patients. *J Am Geriatr Soc* 1975;23:433–441.
197. Foreman M. Reliability and validity of mental status questionnaires in elderly hospitalized patients. *Nursing Res* 1987;36:216–220.
198. Williams MA, Ward SE, Campbell EB. Confusion: testing versus observation. *J Gerontol Nursing* 1986;14:25–30.
199. Miller PS, Richardson JS, Jyu CA, et al. Association of low serum anticholinergic levels and cognitive impairment in elderly presurgical patients. *Am J Psychiatry* 1988;145:342–345.
200. Ingham JM, Brietbart W. Epidemiology and clinical features of delirium. In: Portenoy RK, Bruera E, eds. *Topics in palliative care* New York: Oxford University Press; 7-19. In press.

*Principles and Practice of Supportive Oncology,*
edited by Ann Berger et al.
Lippincott–Raven Publishers, Philadelphia ©1998

CHAPTER 37

# Depression and Anxiety

David K. Payne and Mary Jane Massie

Emotional distress is a normal response to a catastrophic event such as the diagnosis of cancer or other life-threatening medical disease. The diagnosis of cancer induces stresses that are caused by the patient's perceptions of the disease, its manifestations, and the stigma commonly attached to this disease. For most individuals, the primary fear is a painful death. All patients also fear becoming disabled and dependent, having altered appearance and changed body function, and losing the company of those close to them. Each of these fears is accompanied by a level of psychological distress that varies from patient to patient. This variability is related to medical factors (e.g., site and stage of illness at the time of diagnosis, treatments offered, course of the cancer, and the presence of pain); psychological factors (e.g., prior adjustment, coping ability, emotional maturity, the disruption of life goals, and the ability to modify plans); and social factors (e.g., availability of financial support and emotional support from family, friends, and co-workers) (1). Understanding these factors allows the clinician to predict and manage distress that exceeds a threshold arbitrarily defined as normal. The presence of intolerable distress or prolonged distress that compromises the usual function of the patient requires evaluation, diagnosis, and management.

## NORMAL RESPONSES TO THE STRESS OF CANCER

Individuals who receive a diagnosis of cancer, or who learn that relapse has occurred or treatment has failed, show a characteristic emotional response: a period of initial shock and disbelief, followed by a period of turmoil with mixed symptoms of anxiety and depression, irritability, and disruption of appetite and sleep. The ability to concentrate and carry out usual daily activities is impaired, and thoughts about the diagnosis and fears about the future may intrude (2). These normal responses to crisis or transitional points in cancer resemble the response to stress that has been described in relation to other threatened or actual losses (3–6).

These symptoms usually resolve by 7–10 days with support from family and friends, and from the physician who outlines a treatment plan that offers hope. Interventions beyond those provided by physicians, nurses, social workers, and clergy are generally not required, unless symptoms of emotional distress interfere with function or are prolonged or intolerable. Prescribing a hypnotic (e.g., zolpidem or triazolam) to permit normal sleep and a daytime sedative (e.g., a benzodiazepine, such as alprazolam or lorazepam) to reduce anxiety can help the patient through this crisis period.

Some patients continue to have high levels of depression and anxiety (both are usually present, although one may predominate) that persist for weeks or months. This persistent reactive distress is not adaptive and frequently requires psychiatric treatment. These disorders are classified in the current *Diagnostic and Statistical Manual of Mental Disorders (DSM-IV)* (7) as adjustment disorders with depressed mood, anxiety, or mixed anxiety and depressed mood, depending on the major symptoms. For these patients, mental health professionals working in oncology utilize short-term supportive psychotherapy based on a crisis intervention model. This approach offers emotional support, provides information to help the patient to adapt to the crisis, emphasizes past strengths, and supports previously successful ways of coping. Patients and their families are seen at least weekly, and anxiolytic or antidepressant drugs are prescribed as indicated. As symptoms improve, medication can be reduced and discontinued. Having the patient talk with a veteran patient who has been through the same treatment is often a helpful adjunct (8).

D. K. Payne: Psychiatry Service, Memorial Sloan-Kettering Cancer Center, New York, NY 10021.

M. J. Massie: Barbara White Fishman Center for Psychological Counseling, Memorial Sloan-Kettering Cancer Center, and Department of Psychiatry, Cornell University Medical College, New York, NY 10021.

## PREVALENCE OF PSYCHIATRIC DISORDERS IN PATIENTS WITH CANCER

There are many myths about the psychological problems of patients with life-threatening illness, the conclusions of which range from "all patients are distressed and need psychiatric help" to "none are upset and no one needs help." One of the first efforts in the new field of psychooncology was to obtain objective data on the type and frequency of psychological problems in cancer patients. These data are useful to plan for the provision of services and utilization of support staff in cancer centers and oncology units.

Using criteria from the *DSM-III* (9) classification of psychiatric disorders, the Psychosocial Collaborative Oncology Group (PSYCOG) determined the psychiatric disorders in 215 randomly selected hospitalized and ambulatory adult cancer patients in three cancer centers (10). Slightly over half (53%) of the patients evaluated were adjusting normally to stress; the remainder (47%) had clinically apparent psychiatric disorders. Of this 47% with psychiatric disorders, over two thirds (68%) had reactive or situational anxiety and depression (adjustment disorders with depressed or anxious mood), 13% had a major depression, 8% had an organic mental disorder, 7% had a personality disorder, and 4% had a preexisting anxiety disorder. Thus, nearly 90% of the psychiatric disorders observed in this study were reactions to, or manifestations of, disease or treatment. Only 11% represented prior psychiatric problems, such as personality disorders or anxiety disorders. Comparable research in children is lacking, but clinical data appear to reflect a similar spectrum of problems. The physician who treats patients with cancer can expect, for the most part, to find a group of psychologically healthy individuals who are responding to the stresses posed by cancer and its treatment.

### Disorders in Cancer Patients with Pain

In the PSYCOG study (10), 39% of those who received a psychiatric diagnosis experienced significant pain. In contrast, only 19% of patients who did not receive a psychiatric diagnosis had significant pain. The psychiatric diagnosis of the patients with pain was predominately adjustment disorder with depressed or mixed mood (69%); however, it is of note that 15% of patients with significant pain had symptoms of a major depression.

Both data and clinical observation suggest that the psychiatric symptoms of patients who are in pain must initially be considered a consequence of uncontrolled pain. Acute anxiety, depression with despair (especially when the patient believes the pain means disease progression), agitation, irritability, uncooperative behavior, anger, and inability to sleep may be the emotional or behavioral concomitants of pain. These symptoms are not labeled as a psychiatric disorder unless they persist after pain is adequately controlled. Clinicians should manage pain (11) and then reassess the patient's mental state after pain is controlled to determine whether the patient has a psychiatric disorder.

## PREVALENCE OF DEPRESSION IN PATIENTS WITH CANCER

In De Florio and Massie's recent review of 49 studies, the prevalence of depression in cancer patients ranged from 1% to 53% (12). Most of this variance can be attributed to the lack of standardization of methodology and diagnostic criteria. For example, in a study of 152 oncology patients, Kathol and colleagues found a 13% difference (25% versus 38%) in the prevalence of depression depending on the diagnostic system used (13). Although the Research Diagnostic Criteria (RDC), *DSM-III* criteria, and *DSM-III-R* (14) criteria exclude the diagnosis of major depression if organic factors are involved, Kathol et al. did not apply this exclusion. *DSM-III* criteria (38%) yielded an 8% higher rate of depression than the *DSM-III-R* (30%) criteria, which excludes symptoms if they are definitely related to a physical condition, and the Endicott criteria, which substitute cognitive for physical symptoms, demonstrated a prevalence (36%) that approximated the *DSM-III* system. Using the most stringent criteria, the RDC, the lowest prevalence was found (25%). Kathol et al. suggest that different criteria identify different subsets of depressed individuals; the RDC identifies those with the most severe depression.

Using both *DSM-III* criteria, which were modified to eliminate physical symptoms characteristic of cancer, and validated depression rating scales, Bukberg and colleagues found a 42% (24% severe, 18% moderate) prevalence of depression among 62 (30 F, 32 M) patients hospitalized on oncology units (15), and Plumb and Holland found a 33% prevalence of depression among 80 (40 F, 40 M) hospitalized patients with advanced cancer (16). The Bukberg et al. finding of 42% prevalence of depression approximates the Kathol et al. finding of 38%, using the *DSM-III* criteria.

The existing data can answer many of the questions commonly asked about the prevalence of depression in patients with cancer: (a) Are there gender differences? (b) Are hospitalized patients more depressed than ambulatory patients? (c) Are those with advanced disease more depressed? In the aforementioned review of 49 studies (12), 29 included both males and females (12). Six studies did not examine or report gender differences, and the remaining 23 found no significant gender differences in the prevalence of depression.

Many clinicians have believed that hospitalized patients with advanced cancer are more depressed than ambulatory patients. However, as more studies have been done over time, hospitalization status explains little of the large variance. Now, because of insurance restrictions, many seriously ill cancer patients who would have been hospitalized are treated in ambulatory settings.

Advanced disease has been correlated with a higher prevalence of depression in several studies. The reported prevalence of depression in patients with advanced cancer ranges from 23% (16) to 53% (17). Bukberg and colleagues found that greater physical disability measured by the Karnofsky Performance Status Scale was associated with depression in their study of 62 patients with cancer (15). Their 42% overall prevalence of depression reflected a range of 23% in those with Karnofsky scores greater than 60 to 77% in those with Karnofsky scores <40.

Consultation data provide another source of information about depression in patients with cancer. At Memorial Sloan-Kettering Cancer Center, 59% of 546 consultations were requested for evaluation of depression or suicidal risk, or both (18). When the consultant's actual impressions were reviewed, depressive symptoms were by far the most common; adjustment disorders with depressed mood accounted for 54% of diagnoses, and major depression accounted for 9%. Breitbart reviewed data on 1080 consultation requests to the Psychiatry Service at the same institution and observed that evaluation of suicidal risk was the reason for referral in nearly 9% of referrals; suicide risk was found in 71 patients (6.5%) (19). One third of the suicidal patients had a major depression, more than half had an adjustment disorder, and nearly 20% had a delirium or organic brain syndrome.

## DIAGNOSIS OF DEPRESSION IN PATIENTS WITH CANCER

The practice guidelines for depression developed both by the American Psychiatric Association (20) and the Agency for Health Care Policy and Research (21) are practical guides to the management of depression in adults. These guidelines provide an overview of depression in both physically healthy and medically ill patients.

The diagnosis of depression in physically healthy patients depends heavily on the presence of somatic symptoms, including anorexia, fatigue, insomnia, and weight loss. These indicators are of little value as diagnostic criteria for depression in cancer patients, as they are common to both cancer and depression. In cancer patients, the diagnosis of depression must depend on psychological, not somatic, symptoms. These psychological symptoms are dysphoric mood, feelings of helplessness and hopelessness, loss of self-esteem, feelings of worthlessness or guilt, anhedonia, and thoughts of death or suicide (22).

## Mood Disorder Due to Cancer, Other Medical Conditions, or Substances

When evaluating depressed patients, it is imperative to determine whether organic factors underlie the depressive syndrome. A depressive syndrome caused by the direct physiologic effects of cancer is called "mood disorder due to cancer" in the current *DSM-IV* nosology. Although the key feature of this disorder is a prominent and persistent depressed mood that resembles a major depression, the presence of encephalopathy precludes the diagnosis of mood disorder due to cancer unless depression had been diagnosed before confusional symptoms developed. The patient with a mood disorder due to cancer may have mild cognitive deficits, such as poor memory or decreased concentration, and may have decreased control over sexual or aggressive impulses. Tumor involvement of the central nervous system, metabolic disturbances, and the presumed organic processes associated with carcinoma of the pancreas may cause this disorder. The case of pancreatic carcinoma represents a special problem because it is often unclear as to whether depressive symptoms are due to an indirect effect of the cancer on the brain (possibly alteration of serotonergic function) or due to a psychological reaction to this devastating cancer (23).

Among the metabolic causes of mood disorder due to cancer are electrolyte disturbances (e.g., hypercalcemia), endocrinopathies (e.g., hypothyroidism), and nutritional disorders (e.g., vitamin $B_{12}$ deficiency) disorders. Infections may also be responsible (e.g., Epstein-Barr virus infection).

*DSM-IV* defines disturbances in mood due to the direct physiologic effects of a substance (i.e., a drug of abuse or a medication) as a "substance-induced mood disorder." This diagnosis would be appropriate when depression is related to drug therapy such as β-adrenergic antagonists (24) (Table 1) or anticancer drugs, particularly corticosteroids, vinblastine, vincristine, procarbazine, asparaginase (25), tamoxifen (26), and interferon, which can cause depression (25) (Table 2).

In the medically ill, the evaluation of every depressed patient must include a thorough medical, endocrinologic, and neurologic assessment. A cognitive evaluation must be performed. Many clinicians prefer to use at least one easily reproducible instrument (e.g., the Mini-Mental Status Examination) (27) to document the mental status at the time of the initial evaluation and subsequent evaluations. All such brief instruments have limitations because they assess only selected aspects of cognition.

If the depressive disorder is believed to be caused by a medical condition or by a drug, the clinician should first attempt to treat the disorder or change the drug. Often antidepressants are started concurrently in an effort to alleviate symptoms more quickly or because the clinician anticipates that the depression that complicates the

**TABLE 1.** *Drugs that cause depression*

| Generic name | Brand name |
| --- | --- |
| Acyclovir | |
| Amphetamine-like drugs | |
| Anabolic steroids | |
| Anticonvulsants | |
| Baclofen | Lioresal |
| Barbiturates | |
| Benzodiazepines | |
| β-Adrenergic blockers | |
| Bromocriptine | Parlodex |
| Clonidine | Catapres |
| Cycloserine | Seromycin |
| Dapson | |
| Digitalis glycosides | |
| Diltiazem | Cardizem |
| Disopyramide | Norprace |
| Disulfiram | Antabuse |
| Ethionamide | Trecator-SC |
| Etretinate | Tegison |
| HMG-CoA reductase inhibitors | |
| Isoniazid INH | |
| Isosorbide dinitrate | Isordil |
| Isotretinoin | Accutance |
| Levodopa | Dopar |
| Mefloquine | Lariam |
| Methyldopa | Aldomet |
| Metoclopramide | Reglan |
| Metrizamide | Amipaque |
| Metronidazole | Flagyl |
| Nalidixic acid | Neggram |
| Narcotics | |
| Nifedipine | Procardia |
| Nonsteroidal antiinflammatory drugs | |
| Norfloxacin | Noroxin |
| Ofloxacin | Floxin |
| Phenylephrine | NeoSynephrine |
| Procaine derivatives | |
| Reserpine | Serpasil |
| Sulfonamides | |
| Thiaziades | |
| Thyroid hormones | |
| Trimethoprim-sulfamethoxazole | Bactrim |

Adapted from ref 24.

**TABLE 2.** *Anticancer drugs associated with depression*

| Drug | Cancer |
| --- | --- |
| Corticosteroids | |
| Vinblastine | Breast, lung |
| Vincristine | All, brain |
| Interferon | Renal, KS |
| Procarbazine | Brain |
| Asparaginase | All |
| Tamoxifen | Breast |
| Cyproterone | Prostate |

KS, Kaposi's sarcoma.
Adapted from ref 25.

underlying disorder will not be relieved by addressing the medical condition alone. When the primary cause of the depression cannot be corrected (e.g., the chemotherapeutic agent must be continued, as it usually must), antidepressant therapy is also initiated.

## Depression with Psychotic Features

Although rare, depression accompanied by delusions, hallucinations, or grossly disorganized behavior is sometimes encountered in medically ill patients. In this population, the presence of depressive symptoms (e.g., flat affect, lack of interest in daily activities), coupled with psychotic symptoms, more often reflects a delirium, and before the diagnosis of depression with psychotic fea-

tures is made, the presence of underlying organic causes for these mental status changes should be explored. When psychotic features are present, an antipsychotic and an antidepressant are usually started concurrently. High-potency neuroleptics (e.g., haloperidol, trifluoperazine, and fluphenazine) are usually preferred because of their low anticholinergic potential, which reduces the risk of delirium and other anticholinergic side effects (e.g., cardiac arrhythmias, constipation, urinary retention, and blurred vision). These high-potency neuroleptics also lower seizure threshold less than low-potency neuroleptics (e.g., chlorpromazine and thioridazine) and are preferable when the risk of seizures is a concern. Molindone, an intermediate potency neuroleptic, has been reported to have the lowest epileptogenic potential and may also be a good choice for a patient with psychotic symptoms and seizures that are difficult to control with anticonvulsants (28).

## Depression in the Elderly

Older individuals are at greater risk for depression and suicidal acts, whether physically healthy or not. In addition to the loss of good health, the elderly cancer patient often has sustained other losses, including physical ability (e.g., hearing loss) and financial stability. Grief following the death of a spouse or friends may be unresolved, and self-esteem may be damaged through retirement or changed social standing. Although the clinical presentation of depression can be similar to that described for younger adult patients, other presentations are more typical of this phase of life (29). For example, the chief complaints may be cognitive, such as poor memory or concentration. By taking a thorough history and by interviewing relatives or friends to document the patient's history, the clinician learns that depressive features may antedate the cognitive complaints. When asked specific questions, the patient often says "I don't know" instead of attempting to answer. Objective testing (e.g., with the Mini-Mental Status Examination) often reveals better results than those expected based on subjective complaints. This constellation is typical of the clinical syndrome *depressive pseudodementia*.

## Suicide

Suicidal ideation requires careful assessment to determine whether the patient has a depressive illness or is expressing a wish to have ultimate control over intolerable symptoms. Thoughtful clinical judgment is required to make this differentiation, especially in the patient with advanced disease. Breitbart (19) has outlined factors that place a cancer patient at a high risk for suicide: poor prognosis and advanced illness, depression and hopelessness, uncontrolled pain, delirium, prior psychiatric history, history of previous suicide attempts or family history of suicide, history of recent death of friends or spouse, history of alcohol abuse, and few social supports. Other risk factors include male sex; advanced age (sixth and seventh decades); presence of fatigue; and oral, pharyngeal, lung, gastrointestinal, urogenital, and breast cancers (Table 3).

Cancer patients have twice the risk of actually committing suicide as the general population (31,32). Many factors, such as poor prognosis, delirium, uncontrolled pain, depression, and hopelessness, are often linked in a patient with advanced disease, together increasing the risk of suicide. Hopelessness is an even stronger predictive factor than depression itself (33). Cancer patients usually commit suicide by overdosage with analgesics or sedative drugs prescribed by their doctors. Men use violent means, such as hanging or gunshot, more often than women.

**TABLE 3**. *Suicide risk factors in cancer patients*

Related to mental status
  Suicidal ideations
  Lethal plans (medications)
  Depression and hopelessness
  Delirium and disinhibition
  Psychotic features (hallucinations and delusions)
  Loss of control and impulsivity
  Irrational thinking
Related to cancer
  Uncontrolled pain
  Advanced disease and poor prognosis
  Site (oral pharyngeal, lung, gastrointestinal, urogenital, breast)
  Exhaustion and fatigue
  Use of steroids (mood changes)
Related to history
  Prior suicidal attempts
  Psychopathology
  Substance abuse (alcohol)
  Recent loss (spouse or friends)
  Poor social support
  Older male
  Family history of suicide

The management of the suicidal cancer patient includes maintaining a supportive therapeutic relationship; conveying the attitude that much can be done to improve the quality, if not the quantity, of life even if the prognosis is poor; and actively eliciting and treating specific symptoms (e.g., pain, nausea, insomnia, anxiety, and depression). The most useful psychotherapeutic modalities are based on a crisis intervention model using cognitive techniques (e.g., giving back a sense of control by helping the patient to focus on that which can still be controlled) and supportive methods, usually involving family and friends. One should keep in mind that the spouse and other family members are also at increased risk for suicide and that they also often require evaluation and support (1).

At Memorial Sloan-Kettering Cancer Center, virtually all hospitalized patients who have attempted suicide have had poorly controlled pain, mild encephalopathy, disinhibition secondary to drugs, and hopelessness combined with distress about the inability to communicate their concerns about their discomfort to caregivers. If a patient is suicidal, a 24-hour companion is provided to establish constant observation, monitor the suicidal risk, and reassure the patient. Need for observation is evaluated daily; companions are discontinued when the patient is no longer suicidal and is judged to be in control and able to act rationally.

## TREATMENT OF DEPRESSION

Before planning an intervention, the patient should be evaluated for a history of previous depressive episodes and substance (including alcohol and cocaine) abuse, family history of depression and suicide, concurrent life stresses, losses secondary to cancer (e.g., financial, social, and occupational), and the availability of social support. An assessment of the meaning of illness to the patient and his or her understanding of the medical situation (including prognosis) is essential. Depressed patients with cancer are usually treated with a combination of supportive psychotherapy and antidepressants (8,22); electroconvulsive therapy is utilized less often.

### Psychological Treatment

The goals of psychotherapy are to reduce emotional distress and to improve morale, coping ability, self-esteem, sense of control, and resolution of problems (34). Cancer patients are often referred for, or request, psychiatric consultation at times of crisis in illness: at the time of diagnosis or diagnosis of recurrence, at the beginning of any new treatment, when standard or experimental treatments fail, or when patients perceive themselves as terminal. The referral is often an emergency and, because of the acute crisis, the patient often readily accepts an intervention.

Various models of intervention for the acutely or chronically medically ill have been described, including time-limited dynamic psychotherapy or short-term dynamic therapy (35) and cognitive–behavioral therapy (36). Often 4–15 sessions is required to treat the acute problem. The patient considers his or her recent losses (good health, body integrity, self-esteem, family support, presumed longevity, financial security, and opportunity for job satisfaction) in the context of a past history of loss or success, and is helped to chart a future direction that incorporates life and body alterations brought on by the diagnosis of a chronic life-threatening illness. As mentioned above, the most useful model is based on a crisis intervention model that involves an active therapeutic role. Educational interventions, such as clarifying information and explaining emotional reactions to the patient, family, and staff, are useful. Cognitive techniques are also useful to help the patient correct misconceptions and exaggerated fears. Patients are encouraged to consider an array of different possible explanations or outcomes for their situation and then to determine which aspects they can still improve. This approach provides the patient with a sense of control over his or her situation and helps the individual to avoid focusing only on the worst eventualities.

Emotional support is also provided. Listening to the patient carefully and allowing him or her to express all feelings, fears, and anger in a nonjudgmental setting is often therapeutic in itself. Legitimization of the difficulty of the situation and of the right to be upset reduces the fear of being perceived as weak or inappropriate. Reassurances should be realistic and consistent with the available knowledge of the situation. The desire of patients to maintain hope is, of course, respected, as are the defense mechanisms of denial, repression, and regression, as long as these do not interfere with diagnostic or therapeutic processes or with important personal matters that must be addressed. As the patient's history of loss is explored, the clinician identifies and reinforces his or her successful ways of coping. At the termination of psychotherapy, patients are reassured to hear that the clinician is available for future visits if symptoms recur or if the disease worsens (1).

Another important aspect of the treatment of the depressed cancer patient is social support provided by family, friends, and community or religious groups. Although family is enlisted to provide emotional support, family members must be encouraged to minimize family conflicts, which add an additional emotional burden and can be addressed more appropriately after the depression has resolved. This process may also identify vulnerable family members who cannot provide emotional support and indeed may also need psychosocial help. These family members are encouraged to seek individual or group support for themselves.

## Drug Therapies

### Antidepressants

Although there are many reports of the efficacy of antidepressants in depressed patients with cancer (37–39), there is only one double-blind, placebo-controlled study (40) demonstrating efficacy. This observation reflects the difficulty in conducting controlled studies of drugs in medically ill cancer patients. Nonetheless, there is much clinical experience with antidepressant drugs in this population. The antidepressant agents that can be considered for use in cancer patients are (a) the newer agents, including selective serotonin reuptake inhibitors; (b) the tricyclic antidepressants; (c) the psychostimulants; (d) lithium carbonate; and (e) the monoamine oxidase inhibitors (41) (Table 4).

### Newer Antidepressants

The selective inhibitors of neuronal serotonin uptake (SSRIs), fluoxetine, sertraline, and paroxetine, are often prescribed first because they have fewer sedative and autonomic effects than the tricyclic antidepressants (TCAs). The most common side effects are nausea, headache, somnolence or insomnia, and a brief period of increased anxiety; hyponatremia is an uncommon adverse effect (42). These drugs can cause appetite suppression that usually lasts a period of several weeks. Some cancer patients experience transient weight loss, but weight usually returns to baseline level, and the anorectic properties of these drugs have not been a limiting factor in this population. Paroxetine has no active metabolites, and sertraline has fewer than fluoxetine; both have a shorter half-life. Their characteristics reduce the risk of accumulation during dose finding and allow more precise titration.

Bupropion, trazodone, maprotiline, amoxapine, venlafaxine, and nefazodone are prescribed less frequently than the SSRIs. Bupropion is considered if patients have a poor response to a reasonable trial of other antidepressants. It may be somewhat activating in medically ill patients and should be avoided in patients with seizure disorders, brain tumor or other factors that predispose to seizures, or malnutrition. Trazodone is strongly sedating and in low doses (100 mg at bedtime) is helpful in the treatment of the depressed cancer patient with insomnia. Effective antidepressant doses are often greater than 300 mg/day. Trazodone has been associated with priapism and should therefore be used with caution in male patients. Maprotiline also should be avoided in patients who are at high risk for seizures. Amoxapine has strong dopamine-blocking activity. Hence, patients who are taking other dopamine blockers (e.g., antiemetics) have an increased risk of developing extrapyramidal symptoms

**TABLE 4.** *Antidepressant medications used in cancer patients*

| Drug | Starting daily dosage, mg (PO) | Therapeutic daily dosage, mg (PO) |
|---|---|---|
| Newer agents | | |
|   Serotonin reuptake inhibitors | | |
|     Fluoxetine | 20 | 20–60 |
|     Sertraline | 50 | 50–150 |
|     Paroxetine | 10 | 10–50 |
|   Others | | |
|     Amoxapine | 25 | 100–150 |
|     Maprotiline | 25 | 75–150 |
|     Trazodone | 50 | 150–300 |
|     Bupropion | 75 | 200–300 |
|     Venlafaxine | 18.75 | 75–225 |
|     Nefazodone | 50 | 50–300 |
| Tricyclic antidepressants | | |
|   Amitriptyline | 25 | 50–150 |
|   Doxepin | 25 | 50–200 |
|   Imipramine | 25 | 50–200 |
|   Desipramine | 25 | 50–150 |
|   Nortriptyline | 25 | 20–100 |
|   Protriptyline | 20 | 10–30 |
| Psychostimulants | | |
|   Dextroamphetamine | 2.5 at 8 a.m. and noon | 5–30 |
|   Methylphenidate | 2.5 at 8 a.m. and noon | 5–30 |
|   Pemoline | 18.75 in a.m. and noon | 37.5–150 |
| Monoamine oxidase inhibitors | | |
|   Isocarboxazide | 10 | 20–40 |
|   Phenelzine | 15 | 30–60 |
|   Tranylcypromine | 10 | 20–40 |
| Lithium carbonate | 300 | 600–1200 |
| Benzodiazepine | | |
|   Alprazolam | 0.25–1.00 | 0.75–6.00 |

PO, orally.

and dyskinesias. Venlafaxine is a selective inhibitor of uptake pumps for both serotonin and norepinephrine and requires a twice-a-day dosing schedule. Nefazodone is structurally similar to trazodone and requires a twice-a-day dosing schedule.

When treating depression in the elderly, medications are started at a low dose, and the dosage is increased more slowly than with a younger adult patient. Also, drugs with few anticholinergic effects are preferred due to greater sensitivity of the elderly to anticholinergic complications (e.g., delirium, urinary retention, and cardiac arrhythmias) (43).

In contrast to adults, there are no clear data to support the efficacy of antidepressants in children (44). Nevertheless, clinicians often find it helpful to prescribe antidepressants to treat specific symptoms associated with depression. When the target symptoms are insomnia, poor appetite, or anxiety, a sedative tricyclic antidepressant (e.g., amitriptyline or doxepin) is usually prescribed. When the clinical picture is dominated by lack of energy or motivation, a serotonin reuptake inhibitor or an energizing tricyclic, such as desipramine, may be selected. As in the elderly, these drugs are started at a low dose.

*Tricyclic Antidepressants (Amitriptyline, Imipramine, Doxepin, etc.)*

Tricyclic antidepressants are still used in the oncology setting for both adults and children with cancer. Dosing is typically initiated at 10–25 mg at bedtime, especially in debilitated patients, and the dose is increased by 25 mg every 1–2 days until beneficial effect is achieved. For reasons that are unclear, depressed cancer patients often show a therapeutic response to a tricyclic at much lower doses (75–125 mg daily) than are usually required in physically healthy depressed patients (150–300 mg daily). Patients are usually maintained on a TCA for 4–6 months after symptoms improve, after which time the dose is gradually lowered and discontinued (41). The effects on appetite and sleep are frequently immediate; the effects on mood may be delayed.

The choice of TCA depends on the nature of the depressive symptoms, medical status, and side effects of the specific drug. The depressed patient who is agitated and has insomnia will benefit from the use of a TCA that has sedating effects, such as amitriptyline or doxepin. Patients with psychomotor slowing will benefit from use of the compounds with the least sedating effects, such as protriptyline or desipramine. The patient who has stomatitis secondary to chemotherapy or radiotherapy, or who has slow intestinal motility or urinary retention, should receive a TCA with the least anticholinergic effects, such as desipramine or nortriptyline.

Patients who are unable to swallow pills may be able to take an antidepressant in an elixir (amitriptyline, nortriptyline, or doxepin) or in an intramuscular form (amitriptyline or imipramine). Hospital pharmacies can prepare some TCAs (e.g., amitriptyline) in rectal suppository form, but absorption by this route has not been studied in cancer patients. Intramuscular (IM) administration causes discomfort because of the volume of the vehicle; hence, 50 mg is usually the maximum dosage that can be delivered per IM injection. Parenteral administration of TCAs may be considered for the cancer patient who is unable to tolerate oral administration because of impaired swallowing, the presence of gastric or jejunal drainage tubes, or intestinal obstruction. Although three TCAs (amitriptyline, imipramine, and clomipramine) are available in injectable form, the U.S. Food and Drug Administration has approved imipramine and amitriptyline for oral and muscular administration and clomipramine for oral use only. Formal informed consent and close monitoring of the electrocardiogram is recommended when these medications are used intravenously. Santos and colleagues have reviewed the few studies of parenteral TCA use (45) and have observed that therapeutic serum levels are more rapidly attained due to the lack of first-pass metabolism. A dose of imipramine administered intramuscularly yields twice the plasma concentration of the same dose administered orally. Route of administration also affects the pharmacologic action. With oral administration of imipramine, the demethylated metabolite (desipramine), a potent inhibitor of norepinephrine uptake, predominates in the plasma, whereas intramuscular imipramine administration yields a preponderance of imipramine, a serotonergic drug, in the plasma.

Imipramine, doxepin, amitriptyline, desipramine, and nortriptyline are used frequently in the management of neuropathic pain in cancer patients. Dosing is similar to that in the treatment of depression. Analgesic efficacy, if it occurs, is usually observed at a dose of 50–150 mg daily; higher doses are needed occasionally. Although the initial assumption was that analgesic effect resulted indirectly from the effect on depression, it is now clear that these tricyclics have a separate specific analgesic action, which is probably mediated through several neurotransmitters, most prominently norepinephrine and serotonin (46).

### Lithium Carbonate

Patients who have been receiving lithium carbonate for bipolar affective disorder prior to cancer should be maintained on it throughout cancer treatment, although close monitoring is necessary when the intake of fluids and electrolytes is restricted, such as during the preoperative and postoperative periods. The maintenance dose of lithium may need reduction in seriously ill patients. Lithium should be prescribed with caution in patients receiving cisplatin due to potential nephrotoxicity of both drugs.

Although several authors have reported that the leukocytosis produced by lithium could be beneficial in neutropenic cancer patients (47,48), the functional capabilities of these leukocytes have not been determined. The bone marrow stimulation appears to be transient. In patients without prior affective disorder, lithium does not produce mood changes.

### Monoamine Oxidase Inhibitors

If a patient has responded well to a monoamine oxidase inhibitor (MAOI) for depression prior to treatment for cancer, its continued use is warranted. Most psychiatrists, however, are reluctant to start depressed cancer patients on MAOIs because the need for dietary restriction is poorly received by patients who already have dietary limitations and nutritional deficiencies secondary to cancer illness and treatment.

### Psychostimulants

In cancer patients, the psychostimulants (i.e., dextroamphetamine, methylphenidate, and pemoline) promote a sense of well-being, decrease fatigue, and stimulate appetite (49–51). An advantage of these drugs is a rapid onset of antidepressant action compared with that of the TCAs. Psychostimulants can potentiate the analgesic effects of opioid analgesics and are commonly used to counteract opioid-induced sedation. Occasionally they can produce nightmares, insomnia, and even psychosis.

Treatment with dextroamphetamine and methylphenidate is usually initiated at a dose of 2.5 mg at 8 a.m. and noon. Pemoline, a chewable and less potent psychostimulant, is usually initiated at a dose of 18.75 mg at 8 a.m. The dose and dosing interval should be adjusted to optimize effects. Typically, patients are maintained on a psychostimulant for 1–2 months, after which time approximately two thirds will be able to be withdrawn without a recurrence of depressive symptoms (52). Those who develop recurrence of depressive symptoms can be maintained for long periods (e.g., >1 year). Tolerance may develop, and late adjustment of the dose may be necessary. Pemoline should be used with caution in patients with renal impairment; liver function tests should be monitored periodically with longer term treatment (53).

### Electroconvulsive Therapy

Occasionally, it is necessary to consider electroconvulsive therapy (ECT) for medically ill patients who are depressed and are refractory to antidepressants, or have depression with psychotic or dangerously suicidal features. Patients who have significant contraindications to treatment with antidepressant drugs are also considered for this approach. The safe and effective use of ECT in the medically ill has been reviewed by others (54).

## PREVALENCE OF ANXIETY IN PATIENTS WITH CANCER

Cancer disrupts the social roles of patients, their interpersonal relationships, and the ways in which they view their future (55); most people who have cancer are both fearful and sad. In the general population, anxiety is associated with female gender, younger age, and lower socioeconomic status (56). These patterns do not appear in cancer patients, suggesting that demographic factors may become less important in disease-related anxiety. Evaluation of anxiety symptoms is a frequent reason for psychiatric consultation in the oncology setting, accounting for 16% of requests in one study (18). In this study (18), 25% of patients were diagnosed as having either an anxiety disorder (4%) or an adjustment disorder with anxious mood (21%); in contrast, 57% were diagnosed as having either major depression (9%) or an adjustment disorder with depressed mood (48%). In the PSYCOG study, about 21% of the sample had symptoms of anxiety (10), and in several controlled studies cancer patients have been found to have higher levels of anxiety than healthy individuals. Maguire et al. (57) reported that 27% of women undergoing mastectomy had moderate to severe anxiety, compared to 14% of controls; and Brandenberg et al. (58) reported that 28% of advanced melanoma patients were anxious in comparison to 15% of controls.

Most studies of psychiatric symptoms in cancer patients have reported a higher prevalence of mixed anxiety and depressive symptoms than anxiety alone (10). Correlations between measures of depression and anxiety on both clinician-rated (59) and self-report measures (60) are high. In all likelihood, this observation indicates that these measures tap a common psychological trait: negative affect (61).

Maguire et al. reported that anxiety increases with the diagnosis of cancer, peaks prior to surgical interventions, and frequently remains high thereafter, declining gradually during the first postoperative years (57). Others have reported that anxiety increases as cancer progresses, and psychological health declines along with the decline in physical status (60,62). Chemotherapy administration is a source of anxiety that may develop into a conditioned anticipatory response, which may persist for years following the cessation of the chemotherapy (63–65). Radiotherapy treatment is also associated with increased anxiety, accompanied by concerns about increased bodily vulnerability and worries about whether the radiation will cause further body damage (66). The anxiety experienced during chemotherapy and radiation therapy may paradoxically increase at the termination of treatment, as patients feel unprotected, see their physician(s) less often, and worry about the effectiveness of treatment. Patients who are participating in clinical trials and feel that they have been randomized to a less aggressive treatment modality may also experience increased anxiety (67).

## DIAGNOSIS OF ANXIETY IN PATIENTS WITH CANCER

A small percentage of cancer patients have anxiety disorders that antedate the diagnosis of cancer and are exacerbated by the stress associated with cancer diagnosis or treatment (68). For most patients, anxiety symptoms are reactions to cancer and its treatment and are associated with feelings of foreboding, apprehension, or dread. Although anxiety symptoms can be either cognitive or somatic, the most salient symptoms are usually somatic and include tachycardia, shortness of breath, sweating, abdominal distress, and nausea. Loss of appetite, diminished libido, and insomnia, symptoms also associated with depression, are common in patients with anxiety, as are feelings of hyperarousal and irritability. In patients with panic attacks, symptoms related to increased autonomic discharge increase dramatically.

In addition to somatic symptoms, the anxious cancer patient is often plagued with recurrent unpleasant thoughts about cancer, including fears of death, disfigurement, disability, and dependency on others. The thinking style of the anxious patient is characterized by overgeneralization and catastrophizing; negative outcomes seem inevitable, and patients view themselves as helpless in a hopeless situation. Anxious patients may see their environment as threatening and often are motivated to flee, a reaction that commonly precipitates treatment refusals or demands for premature hospital discharge (69).

Although the diagnosis of anxiety in the cancer patient usually is determined by a clinical interview, the use of assessment instruments adds specificity to the diagnosis and facilitates the monitoring of treatment progress. Several instruments have been used to measure anxiety in cancer patients: the Profile of Mood States (70), the Symptom Checklist—90 (17), the Hospital Anxiety and Depression Scale (71), and the Rotterdam Symptoms Checklist (72). The Hospital Anxiety and Depression Scale (HADS) is a self-report measure that assesses the cognitive items associated with depression and anxiety and thus avoids the confound of physical symptoms in medically ill patients (71). The HADS has demonstrated validity in assessing mood disturbances in cancer patients (73). The Rotterdam Symptoms Checklist is a self-report scale that measures both psychological and physical distress in cancer patients (72). Although the Rotterdam Symptoms Checklist measures anxiety and depression in its psychological distress scale as a unitary phenomenon, the psychological distress scale does contain items associated with anxiety.

## Phobia, Panic Disorders, Generalized Anxiety Disorder, and Posttraumatic Stress Disorder

Phobias, panic disorder, posttraumatic stress disorder, and generalized anxiety disorder may antedate the diagnosis of cancer or first appear as patients are diagnosed and undergo cancer treatment. Because they cause extreme distress and have the potential to interfere with adequate medical management of the patient, it is important to accurately diagnose and treat these anxiety disorders (74).

There are a range of phobias that can be exacerbated by exposure to the medical environment; phobias about needles, blood, hospitals, and doctors are common. The common characteristic of all phobias is extreme anxiety on exposure to a feared object(s) or situation(s), and a persistent anxiety in the anticipation of these situations. Agoraphobia, the most common phobia in the general population, and claustrophobia may appear to present *de novo* in patients who are confined in the frightening hospital environment without their usual environmental supports. Patients who require magnetic resonance imaging or radiation therapy, or who must be confined in intensive care or reverse-isolation settings, frequently experience increased anxiety (75).

In contrast to phobias, in which there is a clearly defined situation or object of dread, panic disorder often presents as sudden, unpredictable episodes of intense discomfort and fear, accompanied by shortness of breath, diaphoresis, tachycardia, feelings of choking or being smothered, and thoughts of impending doom. Symptoms of a pre-existing panic disorder may intensify during cancer treatment; severe untreated symptoms may result in abrupt termination of cancer treatment. In contrast to panic disorder, generalized anxiety disorder is characterized by continuous and pervasive worry, difficulty in controlling the worry or apprehension, and the presence of symptoms of autonomic hyperactivity and hypervigilance.

In addition to heightened psychological distress associated with cancer treatment, cancer patients may experience the symptoms characteristic of posttraumatic stress disorder (PTSD) following the completion of their treatment. This disorder is similar to that reported by individuals who have been subjected to other types of trauma (e.g., combat, rape, or natural disaster) (76). Alter et al. reported that almost half (48%) of a group of cancer survivors reported symptoms related to PTSD, with 4% meeting the criteria for current PTSD diagnosis and 22% meeting the criteria for a lifetime diagnosis of PTSD (77). Patients with this disorder may repeatedly re-experience frightening events associated with their cancer diagnosis or treatment and have a chronic exaggerated startle response, nightmares, or autonomic hyperactivity.

## Anxiety Disorder Due to Cancer and Substance-Induced Anxiety Disorder

Anxiety in cancer patients may also be caused or exacerbated by medications used to treat cancer or other conditions, abnormal metabolic states, or uncontrolled pain. Anxiety may also be conditioned by events related to chemotherapy or radiation therapy. Although previous diagnostic nosologies did not allow for the classification of anxiety symptoms resulting from medically related causes, the *DSM-IV* (7) has included the diagnostic categories of anxiety disorder due to a medical condition (such as cancer) and substance-induced anxiety disorder.

Some drugs, such as the corticosteroids, can produce anxiety, and others can cause restlessness and agitation that is described as anxiety by the patient. The akathisia produced by neuroleptics (e.g., metoclopramide and prochlorperazine), for example, is frequently misdiagnosed as anxiety (78). Drug intoxication (e.g., cocaine) and withdrawal symptoms (e.g., from alcohol, benzodiazepines, or opioids) also have anxiety as a common symptom. Bronchodilators, β-adrenergic drugs, and psychostimulants (including caffeine) can cause anxiety, irritability, and tremulousness. Thyroid replacement medication can produce symptoms of anxiety, especially when the dosage is being adjusted (79).

Metabolic disturbances, such as hypoglycemia, hypoxia, and undetected anemia, may be manifested by symptoms of anxiety, restlessness, and agitation followed by confusion and disorientation. Encephalopathy associated with systemic infection and the remote effects of specific tumors (pancreatic [80], thyroid [81], pheochromocytomas [82], and parathyroid [83]) may also result in high levels of anxiety. Some patients with central nervous system neoplasms report anxiety as a prominent symptom (84).

One of the most common causes of anxiety is poorly controlled pain. The individual in pain may appear mildly to moderately anxious (85), and if no relief is available, the patient's level of anxiety and agitation may increase. Not uncommonly, patients express suicidal ideation in the context of uncontrolled pain. The existence of an anxiety disorder, like a depressive disorder, cannot be confirmed in the context of uncontrolled pain (86).

Chemotherapy and radiation therapy also can be associated with increased anxiety. Repeated exposures to highly emetogenic chemotherapeutic agents may lead to the development of anticipatory nausea and vomiting (ANV), a conditioned response to environmental cues (such as the sight of the hospital or the smell of the alcohol swabs) that surround the chemotherapy experience. There is evidence that ANV may be linked to a preexisting anxiety diathesis and that it may persist for years following the cessation of chemotherapy (65,87). Patients undergoing radiation therapy also feel apprehensive and anxious (88), and this affect may not decline as treatment progresses. Worsening side effects and the fear associated with the cessation of treatment may help perpetuate the anxiety. The psychological distress associated with radiation therapy may exceed the physical distress resulting from the treatment itself (89–91).

## Anxiety as a Manifestation of Other Psychiatric Disorders

In the medically ill, anxiety may be a manifestation of either depression or delirium. Increasingly, depression and anxiety are viewed as syndromes existing on a continuum; there is an overlap in the symptomatology between these two mood states. Depression may be distinguished from anxiety by the presence of the psychological symptoms of depression, such as hopelessness, anhedonia, worthlessness, and suicidal ideation. Delirium frequently has anxiety or restlessness as a prominent feature but is distinguished from anxiety by the presence of disorientation; impaired memory and concentration; fluctuating level of consciousness; and altered perceptions, including hallucinations and delusions (92).

## TREATMENT OF ANXIETY

The most effective management of anxiety in cancer patients is multimodal and usually involves psychotherapy, behavioral therapy, and pharmacologic management. During the initial evaluation of the patient's symptoms, both emotional support and information is given to the patient (93). Exploration of the patient's fears and apprehensions about disease progression, upcoming procedures, or psychosocial concerns often alleviate a substantial degree of the anxiety. Patient concerns usually include death, physical suffering, increased dependence, changes in social role functioning, spiritual matters, and worry about finances or employment (94).

### Psychological Treatment

Relatively short-term psychological interventions have proven to be effective in reducing the distress associated

with cancer (95). The efficacy of psychological treatments without the use of drugs depends upon the duration and severity of the patient's anxiety. In the case of mild to moderate anxiety, the use of psychological techniques alone may be sufficient (96).

Careful patient selection is important for the success of psychological approaches. Cancer patients who are most likely to benefit from psychological interventions are those who have anxiety that has not been controlled by other means; who have a need for self-control and are reluctant to take medication; and who have experienced or acknowledge the efficacy of such approaches. Individuals who are poor candidates for psychological approaches are those who have delirium or dementia; who are disinterested or demonstrate non-compliance in learning to use psychological techniques; and who have a history of serious psychiatric illness (97).

The psychological interventions for anxiety in cancer patients comprise four categories: psychoeducational, behavioral, cognitive–behavioral, and group interventions (98). Psychoeducational interventions are particularly useful for anxious cancer patients who have difficulty understanding medical information about their prognosis and planned procedures and treatments. As patients begin surgical, chemotherapeutic, or radiotherapeutic interventions, providing information about predictable side effects helps to normalize the experience and reduce anxiety (99,100). Similarly, explaining the predictable emotional phases associated with cancer may also alleviate anxiety. Providing information to a patient's family can improve the coping of family members, which in turn enhances the patient's sense of support (2,101).

The rationale for all behavioral techniques is the substitution of more adaptive behavior (e.g., increased coping ability) for less adaptive behavior (e.g., anxiety). Behavioral approaches to the management of anxiety are more useful than standard psychodynamic approaches for adults who do not think psychologically and for children. Progressive muscle relaxation has been demonstrated to be effective in the management of anxiety in cancer patients (102,103). In a study comparing the efficacy of relaxation and alprazolam in cancer patients, both treatments were shown to be effective for mild to moderate anxiety, with alprazolam having a slight advantage over relaxation training alone (104). Progressive relaxation involves instructing the patient to sequentially relax parts of the body through either tensing and relaxing the muscle groups (active muscle relaxation) or through concentrating on relaxing parts of the body without tensing the muscles (passive muscle relaxation). Both approaches are effective in reducing anxiety, although in medically debilitated patients passive relaxation may be more manageable (105). Frequently, guided imagery is a component of a progressive relaxation training program, and a behavioral treatment that includes both guided imagery and relaxation has been demonstrated to be more effective in lowering distress than either component alone (106,107). Hypnosis can be effective in the management of psychological distress associated with procedures (108) and in the management of treatment-related side effects such as ANV and pain. Desensitization, response prevention, thought stopping, modeling, and distraction are other behavioral techniques that may be useful in the management of anxiety and phobias (97).

Behavioral techniques have also been demonstrated to be effective in the treatment of anticipatory nausea and vomiting. As noted previously, ANV appears to be correlated with preexisting trait anxiety (87) and with state anxiety at the time of the chemotherapy infusions (109). Progressive muscle relaxation has been shown to decrease both nausea and vomiting, as well as anxiety, in patients who are receiving emetogenic chemotherapy (102,106, 110). Watson and Marrell have described an approach to ANV that combines behavioral approaches and a cognitive approach in which the patient's thoughts and feelings about chemotherapy are explored and modified (111).

Individual psychotherapy (98), including cognitive behavioral approaches (112), can be effective in the treatment of cancer-related anxiety. According to the cognitive–behavioral model, emotional distress arises or continues because of maladaptive beliefs and thinking patterns. Patients are encouraged to identify these maladaptive thoughts, reconsider them more logically, and experiment with alternative viewpoints and behaviors that give them greater control over their situation. Using this model to develop an intervention designed to address issues associated with cancer, Moorey and Greer (113) teach patients to identify negative thoughts, rehearse impending stressful events, implement ways of handling them more effectively, plan and carry out practical activities that create a sense of mastery, express feelings openly to one's partner, and increase both self-esteem and a fighting spirit by identifying and fostering personal strengths. Follow-up studies of this intervention have consistently demonstrated significantly lower scores on anxiety and psychological distress as compared to controls (113,114).

Group interventions have also been shown to reduce psychological distress in cancer patients (98). These interventions have benefited patients with a variety of cancer diagnoses (115) and stages of cancer (116). In one study, patients who participated in support groups for at least a year reported less tension than did controls (116). The techniques employed in these groups included fostering a sense of supportive commonality among the members, education, emotional support, stress management, coping strategies, and behavioral training.

## Pharmacologic Treatment

One quarter to one third of patients with advanced cancer receive antianxiety drugs during hospitalization (117). The severity of symptoms is the most useful guide in deciding whether a pharmacologic approach to the management of anxiety should be tried. Patients with mild reactive anxiety may benefit from either supportive measures or behavioral measures alone.

For patients who experience persistent apprehension and anxiety, the first-line drugs are the benzodiazepines. Lorazepam (0.25–2 mg four times daily) and alprazolam (0.25–1 mg three times daily) are useful for anxiety and other indications, such as nausea (lorazepam) and panic (alprazolam). Both lorazepam and alprazolam have been shown in controlled trials to reduce postchemotherapy nausea and vomiting and ANV (118,119). Lorazepam also has amnestic properties; when given prior to chemotherapy or a procedure, this effect may reduce the likelihood that a conditioned aversion will develop (120). A longer-acting benzodiazepine, such as clonazepam (0.5–1 mg), may provide more consistent relief of anxiety symptoms and have mood stabilizing effects as well. For insomnia, the benzodiazepines temazepam (15–30 mg at night) and triazolam (0.25–0.5 mg at night), as well as the nonbenzodiazepine hypnotic zolpidem (10–20 mg at night), may be effective. A nonsedating neuroleptic such as haloperidol (5 mg at night) or a sedating neuroleptic such as thioridazine (25–50 mg three times daily) may be more effective for the patient who is both anxious and confused. For patients with compromised hepatic function, the use of shorter-acting benzodiazepines, such as lorazepam, oxazepam, and temazepam, is preferred; these drugs are metabolized by conjugation with glucuronic acid and have no active metabolites.

Drowsiness and somnolence are the most common adverse effects of benzodiazapines. Reductions in dose and the passage of time eliminates these effects. Mental status changes, such as impaired concentration, memory, or recall, may result from benzodiazepine usage and are more common in elderly patients, those with advanced disease, and those patients with impaired hepatic function.

Structurally unlike other anxiolytics, buspirone (5–20 mg three times daily) is useful for patients with generalized anxiety disorder and those in whom there is the potential for benzodiazepine abuse. Buspirone is not effective on an as-needed basis, and its effects are not apparent for 1–2 weeks. Additionally, patients who have been prescribed benzodiazepines in the past may find that buspirone does not alleviate their anxiety as effectively as benzodiazepines.

For the treatment of panic disorder and agoraphobia, the benzodiazepine alprazolam and antidepressant medications (tricyclic antidepressants, serotonin reuptake inhibitors, and monoamine oxidase inhibitors) have demonstrated effectiveness. Although alprazolam rapidly blocks panic attacks, withdrawal can be difficult after prolonged use. The tricyclic antidepressant imipramine is often used for panic disorder; its anticholinergic side effects, however, are not well tolerated by debilitated cancer patients. In the oncology setting, the serotonergic reuptake inhibitors sertraline and paroxetine, which have

**TABLE 5.** *Antianxiety medications used in cancer patients*

| Drug | Approximate dose equivalent | Starting daily dosage, mg (PO) | Absorption | Metabolites |
|---|---|---|---|---|
| Benzodiazepines | | | | |
| Alprazolam | 0.5 | 0.25–1 t.i.d. | Intermediate | Yes |
| Oxazepam | 10 | 10–15 t.i.d. | Slow-Intermediate | No |
| Lorazepam | 1 | 0.5–2 t.i.d. | Intermediate | No |
| Chlordiazepoxide | 10 | 10–25 t.i.d. | Intermediate | Yes |
| Diazepam | 5 | 2–10 b.i.d. | Fast | Yes |
| Chlorazepate | 7.5 | 7.5–15 b.i.d. | Fast | Yes |
| Clonazepam | 0.25 | 0.25–1 b.i.d. | Intermediate | Yes |
| Temazepam | 30 | 15–30 qhs | Intermediate | No |
| Triazolam | 0.25 | 0.25–0.5 qhs | Intermediate | No |
| Antihistamines | | | | |
| Hydroxyzine | 10 | 10–50 t.i.d. | | |
| Diphenhydramine | 25 | 25–50 t.i.d. | | |
| Neuroleptics | | | | |
| Haloperidol | 0.5 | 0.5–2 b.i.d. | | |
| Thioridazine | 10 | 10–50 t.i.d. | | |
| Other | | | | |
| Zolpidem | 10 | 10–20 qhs | | |

fewer side effects than the tricyclic antidepressants, are effective in the management of both depression and panic disorder. Although monoamine oxidase inhibitors are effective in the management of panic disorder and depression, the risk of hypertensive crisis from concomitant ingestion of drugs or tyramine-containing foods make these medications less desirable for cancer patients.

In anxious patients with severely compromised pulmonary function, the use of benzodiazepines that suppress central respiratory mechanisms may be unsafe. A low dose of an antihistamine (e.g., hydroxyzine 10–50 mg three times daily) can be useful for these individuals.

## CONCLUSION

Depression and anxiety are common symptoms in cancer patients. These symptoms warrant evaluation and the use of pharmacologic and psychosocial interventions to relieve suffering. Psychologic distress should not be regarded as an unavoidable consequence of cancer.

## REFERENCES

1. Massie MJ, Gagnon P, Holland JC. Depression and suicide in patients with cancer. *J Pain Sympt Manage* 1994;9:325.
2. Massie MJ, Holland JC. Overview of normal reactions and prevalence of psychiatric disorders. In: Holland JC, Rowland JH, eds. *Handbook of psychooncology: psychological care of the patient with cancer.* New York: Oxford University Press, 1989;273.
3. Hamburg D, Hamburg B, de Goza S. Adaptive problems and mechanisms in severely burned patients. *Am J Psychiatry* 1953;16:1.
4. Horowitz M. *Stress response syndromes.* New York: Jason Aronson, 1976.
5. Lifton RJ. *Death in life: survivors of Hiroshima.* New York: Random House, 1967.
6. Lindemann L. Symptomatology and management of acute grief. *Am J Psychiatry* 1944;101:141.
7. American Psychiatric Association. *Diagnostic and statistical manual of mental disorders,* 4th ed. Washington, DC, 1994.
8. Massie MJ, Holland JC, Straker N. Psychotherapeutic interventions. In: Holland JC, Rowland JH, eds. *Handbook of psychooncology: psychological care of the patient with cancer.* New York: Oxford University Press, 1989;455.
9. American Psychiatric Association. *Diagnostic and statistical manual of mental disorders,* 3rd ed. Washington, DC, 1980.
10. Derogatis LR, Morrow GR, Fetting J, et al. The prevalence of psychiatric disorders among cancer patients. *JAMA* 1983;249:751.
11. American Pain Society. Principles of analgesic use in the treatment of acute pain and cancer pain. *Clin Pharmacol* 1990;9:601.
12. DeFlorio M, Massie MJ. Review of depression in cancer: gender differences. *Depression* 1995;3:66.
13. Kathol R, Mutgi A, Williams J, Clamong G, Noyes R. Diagnosis of major depression according to four sets of criteria. *Am J Psychiatry* 1990;147:1021.
14. American Psychiatric Association. *Diagnostic and statistical manual of mental disorders,* 3rd ed. Revised. Washington, DC, 1987.
15. Bukberg J, Penman D, Holland JC. Depression in hospitalized cancer patients. *Psychosom Med* 1984;46:199.
16. Plumb M, Holland JC. Comparative studies of psychological function in patients with advanced cancer. 1. Self-reported depressive symptoms. *Psychosom Med* 1977;39:264.
17. Craig TJ, Abeloff MD. Psychiatric symptomatology among hospitalized cancer patients. *Am J Psychiatry* 1974;131:1323.
18. Massie MJ, Holland JC. Consultation and liaison issues in cancer care. *Psychiatr Med* 1987;5:343.
19. Brietbart W. Suicide in cancer patients. *Oncology* 1987;1:49.
20. American Psychiatric Association. Practice guideline for major depressive disorders in adults. *Am J Psychiatry* 1993;150(Suppl):4.
21. Depression Guideline Panel. *Depression in primary care,* vol 2. Treatment of major depression. Clinical practice guideline, number 5, Rockville, MD: US Department of Health and Human Services, Public Health Service, Agency for Health Care Policy and Research. AHCPR Publ 93-0551, April 1993.
22. Massie MJ. Depression. In: Holland JC, Rowland JH, eds. *Handbook of psychooncology: psychological care of the patient with cancer.* New York: Oxford University Press, 1989;283.
23. Green AI, Austin PC. Psychopathology of pancreatic cancer: a psychobiologic probe. *Psychosomatics* 1993;34:208.
24. Drugs that cause psychiatric symptoms. *Med Lett* 1993;35:65.
25. Drugs of choice for cancer chemotherapy. *Med Lett* 1993;35:43.
26. Jones S, Cathcart C, Pumroy S, et al. Frequency, severity and management of tamoxifen-induced depression in women with node-negative breast cancer. *Proc Am Soc Clin Oncol* 1993;12:78.
27. Folstein MF, Folstein S, McHugh PR. Minimental state: a practical method for grading the cognitive state of patients for the clinician. *J Psychiatr Res* 1975;12:189.

28. Oliver AP, Luckins DJ, Wyett RJ. Neuroleptic induced seizures. *Arch Gen Psychiatry* 1982;39:206.

29. Magni G, Schafino F, DeLeo D. Assessments of depression in an elderly medical population. *J Affect Dis* 1986;11:121.

30. Breitbart W. Suicide in cancer patients. In: Holland JC, Rowland JH, eds. *Handbook of psychooncology: psychological care of the patient with cancer.* New York: Oxford University Press, 1989;291.

31. Fox BH, Stanek EJ, Boyd SC, Flannery JT. Suicide rates among women patients in Connecticut. *J Chronic Dis* 1982;35:85.

32. Louhivuori KA, Hakama M. Risk of suicide among cancer patients. *Am J Epidemiol* 1979;109:59.

33. Kovacs M, Beck AT, Weissman A. Hopelessness: an indication of suicide risks. *Suicide* 1975;5:98.

34. Worden JW, Weisman AD. Preventive psychosocial intervention with newly diagnosed cancer patients. *Gen Hosp Psychiatry* 1984;6:243.

35. Levenson H, Hales RE. Brief psychodynamically informed therapy for medically ill patients. In: Stoudemire A, Fogel BS, eds. *Medical psychiatric practice,* vol 2. Washington, DC: American Psychiatric Press, 1993;3.

36. Beck A, Rush AJ. Cognitive approaches to depression and suicide. In: Serban G, ed. *Cognitive defects in the development of mental illness.* New York: Brunner/Mazel, 1978;235.

37. Rifkin A, Reardon G, Siris S, Karagji B, Kim Y, et al. Trimipramine in physical illness with depression. *J Clin Psychiatry* 1985;46(2, sec 2):4.

38. Purohit DR, Navlakha PL, Modi RS, Eshpumiyani R. The role of antidepressants in hospitalized cancer patients. *J Assoc Phys India* 1978; 26:245.

39. Popkin MK, Callies AL, MacKenzie TB. The outcome of antidepressant use in the medically ill. *Arch Gen Psychiatry* 1985;42:1160.

40. Costa D, Mogos I, Toma T. Efficacy and safety of mianserin in the treatment of depression of women with cancer. *Acta Psychiatr Scand* 1985;72(Suppl 320):85.

41. Massie MJ, Lesko L. Psychopharmacological management. In: Holland JC, Rowland JH, eds. *Handbook of psychooncology: psychological care of the patient with cancer.* New York: Oxford University Press, 1989;470.

42. Vishwanath BM, Navalgund AA, Cusano W, Navalgund KA. Fluoxetine as a cause if SIADH. *Am J Psychiatry* 1991;148:542.

43. Salzman C. Practical considerations on the pharmacological treatment of depression and anxiety in the elderly. *J Clin Psychiatry* 1990; 51(Suppl):40.

44. Ambrosini PJ, Bianchi MD, Rabinovich HD, Elia J. Antidepressant treatments in children and adolescents: affective disorders. *J Am Acad Child Adolesc Psychiatry* 1993;32:1.

45. Santos AB, Beliles KE, Arana GW. Parental use of psychotropic agents. In: Stoudemire A, Fogel BS, eds. *Medical psychiatric practice,* vol 2. Washington, DC: American Psychiatric Press, 1993;113.

46. France RD. The future for antidepressants: treatment of pain. *Psychopathology 1987;20:99.*

47. Cantane RL, Kaufman J, Mittelman A, Murphy GP. Attenuation of myelosuppression with lithium. *N Engl J Med* 1977;297:452.

48. Lyman GH, Williams CC, Preston D. The use of lithium carbonate to reduce infection and leukopenia during systemic chemotherapy. *N Engl J Med* 1980;302:257.

49. Woods SW, Tesar GE, Murray GB, Cassem NH. Psychostimulant treatment of depressive disorders secondary to medical illness. *J Clin Psychiatry* 1986;47:12.

50. Fernandez F, Adams F, Holmes VF, et al. Methylphenidate for depressive disorders in cancer patients. *Psychosomatics* 1987;28:455.

51. Bruera E. Use of methylphenidate as an adjuvant to narcotic analgesics in patients with advanced cancer. *J Pain Sympt Manage* 1989;1:3.

52. Chiarello RJ, Cole JO. The use of psychostimulants in general psychiatry: a reconsideration. *Arch Gen Psychiatry* 1987;44:286.

53. Breitbart W, Mermelstein H. Pemoline, an alternative psychostimulant for the management of depressive disorders in cancer patients. *Psychosomatics* 1992;33:352.

54. Weiner RD, Caffey CE. Electroconvulsive therapy in the medical and neurologic patient. In: Stoudemire A, Fogel BS, eds. *Psychiatric care of the medical patient.* New York: Oxford University Press, 1993;207.

55. Derogatis L, Wise T. *Anxiety and depressive disorders in the medical patient.* Washington, DC: American Psychiatric Press, 1989.

56. Kessler R, McGonagle K, Zhao S, et al. Lifetime and 12 month prevalence of DSM III-R psychiatric disorders in the United States. *Arch Gen Psychiatry* 1994;51:8-19.

57. Maguire GP, Lee E, Bevington D, Kuchman C, Crabtree R, Cornell C. Psychiatric problems in the first year after mastectomy. *Br Med J* 1978;1:963.

58. Brandenberg Y, Bolund C, Sigurdardottir V. Anxiety and depressive symptoms at different stages of malignant melanoma. *Psychooncology* 1992;1:71.

59. Moorey S, Greer S, Watson M, et al. The factor structure and factor stability of the Hospital Anxiety and Depression Scale in patients with cancer. *Br J Psychiatry* 1991;158:255.

60. Cassileth BR, Lusk E, Huter R, Strouse T, Brown L. Concordance of depression and anxiety in patients with cancer. *Psychol Rep* 1984;54: 588.

61. Zinberg R, Barlow D. Mixed anxiety-depression. A new diagnostic category. In: Rapee R, Barlow D, eds. *Chronic anxiety: generalized anxiety disorder and mixed anxiety-depression.* New York: Guilford Press, 1991;136.

62. Weisman A, Worden J. The emotional impact of recurrent cancer. *J Psychosoc Oncol* 1986;3:5.

63. Holland J. Anxiety and cancer: the patient and the family. *J Clin Psychiatry* 1989;. 50:20.

64. Olafsdottir M, Sjoder P, Westling B. Prevalence and prediction of chemotherapy-related anxiety, nausea and vomiting in cancer patients. *Behav Res Ther* 1986;24:59.

65. Kvale G, Glimelius B, Hoffman K, Sjoden P. Pre-chemotheapy nervousness as a marker for anticipatory nausea: a case of a non-causal predictor. *Psychooncology* 1993;2:33.

66. Peck A, Boland J. Emotional reactions to radiation treatment. *Cancer* 1977;40:180.

67. Cassileth B, Knuiman M, Abeloff G, et al. Anxiety levels in patients randomized to adjuvant therapy versus observation for early breast cancer. *J Clin Oncol* 1986;4:972.

68. Sharer A, Schreiber S, Galai T, McLoud R. Posttraumatic stress disorder following medical events. *Br J Clin Psychol* 1993;32:247.

69. Braun P, Greenberg D, Dasberg H, Lerer B. Core symptoms of PTSD improved by alprazolam treatment. *J Clin Psychiatry* 1990;51:236.

70. Cella D, Jacobsen P, Orav E, Holland J, Silberfarb P, Rafla S. A brief POMS measure of distress in cancer patients. *J Chronic Dis* 1987;40: 939.

71. Zigmond A, Snaith R. The Hospital Anxiety and Depression Scale. *Acta Psychiatr Scand* 1983;67:361.

72. de Haes J, van Knippenberg F, Neijut J. Measuring psychological and physical distress in cancer patients: structure and application of the Rotterdam Symptom Checklist. *Br J Cancer* 1990;62:1034.

73. Ibbotson T, Maguire P, Selby T, Priestman T, Wallace L. Screening for anxiety and depression in cancer patients: the effects of disease and treatment. *Eur J Cancer* 1994;30A:37.

74. Massie M. Anxiety, panic, and phobias. In: Holland JC, Rowland, JH, eds. *Handbook of psychooncology: psychological care of the patient with cancer.* New York: Oxford University Press, 1989;300.

75. Brennan S, Redd W, Jacobsen P, et al. Anxiety and panic during magnetic resonance scans. *Lancet* 1988;2:512.

76. Hamner M. Exacerbation of posttraumatic stress disorder symptoms with medical illness. Gen Hosp Psychiatry. 1994;16:135.

77. Alter CL, Pelcovitz D, Axelrod A, et al. The identification of PTSD in cancer survivors. *Psychosomatics* 1996;37(2):137–143.

78. Fleishman S, Lavin M, Sattler M, Szarka H. Antiemetic-induced akathisia in cancer patients. *Am J Psychiatry* 1994;151:763.

79. Hall R. Psychiatric effects of thyroid hormone disturbance. *Psychosomatics* 1983;27:7.

80. Holland J, Hughes A, Korzan A, et al. Comparative psychological disturbance in patients with pancreatic and gastric cancer. *Am J Psychiatry* 1986;143:982.

81. Kathol R, Dalahunt J. The relationship of anxiety and depression to symptoms of hyperthyroidism using operational criteria. *Gen Hosp Psychiatry* 1986;8:23.

82. Starkman M, Zelnik T, Nesse R, et al. Anxiety in patients with pheochromocytomas. *Arch Intern Med* 1985;145:248.

83. Lawlor B. Hypocalcemia, hypoparathyroidism, and organic anxiety syndrome. *J Clin Psychiatry* 1988;49:317.

84. Strain F, Ploog R Anxiety related to nervous system dysfunction. In: Noyes R, Roth M, Burrows G, eds. *Handbook of Anxiety,* vol 2. Amsterdam: Elsevier, 1988;431.

85. Sternbach R. *Pain patients: traits and treatments.* New York: Academic Press, 1974.

86. Massie MJ, Holland J. The cancer patient with pain: psychiatric complications and their management. *Med Clin North Am* 1987;71:243.

87. Jacobsen P, Bovberg D, Redd W. Anticipatory anxiety in women receiving chemotherapy for breast cancer. *Health Psychol* 1993;12:469.

88. Forester B, Kornfeld D, Fleiss J. Psychiatric aspects of radiotherapy. *Am J Psychiatry* 1978;135:960.

89. Anderson B, Karlson J, Anderson B, Tewfik H. Anxiety and cancer treatment: response to stressful radiotherapy. *Health Psychol* 1984; 3:535.

90. Holland J, Rowland J, Lebovits A, et al. Reactions to cancer treatment: assessment of emotional response to adjuvant radiotherapy as a guide to planned intervention. *Psychiatr Clin North Am* 1979;2: 347.

91. Munro A, Biruls R, Griffin A, Thomas H, Vallis K. Distress associated with radiotherapy for malignant disease: A quantitative analysis based on patients perceptions. *Br J Cancer* 1989;60:370.

92. Wise M, Rieck S. Diagnositic considerations approaches to underlying anxiety in the medically ill. *J Clin Psychiatry* 1993;54:22.

93. Massie M, Shakin E. Management of depression and anxiety in cancer patients. In: Breitbart W, Holland J, eds. *Psychiatric aspects of symptom management in cancer patients*. Washington, DC: American Psychiatric Press, 1993;1.

94. Maguire P, Faulkner A, Regnard C. Eliciting the current problems of the patient with cancer. *Palliat Med* 1993;7:63.

95. Trijsburg R, Van Knippenbert F, Rijpma W. Effects of psychological treatment on cancer patients: a critical review. *Psychosom Med* 1992;54:489.

96. Maguire P, Faulkner A, Regnard C. Managing the anxious patient with advancing disease—a flow diagram. *Palliat Med* 1993;7:239.

97. Mastrovito R. Behavioral Techniques. In: Holland JC, Rowland JH, eds. *Handbook of psychooncology: psychological care of the patient with cancer*. New York: Oxford University Press, 1989;492.

98. Fawzy F, Fawzy N, Arndt L, Pasnau R. Critical review of psychosocial interventions in cancer care. *Arch Gen Psychiatry* 1995;52:100.

99. Ali N, Khalil H. Effect of psychoeducational intervention on anxiety among Egyptian bladder cancer patients. *Cancer Nursing* 1989;12:236.

100. Jacobs C, Ross R, Walker I, Stockdale F. Behavior of cancer patients: a randomized study of the effects of education and peer support groups. *Am J Clin Oncol* 1983;6:347.

101. Wellisch D, Moster M, Van Scoy C. Management of family emotional stress: family group therapy in a private oncology practice. *Int J Group Psychother* 1978;28:225.

102. Burish T, Tope D. Psychological techniques for controlling adverse side effects of cancer chemotherapy: Findings from a decade of research. *J Pain Sympt Manage* 1992;7:287.

103. Fleming U. Relaxation therapy for far-advanced cancer. *Practitioner* 1987;229:471.

104. Holland J, Morrow G, Schmale A, et al. A randomized clinical trial of alprazolam versus progressive muscle relaxation in cancer patients with anxiety and depressive symptoms. *J Clin Oncol* 1991;9:1004.

105. Ferguson J, Marquis J, Taylor C. A script for deep muscle relaxation. *Dis Nerv Syst* 1977;38:703.

106. Burish T, Carey M, Krozely M, Greco F. Conditioned side effects induced by cancer chemotherapy prevention through behavioral treatment. *J Consult Clin Psychol* 1987;55:42.

107. Gruber B, Hersh S, Hall N, et al., Immunological responses of breast cancer patients to behavioral interventions. *Biofeedback Self Regul* 1993;18:1.

108. Wilson-Barnet, J. Psychological reaction to medical procedures. *Psychother Psychosom* 1992;57:118.

109. Andrykowski, M. The role of anxiety in the development of anticipatory nausea in cancer chemotherapy: a review and synthesis. *Psychosom Med* 1990;52:458.

110. Vasterling J, Jenkins R, Tope D. Burish T. Cognitive distraction and relaxation training for the control of side effects due to cancer chemotherapy. *J Behav Med* 1993;16:65.

111. Watson M, Marvell C. Anticipatory nausea and vomiting among cancer patients: A review. *Psychology Health* 1992;6:97.

112. Moorey S, Greer S. *Psychological therapy for patients with cancer: a new approach*. Oxford: Heinemann, 1989.

113. Greer S, Moorey S, Baruch J, et al. Adjuvant psychological therapy for patients with cancer: a prospective randomized trial. *Br Med J* 1992;304:675.

114. Moorey S, Greer S, Watson M, et al. Adjuvant psychological therapy for patients with cancer: outcome at one year. *Psychooncology* 1994; 3:39.

115. Cain D, Kohorn E, Quinlan D, Latimer K, Schwartz P. Psychosocial benefits of a cancer support group. *Cancer* 1986;57:183.

116. Spiegel D, Bloom J, Yalom I. Group support for patients with metastatic cancer. *Arch Gen Psychiatry* 1981;38:527.

117. Stiefel F, Kornblith A, Holland J. Changes in the prescription patterns of psychotropic drugs for cancer patients during a 10 year period. *Cancer* 1990;65:1048.

118. Triozzi P, Goldstein D, Laszlo J. Contributions of benzodiazepines to cancer therapy. *Cancer Invest* 1988;6:103.

119. Greenberg D, Surman O, Clarke J, et al. Alprazolam for phobic nausea and vomiting related to cancer chemotherapy. *Cancer Treat Rep* 1987;71:549.

120. Klein D. Prevention of claustrophobia induced by MR imaging: use of alprazolam. *AJR* 1991;156:633.

*Principles and Practice of Supportive Oncology,*
edited by Ann Berger et al.
Lippincott–Raven Publishers, Philadelphia ©1998

CHAPTER 38

# Substance Abuse Issues in Palliative Care

Steven D. Passik and Russell K. Portenoy

Nearly one third of the United States population has used illicit drugs and an estimated 6–15% have a substance use disorder of some type (1–3). As a result of this high prevalence, and the association between drug abuse and life-threatening diseases such as AIDS, cirrhosis, and some types of cancer (4), problems related to abuse and addiction are commonly encountered in palliative care settings. In diverse patient populations with progressive life-threatening diseases, a remote or current history of drug abuse presents a constellation of physical and psychosocial issues that can both complicate the management of the underlying disease and undermine palliative therapies. The stigma associated with drug abuse is profound, and fear of addiction can also adversely influence the management of patient populations, including those with no prior history of drug abuse or addiction. Clearly, the interface between the therapeutic use of potentially abusable drugs and the abuse of these drugs is complex and must be understood to optimize palliative care.

Patients who have a history of abuse or addiction are extremely heterogeneous and the concerns central to palliative care may vary with the status of the patient. Although empirical data that define group differences are lacking, it is evident that patients who are actively abusing illicit drugs, alcohol, or prescription drugs present a spectrum of problems distinct from patients in drug-free recovery and those in methadone maintenance programs. This distinction is useful but still oversimplifies the variation in these populations. Among those who are actively abusing, for example, the clinical issues associated with heroin addiction are different from those that attend alcoholism; and for both disorders, the problems associated with frequent daily use may be different from those associated with more occasional use. In all cases, appropriate diagnosis of the patient may be challenging because of the variability over time in abuse behaviors, the changes in comorbid physical and psychosocial factors that influence drug use, and the problems inherent in the nomenclature of drug abuse in the medically ill.

There is similar complexity in the range of clinical problems presented by patients with substance abuse histories. Clinicians must control and monitor drug use in all patients, a daunting task in some active abusers. In some cases, a major issue is compliance with treatments for the underlying disease, which may be so poor that the substance abuse actually shortens life expectancy by preventing the effective administration of primary therapy. Prognosis may also be altered by the use of drugs in a manner that negatively interacts with therapy or predisposes to other serious morbidity. The goals of care can be very difficult to define when poor compliance and risky behavior appears to contradict a reported desire for disease-modifying therapies.

A remote or current history of substance abuse also may weaken already fragile social support networks that are crucial for mitigating the chronic stressors associated with cancer and cancer treatment. Among these supports is the relationship to the treatment team. Concerns about drug abuse may lead clinicians to doubt the veracity of the history, the report of symptoms, and the compliance with therapy. A desire to build trust may lead clinicians to hide these concerns from the patient, which reduces the opportunity for resolution and further undermines the therapeutic alliance with staff. Patients with a history of substance abuse, who often come from backgrounds characterized by exploitation and neglect, may sense the mistrust, question the team's good will, and harbor negative expectations that become self-fulfilling prophesies. The lack of mutual trust that can characterize the relationships between the patients and members of the treatment team can disrupt the assess-

S. D. Passik: Community Cancer Care, Inc., Indianapolis, IN 46202.

R. K. Portenoy: Department of Pain Medicine and Palliative Care, Beth Israel Medical Center, New York, NY 10003.

ment, management, and follow-up of these patients and result in the failure of therapies intended to improve quality of life. If illicit or manipulative behaviors occur, extraordinary efforts by the treatment team may be required to avoid a vicious cycle of undertreatment, drug abuse, and diminished trust.

Thus, a history of substance abuse can undermine palliative care and increase the risk of morbidity, and even early mortality, among those with progressive life-threatening diseases. This potential can only be mitigated by a therapeutic strategy that addresses drug taking behavior while implementing other therapies. Clinicians who provide palliative care must be knowledgeable about the basic concepts of addiction medicine to organize this strategy.

## PREVALENCE OF SUBSTANCE USE DISORDERS IN THE MEDICALLY ILL

There have been few studies that evaluate the epidemiology of substance abuse in patients with progressive medical illnesses. Most of the extant data originate from the cancer population. Substance abuse appears to be very uncommon within the large population with cancer. In 1990, only 3% of inpatient and outpatient consultations performed by the Psychiatry Service at Memorial Sloan-Kettering Cancer Center were requested for management of issues related to drug abuse. This prevalence is much lower than the prevalence of substance use disorders in society at large, in general medical populations, and in emergency medical departments (1–3,5,6). This relatively low prevalence was also reported in the Psychiatric Collaborative Oncology Group study, which assessed psychiatric diagnoses in ambulatory cancer patients from several tertiary care hospitals (6): Following structured clinical interviews, <5% of 215 cancer patients met the *Diagnostic and Statistical Manual for Mental Disorders,* 3rd ed. *(DSM-III)* criteria for a substance use disorder (7).

The relatively low prevalence of substance abuse among cancer patients treated in tertiary care hospitals may reflect institutional biases or a tendency for patient underreporting in these settings. Many drug abusers are poor, feel alienated from the health care system, and may not seek care in tertiary centers. Those who are treated in these centers may be disinclined to acknowledge the stigmatizing history of drug abuse. For these reasons, the low prevalence of drug abuse in cancer centers may not be representative of the true prevalence in the cancer population overall. In support of this conclusion, a recent survey of patients admitted to a palliative care unit observed findings indicative of alcohol abuse in >25% (8). Additional studies are needed to clarify the epidemiology of substance abuse and addiction in cancer patients and others with progressive medical diseases.

## DEFINING ABUSE AND ADDICTION IN THE MEDICALLY ILL

Both epidemiologic studies and clinical management depend on an accepted, valid nomenclature for substance abuse and addiction. Unfortunately, this terminology is highly problematic. The pharmacologic phenomena of tolerance and physical dependence are commonly confused with abuse and addiction, and all of the definitions applied to medical patients have been developed from addict populations without medical illness. The use of terms is also strongly influenced by sociocultural considerations, which may lead to mixed messages in the clinical setting. The clarification of this terminology is an essential step in improving the diagnosis and management of substance abuse in the palliative care setting.

### Definition of Tolerance and Physical Dependence

Tolerance and physical dependence can occur during long-term therapy with opioids and other drugs. The defining characteristics of these phenomena must be understood to appropriately distinguish them from abuse and addiction (Table 1).

**TABLE 1.** *Proposed terminology of substance abuse*

| Term | Definition |
|---|---|
| Physical Dependence | Pharmacologic property of some drugs defined solely by the occurrence of abstinence on abrupt dose reduction, discontinuation of dosing, or administration of an antagonist drug. |
| Tolerance | Diminution of one or more drug effects (either favorable effects or adverse effects) caused by exposure to the drug; may be pharmacologic or associative (related to learning). |
| Substance Abuse | Use of a substance in a manner outside of sociocultural conventions; according to this definition, all use of illicit drugs is abuse and use of a licit drug in a manner not dictated by convention (e.g., according to physician's orders) is abuse. |
| Addiction | Commonly used term that does not appear in current psychiatric nosologies but can be taken to mean the aberrant use of a substance in a manner characterized by loss of control, compulsive use, preoccupation, and continued use despite harm. |

### Tolerance

Tolerance, a pharmacologic property defined by the need for increasing doses to maintain effects (9,10), has been a particular concern during opioid therapy. Clinicians and patients alike commonly express concern that tolerance to analgesic effects may compromise the benefits of therapy and lead to the requirement for progressively higher, and ultimately unsustainable, doses. In addition, the development of tolerance to the reinforcing effects of opioids, and the consequent need to increase doses to regain these effects, has been speculated to be an important element in the pathogenesis of addiction (11).

Notwithstanding these concerns, an extensive clinical experience with opioid drugs in the medical context has not confirmed that tolerance causes substantial problems (12,13). Although tolerance to a variety of opioid effects can be reliably observed in animal models (14) and tolerance to *nonanalgesic* effects, such as respiratory depression and cognitive impairment (15), occurs routinely in the clinical setting, *analgesic* tolerance does not appear to routinely interfere with the clinical efficacy of opioid drugs. Numerous surveys have demonstrated that most patients can attain stable doses associated with a favorable balance between analgesia and side effects for prolonged periods; dose escalation, when it is required, usually heralds the appearance of a progressive painful lesion (16–22). Unlike tolerance to the side effects of the opioids, clinically meaningful analgesic tolerance appears to be a rare phenomenon and is rarely the driving force for dose escalation.

Clinical observation also fails to support the conclusion that analgesic tolerance is a substantial contributor to the development of addiction. It is widely accepted that addicts without a medical disorder may or may not have any of the manifestations of analgesic tolerance, and the occasional opioid-treated patient who presents findings consistent with analgesic tolerance typically does so without evidence of abuse or addiction.

### Physical Dependence

Physical dependence is defined solely by the occurrence of an abstinence syndrome (withdrawal) following abrupt dose reduction or administration of an antagonist (9,10,23).

Neither the dose nor the duration of administration required to produce clinically significant physical dependence in humans is known, and most practitioners assume that the potential for abstinence exists after opioids have been administered repeatedly for only a few days.

Physical dependence is inapparent unless abstinence is induced. In the clinical setting, physical dependence to an opioid is not considered to be a problem as long as patients are told to avoid abrupt discontinuation of ther-

apy and inadvertent administration of an opioid antagonist (including an analgesic from the agonist-antagonist class) is avoided.

There is great confusion among clinicians about the differences between physical dependence and addiction. Physical dependence, like tolerance, has been suggested to be a component of addiction (24,25), and the avoidance of withdrawal has been postulated to create behavioral contingencies that reinforce drug-seeking behavior (11). These speculations, however, are not supported by experience acquired during opioid therapy for chronic pain. Physical dependence does not preclude the uncomplicated discontinuation of opioids during multidisciplinary pain management of nonmalignant pain (26), and opioid therapy is routinely stopped without difficulty in the cancer patients whose pain disappears following effective antineoplastic therapy. Indirect evidence for a fundamental distinction between physical dependence and addiction is even provided by animal models of opioid self-administration, which have demonstrated that persistent drug-taking behavior can be maintained in the absence of physical dependence (27).

### Deficiencies in the Current Nomenclature

These definitions of tolerance and physical dependence highlight deficiencies in the current nomenclature applied to substance abuse. The terms addiction and addict are particularly troublesome. In common parlance, these labels are often inappropriately applied to describe both aberrant drug use (reminiscent of the behaviors that characterize active abusers of illicit drugs) and phenomena related to tolerance or physical dependence. Clinicians and patients may use the word "addicted" to describe compulsive drug taking in one patient and nothing more than the possibility for withdrawal in another. It is not surprising, therefore, that patients, families, and staff become very concerned about the outcome of opioid treatment when this term is applied.

The labels "addict" and "addiction" should never be used to describe patients who are only perceived to have the capacity for abstinence. These patients must be labeled "physically dependent." Use of the word "dependent" alone also should be discouraged because it fosters confusion between physical dependence and psychological dependence, a component of addiction. For the same reason, the term "habituation" should not be used.

The psychiatric terminology applied to drug abuse and addiction, which has been codified in the *DSM-IV,* is also very problematic (25). The *DSM-IV* eschews the term "addiction" altogether and offers definitions of two types of substance use disorders: substance abuse and the more serious substance dependence (Table 2). The criteria for substance abuse are focused on the negative psychosocial sequelae of drug use rather than the pattern of use. In

**TABLE 2.** *Definitions of substance dependence and substance abuse recommended by DSM-IV (25)*

*Substance Dependence*

A maladaptive pattern of substance abuse, leading to clinically significant impairment or distress, as manifested by three or more of the following occurring at any time in the same 12-month period:

  A. Tolerance, as defined by either of the following:
    1. a need for markedly increased amounts of substance to achieve intoxication or desired effect.
    2. markedly diminished effect with continued use of the same amount of the substance.
  B. Withdrawal, as manifested by either of the following:
    1. the characteristic withdrawal syndrome for the substance.
    2. the same (or closely related) substance is taken to relieve or avoid withdrawal symptoms.
  C. The substance is often taken in larger amounts or over a longer period than was intended.
  D. There is a persistent desire or unsuccessful efforts to cut down or control substance use.
  E. A great deal of time spent in activities necessary to obtain the substance (e.g., visiting multiple doctors or driving long distances), use the substance (e.g., chain smoking), or recover from its effects.
  F. Important social, occasional, or recreational activities are given up or reduced because of substance use.
  G. The substance use is continued despite knowledge of having a persistent or recurrent physical or psychological problem that is likely to have been caused or exacerbated by the substance (e.g., current cocaine use despite recognition of cocaine-induced depression, or continued drinking despite recognition that an ulcer was made worse by alcohol consumption).

*Substance Abuse*

A maladaptive pattern of substance abuse leading to clinically significant impairment or distress, as manifested by one (or more) of the following, occurring within a 12-month period:

  A. Recurrent substance use resulting in a failure to fulfill major role obligations at work, school, or home (e.g., repeated absences or poor work performance related to substance use; substance related absences, suspensions, or expulsions from school; neglect of children or household).
  B. Recurrent substance use in situations in which it is physically hazardous (e.g., driving an automobile or operating a machine when impaired by substance use).
  C. Recurrent substance-related legal problems (e.g., arrests for substance-related disorderly conduct).
  D. Continued substance use despite having persistent or recurrent social or interpersonal problems caused or exacerbated by the effects of the substance (e.g., arguments with spouse about consequences of intoxication, physical fights).
  E. The symptoms have never met the criteria for substance dependence for this class of substance.

contrast, a pattern of use outside of sociocultural convention is considered to be the most important criterion for abuse in other definitions (28,29) (see Table 1). The disparity in these definitions of abuse is confusing and underscores the challenge in labeling drug taking behaviors in patients who are receiving potentially abusable drugs for legitimate medical purposes.

The *DSM-IV* criteria for substance dependence highlight chronicity and add the dimensions of physical dependence and tolerance. This is perhaps the most striking example of the nomenclatural problems that occur when criteria developed in substance abusers without medical illnesses are applied in a different context (30). Most of the criteria for substance dependence disorder indicate that the term is meant to be used in a manner synonymous with addiction. The criteria of tolerance and physical dependence therefore are inappropriate and preclude the use of this terminology in the medically ill, who may develop these phenomena as expected consequences of therapeutic drug use.

Thus, the existing terminology can complicate the effort to characterize the drug taking behavior of a patient with a medical illness that is appropriately treated with a potentially abusable drug. Problems with nomenclature impede the communication that is essential for palliative care. This communication depends on the use of appropriate, clearly defined terms and a strategy for diagnosis

that recognizes the complexity of the clinical setting (see below).

## Conceptual Issues in Defining Terms for the Medically Ill

The problems with inappropriate terminology are compounded by other concerns that increase the difficulty in assessing drug taking behavior and rendering a diagnosis of abuse or addiction (substance dependence in *DSM-IV* terminology) when the label would truly be clinically meaningful. These concerns relate to (a) the problem of undertreatment, (b) the sociocultural influence on the definition of aberrancy, and (c) the importance of disease-related variables.

### The Problem of Undertreatment

Clinical observation suggests that the inadequate management of symptoms may be impetus for aberrant drug-related behaviors. This concept has been most explored in the area of cancer pain. There is compelling evidence that pain is undertreated in populations of medically ill patients, including cancer and AIDS (31,32). The term "pseudo-addiction" was coined to depict the distress and drug seeking that can occur in the context of unrelieved cancer pain (33). The cardinal feature of this syndrome is that the aberrant behaviors disappear when an effective analgesic intervention is administered; in the cancer population, the first-line intervention is often a higher dose of an opioid.

The potential for pseudoaddiction poses a very challenging assessment in the population of known substance abusers who develop painful medical disease. Clinical experience suggests that aberrant behaviors driven by unrelieved pain can become dramatic or particularly worrisome in this population. Some patients appear to return to illicit drug use as a means to self-medication, at least in part. Others adopt patterns of behavior with health care providers that also generate intense concerns about the possibility of true addiction. Although it may be clear that the drug-related behaviors are aberrant, the meaning of these behaviors may be difficult to discern in the context of unrelieved symptoms. Management strategies must reflect the diagnostic complexity.

### Sociocultural Influences

By definition, the use of an illicit drug, or the use of a prescription drug without a medical indication, is abuse. If either type of drug is used in a compulsive manner that continues despite harm to the user or others, a diagnosis of addiction may be appropriate (see Table 1). These definitions are consonant with the social and cultural norms of drug taking.

When a drug is prescribed for a legitimate medical purpose, however, there is less certainty about the behaviors that could be characterized as aberrant and potentially diagnosed as abuse or addiction. Although the aberrancy of some behaviors would not be argued, such as prescription forgery or the intravenous injection of an oral formulation, many other behaviors are less clear cut. For example, is it aberrant for the patient with unrelieved pain to consume a few extra doses of a prescribed opioid, particularly if this behavior was not specifically proscribed by the clinician? Is it aberrant to use an opioid drug prescribed for pain as a nighttime hypnotic?

The ability to categorize such questionable behaviors as outside the social or cultural norm also presupposes that there is certainty about the parameters of normative behavior. In the area of prescription drug use, there are no empirical data that define these parameters. If a large proportion of patients were discovered to engage in a specific behavior, it may be normative and judgments about deviance would be influenced accordingly. This issue was recently highlighted in a pilot survey performed at Memorial Sloan-Kettering Cancer Center, which revealed that 26% of inpatients with cancer admitted borrowing an anxiolytic from a family member at some time. The prevalence of this behavior among the medically ill raises concern about its predictive validity as a marker of any diagnosis related to substance abuse. Clearly, there is a need for empirical data that illuminate the prevalence of drug taking attitudes and behaviors in different populations of medically ill patients.

The importance of social and cultural norms, in turn, raises the inevitable possibility of bias in determinations of aberrancy. Bias against a social group, even if subtle, could influence the willingness of clinicians to label a questionable drug-related behavior as aberrant when performed by a member of that group. Clinical observation suggests that this type of bias is common in the assessment of drug-related behaviors of patients with substance abuse histories. Questionable behaviors by such patients may be promptly labeled as abuse or addiction, even if the drug abuse history was in the remote past. In a similar way, the possibility of bias in the assessment of drug-related behaviors exists for patients who are members of racial or ethnic groups different from that of the clinician.

### Disease-Related Variables

The core concepts used to define addiction may also be problematic as a result of changes induced by a progressive disease. Deterioration in physical or psychosocial functioning caused by the disease and its treatment may be difficult to separate from the morbidity associated with drug abuse. This may particularly complicate efforts to evaluate the concept of use despite harm, which is critical to the diagnosis of addiction. For example, the nature of questionable drug-related behaviors can be difficult to discern in the patient who develops social withdrawal or cognitive changes following brain irradiation for metastases. Even if impaired cognition is clearly related to the drugs used to treat symptoms, this outcome might only reflect a narrow therapeutic window, rather than a desire on the patient's part for these psychic effects.

The accurate assessment of drug-related behaviors in patients with advanced medical disease usually requires detailed information about the role of the drug in the patient's life. The existence of mild mental clouding or the time spent of out of bed may be less meaningful than other outcomes, such as noncompliance with primary therapy related to drug use, or behaviors that jeopardize relationships with physicians, other health care providers, or family members.

## Operationalizing the Definitions of Abuse and Addiction

The foregoing discussion emphasizes the difficulties inherent in formulating and applying a nomenclature that would allow appropriate diagnosis of drug-related phenomena in the medically ill. Previous definitions that include phenomena related to physical dependence or tolerance cannot be the model terminology for medically ill populations who receive potentially abusable drugs for legitimate medical purposes. A more appropriate model definition of addiction notes that it is a chronic disorder characterized by "the compulsive use of a substance resulting in physical, psychological or social harm to the user and continued use despite that harm" (29). Although this definition was developed from experience in addict populations without medical illness, it appropriately emphasizes that addiction is fundamentally a psychological and behavioral syndrome. Any appropriate definition of addiction must include several important characteristics, including (a) loss of control over drug use, (b) compulsive drug use, and (c) continued use despite harm.

Even appropriate definitions will have limited utility, however, unless operationalized for a clinical setting. The concept of aberrant drug-related behavior is a useful first step in operationalizing the definitions of abuse and addiction, and recognizes the broad range of behaviors that may be considered problematic by prescribers (Table 3). Although the assessment and interpretation of these behaviors can be challenging, as discussed previously, the occurrence of aberrant behaviors signals the need to reevaluate and manage drug taking, even in the context of an appropriate medical indication for a drug.

If drug taking behavior in a medical patient can be characterized as aberrant, a "differential diagnosis" for this behavior can be explored (Table 4). A true addiction (substance dependence) is only one of several possible explanations. The challenging diagnosis of pseudoaddiction must be considered if the patient is reporting distress associated with unrelieved symptoms. Alternatively, impulsive drug use may indicate the existence of another psychiatric disorder, diagnosis of which may have therapeutic implications. Occasionally, aberrant drug-related behavior appears to be causally related to a mild encephalopathy, with confusion about the appropriate therapeutic regimen; rarely, problematic behaviors indicate criminal intent. These diagnoses are not mutually exclusive.

It may be difficult to apply appropriate labels until sufficient time has passed to allow observations that are both varied and repeated. Astute psychiatric assessment is essential and may require evaluation by consultants who can clarify the complex interactions among personality factors and psychiatric illnesses. Some patients may be self-medicating symptoms of anxiety or depression, insomnia, or even problems of adjustment (such as boredom due to diminished ability to engage in usual activities and hobbies). Others have character pathology that may be the more salient determinant of drug taking behavior. For example, patients with borderline personality disorder may use prescribed drugs in a chaotic and impulsive manner that regulates inner tension; expresses anger at doctors, friends, or family; or ameliorates chronic emptiness or boredom. This psychiatric assessment is critically important both in the population without a prior history of substance abuse and the population of known abusers, who have a high prevalence of psychiatric comorbidity (34).

In assessing the differential diagnosis for drug-related behavior, it is useful to consider the degree of aberrancy (see Table 3). The less aberrant behaviors (such as aggressively complaining about the need for medications) are more likely to reflect untreated distress of some type rather than addiction-related concerns. Conversely, the more aberrant behaviors (such as injection of an oral formulation) are more likely to reflect true addiction.

**TABLE 3.** *Spectrum of aberrant drug-related behaviors encountered during treatment of the medically ill with prescription drugs*

---

*More Suggestive of Addiction*
 Selling prescription drugs
 Prescription forgery
 Stealing of drugs from others
 Injecting oral formulations
 Obtaining prescription drugs from nonmedical sources
 Concurrent abuse of alcohol or illicit drugs
 Repeated dose escalations or similar noncompliance despite multiple warnings
 Repeated visits to other clinicians or emergency rooms without informing prescriber
 Drug-related deterioration in function at work, in the family, or socially
 Repeated resistance to changes in therapy despite evidence of adverse drug effects
*Less Suggestive of Addiction*
 Aggressive complaining about the need for more drugs
 Drug hoarding during periods of reduced symptoms
 Requesting specific drugs
 Openly acquiring similar drugs from other medical sources
 Occasional unsanctioned dose escalation or other noncompliance
 Unapproved use of the drug to treat another symptom
 Reporting psychic effects not intended by the clinician
 Resistance to a change in therapy associated with tolerable adverse effects
 Intense expressions of anxiety about recurrent symptoms

---

**TABLE 4**. *Differential diagnosis for aberrant drug-related behaviors*[a]

Addiction (Substance Dependence Disorder)
"Pseudoaddiction"
Psychiatric disorder associated with impulsive or aberrant drug taking
Personality disorders, including borderline and psychopathic personality disorders
Depressive disorder
Anxiety disorder
Encephalopathy with confusion about appropriate therapeutic regimen
Criminal intent

[a]Categories are not mutually exclusive.

Although empirical studies are needed to validate this conceptualization, it may be a useful model when evaluating aberrant behaviors.

## RISK OF ABUSE AND ADDICTION

An accepted nomenclature for abuse and addiction and an operational approach to the assessment of patients with medical illness are prerequisite to an accurate definition of risk in populations with and without histories of substance abuse. Unfortunately, there are very limited data relevant to risk assessment in the medically ill. Most data relate to the risk of serious abuse or addiction during long-term opioid treatment of chronic pain in patients with no history of substance abuse. There is almost no information about the risk of less serious aberrant drug-related behaviors, the risk of these outcomes in populations that do have a history of abuse, or the risk associated with the use of potentially abusable drugs other than opioids.

### Risk of Abuse and Addiction in Populations Without Prior Drug Abuse

An extensive worldwide experience in the long-term management of cancer pain with opioid drugs has demonstrated that opioid administration in cancer patients with no prior history of substance abuse is only rarely associated with the development of significant abuse or addiction (35–47). Indeed, concerns about addiction in this population are now characterized by an interesting paradox: Although the lay public and inexperienced clinicians still fear the development of addiction when opioids are used to treat cancer pain, specialists in cancer pain and palliative care widely believe that the major problem related to addiction is not the phenomenon itself, but rather the persistent undertreatment of pain driven by inappropriate fear that it will occur.

The very sanguine experience in the cancer population has contributed to a desire for a reappraisal of the risks and benefits associated with the long-term opioid treatment of chronic nonmalignant pain (48,49). The traditional view of this therapy is negative and early surveys

of addicts, which noted that a relatively large proportion began their addiction as medical patients administered opioid drugs for pain (50–52), provided some indirect support for this perspective. The most influential of these surveys recorded a history of medical opioid use for pain in 27% of white male addicts and 1.2% of black male addicts (52).

However, surveys of addict populations do not provide a valid measure of the addiction liability associated with chronic opioid therapy in populations without known abuse. Prospective patient surveys are needed to define this risk accurately. The Boston Collaborative Drug Surveillance Project evaluated 11,882 inpatients who had no prior history of addiction and were administered an opioid while hospitalized; only four cases of addiction could be identified subsequently (53). A national survey of burn centers could find no cases of addiction in a sample of more than 10,000 patients without prior drug abuse history who were administered opioids for pain (54), and a survey of a large headache clinic identified opioid abuse in only 3 of 2369 patients admitted for treatment, most of whom had access to opioids (55).

Other data suggest that the typical patient with chronic pain is sufficiently different from the addict without painful disease that the risk of addiction during therapy for pain is likely to be low. For example, surveys of cancer patients and postoperative patients indicate that euphoria, a phenomenon believed to be common during the abuse of opioids, is extremely uncommon following administration of an opioid for pain; dysphoria is observed more typically, especially in those who receive meperidine (56). Although the psychiatric comorbidity identified in addict populations could be an effect, rather than a cause, of the aberrant drug taking, the association suggests the existence of psychological risk factors for addiction. The likelihood of genetically determined risk factors for addiction also has been suggested by a twin study that demonstrated a significant concordance rate for aberrant drug-related behaviors (57).

Of course, favorable surveys of pain patients are not definitive, and there are conflicting data collected by multidisciplinary pain management programs that suggest a high prevalence of abuse behaviors among the patients referred to this setting (58–66). The latter surveys, however, are subject to an important selection bias, and this bias, combined with other methodologic concerns (67), limits the generalizability of these data to the large and heterogeneous populations with chronic nonmalignant pain.

Overall, the evidence generally supports the view that opioid therapy in patients with chronic pain and no history of abuse or addiction can be undertaken with a very low risk of these adverse outcomes. This is particularly so in the older patient, who has had ample time to reveal a propensity for abuse. There is no substantive support for the view that large numbers of individuals with no personal or family history of abuse or addiction, no affiliation with a substance abusing subculture, and no significant premorbid psychopathology, will develop abuse or addiction *de novo* when administered potentially abusable drugs for appropriate medical indications.

The inaccurate perception that opioid therapy inherently yields a relatively high likelihood of addiction has encouraged assumptions that are not supportable in populations without a prior history of substance abuse. For example, agonist-antagonist opioid analgesics are less likely to be abused by addicts than pure mu agonist opioids, and consequently, some clinicians view the agonist-antagonist drugs as safer in terms of addiction liability. There is no evidence for this conclusion in populations without drug abuse histories, and the extensive experience with long-term opioid therapy for cancer pain and chronic nonmalignant pain (49,68–73) has relied on the pure μ agonists. Similarly, there is a common perception that short-acting oral opioids and opioids delivered by the parenteral route carry a relatively greater risk of addiction because of the rapid delivery of the drug. Again, these perceptions derive from observations in the healthy addict population and are not relevant to the treatment of pain in medical patients with no prior history of substance abuse.

### Risk of Abuse and Addiction in Populations with Current or Remote Drug Abuse

There is very little information about the risk of abuse or addiction during or after the therapeutic administration of a potentially abusable drug to patients with a current or remote history of abuse or addiction. Anecdotal reports have suggested that successful long-term opioid therapy in patients with cancer pain or chronic nonmalignant pain is possible, particularly if the history of abuse or addiction is remote (74–76).

Notwithstanding the lack of empirical information, it is generally accepted that the risk of aberrant drug-related behaviors during treatment for a medical disorder is higher among the population with a remote or current history of substance abuse. Given this risk, it is reasonable to consider the common clinical lore concerning the likelihood of abuse behaviors when different types of therapies are implemented. For example, although there is no empirical evidence that the use of short-acting drugs or the parenteral route is more likely to lead to problematic drug-related behaviors than other therapeutic approaches, it may be prudent to avoid such therapies in patients with histories of substance abuse.

The most prudent actions cannot obviate risk, and clinicians must recognize that virtually any drug that acts on the central nervous system, and any route of drug administration, can be abused. The effective management of patients with substance abuse histories necessitates a more comprehensive approach that recognizes the biological, chemical, social, and psychiatric aspects of substance abuse and addiction, and provides practical means to manage risk.

## CLINICAL MANAGEMENT OF PATIENTS WITH SUBSTANCE ABUSE HISTORIES

As described previously, the population of patients with substance abuse histories is extremely heterogeneous. The most difficult issues in palliative care typically present in those who are actively abusing alcohol or other drugs. Although the following principles can also apply to patients who are in drug-free recovery and those who are in methadone maintenance programs, they are likely to be most helpful in the management of the active drug abuser.

### General Guidelines

Recommendations for the long-term administration of potentially abusable drugs, such as the opioids, to patients with histories of substance abuse are based solely on clinical experience. Studies are needed to determine the most effective therapeutic strategies and to empirically define patient subgroups that may be most amenable to different approaches. The following guidelines broadly reflect the types of interventions that might be considered in this clinical context.

#### Involve a Multidisciplinary Team

In the population of patients with progressive medical disorders and substance abuse, palliative care often must contend with multiple medical, psychosocial, and administrative problems. A team approach can be very useful in addressing these problems. The most knowledgeable team may involve one or more physicians with expertise in palliative care, nurses, social workers, and, if possible, one or more mental health care providers with expertise in addiction medicine.

### Set Realistic Goals for Therapy

Drug abuse and addiction often remit and relapse. The risk of relapse is likely to be enhanced because of the heightened stress associated with life-threatening disease and the ready availability of centrally acting drugs prescribed for symptom control. Preventing relapses may be impossible in such a setting. Conflict with staff may be lessened if there is a general understanding that unerring compliance is not a realistic goal of management. Rather, the goal might be viewed as the creation of a structure for therapy that includes sufficient social and emotional support, and limit setting, to contain the harm done by occasional relapses.

A small subgroup of patients may be incapable of complying with the requirements of therapy because of a severe substance-use disorder and associated psychiatric comorbidity. To establish the intractability of the problem, clinicians must reestablish limits on multiple occasions and attempt to develop an increasing variety and intensity of supports. Frequent team meetings and consultations with other clinicians who have expertise in palliative care and addiction medicine may be needed. Ultimately, however, appropriate expectations must be clarified and therapy that is failing cannot be continued in the same way. The success rate for converting highly problematic therapies into those that can be managed over time is unknown.

### Evaluate and Treat Comorbid Psychiatric Disorders

The comorbidity of personality disorder, depression, and anxiety disorders in alcoholics and other patients with substance abuse histories is extremely high (34). The treatment of anxiety and depression can increase patient comfort and possibly diminish the likelihood of relapse.

### Prevent or Minimize Withdrawal Symptoms

Clinicians must be familiar with the signs and symptoms associated with abstinence from opioids and other drugs. Many patients with a history of drug abuse consume multiple drugs and a complete drug use history must be elicited to prepare for the possibility of withdrawal. Delayed abstinence syndromes, such as may occur following abuse of some benzodiazepine drugs, may pose a particular diagnostic challenge.

### Consider the Impact of Tolerance

Patients who are actively abusing drugs may have sufficient tolerance to influence the use of prescription drugs subsequently administered for an appropriate med-

ical indication. As mentioned previously, tolerance is a complex phenomenon (13,14) and its impact on clinical management in this context is likely to be highly variable.

Tolerance to adverse effects can increase the safety of therapy. Obviously, this outcome is not a concern. The more relevant possibility is that exposure to a drug of abuse will induce sufficient tolerance to the desired therapeutic effects that management becomes more difficult. There has been no systematic investigation of this phenomenon and observations in the clinical setting are difficult to interpret. Although one survey failed to identify any difference in the need for postoperative analgesics between those with and without a substance abuse history (77), anecdotal experience suggests that some actively abusing patients who develop a therapeutic need for an opioid or a sedative-hypnotic drug do require relatively high initial doses, or a need for rapid dose escalation to establish, or retain, therapeutic effects. Similarly, clinical observation suggests that some patients receiving methadone maintenance require relatively higher opioid doses to treat acute pain and relatively rapid dose escalation at the start of therapy to identify a useful dose for chronic pain management.

These phenomena could indeed reflect the impact of pharmacologic tolerance on the ability to produce therapeutic effects. Alternatively, they could represent rapidly worsening pain, such as occurs in the nonabusing population, or, possibly, aberrant drug-related behavior attributable to addiction itself. From a practical perspective, the clinician must be cautious in estimating the degree to which tolerance may be operating but also cognizant of the potential need for relatively higher doses. The starting dose of a therapeutic drug should be conservative and rapid dose titration with careful monitoring should be available.

### Apply Appropriate Pharmacologic Principles to Treat Chronic Pain

To optimize long-term opioid therapy, well-accepted guidelines for cancer pain management must be applied (44,46). These guidelines emphasize the importance of patient self-report as the basis for dosing, individualization of therapy to identify a favorable balance between efficacy and side effects, and monitoring over time. They also strongly indicate the concurrent treatment of side effects as the basis for optimizing the balance between analgesic and adverse effects (78).

The most important guideline for long-term opioid therapy, individualization of the dose without regard to its size, can be problematic in populations with histories of substance abuse. Although it may be appropriate to exercise caution in prescribing potentially abusable drugs to these populations, the decision to forego the principle of dose individualization without regard to

**TABLE 5.** *Guidelines for the management of patients with substance abuse disorders*

Involve a multidisciplinary team
Set realistic goals for therapy
Evaluate and treat comorbid psychiatric disorders
Prevent or minimize withdrawal symptoms
Consider tolerance when prescribing medications for pain and symptom control
Apply accepted guidelines for opioid therapy[a]
Accept patients' self-report of distress
Frequently reassess the adequacy of pain and symptom control
Recognize specific drug abuse behaviors
Use nonopioids and psychological techniques as indicated, but not as substitutes

[a]Recently published guidelines for long-term opioid pharmacotherapy are available (see refs 41, 43, and 45).

absolute dose may increase the likelihood of undertreatment (31,32). The unrelieved pain that results can in turn lead to the development of aberrant drug-related behaviors. Although these behaviors might be best understood as pseudoaddiction, their occurrence confirms the clinician's fears and encourages even greater caution in prescribing.

This cycle must be recognized and openly acknowledged to the patient and the staff. The request for dose escalation should not by itself be viewed as aberrant drug-related behavior, but the concerns it generates should be discussed. If the clinician perceives that limits on prescribing are necessary to assess, or manage, a problematic therapy, frequent monitoring and alternative approaches to pain control might be offered. The patient should be given clear guidelines for responsible drug taking behaviors, with the expectation that responsible drug taking on the part of the patient will reassure the physician that dose escalation is appropriate.

Given the dual role of methadone as a treatment for opioid addiction (79) and an analgesic (80), clinicians who manage patients with substance abuse histories must understand the pharmacology of this drug. The use of methadone for the management of opioid addiction is subject to federal regulation. Prescribers must have a specific license, treatment is based on a single dose per day, and the parameters for acceptable monitoring are closely defined. When used as an analgesic, however, no special license is required, therapy almost always requires multiple doses per day, and monitoring can be undertaken in a manner consistent with conventional medical practice.

The differences in the dosing of methadone for its two indications are striking. Abstinence can be avoided and opioid craving reduced with a single daily dose. This is consistent with the long elimination half-life of this drug. Analgesic effects after a dose, however, are usually much briefer than would be expected given the half-life. Indeed, one double-blind study demonstrated that the duration of analgesia after a single dose of methadone is comparable to that of morphine, a short half-life opioid (81). Although there are exceptions, most patients appear to require a minimum of four doses per day to achieve sustained analgesia with methadone.

Patients who are receiving methadone maintenance as a treatment for opioid addiction can be administered methadone as an analgesic outside the guidelines of the addiction treatment program. This typically requires a substantial change in therapy, including dose escalation and multiple daily doses. Although the management of such a change does not pose difficult problems from a pharmacologic perspective, it can create considerable stress for the patient and the clinicians involved in the treatment of the addiction disorder. Some patients express a lack of faith in the analgesic efficacy of methadone because the drug has been labeled as addiction therapy rather than pain therapy. Others wish to continue the morning dose for addiction even if treatment during the rest of the day uses the same drug at an equivalent or higher dose. Some physicians who work at methadone clinics are willing to stay involved and prescribe opioids, including methadone, outside of the program, and others wish to relinquish care.

In some cases, the psychosocial problems associated with the use of methadone as an analgesic overwhelm the advantage of simplicity and it is preferable to treat the chronic pain with an alternative drug. Again, some patients request continuation of the daily methadone despite the lack of a medical indication once chronic therapy is begun with a different opioid. Some, but not all, methadone programs are willing to comply with this request. The variety of possible management strategies and the common confusion surrounding these different uses for methadone indicate the need to assess the utility of this drug on a case-by-case basis. In all situations, the clinicians involved in palliative care must contact those involved in the management of the substance abuse so that care can be coordinated appropriately.

## Select Drugs and Routes of Administration for the Symptom and Setting

As discussed previously, there is little reason to believe that the common clinical lore about the differences in addiction liability between short-acting and long-acting drugs, or among different routes of administration, is relevant to the management of palliative therapies in populations without substance abuse. In the population of known substance abusers, however, it may indeed be prudent to consider these observations. There is no disadvantage to the use of a long-acting preparation, and it is possible on theoretical grounds that the rapid onset and decline of effects associated with short-acting drugs could contribute to the development of aberrant drug-related behaviors. Accordingly, it is appropriate during opioid therapy to rely, if possible, on the use of oral methadone, oral-controlled release or sustained-release opioid formulations, and transdermal formulations for long-term therapy. For pain that is moderate but exceeds the maximal efficacy of nonsteroidal anti-inflammatory drugs, the use of lower doses of the long-acting opioids or the use of tramadol might be preferable if there is concern about the use of the short-acting analgesics conventionally used for pain of this type (such as acetaminophen-codeine preparations). Tramadol is a unique opioid compound that has been demonstrated to have a relatively low abuse potential.

## Recognize Specific Drug Abuse Behaviors

All patients who are prescribed potentially abusable drugs must be carefully monitored over time for the development of aberrant drug-related behaviors. The need for this monitoring is especially strong when patients have a remote or current history of substance abuse, including alcohol abuse. If there is a high level of concern about such behaviors, monitoring may require relatively frequent visits and regular discussions with family members, significant others, and friends who can provide observations about patients' drug use.

To facilitate the early recognition of aberrant drug-related behaviors in those patients who have been actively abusing drugs in the recent past, regular screening of urine for illicit or licit but unprescribed drugs may be appropriate. The patient should be informed about this approach, which should be explained as a method of monitoring that can be reassuring to the clinician and provide a foundation for aggressive symptom-oriented treatments. Viewed in this light, it is a technique that enhances rather than threatens the therapeutic alliance with the patient. Patients who protest excessively may be unwilling or unable to enter a collaborative relationship in which the clinician can be confident of responsible drug taking by the patient and the patient can be confident that the clinician will respond to unrelieved symptoms with aggressive therapies. Such patients cannot be treated with the same willingness to use potentially abusable drugs for symptom control.

## Utilize Nondrug Approaches as Appropriate

A variety of nondrug interventions may be useful in helping patients cope with the rigors of medical treatments. These include educational interventions designed to assist patients in communicating with staff and negotiating the complexities of the medical system, and numerous cognitive techniques that enhance relaxation and aid in coping. Nondrug interventions may be helpful adjunctive therapies but should not be seen as substitutes for drugs targeted to pain, depression, anxiety, or other physical or psychological symptoms.

## Taking a Substance Use History

Clinicians often avoid asking patients about drug abuse (and other socially undesirable behaviors) for fear that patients will be offended, or feel angry or threatened. Often there is the expectation that the patient will not respond truthfully. These attitudes are self-defeating. They may reduce the likelihood of truthful communication and increase the problems associated with the monitoring of therapy over time.

The clinician must be nonjudgmental when taking the patient's history of substance use. Adopting a professional and caring demeanor often necessitates some degree of self-observation and exploration of one's attitudes about members of subcultures who hold different values.

The clinician should anticipate defensiveness on the part of the patient. It can be helpful to mention that patients often misrepresent their drug use for valid reasons: stigmatization, mistrust of the interviewer, or concern about fears of undermedication. Clinicians must tell the patient that they need accurate information about drug use to help keep the patient as comfortable as possible by avoiding withdrawal states and prescribing adequate medication for pain and symptom control.

The clinician must be inquisitive and knowledgeable about drug abuse. The use of street names for drugs should be avoided unless the clinician has current knowledge of the names in use. The interview should include a review of all drugs taken, including the chronology of use over time, the current frequency of use, and triggers that initiate use. The so-called "pyramid" interview can be a useful way to slowly introduce the subject of drug use. This style of interviewing begins with broad and general questions about the role of substances in one's life, beginning with licit ones such as caffeine and nicotine. It then proceeds to more specific questions about illicit substances.

In the palliative care setting, it is very important to inquire about the desired effects of all drugs used. This question can often lead to very valuable information about comorbid mood disturbances or unrelieved symptoms that require treatment. The answers may provide a key to helping patients with control of symptoms they find particularly noxious and diminish the need for drugs of abuse.

### Inpatient Management Plan

Specific guidelines may be helpful in planning the inpatient management of the actively abusing patient who is admitted to a medical setting for treatment of the disease or symptom control. Although these guidelines have not been tested empirically and are more or less applicable to different inpatient settings, they offer a set of approaches that can ensure the safety of the patient and staff, provide control of manipulative behaviors by patients, maintain surveillance of illicit drug use, avoid conflicts surrounding the use of medications appropriately used for pain and symptom control, and communicate knowledge of pain and substance abuse management.

The proactive use of specific guidelines in anticipation of potential problems with drug use should be discussed with the patient. When feasible, the possible use of these strategies should be addressed in the outpatient setting prior to admission. Whether at this meeting or on admission, the discussion should focus on the need to approach the patient's drug use with the staff in an open manner. The patient must be reassured about the staff's desire to avoid aversive experiences related to withdrawal or unrelieved symptoms. In essence, the patient is offered a consistent approach focused on treatment goals in return for compliance with the treatment plan. The details of the plan should be presented, including policies for violations of the plan. Depending on the severity of recent drug abuse, it may be necessary to inform patients that medical treatment is contingent on compliance with the treatment plan.

If possible, actively abusing patients who are scheduled for a surgical procedure should be admitted to the hospital several days early to permit stabilization of the drug regimen. This period can be used to prevent withdrawal and provide an opportunity to judge the need for alteration of the plan established on admission.

A variety of actions can be considered in developing appropriate guidelines for the specific concerns posed by the patient (Table 6). Some patients should be given a private room close to the nursing station to allow for monitoring. The patient may be restricted to his or her room or floor until the danger of withdrawal or illicit drug use is judged to be diminished. It can be appropriate to require hospital pajamas to reduce the risk of departure from the hospital to buy drugs. The patient's visitors can be limited

to family and friends known to be drug-free. Visitors can be told that check-in with the staff is required before contact with the patient is made.

Some patients should undergo one or more searches of the hospital room. This search, which should be conducted by a minimum of two staff members (security guards, nurses, physicians, administrators, or others), is within the rights and responsibilities of the hospital. If an illicit drug, previously prescribed medication, or alcohol is discovered, it should be removed from the room and discarded as per hospital protocol. Packages brought to the hospital by family members and friends can be searched by responsible staff to ensure that they do not contain illicit drugs or alcohol.

In some cases it is useful to require periodic urine drug screens. To simplify this process, the patient can be instructed to provide a daily specimen. Some of these specimens are sent for analysis and others are discarded. The frequency of screening depends on the behaviors observed in the hospital. This approach establishes the concept of regular surveillance for the patient, without excessive use of the laboratory.

Again, this plan must be tailored to reflect the degree of risk perceived by the staff. In some cases, no special requirements are needed, and in others, the severity of recent abuse indicates the need for maximal caution. The plan may evolve in the hospital depending on the occurrence of aberrant drug-related behaviors and the changing medical status of the patient. In the discussion with the patient, it is often useful to emphasize that the implementation of these guidelines is truly in the best interest of the patient and institution. Aggressive medical management unencumbered by doubts about the history and concerns regarding ongoing drug use is possible only if the staff can be reassured that drug abuse is not occurring. Open discussion about guidelines that provide this reassurance will allow optimal treatment for the disease and the most sensitive palliative care possible.

Once a structure is established to control drug use, the medical management of the active abuser must proceed attentively. Frequent visits are usually needed to assess and manage symptoms. Drug withdrawal should be prevented and prescribed drugs for symptom control should be administered on a regularly scheduled basis to the extent possible. This avoids frequent encounters with staff that focus on the desire to obtain a drug.

Some patients may be incapable of abiding by these guidelines after admission. Most clinicians will offer a patient several chances and attempt to increase the extent and rigidity of the plan in an effort to encourage compliance. Patients who continue to actively abuse drugs and are unwilling to abide by hospital policy should be discharged from the hospital and offered a drug rehabilitation program. The ethical and legal implications of this action, like the inpatient plan itself, should be discussed

**TABLE 6.** *Management strategies for inpatients who require palliative care and are actively abusing drugs at the time of admission*

Have regular contact with floor staff and facility administrators to apprise them of necessary strategies
Document strategies in the medical record and note justification
Obtain private room close to nursing station
Search possessions and packages brought by visitors
Restrict patient's mobility (to room, floor, etc.)
Collect urine for toxicology screens daily

in detail by members of hospital administration, the ethics committee, and senior clinicians, depending upon the setting.

Discharge planning for those patients who do comply with the inpatient program should be initiated as early as possible. Some patients may be able to undergo dose tapering of opioids and other drugs. The considerations that guide the selection of drugs and routes of administration for outpatient management were discussed previously. Many patients return home receiving drugs that will require close monitoring and a structured outpatient treatment plan.

## Outpatient Management Plan

Other guidelines may apply to the management of the actively abusing outpatient who is undergoing outpatient treatment (Table 7). Occasionally, this plan can be coordinated with referral to a drug rehabilitation program. Patients with advanced medical illnesses may find it difficult to obtain entry into such programs, however, and often the outpatient management of drug abuse is left to the clinician who is also attempting to optimize palliative care and, perhaps, offer whatever primary disease-oriented treatments remain.

### Written Contracts

The use of written contracts that clearly state the roles of the team members and the rules and expectations for the patient can be helpful in structuring outpatient treatment. The contract should explicitly state the consequences of aberrant drug use. It is best to tailor the contract to the level of concern about the patient's behavior. Clinicians who treat many patients who are actively abus-

**TABLE 7.** *Management strategies for outpatients who require palliative care and are actively abusing drugs*

Use written contracts
Use frequent clinic visits
Give small quantities of medications per prescription
Renew prescriptions contingent on clinic attendance
Use 12-step programs where possible
Use spot urine toxicology screens
Involve family in treatment planning

ing may find it efficient to prepare a group of contracts, each incorporating guidelines with varying rigidity. The appropriate contract can then be selected on the basis of the assessment of patient risk.

### Guidelines for Prescribing

Patients must be given detailed instructions about the parameters of responsible drug taking. The goal is to prevent the use of illicit drugs, if possible, and to eliminate abuse of the prescribed drug regimen. The actively abusing patient must be seen frequently in the outpatient department. Weekly visits are common. Frequent visits help establish close ties with staff and allow evaluation of both symptom control and addiction-related concerns. Frequent visits also allow the prescription of small quantities of drugs, which may diminish the temptation to divert and provide an incentive for keeping appointments.

The clinician's response to lost prescriptions, requests for early refills, and other aberrant behaviors should be decided in advance, to the extent possible, and explicitly explained to the patient. There can be no prescription renewals if appointments are missed. The patient should be told that dose changes require a contact with the clinician or designee. It may be useful to reassure the patient that dose escalation of drugs used for symptom control is common and acceptable, if the clinical evaluation supports this course and the patient deals with the need for a change in drug regimen without relying on aberrant behaviors.

The rigidity of the plan to deal with lost prescriptions or the need for early refills due to unsanctioned dose escalation again depends on the clinician's assessment of the degree of abuse. In some cases, it is appropriate to stipulate at the outset that early refills for prescription loss will not be provided unless the patient presents a police report that documents the event. In other cases, it may be sufficient to inform the patient that the behavior is unacceptable and may lead to an inability to provide uninterrupted treatment. Subsequent decisions about the response to aberrant behavior can then be made based on observation of the patient's response to these guidelines.

To avoid conflicts after hours or during holiday periods, clinicians who cover for the primary caregiver must be informed about the guidelines that have been established for each patient with a history of abuse. Again, the restrictions should be made more or less stringent based on the level of concern about aberrant behaviors.

### 12-Step Programs

Some patients can be referred to a so-called 12-step program as a means for helping curtail drug abuse during palliative treatment of a progressive medical disease. Patients can document their attendance at meetings to further reassure the clinician about the effort to comply with therapy. Patients who enter a program and are assigned a sponsor may be allowed contact with the sponsor, who may also help support the clinical plan. This type of contact also helps to prevent the patient's ostracism by others in the program when they attend while receiving controlled prescription drugs.

Although there may be clear benefits for the patient who is able to successfully use a 12-step program while receiving potentially abusable drugs as prescribed therapy, there are potential problems. These programs usually endorse drug-free recovery in very strong terms and it may not be possible for the patient to maintain comfortable contacts while using opioids or other prescription drugs. The response of those in the program to a request for dose escalation may be quite different from that of the clinician, and this disparity may compound the patient's stress or lead to underreporting of symptoms. As a result of these problems, the patient may not be able to identify a program that will allow long-term involvement during treatment.

### Urine Toxicology Screens

To promote compliance and detect the concurrent use of illicit substances, most patients should be periodically asked to submit urine specimens for drug screening. The patient should be informed at the start of outpatient therapy that this request will be made from time to time. The patient should also be apprised of the clinician's response to positive screens. This response usually involves increasing the guidelines for continued treatment, including greater frequency of visits, smaller quantities of prescribed drugs, and other measures. In the case of repeated violations, referral for concurrent drug rehabilitation may be the most appropriate course. Rarely, the abuse is so extreme and unremitting that ongoing treatment cannot be justified.

### Family Sessions and Meetings

Many drug-abusing patients come from dysfunctional families. Family meetings may identify family members who are using alcohol or illicit drugs. Referral of family members to drug treatment can be offered and portrayed as a way of marshaling support for the patient. The patient should be prepared to cope with friends or family members who may try to buy or steal prescribed drugs. Identifying reliable individuals who can be sources of strength and support for the patient can be extremely valuable.

### Establishing and Revising the Team

In many settings, outpatient management begins with the individual practitioner as the sole caregiver. For some patients, this treatment model may be sufficient, at least for a time. The individual prescriber must be able to coordinate multimodality treatment designed to address palliative care needs and the potential for substance abuse.

The complexity of both palliative care and substance abuse treatment suggests the value of a treatment team, and the isolated clinician is often a poor substitute for an interdisciplinary model of care. The treatment team for the active drug abuser with a progressive medical disease may include a specialist in addiction medicine as well as others who can address diverse palliative care needs.

### Staff Issues

The adoption of structured management plans for inpatients or outpatients may temper staff anger and mistrust, as well as avoid the self-defeating cycle in which wariness on the part of clinicians leads to undertreatment and the unrelieved symptoms that result lead to aberrant behaviors that reinforce this wariness. The plan helps staff members maintain a sense of control and channel hostile feelings sometimes evoked by uncooperative patients into a productive direction.

Several common reactions by staff can be particularly problematic in implementing and maintaining the management plan. Some individuals react negatively to aspects of the plan, perceiving them as excessively harsh in the context of medical disease. Staff members sometimes feel that it is unethical to deprive patients with life-threatening illness of visits with friends or other privileges, even if the friends may be supplying the patient with illicit substances. In some cases, there is disagreement about the ethical and legal nature of the restrictive aspects of the management plan. Inexperienced staff members may erroneously believe that restrictions are illegal or outside the authority of the hospital. This is clearly untrue when staff and patient safety are at issue.

Occasionally, members of the staff react to a structured management plan as if it indicates that the patient is dangerous. The impulsivity of drug-abusing patients can make staff fearful of violence and even the spread of AIDS. This misinterpretation must be addressed openly with reassurance about the true risks involved in management of the patient.

Doubt and conflict among the staff can confuse the patient and undermine the goals of therapy. The primary treatment team must continually communicate with all of the clinicians who come into contact with the patient, including consulting physicians, staff nurses, pharmacists, and others, to clarify the nature of the treatment plan, provide reassurance that the plan is neither unethical nor illegal, support the need for compassion and understanding within the structure of the drug treatment plan, and identify problems that must be addressed by changes in the approach. Special efforts are needed to educate those staff members who are so troubled by the structure of the treatment plan that they subtly bend the rules or allow themselves to become the main recipient of the patient's complaints about other clinicians.

The ability to provide optimal palliative care to the patient who has been recently abusing licit or illicit drugs is a labor-intensive endeavor predicated on continuing communication and education between members of the primary treatment team and the patient, family, and many other clinicians. Regular team meetings can be an efficient approach to maintaining communication among the professionals involved and identifying problems early. Such meetings are beneficial in that they maintain consistency, and allow staff to express feelings and concerns and discuss ethical and legal issues. In the inpatient setting, it may be helpful to invite a hospital administrator, who can clarify the legality and policy implications of any measures. Regardless of the setting, meetings between selected members of the team and the patient's caregivers in the home can similarly preempt problems related to unmet needs or an incipient problem with abuse. It may be valuable to have the patient attend occasional family meetings to reconcile any disparate observations concerning symptom control or the use of drugs.

## Concerns of Patients in Drug-Free Recovery

The provision of optimal palliative care to patients with a remote history of alcoholism or drug addiction may present special needs for patient support and education. Irrespective of ongoing involvement with 12-step or other programs, patients may harbor great concerns about the power of drugs in their lives. They may be rightly proud of their ability to remain drug-free and have great fear that the use of drugs for pain or other symptoms could "readdict" them and lead to cravings for illicit or licit drugs. They may worry that family or friends could view the use of therapeutic drugs as abuse and this perception could jeopardize family or social support. Some may be afraid that friends or others who are actively using drugs will attempt to gain access to their prescribed drugs.

The clinician should acknowledge these concerns, offer reassurance, and attempt to address practical matters, such as security of prescribed drugs in the home or the need for contact between the treatment team and family members. The social context in which palliative care is offered is strikingly different from that which surrounds substance abuse. The readdiction concern expressed by some patients appears to be a very uncommon phenomenon among patients with a remote history of drug abuse who receive prescribed drugs under medical guidance for the control of symptoms associated with progressive medical disease. Indeed, it is sometimes observed that addicts in recovery express the opinion that the opioids given for pain control produce an entirely different subjective experience (e.g., no euphoria, even with intravenous injection) than the opioids taken during a period of addiction. These reports may reflect the power of social forces, the physiologic or psychological effect of the painful lesion, the influence of the clinician, or other factors that somehow change the nature of drug use for such patients.

Regardless, some patients are so concerned about the potential for adverse effects of opioids or other potentially abusable drugs that compliance with therapy is threatened. It may be helpful to emphasize nonpharmacologic means of symptom control and offer the patient a detailed structure for the administration of prescribed drugs. It is ironic that some patients prefer the type of rigid guidelines described previously because of an enhanced sense of control over drugs. In discussing the need for compliance, it is also important to have the patient realize that there may be a risk of readdiction associated with uncontrolled pain or other symptoms. Counseling can also help patients identify possible triggers to drug and alcohol abuse that they might encounter during treatment and develop strategies for avoiding illicit drug use or uncontrolled use of prescribed drugs at those times.

## CONCLUSION

The diagnosis of abuse and addiction during palliative treatment of symptoms with potentially abusable drugs can be challenging, particularly in the population with a remote or current history of drug abuse. Although addiction appears to a very rare phenomenon during treatment of patients with no such history, the possibility of aberrant drug-related behavior must be acknowledged. Clinicians must recognize that aberrant drug-related behaviors have a differential diagnosis that can only be clarified by careful assessment of the physical and psychosocial influences on drug taking. The monitoring of drug taking to ensure that it remains responsible and the management of aberrant behaviors if they occur are obligations of the prescriber that are as important as individualization of the dose and the management of side effects.

Patients with a history of abuse and addiction pose numerous problems in assessment and management. Clinicians must recognize the heterogeneity in the population of patients with a history of abuse or addiction, and understand the complexity of the issues associated with palliative care. These issues may relate to assessment of symptoms and drug taking behaviors, difficulties in maintaining symptom control, management of drug use and prevention of drug abuse, education and communication among the treatment team and other clinicians, and the need to address the unique fears of patients who may be stigmatized by a history of socially unacceptable behavior.

The practical management of prescribed drugs for symptom control is particularly challenging among those with a current history of abuse. A treatment team that includes a clinician with experience in addiction medicine may be the most efficient structure for implementing a detailed plan for outpatient and inpatient management that offers security to the patient and staff, as well as allowing the staff to address the medical issues without undue concern about the problems associated with aberrant drug taking.

The interface between the therapeutic use of potentially abusable drugs for symptom control and the multifaceted nature of abuse and addiction is extraordinarily complex. Research into the nature of this interface and its clinical implications has only recently begun. Practical management is yet based largely on clinical experience and anecdotal observations. As progress in providing a scientific basis for this endeavor proceeds, clinicians must attempt to provide consistent and sensitive treatment that addresses the potential problems while ensuring humane and compassionate treatment for patients with progressive medical diseases.

## REFERENCES

1. Colliver JD, Kopstein AN. Trends in cocaine abuse reflected in emergency room episodes reported to DAWN. *Publ Health Rep* 1991;106:59–68.
2. Groerer J, Brodsky M. The incidence of illicit drug use in the United States, 1962–1989. *Br J Addict* 1992;87:1345.
3. Regier DA, Meyers JK, Dramer M, et al. The NIMH epidemiologic catchment area program. *Arch Gen Psychiatry* 1984; 41:934.
4. Wells KB, Golding JM, Burnam MA. Chronic medical conditions in a sample of the general population with anxiety, affective, and substance use disorders. *Am J Psychiatry* 1989;146:1440.
5. Burton RW, Lyons JS, Devens M, Larson DB. Psychiatric consults for psychoactive substance disorders in the general hospital. *Gen Hosp Psychiatry* 1991;13:83.
6. Derogatis LR, Morrow GR, Fetting J, et al. The prevalence of psychiatric disorders among cancer patients. *J Am Med Assoc* 1983;249:751.
7. American Psychiatric Association. *Diagnostic and statistical manual for mental disorders,* 3rd ed. Revised. Washington, DC, 1983.
8. Bruera E, Moyano J, Seifert L, Fainsinger RL, Hanson J, Suarez-Almazor M. The frequency of alcoholism among patients with pain due to terminal cancer. *J Pain Sympt Manage* 1995;10(8):599.
9. Dole VP. Narcotic addiction, physical dependence and relapse. *N Engl J Med* 1972;286:988.
10. Martin WR, Jasinski DR. Physiological parameters of morphine dependence in man—tolerance, early abstinence, protracted abstinence. *J Psychiatr Res* 1969;7:9.
11. Wikler A. *Opioid dependence: mechanisms and treatment.* New York: Plenum Press, 1980.
12. Portenoy RK. Opioid tolerance and efficacy: basic research and clinical observations. In: Gebhardt G, Hammond D, Jensen T, eds. *Proceedings of the VII World Congress on Pain.* Progress in Pain Research and Management, vol 2. Seattle: IASP Press, 1994;595.
13. Foley KM. Clinical tolerance to opioids. In: Basbaum AI, Besson J-M, eds. *Towards a new pharmacotherapy of pain.* Chichester: John Wiley and Sons, 1991;181.
14. Ling GSF, Paul D, Simantov R, Pasternak GW. Differential development of acute tolerance to analgesia, respiratory depression, gastrointestinal transit and hormone release in a morphine infusion model. *Life Sci* 1989;45:1627.
15. Bruera E, Macmillan K, Hanson JA, MacDonald RN. The cognitive effects of the administration of narcotic analgesics in patients with cancer pain. *Pain* 1989;39:13.
16. Twycross RG. Clinical experience with diamorphine in advanced malignant disease. *Int J Clin Pharmacol Ther Toxicol* 1974;9:184.
17. Kanner RM, Foley KM. Patterns of narcotic drug use in a cancer pain clinic. *Ann NY Acad Sci* 1981;362:161.
18. Chapman CR, Hill HF. Prolonged morphine self-administration and addiction liability: evaluation of two theories in a bone marrow transplant unit. *Cancer* 1989;63:1636 .
19. France RD, Urban BJ, Keefe FJ. Long-term use of narcotic analgesics in chronic pain. *Soc Sci Med* 1984;19:1379.
20. Portenoy RK, Foley KM. Chronic use of opioid analgesics in nonmalignant pain: report of 38 cases. *Pain* 1986;25:171.
21. Urban BJ, France RD, Steinberger DL, Scott DL, Maltbie AA. Long-term use of narcotic-antidepressant medication in the management of phantom limb pain. *Pain* 1986;24:191.
22. Zenz M, Strumpf M, Tryba M. Long-term opioid therapy in patients with chronic nonmalignant pain. *J Pain Sympt Manage* 1992;7:69.
23. Redmond DE, Krystal JH. Multiple mechanisms of withdrawal from opioid drugs. *Annu Rev Neurosci* 1984;7:443–478.
24. World Health Organization. Technical report no. 516, youth and drugs. Geneva, 1973.
25. American Psychiatric Association. *Diagnostic and statistical manual for mental disorders*, 4th ed. Washington, DC, 1994.
26. Halpern LM, Robinson J. Prescribing practices for pain in drug dependence: a lesson in ignorance. *Adv Alcohol Subst Abuse* 1985;5:184.
27. Dai S, Corrigal WA, Coen KM, Kalant H. Heroin self-administration by rats: influence of dose and physical dependence. *Pharmacol Biochem Behav* 1989;32:1009.
28. Jaffe JH. Current concepts of addiction. *Res Publ Assoc Res Nerv Mental Dis* 1992;70:1.
29. Rinaldi RC, Steindler EM, Wilford BB, Goodwin D. Clarification and standardization of substance abuse terminology. *J Amer Med Assoc* 1988;259:555.
30. Sees KL, Clark HW. Opioid use in the treatment of of chronic pain: assessment of addiction. *J Pain Sympt Manage* 1993;8:257.
31. Breitbart W, Rosenfeld BD, Passik SD, McDonald MV, Thaler H, Portenoy RK. The undertreatment of pain in ambulatory AIDS patients. *Pain* 1996;65:239.
32. Cleeland C, Gonin R, Hatfield A, et al. Pain and its treatment in outpatients with metastatic cancer. *N Engl J Med* 1994;330;592.
33. Weissman DE, Haddox JD. Opioid pseudoaddiction—an iatrogenic syndrome. *Pain* 1989;36:363.
34. Khantzian EJ, Treece C. DSM-III psychiatric diagnosis of narcotic addicts. *Arch Gen Psychiatry* 1985;42:1067.
35. Jorgensen L, Mortensen M-J, Jensen N-H, Eriksen J. Treatment of cancer pain patients in a multidisciplinary pain clinic. *Pain Clin* 1990;3:83.
36. Moulin DE, Foley KM. Review of a hospital-based pain service. In: Foley KM, Bonica JJ, Ventafridda V, eds. *Advances in pain research and therapy,* vol 16. Second International Congress on Cancer Pain. New York: Raven Press, 1990;413.
37. Schug SA, Zech D, Dorr U. Cancer pain mangement according to WHO analgesic guidelines. *J Pain Sympt Manage* 1990;5:27.
38. Schug SA, Zech D, Grond S, Jung H, Meurser T, Stobbe B. A long-term survey of morphine in cancer pain patients. *J Pain Sympt Manage* 1992;7:259.
39. Ventafridda V, Tamburini M, DeConno F. Comprehensive treatment in cancer pain. In: Fields HL, Dubner R, Cervero F, eds. *Advances in pain*

*research and therapy,* vol 9, Proceedings of the Fouth World Congress on Pain. New York: Raven Press, 1985;617.

40. Ventafridda V, Tamburini M, Caraceni A, et al. A validation study of the WHO method for cancer pain relief. *Cancer* 1990;59:850.

41. Walker VA, Hoskin PJ, Hanks GW, White ID. Evaluation of WHO analgesic guidelines for cancer pain in a hospital-based palliative care unit. *J Pain Sympt Manage* 1988;3:145.

42. World Health Organization. *Cancer pain relief and palliative care.* Geneva, 1990.

43. Health and Public Policy Committee, American College of Physicians. Drug therapy for severe chronic pain in terminal illness. *Ann Intern Med* 1983;99:870.

44. Agency for Health Care Policy and Research. *Clinical practice guideline number 9: management of cancer pain.* Washington, DC: U.S. Dept. of Health and Human Services, 1994.

45. Ad Hoc Committee on Cancer Pain, American Society of Clinical Oncology. Cancer pain assessment and treatment curriculum guidelines. *J Clin Oncol* 1992;10:1976.

46. American Pain Society. *Principles of analgesic use in the treatment of acute pain and cancer pain.* Skokie, IL: American Pain Society, 1992.

47. Zech DFJ, Grond S, Lynch J, Hertel D, Lehmann KA. Validation of the World Health Organization Guidelines for cancer pain relief: a 10 year prospective study. *Pain* 1995;63:65.

48. Portenoy RK. Opioid therapy for chronic nonmalignant pain: current status. In: Fields HL, Liebeskind JC, eds. *Progress in pain research and management,* vol. 1. *Pharmacological approaches to the treatment of chronic pain: new concepts and critical issues.* Seattle: IASP, 1994; 247.

49. Zenz M, Strumpf M, Tryba M. Long-term opioid therapy in patients with chronic nonmalignant pain. *J Pain Sympt Manage* 1992;7:69.

50. Kolb L. Types and characteristics of drug addicts. *Ment Hyg* 1925;9: 300.

51. Pescor MJ. The Kolb classification of drug addicts. Washington, DC: *Public Health Rep* (Suppl 155), 1939.

52. Rayport M. Experience in the management of patients medically addicted to narcotics. *JAMA* 1954;156:684.

53. Porter J, Jick H. Addiction rare in patients treated with narcotics. *N Engl J Med* 1980;302:123.

54. Perry S, Heidrich G. Management of pain during debridement: a survey of U.S. burn units. *Pain* (1982);13:267.

55. Medina JL, Diamond S. Drug dependency in patients with chronic headache. *Headache* 1977;17:12.

56. Kaiko RF, Foley KM, Grabinski PY, et al. Central nervous system excitatory effects of meperidine in cancer patients. *Ann Neurol* 1983;13: 180.

57. Grove WM, Eckert ED, Heston L, Bouchard TJ, Segal N, Lykken DT. Heritability of substance abuse and antisocial behavior: a study of monozygotic twins reared apart. *Biol Psychiatry* 1990;27:1293.

58. Buckley FP, Sizemore WA, Charlton JE. Medication management in patients with chronic non-malignant pain. A review of the use of a drug withdrawal protocol. *Pain* 1986;26:153.

59. Finlayson RD, Maruta T, Morse BR. Substance dependence and chronic pain: profile of 50 patients treated in an alcohol and drug dependence unit. *Pain* 1986;26:167.

60. Finlayson RD, Maruta T, Morse BR, Martin MA. Substance dependence and chronic pain: experience with treatment and follow-up results. *Pain* 1986;26:178.

61. Maruta T. Prescription drug-induced organic brain syndrome. *Am J Psychiatry* 1978;135:376.

62. Maruta T, Swanson DW, Finlayson RE. Drug abuse and dependency in patients with chronic pain. *Mayo Clin Proc* 1979;54:241.

63. Maruta T, Swanson DW. Problems with the use of oxycodone compound in patients with chronic pain. *Pain* 1981;11:389.

64. McNairy SL, Maruta T, Ivnik RJ, Swanson DW, Ilstrup DM. Prescription medication dependence and neuropsychologic function. *Pain* 1984;18:169.

65. Ready LB, Sarkis E, Turner JA. Self-reported vs. actual use of medications in chronic pain patients. *Pain* 1982;12:285.

66. Turner JA, Calsyn DA, Fordyce WE, Ready LB. Drug utilization pattern in chronic pain patients. *Pain* 1982;12:357.

67. Fishbain DA, Rosomoff HL, Rosomoff RS. Drug abuse, dependence, and addiction in chronic pain patients. *Clin J Pain* 1992; 8:77.

68. Gardner-Nix JS. Oral methadone for managing chronic nonmalignant pain. *J Pain Sympt Manage* 1996;11:321.

69. Tennant FS, Uelman GF. Narcotic maintenance for chronic pain: medical and legal guidelines. *Postgrad Med* 1983;73.

70. Taub A. Opioid analgesics in the treatment of chronic intractable pain of non-neoplastic origin. In: Kitahata LM, Collins D, eds. *Narcotic analgesics in anesthesiology.* Baltimore: Williams and Wilkins, 1982; 199.

71. France RD, Urban BJ, Keefe FJ. Long-term use of narcotic analgesics in chronic pain. *Soc Sci Med* 1984;19:1379.

72. Portenoy RK, Foley KM. Chronic use of opioid analgesics in nonmalignant pain: report of 38 cases. *Pain* 1986;25:171.

73. Urban BJ, France RD, Steinberger DL, Scott DL, Maltbie AA. Longterm use of narcotic-antidepressant medication in the management of phantom limb pain. *Pain* 1986;24:191.

74. Macaluso C, Weinberg D, Foley KM. Opioid abuse and misuse in a cancer pain population (Abstract). *J Pain Sympt Manage* 1988;3:S24.

75. Gonzales GR, Coyle N. Treatment of cancer pain in a former opioid abuser: fears of the patient and staff and their influence on care. *J Pain Sypmt Manage* 1992;7:246.

76. Dunbar SA, Katz NP. Chronic opioid therapy for nonmalignant pain in patients with a history of substance abuse: report of 20 cases. *J Pain Sympt Manage* 1996;11:163.

77. Kantor TG, Cantor R, Tom E. A study of hospitalized surgical patients on methadone maintenance. *Drug Alcohol Depend* 1980;6:163.

78. Portenoy RK. Management of common opioid side effects during long-term therapy of cancer pain. *Ann Acad Med Singapore* 1994;23: 160.

79. Lowinson JH, Marion IJ, Joseph H, Dole VP. Methadone maintenance. In: Lowinson JH, Ruiz P, Millman RB, eds. *Substance abuse: a comprehensive textbook.* Baltimore: Williams and Wilkins, 1992;550.

80. Fainsinger R, Schoeller T, Bruera E. Methadone in the management of cncer pain: a review. *Pain* 1993;52:137.

81. Grochow L, Sheidler V, Grossman S, Green L, Enterline J. Does intravenous methadone provide longer lasting analgesia than intravenous morphine? A randomized, double blind study. *Pain* 1989;38:151–157.

*Principles and Practice of Supportive Oncology,*
edited by Ann Berger et al.
Lippincott–Raven Publishers, Philadelphia ©1998

CHAPTER 39

# Psychosocial Consequences of Advanced Cancer

James R. Zabora and Matthew J. Loscalzo

## OVERVIEW

Despite significant progress in research and treatments, the diagnosis of cancer creates fear and turmoil in the lives of every patient and family. In many respects, cancer generates a greater sense of dread than other life-threatening illnesses with similar prognoses (1). Some studies have found that cancer patients are sicker and have more symptoms than noncancer patients in the year prior to death (2).

Cancer disrupts all components of social integration—family, work, finances, friendships—as well as patients' psychological status. Most patients enter the cancer experience as a vital member of a family system that simultaneously attempts to adjust and respond to the diagnosis and its challenges. Over the extended course of the illness, physical changes and deterioration create multiple and complex demands on the family. These demands, in conjunction with financial burdens, generate a negative synergy that is often ignored in the care of patients with advanced disease.

Frequently, cancer patients' greatest concern is not death, pain, or physical symptoms, but rather the impact of the disease on their families (3). According to the World Health Organization (4), "family" refers to those persons who are either relatives or other significant individuals as defined by the patient. Health care professionals must acknowledge the role of the family to maximize treatment outcomes. If the family is actively incorporated into the patient care, the health care team gains valuable allies and resources. Families are the primary source of support and also provide the caregiving roles for persons with cancer. Of note, women comprise the majority of individuals who serve in these caregiving roles (5,6).

Although access to ongoing palliative care could potentially provide needed support for both patient and family, resources for palliative care are consistently limited. In the United States, most palliative care is invested in hospice programs, and only one third of all cancer patients receive formal hospice care, often only in the final days of life (7,8). Furthermore, a discussion concerning a referral to hospice can seem quite sudden and may be experienced as rejection by the patient and family. Despite the sobering survival statistics for many cancers, relatively few hospitals have developed a continuum of cancer care that informs patients and families that most antineoplastic therapy is palliative, not curative. The transition from a period of primary therapy to a period without such therapy can be very difficult, and it may be surmised that the situation is worse for other chronic life-threatening diseases. At present, patients and family members enter hospice care, which is the primary deliverer of comprehensive palliative care services, and attempt to accept that prolongation of life is no longer the goal of care. In addition to the shift in the focus from cure to care, the patient and family experience the loss of the health care team with whom trust has been imbued over months and sometimes many years. The loss occurs simultaneously at multiple levels. Only one third of all cancer patients receive formal hospice care and often only in the final days of life. Although palliative care at the end of life should be a time of refocusing and resolution, the referral process may cause an iatrogenic crisis rather than comfort.

The psychological impact of cancer and its treatments is directly influenced by the interactions between the degree of physical disability, internal resources of the patient, the intensity of the treatment, side effects and other adverse reactions, and the relationship with the health care team. In addition, two salient timelines or continua related to patient and family adaptation must be considered. The level of psychological distress forms the

J.R. Zabora (The Johns Hopkins Oncology Center) and M.J. Loscalzo (Department of Oncology): The Johns Hopkins University School of Medicine, Baltimore, MD 21287-8391.

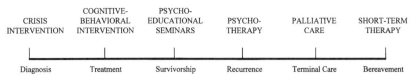

**Disease Continuum**

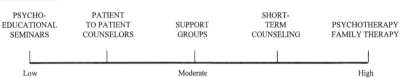

**Distress Continuum**

**FIG. 1.** Continuums of care for cancer patients and their families.

first continuum and the second consists of the predictable and transitional phases of the disease process.

Patients with a preexisting high level of psychological distress can experience significant difficulty with any attempt to adapt to the stressors associated with a cancer diagnosis. Although most patients experience significant distress at the time of their diagnosis, the majority of patients gradually adjust during the following 6 months (9).

Figure 1 details potential interventions along the disease and distress continua. The level of psychological vulnerability also falls along a continuum from low to high distress and should guide this selection of interventions. Prevalence studies demonstrate that one of every three newly diagnosed patients (regardless of prognosis) need psychosocial or psychiatric intervention (10–12). As disease advances, a positive relationship exists between the increase in the occurrence and severity of physiologic symptoms and the patient's level of emotional distress and overall quality of life. For example, a study of 268 cancer patients with recurrent disease observed that patients with higher symptomatology, greater financial concerns, and a pessimistic outlook experience higher levels of psychological distress and lower levels of general well-being (13).

If distress levels can be identified through techniques such as psychosocial screening, patients can then be intro-

duced into supportive care systems earlier in the treatment process. Accordingly, any attempt to identify vulnerable patients and families in a prospective manner is worthwhile. Screening techniques are available through the use of standardized instruments that are capable of prospectively identifying the patients and families who may be more vulnerable to the cancer experience. Preexisting psychosocial resources are critical in any predictive or screening process. In one approach, Weisman et al. (14) delineated key psychosocial variables in the format of a structured interview accompanied by a self-report measure (Table 1). However, in hospitals, clinics, or community agencies that provide care to a high volume of patients and their families, a structured interview by a psychosocial provider is seldom feasible. Consequently, brief and rapid methods of screening are necessary. Brief screening techniques that examine components of distress such as anxiety or depression can be incorporated into the routine clinical care of the patient. Early psychosocial interventions may be less stigmatizing to the patient and more readily accepted by patients, families, and staff if screening identifies the management of distress as one component of comprehensive care (15). Screening is also a cost-effective technique for case identification in comparison to an assessment of all new patients (16).

The second continuum relates to the predictable phases of the disease process. This disease continuum extends

**TABLE 1.** *Variables associated with psychosocial adaptation (14)*

| Social support | Past history | Current concerns | Other variables |
|---|---|---|---|
| Marital status | Substance abuse | Health | Education |
| Living arrangements | Depression | Religion | Employment |
| Number of family members and relatives in vicinity | Mental health | Work–finance | Physical symptoms |
| Church attendance | Major illness | Family | Anatomic staging |
| | Past regrets | Friends | |
| | Optimism vs. pessimism | Existential | |
| | | Self-appraisal | |

**TABLE 2.** *Advancing disease and psychosocial treatment*

| Crisis event | Personal meaning | Manifestation | Coping tasks | Survivor goals | Professional interventions |
|---|---|---|---|---|---|
| Recurrence/ new primary | What did I do wrong? Was it my negative attitude? Was I foolish to hope this was over forever? God has failed me. I beat this last time; I will beat it again. Nothing ever works out well for me. They said I was okay but I'm not. Do I have to start all over again? | Anger Fear Depression Anxiety Shock Loss of hope Denial Guilt Loss of trust Feelings of alienation Increased vulnerability Loss of control Confronting mortality Search for meaning | Reestablish hope. Accept the uncertainty about the future. Understand information about new situation. Regain a life focus and time perspective appropriate to the changed prognosis. Communicate new status to others. Make decisions about the new treatment course. Integrate reality of ongoing nature of disease to probable death from cancer. Tolerate changes in routine and roles again. Adjust to increased dependency again. Reinvest in treatment. | Integrate reality with family functioning, maintain self-worth. | Information Support Education Cognitive/ behavioral skills training Physical availability Supportive psycho- therapy Resource provision/ referral |
| Advanced disease | I'm out of control. Will they offer new treatment? What am I doing wrong? Will it be as bad as the last time? Will I go broke? | Depression  Anxiety Demoralization Fear Denial Anger Fear of intimacy | Maintain hope and direction. Tolerate medical care. Enhance coping skills. Maintain open communication with family, friends and health care professionals. Assess treatment and care options. Maintain relationships with medical team. | Dignity Direction Role in work, family, and community | Support Cognitive/ behavioral skills training Supportive psycho- therapy Physical availability Resource provision/ referral Information Education |
| Terminal | When am I going to die? Does dying hurt? What happens after you die? Why me? Why now? What did I do to deserve this? What will happen to my family? Will I be remembered by my family and friends? What if I start to die and I'm all alone? Can't the doctors do something else, are they holding back on me, have they given up on me? | Depression Fear Anxiety Denial Demoralization Self-destructive behavior Loss of control Guilt Anger Fear of abandonment Fear of isolation Increased dependency Acceptance Withdrawal Search for meaning in past as well as present Pain/suffering Need to discuss afterlife | Maintain a meaningful quality of life. Adjust to physical deterioration. Plan for surviving family members. Accept reality of prognosis. Mourn actual losses. Mourn the death of dreams. Get things in order. Maintain and end significant relationships. Say good-bye to family and friends. Accept impending death. Confront the relevant existential and spiritual issues. Talk about feelings. Review one's life. | Dignity Family support and bereavement | Physical availability Support Cognitive/ behavioral skills training Therapeutic rituals Coordination of services Advocacy Information |

The authors acknowledge the assistance of Karlynn Brintzenhofeszoc, DSW and the Department of Oncology Social Work of The Johns Hopkins Oncology Center in the development of this table.

from the point of diagnosis to cancer therapies and beyond. As patients move across this continuum, they may acquire experiences, knowledge, and skills that enable them to respond to the demands of their disease. The needs of a newly diagnosed patient with intractable symptoms differ significantly from those of a patient who has advanced disease and no further options for curative treatments.

Recurrent disease challenges the adaptive resources of any patient and family. Relapse may greatly intensify the focus on death. However, as with the newly diagnosed patient, adaptation to recurrent disease does occur. Many of the same variables promote adaptation at this difficult phase on the disease continuum. In many respects, patients with recurrent disease become both chronically and terminally ill. For these patients, the hope for cure of their disease is unrealistic, but life expectancy is usually unknown. Death could occur within 6 months, or the time remaining could be considerably longer. Consequently, the demands on family caregivers who provide terminal care may be quite demanding and prolonged.

The patient and family may be supported throughout the illness process and the family requires continuing support following the death of the patient. At times, families are overwhelmed by the illness and as a result are unable to respond effectively. For some families, a death may represent a loss of the family's identity and may paralyze the family's coping and problem-solving responses. Failure to respond and problem-solve leads to a lack of control and may generate a significant potential for a chronic grief reaction (17). Although the disease continuum consists of specific points, Table 2 identifies a series of predictable and relevant crisis events and psychosocial challenges that occur as patients and families confront advanced disease.

## KEY PSYCHOSOCIAL VARIABLES AND CONSTRUCTS

Weisman et al. (14) defined the critical variables that influence adaptation as past history of functioning; social support; and current concerns such as health, work-finance, and family (see Table 1). In part, adjustment to illness is determined by social support and the patient's past history of functioning. Most often, the family is the core of social support. Marital status, living arrangements, and number of family members in the immediate geographic area indicate the availability of the family as a potential source of support.

Another social support variable is "church attendance," which may be a proxy for spirituality as a source of potential support. Quality-of-life studies only recently began to consider this concept, and health care providers frequently ignore the spiritual domain (18). A cancer diagnosis stimulates an exploration of the meaning of life

and death. Traditional values and belief systems are questioned and challenged. If a patient and family can achieve a different perspective of death, a new level of comfort may be attained. Evidence indicates that spirituality decreases psychological distress (19).

The impact of the family as a primary source of social support must be assessed on the basis of availability and adequacy. Although family composition and size determines the potential for multiple family members to be available to the patient, it is a common misperception that large families automatically provide an appropriate level of support. Neither composition nor size can be equated with a family's capability and willingness to provide necessary support and care. In many respects, each family varies in its ability and willingness to be a consistent source of support (20).

## FAMILY ADAPTABILITY AND COHESION

The circumplex model of family functioning, as developed by Olson et al. (21), categorizes families in a manner that explains the variations in their behavior. Although not specifically developed for cancer, this model conceptualizes families' responses to stressful events based on two constructs: adaptability and cohesion. Adaptability reflects the capability of a family to reorganize internal roles, rules, and power structure in response to a significant stressor. Given the impact of advancing cancer on the total family unit, families must frequently reassign roles, alter rules for daily living, and revise long-held methods for problem solving. Dysfunction in the family can relate to either low adaptability (rigidity) or excessively high adaptability (chaotic). A family characterized as rigid in its adaptability persists in the use of specific coping behaviors even when they are ineffective. Those that exhibit adaptability create a chaotic response within the power structure, roles, and rules of the family; such families lack structure in their responses and attempt different coping strategies with every new stress. Although the majority of families are in the more functional category of "structured adaptability," 30% are rigid or chaotic. These families are likely to exhibit problematic behaviors (Table 3) that the health care team may find difficult to manage (22).

The second construct of Olson et al.—cohesion—is indicative of the family's ability to provide adequate support. Cohesion is the level of emotional bonding that exists among family members and is also conceptualized on a continuum from low to high. Low cohesion (disengagement) suggests little or no connectedness among family members. A commitment to care for other family members is not evident and, as a result, these families are frequently unavailable to the medical staff for support of the patient or the decision-making process. At the other extreme, high cohesion (enmeshment) blurs the bound-

**TABLE 3.** *Problematic family behaviors*

Direct interference with the delivery of medical care
Excessive demands of staff time
Alliances with other families against the health care team
Inability to follow guidelines or noncompliance with directives
Encouragement of the patient to be noncompliant
Unrealistic expectations of the health care team
Unavailability to patient or team concerning decision making or support
Dysfunctional or potentially destructive home environment that inhibits effective management of the patient

aries among family members. This results in the perception by health care providers that some family members seem to be just as affected by the diagnosis or treatment, or by each symptom, as the patient. Enmeshed families may demand excessive amounts of time from the health care team and be incapable of following simple medical directives. These families are not able to objectively receive and comprehend information that may be in the best interest of the patient. Also, these families may assume an overprotective position in relation to the patient and may speak for the patient even when the patient's self-expression could be encouraged.

As a result of social demands, threats to the integrity of the family structure, noxious symptoms, and the patient's physical deterioration and disfigurement, patients and families struggle to maintain a meaningful life. Within the context of advancing cancer, the extreme types of family behaviors are likely to occur.

In the Weisman et al. (14) framework, the patient's past history of functioning may illuminate the response to the demands of the illness and treatments. However, individual disturbances are deeply intertwined with family interaction, and it may be difficult distress related to a previous history of psychiatric illness, substance abuse, or other mental health problems. Families possess significant power through their ability to encourage, coerce, reinforce, or shame. For example, it is quite difficult for a patient to maintain his or her social isolation without direct or indirect reinforcement by family members.

Patients may bring to their cancer treatment life experiences that breed mistrust and turmoil. Patients may emerge from problematic family situations to receive treatment from caring strangers. Although most people experience support as comforting, vulnerable patients may be unable to accept support and families may feel threatened. Some patients unconsciously reconstruct their familial relationships with the health care team and staff may sense rejection from these families. Health care professionals who do not anticipate these possibilities may maintain unrealistic expectations of families and react in an inappropriate and maladaptive manner.

When engaging families, it is necessary to gain an appreciation for the rules and regulations of particular families. Each family has its own rules, regulations, and communication styles. In gaining an understanding of the role of the patient in the family, it is helpful to ask the patient to describe the specific responsibilities he or she performs in the family, especially during a crisis. Generalities are less informative than descriptions of the specific experiences and duties of each family member during a crisis. These queries enable the patient to openly communicate and objectively evaluate his or her role and importance in the family system and provides a clinical opportunity to assess ongoing progress or deterioration. Patients and families can usually tolerate even the worst news or the most dire prognosis as long as it is framed within a context in which both patient and family know how they are expected to respond and that the health care team will not abandon them.

## PSYCHOSOCIAL SCREENING

As noted, there are many potential advantages to efficiently screen for psychosocial distress. Standardized measures such as the Brief Symptom Inventory (23) or the General Health Questionnaire (24) can be employed to prospectively identify patients who experience significantly elevated levels of distress at the time of the diagnosis. Distress is often directly related to inadequate social support. A history of mental health difficulties, substance abuse, or other major illnesses may indicate that the patient or family will experience significant difficulty with a cancer diagnosis. Fifteen to eighteen percent of newly diagnosed patients have a psychiatric or substance abuse history, severe family dysfunction, or a history of physical or sexual abuse (25), and may be particularly vulnerable to the physical impact of the illness and the rigors of cancer therapies. For the homebound patient, screening can be administered by the visiting nurse or social worker. If possible, family members should also be screened.

A standardized measure of psychological distress such as the Brief Symptom Inventory can differentiate patients into low, moderate, or high degree of vulnerability. Patients with a low level of distress may benefit from a psychoeducational program that can enhance adaptive capabilities and problem-solving skills; high-distress patients may possess psychosocial needs that require individual psychotherapy or family therapy along with psychotropic drug therapy for the patient. For some patients, ongoing mental health services are essential, whereas other patients may require assistance only at critical transition points. Clinical practice suggests that virtually all patients could benefit from some type of psychosocial intervention at some point along the disease continuum. Psychosocial interventions include educational programs, support groups, cognitive-behavioral techniques, and psychotherapy (26).

## PSYCHOLOGICAL IMPACT OF PAIN AND OTHER NOXIOUS SYMPTOMS

Patients with advanced illness experience pain, dyspnea, fatigue, nausea, anxiety, depression, sleeplessness, and many other symptoms that impair quality of life. These noxious symptoms also compromise cognition, concentration, and memory (27) and override the underlying mental schema of patients. For the person in pain or acute physical distress, perception is confined to only the most immediate and essential elements of his or her sensory experience and there is only a fragmented, distant remnant of a past or future. The immediate need and goal is to stop or minimize the noxious experience. In some sense, pain and other symptoms absorb the limited psychic energy of the patient, and valuable energy can only be made available if physical distress is effectively managed. The psychic life is subservient to and dependent on the bodily experience.

Family members of patients with advancing disease are often bewildered and frightened by the dramatic changes they perceive in the person they have known throughout their lives. This is especially true if the person has been a nurturing figure who provided support and sustenance.

Moderate to severe pain is reported by 30–45% of patients undergoing (28) cancer treatments and 75–90% of patients with advanced disease (29). Pain seems to stand alone in its ability to gain the active attention of others while dramatically demonstrating a person's being alone and vulnerable. This is especially true of patients with advanced disease and their families. While a patient is experiencing pain, another person only inches away is incapable of truly understanding what is so central and undeniable to the patient. This invisible and almost palpable boundary between the person in pain and his or her caregivers has significant implications for the quality and effectiveness of the therapeutic relationship (30).

It is generally accepted that pain is poorly managed despite the availability of effective therapies. Patients, families, and professional staff may share a reluctance to use opioid analgesics even when life expectancy is quite limited. The circumstances that surround a primordial evolutionary process enable patients to accept suffering and allow the health care team to permit the unnecessary pain to continue. Although most cancer patients are psychologically healthy (10,31), inadequately managed cancer pain and other symptoms can produce a variety of

"pseudopsychiatric" syndromes that are anxiety-provoking and confusing to patients, families, and clinicians. Cancer patients with pain are also more likely to develop psychiatric disorders than cancer patients without significant pain (32). In the short term, pain provokes anxiety; over the long term, it may generate depression and demoralization.

At present, the differences between depression and demoralization as clinical constructs have yet to be empirically explored. Depression is significantly related to higher levels of cancer pain, and pain is likely to play a causal role related to depression. Overall depression rates for cancer patients are 20–25% (32), and estimates as high as 50–70% have been applied to populations with advanced disease (33). There is a significant correlation between affective disorders and pain, and among the negative emotional states associated with pain (dysphoria, hopelessness, guilt, suicidal ideation, etc.). Anecdotal clinical experience consistently demonstrates that once pain and related distressing physical symptoms are relieved, suffering, anxiety, depression, demoralization, and suicidal ideation are ameliorated. The impact on the family is equally significant.

Depressed patients distort reality and grossly minimize their perceived abilities in managing the demands of the illness and its treatment. Furthermore, depressed cancer patients with inadequately controlled pain are at increased risk of suicide (34). For the depressed patient, acute sensitivity to physical sensations may lead to or exaggerate pre-existing morbid or catastrophizing thoughts. The complex and interactive associations among physical sensations (neutral or noxious sensations), mentation (personal meaning given to the sensations), and behaviors (attempts to minimize threat and regain control) are all negatively influenced by depression. The destructive synergy of unrelieved pain and depression may lead to overwhelming suffering in patients and families, and to a shared sense of hopelessness and helplessness. Consequently, a patient or family may develop the faulty perception that suicide is their only remaining vestige of control. From this perspective, the value of a multimodality approach that combines pharmacology, supportive psychotherapy, and cognitive-behavioral skills training is clear (35). From a psychological perspective, promotion of compliance with medical regimens, correction of distorted cognitive perceptions, acquisition of coping skills to manage physical tension/stress/pain, and the effective use of valuable physical energy to maximize engagement of life become the focus of care.

## SOCIOCULTURAL INFLUENCES ON PATIENT AND FAMILY ADAPTATION

Perceptions of illness and death can be conceptualized as experiences with both conscious and unconscious associations. These perceptions include concerns and fears that are beyond the limits of objective knowledge. Sociocultural beliefs may sooth anxiety or fear by providing comfort when a vacuum exists due to a lack of experience in a particular area, and sociocultural attitudes exert considerable influence as patients approach the ends of their lives (36,37). These beliefs and attitudes are evident in direct observations of how the family cares for the patient, views of an afterlife, or rituals related to how the corpse is to be managed.

Although there have been efforts to increase sensitivity about the importance of integrating sociocultural influences into an overall assessment of the cancer patient and family, readily accessible tools, methods, and instruments are still virtually absent. In addition, under certain circumstances, culturally sensitive labels have devolved into stereotyping by age, gender, race, religion, or economic status. Clearly, the role of sociocultural influences is complex and cannot be placed simply into a formula or compartment.

Koenig and Williams (38) offer a framework to assess cultural responses relevant to palliative care. This framework, which is consistent with a comprehensive psychosocial assessment, posits that "culture is only meaningful when interpreted in the context of a patient's unique history, family constellation, and socioeconomic status. . . . Dangers exist in creating negative stereotypes—in simply supplying clinicians with an atlas or map of "cultural traits" common among particular ethnic groups" (p. 244).

Difficulties notwithstanding, patients and their families cannot be adequately understood without knowledge of their sociocultural backgrounds (Table 4) (39). Patients and families vary according to interests, beliefs, values, and attitudes. Individuals learn attitudes or values through family interactions, and these patterns influence how patients respond to the heath care team. Although the health care team represents expertise, safety, and authority, it is also an external and foreign force that only through necessity has gained influence and power within the family system. In stressful situations, the patient and family may project their own perceptions about themselves onto the health care team. For example, family members may feel angry, frustrated, and exhausted by the demands of caring for a dying loved one. This emotional and distressing experience can be projected onto the medical staff, which may come to be perceived negatively as a result. It is essential that the team be aware of this process and directly correct any distorted and maladaptive perceptions by the patient or family. How the health care team role models deal with communication and support problems can significantly influence how the family will integrate this outside force.

Although cultural characteristics are important, these influences often diminish over time as families are assimilated into the predominant culture. Second-generation families are more similar to the host country than to the country of origin. First-generation immigrants may possess old-world attitudes and values about authority and illness, whereas the perspectives of their offspring may be more consistent with the health care team. In this case, everyone may experience estrangement. A brief case example will illustrate this potential dilemma.

An 80-year-old Russian emigre developed widely metastatic colon cancer and approached his disease with stoic submission as he surrendered treatment decisions to his physician. The patient's middle-aged sons reacted differently, experiencing distress because of the health care team's reluctance to confront the patient with the reality of his illness and prognosis. The simmering conflict

**TABLE 4.** *Family characteristics susceptible to cultural influences (39)*

| Characteristics | Definition |
| --- | --- |
| 1. Value System | The family's rules and norms for daily living and how family life is structured. |
| 2. Mobility | The concept of "home" may be more than a fixed address. "Home" may connote relationships, goals, and needs among family members. |
| 3. Socialization | Implies the level of interaction with the world external to the family, such as utilization of community resources, openness to social opportunities, financial means to afford social outlets, etc. |
| 4. Parent–Child Interaction | Specific cultural norms may be intimately woven into the frequent interactions between parents and children. An example is the expectation that women devote themselves to the care of their children. |
| 5. Kin Network | Family relationships among in-laws, visiting relatives, and other extended members. In some cultures, families choose to live close to other relatives as an indication of solidarity rather than enmeshment. |
| 6. Family Orientations | Commitment to work is highly valued. Religious orientations often provide a consistent source of moral support and standards. |
| 7. Parental Roles | Roles within the family and in relation to children are clearly demarcated. Mutuality and shared tasks may be preferred. |

Adapted from Power PW, Dell Orto AE. Understanding the family. In: PW Power, Dell Orto AE, eds. *Role of the family in the rehabilitation of the physically disabled.* Baltimore: University Park Press, 1980.

between the sons and the team heightened the patient's fear of abandonment and rejection by the health care staff. As the health care team continued to respect the patient's request that the doctor make the decisions, the sons felt excluded from the process. When the patient requested to die at home, his sons opposed his wishes due to their concern about the impact of the physical demands on their mother. Again, the sons felt that the staff were being irresponsible by not keeping their father in the hospital for terminal care. When the staff suggested a family meeting to openly discuss the options, the sons perceived this request as a betrayal.

This case illustrates the clash of three systems with distinct perceptions and values that guide their behavior. The patient perceived questioning of authorities as an indication of mistrust. The sons desired to protect their vulnerable father from a staff that they perceived as irresponsible. Finally, the staff valued open communication and interaction with the patient concerning treatment decisions and wished to respect his wishes. Within this complex set of interactions, it was too simplistic to select one system as being the only correct one. The most appropriate intervention was to unify forces, accept each system's limitations, and develop a specific plan of action focusing on optimizing physical comfort and open communication.

## PRINCIPLES OF EFFECTIVE PATIENT AND FAMILY MANAGEMENT

The family as defined by the patient is virtually always the primary supportive structure for the patient. The family serves as a supportive environment that provides instrumental assistance, psychological support, and consistent encouragement so that the patient seeks the best available medical care. Early in the diagnostic and treatment planning phases, a family's primary functions are to instill hope and facilitate communication. For the patient whose disease is beyond life-prolonging therapy, caregiving becomes the primary focus for the family. In the latter situation, families must prepare psychologically and financially for the experience of life without the patient. Cancer and its treatments are always a crisis and an assault on the family system. As an uninvited intruder, cancer challenges the viability of the family structure to tolerate and integrate a harsh and threatening reality that cannot be overcome by force, denial, or even joint action. Joint action, however, can be successful in terms of adaptation, and if the goals are clearly defined, there is an ongoing plan that promotes the optimal opportunity for successful goal attainment.

The health care team can guide the family in developing a problem-solving approach to the demands of the illness. The plan must be clearly communicated because it delineates each individual's responsibility, so that the potential for goal attainment is maximized. For many families with histories of effective functioning, the cancer experience represents the first time that their joint action may not overcome an external threat. Consequently, the cancer experience must be reframed into more realistic terms so that the threat can be perceived as manageable rather than destructive. If this is not achieved, the family can manifest anger, avoidance, displacement, or another form of regressive behavior. For the family with a history of multiple defeats and failures, the cancer experience may be perceived by a family as more evidence that they are incapable of managing the demands of an overwhelming world. The cancer experience temporarily alters the family structure, but it has the potential to inflict permanent change. The health care team can significantly influence how these changes are interpreted and integrated into family life.

Patients often identify the effect on the family as the most upsetting repercussion of the cancer (3). Therefore, any effective intervention must include the patient, the family, and other social support networks. When patients consider their families, they may experience guilt, shame, anger, frustration, and fear of abandonment. Family members may experience anger, fear, powerlessness, survivor guilt, and confusion as they attempt to care for the patient. Family members may demonstrate the defense mechanism of displacement, transferring emotion from one person or situation to another and potentially confusing health care professionals. This confusion can create tension for family members and providers at a time when clarity and effective interactions are essential.

As the role and presence of the family changes, other supportive networks can also play a significant function. Resources such as religious groups, social clubs, and occupationally oriented groups should not be overlooked as efforts are made to assess and manage psychosocial distress.

With little exception, assessment of the primary players in the family system is a rather straightforward process. The patient can be asked directly: "Whom do you rely on most to assist you in relation to the practical needs of your illness, such as transportation and insurance transactions? When you get scared or confused, with whom in your family are you most able to talk? Who in your family most concerns you? Is anyone in your family overwhelmed with your ongoing medical and practical needs? Who in your family is coping least well with your illness? Is anyone in your family openly angry with you because of your illness? Are you particularly worried about how a specific person in your family is coping? Are you ever concerned that the demands of your illness will be too much for your family? Who is most dependent on you in your family? For what are they dependent on you? What would happen to your family if you were unable to maintain your present level of functioning?"

The answers to these questions communicate to the patient and family that it is appropriate and necessary to gauge the impact of the cancer and its treatment on their lives, and also provides the groundwork for the coordination of patient and family functions. In addition, role modeling of open communication provides an environment of emotional support, flexibility in roles, and the implied and spoken promise never to abandon each other. This cannot be achieved unless the patient and family accept that some treatment effects and life events are beyond their control and there are limits to what is possible. The medical team has the responsibility to manage the physical aspects of the disease, whereas the patient and family actively strive to integrate change, maintain normalcy, and accept the reality of the illness. The course of the illness, including death, must be identified as one of the potentially uncontrollable issues so that the patient and family can focus on areas that are amenable to their influence.

Financial resources are virtually always a major concern of patients and families. When discussions of money and resources occur within the family system, shame and guilt are common. These emotions are frequently alluded to but not openly discussed. This can be a barrier to open communication and can lead to patient fears and fantasies of abandonment. This is especially true for patients with advancing disease. Simultaneously, the family may have concerns about life goals after the patient's acute need is past or death occurs. The expected range of emotional reactions in the family includes anger, fear, guilt, anxiety, frustration, powerlessness, and confusion. Cancer confronts people with the reality of limitations.

In addition to the increasing costs of health insurance and home care, there are a wide variety of nonreimbursable illness-related costs that can be financially devastating to patients and families. Transportation, nutritional supplements, temporary housing, child care, and lost work days are but a few examples of costs borne almost totally by patients and families, for which there is seldom any form of reimbursement (40). Schulz et al. (41) found that respondents spent more than $200 per month on health-related expenses and reported significant negative effects on amount of time spent working. Other studies have confirmed the negative financial impact of advanced cancer (42,43).

Money is also a metaphor for value, control, and power (44). How patients and family members communicate about money can be an indication of their perceptions of whether treatment is progressing or not. Thus, interchanges about financial matters can actively represent latent communications about the perceived but unexpressed value of care and its potential outcome. For example, the patient and family may at the beginning of treatment state that money is no object and all must be done to save the patient. By the end of treatment, however, a much more sober and realistic view concerning valuable and vanishing resources may become evident, and a greater discussion of investment and return may ensue. At this point, both patient and family may actually be talking about their ability to persevere. Concerns about money may then be an expression of exhaustion, diminishing hope, or anger. It is important that this metaphorical communication be seen as inadequate for open and direct communication. A metaphor is a signal and a cue that indicates the need for open discussion. Openness is essential for the patient and family to discuss both their common and their increasingly diverging needs. Patients and families must discuss their physical and spiritual fatigue, as well as specific financial concerns related to diminishing resources as a result of their struggle with cancer. The following clinical example illustrates a number of these points.

A 54-year-old married woman with three adolescent daughters expressed concern to the team about the ongoing cost of care for her terminally ill husband. The team felt that she was selfish and that it was unethical for them to consider the financial impact on the family in caring for the patient. Sensing their resistance to her plight, she felt rejected and became irate. A meeting with the patient, family, and relevant staff was organized by the social worker to openly address her financial concerns. The family had existing financial debts due to past medical treatments and consequently had ample reason for their concern related to the additional costs of care. Once this meeting resolved concerns over additional unneeded expenditures, the focus shifted to the much more emotionally laden issues related to the slow deterioration of the patient and the family's intense grief over the impending loss. It became evident that money for the family represented the loss of "everything."

In some cases, the family may begin to perceive the dying patient as already being deceased. Anticipatory grief and premature emotional withdrawal from the dying patient creates confusion and a sense of terror in the patient. As a result, the family experiences guilt and shame because they are prepared for the loss, but the patient is still alive.

Physical exhaustion originates from diverse sources, such as multiple and complex physical demands, emotional distress, poor mental health, inadequate coping skills, social isolation, depression, anxiety, insomnia, powerlessness, helplessness, hopelessness, fear, divided loyalties, financial limitations, etc. These common factors, endemic to chronic illness, generate long-term demands that the family may find overwhelming. Extreme family types will select ineffective coping strategies (e.g., isolation, projection, regression, denial, etc.) in their attempts to resolve these problems. Substance abuse, mental illness, history of poor relationships, dependency, poverty, isolation, few family members in the geographic area, and a previous medical or psychiatric history may each act in synergy to exhaust and immobilize families. A supportive environment within the palliative model can reframe an overwhelming situation into an effective response that provides comfort and the potential for psychological growth.

## SPECIFIC PROBLEMATIC PATIENT AND FAMILY BEHAVIORS

In the context of the family milieu, conflicts with staff may be unavoidable. It is the management of these conflicts that will determine the quality of the relationship between the patient, family, and professional staff. Conflicts may result if a family cannot follow simple guidelines or is intolerant of any physical discomfort that the patient may experience. Families who are critical of staff frequently may be held to rigid standards of behavior. Unit guidelines become laws and the struggle for control results in fear and mistrust. Conversely, patients and families who endear themselves to staff through verbal praise of the quality of care often receive warmth and flexibility, and as a result unit guidelines, such as visiting hours or number of visitors, may be relaxed.

The professional staff must be flexible in their communication styles or they may be perceived as violating family boundaries. This type of interaction can devolve into a battle for power and control. Conflicts that remain at the level of power and control make it virtually impossible to work with the patient and family to develop action-oriented, problem-solving strategies that unite all in a common set of values and goals. The following case illustrates this problem.

A 69-year-old retired history professor with metastatic colon cancer guarded his privacy and attempted to maintain independence by ignoring his pain. He routinely delayed his requests for medication until the pain became intolerable. He perceived any delay in the staff's response to his agitated demands as punishment for his being weak. His responses to dependence on staff and delays in dispensing medications, which were reinforced by his wife, bred mistrust and created barriers between patient, spouse, and staff. As a result, staff were not prone to empathic responses. The staff defined the patient's demands as inappropriate. The wife perceived herself as being marginalized, and the patient felt out of control.

Effective symptom management is essential to engage the patient, family, and the staff toward a common goal. Poor management can lead to estrangement and abandonment (45). Open communication can establish goals in the context of the family and significantly reduce the strain. However, health care providers must accept that at times any approach may be ineffective because the family structure cannot tolerate the influence of external forces. When this occurs, a continued attempt at open communication is the only alternative that can achieve some sense of mutual understanding and trust.

Families can exhibit a range of behaviors (see Table 3) that the health care team defines as problematic and can potentially interfere with the delivery of medical care. Families can delay or prevent the completion of a procedure, verbally abuse the staff, or divide the team. Families may demand excessive staff time, repeatedly requesting sessions to review the same information. Although confusion may reflect intense anxiety and the overwhelming nature of this experience for caregivers, these outcomes can disrupt treatment. Some families have unrealistic expectations and compare the responses of staff members, searching for inconsistencies. Others fail to follow unit guidelines, consistently arriving well before visiting hours or delaying their departure from the hospital at the end of the day. Families may encourage patients to refuse medical recommendations or directives. Family members may at times speak for the patient and encourage the patient to withdraw and regress. Families may also possess unrealistic expectations of staff. Family members may perceive the staff as their own medical providers and seek personal care from the team.

Problematic families may find each other in waiting rooms, family groups, or other events. These families may form alliances against the staff. Together they may identify inconsistencies in medical care, availability of staff, and access to information. Instead of one family, the staff may be confronted by a number of families who together approach the staff with similar concerns or complaints.

Family functions include facilitation of medical decision making, reduction of stress, initiation of effective problem solving, and provision of comfort to the patient. If the family cannot provide these functions or is unavailable to the patient and staff, the staff may need to assume and fulfill these roles. At times, the staff may be resentful when families are unavailable or withdraw from participation. The burden on staff to care for these patients can be dramatically increased.

## SPECIAL PATIENT AND FAMILY ISSUES

### Children in the Home

Children of adult cancer patients may be an unseen and forgotten population. In acute clinical settings, children are not observed due to the patients' daytime appointments or policies that prohibit visits to inpatient units. Within the palliative setting, however, children and grandchildren are often present and may play an active role in the caregiving process.

Although salient developmental differences exist among children of different ages, those 3 years or older are usually able to verbalize their concerns so that ongoing communication can take place. Highly sensitive to emotional and physical changes, children benefit most from an environment where they are continually given information in a manner in which they can understand it and are encouraged to ask questions. Adults should be prepared for questions to be somewhat concrete and egocentric, centered around the immediate needs of the child and any potential change in the immediate family. Children are specifically concerned about the continued presence of parents and their own safety. Questions from children usually come one or two at a time. Children often need time to interpret and integrate the adult responses before returning for additional information, which may occur days or weeks later.

Methods to deliver medical information or relieve distress must vary according to each child's developmental stage. Children have fantasies about the etiology, meaning, and duration of a parent's illness. Young children need consistent information about the chronic nature of the disease so that they can anticipate changes and incorporate an understanding of these medical events into their world. Young children cannot fully appreciate the concept of permanence. The permanence of death or abstract terms such as "forever" are beyond their ability to integrate. Children need consistent support, measured doses of information, and an environment in which their questions can be addressed.

Developmentally, adolescence is the time for resolution of conflicts with parents as well as a quickened pace to individuation from the family. These processes can be delayed or significantly complicated by the family's focus on a loved one who is slowly deteriorating and dying. Competitiveness, sexuality, aggression, and peer relationships may compound and confuse attempts to cope with a loss and the end of a specific relationship.

Familial roles can be disrupted or confused during a parent's illness and as a result adolescents may be required to assume adult responsibilities. There is a danger in treating an adolescent as an adult. The demands of adolescence under normal circumstances generate numerous stressors for the family and a chronic illness at this point in the life cycle can significantly exacerbate the family's level of distress. Of particular concern, adolescents may be "parentified." Physical maturity should not be equated with emotional, intellectual, or spiritual development. Adolescents can easily be overwhelmed with guilt and shame when their normal sense of power and grandiosity cannot control symptoms or death. This may have a long-term negative effect on the ability to tolerate emotional relationships. If the death of a parent or grandparent is to occur in the home, children must be carefully assessed and appropriate interventions and support should be offered.

## Psychiatric Illness

Histories of psychiatric disorders present further challenges in the effective management of patients and families. Psychiatric symptoms must be assessed and appropriately managed if the patient is to truly benefit from supportive care interventions. For example, symptoms such as severe depression may dramatically influence a patient's perception of pain and the ability of the health care team to control it. Furthermore, psychiatric symptoms of a family member can also cause a significant concern given the health care team's expectations concerning caregiving in the home by family members. Frequently, expectations of family members as caregivers are relatively uniform despite the significant variation that exists in each family's level of functioning. Families must be assessed not only for their availability but for their ability to provide adequate supportive care.

Patients or family members with a history of physical or sexual abuse may exhibit significant difficulty in the ability to develop a trusting relationship with the health care team and may require psychiatric management. Families with a history of abuse may try to withhold information related to the abuse and perceive any attempt to assess the patient or family as an intrusion. Trust can only be developed over time as the health care team members consistently verbalize their concern for patient and family, as well as their availability for support and intervention. Families with severe dysfunction isolate and protect themselves from the outside world with rigid outer boundaries. Health care providers may define such a family as problematic when initial offers of assistance are refused. The team may experience frustration and rejection, which is inevitably communicated directly to the patient and family. Consequently, the family is lost as an ally and resource and, as a result, the patient's isolation from the team is increased. Although few in number, timely psychiatric referrals for these patients and family members are essential.

## Addictions

The history of substance abuse or an active addiction on the part of the patient or in the family creates a sense of alarm within the health care team. For example, the patient with a history of addiction may not be trusted by health care providers. The patient's behavior may be viewed as manipulative, and if pain is a problem, there may be reticence to prescribe higher opioid doses even if the patient is in pain or is terminally ill.

Patients should not suffer needlessly as a result of a prior history of opioid abuse or their current treatment in a methadone clinic. Patients with a history of opioid addiction that is remote or has been effectively managed in a drug treatment program may be at much greater risk of undertreatment. Consultation with a drug treatment facility may be necessary to plan effective management strategies.

Family members of a substance abuser can negatively influence or reinforce the patient's drug seeking behavior, if this type of behavior is occurring. These families frequently possess a high level of cohesion, which can be characterized as enmeshed. Within this type of family, boundaries between family members are nebulous and, as a result, family members may appear to be equally affected by the status of the patient. The care provided the patient may be sporadic or inconsistent because the family may be overwhelmed by the severity of the illness. Careful medical and psychosocial coordination between patient, family, staff, and, when appropriate, a drug treatment center are necessary to maximize cooperation and to maintain quality care. Despite the level of frustration associated with this group of patients, dignified care is possible and attainable.

## Intimacy and Sexuality

Advanced disease always affects sexuality and sexual functioning. Notwithstanding, the lack of libido and impaired sexual functioning are frequently overlooked or ignored as a concern of the patient. Open discussion of intimacy and sexuality with the team can actually result in enhancement of emotional vitality. In fact, an increase in intimacy can evolve as closeness is redefined and openly discussed. Patients' needs for intimacy and sexual activity must be examined and supported. A couple's expression of intimacy, even during terminal care, can create a sense of normalcy and relief in the midst of a highly traumatic course of medical events. As patients enter the terminal phase, these discussions require a high level of sensitivity. Most patients long to be touched and held, and it is not uncommon for spouses or children to lie in bed with a dying patient in order to provide comfort and experience closeness or intimacy.

## Dying at Home

Although many patients and families describe a preference for death to occur in the comfort of their homes, this goal is not always attainable. Approximately 76–80% of patient deaths occur in medical institutions; only 10–14% of patients die in hospices and the remaining 5–10% die in nursing homes or in their own homes (46–48). The return to home, nursing homes, or hospices as the chosen places of death continues to increase, primarily as a result of the Medicare Hospice Benefit (49). A number of key psychosocial variables (see Table 2) may inhibit or prevent the occurrence of death in the home even with the highest level of supportive care or hospice services. Families must be carefully assessed and prepared for the death event. Key family members can be specifically questioned concerning their level of comfort or toleration for stressful events in the home. Preparations, including advance directives, wills, and do-not-resuscitate orders, should begin as early as possible to resolve all questions and informational needs that the family may possess. Often hospice services are only in the home for a fraction of each day. Consequently, the patient's death will probably occur when the family is alone.

A family that wants to maintain a dying member at home despite complex needs may suddenly request that the patient die in the hospital. Reasons for rapid changes may be obvious and practical or may be irrational and unconscious. Either way, the resources and limitations of the family must be assessed and supported. Many terminally ill patients possess acute care needs (e.g., pain control, mental status changes), and admission may be warranted to provide brief respite for the family or to actually manage the death event.

## When the Patient Dies

The final hours of a patient's life have significant meaning for the family and offer an opportunity for closure. The ritualistic need to be present at the exact moment of death can be very powerful for family members. The desire to be present for the death event is common, and for family members who are absent, significant regrets may result (50). Unexpected deaths occur in about 30% of patients; attempts to notify the family of the impending event is possible in 70% of cases (51)..

Family members may require objective information concerning the cause of death, especially if the death was unexpected. Despite the terminal prognosis, many families need to understand why the patient died when he or she did. This information can mitigate the high level of distress and address any irrational concerns and fears associated with the death as it is happening.

Interactions with staff that occur immediately following the death can have a long-term effect. Emotional reactions of family members are expected, and crying, sobbing, and wailing are common. The therapeutic demands associated with the provision of terminal care challenges the health care professional to communicate with empathy while facilitating the initiation of essential tasks such as removal of the body and funeral arrangements. Families vary in their ability to receive information and emotional support during this time. The relationship between the family and the health care team influences how much of the necessary preparations can be made prior to the death event and how much clinical intervention the family requires and can tolerate. Generally, families elect a spokesperson to provide and receive information, but care must be taken to assess other members of the family. A follow-up meeting with the family by a social worker or nurse in the home can be very helpful to identify any family member who may be at risk for an abnormal grief response.

## Bereavement

Bereavement represents the end of the care cycle. At diagnosis, the primary focus is to save the patient from the immediate threat of disease. As disease progresses, the focus of care increasingly shifts to the needs of patients and families. As death approaches, attention is focused on the family and their efforts to cope with the demands of advanced disease. Generally, nurses, social workers, and chaplains are responsible for the provision of emotional support and bereavement counseling. Anecdotal reports, in conjunction with well-designed research studies, have established an increased risk for morbidity and mortality among bereaved spouses (52).

Most often, the social tolerance for a grieving family is brief and intense. Following a significant level of attention and care, family members find themselves in an emotional turmoil after the loss. Once the funeral and burial rituals are completed, the full and true impact of the loss is experienced. The central issue—caring for the patient—is now gone and little can replace this demanding, meaningful, and intense experience. This void is filled with a longing for the patient, periodic or sustained loneliness, and ambivalence associated with an uncertain future. Many families experience a sense of abandonment by the health care team following the death of the patient and may also experience the termination of their relationship with the health care team as an additional significant loss.

Although most families cope and adapt to the loss, an integral role exists for health care professionals. Periodic or regularly scheduled telephone contact provides an excellent mechanism to provide support and to assess the family's return to a sense of normalcy. The family can be actively encouraged to contact members of the team with specific concerns or unanswered questions.

The focus on these interactions should guide the family to a return to social functioning and resumption of a future-oriented life. It is not unusual for family members (especially spouses and parents) to believe that they see the deceased in a crowd, hear his or her voice, or sense his or her presence. Vivid nocturnal dreams, nightmares, insomnia, intense sorrow, and social withdrawal are components of the grief process.

Many family members and close friends find it helpful to talk to a social worker, psychologist, or psychiatrist to gain support and direction during this period. Family members need to understand that the intensity of their emotional reactions will subside following an acute phase of 3–6 months. For some families, a sense of fear is present that is related to their belief that the absence of sadness disconnects them from memories of the deceased. Families must be assured that once the acute phase of the loss passes, they will still be connected with the deceased because nothing can remove their memories and the life they shared.

Anniversaries and other significant dates such as holidays are a time to remember and reflect on the family's loss. Family members may wish to contact those professionals who cared for the deceased. This healthy response represents a time to emotionally connect with the deceased and to make contact with the caring support of the living. The following case example illustrates the needs of the bereaved at this point.

A 59-year-old book designer cared for her father for 3 years until his death occurred in her home. Motherless since the age of 5, this bereaved daughter perceived her father as a loving and kind source of support throughout her life. Although quite saddened and depressed following his death, she was able to enter weekly counseling until she returned to normal functioning about 4 months later. At each anniversary of his death for 8 years thereafter, the daughter returned to the hospital to sit quietly in the lobby for one hour. This ritual enables her to feel "connected and healed." Although she continued to miss her father, her level of functioning did not diminish.

## CONCLUSIONS

All patients and families possess a personal meaning of disease, prolonged illness, and death. These meanings are influenced over time by numerous factors. A clear understanding of these meanings, associated emotions, and their antecedents enhances the health care team's ability to provide care and anticipate potential problems. Information and education must be consistently available as the patient and family move across the disease continuum toward the death event.

Approximately 30% of patients and families need social work or psychiatric intervention at any point on the disease continuum. Psychosocial screening offers the capability to prospectively identify vulnerable patients and families with a high degree of accuracy. These predictive techniques can also be employed to identify high-risk families who may experience a chronic grief reaction. As a result, assessments can then be targeted to patients and families who may be at a higher level of psychological risk. This process enables the team to maximize its psychosocial resources in the most cost-effective manner.

Comprehensive psychosocial assessments of the patient must move beyond traditional considerations and include intimacy and sexuality, as well as a realistic appraisal of the capabilities and limitations of each family. Health care providers can no longer maintain equal expectations of families in terms of their level of caregiving. Because of the ongoing trend to reduce the inpatient length of stay, families must be carefully assessed to determine if the level of care for the patient is adequate.

If indications of marginal or inadequate care exist, the patient may require additional supportive services or an inpatient admission.

Variables such as cohesion describe the quality and intensity of relationships in the family. High-cohesion or enmeshed families lose more than a family member when the patient dies. For these families, part of their identity is also lost. Given their extreme level of dependence, these families may experience the death as catastrophic, which prevents the effective resolution of the loss. Chronic grief can exacerbate current psychological symptoms and influence health care practices. Bereavement follow-up among high-risk families is essential as a means to develop psychosocial prevention programs. The psychosocial obligation to the family does not end with the patient's death and some families may require follow-up beyond the customary 1-year period. Given the intensity of the loss and the family's level of risk, grief must be monitored and resolved.

## REFERENCES

1. Mishel M, Hostetter T, King B, et al. Predictors of psychosocial adjustment in patients newly diagnosed with gynecological cancer. *Cancer Nursing* 1984;7(8):291.
2. Seale C, Cartwright A. *The year before death.* Brookfield: Ashgate, 1994.
3. Levin DN, Cleeland CS, Dar R. Public attitudes toward cancer pain. *Cancer* 1985;56:2337–2339.
4. World Health Organization. *Cancer pain and palliative care.* Technical Report 804. Geneva, 1990.
5. Zarit SH, Todd PA, Zarit JM. Subjective burdens of husbands and wives as caregivers: a longitudinal study. *Gerontologist* 1986;26:260.
6. Brody EM. Women in the middle and family help to older people. *Gerontologist* 1981;21:471.
7. Gochman DS, Bonham GS. Physicians and the hospice decision: awareness, discussion, reasons and satisfaction. *Hospice J* 1988;4(1): 25–53.
8. Hyman RB, Bulkin W. Physician reported incentives and disincentives for referring patients to hospice. *Hosp J* 1990; 6(4):39–64.
9. Weisman AD, Worden JW. The existential plight in cancer: significance of the first 100 days. *Int J Psychiatry Med* 1976/77;7:1.
10. Derogatis LR, Morrow GR, Fetting J. The prevalence of psychiatric disorders among cancer patients. *JAMA* 1983;249(6):751.
11. Farber JM, Weinerman BH, Kuypers JA. Psychosocial distress in oncology outpatients. *J Psychosoc Oncol* 1984;2:109.
12. Stefanek M, Derogatis L, Shaw A. Psychological distress among oncology outpatients. *Psychosomatics* 1987;28:530.
13. Schulz R, Williamson GM, Knapp JE, Bookwala J, et al. The psychological, social, and economic impact of illness among patients with recurrent cancer. *J Psychosoc Oncol* 1995;13(3):21.
14. Weisman AD, Worden JW, Sobel HJ. *Psychosocial screening and interventions with cancer patients: a research report.* Boston: Harvard Medical School and Massachusetts General Hospital, 1980.
15. Fawzy, FI, Fawzy NW, Arndt LA, Pasnau RO. Critical review of psychosocial interventions in cancer care. *Arch Gen Psychiatry* 1995;52: 100.
16. Zabora JR, Smith-Wilson R, Fetting JH, et al. An efficient method for the psychosocial screening of cancer patients. *Psychosomatics* 1990; 31(2):192.
17. BrintzenhofeSzoc KM. Family functioning and psychosocial distress as related to special grief reaction following the death of a cancer patient (abstract). *Abstracts of the Annual Conference of the Association of Oncology Social Work,* 1996.
18. Donovan K, Sanson-Fisher RW, Redman S. Measuring quality of life in cancer patients. *J Clin Oncol* 1989;7(7):959.
19. Smith ED, Stefanek ME, Joseph MV, et al. Spiritual awareness, personal perspective on death, and psychosoical distress among cancer patients. *J Psychosoc Oncol* 1993;11(3):89.
20. Zabora JR, Smith ED. Family dysfunction and the cancer patient: early recognition and intervention. *Oncology* 1992;5(2):31.
21. Olson DH, McCubbin HI, Barnes HL, et al. Predicting conflict with staff among families of cancer patients during prolonged hospitalizations. *J Psychosoc Oncol* 1989;7(3):103.
22. Zabora JR, Fetting JH, Shaley VB, et al. Predicting conflict with staff among families of cancer patients during prolonged hospitalization. *J Psychosoc Oncol* 1989;7(3):103.
23. Derogatis LR, Melisaratos N. The brief symptom inventory: an introductory report. *Psychol Med* 1983;13:595.
24. McDowell I, Newell C. *Measuring health: a guide to rating scales and questionnaires.* New York: Oxford University Press, 1987.
25. Seddon CF, Zabora JR. Psychotherapy needs of cancer patients and their families (abstract). *Abstracts of the Association of Oncology Social Work,* May 1995.
26. Zabora JR, Loscalzo MJ. Comprehensive psychosocial programs: a prospective model of care. *Oncol Issues* 1996;11(1):14.
27. Jamison RN, Sbrocco T, Parris W. The influence of problems in concentration and memory on emotional distress and daily activities in chronic pain patients. *Int J Psychiatry Med* 1988;18:183.
28. Daut RL, Cleeland CS. The prevalence and severity of pain in cancer. *Cancer* 1982;50(9):1913.
29. Bond MR, Pearson IB. Psychological aspects of pain in women with advanced cancer of the cervix. *J Psychosom Res* 1969;13:13.
30. Cleeland CS. The impact of pain on the patient with cancer. *Cancer* 1984;54:2635.
31. Spiegel D, Sands SS, Koopman C. Pain and depression in patients with cancer. *Cancer* 1994;74:2570–2578.
32. Razavi D, Delvaux N, Farvacques C, et al . Screening for adjustment disorders and major depressive disorders in cancer inpatients. *Br J Psychiatry* 1990;156;79.
33. Shacham S, Reinhart LC, Raubertas RF, Cleeland CS Emotional States and pain: intraindividual and interindividual measures of association. *J Behav Med* 1983;6:405.
34. Bolund C. Suicide and cancer II: Medical and care factors in suicide by cancer patients in Sweden, 1973–1976. *J Psychosoc Oncol* 1985;3:17.
35. Massie MJ, Holland JC. Depression and the cancer patient. *J Clin Psychiatry* 1990;51(Suppl):12.
36. Kagawa-Singer M. Diverse cultural beliefs and practices about death and dying in the elderly, In: Wieland DM, ed. *Cultural diversity and geriatric care.* New York: McGraw-Hill, 1994.
37. Hellman C. *Culture, health and illness,* 3rd ed. Newton, MA: Butterworth, Heinemann, 1995.
38. Koenig BA, Gates-Williams J. Understanding cultural difference in caring for dying patients. In: Caring for patients at the end of life. (Special Issue) *World J Med* 1995;163(3):244.
39. Power PW, Dell Orto AE. Understanding the family. In: Power PW, Dell Orto AE, eds. *Role of the family in the rehabilitation of the physically disabled.* Baltimore: University Park Press, 1980.
40. Lansky SB, Cairns N, Lowman J, et al. Childhood cancer: non-medical costs of the illness. *Cancer* 1979;43(1):403.
41. Schultz R, Williamson GM, Knapp JE, Bookwala MS, Lave J, Fello M. The psychological, social, and economic impact of illness among patients with recurrent cancer. *J Psychosoc Oncol* 1995;13(3):21.
42. Houts PS, Lipton A, Harvey HA, Martin B, Simmonds MA, Dixon R, et al. Nonmedical costs to patients and their families associated with outpatient chemotherapy. *Cancer* 1984;53, 2388.
43. Mor V, Guadagnoli E, Wool M. An examination of the concrete service needs of advanced cancer patients. *Psychosoc Oncol* 1987;5(1): 1.
44. Farkas C, Loscalzo M. Death without indignity. In: Kutscher AH, Carr AC, Kutscher LG, eds. *Principles of thanatology.* New York: Columbia University Press, 1987;133.
45. Loscalzo M, Amendola J. Psychosocial and behavioral management of cancer pain: the social work contribution. In: Foley KM, Bonica JJ, Ventafridda V, eds. *Advances in pain research and therapy,* New York: Raven Press, 1990;(16)429.
46. McCusker J. Where cancer patients die: an epidemiological study. *Public Health Rep* 1983;98:170.
47. Merrill D, Mor V. Pathways to hospital death among the oldest old. *J Aging Health,* 1993;8:206.
48. Sager M, Easterling D, Kindig D, Anderson O. Changes in the location

of death after passage of Medicare's prospective payment system. *N Engl J Med* 1989;320,1101.

49. McMullan A, Mentnech R, Lubitz J, McBean AM, Russell D. Trends and patterns in place of death for Medicare enrollees. *Health Care Finance Rev* 1990;12:107.

50. Tolle SW, Bascom PB, Hickam DA, Benson JA. Communication between physicians and surviving spouses following patient death. *J Gen Intern Med* 1986;1:309.

51. Tolle SW, Girard DW. The physician's role in the events surrounding patient death. *Arch Intern Med* 1982;143:1447.

52. Helsing KJ, Szklo M. Mortality after bereavement. *Epidemiol Rev* 1981; 114:41.

# SECTION II

# Special Interventions

*Principles and Practice of Supportive Oncology,*
edited by Ann Berger et al.
Lippincott–Raven Publishers, Philadelphia ©1998

## CHAPTER 40

# The Hematologic Support of the Cancer Patient

Eileen Johnston and Jeffrey Crawford

## MALIGNANCY ASSOCIATED CYTOPENIAS

Anemia, thrombocytopenia, and leukopenia are common complications of malignancy and its treatment. Appropriate supportive care for the oncology patient requires an understanding of the many mechanisms for the development of cytopenia as well as the judicious use of appropriate transfusion products and growth factors.

Disease-related pancytopenia may be due to myelophthisic disease (characterized by a leukoerthythroblastic peripheral smear), splenomegaly with resulting sequestration, or immune-mediated destruction of blood cells. Microangiopathic hemolytic anemia and thrombocytopenia (with a clinical picture resembling that of thrombotic thrombocyterpenic purpura [TTP]) have been linked to various mucin-secreting adenocarcinomas including gastric, breast, pancreatic, colon, and lung cancer (1). Treatment-related cytopenia is common. Bone marrow stem cells have a poor capacity for repair of sublethal radiation damage; thus, fractionation of radiation dose (which is useful in avoiding toxicity to visceral organs) is not helpful in avoiding toxicity to the bone marrow in irradiated fields. Chemotherapy can cause both transient and sustained cytopenia. The storage compartment of the marrow contains enough maturing cells to maintain peripheral counts for approximately 8–10 days after stem cell production ceases; thus, the effect of cell cycle specific chemotherapy will be notable by the tenth day after treatment, nadir counts are manifest between days 14 and 18, and recovery between days 21 and 28. In contrast, $G_0$ active agents are characterized by delayed nadir counts (4 weeks) and prolonged recovery time (6 weeks) owing to the preferential effect on resting stem cells. Repeated dosing of chemotherapy, especially during early marrow recovery, may result in sustained toxicity and persistent pancytopenia. This effect is perhaps most notable with the alkylating agents owing to cumulative DNA damage. Potentially reversible causes of anemia should be sought. These include various nutritional deficiencies, chronic blood loss, and subclinical disseminated intravascular coagulopathy (DIC). Medications induced immunologic destruction of red cells and platelets should be excluded as a cause of persistent cytopenias.

Unfortunately, identification of the cause of leukopenia, thrombocytopenia, and/or anemia does not guarantee its reversibility. Historically, many oncology patients became reliant on blood product transfusion. Recently, advances in biotechnology have made cytokine support available to this population. We will discuss the current indications for transfusion of red cells, platelets, and granulocytes. In addition, we will comment on the use of growth factor support for each cell line as well as the development of artificial blood products. Product specific complications of transfusion are discussed in each section with a review of the general complications of transfusion at the conclusion of the chapter.

## ANEMIA

The clinical symptoms of the anemic patient vary with the rapidity of onset, patient age, plasma volume, and comorbid illness. Tachycardia, orthostatic hypotension, acute dyspnea, and lightheadedness are manifestations of acute blood loss. In the chronically anemic patient com-

E. Johnston and J. Crawford: Duke University Medical Center, Durham, NC 27710.

pensatory mechanisms maintain blood volume through plasma expansion; thus tachycardia and hypotension are less frequent signs. These patients more often complain of fatigue, dyspnea on exertion, anginal chest pain, palpitations, and decreased exercise capacity. The elderly can manifest confusion as the only complaint. Physical exam may reveal pallor, a hyperdynamic precordium, and a systolic ejection murmur; in severe cases signs of high output cardiac failure, including peripheral edema and an $S_3$ gallop, may become evident.

Anemia is a prevalent clinical syndrome in the patient with cancer and is most often multifactorial. In addition to the causes outlined above, the anemia of chronic disease (characterized by normal morphology on peripheral and bone marrow exam, low serum iron and iron binding capacity, and normal or increased marrow iron stores) may be an important contributor. Approximately 20% of all patients undergoing chemotherapy will require red blood cell (RBC) transfusion, whereas >50% of all cancer patients will be anemic regardless of treatment received.

When transfusion is used as a temporary means of sustaining the patient during recovery from an acute insult its role is fairly straightforward. In this situation the primary goal for transfusion is the maintenance of adequate tissue oxygenation. Oxygen consumption can be approximated by calculating the difference in oxygen saturation between arterial and venous blood, the oxygen extraction. Under normal conditions this difference is approximately 25% but can increase to 50% before cells must turn to anaerobic metabolism. Thus it is clear that a decrease in oxygen carrying capacity via hemoglobin reduction will not necessarily compromise the host under no or minimal physiologic stress. Oxygen delivery is maximized at hematocrits between 30% and 40%, however, many observational studies of patients refusing transfusion after surgery, trauma, or acute GI hemorrhage have shown that morbidity and mortality are not increased by hematocrits as low as 10% as long as adequate plasma volume is maintained.

It is clear that chronically anemic patients fare better than those rendered acutely anemic because of compensatory mechanisms including maintenance of plasma volume, increased cardiac output, and shifts in the oxygen–hemoglobin dissociation curve secondary to 2,3-diphosphoglycerate (2,3-DPG) production. The decision to transfuse a patient with RBCs must encompass a multitude of clinical features including the degree of physiologic stress, comorbid illness, the anticipated recovery time of hematocrit without transfusion, and the risks of transfusion. Thus there is no clear "trigger" hematocrit as an indicator for transfusion. It is common practice to routinely transfuse patients for hemoglobin at or below 7 g/dl when imminent recovery is not anticipated. However, there are clearly patients who become symptomatic from anemia at hemoglobins above 7 g/dl, especially the elderly or those with cardiac disease. For these patients a much more liberal transfusion threshold may be appropriate and should be guided by symptomatic improvement with administration of packed red cells. Individuals with chronic anemia may become hypervolemic with transfusion due to the expanded plasma volume such that concomitant diuresis may be appropriate.

A more controversial area is the use of packed red blood cell (PRBC) transfusion for improvement in quality of life. In patients with chronic illnesses, including malignancy, it is difficult to define which symptoms are attributable to the anemia and which to the underlying disease. However, Gleeson has shown that quality of life can be improved by PRBC transfusion in patients with advanced malignancy as measured by visual analog scales assessing subjective dyspnea, weakness, and sense of well-being (2). The improvement in quality of life was sustained for at least 2 weeks after single transfusion and was seen even in patients with pretransfusion hemoglobin above 7.9 who displayed symptoms compatible with anemia. This is a fertile ground for outcomes research in assessing societal and personal costs of transfusion therapy given to improve quality of life especially in comparing such a practice to alternative approaches such as the use of erythropoietin therapy.

## COMPLICATIONS OF RED CELL TRANSFUSION

### Hemolytic Transfusion Reaction

Under normal physiologic conditions a single unit of packed RBCs can be expected to increase the hemoglobin by 1 g/dl measured 24 hours after the completion of transfusion. An increment less than this should prompt a search for obvious causes such as blood loss, microangiopathy, or splenomegaly but in the absence of these factors must raise the concern for a clearing antibody resulting in a hemolytic transfusion reaction.

Acute intravascular hemolytic transfusion reactions are not usually subtle and most frequently are manifest as fever, hypotension, DIC, renal failure, hemoglobinuria, hemoglobinemia, decreased haptoglobin and schistocytes on peripheral smear. The most common precipitating cause is the infusion of ABO mismatched blood, most often as a result of errors occurring outside the blood bank such as misidentification of the cross-match specimen or failure to compare the identity of the recipient with the label on the released product. Other causes may include transfusion of glucose-6-phosphate dehydrogenase (G6PD)-deficient blood into a patient receiving sulfa-based drugs, thermal injury to the unit of blood, or mechanical destruction related to pressurized infusion through small-bore needles. Treatment is preventative and supportive consisting predominantly of maintaining intravascular volume and renal perfusion. Fatality is related to the quantity of transfused blood with the majority of deaths occurring in patients receiving more than 100 ml of mismatched blood.

These acute, immunologically mediated hemolytic reaction are almost always attributable to preexisting, naturally occurring IgM antibodies to major blood group antigens. Complement-mediated RBC destruction results in release of intravascular free hemoglobin and the components of the complement cascade cause mast cell degranulation, bronchospasm, and hypotension. Recently, it was shown that the addition of non O group red cells to whole, group O blood results in a rapid rise in plasma tumor necrosis factor (TNF) and an increase in the mononuclear cell production of mRNA for TNF (3). A case report detailed a rapid rise in circulating TNF in an operative patient who accidentally received 100 ml of mismatched blood in the operating room (TNF levels were being monitored to investigate inflammatory response resulting from cardiopulmonary bypass but none of the other patients in the study showed elevation in their TNF levels) (4). TNF release results in fever, hypotension, and capillary leak in a clinical scenario similar to that of septic shock. TNF also results in activation of the common pathway of coagulation, increases tissue factor release, and decreases thrombomodulin—all factors that might contribute to the development of DIC.

Transient renal failure is almost universal in patients with acute hemolytic transfusion reaction and is likely multifactorial. The hemodynamic compromise noted above is a contributor to renal ischemia; in addition, free hemoglobin is felt to bind to nitric oxide and thus inhibit vascular smooth muscle relaxation. Precipitation of free hemoglobin in renal tubules may further contribute to the development of acute tubular necrosis.

Delayed hemolytic transfusion reactions tend to be less fulminant and manifest by a dropping hematocrit associated with positive direct Coombs, elevated bilirubin, fever, hemoglobinuria, and varying degrees of renal insufficiency occurring 7–14 days after transfusion. The precipitating event in this case is either an amnestic response to RBC antigens or the de novo development of IgG antibodies to non-ABO antigens. When studied prospectively the incidence of delayed serologic transfusion reaction can be as high as 0.5%, but only one in 10,000 transfusions will result in a symptomatic reaction. Predictors of clinically evident reaction include antibody specificity (Kidd and Duffy system antibodies are more likely to result in symptomatic reaction) and the thermal range of the antibody. Treatment again is symptomatic but in the case of massive precipitating transfusion may require exchange transfusion to avoid life-threatening decline in the hemoglobin. Delayed hemolytic transfusion reactions are more difficult to prevent than are immediate hemolytic reactions but communication with a previously transfusing blood bank for the results of prior type and screens is especially useful.

## Iron Overload

Secondary hemosiderosis is common in patients with marrow failure states such as aplastic anemia or severe myelodysplasia and in patients with significant hemoglobinopathies. However, it is much less common in the patient with anemia secondary to malignant disease because of a lower transfusion requirement. Each unit of RBCs contains approximately 200 mg of iron and it is generally accepted that clinically significant hemosiderosis requires an iron intake exceeding output by 2 g (or 100 transfusion products in the absence of continued bleeding). Clinical manifestations of iron overload are the direct result of iron deposition in the affected organ and most commonly include skin discoloration, gonadal failure, liver dysfunction, and diabetes. Less frequently, patients may display signs of cardiac failure or arrhythmia, arthropathy, and personality changes. Because the liver is often the first organ to be severely affected, observation for evidence of rising transaminases or declining synthetic function is warranted. If left untreated iron deposition in the hepatocytes will cause fibrosis and cirrhosis sometimes complicated by hepatocellular carcinoma.

Treatment of the transfusion dependent patient with evidence of significant iron overload should be initiated only in those patients who have a good prognosis with regard to the underlying disease and consists of chelation therapy with desferrioxamine. At this time no effective oral chelation agent is available and desferrioxamine must be administered by slow subcutaneous or intravenous infusion over approximately 10 hours/day. The drug itself is generally well tolerated although the administration regimen is not. Side effects may include severe allergic reaction, auditory and visual abnormalities, as well as infectious complications are more common.

## IMMUNOLOGIC EFFECTS OF RED BLOOD CELL TRANSFUSION

The effect of transfusion on immunologic function has been debated since Opelz first described improvement of renal allograft survival in patients who had received allogeneic blood in 1973 (5). Since the time of this initial report, allogeneic transfusion has proven beneficial in promoting disease regression in patients with inflammatory bowel disease and in allowing for term pregnancy in women with a history of multiple miscarriages on the basis of immunologic rejection of human leukocyte antigen (HLA) antigens of paternal origin carried by the fetus. The potential immunologic benefits of transfusion therapy have been balanced by concern for a possible negative impact of this immunosuppressive therapy with regard to infection and tumor recurrence after oncologic surgery with curative intent.

It was anecdotally noted in the 1980s that patients who received whole-blood transfusions perioperatively during resection of colon cancer had a higher incidence of tumor recurrence and perioperative infection than those who remained untransfused. More than 20 retrospective analyses were published in an attempt to verify the validity of this observation. Most of the trials showed higher rates of cancer recurrence and disease-specific and/or overall mortality in transfused patients, but several trials showed no statistical difference in patient outcome between the groups. Interpretation of the studies is difficult as they represent retrospective, nonrandomized data and it has been unclear if adverse outcomes were causally related to transfusion or if in fact transfusion was a surrogate marker for outcome reflecting severity of disease or comorbid conditions. Many of the authors attempted to eliminate the effect of confounding variables with multivariate analysis but the interpretation of these trials remains controversial. Furthermore, the characteristics of transfused products were variable between studies in that some groups employed whole-blood transfusions and others used packed red cell preparations; in addition, some products were leukocyte depleted, others had the buffy coat removed, and still others were unaltered in terms of contaminating leukocytes. Nonetheless, additional studies have claimed similar adverse outcomes in transfused patients with other solid tumors, most notably head and neck carcinoma.

Recently, several meta-analyses of the above data have been reported despite the limitations imposed by the variability of study design and treatment practice (6–8). The meta-analysis reported by Chung included over 5000 patients undergoing surgery for colorectal carcinoma and concluded that the overall odds ratio for adverse outcome (death, cancer death, or recurrence) in the transfused group was 1.69 with a 95% confidence interval of 1.31–2.19. The authors expressed concern for the possibility of publication bias affecting the availability of data as well as concerns for the retrospective nature of the vast majority of these studies. The analysis of outcome in patients with colorectal carcinoma reported by Vamvakas concluded that the relative risk for recurrence of disease or cancer-related death was 1.37 with a 95% confidence interval of 1.2–1.56; however, the authors concluded that this modest increase in adverse outcome could be accounted for by confounding variables such as those noted above. Furthermore, if an effect exists it must be small. The authors also point out that inclusion criteria for their analysis may have been biased toward the null as 63% of the patients included were from trials unable to display transfusion effect.

Two large, randomized, controlled trials have attempted to address the issues of transfusion associated tumor recurrence and infection (9,10). Busch et al. evaluated 475 patients meeting established criteria for autologous blood banking who were randomized between autologous and allogeneic transfusion perioperatively for colorectal carcinoma resection. Criteria for transfusion were at the discretion of the attending physician; no patients received adjuvant therapy. There were no differences between the groups with regard to postoperative mortality, infectious complications, recurrent disease, or disease-free survival. However, the disease-free survival of patients who received no transfusions was significantly superior to that of transfused patients of both groups (73% and 59%, respectively). The number of autologous transfusions was limited to two thus 28% of patients in the autologous transfusion group actually received allogeneic blood in addition to their own prestored units and this may have been a significant detriment to uncovering a difference in the groups as randomized. The second trial was predicated on the observed absence of immunosuppressive effect in solid organ transplantation when leukocyte-depleted blood products were used. This trial compared leukocyte-depleted blood against the standard RBC preparation in that region, specifically buffy coat–depleted blood. The conclusion supported those of the Busch study showing no difference in cancer recurrence rates between the randomized groups but again indicating that patients who required no transfusion support fared better in terms of 3-year survival and postoperative infection rate. The authors conclude that differences between the transfused and nontransfused patients are probably the result of other prognostic factors for which transfusion is a surrogate marker.

As noted above, there are anecdotal reports of higher rates of postoperative infection in transfused patients. Two randomized trials supporting this contention have shown a significant increase in postoperative infection rates in patients receiving allogeneic versus autologous transfusion in one case (11) and between patients receiving unaltered whole blood versus prestorage leukocyte-depleted blood in the other (12). The clinical implications of this finding remain unclear but there is the suggestion that donor leukocytes may be responsible for the mediation of this effect.

Attempts to define the physiology responsible for the possible increase in tumor recurrence in transfused patients has resulted in the development of animal models. These models have shown a significantly increased rate of pulmonary metastasis in mice and rabbits subjected to tail vein injections of tumor cells in the setting of allogeneic whole-blood transfusion as compared to animals transfused with syngeneic blood. Furthermore, leukodepletion of blood products resulted in a metastatic rate equivalent to the syngeneically transfused animals. The tumor growth propensity observed in allogeneically transfused animals was transferable passively to additional animals via spleen cell infusion (13).

Allogeneic blood transfusion has been shown to decrease the T-helper/suppressor lymphocyte ratio, depress delayed hypersensitivity reactions, decrease antigen presentation, decrease natural killer cell function, and upregulate some types of humoral immunity including anti-HLA allo-antibody formation. Attempts have been made to correlate these observed changes with clinical outcomes of increased infection, increased rates of tumor recurrence and improved allograft survival in transfused hosts. The current hypothesis of immunogenic reaction in this situation invokes donor leukocytes acting as antigen presenting cells, presenting major histocompatibility complex (MHC) class II molecules to recipient lymphocytes. Depending on the type of cytokine present, the T cells are induced to differentiate into either T-helper 1 cells (IL-2-mediated) which are involved in cell-mediated immunity, or T-helper 2 cells (IL-4-, IL-6-, IL-5-, IL-10- mediated) which control antibody production by B cells. Although controversial, Blumberg and Heal have postulated that allogeneic transfusion as well as the stresses of surgery and anesthesia act to alter cytokine production and result in a shift from predominance of T-helper 1 differentiation to increased T-helper 2 production. They strengthen their argument by noting that Il-2 production is blunted in transfused patients and in those undergoing surgery; this decreased IL-2 production may result in T-cell anergy and account for the noted decline in hypersensitivity reactions in these patients. In addition, a relative upregulation of IL-10 and IL-4 have been noted in this population potentially resulting in the postulated shift to T-helper 2 differentiation and consequent enhanced humoral immunity. The downregulation of cell-mediated immunity as proposed in this model could account for enhanced tumor survival, the improvement in autoimmune disease such as inflammatory bowel disease, the allowance of term pregnancy in patients with recurrent HLA-mediated fetal rejection, and improved survival of transplanted organs (14).

## ALTERNATIVES TO RED BLOOD CELL TRANSFUSION

### Erythropoietin

The etiology of anemia in most cancer patients is multifactorial with a significant contributing factor being the anemia of chronic disease. Physiologic characterization of this entity has been difficult but it is generally felt that anemia of chronic disease is defined by some degree of erythroid hypoplasia, normal RBC morphology, decreased RBC survival, decreased reticulocytosis, and inappropriately low erythropoietin levels for the degree of anemia. Erythropoietin is produced in the peritubular interstitial cells of the kidney and in the hepatocytes; it is tightly regulated in any one individual although "normal" serum levels display a broad range. It is responsible for enhancing proliferation and maintaining the viability of erythroid progenitor cells in the bone marrow. Erythropoietin production is enhanced in the presence of tissue hypoxia but the exact mechanism is unknown; in the kidney, hypoxia results in the recruitment of additional cells in the production of the hormone but in the liver upregulation is accomplished within each hormone producing cell. The absolute erythropoietin level is inversely related to hemoglobin in patients with iron deficiency anemia but in several studies this inverse relationship has not been demonstrated for patients with anemia resulting from cancer/chronic disease. IL-1 and TNF levels are elevated in many patients with chronic inflammatory states including malignancy; it is postulated that elevated levels of these cytokines may be indirectly responsible for depressed erythropoietin production and responsiveness in these patients. IL-1 stimulates T lymphocytes to produce γ-interferon and TNF stimulates production of β-interferon in the marrow stromal cells. The interferons in turn suppress erythroid and myeloid precursors in the marrow, effects that can be overcome in vitro by the addition of G-CSF, GM-CSF, and erythropoietin. Many investigators have investigated the potential role of erythropoietin in overcoming anemia in cancer patients whether it be attributed to the anemia of chronic disease or the result of chemo-/radiotherapy.

In 1990 the first nonrandomized phase II trials of erythropoietin use in cancer patients were published. The patient populations were quite variable with some groups receiving chemotherapy and others receiving only supportive care; the presence or absence of marrow involvement was also variable. Overall these early trials demonstrated that erythropoietin was effective in reducing or eliminating transfusion requirements in many but not all patients studied. Furthermore, no reliable predictors of response were elucidated including pretreatment erythropoietin levels, pretreatment hemoglobins, or type of malignancy.

Randomized trials of erythropoietin use remain few in number but are well represented by the following examples. The first randomized study was a small trial (21 patients) and involved ovarian cancer patients receiving platinum based chemotherapy randomized to receive three times per week subcutaneous erythropoietin versus no growth factor support. At the end of 3 months the average hemoglobin in the control group was 10 g/dl but in the erythropoietin group had reached 14 g/dl. A higher percentage of the control group (46%) required transfusion than did the treatment group (10%) (15).

Abels studied 413 patients with advanced malignancy (excluding myeloid malignancy) and hematocrit less than 32%, divided into those receiving no chemotherapy, those receiving non-platinum-based chemotherapy and those receiving platinum compounds with randomization to erythropoietin versus placebo (16). Patients not receiving chemotherapy had growth factor dosed at 100 U/kg subcutaneously three times per week while those on chemotherapy regimens were administered 150 U/kg on the same schedule with titration of dose if hematocrit exceeded 38%. Endpoints were transfusion requirement, hemoglobin level, and quality of life as measured on a visual analog scale for energy level, performance of daily activities, and overall quality of life. Response was defined as elevation in hematocrit of six or more percentage points. In the nonchemotherapy group 32% of patients were responders versus 10% in the placebo group; the difference in transfusion requirement did not reach statistical significance in the blinded portion of the trial but did in fact become significantly different in the open label follow-up portion of the trial. For those patients receiving non platinum based chemotherapy the erythropoietin group showed a 58% response rate versus 13% in the placebo population and by the second month of therapy there was a significant difference in transfusion requirement between the cohorts. Similarly, in the cisplatin-treated patients response to erythropoietin was 48 versus 6% in treatment versus placebo subjects with a decline in transfusion requirement in the treatment group after month 2 of therapy. All quality-of-life parameters improved in the patients responding to erythropoietin regardless of chemotherapy status. No reliable predictors of response were identified (including evaluation by tumor type) and no excess of adverse effects was seen in the treatment arm as compared to placebo. At the end of the 6-month, open label portion of the trial (which allowed for dose escalation of erythropoietin), the response rates in the three treatment groups were 40%, 56%, and 58% with residual transfusion requirement in 10%, 13%, and 12% in the no-chemotherapy, nonplatinum chemotherapy, and platinum chemotherapy cohorts, respectively (17).

Erythropoietin therapy has also been studied in an attempt to delay or prevent the development of anemia in patients beginning intensive chemotherapy regimens. A three-armed randomized trial comparing 300 U/kg three times per week versus 150 U/kg three times per week versus no growth factor was conducted in patients receiving ifosfamide, carboplatin, etoposide, and vincristine for small cell lung cancer. All groups ultimately developed anemia but this was delayed in the erythropoietin groups. Furthermore, transfusion requirement was 100% in the no-growth-factor group, 85% in the low-dose erythropoietin group, and 50% in those on higher dose erythropoietin (18). Interestingly, a nonsignificant trend in decreased platelet transfusion requirement was also seen in the treated patients.

The concomitant use of granulocyte growth factor with chemotherapy and radiation therapy has been complicated by an initially unexpected worsening of hematologic toxicity in some patients. This has not been the case with erythroid growth factor. Several studies have shown that progressive anemia resulting from irradiation can be eliminated or diminished by the initiation of erythropoietin at the outset of radiation (19,20).

It is difficult to study quality of life in patients with advanced malignancy because there are many sources of bias and confounding in the data collection. Despite the difficulties in obtaining accurate information, Leitgeb et al. (21) have studied the impact of erythropoietin on patients with advanced malignancies. Evaluation employed a questionnaire assessing sense of well-being, mood, level of activity, pain, appetite, physical ability, social activities, anxiety, and an assessment by the patient as to whether the therapy was helping. Response (defined as an increase in the hemoglobin level of 2 g/dl by the twelfth week of therapy) was 41% and was accompanied by improvement in all quality-of-life measures over pretreatment scores. Patients without objective response showed trends of lower magnitude in improved quality of life for some measured parameters. Survival was also significantly prolonged in responders prompting the authors to conclude that patients with evidence of response were likely in a more favorable pretreatment prognostic category but that this fact does not mitigate the importance of the effect of the drug on functional status (21).

The beneficial effects of erythropoietin have clearly been demonstrated in the subset of cancer patients who respond to the therapy as defined by increase in hemoglobin by 2 g/dl or improvement in hematocrit by 6%. What remains elusive is a means by which the likely responders can be identified pretreatment so as to spare the nonresponders the inconvenience and expense of this treatment. Analysis of studies to date shows that no reliable prediction of response can be made based on pretreatment erythropoietin level alone or by pretreatment hemoglobin, age, gender, tumor type, marrow involvement, stage of disease, or treatment modality. In addition, the expected time to response and required dose for response are variable and unpredictable. Thus far the best model for predicting response to therapy is applied 2 weeks after initiation of treatment and involves measurement of serum erythropoietin levels, hemoglobin, and ferritin. If the erythropoietin level is over 100 mU/ml and hemoglobin has not risen by 0.5 g/dl, the negative predictive value of response is 93%. If, on the other hand, the erythropoietin levels are <100 mU/ml and hemoglobin has risen by 0.5 g/dl or more, the positive predictive value of response is 95%. Serum ferritin level over 400 ng/ml carries a 88% negative predictive value but levels below this predict a 75% response rate (22). Although somewhat useful, this schema does not avoid the need to initiate therapy in patients who will ultimately show themselves to be nonresponders.

The utility of erythropoietin in the supportive care of cancer patients receiving chemotherapy has recently been corroborated in an open label, nonrandomized, community-based study published by Glaspy et al. (23). More than 500 oncologists enrolled 2342 patients with hematologic malignancy or solid tumor to receive erythropoietin at a dose of 150 U/kg subcutaneously three times weekly with a suggested doubling of the dose for lack of response at 8 weeks. As in previous trials, response was defined as a rise in hemoglobin 2 g/dl or greater. Evaluated endpoints included hemoglobin response; transfusion requirement; and patient recorded quality of life as measured by visual analog scales of energy, daily activity, and overall quality of life. The drug was well tolerated with only 3% of patients discontinuing therapy due to adverse effect of the drug. Among the 2019 evaluable patients a mean increase in hemoglobin of 1.8 g/dl was observed with 53% of patients experiencing increases of 2.0 g/dl or more. Statistically significant increases in all measured quality-of-life parameters were noted, the magnitude of which correlated with increase in hemoglobin from baseline. The only subgroup showing no improvement in quality of life was patients with decrease in hemoglobin on erythropoietin therapy. The authors attempted to determine the contributions of erythropoietin therapy as opposed to tumor response in improving quality of life through a retrospective review of tumor response. Unfortunately, data were available on only 759 patients. However, energy, daily activity, and overall quality-of-life scores were improved for patients manifesting complete response, partial response, no response, and stable disease. For those with progressive disease energy, but not daily activity or overall quality of life, was improved over baseline scores. In regression analysis, hemoglobin response as well as tumor response were independent predictors of improved quality of life. Finally, erythropoietin therapy resulted in a 50% reduction in both the number of patients requiring red cell transfusion and the number of units transfused. This improvement was evident in the second month of treatment and maintained statistical significance through the planned 4 months of therapy regardless of tumor type (hematologic versus solid). As in other trials, no clear predictors of hemoglobin response were discernible.

Erythropoietin has proven to be extremely safe with no report of significant adverse effect in clinical trials involving patients with cancer. Some patients receiving the drug for anemia due to renal failure have experienced significant hypertension and seizures, but these effects seem unique to that population of patients. As noted above, erythropoietin appears safe when used concomitantly with chemotherapy or radiation therapy and has not shown clinical evidence of enhancing tumor growth. The usual starting dose is 150 U/kg subcutaneous TIW with escalation by 50 U/kg/dose to a total dose of 300 U/kg if no response is evident after 2 weeks on any one dose (early response evidenced by rising reticulocyte count). Most authors advocate discontinuation of the drug if there is no improvement by weeks 8–12 of therapy. Supplemental iron has been effective in maximizing response to erythropoietin in dialysis patients as this population has a high incidence of iron deficiency. The iron status of all patients maintained on erythropoietin therapy should be monitored closely.

## Blood Substitutes

The concept of developing an effective blood substitute is attractive for many reasons, including a potential reduction in the risk of transmitted infection; decreased provocation of HLA antibody formation; rapid and wide availability in cases of sudden, massive hemorrhage when time for cross-matching is limited; decrease in allergic reactions; and mitigation of any immunosuppressive effects of allogeneic transfusion.

Recent efforts at developing an effective blood substitute have focused on the modification of free hemoglobin of human or bovine source, an attractive approach because free hemoglobin retains its ability to bind oxygen. However, development of these agents has been hampered by rapid destruction of free hemoglobin tetramer to constituent dimers, which are rapidly cleared by the kidneys resulting in renal tubular damage. In addition, without intracellular 2,3-DPG, oxygen affinity is enhanced and tissue delivery of oxygen inhibited. Attempts have been made at overcoming these limitations. For instance, the introduction of oxygen affinity modifiers has met with some success in increasing release of oxygen at the tissue level while placement of site specific crosslinks can prevent dissociation of the hemoglobin tetramer. Others have attempted encapsulation of hemoglobin into phospholipid vesicles to prevent rapid clearance of the molecule; however, efficiency and size consistency of these liposome preparations remain problematic.

Toxicity of modified free hemoglobin products is significant and includes vasoconstriction with increased blood pressure and decreased cardiac output; the mechanism of this response is postulated to be interference by free hemoglobin with the action of nitric oxide in relaxing vascular smooth muscle. Complaints of shortness of breath, abdominal and chest pain are not uncommon and may be mediated in a similar fashion. Furthermore, the breakdown products consist of free iron, which can participate in the development of free radicals and may increase host susceptibility to infection. Despite the above limitations, there are at least seven products in phase I/II clinical trials, almost exclusively in surgical patients. The half-life of the products currently in use in early clinical trials is in the range of 5–20 hours; therefore, these substances have their greatest potential utility in the resuscitation of trauma victims. Utility in the chronic support of patients with malignancy associated anemia remains a goal for the future.

## NEUTROPENIA

Acquired neutropenia may result from underproduction or increased destruction of leukocytes as well from migration from the circulatory pool to the tissue pool in response to an inflammatory process. Neutrophil production may be impaired by a myelophthisic process, chemotherapy or other drug administration, or by previous radiation therapy. Unlike patients with chronic neutropenia, patients with acute forms of neutropenia (most often chemotherapy-induced) may suffer from fulminant, life-threatening pyogenic infection. The propensity for infection in this population rises with declining neutrophil count (a sharp rise in infectious complications occurs with absolute neutrophil count <500/mm$^3$). Common pathogens are colonizing host bacteria including skin saprophytes and enteric gram-negative rods. Isolated bacteremia is a common cause of neutropenic fever but pneumonia, perirectal abscess, central venous access catheter infection, and prostatitis are also frequently identified. No infectious etiology will be identified in half of cases. Because inflammatory cells are lacking, many of the common signs of inflammation may not be manifest; thus, the empiric treatment of neutropenic fever with broad spectrum antibiotics is mandatory. Prolonged neutropenic fever (>5–7 days) warrants a trial of antifungal therapy in addition to antibiotics. Historically, the presence of neutropenic fever has been an indication for hospitalization but current efforts are ongoing to assess the safety and cost savings of outpatient therapy for those with uncomplicated, transient, chemotherapy-induced neutropenia accompanied by fever.

## Granulocyte Transfusion

Granulocytes collected from patients with chronic myelogenous leukemia were first transfused into neutropenic hosts more than 30 years ago. Since that time much effort has gone into the development of techniques for the procurement of granulocytes and debate has persisted as to the utility of this transfusion practice. The first hurdle in procurement of granulocytes is donor selection. Because there is a high rate of contaminating RBCs in the final product, it is clear that donor and recipient must be ABO-compatible. What is less clear is whether there is a need for HLA compatibility of donor and recipient as it appears that a failure to account for HLA type may result in rapid alloimmunization and subsequent refractoriness to both granulocyte and platelet transfusion. Cytomegalovirus transmission may be diminished by matching donor and recipient for serologic evidence of previous infection.

Current technology for the collection of granulocytes for transfusion employs a preparative regimen for the donor designed to cause demargination of neutrophils; most commonly this is accomplished with oral steroids given several hours prior to collection although other methods have been utilized including administration of epinephrine and, more recently, G-CSF. The donor then undergoes leukopheresis with the processing of 7–10 L of blood during which time neutrophils are separated from red cells by centrifugation. The separation of white and red cells requires the addition of a red cell sedimenting agent, most commonly hydroxyethyl starch; this is rarely complicated by allergic reaction in the donor. Collected granulocytes undergo rapid deterioration of functional capacity and should be transfused within hours of collection.

Granulocyte concentrations are not currently licensed by the U.S. Food and Drug Administration (FDA) and thus product specifications are lacking. However it is generally accepted that the minimum concentration of granulocytes be $1 \times 10^{10}$ cells with a desirable level being twice this number. The expensive and labor-intensive nature of this process as well as the inconvenience for donors makes studies of utility paramount in importance.

The use of granulocyte transfusion in the treatment of bacterial sepsis was met with great enthusiasm in the 1960s and 1970s owing to more than 30 published reports showing promise for this approach when combined with standard antibiotics. However, meaningful interpretation of these data is difficult as the vast majority of trials were uncontrolled; furthermore, there was great diversity of underlying illness, treatment modality, and granulocyte collection/infusion protocol. Controlled trials were undertaken in ensuing years but the aforementioned enthusiasm began to wane as myeloid growth factors and immune globulin became available concomitantly with improvements in antibiotic and antifungal therapy. With the enhancement of these effective supportive measures the potential utility of granulocyte transfusion has become limited to the patient population with prolonged neutropenia and/or severe infections not responsive to standard antibiosis. More recent work has therefore focused on the use of granulocyte transfusion in patients receiving myeloablative therapy, specifically acute leukemics and bone marrow transplant recipients.

The role of prophylactic granulocyte transfusion in patients with acute myelogenous leukemia (AML) undergoing induction chemotherapy has been investigated in several controlled trials (24–26). Although some decrease in the incidence of bacteremia was demonstrated, there was no impact on remission rate, marrow recovery, or overall survival in those patients receiving transfusion. In addition, granulocyte transfusion was associated with significant toxicity including, most notably, pulmonary edema/infiltrates (which were associated with 35% mortality in one study) and CMV infection. The risk/benefit ratio does not support the use of granulocyte transfusions on a prophylactic basis in this clinical scenario.

To date, seven controlled trials of antibiotic therapy with or without the addition of granulocyte transfusion in neutropenic, febrile patients have been published (27–33). Overall survival advantage was demonstrated in three of these trials all of which required documentation of infection in the setting of neutropenia prior to enrollment (27–29). Patients with prolonged marrow suppression showed the greatest benefit. Two additional trials showed no overall survival benefit for transfused patients but did show a positive trend in one trial and advantage for certain subgroups of patients in the other. The trial by Graw et al. showed a nonsignificant trend in improved overall survival for transfused patients despite the fact that the granulocytes were obtained by leukofiltration (a method now known to produce functionally impaired granulocytes) and were administered in what are now considered subtherapeutic doses (30). A study by Alavi et al. included febrile neutropenic patients whether or not infection was documented. Again, no overall survival advantage was demonstrated for transfused patients but analysis of patients with documented infection or prolonged marrow failure did show prolonged survival with this modality (31). The remaining two trials showed no benefit to granulocyte transfusions but have been criticized for the administration of relatively low doses of granulocytes and for failure to provide HLA-compatible granulocytes (32,33). Perhaps most importantly, it should be noted that the combination of all seven trials provides data on only 163 evaluable patients in the treatment groups and 171 patients in the control arms; in addition, the data are dated and did not employ optimal granulocyte support by current standards. Finally, although there is some evidence of advantage to recipients of transfusion, the benefit was in a small subset of oncologic patients and was not compared with antiinfective modalities available at the current time including growth factor support.

Barring further data supporting this treatment modality, it is difficult to recommend granulocyte transfusion in the care of infected, neutropenic patients. However, a renewed interest has been fostered by the discovery that small doses of G-CSF administered to normal, healthy granulocyte donors can dramatically improve granulocyte recovery during leukopheresis. There is hope that higher transfused doses of functional granulocytes may improve outcome in severely neutropenic patients but controlled trials are ongoing to document patient outcome and donor safety.

## COMPLICATIONS OF GRANULOCYTE TRANSFUSION

Granulocyte transfusions are associated with significant side effects. Among the adverse effects are included a high rate of febrile reactions and hypervolemia due to the large volume of each transfusion and the need for repeated administration. Less commonly reported effects include pruritus, urticaria, hypertension, hypotension, and vomiting. A more serious side effect of pulmonary infiltrates and hypoxemia has also been reported with varying frequency. The physiology of the latter complication may be related to white blood cell (WBC) aggregation with resulting leukostasis or may be an immunologically mediated reaction against HLA or granulocyte specific antigens with resultant cytokine release and inflammation in the lungs. Appropriate migration of transfused granulocytes to an infected pulmonary bed may also produce local inflammation and transient worsening of the pulmonary examination and radiographs.

Many infectious complications of blood product administration are due to pathogens that are transfused within white blood cells. The possibility of transmission of infection to an already seriously immunocompromised host is a significant concern with perhaps the most worrisome pathogen being CMV.

The immunology of granulocyte transfusion is a complex issue. It is clear that granulocytes carry HLA antigens but that they also possess granulocyte specific antigens that are inherited independently from HLA antigens. It is known that, at least initially, granulocytes obtained from RBC-compatible donors will migrate to sites of infection in the non-alloimmunized recipient (34), but there is considerable concern that rapid alloimmunization may limit the duration of effective transfusion unless the product is also HLA-compatible with the recipient. This theoretical concern is supported by the work of Dutcher et al. who demonstrated a dramatic reduction in migration to known sites of infection of indium-labeled granulocytes in the alloimmunized host (as defined by a need for HLA-matched platelet transfusion) (35). Some have proposed that in vitro cross-matching of granulocytes may be necessary to ensure sustained response although technology for this approach is lacking. Additionally, there is some evidence that the transfusion of granulocytes results in a high incidence of lymphocytotoxic antibody production and resultant refractoriness to platelet transfusions (36).

Granulocyte transfusions are contaminated by significant numbers of RBCs and nongranulocytic leukocytes as well as by donor plasma. Because these transfusions are administered to severely immunocompromised patients there is a considerable risk for the development of fatal graft vs. host disease resulting from transfusion of immunocompetent donor lymphocytes. This complication is avoidable by low-dose γ-irradiation not affecting granulocyte function.

## MYELOID GROWTH FACTORS AS ALTERNATIVES TO GRANULOCYTE TRANSFUSION

Until recently, the management of the infectious complications of malignancy and chemotherapy had consisted of antibiotics and general supportive measures with or without the addition of granulocyte transfusion. However, with the advent of myeloid growth factors a new class of agents is available to the oncologist. Currently there are three growth factors with demonstrated efficacy in enhancing proliferation and maturation of myeloid cells, specifically filgrastim (G-CSF, *E. coli*-derived), sargramostim (yeast-derived GM-CSF), and molgramostim (*E. coli*-derived GM-CSF).

G-CSF was purified by investigators at Memorial Sloan Kettering in the 1980s and is a lineage-specific growth factor that hastens maturation of the committed progenitor pool and prolongs circulation of released granulocytes. The growth factor also has a role in enhancing efficacy of neutrophils by increasing chemotaxis and phagocytosis as well as priming granulocytes for respiratory burst. GM-CSF is a lineage-nonspecific factor that seems to act synergistically with other cytokines to enhance erythroid and multipotent colonies. Clinical effects include expansion of the myeloid, eosinophil, and monocyte/macrophage pools. Enhancement of effector functions has also been demonstrated.

G-CSF and GM-CSF are administered subcutaneously at standard doses of 5 µg/kg/day and 250 µg/m²/day, respectively. Use of these growth factors concomitantly with radiation or chemotherapy may enhance hematologic toxicity and is not currently recommended. The optimal timing for initiation and duration of therapy is not completely clear but typically growth factor is begun 24–72 hours after completion of chemotherapy and continued until the absolute neutrophil count exceeds 10,000/mm³.

Toxicity related to G-CSF is rare and generally mild, with the most prominent reaction being medullary bone pain experienced by up to 40% of patients but generally relieved by nonsteroidals. Less common side effects include allergic reaction; Sweet's syndrome; injection site reaction; elevated LDH, uric acid and alkaline phosphatase; and reduction in platelet counts. GM-CSF is more frequently associated with symptomatic side effects such as fever, nausea, headache, bone pain, diarrhea, hypotension, thrombosis, injection site reactions, and anorexia, not infrequently necessitating cessation of therapy. Neutralizing antibodies to GM-CSF but not to G-CSF have been reported.

Fligrastim is FDA-approved for protection against chemotherapy-induced neutropenic fever, for reduction in duration of neutropenia and fever following bone marrow transplant, and for use in chronic neutropenia. Sargramostim is approved for enhancement of neutrophil recovery following bone marrow transplant in patients with lymphoid malignancy. Despite the limited basis of FDA approval for these agents, there are data supporting their use in other clinical settings. The data publication has been explosive in speed and volume making adequate interpretation difficult for the practicing oncologist. A set of clinical guidelines as proposed by a panel of experts has been adopted by the American Society of Clinical Oncology and provides a useful summary of clinical trials to date (37,38).

Three prospective, randomized, placebo-controlled trials have shown efficacy for primary G-CSF administration (initiation of G-CSF therapy with the first cycle of chemotherapy) in reducing the incidence of febrile neutropenia by approximately 50% in patients receiving cytotoxic chemotherapy with an expected rate of febrile neutropenia of at least 40% in the control arm (39–41). The use of growth factor resulted in greater dose density of chemotherapy, shorter hospitalization, and decreased usage of antibiotics but did not impact on response rate or overall survival in the study populations, which consisted of patients with small cell lung cancer and non-Hodgkin's lymphoma.

Primary GM-CSF therapy has been studied in five prospectively randomized trials of patients receiving chemotherapy for small cell lung cancer, germ cell carcinoma, or non-Hodgkin's lymphoma. One of these trials reported no benefit to the addition of growth factor in reducing infection or antibiotic use; disease response and survival were not reported (42). The trial by Nichols et al. preliminarily shows fewer infections and less antibiotic use in the growth factor arm after two cycles of chemotherapy (43). The third trial employed GM-CSF in the setting of chemotherapy and radiotherapy for small cell lung cancer. This trial was stopped early because of enhanced toxicity in the GM-CSF arm in terms of thrombocytopenia, anemia, and infections (43). One of the two trials in patients with lymphoma demonstrated less severe neutropenia, decreased neutropenic fever, decreased antibiotic use, and less hospitalization in the subset of patients who were able to tolerate the growth factor (72% of patients) (45). The final study was conducted in HIV-positive patients with non-Hodgkin's lymphoma receiving cyclophosphamide, adriamycin, vincristine and predmisone chemotherapy and showed improvement in neutropenia, neutropenic infection, and length of hospitalization. Again there was no improvement in disease response or overall survival (46).

The use of colony stimulating factors in patients with myeloid malignancies has been approached with some trepidation because of reports that these agents can stimulate leukemic blast proliferation in vitro. Nonetheless, at least five trials of placebo-controlled administration of G-CSF in patients with acute myelogenous leukemia have been conducted, none has shown enhancement of leukemic growth in the treatment arm (47–51). The studies have uniformly demonstrated decreased duration of neutropenia but have been variable in terms of effect on documented infection, hospitalization time, and antibiotic use. A single trial reported enhanced complete response rate (47) but all trials demonstrated equal overall survival. Even more contradictory are results of trials using GM-CSF in the same patient population with divergent reports of both increased median survival and decreased complete response rate in the treatment arms; there was no consistent effect on duration of neutropenia or rate of infection (52–55).

The secondary use of growth factors (administration of growth factor in a patient who has experienced neutropenic fever or dose delay due to prolonged neutropenia on a previous cycle of chemotherapy) has not been studied thoroughly. However, in the Crawford trial noted above (38), patients in the placebo group who experienced febrile neutropenia were crossed over into the growth factor arm with subsequent reduction in the duration of neutropenia and episodes of febrile neutropenia. Utilization of growth factor to prevent recurrent neutropenic fever and to preserve dose density is a common practice despite the limited evidence.

The initiation of growth factor after documentation of neutropenic fever remains a controversial topic. Randomized trails in the nontransplant setting have consistently shown a decrease in the duration of neutropenia by approximately 1 day if either G-CSF or GM-CSF is added at the time of initiation of antibiotic therapy, but this difference has not reached statistical significance in all trials (56–59). However, these trials have failed to document improvement in clinical outcomes such as duration of fever and antibiotics. Effects on length of hospitalization were variable and most likely represent different criteria for hospital discharge among the protocols, although there is a suggestion that growth factors may shorten hospitalization in those patients in whom prolonged neutropenia can be anticipated. Subset analyses did suggest that patients with tissue infection or signs of bacteremia may benefit from CSF treatment in this setting (56).

# THROMBOCYTOPENIA

Thrombocytopenia is a common hematologic disorder in the patient with malignancy and is often multifactorial. In many cases it is the disease itself causing decreased platelet production through marrow infiltration or replacement. Nutritional factors and marrow suppression by drugs or infection are other likely contributors. There are treatment-associated causes of poor platelet production including marrow toxic chemotherapy and irradiation; mitomycin C is associated with the development of hemolytic uremic syndrome. Finally, many malignancies are associated with immune destruction of hematologic cells.

Persistent thrombocytopenia impacts on patient quality of life in a significant manner. In the clinical setting health care providers appropriately focus on avoidance and treatment of life-threatening consequences of thrombocytopenia, including intracerebral or GI hemorrhage. Minor bleeding episodes tend to be viewed as a nuisance and are often minimized in treatment strategies. Patients, however, are plagued by recurrent gingival bleeds, epistaxis, menorrhagia, and more cosmetic issues such as petechiae or excessive bruisibility, all of which can adversely affect social and professional functioning.

Oncologic services are the prime consumers of platelet transfusions in most hospitals. Cancer patients undergoing active treatment or supportive care can be expected to require repeated platelet transfusion support with all the attendant risks and complications. Establishing appropriate guidelines for transfusion, identification of the appropriate product for transfusion, and recognition of alternatives to transfusion is often surprisingly difficult.

## Indications for Platelet Transfusion

Management of thrombocytopenia in the cancer patient has been a controversial area of transfusion medicine in recent years. The majority of literature addressing this issue has focused on the leukemic population and was spearheaded by Gaydos in an oft-cited 1962 publication (60). Prior to the 1960s hemorrhage was the most common cause of death in this population of patients and it became rapidly evident that platelet transfusion could prevent or delay such deaths. Gaydos's study was an observational attempt to define a platelet "threshold" above which patients did not experience significant hemorrhage; in this regard the study was not a success in that the authors drew the conclusion that no threshold was definable. They were able to document that many factors besides thrombocytopenia were important in predicting bleeding risk including fever, rapid fall in platelet count, coagulation defects, trauma, and the presence of "blast crisis." However, the authors made the important observation that the frequency and severity of hemorrhage increased in a non-threshold manner with lower platelet counts; furthermore, they noted that a grossly visible hemorrhage occurred rarely (on <1% of days) with platelet counts above 20,000 per mm$^3$. It was this statement that established the standard practice of transfusing patients prophylactically when platelet counts dipped below 20,000. In fact, further evaluation of the data collected in this study of 92 patients shows that life-threatening hemorrhage was rare at platelet counts between 10,000 and 20,000 but rose sharply below 5000. Furthermore, the effect of aspirin on platelet function was not known until the late 1960s, so that the majority of patients observed during the study period were receiving aspirin on a regular basis for antipyretic and analgesic effect. These issues have led to a recent reevaluation of the role of platelet transfusions in patients with thrombocytopenia resulting from marrow underproduction.

The definition of a "threshold" platelet count remains an elusive goal because the population of patients with malignancy suffers from a number of insults to platelet function and compromise of mucosal boundaries compounding the already depressed numbers of platelets. These abnormalities include fever/infection, excess fibrinolysis, mucositis, and drug use (including nonsteroidal antiinflammatory drugs and semisynthetic penicillins). Several studies have attempted to better define bleeding risk for patients with platelet underproduction and varying degrees of thrombocytopenia. A study examining 20 patients with aplastic anemia and thrombocytopenia for occult fecal blood loss by chromium-labeled RBCs demonstrated that average blood loss was <5 ml/day, 9 ml/day, and >50 ml/day in patients with platelet counts above 10,000, between 5000 and 10,000, or <5000, respectively (61).

The data among solid tumor patients have been less conclusive, with one study showing clinically significant increases in bleeding only when platelet counts fell below 10,000 (62). An alternative conclusion comes from Dutcher who reported that >5% of severe bleeding episodes in patients with solid tumors in his cohort occurred with platelet counts above 20,000 with most of these bleeds originating at the site(s) of tumor (63).

Prospective trials of prophylactic platelet transfusion versus transfusion for specific indications in adults have been undertaken in leukemic patients only. Two randomized trials in the 1970s (64,65) indicated no survival benefit for prophylactic transfusion, although one trial reported decreased "clinically significant" bleeding in the prophylactically transfused population despite no significant difference in platelet count between the two groups. The other trial reported a slight decrease in the number of required RBC transfusions in the prophylactically platelet transfused group.

More recently, a trial assessing the practicality and safety of more stringent guidelines for platelet transfusion was undertaken (66). Transfusion was given for platelets <5000 in all patients except when HLA-matched platelets were unavailable for a patient known to be refractory to random donor platelets. Patients with counts between 5000 and 10,000 received platelets if there were hemorrhagic signs or if the temperature exceeded 38.0°C; platelets between 11,000 and 20,000 mandated transfusion if abnormal coagulation studies were documented or if a minor invasive procedure was planned; patients with platelets >20,000 were transfused to control major bleeding or in anticipation of surgical procedures/arterial punctures. With a total of 6002 patient-days characterized by platelets below 100,000, the authors' recorded 31 major bleeds, 3 of which were fatal. One fatal bleed was in a patient with platelets <1000 who was known to be refractory to random donor transfusion; the other two patients had platelets in excess of 50,000 but had evidence of DIC. Of the 31 significant bleeding episodes, 18 occurred with platelets >10,000 and were associated with other predisposing conditions such as fever, DIC, and/or mucositis. The authors concluded that this strategy of transfusion was not only safe but more cost-effective than a strategy of prophylactic transfusion for platelets <20,000. Furthermore, they felt that the serious bleeding complications would not have been prevented by a more aggressive transfusion protocol because events were infrequent, responsive to clinically directed transfusion, and often occurred in patients with platelets above the more commonly accepted threshold of 20,000.

A NIH Consensus Conference with regard to platelet transfusion was convened in the late 1980s. Interestingly, the committee avoided specific guidelines for the administration of prophylactic platelet transfusion but concluded that more stringent transfusion practices may be appropriate in light of recent data regarding bleeding risks in thrombocytopenic patients (67). Likewise the College of American Pathologists in its recent task force recommendations suggested transfusion for platelets below 5000 but leave open to clinical judgment the use of prophylactic transfusion for patients with platelet counts between 5000 and 30,000 (67).

The most practical approach to the patient with malignancy-associated thrombocytopenia would reflect the strategy suggested by Gmur and by the College of American Pathologists. Patients with platelet counts <5000 should receive prophylactic transfusion but asymptomatic patients with an uncomplicated clinical course are likely to be relatively safe from spontaneous life-threatening bleeds with platelets 5-10,000. The old standard of prophylactic transfusion to maintain platelets above 20,000 should be reserved for patients with other risk factors including fever, infection, elevated blast count, trauma, splenomegaly, precipitous fall in platelets, other coagulopathy, or mucositis. Patients expected to undergo invasive procedure other than simple phlebotomy or bone marrow biopsy are by custom transfused to achieve a platelet count of 50,000, though there are few data to support or refute this approach.

## Platelet Transfusion Refractoriness

Refractoriness to platelet transfusion is a common occurrence in the frequently transfused population with malignancy (20–50% of leukemics) and is even more common in patients receiving chronic transfusions for non malignant conditions (in excess of 80% in patients with aplastic anemia). A patient is usually considered refractory if the 1-hour posttransfusion platelet count increases by $<5 \times 10^9/L$. Although a patient showing a platelet increment less than this stated value is often assumed to be alloimmunized against HLA antigens, it is important to realize that there may be factors inherent in the platelet product or clinical circumstances that are contributing to or accounting for the suboptimal transfusion response. In addition, there are immune mechanisms other than HLA alloimmunization that are active in these circumstances. Important blood banking issues include the fact that platelets have a relatively short storage life (5 days) and must be maintained at room temperature with constant agitation; furthermore, recovery of platelets from a single random donor unit of whole blood is variable. Clinical circumstances affecting in vivo platelet survival are outlined above.

Immune mechanisms of platelet destruction are varied and include drug-mediated antiplatelet antibody production as well as idiopathic direct antiplatelet antibodies common in patients with hematologic malignancy. Transfusion-specific immunologically mediated platelet destruction may be related to ABO incompatibility as it has been shown that donors have varying degrees of ABH expression on platelets (69) and that transfusion of ABO-matched products may enhance posttransfusion counts (70). A small but important group of transfusion refractory patients are those without clinical circumstances expected to adversely affect platelet survival who have no discernible HLA alloimmunization. This population is likely to have developed antibodies to platelet-specific antigens and may benefit from platelet cross-matching.

Those patients whose refractory status is not accounted for by one of the above-noted processes has likely developed anti-HLA antibodies. The mechanism of HLA alloimmunization is not completely clear but most believe that it does not represent a response against transfused platelets alone as they do not carry class II major histocompatibility antigens necessary for recognition and processing of other antigens. The process is felt to require MHC class II antigens on cotransfused WBCs in order to generate an antibody capable of destroying both platelets and WBCs via recognition of class I antigens. Furthermore, it seems that these antigens must be present on intact, viable lymphocytes as the transfusion of WBC membrane fragments is inadequate to generate a response. It is felt that at least $10^3$ contaminating leukocytes are necessary to result in alloimmunization. Because the development of anti-HLA antibodies has been described after transfusion of platelets devoid of WBCs, it has been postulated that a less efficient mechanism of immunogenesis may directly result from the class I antigens present on platelets but conclusive evidence is lacking. The development of an anti-HLA response takes on the order of 10 days to 3 weeks such that a more rapid development of refractoriness should prompt an investigation of alternative explanations.

The presence of HLA antigens as well as the strength of this antibody response can be assayed by an in vitro complement-dependent microlymphocytotoxicity panel in which the patients serum is reacted against a wide panel of lymphocytes with determination of the percent of samples showing cytotoxicity. The strength of a positive reaction is graded by the percentage of lymphocytes killed in the sample. By convention a sample with 10–20% kill is considered positive. However, this test is cumbersome, time consuming, and expensive; an alternative means of predicting HLA alloimmunization would be of more clinical utility. It has been shown repeatedly that platelets destroyed by alloantibodies or splenomegaly are destroyed more rapidly than those destroyed by other mechanism such as drug-mediated antibody destruction, infection, DIC, etc. It has been suggested by several authors that a 1-hour posttransfusion platelet count with suboptimal response is indicative of alloimmunization or

splenomegaly, whereas a more hearty response with subsequent rapid decline (over 18–24 hours) is indicative of an alternate means of platelet loss. This distinction is important in that the appropriate intervention for the alloimmunized patient is the use of HLA-matched platelets, which is an expensive undertaking, whereas the alternate population of patients will not show any better response to HLA-matched as compared to random donor platelets.

It is clear that a large portion of patients with malignancy who are heavily transfused will not become immunized against HLA antigens. In contrast, there are many patients with preexisting HLA alloimmunization from prior pregnancy or transfusion who may display amnestic immune response and therefore seem to develop rapid immunization. It is generally felt that disease- and/or therapy-induced immunosuppression are responsible for the lower incidence of immunization in cancer patients. An alternative theory is the induction of tolerance to HLA antigens in these patients. Many trials have attempted to define risk factors for alloimmunization but the results are disappointingly contradictory. Controversy exists as to whether there is a dose–response curve between number of platelet transfusions and the development of alloimmunization with several studies reporting both positive and negative correlations. None of these studies controls for the number of PRBC transfusions which also carry immunogenic WBCs. The loss of anti-HLA antibodies despite continued transfusion stimulation has been reported and has been associated with the development of antiidiotype antibodies directed against the anti-HLA antibodies. Current standard of care calls for the use of random, pooled platelets followed in turn by the use of single-donor, pheresed platelets; HLA-matched products; family member–donated products; and ultimately cross-matched products. Up to one third of patients repeatedly receiving fully HLA-matched platelets from unrelated donors are unresponsive to these transfusions.

Even with no clear predictors for the development of alloimmunization, trials have been undertaken to attempt to prevent this occurrence. The funding of such trials is in itself controversial since any defined means by which the immune response can be mitigated or eliminated will no doubt be expensive and will be utilized in a large number of patients who would never have developed this complication regardless of intervention. The unanswerable question at this point is whether the cost of preventative measures applied to all patients will outweigh the cost of HLA matched platelets in the population that becomes refractory to transfusion.

Many methods of avoiding alloimmunization have been studied without much success including immunosuppression, IV gamma globulin, plasma exchange and massive platelet transfusion. Still under investigation is the primary use of single-donor pheresed platelets, the use of leukoreduction filters and the UV irradiation of blood products. Each of these methods is an attempt to decease antigenic stimulation with resultant decrease in antibody formation.

The use of single random donor pheresed platelets at the inception of transfusion support has been prospectively compared to the use of random pooled donor platelets in assessing sustained transfusion response. Again, the results are disparate with two studies showing reduced rates of alloimmunization for those receiving single-donor products (71,72) but at least one trial showing no significant difference in the two groups (73). This approach is expensive and of questionable benefit, and thus has not been adopted into general practice.

In the dog model Slichter transfused recipients with single random donor, pooled random donor, DLA-mismatched siblings, DLA-matched siblings, or pooled donor followed by DLA-matched sib once the recipient animal has been sensitized (74). This study showed a longer period of adequate platelet support from random pooled donor than from single random donor platelets (7.4 versus 2.7 transfusions prior to sensitization); however, sequential single random donors was superior to pooled random donors. Single-donor platelets from a matched sibling provided the longest period of support. Interestingly, DLA match did not prevent alloimmunization in all dogs, supporting the theory that other, non-DLA-associated antigens can be mechanisms of immunization. The rate of alloimmunization in dogs receiving only DLA-matched platelets and those receiving DLA matches only when sensitized to random pooled donors was not significantly different implying that the reservation of HLA-matched platelets for those patients who develop refractoriness is not a compromise of care. However, the generalizability of this data to humans remains a valid question.

Leukocyte depletion shows promise as a means of reducing the rates of alloimmunization because it is felt that the primary immune response is mediated against the HLA antigens on WBCs, not on platelets, and that platelets are destroyed by a crossover immune reaction. The literature with regard to the success of this practice is difficult to interpret because leukoreduction filters have evolved over recent years and the varying results of clinical trails may be attributable in large part to varying success in leukoreduction. It is, however, an important issue to resolve as the use of these filters results in a reduction in platelet delivery by approximately 10%. On the other hand, the removal of white cells is helpful in mitigating febrile and allergic transfusion reactions. The success of this approach requires the use of leukoreduction filters for the administration of RBCs as well as platelet transfusions.

The first randomized trial attempting leukoreduction for transfused platelets employed centrifugation techniques (now known to be less effective than filtration). It was not supportive of leukoreduction as a means of reducing alloimmunization, although the negative result may be an issue of statistical power rather than true lack of effect (there was a difference in the rates of alloimmunization of 20% versus 41% in the control versus leukoreduced groups, a difference that did not achieve statistical significance) (75). With more modern techniques of WBC filtration, results have been more promising. Andreu showed a reduction of alloimmunization rate from 31% to 11% in control leukemic patients versus those transfused with leukofiltered platelets and RBCs (76). It is important to note that in this trial leukocyte contamination was reduced to one half of that seen it the above-noted centrifugation trial. This approach has the advantage of simplicity and wide availability via almost any blood bank.

Several groups have shown that UV irradiation prevents peripheral blood lymphocytes from stimulating or responding in a mixed lymphocyte reaction. The mechanism for this phenomenon remains obscure with main theories being the shedding of MHC antigens upon exposure to UV light versus a qualitative effect on MHC antigen presentation. Since transfusion is essentially an in vivo mixed lymphocyte reaction the approach of UV irradiation of transfused products has been postulated either alone or as an adjunct to leukofiltration as a means of decreasing the rate of sensitization. Indeed, this approach has been successful in enhancing the rate of marrow engraftment in dogs who were first transfused with irradiated whole blood and subsequently received bone marrow transplants from the donor of these blood products. The major concerns in applying this approach to humans have been that the irradiation may inactivate or shorten survival time for platelets and that it is difficult to deliver a homogeneous radiation dose to a bag of platelets due to issues of radiation penetration through the bag and the blood product.

Despite the promise of the above data there are two recently published trials that fail to show benefit to irradiated platelets in terms of the development of HLA antibodies. The first trial was performed in cardiac patients who were randomized to irradiated or nonirradiated platelets perioperatively during cardiopulmonary bypass (77). All patients received leukofiltered PRBCs; the rates of HLA antibody detection were not significantly different between the groups but may be a reflection of the short duration of platelet support. Similarly, Blundell examined the impact of platelet irradiation in patients with hematologic malignancy in a randomized fashion (78). Posttransfusion increments were similar in the two groups as was the need for PRBC and platelet transfusion; the rate of HLA antibody formation was 13% in the irradiation group and 25% in the control group, a difference not reaching statistical significance. There was no difference in clinically evident platelet refractoriness in the two groups; it should be noted that the study may have been underpowered with only 50 patients. Currently the data do not support the role of irradiation of blood products in an effort to decrease rates of alloimmunization.

## Alternatives to Platelet Transfusion

The provision of platelet transfusion support for patients with malignancy is fraught with complications such as transfusion reaction, infection, and transfusion refractoriness; therefore it is logical to pursue alternatives to platelet transfusion. At the current point in time this research has taken two main directions, specifically the search for a safe and effective platelet growth factor and the search for synthetic platelet substitutes.

## Thrombopoietin

For almost 40 decades the research community has sought the identification of a humoral substance capable of inducing megakaryocyte development and the generation of active platelets. Of course, this search has been augmented by the success of granulocyte growth factors in diminishing neutropenia and its complications. Several investigators reported on the ability of the serum of thrombocytopenic animals to induce thrombocytosis in recipients and much effort was focused in the 1980s on the recovery of the responsible substance from blood, urine, and conditioned culture media. In 1990 a murine retrovirus was discovered that induced a myeloproliferative disease in mice (79). The virus was cloned and the transforming gene was identified as v-mpl. A homologous gene was cloned from a human erythroleukemia line and called c-mpl (79); the gene sequence for this receptor had distinct characteristics shared with known cytokines and growth factors. Almost simultaneously the ligand was identified and cloned by four different research groups and has since entered preclinical and, now, clinical trials.

The newly discovered growth factor has been referred to by several names with the most common being megakaryocte growth and development factor (MGDF) and thrombopoietin (TPO). The gene has been mapped to the long arm of chromosome 3 and codes for five exons. The mRNA is located primarily in liver, kidney, spleen, and marrow. Levels of this cytokine are known to vary inversely with platelet count but it is not clear whether this is due to feedback regulated production of mRNA or the rate of receptor-mediated uptake. The c-mpl ligand has been shown to increase megakaryocyte number and ploidy, increase mean platelet volume, alter megakaryocyte expression of platelet-specific membrane proteins (increase Gp Ib, IIb, and IIIa expression), and induce maturation of the megakaryocytes ultrastructure. Platelets released from these megakaryocytes have normal function. Knockout mice for either c-mpl loss or c-mpl ligand loss have shown circulating platelet counts approximately 15% of normal but have not been lethal mutations, thus raising the question of whether this growth factor is absolutely necessary to platelet production or alternately represents the most efficient mechanism of production (80,81).

As was the case with G-CSF and GM-CSF there has been theoretical concern for a positive growth effect of TPO on abnormal marrow cells including leukemic cells. At least one study showing enhanced proliferation of AML cells in culture (regardless of FAB classification) has been published and will require further investigation (83).

Animal studies employing mice and subhuman primates pretreated with chemotherapy and radiation followed by thrombopoietin or vehicle alone have shown decreased mortality, higher platelet nadirs, and shortened time to platelet recovery in the drug-treated groups. Platelet counts begin to rise 3 days after administration and reach a peak by day 9; no effect on WBC count or hematocrit has been noted. Recombinant human megakaryocyte growth and development factor (rHuMGDF) has recently entered clinical trials in patients with malignancy with initial reports showing promise. Fanucchi et al. have done a randomized phase I dose escalation trial of pegylated rHuMGDF in patients with advanced non–small cell lung cancer receiving carboplatin and paclitaxel. This trial has shown a reduction in severity and duration of platelet nadir counts in patients receiving drug as compared to controls with two thrombotic complications in the treatment arm (not statistically different from controls). This effect was shown over broad ranges of dose and duration of therapy (84).

## Other Thrombopoietic Agents

Many other cytokines have been investigated for their role in platelet production and maturation, most notably IL-3, IL-6, and IL-11. It appears that IL-3 exerts its main effect early in the development of megakaryoctes but that it is not sufficient alone to produce normal, functional platelets. IL-6 and IL-11 have more of an effect of enhancing platelet maturation and release. It seems likely that the above-mentioned knockout mice produce what few platelets they can via a pathway involving these interleukins in combination. Trials of IL-6 have shown limited clinical benefit, but initial studies of IL-11 have suggested a 26% reduction in platelet transfusions in cancer chemotherapy patients (85). Randomized clinical trials with IL-11 continue to try to define the efficacy and safety of IL-11 in a larger population.

## Platelet Substitutes

Refractoriness to platelet transfusion, cost of transfusion, and infection risk have been driving a search for an effective platelet substitute. Unfortunately, the complex physiology of functional platelets has made this endeavor exceedingly difficult. Recently, liposome-based "platelet-somes" have been manufactured and consist of a unil-amellar vesicle containing many specific platelet glyco-proteins. In animal studies these products have shown promise in decreasing bleeding after acute injury to the thrombocytopenic or thrombocytopathic mouse; how-ever, difficulties with adequate delivery of the platelet-some and mechanistic uncertainties will require further investigation and refinement (86). Phase I trials have begun in humans but are too immature for comment at this time.

## COMPLICATIONS OF BLOOD TRANSFUSION

### Infectious Complications

#### Bacterial Contamination

Bacterial infection accounts for approximately 15% of reported transfusion-related mortality despite the fact that it is felt to be underrecognized (29 deaths reported to the FDA between 1986 and 1991). Bacterial contamina-tion of blood products occurs most commonly at the time of collection either from inadequate cleansing of the venipuncture site or from asymptomatic bacteremia in the donor. Both red cell and platelet transfusions have resulted in sepsis, although the incidence is much higher with platelet products, especially pooled donor units. Platelet units are usually contaminated by skin sapro-phytes that grow well at room temperature as platelets are stored at ambient temperature. This infectious risk is the main reason that platelet storage life is limited to 5 days. RBC products are usually contaminated by organisms that can survive the cold temperatures at which these products are stored, specifically *Yersinia, Serratia, Pseudomonas* and *Enterobacter* species.

The prominent clinical manifestation of transfusion-related bacterial sepsis is fever which can occur shortly after the initiation of transfusion secondary to accumulated endotoxin, or sepsis may become manifest several hours after completion of transfusion when it is often not attrib-uted to the transfusion by the treating clinician. In some instances hypotension and shock may also be present.

Prevention of bacterial contamination of blood prod-ucts has been aimed mainly at improved collection sys-tems and better sterile technique. Somewhat counterintu-itively, prestorage leukocyte depletion has been shown to decrease the rate of *Yersinia* contamination in RBC prod-ucts (but not consistently for platelets). The greatest reduction in culture positivity of the units occurs when leukocyte depletion is done between 2 and 12 hours post collection and likely results from removal of WBCs that have engulfed the bacteria as well as from direct bacter-ial adhesion to the filter. Thermal inactivation of bacteria is not possible with cellular blood products. UV light, γ-irradiation, and laser inactivation with or without sensi-tizing compounds are limited to products that are nonopaque and are not generally employed because of the theoretical risk of mutagenicity or compromise of cellu-lar function.

### Viral Infection

The safety of the U.S. blood supply has improved over recent years such that the risk of transmission of a serious viral pathogen is approximately 29 per million units (87), yet fear of this complication is often the greatest concern of blood product recipients. Failure to detect the presence of virus in the contaminated units is largely the result of donation and testing during the "window period" shortly after the donor has acquired the infection and before sero-logic conversion.

The screening of blood products for the presence of human immunodeficiency virus–1 (HIV-1) antibodies began in the United States in 1985; in 1992 antibody test-ing for HIV-2 was also applied routinely. More recently, since March 1996, products have been screened for the presence of HIV-1 p24 antigen with a consequent decrease in the duration of the window period from 55 days in 1985 to 16 days in 1996. The current estimated risk of transmission of HIV via blood product transfusion is estimated to be <1 in 493,000 (87).

Infection with human t-cell lymphotrophic virus (HTLV-1) is associated with the clinical syndromes of adult T-cell leukemia/lymphoma and tropical spastic paraparesis. There is no clear clinical disease imparted by infection with HTLV-2 virus but there is suggestion of a neurologic condition similar to that of HTLV-1-infected persons. Transfusion-related tropical spastic paraparesis has been described with an incubation period of approximately 3 years. Recipient seroconversion following transfusion of a cellular blood component seropositive for HTLV is approximately 40% and is diminished with increasing age of the transfused component. Assays for the presence of envelope proteins common to the two viruses are used to detect contaminated units with an estimated risk of trans-mission of approximately 1 in 641,000 (87).

Hepatitis B infection becomes chronic in approxi-mately 10% of infected persons, usually with no symp-toms. A percentage of these asymptomatic carriers have undetectable levels of hepatitis B surface antigen (HBsAg) and anti-hepatitis B core antigen (anti-HBc) such that their donated units will escape detection with an estimated risk of posttransfusion hepatitis B of approxi-mately 1 in 63,000 (87). It is possible that this represents an overestimate and that many of these infections are acquired independently of the transfusion given the high seroconversion rate in the general public.

Hepatitis C virus was first characterized molecularly in 1989; current immunoassays are directed against various viral epitopes resulting in a 70-day window for detectability. During this time period some units are excluded from transfusion on the basis of elevated alarine aminotransferase (ALT) levels, which rise approximately 2 weeks before one becomes seropositive. However, ALT measurement is no longer required by the FDA (since the development of enzyme immunoassays for hepatitis C) and many blood banks do not perform this laboratory. Transfusion with an infected unit of blood results in a 90% seroconversion rate with at least 65% of patients developing chronic infection. In one study, clinical evidence of liver failure was present in 18% of patients 16 years after transfusion-related seroconversion (88). A current estimate for the risk of transmission with transfusion is 1 in 103,000 (87).

Many other clinical infections have been related to blood transfusion including common pathogens such as Epstein-Barr virus and parvovirus as well as rarer illnesses including Chagas's disease, Creutzfeldt-Jakob disease, malaria, babesiosis, and syphilis. Fortunately, the transfusion-related incidence of these diseases is uncommon. CMV deserves special note because of the high seroprevalence in the United States (35–80% varying by region) and the potentially devastating effects on the immunosuppressed host who acquires the infection. CMV is a leukocyte-associated virus; thus any blood product contaminated with WBCs is capable of transmitting infection. Several studies have shown decreased rates of CMV infection in patients receiving leukodepleted blood products but prospective trials comparing leukocyte reduced versus CMV seronegative transfusions are limited. Thus CMV negative donors are still used as the standard of care for those patients in whom CMV infection could be devastating including seronegative bone marrow transplant patients.

## Noninfectious Complications

### Febrile Nonhemolytic Transfusion Reactions

Febrile nonhemolytic transfusion reactions (FNHTRs) have been associated with approximately 30% of platelet transfusions and 7% of PRBC transfusions. FNHTRs are defined by a temperature elevation of at least 1°C during transfusion with no other discernible cause for fever; occasionally such reactions are accompanied by chills and hypertension. Cytokine release from leukocytes during product storage is felt to be one of the mechanisms for this reaction, a theory that is supported by the fact that the age of the transfused product is the best predictor of an FNHTR. Increasing concentrations of IL-1, TNF, IL-6, and IL-8 with increasing storage time of the product have been reported (89); furthermore, prestorage leukoreduction prevents accumulation of these cytokines. The

efficacy of prestorage leukodepletion in preventing clinical reactions has not yet been explored. Alternately, reactions may result from recipient antibodies directed against donor WBCs or platelets with resultant complement activation and release of cytokines from both donor and recipient leukocytes. FNHTRs are most common in multiply transfused persons and in multiparous women. Both of these populations have an increased incidence of HLA alloimmunization, lending credence to the proposed physiologic mechanism. The final common pathway of both proposed mechanisms is of IL-2 production in turn stimulating prostaglandin $E_2$ release, which acts directly on the hypothalamus to induce fever. Many patients display repeated reactions and are likely alloimmunized against HLA antigens which are common in the donor population. Treatment involves at least temporary discontinuation of the transfusion while an evaluation is undertaken to exclude hemolytic reaction. Administration of acetaminophen is usually adequate antipyresis, and patients with a history of repeated febrile reactions may benefit from prophylactic acetaminophen prior to transfusion.

### Allergic Transfusion Reaction

Allergic transfusion reactions are felt to be mediated by recipient antibodies to foreign plasma proteins, drugs, or food products of donor origin in the transfused product. The transfused antigen binds to IgE on mast cells resulting in their degranulation with histamine release and leukotriene production. The clinical syndrome of allergic transfusion reaction occurs after approximately 2% of transfusions and is variable in severity ranging from a pruritic urticarial reaction to fulminant anaphylaxis. The best documented variety of allergic reaction occurs in IgA-deficient patients with naturally occurring IgG anti-IgA antibodies. Such a reaction occurs in 1 in 20,000–30,000 patients and causes complement activation with subsequent mast cell degranulation. True anaphylactic reaction is not uncommon in this situation. These patients should be given blood products from IgA-deficient donors for all future transfusions. Patients without IgA deficiency who display repeated, severe allergic reactions after transfusion may benefit from washed products in an effort to minimize exposure to plasma proteins; however, this process results in loss of 20–30% of platelets and is expensive warranting discretion in its use. For repeated mild allergic reactions, prophylactic antihistamines are adequate therapy.

### Transfusion-Related Acute Lung Injury

Acute pulmonary insufficiency is a rare (<1%) but potentially fatal complication of the transfusion of plasma-containing products. The purported mechanism of this phenomenon is the transfusion of donor antibodies (anti-HLA and neutrophil-specific antibodies have been identified) against recipient WBCs with agglutination of the recipient leukocytes and trapping of these aggregates in the lungs. The release of proteases and complement activation cause pulmonary damage and capillary leak with resultant noncardiogenic pulmonary edema. Multiparous and previously transfused donors are the most common sources for units that result in such reactions. No prospective trials of treatment have been undertaken owing to the rarity of this reaction but the use of steroids and aggressive respiratory support is the accepted standard. Recovery is usually rapid and complete. Because the antibody is felt to be of donor origin the recurrence of this syndrome in any one patient is unlikely and requires no specific prophylactic intervention. However, there are some investigators who believe that recipient antibody against donor leukocytes may occasionally be the cause of this process; in this case the risk for recurrence depends on the frequency of the particular antigen in the donor population.

### Graft vs. Host Disease

Transfusion associated graft vs. host disease (GVHD) is a result of the transfusion of immunocompetent lymphocytes into an immunodeficient host (incapable of destroying transfused WBCs) with subsequent engraftment of the donor lymphocytes. The newly engrafted cells then recognize the host as foreign and mount an immunologic response against host tissues. Resultant clinical symptoms and signs include fever, diffuse maculopapular rash, jaundice, alopecia, vomiting, diarrhea, bone marrow hypoplasia, and pancytopenia. Karyotype analysis may demonstrate different populations among the circulating lymphocytes and host tissues. Whole-blood, PRBC, granulocyte, platelet, and fresh plasma transfusions have all resulted in GVHD. Onset after transfusion is rapid (median 8 days) and often fatal. The potential for GVHD is enhanced when a donor is homozygous for an HLA haplotype for which the recipient is heterozygous. In this situation the recipient is unable to recognize the transfused cells as foreign and the resulting tolerance enhances the likelihood of donor engraftment. The chance that a random homozygous donor product will be transfused to a haploidentical patient is estimated to be 1 in 500 but this risk is increased if a family member serves as directed donor. The overall estimated risk of transfusion associated GVHD is 0.1%. Leukocyte reduction is inadequate prevention of GVHD in the immunocompromised host and therapy is uniformly disappointing with a >90% mortality. Gamma irradiation (25 Gy) prior to transfusion is effective prophylaxis but the risk for this complication must be recognized so that appropriate patients will receive such units. Gamma irradiation causes single-strand breaks in DNA via the liberation of hydroxyl free radicals as well as the disruption of peptide bonds and disulfide bridge formation. Lymphocytes are

thus rendered incapable of blast transformation and replication. The irradiation of RBCs results in membrane damage that is subsequently repaired; however, with prolonged storage post irradiation the RBC recovery is decreased. Irradiated platelet recovery may also be diminished slightly and there is some concern that irradiated platelets are less effective at compensating for aspirin-related defects in the transfused patient.

## SUMMARY

The evolution of hematologic support of the cancer patient has been dramatic in the last decade with refinement of transfusion products and practice and by the advent of hematologic growth factors. Randomized trials have clearly demonstrated beneficial effects of erythropoietin in reducing red cell transfusions and of colony-stimulating factors in reducing the morbidity of neutropenia. Preliminary trials of thrombopoietin/MGDF suggest that reduction in platelet transfusions may also be possible. The task now is to increase our understanding of these powerful biological agents and optimize their use by carefully designed clinical investigation.

## REFERENCES

1. Brain MC, Azzapardi JG, Baker LR, Pineo GF, Roberts PD, Dacie JV. Microangiopathic haemolytic anemia and mucin forming adenocarcinoma. *Br J Haematol* 1970;18(2):183–193.
2. Gleeson C, Spencer D. Blood transfusion and its benefits in palliative care. *Palliat Med* 1995;9:307–313.
3. Davenport RD, Streiter RM, Kunkel SL. Red cell ABO incompatibility and production of tumour necrosis factor-alpha. *Br J Haematol* 1991; 78:540–544.
4. Butler J, Parker D, Pillai R, Shale DJ, Rocker GM. Systemic release of neutrophil elastase and tumour necrosis factor alpha following ABO incompatible blood transfusion. *Br J Haematol* 1991;79(3):525–526.
5. Opelz G, Sengar DP, Mickey MR, Terasaki PI. Effect of blood transfusions on subsequent kidney transplants. *Transplant Proc* 1973;5: 253–259.
6. Chung M, Steinmetz OK, Gordon PH. Perioperative blood transfusion and outcome after resection for colorectal carcinoma. *Br J Surg* 1993; 80:427–432.
7. Vamvakas E, Moore SB. Perioperative blood transfusion and colorectal cancer recurrence: a qualitative statistical overview and meta-analysis. *Transfusion* 1993;33(9):754–765.
8. Vamvakas EC. Perioperative blood transfusion and cancer recurrence: meta-analysis for explanation. *Transfusion* 1993;35(9):760–768.
9. Busch ORC, Hop WCJ, Hoynck van Papendrecht MAW, Marquet RL, Jeekel J. Blood transfusions and prognosis in colorectal cancer. *N Engl J Med* 1993;328(19):1372–1376.
10. Houbiers JGA, Brand A, van de Watering LMG, Hermans J, Verwey PJM, Bijnen AB, Pahlplatz P, Eiftinck Schattenkerk M, Wobbes T, de Vries JE, Klementschitsch P, van de Maas AHM, van de Velde CJH. Randomised controlled trial comparing transfusion of leukocyte-depleted or buffy-coat-depleted blood in surgery for colorectal cancer. *Lancet* 1994;344:573–578.
11. Heiss MM, Mempel W, Jauch KW, Delanoff C, Mayer G, Mempel M, Eissner HJ, Schildberg FW. Beneficial effect of autologous blood transfusion on infectious complications after colorectal cancer surgery. *Lancet* 1993;342(27):1328–1333.
12. Jensen LS, Anderson AJ, Christiansen PM, Hokland P, Juhl CO, Madsen G, Mortensen J, Moller-Nielsen C, Hanberg-Sorensen F, Hokland M. Postoperative infection and natural killer cell function following

blood transfusion in patients undergoing elective colorectal surgery. *Br J Surg* 1992;79(6):513–516.

13. Blajchman MA, Bardossy L, Carmen R, Sastry A, Singal DP. Allogeneic blood transfusion-induced enhancement of tumor growth: two animal models showing amelioration by leukodepletion and passive transfer using spleen cells. *Blood* 1993;81(7):1880–1882.

14. Blumberg N, Heal J. Immunomodulation by blood transfusion: an evolving scientific and clinical challenge. *Am J Med* 1996;101:299–308.

15. James RD, Wilkinson PM, Belli F, Welch R, Cowan R. Recombinant human eryhtropoietin in patients with ovarian carcinoma and anaemia secondary to cisplatin and carboplatin chemotherapy: preliminary results. *Acta Haematol* 1992;87(Suppl 1):12–15.

16. Abels RI. Use of recombinant human erythropoietin in the treatment of anemia in patients who have cancer. *Semin Oncol* 1992;19(3 Suppl 8):29–35.

17. Henry DH, Abels RI. Recombinant human erythropoietin in the treatment of cancer and chemotherapy-induced anemia: results of a double-blind and open-label follow-up studies. *Semin Oncol* 1994;21(2 Suppl 3):21–28.

18. deCampos E, Radford J, Steward W, Milroy R, Dougal M, Swindell R, Testa N, Thatcher N. Clinical and in vitro effects of recombinant human erythropoietin in patients receiving intensive chemotherapy for small-cell lung cancer. *J Clin Oncol* 1995;13(7):1623–1631.

19. Lavey RS, Dempsey WH. Erythropoietin increases hemoglobin in cancer patients during radiation therapy. *Int J Radiat Oncol Biol Phys* 1993;27(5):1147–1152.

20. Vijayakumar S, Roach M, Wara W, Chan SK, Ewing C, Rubin S, Sutton H, Halpern H, Awan A, Houghton A, et al. Effect of subcutaneous recombinant human eryhtropoietin in cancer patients receiving radiotherapy: preliminary results of a randomized open-labeled, phase II trial. *Int J Radiat Oncol Biol Phys* 1993;26:721–729.

21. Leitgeb C, Pecherstorfer M, Fritz E, Ludwig H. Quality of life in chronic anemia of cancer during treatment with recombinant human erythropoietin. *Cancer* 1994;73(10):2535–2542.

22. Ludwig H, Fritz E, Leitgeb C, Pecherstorfer M, Samonigg H, Schuster J. Prediction of response to erythropoietin treatment in chronic anemia of cancer. *Blood* 1994;84(4):1056–1063.

23. Glaspy J, Bukowski R, Steinberg D, Taylor C, Tchekmedyian S, Vadhan-Raj S. Impact of therapy with Epoetin Alfa on clinical outcomes in patients with nonmyeloid malignancies during cancer chemotherapy in community oncology practice. *J Clin Oncol* 1997;15:1218–1234.

24. Strauss RG, Connett JE, Gale RP, Bloomfield CD, Herzig GP, McCullough J, Maguire LC, Winston DJ, Ho W, Stump DC, Miller WV, Koepke JA. A controlled trial of prophylactic granulocyte transfusions during initial induction chemotherapy for acute myelogenous leukemia. *N Engl J Med* 1981;305(11):597–603.

25. Winston DJ, Ho WG, Gale RP. Prophylactic granulocyte transfusions during chemotherapy of acute nonlymphocytic leukemia. *Ann Intern Med* 1981;94:616–622.

26. Ford JM, Cullen MH, Roberts MM, Brown LM, Oliver RTD, Lister TA. Prophylactic granulocyte transfusions: results of a randomized controlled trial in patients with acute myelogenous leukemia. *Transfusion* 1982;22:311–316.

27. Vogler WR, Winton EF. A controlled study of the efficacy of granulocyte transfusions in patients with neutropenia. *Am J Med* 1977;63:548–555.

28. Herzig RH, Herzig GP, Graw RG, Bull MI, Ray KK. Successful granulocyte transfusion therapy for gram negative septicemia. *N Engl J Med* 1977;296(13):701–705.

29. Higby DJ, Yates JW, Henderson ES, Holland JF. Filtration leukapheresis for granulocyte transfusion therapy. Clinical and laboratory studies. *N Engl J Med* 1975;292(15):761–766.

30. Graw RG, Herzig G, Perry S, Henderson ES. Normal granulocyte transfusion therapy: treatment of septicemia due to gram-negative bacteria. *N Engl J Med* 1972;287(8):367–371.

31. Alavi JB, Root RK, Djerassi I, Evans AE, Gluckman SJ, MacGregor RR, Guerry D, Schreiber AD, Shaw JM, Kpoch P, Cooper RA. A randomized clinical trial of granulocyte transfusions for infection in acute leukemia. *N Engl J Med* 1977;296(13):706–711.

32. Fortuny IE, Bloomfield CD, Hadlock DC, Goldman A, Kennedy BJ, McCullough JJ. Granulocyte transfusion: a controlled study in patients with acute nonlymphocytic leukemia. *Transfusion* 1975;15(6):548–558.

33. Winston DJ, Ho WG, Gale RP. Therapeutic granulocyte transfusions for documented infections. A controlled trial in ninety-five infectious granulocytopenic episodes. *Ann Intern Med* 1982;97(4):509–515.

34. Dutcher JP, Schiffer CA, Johnston GS. Rapid migration of 111indium-labeled granulocytes to sites of infection. *N Engl J Med* 1981;304(10):586–589.

35. Dutcher JP, Schiffer CA, Johnston GS, Papenburg D, Daly PA, Aisner J, Wiernik PH. Alloimmunization prevents the migration of transfused indium-111-labeled granulocytes to sites of infection. *Blood* 1983;62(2):354–360.

36. Schiffer CA, Aisner J, Daly PA, Schimpff SC, Wiernik PH. Alloimmunization following prophylactic granulocyte transfusion. *Blood* 1979;54(4):766–774.

37. ASCO Ad Hoc Colony-Stimulating Factor Guidelines Expert Panel. American Society of Clinical Oncology Recommendations for the Use of Hematopoietic Colony-Stimulating Factors: evidence based, clinical practice guidelines. *J Clin Oncol* 1994;12(11):2471–2508.

38. ASCO Ad Hoc Colony-Stimulating Factor Guidelines Expert Panel. Update of recommendations for the use of hematopoietic colony-stimulating factors: evidence-based clinical practice guidelines. *J Clin Oncol* 1996;14(6):1957–1960.

39. Crawford J, Ozer H, Stoller R, Johnson D, Lyman G, Tabbara I, Kris M, Grous J, Picozzi V, Rausch G, Smith R, Gradishar W, Yahanda A, Vincent M, Stewart M, Glaspy J. Reduction by granulocyte colony-stimulating factor of fever and neutropenia induced by chemotherapy in patients with small-cell lung cancer. *N Engl J Med* 1991;325(3):164–170.

40. Trillet-Lenoir V, Green J, Manegold C, Von Pawel J, Gatzemeier U, Lebeau B, Depierre A, Johnson P, Decoster G, Tomita D. Recombinant granulocyte colony stimulating factor reduces the infectious complications of cytotoxic chemotherapy. *Eur J Cancer* 1993;29A(3):319–324.

41. Pettengell R, Gurney H, Radford JA, Deakin DP, James R, Wilkinson PM, Kane K, Bentley J, Crowther D. Granulocyte colony-stimulating factor to prevent dose-limiting neutropenia in non-Hodgkin's lymphoma: a randomized controlled trial. *Blood* 1992;80(6):1430–1436.

42. Hamm JT, Schiller JH, Oken MM, Gallmeier WM, Rusthoven J, Israel RJ. Granulocyte-macrophage colony-stimulating factor (GM-CSF) in small cell carcinoma of the lung (SCCL): preliminary analysis of a randomized controlled trial. *Proc Am Soc Clin Oncol* 1991;10:255 (Abstr).

43. Nichols C, Bajorin D, Schmoll HJ, Pizzocaro G, Bosl GJ, Einhorn LH, Israel RJ. VIP chemotherapy with/without GM-CSF for poor risk, relapsed, or refractory germ cell tumors (GCT): preliminary analysis of a randomized controlled trial. *Proc Am Soc Clin Oncol* 1991;10:167 (Abstr).

44. Bunn PA, Crowley J, Hazuka M, Tolley R, Livingston R. The role of GM-CSF in limited stage SCLC: a randomized phase III trial of the Southwest Oncology Group (SWOG). *Proc Am Soc Clin Oncol* 1992;11:292 (Abstr).

45. Gerhartz HH, Engelhard M, Meusers P, Brittinger G, Wilmanns W, Schlimok G, Mueller P, Huhn D, Musch R, Siegert W, Gerhartz D, Hartlapp JH, Eckhard T, Huber C, Peschl C, Spann W, Emmerich B, Schadek C, Westerhausen M, Pees HW, Radtke H, Engert A, Terhardt E, Schick H, Binder T, Fuchs R, Hasford J, Brandmaier R, Stern A, Jones T, Ehrlich HJ, Stein H, Parwaresch M, Tiemann M, Lennert K. Randomized, double-blind, placebo-controlled, phase III study of recombinant human granulocyte-macrophage colony-stimulating factor as adjunct to induction treatment of high-grade malignant non-Hodgkin's lymphomas. *Blood* 1993;82(8):2329–2339.

46. Kaplan LD, Kahn JO, Crowe S, Northfelt D, Neville P, Grossberg H, Abrams DI, Tracey J, Mills J, Volberding PA. Clinical and virologic effects of recombinant human granulocyte-macrophage colony-stimulating factor in patients receiving chemotherapy for human immunodeficiency virus associated non-Hodgkin's lymphoma: results of a randomized trial. *J Clin Oncol* 1991;9(6):929–940.

47. Dombret H, Chastang C, Fenaux P, Reiffers J, Bordesoule D, Bouabdalla R, Mandelli F, Ferrant A, Auzanneau G, Tilly H, Yver A, Degos L. A controlled study of recombinant human granulocyte colony-stimulating factor in elderly patients after treatment for acute myelogenous leukemia. *N Engl J Med* 1995;332(25):1678–1683.

48. Ohno R, Tomanaga M, Tohru K, Kanamura A, Shirakawa S, Masaoka T, Omine M, Oh H, Nomura T, Sakai Y, Hirano M, Yokomaku S, Nakayama S, Yoshida Y, Miura A, Morishima Y, Dohy H, Niho Y, Hamajima N, Takaku F. Effect of granulocyte colony-stimulating factor after intensive induction therapy in relapsed or refractory acute leukemia. *N Engl J Med* 1990;323(13):871–877.

49. Takeshita A, Ohno R, Hirashima K, Toyama K, Okuma M, Saito H, Ikeda Y, Tomonaga M, Asano S. A randomized double-blind controlled study of recombinant human granulocte colony-stimulating factor in

patients with neutropenia induced by consolidation chemotherapy for acute myeloid leukemia. *Jap J Clin Hematol* 1995;36(6):606–614.

50. Heil G, Hoelzer D, Sanz MA, Lechner K, Liu Yin J, Papa G, Noens L, Ho J, O'Brien C, Matchum J, Barge A. Results of a randomized double-blind placebo controlled phase III study of filgrastim in remission induction and early consolidation therapy for adults with de-novo acute myeloid leukemia. *Blood* 1994;86 (Suppl 1):1053 (Abstr).

51. Godwin JE, Kopecky KJ, Head DR, Hynes HE, Balcerak SP, Appelbaum FR. A double-blind placebo controlled trial of G-CSF in elderly patients with previously untreated acute myeloid leukemia. A Southwest Oncology Group Study. *Blood* 1994;86 (Suppl 1):1723 (Abstr).

52. Zittoun R, Suciu S, Mandelli F, de Witte T, Thaler J, Stryckmans P, Hayat M, Peetermans M, Cadiou M, Solbu G, Petti MC, Willemze R. Granulocyte-macrophage colony-stimulating factor associated with induction treatment of acute myelogenous leukemia: a randomized trial by the European Organization for Research and Treatment of Cancer Leukemia Cooperative Group. *J Clin Oncol* 1996;14(7): 2150–2159.

53. Heil G, Chadid L, Hoelzer D, Seipelt G, Mitrou P, Huber C, Kolbe K, Mertelsmann R, Lindemann A, Frisch J, et al. GM-CSF in a double-blind randomized, placebo controlled trial in therapy of adult patients with de novo acute myeloid leukemia (AML). *Leukemia* 1995;9(1): 3–9.

54. Rowe JM, Anderson JW, Mazza JJ, Bennett JM, Paietta F, Hayes FA, Oette D, Cassileth PA, Stadtmauer EA, Wiernik PH. A randomized placebo-controlled phase III study of granulocyte-macrophage colony-stimulating factor in adult patients (>55 to 70 years of age) with acute myelogenous leukemia: a study of the Eastern Cooperative Oncology Group (E1490). *Blood* 1995;86(2):457–462.

55. Stone RM, Berg DT, George SL, Dodge RK, Paciucci TA, Schulman P, Lee EJ, Moore JO, Powell BL, Schiffer CA. Granulocyte-macrophage colony-stimulating factor after initial chemotherapy for elderly patients with primary acute myelogenous leukemia. *N Engl J Med* 1995;332(25):1671–1677.

56. Maher DW, Lieschke GJ, Green M, Bishop J, Stuart-Harris R, Wolf M, Sheridan WP, Kefford RF, Cebon J, Olver I, McKendrick J, Toner G, Bradstock K, Lieschke M, Cruickshank S, Tomita DK, Hoffman EW, Fox RM, Morstyn G. Filgrastim in patients with chemotherapy-induced febrile neutropenia. A double-blind, placebo-controlled trial. *Ann Intern Med* 1994;121:492–501.

57. Mayordoma JI, Rivera F, Diaz-Puente MT, Lianes P, Colomer R, Lopez-Brea M, Lopez E, Paz-Ares L, Hitt R, Garcia-Ribas I, Cubedo R, Alonso S, Cortes-Funes H. Improving treatment of chemotherapy-induced neutropenic fever by administration of colony-stimulating factors. *JNCI* 1995;87(11):803–808.

58. Anaissie EJ, Vartivarian S, Bodey GP, Legrand CL, Kantarjian H, Abi-Said D, Karl C, Vadhan-Raj S. Randomized comparison between antibiotics alone and antibiotics plus granulocyte-macrophage colony-stimulating factor (Escherichia coli-derived) in cancer patients with fever and neutropenia. *Am J Med* 1996;100:17–23.

59. Vallenga E, Uyl-de Groot CA, de Wit R, Keizer HJ, Lowenberg B, ten Haaft MA, de Witte ThJM, Verhagen CAH, Stoter GJ, Rutten FFH, Mulder NH, Smid WM, de Vries EGE. Randomized placebo-controlled trial of granulocyte-macrophage colony-stimulating factor in patients with chemotherapy-related febrile neutropenia. *J Clin Oncol* 1996;14(2):619–627.

60. Gaydos LA, Freireich EJ, Mantel N. The quantitative relation between platelet count and hemorrhage in patients with acute leukemia. *N Engl J Med* 1962;266 (18):905–909.

61. Slichter SJ, Harker LA. Thrombocytopenia: mechanism and management of defects in platelet production. *Clin Hematol* 1978;7:523–539.

62. Belt RJ, Leite C, Haas CD, Stephens RL Incidence of hemorrhagic complication in patients with cancer. *JAMA* 1978;239:2571–2574.

63. Dutcher JP, Schiffer CA, Aisner J, O'Connell BA, Levy C, Kendall JA, Wiernik PH. Incidence of thrombocytopenia and serious hemorrhage among patients with solid tumors. *Cancer* 1984;53:557–562.

64. Higby DJ, Cohen JF, Sinks L. The prophylactic treatment of thrombocytopenic leukemic patients with platelets: a double blind study. *Transfusion* 1974;14(5):440–446.

65. Solomon J, Bofenkamp T, Fahey JL, Chiller RK, Beutel E. Platelet prophylaxis in acute non-lymphoblastic leukemia. *Lancet* 1978; 1(8058):267.

66. Gmur J, Burger J, Schanz U, Fehr J, Schaffner A. Safety of stringent prophylactic platelet transfusion policy for patients with acute leukemia. *Lancet* 1991;338:1223–1226.

67. Platelet Transfusion Therapy Consensus Conference. *JAMA* 1987; 257(13):1777–1780.

68. Fresh Frozen Plasma, Cryoprecipitate and Platelets Administration Practice Guidelines Development Task Force of the College of American Pathologists. Practice parameter for the use of fresh frozen plasma, cryoprecipitate and platelets. *JAMA* 1994;271:777–781.

69. Ogasawara K, Ueki J, Takenaka M, Furihata K. Study on the expression of ABH antigens on platelets. *Blood* 82(3):993–999.

70. Heal JM, Rowe JM, McMican A, Masel D, Finke C, Blumberg N. The role of ABO matching in platelet transfusion. *Eur J Hematol* 1993;50: 110–117.

71. Gmur J, von Felten A, Osterwalder B, Honegger H, Hormann A, Sauter C, Deubelleiss K, Berchtold W, Metaxas M, Scali G, Frick PG. Delayed alloimmunization using random single donor platelet transfusions: a prospective study in thrombocytopenic patients with acute leukemia. *Blood* 1983;62:473–479.

72. Sintnicolaas K, Sizoo W, Haije WG, Abels J, Vriesendorp HM, Stenfert Kroese WF, Hop WC, Lowenberg B. Delayed alloimmunization by random single donor platelet transfusions. A randomized study to compare single donor and multiple donor platelet transfusion in cancer patients with severe thrombocytopenia. *Lancet* 1981;1(8223): 750–754.

73. Murphy MF, Metcalfe P, Thomas H, Eve J, Ord J, Lister TA, Waters AH. Use of leukocyte poor blood components and HLA matched platelet donors to prevent HLA alloimmunization. *Br J Haematol* 1986;62(3):529–534.

74. Slichter SJ, O'Donnell MR, Weiden PL, Storb R, Schroeder ML. Canine platelet alloimmunization: the role of donor selection. *Br J Haematol* 1986;63(4):713–727.

75. Schiffer CA, Dutcher JP, Aisner J, Hogge D, Wiernik PW, Reilly JP. A randomized trial of leukocyte-depleted platelet transfusion to modify alloimmunization in patients with leukemia. *Blood* 1983;64(4): 815–820.

76. Andreu G, Dewailly J, Leberre C, Quarre MC, Bidet ML, Tardivel R, Devers L, Lam Y, Soreau E, Boccaccio C, Piard N, Bidet JM, Genetet B, Fauchet R. Prevention of HLA immunization with leukocyte-poor packed red cells and platelet concentrates obtained by filtration. *Blood* 1988;72(3):964–969.

77. Grijzenhout MA, Aarts-Riemans MI, de Gruijl FR, van Weelden H, van Prooijen HC. UVB irradiation of human platelet concentrates does not prevent HLA alloimmunization in recipients. *Blood* 1994;84 (10):3524–3531.

78. Blundell EL, Pamphilon DH. Fraser ID, Menitove JE, Greenwalt TJ, Snyder EL, Repucci AJ, Hedberg SL, Anderson JK, Buchholz DH, Kagen LR, Aster RH. A prospective, randomized study of the use of platelet concentrates irradiated with ultraviolet-B light in patients with hematologic malignancy. *Transfusion* 1996;36(4):296–302.

79. Wendling F, Varlet P, Charon M, Tambourin P. MPLV: a retrovirus complex inducing an acute myeloproliferative leukemic disorder in adult mice. *Virology* 1986;149(2):242–246.

80. Vigon I, Mornon JP, Cocault L, Mitjavila MT, Tambourin P, Gisselbrecht S, Souyri M. Molecular cloning and characterization of MPL, the human homolog of the v-mpl oncogene: identification of a member of the hematopoietic growth factor receptor superfamily. *Proc Natl Acad Sci USA* 1992;89(12):5640–5644.

81. Gurney AL, Carver-Moore K, de Sauvage FJ, Moore MW. Thrombocytopenia in C-MPL-deficient mice. *Science* 1994;265(5177): 1445–1447.

82. de Sauvage FJ, Carver-Moore K, Luoh SM, Ryan A, Dowd M, Eaton DL, Moore MW. Physiologic regulation of early and late stages of megakaryopoiesis by thrombopoietin. *J Exp Med* 1996;183:651–656.

83. Matsumura I, Kanakura Y, Kato T, Ikeda H, Ishikawa J, Horikawa Y, Hashimoto K, Moriyama Y, Tsujimura T, Nishiura T, Miyazaki H, Matsuzawa Y. Growth response of acute myeloblastic leukemia cells to recombinant human thrombopoietin. *Blood* 1995;86(2):703–709.

84. Fanucchi M, Glaspy J, Crawford J, Garst J, Figlin R, Sheridan W, Menchaca D, Tomita D, Ozer H, Harker L. Effects of pegylated recombinant human megakaryocyte growth and development factor (PEG-rHuMGDF) on platelet counts before and after chemotherapy for carcinoma of the lung. *N Engl J Med* 1997;336:404–409.

85. Tepler I, Elias L, Smith II JW, Hussein M, Rosen G, Chang A Y-C, Moore JO, Gordon MS, Kuca B, Beach KJ, Loewy JW, Garnick MB,

Kaye JA. A randomized placebo controlled trial of recombinant human interleukin-11 in cancer patients with severe thrombocytopenia due to chemotherapy. *Blood* 1996;87(9):3607–3614.

86. Rybak ME, Renzulli LA. A liposome based platelet substitute, the plateletsome, with hemostatic efficacy. *Biomat Artif Cells Immob Biotechnol* 1993;21(2):101–118.

87. Screibner GB, Busch MP, Kleinman SH, Korelitz JJ. The risk of trans-fusion-transmitted viral infections. *N Engl J Med* 1996;334(26):1685–1690.

88. Koretz RL, Abbey H, Coleman E, Gitnick G. Non-A, non-B post-transfusion hepatitis. Looking back in the second decade. *Ann Intern Med* 1993;119(2):110–115.

89. Stack G, Snyder EL. Cytokine generation in stored platelet concen-trates. *Transfusion* 1994;34:20–25.

*Principles and Practice of Supportive Oncology,*
edited by Ann Berger et al.
Lippincott–Raven Publishers, Philadelphia ©1998

# CHAPTER 41

# Nutrition Support

Caroline M. Apovian, Christopher D. Still, and George L. Blackburn

Malignant disease is frequently accompanied by profound weight loss and malnutrition. In fact, cancer patients have the highest prevalence of malnutrition of any hospitalized group of patients (1). In its most severe form, weight loss due to malignancy is termed the "anorexia-cachexia syndrome" and is characterized by anorexia, skeletal muscle atrophy, tissue wasting, and organ dysfunction (2). Malnutrition associated with malignancy is a poor prognostic indicator leading to a higher mortality rate (3) and a higher perioperative morbidity rate (4) in patients who have lost >5% of their body weight and have a reduction in some of the indices of nutritional status. The indications for implementing nutrition support in cancer patients as well as its safety have been established (5–11), although possible benefits of nutritional therapy are still contentious. This chapter will address the following questions: What is the effect of nutritional support on the outcomes of cancer patients undergoing various treatment modalities? What is the role of nutritional support in the treatment of cytokine-mediated cancer anorexia and altered host metabolism? Are there specific nutritional supplements that take on a pharmacologic role by modulating tumor cell growth? Finally, is preservation of quality of life by reduction of fatigue and other effects of malnutrition an adequate outcome of adjuvant nutritional therapy?

Because of the ongoing controversies associated with these issues and ethical issues regarding nonvolitional feeding guidelines, nutritional support of the cancer patient should be emphasized in the clinical setting.

C. M. Apovian: Spence Center for Women's Health, Braintree, MA 02184.

C. D. Still: Department of Internal Medicine, Geisinger Medical Center, Danville, PA 17822.

G. L. Blackburn: Department of Surgery, Nutrition Support Service, Harvard Medical School/Beth Israel Deaconess Medical Center, Boston, MA 02215.

Nutritional support is an integral component of comprehensive cancer care in patients who are carefully selected using nutrition screening tools and for whom appropriate goals of treatment have been established.

## MALNUTRITION IN THE CANCER PATIENT

Malnutrition in the cancer patient can occur secondary to several mechanical and metabolic processes. The cachexia of malignancy is a complex metabolic disorder characterized by involuntary weight loss which, if not treated, often leads to death (3). Certain tumors predispose individuals to cancer cachexia more frequently. Table 1 depicts the frequency of weight loss among approximately 3000 cancer patients studied by the Eastern Cooperative Oncology Group (ECOG). Breast cancer and sarcomas rarely resulted in significant host weight loss compared with cancers involving digestive organs such as stomach and pancreas. Patients with lung and prostate cancer also demonstrated significant weight loss and malnutrition. The ECOG demonstrated a lower morbidity and longer survival in patients without weight loss, except in cases of pancreatic or gastric cancer. Preventing weight loss by nonvolitional feeding does fully restore the difference in outcomes (12,13).

### Causes of Malnutrition

Table 2 lists the potential etiologic factors in the development of cancer anorexia. The development of malnutrition is usually the result of a combination of these mechanisms in any one cancer patient (14).

### Anorexia of Malignancy

A decrease in food intake without a perceived cause can be encountered in the cancer patient and is referred

**TABLE 1.** *Frequency of weight loss in cancer patients*

| Tumor type | Number of patients | Weight loss in the previous 6 months (%) | | | |
|---|---|---|---|---|---|
| | | 0 | 0–5 | 5–10 | >10 |
| Favorable non-Hodgkin's lymphoma | 290 | 69 | 14 | 8 | 10 |
| Breast | 289 | 64 | 22 | 8 | 6 |
| Sarcoma | 189 | 60 | 21 | 11 | 7 |
| Unfavorable non-Hodgkin's lymphoma | 311 | 52 | 20 | 13 | 15 |
| Colon | 307 | 46 | 26 | 14 | 14 |
| Prostate | 78 | 44 | 27 | 18 | 10 |
| Lung, small cell | 436 | 43 | 23 | 20 | 14 |
| Lung, non-small cell | 590 | 39 | 25 | 21 | 15 |
| Pancreas | 111 | 17 | 29 | 28 | 26 |
| Nonmeasurable gastric | 179 | 17 | 21 | 32 | 30 |
| Measurable gastric | 138 | 13 | 20 | 29 | 38 |
| Total | 2918 | 42 | 22 | 18 | 16 |

Data from ref 3.

to as the anorexia-cachexia syndrome. Several factors, including changes in the central nervous system, changes in taste perception due to tumor, and depression and its associated reduced physical activity, have been implicated as causes of cancer anorexia of malignancy. The regulation of appetite is complex and is mediated by blood nutrient levels, host nutrient resources, liver function, gastrointestinal (GI) capacity, and environmental cues such as smell and sight, all of which are processed by the brain (15). Recently, considerable attention has been directed to the role of various cytokines as mediators of the anorexia-cachexia syndrome, particularly tumor necrosis factor (TNF). Cytokines are discussed in detail later in this chapter under mediators of cancer cachexia.

## NUTRITIONAL EFFECTS OF CANCER TREATMENTS

### Radiation

The site, magnitude, and duration of radiation therapy all influence the severity of nutritional injury. This injury

**TABLE 2.** *Etiology of the anorexia-cachexia syndrome*

*Direct and Indirect Tumor Effects*
   Change in taste
   Dysphagia
   Pain
   GI tract obstruction
   Early satiety
   Anorectic factors (cytokines) produced by tumor or host
*Antineoplastic Therapy*
   Chemotherapy
   Radiotherapy
   Anorexia/anosmia
   Nausea
   Mucosal/ulcerations/infections

may be associated with both acute and late effects of radiation therapy (16–19).

After radiotherapy of the oral cavity and pharynx, patients can experience both heightened and suppressed taste sensation. Loss of taste is severe and rapid after oral pharyngeal irradiation as measured by quantitative tests of sensitivity to sour, sweet, and bitter substances. Fortunately, patients often regain pre-irradiation taste sensitivity 60–120 days after therapy is completed.

Radiation to the head and neck may inhibit adequate salivation leading to changes in eating habits. Also, patients may experience increased sensitivity of their teeth to extreme temperature and sweetness. In a study of weight loss during a 6- to 8-week course of external beam radiation therapy to the head and neck regions, 93% of 114 patients lost an average weight of 3.7 kg. In addition, approximately 9% of individuals lost more than one tenth of their body weight during their 6- to 8-week course of radiation (17).

Radiation to the gastric area and small and large intestine is associated with various complications that may influence nutritional status. Low doses of gastric irradiation reduce gastric acidity, whereas higher doses may induce ulcer formation. Nausea, vomiting, and diarrhea are common in individuals undergoing radiation to the small and large bowel. In addition, chronic diarrhea or bowel obstruction may develop due to radiation-induced enteritis following high-dose GI irradiation.

Upper abdominal radiation may produce radiation-induced hepatitis, characterized by anorexia, nausea, vomiting, and abdominal distention, which is usually temporary. Radiation to the pancreas may similarly result in acute anorexia, nausea, and vomiting.

### Chemotherapy

Chemotherapy can affect host tissue in addition to the targeted neoplasm and thus cause short-term nutritional defects. Almost every major class of compound used in chemotherapy and immunotherapy products can produce nausea and vomiting (20) accompanied by anorexia. This often results in reduced dietary intake, electrolyte imbalance, weakness, and progressive weight loss (21).

Mucosal toxicity, manifested as oral ulcerations, cheilosis, glossitis, and pharyngitis, may be inevitable with the use of some chemotherapeutic agents. This often leads to odynophagia and anorexia. Specific agents such as actinomycin D, cytarabine, 5-fluorouracil, hydroxyurea, and methotrexate can produce ulcerations of the entire GI epithelium (22,23). Therapy itself does not induce malabsorption but, because of its side effects, can aggravate the effect of tumor-related malabsorption syndromes (22). Small intestinal absorptive function with either a single agent or combination chemotherapy remains well preserved in most instances. Nutritional support is usually unnecessary in the initially well-nourished patient if the ill effects of chemotherapy are significantly limited in time and intensity.

Many major organ systems are affected by various chemotherapeutic agents, resulting in decreased efficiency of metabolism. The liver is especially vulnerable, and hepatic injury is commonly associated with anorexia. Diffuse hepatocellular damage often results in hypoalbuminemia. Several agents affect specific organ systems. Hydroxyurea may cause renal impairment. Doxorubicin may cause cardiac toxicity leading to congestive heart failure, water retention, and electrolyte imbalance. Ohnuma and Holland (20) and Carter (24) provide extensive discussions of the nutritional consequences of chemotherapy and immunotherapy.

## Surgery

Nutritional depletion can be attributed to surgical intervention in many cancer patients. Nutritional support can be a beneficial tool, as a patient with good nutritional status develops fewer postoperative complications. If nutritional assessment reveals protein calorie malnutrition, elective surgery can even be delayed until nutritional status improves (25). Yamada et al. (26) analyzed the association between nutritional parameters and postoperative complications in 440 patients with gastric cancer. The frequency of postoperative complications was highest in patients with stage IV gastric cancer. A strong interrelationship was found between nutritional status and postoperative complications.

Certain surgical procedures require nutritional intervention. Radical resection of the oropharyngeal area often necessitates postoperative tube feeding (27). Conditions associated with esophagectomy and esophageal reconstruction may include delayed gastric emptying secondary to vagotomy, malabsorption, and the development of a fistula or stenosis. Gastric surgery may result in dumping syndrome, malabsorption, and/or hypoglycemia.

The site and extent of intestinal resection can result in a variety of nutritional complications. Jejunal resection can decrease the efficiency of absorption of many nutrients. Ileum resection commonly results in vitamin $B_{12}$ deficiency and bile salt losses. With extensive small bowel resection, malabsorption leading to malnutrition is common, as reported in jejunoileal bypass (28). Abnormalities in sodium and water balance are commonly associated with ileostomy and colostomy formation. In addition, gastric and intestinal bypass surgery to relieve obstruction can result in a blind loop syndrome with specific nutritional deficiencies.

Individuals with pancreatic cancer should be nutritionally assessed because they frequently lose weight prior to their diagnosis and surgical intervention. After pancreatectomy, malabsorption and endocrine as well as exocrine insufficiency are common problems that may require insulin and pancreatic enzyme replacement. Cancer patients undergoing ureterosigmoidostomy may experience hyperchloremic acidosis and hypokalemia in addition to other more common postoperative problems.

If it is anticipated that nutritional intervention will be required postoperatively, a nasoenteric feeding tube can be placed intraoperatively. In patients in whom a longer recuperative course is anticipated, placement of a gastrostomy tube or jejunostomy tube may be more appropriate.

## Energy Metabolism in the Cancer Patient

Altered metabolism of nutrients is common in cancer anorexia. A wasting of 100 nonprotein calories per day in futile pathways can contribute to major losses in both total weight and lean body mass over the long term. Abnormalities in carbohydrate, protein, and lipid metabolism are common. The inability of cachectic cancer patients to gain lean body mass despite adequate nutritional support is likely due to the effect of the tumor on host metabolism. The Pancreatic Cancer Task Force reported that 80% of 924 patients with pancreatic cancer had weight loss prior to diagnosis (29). Whereas 50% of the pancreatic cancer patients studied had experienced weight loss longer than two months prior to diagnosis, only 26% of these patients reported anorexia during this period.

### Carbohydrate Metabolism

Abnormal glucose metabolism, a major source of caloric wasting, is a hallmark of cancer cachexia (30). Both increased glucose production and utilization, as well as insulin resistance, are characteristic. Glucose intolerance may be attributable to a reduced tissue sensitivity to insulin (31). There may be decreased pancreatic β-cell receptor sensitivity in cancer patients as well, leading to inadequate insulin release in response to a glucose load. Such abnormalities in peripheral glucose metabolism simulate a type II diabetic state but also share elements similar to the stress state (32–36).

An increase in gluconeogenesis in the liver of the cancer patient is a common finding. This can be the result of an increased release of glucogenic fuel substrates, such as lactate and alanine (34,36), as well as an increased induction of hepatic gluconeogenetic enzymes (33). The energy drain created by increased hepatic gluconeogenesis leads to host depletion of protein and calories. Elevation of hepatic glucose production in a tumor-bearing host requires energy; 3 moles of ATP is necessary to convert each mole of lactate to glucose. Therefore, abnormal glucose kinetics can result in calorie-consuming futile metabolic cycles with a drain on host energy. Cancer patients who lose weight may exhibit increases in glucose flux and glucose oxidation rates. This mechanism is central in the development of host depletion in cachexia, although the energy expenditure involved in these processes suggests that they are more likely associative than causative (37,38).

### Protein Metabolism

Cancer anorexia is accompanied by wasting of host protein mass, leading to fatigue, weakness, and altered host cell-mediated immune response. Clinical signs include skeletal muscle and visceral organ atrophy, hypoalbuminemia, and anergy. Host protein wasting results from alterations in total body protein turnover, muscle protein synthesis and catabolism, hepatic protein metabolism, and plasma secretory protein levels. Several studies have shown that cachectic cancer patients have elevated rates of protein turnover and that the normal adaptation of reduced protein metabolism (i.e., protein sparing) in the setting of starvation does not occur (39). With nutritional depletion, patients with cancer anorexia continue to manifest elevated rates of skeletal protein mobilization rather than the normal response of decreased protein turnover and protein sparing. Protein turnover rates in cachectic cancer patients are significantly higher compared to similarly malnourished control patients without cancer. A loss of <100 g of protein nitrogen or 625 g of body protein equal to 2.5 kg of lean body mass can produce mild protein malnutrition, fatigue, weakness, and altered immune response (40). Explanations for this phenomenon of increased nitrogen turnover remain controversial; however, the findings suggest an injury response to cancer with the tumor acting as a "nitrogen sink."

### Lipid Metabolism

The most common impairments in lipid metabolism seen in cancer patients are hyperlipidemia and depletion of fat stores (41–43). Abnormal lipoprotein lipase activity alters the ability of fatty acids to be utilized as protein-sparing energy fuels and is a major cause of protein malnutrition. The hyperlipidemia seen in cancer patients is significant and may play a role in disease outcome. Elevated lipid levels may have an inhibitory effect on monocytes and macrophages. The combination of increased lipolysis, fatty acid recycling via very low density lipoprotein, and the impairment of lipoprotein lipase enzyme activity leading to decreased lipid clearance can be immuno-suppressive.

Suppression of lipoprotein lipase occurs in cancer patients, but the mechanism is different from that which occurs in starvation. In the latter, lipid mobilization occurs despite a decrease in lipoprotein lipase activity because of a 50% decrease in plasma insulin levels. Vlassara et al. (44) have shown that cancer-associated reductions in plasma lipoprotein lipase are accompanied by normal or even increased insulin levels. This represents a maladaptive host response, since insulin promotes lipid storage, not fat oxidation. Impaired glucose and fat oxidation provide a sink for loss of gluconeogenic amino acids, thus producing an energy deficit and malnutrition.

### Biochemical Mediators of the Anorexia-Cachexia Syndrome

The anorexia-cachexia syndrome incorporates a group of symptoms and signs such as inanition, anorexia, weakness, tissue wasting, and organ dysfunction (2,14, 45–47). Potential etiologies of cancer anorexia are listed in Table 2. There has been much interest in the possible role of cytokines in cancer anorexia. Prominent cytokines include tumor necrosis factor (TNF), interleukin-1α and β (IL-1), interleukin-6 (IL-6), interferon-α (IFN-α), and differentiation factor (D factor), also known as leukemia inhibitory factor (48). The peptides are pyrogens, and their administration, with the exception of IL-6, can produce many of the systemic vascular effects seen in sepsis and shock. For example, IL-1 and TNF-α share the capacity to up-regulate gene transcription of endothelial cell adhesion molecules, increase procoagulant activity, promote the transendothelial migration of leukocytes out of the vascular component into the pulmonary epithelium, and activate the release of toxic superoxide and other enzyme products from neutrophils (49).

Features of cancer cachexia can be reproduced by cytokine administration. For example, IL-1 (50) and, to a lesser extent, TNF-α (51) and IFN-α (52) are potent anorexia-producing agents. Some cytokines are mediated through the hypothalamus (53) and others act directly on the GI tract, causing decreased gastric emptying (51). Other cytokines may promote cachexia by increasing resting energy expenditure. Warren et al. (54) reported that cancer patients receiving cytokines as antineoplastic therapy had a dose-dependent increase in resting energy expenditure.

A mechanism proposed by Kern and Norton (2) to explain the anorexia and metabolic derangements of the anorexia-cachexia syndrome is shown in Fig. 1. Some cancers incite a paracrine-induced systemic host response with production of cytokines such as interleukins or cachectin/TNF. These are secreted by immune cells and may be part of the host defense in an attempt to destroy the tumor. However, cytokines have negative secondary effects on host organs, resulting in anorexia and abnormalities in carbohydrate, protein, and lipid metabolism. Mobilization of nutrients from fat and skeletal muscle during the acute phase of sepsis or in trauma patients rapidly provides a physiologic source of nutrients to the liver so that it can synthesize acute injury proteins. In the cancer patient, the low-grade release of cytokines persists because of the metabolic activity of the tumor and eventually causes severe depletion of host cell mass. The anorexia of chemotherapy, radiotherapy, or surgery only exacerbates this process, adding to the net effect of host depletion. The "at-risk" cancer patient can be identified by a rapid weight loss of >10% of usual body weight.

## ADJUNCTIVE NUTRITIONAL SUPPORT DURING ANTINEOPLASTIC TREATMENT

The goal of nutritional care in the cancer patient should always be considered supportive whether the aim of primary therapy is cure or palliation. Nutritional therapy should be aimed at improving metabolic status, body composition, functional status, and, ultimately, quality of life. Nutrition support can prevent further deterioration in all of these parameters; however, because of the metabolic derangements of cancer cachexia, attempts to reverse severe nutritional depletion are almost universally unsuccessful.

Concerns also exist over the risk of disproportionately stimulating tumor growth as well as the ability to replete the malnourished cancer patient (55). Animal studies have been inconclusive concerning this issue. Undoubtedly, in a cachectic non-cancer patient receiving either total parenteral nutrition (TPN) or enteral feeding, nitrogen balance, wound healing, and outcome are improved; however, controversy continues about the role of nutritional support in cancer patients. The use of nonvolitional feeding, particularly intestinal feeding tubes and TPN, is designed to prevent the nutrition-related complications of cancer therapy (5). In the setting of chemotherapy, the risk of providing nutritional support inappropriately must be foremost in clinical decision making. TPN is not indicated for patients with advanced metastatic cancer who

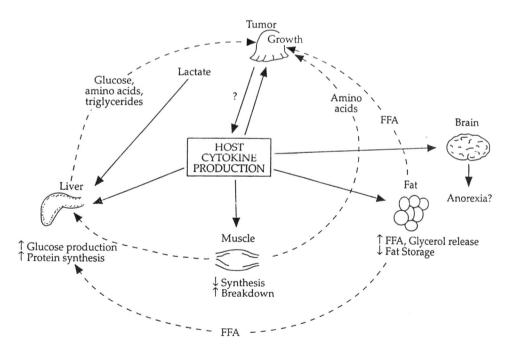

**FIG. 1.** Proposed mechanism of the cancer anorexia syndrome. Tumor–host interaction results in production of metabolically active cytokines that cause anorexia and abnormalities in host intermediary metabolism. (From ref 2.)

are not receiving antineoplastic treatment, and the routine use of TPN in cancer patients who can tolerate enteral nutrition is unjustified. The potential adverse consequences of nutritional support in the setting of cancer makes it important to establish the therapeutic benefits prior to the initiation.

"If the gut works, use it" has become the motto of most nutrition support teams around the country. The use of the GI tract is encouraged whenever possible because it is safe, physiologic, and cost effective. There is also evidence that enteral nutrition may improve visceral protein synthesis. In addition, enteral feeding is superior to TPN in supporting GI mucosal growth and function. This may be important for critically ill patients in whom the gut mucosal barrier may become compromised.

### Nutritional Support in the Perioperative Setting

Prospective randomized clinical trials evaluating the clinical efficacy of nutrition support in cancer patients undergoing surgical therapy were recently reviewed (56). Twenty-seven trials were identified evaluating TPN in cancer patients who underwent surgery (57–84). Only five trials found statistically significant differences in clinical outcomes (59,64,68,69,76). One study reported fewer postoperative complications and decreased mortality in patients with GI carcinoma receiving preoperative TPN (64). Two other trials (59,69) reported decreased postoperative complications in patients receiving preoperative TPN. However, a large multicenter Veterans Administrative cooperative study (76) found similar rates of complications in the TPN and control groups. In addition, they found a statistically significant increase in the infection rate in patients receiving preoperative TPN and concluded that routine use of TPN in the perioperative setting is not indicated. Seven trials reported hospital length of stay (59,68,72,74,75,77,84). Only one of these studies (68) reported a significantly shorter length of stay in patients given TPN perioperatively. There were two meta-analytic reviews of prospective and mixed clinical trials published recently (85,86). Both reviews found that the combined rate of complications or mortality in patients receiving perioperative TPN was one half to two thirds that of the control group.

Klein and Koretz (56) report that data from studies providing at least 7 days of preoperative TPN suggest that the rate of preoperative complications can be decreased by approximately 5%, but that this result may not be justified economically.

Seven trials (82,87–92) investigated the use of enteral nutrition in surgical patients with cancer. Perioperative mortality and length of hospital stay were similar in both enterally fed and control patients. A study looking at the effect of postoperative jejunostomy tube feeding with a formula enriched with arginine, ribonucleic acids, and omega-3 fatty acids in cancer patients reported fewer complications and shortened length of stay compared with patients receiving a standard formula (93).

### Nutrition Support in Patients Treated with Chemotherapy

In recent studies evaluating the use of TPN in patients undergoing chemotherapy (94–118), there was no advantage in overall survival in those receiving nutritional support. Only one trial in patients with squamous cell lung cancer reported an increase in survival of patients given TPN (115). Other trials in patients with colorectal cancer (98) and adenocarcinoma of the lung (118) reported decreased survival in the TPN-treated groups. Two meta-analytic reviews (85,199) concluded that TPN provided no added benefits in terms of survival, tumor response, or chemotherapy toxicity. However, TPN did seem to increase the infection rate.

Studies evaluating enteral nutrition in patients receiving chemotherapy were difficult to evaluate due to differences in composition, timing, and duration of nutritional therapy (56). However, no therapeutic benefit was reported in these trials in terms of survival, tumor response, or chemotherapy toxicity (120–125).

### Nutrition Support in Patients Treated with Radiation Therapy

Four prospective and mixed controlled trials evaluated the effect of TPN in patients undergoing radiation therapy for cancer, with no difference in survival reported between TPN and control subjects (126–130). Moreover, the rate of infection was greater in patients receiving TPN than in controls in one study reporting infection rates (129).

Seven trials reported the outcome of enteral nutrition in patients receiving radiation (131–138). There was no difference in survival noted in the two studies that reported survival rates. Side effects were fewer in nutritionally treated patients receiving radiation for abdominal and pelvic cancer (132–134), but were greater in one study looking at head and neck cancer patients (136).

### Nutrition Support in Patients Treated with Bone Marrow Transplantation

Two studies investigated the use of nutritional support in patients treated with bone marrow transplantation (BMT). BMT requires intensive chemotherapy and, often, radiation, leading to esophagitis and enteritis, resulting in severe nutritional depletion. In one study, Weisdorf et al. (139) reported increased survival in patients who received TPN as compared to controls. In a study by Szeluga et al. (140), patients received either TPN or enteral nutrition post-bone marrow transplantation, and survival did not differ between the two groups. However, the infection rate was higher in patients receiving TPN as compared to those given enteral therapy.

Several studies have evaluated the efficacy of glutamine-enriched TPN in patients undergoing bone marrow transplantation. Glutamine is an important intestinal fuel that attenuates mucosal damage, thereby potentially decreasing bacterial translocation and bacteremia. Glutamine-enriched TPN is hypothesized to decrease the occurrence of systemic infection in those patients who are predisposed. In one study (141), Ziegler et al. reported similar survival but decreased infection rates and shortened length of stay in patients receiving glutamine-TPN versus those receiving standard TPN. However, Schloerb et al. (142) reported similar rates of survival, infections, and length of hospitalization when involving patients with both hematologic and solid tumors.

In conclusion, most clinical trials have failed to demonstrate the clinical efficacy of providing nutritional support to most patients with cancer. However, nutrition support during treatment for cancer should not be denied in patients judged to have life-threatening malnutrition, as is provided for patients with benign disease (143).

## GUIDELINES AND RISK FACTOR ASSESSMENT FOR NUTRITION SUPPORT

### Global Assessment Tools

The implementation of nutritional support teams as well as proper guidelines and protocols for surveillance are the first steps in ensuring that malnourished patients are identified through nutrition screening (Table 3). Three simple assessment measures discussed below can be used initially to screen for protein calorie malnutrition: height and weight to determine body mass index (BMI) (144), percent of regular weight lost, and serum albumin levels. These measures are sensitive enough to identify most patients with protein calorie malnutrition. Other indicators from the Nutrition Screening Initiative (NSI) level II screen (145) include midarm muscle circumference, triceps skinfold, and serum cholesterol. In addition, clinical history, drug use, eating habits, living environment and income, and functional status, as well as mental and cognitive functioning, need to be assessed.

Other indicators are also available (146–150). Buzby et al. (146) developed a Prognostic Nutritional Index (PNI) evaluating serum albumin, serum transferrin, triceps skin fold, and delayed hypersensitivity as a multiparameter index of nutrition status for preoperative nutrition support.

The Prognostic Nutritional Index (PNI) is defined as:

$$PNI\ (\%) = 158 - 16.6\ (Alb) - 0.78\ (TSF) - 0.20\ (TFN) - 5.8\ (DH)$$

**TABLE 3.** *Nutritional assessment parameters*

| | Standards |
|---|---|
| Initial Evaluation | |
| Body mass index (kg/m$^2$) | (see Table 5) |
| Rate weight loss (% weight loss/time) | (see Table 6) |
| Serum Albumin (g/dl) | >3.5 g/dl |
| Comprehensive Evaluation | |
| Anthropometrics | |
| Triceps skinfold (mm) | (see Table 8) |
| Arm muscle circumference | (see Table 8) |
| Biochemical indices | |
| Urine | |
| Creatine height index | (see Table 9) |
| Urine urea nitrogen | 6–7 g/24 hr |
| Nitrogen Balance | 0–1 g/24 hr |
| Catabolic index | (see text) |
| Serum | |
| Transferrin (g/dl) | >170 g/dl |
| Total lymphocyte count | >1500 cell/mm$^3$ |
| Prealbumin | 18–45 mg/dl |
| Immune Function: Delayed Hypersensitivity | |
| Skin Tests | |
| *Candida* | >5 mm induration |
| Mumps | >5 mm erythema/induration |
| Tetanus toxoid | >5 mm induration |

**TABLE 4.** *Patient-generated subjective global assessment of nutritional status*

History

    Weight change:

    I weigh about _____ pounds

    I am about _____ feet and _____ inches tall

    A year ago I weighed about _____ pounds

    Six months ago I weighed about _____ pounds

    During the past 2 weeks by weight has:

    _____ decreased

    _____ not changed

    _____ increased

    I would rate my food intake during the past month (compared to my normal) as:

    _____ no change

    _____ changed

    _____ more than usual

    _____ much less than usual:

    _____ taking little solid food

    _____ taking only liquids

    _____ taking only nutritional supplements

    _____ really taking in very little of anything

    Over the past 2 weeks I have had the following problems that keep me from eating enough (check all that apply):

    _____ no problems eating

    _____ no appetite, just did not feel like eating

    _____ nausea

    _____ vomiting

    _____ diarrhea

    _____ constipation

    _____ mouth sores

    _____ dry mouth

    _____ pain

    _____ things taste funny or have no taste

    _____ smells bother me

    _____ other

    Functional capacity:

    Over the past month I would rate my activity as generally:

    _____ 0 = normal, no limitations

    _____ 1 = not my normal self but able to be up and about with fairly normal activities

    _____ 2 = not feeling up to most things but in bed less than half the day

    _____ 3 = able to do little activity and I spend most of the day in bed or chair

    _____ 4 = pretty much bedridden (rarely out of bed)

    The remainder of this form will be filled in by your doctor, nurse, or therapist. Thank you.

    Disease and its relation to nutrition requirements:

    Primary diagnosis _____

    (stage, if known _____ )*

    Metabolic demand (stress):

    _____ no stress

    _____ low stress

    _____ moderate stress

    _____ high stress

    Physical (for each trait specify: 0 = normal, 1+ = mild, 2+ = moderate, 3+ = severe)

    _____ loss of subcutaneous fat (triceps, chest)

    _____ muscle wasting (quadriceps, deltoid)

    _____ ankle edema

    _____ sacral edema

    _____ ascites

    SGA rating (select one)

    _____ A = well nourished

    _____ B = moderately (or suspected of being) malnourished

    _____ C = severely malnourished

*Modification of the original SGA for oncology patients (154).

where Alb is serum albumin in g/100 ml, TSF is triceps skinfold in mm, TFN is serum transferrin in mg/100 ml, and DH is cutaneous delayed-type hypersensitivity reactivity to any three recall antigens as 0 (nonreactive), 1 (<5 mm induration), or 2 (>5 mm induration) (19). A PNI of <40% is categorized as low risk, 40–49% intermediate risk, and >50% high risk.

Another index, the Nutritional Risk Index (NRI), was developed by the Veterans Affair TPN Cooperative Study Group (11). This index approximates the degree of malnutrition based on a specific constant, serum albumin levels, and percent weight loss.

Perhaps the most beneficial tool for nutritional screening in the oncology patient is the Subjective Global Assessment (SGA) (Table 4) modified by Ottery (151,152) for the practicing oncologist and other health care providers. The original SGA (153) estimates nutritional status on the basis of medical history (i.e., weight and weight history,

dietary intake, GI symptoms with >2 weeks duration, functional status, and metabolic demands) and physical examination (five determinations of muscle, fat, and fluid status) (154). On the basis of these features, the patient is categorized as (a) well nourished, (b) having moderate or suspected malnutrition, or (c) having severe malnutrition (155). Two modifications of the SGA have been developed specifically for use in oncology patients (151,152). Figure 2 (156) demonstrates an algorithm for optimal nutritional oncology intervention based on the SGA.

**Individual Screening Tools**

*Body Mass Index*

The body mass index (BMI) (144) may be a useful tool to identify individuals at risk for protein calorie malnutrition (Table 5).

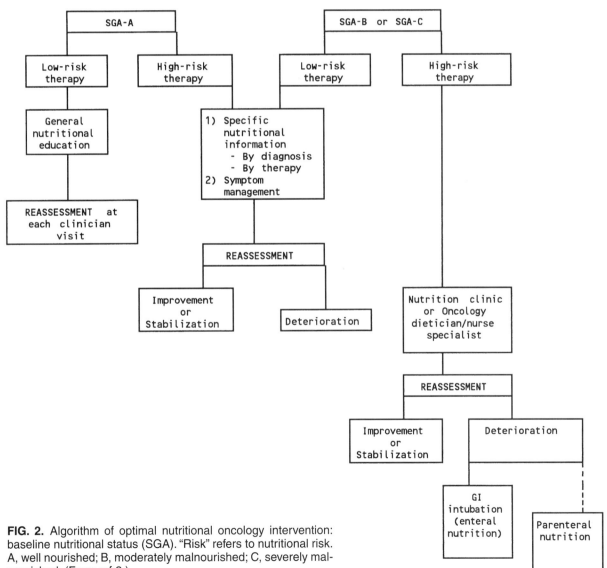

**FIG. 2.** Algorithm of optimal nutritional oncology intervention: baseline nutritional status (SGA). "Risk" refers to nutritional risk. A, well nourished; B, moderately malnourished; C, severely malnourished. (From ref 2.)

**TABLE 5.** *Body mass index table*

| Height (inches) | 19 | 20 | 21 | 22 | 23 | 24 | 25 | 26 | 27 | 28 | 29 | 30 | 35 |
|---|---|---|---|---|---|---|---|---|---|---|---|---|---|
| | | | | | | Body weight (pounds) | | | | | | | |
| 58 | 91 | 96 | 100 | 105 | 110 | 115 | 119 | 124 | 129 | 134 | 138 | 143 | 167 |
| 59 | 94 | 99 | 104 | 109 | 114 | 119 | 124 | 122 | 133 | 138 | 143 | 148 | 173 |
| 60 | 97 | 102 | 107 | 112 | 118 | 123 | 128 | 133 | 138 | 143 | 148 | 153 | 179 |
| 61 | 100 | 106 | 111 | 116 | 128 | 127 | 132 | 137 | 143 | 148 | 153 | 158 | 185 |
| 62 | 104 | 109 | 115 | 120 | 126 | 131 | 136 | 142 | 147 | 153 | 158 | 164 | 191 |
| 63 | 107 | 113 | 118 | 124 | 130 | 135 | 141 | 146 | 152 | 158 | 163 | 169 | 197 |
| 64 | 110 | 116 | 122 | 128 | 134 | 140 | 145 | 151 | 157 | 163 | 169 | 174 | 204 |
| 65 | 114 | 120 | 126 | 132 | 138 | 144 | 150 | 156 | 162 | 168 | 174 | 180 | 210 |
| 66 | 118 | 124 | 130 | 136 | 142 | 148 | 155 | 161 | 167 | 173 | 179 | 186 | 216 |
| 67 | 121 | 127 | 134 | 140 | 146 | 153 | 159 | 166 | 172 | 178 | 185 | 191 | 223 |
| 68 | 125 | 131 | 138 | 144 | 151 | 158 | 164 | 171 | 177 | 184 | 190 | 197 | 230 |
| 69 | 128 | 135 | 142 | 149 | 155 | 162 | 169 | 176 | 182 | 189 | 196 | 203 | 236 |
| 70 | 132 | 139 | 146 | 153 | 160 | 167 | 174 | 181 | 188 | 195 | 202 | 207 | 243 |
| 71 | 136 | 143 | 150 | 157 | 165 | 172 | 179 | 186 | 193 | 200 | 208 | 215 | 250 |
| 72 | 140 | 147 | 154 | 162 | 169 | 177 | 184 | 191 | 199 | 206 | 213 | 221 | 258 |
| 73 | 144 | 151 | 159 | 166 | 174 | 182 | 189 | 197 | 204 | 212 | 219 | 227 | 265 |
| 74 | 148 | 155 | 163 | 171 | 179 | 186 | 194 | 202 | 210 | 218 | 225 | 233 | 272 |
| 75 | 152 | 160 | 168 | 176 | 184 | 192 | 200 | 208 | 216 | 224 | 232 | 240 | 279 |
| 76 | 156 | 164 | 172 | 180 | 189 | 197 | 205 | 213 | 221 | 230 | 238 | 246 | 287 |

Body mass index measured as weight divided by height squared ($W/H^2$ (kg/m$^2$)).

$$BMI = weight\ (kg)/height\ (m^2)$$

A BMI of <22 may be indicative of possible protein calorie malnutrition, especially among cancer patients.

### Weight Loss

Documentation of the patient's weight history is an important and easily obtainable index for the suspected presence or progression of malignancy. There are several parameters available to interpret weight measurements including the weight/height index and the percentage of weight lost. Since the patient's height remains essentially constant, the weight/height index remains a reliable tool for estimating nutritional status. An index <90% of standard would suggest moderate nutritional risk whereas a weight/height index <75% of standard suggests severe malnutrition.

Table 6 focuses on the percentage of regular weight lost. This too can be a good indication of the severity of nutritional deficiency. For example, "severe" weight loss should be considered with a 5% loss of body weight in 1 month or a 10% loss within 6 months (157).

Fluid balance or degree of hydration also affects the accuracy of the change in weight. Fluid retention or loss can account for significant weight shifts rather than changes in body cell mass or protein content; therefore, fluid balance should be closely monitored.

### Serum Albumin

Serum albumin concentration is a commonly used index of nutritional status. Albumin, synthesized in the liver, has a half-life of approximately 20 days with normal serum concentrations of greater than 3.5 g/dl (see Table 3).

As a nutritional marker, serum albumin concentrations may be beneficial for detecting malnutrition. Table 7 demonstrates that in hospitalized patients hypoalbuminemia is associated not only with anergic immune status but with increased morbidity and mortality, and is a poor prognostic indicator (158).

There are, however, limitations to the use of serum albumin concentration as a nutritional index for stressed

**TABLE 6.** *Evaluation of weight change*

| | Significant weight loss (%) | Severe weight loss (%) |
|---|---|---|
| 1 week | 1–2[a] | >2 |
| 1 month | 5 | >5 |
| 3 months | 7.5 | >7.5 |
| 6 months | 10 | >10 |

[a]Percent weight change = (usual weight − actual weight) × 100
(usual weight)
From ref 157, with permission.

**TABLE 5.** *(continued)*

| | 40 | 41 | 42 | 43 | 44 | 45 | 46 | 47 | 48 | 49 | 50 | 51 | 52 | 53 | 54 |
|---|---|---|---|---|---|---|---|---|---|---|---|---|---|---|---|
| Height (inches) | | | | | | | Body weight (pounds) | | | | | | | | |
| 58 | 191 | 196 | 201 | 205 | 210 | 215 | 220 | 224 | 229 | 234 | 239 | 244 | 248 | 253 | 258 |
| 59 | 198 | 203 | 208 | 212 | 217 | 222 | 227 | 232 | 237 | 242 | 247 | 252 | 257 | 262 | 267 |
| 60 | 204 | 209 | 215 | 220 | 225 | 230 | 235 | 240 | 245 | 250 | 255 | 261 | 266 | 271 | 276 |
| 61 | 211 | 217 | 222 | 224 | 232 | 238 | 243 | 248 | 254 | 259 | 264 | 269 | 275 | 280 | 285 |
| 62 | 218 | 224 | 229 | 235 | 240 | 246 | 251 | 256 | 262 | 267 | 273 | 278 | 284 | 289 | 295 |
| 63 | 225 | 231 | 237 | 242 | 248 | 254 | 259 | 265 | 270 | 276 | 282 | 287 | 293 | 299 | 304 |
| 64 | 232 | 238 | 244 | 250 | 256 | 262 | 267 | 273 | 279 | 285 | 291 | 296 | 302 | 308 | 314 |
| 65 | 240 | 246 | 252 | 258 | 264 | 270 | 276 | 282 | 288 | 294 | 300 | 306 | 312 | 318 | 324 |
| 66 | 247 | 253 | 260 | 266 | 272 | 278 | 284 | 291 | 297 | 303 | 309 | 315 | 322 | 328 | 334 |
| 67 | 255 | 261 | 268 | 274 | 280 | 287 | 293 | 299 | 306 | 312 | 319 | 325 | 331 | 338 | 344 |
| 68 | 262 | 269 | 276 | 282 | 289 | 295 | 302 | 308 | 315 | 322 | 328 | 335 | 341 | 348 | 354 |
| 69 | 270 | 277 | 284 | 291 | 297 | 304 | 311 | 318 | 324 | 331 | 338 | 345 | 351 | 358 | 365 |
| 70 | 278 | 285 | 292 | 299 | 306 | 313 | 320 | 327 | 334 | 341 | 348 | 355 | 362 | 369 | 376 |
| 71 | 286 | 293 | 301 | 308 | 315 | 322 | 329 | 336 | 343 | 351 | 358 | 365 | 372 | 379 | 386 |
| 72 | 294 | 302 | 309 | 316 | 324 | 331 | 338 | 346 | 353 | 361 | 368 | 375 | 383 | 390 | 397 |
| 73 | 302 | 310 | 318 | 325 | 333 | 340 | 348 | 355 | 363 | 371 | 378 | 386 | 393 | 401 | 408 |
| 74 | 311 | 319 | 326 | 334 | 342 | 350 | 358 | 365 | 373 | 381 | 389 | 396 | 404 | 412 | 420 |
| 75 | 319 | 327 | 335 | 343 | 351 | 359 | 367 | 375 | 386 | 391 | 399 | 407 | 415 | 423 | 431 |
| 76 | 328 | 336 | 344 | 353 | 361 | 369 | 377 | 385 | 394 | 402 | 410 | 418 | 426 | 435 | 443 |

Body mass index measured as weight divided by height squared ($W/H^2$ (kg/m$^2$)).

and critically ill patients. During an acute illness or stress, such as injury, infection, or surgery, serum albumin synthesis decreases and hypoalbuminemia ensues. In addition, due to the long half-life, serum albumin does not respond on a daily or weekly basis to nutritional support. Lastly, serum albumin concentrations can be affected by fluid status and volume repletion.

### Anthropometrics

Anthropometric techniques are tools that may be beneficial in defining fat stores in the patient with cancer. One of the major sites of fat deposition in the human body is the subcutaneous space (19). Subcutaneous fat represents approximately 30% and 33% of total body fat in men and women, respectively, although these numbers vary according to age, level of obesity, and measurement techniques (12).

A useful anthropometric assessment of body fat mass is the triceps skinfold measurement (TSF). This is per-

formed by using large calipers at the upper left arm. Knowing the TSF, one can derive the more valuable arm muscle circumference (AMC):

$$AMC = arm\ circumference - TSF$$

The AMC is compared with standard tables (Table 8), and values <60% of standard are consistent with protein depletion (19). As with all anthropometric techniques, interobserver and intraobserver variation ranges from 15% to 20%, and the exact correlation between upper arm circumference and total body protein stores is unknown.

### Transferrin

Transferrin is a 90-kd globulin that binds and transports iron. The half-life of transferrin, which is primarily synthesized in the liver, is 8–10 days. Visceral protein depletion is reflected with transferrin levels <170 g/dl. This makes it more sensitive than albumin as an index of

**TABLE 7.** *Probability estimates using serum albumin*

| | <10% | <25% | 50% | >75% | >90% |
|---|---|---|---|---|---|
| Anergy | 5.2 | 4.2 | 3.2 | 2.2 | 1.2 |
| Sepsis | 4.3 | 3.7 | 3.1 | 2.5 | 1.9 |
| Death | 4.9 | 4.0 | 3.2 | 2.3 | 1.5 |

From ref 184, with permission.

**TABLE 8.** *Midarm muscle circumference in adults (18–74 years), United States*[a]

| Age group (years) | Sample size | Estimated population (millions) | Mean (cm) | Percentile | | | | | | |
|---|---|---|---|---|---|---|---|---|---|---|
| | | | | 5th | 10th | 25th | 50th | 75th | 90th | 95th |
| Men | | | | | | | | | | |
| 18–74 | 5261 | 61.18 | 28.0 | 23.8 | 24.8 | 26.3 | 27.9 | 29.6 | 31.4 | 32.5 |
| 18–24 | 773 | 11.78 | 27.4 | 23.5 | 24.4 | 25.8 | 27.2 | 28.9 | 30.8 | 32.3 |
| 25–34 | 804 | 13.00 | 28.3 | 24.2 | 25.3 | 26.5 | 28.0 | 30.0 | 31.7 | 32.9 |
| 35–44 | 664 | 10.68 | 28.8 | 25.0 | 25.6 | 27.1 | 28.7 | 30.3 | 32.1 | 33.0 |
| 45–54 | 765 | 11.15 | 28.2 | 24.0 | 24.9 | 26.5 | 28.1 | 29.8 | 31.5 | 32.6 |
| 55–64 | 598 | 9.07 | 27.8 | 22.8 | 24.4 | 26.2 | 27.9 | 29.6 | 31.0 | 32.8 |
| 65–74 | 1657 | 5.50 | 26.8 | 22.5 | 23.7 | 25.3 | 26.9 | 28.5 | 29.9 | 30.7 |
| Women | | | | | | | | | | |
| 18–74 | 8410 | 67.84 | 22.2 | 18.4 | 19.0 | 20.2 | 21.8 | 23.6 | 25.8 | 27.4 |
| 18–24 | 1523 | 12.89 | 20.9 | 17.7 | 18.5 | 19.4 | 20.6 | 22.1 | 23.6 | 24.9 |
| 25–34 | 1896 | 13.93 | 21.7 | 18.3 | 18.9 | 20.0 | 21.4 | 22.9 | 24.9 | 26.6 |
| 35–44 | 1664 | 11.59 | 22.5 | 18.5 | 19.2 | 20.6 | 22.0 | 24.0 | 26.1 | 27.4 |
| 45–54 | 836 | 12.16 | 22.7 | 18.8 | 19.5 | 20.7 | 22.2 | 24.3 | 26.6 | 27.8 |
| 55–64 | 669 | 9.98 | 22.8 | 18.6 | 19.5 | 20.8 | 22.6 | 24.4 | 26.3 | 28.1 |
| 65–74 | 1882 | 7.28 | 22.8 | 18.6 | 19.5 | 20.8 | 22.5 | 24.4 | 26.5 | 28.1 |

[a]Measurements made in the right arm.
Data compiled by Friasancho (*Am J Clin Nutr* 1984;40:808–819) from NHANES I and II.
From Bishop CW, Bowen PE, Ritchey SJ. *Am J Clin Nutr* 1981;34:2530–2539 (NHANES 1).

improvement in nutritional status. There are, however, two instances when transferrin levels are unreliable for nutritional status: in iron-deficient or iron-overloaded patients who tend to show high and low transferrin levels, respectively, and in patients who have had multiple transfusions (7).

### *Delayed Hypersensitivity*

Assessment of the function of the cellular immune system through delayed hypersensitivity testing to common skin antigens can be a marker of nutritional status. Anergy has been correlated with an increased incidence of postoperative morbidity and mortality (159). The common recall antigens used are *Candida*, mumps, dermatophytes, or tetanus toxoid. After 24–48 hours, 5 mm or greater of induration is considered a positive response. Cellular immunity is most sensitive to malnutrition but protein deficiency also reflects leukocyte function, particularly immune cell activation and cytokine release.

### Evaluation of Ongoing Nutritional Support

Patients undergoing administration of nutritional support require assessment of several parameters to tailor daily requirements of specific nutrients. Many of these parameters, notably serum albumin, arm muscle circumference, and body mass index, are not sensitive enough to detect the short-term effects of nutritional support. In addition to daily electrolyte determinations, physical examination, and accurate body weights, other parameters such as nitrogen balance may be more beneficial in assessing the impact of nutritional therapy on a short-term basis.

Health care providers must, however, differentiate an increase in weight caused by fluid retention from lean body mass. Malnourished patients who are suddenly overfed can develop an increase in intravascular volume, congestive heart failure, and electrolyte abnormalities, which can be fatal (160).

### Nitrogen Balance

The nitrogen balance determination is a dependable measure that can reflect the influence of nutritional support on lean body mass. Nitrogen balance reflects the difference between nitrogen intake versus output over a 24-hour period. With 1 g of nitrogen representing 6.25 g of protein, the nitrogen balance is calculated as:

$$\text{Nitrogen balance} = \text{protein intake (g)} + 6.25 - (24\text{-hour urine urea nitrogen} + 4 \text{ g})$$

The principal form of urine nitrogen is called urine urea nitrogen, which can be easily measured. Urea excreted in the urine reflects protein degradation. In addition to urea, other forms of nitrogen are excreted including nonurea urine nitrogen, fecal nitrogen, and integumental nitrogen. These are lost at a fairly constant rate except when diarrhea is present. In calculating nitrogen loss, 4 g is added to the nitrogen output as an estimate of fecal and integumental losses.

## NUTRITIONAL SUPPORT

### Parenteral Nutrition Requirements

#### Caloric Requirements

The "gold standard" for estimating basal energy requirements was derived by Harris and Benedict around the turn of the century (161). Basal metabolic requirements (BMRs) can be calculated using the Harris–Benedict equations:

$$\text{BMR for males} = 66.4730 + (13.7516W) + (5.0033H) - (6.7550A)$$

$$\text{BMR for females} = 65.5095 + (9.563W) + (1.8496H) - (4.6756A)$$

where $W$ is weight in kilograms, $H$ is height in centimeters, and $A$ is age in years.

The primary goal of parenteral and enteral nutrition support is to supply adequate protein and nonprotein calories to prevent further catabolism and promote the accrual of protein. The mild to moderately stressed patient usually requires 25–35 kcal/kg and 1.5 g of protein/kg of ideal body weight in order to maintain positive nitrogen balance. Nonprotein calories are supplied by both carbohydrates and lipids, with glucose being the major energy source for the central nervous system, red blood cells, and renal medulla. These organ systems require a minimum of 100–150 g/day (19). The maximal infusion of dextrose given should be 5 mg/kg/minute. Exceeding this rate may lead to hepatic steatosis and excess fat synthesis and carbon dioxide production (19). The caloric density of glucose is 3.4 kcal/g; approximately 60–70% of nonprotein calories should be provided as dextrose (162).

#### Lipid Requirements

Fat emulsions, derived from soybean or safflower oil, provide 2.0 kcal/ml in standard 20% solutions. The usual dose of lipid is 0.5–1.0 g/kg/day, with the maximum of 2.5 g/kg/day (163). Lipid emulsions are usually formulated to provide approximately 30% of total nonprotein calories. However, a minimum of 0.5 mg/kg/day is sufficient to prevent essential fatty acid deficiency.

#### Protein Requirements

The protein requirements for a mild to moderately stressed patient may be estimated at 1.5–2.0 g protein/kg based on ideal body weight. Although nonprotein calories may spare nitrogen retention in the non-stressed state, patients with cancer usually require an infusion of 0.2–0.3 g nitrogen/kg/day to maintain a positive nitrogen balance (164).

#### Fluid Requirements

Fluid requirements depend on baseline requirements, losses, and fluid deficits. Fluid status is dynamic and should be monitored on a constant basis by physical examination and accurate daily weights. The average fluid requirement varies from 1250 to 3000 ml/day, depending on body habitus. The average semistressed patient requires approximately 35 ml/kg/day. A wide array of fluid abnormalities can be seen in cancer patients due to the disease process and therapies such as surgery, radiation therapy, and chemotherapy.

#### Electrolytes

Electrolytes are included in all parenteral nutrition solutions. Electrolyte requirements for patients with cancer are essentially the same as for patients with nonmalignant forms of disease. The electrolyte composition of TPN will be dependent on the hormonal milieu, GI and pulmonary losses, disease state, and renal and hepatic function (19). In addition, treatment modalities (i.e., amphotericin B administration) can alter electrolyte requirements. Daily serum electrolyte measurements are important to customize the patient's daily nutrition prescription. Limitations exist for calcium, phosphorus, and magnesium in parenteral nutrition solutions. Calcium and phosphorus can form a precipitate if they are not compounded properly or if excessive amounts are added to the solution (165). The pH, temperature, and type of amino acid solution will also affect the compatibility of calcium and phosphorus (166). Hypophosphatemia may result from hyperalimentation without adequate supplementation. A minimum of 20 meq of potassium phosphate per 1000 kcal will usually prevent hypophosphatemia (167).

### ENTERAL FEEDINGS

If the GI tract is intact and functioning, liquid formula diets are preferred. Oral supplements provide an excellent source of calories and protein to bolster a modest PO intake or as an adjunct to hyperalimentation. Unfortunately, cancer patients often suffer from anorexia, nausea, oropharyngeal obstruction, or central nervous system pathology and cannot meet their caloric needs despite a functioning intestinal tract. These individuals can benefit from tube feeding. Small pliable nasogastric tubes are available and well tolerated by most patients. Delivery methods can be by either bolus feeding, gravity, or mechanical pump systems. In the critically ill patient, the literature supports the use of continuous rather than intermittent tube feeding. In this population, continuous tube feedings have been associated with positive nitrogen balance and weight gain as compared to intermittent tube feedings (168). Continuous tube feedings require less energy expenditure because of diet-induced thermogenesis and have been shown to be effective in the prevention of stress ulceration (169,170).

Although most patients' needs can be met with one or two enteral formulations, there are a myriad of disease-specific products available. Slow rates should be initiated at 10–20 ml/hour and then increased 10 ml every 8–12 hours until full flow rates are obtained. There is usually no reason to dilute low-fat, well-tolerated formulas such as Peptamen, Vital, or Vivonex. The patient's head should be maintained at a 30° elevation with nasogastric and nasoduodenal feedings to avoid aspiration. For patients needing chronic enteral feedings, surgical or endoscopically placed gastrostomy or jejunostomy tubes may be beneficial.

## Nutritional Adjuncts

Insulin has been investigated as an anabolic agent in the treatment of cancer cachexia because of the tumor-associated alterations in carbohydrate metabolism and insulin resistance demonstrated in cancer patients.

Studies have shown that parenteral nutrition administered with insulin to cancer patients results in improved skeletal muscle protein synthesis and whole-body protein net balance compared with standard TPN (171). The use of insulin as an anabolic adjunct to TPN appears promising, but further trials examining clinical outcomes are needed.

Growth hormone has been shown to attenuate the loss of body protein when administered to patients without cancer (172). There has been little study of growth hormone as a nutritional adjunct in patients with cancer because of the fear of stimulating tumor growth. In animals studies and in vivo human tumor studies, no increase in tumor volume has been reported (173,174). Further studies will be needed to outline a potential role for growth hormone in the nutritional therapy of cancer patients.

Glutamine is a nonessential amino acid that has been noted to be depleted in patients with cancer. Standard TPN solutions do not contain glutamine because of instability issues. Addition of glutamine to TPN formulations has been shown to improve nitrogen balance and promote protein synthesis without stimulating tumor growth (175). Ziegler and colleagues in a double-blinded prospective trial found that patients receiving glutamine-enriched TPN had an improved nitrogen balance, fewer infections, and shortened length of hospitalization compared with controls (176). Further clinical studies using glutamine are ongoing, as it may be potentially beneficial as an adjunct to conventional TPN in cancer patients.

## Home Parenteral and Enteral Nutrition

Oral or tube feedings in the home setting are both financially and physiologically preferred over parenteral nutrition. However, patients who cannot tolerate oral or tube feedings may benefit from home TPN. The technology and science of nutrition support has flourished in the last 20 years but not without a significant increase in costs. It has been estimated that nutrition support accounts for approximately 1% of all health care dollars (177,178). As expected, most of these dollars are spent on hospitalized patients but approximately 20% are spent on patients living outside the hospital (177). Half of these patients are nursing home residents and half reside at home. Twenty percent of home patients receive parenteral nutrition support and 80% receive enteral nutrition support (177). The cost for enteral feeding is estimated at $15,000/year with home parenteral nutrition support being at least 10 times as costly (178).

Patients with a curable malignancy, who require aggressive primary treatment causing anorexia, nausea, and/or ileus, may benefit from home nutrition support. Other indications for home nutrition support are patients who are "cured" from their primary cancer but are left with bowel dysfunction from irradiation or resection.

A voluntary patient registry, the North American Home Parenteral and Enteral Patient Registry, was formed in 1984 to follow clinical outcomes of home patients receiving home parenteral or enteral nutrition. There are approximately 204 programs with more than 10,000 home nutrition patients registered. The Oley Foundation has published outcomes information on patients registered to date (179).

**TABLE 9.** *Ideal urinary creatinine values*

| Men | | Women | |
|---|---|---|---|
| Height (cm) | Ideal creatinine (mg) | Height (cm) | Ideal creatinine (mg) |
| 157.5 | 1288 | 147.3 | 830 |
| 160.0 | 1325 | 149.9 | 851 |
| 162.6 | 1359 | 152.4 | 875 |
| 165.1 | 1386 | 154.9 | 900 |
| 167.6 | 1426 | 157.5 | 925 |
| 170.2 | 1467 | 160.0 | 949 |
| 172.2 | 1513 | 162.6 | 977 |
| 175.3 | 1555 | 165.1 | 1006 |
| 177.8 | 1596 | 167.6 | 1044 |
| 180.3 | 1642 | 170.2 | 1076 |
| 182.9 | 1691 | 172.7 | 1109 |
| 185.4 | 1739 | 175.3 | 1141 |
| 188.0 | 1785 | 177.8 | 1174 |
| 190.5 | 1831 | 180.3 | 1206 |
| 193.0 | 1891 | 182.9 | 1240 |

From ref 157.

For the individual deemed a candidate for home nutrition support, techniques used at home and in the hospital are essentially similar. In the home setting the patient and the patient's family may take responsibility for solutions administered (180). For parenteral nutrition, central catheter administration is the preferred route for hyperalimentation. This allows provision of adequate calories and protein without large fluid volumes. If possible, a Hickman catheter is preferred because it has two Dacron cuffs that help secure placement and reduce the risk of ascending bacterial infection. Strict sterile technique is essential to reduce the risk of catheter infection and sepsis. Even with precautionary measures, the incidence of catheter-related sepsis is 4.5–11% (181). In addition to the traditional subclavian or internal jugular central venous access, peripherally inserted central catheters (PICCs) (182,183) can be inserted into the basilic or cephalic vein in the antecubital fossa and threaded into the superior vena cava. PICC lines are safe and reliable central venous access routes for patients receiving parenteral nutrition, long-term antibiotics, and chemotherapy without the complications of pneumothorax or hemopneumothorax. For all patients with intravenous lines, close follow-up with a nutrition support team is important to monitor fever, fluid status, and electrolyte abnormalities. To improve quality of life, patients can have enteral or parenteral feeding cycled at night to allow mobility during the day.

## CONCLUSIONS

It is well known that patients with malignancy have a high incidence of malnutrition and cachexia resulting from decreased intake as well as metabolic alterations due to the influence of the tumor. The clinician must not only identify those patients at risk for malnutrition but must also identify those who will benefit from nutrition support.

Routine use of TPN in patients with cancer has not been substantiated in the literature. The clinician must carefully assess the severity of malnutrition, treatment options, and potential quality of life in the cancer patient before opting to use nutritional support as an adjunctive therapy. Decisions regarding methods and aggressiveness of the nutritional intervention should be based on these issues as well. The enteral route is always preferable to TPN in terms of physiologic response, immune competence, quality of life, and cost.

## REFERENCES

1. Bistrian BR, Blackburn GL, Vitale J, et al. Prevalence of malnutrition in general medical patients. *JAMA* 1976;235:1567.
2. Kern KA, Norton JA. Cancer cachexia. *J Parent Enteral Nutr* 1988;12:286-298.
3. DeWys WD, Begg C, Lavin PT, et al. Prognostic effect of weight loss prior to chemotherapy in cancer patients. *Am J Med* 1980;69:491-497.
4. Nixon DW, Heymsfield SB, Cohen AE, et al. Protein-calorie undernutrition in hospitalized cancer patients. *Am J Med* 1989;68:683-690.
5. Klein S, Simes J, Blackburn GL. Total parenteral nutrition and cancer clinical trials. *Cancer* 1986;58:1378–1386.
6. Detsky AS, Baker JP, O'Rourke K, Goel V. Perioperative parenteral nutrition: a meta-analysis. *Ann Intern Med* 1987;107:195–203.
7. McGeer AJ, Detsky AS, O'Rourke K. Parenteral nutrition in patients undergoing cancer chemotherapy: a meta-analysis. *Nutrition* 1990;6:233–240.
8. Kaminski MV, Hasse D, Rosas M, et al. Letter to the editor. *Nutrition* 1990;6:336–337.
9. Buzby GP, Williford WO, Petterson DL, et al. A randomized clinical trial of parenteral nutrition in malnourished surgical patients: the rational and impact of previous clinical trials and pilot study on protocol design. *Am J Clin Nutr* 1988;47:357–365.
10. Buzby GP, Knox LS, Crosby LO, et al. Study protocol: A randomized clinical trial of total parenteral nutrition in malnourished surgical patients. *Am J Clin Nutr* 1988;47:366–381.
11. Veterans Affairs Total Parenteral Nutrition Co-operative Study Group. Perioperative total parenteral nutrition in surgical patients. *N Engl J Med* 1991;325:525–532.
12. Brennan MF. Total parenteral nutrition in the cancer patient. *N Engl J Med* 1981;305:375.
13. Hill GL, Church J. Energy and protein requirements of general surgical patients requiring intravenous nutrition. *Br J Surg* 1984;71:1.
14. Langstein HN, Norton JA. Mechanisms of cancer cachexia. *Hematol Oncol Clin North Am* 1991;5:103–123.
15. Norton JA, Peacock JL, Morrison SD. Cancer cachexia. *Crit Rev Oncol Hematol* 1987;7:289–327.
16. Donaldson SS. Nutritional consequences of radiotherapy. *Cancer Res* 1977;37:2407.
17. Donaldson SS. Nutritional problems associated with radiotherapy. In: Newell GR, Ellison NM, eds. *Nutrition and cancer: Etiology and treatment.* New York: Raven Press, 1981.
18. Donaldson SS, Leon RA. Alterations of nutritional status: Impact of chemotherapy and radiation therapy. *Cancer* 1979;43:2037.
19. Harrison LE, Brennan MF. The role of total parenteral nutrition in the patient with cancer. In: Wells, ed. *Curr Prob Surg* 1995;32(10):833–924.
20. Ohnuma T, Holland JS. Nutritional consequences of cancer therapy and immunotherapy. *Cancer Res* 1977;37:2395.
21. Kokal WA. The impact of antitumor therapy on nutrition. *Cancer* 1985;55:273–278.
22. Mitchell EP, Schein PS. Gastrointestinal toxicity of chemotherapeutic agents. *Semin Oncol* 1982;9:52.
23. Souchan EA, Copeland EM, Watson P. Intravenous hyperalimentation as an adjunct to chemotherapy with 5-fluorouracil. *J Surg Res* 1975;18:451–454.
24. Carter SK. Nutritional problems associated with cancer chemotherapy. In Newell GR, Ellison NM, eds. *Nutrition and cancer: Etiology and treatment.* New York: Raven Press, 1981.
25. Blackburn GL, Harvey KB. Nutrition in surgical patients. In: Hardy JD, ed. *Surgery: Basic principles and practice,* 2nd ed. Philadelphia: JB Lippincott, 1988.
26. Yamada N, Koyama H, Hioki K, et al. Effect of postoperative total parenteral nutrition (TPN) as an adjunct to gastrectomy for advanced gastric carcinoma. *Br J Surg* 1983;70:267.
27. Goodwin WJ, Byers PM. Nutritional management of the head and neck cancer patients. *Med Clin North Am* 1993;77:597–610.
28. Bray GA. Intestinal bypass operation and the treatment for obesity. *Ann Intern Med* 1976;85:97.
29. Pollard HM. The Pancreatic Cancer Task Force: staging of cancer of the pancreas. *Cancer* 1981;47:1631.
30. Kokal WA, McCulloch A, Wright PD, et al. Glucose turnover and recycling in colorectal cancer. *Ann Surg* 1983;198:601–604.
31. Lundholm K, Hom G, Schersten T: Insulin resistance in patients with cancer. *Cancer Res* 1978;38:4665.
32. Heber D, Byerly LO, Chlebowski RT, et al. Medical abnormalities in glucose and protein metabolism in non-cachectic lung cancer patients. *Cancer Res* 1982;42:4815.
33. Heber D, Byerly LO, Chlebowski RT, et al. Medical abnormalities in the cancer patient. *Cancer* 1985;55:225.
34. Lundholm K, Edstrom S, Karlberg I, et al. Glucose turnover, gluconeogenesis from glycerol in estimation of net glucose cycline in cancer patients. *Cancer* 1982;50:1142.
35. Tayek JA, Bistrian BR, Hehir DJ, et al. Improved protein kinetics

and albumin synthesis by branch chain amino acid enriched total parenteral nutrition in cancer cachexia. *Cancer* 1986;58:147.

36. Waterhouse C: Lactate metabolism in patients with cancer. *Cancer* 1974;33:66.

37. Norton JA, Burt ME, Brennan MF. In vivo utilization of substrate by human sarcoma-bearing limbs. *Cancer* 1980;45:2934.

38. Warnold I, Lundholm K, Schersten T. Energy balance and body composition in cancer patients. *Cancer Res* 1978;38:1801.

39. Shaw JHF, Humberstone DM, Douglas RG, et al. Leucine kinetics in patients with benign disease, non-weight losing cancer, and cancer cachexia: studies at the whole body and tissue level and the response to nutritional support. *Surgery* 1991;109:37–50.

40. Blackburn GL, Wolfe RR. Clinical biochemistry in intravenous hyperalimentation. In: Alberti KGMM, Price CP, eds. *Recent advances in biochemistry.* Edinburgh: Churchill Livingstone 1981, 217–223.

41. Kralovic RC, Zepp A, Canedella RJ. Studies of the mechanism of carcus fat depletion in experimental cancer. *Eur J Cancer* 1977;13:1071.

42. Legaspi A, Jevanandam M, Staves HF, et al. Whole body lipid and energy metabolism in the cancer patient. *Metabolism* 1987;36:958–963.

43. Beck SA, Tisdale MJ. Production of lipolytic and proteolytic factors by a Murine tumor producing cachexia in the host. *Cancer Res* 1987; 47:S919–923.

44. Vlassara H, Spiegel RJ, Doval DS, et al. Reduced plasma lipoprotein lipase activity in patients with malignancy-associated weight loss. *Horm Metab Res* 1986;18:698.

45. Daly JM, Redmon HP, Gallagher H. Perioperative nutrition in cancer patients. *J Parenter Enter Nutr* 1992;16:100S–105S.

46. Norton JA, Peacock JL, Morrison SD. Cancer cachexia. *Crit Rev Col Hematol* 1987;7:289–327.

47. Nelson KA, Walsh D, Sheehan FA. The cancer anorexia-cachexia syndrome. *J Clin Oncol* 1994;12:213–225.

48. McNamara MJ, Alexander HR, Norton JA. Cytokines and their role in the pathophysiology of cancer cachexia. *J Parenter Enter Nutr* 16: 50S-55, 1992.

49. Moldawer LL, Rogy MA, Flowery SF: The role of cytokines in cancer cachexia. *J Parenter Enteral Nutr* 16:43S–49S.

50. Hellerstein MK, Meydani SN, Meydani M, et al. Interleukin-1 induced anorexia in the rat. Influence of prosthetic glandins. *J Clin Invest* 1989;84:228–235.

51. Bodnar RJ, Pasternak GW, Mann PE, et al. Mediation of anorexia by human recombinant tumor necrosis factor through a peripheral action in the rat. *Cancer Res* 1989;49:6280–6284.

52. Langstein HN, Doherty GM, Frajer DL, et al. The role of alpha interferon and tumor necrosis factor in an experimental rat model of cancer cachexia. *Cancer Res* 1991;51:2302–2306.

53. Uehara A, Sekya C, Takasugi Y, et al. Anorexia induced by interleukin-1: involvement of corticotropin-releasing factor. *Am J Physiol* 1989;257:R613–R617.

54. Warren RS, Starnes HF. Gabrilove JL, et al. The acute metabolic effects of tumor necrosis factor administration in humans. *Arch Surg* 1987;122:1396–1400.

55. Torosian MH. Stimulation of tumor growth by nutrition support. *J Parenter Enter Nutr* 1992;16:72S–75S.

56. Klein S, Koretz RL. Nutrition support in patients with cancer: What do the data really show? *Nutr Clin Pract* 1994;9:91–100.

57. Moghissi K, Hornshaw J, Teasdale PR, et al. Parenteral nutrition in carcinoma of the oesophagus treated by surgery: nitrogen balance and clinical studies. *Br J Surg* 1977;64:125–128.

58. Holter AR, Rischer JE. The effects of perioperatie hyper-alimentation on complications in patients with carcinoma and weight loss. *J Surg Res* 1977;23:31–34.

59. Heatley RV, Williams RH, Lewis MH. Preoperative intravenous feeding: a controlled trial. *Postgrad Med J* 1979;55:541–545.

60. Preshaw RM, Attisha RP, Hollingsworth WJ, et al. Randomized sequential trial of parenteral nutrition in healing of colonic anastomoses in man. *Can J Surg* 1979;22:437–439.

61. Lim STK, Choa RG, Lam KH, et al. Total parenteral nutrition versus gastrostomy in the preoperative preparation of patients with carcinoma of the oesophagus. *Br J Surg* 1981;68:69–72.

62. Thompson BR, Julian TB, Stremple JF. Perioperative total parenteral nutrition in patients with gastrointestinal cancer *J Surg Res* 1981; 80(5):497–500.

63. Sako K, Lore JM, Kaufman S, et al. Parenteral hyperalimentation in surgical patients with head and neck cancer: a randomized study. *J Surg Oncol* 1981;16:391–402.

64. Muller JM, Brenner U, Dienst C, et al. Preoperative parenteral feeding in patients with gastrointestinal carcinoma. *Lancet* 1982;1: 68–71.

65. Yamada N, Koyama H, Hioki K, et al. Effect of postoperative total parenteral nutrition (TPN) as an adjunct to gastrectomy for advanced gastric carcinoma. *Br J Surg* 1983;70:267–274.

66. Bonau RA, Ang SD, Jeevanandam M, et al. High-branched chain amino acid solutions: relationship of composition to efficacy. *J Parenter Enter Nutr* 1984;8:622–627.

67. Jensen S. Clinical effects of enteral and parenteral nutrition preceding cancer surgery. *Med Oncol Tumor Pharmacother* 1985;2: 225–229.

68. Askanazi J, Hensle TW, Starker PM, et al. Effect of immediate postoperative nutritional support on length of hospitalization. *Ann Surg* 1986;203:236–239.

69. Muller JM, Keller HW, Brenner U, et al. Indications and effects of preoperative parenteral nutrition. *World J Surg* 1986;10:53–63.

70. Bellantone R, Doglietto GB, Bossola M, et al. Preoperative parenteral nutrition in the high risk surgical patient. *J Parenter Enter Nutr* 1988;12:195–197.

71. Bellantone R, Doglietto G, Bossola M, et al. Preoperative parenteral nutrition of malnourished surgical patients. *Acta Chir Scand* 1988; 154:249–251.

72. Smith RC, Hartemink R. Improvement of nutritional measures during preoperative parenteral nutrition in patients selected by the prognostic nutritional index: a randomized controlled trial. *J Parenter Enter Nutr* 1988;12:587–591.

73. Fan ST, Lau WY, Wong KK, et al. Pre-operative parenteral nutrition in patients with oesophageal cancer: a prospective, randomized clinical trial. *Clin Nutr* 1989;8:23–27.

74. Woolfson AM, Smith JA. Elective nutritional support after major surgery: a prospective randomized trial. *Clin Nutr* 1989;8:15–21.

75. Hansell DT, Davies JW, Shenkin A, et al. The effects of an anabolic steroid and peripherally administered intravenous nutrition in the early postoperative period. *J Parenter Enter Nutr* 1989;13:349–358.

76. The Veterans Affairs Total Parenteral Nutrition Cooperative Study Group. Perioperative total parenteral nutrition in surgical patients. *N Engl J Med* 1991;325:525–532.

77. Sandstrom R, Drott C, Hyltander A, et al. The effect of postoperative intravenous feeding (TPN) on outcome following major surgery evaluated in a randomized study. *Ann Surg* 1993;217:185–195.

78. Simms JM, Oliver E, Smith JA. A study of total parenteral nutrition (TPN) in major gastric and esophageal resection for neoplasia (Abstract). *J Parenter Enter Nutr* 1980;4:42.

79. Simms JM, Smith JAR. Intravenous feeding after total cystectomy: a controlled trial (Abstract). *J Parenter Enter Nutr* 1981;5:357.

80. Schildt B, Groth O, Larsson J, et al. Failure of preoperative TPN to improve nutritional status in gastric carcinoma (Abstract). *J Parenter Enter Nutr* 1981;5:360.

81. Moghissi K, Teasdale P, Dench M. Comparison between preoperative enteral (nasogastric tube) and parenteral feeding in patients with cancer of the esophagus undergoing surgery (Abstract). *J Parenter Enter Nutr* 1982;6:335.

82. von Meyenfeldt MF, Meyerink WJ, Soeters PB, et al. Perioperative nutritional support results in a reduction of major postoperative complications especially in high risk patients (Abstract). *Gastroenterology* 1991;100:A553.

83. Cromack D, Moley J, Pass H, et al. Prospective randomized trial of parenteral nutrition (TPN) compared to ad lib oral nutrition in patients with upper GI cancer and weight loss undergoing surgical treatment. Presented at the Association of Academic Surgery Meeting, November 1988, Salt Lake City, UT.

84. Sclafani LM, Shike M, Quesada E, et al. A randomized prospective trial of TPN following major pancreatic resection or radioactive implant for pancreatic cancer. Presented at the Society of Surgical Oncology, March 1991, Orlando, FL.

85. Klein S, Simes J, Blackburn G. Total parenteral nutrition and cancer clinical trials. *Cancer* 1986;58:1378–1386.

86. Detsky AS, Baker JP, O'Rourke K, et al. Perioperative parenteral nutrition: a meta-analysis. *Ann Intern Med* 1987;107:195–203.

87. Sagar S, Harland P, Sheilds R. Early postoperative feeding with elemental diet. *Br Med J* 1979;1:293–295.

88. Ryan JA, Page CP, Babcock L. Early postoperative jejunal feeding of elemental diet in gastrointestinal surgery. *Am Surg* 1981;47:393–403.

89. Shukla HS, Rao RR, Banu N, et al. Enteral hyperalimentation in malnourished surgical patients. *Indian J Med Res* 1984;80:339–346.

90. Smith RC, Hartemink RJ, Hollinshead JW, et al. Fine bore jejunostomy feeding following major abdominal surgery: a controlled randomized clinical trial. *Br J Surg* 1985;72:458–461.

91. Foschi D, Cavagna G, Callioni F, et al. Hyperalimentation of jaundiced patients on percutaneous transhepatic biliary drainage. *Br J Surg* 1986; 73:716–719.

92. Flynn MB, Leightty FF. Preoperative outpatient nutritional support of patients with squamous cancer of the upper aerodigestive tract. *Am J Surg* 1987;154:359–362.

93. Daly JM, Lieberman MD, Goldfine J, et al. Enteral nutrition with supplemental arginine, RNA, and omega-3 fatty acids in patients after operation: immunologic, metabolic and clinical outcome. *Surgery* 1982;112:56–67.

94. Popp MB, Fisher RI, Wesley R, et al. A prospective randomized study of adjuvant parenteral nutrition in the treatment of advanced diffuse lymphoma: influence on survival. *Surgery* 1981;90:195–203.

95. Popp MB, Fisher RI, Simon RM, et al. A prospective randomized study of adjuvant parenteral nutrition in the treatment of diffuse lymphoma: effect on drug tolerance. *Cancer Treat Rep* 1981;65(suppl 5):129–135.

96. Coquin JY, Maraninchi D, Gastaut JA, et al. Influence of parenteral nutrition (P.N.) on chemotherapy and survival of acute leukemias (A.L.): preliminary results of a randomized trial (Abstract). *J Parenter Enter Nutr* 1981;5:357.

97. Hays DM, Merritt RJ, White L, et al. Effect of total parenteral nutrition on marrow recovery during induction therapy for acute nonlymphocytic leukemia in childhood. *Med Pediatr Oncol* 1983;11:134–140.

98. Nixon DW, Moffitt S, Lawson DH, et al. Total parenteral nutrition as an adjunct to chemotherapy of metastatic colorectal cancer. *Cancer Treat Rep* 1981;65(suppl 5):121–128.

99. Nixon DW, Heymsfield SB, Lawson DH, et al. Effect of total parenteral nutrition on survival in advanced colon cancer. *Cancer Detect Prev* 1981;4:421–427.

100. Samuels ML, Selig DE, Ogden S, et al. IV hyperalimentation and chemotherapy for stage III testicular cancer: a randomized study. *Cancer Treat Rep* 1981;65:614–627.

101. Hickey AJ, Toth BB, Lindquist SB. Effect of intravenous hyperalimentation and oral care on the development of oral stomatitis during cancer chemotherapy. *J Prosthet Dent* 1982;47:188–193.

102. Drott C, Unsgaard B, Schersten T, et al. Total parenteral nutrition as an adjuvant to patients undergoing chemotherapy for testicular carcinoma: protection of body composition-a randomized, prospective study. *Surgery* 1988;103:499–506.

103. Shamberger RC, Rennan MF, Goodgame JT, et al. A prospective, randomized study of adjuvant parenteral nutrition in the treatment of sarcoma: results of metabolic and survival studies. *Surgery* 1984;96:1–12.

104. Shamberger RC, Pizzo PA, Goodgame JT, et al. The effect of total parenteral nutrition on chemotherapy-induced myelosuppression. *Am J Med* 1983;74:40–48.

105. Van Eys J, Copeland EM, Cangir A, et al. A clinical trial of hyperalimentation in children with metastatic malignancies. *Med Pediatr Oncol* 1980;8:63–73.

106. Shike M, Feld R, Evans WK, et al. Long-term effect of TPN on body composition of patients with lung carcinoma (Abstract). *J Parenter Enter Nutr* 1981;5:564.

107. Russell DM, Shike M, Marliss EB, et al. Effects of total parenteral nutrition and chemotherapy on the metabolic derangements in small cell lung cancer. *Cancer Res* 1984;44:1706–1711.

108. Serrou B, Cupissol D, Plagne R, et al. Effects of total parenteral nutrition and chemotherapy on the metabolic derangements in small cell lung cancer. *Cancer Res* 1984;44:1706–1711.

109. Valdivieso M, Frankmann C, Murphy WK, et al. Long-term effects of intravenous hyperalimentation administered during intensive chemotherapy for small cell bronchogenic carcinoma. *Cancer* 1987;59: 362–369.

110. Valdivieso M, Bodey GP, Benjamin RS, et al. Role of intravenous hyperalimentation as an adjunct to intensive chemotherapy for small cell bronchogenic carcinoma. *Cancer Treat Rep* 1981;65(Suppl 5): 145–150.

111. Clamon GH, Feld R, Evans WK, et al. Effect of adjuvant central IV hyperalimentation on the survival and response to treatment of patients with small lung cancer: a randomized trial. *Cancer Treat Rep* 1985;69: 167–177.

112. Weiner RS, Kramer BS, Clamon GH, et al. Effects of intravenous hyperalimentation during treatment in patients with small-cell lung cancer. *J Clin Oncol* 1985;3:949–957.

113. Lanzotti V, Copeland EM, Bhuchar V, et al. A randomized trial of total parenteral nutrition (TPN) with chemotherapy for non-oat cell lung cancer (NOCLC) (Abstract). Proceedings of the American Association of Cancer Research/American Society of Clinical Oncology. 1980;21:377.

114. Issell BF, Valdivieso MD, Zaren HA, et al. Protection against chemotherapy toxicity by IV hyperalimentation. *Cancer Treat Rep* 1978;62:1139–1143.

115. Serrou B, Cupissol D, Favier F, et al. Opposite results in two randomized trials evaluating the adjunct value of peripheral intravenous nutrition in lung cancer patients. In: Salmon SE, Jones SE, eds. *Adjunctive therapy of cancer III*. New York: Grune and Stratton, 1981;255–263.

116. Moghissi K, Teasdale P. Supplementary parenteral nutrition in disseminated cancer of the lung treated by surgery (Abstract). *J Parenter Enter Nutr* 1979;3:292.

117. Jordan WM, Valdivieso M, Frankman C, et al. Treatment of advanced adenocarcinoma of the lung with ftorafur, doxorubicin, cyclophosphamide, and cisplatin (FACP) and intensive IV hyperalimentation. *Cancer Treat Rep* 1981;65:197–205.

118. DeCicco M, Panarello G, Fantin D, et al. Parenteral nutrition in cancer patients receiving chemotherapy: effects on toxicity and nutritional status. *J Parenter Enter Nutr* 1993;17:513–518.

119. McGeer AJ, Detsky AS, O'Rourke KO. Parenteral nutrition in cancer patients undergoing chemotherapy: a meta-analysis. *Nutrition* 1990;6: 233–240.

120. Elkort RJ, Baker FL, Vitale JJ, et al. Long-term nutritional support as an adjunct to chemotherapy for breast cancer. *J Parenter Enter Nutr* 1981;5:385–390.

121. Lipschitz DA, Mitchell CO. Enteral hyperalimentation and hematopoietic toxicity caused by chemotherapy of small cell lung cancer (Abstract). *J Parenter Enter Nutr* 1980;4:593.

122. Evans WK, Nixon DW, Daly JM, et al. A randomized study of oral nutritional support versus ad lib nutritional intake during chemotherapy for advanced colorectal and non-small cell lung cancer. *J Clin Oncol* 1987;5:113–124.

123. Tandon SP, Gupta SC, Sinha SN, et al. Nutritional support as an adjunct therapy of advanced cancer patients. *Indian J Med Res* 1984; 80:180–188.

124. Bounous G, Gentile JM, Hugon J. Elemental diet in the management of the intestinal lesion produced by 5-fluorouracil in man. *Can J Surg* 1971;14:312–324.

125. Cousineau L, Bounous G, Rochon M, et al. The use of an elemental diet during treatment with anticancer agents (Abstract). *Clin Res* 1973; 21:1067.

126. Solassol C, Joyeux J, Dubois JB. Total parenteral nutrition (TPN) with complete nutritive mixtures: an artificial gut in cancer patients. *Nutr Cancer* 1979;1:13–18.

127. Kinsella TJ, Malcolm AW, Bothe A, et al. Prospective study of nutritional support during pelvic irradiation. *Int J Radiat Oncol Biol Phys* 1981;7:543–548.

128. Valerio D, Overett L, Malcolm A, et al. Nutritional support for cancer patients receiving abdominal and pelvic radiotherapy: a randomized prospective clinical experiment of intravenous versus oral feeding. *Surg Form* 1978;29:145–148.

129. Ghavimi F, Shils ME, Scott BF, et al. Comparison of morbidity in children requiring abdominal radiation and chemotherapy, with and without total parenteral nutrition. *J Pediatrics* 1982;101:530–537.

130. Donaldson SS, Wesley MN, Ghavimi F, et al. A prospective randomized clinical trial of total parenteral nutrition in children with cancer. *Med Pediatr Oncol* 1982;10:129–139.

131. Douglass HO, Milliron S, Nava H, et al. Elemental diet as an adjuvant for patients with locally advanced gastrointestinal cancer receiving radiation therapy: a prospectively randomized study. *J Parenter Enter Nutr* 1978;2:682–686.

132. Brown MS, Buchanan RB, Karran SJ. Clinical observations on the effects of elemental diet supplementation during irradiation. *Clin Radiol* 1980;31:19–20.

133. Foster KJ, Brown MS, Alberti GMM, et al. The metabolic effects of abdominal irradiation in man with and without dietary therapy with an elemental diet. *Clin Radiol* 1980;31:13–17.

134. Bounous G, LeBel E, Shuster J, et al. Dietary protection during radiation therapy. *Strahlentherapie* 1975;149:476–483.
135. Nayel H, El-Ghoneimy E, El-Haddad S. Impact of nutritional supplementation on treatment delay and morbidity in patients with head and neck tumors treated with irradiation. *Nutrition* 1992;8:13–18.
136. Daly JM, Hearne B, Dunaj J, et al. Nutritional rehabilitation in patients with advanced head and neck cancer receiving radiation therapy. *Am J Surg* 1984;148:514–520.
137. Moloney M, Moriarty M, Daly L. Controlled studies of nutritional intake in patients with malignant disease undergoing treatment. *Hum Nutr Appl Nutr* 1983;37A:30–35.
138. Besser PM, Bonau RA, Erlandson RA, et al. Can enteral elemental diets (ED) protect the G-I tract from acute radiation enteritis? (Abstract). *J Parenter Enter Nutr* 1986;10(suppl):4S.
139. Weisdorf SA, Lysne J, Wind D, et al. Positive effect of prophylactic total parenteral nutrition on long-term outcome of bone marrow transplantation. *Transplantation* 1987;43:833–838.
140. Szeluga DJ, Stuart RK, Brookmeyer R, et al. Nutritional support of bone marrow transplant recipients: a prospective randomized clinical trial comparing total parenteral nutrition to an enteral feeding program. *Cancer Res* 1987;47:3309–3316.
141. Ziegler TR, Young LS, Benfell K, et al. Clinical and metabolic efficacy of glutamine-supplemented parenteral nutrition after bone marrow transplantation. *Ann Intern Med* 1992;116:821–828.
142. Schloerb PR, Amare M. Total parenteral nutrition with glutamine in bone marrow transplantation and other clinical applications (a randomized double-blind study). *J Parenter Enter Nutr* 1993;17:407–413.
143. American College of Physicians. Parenteral nutrition in patients receiving cancer chemotherapy. *Ann Intern Med* 1989;110:734.
144. Ferro-Luzzi A, Sette S, Franklin M, et al. A simplified approach of assessing adult chronic energy deficiency. *Eur J Clin Nutr* 1992;46(3):173–186.
145. Nutrition Screening Initiative: Nutrition Intervention Manual for Professionals Caring for Older Americans. Washington, DC: Nutrition Screening Initiative (2626 Pennsylvania Avenue NW, Suite 301, Washington, DC 20037), 1992.
146. Buzby GP, Mullen JL, Matthews DC, et al. Prognostic nutritional index in gastrointestinal surgery. *Am J Surg* 1980;139:160–167.
147. Hickman DM, Miller RA, Rombeau JL, et al. Serum albumin and body weight as predictors of postoperative course in colorectal cancer. *J Parenter Enter Nutr* 1980;4:314–316.
148. Klidjian AM, Archer TJ, Foster KJ, et al. Detection of dangerous malnutrition. *J Parenter Enter Nutr* 1982;6:119–121.
149. Seltzer MH, Bastidas JA, Cooper DM, et al. Instant nutritional assessment. *J Parenter Enter Nutr* 1979;3:157–159.
150. Seltzer MH, Slocum BA, Cataldi-Betcher EL, et al. Instant nutritional assessment: absolute weight loss and surgical mortality. *J Parenter Enter Nutr* 1982;6:218–221.
151. Ottery FD. Rethinking nutritional support of the cancer patient: a new field of nutritional oncology. *Semin Oncol* 1994;21:770–778.
152. Ottery FD. Modification of subjective global assessment (SGA) of nutritional status (NS) for oncology patients. 19th Clinical Congress, American Society for Parenteral and Enteral Nutrition, Miami, FL, January 15–18, 1995 (Abstr 119).
153. Detsky AF, McLaughlin JR, Baker JP, et al. What is subjective global assessment of nutritional status? *J Parenter Enter Nutr* 1987;11:8–13.
154. Ottery FD. Supportive nutrition to prevent cachexia and improve quality of life. *Semin Oncol* 1995;22:98–111.
155. Sluys TEMS, van de Ende ME, Swart GR, et al. Body composition in patients with acquired immunodeficiency syndrome: a validation study of bioelectrical impedance analysis. *J Parenter Enter Nutr* 1993;17:404–406.
156. Ottery FD. Cancer cachexia: Prevention, early diagnosis, and management. *Cancer Pract* 1994;2:123–131.
157. Blackburn GL, Harvey KB. Nutritional assessment as a routine in clinical medicine. *Postgrad Med* 1982;71:46.
158. Herrmann FR, Safran C, Levkoff SE, et al. Serum albumin level on admission as a predictor of death, length of stay, and readmission. *Arch Intern Med* 1992;152:125–130.
159. Pietsch JB, Meakins JL, MacLean LD. The delayed hypersensitivity response: application in clinical surgery. *Surgery* 1977;82:349–355.
160. Apovian CM, McMahon MM, Bistrian BR. Guidelines for refeeding the marasmic patient. *Crit Care Med* 1990;18:1030–1033.
161. Harris JA, Benedict FG. A biometric study of basal metabolism in man. Carnegie Institute of Washington, Washington, DC, 1919, publication no. 279.
162. Grant JP. *Handbook of total parenteral nutrition,* 2nd ed. Philadelphia: WB Saunders, 1992;208–209.
163. Aspen Board of Directors. Guidelines for the use of total parenteral nutrition in the hospitalized patient. *J Parenter Enter Nutr* 1986;10:441–444.
164. Lowry SF, Brennan MS. Intravenous feeding in the cancer patient. In: Rombeau JL, Caldwell MD, eds. *Parenteral nutrition.* Philadelphia: WB Saunders, 1986;445–470.
165. American Medical Association, Department of Food and Nutrition. Multivitamin Preparations for parenteral use: a statement by the nutrition advisory group. *J Parenter Enter Nutr* 1986;10:441–445.
166. Brown R, Querchia RA, Sigman R. Total nutrient admixture: a review. *J Parenter Enter Nutr* 1986;10:650–658.
167. Rombeau JL, Rolandelli RH, Wilmore DW. Nutritional support. In: Wilmore DW, Brennan MF, Harken AH, Holcroft JW, Meakins JL, eds. American College of Surgeons. *Care of the surgical patient.* New York: Scientific American, 2994;1–40.
168. Parker P Stroop, Greene H. A controlled comparison of continuous versus intermittent feeding in the treating of infants with intestinal disease. *J Pediatrics* 1981;99:360–364.
169. Heymsfield S, Casper K, Grossman G. Bioenergetic and metabolic response to continuous versus intermittent nasogastric feeding. *Metabolism* 1987;36:570–575.
170. Zarling EJ, Parmar JR, Mobarhan S, et al. Effective enteral formula infusion rate, osmolality and chemical composition upon clinical tolerance and carbohydrate absorption in normal subjects. *J Parenter Enter Nutr* 1986;10:588–590.
171. Pearlstone DB, Wolf RF, Berman RS, Burt ME, Brennan MF. Effect of systemic insulin on protein kinetics in postoperative cancer patients. *Ann Surg Oncol* 1992;1:257–267.
172. Ziegler TR, Young LS, Manson JM, Wilmore DW. Metabolic effect of recombinant human growth hormone in patients receiving parenteral nutrition. *Ann Surg* 1988;208:6–16.
173. Wolf RF, Nag B, Weksler B, Burt ME, Brennan MF. Effect of growth hormone on tumor and host in an animal model. *Ann Surg Oncol* 1994;1:314–320.
174. Harrison LE, Blumberg D, Berman RS, et al. Exogenous human growth hormone does not influence growth, protein kinetics, or cell cycle kinetics of human pancreatic carcinoma in vivo. *Surg Forum* 1994;65:469–471.
175. Klimberg VS, Souba WW, Salloum RM, et al. Glutamine enriched diets support muscle glumtamine metabolism without stimulating tumor growth. *J Surg Res* 1990;48:319–323.
176. Ziegler, TR, Young LS, Benfell K. Glutamine-supplemented parenteral nutrition improves nitrogen retention and reduces hospital mortality versus standard parenteral nutrition following bone marrow transplantation: a randomized, double-blinded trial. *Ann Intern Med* 1992;116:821–828.
177. Howard L. Home enteral and parenteral nutrition in cancer patients. *Cancer* 1993;72:3531–3541.
178. Howard L. Parenteral and enteral nutrition therapy. In: Wilson JD, Braunwald E, Isselbacher KJ, et al, eds. *Harrison's principles of internal medicine,* 12th ed. New York: McGraw-Hill, 1990;434.
179. North American Home Parenteral and Enteral Nutrition Patient Registry. *Annual Report 1985–1990.* Albany, NY: Oley Foundation, 12208, 1987–1992.
180. Bothe A, Orr G, Bistrian BR, Blackburn GL. Home hyperalimentation. *Compreh Ther* 1979;5:54.
181. Flowers JF, Ryan JA, Gough JA. Catheter-related complications of total parenteral nutrition. In: Fischer JE, editor. *Total parenteral nutrition.* Boston: Little, Brown, 1991;25–45.
182. Rogers JZ, McKee K, McDermott E. Peripherally inserted central venous catheters. In: Fish J, ed. *Support line* 1995;27(5):6–10.
183. Loughran SC, Borzatta M. Peripherally inserted central catheters: a report of 2506 catheter days. *J Parenter Enter Nutr* 1995;19:133–136.
184. Harvey KB, Moldwater LL, Bistrian BR, et al. Biological measures for the formulation of a hospital prognostic index. *Am J Clin Nutr* 1981;34:2013.

*Principles and Practice of Supportive Oncology,*
edited by Ann Berger et al.
Lippincott–Raven Publishers, Philadelphia ©1998

CHAPTER 42

# Dehydration

J. Andrew Billings

## THE CONTROVERSY ABOUT HYDRATION IN TERMINAL ILLNESS

Dehydration is a common clinical condition and a regular accompaniment to the dying process. As a prominent feature of the "final common pathway" (1) to death that so many dying persons follow, as they become weak, bedbound, unable to take fluids without assistance, and even unable to drink, dehydration may play a role in both aggravating and alleviating the discomfort of terminal disease, and may hasten dying or cause death.

Although fluid deficits should be prevented and treated in most clinical settings, the appropriateness of rehydration in late stages of terminal illness is debatable. In conventional medical management, dehydration is routinely avoided or reversed with fluid and electrolyte replacement, typically administered by an oral or parenteral route. Similarly, whenever a terminally ill patient seeks to prolong life and when the goals of treatment are to cure or to sustain life, maintaining adequate hydration is accepted medical management. For example, fluid replacement may be desirable for a dying patient who enjoys a reasonable quality of life but is unable to swallow, retain, or absorb oral fluids due to a condition affecting the mouth or gastrointestinal tract. Conversely, when a patient does not wish to delay death or even seeks to hasten dying, fluid replacement is generally inappropriate.

In terminally ill patients for whom the goal of treatment is primarily to assure comfort, the clinical significance of dehydration, particularly in the final few days and weeks of life, and the appropriateness of preventing this condition or of providing rehydration has been a controversial subject over the past two decades. Uncertainty exists both about the discomfort associated with different states of fluid balance, as well as whether symptoms are

best managed through hydration or through other palliative measures. The paradigmatic case in palliative care is the dying cancer patient who simply becomes too weak or too obtunded to maintain normal fluid intake, who will surely die soon but may die less comfortably or more quickly without rehydration. Similar issues commonly arise in managing terminal cancer patients with intestinal obstruction or noncancer patients with end-stage dementia and other debilitating neurologic conditions that affect the ability to maintain a normal fluid balance. When dehydration is precipitated by or at least partially the result of palliative medical management, such as the administration of analgesics and sedatives, clinicians often are particularly troubled or uncertain about the correct ethical course.

Palliative care clinicians, relying on extensive clinical experience with end-of-life care, have generally stated that the symptoms of dehydration in terminal illness are mild and readily treated through simple mouth care, making rehydration unnecessary in the final days of life (2–6). A small amount of empirical evidence supports this stance (5,7). The hospice literature has also stressed the discomfort, psychological distress, and even overt harm associated with fluid replacement, asserting that physical symptoms can be worsened through treatment and that intravenous lines or feeding tubes significantly diminish the quality of life for the dying patient and family. Recently, however, other members of the palliative medicine community have put forth concerns about undesirable consequences of terminal dehydration, new theories about the value of rehydration, and a few instances of apparent benefit from fluid replacement (8–13).

Unfortunately, few of these issues have been clarified through clinical research (9). Indeed, studies of fluid and electrolyte disorders in the final days of life are rare and difficult to carry out, and research on normal volunteers or patients at other phases of illness cannot readily be applied to the care of the dying. This chapter reviews the controversy about dehydration, focusing on terminally ill

J. A. Billings: Palliative Care Service, Massachusetts General Hospital, Boston, MA 02114.

patients for whom rehydration to prolong life is not a clearly desirable or achievable goal but for whom comfort is the prime concern. Relevant studies are interpreted in order to address many partially answered questions: What are current practices with regard to managing terminal hydration and how are these clinical strategies justified? How are fluid and electrolyte balance normally maintained? What problems and benefits are associated with fluid and electrolyte imbalance? How is dehydration clinically recognized? Should terminal dehydration be treated? If so, how?

## ETHICAL DECISION MAKING

Inextricably mixed with clinical discussions about the pathophysiology of terminal dehydration and the effects of alternate management strategies on the patient and family are important ethical and emotional issues that will only be touched on briefly here. Clearly, a host of psychological, social, ethical, moral, religious, and legal issues may influence views about dehydration and its management for patients, families, and clinicians. Cranford states that "for the most part, the use of artificial nutrition and hydration in the imminently dying is not a major ethical dilemma" (14), but the definition of imminently dying may be problematic, whereas moral and legal issues and clinical uncertainties may render clinicians unable to treat these matters as straightforward.

While the decision about administering fluids and electrolytes to a dehydrated, terminally ill patient may be treated as primarily an ethical matter (15,16), and even based on *a priori* or absolute principles, this chapter takes an individualistic, utilitarian approach to the controversy (17), seeking empirical evidence to understand the benefits and burdens for the patient of any action. The guiding principle is that "everything in the terminal phase of an irreversible illness should be clearly decided on the basis of whether it will make the patient more comfortable and whether it will honor his or her wishes" (18). We assume that the patient and his or her expressed values provide the core foundation for all medical decisions and that treatments are evaluated principally according to their consequences—benefits and burdens, both physical and psychosocial, weighed within the patient's value framework (19). We judge the merit of any intervention primarily by the subjective outcome for patient and, secondarily, for the family. No treatment is absolutely required—fluid administration is viewed as an elective medical regimen (15,16,20). Thus, dehydration per se does not require treatment, although symptoms associated with it may deserve palliation through either symptomatic measures or partial reversal of the underlying fluid or electrolyte imbalance. Such an approach has generally been supported in the courts (19), at least in the United States (21).

When a patient is unable to express his or her wishes, advanced directives will be followed. If relatives disagree with these advanced directives, physicians have a professional duty to comfort distressed family members, but the family's role in decision making is primarily to assist in providing substituted judgment, i.e., figuring out what the patient would have wanted if he or she could express his or her wishes, not in expressing the relatives' personal preferences for management. At the same time, a focus on patient autonomy should not lead clinicians to ignore the family: attention to their wishes is often a significant and even overriding factor when patients make decisions (19). Thus, in select circumstances, fluids might be administered to comfort family members who do not appreciate or accept the clinician's view that such treatment is unnecessary or even potentially harmful.

## EMPIRICAL STUDIES OF CLINICAL PRACTICE: TERMINAL HYDRATION AS A "MEDICAL LAST RITE"

Conventional medical teaching suggests that dehydration is a disagreeable, perhaps even very painful, state that should be alleviated by replacement of fluid and electrolytes, and that rehydration produces significant benefit and little harm. Indeed, the development of dehydration may be viewed as a sign of medical neglect in some populations, particularly in the nursing home (22,23).

Such an approach is often carried over into the management of terminal illness, where rehydration has been described as a "medical last rite" (24). In Micetich's study from the early 1980s of how doctors would hypothetically manage a comatose dying cancer patient with widespread metastases, 73% of physicians indicated that they would order an intravenous infusion at a "physiologically rehydrating rate." If a peripheral route were not available, 40% would start a central venous line or perform an intravenous "cutdown." The remaining 27% of physicians would replace fluids but at a lesser rate. About a third of these doctors would maintain the intravenous infusion after 3 days, regardless of whether clinical improvement was noted (15). Similar results were reported from Wales in 1989 by Marin (25), who also noted that house officers were more likely than senior physicians to administer fluids, though all based their decision on the patient's comfort. Penn's 1992 study from the United Kingdom revealed fewer doctors— slightly less than half of either senior or junior staff— who would prescribe intravenous fluids in such a setting (26). In Burge's Canadian study, 81% of cancer patients dying in a tertiary care facility received intravenous fluids within the last 30 days of life, and 69% died with fluids being infused (24). Nurses based in general hospitals similarly view dehydration as unpleasant and hence deserving of treatment (6). While the reasons for administering fluids are not always clear—and some treatment might simply be viewed as an ethical imperative—physicians often noted concerns with discomfort or thirst from dehydration, even though a significant minority of doctors would neither monitor the patient's condition for the adequacy of rehydration nor replace fluids at a rate sufficient to restore normal fluid balance. In other words, some physicians provide fluids at a rate that does not produce rehydration, suggesting either that the intravenous line is meant as a symbolic gesture, perhaps applied somewhat deceptively insofar as it implies that the patient is being rehydrated, or that some treatment, albeit ineffective, rather than no treatment, is viewed as morally necessary.

In contrast, 85% of hospice physicians in Miller's study reported that death "without artificial nutritional/hydration support" is "peaceful/comfortable," whereas only 4% noted painful thirst and starvation, and 11% were unsure (27).

## NORMAL FLUID HOMEOSTASIS AND CHANGES WITH AGING

### Osmoregulation

Water homeostasis is maintained through parallel neuroendocrine influences on excretion (via the kidneys) and on intake (via thirst). Renal excretion of free water is primarily influenced by pituitary excretion of arginine vasopressin (AVP). This hormone, also known as antidiuretic hormone (ADH), increases water reabsorption in the collecting ducts of the kidney. Two major inputs—osmotic and hemodynamic—contribute both to the production of arginine vasopressin and the generation of thirst: (a) osmoreceptor neurons in the hypothalamus, which respond to hyperosmolality and communicate with cells producing AVP in the posterior pituitary; and (b) extracellular fluid (ECF) sensors—baroreceptors in the aortic arch, cardiac atria, and carotid sinus—that respond to diminished ECF, transmitting information to the brainstem via cranial nerves (vagal and glossopharyngeal) and from the brainstem to the hypothalamus by ascending noradrenergic pathways. An additional contribution may possibly be made by angiotensin II responding to the blood or brain renin-angiotensin system.

Increased osmotic pressure is the prime stimulus for thirst, and appears with 1.23% osmotic cellular dehydration in male medical students (28). Vasopressin is released at osmolality levels of 280–287 mOsm/kg, but thirst appears simultaneously or even earlier (at 296–299 mOsm/kg) in some studies, even before urine is maximally concentrated and renal mechanisms are saturated. In studies of thirst from hypertonic saline infusion, thirst appeared with an increase of 7 mOsm/kg and an increase of serum sodium of 4.2 meq/L.

### Thirst

While thirst is believed to be controlled by similar mechanisms as have been demonstrated to control renal water excretion, it may sometimes behave independently. For example, common experience tells us that certain fluids are more effective than others in quenching thirst and that cold liquids are preferable to warm ones, yet the salt and water content of these drinks and their immediate physiologic effects on salt and water homeostasis may be identical (29).

In healthy individuals who become dehydrated and then replenish body water, the subsequent inhibition of thirst and of vasopressin secretion occurs in two stages: first, within minutes of drinking, thirst and AVP secretion are promptly inhibited; later, water is absorbed, hypertonicity is corrected, and the ECF volume is restored, abolishing the original stimuli to thirst and retention of free water. Dehydrated subjects experience prompt (within 2.5 minutes) relief of thirst from drinking fluids, well before plasma dilution is evident (occurring as early as 12.5 minutes) or before plasma volume had been restored (occurring as early as 7.5 minutes). Similarly, after 24 hours of water deprivation, healthy young subjects experience thirst, increased pleasantness of the taste of water, dryness of the mouth, and an unpleasant taste in the mouth, but all sensations return to normal levels with 2.5–5 minutes after the onset of drinking, and the rate of drinking slows markedly after this initial period (30). The availability of food or other osmolar substances may normally be required for achieving full rehydration.

Preabsorptive oropharyngeal factors can reduce thirst and AVP secretion and may increase atrial natriuretic peptide (ANP) immediately upon drinking water and well before correction of water deficits, thus discouraging overcompensation (overhydration). In some animals, satiety for fluids may be related to gastric distention, but similar phenomena have not been demonstrated in humans. Oropharyngeal factors (presumably related at least partly to local osmotic dehydration) are associated with thirst, and may also be affected by disease processes and various treatments. Inhibition of thirst is accomplished more effectively with cold liquid—ice works well—and may be unrelated to the tonicity of fluids being used for replenishment or even the palatability of oral fluids (31). Thus, as noted in the hospice literature, relief of thirst may be provided by amounts of liquid too small to correct fluid deficits.

### Sodium Homeostasis and Extracellular Fluid Volume Control

Osmoregulation is primarily determined by water intake and excretion, but sodium regulation (and hence, extracellular fluid volume or effective circulating volume) is primarily controlled through sodium excretion via the renin-angiotensin-aldosterone system (32). Additionally, plasma atrial natriuretic peptide (ANP) responds to volume expansion and has prompt, potent diuretic and natriuretic actions that may also play a role in volume regulation. ANP falls with dehydration, reducing renal water loss (28). There is no predictable relationship between the plasma sodium concentration and the extracellular fluid volume or urinary sodium excretion (33). The control of sodium excretion differs from the control of water excretion, except insofar as hypovolemia can be a stimulus to ADH release and thirst.

## Homeostasis and Aging

The pathophysiology of dehydration and the response of dehydrated persons to fluid replenishment has been studied almost entirely in healthy young subjects, including soldiers and athletes, and not in ill or dying patients. However, research on the elderly suggests that aging is associated with disturbances in homeostatic capacity, reflected both in control of water intake and in excretion, predisposing the elderly to disturbances in salt and water balance. Similar alterations in fluid balance regulation may occur in medically ill persons.

Elderly men show less thirst than younger men, just as they exhibit less sense of taste. They have a higher threshold before developing thirst in response to dehydration or hypertonicity, suggesting a deficit in responsiveness to dehydration in bringing thirst to consciousness. They also generally show decreased water intake in response to dehydration. Some elderly—and this also appears true of many dying persons—have a reduced ability to seek water or communicate a need for water.

Altered neuroendocrine controls of salt and water balance also make the elderly more susceptible to fluid and electrolyte disturbances. Aged kidneys are less able to retain water, although the AVP response to dehydration is probably normal in the elderly, suggesting renal resistance to vasopressin. Reduced sensitivity of baroceptors has also been reported, as well as diminished renin-angiotensin-aldosterone. The elderly do inhibit thirst with fluid replacement, but do not inhibit AVP secretion as do younger patients, and plasma AVP does not fall as immediately as with younger patients after water replacement (34). The elderly are more susceptible to fluid overload due to blunted inhibition of dehydration-induced AVP secretion (31).

The elderly also exhibit reduced renal sodium and water conservation, indicating diminished renal concentrating ability (35–39). Additionally, the elderly do not rehydrate adequately when offered free access to water. They do not excrete water as effectively as younger subjects, predisposing them to overhydration and hyponatremia. Their osmostat may be reset to a higher osmolality when they encounter stressful settings or other chronic conditions (40,41).

## Pathophysiology and Symptoms of Dehydration (5,42)

Dehydration is a loss of normal body water. Classic studies of short-term, experimentally induced dehydration in small series of normal subjects (42–45) suggest that quite different clinical syndromes can be associated with two prototypical forms of dehydration: sodium depletion (or hyponatremic dehydration) and pure water loss (or hypernatremic dehydration). Few commentators on the symptoms associated with terminal hydration have taken this research into account or provided clear data about the type and degree of dehydration being studied.

*Hyponatremic dehydration* occurs experimentally when subjects undergo salt and water depletion but only water is restored. Clinically, the condition results from loss of sodium and water but with relatively greater sodium loss or when relatively hypotonic solutions are used for replenishment. Common causes of predominant sodium loss include diuretic use, vomiting, diarrhea, osmotic diuresis (e.g., from hyperglycemia), salt-wasting renal conditions, third spacing (ascites), and adrenal insufficiency.

Sodium is the principal cation of the extracellular fluid compartment. Salt depletion is associated with loss of salt and water primarily from the intravascular and interstitial fluid compartments. Predominant clinical signs are those associated with *volume depletion*: weight loss, diminished skin turgor, dry mucus membranes, reduced sweat, and orthostatic hypotension, perhaps accompanied by near-faint or syncope. Laboratory correlates include azotemia (with a disproportionate increase in BUN compared to creatinine), hyponatremia, hemoconcentration, and high urine osmolality with low sodium concentration. Neuropsychiatric manifestations—weakness, apathy, lethargy, restlessness, confusion, stupor, coma, and seizures—have been related to cerebral edema and particularly occur when hyponatremia is severe or develops rapidly. Less commonly reported symptoms of hyponatremia include psychosis and localized neurologic findings. Persons engaged in physical labor describe muscle cramps. Symptoms reported in the elderly included anorexia, nausea, vomiting, drowsiness, confusion, and sometimes weakness, coma, seizures, and death (46).

Anorexia, nausea, vomiting, and loss of taste have been reported in experimental and clinical subjects with hyponatremic dehydration. These gastrointestinal symptoms may lead to diminished salt intake or further salt loss, leading to a vicious cycle of worsened salt depletion (42). Aberrations in flavor and taste generally do not occur until severe ECF volume depletion has developed (43).

Notably, thirst, which is provoked primarily by hyperosmolar states, may be absent or mild in patients with hyponatremic dehydration, although marked volume loss and hypotension may stimulate ADH and water craving.

*Hypernatremic dehydration* occurs when water loss is proportionally greater than sodium loss or replenishment is provided with relatively hypertonic fluids. Experimentally, this condition occurs when subjects lose salt and water but are given limited access to water while continuing to ingest salt. Thirst is a powerful sensation, and normal adult subjects with access to water—persons capable of experiencing thirst and ingesting fluids—generally do not become hypernatremic under a variety of conditions (33). Clinically, this pattern of dehydration develops in confused or somnolent persons or those unable to drink without assistance who are losing water disproportionately to salt or for whom water is inadequately replaced. The precipitating event may be fever, increased insensible fluid loss in a hot climate, vomiting, diarrhea, diuretic or laxative use, or just insensitivity to thirst. Less commonly, solute loading from intravenous or feeding tubes and adrenal hyperfunction (Cushing's syndrome, or hyperaldosteronism) or corticosteroid treatment can produce this syndrome. It is also observed in patients undergoing an osmotic or postobstructive diuresis or fluid loss from burns.

Two thirds of body water resides in the intracellular fluid compartment, so that equilibration from losses of extracellular fluid will result in water loss from cells, which is a potent trigger for thirst and ADH release. Intense thirst is a key symptom of hypernatremic dehydration, whereas extracellular fluid volume may be well maintained, so that skin turgor, blood pressure, and pulse may be relatively normal. The only major laboratory finding is hypernatremia. As pure water loss worsens, mental status changes ensue, including confusion, progressing to obtundation and coma, presumably related to cerebral shrinkage. Profound neurologic damage has been reported in children. These neuropsychiatric symptoms may hinder the ability to replace fluids. Fatigue and muscular weakness have also been reported.

### Mixed Dehydration Disorders

Dehydrated, terminally ill patients (and many other clinical and experimental subjects with dehydration) present with mixed disorders of fluid and salt loss. Isotonic dehydration may occur. Indeed, a few studies of electrolytes, osmolality, BUN, and creatinine in terminal illness indicate relatively minor or no abnormalities (47–50), as well as uncertain benefits of intravenous fluid treatment in terms of metabolic changes or improved consciousness (51).

A variety of studies of normal subjects undergoing experimental dehydration—including healthy workers, or soldiers in hot environments, or athletes—reveal that even persons who have free access to fluids during activities that are associated with fluid and electrolyte loss develop progressive fluid loss, termed "voluntary" dehydration. The perception of effort during exercise increases in proportion to fluid deficits. Subjects are described as morose, aggressive, demoralized, apathetic, and uncoor-

dinated. Remarkably, feelings of well-being return within minutes of the resumption of drinking (52).

### Additional Influences on Fluid Homeostasis

As described above, healthy elderly subjects respond somewhat differently to dehydration and rehydration than do healthy younger subjects. These differences and others may be reflected in the general palliative care population. Disease-specific susceptibility to fluid and electrolyte disorders may also occur, as, for instance, has been noted in Alzheimer's disease (53) and stroke in the elderly (54).

Opioid peptides are involved in the control of fluid ingestion (55). The endogenous opioid system may influence the drinking response and play a role in the hypodipsia of the elderly (56), whereas exogenous opioids, including opioid antagonists, may modulate various ingestive behaviors, though their influence on thirst and drinking behavior is uncertain.

### CLINICAL ASSESSMENT OF DEHYDRATION (57)

How does one identify a patient as being dehydrated? The sensitivity and specificity of various clinical methods for assessing fluid balance have not been rigorously determined. Clinical teachings point to the following:

1. Thirst and a *history* of diminished intake or increased fluid loss;
2. *Physical findings*, such as weight loss, dry mouth, dry tongue, reduced axillary sweat, dry skin, reduced skin turgor, and postural hypotension and/or acceleration of the pulse upon rising; and
3. *Laboratory tests*, including concentrated urine, hyperosmolality, increased hematocrit, hypernatremia, and azotemia with a disproportionate rise in the BUN in relation to creatinine.

No physical findings offer conclusive evidence of dehydration. In a study of elderly patients presenting to an emergency ward, indicators that correlated best with dehydration severity (generally hypernatremic dehydration) and that were not age-related included tongue dryness, longitudinal tongue furrows (58), dryness of the mucus membranes of the mouth, upper body muscle weakness, confusion, speech difficulty, and sunkenness of eyes, but not sensations of thirst or dryness (59).

A moist mouth is unlikely with significant dehydration, but oral dryness may be related to dehydration, mouth breathing, Sjogren's syndrome, and various drugs, particularly those with anticholinergic properties. Reduced skin turgor may be difficult to judge in the elderly. The presence of axillary sweating in ill elderly has a high negative predictive value for dehydration, but reduced sweating has only a modest positive predictive value (60). Pediatricians assess dehydration with capillary refilling (carefully measured with some standardization of technique) and elasticity (tenting) (61), but these measures have not been examined in a medically ill adult population. Postural hypotension may occur for a variety of reasons unrelated to fluid status in elderly and ill persons, and reflex tachycardia may be absent in the setting of cardiac conduction abnormalities, pacemakers, or beta blockade. Confusion is common in dehydrated elderly patients, but may be a cause rather than a consequence of fluid imbalance (62).

As noted above, dehydration may be isotonic, and significant fluid loss may occur without notable elevations of the BUN and creatinine.

## DOES DEHYDRATION CAUSE SYMPTOMS IN TERMINAL ILLNESS?

Experienced hospice clinicians have repeatedly stated that dehydration is usually not associated with disagreeable symptoms in the late stages of terminal illness, that dying patients generally do not complain of thirst, and that dry mouth can be relieved readily with proper mouth care, sips of water, or other methods of maintaining oral moisture. There has been little clinical research to support or contradict these assertions. Certainly, the development of terminal dehydration may be evidence that thirst is inactive in many of these patients. Intentional dehydration has even been proposed as an ethically acceptable and physically comfortable form of suicide for terminally ill patients eager to hasten death without imposing on their physicians (63,64).

### Studies in Healthy Subjects

As noted above, studies in healthy subjects have generally reported troublesome symptoms with dehydration. Adolph's research on soldiers in the desert indicates that thirst and dry mouth are relatively minor problems during periods of mild dehydration (loss of 1–5% of body water) and often abate after a while. Soldiers predominantly complained of muscular fatigue while walking but also noted intestinal ache, nausea, headache, and irritability or drowsiness, along with a lack of interest in food. Worsened thirst was noted at higher (6–10%) deficits, whereas progressive obtundation or delirium was seen at these and greater levels of dehydration. Decreased salivary flow was seen with even small water deficits, was pronounced at 4% or more, and was not relieved with pilocarpine (65). Even in young army subjects, thirst was not a perfect indication of fluid imbalance, and "voluntary dehydration"—a loss of normal body water despite the availability of water for oral rehydration—occurred at a level of 2–5% (66).

Similarly, thirst has been shown to increase with water deficits ranging from 1% to 7% of total body water in normal volunteers (67). Subjects noted mouth dryness and irritation; thirst; bad and chalk-like taste in mouth; dry, scratchy, warm throat; chapped lips; feeling weary, dizzy, lightheaded, sleepy, tired, or irritable; headache; and loss of appetite. Volunteers with severe (7%) water deficits had trouble sleeping and noted trembling. Significant other gastro-intestinal sensations were not reported.

### Studies in the Terminally Ill (see Table 1)

Terminally ill patients suffer a plethora of disagreeable symptoms, many of which might be attributed to or related to dehydration, and some of which may foster fluid imbalance. Vomiting, anorexia, confusion, drowsiness, and dry mouth/thirst each occur in at least one third of patients, often in one half or three quarters (68–72). However, a cause-and-effect relationship between dehydration and these symptoms has not been established. Even dry mouth may be related to medications, mouth breathing, and other factors unrelated to water balance. In one study, the state of consciousness of terminal cancer patients was inversely correlated with serum sodium and urine osmolality, but not clearly with plasma osmolality (49).

Healthy persons who become dehydrated in a research study or while working in a hot climate or exercising may be bothered by water deficits in a fashion different from that experienced by terminally ill persons or other patients, who often become dehydrated in part because of physical deficits related to their terminal illness. Also, some of the consequences of dehydration in normal volunteers, such as reduced exercise capacity, probably have little clinical significance for terminally ill patients.

Burge performed a careful study of symptoms associated with dehydration in terminally ill cancer patients (47). In a sample population drawn from an inpatient palliative care service, he (a) estimated 24-hour fluid intake; (b) described mouth care; (c) reviewed charts to determine whether the patient had oral disease or was receiving medications that could produce dry mouth; (d) asked patients about seven symptoms that might be associated with dehydration, quantifying their responses with a 100-mm visual analog scale; and (e) measured serum sodium, urea, and osmolality. Half of patients who were approached had to be excluded because of confusion, drowsiness, or weakness. He found a high incidence of apparently bothersome symptoms, including thirst (mean visual analog scale rating=54 mm), dry mouth (60 mm), bad taste in mouth (47 mm), fatigue, and increased pleasure in drinking (62 mm), compared to nausea (24 mm) and pain (35 mm). There was no correlation between these symptoms and various predictors or confounding variables, including measures of fluid intake, metabolic abnormalities, or use of drying medications. Mean and median serum sodium, osmolality, and urea were within normal range, though almost half of study patients were felt to be taking <750 cm$^3$ of fluid a day. Thirst seemed to decrease with age and was more apparent in patients who lived for briefer periods (<14 days). Although these data are difficult to interpret, it appears that significant thirst and the desire for fluids are common in the terminally ill but that a clear association between these symptoms and dehydration, either as cause or effect, is lacking.

Ellershaw followed 82 dying hospice patients with diminished oral intake who were not receiving artificial fluid replacement (50). One serum sample was obtained on entry (1–5 days prior to death). Mean osmolality was 298 mOsm/kg with half of values below 295 mOsm/kg. The mean serum sodium and potassium levels were normal. Mean urea was 15.5 mmol/L with a range of 2.9–8304 mmol/L (normal 2.5–6.5 mmol/L) and the mean creatinine was 177.3 mol/L with a range of 32–1416 mol/L (normal 60–120 mol/L). Despite many patients having relatively normal chemistries, 87% noted thirst and 83% a dry mouth. The more dehydrated patients complained more frequently of dry mouth but less frequently of feeling thirst. No statistical difference was noted in terms of respiratory tract secretions (as indicated by audible airway sounds or the need for hyoscine hydrobromide or the expectoration of purulent sputum) between patients identified as dehydrated or not dehydrated, though both groups had high levels of thirst. Ninety-one percent of patients were receiving drugs that might cause a dry mouth.

In the most important study so far on the discomfort of terminal dehydration, McCann followed 32 terminally ill patients who were initially able to report symptoms of hunger, thirst, and dry mouth (7). Treatment consisted of comfort measures only, including offering (but not forcing) nutrition and liquids, as well as opioids for pain and dyspnea, and careful mouth care. Practically all (84%) patients were judged to have died comfortably, whereas 13% experienced some discomfort. Thirst or dry mouth were absent in about a third, present only initially in about a third, and present until death in the remaining third. All symptomatic patients were relieved with food and fluids, ice chips, and mouth care. Relief lasted between one and several hours.

Reduced intravascular volume and glomerular filtration associated with dehydration may lead to renal failure and to the accumulation of drug metabolites. Relatively scant pharmacokinetic data are available to anticipate the effect of mild or moderate dehydration on the metabolism of various commonly used medicines in palliative care, the clinical consequences of these alterations in drug metabolism, the need for adjusting dosages, or the effects of rehydration. In the case of opioids, renal failure is associated with instances of confusion, myoclonus, and seizures, probably related to accumulation of toxic metabolites (73–75). Fainsinger noted a decrease in the need for terminal sedation in a population of patients who received, among other interventions, hypodermoclysis. Clearly, serious dehydration causes confusion and restlessness in nonterminal patients, symptoms that are often reported in the terminally ill (76–79), many of whom are also receiving sedating medications. Confusional states could be caused or aggravated by dehydration. The role of sedating medications in producing symptoms in the final days of life deserves careful study.

**The Burden of Treating Dehydration**

Some commentators particularly stress the burden of treatment for dehydration: pain and complications from inserting intravenous lines; infections, phlebitis, and other problems with the infusion sites; immobilization of limbs and other curtailment of movement or requirement for restraints; discomfort and aspiration from nasogastric tubes; and fluid overload. A high incidence of complications from nasogastric tubes or gastrostomy are reported from skilled nursing facilities (80,81). Little convincing information is available about how an intravenous line or feeding tube influences the personal comfort, mobility, anxiety level, sense of depersonalization, or ability to enjoy physical contact of patients and families.

**TREATMENT OF THIRST AND OTHER POSSIBLE SYMPTOMS OF DEHYDRATION**

Treatment of thirst does not require rehydration, nor is dehydration invariably associated with troubling thirst. Rehydration can abolish thirst, even before enough water and electrolytes have been absorbed to correct osmolality, serum sodium, or extracellular fluid volume. Relief of thirst may be provided by amounts of liquid too small to correct fluid deficits. Other factors may influence the perception of thirst, such as immersion in cool water (82) and ingestion of a variety of "antidipsogens"—substances that suppress thirst (83). At the same time, thirst is not merely a reflection of a dry mouth and may not be entirely relieved by oral fluids (28,84) or substances increasing salivary flow.

Mouth care to relieve dry mouth and thirst is discussed elsewhere in this book and includes stopping or reducing medications that reduce salivation, which may include opioids (85); encouragement of fluid intake; moistening of the lips with liquids or lubrication with petroleum jelly; moistening of the mouth with fluids, ice chips, popsicles, or lubricants; and attention to oral hygiene (including mouth rinses and treatment of specific infections). Hospice texts commonly admonish against the drying effects of glycerin swabs, and patients seem to prefer solutions containing carboxycellulose or mucin to plain water, though only mucin-based substitutes have demonstrated advantages (86,87). Pilocarpine has effectively alleviated radiation-induced xerostomia in head-and-neck cancer patients and in other patients with dry mouth, as long some residual salivary gland function is present (88–90).

Additional attention to skin care may be required in dehydrated patients. Care in positioning, transferring, and ambulation should be taken to avoid postural symptoms. Nausea and vomiting, if present, are treated with standard antiemetics, whereas muscular twitching and other neuropsychiatric manifestations can be managed, when bothersome, with opioid rotation or sedatives. Medications may often be discontinued in the final days of life, and reduction of the dosage for essential medications may also be considered to avoid toxicity associated with renal failure and altered drug metabolism.

## HOW SHOULD FLUID AND ELECTROLYTES BE ADMINISTERED?

In the absence of abnormal water and electrolyte losses (e.g., from insensible, gastrointestinal, urinary, or wound losses and internal fluid shifts), a standard goal for fluid intake in a normal subject is 1500–3000 ml of water daily or 8–10 glasses of fluid a day. This should produce a urine output of 1000–1500 ml/day (91). Less vigorous hydration is often sufficient in older, ill persons. Although special rehydration solutions have been devised for athletes, their potential benefit has only been demonstrated in exercise-induced dehydration in healthy, young volunteers. Commercial preparations are not reimbursed by Medicare or Medicaid, though they may be more palatable than plain water or other solutions (57).

When oral intake appears to be insufficient to maintain fluid balance and when avoidance of dehydration is desirable, a first step may include the stopping of diuretics. Standard methods of fluid and electrolyte replenishment include administration through intravenous lines and enteral feeding tubes. Bruera and associates have described the advantages of hypodermoclysis—subcutaneous fluid infusion—in palliative medicine (92,93), noting ease of access compared to intravenous administration, absence of need to monitor for clotting in the needle or even cessation of the infusion, relatively minor local complications, and infrequent need to change the insertion site. Hypodermoclysis may be easier to manage (and less subject to regulation) in the home or nursing home than intravenous therapy (57,94). Further studies are needed on the appropriate use of hyaluronidase or corticosteroids in the infusate, choice of electrolyte solutions, and concomitant administration of medications (95–97).

Rectal instillation of fluids has also been described as a useful, convenient measure in palliative care; a liter of fluids can be instilled over 6–8 hours (98,99).

Feeding tubes inserted through the mouth or nose are generally uncomfortable for patients and may cause complications, though researchers have had difficulty distinguishing some complications attributable to the tube from those associated with the condition that led to the insertion of the tube. Among complications are agitation, self-extubation, aspiration, and tube dysfunction. In the first 2 weeks with an nasogastric tube, 67% of patients extubated themselves and developed agitation. Percutaneous endoscopic gastrostomy has largely replaced operative gastrostomy and may be better tolerated than peroral tubes; it should be considered in patients requiring sustained fluid and nutritional replacement.

## ARE THERE BENEFITS TO DEHYDRATION?

A variety of clinicians have sung the virtues of dehydration in terminal illness and speculated on various salutary neuroendocrine consequences (100–103) (see Table 1). Among the likely benefits are a decreased need to void (and reduced need for catheterization and fewer difficulties associated with moving to the bathroom or commode or getting on a bedpan) and decreased urinary incontinence; decreased gastrointestinal secretions, possibly leading to reduced nausea, vomiting, cramps, and diarrhea; diminished pulmonary secretions, possibly reducing congestion, cough, dyspnea, terminal "death rattle," and the need for suctioning; and reduced ascites and pleural or pericardial effusions, and reduced cerebral edema, tumor edema, and peripheral edema, as well as their associated symptoms. More theoretical benefits include electrolyte imbalance and hypovolemia producing a desirable altered consciousness (lethargy, coma) with associated analgesia (104,105); ketosis, which may be associated with anesthesia (104,106); and increased production of endogenous opioid peptides in malnutrition and dehydration (104,107,108). A number of clinicians have noted that treatment of dehydration in small bowel obstruction only leads to worsened vomiting (109,110).

By accepting dehydration, painful procedures are avoided. Intravenous lines or feeding tubes may be associated with various complications, discomforts, nuisances, and costs from their placement, maintenance, and need for replacement. Disagreeable venipunctures may be required when fluid and electrolyte therapy is closely monitored. Reportedly, "tubes make a cuddle almost impossible" (111).

Dehydration is sometimes compared with overhydration rather than with maintenance of good fluid balance (see Table 1). Certainly, any attempt at maintaining hydration runs the risk of producing overhydration. Overhydration may cause or worsen peripheral or pulmonary edema, ascites, pleuropericardial fluid, and tumor swelling and weeping, and may increase oral, gastrointestinal, and pulmonary secretions and urinary output. Terminally ill patients often are malnourished and have low serum albumins, which may predispose them to developing symptomatic fluid overload (112).

**TABLE 1.** *Possible effects of fluid balance on comfort in terminal illness*

| Body system | Consequences of dehydration | Beneficial effects of rehydration for a dehydrated patient | Undesirable effects of rehydration or excess hydration |
|---|---|---|---|
| General appearance | Sunken eyes, wasted appearance | Improved appearance | Uncomfortable and unwelcome procedures to provide, maintain, and monitor hydration:venipunctures; insertion and maintenance of intravenous lines or enteral feeding devices<br>Immobility and awkwardness due to lines or tubes; need for restraints<br>Increased demands on family and heightened anxiety related to care for medical apparatus<br>Increased nursing needs<br>Expense |
| Mouth | Reduced salivation, dry mouth, difficulty talking<br>Thirst<br>Bad taste, reduced taste<br>Dry, cracked lips<br>Predisposition to oral infections, sores | Normal oral moisture, improved oral comfort, clearer speech<br>Relief of thirst<br>Improved taste, enjoyment of food | Excess secretions, drooling, need for suctioning |
| Skin | Poor turgor, predisposition to bed sores<br>Diminished swelling/weeping from wounds<br>Reduced sweating, impaired thermoregulation, fever, sweats | Healthier skin<br><br>Normal sweating, improved thermoregulation | Recurrence or development of edema<br>Weeping and swelling of wounds<br>Sweating<br>Pain, inflammation, phlebitis, infections from intravenous or subcutaneous lines |
| Pulmonary | Dry airway, viscous secretions, difficulty clearing secretions; reduced death rattle<br><br>Reduced secretions with concomitant reduced cough and reduced need for suctioning<br>Reduced congestion, wheezing, dyspnea<br>Reduced pleural effusions with reduced dyspnea | Normal or increased secretions<br><br><br>Facilitates productive cough, clearing of secretions | Increased secretions, cough, congestion, dyspnea, death rattle; need for pulmonary toilet, suctioning<br>Aspiration provoked by feeding tubes and increased GI fluids<br><br><br>Recurrence or development of pleural effusion and its consequences |
| GI tract | Constipation<br>Reduced secretions (advantageous with obstruction, vomiting, diarrhea)<br>Reduced cramps, pain, and vomiting in patient with bowel obstruction<br>Possible nausea, vomiting, anorexia<br>Reduced ascites | Normal bowel function<br><br><br><br><br><br>Ascites | Excess GI secretions<br>Probable worsened GI obstruction<br>Normal secretions may be troublesome for patient with bowel obstruction, and may aggravate nausea and vomiting<br>Increased ascites |
| Urinary tract | Reduced glomerular filtration, reduced clearance of normal metabolic products, azotemia; when severe, may cause fatigue, nausea, somnolence, etc.<br>Reduced drug clearance, possible accumulation of metabolites, possible prolonged action of agents with reduced need for dosing and potential for overdosing | Normal renal function; resolution of azotemic symptoms<br><br><br>Improved renal drug clearance with reduction of toxic metabolites or enhanced clearance of toxic levels | Edema, other sequelae of fluid overload<br><br><br>Improved renal function implies need for more frequent dosing of some drugs |

**TABLE 1.** *Continued.*

| Body system | Consequences of dehydration | Beneficial effects of rehydration for a dehydrated patient | Undesirable effects of rehydration or excess hydration |
|---|---|---|---|
| Urinary tract (continued) | Reduced urine output; reduced need to void or be catheterized, reduced incontinence and associated care needs<br>Possible increased urinary tract infections | Normal voiding | Excess voiding, incontinence, associated care problems |
| Cardiovascular | Hypotension, postural hypotension, tachycardia, dizziness, syncope, fatigue<br>Possibly reduced pericardial fluid | Resolution or improvement of postural symptoms | Congestive heart failure<br><br>Recurrence or development of pericardial effusion |
| Neuromuscular and neuro-psychiatric | Fatigue, asthenia, ataxia<br>Headache<br>Muscle cramps<br>Neuromuscular irritability, myoclonus<br>Personality and mood changes, apathy, lethargy, restlessness<br>Confusion, obtundation, coma; perhaps less pain and suffering<br>Reduced cerebral edema and associated headache, confusion, etc.<br>Seizures | Resolution or improvement of neuromuscular symptoms | Agitation associated with invasive procedures, immobility<br>Worsened cerebral edema and associated headache, confusion, etc. |
| Metabolic | Hypernatremia, hyponatremia<br>Hypercalcemia<br>Hemoconcentration, thrombotic diathesis | Improved general comfort from correction of fluid and electrolyte disorders | Fluid and electrolyte disorders may be aggravated |
| Psychosocial and family | Concerns about neglect, deprivation, starvation | Sense of providing caring, comfort, and nourishment | Meddling, fostering inappropriate interventions; medicalization of death: focussing on laboratory tests and other medical outcomes rather than on comfort and psychosocial support support<br>Failing to acknowledge imminence of death |
|  | May postpone or hasten death | Postpone or hasten death | May hasten or postpone death |

## CONCLUSION

Polarized arguments around the supportive use of fluids and nutrition in terminal illness are common within clinical medicine, as well as in ethics and law. A host of anecdotal and sometimes cloyingly romantic or prejudicial observations and gross exaggerations have been seized on to justify administration or withholding of fluids, and the debate has been marred by the use of provocative, emotion-laden, and often confusing terms or slogans (113): abandonment, artificial, barbaric custom (114), basic care, cruelty, dignity, forced, natural, neglect, overload, sanctity of life, starvation, and so forth. Moreover, at least in the United States where hospices are typically reimbursed at a daily rate that must include all mandated services, eagerness in arguing against potentially expensive rehydration methods and their monitoring might be construed as reflecting fiscal rather than clinical concerns.

In the last hours of life, few would argue that rehydration has any justification unless specific, troubling symptoms fail to respond to simpler palliative measures and these troubling symptoms are likely to be ameliorated by fluid replacement. In late phases of terminal illness—when death is near but not certain within hours or days—indications for treating dehydration are not entirely clear. Limited research is available, and studies are difficult to perform. As with other difficult decisions about intervening in terminal illness, a therapeutic trial of hydration may be considered if troubling target symptoms do not respond to simple comfort measures. Rehydration should not be continued if subjective improvement does not occur.

Careful studies of healthy persons document many disagreeable symptoms associated with dehydration. Some palliative care programs have reported a "crescendo of pain" in the last 48 hours of life when dehydration is common, and certainly dying patients experience a multitude of symptoms, some of which might be caused or aggravated by dehydration and relieved by fluid replacement. However, the best studies of terminally ill persons and the bulk of clinical experience with end-of-life care suggest that the vast majority of dying persons can be kept comfortable by taking in small amounts of fluid as they approach death. Many patients will not experience troubling thirst or dry mouth, but those who do can almost always be readily relieved by simple mouth care: cleaning the mouth and frequently offering lubricants, such as ice chips or artificial saliva. Thus, treatment for terminal dehydration should generally be confined to encouraging fluid intake and regularly offering mouth care. In the absence of clear data supporting the routine use of hydration, such treatment should generally be foregone.

More vigorous rehydration, beginning with encouraging oral fluids but perhaps including parenteral or artificial enteral means, has a clear role in earlier phases of illness and perhaps in selected patients in the final days of life. Even in advanced terminal disease, patients who are able to enjoy a meaningful and satisfying existence but are unable to maintain adequate fluid balance through oral intake may want to consider hydration through parenteral or enteral means. In particular, patients with oropharyngeal and gastrointestinal conditions that prevent oral hydration may benefit from feeding tubes or parenteral (subcutaneous or intravenous) alimentation. Selected patients with hypercalcemia may benefit from maintaining normal or even enhanced fluid intake, though careful consideration should first be given to whether this condition should be treated (115,116). Situations in which improvement in renal failure might lower the toxicity of medication regimens, particularly situations in which opioid toxicity is presumed to be caused by metabolites poorly cleared by the kidneys, might be such an instance. The benefits of maintaining adequate hydration need to be weighed against the harm of such measures (e.g., worsening of vomiting from small bowel obstruction). Certainly, overhydration should be avoided.

Regardless of clinical research on the benefits and harms of rehydration, patients, families, and health professionals may have strong feelings about the necessity of artificial hydration and nutrition (117) and its symbolic (rather than physiologic) role (118), perhaps viewing such treatment as basic care that should never be foregone (119). In general, commentators from a variety of philosophical and religious backgrounds have concluded that hydration is a treatment that can be withheld or withdrawn when medically and ethically appropriate (120), but popular and professional consensus on this issue is lacking (117,121). State regulations may characterize artificial hydration as different from other potential medical interventions that may be foregone (122), and institutional policies, particularly in nursing homes, may not support good clinical judgment or management. Moreover, even clinicians who accept withholding or with-

drawing of treatments as ethically appropriate may find such procedures upsetting and difficult (123) and may not act entirely logically (124).

Finally, careful clinical judgment about the use of fluids in the terminally ill is preferable to any simple formula for care (125). We cannot say for sure that various degrees of dehydration will definitely produce particular symptoms, nor can we anticipate the severity of such symptoms. We are also uncertain about the value of various interventions, both fluid replacement and symptomatic. In general, the harm or lack of benefit from rehydration outweighs any potential benefit in the final few days of life, and the onus is placed on the clinician to justify fluid replacement in terms of patient comfort. Treatment that promotes comfort can be justified, but we should beware of increasing suffering or simply meddling or prolonging dying.

The decision about whether to institute fluid and electrolyte replacement in a terminally ill patient can best be carried out when decision makers are clear about the goals of treatment and the potential value or cost of various management options. Helping the patient and family understand the benefits and harm of dehydration and its treatment can be time consuming and difficult because fluids, like feeding, have a symbolic meaning, so that foregoing this treatment may be equated with neglect, cruelty, or punishment. Withholding fluids and nourishment should not be confused with or lead to neglect, inattention, or withholding optimal care. Physicians' attitudes and behaviors in presenting such decisions can have a profound influence on patients and families, who are often desperate for straightforward guidance (126). Often the underlying issue in discussions of whether to institute fluid replacement for a terminally ill patient and instances of "psychological palliation" through fluid administration is the acceptance of the inevitability of imminent demise by the patient, family, and professional staff.

## REFERENCES

1. Wachtel T, Allen-Masterson S, Reuben D, Goldberg R, Mor V. *The end stage cancer patient: terminal common pathway.* Hospice J 1988; 4(4):43–80.
2. Baines MJ. Control of other symptoms. In: Saunders CM ed. *The management of terminal disease.* Chicago: Year Book, 1978;99–100.
3. Andrews MR, Levine AM. Dehydration in the terminal patient: perception of hospice nurses. *Am J Hospice Care* 1989;6(1):31–34.
4. Twycross RG, Lack SA. *Control of alimentary symptoms in far advanced cancer.* New York: Churchill Livingstone, 1986;86–87.
5. Billings JA. Comfort measures for the terminally ill: is dehydration painful? *J Am Geriatr Soc* 1985;33:808–810.
6. House N. The hydration question: hydration or dehydration of terminally ill patients. *Professional Nurse 1992* (October);8(1):44–48.
7. McCann RM, Hall WJ, Groth-Juncker A. Comfort care for terminally ill patients: the appropriate use of nutrition and hydration. *JAMA* 1994;272:1263–1266.
8. Fainsinger R, Bruera E. The management of dehydration in terminally ill patients. *J Palliat Care* 1994;10:55–59.
9. Yan E, Bruera E. Parenteral hydration of terminally ill cancer patients. *J Palliat Care* 1991;7(3):40–43.

10. Bruera E, Franco JJ, Maltoni M, Watanabe S, Suarez-Almazor M. Changing pattern of agitated impaired mental status in patients with advanced cancer: association with cognitive monitoring, hydration, and opioid rotation. *J Pain Sympt Manag* 1995;10:287–291.

11. Dunphy K, Finlay I, Rathbone G, Gilbert J, Hicks F. Rehydration in palliative and terminal care: if not—why not? *Palliat Med* 1995;9:221–228.

12. McQuillan R, Finlay I. Dehydration in dying patients. *Palliat Med* 1995;9:341–342.

13. Andrews M, Bell ER, Smith SA, Tischler JF, Veglia JM. Dehydration in terminally ill patients: is it appropriate palliative care? *Postgrad Med* 1993;93(1):201–203,206,208.

14. Cranford RE. Neurologic syndromes and prolonged survival: when can artificial nutrition and hydration be forgone? *Law Med Health Care* 1991;19(1–2):3–22.

15. Micetich KC, Steinecker PH, Thomasma DC. Are intravenous fluids morally required for a dying patient? *Arch Intern Med* 1983;143: 975–978.

16. Lynn J, Childress JF. Must patients always be given food and water? *Hastings Center Rep* 1983;13:17–21.

17. Churchill LR. Theories of justice. In: Kjellstrand CM, Dossetor KB, eds. *Ethical problems in dialysis and transplantation.* Netherland: Kluwer Academic, 1992;21–34.

18. Wanzer SH, Adelstein SJ, Cranford RE, Federman DD, Hook ED, Moertel CG, Safar P, Stone A, Taussig HB, vanEys J. The physician's responsibility toward hopelessly ill patients. *N Engl J Med* 1984;310: 955–959.

19. Miles SH. Futile feeding at the end of life: family virtues and treatment decisions. *Theoret Med* 1987;8:293–302.

20. Presidents Commission for the Study of Ethical Problems in Medicine and Biomedical and Behavioral Research. *Deciding to forego life sustaining treatment: ethical, medical, and legal issues in treatment decisions.* Washington, DC: U.S. Printing Office, 1983.

21. Craig G. Is sedation without hydration or nourishment in terminal care lawful? *Medico-Legal J* 1994;62(4):198–201.

22. Himmelstein DU, Jones AA, Woolhandler S. Hypernatremic dehydration in nursing home patients. An indicator of neglect. *J Am Geriatr Soc* 1983;31:466–471.

23. Mahowald JM, Himmelstein DU. Hypernatremia in the elderly: relation to infection and mortality. *J Am Geriatr Soc* 1981;29:177–180.

24. Burge FI, King DB, Willison D. Intravenous fluids and the hospitalized dying: a medical last rite? *Can Fam Physician* 1990;36:883–886.

25. Marin PP, Bayer AJ, Tomlinson A, Pathy MSJ. Attitudes of hospital doctors in Wales to use of intravenous fluids and antibiotics in the terminally ill. *Postgrad Med J* 1989;65:650–652.

26. Penn K. Passive euthanasia in palliative care. *Br J Nursing* 1992;1(9): 462–466.

27. Miller RJ. Ethics and hospice physicians. *Am J Hospice Palliat Care* 1991 (Jan/Feb):8(1):17–26.

28. Rolls BJ. Physiological determinants of fluid intake in humans. In: Ramsay DJ, Booth D, eds. *Thirst: physiological and psychological aspects.* New York: Springer-Verlag, 1991;391–399.

29. Rolls BJ, Phillips PA. Aging and disturbances of thirst and fluid balance. *Nutr Rev* 1990;48(3):137–144.

30. Rolls BJ, Wood RJ, Rolls ET, Lind H, Lind W, Ledingham JGG. Thirst following water deprivation in humans. *Am J Physiol* 1980;239 (Regulatory Integrative Comp. Physiol 8):R476–R482.

31. Phillips PA, Johnston CI, Gray L. Disturbed fluid and electrolyte homeostasis following dehydration in elderly people. *Age Aging* 1993; 22:26–33.

32. Rose BD. *Clinical physiology of acid–base and electrolyte disorders,* 4th ed. New York: McGraw-Hill, 1994;235–236.

33. Rose BD, Rennke HG. *Renal pathophysiology.* Baltimore: Williams and Wilkins, 1994;29–66.

34. Phillips PA, Bretherton M, Risvanis J, Casley D, Johnston C, Gray L. Effects of drinking on thirst and vasopressin in dehydrated elderly men. *Am J Physiol* 1993;264 (Regulatory Integrative Comp Physiol 33):R877–R881.

35. Phillips PA, Rolls BJ, Ledingham JGG, Forsling ML, Morton JJ, Crowe MJ, Wollner L. Reduced thirst after water deprivation in healthy elderly men. *N Engl J Med* 1984;311:753–759.

36. Phillips PA, Bretherton M, Johnston CI, Gray L. Reduced osmotic thirst in healthy elderly men. *Am J Physiol* 1991;261:R166–171.

37. Weinberg AD, Pals JK, McGlinchey-Berroth R, Minaker KL. Indices of dehydration among frail nursing home patients: highly variable but stable over time. *J Am Geriatr Soc* 1994;42:1070–1073.

38. Phillips PA, Johnston C, Gray L. Reduced oropharyngeal inhibition of AVP secretion in dehydrated elderly men. *Ann NY Acad Sci* 1993 (July 22);689:651–655.

39. Mack GW, Weseman CA, Langans GW, Scherzer H, Gillen CM, Nadel ER. Body fluid balance in dehydrated healthy older men: thirst and renal osmoregulation. *J Appl Physiol* 1994;74(4):1615–1623.

40. Mack GW, Weseman CA, Langans GW, Scherzer H, Gillen CM, Nadel ER. Body fluid balance in dehydrated healthy older men: thirst and renal osmoregulation. *J Appl Physiol* 1994;74(4):1615–1623.

41. Kirkland J, Lye M, Goddard C, Vargas E, Davies I. Plasma arginine vasopressin in dehydrated elderly patients. *Clin Endocrinol* 1984;20: 451–456.

42. Leaf A. The clinical and physiologic significance of the serum sodium concentration. *N Engl J Med* 1962;267:24–30.

43. McCance RA. Experimental sodium chloride deficiency in man. *Proc R Soc Lond* 1936;119(series B):245–268.

44. Nadal JW, Pedersen S, Maddock WG. A comparison between dehydration from salt loss and from water deprivation. *J Clin Invest* 1941; 20:691–703.

45. Adolph EF and associates, eds. *Physiology of man in the desert.* New York: Interscience, 1947;142,212,208–240.

46. Booker JA. Severe symptomatic hyponatremia in elderly outpatients: the role of thiazide therapy and stress. *J Am Geriatr Soc* 1984;32: 108–111.

47. Burge FI. Dehydration symptons of palliative care cancer patients. *J Pain Sympt Manag* 1993;8:454–464.

48. Oliver D. Terminal dehydration. *Lancet* 1984;2:631.

49. Waller A, Hershkowitz M, Adunsky A. The effect of intravenous fluid infusion on blood and urine parameters of hydration and on state of consciousness in terminal cancer patients. *Am J Hospice Palliat Care* 1994;11(6):22–27.

50. Ellershaw JE, Sutcliffe JM, Saunders CM. Dehydration and the dying patient. *J Pain Sympt Manag* 1995;10:192–197.

51. Waller A Adunski A, Hershkowitz M. Terminal dehydration and intravenous fluids. *Lancet* 1991;337(8747):981–982.

52. Noakes TD. Fluid replacement during exercise. *Exercise and Sport Sci. Rev.* 1993;21:297–330.

53. Albert SG, Nakra BR, Grossberg GT, Caminal ER. Vasopressin response to dehydration in Alzheimer's disease. *J AM Geriatr Soc* 1989;37:843–847.

54. Miller PD, Krebs RA, Neal BJ, McIntyre DO. Hypodipsia in geriatric patients. *Am J Med* 1982;73:354–356.

55. Silver AJ. Aging and risks for dehydration. *Cleve Clin J Med* 1990;57: 341–344.

56. Silver AJ, Morley JE. Role of the opioid system in the hypodipsia associated with aging. *J Am Geriatr Soc* 1992;40:556–560.

57. Weinberg AD, Minaker KL, and the Council on Scientific Affairs, American Medical Association. Dehydration: evaluation and management in older adults. *JAMA* 1995;274:1552–1556.

58. Lapides J, Bourrie RB, MacLean LR. Clinical signs of dehydration and fluid loss. *JAMA* 1965;191:413–415.

59. Gross CR, Lindquist RD, Woolley AC, Granieri R, Allard K, Webster B. Clincal indicators of dehydration severity in elderly patients. *J Emerg Med* 1992;10:267–274.

60. Eaton D, Bannister P, Mulley GP, Connolly MJ. Axillary sweating in clinical assessment of dehydration in ill elderly patients. *Br Med J* 1994;308:1271.

61. Saaverda JM, Harris GD, Li S, Finberg L. Capillary refilling (skin turgor) in the assessment of dehydration. *Am J Dis Child* 1991;145: 296–298.

62. Seymour DG, Henschke PJ, Cape RD, Campbell AJ. Acute confusional states and dementia in the elderly: the role of dehydration/volume depletion, physical illness and age. *Age Aging* 1980;9: 137–146.

63. Sullivan RJ. Accepting death without artificial nutrition or hydration. *J Gen Intern Med* 1993;8:220–227.

64. Bernat JL, Gert B, Mogielnicki RP. Patient refusal of nutrition and hydration: an alternative to physician-assisted suicide or voluntary active euthanasia. *Arch Intern Med* 1993;153:2723–2727.

65. Adolph EF, Wills JH. Thirst. In:Adolph EF and associates, eds. *Physiology of man in the desert.* New York:Interscience, 1947; 241–253.

66. Rothstein A, Adolph EF, Wills JH. Voluntary dehydration. In: Adolph EF and associates, eds. *Physiology of man in the desert.* New York: Interscience, 1947;254–270.

67. Engell DB, Maller O, Sawaka MN, Francisco RN, Drolet L, Young AJ. Thirst and fluid intake following graded hypohydration levels in humans. *Physiol Behav* 1987;40(2):229–236.

68. Coyle N, Adelhardt J, Foley KM, Portenoy RK. Character of terminal illness in the advanced cancer patient: pain and other symptoms during the last four weeks of life. *J Pain Sympt Manag* 1990;5:83–93.

69. Dunlop GM. A study of the frequency and importance of gastrointestinal symptoms and weakness in patients with far advanced cancer (student paper). *Palliat Med* 1989;4(1):37–43.

70. Reuben DB, Mor V, Hiris J. Clinical symptoms and length of survival in patients with terminal cancer. *Arch Intern Med* 1988;148: 1586–1591.

71. Seale C, Cartwright A. *The year before death.* Brookfield, CT: Avebury, 1994;90,115.

72. Reuben DB, Mor V. Nausea and vomiting in terminal cancer patients. *Arch Intern Med* 1986;146:2021–2023.

73. Hagen NA, Foley KM, Cerbone DJ, Portenoy RK, Inturrisi CE. Chronic nausea and morphine 6-glucuronide. *J Pain Sympt Manag* 1991;6(3):125–128.

74. Sear JW, Hand CW, Moore RA, McQuay HJ. Studies on morphine disposition: influence of renal failure on the kinetics of morphine and its metabolites. *Br J Anaesth* 1989;62:28–32.

75. Peterson GM, Randall CT, Paterson J. Plasma levels of morphine and morphine-glucuronides in the treatment of cancer pain: relationship to renal function and route of administration. *Eur J Clin Pharmacol* 1990;38:121–124.

76. Back IN. Terminal restlessness in patients with advanced malignant disease. *Palliat Med* 1992;6:293-298.

77. Dunlop RI. Is terminal restlessness sometimes drug induced? *Palliat Med* 1989;3:65–66.

78. Lichter I, Hunt E. The last 48 hours of life. *J Palliat Care* 1990; 6(4):7–15.

79. Ventafridda V, Ripamonti C, DeConno F, Tamburini M, Cassileth BR. Sympton prevalence and control during cancer patients last days of life. *J Palliat Care* 1990;6(3):7–11.

80. Ciocon JO, Silverstone FA, Graver LM, Foley CJ. Tube feeding in elderly patients. Indication, benefits, and complications, *Arch Intern Med* 1988;148:429–433.

81. Quill TE. Utilization of nasogastric feeding tubes in a group of chronically ill, elderly patients in a community hospital. *Arch Intern Med* 1989;149:1937–1941.

82. Sagawa S, Miki K, Tajima F, Tanaka H, Choi JK, Keil LC, Shiraki K, Greenleaf JE. Effect of dehydration on thirst and drinking during immersion in men. *J Appl Physiol* 1992;72(1):128–134.

83. Epstein AN. Thirst and salt intake: a personal review and some suggestion. In: Ramsay DJ, Booth D, eds. *Thirst: physiological and psychological aspects.* New York: Springer-Verlag, 1991; 481–501.

84. McQuillan R, Finlay I. *Dehydration in dying patients.* Palliat Med 1995;9:341.

85. White ID, Hoskin PJ, Hanks GW, Bliss JM. Morphine and dryness of the mouth. *Br Med J* 1989;298:1222–1223.

86. Xerostomia. [Editorial] *Lancet* 1989;1(8643):884–885.

87. Treatment of xerostomia. *Med Lett Drugs Therapeut* 1988;30(771): 74–76.

88. Rousseau P. Pilocarpine in radiation-induced xerostomia. *Am J Hospice Palliat Care* 1995;12(March/April):38–39.

89. Johnson JT, Ferretti GA, Nethery WJ, Valdez IH, Fox PC, Ng D, Muscoplat CC, Gallagher SC. Oral pilocarpine for post-irradiation xerostomia in patients with head and neck cancer. *N Engl J Med* 1993;329: 390–395.

90. Oral pilocarpine for xerostomia. *Med Lett Drugs Therapeut* 1994;36 (929):76.

91. Lippman BJ. Fluid and electrolyte management. In: Eward GA, McKenzie CR, eds. *Manual of medical therapeutics, 28th ed.* Boston: Little, Brown, 1995;43–64.

92. Fainsinger R, Bruera E. Hypodermoclysis for symptom control vs the Edmonton injector. *J Palliat Care* 1991;7:5–8.

93. Fainsinger R, MacEachern T, Miller MJ, et al. The use of hypodermoclysis for rehydration in terminally ill cancer patients. *J Pain Sympt Manag* 1994;9(5):298–302.

94. Berger EY. Nutrition by hypodermoclysis. *J Am Geriatr Soc* 1984;32: 199–203.

95. Bruera E, Legris MA, Kuehn N, Miller MJ. Hypodermoclysis for the administration of fluids and narcotic analgesics in patients with advanced cancer. *J Pain Sympt Manag* 1990;5:218–220.

96. Schen RJ, Singer-Edelstein M. Subcutaneous infusions in the elderly. *J Am Geriatr Soc* 1981;24:583–585.

97. Schen RJ, Singer-Edelstein M. Hypodermoclysis (letter). *JAMA* 1983; 250:1694.

98. Lamerton R. *Care of the dying* (revised and expanded edition). New York: Penguin Books, 1980;84.

99. Bruera E, Schoeller T, Pruvost M. Proctoclysis for hydration of terminal cancer patients. *Lancet* 1994;344:1699.

100. Printz LA. Terminal dehydration, a compassionate treatment. *Arch Intern Med* 1992;152:697–700.

101. Zerwekh JV. Should fluid and nutritional support be withheld from terminally ill patients? Another opinion. *Am J Hospice Care* 1987 (July/August);4(4):37–38.

102. Zerwekh JV. The dehydration question. *Nursing* 1983;13:47–51.

103. Sutcliffe J, Holmes S. Dehydration: burden or benefit to the dying patient? *J Adv Nursing* 1994;19:71–76.

104. Printz LA. Is withholding hydration a valid comfort measure in the terminally ill? *Geriatrics* 1988;43(11):84–88.

105. Arieff A, Defranzo R. *Fluid, electrolyte and acid–base disorders.* Edinburgh: Churchill Livingstone, 1985.

106. Elliot J, Haydon D, Hendry B. Anaesthetic action of esters and ketones evidence for an interaction with the sodium channel protein in squid axons. *J Phys(London)* 1984;354:407–418.

107. Majeed N, Lason N, Przewlocka B. Brain and peripheral opioid peptides after changes in ingestive behavior. *Neuroendocrinology* 1986; 42:267–276.

108. Takahashi M, Motomatsu T, Nobunage M. Influence of water deprivation and fasting on hypothalamic, pituitary and plasma opioid peptides and prolactin in rats. *Physio Behav* 1986;37:603–608.

109. Ventafridda V, Ripamonti E, Caraceni A, Spoldi F, Messina L, DeConno F. The management of inoperable gastrointestinal obstruction in terminal cancer patients. *Tumori* 1990;76:389–393.

110. Baines M, Oliver DJ, Carter RL. Medical management of intestinal obstruction in patients with advanced malignant disease: a clinical and pathological study. *Lancet* 1985;2(8462):990–993.

111. Lamerton R. Dehydration in dying patients. *Lancet* 1991;337: 981–982.

112. Dunlop RJ, Ellershaw JE, Baines MJ, Sykes N, Saunders CM. On withholding nutrition and hydration in the terminally ill: has palliative medicine gone too far? A reply. *J Med Ethics* 1995;21:141–143.

113. Aronheim JC, Gasner MR. The sloganism of starvation. *Lancet* 1990; 335:278–279.

114. Storey P. Artificial feeding and hydration in advanced illness. In: Wildes KW, eds. *Birth, suffering and death.* Netherlands: Kluwer Academic, 1992; 67–75.

115. Ralston SH, Gallagher SJ, Campbell J, Boyle IT. Cancer-associated hypercalcemia: morbidity and mortality—clinical experience in 126 treated patients. *Ann Intern Med* 1990;112:499–504.

116. Kovacs CS, MacDonald SM, Chik CL, Bruera E. Hypercalcemia of malignancy in the palliative care patient: a treatment strategy. *J Pain Sympt Manag* 1995;10:224–232.

117. Slomka J. What do apple pie and mother hood have to do with feeding tubes and caring for the patient? *Arch Intern Med* 1995;155: 1258–1263.

118. McInerney F. Provision of food and fluids in terminal care: a sociological analysis. *Soc Sci Med* 1992;34(11):1271–1276.

119. Craig GM. On withholding nutrition and hydration in the terminally ill: has palliative medicine gone too far? *J Med Ethics* 1994;20:139–143.

120. American Medical Association Council on Ethical and Judicial Affairs. Decision near the end of life. *JAMA* 1992;267:2229–2233.

121. Miller R, Albright P. What is the role of nutritional support and hydration in terminal cancer patients? *Am J Hospice Care* 1989 (Nov/Dec):33–38.

122. Hodges MO, Tolle SW, Stocking C, Cassel C. Tube feeding: internists attitudes regarding ethical obligations. *Arch Intern Med* 1994;154: 1013–1020.

123. Edwards MJ, Tolle SW. Disconnecting a ventilator at the request of a patient who knows he will then die: the doctor's anguish. *Ann Intern Med* 1992;117:254–256.

124. Christakis NA, Asch DA. Biases in how physicians choose to withdraw life support. *Lancet* 1993;342:642–646.

125. Pearlman RA. Forgoing medical nutrition and hydration: An area for fine-tuning clinical skills. *J Gen Intern med* 1993;8:225–227.

126. Tilden VP, Tolle SW, Garland MJ, Nelson CA. Decisions about life-sustaining treatment: Impact of physicians behaviors on the faimly. *Arch Intern Med* 1995;155:633.

*Principles and Practice of Supportive Oncology,*
edited by Ann Berger et al.
Lippincott–Raven Publishers, Philadelphia ©1998

CHAPTER 43

# Palliative Radiation Therapy

Wayne H. Pinover and Lawrence R. Coia

Radiation therapy is a well-established modality for the palliation of distressing symptoms from locally advanced and metastatic malignancies. While most research efforts are directed to improving the curative potential of radiation therapy, some estimate that up to approximately 50% of cancer patients treated with radiation therapy are treated with palliative intent (1). Considering that over 1.3 million cases of cancer are estimated to occur in 1996 and up to 60% of cancer patients will present with or develop metastases during the course of their disease (2,3), the number of patients who may require palliative radiotherapy is staggering. Mindful of these statistics and today's cost-conscious health care environment, the radiation oncologist must provide the best palliative care for patients in the most cost-effective radiotherapeutic treatment program.

Numerous retrospective reviews and randomized prospective studies have demonstrated the benefits of palliative radiotherapy. These benefits include the relief of pain, improvement in function and cosmesis, alleviation of obstruction, and control of bleeding. While lung cancer is the predominant tumor requiring radiotherapeutic palliation for symptoms of locally advanced or metastatic disease, other tumors commonly referred for palliative irradiation include those of the breast, prostate, kidney, gastrointestinal (GI) tract, head and neck, gynecologic areas, non-Hodgkin's lymphomas, and melanomas. The most frequent sites of metastatic or locally advanced disease requiring palliative radiotherapy are the brain, skeleton, lung, liver, gastrointestinal, and genitourinary tracts.

Once it is established that a patient is no longer curable, efforts should proceed to establish the extent of tumor and the tumor- associated symptoms that require palliation. Palliative radiotherapy is most effective when it is considered as part of the overall management of the patient that includes chemotherapy, surgery, pain management, reha-

bilitation, psychosocial intervention, nutritional and nursing support. Patients and their families should have realistic expectations of the goals of treatment. Alternative treatments should be noted. While the relief of troubling symptoms is the primary goal, the avoidance of debilitating radiotherapy side effects is equally important. In addition, prolonged courses of radiotherapy in patients with limited life expectancies and excessive costs associated with complicated treatment programs have no place in the radiotherapeutic management of patients when they are of unproven benefit. It is incumbent on the radiation oncologist to decide whether a patient should receive a course of accelerated fractionation, typically ranging from 1000 cGy in 1 fraction to 2000 cGy in 5 fractions, or a more conventional fractionation scheme of 3000 cGy in 10 fractions. This decision is based on the patient's anticipated life expectancy, extent of disease, rate of disease progression, disease-free interval, functional status, and normal tissue tolerances of those tissues that will receive a dose of radiation. The normal tissue tolerance of critical structures in the treatment field such as brain, spinal cord, kidney, lung, bowel, liver, and skin must be accounted for in the radiation prescription. Radiation side effects are divided into early and late. Early effects are influenced by the fractional dose, total dose, and overall treatment time, whereas late effects are primarily influenced by fractional dose. All of these factors and the fact that there is a discrepancy between early and late effects are taken into consideration in the decision as to which fractionation scheme will produce maximum benefit with minimal complications, cost, and patient inconvenience.

## BONE METASTASES

### Etiology and Epidemiology

Bone metastases occur in 30–70% of patients with cancer (4). The most commonly diagnosed primary

W. H. Pinover: Department of Radiation Oncology, Fox Chase Cancer Center, Philadelphia, PA 19111.

L.R. Coia: Department of Radiation Oncology, Community Medical Center, Toms River, NJ 08755.

tumors—namely, prostate, lung, and breast cancer—account for >75% of bone metastases. Arcangeli et al., in a series of 281 patients with bone metastases, demonstrated the most common primary sites to be breast (50%), prostate (17%), and lung (11%) (5). Primary tumors of the kidney, rectum, pancreas, stomach, colon, and ovary are also associated with bony metastases. Prostate tumors have a predilection for spread to pelvic bones, as well as vertebral bodies, due to Batson's venous plexus. Most solid tumors have similar patterns of spread, most commonly involving the vertebra (69%), pelvis (41%), femur (25%), and skull (14%) (4). The upper extremity is involved in 10–15% of bony metastases. Pathologic fracture, most commonly involving the femur or humerus, occurs in 9% of patients with bony metastases. Breast, kidney, lung, and thyroid carcinomas account for the majority of bone metastases associated with pathologic fracture.

Patients with skeletal metastases present with localized pain. Some patients may be asymptomatic and present with incidentally found X-ray or bone scan abnormalities. Vertebral body involvement may present with back pain or referred pain to the chest wall or lower extremity. Any cancer patient presenting with back pain or possibly referred pain from vertebral body metastases must undergo evaluation for spinal cord compression, as this is an oncologic emergency with dramatic consequences.

## Evaluation

The diagnostic workup of bone pain in the cancer patient should include plain x-rays and a whole-body bone scan. Multiple lesions of the skeleton with involvement of spine, hips, and femur is typical and requires no further diagnostic procedure. Typical radiographic patterns of bony metastases are osteolytic, osteoblastic, and mixed (4). Patients can demonstrate any combination of patterns. Osteoblastic lesions are less common that osteolytic lesions overall and are more commonly seen in patients with bony metastases from prostate and breast primaries (4).

Whole-body bone scans utilizing technetium should be part of the evaluation of patients with bony metastases. Bone scans can detect metastatic disease 2–18 months earlier than plain radiographs (4). Occasionally, bone scans may detect a solitary lesion. Solitary lesions should undergo further evaluation in order to exclude other possibilities. In 273 patients with malignancy, McNeil demonstrated trauma, infection, and other nonmalignant factors to account for solitary bone-scan abnormalities in 25%, 10%, and 10% of patients, respectively (6). Computed tomography (CT) scans, magnetic resonance imaging (MRI) scans, and biopsy are recommended for further evaluation. Bone scans may demonstrate decreased activity in an area of bone metastasis that has been irradiated.

Magnetic resonance imaging is also useful in the early detection of skeletal metastases. Radiographs and bone scans only demonstrate metastases when there are changes in the bone adjacent to a site of metastatic disease and therefore identify lesions already associated with significant bone destruction at the time of diagnosis. MRI is uniquely able to identify bone metastases earlier in their course, prior to the onset of abnormalities seen on plain films and bone scan. Bony metastases are secondary to the hematogenous spread of neoplastic cells from the primary. These neoplastic cells reach the medullary cavity of bone prior to invading the cortex and causing bone destruction. Because fat is a major component of the medullary area, this is typically bright on T1-weighted MRI images. An accumulation of neoplastic cells will have a high water content and appear as a low-signal area on T1-weighted MRI images. Although the role of MRI in the diagnostic workup of patients with bone metastases is not well established, we recommend MRI in those patients with signs and symptoms consistent with bone metastases and negative plain x-rays and whole-body bone scans.

Patients with lytic lesions in weight-bearing bones where there is >50% destruction of the cortex or a lesion 2.5 cm or larger are typically felt to be at high risk for pathologic fracture (7) and should undergo orthopedic evaluation for prophylactic fixation. Indications for prophylactic fixation of an impending fracture include any one of the following: a painful intramedullary osteolytic lesion equal to or larger than 50% of the cross-sectional diameter of the bone, a painful lytic lesion involving a length of cortex equal to or greater than the cross-sectional diameter of the bone or larger than 2.5 cm in axial length, or a lesion of bone in which pain was unrelieved after radiation therapy (4). Others recommend prophylactic fixation based on clinical criteria including anatomic site, pain pattern, type of lesion, and size. Following fixation, patients should receive a course of palliative radiotherapy to the involved area (4). Historically, it has been thought that intramedullary and fixation devices should be included in the radiation field in order to sterilize any microscopic tumor deposits that may have been dislodged at the time of surgery. Practically, this requires rather large radiation fields and is of unproven clinical benefit. The inclusion of intramedullary and fixation devices is not routine and is dependent on the treating radiation oncologist. Adjacent joints should be excluded from the radiation fields, unless involved by tumor. A strip of soft tissue should also be excluded from the radiation field in order to preserve adequate lymphatic drainage.

## Treatment

Patients with skeletal metastases are frequently at risk for other complications from their primary malignancy and treatment and subsequently pose difficult management issues to their health care providers. The goals of radiation therapy in patients with bony metastases are to palliate pain, reduce the need for narcotic analgesics, improve ambulation, and prevent complications of spinal cord compression and pathologic fracture. External beam radiotherapy is well established as the standard of care in providing durable pain relief in the majority of patients with a limited number of metastases, as documented in retrospective studies (8–11). General considerations prior to palliative radiotherapy include the number and location of involved sites, normal tissue tolerances, the patient's ability to undergo multiple fractions of radiotherapy over a short period of time, the acute side effects and long-term morbidity of treatment, and the patient's expected survival.

Palliative radiotherapy does not improve survival in patients with bony metastatic disease. Patients and their families should be aware of this so that their expectations of treatment are realistic. The prognosis for patients is dependent on the location and extent of bony involvement and the presence of extraskeletal metastases. Patients with breast or prostate primary malignancies who have metastatic disease to the bones only may be expected to survive for a relatively longer time than patients with widespread metastatic disease. Radiation therapy must therefore provide durable palliation in these patients.

The radiation portal should include the painful localized site of disease and any nearby adjacent symptomatic sites. Consideration should be given to the inclusion of adjacent asymptomatic sites of disease if the irradiated volume does not become excessive. This will provide prophylactic palliation, possibly avoiding the need to irradiate these areas in the future and prevent the delivery of high doses to normal tissues from unnecessarily overlapping radiation fields. Treating an area near a previously treated site requires gapping the two fields to avoid overlapping. Therefore, doses received by critical structures, such as the spinal cord, should be recorded so that the radiation tolerance of theses structures is not exceeded. Many patients will require further palliative treatment, and knowledge of radiation tolerance doses and the doses previously received by critical structures is essential in preventing late radiation complications.

A wide range of photon energies can be used depending on the depth of the bone to be treated. High-energy electrons or photons may be used to treat superficial bony metastases such as the ribs or scapulae. Other areas are usually treated with parallel opposed fields. External beam radiation therapy can provide durable pain relief in 73–90% of patients (8–11). Analysis of retrospective studies with regard to optimal dose fractionation is complicated by inherent selection bias, differences in patients' extent of disease and location of metastases, primary histologies, and the variable use of systemic therapies.

Prospective studies of different dose fractionation schedules have generally concluded that there is no difference in pain relief using high-dose single fractions compared to fractionated schedules. Tong et al. reported the prospective randomized experience from the Radiation Therapy Oncology Group (RTOG) (12). Patients with solitary bone metastases were stratified by primary site, use of internal fixation, and institution prior to randomization to either 4050 cGy in 15 fractions over 3 weeks, or 2000 cGy in 5 fractions over 1 week. Patients with multiple sites of metastases were similarly stratified prior to randomization to one of four dose fractionation schedules: 300 cGy $\times 10$, 300 cGy $\times 5$, 400 cGy $\times 5$, or 500 cGy $\times 5$. All fractions were given once daily. No difference was noted in the incidence of partial pain relief, complete pain relief, or the duration of pain relief between the various dose fractionation schedules in the solitary or multiple bony metastases groups. Overall, 83% of patients obtained partial relief and 53% obtained complete relief. The median duration of pain relief in the solitary group was approximately 15 weeks for patients with complete relief and 28 weeks for patients with minimal relief. In the multiple metastases group, the corresponding duration of relief was 12 weeks and 20 weeks for those with complete and partial relief, respectively. The overall percentage of relapses in the solitary group was 29% for those with minimal relief and 57% for those with complete relief. In the multiple bone metastases group, the incidence of relapsing pain was 29% and 54%, respectively. The only notable difference by treatment was in the solitary group with an 18% fracture rate compared to 4%, in favor of the group receiving 4050 cGy in 15 fractions. In a reanalysis of this data by Blitzer, the longer fractionation schedules (4050 cGy/15 fractions/3 weeks and 3000 cGy/10 fractions/2 weeks) produced statistically significantly more pain relief than the shorter fractionation schedules (13). Blitzer grouped all solitary and multiple metastases together to increase the statistical power of the study. In addition to pain relief, the reanalysis used endpoints that also accounted for retreatment and the use of narcotics.

Numerous investigators have evaluated different dose fractionation schemes without noting any striking differences in results. Price et al., then at Royal Marsden Hospital, randomized 288 patients to receive either 8 Gy in a single fractions or 30 Gy in 10 daily fractions over 2 weeks (14). No significant differences in the two groups were noted in the onset of pain relief, incidence of complete relief, duration of relief, or incidence of response according to initial pain score. In 1-year survivors, 55–60% of responders demonstrated durable pain relief. Patients responded usually within the first 4 weeks following radiation therapy. Acute morbidity was tolerable and not increased in patients treated with larger fields. Retreatment was required in 11% and 3% of the patients in the single- and multiple-fraction groups, respectively.

Rasmusson et al. prospectively randomized 200 breast cancer patients with bone metastases to receive 30 Gy in 10 daily fractions or 15 Gy in 3 fractions given over 2 weeks (15). Pain relief was equal in both groups at 3 months, with 80% and 75% of patients experiencing relief in the 30-Gy and 15-Gy groups, respectively. Madsen prospectively evaluated 4 Gy ×6 fractions giving two fractions per week versus 10 Gy ×2 fractions giving one fraction per week (16). Approximately 48% of patients in both groups responded with satisfactory pain control and no difference in side effects by field size or dose fractionation was noted.

Single-fraction radiotherapy has the advantages of decreased cost and fewer visits to the radiation department for patients with limited survival. Price et al. demonstrated, as previously mentioned, the effectiveness of 8 Gy in a single fraction compared to 30 Gy in 10 daily fractions (14). In a follow-up study seeking an optimal single dose of radiotherapy, 270 patients at Royal Marsden Hospital were randomized to single fractions of 8 or 4 Gy (17). At 4 weeks, the overall response rates were significantly improved in the 8-Gy arm compared to the 4-Gy arm with 69% and 44% responses in the two groups, respectively. In another prospective trial, no differences in pain relief were noted for patients randomized to 8 Gy in a single fraction or 24 Gy in six fractions, although 25% of patients receiving 8 Gy in a single fraction required retreatment (18). It is evident from the literature that painful bone metastases may be palliated equally well with either large single fractions, a short course of fractionated radiotherapy, or a more protracted course of treatment. Single fractions or accelerated courses of radiotherapy given in 1 week may be appropriate in certain palliative settings, such as (a) rapid tumor progression; (b) early dissemination following definitive treatment; (c) anticipated short survival; and (d) patients with an expected survival <3 months and the inability to return for daily fractionated treatment. Protracted courses of palliative irradiation may be more appropriate for patients with indolent disease, high functional status, life expectancy >3 months, or a solitary bone metastasis with a controlled primary (1).

Acute reactions during palliative local field radiotherapy are usually mild, well tolerated, and easily managed. The acute reactions and long-term complications are restricted to the anatomic structures included in the radiation field. Local fields treating an extremity bone metastasis should produce minimal to no acute side effects and long-term complications, depending on the dose fractionation schedule chosen. Treatment of bone metastases involving the axial skeleton may produce more acute side effects and long-term complications secondary to the inclusion of thoracic, abdominal, and pelvic viscera such as the esophagus, lung, heart, bowel, liver, kidneys, rectum, and bladder. Knowledge of the normal tissue tolerance of these critical organs is essen-

tial in the treatment planning of patients with skeletal metastases. A course of palliative radiation therapy should not be prescribed with the anticipation that the patient will not survive long enough to suffer any toxicity from the treatment (1).

## Retreatment

Despite durable pain relief in the majority of patients, approximately 25–30% of patients will require retreatment (18,19). Initial retreatment, with a variety of dose fractionation schedules, may provide pain relief in up to 84% of the sites retreated. Although the numbers are few, 87% of bone metastases respond to a second retreatment (19). The acute morbidity has been minimal at the low dose levels typically used in the retreatment of bone metastases.

## Hemibody Radiation Therapy

Palliative radiotherapy for bony metastases using relatively small to moderate-sized localized fields is adequate for patients with a limited number of disease sites. The use of numerous localized fields for patients with extensive bony metastatic disease is problematic due to increased daily setup time, patient discomfort, and the risk of overlapping fields. Patients with extensive bony metastatic disease may be more appropriately treated with either hemibody irradiation or systemic radiotherapy.

Single-dose half-body irradiation for the palliation of multiple bone metastases relieved pain in 73% of patients in a large prospective trial by the RTOG (20). Patients receiving upper hemibody irradiation (UHBI) are treated to the head, neck, and torso using the umbilicus as the inferior border. Lower hemibody irradiation (LHBI) extends from the umbilicus inferiorly. The RTOG showed the optimally safe and effective dose delivered in a single fraction in UHBI and LHBI to be 600 cGy and 800 cGy, respectively. Overall, 73% of patients experienced pain relief while 20% had complete relief. The response was rapid and durable with 50% of the responders doing so within 2 days and 80% within a week. Patients with metastatic breast and prostate cancer had higher overall and complete response rates. Pain recurrence at the initial site of disease was noted in only 13% of patients. The acute radiation side effects associated with UHBI are tolerable following effective premedication with antiemetics, steroids, and intravenous fluids.

Investigators at Memorial Sloan-Kettering Cancer Center evaluated fractionated hemibody irradiation in 15 patients receiving 2500–3000 cGy in 9–10 fractions (21). The results in this group were compared to a group of 14 patients receiving single doses of 600 cGy UHBI or 800 cGy LHBI. Twenty-eight of 29 patients achieved a complete or partial response, but 71% of the patients in the single-dose group compared to 13% in the fractionated group required retreatment. The median duration of relief was longer in the fractionated versus the single-dose group, i.e., 8.5 months versus 2.8 months, respectively. Finally, the RTOG randomized 499 patients to receive hemibody irradiation or no further treatment following completion of palliative local field radiation delivering 3000 cGy in 10 fractions (22). Improvements were noted in the time-to-disease progression at 1 year (35% versus 46%), time-to-new disease in the targeted hemibody at 1 year (50% versus 68%), and median time-to-new disease within the targeted hemibody (12.6 months versus 6.3 months) for those patients receiving local field and hemibody irradiation compared to local field irradiation alone, respectively. The need for retreatment was also decreased from 76% to 60% with the addition of single-dose hemibody irradiation. Although there was an increased incidence of hematologic toxicity in the patients receiving hemibody irradiation, this was transient. Hemibody irradiation is an effective, well-tolerated treatment that should be considered for patients with diffuse bony metastatic disease.

### Systemic Radiotherapy

Systemic intravenous radiopharmaceuticals have been demonstrated to relieve pain in patients with multiple skeletal metastases (23–25). Strontium-89 is a β emitter with a half-life of 50 days. Strontium is similar to calcium in the mode in which it is physiologically handled with a 10-fold increased deposition in areas of increased bone metabolism (23). This increased deposition in areas of active bone turnover likely accounts for its efficacy in osteoblastic metastases.

In a phase III trial, 126 patients with hormone refractory metastatic prostate cancer were randomized to receive either a single intravenous injection of 10.8 mCi strontium-89 or placebo following local field radiotherapy (23). There were no significant differences in survival or pain relief between the two groups. However, significantly more patients in the strontium group, 50%, were free of new painful metastases compared to 34% in the placebo group. This translated to a significantly decreased need for and longer time interval to further radiotherapy. Hematologic toxicity was significantly more common in the patients receiving strontium. In particular, 33% in the strontium group experienced grade 3 or 4 thrombocytopenia compared to only 3% in the placebo group. Similar findings were noted by Quilty et al. (26). Patients with hormone refractory metastatic prostate cancer to bone were first stratified accordingly for treatment with either local field or hemibody irradiation. Within those two groups, patients were then randomized to receive external beam radiotherapy or 5.4 mCi strontium-89. Approximately 65% of all patients

experienced at least partial pain relief at 12 weeks of follow-up. In the local and hemibody radiotherapy groups, significantly more patients receiving strontium were free of new pain sites. Grade 3 or 4 thrombocytopenia was noted in 7% and 3% of the strontium and external beam radiotherapy groups, respectively. Thrombocytopenia nadired at 50–60% of baseline values approximately 4–8 weeks following strontium administration. Consequently, strontium-89 should not be used in patients with thrombocytopenia or significant bone marrow depression (27). Additionally, patients with impending spinal cord compression should not receive strontium-89 because of the possibility of a flare phenomenon. Other contraindications include impending pathologic fracture, leukopenia, prior myelosuppressive chemotherapy, and less than 2 months of expected survival (29). In the United States, strontium-89 injection is only approved for use at a dose of 4 mCi. In addition to strontium-89, other radiopharmaceuticals, including phosphorous-32, iodine-131, yttrium-90, samarium-153, and rhenium-186, have been used for the palliation of painful bony metastases (25).

### Summary of Radiation for Bone Metastases

Radiation therapy plays an essential role in the palliation of bone metastases. A wide variety of treatment techniques, including local fields, hemibody irradiation, and the administration of systemic radionuclides, can be utilized. Pain relief is demonstrated in approximately 70–90% of patients receiving palliative radiotherapy and a minority of patients will require retreatment. A variety of dose fractionation schemes, including large single doses, have demonstrated their ability to provide durable palliation. Treatment planning decisions should be based on an individual patient's anticipated survival, number of involved bony sites, his or her ability to undergo a course of fractionated radiotherapy, prior treatments received, and overall extent of metastatic disease.

## BRAIN METASTASES

### Etiology and Epidemiology

Brain metastases are common in cancer patients, with 25–35% of all cancer patients experiencing metastatic spread to the central nervous system (CNS) during the course of their disease (28). Any intracranial involvement is estimated to occur in approximately 25% of patients, with intradural (parenchymal and leptomeningeal) involvement occurring in 20% and parenchymal involvement alone affecting 10%. Estimates in 1992 forecast symptomatic brain metastasis in 152,600 patients, representing 13.5% of the total U.S. cancer population (28).

Clinically, 53% of patients develop multiple deposits, although autopsy series estimate the incidence to be higher (28). Multiple brain metastases are commonly seen in patients with lung cancer, melanoma, and seminoma. Solitary brain metastases are more commonly associated with renal, ovarian, and breast carcinomas and osteogenic sarcomas. In men, lung, GI, and urinary tract primary tumors account for 80% of brain metastases. In women, tumors of the breast, lung, GI tract, and melanoma account for 80% of brain metastases (28). Melanoma has the highest likelihood of brain metastases, with 65% of patients experiencing metastasis during their course. Although brain metastases occur less commonly in breast and lung cancer patients—51% and 41%, respectively—they account for most of the cases of brain metastases secondary to their increased incidence compared to other tumors such as melanoma.

## Clinical Presentation

Eighty percent of metastases occur in the supratentorial compartment. Pelvic and GI primary tumors may have a predilection for the posterior fossa. The presenting signs and symptoms of brain metastases are varied. Focal signs and symptoms such as unilateral headache, weakness, and seizures are a result of direct mechanical distortion and parenchymal injury by a mass lesion. Generalized signs and symptoms of diffuse headache, cognitive or behavioral changes, and papilledema are more typical of cerebral edema, cerebrospinal fluid (CSF) obstruction, or metabolic dysfunction (28). Headache occurs in >50% of patients and is described as occurring in the morning and resolving soon after awakening. With tumor progression, the morning headache increases in duration and frequency (29). Symptomatic focal weakness occurs in 40% and can be found upon examination in 65% of patients. Disturbances of mental function occur in approximately 30% but can be found upon detailed examination in 50–75% of patients. Ataxia due to CSF obstruction and/or cerebellar metastases may be seen in up to 20% of patients. Seizures occur in 15% and are more commonly seen in metastatic melanoma or patients with leptomeningeal disease (28).

## Evaluation

The differential diagnosis of neurologic dysfunction in the cancer patient is extensive and includes other neoplastic processes including infections, toxic/metabolic processes, cerebrovascular events, and paraneoplastic syndromes (28). Biopsy should be performed in patients presenting without a prior diagnosis of malignancy and should be considered in patients presenting with a solitary metastasis or with a long disease-free interval. The diagnostic workup includes CT or MRI of the brain with contrast agents. MRI is more sensitive in detecting smaller metastatic deposits (28). Lumbar puncture is of diagnostic benefit in patients with leptomeningeal spread or patients with infectious meningitis.

## Treatment

The goal of treatment for brain metastases is to maximize and maintain the highest neurologic function attainable (28). Early and appropriate therapeutic intervention can positively influence the patient's quality of remaining life. Standard treatment includes best supportive care, corticosteroids, and radiation therapy. Surgical resection is usually reserved for solitary metastases.

Empiric doses of corticosteroids (16–24 mg/day or higher) reduce cerebral edema with 60–80% of patients noting resolution or improvement in their symptoms in 6–24 hours. Patients presenting with severe symptoms and signs secondary to elevated intracranial pressure should receive further therapy using diuretics, hyperosmolar solutions, or hyperventilation. Patients with brain metastases and the acute onset or rapid progression of neurologic symptoms may be candidates for urgent radiotherapy. Corticosteroids should be tapered following cranial irradiation.

The anticipated expected survival of patients with spread to the brain is an important consideration in choosing the appropriate palliative regimen. Median survival improves from 1 month with no treatment to 2 months with the administration of corticosteroids alone. Cranial irradiation can further improve the median survival to 3–6 months with 1- and 2-year survivals of 15% and 5–10%, respectively. Twenty-five to fifty percent of patients treated with radiotherapy will die of progressive brain metastases (30). Several prognostic factors for survival have been investigated and knowledge of these may aid in determining prognosis and optimum management. Table 1 demonstrates the prognostic factors for survival

**TABLE 1.** *Survival prognosticators in RTOG studies*

|  | Median survival (mos) |
| --- | --- |
| Initial neurologic function class | |
| I | 6.6 |
| II | 4.1 |
| III | 3.4 |
| IV | 1.2 |
| Karnofsky performance status | |
| 70–100 | 4.7 |
| 40–60 | 2.3 |
| Status of primary tumor | |
| Absent | 4.9 |
| Controlled | 3.1 |
| Age | |
| <60 | 4.7 |
| 60+ | 3.3 |
| Metastatic extent | |
| Brain only | 4.8 |
| Brain + other | 3.4 |

**TABLE 2.** *Neurologic function class*

Neurologic functional status:
1. Able to work; neurologic findings minor or absent
2. Able to be at home, although nursing care may be required. Neurologic findings present but not serious
3. Requires hospitalization and medical care with major neurologic findings
4. Requires hospitalization and in serious physical or neurologic state, including coma

along with their corresponding median survivals as identified in large Radiation Therapy Oncology Group studies. Table 2 defines the neurologic functional classes. The neurologic function classes are predictors of survival with classes I, II, III, and IV having median survivals of 27, 17, 14, and 5 weeks, respectively (31). Multivariate analysis has identified Karnofsky performance status 70, an absent or controlled primary, age <60 years, and metastatic spread limited to the brain as the four factors predictive of improved survival. Eleven percent of the study population had these four factors present and had a predicted 200-day survival of 52%. Patients with 3, 2, 1, or none of these factors present had a predicted probability of surviving 200 days of 36%, 24%, and 14%, respectively.

Palliative radiotherapy for brain metastases is delivered to the entire cranial contents through parallel opposed lateral fields. The energy range used includes cobalt-60 through 20-MV x-rays. Lower energies typically result in higher skin doses an acute effects. Higher energies may result in underdosage due to lack of buildup at shallow depths. Parallel opposed lateral whole-brain fields are utilized. Both fields are treated daily. Dose is prescribed at midplane. If a simulator is available, care should be taken to ensure adequate coverage of the mid-

dle cranial fossa. If a simulator is unavailable, a clinical setup can be performed placing the inferior field border on a line that extends from the superior orbital ridge to the tip of the mastoid process. In patients with metastases in the inferior portion of the frontal or temporal lobe, the inferior border should extend from the infraorbital ridge to the external auditory meatus (32). Beam blocks to protect normal tissues such as the orbital structures, pharynx, and neck should be used, if necessary. There should be fall-off of the field on the skull anteriorly, posteriorly, and superiorly. Figure 1A demonstrates MRI findings of multiple brain metastases in a patient with non-small cell lung cancer. Figure 1B demonstrates the typical lateral whole-brain irradiation field described above and used in the palliative treatment of the patient from Fig. 1A.

The palliative effects of cranial irradiation were first noted by Chao et al. in 1954 (33). Palliation of neurologic symptoms was noted in 63% of 38 patients after receiving 3000–4000 cGy in 3–5 weeks. Several prospective randomized studies have attempted to define the optimal dose fractionation schedule for palliative whole-brain irradiation. In their first study of brain metastases, the RTOG randomized 993 patients to one of four arms: 30 Gy in 2 weeks, 30 Gy in 3 weeks, 40 Gy in 3 weeks, and 40 Gy in 4 weeks (33). The second RTOG study random-

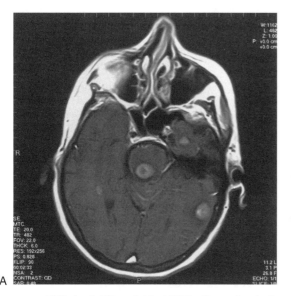
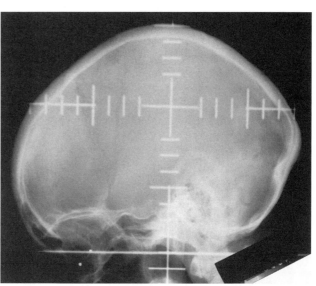

**FIG. 1. A:** T1-weighted MRI with contrast of a patient with non-small cell lung cancer and multiple brain metastases. **B:** The whole brain was treated with parallel opposed lateral fields prescribing 30 Gy in 10 daily fractions to the midplane.

ized patients to shorter time–dose fractionation schemes, including 20 Gy in 1 week, 30 Gy in 2 weeks, and 40 Gy in 3 weeks (33). No differences were noted between the treatment schedules in the first and second RTOG studies with regard to frequency of improvement (56–75%), median time to progression (8–12 weeks), or median survival (15–21 weeks). The percent of survival spent in an improved or stable neurologic state ranged from 72% to 81% without any demonstrable time–dose response effect. Ambulatory patients survived significantly longer than nonambulatory patients (21 weeks versus 12 weeks, respectively). Within each neurologic function class responders survived longer than nonresponders. Approximately 50% and 31% of patients died of brain metastases in the first and second studies, respectively. The overall response rates for the three most common presenting symptoms of headache, motor deficit, and impaired mentation were 82%, 67%, and 70%, respectively. These studies used patient-based assessments of response. Important quality-of-life issues remain to be resolved for patients receiving palliative whole-brain irradiation.

The use of single-dose palliative radiotherapy has been investigated. The Princess Margaret Hospital in Toronto noted no significant difference in survival, response rates, local control, and complications in 101 patients prospectively randomized to receive 10 Gy in a single fraction or 30 Gy in 10 fractions (34). Both of the previously noted RTOG trials included an optional arm into which patients were randomized to receive 10 Gy in one fraction (26 patients) or 12 Gy in two fractions (35). For those patients receiving one of these ultrarapid high-dose radiation schedules, there was no difference in the time to improved neurologic function, acute treatment morbidity, and median survival. However, patients receiving either the 10- or 12-Gy treatment arms had a shorter duration of response, a shorter time to progression of neurologic symptoms, and a lower rate of complete disappearance of neurologic symptoms compared to patients receiving the more protracted schedules. Patients receiving 10 Gy required retreatment more frequently than patients receiving 30 or 40 Gy (19% versus 5%, respectively; $p = 0.025$). It has been subsequently recommended that use of these ultrarapid fractionation schedules be limited to patients with an extremely shortened expected survival and in patients unlikely to tolerate a protracted course of palliative cranial radiation therapy.

At the opposite extreme, it has been postulated that a favorable subgroup of patients with brain metastases may benefit from a high-dose course of radiotherapy (36). Kurtz et al. reported another RTOG prospective trial randomizing a favorable subset of patients with brain metastases to 30 Gy in 2 weeks or 50 Gy in 4 weeks (36). Patients with uncontrolled primary tumors, extracranial metastases, or class IV neurologic function were ineligible. The two treatment arms were similar with respect to palliation of symptoms, improvement rate, median time to progression, cause of death, and median survival. The only notable significant difference was the improved response rate in the neurologic function class II patients treated with 30 Gy in 2 weeks. It therefore does not appear that more aggressive palliative radiotherapy is of benefit, even in a highly selected subset of patients.

Accelerated fractionation has the advantages of a shortened course of treatment and the theoretical benefits of increased acute tumor effects and decreased late complications. The RTOG performed a phase I/II trial of accelerated fractionation in a favorable subset of patients (37). Three hundred forty-five favorable patients with brain metastases (solitary in 50%) received 32 Gy in twenty 1.6-Gy fractions given twice daily with an interfraction interval of 4–8 hours. Patients were then randomized and given additional treatment to a boost field that included the metastatic lesion(s) with a 2.5-cm margin. The boost field was treated at 1.6 Gy given twice daily with a dose escalation to total doses of 48, 54.4, 64, and 70.4 Gy, respectively. Overall, the median survival varied from 4.2 months to 6.4 months without any significant difference noted between the four treatment arms. The median survival was improved in patients with controlled primary tumors, nonlung primaries, and solitary metastases. The 1-year survival was improved for those patients in the arms receiving >54.4 Gy (13% versus 30%). A multivariate analysis of the 153 patients with unresected solitary brain metastases demonstrated a superior survival for these patients receiving >54.4 Gy ($p = 0.05$) (38). No significant difference was found between the dose levels with respect to neurologic improvement, duration of improvement, or percentage of patients dying secondary to brain metastases (38). No increased acute and late toxicity was seen with increasing doses up to 70.4 Gy. Accelerated fractionation for brain metastases is not considered standard of care at present. A prospective randomized trial would have to demonstrate its benefit over standard once-daily fractionation to justify its use.

## Solitary Metastases

The optimal management of patients with solitary brain metastases is controversial. Two prospective randomized trials have compared surgical resection and postoperative whole-brain irradiation with whole-brain irradiation only (39,40). Patchell et al. randomized 48 solitary brain metastasis patients, with no other systemic disease or limited/controllable disease outside of the brain and Karnofsky score >70, to surgical resection and postoperative radiotherapy consisting of 36 Gy in 12 fractions or whole-brain radiotherapy alone by the same treatment schedule (39). An important significant difference was noted in the median duration of functional independence—38 weeks in the surgical arm versus 8 weeks in the radiotherapy-alone arm. Despite a significant improvement in overall survival in the surgical group (40 weeks versus 15 weeks, $p = 0.01$) the survival at 90 weeks was <10% in both arms. The 20% local failure rate in the surgical arm was a significant improvement over the 52% local failure rate in the radiotherapy-alone arm. Surgical resection also prolonged the time to failure at the site of original brain metastasis from a median of 21 weeks to >59 weeks. Although surgery improved the local control rate at the original site of brain metastasis, no difference was shown in the incidence of distant brain metastases or leptomeningeal disease. An unexpected finding was the 11% incidence of nonmetastatic brain lesions found upon resection or biopsy of the lesions. Noordijk et al. similarly compared surgery and radiotherapy to radiotherapy alone in 63 patients with solitary brain metastases. Patients were stratified by primary site and the activity of systemic disease. Radiotherapy in both arms delivered a total dose of 40 Gy given in 2-Gy fractions twice daily over 2 weeks. Overall survival was significantly improved in the surgery and radiation group with a median survival of 10 months compared to 6 months in the radiotherapy-alone group. The most significant difference in survival was noted in the group of patients with stable extracranial disease who had a median survival of 12 months versus 7 months, in favor of surgical resection. All patients with progressive extracranial disease had a 5-month median survival without significant differences for the two treatment arms. The most important predictor of survival was age younger or older than 60 years. Younger patients had a median survival of 19 months compared to 9 months, again favoring surgery and radiation over radiation alone. For the patients older than 60 years, the median survival was approximately 6 months without any significant difference noted between the treatment groups.

Considering these prospective studies, surgery and postoperative whole-brain radiotherapy is an appropriate treatment for selected patients with operable solitary brain metastases. The quality and duration of survival can be improved in those patients with surgically accessible solitary lesions with no leptomeningeal spread, good performance status, young age, a nonradiosensitive histology, and no active disease outside of the CNS. Patients with solitary brain metastases on MRI should receive prompt evaluation by the radiation oncologist, medical oncologist, and neurosurgeon.

The role of adjuvant whole-brain radiation therapy following resection of a solitary metastasis has been questioned and reported in several retrospective studies (41–43). In a review from the Mayo Clinic of 85 patients receiving surgical resection with or without adjuvant whole-brain radiotherapy, the brain relapse rate was 21% in the adjuvant radiation group compared to 85% in the surgery-alone group (41). An additional finding arguing for the use of adjuvant radiation was the improved median survival of 21 months in the radiotherapy group

versus 12 months in the surgery-alone group. This study also suggested that a dose response exists. Failure in the brain occurred in 31% of the patients receiving <39 Gy and 11% of those receiving >39 Gy. A similar improvement in the 1-year recurrence rate from 46% to 22% was noted in the adjuvant whole-brain radiotherapy group as described in a report from investigators at Memorial Sloan-Kettering Cancer Center (42). Adjuvant radiation also significantly prolonged the disease-free interval but did not significantly improve the median or 1-year survival. In a more recent report from Memorial Sloan-Kettering Cancer Center, 185 patients with lung cancer and a solitary brain were reviewed to evaluate the impact of postoperative whole-brain radiotherapy following resection of a single brain metastasis (43). In an attempt to remove the inherent selection bias, those patients receiving postoperative irradiation were prognostically matched to those patients undergoing surgery alone. The use of postoperative whole-brain radiotherapy did not appear to influence survival or the overall brain failure rate, although the failure rate in the brain adjacent to the site of the resected brain metastasis (focal failure) was improved (34% versus 23%, $p = 0.07$). Upon subset analysis, it was noted that postoperative whole-brain radiotherapy significantly decreased the focal failure rate for patients with adenocarcinoma histology from 33% to 14%.

The true impact of postoperative whole-brain radiotherapy following resection of a single brain metastasis can only be determined in a prospective randomized study. Unfortunately, a phase III RTOG trial investigating the role of postoperative whole-brain radiotherapy was closed early due to poor accrual.

In patients with unresected solitary brain metastases, the role of a boost dose of radiation following whole-brain irradiation has been questioned. Conventional once-daily fractionated boost doses of radiation in patients with solitary metastases has been reported by Hoskin et al. (17). All patients received 35 Gy in 15 fractions over 3 weeks. In a nonrandomized fashion, patients with solitary brain metastases, who either had no extracranial metastases or had primary breast cancer with only bone metastases, received an additional boost of 15 Gy in 8 daily fractions. No difference was noted in overall survival or the incidence of death from progressive brain metastases for those highly selected solitary brain metastases patients receiving a boost and those patients with multiple brain metastases not receiving a boost. The only factor predictive of improved survival was the 3- and 6-week response to treatment. In the phase I/II RTOG study of accelerated fractionation for brain metastases previously noted (37), a subset of solitary brain metastases patients were treated as previously described with a boost dose to the lesion to increase the total doses to 48, 54.4, 64, and 70.4 Gy. No dose response was seen with regard to duration of stable or improved neurologic function, death from brain metastases, or survival. However, a multivariate analysis of prognostic factors demonstrated a superior survival time of borderline statistical significance for the upper three dose treatment arms compared to the 48-Gy treatment arm ($p = 0.05$). It is difficult to make any definite recommendations regarding the benefit of boosting the dose to unresected solitary metastases beyond the dose given with whole-brain irradiation. Again, patient-based endpoints were used and quality-of-life issues have not been well addressed.

## Complications

The acute complications of whole-brain radiotherapy are a function of dose fractionation and are usually mild and well tolerated, although they can occasionally be severe (30). Dry desquamation occurs early in the course of radiotherapy followed by hair loss beginning 2 weeks after the start of irradiation. The large majority of patients experience almost complete alopecia with subsequent hair growth appearing a few months after completion of radiation. Headaches, nausea, lethargy, and otitis media can be seen. Dermatitis, alopecia, and otitis media are complications that may last for a prolonged time following whole-brain irradiation (30). Patients should be taking dexamethasone by the time radiotherapy begins to prevent any increased intracranial pressure during treatment. If any bothersome signs or symptoms of increased intracranial pressure, such as headache or nausea, appear during treatment, they can usually be managed with an increased dose of dexamethasone. Worrisome signs and symptoms including progressive motor loss or mental status deterioration should prompt a diagnostic investigation. The somnolence syndrome of increased fatigue and lethargy can occur 1–4 months after cranial irradiation but usually resolves spontaneously. Cranial irradiation can also cause myelosuppression, which may necessitate dose reduction in patients also receiving chemotherapy (30).

Long-term survivors following cranial irradiation are at risk for suffering severe and debilitating late complications. These include brain atrophy, necrosis, leukoencephalopathy with neurologic and mental deterioration and dementia (30). The incidence of late complications is most dependent on the fractional dose, but total dose and the use of chemotherapy must also be considered. Clinically apparent dementia can be seen following 30-Gy whole-brain irradiation given in 10 fractions. DeAngelis et al. reported an incidence of radiation-induced dementia in 1.9–5.1% of long-term survivors following whole-brain irradiation (44). A variety of dose fractionation schedules were used, but most patients received fractional doses >300 cGy. The affected patients developed progressive dementia, ataxia, and urinary incontinence at a median of 14 months following treatment. There was no

evidence of tumor recurrence when neurologic symptoms began. CT imaging demonstrated ventricular dilatation, atrophy, and hypodense white matter in all patients. Retrospective studies of prophylactic whole-brain radiotherapy in small-cell lung cancer patients have shown late complications of memory loss with moderate to severe neuropsychologic impairment in up to half of patients (45,46). However, a prospective study of prophylactic cranial irradiation in 229 small-cell lung cancer patients receiving 24-Gy whole-brain irradiation in eight fractions over 12 days or no prophylactic cranial irradiation failed to demonstrate any difference in the 2-year cumulative incidence of neuropsychological changes between the two groups (47). Brain necrosis occurs in <1% of patients receiving standard fractionation to 52 Gy (30).

## Reirradiation

The role of repeat whole-brain irradiation for patients with recurrence or progression of brain metastasis is not clear. Less than half of the patients with symptomatic recurrences undergo a second course of radiation therapy (30). Cooper et al. demonstrated improvement in symptoms and at least one neurologic functional level in 42% of patients undergoing reirradiation (48). The patients more likely to benefit from reirradiation, as noted by these authors, are those patients who are in good general condition and suffer neurologic deterioration 4 or more months after a satisfactory response to initial whole-brain radiation therapy. Care must be taken not to exceed the brain tolerance dose when determining the total and fractional doses of reirradiation.

## Stereotactic External Beam Irradiation and Brachytherapy

Stereotactic radiosurgery is able to accurately and precisely deliver a high dose of radiation to a limited volume. Treatment is usually delivered in one fraction by a small field using an arc rotation with a linear accelerator or a focused multiple source cobalt-60 unit (gamma knife). The tumor is localized by the use of a fixation device and a system of coordinates that are determined by stereotactic computed tomography. Typically, stereotactic radiosurgery has been used to treat solitary brain metastases or for salvage of recurrent or persistent brain metastases (49–54). Flickinger et al. reported a multiinstitutional experience of gamma knife stereotactic radiosurgery in 116 patients with solitary brain metastases (49). The 2-year actuarial local control rate was 67% with documented radiation necrosis in only one patient. In addition to radiosurgery, 65 patients received fractionated large-field irradiation and were noted to have improved local control, although this improvement was not statistically significant. The median survival for the entire group of patients was 11 months, which is similar to the median survival in solitary brain metastasis patients treated with surgical resection and whole-brain radiotherapy (39,40).

Results of a multiinstitutional experience using linear accelerator-based stereotactic radiosurgery followed by whole-brain irradiation in patients considered to have resectable solitary brain metastases have been reported (55). The median survival for patients with solitary brain metastases treated with radiosurgery and whole-brain irradiation was 56 weeks with an 85% local control rate. The only significant predictors for improved survival were baseline Karnofsky performance score and the absence of other metastases. These results are comparable with those of surgical resection for solitary brain metastases. To determine the benefit of stereotactic radiosurgery and whole-brain irradiation over whole-brain irradiation alone, the RTOG is presently conducting a prospective randomized trial comparing whole-brain irradiation to whole-brain irradiation followed by stereotactic radiosurgery for patients with one to three brain metastases. While the role of stereotactic radiosurgery in the palliation of brain metastases continues to be more clearly defined, these results demonstrate its effectiveness in untreated, recurrent, or persistent solitary brain metastases. Stereotactic interstitial radiation with or without whole-brain radiotherapy has been used in the palliation of initial and recurrent brain metastases. Prados et al. reported an 80-week median survival in 14 patients with progressive brain metastases treated with the temporary implantation of radioactive iodine sources (56). In 21 patients with recurrent cerebral metastases treated with interstitial radiosurgery (iodine-125), the median survival was 6 months (57).

## Summary of Radiation for Brain Metastases

Whole-brain radiotherapy remains the standard of care in the palliation of patients with brain metastases. Approximately 70–90% of patients will experience a symptomatic response, although up to 50% will eventually die of failure in the brain. For this reason, entry of patients with brain metastases into investigational trials is essential for continued progress in the management of this problem. Off protocol, 20 Gy in 1 week or 30 Gy 2 two weeks provides as effective palliation as more prolonged courses of treatment. Shorter courses of radiotherapy should be considered for symptomatic patients with an anticipated life expectancy of 1–2 months. Patients with solitary brain metastases and stable or minimal extracranial disease should be considered for surgical resection and adjuvant whole-brain irradiation. Stereotactic radiosurgery will likely have an important role in the management of patients with one to three brain metastases or recurrent brain metastases.

## Meningeal Metastases

Patients with meningeal metastases demonstrate a uniformly poor prognosis, with <10% of patients surviving for 1 year. Up to 50% of patients with meningeal metastases secondary to breast or lung cancer may improve with standard treatment. Patients with leukemia or lymphoma usually respond well to treatment (58). A recent review of 35 patients with carcinomatous meningitis from breast cancer demonstrated meningeal metastasis to complicate <3.5% of cases of metastatic breast cancer. The majority had primary tumors that were of lobular or combined lobular/ductal histology. The median time from recurrence in the meninges to death was 15 months. The Karnofsky performance status was noted to be the most significant prognostic factor for improved survival (1). Patients with meningeal metastases usually die of progressive systemic disease with controlled CNS disease. Standard treatment involves the intrathecal administration of methotrexate, ARA-C, or thiotepa, usually in single-drug regimens, delivered through an Ommaya reservoir or lumbar puncture.

The Eastern Cooperative Oncology Group (ECOG) reported results of a prospective randomized trial of intrathecal methotrexate or thiotepa given twice weekly every 8 weeks in patients with neoplastic meningitis (59). Concomitant cranial irradiation delivered 30 Gy in 10 fractions to those patients with cranial nerve palsies, cortical dysfunction, or concomitant brain metastases. No patient experienced significant neurologic improvement with therapy and 75% deteriorated neurologically within 8 weeks of the start of treatment. The median survival in both arms was approximately 15 weeks. The predictors for decreased survival were progressive systemic disease, poor performance status, and cranial nerve palsies. It is likely that early intervention is necessary for there to be any benefit in the treatment of neoplastic meningitis. Radiation oncologists are always concerned regarding the added toxicity of concomitant cranial irradiation and intrathecal chemotherapy, especially regarding the incidence of leukoencephalopathy. While only about 50% of patients on the ECOG study received concomitant intrathecal chemotherapy and cranial irradiation, a direct comparison of toxicity between those patients receiving and not receiving radiation was not reported. Only one case of necrotizing leukoencephalopathy was seen in this study. However, there was a 4% incidence of lethal toxicity in both arms and a 54% and 30% incidence of severe or life-threatening toxicity in the methotrexate and thiotepa arms, respectively (59). Intrathecal chemotherapy with or without concomitant cranial irradiation is associated with significant toxicity and should only be given to patients expected to benefit from treatment, namely, those without progressive systemic disease, with a good performance status (0, 1, or 2), and with no severe cranial nerve deficits. The concomitant delivery of cranial irradiation with intrathecal chemotherapy is recommended in those patients with neoplastic meningitis associated with brain metastases, cranial nerve palsies, or cortical dysfunction. Although there is a risk of leukoencephalopathy, the incidence is not known secondary to the short survival time of these patients.

Craniospinal irradiation is not recommended secondary to the large amount of bone marrow, up to 40%, that can be included in the craniospinal radiation field (58). Patients with cranial nerve palsies can be treated with whole-brain irradiation or a helmet brain portal that extends inferiorly to the bottom of the C2 vertebral body and includes the reflections of the temporal meninges and the retro-orbital regions. The typical dose fractionation scheme delivered to these fields is 3000 cGy in 10 fractions given over 2 weeks.

There may also be a role for the use of partial brain portals to areas of CSF obstruction. Using technetium-99m DTPA ventriculography, Glantz et al. demonstrated obstruction of CSF flow in 61% of patients (60). Focal radiotherapy to the site of the CSF block was able to restore flow in 11 of 19 patients. Improved survival was noted in those patients whose abnormal CSF flow was correctable with focal radiotherapy. The median survival of patients with normal CSF flow, abnormal flow that was corrected with radiotherapy, and abnormal flow that was not correctable with radiotherapy was 7 months, 13 months and 0.7 months, respectively. This approach, using focal radiotherapy to relieve obstruction of CSF flow, improved the survival of patients with leptomeningeal metastasis and decreased the morbidity, neurotoxicity, and systemic toxicity of intrathecal chemotherapy.

Complications of the treatment of leptomeningeal metastasis include aseptic meningitis, necrotizing leukoencephalopathy, or infection secondary to the CSF reservoir placement. Necrotizing leukoencephalopathy occurs most frequently in patients receiving intraventricular or high-dose systemic methotrexate (58). It is difficult to recommend palliative radiotherapy for patients with meningeal metastasis and a poor performance status. Those patients with a good Karnofsky performance status should be treated aggressively with attention to the dose fractionation of radiotherapy and dose of concurrent intrathecal chemotherapy to avoid unnecessary complications in patients with limited survival.

## SPINAL CORD COMPRESSION

### Etiology and Epidemiology

Spinal cord or cauda equina compression is a medical emergency with severe and debilitating consequences. Delay in treatment results in irreversible paralysis and loss of sphincter control. Eighteen thousand new cases have been estimated to occur annually in the United States (61). An autopsy series documented spinal cord compression in 5% of patients with malignancies (62).

Compression of the spinal cord or cauda equina usually arises from extradural metastases rather than intradural metastases (63). Tumor most commonly arises in the vertebral body and compresses the dural sac anteriorly. Neurologic impairment results from progressive tumor expansion posteriorly that compresses the spinal cord. The cauda equina is compressed from lesions arising below the L1–L2 vertebral level. The treatment and functional outcomes of cauda equina compression are similar to those of spinal cord compression. Metastases can arise in the epidural space without prior bone involvement. Spinal cord compression can also result from paraspinal tumors such as lymphoma or neuroblastoma, invading through the intervertebral foramen. Animal models of spinal cord compression have demonstrated spinal cord edema and histologic evidence of neuronal injury (64). Steroids have been shown to decrease cord edema but did not delay the onset of paraplegia (65).

Spinal cord compression most commonly occurs in patients with previously diagnosed malignancies, although 8–47% of patients present initially with spinal cord compression without a prior diagnosis of malignancy (63). Lung and breast cancers, unknown primaries, and lymphoma account for spinal cord compression in 16%, 12%, 11% and 11% of the cases, respectively. The remainder of the cases are secondary to a variety of malignancies including malignancies of the GI tract (4%), thyroid (3%), kidney (6%), prostate (7%), sarcoma (8%), and myeloma (9%) (66). The interval from diagnosis of the primary tumor to presentation with spinal cord compression is variable, averaging 6 months in lung cancer patients and 4 years in women with breast cancer (63). The cervical, thoracic, and lumbosacral spinal cord levels are involved in approximately 10%, 70%, and 20%, respectively, of the patients with spinal cord compression. Metastatic disease from breast cancer, prostate cancer, and myeloma can involve more than one site of epidural metastasis. A second site of epidural metastases occurs in 8–37% of patients.

### Clinical Presentation

Over 90% of patients presenting with spinal cord compression complain of back pain (63). Back pain may be present without neurologic symptoms for days to months. The pain may be worsened by movement or straining or it may be radicular in nature. Radicular pain can aid in localizing the level of vertebral involvement. Following back pain, patients can develop weakness, sensory loss, and autonomic dysfunction. The progression to irreversible paraplegia can be complete within hours to days.

This rapid progression to paraplegia makes this complication of malignancy a medical emergency requiring early recognition and early treatment. Any patient with a known cancer diagnosis presenting with back pain must be evaluated immediately and with a high index of suspicion for spinal cord compression because the consequences are frequently preventable and certainly devastating.

The patient's neurologic status at the start of treatment is the most important predictor of neurologic outcome. Patients who are ambulatory at the start of treatment usually remain ambulatory, whereas nonambulatory patients are less likely to regain ambulatory abilities following treatment. This reinforces the need for early intervention. Physical examination may demonstrate percussion tenderness over the involved spine. Straight leg raising or neck flexion can exacerbate pain over the involved vertebrae. Neurologic examination can demonstrate motor deficits including weakness, spasticity, abnormal deep tendon reflexes, and extensor plantar responses (63). Sensory loss usually begins distally and ascends proximally to the level of involved spinal cord. The sensory loss tends to be more marked distally. A sensory level on the trunk, the level at which abnormal sensation becomes normal, roughly indicates the level of cord compression. Autonomic dysfunction may manifest as urinary retention and constipation. Patients with autonomic dysfunction may present with a palpable bladder, a large postvoid urinary residual, or decreased anal tone.

### Diagnostic Evaluation

Patients with spinal cord compression should be evaluated by a neurosurgeon in addition to medical and radiation oncologists. High-dose intravenous dexamethasone (10 mg intravenously, then 4 mg every 6 hours) should be started to decrease cord edema (67), relieve pain and improve function (68). Corticosteroids should be tapered following treatment to prevent associated complications of infection, myopathy, and ulcer (63).

More than two-thirds of patients will have radiographic bony abnormalities, including possible pedicle erosion, vertebral body compression, or paraspinal soft tissue mass, but the absence of abnormalities does not exclude epidural metastases (63). Myelography has historically been the standard imaging modality for diagnosing and localizing epidural spinal cord compression. Presently, MRI offers advantages over myelography including the lack of a need for a lumbar puncture, less time and patient discomfort, and fewer neurologic and bleeding complications (63). Carmody et al. demonstrated similar sensitivities of 92% and 95% for MRI and myelography, respectively (69). The specificities were also similar at 90% and 88%, respectively. Li et al. also showed a similar sensitivity of 93% and a high specificity of 97% for MRI (70). When available, MRI has been estimated to be more cost-effective than myelography (71). MRI also aids in the treatment planning for radiation therapy and planning surgery because of its ability to identify paravertebral tumor extensions and other areas of spinal cord compression that may arise between myelographic blocks. MRI can also differentiate extradural from extramedullary and intramedullary intradural lesions (63). If a nondiagnostic MRI is obtained in a patient with malignancy and neurologic signs and symptoms consistent with spinal cord compression, a CT myelogram should be sought.

### Treatment

The goal of palliative radiation therapy or surgery for spinal cord compression is to relieve pain, preserve or improve neurologic function, provide local tumor control, and stabilize the spine. As previously stated, the most important factor predicting neurologic status after treatment is the neurologic status prior to treatment. Most ambulatory patients will remain ambulatory following radiation or surgery. Approximately 40–60% of patients overall remain ambulatory following treatment (63). Table 3 demonstrates the improved neurologic outcome according to pretreatment neurologic condition in patients treated with irradiation alone or laminectomy and irradiation. Less than 10% of patients who are paraplegic prior to therapy become ambulatory after therapy.

Historically, a decompressive laminectomy was performed for metastatic spinal cord compression regardless of whether the tumor was anterior or posterior to the spinal cord (61). Following laminectomy, only 30% of patients improved, whereas 12% worsened. However, the operative mortality rate was 9% with an 11% incidence of nonfatal complications. By the 1980s, retrospective stud-

**TABLE 3.** *Effect of pretreatment motor function on treatment outcome*

| Pretreatment condition | Laminectomy and irradiation | | Irradiation only | |
|---|---|---|---|---|
| | No. ambulatory/ no. treated | Percent ambulatory | No. ambulatory/ no. treated | Percent ambulatory |
| Ambulatory | 14/22 | 64 | 46/58 | 79 |
| Paraparetic | 15/33 | 45 | 37/83 | 45 |
| Paraplegic | 1/10 | 10 | 1/29 | 3 |

ies were demonstrating superior or similar results using radiotherapy in comparison to decompressive laminectomy (63). Radiotherapy was associated with less morbidity and mortality than laminectomy and is presently considered to be the standard of care for patients initially presenting with spinal cord compression. Recent studies have demonstrated superior results for aggressive surgical procedures based on the site of tumor involvement in the spinal column, as opposed to decompressive laminectomy for all metastatic epidural cord compressions (72–74). While the newer improvements in the surgical management of cord compression are promising, many patients are medically inoperable due to the presence of advanced metastatic disease and other comorbidities or may not be considered candidates for an extensive surgical procedure for various other reasons. There are no prospective randomized trials of surgery and radiation therapy. The choice of surgery, radiation therapy, or the combination of both depends on each patient's clinical presentation, rate of progression, availability of a prior tissue diagnosis, tumor type, site of spinal involvement, stability of the spine, and any prior treatment received (63). Currently, radiotherapy and corticosteroids are the standard of care for the palliation of most patients with epidural spinal cord compression. Surgery is recommended for patients without a prior tissue diagnosis of malignancy, progressive neurologic dysfunction during radiation therapy, or recurrent cord compression after prior radiotherapy (63). Surgery should also be considered for younger patients with minimal metastatic disease, a good performance status, a stable spine above and below the lesion, and for those patients with a relatively longer expected survival.

Energies used to treat spinal cord compression are varied, but typically lower energies such as cobalt-60 4- or 6-MV linear accelerators are used. The treatment volume includes sites of symptomatic disease as determined by MRI or myelography plus one vertebral body above and below the metastasis. If the patient has an anticipated survival >6 months, consideration should be given to including two vertebral bodies above and below the site of disease. Depending on the energy used and depth to the vertebral body, patients can be treated with either a posterior field only or parallel opposed anterior–posterior fields. Cervical spine lesions should be treated with parallel opposed lateral fields to avoid irradiating the larynx unnecessarily. Thoracic and lumbar spine lesions should be treated with a posterior spine field if the depth is <6–8 cm. Otherwise, thoracic and lumbar spine lesions are usually treated with parallel opposed anterior and posterior fields. Figure 2 demonstrates the MRI findings of spinal cord compression and the radiation portal used to palliate this patient. The optimal total dose and dose fractionation schedule have not been determined in a prospective randomized fashion. Usual dose fractionation schemes employed are 2000 cGy in 1 week or 3000 cGy in 2

weeks. Occasionally, longer fractionation schedules, such as 4000 cGy given over 3–4 weeks, may be used. Care must be taken not to exceed spinal cord tolerance, which is typically considered to be 45 Gy in 22–25 fractions. Although the dose resulting in a 5% incidence of radiation myelopathy is likely in the range of 57–61 Gy, based on analysis of retrospective data, this dose level is not justified in the palliative irradiation of spinal cord compression (75).

## Treatment Results

Black reviewed reports prior to 1979 of palliative treatment for spinal cord compression (61). The overall incidence of maintaining ambulatory function after laminectomy, radiotherapy, or laminectomy plus radiotherapy was 31%, 45%, and 51%, respectively. Gilbert et al. at Memorial Sloan-Kettering Cancer Center similarly showed that 49% of patients were ambulatory after radiotherapy alone, which was similar to 46% of those patients receiving surgery and postoperative radiotherapy (76). The pretreatment neurologic status, not the type of treatment received, was the most important determinant of neurologic outcome. The ability to walk posttreatment was retained in 73%, 36%, and 3% of those patients who were ambulatory, paraparetic, or paraplegic prior to treatment. Patients with more radioresistant tumors or autonomic dysfunction had a worse outcome than patients with radioresponsive tumors or no evidence of autonomic dysfunction. Interestingly, patients with rapid progression of spinal cord dysfunction, usually an indication for surgery, had a more improved outcome following radiation therapy than after surgery and postoperative irradiation. The surgery performed in all patients was a decompressive laminectomy no matter the site of tumor in the spinal column. In a small prospective study, no significant difference in pain relief, ambulatory status, or sphincter function was noted between the 16 patients randomized to laminectomy with postoperative irradiation and the 13 patients randomized to radiation alone (77). While the final outcome of patients receiving surgery or radiotherapy is similar, radiotherapy patients may be more likely to deteriorate during the course of irradiation. Cobb et al. demonstrated the importance of frequent neurologic examinations during treatment in order to identify those patients with neurologic deterioration during radiotherapy, an indication for surgical intervention (78).

Maranzano and Latini recently published results of a prospective trial of radiation and steroids in 275 patients with metastatic spinal cord compression (79). Only 7% of the patients received surgery prior to irradiation. Patients were referred for surgery if the diagnosis was in doubt, if there was evidence of vertebral body collapse with resultant bone impinging on the spinal cord, if the vertebral column required stabilization, and/or if there was prior

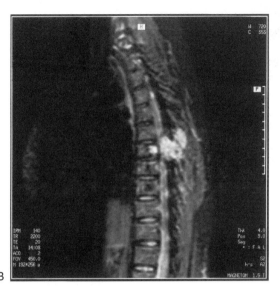
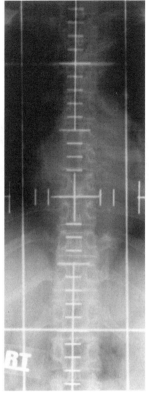

**FIG. 2. A:** T2-weighted MRI demonstrating spinal cord compression at T6–T8 secondary to multiple myeloma with multiple vertebral body metastases throughout the spine. **B:** The T4–T12 spine was treated with parallel opposed anterior and posterior fields prescribing 24 Gy in 8 daily fractions prescribed to the midplane. Erosion of the pedicle on the right side of T7 is seen.

irradiation in the same area. Considering the 209 patients treated with radiation and steroids, 94%, 60%, and 11% of the patients who were ambulatory, non-ambulatory, or paraplegic prior to treatment, respectively, maintained the ability to walk posttreatment. Overall, 76% of patients were ambulatory following irradiation. These results are similar to those of Gilbert et al. (76). In those paraparetic and paraplegic patients, those with favorable histologies (breast and prostate carcinoma, myeloma, and lymphoma) had an improved ambulatory outcome compared to those patients with unfavorable histologies. In those patients with autonomic dysfunction and requiring a bladder catheter, 44% regained urinary function. The median survival for the entire group was 6 months with a 1-year actuarial survival of 28%. The median survival was significantly improved in patients who were ambulatory versus non-ambulatory pretreatment (8 months versus 4 months, $p = 0.02$), ambulatory versus nonambulatory post-treatment (9 months versus 1 month, $p < 0.001$), and in those with favorable versus unfavorable histologies (10 months versus 3 months, $p < 0.001$). Patients with favorable histologies also had a longer duration of response (11 months versus 3 months, $p < 0.001$). Primary histology was an important predictor of outcome only in patients with paraparesis, paraplegia, or bladder dysfunction. Long-term survival was rare, with only 9% of patients surviving longer than 3 years without pain or neurologic dysfunction. The local recurrence rate was 3%, all of whom were inoperable and died within 3

months. A second site of cord compression developed in 4% of patients. All received radiotherapy and 66% responded. The authors concluded that early diagnosis was an important predictor of outcome and primary histology was only important in patients with paraparesis, paraplegia, or bladder dysfunction. In this large prospective report, the authors have minimized the inherent variables present in retrospective reports and have more clearly defined the criteria for considering radiation therapy or surgery in the treatment of spinal cord compression (80).

Interesting results of spinal cord compression due to specific histologies, melanoma, and renal cell carcinoma in particular have been reported (81,82). In a retrospective review of patients with spinal cord compression due to metastatic melanoma, Herbert et al. demonstrated a dose response (81). Sixty-two percent of patients receiving 3000 cGy or greater had a symptomatic complete response compared to 20% of patients receiving less than 3000 cGy. However, the overall palliative response rate of 71%, in patients with spinal cord compression due to melanoma, was noted to be independent of fractional dose and total dose by Rate et al. (83). In a retrospective report, Sundaresan et al. demonstrated improved response and survival in renal cell carcinoma patients with spinal cord compression treated with surgery as compared to radiotherapy alone (82). Generally, radiosensitive tumors such as myeloma, lymphoma, and seminoma have excellent response rates following irradiation (63). Prostate, breast, and renal cell carcinomas have intermediate prognoses compared to the poor outcome of lung cancers. In the large prospective study by Maranzano, the response rate for breast cancer, myeloma, and lymphoma ranged from 80% to 88% (79). The response rate for primary tumors of the lung, prostate, kidney, and bladder was approximately 70% compared to 43% for hepatic primaries.

Local recurrence and second metastatic deposits causing spinal cord compression are uncommon given the shortened survival of patients with spinal cord compression. Local recurrence within the radiation field occurs in 3% of patients (79). This figure appears low and is likely due to the limited 6-month median survival of these patients. Kaminski et al. reported a 16% recurrence rate with recurrences occurring within three vertebral bodies of the initial site (84). Early recurrences tended to develop within two vertebral bodies of the original metastatic site, whereas later recurrences were more likely to be three or more vertebral bodies apart. In contrast to Kaminski et al., others were unable to demonstrate any relationship between time to a second spinal cord compression and location within the vertebral column (28). Helweg-Larsen et al. investigated second spinal cord compression and location within the vertebral column (85). However, these investigators did demonstrate a 7% symptomatic recurrence rate outside of the radiation port. This group of patients with second symptomatic recurrences had a longer median survival of 9 months compared to the 3-month median survival of the entire group. Patients with a longer survival time are at an increased risk for developing a second spinal cord compression.

In addition to documenting improvement or stabilization of neurologic function and pain, the myelographic changes following radiation have been reported. In a small retrospective report of 50 cases of epidural spinal cord compression treated with radiation therapy, follow-up myelography was normal in 58%, improved in 25%, and unchanged in 18% (86). High-grade compression fractures predicted for poor tumor response on myelography. The posttreatment myelogram results, in addition to the pretreatment ambulatory status, were the most important predictors of response to radiation therapy.

Radiation oncologists frequently encounter patients with multiple sites of epidural or spinal cord compression and must consider irradiating extensive spinal fields with the attendant acute side effects or withholding treatment until those asymptomatic sites become symptomatic. Helweg-Larsen et al. demonstrated multiple spinal epidural metastases in 35% of 107 patients (85). In 23 patients, only neurologically symptomatic lesions were treated, whereas any additional asymptomatic minor epidural metastases were not irradiated. Only 8% of these untreated epidural metastases ever became symptomatic and required irradiation. Follow-

ing a detailed history and physical examination and careful review of the imaging studies, one may not need to extend the radiation field in order to include all asymptomatic small epidural metastases, as long as the patient is followed closely for new onset back pain or neurologic findings.

## Summary of Radiation for Spinal Cord Compression

The role of radiation therapy in the palliation of spinal cord compression is well established. Spinal cord compression is an oncologic emergency requiring a high index of suspicion and immediate evaluation in any cancer patient presenting with back pain. Early intervention with corticosteroids and radiation therapy can prevent progression to paraparesis and paraplegia. Following irradiation, 65–95% of patients who are ambulatory or nonambulatory prior to treatment will be able to ambulate, but only approximately 10% of patients paraplegic prior to irradiation will have significant improvement following treatment. Radiotherapy results in relief of back pain in most patients, approximately 70–85%. Newer, more promising aggressive surgical techniques will likely play a greater role in the palliation of a subset of patients with spinal cord compression in the future.

## SUPERIOR VENA CAVA SYNDROME

Superior vena cava syndrome (SVCS) is a constellation of signs and symptoms resulting from the obstruction of blood flow in the superior vena cava. This causes an increase in the venous pressures in the upper extremities and head and neck. Superior vena cava syndrome was first described in 1757, associated with a case of syphilitic aortic aneurysm (87). In 1957, Schecter reviewed 274 cases of superior vena cava syndrome and noted that 40% were secondary to syphilis or tuberculosis. Presently, benign causes of SVCS are uncommon and malignancy accounts for 75–85% of the cases (87).

### Etiology and Epidemiology

Lung cancer is the most common cause of SVCS. In four series with a total of 415 patients, the etiology of SVCS was noted to be lung cancer and lymphoma in 65% and 8%, respectively (87). Other malignancies and nonneoplastic causes were associated with SVCS in 10% and 12% of the cases, respectively. Of lung cancer patients, 2.5–4.2% of those with non-small cell lung cancer developed SVCS (88,89). Of those patients with small cell lung carcinoma, 6.6–11.5% present with or develop SVCS at some time in their course (90–92). On the other hand, small cell lung carcinoma was present in 38% of 370 patients with lung cancer and SVCS, whereas squamous cell and adenocarcinoma histologies were present in 26% and 14%, respectively. Large cell histology and other unclassified histologies were present in 12% and 9%, respectively.

Following lung cancer, non-Hodgkin's lymphoma is the next most common primary malignancy accounting for SVCS (87). Data from Mallinckrodt and MD Anderson demonstrate SVCS in 2–4% of patients with non-Hodgkin's lymphoma (88,93). The lymphoma histologies associated with SVCS were diffuse large cell in 64%, lymphoblastic in 33%, and follicular in 3% (93). Of the patients with diffuse large cell lymphoma, 7% were noted to develop SVCS whereas 21% of those with lymphoblastic lymphoma developed SVCS. Other malignant etiologies of SVCS include Hodgkin's disease, germ cell tumors, thymoma, and metastatic disease. Breast cancer is the most common metastatic cause of SVCS (87). Nonmalignant causes of SVCS include central venous catheters, pacemakers, tuberculosis, and histoplasmosis (87).

Anatomically, the superior vena cava lies in the right side of the mediastinum and can become obstructed secondary to compression, invasion, or thrombosis. The azygos venous system is the most important alternate collateral pathway for the return of venous blood from the upper extremities and head and neck in a patient with superior vena cava obstruction.

## Presentation

The most common presenting symptoms of SVCS are dyspnea and facial swelling/head fullness in 63% and 50%, respectively (87). Other presenting symptoms include cough, arm swelling, chest pain, and dysphagia. Physical examination findings, including neck vein distention, chest wall vein distention, and facial edema, are seen in 66%, 54%, and 46%, respectively, of patients with SVCS. Cyanosis, facial plethora, and arm edema may also be seen.

Although the signs and symptoms of SVCS can be very distressing for the patient and physician, SVCS is rarely life threatening. In animal studies, Carlson demonstrated that following ligation of the superior vena cava the signs and symptoms of SVCS were relieved in 1 week due to the formation of collateral blood flow (94). Although the signs and symptoms of SVCS returned with ligation of the azygos vein, all dogs recovered eventually without sequelae. In a review of almost 2000 cases of SVCS, Ahmann demonstrated that SVCS rarely resulted in patient mortality (95). One documented case of a patient with SVCS dying from aspiration of epistaxis was noted, whereas three other deaths could not convincingly be attributed to SVCS.

## Evaluation

Following a thorough history and physical examination, the diagnostic evaluation includes a chest x-ray, which may demonstrate widening of the superior mediastinum in 64% of patients, a pleural effusion in 26%, and a right hilar mass in 12% (87). A normal chest x-ray has been noted in 16% of patients with SVCS. Additional evaluation should include CT and/or MRI scans, as these can provide detailed information regarding the location and extent of obstruction of the superior vena cava and whether the obstruction is due to thrombus, external compression, or invasion by a mediastinal mass. This information obtained is critical for the radiation oncologist in order to tailor fields that will fully encompass the disease. The use of contrast venography may be beneficial in detailing the extent and location of thrombosis. The use of venography was previously considered controversial because of the theoretical risk of increased bleeding following puncture of a vein under pressure. Ahmann demonstrated this risk to be small (95). In a review of 843 invasive or semiinvasive procedures in patients with SVCS, Ahmann found only 10 nonfatal complications and only 3 of these 10 complications were bleeding episodes.

## General Measures

The goal in the treatment of SVCS is to provide rapid palliation of distressing symptoms and improve the patient's likelihood for cure. General measures that should be used in all patients initially include bedrest and elevation of the head of the bed to decrease the venous pressures in the upper extremities and head and neck. Additionally, oxygen, diuretics, and a low-salt diet may also improve symptoms by decreasing the venous pressures (87). Corticosteroids are also begun at the time of presentation to reduce any inflammatory component associated with the process and improve venous blood flow through the superior vena cava [87].

## Radiation Therapy

Although SVCS is no longer considered an oncologic emergency, external beam irradiation continues to be considered the standard of care for the palliation of the signs and symptoms of SVCS in patients with non-small cell lung cancer. Patients with small cell lung cancer or malignant lymphoma who present with SVCS may be palliated with the appropriate curative chemotherapy with or without the addition of radiation. Armstrong and Perez reported the results of 125 cases of SVCS receiving radiation therapy at Mallinckrodt Institute of Radiology (88). Non-small cell lung cancer was the most common primary histology, followed by small cell lung cancer and non-Hodgkin's lymphoma. A variety of radiation fractionation schemes were used, including a high initial dose of 300–400 cGy fractions daily for the first 3 days. Thirty-nine patients received a combination of radiation and chemotherapy. The radiation volume included the tumor with an adequate margin, mediastinum, ipsilateral hilum, and supraclavicular fossa. The overall median survival was 5.5 months with 24% and 9% of all patients surviving at 1 year and 5 years, respectively. The 5-year survival of the non-Hodgkin's lymphoma patients was 41%, a marked improvement compared to the 5-year survival of patients with small cell and non–small cell lung cancer—5% and 2%, respectively. The evaluation of the patterns of failure demonstrated that the majority of patients died secondary to distant metastatic disease. Recurrent SVCS developed in 14% of lung cancer patients and 6% of patients with lymphoma. A trend in an improved response rate was noted in favor of the high-initial-dose fractionation scheme. There also appeared to be a dose response with an improved response rate for those patients receiving >2000 cGy (87% versus 50%). Davenport et al. also evaluated the use of high initial fractional doses initially in the treatment of 19 patients with SVCS, the majority of whom had small cell lung cancer (96). Patients received 4 Gy ×3 fractions followed by 1.5 Gy daily to a total dose of 30–50 Gy. Response was noted in 89% of patients within 3 days, and within 2 weeks 95% of patients demonstrated an objective improvement in their signs and symptoms of SVCS. The presence of SVCS in patients with non-small cell lung cancer has not been shown to be a poor prognostic factor for survival and these patients should be treated aggressively with radiotherapy alone or combined chemoradiation if they are appropriate candidates.

In small cell lung cancer patients with SVCS, excellent results have been demonstrated using chemotherapy with or without radiation therapy. Dombernowsky demonstrated a complete response in 22 patients with small cell lung cancer and SVCS within a median of 7 days with the use of combination chemotherapy (90). In a retrospective review of 37 patients, Spiro compared the local control and survival rates of small cell lung carcinoma patients with SVCS receiving chemotherapy or chemotherapy with radiation therapy (97). No improvement in the local control or survival rates could be demonstrated with the addition of radiation therapy. In a retrospective multivariate analysis for survival of patients with SVCS treated with chemotherapy alone, radiation alone, or chemoradiation at the M.D. Anderson Cancer Center, the presence of SVCS was not an adverse prognostic factor (91). While these studies demonstrate the outcome of SVCS in a chemosensitive malignancy such as small cell lung cancer, it is difficult to draw any conclusions given the small number of patients and retrospective nature of these reports.

Other investigators have also demonstrated that the presence of SVCS does not impact on the survival of patients with small cell lung cancer (92,98). Sculier et al.

demonstrated that induction chemotherapy provided relief of SVCS in 73% of patients, as opposed to 43% of patients receiving induction radiation (92). Relief of symptoms was generally noted within 7–10 days and no survival differences were noted between patients with or without SVCS. Van Houtte et al. also reported a high response rate of 80% following chemoradiation in patients with limited stage small cell lung cancer and SVCS (98). Again, no survival differences were noted between patients with or without SVCS. Radiation therapy may not be necessary for mildly symptomatic patients with SVCS and limited stage small cell lung cancer receiving chemotherapy, but considering the evidence of improved survival for limited stage small cell lung cancer patients receiving combined chemoradiation, radiation is routinely recommended for these patients as part of their definitive management (99).

The use of hypofractionated irradiation has also been investigated in the treatment of SVCS (100). Rodrigues retrospectively reviewed 46 patients with SVCS; most patients had a primary lung carcinoma or metastatic disease as the cause of their SVCS. Patients had received one- or two-dose fractionation schemes: 16 Gy in two fractions given over 1 week, or 24 Gy in three fractions delivered over 2 weeks. Response rates and survival were noted to be improved in those patients receiving 24 Gy in three fractions. Firm conclusions regarding the optimal dose fractionation for SVCS cannot be made from this study or other retrospective studies on account of possible selection bias and small patient numbers.

Non-Hodgkin's lymphoma patients who present with or develop SVCS can be treated with chemotherapy alone, radiation therapy alone, or combined chemoradiation. Perez-Soler et al. from the M.D. Anderson Cancer Center evaluated the local control and survival of patients with non-Hodgkin's lymphoma and SVCS treated with one of the three modalities mentioned above (93). All three modalities produced complete relief of SVCS symptoms within 2 weeks of the onset of treatment. Relapse-free survival and overall survival were improved with the use of chemotherapy alone or in combination with radiation therapy compared to radiation therapy alone. The addition of consolidative radiotherapy appeared to improve the local control in the subgroup of patients with large cell lymphomas. The presence of dysphagia, hoarseness, or stridor, not SVCS, was identified as adverse prognostic factors for relapse-free and overall survival. In patients with non-Hodgkin's lymphoma and SVCS, the signs and symptoms of SVCS can be relieved equally well with radiation therapy, chemotherapy, or combined chemoradiation, but the treatment of choice should be dictated by the histology, stage of disease, degree of patient discomfort, and response to chemotherapy if this was chosen as the initial therapy.

Patients with non-small cell lung cancer, limited stage small cell lung cancer, and non-Hodgkin's lymphoma who are free of metastatic disease are treated with definitive intent. Lung cancer patients should be treated to the primary tumor with adequate margin, the ipsilateral hilum, and the mediastinum. Inclusion of the supraclavicular areas is typically included for upper lobe lung tumors or evidence of superior mediastinal adenopathy. Customized cerrobend blocks should be used to spare uninvolved areas of lung or regional spread. The initial volumes are treated with parallel opposed fields to spinal cord tolerance and are then shifted off cord to an oblique or three-field plan to limit any further irradiation of the spinal cord beyond its normal tolerance level. Most patients respond well to conventional fractionation schemes, but large initial fractional doses of 300–400 cGy can be delivered for severely distressing symptoms of SVCS (88). Typical total doses are approximately 5000–6000 cGy. Non-Hodgkin's lymphoma patients presenting with SVCS due to bulky mediastinal adenopathy are best treated with consolidative involved field radiotherapy following a course of chemotherapy (101). Total doses are 3000 or 4000 cGy for patients with a complete or partial response to chemotherapy, respectively. Early stage low-grade non-Hodgkin's lymphoma patients experience 50–85% disease-free survival rates at 10 years following involved or extended field radiotherapy (102). Total doses range from 2500 to 4000 cGy. Advanced stage non-Hodgkin's lymphomas can be palliated with involved field radiotherapy alone, but improved survival rates are seen following combination chemotherapy regimens or combined modality treatment (102,103).

Many patients with malignancy receive prolonged chemotherapy and require indwelling central venous catheters. Central venous catheters can act as a nidus for thrombus formation and result in SVCS. This benign cause of SVCS should be treated primarily by removal of the catheter. Barring any contraindications, patients with SVCS secondary to thrombosis may then require anticoagulation or thrombolytic therapy with streptokinase, urokinase, or tissue plasminogen activator (87,104). Repeated angioplasty has also been demonstrated to provide prolonged symptomatic relief in patients with obstruction of the superior vena cava and its major tributaries (105). The placement of intraluminal mechanical stents has been used successfully to relieve symptoms in patients with SVCS that is recurrent following chemotherapy or radiation therapy, or in patients who fail to respond to the initial treatment (106–109). Improvement in survival has not been demonstrated following surgical bypass in patients with malignancy-associated SVCS, although improvement in symptoms has been reported (110). Surgical bypass of superior vena cava obstruction is usually not undertaken in patients with SVCS secondary to malignancy, as most of these patients are not surgical candidates. Patients with benign causes of SVCS have been reported to have long survivals following surgical bypass (110).

## Summary of Radiation Therapy for Superior Vena Cava Syndrome

Superior vena cava syndrome is a distressing but rarely life-threatening complication of malignant obstruction of the superior vena cava. Non-small cell and small cell lung carcinoma in addition to non-Hodgkin's lymphoma are the most common causes of superior vena cava syndrome. Because the prognosis and optimal treatment is dependent on the primary histology, it is important to obtain a tissue diagnosis. Urgent radiotherapy is indicated in the presence of distressing respiratory symptoms. Radiotherapy is the standard treatment for non-small cell lung cancer with SVCS. The addition of chemotherapy may be indicated in certain patient subsets. Palliative radiotherapy has also demonstrated its role in relieving the signs and symptoms of SVCS associated with small cell lung cancer and non-Hodgkin's lymphoma. In patients who are unresponsive to aggressive standard treatment or demonstrate recurrent SVCS following maximal treatment, thrombolytic therapy, intravascular stenting, and angioplasty should be considered, as these can provide further palliative benefit.

## PALLIATION OF THORACIC SYMPTOMS

Patients with thoracic malignancies, especially lung and esophageal carcinomas, commonly present with locally advanced or metastatic disease requiring palliation of thoracic symptoms. Approximately 180,000 new lung cancers were diagnosed in 1995, the majority of which presented as advanced or metastatic disease. These patients frequently require palliative radiotherapy (16). Additionally, the lung is the second most common site of metastatic disease for all histologic types of malignancies (111).

Common signs and symptoms of locally advanced lung carcinoma or thoracic metastatic disease include airway obstruction, hemoptysis, cough, dyspnea, or chest pain. These tend to be more common in patients with centrally located tumors. Patients presenting with locally advanced lung cancer frequently require palliative radiotherapy during the course of their disease. In a study of 134 inoperable non-small cell lung carcinoma patients, 36% did not require immediate irradiation (112). Of those patients observed, 54% developed intrathoracic symptoms requiring palliative radiotherapy at some point during their illness. The median symptom-free survival of these patients was 10 months. Ultimately, only 16% did not require palliative radiotherapy at any stage in their disease.

Palliative radiotherapy does not extend survival, but it does improve the quality of life for lung cancer patients. Investigators from the University of Maryland demonstrated excellent symptomatic improvement in lung cancer patients receiving palliative radiotherapy (113). The ability of radiotherapy to improve obstructive atelectasis is most likely dependent on the duration of atelectasis, with the earlier the atelectasis treatment, the more likely that reexpansion will occur (1).

Simpson reported results from the RTOG in which lung cancer patients were randomized to receive 40 Gy split course irradiation, 30 Gy continuous course irradiation, or 40 Gy continuous course radiation (114). Palliation of symptoms was noted in 60% of patients with 25% of patients remaining symptom-free for the duration of their disease. No difference in palliation was noted for the three different dose fractionation schemes. Significant toxicity was noted in 6% of patients. Investigators from Hong Kong randomized 273 patients with locally advanced inoperable non–small cell lung carcinoma to 45 Gy in 18 fractions given over 4.5 weeks, or 31.2 Gy in 4 fractions given over 4 weeks (115). More effective palliation was noted for the patients receiving 45 Gy compared to those receiving 31.2 Gy, 71% versus 54%, respectively. Others have demonstrated palliation in 65–86% of patients randomized to 17 Gy in 2 fractions given over 1 week compared to 30 Gy in 10 fractions, or 27 Gy delivered in 6 fractions (116). The median duration of palliation was 50% or more of survival and there were no differences noted between the two treatment groups. Investigators recommended two fractions of 8.5 Gy given 1 week apart. It was noted, though, that patients receiving 10 Gy in a single fraction or 17 Gy in two fractions 1 week apart experienced transient acute side effects including acute chest pains, fevers, sweats, and rigors during the first 24 hours following radiotherapy (117). Based on the RTOG data, patients requiring thoracic palliation are typically treated with 30 Gy given in 10 fractions over 2 weeks. Patients with significantly compromised performance status or comorbidities are typically treated with 20 Gy delivered in 5 fractions given over 1 week. A repeat course of irradiation can provide symptomatic benefit in approximately half of those patients with recurrent symptoms (118).

Patients receiving palliative chest radiotherapy are typically treated with parallel opposed anterior–posterior fields encompassing the tumor and involved lymph nodes with an adequate margin. Care should be taken to minimize the volume of irradiation to decrease the risks of radiation pneumonitis and fibrosis. The dose that the spinal cord will receive during treatment should be recorded to prevent exceeding the spinal cord tolerance dose, possibly resulting in radiation myelitis.

Endobronchial disease is a common cause of symptoms in patients with locally advanced lung cancer. Many investigators have demonstrated the efficacy of endobronchial irradiation to improve symptoms in 50–100% of patients. Speiser and Spratling demonstrated the palliative benefit of endobronchial high-dose-rate brachytherapy (119). Hemoptysis and obstructive pneu-

monia were improved remarkably well following three treatments of 750-cGy high-dose-rate brachytherapy prescribed at a depth of 10 mm. These investigators also described an entity of radiation bronchitis and stenosis in 12% of patients following high-dose-rate endobronchial irradiation (120). Fatal hemoptysis was noted to occur in 7% of patients. Huber et al. prospectively randomized patients to receive four weekly fractions of 3.8 Gy prescribed to a depth of 10 mm or two fractions of 7.2 Gy prescribed to a depth of 10 mm given 3 weeks apart (121). No differences were noted with respect to survival, local control, or side effects with either of these treatments. Fatal hemoptysis was noted in 22% of patients and was similar between the two arms. Nori et al. demonstrated the palliative benefit of endobronchial irradiation utilizing three weekly fractions of 5 Gy prescribed to a depth of 10 mm without a significant incidence of fistula formation or fatal hemoptysis (122).

Endobronchial placement of the high-dose-rate catheter is performed jointly by the bronchoscopist and radiation oncologist. Patients at our institution typically receive 750 cGy prescribed to a depth of 1 cm to the entire length of high-grade obstruction. Patients with complete obstruction of a central airway bronchus may require initial external beam irradiation to provide some relief and shrinkage of the obstruction so that an endobronchial catheter can be placed.

Esophageal carcinoma patients frequently present with signs and symptoms of esophageal obstruction. Radiation therapy with or without chemotherapy is a well-established palliative modality to relieve esophageal obstruction and improve swallowing symptoms (29,123,124). In a phase II study by Coia et al. patients with stage III or IV esophageal carcinoma received combination chemotherapy with 5-fluorouracil (5-FU) and mitomycin given concurrent with 50 Gy radiotherapy (29). Seventy-seven percent of patients were free of dysphagia following radiation and 60% were dysphagia-free until death or last follow-up. The improvement in swallowing began 2 weeks into treatment and the median duration of response was approximately 5 months. The median survival of stage III and IV patients was 9 months and 7 months, respectively. Burmeister et al. reported the results of a large Australian multicenter study in which 79 patients with extensive locally advanced or metastatic esophageal carcinoma received combination chemotherapy with cisplatin and 5-FU given concurrently with 30–35 Gy of radiotherapy (124). The median dysphagia-free survival was 8 months, and 22% of those patients surviving 3 years remained free of local recurrence or benign stricture requiring repeated dilatation. The volume irradiated is typically the tumor with 5 cm proximal and distal margins and the draining lymph nodes. At our institution, this volume is typically treated with anterior and posterior fields to a dose of 30 Gy. The same volume is then treated with a three-field off-cord cone down to 40 Gy, which is then followed by a three-field boost to the tumor with a 2- to 3-cm margin to a total of 50 Gy. Those patients with severely compromised performance status, weight loss, and comorbidities can also be treated with 30–35 Gy delivered in 15 fractions through anteroposterior–posteroanterior fields. Appropriate candidates should receive combined chemoradiation using 5-FU and cisplatin. Mitomycin may be used for patients with poor renal function or the elderly.

## HEMORRHAGE AND OBSTRUCTION

Patients with moderate hematemesis from esophageal or gastric cancer, hemoptysis from lung cancer, or bleeding secondary to advanced pelvic malignancies can benefit from palliative radiotherapy. For pelvic malignancies, standard fractionated radiotherapy to a total dose of 50 Gy in patients with rectal or vaginal hemorrhage or discharge secondary to recurrent rectal carcinoma can provide adequate palliation in approximately 69% of patients (125). In patients with advanced pelvic malignancies, Boulware et al. demonstrated the benefits of hypofractionated radiotherapy using fractionated doses of 1000 cGy once, twice, or three times at intervals of 3–4 weeks (126). The initial 1000 cGy was delivered through parallel opposed anterior and posterior pelvic fields measuring $15 \times 15$ cm up to $18 \times 18$ cm. The second and third doses were delivered with the same technique, but reduced fields of $12 \times 12$ cm. Pelvic pain was palliated in 45%, 59%, and 63% of patients receiving 1, 2, or 3 fractions, respectively. Additionally, edema and uremia were relieved in 24%, 75%, and 75% of patients receiving one, two, or three fractions, respectively. Treatment was well tolerated and the median survival of patients was 3 months, 7 months, and 9 months for those patients receiving one, two, or three fractions, respectively. Canadian investigators also demonstrated satisfactory palliation in 38 patients with GI and uterine tumors treated with 30 Gy delivered in three monthly fractions, delivered through parallel opposed anterior–posterior fields (127). In a prospective phase I/II study by the RTOG, patients were treated to 3000 cGy total dose in 1000 cGy fractions repeated at 4-week intervals (128). The overall response rate was 41%, but the incidence of late grade 3 and 4 toxicities was 41% for those patients completing all three fractions. A follow-up RTOG study treated patients with advanced pelvic malignancies with 370 cGy fractions twice daily to 1480 cGy (129). This was then repeated at 4–week intervals for three courses to a total dose of 4440 cGy. Although 41% of patients could not complete all three courses due to secondary death or disease progression, there was a significant improvement in the overall response rate (42%) compared to those not completing three courses. The overall response rate was not improved for patients randomized to have a 2-week treatment break compared to a 4-week break. The Karnofsky performance score was an important predictor for survival and the number of courses of radiation completed. The 7% late complication rate in this radiation schedule is tolerable and much improved over that of the prior RTOG study delivering 1000 cGy fractions.

Advanced abdominal and pelvic malignancies causing pain, bleeding, or partial obstruction can be palliated with radiotherapy delivered to the tumor mass with a 1- to 2-cm margin. Typical doses used are 30 Gy in 10 fractions, or 40 Gy in 16 fractions, depending upon the field size used and the amount of small bowel in the field. Hypofractionated radiotherapy, as given in the RTOG study, can be used for those patients with severely compromised performance status, weight loss, and comorbidities. For patients with more profuse bleeding from locally advanced malignancies, large initial fractional doses for the first one to three fractions may provide adequate palliation.

## HEPATIC METASTASES

Liver metastases are commonly seen in the course of many malignancies. Up to 50% of patients with colorectal carcinoma develop liver metastases during the course of their disease. Other non-colorectal malignancies metastasizing to the liver include primaries of the stomach, pancreas, breast, ovaries, uterus, and cervix. Surgery is the only potentially curative procedure with limited metastatic spread to the liver (130). Unfortunately, only 10% of patients with hepatic metastases are surgical candidates. The 5-year survival of patients who do not undergo surgery is typically <5% compared to the 23–40% 5-year survival seen in carefully selected patients undergoing surgical resection of liver metastases.

Radiation therapy alone is indicated only for the palliation of painful hepatomegaly. Radiation produces improvement in hepatomegaly and liver function tests in 55–95% of patients (1). Sherman et al. reviewed the results of palliative hepatic irradiation to 24 Gy given in eight fractions to a total of 55 patients. Significant symptom palliation was noted in 90% of patients. The overall median survival was 4.5 months but was noted to improve to 9 months in those patients experiencing an excellent response to hepatic irradiation. Pain relief was noted to last for the duration of the patient's survival and most patients failed with progressive liver disease (131). Prasad et al. reviewed the results of palliative hepatic irradiation in 20 patients receiving an average dose of 2500 cGy over 3–3.5 weeks (132). Seven other patients received 600–1600 cGy over 1–2 weeks because of the terminal stage of their disease. Symptomatic pain relief was provided in 70% of all 27 patients. Excluding the seven patients in whom therapy was discontinued, 95% of patients demonstrated symptomatic improvement in pain. The average survival was 4 months.

The typical volume to be irradiated includes the whole liver unless the metastatic deposit is limited in its size and extent. Typical doses used range from 2100 to 2400 cGy given in seven to eight fractions over 2 weeks to doses as high as 2800 cGy given in 14 fractions over 3 weeks. For those patients with limited liver metastases, focal external beam radiation therapy utilizing conformal or three-dimensional technique can be used to deliver higher doses to smaller hepatic volumes. Lawrence et al., utilizing dose volume histograms to protect radiation hepatitis, demonstrated that high doses of radiation therapy can be safely delivered if whole-liver treatment is omitted (133). Although the median survival following palliative hepatic irradiation is 4–6 months, responders can have a median survival of 9 months as demonstrated by Sherman (131). Several efforts have been made to improve the palliative effect and objective response rate for radiation therapy. The combined use of intra-arterial chemotherapy with total hepatic irradiation has had some encouraging results (134-136). Hepatic arterial chemotherapy infusion using 5-FU or 5-FUDR along with 21–30 Gy of whole-liver irradiation has demonstrated responses in 33–83% of patients. The median survival of patients treated with intraarterial chemotherapy and total hepatic irradiation is in the range of 8 months for all treated patients. The benefits of this approach compared to hepatic irradiation alone can only be determined in a prospective randomized setting.

## REFERENCES

1. Richter MP, Coia LR. Palliative radiation therapy. *Semin Oncol* 1985; 12:375.
2. Rubin P, Cooper R. Statement of the clinical oncologic problem. In: Rubin P, ed. *Clinical oncology: a multidisciplinary approach for medical students and physicians.* Philadelphia: WB Saunders, 1993;13.
3. Parker S, Tong T, Bolden S, Wingo P. Cancer statistics, 1996. *Ca--A Cancer Journal for Clinicians* 1996;46:5.
4. Malawer MM, Delaney TF. Treatment of metastatic cancer to bone. In: DeVita VT HS, Rosenberg SA, ed. *Cancer: Principles and Practice of Oncology.* Philadelphia: JB Lippincott, 1993;2225.
5. Arcangeli G, Micheli A, Arcangeli G, et al. The responsiveness of bone metastasis to radiotherapy: the effect of site, histology and radiation dose on pain relief. *Radiother Oncol* 1989;14:95.
6. McNeil BJ. Value of bone scanning in neoplastic disease. *Semin Nucl Med* 1984;14:277.
7. Fidler M. Incidence of fracture through metastasis in long bones. *Acta Orthop Scand* 1981;52:623.
8. Gilbert HA, Kagan AR, Nussbaum H, et al. Evaluation of radiation therapy for bone metastases: pain relief and quality of life. *AJR* 1977; 129:1095.
9. Trodella L. Pain in osseous metastases: results of radiotherapy. *Pain* 1984;18:387.
10. Vargha ZO, Glicksman AS, Boland J. Single-dose radiation therapy in the palliation of metastatic disease. *Radiology* 1969;93:1181.
11. Qasim MM. Single dose palliative irradiation for bone metastasis. *Strahlentherapie* 1977;153:531.
12. Tong D, Glick L, Hendrickson F. The palliation of osseous metastases—final results of the study by the Radiation Therapy Oncology Group. *Cancer* 1982;50:893.
13. Blitzer PH. Reanalysis of the RTOG study of the palliation of symptomatic osseous metastasis. *Cancer* 1985;55:1468.
14. Price P, Hoskin PJ, Easton D, Austin D, Palmer SG, Yarnold JR. Prospective randomised trial of a single and multifraction radiotherapy schedules in the treatment of painful bony metastases. *Radiother Oncol* 1986;6:247.
15. Rasmusson B, Vejborg I, Jensen AB, et al. Irradiation of bone metastases in breast cancer patients: a randomized study with 1 year follow-up. *Radiother Oncol* 1995;34:179.
16. Madsen EL. Painful bone metastasis: efficacy of radiotherapy assessed by the patients—a randomized trial comparing 4 Gy × 6 versus 10 Gy × 2. *Int J Radiat Oncol Biol Phys* 1983;9:1775.
17. Hoskin PJ, Crow J, Ford HT. The influence of extent and local management on the outcome of radiotherapy for brain metastases. *Int J Radiat Oncol Biol Phys* 1990;19:111.
18. Cole DJ. A randomized trial of a single treatment versus conventional fractionation in the palliative radiotherapy of painful bone metastases. *Clin Oncol* 1989;1:59.
19. Mithal NP, Needham PR, Hoskin PJ. Retreatment with radiotherapy for painful bone metastases. *Int J Radiat Oncol Biol Phys* 1994;29:1011.
20. Salazar OM, Rubin P, Hendrickson F, et al. Single dose half body irradiation for palliation of multiple bone metastases from solid tumors. Final Radiation Therapy Oncology Group report. *Cancer* 1986;58:29.
21. Zelefsky MJ, Scher HI, Forman JD, Linares LA, Curley T, Fuks Z. Palliative hemiskeletal irradiation for widespread metastatic prostate cancer: a comparison of single dose and fractionated regimens. *Int J Radiat Oncol Biol Phys* 1989;17:1281.
22. Poulter CA, Cosmatos D, Rubin P, et al. A report of RTOG 8206: a phase III study of whether the addition of single dose hemibody irradiation is more effective than local field irradiation alone in the treatment of syptomatic osseous metastases. *Int J Radiat Oncol Biol Phys* 1992;23:207.
23. Porter AT, McEwan AJ, Powe JE, et al. The results of a randomized phase-III trial to evaluate the efficacy of strontium-89 adjuvant to local field external beam irradiation in the management of endocrine resistant metastatic prostate cancer. *Int J Radiat Oncol Biol Phys* 1993;25:805.
24. Silberstein EB. The treatment of painful osseous metastases with phosphorous-32-labeled phosphates. *Semin Oncol* 1993;20:10.
25. Serafini AN. Current status of systemic intravenous radiopharmaceuticals for the treatment of painful metastatic bone disease. *Int J Radiat Oncol Biol Phys* 1994;30:1187.
26. Quilty PM, Kirk D, Bolger JJ, et al. A comparison of the palliative effects of strontium-89 and external beam radiotherapy in metastatic prostate cancer. *Radiother Oncol* 1994;31:33.
27. Ackery D, Yardley J. Radionuclide-targeted therapy for the management of metastatic bone pain. *Semin Oncol* 1993;20:32.
28. Wright DC, Delaney TF, Buckner JC. Treatment of metastatic cancer to the brain. In: DeVita VT, Hellman S, Rosenberg SA, eds. *Cancer: principles and practice of oncology.* Philadelphia: JB Lippincott, 1993; 2170.
29. Coia LR. Palliation. In: Coia LR, Moylan DJ, eds. *Introduction to clinical radiation oncology.* Madison, WI: Medical Physics, 1994;455.
30. Coia LR. The role of radiation therapy in the treatment of brain metastases. *Int J Radiat Oncol Biol Phys* 1992;23:229.
31. Hendrickson FR. The optimum schedule for palliative radiotherapy for metastatic brain cancer. *Int J Radiat Oncol Biol Phys* 1977;2:165.
32. Kagan AR. Radiation therapy in palliative cancer management. In: Perez CA, Brady LW, eds. *Principles and practice of radiation oncology.* Philadelphia: JB Lippincott, 1993;1499.
33. Borgelt B, Gelber R, Kramer S, et al. The palliation of brain metastases: final results of the first two studies by the Radiation Therapy Oncology Group. *Int J Radiat Oncol Biol Phys* 1980;6:1.
34. Harwood AR, Simpson WJ. Radiation therapy of cerebral metastases: a randomized prospective trial. *Int J Radiat Oncol Biol Phys* 1977;2:1091.
35. Borgelt B, Gelver R, Larson M, Hendrickson F, Griffin T, Roth R. Ultra-rapid high dose irradiation schedules for the palliation of brain metastases: final results of the first two studies by the Radiation Therapy Oncology Group. *Int J Radiat Oncol Biol Phys* 1981;7:1633.
36. Kurtz JM, Gelber R, Brady LW, Carella RJ, Cooper JS. The palliation of brain metastases in a favorable patient population: a randomized clinical trial by the Radiation Therapy Oncology Group. *Int J Radiat Oncol Biol Phys* 1981;7:891.
37. Sause WT, Scott C, Krisch R, et al. Phase I/II trial of accelerated fractionation in brain metastases RTOG 85-28. *Int J Radiat Oncol Biol Phys* 1993;26:653.

38. Epstein BE, Scott CB, Sause WT, et al. Improved survival duration in patients with unresected solitary brain metastasis using accelerated hyperfractionated radiotherapy at total doses of 54.4 Gray and greater. *Cancer* 1993;71:1362.
39. Patchell RA, Tibbs PA, Walsh JW, et al. A randomized trial of surgery in the treatment of single metastases to the brain. *N Engl J Med* 1990;322:494.
40. Noordijk EM, Vecht CJ, Haaxma-Reiche H, et al. The choice of treatment of single brain metastases should be based on extracranial tumor activity and age. *Int J Radiat Oncol Biol Phys* 1994;29:711.
41. Smalley SR, Schray MF, Laws ER, O'Fallon JR. Adjuvant radiation therapy after surgical resection of solitary brain metastasis: association with pattern of failure and survival. *Int J Radiat Oncol Biol Phys* 1987;13:1611.
42. DeAngelis LM, Mandell LR, Thaler HT, et al. The role of postoperative radiotherapy after resection of single brain metastases. *Neurosurgery* 1989;24:798.
43. Armstrong JG, Wronski M, Galicich J, Arbit E, Leibel SA, Burt M. Postoperative radiation for lung cancer metastatic to the brain. *J Clin Oncol* 1994;12:2340.
44. DeAngelis LM, Delattre JY, Posner JB. Radiation-induced dementia in patients cured of brain metastases. *Neurology* 1989;39:789.
45. Johnson B, Becker B, Goff II W, et al. Neurologic, neuropsychologic, and computed tomography scan abnormalitites in 2 to 10 year survivors of small cell lung cancer. *J Clin Oncol* 1985;3:1659.
46. Laukkanen E, Klonoff H, Allan B, Graeb D, Murray N. The role of prophylactic brain irradiation in limited stage small cell lung cancer: clinical, neuropsychologic and CT sequelae. *Int J Radiat Oncol Biol Phys* 1988;14:1109.
47. Arriagada R, Le Chevalier T, Borie F, et al. Prophylactic cranial irradiation for patients with small cell lung cancer in complete remission. *JNCI* 1995;87:183.
48. Cooper J, Steinfeld A, Lerch I. Cerebral metastases: value of re-irradiation in selected patients. *Radiology* 1990;174:883.
49. Flickinger JC, Kondziolka D, Lunsford LD, et al. A multi-institutional experience with stereotactic radiosurgery for solitary brain metastasis. *Int J Radiat Oncol Biol Phys* 1994;28:797.
50. Davey P, O'Brien PF, Schwartz ML, Cooper PW. A phase I/II study of salvage radiosurgery in the treatment of recurrent brain metastases. *Br J Neurosurg* 1994;8:717.
51. Mehta MD, Rozental JM, Levin AB, et al. Defining the role of radiosurgery in the management of brain metastases. *Int J Radiat Oncol Biol Phys* 1992;24:619.
52. Engenhart R, Kimmig BN, Hover KH, et al. Long-term follow-up of brain metastases treated by percutaneous stereotactic single high-dose irradiation. *Cancer* 1993;71:1353.
53. Kihlstrom L, Karlsson B, Lindquist C, Noren G, Rahn T. Gamma knife surgery for cerebral metastases. *Acta Neurochisurgica* (Suppl) 1991;352:87.
54. Loeffler JS, Kooy HM, Wen PY, et al. The treatment of recurrent brain metastases with stereotactic radiosurgery. *J Clin Oncol* 1990;8:576.
55. Auchter RM, Lamond JP, Alexander E, et al. A multi-institutional outcome and prognostic factor analysis of radiosurgery (RS) for resectable single brain lesions. *Int J Radiat Oncol Biol Phys* 1995;32:145 (Abstr).
56. Prados M, Leibel S, Barnett CM, Gutin P. Interstitial brachytherapy for metastatic brain tumors. *Cancer* 1989;63:657.
57. Kreth FW, Warnke PC, Ostertag CB. Stereotactic interstitial radiosurgery and percutaneous radiotherapy in treatment of cerebral metastases. *Nervenarzt* 1993;64:108.
58. Ginsberg RJ, Kris MG, Armstrong JG. Cancer of the lung. In: DeVita VT, Hellman S, Rosenberg SA, eds. *Cancer: principles and practice of oncology.* Philadelphia: JB Lippincott, 1993;746.
59. Grossman SA, Finkelstein DM, Ruckdeschel JC, Trump DL, Moynihan T, Ettinger DS. Randomized prospective comparison of intraventricular methotrexate and thiotepa in patients with previously untreated neoplastic meningitis. *J Clin Oncol* 1993;11:561.
60. Glantz MJ, Hall WA, Cole BF, et al. Diagnosis, management, and survival of patients with leptomeningeal cancer based cerebrospinal fluid-flow status. *Cancer* 1995;75:2919.
61. Black P. Spinal metastasis: current status and recommended guidelines for management. *Neurosurgery* 1979;5:726.
62. Barrons KD, Hirano A, Araki S, Terry RD. Experiences with metastatic neoplasms involving the spinal cord. *Neurology* 1959;9:91.
63. Delaney TF, Oldfield EH. Spinal cord compression. In: DeVita VT, Hellman S, Rosenberg SA, eds. *Cancer: principles and practice of oncology.* Philadelphia: JB Lippincott, 1993;2118.
64. Ushio Y, Posner R, Posner JB, Shapiro WR. Experimental spinal compression by epidural neoplasms. *Neurology* 1977;27:422.
65. Siegal T, Siegal TZ. Current considerations in the management of neoplastic spinal cord compression. *Spine* 1989;14:223.
66. Bruckman JE, Bloomer WD. Management of spinal cord compression. *Semin Oncol* 1978;5:135.
67. Ushio Y, Posner R, Kim J, Shapiro WR, Posner JB. Treatment of experimental spinal cord compression caused by extradural neoplasms. *J Neurosurg* 1977;47:380.
68. Greenberg HS, Kim JH, Posner JB. Epidural spinal cord compression from metastatic tumor: results with a new treatment protocol. *Ann Neurol* 1980;8:361.
69. Carmody RF, Yang PJ, Seely GW, Seeger GW, Unger EC, Johnson JE. Spinal cord compression due to metastatic disease: diagnosis with MR versus myelography. *Radiology* 1989;173:225.
70. Li KC, Poon PY. Sensitivity and specificity of MRI in detecting malignant spinal cord compression and distinguishing malignant from benign compression fractures of vertebrae. Magnetic resonance imaging in diagnosing cord compression. *Cancer* 1988;75:2579.
71. Jordan JE, Donaldson SS, Enzmann DR. Cost effectiveness and outcome assessment of magnetic resonance imaging in diagnosing cord compression. *Cancer* 1995;75:2579.
72. Harrington KD. Anterior cord decompression and spinal stabilization for patients with metastatic lesions of the spine. *J Neurosurg* 1984;61:107.
73. Sundaresan N, Digiacinto GV, Hughes JEO, Cafferty M, Vallejo A. Treatment of neoplastic spinal cord compression: results of a prospective study. *Neurosurgery* 1991;29:645.
74. Siegal T, Siegal TZ. Surgical decompression of anterior and posterior malignant epidural tumors compressing the spinal cord: a prospective study. *Neurosurgery* 1985;17:424.
75. Schultheiss TE, Kun LE, Ang KK, et al. Radiation response of the central nervous system. *Int J Radiat Oncol Biol Phys* 1995;31:1093.
76. Gilbert RW, Kim JH, Posner JB. Epidural spinal cord compression from metastatic tumor: diagnosis and treatment. *Ann Neurol* 1978;3:40.
77. Young RF, Post EM, King GA. Treatment of spinal epidural metastases: randomized prospective comparison of laminectomy and radiotherapy. *J Neurosurg* 1980;53:741.
78. Cobb III CA, Leavens ME, Eckles N. Indications for nonoperative treatment of spinal cord compression due to breast cancer. *J Neurosurg* 1977;47:653.
79. Maranzano E, Latini P. Effectiveness of radiation therapy without surgery in metastatic spinal cord compression: final results from a prospective trial. *Int J Radiat Oncol Biol Phys* 1995;32:959.
80. Scarantino CW. Metastatic spinal cord compression: criteria for effective treatment—regarding Maranzano et al., *Int J Radiat Oncol Biol Phys* 1995;32:959–967. *Int J Radiat Oncol Biol Phys* 1995;32:11259.
81. Herbert SH, Solin LJ, Rate WR, Schultz DJ, Hanks GE. The effect of palliative radiation therapy on epidural compression due to metastatic malignant melanoma. *Cancer* 1991;67:2472.
82. Sundaresan N, Scher H, Digiacinto GV, Yagoda A, Whitmore W, Choi IS. Surgical treatment of spinal cord compression in kidney cancer. *J Clin Oncol* 1986;4:1851.
83. Rate WR, Solin LJ, Turrisi AT. Palliative radiotherapy for metastatic malignant melanoma: brain metastases, bone metastases, and spinal cord compression. *Int J Radiat Oncol Biol Phys* 1988;15:859.
84. Kaminski HJ, Diwan VG, Ruff RL. Second occurrence of spinal epidural metastases. *Neurology* 1991;41:744.
85. Helweg-Larson S, Hansen SW, Sorensen PS. Second occurrence of symptomatic metastatic spinal cord compression and findings of multiple spinal epidural metastases. *Int J Radiat Oncol Biol Phys* 1995;33:595.
86. Zelefsky MJ, Scher HI, Krol G, Portenoy RK, Leibel SA, Fuks ZY. Spinal epidural tumor in patients with prostate cancer. Clinical and radiographic predictors of response to radiation therapy. *Cancer* 1992;70:2319.
87. Yahalom J. Superior vena cava syndrome. In: DeVita VT, Hellman S, Rosenberg SA, eds. *Cancer: principles and practice of oncology.* Philadelphia: JB Lippincott, 1993;2225.
88. Armstrong B, Perez C, Simpson J, Hederman M. Role of irradiation

in the management of superior vena cava syndrome. *Int J Radiat Oncol Biol Phys* 1987;13:531.

89. Salsali M, Cliffton EE. Superior vena caval obstruction in carcinoma of lung. *NY State J Med* 1969;69:2875.

90. Dombernowsky P, Hansen HH. Combination chemotherapy in the management of superior vena caval obstruction in small-cell anaplastic of the lung. *Acta Med Scand* 1978;204:513.

91. Maddox A, Valdivieso M, Lukeman J, et al. Superior vena cava obstruction in small cell bronchogenic carcinoma. *Cancer* 1983;52:2165.

92. Sculier J, Evans W, Feld R, et al. Superior vena caval obstruction syndrome in small cell cancer. *Cancer* 1986;57:847.

93. Perez-Soler R, McLaughlin P, Velaspuez W, et al. Clinical features and results of management of superior vena cava syndrome secondary to lymphoma. *J Clin Oncol* 1984;2:260.

94. Carlson HA. Obstruction of the superior vena cava: an experimental study. *Arch Surg* 1934;29:669.

95. Ahmann F. A reassessment of the clinical implications of the superior vena caval syndrome. *J Clin Oncol* 1984;2:961.

96. Davenport D, Ferree C, Blake D, Raben M. Response of superior vena cava syndrome to radiation therapy. *Cancer* 1976;38:1577.

97. Spiro SG, Shah S, Harper PG, Tobias JS, Geddes DM, Souhami RL. Treatment of obstruction of the superior vena cava by combination chemotherapy with and without irradiation in small-cell carcinoma of the bronchus. *Thorax* 1983;38:501.

98. Van Houtte P, R. D, Lustman-Marechal J, Kenis Y. Prognostic value of the superior vena cava syndrome as the presenting sign of small cell anaplastic carcinoma of the lung. *Eur J Cancer* 1980;16:1447.

99. Pignon JP, Arriagada R, Ihde DC, et al. A meta-analysis of thoracic radiotherapy for small-cell lung cancer. *N Engl J Med* 1992;327:1618.

100. Rodrigues CE, Njo KH, Karim ABMF. Hypofractionated radiation therapy in the treatment of superior vena cava syndrome. *Lung Cancer* 1993;10:221.

101. Glick J, Kin K, Earle J, O'Connell M. An ECOG randomized phase III trial of CHOP versus CHOP:radiotherapy (XRT) for intermediate grade early stage non-Hodgkin's lymphoma (NHL). *Proc ASCO* 1995;14:391.

102. Mendenhall N, Lynch J. The low-grade lymphomas. *Semin Radiat Oncol* 1995;5:254.

103. Shafman T, Mauch P. The large-cell lymphomas. *Semin Radiat Oncol* 1995;5:267.

104. Gray BH, Olin JW, Graor RA, Young JR, Bartholomew JR, Ruschhaupt WF. Safety and efficacy of thrombolytic therapy for superior vena cava syndrome. *Chest* 1991;99:54.

105. Wisselink W, Money S, Becker M, et al. Comparison of operative reconstruction and percutaneous balloon dilatation for central venous obstruction. *Am J Surg* 1993;166:200.

106. Oudkerk M, Heystraten FMJ, Stpter G. Stenting in malignant vena caval obstruction. *Cancer* 1993;71:142.

107. Gaines PA, Belli AM, Anderson PB, McBride K, Hemingway AP. Superior vena caval obstruction managed by the Gianturco Z stent. *Clin Radiol* 1994;49:202.

108. Dyet JF, Nicholson AA, Cook AM. The use of the wall stent endovascular prosthesis in the treatment of malignant obstruction of the superior vena cava. *Clin Radiol* 1993;48:381.

109. Putnam JS, Uchida BT, Antonovic R, Rosch J. Superior vena cava syndrome associated with massive thrombosis: treatment with expandable wire stents. *Radiology* 1988;167:727.

110. Doty DB, Doty JR, Jones KW. Bypass of superior vena cava syndrome. Fifteen years experience with spiral vein graft for obstruction of superior vena cava caused by benign disease. *J Thorac Cardiovasc Surg* 1990;99:889.

111. Pass HI. Treatment of metastatic cancer to the lung. In: DeVita VT, Hellman S, Rosenberg SA, eds. *Cancer: principles and practice of oncology.* Philadelphia: JB Lippincott, 1993;2186.

112. Carroll M, Morgan SA, Yarnold JR, Hill JM, Wright NM. Prospective evaluation of a watch policy in patients with inoperable non-small cell lung cancer. *Eur J Cancer Clin Oncol* 1986;22:1353.

113. Slawson R, Scott R. Radiation therapy in bronchogenic carcinoma. *Radiology* 1979;132:175.

114. Simpson JR, Francis ME, Perez-Tamayo R, Marks RD, Rao DV. Palliative radiotherapy for inoperable carcinoma of the lung: final report of a RTOG multi-institutional trial. *Int J Radiat Oncol Biol Phys* 1985;11:751.

115. Teo P, Tai TH, Choy D, Tsui KH. A randomized study on palliative radiation therapy for inoperable non small cell carcinoma of the lung. *Int J Radiat Oncol Biol Phys* 1988;14:867.

116. Anonymous. Inoperable non-small-cell lung cancer (NSCLC): a Medical Research Council randomised trial of palliative radiotherapy with two fractions or ten fractions. Report to the Medical Research Council by its Lung Cancer Working Party. *Br J Cancer* 1991;63:265.

117. Omand M, Meredith C. A study of acute side-effects related to palliative radiotherapy treatment of lung cancer. *Eur J Cancer Clin Oncol* 1994;3:149.

118. Jackson MA, Ball DL. Palliative retreatment of locally recurrent lung cancer after radical radiotherapy. *Med J Aust* 1987;147:391.

119. Speiser BL, Spratling L. Remote afterloading brachytherapy for the local control of endobronchial carcinoma. *Int J Radiat Oncol Biol Phys* 1993;25:579.

120. Speiser BL, Spratling L. Radiation bronchitis and stenosis secondary to high dose rate endobronchial irradiation. *Int J Radiat Oncol Biol Phys* 1993;25:589.

121. Huber RM, Fischer R, Hautmann H, et al. Palliative endobronchial brachytherapy for central lung tumors. A prospective, randomized comparison of two fractionation schedules. *Chest* 1995;107:463.

122. Nori D, Allison R, Kaplan B, Samala E, Osian A, Karbowitz S. High dose-rate intraluminal irradiation in bronchogenic carcinoma. Technique and results. *Chest* 1993;104:1006.

123. Herskovic A, Martz K, Al-Sarraf M, et al. Combined chemotherapy and radiotherapy compared with radiotherapy alone in patients with cancer of the esophagus. *N Engl J Med* 1992;326:1593.

124. Burmeister BH, Rad FF, Denham JW, et al. Combined modality therapy for esophageal carcinoma: preliminary results from a large Australian multicenter study. *Int J Radiat Oncol Biol Phys* 1995;32:997.

125. Gallagher MJ, Richter MP. Radiotherapeutic management of pelvic recurrence in patients with rectal and rectosigmoid carcinoma. *Am J Clin Oncol* 1984;7:115.

126. Boulware RJ, Caderao JB, Delclos L, Wharton JT, Peters LJ. Whole pelvis megavoltage irradiation with single doses of 1000 rad to palliate advanced gynecologic cancers. *Int J Radiat Oncol Biol Phys* 1979;5:333.

127. Hodson DI, Malaker K, McLellan W, Meikle AL, Gillies JM. Hypofractionated radiotherapy for the palliation of advanced pelvic malignancy. *Int J Radiat Oncol Biol Phys* 1983;9:1727.

128. Spanos WJ, Wasserman T, Meoz R, Sala J, Kong J, Stetz J. Palliation of advanced pelvic malignant disease with large fraction pelvic radiation and misonidazole: final report of RTOG phase I/II study. *Int J Radiat Oncol Biol Phys* 1987;13:1479.

129. Spanos WJ, Perez CA, Marcus S, et al. Effect of rest interval on tumor and normal tissue response. A report of phase III study of accelerated split course palliative radiation for advanced pelvic malignancies (RTOG-8502). *Int J Radiat Oncol Biol Phys* 1993;25:399.

130. Niederhuber JE, Ensminger WD. Treatment of metastatic cancer to the liver. In: DeVita VT, Hellman S, Rosenberg SA, eds. *Cancer: principles and practice of oncology.* Philadelphia: JB Lippincott, 1993;2201.

131. Sherman DM, Weichelsbaum R, Order SE, Cloud L, Trey C, Piro AJ. Palliation of hepatic metastasis. *Cancer* 1978;41:2013.

132. Prasad B, Lee MS, Hendrickson FR. Irradiation of hepatic metastases. *Int J Radiat Oncol Biol Phys* 1977;2:129.

133. Lawrence TS, Dworzanin LM, Walker-Andrens SC, et al. Treatment of cancers involving the liver and porta hepatis with external beam irradiation and intraarterial hepatic fluorodeoxyuridine. *Int J Radiat Oncol Biol Phys* 1991;20:555.

134. Webber BM. A combined treatment approach to the management of hepatic metastases. *Cancer* 1978;24:1087.

135. Herbsman H. Treatment of hepatic metastases with a combination of hepatic artery infusion chemotherapy and external radiation therapy. *Surg Gynecol Obstet* 1978;147:13.

136. Kinsella T. The role of radiation therapy alone and combined with infusion chemotherapy for treating liver metastases. *Semin Oncol* 1983;10:215.

*Principles and Practice of Supportive Oncology,*
edited by Ann Berger et al.
Lippincott–Raven Publishers, Philadelphia ©1998

CHAPTER 44

# Palliative Surgery

Brian P. Whooley and Kevin C. Conlon

The primary aim of any palliative surgery is the relief of symptoms, with preservation or improvement in the quality of life. In oncologic practice, palliative surgery in the broadest sense refers to surgery that is by nature noncurative. A palliative resection is generally defined as the surgical extirpation of a primary tumor without removal of all grossly identifiable disease or in the presence of positive resection margins. Palliative surgery also encompasses surgical procedures that are aimed primarily at the treatment of symptoms or complications associated with a tumor. It is this latter aspect of palliative surgery that will form the focus of this chapter, with particular reference to gastric, pancreatic, and colorectal carcinomas.

## SYMPTOMS AND OTHER COMPLICATIONS

An estimated 223,000 new cases of gastrointestinal (GI) cancers will be diagnosed in the United States in 1995 (1). Taken together, colorectal, gastric, and pancreatic cancers account for 83% of the total. The majority of these patients will not be cured and will ultimately die of their disease. Colorectal cancer is the second leading cause of cancer death in the United States, with an estimated 55,000 deaths annually. Pancreatic cancer is the fifth leading cause of cancer death, with an estimated 27,000 deaths annually, whereas gastric cancer accounts for an estimated 15,000 deaths.

The usual presenting symptoms and complications requiring palliative surgical intervention for patients with gastric, pancreatic, and colorectal cancer are detailed in Table 1. Pain is a particularly distressing symptom for patients with GI malignancies and generally is indicative of local and perineural invasion. Lillemoe noted that 37 of 137 patients with unresectable pancreatic carcinoma

reported significant pain (2). Hudis reported similar data, with 37 of 77 pancreatic cancer patients having moderate to severe pain at the time of initial referral (3). The majority were considered to have pain secondary to extensive local disease. Locally advanced rectal cancer also commonly presents with pain because of invasion of the pelvic floor, sacral plexus, or nerve roots. Moran and colleagues reported significant pain at presentation in 37 of 125 patients who underwent palliative resections for rectal cancer (4). Longo and co-workers reported significant rectal or pelvic pain in 12 of 103 patients with advanced rectal cancer (5).

Patients with advanced-stage GI malignancies can present with bowel obstruction. Meijer and co-workers at Free University Hospital in Amsterdam reported on a consecutive series of 204 patients with gastric carcinoma (6). Twenty-six patients underwent a palliative resection, and obstruction was the primary presentation in 14 of these patients. An additional 25 patients were unresectable and underwent a palliative bypass gastrojejunostomy.

Obstruction can also be seen as the primary presentation of advanced-stage colorectal cancer. Garcia-Valdecasas and colleagues reported on a series of 53 patients with colorectal cancer who presented with obstruction over a 4-year period (7). Tumor staging was significantly more advanced in these patients compared to 135 patients with colorectal cancer who underwent elective operation over the same time period (34% Dukes stage D versus 17%). Similarly, Gandrup and colleagues reported that 59

**TABLE 1.** *Indications for palliative intervention*

| |
|---|
| Pain |
| Gastrointestinal obstruction |
| Biliary obstruction |
| Hemorrhage |
| Perforation |
| Malignant ascites |

B. P. Whooley and K. C. Conlon: Department of Surgery, Memorial Sloan-Kettering Cancer Center, New York, NY 10021

of 156 consecutive patients who were operated on for obstructing primary colorectal cancers were unresectable and required either a bypass or a diversion procedure (8).

Extensive intraperitoneal disease can also lead to GI obstruction requiring surgical intervention. Turnbull reviewed 356 patients who presented over a 9-year period to Memorial Sloan-Kettering Cancer Center with obstruction and who previously had undergone surgery for an intraabdominal cancer (9). He identified 89 patients who had obstructing carcinomatosis confirmed at operation and noted that the tumor originated in the colon in 59 patients and in the stomach in 19 patients.

Gastrointestinal hemorrhage may also be seen as a complication in patients with GI tumors. Moreno-Otero and co-workers reviewed 427 patients with gastric cancer and reported 36 who presented with acute upper GI bleeding (10). Fox et al. reported that gastric malignancy was the cause of bleeding in 35 of a consecutive series of 2260 patients (1.5%) treated for upper GI hemorrhage (11).

Bleeding is a common symptom of advanced rectal cancer. In a review of 103 patients with advanced rectal cancer, Longo and colleagues reported that bleeding was the most common presenting symptom, occurring in 45% of patients (5). Similarly, Bordos reviewed 34 patients who underwent palliative abdominoperineal resection and noted that bleeding was a presenting symptom in 74% (12).

Perforation is a less common complication of advanced GI cancers. Free perforation of gastric cancer is rare and occurs in 0.9–4% of cases (13). Starnes reviewed colorectal emergencies treated at Memorial Sloan-Kettering Cancer Center over a 5-year period and reported only six patients with spontaneous perforation of a carcinoma (14).

Malignant ascites is a serious complication and portends an extremely short life expectancy. It occurs at a rate of 10–15% with carcinoma of the stomach, pancreas, and large intestine (15). These patients are often very symptomatic because of GI and respiratory compromise associated with markedly increased intraabdominal pressure. Effective palliation of malignant ascites remains a difficult problem. Peritoneovenous shunts were introduced in 1974 by LeVeen and co-workers for the palliation of intractable ascites (16). Early concerns about postshunt coagulopathy and disseminated metastases appear unfounded, and these complications are rare in clinical practice. In 1992, Gough and colleagues in a prospective but nonrandomized study reported on 47 patients who were palliated with shunts (17). The shunt controlled malignant ascites in two thirds of patients, but there was no difference in survival or quality of life when compared to patients who were treated by repeated paracentesis, without surgical intervention. However, a recent report by Schumaker and colleagues, which reported on 116 shunts in 89 patients, determined that the shunts were associated with substantial morbidity and mortality and a brief and only fair relief of symptoms (18). Specifically,

shunt-related complications occurred in 49% of cases. Perioperative mortality was 43%, and the authors considered that 13% was directly related to shunt-associated complications. In addition, flow had stopped in 50% of shunts within 30 days. This controversy can only be resolved by a prospective randomized trial.

## SPECIFIC TUMOR SITES

### Gastric Cancer

The incidence of gastric cancer, which had been on the decline for many decades, plateaued during the last two decades. Nonetheless, gastric cancer continues to be a significant public health problem. An estimated 22,800 new cases were diagnosed in the United States in 1995, with an estimated 14,700 deaths (1). The high mortality associated with gastric cancer is related to both the advanced stage of the disease at presentation and also to a lack of effective adjuvant therapies. As a result, the majority of patients with gastric cancer require some form of palliative surgery during the course of their illness. Determination of resectability frequently requires assessment at laparotomy, and about 85% of patients undergo surgical exploration. At laparotomy, about half of the patients will be resected and of these about 40% are considered palliative at the outset (19).

#### Obstruction

Many authors suggest that when technically feasible gastric resection offers the best palliation of symptoms and other complications caused by the neoplasm (6,19,20). Resection relieves symptoms of obstruction, contributes significantly to improving quality of life, and may also give some survival benefit (6,21). Figure 1 outlines an approach to gastric outlet obstruction due to obstructing gastric cancer.

The early Memorial Sloan-Kettering Cancer Center experience, reported by El-Domeiri and colleagues in 1972, noted that of 80 patients who underwent palliative resections, 9% experienced good palliation until their demise and 76% achieved satisfactory palliation for an average duration of 6½ months (22). Meijer and co-workers reported on 26 patients with stage IV disease who had palliative resections, including 14 total and 12 subtotal gastrectomies. Obstruction and pain were the major symptoms in 20 of the patients. Fifty percent had good palliation of symptoms, whereas a further 27% had moderate palliation (6). The Norwegian Stomach Cancer Trial reported in 1989 was a prospective but nonrandomized trial, and included 1165 patients with stomach cancer, of whom 182 were recorded as undergoing a palliative resection (21). Having stratified patients according to age, debility, and stage of disease, they identified opera-

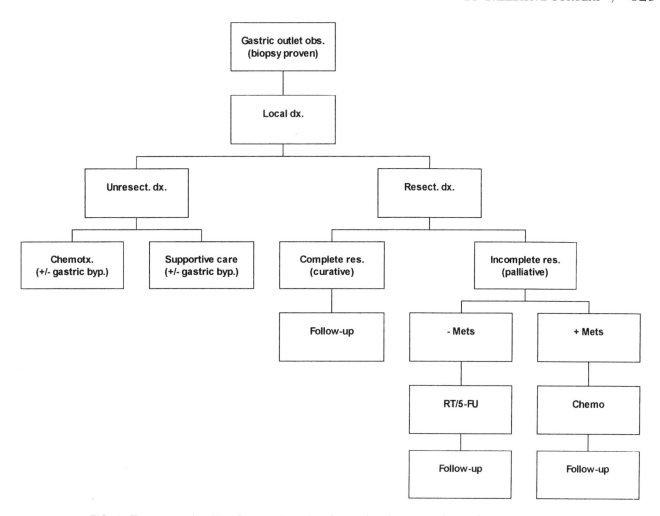

**FIG. 1.** Treatment algorithm for gastric outlet obstruction due to an obstructing gastric cancer.

tive treatment (resection versus nonresection) as an independent prognostic determinant of survival by multivariate analysis. In all of these studies, the reported morbidity and mortality rates for curative and palliative resections are comparable. Five-year survival rates of 6–12% may be realized in these patients (19).

For most lesions a subtotal gastrectomy without an extensive lymphadenectomy is preferable. The role of total gastrectomy in this setting is controversial. In the past, palliative total gastrectomy and esophagogastrectomy, particularly for proximally located tumors, were discouraged due to a prohibitively high perioperative mortality rate ranging between 20% and 30%, and also because there was a suggestion that the quality of life of survivors was reduced (20). However, with improvements in surgical techniques and postoperative care, total gastrectomy has been increasingly performed for palliation. In recent series total gastrectomy comprises as many as one third of cases. In 1991 Monson et al. retrospectively reviewed the Mayo Clinic experience with 53 consecutive total gastrectomies for advanced disease (23). Operative mortality was 8%, and a median survival of 19 months

and good or satisfactory quality of life was achieved in 87% of patients. Butler and co-workers in 1989 described 27 patients who underwent total gastrectomy for palliation of advanced gastric cancer, with an operative mortality of only 4%, and the median survival was an impressive 15 months (24). Twenty-five of 26 patients left the hospital tolerating a solid diet. Total gastrectomy is also the operation of choice for linitus plastica.

When advanced local disease is discovered at operation, with invasion of adjacent organs, an en-bloc resection is indicated in good-risk patients. In the Norwegian Stomach Cancer Trial, 182 patients had palliative resection. Fifty-nine percent of these patients also underwent splenectomy; resection of the pancreatic tail, transverse colon, and liver was added in 7%, 4%, and 2%, respectively (21). In a patient care study conducted by the American College of Surgeons and reported in 1993, 13,295 patients with gastric cancer were treated surgically (25). Extragastric extension was documented in 38% of patients and required an extended resection. Organs involved included the colon (3%), omentum (14%), spleen (2%), pancreas (2%), and esophagus (17%).

In patients with gastric outlet obstruction secondary to an unresectable tumor, a bypass gastrojejunostomy may be performed. However, this procedure is not without risk. Ekbom reviewed 20 patients who underwent palliative gastrojejunostomy and reported a 25% mortality and a 20% incidence of GI complications postoperatively (26). Eighty percent of survivors obtained relief of preoperative symptoms for a mean interval of 5.9 months and no patient was alive at 1 year. Similarly, Bozzetti reported a 10% mortality for 80 patients who underwent palliative gastrojejunostomy and the median survival after bypass was 3.5 months (19). Delayed gastric emptying is a significant problem in as many as 20% of these patients (27). The factors that contribute to delayed gastric emptying include infiltration of the gastric wall by tumor, disturbance of autonomic function, and the frequent inability to place the stoma in a dependent position on the stomach. An alternative to gastrojejunostomy is the Devine antral exclusion procedure. The stomach is transected just proximal to the tumor and a jejunal loop is anastomosed to the proximal stomach. Kwok reported on 20 patients with unresectable antral carcinomas which were locally advanced and infiltrating the head of pancreas or the porta hepatis (28). All were treated by antral exclusion. There was no hospital mortality, and 17 patients were able to tolerate a diet until their demise.

Patients with gastric outlet obstruction who are not candidates for surgical intervention because of associated medical risks may be palliated by percutaneous endoscopic gastrostomy tube drainage (PEG). This can also be converted to a jejunostomy tube (PEJ) for the delivery of enteral nutrition. Alternatively, some patients may be suitable for endoscopic placement of a stent across the obstruction (29).

For unresectable tumors of the cardia, the management options include endoprosthesis placement, endoscopic laser ablation, radiotherapy, or surgical bypass. Endoscopic endoprosthesis placement has a reported mortality rate of 15–45% and a 10% perforation rate (30). Other complications include blockage and displacement. Recent series using improved stents report lower risks of complications and mortality (31). Nd:YAG laser ablation is safe and particularly suited to exophytic lesions involving the distal esophagus. The ability to swallow liquids and semisolids is restored in 60–90% patients, but repeated treatment may be required to maintain patency (32). Radiation treatment has also been used with comparable success (33). Surgical bypass is performed by anastomosing a Roux limb of jejunum to the distal esophagus above the level of the tumor. Good palliation has been reported (34).

### Hemorrhage

Acute GI hemorrhage is an uncommon presentation of gastric cancer. The diagnosis is made by early endoscopy but is frequently difficult to control endoscopically. Loftus and colleagues reported on the Mayo Clinic experience with 15 gastric cancer patients who underwent endoscopic therapy for acute major upper GI hemorrhages (353). They noted that 13 of the 15 patients continued to bleed after treatment. Moreno-Otero reported on 36 patients presenting with bleeding gastric cancers (10). The bleeding was self-limited in 44%; but persistent or massive in 56%. Early emergency surgical intervention in the latter group was associated with a 23% mortality. Cheung and Branicki in 1991 reported on 52 patients of whom 30 underwent elective and 14 emergency surgery (36). The mortality rate for emergency surgery was 42.9% compared to 13.3% for elective surgery. The authors attributed the high mortality rate for emergency surgery to delay in operative intervention. Patients with a self-limited hemorrhage should have early elective surgical intervention, whereas patients with persistent bleeding should have early emergency surgery. A palliative resection is performed when feasible.

### Perforation

Free perforation of gastric carcinoma is rare. It occurs in an ulcerated tumor and is usually associated with advanced stage of disease. In older series, simple closure of the perforation was performed in the great majority of cases but was associated with a mortality rate as high as 68% (37). Recently, Gertsch et al. reported on 34 perforated gastric cancers. Eighty-eight percent of patients underwent emergency gastrectomy and 88% had stage III or IV tumors. The 30-day mortality was 16% in the resected group and the median survival was 10 months (13). Therefore, optimal palliation is achieved by early surgical intervention and by palliative resection when feasible.

### Pancreatic Cancer

An estimated 28,000 new cases of pancreatic cancer occur each year in the United States (38). The incidence appears to be increasing, with most cases occurring in the seventh or eighth decade of life. Over 25,000 deaths per year are due to the disease, making it the fourth leading cause of cancer related mortality, surpassed only by lung, colorectal, and breast cancers. The prognosis is bleak, with an overall 5-year survival of 2–3%. Surgical resection offers the only prospect of cure. However, symptomatology is often vague, and the majority of patients present with advanced disease, which precludes potentially curative therapy (39,40).

Despite recent advances in pancreatic imaging (41–43) and the development of nonoperative techniques for the relief of biliary obstruction, the majority of patients still require an exploratory laparotomy for accurate staging and palliation (44). The most common indication for palliative intervention in this group of patients is for biliary and/or gastric outlet obstruction. For those who do not require a palliative procedure, exploration does not confer any benefit, and is associated with significant morbidity and mortality affecting both the quality and duration of survival (44,45).

### Biliary Obstruction

Between October 1983 and October 1995, 1528 patients were admitted to Memorial Sloan-Kettering Cancer Center with a diagnosis of invasive adenocarcinoma of the pancreas. Of these, 40% were jaundiced and 28% had undergone some form of biliary drainage procedure prior to presentation.

For patients with an unresectable pancreatic tumor, the ideal palliative procedure for biliary obstruction should be effective in relieving jaundice, have minimal morbidity, be associated with a short hospital stay, have a low symptomatic recurrence, and maintain quality of life. In recent years there has been a trend toward nonoperative biliary drainage by either endoscopic or transhepatic routes (44,46–53). Randomized trials have demonstrated a reduced hospital stay and similar early morbidity and mortality with endoscopic stent placement compared to surgical bypass (54,55). However, long-term complications appear to increase, with recurrent jaundice due to occluded or dislodged prosthesis and cholangitis occurring in between 13% and 60% of cases (46,47,50,56). In patients who are expected to live longer than a few months these complications make endoscopic palliation less than optimal.

Prior to the advent of minimal access surgical (MAS) procedures, open surgical drainage was the only other palliative option. Surgical drainage provides excellent relief of jaundice (45,57). Despite extensive controversy in the literature (44–46,48,57), both choledochoenteric and cholecystoenteric bypasses, if selected appropriately, have similar results with regards to reducing serum bilirubin. In a recent analysis of our experience, we were unable to demonstrate any difference between these two methods of biliary diversion (45). Both procedures were associated with considerable morbidity, with complications occurring in 18%. Others have reported similar figures (44,57). It is our clinical impression that particularly after a complicated postoperative course some patients never regain their preoperative performance status and commence a slow inexorable slide in their quality of life until death.

Minimal access surgery offers a new approach to this problem (58,59,60,61). In theory, the reduced operative morbidity in combination with a surgical drainage procedure would be of benefit to the patient expected to live longer than a few months. Figure 2 details our current approach to the jaundiced patient with a peri-pancreatic mass.

### Gastric Outlet Obstruction

The role of prophylactic gastroenteric bypass in the management of patients with unresectable pancreatic cancer is controversial (45). Only 5% of patients will have signs and symptoms of gastric outlet obstruction at the time of presentation; of the remainder, 8–28% will subsequently develop this complication if a gastric bypass has not been performed at the time of the initial operation (62–64). Because of this risk and subsequent need for further surgery, many authors have liberally advocated the use of gastric bypass at the time of initial exploration. Proponents of this approach contend that the mortality of the initial surgical procedure is not increased by the addition of a gastroenteric bypass (63–65).

In contrast, some authors have reported a high mortality and morbidity, including an increased rate of delayed gastric emptying (DGE) in patients undergoing gastrojejunostomy, resulting in poor palliation and prolonged hospitalization (45,66–70). Jacobs and colleagues reported a 29% incidence of DGE in patients who underwent both gastric and biliary bypass, whereas no DGE occurred in the group undergoing biliary bypass alone (69). Welvaart noted that DGE occurred in 67% of 37 patients undergoing both biliary and gastric bypass (70). A recent retrospective review from this institution of 297 patients with unresectable disease demonstrated that a prophylactic gastric bypass was associated with a significantly increased morbidity without improving survival (45). Only 3 of 38 patients who did not receive a gastroenteric bypass at their initial procedure required one subsequently. In all cases duodenal obstruction was a preterminal event.

Currently, we reserve gastric bypass for the subset of patients who are symptomatic at presentation. We believe that in order to determine objective criteria for the selection of patients who would benefit from a prophylactic gastric bypass, a prospective randomized trial is required. In general, we consider those patients who present with obstruction subsequent to their initial presentation, or after therapy (i.e., following resection with recurrent disease) (Fig. 3) as good candidates for a gastric bypass either by the open approach or laparoscopically. The relative merits of one method versus another remain to be determined. In the group of patients in whom gastric outlet obstruction is but one manifestation of their terminal illness, supportive care measures alone are instituted. It is important to identify this group of patients so as to avoid unnecessary pain and suffering.

### Pain

Abdominal or back pain is a major symptom in a significant proportion of patients with unresectable or recurrent pancreatic cancer. Often this is poorly managed, leading to distress and resulting in a major diminution in the patient's

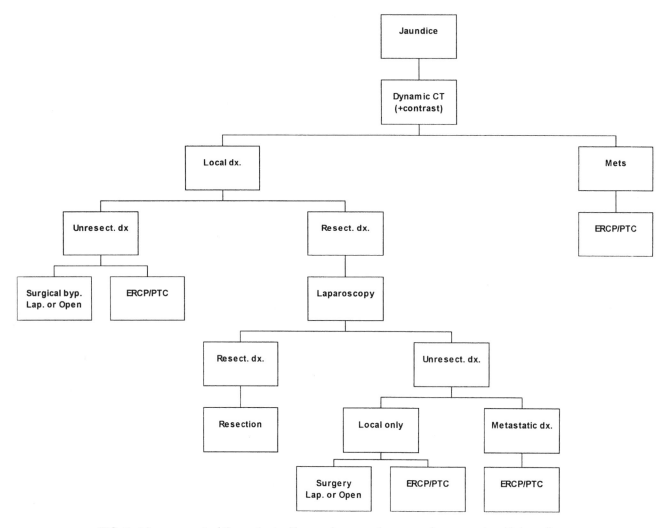

**FIG. 2.** Management of the patient with a peripancreatic mass who presents with jaundice.

quality of life. The primary modalities in the management of pain remain pharmacologic and percutaneous celiac axis blockade. In patients undergoing surgery, however, intraoperative chemical splanchnicectomy should be considered. Celiac plexus blockade has been demonstrated to be effective in providing pain relief from a variety of GI malignancies (71). In 1969, Copping and colleagues first reported the technique for the relief of upper abdominal pain due to pancreatic cancer (72). Recently, Lillemoe and co-workers from the Johns Hopkins Hospital reported a prospective, randomized, double-blind study that compared intraoperative chemical splanchnicectomy with 50% alcohol to saline injection (2). The group receiving the chemical block had significantly reduced pain scores. Those patients without pain at the time of surgery had a significantly delayed onset of pain. In addition, patients with preexisting pain who received the alcohol blockade had improved survival compared to the control group. This exciting study awaits confirmation. Nonetheless, patients with pain who undergo an operative procedure should be considered for a chemical splanchnicectomy.

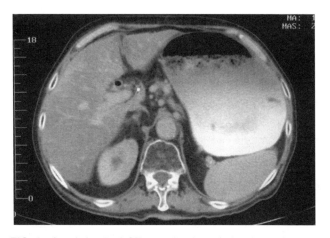

**FIG. 3.** An abdominal CT examination of a patient with gastric outlet obstruction 15 months following pancreatoduodenectomy for a T2 N1 M0 adenocarcinoma of the pancreas. At laparotomy, recurrent disease was noted at the gastroenteric anastomosis.

## Colorectal Cancer

An estimated 138,200 new cases of colorectal cancer will occur in 1995 in the United States (100,000 colonic and 38,200 rectal) (1). The overall 5-year survival is approximately 50%. This survival statistic has not changed significantly over the past 20 years. One third of patients are known to be incurable at presentation because of the presence of extensive local-regional or distant metastatic disease. When patients present with complications of advanced disease, or when patients present with recurrence of disease, an aggressive surgical approach is warranted in properly selected patients. The type of palliative procedure performed will depend on the symptomatology, tumor location, and performance status of the patient.

### Obstruction

Figure 4 outlines our approach to malignant colorectal obstruction. Apart from the patient whose colonic obstruction is a preterminal event, the majority of patients will be eligible and will benefit from some form of surgical procedure.

Approximately 20% of patients with colorectal carcinoma present as emergencies, most commonly obstruction (73). Gandrup reported that 95 of 156 consecutive patients operated on for obstructing colorectal cancers had advanced disease (Dukes stage C and D) (8). Ninety-seven patients had the obstructing lesion resected, with a 30-day mortality of 5%. Fifty-nine patients had palliative non-resective operations (diversion or bypass) and in 39 patients the tumor was completely unresectable. Complication rates were lower in patients who had primary resection of the tumor.

Patients who present with locally advanced or recurrent disease that is resectable are preferably treated by palliative resection, provided that there are no medical contraindications to resection and provided that they do not have widespread disease or very limited life expectancy (74).

The management of the patient with obstruction secondary to widespread recurrence or carcinomatosis is a particularly challenging problem. Most patients are initially treated with a trial of tube decompression. Turnbull and colleagues reviewed the Memorial Sloan-Kettering experience of 144 patients with obstructing carcinomato-

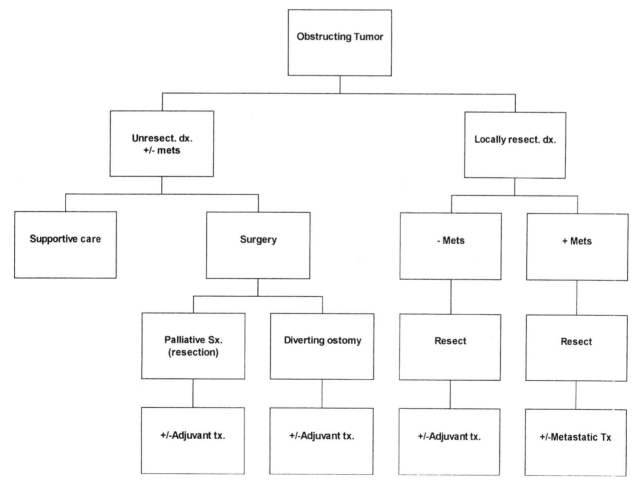

**FIG. 4.** Management of colorectal obstruction.

sis (9). Fifty-five patients with presumed carcinomatosis were treated conservatively. The remaining 89 patients required exploration. Fifty-nine patients had a colonic primary. Enteric bypass was the most common surgical procedure performed. Forty-eight of the 59 colon cancer patients (81%) were improved after surgery, and the mean duration of functioning bowel was 115 days. Lau reported similar results with 30 patients who underwent laparotomy for advanced unresectable, recurrent colorectal cancer (75). Normal bowel function was restored in 19 patients. The types of surgery performed included colonic bypass in 14, resection in 4, and defunctioning colostomy in 4 patients. For patients in whom either resection, diversion, or bypass is not an option, the permanent placement of a long intramural decompressive tube passed across the abdominal wall is an option. McCarthy reviewed 12 patients treated by this procedure and reported that 6 patients left hospital and were capable of fluid ingestion (76).

For patients with widespread disease and limited life expectancy, who are medically unfit to undergo surgery, supportive measures are appropriate (77). Baines published the first study on a pharmacologic approach to treating nausea, vomiting, pain, and other symptoms due to inoperable bowel obstruction in advanced cancer patients (78). Since then, this approach has been used in palliative care units worldwide. Octreotide has recently been introduced as an effective treatment for nausea and vomiting due to malignant bowel obstruction (79).

### Surgical Palliation of Rectal Cancer

Palliation of advanced rectal cancer requires special consideration. Locally invasive rectal cancers can present with complications of pain, hemorrhage, and ureteral obstruction (12). Pain can be a very debilitating problem for these patients. Deland wrote in 1936 (80), "there is hardly a more miserable man alive than the one with advanced rectal cancer." Not infrequently, with sphincter muscle invasion, these patients also suffer from incontinence. The preferred palliation if feasible is surgical resection.

For low-lying lesions within 5 cm of the anal verge, an abdominoperineal resection is appropriate. Bordos and colleagues reported on their experience with 34 patients who underwent palliative abdominoperineal resection (12). The postoperative mortality was 3%, which was the same as for curative resection. Local symptoms were initially relieved in all patients undergoing palliative resection. More than half of these patients survived for 1 year, at which time less than one quarter had perineal symptoms related to recurrent tumor.

For lesions further than 5 cm from the anal verge, a low anterior resection with primary anastomosis is appropriate. Several authors have confirmed that primary anastomosis is safe deep in the pelvis, even in the presence of residual disease, with a low incidence of anastomotic leakage or recurrence with obstruction. In 1987, Moran et al. reported on 57 patients who had palliative low anterior resection and observed only one colonic obstruction secondary to local recurrence and one anastomotic leak (4). Longo and co-workers in 1988 described 33 patients who had palliative low anterior resection and reported one patient (3%) who required reoperation because of an anastomotic leak and two patients (6%) who developed colonic obstruction because of recurrent disease (5). If there are any concerns about the safety of performing a primary anastomosis, a Hartman's pouch and end colostomy is an alternative. A multimodality approach using either preoperative or postoperative radiotherapy might also be indicated.

It is important to differentiate a subgroup of patients with locally advanced colorectal cancer and infiltration of adjacent organs who otherwise have no other evidence of regional or distant metastases. This subgroup of patients, comprising approximately 10% of patients with locally advanced cancer, are node-negative and have a biologically indolent tumor. By extended en-bloc resection, provided that negative resection margins are obtained, these patients can be potentially cured (81).

For patients who are found to be unresectable at laparotomy, a diverting colostomy may be required. However, the palliation achieved is inferior to that of resection. Incapacitating local symptoms of pain, tenesmus, incontinence, and hemorrhage commonly develop prior to the patient's demise. In the series reported by Moran, there were 17 diverting colostomies and the median survival was 6.4 months (4). There were 28 diverting colostomies in the series reported by Longo. Postoperative mortality was 3.8% and the median survival was 5 months (5).

**TABLE 2.** *Results of palliative resection for rectal cancer*

| Author | Year | Number of patients | Operation | Morbidity (%) | Mortality (%) | Overall survival at 1 yr (%) |
|---|---|---|---|---|---|---|
| Bordos et al. | 1974 | 34 | APR | 50 | 2.9 | 58 |
| Moran et al. | 1987 | 95 | Resection[a] | 18 | 1 | 50–60 |
| Longo et al. | 1988 | 68 | Resection[b] | 26 | 4.3 | 65 |

[a]Abdominoperineal resection.
[b]Colonic resection, low anterior resection or abdominoperineal resection.

In high-risk patients who are deemed unfit for major palliative resection of advanced rectal cancer, transanal excision may be an option. For lesions below the peritoneal reflection, electro-desiccation through an anoscope may be performed (82). Nd:YAGq laser therapy has been reported to achieve effective palliation in debilitated patients with disseminated disease (83). Eckhauser reported on 24 patients with unresectable rectal cancer who were palliated by endoscopic laser therapy (84). Seventeen patients presented with obstruction and seven with bleeding. Successful palliation and improvement in quality of life was achieved in all patients. The median survival was 15 months.

### Surgical Palliation of Local Recurrence

Local recurrence occurs in 10–40% of colorectal adenocarcinomas treated for cure, and most appear within 2 years of surgery for the primary lesion (74). These local recurrences represent initial inadequate resection and occur in the pericolic fat and mesentery (85). Untreated, prognosis is poor and death is usually rapid either from continued local extension, with the development of bowel or urinary obstruction, sepsis, perforation or bleeding, or as part of a disseminated disease pattern (86). Palliation of intractable pain and prevention and treatment of these complications are clear-cut indications for operative intervention, and often improve the quality of life for these patients. These recurrent tumors often involve contiguous structures and require extended surgical resection. Pelvic exenteration has produced significant palliation and extended survival in some selected patients. Brophy et al. in 1994 reported on 35 such patients treated by pelvic exenteration for symptom palliation. Operative mortality was 3%, and overall morbidity was 47%. Quality of life was improved in 88% and median survival was 20 months (87).

## SUMMARY

Palliative surgery in patients with GI malignancies represents a particular challenge to the surgeon. As demonstrated for gastric, pancreatic, or colorectal cancer, a properly planned surgical procedure may have a significant benefit for the patient. However, as the aim of surgery differs from a curative resection, it is imperative that the rationale for the procedure and realistic expected outcomes be explained in detail to the patient and family. It must be emphasized that any intervention has as its primary aim an improvement in the patient's quality of life. This is particularly important in cases where survival is expected to be limited.

It is the improvement in the patient's quality of life that makes this form of surgery particularly rewarding to the surgeon who takes care of the terminally ill patient.

## REFERENCES

1. American Cancer Society. Cancer Statistics 1995. *CA Cancer J Clin* 1995;45:8–30.
2. Lillemoe KD, Cameron JL, Kaufman HS, Yeo CJ, Pitt HA, Sauter PK. Chemical splanchnicectomy in patients with unresectable pancreatic cancer. Ann Surg 1993;217: 447–457.
3. Hudis C, Kelsen D, Niedzwiecki D, Banks W, Portenoy R, Foley K. Pain is not a prominent symptom in patients with early pancreas cancer. *Proc Am Soc Clin Oncol* 1991;10:3263.
4. Moran MR, Rothenberger DA, Lahr CJ, Buls JG, Goldberg SM. Palliation for rectal cancer. Resection? Anastomosis. *Arch Surg* 1987;122: 640–643.
5. Longo WE, Ballantyne GH, Bilchik AJ, Modlin IM. Advanced rectal cancer. What is the best palliation. *Dis Colon Rectum* 1988;31: 842–847.
6. Meijer S, DeBakker OJGB, Hoitsma HFW. Palliative resection in gastric cancer. *J Surg Oncol* 1983;23:77–80.
7. Garcia-Valdecasas JC, Llovera JM, deLacy AM, Reverter JC, Grande L, Fuster J, Cugat E, et al. Obstructing colorectal carcinomas. *Dis Colon Rectum* 1991;34:759–762.
8. Gandup P, Lund L, Balsleve I. Surgical treatment of acute malignant large bowel obstruction. *Eur J Surg* 1992;158:427–430.
9. Turnbull ADM, Guerra J, Starnes FH. Results of surgery for obstructing carcinomatosis of gastrointestinal, pancreatic or biliary origin. *J Clin Oncol* 1989;7:381–386.
10. Moreno-Otero R, Rodriguez S, Cabro J, Mearin F, Pajares JM. Acute upper gastrointestinal bleeding as primary symptom of gastric carcinoma. *J Surg Oncol* 1987;36:130–133.
11. Fox JG, Hunt PS. Management of acute bleeding gastric malignancy. *Aust N Z J Surg* 1993;63: 462–465.
12. Bordos DC, Robinson R, Baker R, Cameron JC. An evaluation of palliative abdominoperineal resection for carcinoma of the rectum. *Surg Gynecol Obstet* 1974;139:731–733.
13. Gertsch P, Yip KH, Chow LWC, Lauder IJ. Free perforation of gastric carcinoma. Results of surgical treatment. *Arch Surg* 1995;130: 177–181.
14. Starnes HF, Turnbull ADM, Daly JM. Colon and rectal emergencies. In: Turnbull ADM, ed. *Surgical emergencies in the cancer patient.* Chicago: Year Book, 1987;195–204.
15. LeVeen EG, LeVeen HH. Peritoneovenous shunt in the treatment of malignant ascites. In: Economou SG, Wilt TR, Deziel DJ, Saclarides TJ, Staren ED, Bines SD, eds. *Adjuncts to cancer surgery.* Philadelphia: Lea and Febiger, 1991;339–343.
16. LeVeen HH, Christoudias G, Moon IP, Luft R, Falk G, Grosberg S. Peritoneovenous shunting for ascites. *Ann Surg* 1974;180:580–590.
17. Gough IR, Balderson GA. Malignant ascites. A comparison of peritoneovenous shunting and nonoperative management. *Cancer* 1993;71: 2377–2382.
18. Schumacher DL, Saclarides TJ, Staren ED. Peritoneovenous shunts for palliation of the patient with malignant ascites. *Ann Surg Oncol* 1994; 1:378–381.
19. Bozzetti G, Audisio RA, Doci R, et al. Prognosis of patients after palliative surgical procedures for carcinoma of the stomach. *Surg Gynecol Obstet* 1987;164:151–154.
20. ReMine WH. Palliative operations for incurable gastric cancer. *World J Surg* 1979;3:721–729.
21. Haugstuedt T, Vist A, Eide GE, Soreide O. The survival benefit of resection in patients with advanced stomach cancer: the Norwegian multi center experience. *World J Surg* 1989;13:617–622.
22. El-Domeiri AA, Knapper WH, Fortner JG. A comparative study of palliative resections for gastric carcinoma. *J Surg Oncol* 1972;460–465.
23. Monson JRT, Donohue JH, Mcllrath DC, Farnell WB, Ilstrup DM. Total gastrectomy for advanced cancer. A worthwhile palliative procedure. *Cancer* 1991;64:1863–1868.
24. Butler JA, Dubrow TJ, Trezona T, Klassen M, Nejdl RJ. Total gastrectomy in the treatment of advanced gastric cancer. *Am J Surg* 1989;158: 602–605.
25. Wanebo HJ, Kennedy BJ, Chmiel J, Steele G, Winchester D, Osteen R. Cancer of the stomach: a patient care study by the American College of Surgeons. *Ann Surg* 1993;218:583–592.
26. Ekbom GA, Gleysteen JJ. Gastric malignancy: resection for palliation. *Surgery* 1980;88:476–481.
27. Lo NN, Kee SG, Nambiar R. Palliative gastro-jejunostomy for

advanced carcinoma of the stomach. *Ann Acad Med Singapore* 1991; 20:356–358.

28. Kwok SP, Chung SCS, Griffen SM, Li AKC. Devine exclusion for unresectable carcinoma of the stomach. *Br J Surg* 1991;78:684–685.

29. Solt J, Papp Z: Strecker stent implantation in malignant outlet stenosis. *Gastrointest Endosc* 1993;39:442–444.

30. DeMeester TR, Barlow AP. Surgery and current management for cancer of the esophagus and cardia. *Curr Probl Cancer* 1988;12: 243–327.

31. Ell C, Hockberger J, May A, Fleig WE, Hahn EG. Coated and uncoated self-expanding metal stents for malignant stenosis in the upper GI tract: preliminary clinical experience with Wallstents. *Am J Gastroenterol* 1994;89:1496–1500.

32. Naveau S, Chiesa A, Poynard T, Chaput JC. Endoscopic Nd-Yag laser therapy as palliative treatment for esophageal and cardial cancer. Parameters affecting long-term outcome. *Dig Dis Sci* 1990;35: 294–301.

33. Welvaart K, Caspers RJL, Verhes RJ, Hermans JO. The choice between surgical resection and radiation therapy for patients with cancer of the esophagus and cardia: a retrospective comparison between two treatments. *J Surg Oncol* 1991;47:225–229.

34. Ng WD, Chan YT, Ho KK. Stapled bypass for nonresectable carcinoma located in the upper part of the stomach. *Surg Gynecol Obstet* 1991; 172:234–235.

35. Loftus EV, Glenn GL, Ahlquist DA, Balm RK. Endoscopic treatment of major bleeding from advanced gastroduodenal malignant lesions. *Mayo Clin Proc* 1994;69:736–740.

36. Cheung WL Branicki FJ. Risk factors for mortality in patients with gastric adenocarcinoma presenting with acute hemorrhage. *Eur J Surg Oncol* 1991;17:270–275.

37. Stechenberg L, Bunch RH, Anderson MC. The surgical therapy for perforated gastric cancer. *Am Surgeon* 1981;47:208–210.

38. Boring CC, Squires TS, Tong T. Cancer statistics, 1992. *CA Cancer J Clin* 1992;42:19–38.

39. Brennan MF, Kinsella TJ, Casper ES. Cancer of the pancreas. In: DeVita VT Jr, Hellman S, Rosenberg SA, eds. *Cancer: principles and practice of oncology,* 4th ed. Philadelphia: JB Lippincott, 1993.

40. Carter DC. Cancer of the pancreas. *Gut* 1990;31:494–496.

41. Plainfosse MC, Bouillot JL, Rivaton F, Vaucamps P, Hernigou A, Alexandre JH. The use of operative sonography in carcinoma of the pancreas. *World J Surg* 1987;11:654–658.

42. Yasuda K, Mukai H, Fujimoto S, Nakajima M, Kawai K. The diagnosis of pancreatic cancer by endoscopic ultrasonography. *Gastrointest Endosc* 1988;34:1–8.

43. Palazzo L, Roseau G, Gayet B, Vilgrain V, Belghiti J, Fekete F, Paolaggi J-A. Endoscopic ultrasonography in the diagnosis and staging of pancreatic adenocarcinoma. *Endoscopy* 1993;25:143–150.

44. Watanapa P, Williamson RCN. Surgical palliation for pancreatic cancer: developments during the past two decades. *Br J Surg* 1992;79: 8–20.

45. DeRooij PD, Rogatko A, Brennan MF. Evaluation of palliative surgical procedures in unresectable pancreatic cancer. *Br J Surg* 1991;78: 1053–1058.

46. McGrath PC, McNeill PM, Neifeld JP, Bear HD, Parker GA, Turner MA, Horsley JS, Lawrence W. Management of biliary obstruction in patients with unresectable carcinoma of the pancreas. *Ann Surg* 1989; 209:284–288.

47. Brandabur JJ, Kozarek RA, Ball TJ, Hofer BO, Ryan JA, Traverso LW, Freeny PC, Lewis GP. Nonoperative versus operative treatment of obstructive jaundice in pancreatic cancer: Cost and survival analysis. *Am J Gastroenterol* 1988;83:1132–1139.

48. Potts JR, Broughan TA, Hermann RE. Palliative operations for pancreatic carcinoma. *Am J Surg* 1990;159:72–78.

49. Soehendra N, Grimm H, Berger B, Nam VC. Malignant jaundice: Results of diagnostic and therapeutic endoscopy. *World J Surg* 1989;13: 171–177.

50. Hyoty MK, Nordback IH. Biliary stent or surgical bypass in unresectable pancreatic cancer with obstructive jaundice. *Acta Chir Scand* 1990;156:391–396.

51. Welvaart K. Operative bypass for incurable cancer of the head of the pancreas. *Eur J Surg Oncol* 1992;18:353–356.

52. Gordon RL, Ring EJ, LaBerge JM, Doherty MM. Malignant biliary obstruction; treatment with expandable metallic stents—follow-up of 50 consecutive patients. *Radiology* 1992;182:697–701.

53. Speer AG, Cotton PB, Russell RCG, Mason RR, Hatfield ARW, Leung JWC, MacRae KD, Houghton J, Lennon CA. Randomised trial of endo-scopic versus percutaneous stent insertion in malignant jaundice. *Lancet* 1987;2:57–62.

54. Shepherd HA, Royle G, Ross APR, Diba A, Arthur M, Colin-Jones D. Endoscopic biliary endoprosthesis in the palliation of malignant obstruction of the distal common bile duct: a randomized trial. *Br J Surg* 1988;75:1166–1168.

55. Andersen JR, Sorensen SM, Kruse A, Rokkjaer M, Matzen P. Randomised trial of endoscopic endoprosthesis versus operative bypass in malignant obstructive jaundice. *Gut* 1989;30:1132–1135.

56. Frakes JT, Johanson JF, Stake JJ. Optimal timing for stent replacement in malignant biliary tract obstruction. *Gastrointest Endosc* 1993;39:164–167.

57. Pretre R, Huber O., Robert J, Soravia C, Egeli RA, Rohner A. Results of surgical palliation for cancer of the head of the pancreas and peri-ampullary region. *Br J Surg* 1992;79: 795–8.

58. Nathanson LK, Shimi S, Cuschieri A. Sutured laparoscopic cholecystojejunostomy evolved in an animal model. *J R Coll Surg Edinb* 1992; 37:215–220.

59. Fletcher DR, Jones RM. Laparoscopic cholecystojejunostomy as palliation for obstructive jaundice in inoperable carcinoma of pancreas. *Surg Endosc* 1992;6:147–149.

60. Shimi S, Banting S, Cuschieri A. Laparoscopy in the management of pancreatic cancer: endoscopic cholecystojejunostomy for advanced disease. *Br J Surg* 1992;79:317–319.

61. Wilson RG, Varma JS. Laparoscopic gastroenterostomy for malignant duodenal obstruction. *Br J Surg* 1992;79:1348.

62. Collure DWD, Burns GP, Schenk WG Jr. Clinical, pathological, and therapeutic aspects of carcinoma of the pancreas. *Am J Surg* 1974;128: 683.

63. Sarr MG, Cameron JL. Surgical management of unresectable carcinoma of the pancreas. *Surgery* 1982;91:123–133.

64. Singh SM, Longmire WP, Reber HA. Surgical palliation for pancreatic cancer. *Ann Surg* 1990;212:132–139.

65. Potts JR, Broughan TA, Hermann RE. Palliative operations for pancreatic carcinoma. *Am J Surg* 1990;159:72–78.

66. Schantz SP, Schickler W, Evans TK, Coffey RJ. Palliative gastroenterostomy for pancreatic cancer. *Am J Surg* 1984;147:793–796.

67. Doberneck RC, Berndt GA. Delayed gastric emptying after palliative gastrojejunostomy for carcinoma of the pancreas. *Arch Surg* 1987;122: 827–829.

68. Weaver DW, Wienek R, Bouwman DL, Walt AJ. Gastrojejunostomy: is it helpful for patients with pancreatic cancer. *Surgery* 1987;102: 608–613.

69. Jacobs PPM, van der Sluis, Wobbes T. Role of gastroenterostomy in the palliative surgical treatment of pancreatic cancer. *J Surg Oncol* 1989; 42:145–149.

70. Welvaart K. Operative bypass for incurable cancer of the head of the pancreas. *Eur J Surg Oncol* 1992;18:353–356.

71. Jones J, Gough D. Celiac plexus block with alcohol for the relief of upper abdominal pain due to cancer. *Ann R Coll Surg Eng* 1977;59:46–49.

72. Copping J, Willix R, Kraft R. Palliative chemical splanchnicectomy. *Arch Surg* 1969;98:418–420.

73. Anderson JH, Hole D, McArdle CS: Elective versus emergency surgery for patients with colorectal cancer. *Br J Surg* 1992;79:706–709.

74. Austgen TR, Souba WW, Bland MI. Reoperation for colorectal carcinoma. *Surg Clin North Am* 1991;71:175–192.

75. Lau PWK, Lorentz TG: Results of surgery for malignant bowel obstruction in advanced unresectable, recurrent colorectal cancer. *Dis Colon Rectum* 1993;36:61–65.

76. McCarthy JD. A strategy for intestinal obstruction of peritoneal carcinomatosis. *Arch Surg* 1986;121:1081–1082.

77. Ripamonti C. Management of bowel obstruction in advanced cancer. *Curr Opin Oncol* 1994;6:351–357.

78. Baines M, Oliver DJ, Carter RL. Medical management of intestinal obstruction in patients with advanced malignant disease: a clinical and pathological study. *Lancet* 1985;2:990–993.

79. Khoo D, Hall E, Motson R, Riley J, Denman K, Waxman J. Palliation of malignant intestinal obstruction using octreotide. *Eur J Cancer* 1994;30:28–30.

80. Deland EM, Welch CE, Nathanson I: One hundred untreated cancers of the rectum. *N Engl J Med* 1936;10:451–458.

81. Lopez MJ, Monato WW: Role of extended resection in the initial treatment of locally advanced colorectal carcinoma. *Surgery* 1993;113: 365–372.

82. Salvati EP, Rubin RJ. Electrocoagulation as primary therapy for rectal carcinoma. *Am J Surg* 1976;132:583–586.

83. Faintuch JS. Better palliation of colorectal carcinoma with laser therapy. *Oncology* 1988;2:33–38.
84. Eckhauser MH, Mansour EG. Endoscopic laser therapy for obstructing and/or bleeding colorectal carcinoma. *Am Surgeon* 1992;58: 358–363.
85. Quirtie P, Durdey P, Dixon MF, et al. Local recurrence of rectal adenocarcinoma due to inadequate surgical resection. Histopathological study of lateral tumor spread and surgical excision. *Lancet* 1986;1:996–999.
86. Welch JP, Donaldson GA. Detection and treatment of recurrent cancer of the colon and rectum. *Am J Surg* 1978;135:505–510.
87. Brophy PF, Hoffman JF, Eisenberg BC. The role of palliative pelvic exenteration. *Am J Surg* 1994;167:386–390.
88. Cook-Gotay C, Korn EL, McCabe MS, Moore TD, Cheson BD. Quality-of-life assessment in cancer treatment protocols: research issues in protocol development. *JNCI* 1992;84:575–579.

*Principles and Practice of Supportive Oncology,*
edited by Ann Berger et al.
Lippincott–Raven Publishers, Philadelphia ©1998

CHAPTER 45

# Palliative Orthopedic Surgery

Richard G. Schmidt and Gabor A. Winkler

The American Cancer Society estimates that approximately 800,000 new carcinomas will be diagnosed in the United States each year. Many of these patients will develop metastatic disease. Metastatic cancer to bone is one of the primary sites of metastatic cancer and creates its own set of problems, which have to be addressed accordingly. Unfortunately, metastatic cancer of bone is often not emphasized or is given low priority in the overall treatment regimen of cancer patients. Today the subspecialty of orthopedic oncology has developed within orthopedic surgery, and it concentrates on cancers of the bone. Therefore, patients with metastatic cancer to bone deserve an evaluation by an orthopedic oncologist who is familiar with their treatment. Patients with metastatic cancer to the bone cannot be expected to perform as well metabolically as regular orthopedic patients and should be treated differently.

Metastatic cancer to the bone is the most common malignancy of bone, affecting more than 40 times as many patients as all other types of bone cancer combined. The true incidence of skeletal metastases in patients who die of cancer approaches approximately 70%. Despite the fact that metastatic cancer to bone is common, the complications surrounding metastases to bone are quite serious. Patients with metastatic disease can die of complications of bone metastases. In the past, it was assumed that patients with metastatic cancer to bone, and particularly those with pathologic fractures, had very short life spans and therefore an aggressive approach was not pursued. This assumption does not apply today due to advanced adjuvant therapies. Patients with metastatic cancer to bone, even those with multiple lesions, can enjoy a prolonged survival with improved quality of life if modern and aggressive approaches are pursued.

This chapter will explore the different issues surrounding metastatic cancer of bone and introduce the different treatment options available for this special group of patients.

## EPIDEMIOLOGY

Most cases of metastatic cancer of bone derive from carcinomas of four organs—breast, prostate, lung, and kidney—followed by thyroid, gastric, colon and rectum, pancreas, and all other carcinomas. Breast cancer, diagnosed in approximately 184,000 women each year, does indeed have the highest incidence of associated metastatic bone disease among all cancers. It is estimated that there are currently approximately 100,000 breast cancer patients living with metastatic cancer of bone. The incidence of metastatic cancer of bone is slightly greater in males than in females, with a ratio of 1.5:1. The highest incidence is between ages 40 and 70. It is not exceptional, however, to see metastatic cancer of bone in young patients (30–40 years of age), particularly metastatic pulmonary carcinoma and metastatic renal cell carcinoma. Metastases of thyroid carcinoma have even been observed in 20- to 30-year-old patients. Metastatic cancer of bone commonly occurs in the pelvis and the femur, which is the most common long bone to be involved by metastases, followed by the humerus. Although any bone in the body can be involved in metastatic cancer of bone, lesions occurring distal to the knee and elbow are very rare.

## PATHOPHYSIOLOGY OF BONE METASTASES

To understand why metastatic disease of bone is such a problem for the cancer patient, it is important to understand the different problems that metastatic disease of bone can cause. Pain represents the most signif-

R. G. Schmidt and G. A. Winkler: The Musculoskeletal Tumor and Limb Reconstruction Center, Bala Cynwyd, PA 19004.

icant problem for a cancer patient with bone involvement, followed by severe ambulation dysfunctions.

A patient with metastatic cancer of bone can essentially become bedridden, particularly if the disease is to the lower extremities. This can necessitate significant narcotic ingestion on the part of the patient, which can lead to a whole host of additional problems, including constipation and urinary retention. Lack of ambulation can also precipitate or exacerbate hypercalcemia or predispose to venous thrombosis with subsequent pulmonary embolisms and pneumonia. Most of these cancer patients lose their independence because of their bony involvement and require placement into a nursing home. This can have tremendous socioeconomic ramifications, not only for the patient but for their families as well.

Patients with metastatic cancer to bone who are confined to a hospital bed and have even been declared nonresuscitative candidates because of their obtunded state secondary to narcotic ingestion can often be reversed by managing the patient's bone disease by surgical intervention. Internal fixation of their pathologic fractures or prophylactic stabilization of their impending pathologic fractures usually can get the patients out of bed and off heavy doses of narcotics. Their mental status will often clear to the point at which they can be discharged home and once again resume independence. It has been reported that 40% of the patients with pathologic fractures caused by metastatic carcinoma will survive for 6 months or longer following the fracture and 30% of the patients even survive for 1 year or longer (1). These numbers justify an early aggressive approach in the palliative orthopedic treatment of patients with metastatic cancer to bone in order to prevent the above-described typical scenario (2).

In the management of patients with metastatic cancer to bone, basic understanding of the pathophysiology of the healing of normal bone and bone with metastatic cancer is critical. A pathologic fracture is defined as a fracture occurring in previously weakened bone by either a metabolic process or a neoplastic condition. The force, which causes a pathologic fracture, would not be adequate to cause a fracture in normal bone. In other words, a typical scenario would be a patient who bends over to put on a pair of socks, suddenly feels a crack in his thigh, has severe pain, and is unable to bear weight on that leg. The healing response in traumatic fractures is different from that of pathologic fractures. When a normal bone, particularly a long bone, fractures as a result of trauma, a typical cascade of events ensues. Within 48 hours of the fracture, a hematoma develops and begins to organize.

The callus then matures by vascular capillary proliferation. Mesenchymal cells differentiate into osteoblasts (the cells, responsible for making bone), which lay down seams of new bone in the area of the fracture, which then undergo mineralization. Generally, within 2 weeks of the fracture, a radiographically apparent callus develops. At this time, the fracture becomes somewhat "sticky." Over the next 4–6 weeks, the callus undergoes additional maturation and ossification, and the bone approaches normal strength. This callus then undergoes remodeling, as a result of osteoclastic activity, into a stronger structure. Most fractures typically heal this way within 8–10 weeks, in younger patients, eventually even faster.

Fracture healing in a patient with metastatic cancer to bone is quite different. The metastatic lesion stimulates the production and formation of osteoclasts (the cells responsible for bone digestion and resorption). Osteoclasts are currently the only cells in the body known to be capable of performing this task. Bone destruction does not occur directly as a result of the metastatic cancer cells but as a result of the osteoclast being recruited by the metastatic focus to destroy bone. Osteoclastic bone resorption is more powerful than osteoblastic bone formation. It takes basically 20 osteoblasts to equal the biological activity of one osteoclast.

Therefore, even when a pathologic fracture occurs and there is some stimulation of osteoblastic activity, the osteoclasts that are already present in the site overwhelm the ability of the osteoblast to form any significant callus. As a result, pathologic fractures of bone generally will not heal by themselves. It was reported that only 5% of pathologic fractures of the hip will heal (3).

The intrinsic healing ability of metastatic bone lesions is further complicated by the fact that these patients are often malnourished and their overall physical status is compromised by their primary disease. Chemotherapy has a direct effect on the ability of the osteoblasts to form new bone tissue. The overall bone stock of these patients is another issue that further complicates the situation. Often these patients will suffer from diffuse osteoporosis and osteomalacia in addition to the pathologic fracture or impending fracture.

In the typical healthy patient who sustains a fracture, internal fixation is often elected to treat that fracture to keep the different fracture fragments aligned and in good position (serving as a splint) until the body's normal healing mechanism can take over and heal the fracture. Once the fracture is healed, the internal fixation device is no longer needed to maintain the strength and integrity of the broken bone.

In contrast, in the patient with metastatic cancer of bone, the internal fixation device will be needed as a permanent fixation system. This has obvious direct ramifications with regard to surgical technique. In a typical nontumor patient who fractures a long bone, a plate and screw system can be used. This type of internal fixation system relies on good, healthy bone above and below the fracture to actually seat and secure the device.

The following principles for surgical treatment of pathologic fractures were outlined (4):

1. Proceed with the most advantageous procedure initially and try to eliminate the possibility of a second procedure.
2. Replace as much of the bone destroyed by the tumor as possible.
3. Minimize hospitalization, realizing that the patient's life expectancy is short.
4. Attempt early functional rehabilitation, considering that long periods of immobilization in this group of patients are not well tolerated.

If these principles are followed, patients with metastatic cancer to the bone will experience significant improvement of their quality of life for their remaining life span.

## INTRAMEDULLARY FIXATION OF LONG BONES

Whereas plates and screws are an excellent system for fixing normal fractures, they can have disastrous results in patients with metastatic bone cancer. A plate and screw type of device is a mechanical load-bearing device. This means that the plate and screw system will bear all of the stresses at the level of bone where it is applied. Where the plate and screw system begins and ends, the stress will then be transferred to the remaining bone. If that bone is osteoporotic or weakened by a metastatic lesion, the patient with a pathologic fracture will develop a second fracture where the load is transferred from the plate and screw system to the remaining bone stock. Once again, this is not a problem in a healthy patient because that bone stock is adequate. For this reason, the fixation device typically used in orthopedic oncology in patients with metastatic bone cancer is a rod fixation. An intramedullary rod is not a load-bearing but actually a load-sharing device. An intramedullary rod will transfer some stress onto the remaining bone in a gradual or graduated fashion.

Intramedullary rod fixation of a bone is an excellent way of stabilizing the long bones in patients with either pathologic fractures or impending pathologic fractures. Practically all of the long bones in the body are amenable to intramedullary rod fixation. The femur is the most common long bone involved with malignant fractures. Others include the humerus, tibia, radius, and ulna. The fibula is not typically involved with metastatic bone cancer, and because the shaft of the fibula is not a main structural member, pathologic fractures of the fibula rarely require intramedullary fixation.

Intramedullary fixation of bone was a technique first developed by Küntschner in the early 1940s (5). The technique was initially used in patients with long-bone injuries as a result of trauma and has been extrapolated to the patient with metastatic cancer to bone (6). Intramedullary fixation of bone works best in patients with impending pathologic fractures. It is technically much easier to treat a bone before it breaks, and the patient benefits from this. The adage "A stitch in time saves nine" applies to the patient with metastatic cancer to bone. Therefore, it is important to follow a clinical algorithm for evaluating patients with primary or metastatic bone cancer to evaluate their skeletal systems on a routine basis. If a cancer patient develops bone pain, the treating physician should be worried enough to order plain x-rays and a bone scan. Nocturnal pain is an important indicator of a metastatic lesion to bone. Often, the patient will attribute the symptoms to a muscle strain or soft tissue injury.

The bone scan most of the time will identify the metastasis before the bone fractures. This is not true in patients with multiple myeloma, the one situation where a skeletal survey will be of more help. A bone scan, however, is not always accurate in terms of picking up different types of metastatic lesions. A bone scan relies on the reactive osteoblastic formation around a tumor and the uptake of the technetium-labeled phosphate in the osteoid materials being laid down in response to the metastatic lesion. If a patient has an aggressive metastatic lesion, this reactive zone will not exist and the bone scan will not be hot in the area of metastasis. Therefore, plain x-rays in two planes (anteroposterior and lateral) should be taken of the involved extremity in a routine fashion if a cancer patient develops bone pain. Sometimes an additional, oblique view is necessary to show a lesion. It is important to remember that in this day and age this simple diagnostic test is still of utmost importance and extremely useful in evaluating a patient with metastatic cancer to bone. Another diagnostic tool that is sometimes helpful in localizing metastatic lesions is the magnetic resonance imaging (MRI) examination. This test enables the orthopedic oncologist to exactly define the extent of the metastatic lesion, especially if the lesion is close to a joint line.

When is a prophylactic fixation of a long bone indicated? In general, a low threshold for prophylactic long bone fixation is recommended. There is still some debate concerning the management of impending pathologic fractures. If discovered and treated early, these lesions are sometimes satisfactorily controlled with a short course of radiation therapy. Griessmann and Schüttmeyer first described prophylactic fixation of large lytic lesions in the femur (6). Parrish and Murray believed that pain, together with involvement of half of the cortex, was a definite indication for prophylactic operative intervention (7). Fiedler confirmed that lesions in the long bone involving at least 50% of the cortex have at least a 50% chance for spontaneous fracture if not prophylactically reinforced (8).

The indications for prophylactic fixation of a long bone should not be absolutely rigid. Certainly variations exist that defy a rigid standard for prophylactic internal fixation of long bones. The location of the lesion is of great importance. A large pathologic lesion of the bone may not fracture, whereas patients with small cortical lesions can develop spiral fractures of the bone. This situation will vary from patient to patient. The situation will also depend on the location of the lesion. The stresses that exist normally along the femur will vary depending on the location once it travels down the femoral cortex. The highest areas of stress in the femur are in the subtrochanteric level, approximately 2–3 in. below the lesser trochanter. Small lesions in this particular area should be treated with early internal fixation.

Pain is another important clinical feature to analyze in patients with an impending pathologic fracture of bone. This is particularly true in the patient who has already undergone radiation therapy and has not experienced a subjective improvement as a result of that treatment. It cannot be emphasized enough how much easier it is to treat an impending pathologic fracture than a complete pathologic fracture of a long bone. In general, however, prophylactic internal fixation for a patient with a long-bone lesion is recommended when that lesion compromises one third to one half of the cortical diameter of the bone. In patients with smaller lesions, radiation therapy can be tried initially to arrest the lesions satisfactorily. It is important, however, to have this particular patient on crutches or a walker with non-weight-bearing of the involved lower extremity, or in a sling and non-weight-bearing of the involved upper extremity, in order to decrease the anatomic forces across the lesion while the effects of radiation therapy develop.

It is important for the nonorthopedic oncologist to understand basic principles of intramedullary fixation from a technical perspective. Often, the nonsurgical clinician will not be aware of the option of intramedullary fixation because he or she is not familiar with the basic technical aspects that surround this procedure. Knowing the basic techniques of intramedullary rod fixation also enables the nonsurgical clinician to recommend this option to the patient or consult the orthopedic oncologist.

### Femur

The most common long bone involved with metastatic cancer to bone is the femur. This is the bone that is most often treated with intramedullary fixation (Fig. 1). The normal anatomy of the femur is very amenable to rod fixation. The medullary canal of the femur in an adult is generally filled with normal marrow fat and is generally very easy to enter. The medullary canal of the femur can be entered either proximally through the pyriformis fossa or distally through the intercondylar notch. The pyri-

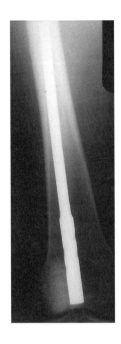

**FIG. 1.** Status postprophylactic rodding of the femur using a distal approach and polymethyl methacrylate (PMMA). The indication was a small lesion in the midshaft area, discovered in a patient with known history of metastatic breast cancer, who had been complaining of severe pain in both legs.

formis fossa represents a small notch at the level of the femoral neck, just medial to the greater trochanter. The pyriformis muscle is a short external rotator muscle of the hip. The decision whether to proceed with intramedullary fixation of the femur through the hip or knee is often determined by the general medical status of the patient and the location of the metastatic disease. If the metastatic lesion is located more proximally, a proximal entry will be chosen. This is performed with the patient in the lateral or sometimes the supine position. An incision is made over the greater trochanter, and dissection is carried through the muscle fibers of the gluteus medius muscle, using a muscle-sparing approach. A drill bit or Hall-type of device is then used to enter the medullary canal. Once the medullary canal has been entered, a guide pin is then placed down the medullary canal and is visualized during the procedure with a C-arm fluoroscopic radiograph. Biplanar imaging will verify that the guide pin is down the medullary canal and has not perforated the cortex. Cortical perforation can occur in patients with metastatic cancer to bone either because of the presence of multiple lesions or because the overall bone stock is poor secondary to osteomalacia or osteoporosis. Once the guide pin is in appropriate positioning, reaming of the medullary canal is performed with flexible intramedullary reamers. This will remove a significant amount of metastatic disease from the femur for pathologic evaluation. Additional studies, such as of estrogen and progesterone receptors in the case of patients with metastatic breast cancer, can also be performed using this additional histologic material. Once reaming has been done to allow entry of a rod, the rod is placed by gentle hammering down the medullary canal over the guide pin. It is important before surgery to make sure that the patient has enough blood products available for potential transfusion. This is particularly true in patients with metastatic thyroid or renal cell carcinoma. These lesions can be quite vascular and can lead to profuse bleeding in a patient. Sometimes such bleeding can be controlled quite satisfactorily with the addition of intramedullary bone cement.

The other available option is intramedullary fixation of the femur through a distal approach. This is particularly useful if the patient has distally placed metastatic lesions down the femur and proximal sparing of the femur. This technique can be used as well in patients who are quite sick overall as a result of their metastatic disease. Intramedullary rodding of the femur through the knee is a relatively easy and quite rapid technique of stabilizing the femur. It is typically done using a tourniquet (sterile or nonsterile), through a small incision just medial to the patella. A small arthrotomy is performed, and the patella is subluxed or everted laterally. This technique exposes the intercondylar notch of the femur, which lies approximately 1–2 cm below the surface of the skin, excluding the depth of the patella. This technique allows the patient to be placed in a supine position and also allows the addition of a sterile tourniquet. Using a tourniquet can be quite useful for purposes of decreasing the amount of bleeding that occurs. Often using this technique, the bleeding can be kept to <100 ml. Most patients who receive intramedullary fixation of the femur through the intercondylar notch, in fact, do not require a transfusion. Once again, C-arm visualization is used for appropriate placement of the guide pin and the reaming with subsequent placement of the rod. Rod fixation of the femur through the knee can be done in <45 minutes.

Postoperatively, a patient with an impending pathologic fracture of the femur treated with prophylactic rod fixation can demonstrate a dramatic improvement. The patient can be progressed to immediate weight bearing the day after surgery. It is often dramatic how the patient will experience significant pain relief as a result of the rod placement.

Of course, patients with complete pathologic fractures of the bone are still amenable to rod fixation. However, these patients will often require another incision to be made directly over the actual fracture itself. This is necessary to align the bone and at the same time add bone cement, polymethyl methacrylate (PMMA), for additional stabilization. The additional incision will increase the length of the operative procedure and often leads to an increased morbidity of the patient. In addition, a patient who has gone on to fracture the bone completely is at risk for experiencing complications of a fracture that could have been avoided with prophylactic internal fixation.

Fractures of the femur can be significant events even in healthy individuals. An adult can easily lose two or three units of blood within the soft tissues of the thigh around a posttraumatic fracture. The situation is further compli-cated in patients with vascular metastatic lesions, such as thyroid and renal cell carcinoma. Patients who go on to have fractures of the femur are also at risk for developing fat embolism and respiratory distress syndrome. For all of these reasons, prophylactic internal fixation of the long bones is generally recommend when possible.

Prophylactic stabilization of a long bone can be readily combined with postoperative radiation therapy. This is particularly true with the femur. The use of a proximal or distal approach will often result in the incision being placed away from the actual site of metastatic involvement. Currently, patients who receive intramedullary fixation of the femur undergo postoperative radiation therapy starting the day after surgery. Therefore, prophylactic internal fixation of the femur does not generally interfere with postoperative radiation therapy. Postoperative radiation therapy is almost always used in conjunction with internal fixation.

The use of internal fixation devices is not combined with cast immobilization. Cast immobilization is an excellent option in many cases for nontumor patients with fractures; however, it is very seldom used for patients with metastatic cancer to bone. The reasons for this become obvious when one understands the basic pathophysiology of metastatic disease to the bone, as earlier delineated.

## Tibia

The tibia is another long bone that is most amenable to intramedullary fixation (Fig. 2). It could be approached surgically through either the same small incision just medial to the patella, as described above for the femur, followed by a small arthrotomy, or by an incision through the patellar tendon. In both cases the patient is again in a supine position and a tourniquet is applied to minimize blood loss. A drill is then used to enter the medullary canal just above the tibial tubercle and anterior to the anterior cruciate ligament. Once the medullary canal is entered, a guide pin can be placed down the medullary canal, and appropriate reaming can be performed under C-arm visualization. In fact, using the incision of the knee, a femur and tibia can be rodded at the same time. A patient's femurs and tibias can actually be rodded simultaneously, thus achieving four bone intramedullary fixations at the same surgical sitting. Although this is certainly not common, it demonstrates the ability to prophylactically fix the lower extremity bones in a patient who is at risk for fractures rapidly and easily with minimal blood loss.

## Humerus

The humerus is also typically involved with metastatic lesions to bone (Fig. 3). It is readily amenable to rod fixation. Surgically, the humerus is approached through a

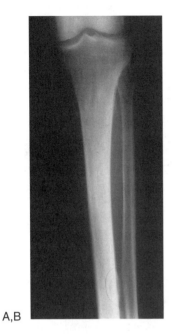 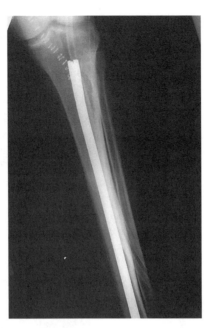

A,B

**FIG. 2. A:** Patient with known history of metastatic lung cancer presents with pain in the left lower leg. On plain x-ray a metastatic lesion of the distal tibia is seen. **B:** Status postprophylactic intramedullary rodding of the left tibia.

proximal incision, just anterior to the acromion. The greater tuberosity can be exposed and the rotator cuff tendon split in line with its fibers. Using a relatively small incision (approx. 2 in.), the entire medullary fixation of the humerus can be instrumented. Because of the distal flare of the humerus and the narrowing of the medullary canal distally, it is not recommended to rod the humerus from a distal approach. As with the femur and tibia, the humerus is better fixed prophylactically than with a completed pathologic fracture. A pathologic fracture of the humerus, again, will often require direct exposure of the fracture fragments so that the cortex can be reconstituted with additionally placed bone cement.

## Radius and Ulna

The radius and ulna, although not common sites for metastatic spread, are also amenable to rod fixation, which can be placed either distally or proximally.

## Metastatic Dissemination

A question that sometimes arises with intramedullary fixation is whether intramedullary fixation and reaming cause clinical evidence of metastatic dissemination of the tumor. There is no clinical evidence to suggest that any spread of tumor occurs as a result of the intramedullary

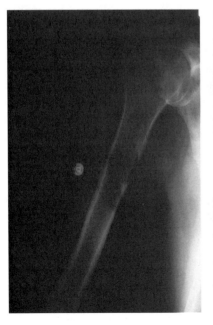 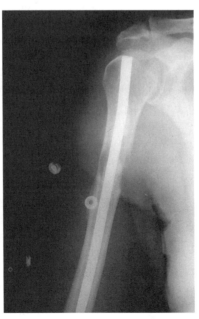

A,B

**FIG. 3. A:** Patient with known history of metastatic renal cell carcinoma presented with severe pain in the right upper arm. The plain x-ray shows a large lesion in the right proximal humerus. **B:** Status postintramedullary rodding of the right humerus using PMMA.

fixation process (9). Clinically, metastatic carcinoma to bone does not undergo transplantation as a result of the intramedullary fixation.

## BONE CEMENT

Bone cement, or polymethyl methacrylate (PMMA), has been used extensively since 1966 in managing patients with metastatic lesions, pathologic fractures, and impending pathologic fractures (10,11). The term "bone cement" is somewhat misleading because it implies the use of an adhesive material. Bone cement is not an adhesive device but a strong filler type of material. It serves well under compressive forces in bony fixation.

The use of PMMA first originated in orthopedics with total hip replacements. However, it has more recently taken on a significant role in treating patients with metastatic cancer to bone. One advantage of bone cement is that it allows immediate and rigid fixation. It is also easily used in conjunction with an intramedullary rod system of fixation. PMMA will generally take approximately 5–8 minutes to set in the operating room. Once it is hardened, it allows immediate fixation for a patient when using combination with an internal fixation device. Therefore, from a clinical standpoint, it avoids the issue of actual fracture healing for the patient with metastatic cancer to bone.

Bone cement also offers other clinical advantages for the patient with bone metastases. Bone cement, because of its filling properties, dramatically decreases intraoperative and postoperative bleeding. This is particularly true in a patient with a vascular lesion such as metastatic renal cell or thyroid carcinoma. The bleeding that occurs with intramedullary fixation of a long bone in metastatic thyroid or renal cell carcinoma can be quite brisk and at times intraoperatively quite intimidating. It is often dramatic how the bleeding stops suddenly and completely when the bone cement is injected into the intramedullary space.

The other potential benefit of bone cement is the cytotoxic effect of the material as it polymerizes. The polymerization process gives off considerable heat in the area of application, which may have some benefits from the standpoint of tumor necrosis. The results of intramedullary fixation with PMMA were compared to the results of conventional internal fixation without additional bone cement (11). This study analyzed pain relief, ambulatory status, and survival time in patients treated with and without additional bone cement. The study included 283 pathologic fractures and 23 impending bone fractures of the femur during a 15-year period. In 196 of these patients the device was cemented, and in 110 the device was not cemented. Complete pain relief could be demonstrated for 97% of the patients who received additional bone cement for 83% of the patients who did not. The ambulatory ability of the patients was also dramatically affected by the use of bone cement. Of the patients treated with bone cement, 95% eventually demonstrated an excellent independent ambulation ability, compared to 75% of those who not receive additional cement. A survival benefit for patients treated with cement was also reported (11). According to unpublished observations in Europe, investigators are currently studying the effects of insertion of anticancer chemotherapeutic agents into PMMA to determine the rates of release of these agents from the cement .

There is no question that supplemental bone cement can have a tremendous beneficial effect on stabilizing patients with metastatic cancers to bone. It is not recommended for those patients who have routine fractures without cancer. The addition of bone cement to an intramedullary rod basically causes the rod to be a permanent implant device. The addition of bone cement would make removal of the rod subsequently extremely difficult if not impossible.

Bone cement can be added both with prophylactic fixation and fixation for patients who have already fractured. Prophylactic rod fixation is easily combined with bone cement. The bone cement can be introduced down the medullary canal while in a very liquid, nonviscous form using a cement gun with a long nozzle or a chest tube. A chest tube can be used in many cases of femur fixation because of its length and reach down the medullary canal.

It is important, however, when using bone cement in intramedullary fixation that the rod be introduced before the cement hardens. If the cement hardens before rod fixation, it is impossible to introduce the rod fixation device.

Bone cement is also used extensively in the spine for fixation of compression injuries and pathologic fractures.

## PROSTHETIC REPLACEMENT OF LESIONS CLOSE TO THE ARTICULAR SURFACES

Prosthetic or joint replacement has, of course, been used for many years in patients with degenerative arthritis of the hip, knee, and shoulder. However, prosthetics is also necessary in treatment of patients with large metastatic lesions of the hip joint, knee joint, or shoulder joint area. Lesions occurring in the periarticular regions of long bones are not manageable with intramedullary rod fixation. In order to prevent stability, healthy bone substance is necessary at both the proximal and distal end of the intramedullary rod. This would not be the case in periarticular lesions. In these cases the joint has to be reconstructed in order to provide sufficient function and pain relief for the patient.

## Hip Joint

The hip joint area, including the acetabulum, the femoral head, and the femoral neck, is a prime site of metastatic cancer to bone. Metastatic lesions of the femoral head are naturally treated with routine prosthetic reconstruction, just as in patients with osteoarthritis of the hip.

Patients with femoral neck lesions are preferably treated with prosthetic reconstruction as well, using the same devices as for femoral head lesions (Fig. 4). Some nonpathologic fractures of the femoral neck, especially the basocervical fractures, can be treated with internal fixation devices, using plates and dynamic screws. This is not feasible in patients with metastatic cancer to the femoral neck, again, considering the pathophysiology of metastatic cancer to the bone. Hip replacement, however, offers the patient a quick recovery and avoids the risk of supplemental fixation failure of the bone. This prevents the necessity of additional surgery. Cement fixation of the prosthesis into the proximal femur is the standard way of treatment.

The acetabulum is also a common site of metastatic spread. Metastatic lesions to the acetabulum should be treated with great vigilance. Patients with metastatic lesions of the acetabulum are best treated prophylactically and as early as possible. From a surgical standpoint, it is very difficult to treat patients with fractures involving the acetabulum and collapse of the pelvis. Radiation therapy can be extremely useful in treating patients with acetabular lesions before they become structurally unstable. If a patients's pain persists after radiation therapy, a surgical option available to that patient is to fix the acetabulum and neck of the ilium with a prosthetic cup component. This can be either cemented in place or fixated with screws to healthy bone in the remaining ilium. Many times a combination of screw fixation and supplemental cement fixation is necessary. Additional devices are available to further fix the acetabulum and pelvis in order to prevent fracture of the femoral head or ball through the acetabulum. This particular situation is called an acetabular protrusion. A patient with a fractured acetabulum with medial displacement of the femoral head into the pelvis will experience a dramatic reduction in ambulation and increase in pain. Therefore, it is generally best to treat these patients before acetabular fracture and protrusion (Fig. 5).

In all cases, rehabilitation can begin on the first postoperative day with the patient bearing full weight or weight as tolerated on the involved leg.

## Knee Joint

Routine prosthetic replacement of the knee joint, for reasons such as degenerative osteoarthritis, is more a retread of the joint surface. Unlike routine hip replacement, where the whole femoral head and the largest part of the femoral neck are replaced by a metal prosthesis, knee replacement does not replace significant parts of the bone. In this case only the worn-out articular cartilage is removed and a retread type of metal implant takes over the function of the articulating surface. The cuts are limited to the epiphysis and hardly ever extend into the metaphysis. The vast majority of metastatic cancer to the bone in the knee joint area, however, occurs in the metaphysis of the distal femur or the proximal tibia. Obviously, the techniques developed for routine knee joint replacement will not be sufficient to address these

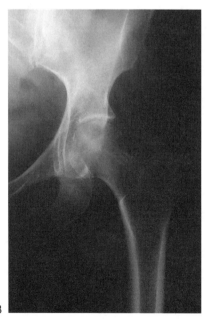 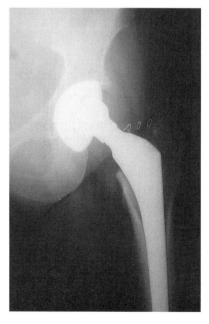

A,B

**FIG. 4. A:** Patient with known history of breast cancer is presenting with ambulatory dysfunction due to pain in the left leg. Plain x-ray shows a lytic lesion in the left femoral head, in the base of the left femoral neck and the greater trochanter. **B:** Status post-left total hip arthroplasty using PMMA.

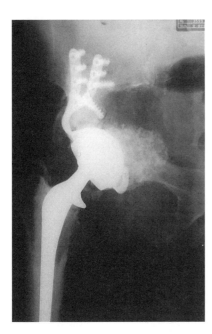

**FIG. 5.** A gap ring fixated with screws into the ilium of a patient with metastatic renal cell carcinoma of the right acetabulum. The procedure became necessary because a previously performed total-hip arthroplasty failed to prevent the acetabular protrusion.

lesions. A segmental replacement type of prosthetic device will be necessary for these conditions. The use and role of these types of devices will be delineated below.

### Shoulder Joint

Pathologic fractures or impending pathologic fractures of the humeral head are often very amenable to treatment with prosthetic reconstruction using a humeral metallic component (Fig. 6). These reconstructions are performed through an anterior incision going through the deltopectoral groove. These patients can experience dramatic reduction of pain and improvement of function with prosthetic reconstruction of the humeral head. The prosthesis is cemented in place; therefore, the patients can begin a physical therapy program the day after surgery. Pathologic fractures of the humeral head are quite painful and will interfere dramatically with remaining limb function. Often patients with metastatic cancer to bone will have lesions of both the upper and lower extremities and will need their upper extremities for independent ambulation with crutches or a walker. It is difficult to use an overhead trapeze successfully for orthopedic patients unless they have satisfactory function of the upper extremity. Therefore, it is important to address both upper and lower extremity lesions.

### MODULAR ONCOLOGY PROSTHETIC REPLACEMENT SYSTEMS

So far we have discussed appropriate orthopedic oncologic interventions for patients with shaft lesions of the long bones as well as patients with lesions of the areas around the articular surfaces. These situations, as discussed, generally can be successfully addressed with rod and prosthetic reconstruction, respectively. However, how does one address those patients who have both, i.e., a patient with a large shaft lesion that also migrates proximally or distally to violate the joint itself? Until recently, this has been a significant problem in the orthopedic oncologic management of patients with extensive localized bony metastatic disease. In the past, these patients were treated surgically with devices called custom prosthetic devices. In other word, a radiograph would be taken of the patient with such a lesion, and the radiograph would be sent to an implant manufacturer so that a custom implant

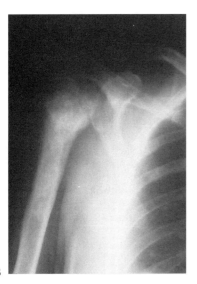 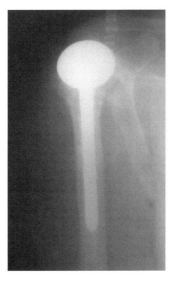

A,B

**FIG. 6. A:** Patient with history of prostate cancer is presenting with severe pain of the right shoulder. Plain x-ray demonstrates a lesion of the proximal humerus. **B:** Status post-right shoulder hemiarthroplasty with Neer prosthesis.

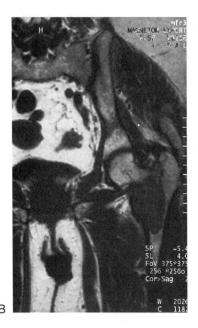
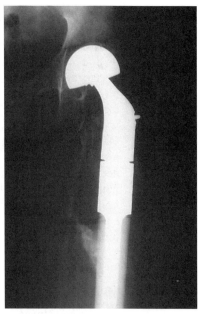

A,B

**FIG. 7. A:** An MRI picture of the left hip of a patient with metastatic breast cancer is seen. A large lytic lesion can be seen in a very strategic location, surrounding the lesser trochanter area, the base of the femoral neck, and the subtrochanteric area. **B:** A postoperative x-ray on the same patient demonstrates the replacement of the proximal femur with a modular oncology system, along with a bipolar hip replacement.

could be built, generally from cobalt chrome. This device would take approximately 6–7 weeks to manufacture. In addition, the devices are expensive and require a significant amount of time, both for the surgeon and for the manufacturer to plan and construct. This type of approach has posed several significant problems in the past. It was very hard for a patient with such an extensive lesion to wait for 6 weeks until the device was ready. Often the patient would be treated with 6 weeks of bedrest and develop other significant complications as a result of the immobility. By the time the device was available, the patient was in such an unstable situation that he or she could not receive the device. Even though the device was not implanted for that

reason, the hospital would bear the cost for the manufacturer of the implant. This created a difficult situation between the surgeon and the associated hospital.

Sometimes the actual implants would not be the right dimensions as determined at the time of the surgery with the patient opened. The device would be either too small or too large. If the volume of the implant is determined by the radius of that implant cubed, a small differential in the measurement and manufacture of the device can have significant ramifications from the standpoint of the volume that it occupies in the leg. Obviously, not being able to close the wound of the patient on implantation of the device creates a disastrous surgical situation.

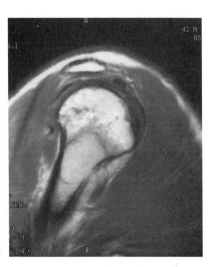
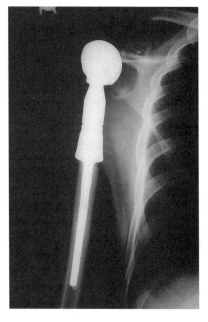

A,B

**FIG. 8. A:** This patient had a known history of metastatic lung cancer and developed severe pain of the right shoulder. The MRI of the right proximal humerus shows a large lesion involving the entire proximal shaft of the humerus and extending into the humeral head. **B:** A postoperative x-ray performed on the same patient shows a proximal humeral replacement with a modular oncology prosthesis in place.

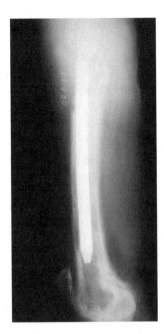

**FIG. 9.** The intramedullary rod in the femur, inserted through a proximal approach. The fracture site can be seen in the midshaft area, at the top of the picture. The entire femur became contaminated with the sarcoma during the reaming of the canal.

Because of these problems, which were frequently encountered, a solution was sought. The modular oncology systems that are available now in orthopedics have been developed to avoid these problems. The device basically combines a joint reconstruction replacement system with a shaft replacement system that can be connected by virtue of tapered ends. This basically allows an erector set system to be used in the operating room. This system has obvious dramatic advantages. It can be obtained for the patient generally within 24 hours of the manufacturer being aware of the need for the implant system. The modular oncology system is sized so as to allow the surgeon to make adjustments in the operating room in terms of how much of the bone needs to be replaced and how large a system is needed. It is theoretically possible to replace most of the femur (Fig. 7), tibia, or humerus (Fig. 8) using such a system. In fact, the replacement of the total femur along with replacement of the proximal tibia is possible as well (Figs. 9 and 10).

In the past, patients with large skeletal metastatic lesions involving the shaft and the joint were often maintained on bedrest, treated with radiation therapy, and considered not salvageable. These patients can often be salvaged quite satisfactorily with the use of a modular oncology system. Many of these patients will regain independent ambulation and often be able to manage themselves and their affairs at home. The modular oncology systems are the latest, most significant development in orthopedic oncology for managing patients with large metastatic lesions of the bone. Unfortunately, however, most clinicians are not familiar with their availability and use. Patients with large segmental lesions of bone involving the shaft and the joint often are the most apparent failures of radiation therapy. The modular oncology systems are secured with the remaining bone by use of intramedullary bone cement. These patients are typically mobilized the day after surgery with physical therapy and rehabilitation. The use of such a large prosthetic reconstruction of the bone does not

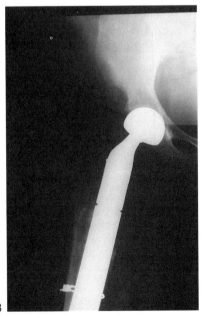
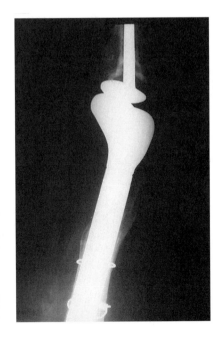

A,B

**FIG. 10. A, B:** Two views of a total femur replacement using a modular oncology system, along with a bipolar hip replacement and a total knee replacement using a kinematic hinge knee. This became necessary because of contamination of the entire femur with the preexisting osteogenic sarcoma.

interfere with radiation therapy once the wound has had a short time (5–7 days) to heal. Physical therapy and rehabilitation with full weight bearing on the involved extremity can start the day after surgery.

## ALL THAT GLITTERS IS NOT GOLD!

*Case Report:* A 70-year-old man with a known history of prostate cancer presents to a community hospital with sudden severe pain in the left femur and significant ambulatory dysfunction. The patient also is known to have had a history of Paget's disease in the left femur for many years. The x-rays taken on arrival at the emergency room demonstrate a fracture of the midshaft of the left femur through an obviously abnormal part of the femur. Also, characteristic chronic changes of the left femur are visible, consistent with the patient's long-standing history of Paget's disease. The orthopedic surgeon on call is aware of the patient's history of prostate carcinoma and, assuming that the lesion in the left femur is a sign of metastatic prostate cancer to the bone, schedules an intramedullary rod fixation of the left femur for the next day. During surgery the guide pin is inserted into the femur, just as described above, and the medullary canal is reamed over the guide pin. Usually at this part of the surgery significant amounts of tumor tissue are being removed with the reamer. The orthopedic surgeon sends the intramedullary tissue for a frozen section in a routine fashion. While the surgeon is closing the wound toward the end of the surgery, the pathologist calls back and announces his surprising preliminary diagnosis: osteogenic sarcoma arising in Paget's disease. After a repeat biopsy is performed in order to verify the preliminary diagnosis, the patient is referred to a multispecialty cancer center. Systemic staging at this point does not demonstrate any metastases of the osteogenic sarcoma or any signs of metastatic prostate carcinoma. For these reasons, limb salvage surgery with radical excision of the sarcoma is indicated. Since the entire femur and the soft tissue surrounding the proximal approach site are contaminated with sarcoma (see Fig. 9), a radical excision of the entire femur is necessary, along with the prosthetic replacement of the complete femur, the hip joint, and the knee joint. This is performed using a modular oncology system (see Fig. 10). Three weeks after surgery the patient is fully mobilized in a hip brace and is walking very well on his own with a walker. One year later the patient is back home and walking with a cane around the house and a walker outside of the house. This case report demonstrates the fact that not every abnormality of bones in a patient with a known history of cancer can be assumed to be an obvious sign for metastatic cancer to bone. It also underlines the fact that patients with a known history of cancer who develop an abnormality of the bone need to be evaluated by a specialist, namely, an orthopedic oncologist.

## SUMMARY

It is important to have an aggressive and appropriate treatment program for patients with metastatic cancer to bone. The specific goals of early aggressive operative management are to give adequate pain relief, to increase the functional mobility of the patient, to facilitate nursing care of the cancer patient, and to improve the patient's mental status for the remaining life span.

Metastasis to bone should no longer be considered the beginning of the end. It should be an invitation for appropriate orthopedic oncologic involvement and management.

Impending pathologic fractures of the long bones can be quickly and relatively easily stabilized with intramedullary rod fixation. Patients with carcinoma should be monitored periodically to identify the focus of metastatic lesions early. Patients with large lesions, which previously were considered disastrous, can be managed successfully today using modular oncology systems. Patients with metastatic cancer to bone deserve evaluation and management by orthopedic oncologists familiar with their treatment options. Managing patients with cancer is today more than ever a team effort.

## REFERENCES

1. Marcove RC, Young DJ. Survival times after treatment of pathologic fractures. *Cancer* 1967;20:2154–2158.
2. Tachdjian MO, Compere CL, Davis PH. Pathologic fractures of the hip. *Surg Gynecol Obstet* 1959;109:13–26.
3. Clain A. Secondary malignant disease of bone. *Br J Cancer* 1965;19:15.
4. Levy RN, Sherry, HS, Siffert RS. Surgical management of metastatic disease of bone at the hip. *Clin Orthop* 1982;169:62.
5. Küntscher G. The intramedullary nailing of fractures. *Arch Klin Chir* 1940;200:443.
6. Griessmann H, Schüttmeyer W. Weitere Erfahrungen mit der Marknagelung nach Küntscher an der Chirurgischen Universitätsklinik Kiel. *Chirurg* 1947;17/18:316.
7. Parrish F, Murray JA. Surgical treatment for secondary neoplastic fractures. *J Bone Joint Surg (Am)* 1970;52:665.
8. Fiedler M. Prophylactic internal fixation of secondary neoplastic fractures. *J Bone Joint Surg (Am)* 1970;52:665.
9. Simm FH. Pathological fractures. *Orthopaedic Surgical Update,* Series 2. Lesson 1982;14:1.
10. Harrington KD. The management of acetabular insufficiency secondary to metastatic malignant disease. *J Bone Joint Surg (Am)* 1981; 63:653.
11. Habermann ET, Sachs R, Stern RE, Hirsh DM, Anderson WJ. The pathology and treatment of metastatic disease of the femur. *Clin Orthop* 1982;169:70.

*Principles and Practice of Supportive Oncology,*
edited by Ann Berger et al.
Lippincott–Raven Publishers, Philadelphia ©1998

CHAPTER 46

# Palliative Endoscopic and Interventional Radiologic Procedures

## Michael L. Kochman, Michael C. Soulen, and Rosemary C. Polomano

Palliation of symptoms associated with advanced cancer can be accomplished through less invasive and more cost-efficient endoscopic and radiologic methods when compared with standard open surgical procedures. Specialization in oncology by gastroenterologists and interventional radiologists has spared many patients additional loss of time and postoperative pain often associated with aggressive surgical interventions (1–3). Technological advances and refinements in endoscopic and interventional radiologic procedures have eliminated the need for extensive surgeries and possibly lengthy recuperation in these systemically ill patients, and have decreased the risks of complications. Patency of the gastrointestinal (GI) tract affected by cancerous tumor growth or strictures caused by radiotherapy can be restored with minimal discomfort and without significant threat to the patient's well-being. Internal and external drainage systems can be placed to relieve organ obstruction pain, and inanition, and to prevent life-threatening end-organ dysfunction. Table 1 outlines palliative endoscopic and interventional procedures, as well as implications associated with patient management.

### GASTROINTESTINAL TUBES FOR DECOMPRESSION AND NUTRITION

Close to half of all patients undergoing gastrostomy and jejunostomy have cancer. Although the majority require GI tubes for enteral nutrition, gastrostomies and jejunos-

tomies are inserted in a select group of patients for the purposes of decompression and drainage of intestinal obstructions. About 40% of patients with ovarian cancer and as many as 28% of patients with colorectal cancer are at risk for developing bowel obstruction (4). Isolated malignant foci or widespread carcinomatosis of the abdomen causing external compression of GI structures are frequently the cause of obstruction. Occlusion of the gastric outlet or intestine by tumor and adhesions from prior surgery, radiotherapy, and intraperitoneal chemotherapy are other mechanisms for gastric and intestinal blockages. Cramping and intestinal distention may be transiently relieved by vomiting, belching, flatus, and defecation; however, the unremitting cycle of these symptoms is often physically and emotionally intolerable. When initial management with aggressive pharmacotherapy, bowel rest, and temporary nasogastric decompression fails, GI decompression should be considered. Intolerable pain, fecal vomitus, intractable nausea or emesis, and esophageal ulceration are clear indications for venting gastrostomies or jejunostomies, which are associated with significant improvements in symptoms and overall quality of life (5–7).

Gastrostomy and jejunostomy, whether intended for venting purposes or for feeding, can be accomplished through surgical, radiologic, or endoscopic techniques. A recent meta-analysis was conducted to determine the efficacy and safety of each technique (8). Investigators were able to evaluate 5680 controls from the literature dating back to 1980 plus 72 subjects from their institution totaling 741 surgical insertions, 837 radiologic placements, and 4194 cases involving percutaneous endoscopic gastrostomy (PEG). The 30-day mortality rate (8%) was the same for both radiologic and percutaneous endoscopic approaches. Statistical analyses revealed significantly fewer complications ($p < 0.001$) and decreased mortality

M. L. Kochman: Department of Medicine, Gastroenterology Division, University of Pennsylvania, Philadelphia, PA 19104.

M.C. Soulen: Department of Interventional Radiology, University of Pennsylvania, Philadelphia, PA 19104.

R. C. Polomano: Department of Surgical Nursing, University of Pennsylvania Medical Center, Philadelphia, PA 19465.

**TABLE 1.** *Common endoscopic and interventional procedures for oncology patients*

| Type of procedure | Indication | Description of procedure | Considerations for oncology care (preprocedure/pain management/follow-up care) |
|---|---|---|---|
| Enteral tube placement for feeding PEG/decompression | Enteral feedings in the absence of the ability to self-feed; decompression of GI obstruction; nutritional support to prevent inanition and to improve sense of well-being and functional status | The stomach of jejunum is punctured through the skin using x-ray guidance. The tract is dilated and an 18- to 20-Fr tube is placed into the stomach and secured at the exit site of the skin. | Preprocedure: antibiotics, coagulation and platelet determinations. Postprocedure: local wound care, possible need for temporary pain management |
| Tracheobronchial or esophageal stenting | Airway or esophageal intrinsic obstruction, extrinsic compression, or tracheoesophageal fistula; relief of obstruction or fistula closure to allow oral nutrition | Obstruction or fistula crossed with a guidewire under fluoroscopic/endoscopic guidance. Tumor is dilated if needed; expandable stent is placed under fluoroscopic/endoscopic guidance. | Preprocedure: barium study, coagulation and platelet determinations, assurance of patient motivation. Postprocedure: barium study, possible need for temporary pain management, lifelong H2RA therapy, HOB up to 30°, aspiration precautions, modified diet |
| Percutaneous nephrostomy/stent | Ureteral obstruction; preserve renal function and prevent renal infection | Renal calyx is punctured with an 18- to 22-gauge needle through the skin under radiologic guidance. Tract is dilated and the nephrostomy tube is placed. Stricture may be crossed, biopsied, and/or dilated, then stented. | Preprocedure: coagulation, platelet, BUN, and Cr determinations. Postprocedure: local wound care, possible need for temporary pain management, serial BUN and Cr, monitoring of urine output |
| Percutaneous transhepatic biliary drainage (PTBD) and endoscopic retrograde biliary drainage (ERBD) with stent | Obstructive jaundice, cholangitis, and pruritus; relief of pruritus, prevention of systemic sepsis, and improvement in sense of well-being. Literature documents that ERBDE is safer overall because of avoidance of puncture of liver capsule and placement of the catheters through hepatic parenchyma (3) | PTBD: Bile duct is punctured with a 18- to 21-gauge needle under x-ray guidance. Tract is dilated and an 8- to 12-Fr tube is placed into the biliary tree-duodenum. Strictures are biopsied and dilated. Possible interval conversion to purely internal plastic or metal stent. ERBD: Bile duct is cannulated at endoscopic retrograde cholangiopancreatography (ERCP). Strictures are biopsied and dilated. Stricture may be stented with removable plastic or permanent metal stents. NBT may be placed to facilitate/aid PTBD. | Preprocedure: antibiotics, coagulation, platelet, and bilirubin determinations. Postprocedure: possible local wound care, possible need for temporary pain management, serial bilirubin to verify function |
| Embolization/chemoembolization | Treatment of unresectable, locally confined tumor; facilitate surgical resection; decrease tumor burden to improve sense of well-being and functional status | Hepatic artery providing blood supply to the tumor is identified and selectively catheterized. Embolic agents are injected into the vessel to occlude blood flow. Chemotherapeutic agents may be added to the embolic mixture for enhanced local effect. | Preprocedure: coagulation, platelet, BUN and Cr, LFT determinations. Postprocedure: local wound care, possible need for temporary pain management, evaluation for systemic effects. Management of postembolization syndrome (nausea and vomiting, fever, pain) |

Adapted from ref 9, Table 2.

($p$ < 0.001) with radiologic techniques compared to surgery and PEG. These data must be interpreted cautiously, as subset analyses on just cancer patients and reasons for placement (feeding versus venting) were not performed.

## Techniques for Gastrostomy and Jejunostomy Placement

### Endoscopic Placement

Both percutaneous radiologic and endoscopic placement of gastrostomy and jejunostomy tubes for decompression and feeding provide an acceptable alternative to the uncomfortable presence of nasogastric tubes, and eliminate the need for costly operative procedures that pose higher risks for complications for patients with advanced cancer (6,9,10). Insertion of PEG involves a standard upper endoscopic technique with conscious sedation. After endoscopic examination of the stomach and duodenum to exclude significant ulcerations, the anterior gastric body or antrum is transilluminated and the gastric body is fully insufflated. Using the endoscopic light source, a suitable area on the anterior abdominal wall is transilluminated and the suitability of the site for a percutaneous tract is confirmed by gentle external compression at the potential entry site. These maneuvers allow for the determination of a safe site with the absence of any intervening viscera or major blood vessels. With some exceptions dependent on the type of gastrostomy (G) tube to be inserted and operator preference, a needle or trocar is passed into the gastric lumen and a guidewire is then threaded through the hollow needle and retrieved endoscopically (Fig. 1). The guidewire is then pulled up to the patients oropharynx and the G-tube is then passed over the wire into the stomach and out of the anterior abdominal wall. Firm traction is applied to ensure passage of the internal bolster through the esophagus and to allow a traction seal and apposition of the gastric and abdominal walls to minimize the leakage of any gastric contents or feedings.

Recently, endoscopic ultrasound has been used as an adjunct to aid in the placement of endoscopically placed G-tubes when the transillumination and indentation are not optimal (11). The advantage of this technique is that it may be performed in formerly complicated situations including previously operated abdomens and in post-partial gastrectomy patients. The use of endoscopic ultrasound imaging significantly improves visualization of the bowel and gastric viscera that might otherwise be impeded by the formation of adhesions, presence of taut peritoneum or ascites, and diffuse intraabdominal metastases. As a result, risks for inadvertent perforation of bowel, other organs, and metastatic foci are minimized. Studies show promising results over conventional proce-

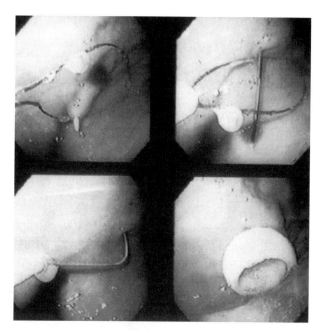

**FIG. 1.** Endoscopic placement of G-tube. (upper left) Initial introduction of trocar into gastric lumen. (upper right) Guidewire passed through trocar and grasped by endoscopy snare. (lower left) Guidewire fed into stomach and withdrawn to allow per os introduction of feeding tube. (lower right) Appearance of gastrostomy after placement.

dures in facilitating ease of insertion and decreasing morbidity associated with the procedure (5).

### Radiologic Placement

Radiologic gastrostomy is performed using fluoroscopic guidance under local anesthetic, with conscious sedation if needed. If swallowing function is intact and there is no GI obstruction, the patient is given oral contrast the night before in order to opacify the transverse colon and splenic flexure the next day. A nasogastric tube is placed and the stomach insufflated with air. Ultrasound is used to mark the left lobe of the liver if it crosses over the stomach. The anterior wall of the stomach is then punctured through the abdominal wall under fluoroscopy, avoiding both the colon and the liver. Aspiration of air and injection of contrast confirm that the needle tip is within the stomach. One or more T anchors are placed for gastropexy; then the puncture tract is dilated over a guidewire and the tube placed. In patients with aspiration risk, the pylorus is crossed and a gastrojejunostomy catheter is placed with the tip beyond the ligament of Treitz. Single- or double-lumen catheters are available, with the second lumen allowing decompression of the stomach as well as jejunal feeding. The catheter is left to external drainage for 24 hours; then it can be capped and used for feeding.

## Complications

Various problems and complications have been associated with gastrostomy inserted by endoscopy and radiologic guidance. Technical difficulties encountered during insertion tend to be relatively low ranging from 4% to 8% (5,7,9,12,13). The inability to implant gastrostomy tubes has been attributed to tumor invasion of anterior gastric wall, anatomic anomalies, and massive ascites (9,14,15). Overall, such difficulties seem to be noted more frequently with PEG placement than for radiologic guidance (8). Complication rates for both procedures vary from study to study, and must be cautiously interpreted in lieu of different methods of placement, operator experience, and diversity among patients. Procedure-related deaths, typically defined as mortality within 30 days of the procedure, have been reported. High mortality rates within 30 days of the procedure may reflect consequences of the underlying disease and the overall poor status of the patients rather than direct causation from the procedure. More importantly, failure to sustain adequate nutrition and fluid replacement following the insertion of venting GI tubes might possibly account for early deaths. Early mortality from PEG placement was assessed by a retrospective review of 416 patients including 44 patients with cancer who had a 50% mortality rate (16). Overall, significant risks for complications included urinary tract infection, previous aspiration, and age >75 years, and patients with all three were 67.1% more likely to die within a month than those without any.

Intestinal (colonic) perforation, peritonitis, and gastric hemorrhage are among the most serious complications. Isolated occurrences of mechanical intraabdominal seeding of tumor (17) and stomal seeding (18) have surfaced in the literature, though for patients undergoing palliation this is not likely to be an issue. While the diameter of the lumen might be expected to increase adverse effects, Cannizzaro et al. found no appreciable differences in symptomatic relief and placement-related complications between patients who received 15- and 20-French lumen catheters (6). Prophylactic use of preprocedure and postprocedure antibiotic administration has been practiced to reduce the incidence of infection. The data are not clear, but it appears that the preprocedure use of antibiotics reduces the postprocedure incidence of tube site cellulitis and fasciitis. Meticulous cleansing of the tube site with an iodine prep or antibacterial soap and application of a sterile gauze dressing will minimize early wound infections. Once the sutures are removed (if used) and the subcutaneous tract has sealed (approximately 3 weeks), no additional care to the site is generally required.

## Considerations with Gastrointestinal Tube Placement

Several factors must be taken into account in order to select the best technology and method of insertion. Feeding gastrostomies are preferred over jejunostomies for patients who may require skilled nursing placement, as jejunostomy tubes tend to fall out and clog more frequently. Venting gastrostomies are indicated for patients with high upper intestinal or gastric outlet obstructions and those who maintain oral intake, whereas venting jejunostomies are more effective for decompression with intestinal obstructions that are more distal. Patients at risk for aspiration via emesis, as opposed to oropharyngeal dysphagia, are better candidates for jejunostomy feeding tubes. Through the use of a dual-lumen gastrojejunostomy tube, an artificial GI bypass can be constructed with a venting gastrostomy above the obstruction enabling enteral feedings via a jejunostomy below the obstruction (19).

Lumen size appears to more of an issue for patients who require intermittent or continuous decompression and wish to ingest soft food and fluids. Modifications in the contour of the tube and outflow portion, rather than lumen size, seem to be most critical in maximizing the flow of GI secretions mixed with semisolid foods and liquids (12). It is necessary to ensure that the tube selected for any patient is appropriate for its intended purpose. Some tubes now have one-way valves built in, which decrease the likelihood of patients expelling gastric contents if the end seal is loose, but these tubes are therefore not suitable for the purpose of gastric decompression. The vast majority of tubes now are designed in such a manner that they may be removed via firm traction and not require a repeat surgery or endoscopic procedure. Replacement button devices and stomal tubes are available, some of which the patients find to be quite comfortable and unobtrusive.

Radiologic and endoscopic placement of jejunostomies are valuable techniques associated with low risks while avoiding the need for surgery. Direct endoscopic jejunostomy is placed using methods similar to PEG placement with low risks (20). The tubes are inserted distal to the ligament of Treitz under conscious sedation. The advantage of this technique is the relative stability of the direct J-tube placement in comparison with a J-tube threaded through a G-tube. Insertion of percutaneous jejunostomy catheters are more easily accomplished when a J-tube has previously been present because the small bowel is adherent to the abdominal wall creating a secure tract. The bowel loop can be punctured under fluoroscopic guidance, the tract dilated, and a new tube placed. The absence of a well-established access site makes the initial percutaneous procedure technically more difficult because of bowel mobility. In these circumstances, a gastrojejunostomy catheter is recommended.

Costs associated with the procedure must also be taken into account. We have found that endoscopically and radiologically placed tubes can avoid the use of the operating room, general anesthesia, and their attendant costs and risks. Charges for PEG placement have been assessed

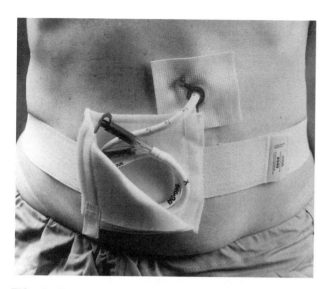

**FIG. 2.** The new Dale gastrostomy tube holder allows patients requiring enteral feeding greater mobility and security and the ability to enjoy a more active, comfortable lifestyle. The tube holder secures percutaneous endoscopic gastrostomy tubes and other abdominal feeding tubes without the discomfort and irritation caused by tape and other adhesive backed holders.

around $2400 and radiologic placement at $4500 (8). Estimated reimbursement for professional fees remains somewhat similar, and for inpatients the hospital reimbursement for the procedure is generally embedded into the fixed rate established for the diagnostic category. Above all, patient and family acceptance, motivation, and ability to care for the tube and empty drainage or administer feedings are critically important in the successful management of GI intubation. Patients and families are instructed to (a) care for the tube exit site; (b) observe the site for any peristomal redness, ulceration, or drainage; and (c) flush, cap, and connect the tube to the appropriate devices. The tube can be anchored to the abdomen with special securing devices (Fig. 2). Arrangements for home health care are coordinated if patients are immediately discharged to home following tube placement, require nutritional support (enteral or total parenteral) or fluid replacement, or need additional teaching following hospitalization. This may be necessary to assist the patient and family with wound care and feedings, and help them select an appropriate drainage container and operate suction devices for venting tubes.

## PALLIATIVE MANAGEMENT OF GASTROINTESTINAL AND BILIARY OBSTRUCTION

Malignant intrinsic obstructions or extrinsic compressions of GI structures can be relieved through the use of endoprostheses made from materials that restore both patency and function of the esophagus, colon, rectum, and biliary and pancreatic ducts. Over the past decade a dramatic improvement in the materials, design, and delivery systems has served to make these procedures both widely disseminated and less dangerous to the patient, thereby bringing additional palliative comfort measures to patients at much lower risk. The insertion of endoprostheses into the esophagus, descending colon, and rectum may obviate the need for more invasive surgical interventions while maintaining normal GI activity. Endoscopically and fluoroscopically guided percutaneous placement of stents into the bile duct relieves narrowing or occlusion of duct and facilitates the flow of bile into the GI tract.

### Esophageal Endoprostheses or Stenting

#### Indications

Esophageal endoprosthetic intubation is used to treat esophageal compression from locally advanced esophageal, mediastinal, or tracheobronchial malignancies and strictures that may result from prior radiotherapy, especially when definitive surgical resection may not be possible or would pose significant risk of postsurgical complications. Endoprostheses also allow for the palliation and occlusion of tracheoesophageal fistula and will allow oral nutrition in those for whom this was not previously possible. The insertion of an artificial tube restores patency of the esophagus and provides relief from dysphagia, pain, and the inability to swallow or effectively clear oral secretions, which if not treated significantly increase the risk for aspiration pneumonia.

Relative contraindications for the placement of esophageal stents include extensive circumferential tumor growth that occludes the lumen and interferes with passage of a guidewire and dilators, necrotic lesions that may hemorrhage, friable tissues increasing the chance for perforation, anticipated discomfort associated with the presence of the stent, and lack of patient acceptance or compliance with dietary modifications and follow-up care. The stents may leave a patient with a persistent globus sensation if placed within 2 cm of the upper esophageal sphincter. The placement of a stent into a fibrotic (posttherapy) stricture or one resistant to dilatation may result in mediastinal pain, as the pressure exerted by the stent in its attempt to deploy will continue until full expansion.

#### Types of Stents

A variety of rigid and metal self-expandable stents are available as endoprosthetic devices. Selection of stents is dependent on several factors such as life expectancy, patterns of tumor growth (i.e., location, orientation of tumor

**TABLE 2.** *Relative indications for rigid and expandable metal endoprostheses*

| Situation | Rigid stents | Expandable metal stents |
|---|---|---|
| Cancer within 2 cm of upper esophageal sphincter | - - | - - |
| Airway compression by tube | - - | - |
| Limited life expectancy | - - | - - |
| Lack of patient motivation | - - | - - |
| Luminal obstruction preventing passage of a guidewire | - - | - - |
| Noncircumferential tumors preventing anchoring of the stent | - - | + |
| Soft or necrotic lesions with poor anchoring qualities | - - | + |
| Profusely bleeding lesions | - | - |
| Horizontal orientation of the malignant lumen | - | + |
| Acutely angulated complex lesions | - | + |

From ref 27.

invasion, extent of invasion, size), anticipated complications, and desired treatment outcomes. Table 2 outlines the relative indications for both types of endoprosthetic stents. Rigid stents have been manufactured from several materials such as polyvinyl tubing, silicone with metal reinforcements (Wilson-Cook, William Cook Europe Limited), radiopaque silicone with metal reinforcements (Key-Med Atkinson), and latex with a nylon spiral (Medoc-Celestin). Promising results have been reported using cuffed rigid stents in managing life-threatening sequelae associated with esophagotracheal fistulas. Patients with these fistulas tend to be poor surgical candidates because of respiratory distress, malnutrition, and debilitation from advanced stages of cancer. Mortality rates as high as 36% have been documented with attempts to surgically repair this type of fistula; however, peroral intubation using a cuffed rigid stent to seal off the fistula has reduced mortality to 24% (21). Expandable cuffs attached to rigid endoprostheses have been successful in occluding fistulas with less patient discomfort and reduced hospitalization compared to surgery, and without the risk of pressure necrosis (22).

The recent introduction of metal self-expanding esophageal stents, patterned after biliary and vascular stents, has minimized problems associated with the rigid polymeric stents and their fixed lumen diameters (Fig. 3). While self-expanding metal stents are approximately 10 times more expensive, their advantages of larger lumen size, ease of insertion, decreased complication rates, and greater success with more stenotic lesions often outweigh any cost expenditures. All of the metal stents share an ability to be placed into a narrow lumen on a small-bore delivery device and then allowed to expand once in correct anatomic position. The Wallstent (Schneider Inc.) is constructed in such a way that its diameter can be reduced during insertion by elongating the tube (23). The Gianturco stent has wires patterned in a zig-zag fashion to expand without shortening in length (24). Some metallic self-expanding stents are covered with a polymeric sheet to inhibit tumor ingrowth and to facilitate occlusion of tracheoesophageal fistula tracts. Unlike rigid stents

that can be taken out, metal self-expanding tubes are virtually impossible to remove short of an open surgical procedure due to the expandable nature of the device. Another endoprosthetic design allows for the insertion of a coil that when released assumes a tightly fitting spiral that may successfully occlude a fistula and restore luminal patency. This device is reported to be endoscopically removable, though large series have not been published to support this.

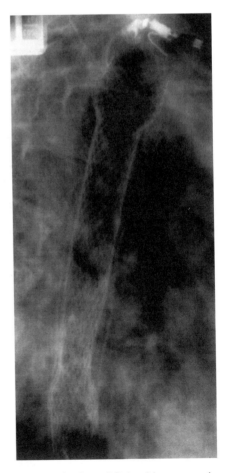

**FIG. 3.** Fluoroscopic view of Schneider-covered esophageal prosthesis at the time of deployment.

### Complications

Perforation, stent migration, and hemorrhage are among the most common complications of rigid stents. Perforation is the most serious complication of esophageal endoprostheses and occurs with a frequency of about 6–8% with the rigid endoprostheses (25,26). The rate of perforation may prove to be <5% with the newer expandable stents, though large datasets are not yet published. Perforation may occur as a result of the endoscopy, esophageal dilatation, or the endoprosthetic placement. Factors associated with a higher incidence of perforation include prior radiotherapy and surgical intervention, sharp angulation from tortuous tumor involvement, and preexisting kyphoscoliosis. In the majority of cases, perforations are easily identified at the time of stent placement by careful inspection of the esophagus and pharynx, the presence of subcutaneous emphysema or crepitation of air, and plain films of the chest and neck areas. Shortly after the procedure, the exact location of a leak can be detected by the use of water-soluble contrast media.

Perforation always carries a risk for accompanying mediastinitis. Once identified, the use of acid-suppressive therapy and intravenous antibiotics are the mainstays of therapy. The stent itself may seal off the site of the perforation, and consideration for the placement of an additional endoprosthetic or surgical repair needs to be entertained for open communicating tracts. Aspiration may occur either during the placement of the endoprosthetic or subsequently due to gastric contents. It is important to instruct patients that they should not lie supine or prone after placement; this is especially important when the endoprosthetic bridges the gastroesophageal junction.

A persistent globus sensation may occur if the stent is placed proximally in the esophagus within 2 cm of the upper esophageal sphincter. Careful preprocedure evaluation is necessary with measurements made both with a barium study and endoscopically, coupled with scrupulous technical placement of the endoprosthetic. Mediastinal pain may occur with placement into a stenotic or fibrotic lesion. The use of additional postprocedure opioids for 10–14 days will suffice in most cases. Stent migration and dislodgement may occur, though currently available expandable designs appear to have a small propensity for this type of movement. Barium studies carried out postprocedure document location of placement and function and are a baseline should migration be suspected in the future.

It is useful to have a preprocedure barium study to assess for sharp angulations, unsuspected perforations, distance from the upper esophageal sphincter, and the presence of fistulas. Despite concerns over complications of esophageal endoprosthetic placement, this procedure is relatively safe and offers considerable benefits for optimizing oral nutrition and improving quality of life. Cusumano and associates evaluated 445 consecutive patients undergoing stent placement for palliation of esophageal cancer and noted a success rate of 92% (409) with 80% of these patients able to resume semisolid feedings at the time of discharge with a complication rate of 3.4% (27). Patients are advised to gradually increase the consistency of their food but to avoid solid meats, breads, and baked products. The time spent counseling patients as to the use of H2 receptor antagonists (H2RAs) to decrease the risk of gastric aspiration, modified diets, and to sleep with the head of the bed raised has resulted in a dramatic improvement in the quality of life in those patients who formerly had a nearly intolerable existence.

## Colorectal Endoprostheses and Stenting

### Indications

The majority of patients with intestinal obstruction from locally advanced colorectal carcinoma are at risk for obstructing lesions in the descending colon, sigmoid colon, or rectum. Neoplasms that narrow the lumen of the colon or rectum not only interfere with passage of stool but cause severe pain and obstruction, and can hemorrhage if untreated. Surgical intervention was until recently the only hope for palliation; however, this was often at a cost of increased surgical morbidity and psychological devastation if a temporary or permanent colostomy was necessary. The introduction of colorectal stents fashioned similarly to esophageal prostheses has successfully relieved colorectal stenosis from obstructing tumors. In some cases, endoprosthetic devices have been implanted for acute management of intestinal obstruction to allow for luminal decompression prior to palliative and definitive surgical resection (28–30). Rupp et al. reported survival following colorectal stents ranging from 1 to 25 months (31), and others have determined that the time to reobstruction varies from 45 to 91 days (32).

### Types of Rectal Stents

The endoprosthesis used to restore and maintain colorectal patency is similar to the metal self-expanding tubes inserted to alleviate esophageal compression. The Wallstent is one of the most popular stents with models that are constructed with diameter of 18–22 mm and a deployed length of 60–90 mm. Plastic stents have been used; however, one study comparing this technology to metal self-expanding stents found a higher incidence of placement failure due to iatrogenic perforation and temporary incontinence with plastic material (31).

### Complications

Mild rectal bleeding is not unanticipated with colorectal stent procedures. More serious complications such as perforation seem to be more prevalent among patients with areas of tumor necrosis. Stent placement failures tend to be related to technical malfunctions or the inability to intubate the obstructed area due to extensive tumor involvement and luminal compromise. In the latter circumstance, surgery is often the only option to alleviate the obstruction. Laser therapy can be tried at intervals to open the lumen to allow placement of a stent and to palliate tumor growth around the proximal and distal margins of the stent.

In a manner analogous to the placement of the esophageal endoprostheses, we have found it beneficial to obtain a preprocedure barium study if possible to rule out any acute angulation that could lead to nonfunctioning of a stent. Following colorectal stent placement, patients are advised to report signs and symptoms of increased pain, rectal bleeding, inability to defecate, abdominal distention, and stent protrusion through the anal opening. Consistent use of laxatives and stool softeners as well as dietary modifications aids in maintaining bowel regularity.

## BILIARY STENTING AND DRAINAGE PROCEDURES

### Indications

Palliative management of biliary obstruction or stenosis in patients with nonresectable hepatic metastases, cholangiocarcinoma, and pancreatic carcinomas is critical to the physical and emotional well-being of patients suffering from intolerable symptomatology. With biliary stenting procedures, dramatic reductions in symptom distress from jaundice, anorexia, pruritus, indigestion, nausea, and vomiting are possible (33–36). A measurable effect on psychosocial outcomes with placement of biliary stents has also been observed (35).

Therapy of malignant biliary obstruction can be approached in a variety of ways. Surgical resection offers the possibility for cure but unfortunately is only possible in 10–15% of cases. Palliation can be achieved by surgical bypass or by endoscopic or percutaneous stenting combined with adjuvant radiation and chemotherapy. Comparative trials have shown no advantage between surgical versus nonsurgical palliation of the obstruction in morbidity and survival. Patients undergoing laparotomy in the hopes of resecting the tumor will have bypass performed at that time, whereas patients who are clearly unresectable can be treated endoscopically or percutaneously. Some surgeons prefer that all patients undergo preoperative biliary drainage, though a clear benefit from preoperative drainage has not been proven.

### Methods of Placement

Endoscopic therapy requires retrograde cannulation of the common bile duct, performance of a sphincterotomy, and placement of a 7- to 11-French plastic endoprosthesis. A successful diagnostic endoscopic retrograde cholangiopancreatography (ERCP) is accomplished 75–90% of the time, after which the technical success rate for performing a sphincterotomy is very high. For low strictures such as pancreatic carcinoma, stent placement after successful cannulation of the duct is achieved 95% of the time, with a morbidity of 10% and a mortality of about 3% (37). Success rates for hilar strictures decline significantly to the 40–60% range, with an increase in morbidity and mortality to 18% and 8%, respectively (38,39). Higher success rates can be obtained using a rendezvous procedure, in which an interventional radiologist passes a guidewire percutaneously down through the biliary tree into the duodenum, and is met by the endoscopist who pulls the guidewire out through the mouth. With this through-and-through approach, an endoprosthesis can be passed retrograde without creating a large transhepatic track. Use of the rendezvous technique increases the success rate for retrograde stenting of hilar strictures to almost 90%.

Percutaneous biliary drainage is successful 95–100% of the time but suffers from an acute, serious complication rate of 15%. Once internal drainage has been achieved, conversion to an endoprosthesis is almost always possible with little added morbidity. Advantages of retrograde endoscopic stenting are its lower morbidity and the ability to change an endoprosthesis if it becomes clogged. On the down side, the endoscopic approach to the bile duct has a lower technical success rate than the percutaneous approach. Endoscopically placed stents are usually smaller than those placed percutaneously. Because of the smaller diameter, and because they protrude into the duodenum and so are exposed to food debris, the occlusion rate for these stents appears to be higher. Hilar lesions are often not well treated from below. Also, it is not possible to administer intracavitary radiation without percutaneous access. Conversely, percutaneous internal–external drainage can almost always be accomplished regardless of the level of obstruction. It allows for larger tubes, which can be changed easily. Access is maintained for brachytherapy or for later interventions as the disease progresses. For some patients, an internal–external tube is their psychological "lifeline" and gives them a sense of managing their own care.

### Types of Stents

Technologic advancements in the perfection of metallic self-expanding implantable stents have maximized the efficiency of stents, but stent malfunction as a result of tumor ingrowth and overgrowth is a significant problem. Percutaneous or endoscopic deployment of these stents (Wallstent; Gianturco-Rosch Z) has been associated with less pain during placement than plastic stents

(39) and appears to be more versatile for either percutaneous or endoscopic techniques. The main advantage of the metal stents appears to be a slightly longer duration of patency of 9–12 months. This is especially important for patients with a limited life span when cost savings in decreased hospital days and repeat procedures are considered. Optimism over these benefits remains guarded due to concerns over stent malfunction from tumor growth and the inability to remove the metal endoprosthetics.

## Complications

Unfortunately, chronic internal–external drainage is associated with late complications in up to 50% of patients, including cholangitis, skin infection, bleeding, leakage of bile and ascites, rib erosion and osteomyelitis, catheter fracture or dislodgement, and seeding of tumor cells along the track. The tubes require regular flushing and dressing, which is difficult for ill or incompetent patients. Even with optimal care, routine tube change is necessary at 8- to 12-week intervals to avoid occlusion, with a cumulative cost and morbidity associated with repeated tube changes. For some, the distortion of their body image is psychologically distressing. Insertion of an endoprosthesis avoids many of the complications of having a chronic percutaneous catheter, but repeat drainage is required if the stent obstructs.

Patency rates are difficult to measure because of the high mortality in this population but appear to run from 68% to 94% at a follow-up of 4–5 months (39,40–43). Occlusion of plastic stents occurs due to a sequence of bacterial adherence, glycoprotein deposition, and encrustation with bile salts. Later series employing longer stents made from new, smooth-surfaced polymers or anti-bacterial coatings show patencies at the higher end of this range, with median patencies of about 6.5 months (41,44). Long-term complications are common, with cholangitis in 20% and an average occlusion rate of 11%. Stents fracture or dislodge in 3–6% of cases. Despite these poor statistics, most patients are reasonably well served. Average survival with malignant biliary obstruction is only 3–5 months, so most patients die of their disease with the stent patent. The stent palliates the symptoms of biliary obstruction without prolonging survival. In the subset of patients with more indolent cholangiocarcinomas, stent placement significantly increases survival to a mean of 8 months. Late complications are more of a problem in these longer living patients.

Several studies have evaluated the efficacy of metal self-expanding stents in the treatment of neoplastic-related biliary obstruction by percutaneous insertion and isolated complication rates in defined populations. Nicholson et al., who placed metal self-expanding stents percutaneously in 77 patients with inoperable biliary obstruction with no evidence of metastatic spread, found serum bilirubin levels returned to normal within 7 days of stent placement in 98.7% of patients (34). Use of metal stents may prove to be advantageous in patients with cholangiocarcinoma when intraductal radiation is administered via an iridium wire prior to stent placement. This may deliver 2000–3000 rads within a 1-cm radius. This can be supplemented by external beam therapy and chemotherapy with 5-fluorouracil (5-FU). This combined modality approach can yield a mean survival of close to 2 years, with mean stent patency of 19.5 months (45). Intraductal brachytherapy does not appear to improve patency in patients with biliary obstruction from other types of tumors. In another series, successful placement and catheter longevity were noted for patients with cholangiocarcinoma ($n = 31$; mean survival 14 months), yet 77% of patients with sclerosing cholangitis from intraarterial chemotherapy ($n = 11$) experienced catheter occlusions (33).

Following catheter or stent placement, patients are followed with an anticipated reduction in serum bilirubin levels and resolution of pruritus over the first 7–10 days. Signs and symptoms of pain, fever, or jaundice at any time may be a signal of stent occlusion or dislocation. Local care to catheter exit site with a sterile dressing is done every day for the first few days, then every 3–4 days. Patients and family members are given instructions for catheter care and when to notify the physician or nurse regarding unusual findings. The site and dressing are continually observed for signs of bile drainage. The catheter is placed to straight drainage with the output emptied and measured as necessary. Temperature is taken at least once a day for about 1 week after insertion. Internal–external catheters can be capped after 24 hours to move the internal flow of bile into the duodenum. Patients with long-term external drainage systems are periodically monitored for electrolyte and bicarbonate depletion. Electrolyte loss can be avoided by reingestion of the bile.

## TUMOR ABLATION TECHNIQUES

### Endoscopic Ablative Palliation

Palliation of GI malignancies may also be achieved through the use of tumor ablative techniques (3). These methods may be applied endoscopically and include thermal debulking techniques (bipolar cautery, monopolar cautery, laser), tissue destruction (alcohol, chemotherapeutic agents, photodynamic therapy), and radiotherapy (afterloading techniques, seed implantation). The use of any of these methods is dependent on the local expertise and resources available, as well as on a multidisciplinary approach to the overall care of the patient.

### Esophagus

The maintenance of esophageal luminal patency is a goal for the palliation of nutritional support, for the prevention of the aspiration of saliva, and allowing the patient to obtain oral gratification. Many different techniques have been used, but relatively long-lasting palliation in the absence of an endoprosthesis or surgical excision will require an ablative technique. The most commonly applied in the past was bipolar cautery, but this has fallen out of favor due to concerns over full-thickness injury, stricture formation, the need for a circumferential tumor, and difficulties in the technical performance of the technique. This technique utilizes a rigid bipolar probe that is inserted into the tumor, and serial applications of current are made as the probe is withdrawn under radiographic or direct visual guidance.

Nd:YAG laser treatment has been the mainstay of the obliterative techniques used recently by gastroenterologists. The technique is relatively fast and inexpensive if the cost of the laser power source is spread over several specialties. Numerous difficulties, including perforation, may be encountered in its application, though careful patient selection may ameliorate these risks (46). Direct EtOH injection into tumor masses has been used with success to debulk lesions and to improve dysphagia, salvage endoprostheses when overgrowth has occurred, and maintain luminal patency. It is clearly the simplest and least expensive of the therapies, though scant data are available on which to base recommendations regarding its efficacy and safety. Current development of chemotherapeutic agents for intratumoral injection is underway in clinical trials and may prove to have long-lasting benefit.

Other techniques include photodynamic therapy, a new technique that is currently Food and Drug Administration-approved for the palliation and restoration of luminal patency in esophageal cancer (47). Further bench and clinical research will most likely lead to better hematoporphyrin derivatives and to better techniques and additional applications. Radiotherapy may be directed and aided by endoscopic techniques including endoscopic ultrasound. Brachytherapy markers and delivery tubes may be placed endoscopically and location of the tumor precisely determined to allow for the accurate delivery of intraluminal and external beam therapy.

### Rectum

The mainstay of endoscopic debulking of colorectal neoplasms has been the use of thermal ablation techniques. Large sessile or pedunculated lesions may be effectively debulked to allow for the passage of stool or to allow for the preparation of the colon for a resection or stent placement. These techniques are relatively easily applied in the rectum below the peritoneal reflection without much concern for the complication of free peritoneal perforation. The use of monopolar cautery snare resection coupled with saline injection is a technique that can be readily mastered and does not require a large investment in capital expenditures. Unfortunately, the lesions that are commonly found in the rectum (and higher in the colon) tend to be circumferential lesions and are not easily dealt with by application of cautery. The majority of lesions require the use of endoscopic laser therapy, most commonly performed with Nd:YAG. The KTP laser (532 nm) is just coming into clinical use and we have found it to quite effective. The laser energy may be applied via a free fiber and allowed to vaporize tissue to open the lumen, or it may be used with contact-type probes to allow for precise delivery of energy and a theoretically more controlled depth of penetration. There is a paucity of data comparing this technique with others, though data that are published support its safety and efficacy when used by those experienced with the equipment and technique.

### Percutaneous Ethanol Injection (PEI) and Other Local Ablation Techniques

Patients with relatively few, small lesions in the liver may be amenable to direct percutaneous ablation of the tumors by application of chemical or physical agents through a needle placed under imaging guidance. Typical selection criteria for percutaneous ablation techniques are patients with one to three tumors <3–5 cm in diameter who nonetheless are unresectable due to location of the tumors or because of inadequate hepatic reserve. Because damage to the liver is minimal, percutaneous ablation techniques can be used even in the setting of severe liver dysfunction precluding embolization. Contraindications are uncontrolled ascites or coagulopathy. Typical side effects are pain due to leakage of chemical agents along the needle tract back to the peritoneum, fever, dose-dependent alcohol intoxication, and, occasionally, vasovagal reaction. Rare complications (<1%) include intraperitoneal bleeding, pleural effusion, hemo- or pneumothorax, and injury to intrahepatic vessels or bile ducts. Treatment is usually performed on an outpatient basis under local anesthesia with or without conscious sedation.

### PEI

Percutaneous ethanol injection can be performed under ultrasound or computed tomography (CT) guidance. A skinny needle is advanced to the back wall of the lesion and slowly retracted to the front wall as

95–100% alcohol is injected. Multiple passes or needles may be necessary to cover the whole lesion, depending on its size and shape. Several outpatient sessions are typically required. Results of PEI for hepatoma have been reported for several hundred patients in Italy and Japan, with long-term survivals equivalent to those achieved by surgical resection (48,49). Small series of tumors that were resected after PEI have revealed 90–100% tumor necrosis in nearly all cases. PEI has been combined with chemoembolization for larger hepatomas, with a suggestion of improved benefit. Results with metastatic lesions have been less satisfying, with incomplete tumor necrosis in both pathologic and clinical studies, although complete responses have been obtained in some patients.

## Tumor Ablation with Physical Agents

The difficulty in achieving dispersion of ethanol through metastatic tumors has led several investigators to evaluate local application of physical energy. Cryosurgery is the prototypical physical ablation technique, but it requires an open surgical procedure. Percutaneous techniques include radiofrequency, microwave, and laser energy applied via fibers introduced through skinny needles placed under CT or ultrasonographic guidance. These technologies are still under development, and whether local destruction of metastatic lesions results in improved survival has yet to be determined.

## Chemoembolization

Malignancies in the liver present one of the most challenging problems in clinical oncology. Other tumors that are less common but frequently develop fatal hepatic metastases despite a resectable primary include ocular melanoma, neuroendocrine tumors, and the rare GI sarcomas. Response rates of hepatoma and metastatic colorectal cancer to a variety of systemic chemotherapeutic agents are no better than 20–40%, and a significant survival benefit has not been demonstrated. Intraarterial chemotherapy delivered by percutaneous catheters or by surgically implanted pumps has remained a popular regional approach to hepatic malignancies, even though none of the phase III trials comparing intraarterial to intravenous chemotherapy for metastatic colorectal cancer has shown a long-term survival benefit for intraarterial infusions (50–53). Response rates of hepatoma to intraarterial chemotherapy are 50–60%, with an increase in survival to 20–60% at 1 year (54,55).

Embolization of the hepatic artery has proven effective for palliation of liver metastases from carcinoid and islet cell tumors with response rates of 80–90% (56,57). Hepatoma has a more modest response to embolization (50–60%), with some increase in short-term survival (58,59). The efficacy of embolization is limited by the liver's ability to develop collateral blood supply when the hepatic artery is occluded. For this reason, benefits from hepatic artery embolization tend to be transient. Embolization has not been shown to extend survival for patients with colorectal metastases (60,61). Chemoembolization combines hepatic artery embolization with simultaneous infusion of a concentrated dose of chemotherapeutic drugs. Theoretical advantages of this technique include the following: (a) embolization renders the tumor ischemic, depriving it of nutrients and oxygen and decreasing drug resistance; (b) tumor drug concentrations are orders of magnitude higher than those achieved by infusion alone (62,63); (c) blood flow is arrested, prolonging the dwelling time of the chemotherapy with measurable drug levels present as long as a month later (64,65); and, (d) most of the drug is retained in the liver, minimizing systemic toxicity.

Critical to the selection of patients for regional therapy is that their tumor is confined to the liver. Patients with minimal or indolent extrahepatic disease may be candidates if the liver disease is considered to be the dominant source of morbidity and mortality for that individual. Tumors that typically meet these criteria include hepatoma, intrahepatic cholangiocarcinoma, and metastases from colorectal cancer, ocular melanoma, neuroendocrine tumors, and sarcomas. Occasionally other cancers will have liver-dominant metastases. When the parenchyma is diseased, the liver becomes more dependent on the hepatic artery for its blood supply. A subgroup of patients have been identified who are at high risk of acute hepatic failure following hepatic artery embolization. They have a constellation of >50% of the liver volume replaced by tumor, LDH >425 IU/L, AST >100 IU/L, and total bilirubin >2 mg/dl (66). The presence of hepatic encephalopathy or jaundice are absolute contraindications to embolization. Biliary obstruction is also a contraindication. Even with a normal serum bilirubin, the presence of dilated intrahepatic bile ducts places the patient at high risk for biliary necrosis in the obstructed segment(s) of the liver.

Preoperative evaluation for chemoembolization includes a tissue diagnosis, cross-sectional imaging of the liver, exclusion of extrahepatic disease, and laboratory studies. Eighty to ninety percent of patients suffer a postembolization syndrome, characterized by pain, fever, and nausea and vomiting. The severity of these symptoms varies tremendously from patient to patient, and they can last from a few hours to several days. Serious complications occur in up to 5% of procedures. Given the significant discomforts, hazards, and expense of this treatment, its palliative role should be clearly understood. After hydration and premedication with antibiotics and antiemetics, diagnostic visceral arteriography is performed to determine the arterial supply to the liver and confirm patency of the portal vein. The origins of vessels supplying the gut, particularly the right gastric and supraduodenal arteries, are carefully noted in order to avoid embolization of the stomach or small bowel. Once the arterial anatomy is clearly understood, a catheter is advanced superselectively into the right or left hepatic artery, depending on which lobe holds the most tumor, and chemoembolization performed. The patient receives intraarterial lidocaine and intravenous fentanyl or morphine to alleviate pain during the embolization. After the procedure, vigorous hydration, intravenous antibiotics, and antiemetic therapy are continued. Opioids, prochlorperazine, and acetaminophen are liberally supplied for control of pain, nausea, and fever. The patient is discharged as soon as oral intake is adequate and parenteral narcotics are not required for pain control. About half of patients are discharged in 1 day, most within 2 days. Oral antibiotics are continued for another 5 days, as well as antiemetics and opioids as needed. Follow-up includes return for a second procedure directed at the other lobe of the liver 3–4 weeks later. Depending on the arterial anatomy, two to four procedures are required to treat the entire liver, after which response is assessed by repeat imaging studies and tumor markers.

Major complications of hepatic embolization include hepatic insufficiency or infarction, hepatic abscess, biliary necrosis, and nontarget embolization to the gut. With careful patient selection and scrupulous technique, the incidence of these serious events collectively is 3–4%. Other complications include renal insufficiency and anemia requiring transfusion, with incidences of <1% each. Thirty-day mortality ranges from 1% to 4%.

Among combined series of 800 patients with unresectable hepatocellular carcinoma treated palliatively with chemoembolization in the Orient, Europe, and the United States, response rates as measured by decreased tumor volume and decreased serum $\alpha$-fetoprotein levels were 60–83% (64,67,68). Cumulative probability of survival ranged from 54% to 88% at 1 year, 33% to 64% at 2 years, and 18% to 51% at 3 years. Survival varies inversely with tumor volume, stage, and Childs class. Despite the large volume of single-institution experiences with chemoembolization of hepatoma published over the past decade, few controlled trials have been reported. A multicenter European trial comparing cisplatin/Lipiodol/gelfoam chemoembolization to no therapy in 100 patients with relatively small tumor burdens (90% stage I) found 1-year survivals of 62% and 43%, respectively, and 2-year survivals of 38% and 26% (69). A French multicenter trial of 127 patients with more advanced disease (62% stage II or III) showed almost identical survival rates in the chemoembolization arm (64% and 38% at 1 and 2 years), with survival in the control arm of only 18% and 6%, respectively ($p < 0.0001$) (70).

## REGIONAL ANALGESIA

Interventional radiologists to a limited extent perform regional anesthetic techniques, such as intercostal and pleural analgesia, that provide superior temporary analgesia during many thoracic and upper abdominal procedures. Intercostal access to the liver and kidney can be extremely painful due to irritation of the pleura and adjacent rib periosteum, especially if a temporary drain remains in place after the procedure. Interpleural analgesia and pleural blocks are especially helpful in controlling pain during procedures that involve the chest wall (i.e., pleural biopsy, thoracentesis, pleural sclerosing) (71), liver and biliary tree (i.e., liver biopsy, percutaneous biliary drainage, and stenting), and kidneys (i.e., renal biopsy, percutaneous nephrostomy), and long-term relief of intractable pain in the thorax and upper abdomen. Temporary pleural blocks may also be considered for patients undergoing radiologic placement of drainage catheters for difficult-to-localize empyemas, and more permanent neurolytic ones for thoracic and lumbosacral pain (72). Interpleural analgesia has demonstrated safety and efficacy in the treatment of both postoperative and diffuse thoracic cancer pain (73,74).

Celiac plexus blocks (CPBs) with local anesthetics have been used to temporarily control pain associated with percutaneous biliary drainage that is performed to gain access to the intrahepatic and extrahepatic tree for the purpose of biopsy, biliary endoscopy, and stent placement (75). This technique has significant advantages in relieving severe visceral pain that arises from biliary tract dilation and manipulation, which can be difficult to manage with sedating agents and opioids alone. Most studies document positive outcomes with CPB during procedures; however, investigators have recently proved that CPB was no better than midazolam and fentanyl in reducing pain (75). The mean elevation in heart rate in this study was significantly lower in the CPB group favoring this form of regional analgesia to intravenous for patients with cardiac disease. For more information on regional analgesic techniques, refer to Table 3.

In addition, neurolytic celiac plexus blockade (NCPB) using a neurolytic agent such as alcohol or phenol is done by both specially trained interventional radiologists and gastroenterologists to gain long-term control of pain from hepatic metastases and pancreatic carcinomas. Unlike surgeons who perform NCPB by visual inspection of the celiac plexus at the time of surgery and anesthesiologists who use a posterior approach under fluoroscopy, interventional radiologists gain anterior access to the nerve plexus aided by fluoroscopy (76). Some gastroenterologists can localize the celiac plexus through endoscopic ultrasound and inject the neurolytic agent through an endoscopic ultrasound needle (Fig. 4).

**TABLE 3.** *Regional analgesia*

| Regional analgesic technique | Indication | Description of procedure | Special care |
|---|---|---|---|
| Intercostal block | Provides short-term relief of pain associated with intercostal placement of catheters and drains into the pleural space, biliary ducts and gallbladder, or through the abdominal wall to drain the kidneys. | Performed by interventional radiologists. Small amount (3–5 ml) of bupivacaine (0.5%) is injected using a 25-gauge needle into the region of the neurovascular bundle posterior to the catheter entry site and 1–2 interspaces above and below the catheter. | 1–2 injections (maximum of 25 ml) can provide pain relief during the procedure. Opioids can be titrated to relieve pain when the anesthetic wears off. Pneumothorax is uncommon but can occur if the needle is advanced too far. |
| Interpleural analgesia | Temporary relief of pain for pleural biopsy, thoracentesis, pleural sclerosing, liver and renal biopsy, percutaneous biliary drains and stenting, renal percutaneous nephrostomy; long-term relief of pleural pain with catheters directly inserted or tunneled subcutaneously for administration of continuous infusions | Performed by interventional radiologists. Approximately 20 ml of 0.5% bupivacaine is injected through a catheter; catheter location confirmed with small amount of x-ray contrast. | Intermittent injections can provide 6–8 hr of pain relief. Pneumothorax and systemic toxicity (risk ↑ when pleura is inflamed or with continuous infusions) from the local anesthetic are uncommon. Continuous infusions are maintained to provide long-term relief. |
| Temporary celiac plexus block (CPB) | Temporary relief of pain accompanying percutaneous biliary drainage, liver biopsy, biliary stent placement, and biliary endoscopy | Performed by interventional radiologists; a 22-gauge needle is inserted anteriorly to the aorta, between the celiac plexus and the superior mesenteric artery under CT or fluoroscopy with the patient in the supine position; 0.25% (10 ml) bupivacaine is injected. | Patients should be NPO after midnight except for analgesics and critical medication. Long-acting opioids should be discontinued if possible, and equianalgesic doses of short-acting medications should be taken 12 hr prior to procedure to control pain and prevent physiologic withdrawal for opioid-dependent patients. Regional analgesia for procedures is preferred for debilitated patients and those with cardiac disease who might not tolerate pain and IV sedation and analgesia. Patients are monitored postprocedure for risks of bleeding. Opioid medications are adjusted for short-term relief of pain. |
| Neurolytic celiac plexus block (NCPB) | Long-term relief (3 months) of pain from liver matastases and pancreatic carcinoma; anterior percutaneous and endoscopic ultrasound (EUS) NCPB are not indicated for extensive tumor infiltration in the area of the celiac plexus. Technical difficulties may be encountered in accurately identifying the celiac plexus. Unsuccessful results may be attributed to inability to penetrate the celiac plexus or progression of the cancer. EUS is thought to be more precise in identifying, characterizing, and sampling abnormalities and vascular structures. | Anterior percutaneous approach is performed by interventional radiologists (see above comments on CPB). Once the celiac plexus is identified 20–30 ml of alcohol and 0.5% bupivacaine are injected. Endoscopic ultrasound (EUS)-guided NCPB is accomplished by specially trained gastroenterologists. The celiac plexus is located by ultrasound and approximately 30 ml of alcohol and 0.5% bupivacaine are injected via a tiny needle inserted through the gastric viscera. | Refer to above comments for CPB. Liberal doses of short-acting opioids are prescribed for pain that may worsen 12–18 hr following the procedure. Patients and families are informed about increased pain as a result of sclerosing of nerves, and they are also cautioned that the patient may feel the systemic effects of the alcohol that may have synergistic effects with IV sedating agents and opioids. Continuous adjustments in long-acting, regularly scheduled opioid medication are made up to 1–2 weeks after the procedure should pain decrease. |

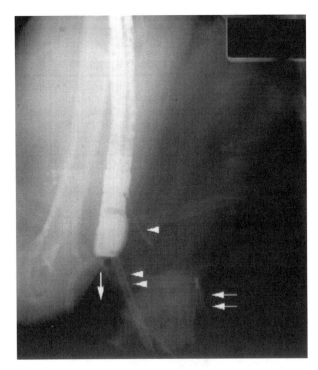

**FIG. 4.** Radiograph demonstrating complete nonsurgical palliation from unresectable pancreatic cancer causing biliary and duodenal obstruction and with accompanying hypercoaguable state with deep venous thrombosis and visceral pain. (*arrowhead*) Needle exiting Pentax endoscopic endoscope at time of celiac axis neurolysis. (*double arrowhead*) Percutaneously placed internal biliary drain. (*arrow*) Schneider-uncovered endoprosthetic in duodenum restoring patency after obstruction (percutaneously placed and endoscopically dilated to full diameter). (*double arrow*) Percutaneously placed vena cava filter.

## CONSCIOUS SEDATION AND ANALGESIA

Interventional techniques for palliation are aimed at relieving pain and improving symptoms. However, in some circumstances these procedures may transiently worsen pain, exacerbate other symptoms, and sometimes create new temporary sources for pain. The need for pain control before, during, and after procedure cannot be overestimated. Uncontrolled pain leads to the release of catecholamines that stimulates the sympathetic nervous system, which can stress the cardiovascular system resulting in tachycardia, cardiac arrhythmias, or cardiac ischemia (77), and elevated blood pressure, which in turn may increase the risk of stroke and potential for hemorrhage at the procedural site (78). Nausea, vomiting, and bradycardia, which are parasympathetic responses, can accompany severe pain originating from the viscera or peritoneum as the result of an invasive procedure.

As areas of the body are manipulated, nociceptors (free nerve endings) are activated, giving rise to various painful sensations that may or may not be similar to the pain of cancer. A painful stimulus to viscera or organ structures, such as inflammation, that is sustained over time increases the vulnerability of visceral nociceptors to stimuli that would not normally evoke pain (79). The slightest manipulation of visceral structures affected by cancer pain can provoke significant pain. Moreover, ischemic pain caused by embolization procedures or damage to vasculature is so severe that adequate pain control during and after remains a clinical priority (80,81).

To some extent, the perception of pain can be diminished by percutaneous and intravascular local anesthetics, regional blocks, and liberal use of systemic opioid analgesics and sedating agents. Non-pharmacologic methods, such as relaxation techniques, can reduce the need for opioids and sedating agents, enhance amnesia, and improve the patient's overall well-being and outlook on the procedure (78). The level of complexity and duration of the procedure have warranted more liberal use of sedating agents and intensive monitoring in endoscopic and interventional radiology procedure units. Specific details are beyond the scope of this chapter and the following recommendations for the selection of sedating agents and opioids to manage procedural pain and anxiety that accompany interventional procedures for cancer (9,82,83).

## CONCLUSION

Decisions for endoscopic and interventional radiologic techniques must be based on available data and sound judgments based on a weighting of potential risks and benefits. The ability to perform some palliative interventions is largely the result of local expertise and the availability of clinical resources. All possible comfort and supportive care measures should be considered or attempted prior to the undertaking of invasive interventions in consultation with patients and their primary care providers. Moral, ethical, and social issues arise if patients are subjected to these procedures only to prolong intense pain and suffering when there is no definitive treatment plan and life expectancy is very limited. On the other hand, withholding therapeutic options for palliation of intolerable and unmanageable symptoms takes hope away from patients for a better quality of life for the remaining weeks or months of life.

Both gastroenterologists and interventional radiologists may overlap in areas of expertise and perform similar procedures; however, each offers unique aspects to the technical performance of the procedure. Careful patient selection and knowledge of the local expertise and areas of interest of each specialist leads to a multidisciplinary effort and more options and opinions in regard to the therapy for the individual patient. Differences in how each specialty approaches an individual clinical situation may be readily evident, but despite these differences, the indications for treatment and the intended outcomes for treatment remain similar. Few data have been published that would justify the preference for the performance of a given procedure by one of the interventional specialists or another.

## REFERENCES

1. Jones SN. Interventional radiology in a palliative care setting. *Palliat Med* 1995;9:319.
2. Rossi P, Bezzi M. Interventional radiology in gastrointestinal neoplasms. *Curr Opin Oncol* 1995;7(4):367.
3. Botet JF. Interventional radiology. In: DeVita VT, Hellman S, Rosenberg SA, eds. *Cancer: Principles and practice of oncology,* 5th ed. Philadelphia: Lippincott-Raven Publishers, 1997;682.
4. Ripamonti C. Management of bowel obstruction in advanced cancer patients. *J Pain Sympt Manage* 1994;9:193.
5. Cannizzaro R, Bortoluzzi F, Valentino M, et al. Percutaneous endoscopic gastrostomy as a decompression technique in bowel obstruction due to abdominal carcinomatosis. *Endoscopy* 1995;27:317.
6. Cunningham MJ, Bromberg C, Kredentser DC, Collins MB, Malfetano JH. Percutaneous gastrostomy for decompression in patients with advanced gynecologic malignancies. *Gynecol Oncol* 1995;59:273.
7. Campagnutta E, Cannizzaro R, Gallo A, et al. Palliative treatment of upper intestinal obstruction by gynecological malignancies: the usefulness of percutaneous endoscopic gastrostomy. *Gynecol Oncol* 1996;62:103.
8. Wollman B, D Agostino HB, Walus-Wigle JR, Easter DW, Beale A. Radiologic, endoscopic, and surgical gastrostomy: an institutional evaluation and meta-analysis of the literature. *Radiology* 1995;197:699.
9. Adelson MD, Kasowitz MH. Percutaneous endoscopic drainage gastrostomy in the treatment of gastrointestinal obstruction from intraperitoneal malignancy. *Obstet Gynecol* 1993;81:467.
10. Pugash RA, Brady AP, Isaacscon S. Ultrasound guidance in percutaneous gastrostomy and gastrojejunostomy. *Can Assoc Radiol J* 1995;46:196.
11. Panzer S, Harris M, Berg W, Ravich W, Kalloo A. Endoscopic ultrasound in the placement of a percutaneous endoscopic gastrostomy tube in the non-transilluminated abdominal wall. *Gastrointest Endosc* 1995;42(1):88-90.
12. Herman LL, Hoskins WJ, Shike. Percutaneous endoscopic gastrostomy for decompression of the stomach and small bowel. *Gastrointest Endosc* 1992;38:314.
13. Marks WH, Perkal MF, Schwartz PE. Percutaneous endoscopic gastrostomy for gastric decompression in metastatic malignancy. *Surg Gynecol Obstet* 1993;177:573.
14. Bell SD, Carmody EA, Yeung EY, Thurston WA, Simons ME, HoCS. Percutaneous gastrostomy and gastrojejunostomy: additional experience in 519 procedures. *Radiology* 1995;194:817.
15. Chait PG, Weinberg J, Connolly BL, et al. Retrograde percutaneous gastrostomy and gastrojejunostomy in 505 children: a 4 1/2-year experience. *Radiology* 1996;201:691.
16. Light VL, Slezak FA, Porter JA, Gerson LW, McCord G. Predictive factors for early mortality after percutaneous endoscopic gastrostomy. *Gastrointest Endosc* 1995;42:330.
17. Becker G, Hess CF, Grund KE, Hoffmann W, Bamberg M. Abdominal wall metastasis following percutaneous endoscopic gastrostomy. *Support Care Cancer* 1995;3:313.
18. Lee DS, Mohit-Tabatabai MA, Rush BF, Levine C. Stomal seeding of head and neck cancer by percutaneous endoscopic gastrostomy. *Ann Surg Oncol* 1995;2:170.
19. Shike M. Percutaneous endoscopic stomas for enteral feeding and drainage. *Oncology* 1995;9:39.
20. Mellert J, Naruhn MB, Grund KE, Becker HD. Direct endoscopic percutaneous jejunostomy (EPJ). Clinical results. *Surg Endosc* 1994;8(8):867-869.
21. Duranceau A, Jamieson GG. Malignant tracheoesophageal fistula: collective review. *Ann Thorac Surg* 1984;37:346.
22. Irving JD, Simson JNL. A new cuffed oesophageal prosthesis for the management of malignant oesophago-respiratory fistula. *Ann R Coll Surg Engl* 1988;70:13.
23. Neuhaus H, Hoffman W, Dittler HJ, Niedermeyer HP, Classen M. Implantation of self-expanding esophageal metal stents for palliation of malignant dysphasia. *Endoscopy* 1992;24:405.
24. Binmoeller K., Maeda M, Lieberman D, Katon RM, Ivancev K, Rosch J. Silicone-covered expandable metallic stents in the esophagus: an experimental study. *Endoscopy* 1992;24:416.
25. Tytgat GNJ, Bartelsman JFWM, Vermeyden JR. Dilation and prosthesis for obstructing esophagogastric carcinoma. *Gastrointest Endosc Clin North Am* 1992;2(3):415.
26. Kadish S, Kochman M. Endoscopic diagnosis and management of gastrointestinal malignancies. *Oncology* 1995;9(10):967.
27. Cusumano A, Ruol A, Segalin A, et al. Push-through intubation: effective palliation in 409 patients with cancer of the esophagus and cardia. *Ann Thorac Surg* 1992;52:1010.
28. Keen RR, et al. Rectosigmoid stent for obstructing colonic neoplasms. *Dis Colon Rectum* 1992;35:912.
29. Mainar A, Tejero E, Maynar M, Ferral H, Castaneda-Zuniga W. Colorectal obstruction: treatment with metallic stents. *Radiology* 1996;198:761.
30. Saida Y, et al. Stent endoprosthesis for obstructing colorectal cancers. *Dis Colon Rectum* 1996;39:552.
31. Rupp KD, Dohmoto R, Meffert R., Holzgreve A, Holbach G. Cancer of the rectum: palliative endoscopic treatment. *Eur J Surg Oncol* 1995;21:644.
32. Rey JF, Romanczyk T, Greff M. Metal stents for palliation of rectal carcinoma: A preliminary report on 12 patients. *Endoscopy* 1995:327:501.
33. Coons H. Metallic stents for the treatment of biliary obstruction: a report of 100 cases. *Cardiovasc Intervent Radiol* 1992;15(6):367.
34. Nicholson AA, Royston CM. Palliation of inoperable biliary obstruction with self-expanding metal endoprostheses: a review of 77 patients. *Clin Radiol* 1993;47(4):245.
35. Ballinger AB, McHugh M, Catnach SM, Alstead EM, Clark ML. Symptom relief and quality of life after stenting for malignant biliary obstruction. *Gut* 1994;35(4):467.
36. Lichtenstein DR, Carr-Locke DL. Endoscopic palliation for unresectable pancreatic carcinoma. *Surg Clin North Am* 1995;75(5):969.
37. Pereira-Lima JC, Jakobs R, Maier M, Benz C, Kohler B, Reimann JF. Endoscopic biliary stenting for palliation of pancreatic cancer: results, survival predictive factor, and complication of 10-French with 11.5-French gauge stents. *Am J Gastroenterol* 1996;9:2179.
38. Magistrelli P, Masetti R, Coppola R, et al. Changing attitudes in the palliation of proximal malignant biliary obstruction. *J Clin Oncol* 1993;3:151.
39. Kauffman SL. Percutaneous palliation of unresectable pancreatic cancer. *Surg Clin North Am* 1995;75(5):989.
40. Huibregtse K, Carr-Locke DL, Cremer W, et al. Biliary obstruction—a problem with self-expanding metal stents. *Endoscopy* 1992;24:391.
41. Speer AG, Cotton PB, Rode J, et al. Biliary stent blockage with bacterial biofilm. *Ann Intern Med* 1988;108:546.
42. Cotton PB. Metallic mesh stents—is the expanse worth the expense? *Endoscopy* 1992;24:421.
43. Uflacker R. Percutaneous biliary procedures. *Gastrointest Endosc Clin North Am* 1996;6(1):177.
44. Seitz U, Vayeyar H, Soehendra N. Prolonged patency with a new design Teflon biliary prosthesis. *Endoscopy* 1994;26(5):478.
45. Eschelman DJ, Shapiro MJ, Bonn J, et al. Malignant biliary duct obstruction: long-term experience with Gianturco stents and combined-modality radiation therapy. *Radiology* 1996;220:717.
46. Lightdale CJ, Heier SK, Marcon NE, McCaughan JS Jr, Gerdes H, Overholt BF, Sivak MV Jr, Stiegmann GV, Nava HR. Photodynamic therapy with porfimer sodium versus thermal ablation therapy with Nd: YAG laser for palliation of esophageal cancer: a multicenter randomized trial. *Gastrointest Endosc* 1995;42(6):507.
47. Overholt BF, Panjehpour M, DeNovo RC, Peterson MG, Jenkins C. Balloon photodynamic therapy of esophageal cancer: effect of increasing balloon size. *Lasers Surg Med* 1996;18(3):248.
48. Livraghi T, Solbiato L. Percutaneous ethanol injection in liver cancer: methods and results. *Semin Intervent Radiol* 1996;10:69.
49. Shiina S, Niwa Y, Osmata M. Percutaneous ethanol injection therapy for liver neoplasms. *Semin Intervent Radiol* 1996;10:57.
50. Chang AE, Schneider PD, Sugarbaker PH, et al. A prospective ran-

domized trial of regional vs. systemic continuous 5-FU chemotherapy in the treatment of colorectal metastases. *Ann Surg* 1987;206:685.

51. Hohn DC, Stagg RJ, Friedman MA, et al. A randomized trial of continuous intravenous versus hepatic intraarterial floxuridine in patients with colorectal cancer metastatic liver: the Northern California Oncology Group trial. *J Clin Oncol* 1989;7:1646.

52. Martin JK, O'Connell MJ, Wieand HS, et al. Intra-arterial floxuridine vs systemic fluorouracil for hepatic metastases from colorectal cancer. *Arch Surg* 1990;125:1022.

53. Kemeny N, Daly JM, Reichman B, et al. Intrahepatic or systemic infusion of fluorodeoxyuridine in patients with liver metastases from colorectal carcinoma: a randomized trial. *Ann Intern Med* 1987;107:459.

54. Onohara S, Kobayashi H, Itoh Y, Shinohara S. Intraarterial cis-platinum infusion with sodium thiosulfate protection and angiotensin II induced hypertension for treatment of hepatocellular carcinoma. *Acta Radiol* 1988;29:197.

55. Doci R, Bignami F, Bozzetti F, et al. Intrahepatic chemotherapy for unresectable hepatocellular carcinoma. *Cancer* 1988;61:1983.

56. Carrasco CH, Charnsangavej C, Ajani J, Samaan NA, Richli W, Wallace S. The carcinoid syndrome: palliation by hepatic artery embolization. *Am J Radiol* 1986;147:149.

57. Ajani JA, Carrasco CH, Charnsangavej C, et al. Islet cell tumors metastatic to the liver: effective palliation by sequential hepatic artery embolization. *Ann Intern Med* 1988;108:340.

58. Lin D-Y, Liaw Y-F, Lee T-U, et al. Hepatic arterial embolization in patients with unresectable hepatocellular carcinoma—a randomized controlled trial. *Gastroenterology* 1988;94:453.

59. Sato Y, Fujiwara K, Ogata I, et al. Transcatheter arterial embolization for hepatocellular carcinoma. *Cancer* 1985;955:2822.

60. Chuang VP, Wallace S. Hepatic artery embolization in the treatment of hepatic neoplasms. *Radiology* 1981;140:51.

61. Clouse ME, Lee RGL, Duszlak EJ. Peripheral hepatic artery embolization for primary and secondary hepatic neoplasms. *Radiology* 1983;147:407.

62. Konno T. Targeting cancer chemotherapeutic agents by use of Lipiodol contrast medium. *Cancer* 1990;66:1897.

63. Egawa H, Maki A, Mori K. Effects of intraarterial chemotherapy with a new lipophilic anticancer agent, estradiol-chlorambucil (KM2210), dissolved in Lipiodol on experimental liver tumor in rats. *J Surg Oncol* 1990;44:109.

64. Nakamura H, Hashimoto T, Oi H, et al. Transcatheter oily chemoembolization of hepatocellular carcinoma. *Radiology* 1989;170:783.

65. Sasaki Y, Imaoka S, Kasugai H, et al. A new approach to chemoembolization therapy for hepatoma using ethiodized oil, cisplatin, and gelatin sponge. *Cancer* 1987;60:1194.

66. Charnsangavej C. Chemoembolization of liver tumors. *Semin Invest Radiol* 1993;10:150.

67. Nakao N, Miura K, Takahashi H, et al. Hepatocellular carcinoma: combined hepatic arterial and portal venous embolization. *Radiol* 1986;161:303–307.

68. Van Beers B, Roche A, Cauquil P, Jamart J, Pariente D, Ajavon Y. Transcatheter arterial chemotherapy using doxorubicin, iodized oil and gelfoam embolization in hepatocellular carcinoma. *Acta Radiol* 1989;30:415.

69. Groupe d'Etude de Traitment du Carcinome Hepatocellulaire. A comparison of lipiodol chemoembolization and conservative treatment for unresectable hepatocellular carcinoma. *N Engl J Med* 1995;332:1256.

70. Bronwicki JP, Vetter D, Dumas F, et al. Transcatheter oily chemoembolization for hepatocellular carcinoma. A 4-year study of 127 French patients. *Cancer* 1994;74:16.

71. Boland GW, Lee MJ, Silverman S, Mueller PR. Interventional radiolgy of the pleural space. *Clin Radiol* 1995;50:205.

72. Quinn SF, Murtagh FR, Chatfield R, Kori SH. CT-guided nerve root block and ablation. *AJR* 1988;151:1213.

73. Myers DP, Lema MJ, de Leon-Casasola OA, Bacon DR. Interpleural analgesia for the treatment of severe cancer pain in terminally ill patients. *J Pain Sympt Manage* 1993;8:505.

74. Waldman SD, Allen ML, Cronen MC. Subcutaneous tunneled interpleural catheters in the long-term relief of right upper quadrant abdominal pain of malignant origin. *J Pain Sympt Manage* 1989;4:86.

75. Savader SF, Bourke DL, Venbrux AC, Trerotola SO, Grass JA, Lund GB, Gittelson AP, Osterman FA. Randomized double-blind clinical trial of celiac plexus block for percutaneous drainage. *J Vasc Intervent Radiol* 1993;4(4):539.

76. Romanelli DF, Beckman CF, Heiss FW. Celiac plexus block: efficacy and safety of the anterior approach. *Am J Radiol* 1993;160:497.

77. Neuhaus C, Leppek R, Christ G, Froelich J, Klose KJ. Monitoring of vital functions in the course of interventional radiology procedures. In: Steinbrich W, Gross-Fengels, eds. *Interventional radiology: adjunctive medication and monitoring.* New York: Springer Publishers, 1993.

78. Lang EV. Overview of conscious sedation. *J Vasc Intervent Radiol* 1996(Suppl)(Part 1):81.

79. Cervero E. Visceral pain: mechanisms of peripheral and central sensitization. *Ann Med* 1995;27:235.

80. Clark BA. A new approach to assessment and documentation of conscious sedation during endoscopy. *Gastroenterol Nursing* 1994;16:199.

81. Rospond RM, Mills W. Hepatic artery chemoembolization for hepatic tumors. *AORN* 1995; 61:573.

82. Molgaard CP, Teitelbaum GP, Pentecost MJ, Flink EJ, Davis SH, Dziubinski JE, Daniels JR. Intraarterial administration of lidocaine for analgesia in hepatic chemoembolization. *J Vasc Intervent Radiol* 1990;1:81.

83. Hiew CY, Hart GK, Thomson KR, Hennessy OF. Analgesia and sedation in interventional radiologic procedures. *Australasian Radiol* 1995;39:128.

84. Polomano R, Soulen M, McDaniels C. Conscious sedation and analgesia with interventional radiologic procedures for oncology patients. *Crit Care Nursing Clin North Am*. In press.

*Principles and Practice of Supportive Oncology,*
edited by Ann Berger et al.
Lippincott–Raven Publishers, Philadelphia ©1998

CHAPTER 47

# Palliative Chemotherapy

Neil M. Ellison

Palliative chemotherapy is a term with many potential meanings. In its broadest sense, it refers to the use of medications to treat an incurable malignancy. Medical literature predominantly reports palliative chemotherapy efficacy results in terms of tumor response rate, duration of response, and survival benefit. Until recently, chemotherapy studies only infrequently described palliation of symptoms as a treatment result. Symptom palliation is becoming a more important aspect in clinical trial evaluation and comprehensive cancer care. An estimated 3000 articles per year describing cancer treatment effects on quality of life will be published by 2002 (1).

"Relief of cancer-induced symptoms" is a more pertinent definition of palliative chemotherapy for this text. It refers to the use of antineoplastic medications to reduce the adverse signs and symptoms directly or indirectly caused by the malignant disease process.

The myriad of cancer-related problems can affect any organ system. Health care providers intuitively realize that significant tumor responses to chemotherapy are usually associated with a decrease in malignancy-induced symptoms. Despite this, common public perception of chemotherapy is that it is extremely toxic and often of little benefit. This chapter will present a broad overview of the use of chemotherapy as a means to alleviate tumor-associated symptoms or to prophylax against their occurrence.

## USUAL RATIONALE FOR CHEMOTHERAPY USE

Chemotherapy or drug treatment of malignancy is used with different intent, depending on the type and stage of malignancy (Table 1). It can be used adjuvantly, primarily (curative), or palliatively. When used in the latter two circumstances, its effect is usually described by response

rate, whereas in all three treatment circumstances changes in median and progression-free survival induced by chemotherapy are possible.

Adjuvant chemotherapy is used as a potentially curative therapy after all gross evidence of disease has been removed by surgery or radiation therapy, but the possibility of cancer recurrence is significant. The benefit-to-toxicity ratio of adjuvant chemotherapy is extremely important (Table 2). Very toxic and potentially lethal chemotherapy would not be advisable if the likelihood of cancer recurrence is low and the percentage of patients to be benefited is also low. In this instance, the treatments may harm more patients than they help. In other adjuvant situations, a temporarily very toxic treatment that provides potential cure for a large percentage of otherwise incurable patients would be of overall value. Various stages of different cancer types are treated with more or less aggressive adjuvant chemotherapy or hormonal therapy regimens based on the likelihood of recurrence and the benefit-to-toxicity ratio of the administered treatment. A comprehensive review of potential situations where adjuvant chemotherapy may be of benefit is beyond the confines of this chapter. Table 3 lists the general cancer types where adjuvant chemotherapy has been proven to be of value in decreasing the likelihood of recurrent disease. Adjuvant chemotherapy that effectively decreases cancer recurrence with its anticipated morbidities can be viewed as prophylactically palliative.

Adjuvant chemotherapy can be used occasionally before primary radiation or surgical therapy and is referred to as neoadjuvant chemotherapy. Potential benefits of this approach are the possibility of determining the cancer's sensitivity to the drug treatment, the shrinkage of the cancer in order to facilitate surgical or radiation control, and the enhanced delivery of drugs because arterial supply has not been compromised by prior surgery or radiation therapy. The survival (benefit) for neoadjuvant chemotherapy remains controversial and unproven at this time.

N. M. Ellison: Geisinger Medical Center, Danville, PA 17822.

**TABLE 1.** *Definitions of chemotherapy-related terms*

| Type of chemotherapy | Description |
|---|---|
| Adjuvant chemotherapy | Chemotherapy administered after all evidence of disease has been surgically removed or controlled with radiation therapy. Used with intention to eradicate any residual but undetectable malignant cells that will eventually cause a disease recurrence. |
| Neoadjuvant chemotherapy | When adjuvant chemotherapy would be used after radiation or surgical treatment but is instead used before these treatments. |
| Primary chemotherapy | Chemotherapy used as the sole modality of treatment to totally eradicate a malignancy and prevent its recurrence. |
| Primary palliative chemotherapy | Use of chemotherapy as a sole modality of treatment to either (a) temporarily control an incurable malignancy or (b) decrease the symptoms caused directly or indirectly by the malignancy. |
| Combined modality chemotherapy | Chemotherapy used in conjunction with either surgery or radiation therapy to enhance the effectiveness of either. This may be given in an adjuvant or palliative fashion. In the palliative approach, cure may or may not be enhanced but end-organ function may be preserved. |

As a primary treatment, chemotherapy may be a curative therapy or it may be a "palliative" therapy when used in instances where there is no chance for cure. Table 3 also lists the malignancies for which chemotherapy has been shown to provide the possibility of cure in the nonadjuvant setting. These metastatic or locally unresectable cancers are considered to be very chemoresponsive and potentially chemotherapy-curable. Chemotherapy should be considered as a treatment option and recommended in most circumstances for these diseases.

Chemotherapy can be considered synergistically curative if its use in conjunction with another anticancer therapy results in less overall treatment-related morbidity with similar chance for cure. For example, anal carcinoma or laryngeal carcinoma can often be locally controlled or cured with aggressive surgery. Surgery alone may be associated in these circumstances with significant morbidity such as the need for a colostomy or the loss of voice, respectively. Often, important cosmetic or organ function can be maintained for patients with these malignancies, even if the disease is incurable, by combined modality treatment with chemotherapy and radiation

therapy (2–5). In the future, it is quite possible that more malignancies will be treated with these organ-sparing techniques and result in less overall morbidity.

Unfortunately, at this time the majority of metastatic malignancies in adults are not curable with chemotherapy. Even for the large number of patients with colon or breast cancer, where adjuvant chemotherapy is generally recommended, the recurrence rate is decreased by only about one third. Thus, many patients will experience recurrent disease, which was not eradicated with the adjuvant treatment, and may thus also receive palliative chemotherapy.

Malignancies that are moderately responsive to chemotherapy are listed in Table 4. Anticipated chemotherapy response rates for these cancers will be in the 25–70% range and cures are not expected. The primary goal of chemotherapy for these metastatic cancers is to obtain a partial or complete tumor response, with few or no side effects, to lengthen life and to maintain or improve the patient's qualify of life. Much of the discussion that follows will define the rationale for treatment of some, but certainly not all, patients with these diseases.

**TABLE 2.** *Examples of possible outcomes of effective and ineffective adjuvant chemotherapy given after surgical resection of a primary cancer in 100 patients*

SURGERY ALONE
Alive and Cured of Cancer: 70     Dead from Cancer: 30
SURGERY PLUS TREATMENT X (Effective and Nontoxic Adjuvant Chemotherapy)
Alive and Cured of Cancer: 85     Dead from Cancer: 15
Note: Recurrence rate decreased by 50% from 30/100 to 15/100, but only 15/100 actually benefited from treatment.
SURGERY PLUS TREATMENT Y (Ineffective and Very Toxic Adjuvant Chemotherapy)
Alive and Cured of Cancer: 60     Dead from Cancer or from Toxic Effects of Chemotherapy: 40
Note: Recurrence rate unchanged from ineffective treatment, but death rate increased from 30/100 to 40/100 secondary to added toxicities from chemotherapy.
SURGERY PLUS TREATMENT Z (Ineffective and Mildly Toxic Adjuvant Chemotherapy)
Alive and Cured of Cancer: 70     Dead from Cancer: 30
Note: No change in cure or recurrence rate. All patients subjected to some possible toxicity and to expense of chemotherapy.

Metastatic or locally advanced cancers that have low expected response rates (<25%) to chemotherapy are listed in Table 5. Partial responses to chemotherapy, usually of short duration (<6 months), have been reported for these malignancies; complete responses are extremely rare. Investigational treatments, single-agent, or combination chemotherapy of proven benefit and non-chemotherapeutic palliative supportive care are all reasonable alternatives for patients with these malignancies. It is noted, however, that most cancer specialists have anecdotal experience of complete or prolonged partial responses for at least one or two patients in their own practices with some of these refractory-to-treatment cancers.

As previously stated, standard chemotherapy should not be offered to every patient with metastatic malignancy. A group of patients for whom the predicted toxicity of treatment should preclude consideration of chemotherapy can be defined. Other patients may fall into a gray zone where the benefit-to-toxicity ratio of treatment may strongly balance toward the toxicity side, but this cannot be predicted as accurately as in the former group. The practice of giving homeopathic (subtherapeutic) doses of chemotherapy, primarily to prevent the patient from believing his or her case is hopeless, should be discouraged. It may be more representative of the discomfort of the physician in dealing with a terminally ill patient than actually attending to the patient's psychological needs. A more humane and ethical approach is to review the medical situation with the patient and family and to provide them with an educated assessment of possible beneficial treatment choices, which may include a nonchemotherapy palliative care approach.

Understanding the art of oncology practice as well as the science of chemotherapy becomes increasingly important as the expected benefit from therapy decreases. If chemotherapy is not recommended to the patient and/or family, they must be fully aware that their physician believes in the adage, "Don't just do something, stand there." Chemotherapy with no proven benefit should not be administered because the patient or physician wants to "try something." Instead, it should be explained to the patient that ineffective treatments may cause more harm than good. In situations like this, fears of abandonment are often a great concern of patients. The patient may believe that "no chemotherapy" means "no need for the physician to follow and treat the patient." If chemotherapy is not recommended, future visits should still be scheduled with the physician who will be supervising the patient's palliative care. The duration of time between visits should be scheduled at intervals that meet the physical and psychological needs of the patient and the family. They must be assured that earlier visits are possible and desirable if problems arise before the scheduled appointment.

## PROGNOSTIC FEATURES FOR POSSIBLE CHEMOTHERAPY RESPONSES

Statistics regarding specific response rates, expected durations of response, and especially duration of expected survivals are often requested or even demanded by the patient or family. Except for the moribund patient, these questions cannot be answered with accuracy. A specific reply based on statistical information may often be misconstrued by the patient or family as extrapolatable to their own situation. A physician statement accurately explaining that studies indicate the median survival is 6 months frequently results in the patient's "parking meter syndrome." The 6-month survival date becomes firmly

**TABLE 3.** *Cancers that are potentially curable with chemotherapy*

**Adjuvant chemotherapy for limited disease**
  Breast cancer
  Colon cancer
  Germ cell tumors
    Choriocarcinoma
    Testicular cancer
  Non-Hodgkin's Lymphoma
  Ovarian cancer
    Ewing's sarcoma
    Osteogenic sarcoma
    Neuroblastoma
**Primary or secondary chemotherapy for metastatic disease**
  Germ cell tumors
    Choriocarcinoma
    Testicular cancers
  Lymphomas
    Hodgkin's Disease
    Intermediate or high-grade non-Hodgkin's
  Acute lymphocytic leukemia
  Acute myelocytic leukemia
  Ewing's sarcoma
  Osteogenic sarcoma
  Rhabdomyosarcoma
  Wilms tumor
  ? Ovarian cancer

**TABLE 4.** *Metastatic incurable cancers with expected frequent response rates (>25–70%) to conventional chemotherapy*

Bladder cancer
Breast cancer
Chronic lymphocytic leukemia
Chronic myelogenous leukemia
Head and neck cancer
Multiple myeloma
Non-Hodgkin's lymphoma (most subtypes)
Non-small cell lung cancer
Ovarian cancer
Prostate cancer (hormone therapy)
Small cell lung cancer
? Cervical/endometrial cancer

**TABLE 5.** *Incurable cancers with low response rates to chemotherapy (<25%)*

Carcinoid tumor
Esophageal cancer
Gastric cancer
Hepatoma/biliary cancer
Melanoma
Prostate cancer
Renal cell cancer
Pancreatic cancer
Colon cancer
Sarcoma in adults
Glioblastoma multiforme

etched in patients' and families' minds, and they may begin to live accordingly. Similarly, an expected "20% response rate to treatment" does not inform the patient that he or she specifically has a 20% chance of responding to treatment. Instead, the patient must be made to realize that statistics refer to groups and not to individuals. A more global discussion between the physician and patient/family is preferable. Data should be reviewed but in the context that each situation is unique and individual patients will fall on either side of the reported response and survival curves. False hope presentations should be avoided. If chemotherapy is decided on by mutual consent of the patient and the physician, even if the response rate is reported to be relatively low, the attitude should be that all will be done to ensure that the particular patient will be one of the responders who does well on treatment with little toxicity. This optimistic approach after a realistic discussion is appropriate and of great psychological benefit to the patient, the family, and also the physician and other members of the health care team.

A composite of patient and disease-related factors will help determine if chemotherapy is a reasonable treatment option. The single most important factor other than tumor type that determines the benefit-to-toxicity ratio of chemotherapy is the performance status (PS) or activity level of the patient. Two measures used to quantitate this are the Eastern Cooperative Oncology Group (ECOG) and Karnofsky scales (Table 6). Regardless of the cause of debility (malignancy or other comorbid medical illness), a severely weakened patient with a restricted PS (ECOG 3 or 4; Karnofsky <50%) is more likely to demonstrate excessive chemotherapy toxicity than a beneficial response. Exceptions occur when the malignancy is causing severe debility and the cancer is exquisitely chemotherapy-sensitive.

Determining the PS of a patient is fraught with difficulty. Differences occur among various health care providers' assessments of a patient's PS with considerable interobserver variability, especially for patients with a poor functional status (6). Even more important is the greater discrepancy that exists between patients' own estimates of their PS and the rating assigned to them by their physicians or nurses. Patients often rate their activity levels and PS as significantly better than the rating given by their health care teams or even their own designated surrogates (7,8).

The sites of metastatic spread may allow better but not totally accurate predictions of the potential initial response to chemotherapy. This varies for different tumor types. For example, metastatic breast cancer to the skin, bone, and lymph nodes is usually more responsive to chemotherapy than when liver or pulmonary lymphangitic metastases are present. Chemotherapy "sanctuary sites," such as the brain and spinal cord, usually respond least well to systemic cytotoxic treatments. However, even these sites of metastatic spread may respond to systemic or locally administered chemotherapy.

Numerous other poor prognostic features exist that are definable for specific malignancies. Examples of prognostic features include the number of sites and size of metastases or absolute value of tumor markers for some testicular cancers, intrathoracic versus extra-thoracic metastatic disease for small cell lung cancer, and bulk of disease remaining after surgery for ovarian cancer. Tumor-specific prognostic factors are important because they may more accurately define an incurable situation. This lack of curability may dictate the use of potentially less toxic treatments. In general, a more toxic chemotherapy regimen is considered if the likelihood of response is high and the possibility of cure or prolonged disease control is present.

Patients whose cancers are refractory to ongoing chemotherapy are less likely to respond to second or subsequent chemotherapy treatment. Cancers that have recurred within 6 months of cessation of adjuvant chemotherapy are less likely to respond to retreatment with the same chemotherapy than those that recur after a more prolonged disease-free period.

Advanced age is reportedly not a prognostic factor in the potential response to chemotherapy as long as there are no significant comorbid medical problems (9,10). Actual biological age may be less important than physiologic age. Pharmacokinetics will change with age secondary to alterations in drug clearance and metabolism, necessitating alteration in drug dose. Older patients agree as readily as younger patients to undergo trials of aggressive chemotherapy for curative or palliative purposes; however, older patients appear less willing to trade significant toxicity for increased survival time (11). Older patients are more likely to shift to a milder, less toxic treatment, even if survival is shorter, than their younger counterparts. A cautionary approach is always wise when considering chemotherapeutic treatments of the elderly, but there is no reason to preclude chemotherapy based solely on age.

**TABLE 6.** *ECOG and Karnofsky performance status scale*

| ECOG | | Karnofsky | |
|---|---|---|---|
| 0 | Fully active, able to carry on all predisease performance without restriction | 100% | Normal, no complaints, no evidence of disease |
| | | 90% | Able to carry on normal activity; minor signs or symptoms of disease |
| 1 | Restricted in physically strenuous activity but ambulatory and able to carry out work of a light or sedentary nature, e.g., light housework, office work | 80% | Normal activity with effort; some signs or symptoms of disease |
| | | 70% | Cares for self; unable to carry on normal activity or to do active work |
| 2 | Ambulatory and capable of all self-care but unable to carry out any work activities; up and about more than 50% of waking hours | 60% | Requires occasional assistance, but is mostly able to care for self |
| | | 50% | Requires considerable assistance and frequent medical care |
| 3 | Capable of only limited self-care, confined to bed or chair more than 50% of waking hours | 40% | Disabled, requires special care and assistance |
| | | 30% | Severely disabled, hospitalization indicated; death not imminent |
| 4 | Completely disabled; cannot carry on any self-care; totally confined to bed or chair | 20% | Very sick, hospitalization necessary, active supportive treatment necessary |
| | | 10% | Moribund, fatal processes, progressing rapidly |
| | | 0% | Dead |

Modified from Karnofsky DA, Abelman WH, Carver LF, et al. *Cancer* 1948;1:634–656; and Oken MM, Creech RH, Tormey DC, et al. *Am J Clin Oncol* 1982;5:649–655.

## QUALITY-OF-LIFE ISSUES

Quality of life (QOL) measurements were infrequently recorded or reported during the first four decades of published contemporary chemotherapy trials. QOL measurements refer to a quantitative evaluation of numerous qualitative parameters that are instrumental in the day-to-day enjoyment of life. QOL assessments are increasingly being measured in clinical trials in addition to the more commonly assessed measures of tumor response, disease-free survival, and overall survival. Multiple QOL systems have been developed with varying degrees of complexity. Simpler methods are more "user-friendly" for the patient and health care team. Examples of parameters measured include pain and pain relief, fatigue, malaise, psychological distress, nausea and vomiting, physical functioning, treatment-related symptoms and toxic effects, body image, sexual functioning, memory, concentration, economic impact of the disease, and global QOL (12–15). These QOL inventories may be used in conjunction with the more commonly used measurements of chemotherapy-induced toxicities to better assess overall patient tolerance to the drug regimen administered.

Quality of life as well as prolongation of life are two important parameters that should be considered when deciding on possible palliative chemotherapy treatments (16). Chemotherapy must be assessed for antitumor effects and toxicities, as well as overall positive or negative impact on the patient's QOL (17–19). A treatment that does not alter survival duration but does improve QOL is usually viewed as beneficial.

A patient's QOL is a subjective parameter that can often be underestimated by the health care provider as well as a patient-appointed surrogate when compared to the patient's self-rating (7). It is certainly possible for a healthy nurse or physician, when evaluating an oxygen- and wheelchair-dependent patient, to assess that individual as having a poor QOL. That same patient may still enjoy many other less active aspects of life and judge his or her QOL to be high. Each individual has unique expectations of "a life worth living." This is a dynamic situation that can change dramatically with time. Malignancy or treatment-induced debilities may possibly be better tolerated by individuals with previous disabilities. For example, a person with severe arthritis may adjust to a more sedentary life due to a newly diagnosed metastatic cancer than a person with no previous problems with ambulation. Younger, more recently active patients may have significant difficulties with a functional compromise. The loss of hair for one patient may be more psychologically debilitating than the loss of mobility for another. Each patient and situation is unique. More research is required to accurately define these complex QOL issues. It appears prudent at this time for the health care team not to judge an individual patient's level of debility or QOL. Consultation for assistance with psychological, spiritual, marital, and other counseling or referral to disease-related support groups can be extremely helpful in allowing patients and their families to maximize their QOL.

An assumption by the health care team that a significant improvement in QOL, with a slight decrease in overall survival, would be in the cancer patient's best interest may, from the patient's point of view, be incorrect. In a study of health values of the seriously ill, patients and their own designated medical decision-making surrogates were interviewed independently (7). The patients had a variety of chronic debilitating diseases with an anticipated median 6-month mortality rate of 50%. All patients had significant disease-related debility. Patients were evaluated for time trade-off—if they could live for 1 year at their current level of function and health, how much time would they trade for a shorter survival in excellent health? About one third of patients would not give up any time at their present level of debility in exchange for a shorter life in excellent health. Nine percent preferred living for 2 weeks or less in excellent health to 1 year in their current state of health. On the average, patients would equate 1 year of their current debilitated condition with 8.8 months of excellent health. Only 2% of patients equated their current health with being equal to or worse than death. In general, patients rated their current state of health as better than the rating given by their designated surrogates. Surrogates were more likely to give up survival time for improved health. This study demonstrated that patients' health values varied widely and could not be accurately predicted by others' perceptions of the patient's current state of health. When sequential interviews with the same patient were possible, health values increased with time. In other words, the longer the patient survived, the less likely they were to trade time alive for better health.

A similar but smaller study was designed to determine how patients with non–small cell lung cancer or prostate cancer evaluated potential survival benefits against potential treatment-related toxicities (20). Patients generally required a lesser survival advantage before accepting more toxic radiation therapy or chemotherapy than medical staff controls. For similar survival advantages, patients would always choose radiotherapy over chemotherapy. Patients were fairly evenly divided regarding whether they desired to take an active role versus a passive role in their medical decision making. Many patients preferred having the health care team make medical decisions for them. Interestingly, no medical personnel desired only to take a passive role. Overall, there was a great variation among patients regarding their therapy risk-taking to benefit ratio.

In summary, cancer treatments can negatively or positively affect a patient's quality of life. Although potential chemotherapy toxicities may adversely affect any organ system, it is also possible that toxicities will not occur or will be mild and readily treatable. The more aggressive/high-dose chemotherapy regimens are associated with significantly greater toxicities. For many types of malignancies it remains to be proven that high-dose or myeloablative chemotherapy is associated with increased duration of disease-free survival or total survival (21–23).

Thus, aggressive high-dose and potentially more toxic treatments should be reserved for use in protocol settings unless definitive data regarding their potential advantage is proven.

## CAN NONCURATIVE CHEMOTHERAPY IMPROVE THE QUALITY OF LIFE?

Relatively few prospective studies address the QOL benefit of only supportive care versus combination palliative chemotherapy plus supportive care for the treatment of incurable metastatic disease. A study of 63 patients with metastatic non-small cell lung cancer reported results of palliative radiation therapy, psychosocial support, analgesics, and nutritional support with or without combination chemotherapy with cisplatin and vinblastine (24). There was a slightly longer but statistically insignificant median survival benefit (20 versus 13 weeks) for the group receiving chemotherapy. The chemotherapy group had more severe toxicity and no improvement in QOL on Karnofsky PS scores.

In a larger study of patients with unresectable metastatic or locally advanced non-small cell lung cancer, 150 patients were prospectively randomized to best supportive care (BSC) or two different chemotherapy regimens (25). Median survival was 8–15 weeks longer for the chemotherapy-treated group (17 weeks versus 24.7 and 32.6 weeks). Improved survival was observed only for those patients initially presenting with an ECOG PS of 0 or 1 and <5 kg weight loss. About 40% of the chemotherapy-treated patients had toxicity judged to be severe, life threatening, or lethal. There were four treatment-related deaths, and the overall impact of treatment on QOL was not reported. Few patients showed improvement in ECOG performance status or gained weight while on treatment.

Several other non-small cell lung cancer studies using different chemotherapy regimens as single-arm studies or compared to a nonchemotherapy or delayed chemotherapy patient group have been reported (26–30). All of these studies reported response rates to chemotherapy in the range of 30–40%. There was a trend toward improved survival in the treated groups. There also appeared to be a longer duration of palliation of cancer-related symptoms in the chemotherapy-treated group.

Meta-analyses of the randomized prospective clinical trials of best supportive care versus initial chemotherapy for unresectable non-small cell cancer have been performed in an attempt to compile other studies' smaller patient populations into a single larger study and therefore allow better determination of statistical significance of treatment effect (31–33). Various chemotherapy regimens were used in individual studies. These meta-analyses supported an overall median and mean survival benefit in the range of 6–10 weeks for the treated group compared to the BSC group. Unfortunately, toxicities, quality of life, and total cost issues could not be accurately addressed by these meta-analyses. Patients with prognostic features such as ECOG PS 3 or 4 had no benefit from chemotherapy. Other reported, but somewhat less dependable, poor prognostic factors were significant weight loss or non-squamous cell carcinoma histology. In general, it appears that there is some survival benefit if chemotherapy is given to selected patients with non-small cell lung cancer, a tumor that is considered only moderately responsive to chemotherapy.

Chemotherapy has been shown to palliate symptoms in some patients with advanced hormone refractory prostate cancer, despite having no impact on overall survival (34,35). A randomized prospective trial confirmed the results of a smaller preliminary study and demonstrated that chemotherapy, when added to prednisone, resulted in decreased pain, decreased use of analgesic medications, and an improvement in overall quality of life for 29% of patients compared to only 12% of patients treated with prednisone alone (36). The use of chemotherapy for hormone-resistant prostate cancer remains a controversial issue for many oncologists, and more effective chemotherapy is certainly desired.

Another small randomized study of 61 patients with advanced gastrointestinal malignancies (gastric, pancreatic or biliary, or colorectal) compared best supportive care to the same therapies given with chemotherapy (37). Improved or prolonged high quality of life was observed in 58% of the chemotherapy group versus 29% in the best supportive group. Survival advantage was only observed in the group with gastric malignancies. Other studies also indicate a symptom-improving role for chemotherapy for patients with gastrointestinal malignancies (38).

Patients with cancer may be more inclined to seek chemotherapy if it were given in less invasive ways. Oral chemotherapy would decrease patient discomfort and stress, be more convenient, and allow chemotherapy to be more easily administered outside the clinic (39,40). About 90% of patients with malignancy would prefer oral over intravenous chemotherapy; however, 70% of studied patients were not willing to sacrifice efficacy or duration of response for the convenience of oral chemotherapy (39). For patients preferring IV chemotherapy, one advantage cited included transferring the responsibility of chemotherapy administration to someone else. Younger males were the group most likely to prefer oral chemotherapy; females and older patients were more likely to defer the choice of administration route to their physicians.

## WHEN TO INITIATE PALLIATIVE CHEMOTHERAPY

When curative therapy is not a realistic goal, as is the case for most adult metastatic malignancies, then multiple factors must be weighed regarding the time to initiate systemic anticancer therapy. The goal of palliative chemotherapy would be to relieve or prevent tumor-induced symptoms and prolong survival.

Since any symptom caused directly or indirectly by the neoplasm can potentially be ameliorated by an effective chemotherapy regimen, patients symptomatic from malignancy or expected to soon become symptomatic should be considered for treatment initiated within a few days to weeks. "Emergency chemotherapy" has been used as the initial sole treatment to effectively palliate emergent oncologic conditions such as superior vena cava syndrome, epidural spinal cord compression, or airway obstruction (42–45). However, local treatment with radiotherapy or surgery may be more appropriate in selected patients.

A more difficult choice is whether to delay noncurative chemotherapy in the asymptomatic patient with relatively low-bulk disease in nonvital areas since some tumor types may display indolent growth. In these circumstances, especially for cancers that respond poorly to chemotherapy, the benefit-to-toxicity ratio of therapy may be more heavily shifted to the toxicity side. Treatment can be withheld with close monitoring of the patient and initiated once symptomatic progression is evident.

A primary concern for this watch-and-wait approach is that a patient can move from "too well to treat" to "too sick to treat" quickly and unexpectedly. This is especially problematic if the patient desires a trial of chemotherapy. It is possible that treatment could be withheld too long and unexpected cancer-related problems could prevent the patient from receiving chemotherapy and thus miss the window of opportunity to treat his malignancy (see Fig. 1). For example, an acute cancer-related bowel, biliary, ureteral, or bronchial obstruction from relative small growth of a cancer in a vital area may have catastrophic consequences that would significantly increase the risk of chemotherapy toxicity. The possibility also exists that a malignancy may demonstrate a decreased response to treatment with increased tumor size (46,47). Delay of chemotherapy theoretically allows for the potential development of more chemotherapy-resistant cells. However, it is assumed that at least some chemotherapy-resistant cells are present in patients with malignancies that are incurable at the time of initial discovery.

There is relatively scant clinical trial information available addressing this specific issue. A prospective study of expectant or delayed chemotherapy versus initial chemotherapy for asymptomatic patients with advanced colorectal cancer indicated an advantage to earlier chemotherapy (48,49). One hundred eighty-three patients with asymptomatic advanced colorectal cancer were randomized to initial chemotherapy for 6 months (unless disease progression occurred or severe toxicity ensued) or to initiation of chemotherapy at a future time when the patient became symptomatic from disease progression. The median survival in the initially treated group was better (14 months) than the delayed treated group (9 months). Median symptom-free survival was 10 months versus 2 months, and progression-free survival was 8

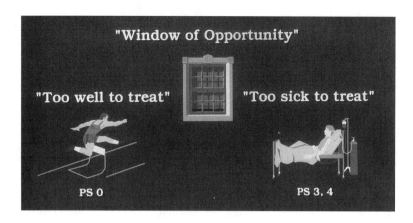

**FIG. 1.** The window of opportunity to treat the asymptomatic patient. A primary concern is that the patient will abruptly change from being asymptomatic to being too sick to treat before chemotherapy can be instituted. (PS = Performance Status)

months versus 3 months in the early versus delayed treated groups, respectively. Some patients in the expectancy group were too ill to receive chemotherapy at the time disease progression was documented (missed the window of opportunity to treat), but some did not require chemotherapy for prolonged asymptomatic periods of time. The survival and progression-free survival curves tended to converge for both groups at about 18 months.

Small cell lung cancer is much more chemotherapy-responsive than colon cancer. A therapeutic watch-and-wait investigative approach for this malignancy similar to that just described for colon cancer has been reported (50). Although the initially treated group had more "adverse reactions" (80% versus 33%), the physicians' assessments of overall quality of life for the chemotherapy group was higher than that of the initially observed group. The initially treated group demonstrated higher activity levels and less breathlessness at follow-up intervals than the delayed treatment group when assessed by the treating physicians.

Indolent B-cell lymphomas, such as follicular small cell lymphoma, have been studied in investigations comparing aggressive chemoradiotherapy with less aggressive treatments or even a watch-and-wait policy (51–54). No survival advantage was found in the groups receiving initial therapies. Other studies even indicate up to a 30% spontaneous regression of untreated follicular small cleaved cell lymphomas, regressions that were usually incomplete and lasted less than 2 years (51).

These prospective trials of treatment versus "watch-and-wait" do not permit a definitive recommendation regarding when to treat the asymptomatic patient with an incurable malignancy. Primary to this decision would be a candid patient–physician discussion of options. Some patients are psychologically distressed with a watch-and-wait policy. They may desire treatment to prevent potential problems or not want to risk the possibility of being too sick to treat when their disease progresses. Patients should make the final decision with advice from their physician.

If there are objective parameters to follow for tumor response to treatment (Table 7), an initial few courses of treatment with reevaluations for tumor response is an acceptable approach. Treatment can be discontinued or changed for tumor progression and continued for stable or regressive disease. If toxicities from treatment are severe or uncontrollable, cessation or attenuation of treatment is appropriate.

The decision to treat the asymptomatic patient becomes even more difficult if there is no disease that can be easily followed for response. Prospective follow-up studies from baseline can then only report on disease progression. Slowly growing tumors refractory to chemotherapy may not demonstrate apparent growth until a few or even many months of treatment. A watch-and-wait policy for the asymptomatic patient, with reservation of treatment until the disease becomes followable or symptomatic, is a reasonable alternative for discussion. The other approach for this asymptomatic group with no evaluable disease is to choose an arbitrary number of chemotherapy cycles (4–8 months) and to stop treatment after this period of time. Reinstitution of treatment can occur later when there is evidence of disease progression. Prospective studies addressing these important issues are needed.

When offered the option of palliative chemotherapy, patients should consider the possible efficacy, benefit, and toxicity of the treatments as well as multiple, uniquely individual, QOL factors. Individuals of any age who are residing in the same dwelling with their children are more likely to accept aggressive treatments, even those with a low probability of success (55). Patients residing with their spouses did not as predictably opt for this same aggressive treatment preference. Patients who had previously received chemotherapy were more likely to accept an aggressive and potentially more toxic form of chemotherapy than a treatment-naive group (11). This finding lends some empirical support to the possibility that actual experience with chemotherapy may not be as difficult as patients' expectations of the difficulties.

The clinician's role in the decision to initiate treatment should not be underestimated. Patients tend overwhelmingly to accept their physician's advice when deciding on treatments for life-threatening illnesses (56). A better informed and educated patient or a patient who believes

**TABLE 7.** *Beneficial results obtainable with palliative chemotherapy*

| | |
|---|---|
| Survival advantage | Improve the expected overall survival or medial survival of a group of patients treated. |
| Tumor response | (A) *Complete:* Total resolution of all evidence of malignancy by any possible criteria that previously documented the malignancy. |
| | (B) *Partial:* ≥50% reduction of the sum of the products of the two greatest perpendicular diameters of lesion sites (indicator) chosen to follow the growth or shrinkage of the cancer. Cannot have any increase in size of other nonindicator lesions. |
| | (C) *Progression:* ≥25% increase of any indicator lesion or appearance of a new lesion. |
| | (D) *Stable:* Lies between partial response and progressive disease. |

that his physician is ambivalent about a recommendation is more likely not to abide by the physician's suggested treatments. Despite this inherent trust by patients, a physician's recommendations for treatment of marginally chemosensitive cancers are often based on beliefs rather than objectively substantiated facts (57).

It is possible to consolidate the findings from the preceding studies in order to develop an overall approach to palliative chemotherapy for the patient with an incurable malignancy. The most problematic situations are the cases with a relatively low response (<25%) rate to chemotherapy. If access to clinical trial protocols is available, they should be recommended. If trials are refused or not available, a limited amount of chemotherapy (such as two or three cycles) can be given with drug attenuation as necessary, depending on the severity of side effects. If a partial or complete response is observed and the patient's PS and QOL are stable or improving, then continuation of treatment to best response or two cycles beyond best response would be reasonable. If the cancer is responding to treatment but the patient is doing poorly with decreasing PS or QOL, the goals of these noncurative therapies must be reassessed and discussed with the patient. Stepwise attenuation of doses, prolonged intervals between chemotherapy cycles, and chemotherapy-free rest and recovery intervals are alternatives to be considered. Paradoxically, the most reasonable patient group for consideration in these trials is composed of those patients who present in the best health. This would include patients with ECOG PS 0, 1, or—infrequently—2, no other cancer-related symptoms such as weight loss, and few if any other significant comorbid medical problems. Unfortunately, this ideal patient group is usually relatively underrepresented in patients presenting with metastatic incurable malignancies.

## DURATION OF CHEMOTHERAPY FOR INCURABLE DISEASE

In the ideal situation, a patient tolerates administered chemotherapy with no adverse effects and the cancer shows a rapid and complete resolution. The patient is cured or the duration of complete remission is long. Unfortunately, this situation is rare for adults with metastatic cancers. More commonly, there are treatment-related toxicities and the cancer demonstrates partial response, remains unchanged, or progresses despite treatment. If a tumor response occurs, a common approach is to treat to best response plus two additional cycles if the therapy is toxic or to treat continuously until disease progression if the treatment is well tolerated with little or no toxicity. The stable disease situation is more problematic. It is impossible to judge if the cancer is just displaying a slow growth phase or if the treatment is keeping the disease in check. One must be dubious of attributing stable disease to chemotherapy "response." Yet if the treatment is not causing significant side effects, it would be reasonable to discuss with the patient the possibility of continued treatment until the time of disease progression versus discontinuing treatment.

Maintenance chemotherapy—treatment that is continued for prolonged or indefinite periods of time after complete response is obtained—has been shown to be of no benefit for a number of chemotherapy-curable or highly chemosensitive cancers (testicular cancer, small cell lung cancer, ovarian cancer, lymphomas, and Hodgkin's disease). Similarly, limited chemotherapy given with curative intent in the adjuvant setting also appears as efficacious as more prolonged treatments (colon cancer, breast cancer, testicular cancer).

Sparse data are available regarding the recommended duration of treatment when curative chemotherapy is not possible. In one study of patients with metastatic breast cancer, patients were randomized to continuous treatment until disease progression or only three cycles of initial chemotherapy and then retreatment with three more cycles at the time of disease progression (58). The group receiving the intermittent therapies had worse outcome self-rating scores for physical well-being, mood, appetite, and overall quality of life. The intermittent treatment group also had a significantly shorter time to disease progression and a trend toward (though not a statistically significantly) shorter overall survival. It should be noted that patients receiving intermittent chemotherapy in this study were not treated to best response as is commonly the case in practice.

A similar approach for treatment of small cell lung cancer used one cycle of initial chemotherapy and then randomized patient groups to continuous chemotherapy or chemotherapy given as needed for symptom control (59). The group of patients given the intermittent chemotherapy received about half as much treatment as the continuously treated group. More importantly, the intermittently treated group scored themselves as having more severe symptoms of pain, nausea, and anorexia than the continuously treated group. They also judged themselves to have poorer sleep, lower mood levels, lower activity levels, and lower levels of general well-being than the continuously treated group. There was no significant difference in survival between the two groups.

Longer initial palliative chemotherapy to allow for a greater tumor response may be of significant benefit. Six courses of initial chemotherapy (cyclophosphamide, doxorubicin, 5-fluorouracil) were given to 250 women with metastatic breast cancer (60). After the induction period, women whose disease regressed or remained stable were randomly assigned to either continued treatment or no further treatment until disease progression. At disease progression, patients were treated with reinstitution of the same chemotherapy regimen. Median time to progression was 9.4 months in the maintenance chemotherapy group and 3.2 months in the observed group, but median survival times were similar in each group, as were changes in performance status. Nausea, vomiting, and mucositis were significantly more common in the maintenance group. This study, as well as others, supports the premise that shorter trials of several courses of initial chemotherapy are not associated with poorer survival for women with metastatic breast cancer than longer or continuous treatment (61,62).

It would appear reasonable to treat a patient with palliative chemotherapy to best clinically objective response plus one or two additional cycles. The additional cycles are necessary because it can not prospectively be determined when best initial response will occur. This approach assumes that the toxicities of the treatment are manageable and do not significantly affect the patient's quality of life. In circumstances where a patient has significant morbidity from an incurable malignancy that is relieved by well-tolerated chemotherapy, maintenance or continued treatment may be beneficial and should be considered. If chemotherapy is discontinued after best response but prior to progressive disease, the same or a similar regimen can usually be reinstituted at the time of disease progression.

## PSYCHOLOGICAL ISSUES FOR THE PATIENT AND FAMILY REGARDING CHEMOTHERAPY

The lay public often has preconceived ideas regarding the potential toxicities of chemotherapy. Patients or their families may state at the initial interview with the medical oncologist that they are not interested in receiving chemotherapy. They may describe a friend or relative who underwent treatments, perhaps long ago, with "terrible side effects." Sometimes they relay third- or fourth-hand information or describe a sensational tabloid report of therapy side effects. In order to allay these fears, the medical oncologist must understand these concerns, correct misconceptions, and ensure adequate attempts to prevent or treat potential chemotherapy-induced side effects. Nurses, social workers, clergy, and other clinic personnel may have special rapport with patients and can be extremely effective patient counselors.

It is very helpful and usually desirable to have a "significant other" (or family member, friend, clergy) accompany the patient for the interview and discussion of planned treatment. Patients should not be given a mandate to choose a treatment at the first discussion of chemotherapy. Only rarely does an emergency situation exist requiring immediate decision making regarding acceptance of chemotherapy. If more time is needed or a second opinion requested, this should be encouraged. Patients or their families may very reasonably want another consultation after they are told that a disease is incurable, progressing, or that beneficial outcome with treatment is uncommon.

The initial recommendation for chemotherapy should include written material describing the drug regimen or investigational protocol to be used and possible therapy-induced toxicities. Methods to control side effects, when to seek help, and the means to contact the health care team at any time if an urgent problem occurs should be reviewed. Written materials or even tapes of the session are extremely helpful and allow the patient and family to review the information at a less stressful time.

## THE DECISION TO ACCEPT, REJECT, OR CONTINUE CHEMOTHERAPY

The diagnosis of cancer is an extremely frightening and anxiety-provoking event. Foremost among patient concerns are the possibility of dying from the disease, the financial burdens that will be incurred, disease-related pain, and the toxicities of treatment. Chemotherapy is often perceived as a very toxic treatment. The patient or family may imagine the emaciated, hairless, bedridden individual lying next to an emesis basin with IV tubes infusing incredibly toxic drugs. This image is a formidable obstacle to overcome. Empathy, patience, and demonstrated concern provided by the oncology team are as important components as treatment-specific education and truly informed consent. In fact, after recovering from the initial shock of cancer diagnosis, patients appear to be quite accepting of possible treatment side effects in an attempt to control the malignancy.

In a study of 100 patients with cancer, Slevin reported on the differences between patients' attitudes to either mild or intensive cancer chemotherapy compared to attitudes of doctors, nurses, and a control group matched for age, sex, and occupation (63). Study participants were asked to consider various probabilities of cure, prolongation of life, and relief of symptoms for mild and aggressive treatments. Patients with cancer were the most likely group to accept intensive and toxic treatments for an extremely small probability of cure, prolongation of life, or symptom relief. The general population control group was less likely to accept the same treatments and wanted more potential benefit for any particular risk. The responses of the medical oncologists, general practitioners, and cancer nurses were intermediate between the population control group and the cancer patient group. Medical oncologists were more likely to accept aggressive treatments than general practitioners. Oncology nurses' scores fell between those of the generalists and the control group. Radiation therapists were the least likely of any group to accept treatment. After 3 months of actual treatment, the same questionnaire was readministered to patients. Their responses were essentially unchanged. This important study indicated that individuals' attitudes change dramatically when they actually receive the diagnosis of cancer. It appears that when the situation is real, more risks are taken. Patients would more likely accept treatments with less potential benefit than any other group that only hypothetically had to consider receiving cancer treatments. A second conclusion is that it is extremely difficult for doctors or nurses to advise patients as to which treatment health care professionals would accept if they were in the cancer patient's position and were asked, "What would you do if this were you?"

Other data regarding oncologists' self-acceptance of chemotherapy for hypothetical diseases also indicated a reluctance to accept treatment. University-affiliated Canadian physicians experienced in the treatment of lung cancer were given open-ended management possibilities and were asked to choose the therapy they would personally accept if they had the disease (64). If the lung cancer were early stage and operable, only 3% of the physicians would elect to undergo adjuvant chemotherapy. This increased to 9% if the disease were operable but locally more extensive and would be only 5% if the cancer were asymptomatic and advanced. Sixteen percent would select chemotherapy for symptomatic metastatic disease. Almost all of the individuals selecting chemotherapy were medical oncologists and most were younger than 40 years of age.

Fifty-one oncologists practicing in the United States (14 surgical, 14 radiation, 23 medical) (65) were asked to choose their own therapy on the basis of being diagnosed with a number of different malignancies. The malignancies varied from those with high cure rates with chemotherapy or radiation therapy to those known to be very refractory to either treatment. The questionnaire

responses were heterogeneous and indicated a lack of agreement on "standard" treatments for various malignancies. Only 37% of cases presented had agreement by 85% or more of the oncologists regarding a treatment they would personally accept or reject. Disparity was particularly common when palliation rather than cure was the goal. For example, 98% of the physicians would "probably or definitely" desire chemotherapy for stage IV Hodgkin's disease, a malignancy with significant curative potential with chemotherapy. This number decreased to 27% for locally advanced (stage III) non-small cell lung cancer and 11% for metastatic melanoma. Both of these cancers are chemotherapy-incurable with relatively low response rates. Surgical oncologists were least likely to accept hypothetical treatment with radiation or chemotherapy for the broad mix of malignancies presented.

Cultural differences may also exist. Japanese doctors were surveyed for their treatment choices for a hypothetical diagnosis of six different stages of non-small cell lung cancer. They indicated a definite preference for surgical resection, even for possibly operable brain metastases (66). Adjuvant chemotherapy for node-positive resected disease was selected by about 40%. About one third would accept chemotherapy for the treatment of metastatic or unresectable disease. Forty percent requested supportive care only in this latter circumstance and no chemotherapy.

A common misconception is that if a chemotherapy regimen is inducing a beneficial tumor response, then toxicities may be more tolerable to the patient. A study of 99 patients refutes this assumption (67). There was little difference in patient side-effects ranking between those patients who thought they were getting better and those who thought that they were the same or worse. Interestingly, nonphysical side effects of treatment such as the inconvenience of coming for appointments, length of treatment, difficulty parking at the clinic, and problems that treatment created for the patient's family or work environment were frequently listed as more bothersome than physical side effects such as vomiting, nausea, hair loss, or fatigue.

Despite the health care providers' best efforts to adequately educate the patient regarding the benefit-to-toxicity ratio of suggested chemotherapy, the overwhelming desire of patients for effective chemotherapy may not allow correct assimilation of the information they are provided. After informed consent was obtained for a phase I trial at a single institution, patients were surveyed regarding their perceptions of the trial (68). It was explained to the patients that the goals of a phase I trial are to determine the toxicities and maximum tolerated dose of an investigational drug and that the doses of drugs are escalated in a stepwise fashion to toxicity. The chance of tumor response to a phase I agent is anticipated to be low, with response rates reported to be only 4–6%

(69,70). Yet, for all the patients electing to participate in a phase I trial, 85% did so for reasons of possible therapeutic benefit, 11% because of advice of their physician, and 4% because of family pressure. Although 93% stated that they understood all or most of the information provided them, only 33% were able to describe the true purpose of a phase I trial. The obvious conclusion was that cancer patients chose to participate in phase I trials because of the strong desire to find a treatment of personal therapeutic benefit. This overwhelming search for an effective anticancer treatment may preclude a truly rational understanding of the treatment being administered. In the actual setting of having the diagnosis of cancer, patients appear to be willing to accept significant risks for relatively low potential likelihood of benefit from proposed anticancer treatments.

## PALLIATIVE CHEMOTHERAPY AND THE ONCOLOGIST

Burnout, the loss of interest in and enthusiasm for one's job, occurs commonly in the oncology practitioner (71). Fifty-six percent of oncologists responding to a mass mailing survey experienced burnout in their professional life. Burnout was more common for private practitioners (63%) than for university-based oncologists (47%). By oncologic subspecialty, burnout was reported by 58% of medical oncologists, 52% of radiation oncologists, 48% of surgical oncologists, and 44% of pediatric oncologists.

The primary reason for burnout in 57% of respondents was insufficient personal or vacation time. Continued exposure to fatal illness (53%) and frustration with limited therapeutic success (45%) were cited as contributing factors. Fifty-six percent of respondents described frustration or sense of failure, and 34% experienced depression.

Coping with the problems of terminal or palliative care was believed to be the single most important qualitative factor related to burnout. Palliative care is just becoming a recognized specialty field in the United States. Until recently, little residency and fellowship training in palliative care was the norm, despite the fact that much of adult oncologic practice is palliative rather than curative chemotherapy. The cancer therapist should recognize the immense benefit patients and their families can derive from a holistic palliative approach. The focus of satisfaction for the practicing oncologist should encompass the delivery of effective palliative care as well as curative and palliative chemotherapy. A current textbook of oncology cites Loeb's rules of therapeutics (72) as described over 70 years ago. These rules succinctly state the essence of palliative chemotherapy and are as follows:

1. If what you are doing is doing good, keep doing it.
2. If what you are doing is not doing good, stop doing it.
3. If you don't know what to do, do nothing.
4. Never make the treatment worse than the disease.

As the specialty of oncologic supportive care matures, the answers to many of the questions regarding how, when, and to what extent palliative chemotherapy should be administered will become more apparent . Until then, a balanced approach to treatment with joint patient and physician-directed decision making regarding quality of life and tumor response issues is recommended.

## REFERENCES

1. Osoba D. Lessons learned from measuring health related quality of life in oncology. *J Clin Oncol* 1994;12:608.
2. Sarraf M. Combinations in the treatment of head and neck cancer. *Semin Oncol* 1994;21(Suppl 5):28.
3. Cummings BJ. Concomitant radiotherapy and chemotherapy for anal cancer. *Semin Oncol* 1992;19:102.
4. Heyn R, Newton W, et al. Preservation of the bladder in patients with rhabdomyosarcoma. *J Clin Oncol* 1997;15:69–75.
5. Bufill JA, Groce WR, Neff R. Intra-arterial chemotherapy for palliation of fungating breast cancer. *Am J Clin Oncol* 1994;17(2);118–124.
6. Sorensen JB, Klee M, Palshof T, Hansen HH. Performance status assessment in cancer patients. An inter-observer variability study. *Br J Cancer* 1993;67:514.
7. Tsevat J, Cook F, Green ML, et al. Health values of the seriously ill. *Ann Intern Med* 1995;122:514.
8. Slevin ML, Plant H, Lynch D, Drinkwater J, Gregory WM. Who should measure quality of life, the doctor or the patient? *Br J Cancer* 1988;57: 109.
9. Conti JA, Christman K. Cancer chemotherapy in the elderly. *J Clin Gastroenterol* 1995;21(1):65–71.
10. Leslie WT. Chemotherapy in older cancer patients. *Oncology* 1992; 6(Suppl2):74–80.
11. Yellen SB, Cella DF, Leslie WT. Age and clinical decision making in oncology patients. *JNCI* 1994;86:1766.
12. Ganz PA, Haskell CM, Figlin RA, LaSoto N, Siau J. Estimating the quality of life in a clinical trial of patients with metastatic lung cancer using the Karnofsky performance status and the functional living index-cancer. *Cancer* 1988;61:649.
13. Moinpour CM. Measuring quality of life: an emerging science. *Semin Oncol* 1994;21(Suppl 5):48.
14. Cella DF. Methods and problems in measuring quality of life. *Suppl Care Cancer* 1995;3:11.
15. Moinpour C, Feigl P, Metch B, Hayden K, Meyskens FL, Crowley J. Quality of life end points in cancer clinical trials: review and recommendations. *JNCI* 1989;81:485.
16. Gough IR, Dalgleish LI. What value is given to quality of life assessment by health professionals considering response to palliative chemotherapy for advanced cancer? *Cancer* 1991;68:220.
17. Presant CA. Quality of life in cancer patients: who measures what. *Am J Clin Oncol* 1984;7:571.
18. Payne SA. A study of quality of life in cancer patients receiving palliative chemotherapy. *Soc Sci Med* 1992;35:1505.
19. Cella DF. Measuring quality of life in palliative care. *Semin Oncol* 1995;22(Suppl 3):73.
20. Brundage M, Davidson J, Maokillop W. Trading treatment toxicity for survival in locally advanced non-small cell lung cancer. *J Clin Oncol* 1997;15:330–340.
21. Jakobsen A, Bertelsen K, Andersen J, et al. Dose-effective study of carboplatin in ovarian cancer: a Danish ovarian cancer group study. *J Clin Oncol* 1997;15:193–198.
22. Peters WB, Ross M, Vredenburgh JJ, et al. High dose chemotherapy and autologous bone marrow support versus consolidation after standard-dose adjuvant therapy for high-risk primary breast cancer. *J Clin Oncol* 1993;11:1132–1143.
23. Biermon PJ, Vose Jm, Anderson JR, et al. High dose therapy with autologous hematopoietic rescue for follicular low-grade non-Hodgkin's lymphoma. *J Clin Oncol* 1997;15:445–450.

24. Ganz PA, Figlin RA, Haskell CM, LaSoto N, Siau J. Supportive care versus supportive care and combination chemotherapy in metastatic non-small cell lung cancer. *Cancer* 1989;63:1271.

25. Rapp E, Pater JL, Willan A, Cormier Y, Murray N, Evans WK. Chemotherapy can prolong survival in patients with advanced non small cell lung cancer—report of a Canadian multicenter randomized trial. *J Clin Oncol* 1988;6:633.

26. Lad TE, Nelson RB, Kiekamp V, et al. Immediate versus postponed combination chemotherapy (CAMP) for non–small cell lung cancer—a randomized trial. *Cancer Treat Rep* 1981;65:973.

27. Cornier Y, Bergerson D, LaForge J, et al. Benefits of polychemotherapy in advanced non small cell bronchogenic carcinoma. *Cancer* 1982;50:845.

28. Woods RL, Levi JA, Page J, et al. Non small cell lung cancer: a randomized comparison of chemotherapy with no chemotherapy. (Abstract) *Proc Am Soc Clin Oncol* 1985;4:177.

29. Tummarello D, et al. Symptomatic Stage IV non small cell lung cancer: response, toxicity, performance status change and symptom relief in patients treated wtih cisplatin, vinblastin and mitomycin C. *Cancer Chemother Pharmacol* 1995;35(3):249–253.

30. Ellis PA, et al. Symptom relief with MVP chemotherapy in advanced non–small cell lung cancer. *Br J Cancer* 1995;71(2):336–370.

31. Grilli R, Oxman AD, Julian JA. Chemotherapy for advanced non-small-cell lung cancer: how much benefit is enough? *J Clin Oncol* 1993;11:1866.

32. Souquet PJ, Chauvin F, Boisel JP, et al. Polychemotherapy in advanced non small cell lung cancer: a meta-analysis. *Lancet* 1993;342:19.

33. Marino R, Pampallona S, Preatoni A, Cantoni A, Invernizzi F. Chemotherapy vs supportive care in advanced non-small-cell lung cancer; results of a meta-analysis of the literature. *Chest* 1994;106:861.

34. Moore MJ, Osoba D, et al. Use of palliative and points to evaluate the effects of mitoxantrone and low dose prednisone in patients with hormonally resistant prostate cancer. *J Clin Oncol* 1994;12(4):689–694.

35. DeLeo A, Bajetta E, et al. Epirubicin plus medroxyprogesterone versus second-line treatment of advanced prostatic cancer. *Am J Clin Oncol* 1995;18(3):239–244.

36. Tannock IF, Osoba D, et al. Chemotherapy with mitoxantrone prednisone or prednisone alone for symptomatic homrmone-resistant prostate cancer: a Canadian randomized trial with palliative end points. *J Clin Oncol* 1996;14(6):1756–1764.

37. Glimelius B, Hoffman R, et al. Cost-effectiveness of palliative chemotherapy in advanced gastrointestinal cancer. *Ann Oncol* 1995;6(3):267–274.

38. Jager, et al. Combination 5FU FA and alpha interferon 2B in advanced gastric cancer: results of a phase II trial. *Ann Oncol* 1995;6(2):153–156.

39. Borst CG, de Kruef AT, von Dom FS, et al. Totally implantable venous access ports: the patients point of view. *Cancer Nursing* 1992;378–381.

40. Claessen KA, DeBries JJ, Heisman SJ, et al. Long term venous access with a Hickman catheter: complications and patient satisfaction. *Neth J Surg* 1990;42:47–49.

41. Lui G, Franssen E, Fitch M, et al. Patient preferences for oral versus intravenous palliative chemotherapy. *J Clin Oncol* 1997;15:110–115.

42. Dombernowsky P, Hansen H. Combination chemotherapy in the management of superior vena caval obstruction in small-cell anaplastic carcinoma of the lung. *Acta Med Scand* 1978;204:513.

43. Hayes A, Thompson EI, Hvizdala E, O'Connor D, Green, AA. Chemotherapy as an alternative to laminectomy and radiation in the management of epidural tumor. *J Pediatrics* 1984;104:221.

44. Sinoff LL, Blumshon A. Spinal cord compression in myelomatosis: response to chemotherapy alone. *Eur J Cancer Clin Oncol* 1989;25:197.

45. Gale GR, O'Connor DM, Chu JY, Tantana S, Weber, TS. Successful chemotherapeutic decompression of epidural malignant germ cell tumor. *Med Pediatr Oncol* 1986;14:97.

46. Goldie JH, Coldman AJ. A mathematic model for relating to drug sensitivity of tumors to their spontaneous mutation rate. *Cancer Treat Rep* 1979;63:1727.

47. Goldie JH, Coldman AJ. Application of theoretic models to chemotherapy protocol design. *Cancer Treat Rep* 1986;70:127.

48. Nordic Gastrointestinal Tumor Adjuvant Therapy Group. Expectancy or primary chemotherapy in patients with advanced asymptomatic colorectal cancer: a randomized trial. *J Clin Oncol* 1992;10:904.

49. Glimelius B, Graf W, Hoffman K, Pahlman L, Sioden P, Wennberg A. General condition of asymptomatic patients with advanced colorectal cancer receiving palliative chemotherapy. *Acta Oncol* 1992;31:645.

50. Lung Cancer Working Party. Survival, adverse reactions and quality of life during combination chemotherapy compared with selective palliative treatment for small cell lung cancer. *Respir Med* 1989;83:51.

51. Horning SJ, Rosenberg SA. The natural history of initially untreated low-grade non-Hodgkin's lymphoma. *N Engl J Med* 1984;311:1471–1475.

52. O'Brien ME, Easterbrook P, Powell J, et al. The natural history of low grade non-Hodgkin's lymphoma and the impact of a no initial treatment policy on survival. *Q J Med* 1991;80:651–660.

53. Young RC, Longo DL, Glatstein E, et al. The treatment of indolent lymphomas: watchful waiting v. aggressive combined modality treatment. *Semin Hematol* 1988;25(Suppl):11–16.

54. Hoppe RT, Kushlan P, Kaplan HS, et al. The treatment of advanced stage favorable histology non-Hodgkin's lymphoma: a preliminary report of a randomized trial comparing single agent chemotherapy, combination chemotherapy, and whole body irradiation. *Blood* 1981;58:592–598.

55. Yellen SB, Cella DF. Someone to live for: social well-being, parenthood status, and decision-making in oncology. *J Clin Oncol* 1995;13:1255.

56. Siminoff LA, Fetting JH. Factors affecting treatment decisions for a life-threatening illness: the case of medical treatment of breast cancer. *Soc Sci Med* 1991;32:813.

57. Raby B, Pater J, Mackillop WJ. Does knowledge guide practice? Another look at the management of non-small-cell lung cancer. *J Clin Oncol* 1995;13:1904.

58. Coates A, Gebski V, Bishop JF, et al. Improving the quality of life during chemotherapy for advanced breast cancer. *N Engl J Med* 1987;317:1490.

59. Earl HM, Rudd RM, Spiro SG, et al. A randomized trial of planned versus as required chemotherapy in small cell lung cancer: a cancer research campaign trial. *Br J Cancer* 1991;64:566.

60. Muss HB, Case D, Richards F, et al. Interrupted versus continuous chemotherapy in patients with metastatic breast cancer. *N Engl J Med* 1991;325:1342.

61. Harris AL, Cantwell BM, Carmichael J, et al. Comparison of short term and continuous chemotherapy (mitoxantrone) for advanced breast cancer. *Lancet* 1990;335:186.

62. Smalley RV, Lefante J, Bartelucci A, Carpenter J. A comparison of cyclophosphamide, adriamycin, and 5-fluorouricil and cyclophosphamide, methotrexate, 5-fluorouracil, vincristine and prednisone in patients with advanced breast cancer. *Breast Cancer Res Treat* 1983;3:209.

63. Slevin ML, Stubbs L, Plant HJ, et al. Attitudes to chemotherapy: comparing view of patients with those of doctors, nurses, and general public. *Br Med J* 1990;300:1458.

64. Mackillop W, O'Sullivan B, Ward G. Non-small cell lung cancer: how oncologists want to be treated. *Int J Radiat Oncol Biol Phys* 1987;13:929.

65. Lind SE, DelVecchio G, Minkovitz L, Good B. Oncologists vary in their willingness to undertake anti-cancer therapies. *Br J Cancer* 1991;64:391.

66. Motohiro A, Hirota N, Komatsu H, Yanai N. Japanese doctors preferred treatment choices for their hypothetical non-small cell lung cancer: how they wished to be treated. *Lung Cancer* 1994;11:43.

67. Coates A, Abraham S, Kaye, SB, et al. On the receiving end—patient perception of the side-effects of cancer chemotherapy. *Eur J Cancer Clin Oncol* 1983;19:203.

68. Dougherty G, Ratain M, Grochowski E, et al. Perceptions of cancer patients and their physicians involved in phase I trials. *J Clin Oncol* 1995;13:1062.

69. VonHoff DD, Turner J. Response rates, duration of response, and dose response effects in phase I studies of antineoplastics. *Invest New Drugs* 1991;9:115.

70. Estey E, Hoth D, Wittes R, et al. Therapeutic response in phase I trials of antineoplastic agents. *Cancer Treat Rep* 1986;70:1105.

71. Whippen DA, Canellos GP. Burnout syndrome in the practice of oncology: results of a random survey of 1,000 oncologists. *J Clin Oncol* 1991;9:1916.

72. Holland James F., Bast RC, Morton DL, Frei E, Kufe DW, Weichselbaum RR, eds. In: *Cancer medicine: principles of medical oncology*, 4th ed. Baltimore: Williams and Wilkens, 1997;761.

*Principles and Practices of Supportive Oncology,*
edited by Ann Berger et al.
Lippincott–Raven Publishers, Philadelphia ©1998

CHAPTER 48

# Rehabilitative Medicine

Richard S. Tunkel and Elisabeth A. Lachmann

Patients with progressive medical diseases often benefit from physical rehabilitation. Referring to the cancer population, Dietz described four levels of rehabilitation: palliative, supportive, restorative, and preventive (1). In palliative rehabilitation, efforts are made to decrease dependence in activities of daily living and to provide comfort and emotional support. This approach is most appropriate for patients with advanced disease and short life expectancies. Supportive rehabilitation is focused on long-term impairments. Efforts are directed at maximizing function at any given level of disability. When impairment is expected to be short term, restorative rehabilitation is appropriate. These techniques, which are intended to return the patient to a previous level of function, may be very useful when function is impaired because of a side effect of treatment (e.g., myopathy caused by corticosteroids). Preventive rehabilitation may be valuable when impairment is anticipated, and interventions are undertaken to prevent impairment from developing. For example, a simple exercise program for the patient fatigued by radiation therapy may prevent deconditioning.

Three terms are commonly used to describe physical, functional, or psychological deficits: impairment, disability, and handicap. Impairment is defined as "any loss or abnormality of psychological, physiological or anatomical structure or function" (2). Disability is "any restriction or lack (resulting from an impairment) of ability to perform an activity in the manner or within the range considered normal for a human being" (2). Handicap is "a disadvantage for a given individual, resulting from an impairment or a disability, that limits or prevents the fulfillment of a role that is normal (depending on age, sex, and social and cultural factors) for that individual" (2).

Thus, an impairment may result in a disability, which in turn may give rise to a handicap.

## THE SPECTRUM OF FUNCTIONAL IMPAIRMENTS

Functional impairment in the patient with cancer may arise from many causes (Table 1). Cancer may directly produce physical impairments that require rehabilitative intervention. A tumor may destroy normal structures, such as long bones or vertebral bodies. Pain from bone metastasis may represent impending or actual pathologic fracture, which can affect a patient's function by decreasing or inhibiting weight-bearing on a limb or functional mobility when the spine is affected. The mass produced by a tumor may cause pressure effects, such as compression of neural structures resulting in focal neurologic deficit. The neurologic consequences of these pressure effects may be even more serious when the damage occurs within the bony confines of the cranium or spinal column. Hemiparesis from unilateral supratentorial lesions, paraparesis or quadriparesis from spinal (usually epidural) lesions, and incoordination or ataxia from cerebellar or brainstem lesions can all pose difficult rehabilitation issues. Similarly, lesions of the peripheral or central nervous system can cause disorders of speech or swallowing, which may require specific attention (3,4). More globally, central nervous system lesions that culminate in specific impairments of higher cerebral function, such as aphasia, or that produce overall cognitive impairment, may complicate rehabilitative efforts at every level. Local pressure may also compromise vascular structures, producing limb edema, and in the case of lung lesions, local mass effect may decrease pulmonary capacity.

Indirect effects of the neoplasm can also cause impairment. Pain may be quite debilitating, and general debility may have additional deleterious effects on function. Pain provoked by movement may produce functional weak-

R. S. Tunkel: Rehabilitation Service, Memorial Sloan-Kettering Cancer Center, New York, NY 10021.

E.A. Lachmann: Department of Rehabilitation Medicine, The New York Hospital–Cornell Medical Center, New York, NY 10021.

**TABLE 1.** *Causes of functional impairments*

Direct effects of cancer
Indirect effects of cancer
    Paraneoplastic syndromes
    Pain
Treatments for malignancy
    Surgery
    Radiation therapy
    Chemotherapy
Deconditioning

ness. Maintenance of a position that decreases pain may result in joint contracture (5). As in the patient who does not have cancer, musculoskeletal pain may result from myofascial pain syndromes, bursitis, tendinitis, or arthritis. At times, successful rehabilitation may help to diminish pain, as in the appropriate application of spinal bracing and improvement through a conditioning program. Various paraneoplastic syndromes associated with neoplasia, such as the cancer-related subtype of polymyositis-dermatomyositis producing weakness, can also produce or worsen impairment (6,7). Sensorimotor paraneoplastic polyneuropathy is only one of a diverse group of paraneoplastic syndromes, which include disorders of the neuromuscular junctions, dorsal root ganglia, or anterior horn cells (7–10). Cancer-associated arthritis may complicate carcinoma, multiple myeloma, or leukemia (11,12). This type of arthritis may resemble rheumatoid arthritis but may have asymmetric involvement, sparing the wrists and small joints. Hypertrophic osteoarthropathy, another paraneoplastic syndrome, may also cause polyarthritis as well as digital clubbing and periostitis. This is most commonly seen with bronchogenic carcinoma (13).

The need for rehabilitation more commonly arises because of impairments resulting from the cancer treatment itself. Surgical resection of a tumor can produce varied impairments, depending on the tissues resected. Focal muscle weakness may result from sacrifice of muscle tissue, as may occur in limb salvage procedures (14). Excision of bone for treatment of sarcoma may require placement of an endoprosthesis or amputation. Sacrifice of nervous tissue often produces an obvious neurologic deficit. Postoperative edema in the central nervous system may produce temporary deficits. Injury or sacrifice of individual peripheral nerves may also have significant consequences. For example, spinal accessory nerve palsy may arise following neck dissection for head and neck cancer or cervical lymph node biopsy (15–17). Patients may experience a depressed, protracted shoulder because of lack of trapezius upward rotation and retraction of the scapula. This results in impaired arm elevation. Shoulder pain may arise when the upper limb is unsupported (18). Resection of lung tissue decreases pulmonary capacity. Creation of ostomies following gastrointestinal or genitourinary surgery requires instruction in their care and use. En-bloc resection of lymphatic structures may give rise to lymphedema.

Radiation therapy may produce relatively acute effects, depending upon the area irradiated. Chronic postradiation changes may evolve months or years later. The persistent impairments related to these effects may be profound. Some chemotherapeutic agents have specific toxicities that affect target organ systems, such as the lungs or peripheral nervous system. Numerous chemotherapeutic agents cause polyneuropathy, with patterns that range from a presentation resembling Guillain-Barré syndrome (suramin) to sensory (cisplatin or paclitaxel) or sensorimotor (vincristine) neuropathy (19–22). Myopathy may result from corticosteroid use, having the predominant feature of proximal limb weakness (23). A so-called pseudorheumatism may occur following the abrupt withdrawal of corticosteroids (24). Avascular necrosis may result from radiation therapy or corticosteroid use. All these measures may produce impairments that require rehabilitative intervention.

## DECONDITIONING

Prolonged bed rest and immobility may produce a multitude of negative effects upon various body systems. Muscle weakness and atrophy can result directly from immobility. As much as 20% of strength may be lost with each week of bed rest; endurance declines at a similar rate (25). The antigravity muscles of the trunk and lower limbs are often the first muscles to atrophy (26). Reconditioning often takes much longer than deconditioning. Strength increases approximately 12% per week until the muscle has three-quarters of its maximal strength (25). Above this level, the rate of strength increase diminishes.

Muscles held in fixed position gradually shorten, especially those that cross two joints. Patients undergoing prolonged bed rest maintain a position of comfort, with the hips and knees held in flexion. This can result in contracture of the psoas and hamstring muscles. The gastrocnemius often shortens as a result of positioning.

Prolonged bed rest may also result in osteopenia, which occurs when bone resorption exceeds bone formation (28). In severe cases, hypercalcemia may result and may worsen the hypercalcemia caused by bone metastases or other processes (29).

Cardiopulmonary deconditioning usually occurs with prolonged immobility. The resting heart rate can increase more than 30 beats per minute after only 2 weeks of bed rest (30). This is a compensatory means of maintaining cardiac output with decreasing stroke volume (29). Stroke volume decreases as immobilization diuresis leads to significant plasma volume loss (30–32). Postural hypotension may be another consequence of plasma loss. While prolonged bed rest has no direct effect on pulmonary function, recumbency impedes diaphragmatic excursion, impairing cough (30,33). This may reduce tidal volume and cause compensatory tachypnea to sustain minute ventilation (31,33).

A hypercoagulable state related to malignancy combined with venous stasis from immobility places the cancer patient at high risk of deep vein thrombosis (DVT) (34). Remobilization of the patient with DVT may increase the risk of pulmonary embolus (35).

Prolonged pressure over bony prominences predisposes to pressure sores. Shearing forces, which are created when the patient slides or is dragged across the bed, may also compromise local blood flow and further increase the risk of pressure sores (36). Moisture from bodily fluids contributes to the formation of pressure sores by skin maceration and chemical irritation.

Finally, prolonged bed rest can lead to decreased gastrointestinal motility, which may predispose to constipation. Bowel dysmotility produced by immobility can augment the constipating effects of other disorders such as hypercalcemia, or treatments, including the opioids.

## THERAPEUTIC INTERVENTIONS

Rehabilitative interventions for the patient with progressive medical disease must be tailored to address the specific deficits of that patient (Table 2). Factors such as life expectancy, living environment, and the availability and capabilities of caregivers must be considered. The potential benefits to the overall quality of life of the patient must be weighed against the real costs in time, discomfort, and money as well as the potential physical, psychological, and psychosocial risks before a specific intervention is begun. Rehabilitation interventions are best provided by a multidisciplinary team because of the diversity of functional impairments (Table 3).

### Therapeutic Exercise

Muscle can be strengthened through isometric, isotonic, or isokinetic exercises (37). Isometric exercise entails muscle contraction without joint movement. This form of exercise can be useful when pain is provoked by joint movement, as in acute joint inflammation. Isometric

**TABLE 2.** *Spectrum of rehabilitative interventions*

Therapeutic exercise
Mobility and gait training
Training in activities of daily living
Cognitive/perceptual rehabilitation
Orthotics and prosthetics
Physical modalities for pain relief
Lymphedema treatment
Chest physical therapy
Bowel and bladder retraining
Speech and swallowing therapies

**TABLE 3.** *Multidisciplinary rehabilitation team*

Physiatrist
Physical therapist
Occupational therapist
Speech pathologist
Palliative care/pain specialist
Nurse specialist
Psychiatrist
Psychologist
Social worker
Clergy

exercise primarily affects strength and has little impact on endurance. Isotonic contraction produces joint movement against a constant force. Walking requires a series of isotonic contractions. Concentric isotonic contraction shortens muscle against constant resistance, whereas eccentric isotonic contraction partially counters a lengthening force upon the muscle. This type of exercise helps to increase both strength and endurance. Isokinetic exercise is muscle contraction at a constant velocity and requires the use of sophisticated, expensive equipment (38).

A typical reconditioning program for debilitated patients with progressive diseases features active range-of-motion exercises aimed at strengthening weak muscle groups (39). Exercises are generally done on an as-tolerated basis. Modifications may be necessary if precautions must be followed because of underlying organic conditions, such as metastatic bone disease or a recent myocutaneous flap. With significant weakness (less than antigravity strength), assisted active range of motion exercises may be needed. The therapist in part assists in moving the limb through its full range of motion. For patients with nonfixed joint immobility secondary to weakness, passive range-of-motion exercises performed by another person may be required.

In general conditioning exercises, low-resistance, high-repetition exercise is used to increase endurance (40). An elastic band may be used to strengthen muscle by providing low to moderate resistance. Patients who are isolated for medical reasons and are unable to walk for endurance training may benefit from the use of bicycle pedals. If feasible, a progressive resistance exercise program is initiated to further strengthen muscle (41).

Range-of-motion and strengthening exercises and compensatory techniques to achieve movement using less affected muscle groups are used in therapy for spastic hemiparesis. Neuromuscular reeducation techniques may facilitate or inhibit spastic synergistic patterns, eventually promoting isolated muscle movement. Neuromuscular reeducation may be facilitated by the use of electromyographic biofeedback (EBF) or functional electrical stimulation (FES) (42–44). For example, FES may improve movement and position of the hemiparetic shoulder (45). Arm positioning is further assisted by use of a sling during ambulation. In the seated or bedbound patient, the sling should be removed and replaced by other supportive devices, such as a lap board or arm trough (46). The paraparetic and quadriparetic patient may benefit from neuromuscular reeducation and sustained muscle stretching. Spasticity may be decreased by physical modalities such as transcutaneous electrical nerve stimulation (TENS), ice, EBF, and FES (47–50). Baclofen, administered orally or intrathecally, is an effective antispasticity agent when physical modalities are not helpful (51). The negative effect of losing what was functional spasticity—for example, quadriceps spasticity maintaining knee extension—must be balanced against the positive effect of increased mobility. When spasticity of an isolated motor group interferes with function, chemical or surgical neurolysis, motor point block, or tenotomy may be considered (50).

When nerve injury or muscle sacrifice has occurred, the goal of physical intervention is to increase active, functional movement. Exercise and FES may be aimed at increasing the strength of the partially sacrificed or partially denervated muscle. Other muscles are strengthened to compensate for the acquired weakness, and instruction in postural and compensatory techniques is given.

In cerebellar disorders, patients lose the smooth coordination of agonist and antagonist motor groups (52). Such incoordination produces intention tremor, ataxia of the limbs, and disturbance of fine and rapid alternating movement. The use of weighted equipment may help decrease tremor amplitude and increase function.

In selected patients, cardiovascular reconditioning may be hastened by appropriate therapeutic exercise. The first aerobic exercises usually recommended may be walking or wheelchair mobility. In order to achieve aerobic benefit, these exercises should be performed for at least 15 minutes, 3 days per week (53). The physical or occupational therapist may use heart and respiratory rate, blood pressure determination, and pulse oximetry to monitor the patient's cardiopulmonary status.

Joint contractures may arise from prolonged immobilization, muscular imbalance, voluntary immobility to maintain a position of comfort, or malignant invasion or high-dose radiation therapy to the joint (5,54). Prevention of contractures is easier than treatment. Once contractures develop, aggressive intervention is required when it is feasible. Range-of-motion exercises with sustained terminal stretch may be effective, especially in mild myogenic contractures (55). Deep heating of tissue may increase the distensibility of collagen and assist in reducing contracture (56). With severe contracture, dynamic splinting or serial casting may be beneficial (57).

In the lower-limb amputee, lying in bed or prolonged sitting can encourage hip and knee flexion contracture. These contractures may not be prevented by ambulation without full joint extension. Lying prone at regular intervals daily may help prevent hip contractures.

## Mobility and Gait Training

Patients with severe debility may benefit from mobility instruction. This begins with bed mobility, such as scooting, rolling, and sitting up; these actions may prevent some of the deleterious effects of bed rest, such as pressure sores. Patients who cannot tolerate upright positions because of orthostatic changes may require progressive upright tolerance training. The hospital bed can be used initially for this training. The patient may next begin sitting with the legs dangling. At times, the seated position cannot be tolerated. A tilt table may be used to gradually incline the patient from a supine position toward a standing position (39). Along with sitting and standing postures, instruction in static and dynamic balance in these positions may be necessary.

A transfer is defined as movement from one surface to another. The most common transfer is a standing transfer, for example, going from a bed to a chair. If patients are unable to transfer, they may require the assistance of another person or the use of an assistive device, such as a walker or sliding board (58). Some patients may require instruction for transfers directly into a chair or wheelchair. Those requiring a wheelchair usually are trained in transfers from a wheelchair to another seating device, such as a commode or car seat (59).

Early progressive ambulation can help prevent the negative effects of deconditioning. A walker or another assistive device may be required. Ambulation training may be facilitated by parallel bars or with support from a rolling pole or wheelchair. These assistive devices widen the base of support and involve the upper limbs in weight bearing (60).

Cerebellar gait ataxia may be associated with limb or truncal incoordination (52). In an effort to decrease the amplitude of the tremor, a weighted walker or limb weights may be beneficial, and other adaptive equipment may also be weighted (61). In some patients, ataxia cannot be improved through rehabilitative interventions.

The pathophysiology of sensory gait ataxia is proprioceptive loss in the lower limbs. The use of an assistive device allows proprioceptive feedback to one or both arms. Impaired joint position sense also may be partially compensated by attention to visual cues. Environmental adaptations should include adequate lighting and unobstructed walkways (62).

The spastic hemiplegic gait often features an extensor synergy pattern in the affected lower limb. The foot and ankle assume an equinovarus posture, with the knee held in extension. The patient may circumduct the affected leg, raise the hip, or lean away from the affected leg to permit foot clearance during the swing phase of gait (63). The use of an ankle foot orthosis (AFO) can assist in foot clearance. A double metal upright AFO may be attached to an orthopedic shoe; a calf band with Velcro closure is attached to the superior portion of the metal uprights.

More often, a custom-molded plastic AFO is prescribed. This AFO extends from the plantar surface of the foot up the posterior aspect of the calf and is secured to the leg by a Velcro closure. Compared with the metal AFO, the plastic AFO is lighter in weight, has a larger area of contact, and offers a better cosmetic appearance. Either AFO may improve speed and decrease energy expenditure, but neither has a significant advantage over the other (64).

Lower limb weakness without spasticity may benefit from different compensatory techniques. Hip extension may be able to compensate for weak knee extensors (65). The knee may also be forcibly extended by the hand pushing backward on the thigh. In either case, genu recurvatum may be the undesirable result. Knee bracing may be required if knee instability persists despite efforts to compensate for the weakness. For example, this may be the case after some limb salvage procedures. Bracing cannot effectively compensate for profound hip flexor or extensor weakness (46). Conversely, weakness localized to all or part of the distribution of the common peroneal nerve may be compensated for with an AFO. This will prevent plantar flexion during the swing phase of gait and lessen the risk of falls associated with foot drop. With the use of effective leg braces, other assistive devices may not be needed.

## Activities of Daily Living (ADLs)

ADLs include dressing, eating, bathing, and writing (66). Coordination and strength training in combination with ADL instruction may be needed for bilateral upper limb weakness. If one or both upper limbs are weak, adaptive equipment may be required for ADLs (67). The use of a rocker knife may assist in one-handed food cutting. Wide-handled utensils, along with fine motor retraining, may be helpful for patients with distal upper limb weakness. Patients with severe, long-term dominant limb weakness may require dominance retraining for many of their ADLs. Bimanual activities should be encouraged in these patients. A long-handled shoe horn and a reacher may help in dressing the lower extremities. Other adaptive equipment may be necessary in the wheelchair-dependent patient, such as a raised toilet seat, a tub chair, and various other environmental adaptations.

## Cognitive/Perceptual Rehabilitation

In the supportive oncology setting, cognitive/perceptual rehabilitation helps improve or maintain the patient's level of daily function, especially with ADLs and social interaction. Simple techniques such as the use of a notebook may be helpful memory aids. The adverse impact of unilateral visual field deficit or neglect may be reduced in part by various occupational therapy exercises, some with computers. Other specific problems may also be helped by tailored strategies, which then require repetitive application.

## Braces and Splints

An orthosis is a device that provides support to a body part and may assist in the function of that part. Orthoses may be used to support fractured long bones or a limb that is paretic or plegic. Functional splinting may be used when some volitional movement remains in the afflicted limb.

Upper extremity bracing includes the resting hand splint for the spastically flexed hand and the cock-up wrist splint. The cock-up splint places the wrist in mild extension, enhancing hand function by placing the finger flexors in a mechanically advantageous position. Lower limb orthoses, which were described previously, include the different AFOs and knee braces.

Spinal orthoses are used to add support to sections of the spine. They are especially useful to decrease pain provoked by movement of the afflicted area. These orthoses help prevent movements, especially forward flexion in the thoracic and lumbar spine, that place additional stress on vertebral bodies compromised by bone disease. Both abdominal binders and lumbosacral corsets provide some support to the spine by increasing intraabdominal pressure. For greater restriction of movement, lumbosacral or thoracolumbosacral orthoses may be prefabricated or custom-made as body jackets (68,69). All spinal orthoses must be used in a manner that avoids direct pressure over ostomy sites, hopefully without compromising the support provided by the orthosis. Patients with pulmonary compromise must be carefully assessed to avoid respiratory compromise caused by lumbar orthoses that increase intraabdominal pressure. Skin lesions may need to be accommodated by relief of pressure directly over the lesion.

Bracing of the cervical spine can provide the greatest restriction of movement (70). A soft cervical collar serves as a reminder, only minimally restricting movement. A more rigid device, such as a Philadelphia or Miami collar, provides some restriction, especially of flexion and extension. More limitation of movement is provided by a four-poster appliance or a sterno-occipito-mandibular immobilizer (SOMI). More complete immobilization is achieved by a Halo vest.

## Prostheses

Sacrifice of the distal portion of a limb may require the use of a functional prosthesis. In the lower limb, the goal is a return to independent ambulation. The more proximal the level of amputation, the greater the increase in energy expenditure for reciprocal gait. The exertion required may preclude the use of prostheses by patients with comorbid cardiopulmonary disorders. Lighter-weight components, improved socket designs, and energy-storing feet whose elasticity allows some energy to be released during toe-off have improved modern-day prostheses (71–73). In all cases, proper care of the distal residual limb and appropriate prosthetic training are required for maximal benefit to be achieved.

Upper limb amputation is much less common. A typical upper limb prosthesis has a socket that serves as an interface between the prosthesis and the residual limb. The most important functional component is the terminal device, which is available in different shapes (including a functional hand). Control of the terminal device may be achieved mechanically by shoulder movement. Following forequarter amputation, a shoulder prosthesis may allow more normal fit of clothing. All prostheses, especially the expensive myoelectric ones, may be impractical for use in the supportive oncology setting.

## Physical Modalities for Pain Relief

Physical therapeutic modalities may be helpful in the cancer patient with pain of muscular origin (74). Both cold and heat have direct effects on local muscle spasm and can provide analgesia. Heat can increase local blood flow and metabolic rate and therefore may be contraindicated in the cancer patient whose pain is at the site of a tumor mass (75). This is especially true with deep heating devices, such as ultrasound diathermy. These and other modalities, such as vigorous electrical stimulation and massage, are avoided in areas of active tumor and over irradiated tissues.

Therapeutic cold causes an initial decrease in temperature through vasoconstriction. Like superficial heat, cold may also be a counterstimulant, tending to inhibit the projection of pain information in the central nervous system and is avoided over irradiated tissues (76).

Electrical stimulation, which may also have a counterstimulating effect, is usually applied superficially for pain via transcutaneous electrical nerve stimulation (TENS). If pain is strictly of myogenic origin, electrical current may also be used to fatigue muscle spasm or relieve muscular tightness from myofascial trigger points (77). Ischemic compression (pressure maintained over a trigger point) or the spray and stretch technique (vapocoolant spray followed by muscle stretch) may also be effective in releasing trigger points. When these methods are insufficient, injection of trigger points with local anesthetic, or dry needling, may be necessary. Whatever method is used, reconditioning of the muscle containing the trigger point is required. Therapeutic exercise should be aimed at recovering full range of movement and strength of the involved muscles.

## Treatment of Limb Swelling

Deep venous thrombosis (DVT) is common in the cancer patient, especially one who is bedridden. In addition to pharmacologic measures, several mechanical methods have been used for prophylaxis of DVT (78–81). These measures include intermittent pneumatic pressure pumping, gradient pressure stockings, and electrical stimulation of calf muscles.

Controversy exists concerning the timing of mobilization of the patient with DVT. Early mobilization may place the patient at risk of embolization, but prolonged bed rest may increase venous stasis and encourage clot formation. The decision when to mobilize the patient is based in part on the location of the lesion, the length of time the patient has undergone anticoagulant therapy, and whether an inferior vena cava filter has been placed (82,83).

Lymphedema is a frequent cause of limb swelling in the cancer patient. Even when mild, lymphedema can produce profound psychological effects in the patient, in addition to physical sequelae (84). When lymphedema is soft and pitting, limb elevation may be helpful. Physical treatment, which has its foundation in the use of static compression garments, may be helpful even when the condition is mild. Most frequently employed are gradient pressure elastic sleeves or stockings. Bandaging techniques, using materials with little compliance, are also used, and a legging orthosis made of noncompliant Velcro straps has been helpful in certain instances (85,86). Static compression facilitates the muscle pump action of muscle contraction. Thus, therapeutic exercise in the affected limb should be performed while the patient is wearing the compression garment.

For more significant lymphedema, two major forms of dynamic limb compression are available. The entire sleeve of a pneumatic compression pump may intermittently inflate, or the sleeve may inflate sequentially, compressing in a distal-to-proximal direction. Each of these techniques is intended to pump fluids from the limb (87–90). A combination of physical therapies (CPT) featuring manual lymphedema treatment (MLT) is another approach that attempts to facilitate flow through residual patent lymphatic channels (85). In principle, MLT helps to enhance lymph drainage from one area of the torso to another. For example, if lymphedema following axillary lymph node dissection is secondary to impaired lymph drainage from both the ipsilateral limb and the upper quadrant of the torso, MLT attempts to enhance lymph flow from the affected upper quadrant to other areas of the torso via the collateral lymph channels. Bandaging the limb between MLT sessions helps to maximize treatment results (91). Active disease is a relative contraindication to any of these dynamic treatments, as may be local infection, congestive heart failure, or acute DVT.

## Chest Physical Therapy

Chest physical therapy assists in mobilizing secretions and enhancing gas exchange in the lungs. Patients who are immobilized in bed should be repositioned every 2 hours (92). This may prevent pooling of secretions in the dependent portions of the lungs. The therapist can administer postural drainage to help remove secretions from specific areas of the lungs (93). Chest vibration or percussion is often used in combination with postural drainage to enhance its effect. A nebulizer may be used prior to chest physical therapy to loosen secretions and deliver a bronchodilator. In selected cases, muscles of ventilation are subjected to specific reconditioning exercises (94). The use of an incentive spirometer between therapy sessions may strengthen the muscles of respiration and help prevent arteriovenous shunting (93).

## Bladder and Bowel Retraining

Bladder incontinence in the cancer patient is usually managed initially with Foley catheterization, either urethral or suprapubic. If practical, intermittent catheterization is preferred because of the decreased risk of bacteriuria and formation of bladder stones (95). Elevated intravesicular pressures can occur in neurogenic bladders with detrusor-sphincter dyssynergia; this may be avoided with appropriate timing of clean intermittent catheterization. Condom catheters are an alternative in the male patient when this increased intravesicular pressure is not a problem (96).

In the patient with spinal cord disease, especially above T6, autonomic dysreflexia may be provoked by noxious stimuli below the level of injury. For example, bladder distension caused by indwelling catheter obstruction may cause headache, flushing, and sweating above the level of injury, as well as hypertension accompanied by bradycardia (97,98). Interventions for autonomic dysreflexia include correction of noxious stimuli and symptomatic therapies, such as elevation of the head of the bed or the use of antihypertensive medications if necessary.

Bladder incontinence may also be treated with drugs. For example, decreased bladder wall contractility in the spastic, reflex bladder may be achieved with anticholinergic agents. Conversely, cholinergic agents, which may increase bladder contractility, should be used cautiously.

A patient with an uninhibited bladder may require a scheduled voiding regimen. Timed voiding combined with such measures as the Valsalva maneuver, suprapubic tapping, and suprapubic pressure (Credé) may be particularly useful when mild urinary retention is present.

Constipation due to bowel dysmotility is a common problem in the medically ill. Many patients find that bowel movements are facilitated by the upright seated position, and this may be an important goal of rehabilitation. Increased mobilization enhances bowel motility and may be a part of a multimodal strategy for constipation, which commonly includes increased fluid intake, fiber consumption, and laxatives (99). Patients with neurogenic

bowel due to a lesion of the spinal cord, cauda equina, or pelvic nerves may benefit from other techniques, such as stimulation of anorectal mucosa and the use of either suppositories or digital stimulation (100,101). With fecal impaction, digital extraction may be necessary (102).

Management of ostomies includes dietary manipulation, control of fluid intake, drug therapies (laxatives or constipating drugs), and appropriate local stoma care. The goal of appropriate care is to produce a controlled effluent and to minimize odor and soiling. A pouch may be worn to prevent soiling of clothes and to collect feces and urine. Patients should avoid wearing constrictive clothing.

## Swallowing and Speech Therapies

The stages of swallowing are the oral phase, the pharyngeal phase, and the esophageal phase, each of which is defined by where the bolus of food is located. A swallowing disorder can arise from neurologic dysfunction or a structural lesion that causes problems with any or all of these stages. A variety of rehabilitative approaches can be used to cope with dysphagia (103–105). The risk of aspiration may be lessened by different textures of food or liquids and by head and body positioning (such as a chin tuck) that help protect the airway.

The manner of oral intake also may be modified to reduce the risk of aspiration. In the supraglottic swallow, the patient holds the breath before and during the swallow and coughs at its completion, decreasing risk of aspiration. The use of a smaller bolus of food or multiple swallows per bolus can help clear the pharyngeal area. Vocal cord adduction exercises may be performed to improve airway closure and protection. Prosthodontic appliances may be required for patients who have undergone resection of part of the oral swallowing mechanism. For example, a palatal augmentation prosthesis adds bulk to the hard palate, which may enhance tongue-to-hard-palate contact following partial glossectomy (106).

Rehabilitative techniques may be used to address disorders of language. Language abilities may be improved by melodic intonation therapy and alternative communication techniques. In melodic intonation therapy, the patient produces verbal communication within the framework of a familiar tune to facilitate word production (107). Alternative communication techniques comprise a variety of nonverbal methods, such as a communication board with pictures, letters, or words.

Dysarthria may arise from neurologic insult or structural damage. Patients with hypernasal speech may benefit from a palatal lift, which decreases nasal air emission. A palatal obturator may be used to fill a surgical defect of the hard palate. Techniques of pausing or rate control may be used to maximize speech production (108). Vocal cord adduction exercises may improve dysphonia after unilateral vocal cord paralysis.

Patients who undergo laryngectomy or tracheostomy may be aphonic or dysphonic. Several methods of voice production are available. An electrolarynx creates vibrations, which can be transmitted to the oral cavity either via an oral tube or by transmission through soft tissue when placed on the neck (109). Tracheoesophageal puncture uses a small voice prosthesis inserted into a fistula between the trachea and esophagus (110). The patient may also be instructed in esophageal speech (111). In all cases, extensive speech therapy is required for proper training.

## THE BENEFITS OF REHABILITATION

Rehabilitation interventions are at times overlooked and underutilized even in the supportive oncology setting. The rehabilitation team may help improve a patient's overall function as well as assist in the management of symptoms. These interventions can have a great impact on the patient's quality of life. Even in the patient with a short life expectancy, functional improvements can also benefit the patient's family and other caregivers. They can also help the patient be more capable of putting personal and social affairs in order at the end of life.

## REFERENCES

1. Dietz JH Jr. *Rehabilitation oncology.* New York: John Wiley & Sons, 1981:1.
2. World Health Organization (WHO). *International classification of impairments, disabilities, and handicaps—a manual of classification relating to the consequences of disease.* Geneva: World Health Organization, 1980:1.
3. Groher ME. Management: general principles and guidelines. *Dysphagia* 1991;6:67.
4. Darley FL, Aronson AE, Brown JR. *Motor speech disorders.* Philadelphia: WB Saunders Co., 1975:1.
5. Akeson WH, Amiel D, Abel MF, Garfin SR, Woo S L-Y. Effects of immobilization on joints. *Clin Orthop Rel Res* 1987;219:28.
6. Cronin ME, Miller FW, Plotz PH. Polymyositis and dermatomyositis. In: Schumacher HR Jr, ed. *Primer on the rheumatic diseases,* 9th ed. Atlanta: Arthritis Foundation, 1988:120.
7. Posner JB. Paraneoplastic syndromes. *Neurol Clinic* 1991;9(4):919.
8. Patchell RA, Posner JB. Neurologic complications of systemic cancer. *Neurol Clin* 1985;3(4):729.
9. Rook JL, Green RF, Tunkel R, Lachmann E. Lower extremity weakness as the initial manifestation of lung cancer. *Arch Phys Med Rehabil* 1990;71:995.
10. Adams RD, Victor M. *Principles of neurology.* 4th ed. New York: McGraw-Hill, 1989:1.
11. Caldwell DS, McCallum RM. Rheumatologic manifestations of cancer. *Med Clin North Am* 1986;70(2):385.
12. Krey PR. *Arthropathies associated with hematologic disease and storage disorders.* In: Schumacher HR Jr, ed. *Primer on the rheumatic diseases.* 9th ed. Atlanta: Arthritis Foundation, 1988:220.
13. Altman RD, Gray RG. Bone disease. In: Katz WA, ed. *Diagnosis and management of rheumatic diseases.* 2nd ed. Philadelphia: JB Lippincott, 1988:620.
14. Simon MA. Limb salvage for osteosarcoma in the 1980's. *Clin Orthop* 1991;270:264.
15. Schuller DE, Reiches NA, Hamaker RC, et al. Analysis of disability resulting from treatment including radical neck dissection or modified neck dissection. *Head Neck Surg* 1983;6:551.
16. Remmler D, Byers R, Scheetz J, et al. A prospective study of shoulder disability resulting from radical and modified neck dissections. *Head Neck Surg* 1986;8:280.
17. Cailliet R. *Shoulder pain.* 3rd ed. Philadelphia: FA Davis, 1991:1.
18. Fialka V, Vinzenz K. Investigations into shoulder function after radical neck dissection. *J Cran Maxillofac Surg* 1988;16:143.
19. Sandler SG, Tobin W, Henderson ES. Vincristine-induced neuropathy. *Neurology* 1969;19:367.
20. LaRocca JV, Meer J, Gilliatt RW, et al. Suramin-induced polyneuropathy. *Neurology* 1990;40:954.
21. Kedar A, Cohen ME, Freeman AI. Peripheral neuropathy as a complication of cis-dichlorodiammineplatinum (II) treatment: a case report. *Cancer Treat Rep* 1978;62:819.
22. Rowinsky EK, Eisenhauer EA, Chaudry V, Arbuck SG, Donehower RC. Clinical toxicities encountered with paclitaxel (Taxol). *Semin Oncol* 1993;20(4 Suppl 3):1.
23. David DS, Grieco MH, Cushman P. Adrenal glucocorticoids after twenty years. A review of their clinically relevant consequences. *J Chron Dis* 1970;22:637.
24. Dorwart BB. Arthropathies associated with endocrine diseases. In: Schumacher HR Jr, ed. *Primer on the rheumatic diseases.* 9th ed. Atlanta: Arthritis Foundation, 1988:217.
25. Vallbona C. Bodily responses to immobilization. In: Kottke FJ, Stillwell GK, Lehmann JF, eds. *Krusen's handbook of physical medicine and rehabilitation.* 3rd ed. Philadelphia: WB Saunders, 1982:963.
26. Halar EM, Bell KR. Contracture and other deleterious effects of immobility. In: DeLisa JA, ed. *Rehabilitation medicine—principles and practice,* 2nd ed. Philadelphia: JB Lippincott, 1993:681.
27. Müeller EA. Influence of training and of inactivity on muscle strength. *Arch Phys Med Rehabil* 1970;51:449.
28. Heaney RP. Radiocalcium metabolism in disuse osteoporosis in man. *Am J Med* 1962;33:188.
29. Mundy GR, Ibbotson KJ, D'Souza SM, Simpson EL, Jacobs JW, Martin TJ. The hypercalcemia of cancer. Clinical implications and pathogenic mechanisms. *N Engl J Med* 1984;310:1718.
30. Saltin B, Blomqvist G, Mitchell JH, Johnson RL Jr, Wildenthal K, Chapmann CB. Response to exercise after bed rest and after training. *Circulation* 38(Suppl VII):1968:1.
31. Halar EM, Bell KR. Rehabilitation's relationship to inactivity. In: Kottke FJ, Lehmann JF, eds. *Krusen's handbook of physical medicine and rehabilitation.* 4th ed. Philadelphia: WB Saunders, 1990:1113.
32. Saltin B, Rowell LB. Functional adaptations to physical activity and inactivity. *Fed Proc* 1980;39:1506.
33. Browse NL. *The physiology and pathology of bed rest.* Springfield, IL: CC Thomas, 1965:1.
34. Naschitz JE, Yerurun D, Lev LM. Thromboembolism in cancer. Changing trends. *Cancer* 1993;71(4):1384.
35. National Institutes of Health Consensus Development Conference. Prevention of venous thrombosis and pulmonary embolism. *JAMA* 1986;256:744.
36. Kosiak M, Kottke FJ. Prevention and rehabilitation of ischemic ulcers. In: Kottke FJ, Lehmann JF, eds. *Krusen's handbook of physical medicine and rehabilitation.* 4th ed. Philadelphia: WB Saunders, 1990:976.
37. deLateur BJ, Lehmann JF. Therapeutic exercise to develop strength and endurance. In: Kottke FJ, Lehmann JF, eds. *Krusen's handbook of physical medicine and rehabilitation.* 4th ed. Philadelphia: WB Saunders, 1990:480.
38. Spielholz NI. Scientific basis of exercise programs. In: Basmajian JV, Wolf SL, eds. *Therapeutic exercise.* 5th ed. Baltimore: Williams & Wilkins, 1990:49.
39. Nagler W. *Manual for physical therapy technicians.* Chicago: Yearbook Medical Publishers, 1974:1.
40. DeLorme TL. Restoration of muscle power by heavy-resistance exercises. *J Bone Joint Surg* 1945;27(A):645.
41. Kendall FP, McKreary EK. *Muscles—testing and function.* 3rd ed. Baltimore: Williams & Wilkins, 1983:1.
42. Davis AE, Lee RG. EMG biofeedback in patients with motor disorders: an aid for co-ordinating activity in antagonistic muscle groups. *J Can Sci Neurol* 1980;7:199.
43. Wolf SL, Baker MP, Kelly JL. EMG biofeedback in stroke: a 1-year follow-up of the effect on patient characteristics. *Arch Phys Med Rehabil* 1980;61:351.
44. Kraft GH. New methods for the assessment and treatment of the hemiplegic arm and hand. *Phys Med Rehabil Clin North Am* 1991;2:579.

45. Baker LL, Parker K. Neuromuscular electrical stimulation of the muscles surrounding the shoulder. *Phys Ther* 1986;66:1930.

46. Garrison SJ, Rolak LA. Rehabilitation of the stroke patient. In: DeLisa JA, ed. *Rehabilitation medicine—principles and practice.* 2nd ed. Philadelphia: JB Lippincott, 1993:801.

47. Shindo N, Jones R. Reciprocal patterned electrical stimulation of the lower limbs in severe spasticity. *Physiotherapy* 1987;73:579.

48. Bajd T, Gregoric M, Vodovinik L, Benko H. Electrical stimulation in treating spasticity resulting from spinal cord injury. *Arch Phys Med Rehabil* 1985;66:515.

49. Basmajian JV. Biofeedback in rehabilitation medicine. In: DeLisa JA, ed. *Rehabilitation medicine—principles and practice.* 2nd ed. Philadelphia: JB Lippincott, 1993:425.

50. Little JW, Massagli TL. Spasticity and associated abnormalities of muscle tone. In: DeLisa JA, ed. *Rehabilitation medicine—principles and practice.* 2nd ed. Philadelphia: JB Lippincott, 1993:666.

51. Ditunno JF, Formal CS. Chronic spinal cord injury. *N Engl J Med* 1994;330:550.

52. Diener HC, Dichgans J. Pathophysiology of cerebellar ataxia [Review]. *Move Disorders* 1992;7(2):95.

53. Torg E, Rogers K, Torg JS. Walking for health. *Contemp Orthop* 1989; 19(3):253.

54. Hicks JE. Exercise for cancer patients. In: Basmajian JV, Wolf SL, eds. *Therapeutic exercise.* Baltimore: Williams & Wilkins, 1990: 351.

55. Kottke FJ, Pauley DL, Ptak RA. The rationale for prolonged stretching for correction of shortening of connective tissue. *Arch Phys Med Rehabil* 1966;47:345.

56. Lehmann JF, Masock AJ, Warren CG, Koblanski JN. Effect of therapeutic temperatures on tendon extensibility. *Arch Phys Med Rehabil* 1970;51:481.

57. Zander CL, Healy NL. Elbow flexion contracture treated with serial casts and conservative therapy. *J Hand Surg [Am]* 1992;17(4):694.

58. Elmwood PM Jr. Transfers—method, equipment, and preparation. In: Kottke FJ, Lehmann JF, eds. *Krusen's handbook of physical medicine and rehabilitation.* 4th ed. Philadelphia: WB Saunders, 1990:529.

59. Pedretti LW, Stone G. Wheelchairs and wheelchair transfers. In: Pedretti LW, Zoltan B, eds. *Occupational therapy—practice skills for physical dysfunction.* 3rd ed. St. Louis: CV Mosby, 1990:380.

60. Joyce BM, Kirby RL. Canes, crutches and walkers. *Am Fam Pract* 1991;43(2):535.

61. Hewer RL, Cooper R, Morgan MH. An investigation into the value of treating intention tremor by weighting the affected extremity. *Brain* 1972;95:579.

62. Nance PW, Kirby RL. Rehabilitation of an adult with disabilities due to congenital sensory neuropathy. *Arch Phys Med Rehabil* 1985;66:123.

63. Esquenazi A, Hirai B. Assessment of gait and orthotic prescription. *Phys Med Rehabil Clin North Am* 1991;2(3):473.

64. Corcoran PJ, Jebsen RH, Brengelmann GL, Simons BC. Effects of plastic and metal leg braces on speed and energy cost of hemiparetic ambulation. *Arch Phys Med Rehabil* 1970;51:69.

65. Steinberg FU. Rehabilitating the older stroke patient: what's possible? *Geriatrics* 1986;41(3):85.

66. Spencer JC. The physical environment and performance. In: Christiansen C, Baum C, eds. *Occupational therapy: overcoming human performance deficits.* Thorofare: Slack Incorporated, 1991:126.

67. Trombly CA. Activities of Daily Living. In: Trombly CA, ed. *Occupational therapy for physical dysfunction.* 2nd ed. Baltimore: Williams & Wilkins, 1983:58.

68. Fidler MW, Plasmans CMT. The effect of four types of support on the segmental mobility of the lumbosacral spine. *J Bone Joint Surg* 1983; 65A:943.

69. Nagel D, Koogle T, Piziali RL, Perkash I. Stability of the upper lumbar spine following progressive disruptions and the application of individual internal and external fixation devices. *J Bone Joint Surg* 1981;63A:62.

70. Fisher SV. Cervical orthotics. *Phys Med Rehabil Clin North Am* 1992; 3:29.

71. Leonard JA Jr, Meier RH III. Upper and lower extremity prosthetics. In: DeLisa JA, ed. *Rehabilitation medicine—principles and practice.* 2nd ed. Philadelphia: JB Lippincott, 1993:507.

72. Michael J. Energy storing feet: a clinical comparison. *Clin Prosthet Orthop* 1987;11:154.

73. Freidmann LW. Rehabilitation of the lower extremity amputee. In:

Kottke FJ, Lehmann JF, eds. *Krusen's handbook of physical medicine and rehabilitation.* 4th ed. Philadelphia: WB Saunders, 1990:1024.

74. Patt RB. Classification of cancer pain and cancer pain syndromes. In: Patt RB, ed. *Cancer pain.* Philadelphia: JB Lippincott, 1993:3.

75. Basford JR. Physical agents. In: DeLisa JA, ed. *Rehabilitation medicine—principles and practice.* 2nd ed. Philadelphia: JB Lippincott, 1993:404.

76. Melzack R, Wall PD. Pain mechanisms—a new theory. *Science* 1965; 150:971.

77. Travell JG, Simons DG. Myofascial pain and dysfunction. *The trigger point manual,* vol I. Baltimore: Williams & Wilkins, 1983:1.

78. Hirsh J. Antithrombotic therapy in deep vein thrombosis and pulmonary embolism. *Am Heart J* 1992;123(4 Pt 2):1115.

79. Hull RD, Raskob GE, Pineo GF, et al. Subcutaneous low-molecular-weight heparin compared with continuous intravenous heparin in the treatment of proximal-vein thrombosis. *N Engl J Med* 1992;326(15):975.

80. Turpie AGG, Hirsch J. Venous thromboembolism: current concepts (Part 2). *Hosp Med* 1984;20:13.

81. Husni EZ, Ximenes JOC, Goyette EM. Elastic support of the lower limbs in hospital patients. *JAMA* 1970;214:1456.

82. Hammond MC, Merli GJ, Zierler RE. Rehabilitation of the patient with peripheral vascular disease of the lower extremity. In: DeLisa JA, ed. *Rehabilitation medicine—principles and practice.* 2nd ed. Philadelphia: JB Lippincott, 1993:1082.

83. Hull RD, Raskob GF, Rosenbloom D, et al. Heparin for 5 days as compared with 10 days in the initial treatment of proximal venous thrombosis. *N Engl J Med* 1990;322(18):1260.

84. Passik S, Newman M, Brennan M, Holland J. Psychiatric consultation for women undergoing rehabilitation for upper extremity lymphedema following breast cancer treatment. *J Pain Sympt Manag* 1993;8(4):226.

85. International Society of Lymphology Executive Committee. The diagnosis and treatment of peripheral lymphedema. *Lymphology* 1995;28: 113–117.

86. Vernick SH, Shapiro D, Shaw FD. Leg orthosis for venous and lymphatic insufficiency. *Arch Phys Med Rehabil* 1987;68:459.

87. Zeissler RH, Rose GB, Nelson PA. Postmastectomy lymphedema: late results of treatment in 385 patients. *Arch Phys Med Rehabil* 1972; 53:159.

88. Zanolla R, Monzeglio C, Balzarini A, Martino G. Evaluation of the results of three different methods of postmastectomy lymphedema treatment. *J Surg Oncol* 1984;26:210.

89. Zelikovski A, Manoach M, Giler SH, Urca I. Lympha-Press: A new pneumatic device for the treatment of lymphedema of the limbs. *Lymphology* 1980;13:68.

90. Klein MJ, Alexander MA, Wright JM, Redmond CK, LeGasse AA. Treatment of adult lower extremity lymphedema with Wright linear pump: statistical analysis of a clinical trial. *Arch Phys Med Rehabil* 1988;69:202.

91. Foldi E, Foldi M, Weissleder H. Conservative treatment of lymphedema of the limbs. *Angiol J Vasc Dis* 1985;36:171.

92. Steinberg FU. *The immobilized patient: functional pathology and management.* New York: Plenum Medical Books, 1980:1.

93. Helmholz HF Jr, Stonnington HH. Rehabilitation for respiratory dysfunction. In: Kottke FJ, Lehman JF, eds. *Krusen's handbook of physical medicine and rehabilitation.* 4th ed. Philadelphia: WB Saunders, 1990:858.

94. Coffin Zadai C. Therapeutic exercises in pulmonary disease and disability. In: Basmajian JV, Wolf SL, eds. *Therapeutic exercise.* 5th ed. Baltimore: Williams & Wilkins, 1990:405.

95. Brechtelsbauer DA. Care with an indwelling urinary catheter. Tips for avoiding problems in independent and institutionalized patients. *Postgrad Med* 1992;92:127.

96. Cancio LC, Sabanegh ES, Thompson IM. Managing the Foley catheter. *Am Fam Pract* 1983;48(5):829.

97. Freed MM. Traumatic and congenital lesions of the spinal cord. In: Kottke FJ, Lehmann JF, eds. *Krusen's handbook of physical medicine and rehabilitation.* 4th ed. Philadelphia: WB Saunders, 1990:717.

98. Naso F. Cardiovascular problems in patients with spinal cord injury. *Phys Med Rehabil Clin North Am* 1992;3(4):741.

99. Portenoy RK. Constipation in the cancer patient. *Med Clin North Am* 1987;71:303.

100. Weingarden SI. The gastrointestinal system and spinal cord injury. *Phys Med Rehabil Clin North Am* 1992;3(4):765.

101. Lennard-Jones JE. Clinical aspects of laxatives, enemas, and suppositories. In: Kamm MA, Lennard-Jones JE, eds. *Constipation*. Petersfield: UK, Wrightson Biomedical, 1994:327.

102. Wrenn K. Fecal impaction. *N Engl J Med* 1989;321:658.

103. Aguilar NV, Olson ML, Shedd DP. Rehabilitation of deglutition problems in patients with head and neck cancer. *Am J Surg* 1979;138:501.

104. Neumann S. Swallowing therapy with neurologic patients: results of direct and indirect therapy methods in 66 patients suffering from neurological disorders. *Dysphagia* 1993;8:150.

105. Linden-Castelli P. Treatment strategies for adult neurogenic dysphagia. *Semin Speech Lang* 1991;12:255.

106. Robbins KT, Bowman JB, Jacob RF. Postglossectomy deglutitory and articulatory rehabilitation with palatal augmentation prostheses. *Arch Otolaryngol Head Neck Surg* 1987;113(11):1214.

107. Sparks RW. Melodic intonation therapy. In: Chapey R, ed. *Language intervention strategies in adult aphasia*. Baltimore: Williams & Wilkins, 1981:265.

108. Yorkston KM, Beukelman DR, Bell KR. Clinical management of dysarthric speaker. Boston: College-Hill Press, 1988:1.

109. Lerman JW. The artificial larynx. In: Salmon SJ, Mount KH, eds. *Alaryngeal speech rehabilitation for clinicians by clinicians*. Austin: Pro-ed, 1991:27.

110. Wenig BL, Mullooly V, Levy J, Abramson AL. Voice restoration following laryngectomy: the role of primary versus secondary tracheoesophageal puncture. *Ann Otol Rhinol Laryngol* 1989;98(1 Pt 1):70.

111. Duguay MJ. Esophageal speech training: the initial phase. In: Salmon SJ, Mount KH, eds. *Alaryngeal speech rehabilitation for clinicians by clinicians*. Austin: Pro-ed, 1991:47.

*Principles and Practice of Supportive Oncology,*
edited by Ann Berger et al.
Lippincott–Raven Publishers, Philadelphia ©1998

CHAPTER 49

# Communication Disorders

Steven B. Leder

Communication, especially verbal communication, receives very little attention in everyday life. Why should attention be directed at something everyone does with such ease? All human societies, in fact, have used speech and found it to be the most convenient form of communication (1). Most people rarely think, however, about not being able to speak, or suddenly having a speech mechanism that does not function as efficiently as it used to, or not being able to hear as well as they did. This, unfortunately, is exactly what happens when a surgical resection involves the structures of the mouth or larynx, a tracheotomy is performed for airway maintenance, or chemotherapy or external beam radiation therapy affects auditory acuity.

Speech communication is far more than just the obvious movement of lips and tongue. It is a highly complex phenomenon that takes place between a speaker and listener. It encompasses linguistic encoding and decoding (the message), physiologic commands (neural and muscle activity), and acoustic features (the sound wave). Overlaid on this system is individual speaker variability, i.e., different people do not produce the same sound waves when pronouncing the same word. In fact, the same speaker does not even produce identical sound waves when pronouncing the same word on different occasions.

How, then, is speech understood? The listener does not rely solely on information from the acoustic features in the sound wave. Knowledge of the rules specific to a particular language and speech system, cues provided by context, and the identity of the speaker are all used to decode the speech signal. Speech communication, therefore, relies on a great number of ambiguous and, most importantly, redundant cues, not on a precise knowledge of a limited number of specific cues (1). This is the only way millions of different speakers producing many mil-

lions of different sound waves can be understood by millions of different listeners.

A basic understanding of speech acoustics and phonology is essential in understanding both the difficulties encountered by cancer patients who, by necessity, have altered speech production mechanisms, and how and why voice and speech restoration rehabilitation are successful.

Communication is the essence of a person's personality and social identity (2). The goal of all communication rehabilitation following cancer treatment is to reinstate, as well as possible, verbal communication so the person can be accepted and not stigmatized by society. Speaking, rather than nonverbal communication (lipreading, communication boards, writing or typing, or computerized augmentative communication systems) is the preferred mode for receptive and expressive communication. Speaking is accepted best by the individual and family, when possible is the most efficient and easiest to use, and maintains a familiar link with the pretreatment life with which the individual was familiar.

Meaningful and understandable communication is greatly needed following a diagnosis of cancer. Communication is critical to a patient's medical care, psychological functioning, and social interactions (3,4). When communication breaks down between the patient and health care professionals, the patient's ability to participate meaningfully in the health care plan is greatly restricted (5,6), and recovery and rehabilitation may be adversely affected (2).

This chapter will review the basic anatomy and physiology of speech production, discuss speech acoustics and phonology, and explore the ways cancer and its treatment affect the individual's ability to maintain verbal communication skills. It will also discuss extensive rehabilitation methods whose goal is to reinstate verbal communication skills for the individual. In addition, the chapter will consider the importance of hearing, its potential loss following cancer therapy, and rehabilitation strategies with the goal of maintaining optimal verbal communication.

S. B. Leder: Department of Surgery, Section of Otolaryngology, Yale University School of Medicine, New Haven, CT 06520-8041.

## THE PRODUCTION AND PERCEPTION OF SPEECH

### Anatomy and Physiology

Speech, swallowing, and breathing are different types of behaviors that share the same anatomical structures. Swallowing and breathing are very old evolutionary behaviors and occur in all animals. Speech is a recent evolutionary behavior and occurs only in humans (7). The shared anatomical structures that move and are involved in speech production are called the articulators: the lips, tongue, teeth, mandible, velum, pharynx, and larynx. Other shared anatomical structures are the oral and nasal cavities, which provide resonance, and the lungs and diaphragm, which provide the air supply and driving force without which normal speech would be impossible. Although the exact neural controls for speech production are not known, the neural controls for swallowing and speech also overlap, and the reader is referred to Chapter 10 on dysphagia for a more detailed discussion of the neural innervation of shared structures.

Speaking is a highly complex motor skill that consists of coordinated movements of the articulators—the lips, tongue, and teeth—upon the air generated from the lungs (7). With reference to speech, the vocal tract is defined by the larynx inferiorly and includes the pharynx, oral cavity, and nasal cavity superiorly. Any mass change, as with a tumor, or insult, as with a surgical resection or denervation, to the vocal tract or articulators may affect voice production (the sound source, voice quality, and resonance) and speech production (consonant and vowel articulation). Depending on the cancer treatment required, the person's ability to communicate verbally will be affected mildly to severely to totally.

The speech-language pathologist's role is to diagnose the communication disorder and provide optimal rehabilitation after treatment, with the goal of having the patient acquire verbal communication skills that are as nearly normal as possible. Realistic goals, sometimes requiring interim steps, are presented to the patient. Success at each step is stressed to help the patient stay motivated and help prevent depression. All types of communication, such as writing or lipreading, are used initially so as to connect the patient to the environment and foster participation in the rehabilitation plan as quickly as possible.

### PHYSIOLOGY OF SOUND

Sound originates from the disturbance of the position of molecules by a vibrating object, which causes a local change in pressure. The vibration of an object is not sound, but rather the source of sound. The local change in pressure produces a pressure differential near the sound source in comparison with the environmental or ambient pressure. This is an unnatural physical situation, which cannot remain. For example, when you clap your hands, a sudden compression of air between your hands is created. The air pressure is higher there than elsewhere. Pressure differences always move from high to low. Because the environmental air pressure will attempt to equalize, the high-pressure area near your hands begins to move rapidly through the surrounding air as a compressional wave. A compressional wave, however, is not the only possible kind of sound wave. It is also possible to have a wave of rarefaction, as is produced when you create a partial vacuum in your mouth and opening your lips with a "kissing" sound. Therefore, sound is a pressure wave propagating through a material medium: solid, liquid, or gas (1). Air is the usual medium that propagates sound from the source, i.e., the speaker, to the receiver, i.e., the listener.

The way in which a sound-pressure wave moves through air is illustrated by a series of connected balls and springs (Fig. 1). Wave motion starts when an outside event causes either a compression or a stretching of one spring. The wave then passes along the ball-and-spring chain. Although the balls move, they stay in the same approximate location and do not get carried along by the wave. A sound wave does not cause a flow of air (wind) but only a temporary local disturbance of air molecules. Sound in speech is due to the action of the vocal folds on the air that is forced out of the lungs. The respiratory muscles compress the air in the lungs. When the vocal folds are adducted, pressure is built up subglottally, and when there is sufficient pressure the vocal folds are forced apart, releasing the lung air. The release of this air acts like a sharp tap on the column of air in the vocal tract and sets it into vibration. It is important to realize that vocal fold vibrations in and of themselves are not sufficient to initiate vibrations that will be heard as sounds. The tap and resultant vibration of the vocal folds in the vocal tract cause the sound. The vocal tract will vibrate,

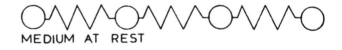

MEDIUM AT REST

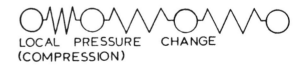

LOCAL PRESSURE CHANGE
(COMPRESSION)

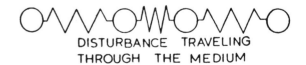

DISTURBANCE TRAVELING
THROUGH THE MEDIUM

**FIG 1.** Sound-pressure wave propagation. (8)

or resonate, at its own natural frequencies: the formant frequencies. This is why male voices are lower in pitch than female voices and also why individuals have specific and easily identifiable voice quality charateristics. The rate at which the vocal folds are blown apart and their tension determine the pitch of the sound, although there will be no change in the resonant or formant frequencies.

When a vowel is produced, the vocal fold vibrations at the glottis produce air molecule disturbances, and the sounds produced by these vibrations are shaped by the vocal tract to produce the desired vowel. When the vocal tract is closed, as with a stop plosive, e.g., /p,d/, or constricted, as with a fricative, e.g., /s,v/, turbulence is created as the air molecules are either forcefully released or directed through a narrower opening. The desired consonant is produced and propagated to the outside air to be decoded by the listener.

A sound with only one frequency is called a pure tone (Fig. 2). The zero line stands for the atmospheric or ambient pressure present before passage of the sound wave. The maximum height the wave rises from the zero line represents the amplitude of the wave. This corresponds to the maximum excess pressure present in the sound wave. A sound wave with a large pressure amplitude exerts a larger force on a receiver (such as a microphone or tympanic membrane) than a wave with a small pressure amplitude, i.e., a louder sound intensity.

Speech sounds are not pure tones but mixtures that consist of many pure tones simultaneously. The acoustic characteristics of these complex sounds are described in terms of the frequencies that are present and their relative amplitudes. When tones of different frequencies are mixed, the sound-pressure wave is no longer a pure sine wave. The sound pressures of the component pure tones add together at each successive instant, making a composite sound-pressure wave (Fig. 3). Notice the instants of time at the dotted lines A and B. At point A the positive pressure (compression) of the top wave is canceled by the negative pressure (rarefaction) of the bottom wave. At point B the waves reinforce each other. The sound-pressure pattern of a complex wave is the sum of the positive and negative pressures of the component frequencies. The components,

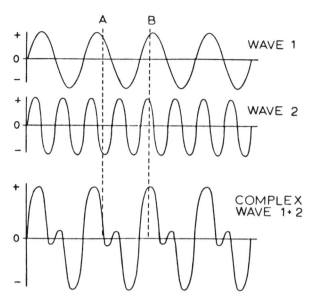

FIG. 3. Composite sound-pressure wave from component sine waves. (From ref. 8.)

when added together, produce a wave identical to the complex wave that makes human speech possible.

## Speech Perception

The frequency components that constitute a complex sound—speech—correspond to specific places on the basilar membrane. Since the cochlea is tonotopically organized, with the high frequencies at the basal turn and low frequencies at the apical turn, different sounds stimulate neurons at different locations. The spectrogram (Fig. 4) shows the frequency (ordinate), time (abscissa), and amplitude (darkness of shading) of the phrase "Say /ikak/ again." This visual representation of the spoken phrase contains the acoustic and phonetic cues that, when combined with the listener's knowledge of the rules of the language, will allow for decoding and understanding of the message. (See refs. 9 and 10 for a more comprehensive discussion of clinical spectrography of speech.)

## Formants and Vowels

In speech, a formant is a local maximum: a frequency at which vocal-tract transmission is more efficient than at nearby frequencies. Formant frequencies are resonances of the vocal tract and are formed by the physical properties of the vocal tract. Formants are numbered from low to high frequencies: first formant (F1), second formant (F2), third formant (F3), etc. The frequency locations and transitions associated with F1 and F2 are determined by the vocal tract length and shape. Vowels are formed by vocal tract shapes and differ by their characteristic areas of high energy at specific frequencies. The formants F1

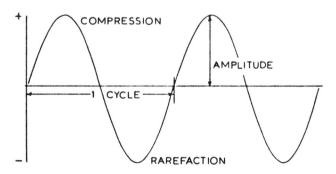

FIG. 2. Sine wave. (From ref. 8.)

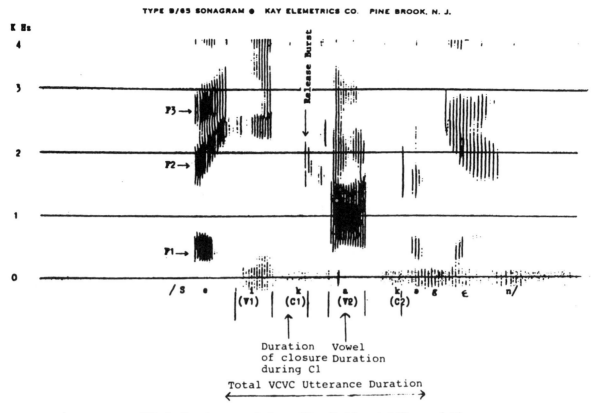

**FIG. 4.** Spectrogram of phrase "Say /ikak/ again." (From ref. 8.)

and F2 and their transitions (movements over time) contribute significantly to both vowel identification and the identification of the preceding stop consonant's place of articulation: /b/ versus /d/ versus /g/ (7,11). The frequency of F3 is related to only a small number of speech sounds, such as the lateral and retroflex glides /l,r/. The higher formants, F4 and F5, maintain a constant position regardless of vocal tract shape.

Vowel-formant-frequency locations for F1 and F2 are determined by the length of the pharyngeal-oral components of the vocal tract, the location of constrictions in the vocal tract, and the degree of narrowness of the constrictions (7,12). Theoretically, a vocal tract has an infinite variety of shapes to produce a given formant frequency. In general, however, five vocal tract shape rules can describe the front and back vowels (9):

1. Length: The longer the vocal tract, the lower the formants.
2. Lip rounding: All formants are lowered by lip rounding.
3. Anterior oral constriction: Anterior lingual elevation lowers F1 and raises F2.
4. Posterior oral constriction: Posterior lingual elevation lowers F2.
5. Pharyngeal constriction: Narrowing the pharynx raises F1.

When the anatomy of the vocal tract is altered, as after surgical resection for cancer, the formants—and therefore the vowels—are affected. The redundacy of the cues inherent in speech permit intelligible verbal communication despite the alteration. The more the vocal tract and articulators are changed, however, the more unintelligible speech becomes.

**Consonants**

Broadly speaking, consonants can be divided into three categories: (a) stop consonants, (b) continuants, and (3) voicing, that is, voiced or voiceless (7). Stop consonants require a complete closure of the vocal tract followed by a release burst as the vocal folds are blown apart by subglottic air pressure. The release burst causes a fast change in amplitude, as is seen in /k/ on the spectrogram (Fig. 4). Continuants, such as /f,l,s/, have only partial closure of the vocal tract, have no sudden release, and have a gradual increase in amplitude. The rate of amplitude increase and the duration of the sound aid in its discrimination.

The time when the vocal folds start their periodic vibrating in relation to the point of constriction in the vocal tract determines the voicing of sounds, for example, /p/ versus /b/. One vocal fold vibration corresponds to one vertical striation on the spectrogram (Fig. 4). The time between the vocal tract release burst and the onset of voicing is called voice-onset-time, and it is an important cue to the recognition of top consonants (13,14). Voiced stop consonants have almost simultaneous voicing and release bursts, while vocal fold vibration in voiceless stop consonants may start 60 msec following the release burst.

No one acoustic feature is necessary or sufficient for discrimination. Rather, the redundancy of the input allows the listener to perceive the correct target sound. The listener hears a sound and, among other acoustic features, is able to discriminate between sudden and gradual amplitude changes, duration differences, periodic versus aperiodic sounds, formant frequency characteristics (positions and transitions), and voice onset time, before determining what phoneme the sound actually represents.

## Phonemes and Allophones

The speech sounds that differentiate words are called phonemes. For example, the three words *pit*, *hit*, and *sit* consist of a sequence of three sounds that differ only by the first sound. However, the initial sound (phoneme) is sufficient to change the meaning of the words. Therefore, a phoneme is the smallest unit of sound that changes the meaning of a word in a language.

If the meaning of the words were not changed, the three sounds /p,h,s/ would be called allophones: variants of the same phoneme. In English, however, /p,h,s/ are not variants of the same phoneme. An example of allophones of the phoneme /t/ is in the words *top*, *stop*, and *pot*. In *top*, the initial /t/ is aspirated slightly. In *stop*, the /st/ blend results in more aspiration of the /t/. In *pot*, the final /t/ is not aspirated at all. However, the aspirated or nonaspirated /t/ is interchangeable in English, as the meanings of the three words are not changed depending on which one is used—for example, it is possible to aspirate the final /t/ in *pot* without changing the meaning of the word. All three productions of /t/ are slightly different acoustically but do not change the meaning of the words. They are, therefore, allophones of the phoneme /t/.

Although phonemes and allophones comprise acoustic features, the acoustic features vary a great deal depending on the context of the adjacent speech sounds. This is called coarticulation (7). Briefly, coarticulation allows for phonemes and allophones to be produced and understood by capitalizing on the redundancy built into the speech code. A speaker rarely produces the articulatory gestures of the ideal phoneme as it would be articulated in isolation. For example, the tongue-tip phoneme /t/ is not produced at the exact same place on the alveolar ridge when it is articulated in the word *top* as it is in *tag* because the tongue is already moving posteriorly to articulate the linguavelar /g/ even before it moves towards the alveolar ridge to articulate the /t/. This is called anticipatory coarticulation. No such lingual anticipatory coarticulation movement is necessary when the next phoneme is the bilabial /p/.

Without the five general vocal tract rule shapes for vowels, consonant coarticulation resulting in the production of phonemes and allophones, and the wonderful redundancy of the encoding and decoding system utilized by the human brain, speech would not be as rapid, fluent, or intelligible as it is.

## Distinctive Features

Different acoustic features correspond to different articulatory features, and the acoustic features form the basis for distinguishing perceptually one phoneme or allophone from another on the basis of their role in the language system, i.e., changing or not changing the meaning of a word. The relations between articulatory, acoustic, and perceptual features form a theory of distinctive features (7). The goal of distinctive features theory is to provide a single consistent framework for delineating the phonology of a language.

Consonants can be broadly categorized by these distinctive features: the place of articulation, the manner of production, and the voicing feature. Place of articulation is where anatomically in the vocal tract the phoneme is produced. Manner of production is how the phoneme is

**TABLE 1.** *Consonant classifications*

| | | | Manner of production | | | |
| | | | Stop | | Fricative | |
| Place of articulation | Glide | Nasal | Voiced | Unvoiced | Voiced | Unvoiced |
| --- | --- | --- | --- | --- | --- | --- |
| Bilabial | w | m | b | p | | |
| Labiodental | | | | | v | f |
| Linguadental | | | | | τ | |
| Lingua-alveolar | j,l | n | d | t | z | s |
| Linguapalatal | r | | | | | |
| Linguavelar | | | g | k | | |
| Pharyngeal | | η | | | | |
| Glottal | | | | | | h |

**TABLE 2.** *Vowel classifications*

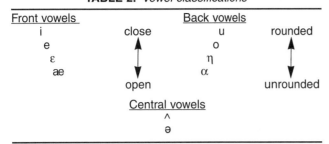

produced, e.g., by a totally constricted vocal tract as in the stop plosive /k/ or by a less constricted vocal tract as in the fricative /s/. Voicing refers to vocal fold vibration and is either voiced, with vibration, or voiceless, without vibration (Table 1). The sound source for consonants is either the vocal folds for voiced sounds or the articulators for voiceless sounds.

Vowels are different from consonants in two main ways: (a) vocal tract shaping and (b) the sound source. Vocal tract shaping is less constricted for vowels than for consonants, and tongue shape and position are critical for vowel production. This is shown in the vowel triangle (Table 2). The sound source for vowels is always periodic, as vocal fold vibration and an open—that is, not constricted—vocal tract is necessary for vowel production. Consonants, however, can be produced with a periodic, an aperiodic, or a combination of periodic and aperiodic waves, depending on the sound sources.

When the vocal tract and articulators are altered by surgical resection or irradiation, the distinctive features that differentiate the consonants and vowels are affected. More change results in greater speech difficulty and requires intensive rehabilitation to restore intelligible verbal communication.

## CLINICAL APPLICATIONS

### Head and Neck Cancer Resections and Reconstructions

The previous discussion regarding the physiology of sound, articulation, phonology of vowels, consonants, phonemes, and allophones, and distinctive features leads to the consequences of head and neck surgery on the vocal tract and articulators. The results of surgery and reconstruction as they affect and change speech production skills, verbal communication, and speech perception acceptability vary, but they affect all cases to some degree.

It should be kept in mind that as long as the intended target phoneme (consonant or vowel) is articulated with enough acoustic and distinctive features to be considered an allophone of the target phoneme, the meaning of the word is not be changed and the verbal message is consid-

ered to be encoded and decoded successfully. Ideally, the surgical resection, subsequent reconstruction, and appropriate rehabilitation will allow for intelligible verbal communication by maintaining at least the minimal redundant cues in the speech signal needed for successful verbal communication.

Unsuccessful verbal communication, however, results when the surgical resection has altered the vocal tract and/or articulators to such a degree that the inherent redundancy built into the speech code is so degraded that the target phoneme is decoded not as an allophone but either as a different phoneme, thus changing the meaning of the intended message, or as an unintelligible sound not considered part of the phonology of the target language, in this case English.

### Counseling

Nothing can fully prepare the patient for the consequences of head and neck cancer surgery. Combined with the emotion and fear inherent in the word *cancer* is the fear of major surgery and its consequences, the fear of losing the ability to communicate effectively, and the fear of becoming a social and psychological burden on the family. An in-depth discussion of the need for counseling, both preoperatively and postoperatively in the long term, appears in reference 2.

The speech-language pathologist offers preoperative counseling to discuss the surgery and its consequences and, just as importantly, the rehabilitation strategies that will be used to restore verbal communication skills to as nearly normal a state as possible. Illustrations and models are helpful in having the individual understand what impact the planned surgery may have on the speech production mechanism.

Counseling does not begin and end preoperatively. The immediate postoperative period, 1 to 14 days, presents problems that will not be encountered later on. Postoperative edema impairs articulation, and the patient should be reassured that this is a temporary condition. Sutures are frequently present, and localized pain may also reduce the proficiency of articulation. If the facial (C-VII), vagus (C-X), or glossopharyngeal (C-XII) nerves were involved in the surgical resection, paresis or numbness may be present, further impairing articulatory precision. Also, the patient's decreased motivation and sadness may make speech production worse in the immediate postoperative period than it will be in a few weeks' time. Counseling should continue postoperatively for as long as the patient needs it (2).

After the 2-week postoperative period, the patient is usually discharged home. Before discharge, the speech-language pathologist determines whether ongoing speech rehabilitation is required. If it is, additional goals are implemented to increase overall speech production skills and the intelligibility of speech, based on the surgical resections and the functioning of the remaining structures in the vocal tract. The patient is assured that articulation and speech intelligibility will improve with therapy. If there is a structural defect that can be compensated for with, for example, a palatal prosthesis, an appropriate referral to a prosthodontist is done as well.

## Speech Articulation Rehabilitation

The ultimate goal of rehabilitation is to return the patient to as nearly normal a life as possible, regardless of the amount of time that remains. Speech articulation rehabilitation following resection of the articulators and vocal tract focuses on compensatory articulation and stresses precise articulation. The goal of speech articulation therapy is to produce either the target phoneme or an allophone of the target phoneme so the word, and therefore the message, will be decoded correctly by the listener.

### Labial Resections

Labial resection can result in decreased lip rounding, affecting vowel production, for example /u/ (see Table 2), and labial closure, affecting articulation of bilabial /b,p,m,w/ and labiodental /f,v/ consonants.

### Anterior Tongue and Floor of Mouth Resections

Resection of the anterior tongue and floor of the mouth can result in decreased lingua-alveolar ridge contact, affecting the production of all consonants with this place of articulation: /t,d,s,z,n,l/, as well as linguadental phonemes /τ, /. The manner of articulation of these phonemes can also be impaired because of poor lingua-alveolar ridge contact. For example, inadequate lingua-alveolar pressure for the stop plosive phoneme /d/ will result in articulation of an /n/ or /l/ phoneme.

### Lateral Tongue Resection

Because of the redundancy built into the speech production mechanism and the decoding ability of the human brain, lateral tongue resections do not usually result in significant articulation errors that impair speech intelligibility. The remaining hemitongue is able to articulate allophones of the target phoneme. Lateral emission of air may occur after more extensive resection, especially if teeth are missing as well.

### Posterior Composite Resections

Posterior composite resections affecting more than one structure, such as the tongue and the mandible, can result in decreased lingual and mandibular range of motion and control, paresis, and decreased sensation, which can

affect vocal tract shape for vowels, and place and manner of articulation for consonants, especially the velar phonemes /k,g,η /.

### Hard and Soft Palate Resection

Hard and soft palate resection affects velopharyngeal closure, resulting in velopharyngeal insufficiency or oronasal fistulas. These defects may cause excessive hypernasal resonance because of the inability to separate the oral from the nasal cavities. The larger the surgical defect, the greater the inappropriate hypernasal resonance. All phonemes are affected, with stop plosive, fricative, and affricate phonemes—the pressure consonants—affected the most because of the inability to build up adequate intraoral air pressure for their articulation. For example, without adequate intraoral air pressure for the release burst, the stop plosive phonemes /p,b/ are articulated and perceived as the phoneme /m/, significantly impairing speech intelligibility.

### Partial Laryngectomy

There are several different types of partial laryngectomies (2). The following are done in the vertical plane: cordectomy via laryngofissure (15), hemilaryngectomy (16), vertical partial laryngectomy (17), anterofrontal and extended anterofrontal laryngectomy (15), and near-total laryngectomy (18,19). Voice production and voice quality following these operations is dependent on the extent of the laryngeal resection and the type of neoglottic reconstruction used (16). Therefore, this population demonstrates a range of vocal capabilities (20).

In general, partial laryngectomy results in hoarseness and possibly breathiness because of the resection, which usually includes one arytenoid cartilage and one true vocal fold, and reconstruction of the neoglottis with mucosa opposing the remaining true vocal fold. The resultant novel vibration of the remaining true vocal fold against mucosa results in a turbulent sound source, changing vocal tract resonance patterns and producing the voice disorder.

### Supraglottic Laryngectomy

The surgical procedure for a supraglottic laryngectomy is done in the horizontal plane. Candidates for a supraglottic laryngectomy are those with cancer of the epiglottis or ventricular vocal fold(s) without cancer extension across or into the ventricle or anterior commissure (15).

Supraglottic laryngectomy does not affect articulation or true vocal fold vibration, but may affect vocal tract resonance and voice quality because it alters the physical characteristics of the vocal tract. Specifically, the removal of the epiglottis, aryepiglottic folds, and false vocal folds in the pharynx alters the length and volume of the vocal tract and may change the resonant characteristics of the vocal tract. Information in this area is scarce. In one of the few studies reporting objective data on the phonatory results following supracricoid partial laryngectomy (21), it was found that the average fundamental frequency for the partial laryngectomy subjects was not significantly different from that for normal speakers. Additional data indicated that partial laryngectomy speech and voice production was less efficient than normal speech and voice production as evidenced by increased jitter, shimmer, and harmonics to noise ratio, and decreased maximum phonation time, speech rate, and phrase grouping.

*Metal and Plastic Tracheotomy Tubes*

The most disruptive change for the posttracheotomized patient is the loss of verbal communication (22–24). There are two major types of tracheotomy tubes: metal (stainless steel) and plastic. A metal (Jackson) tracheotomy tube is always cuffless. Inspiration occurs through the tube. Expiration occurs out of the tube when it is open and via the upper airway and out of the mouth and nose when the tube is occluded (Fig. 5). Plastic tracheotomy tubes can be either cuffed or cuffless. The cuff is an inflatable diaphragm attached around the distal end of the tube. When the cuff is inflated, expiration occcurs out of the tube, and when the cuff is deflated and the tracheotomy tube occluded, expiration must occur via the upper airway and out of the mouth and nose (Fig. 6). Both types of tracheotomy tubes have inner cannulas whose purpose is to facilitate maintaining hygiene and the patency of the tube itself (Figs. 5 and 6). In addition, both

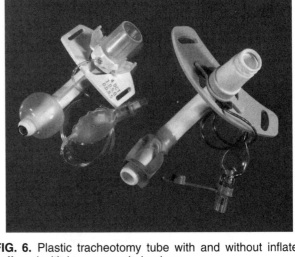

**FIG. 6.** Plastic tracheotomy tube with and without inflated cuff, and with inner cannula in place.

types of tubes can be fenestrated, i.e., by a hole or holes placed on the superior surface of the tracheotomy tube that resides in the trachea to allow for air to pass through into the upper airway.

A tracheotomy tube can be occluded with a finger, cork, or flapper valve. If there is an upper airway problem that prevents easy expiration out the mouth and nose, intermittent finger occlusion is used to allow for inspiration through the tube but then only for selected expiration via the upper airway during speech production. If there is no upper airway problem but a tracheotomy tube is required for airway maintenance, either short-term or long-term occlusion of the tube

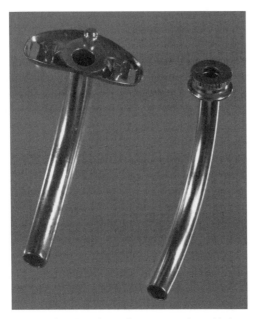

**FIG. 5.** Metal (Jackson) tracheotomy tube with inner cannula.

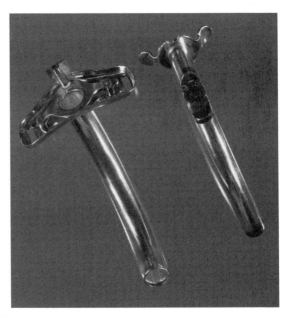

**FIG. 7.** Tucker tracheotomy tube with inner cannula containing one-way flapper valve.

with a cork is appropriate. This eliminates the need for occlusion of the tracheotomy tube with a finger during speech. A special type of metal tracheotomy tube is a Tucker tube (Fig. 7). This is a sterling silver tube with an inner cannula that contains a one-way flapper valve. The flapper valve allows inspiration through the tube but then passively closes during expiration, diverting air around the tube via the upper airway to be used for voice production or simply exhaled. The Tucker tube is used when a tracheotomy tube is required for a longer time.

### "Speaking" Tracheotomy Tube

The primary goal of a speaking tracheotomy tube is to allow cognitively intact ventilator-dependent patients to communicate verbally (22,25,26). The Portex "Talk" tracheotomy tube has been shown to be successful in allowing this population of patients to speak (26). It is a double-lumen, unfenestrated, single-cuffed tube designed with an external airflow line at the 9 o'clock position. Gas travels through the airflow line, exits via a slit just superior to the cuff, and then continues up through the glottis and vocal tract to allow for speech production (Fig. 8). The user can occlude the airflow line for independent speech production, or, if upper extremity paralysis or weakness prevents self-use, the listener can occlude the airflow line to allow for verbal communication.

### One-Way Tracheotomy Speaking Valves

A one-way tracheotomy speaking valve attaches to the external hub of a tracheotomy tube, usually plastic, and permits inspiration through the tracheotomy tube, but upon exhalation the tube is blocked and air must exit through the larynx and out the mouth or nose. The one-way valves eliminates the need for finger occlusion. It circumvents the problem of a patient not tolerating permanent occlusion of the tracheotomy tube with a cork when he or she has an upper airway restriction such as tracheal stenosis, laryngeal web, laryngomalacia, or arytenoid edema (27).

Rehabilitation with a one-way tracheotomy speaking valve is straightforward. The tracheotomy tube cuff, if present, must always be deflated with valve use to allow for expiration around the tube and through the glottis and upper airway. Most patients require only a short acclimation period with the valve. During this trial period, the patient is told that breathing, especially expiration, may feel different because of the valve. If the patient experiences difficulty in breathing, continued trial periods of valve use, increasing in length, should be done to habituate the patient to the valve. A pulse oximeter can be used to monitor arterial oxygen percent saturation (27).

There are four different commercially available one-way speaking tracheotomy valves: Kistner, Montgomery, Olympic, and Passy-Muir (Fig. 9). All have similar basic components, but they differ in their engineering and design. Each has a diaphragm that is either bias open (open at all times and closed only upon expiration) or bias closed (closed at all times, inspiratory effort being needed for opening). All diaphragms close upon expiration, and all valves attach to the hub of a tracheotomy tube. In addition, the Passy-Muir valve comes in two types, one for patients who are ventilator dependent and one for those who are not. The Passy-Muir valve has been identified with the best speech quality most often by both

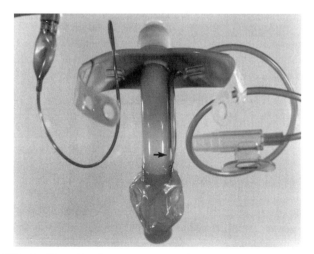

**FIG. 8.** "Speaking" tracheotomy tube with external airflow line. Arrow shows slit where air exits.

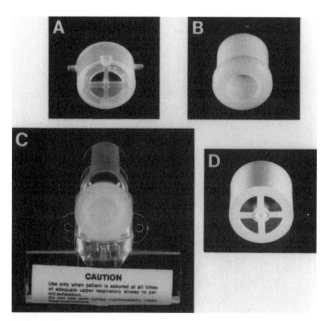

**FIG. 9.** The four one-way tracheotomy speaking valves. **A:** Kistner, **B:** Montgomery, **C:** Olympic, **D:** Passy-Muir. (From ref. 27.)

listeners and users, and it has also exhibited the fewest clinically relevant mechanical problems (27).

### Total Laryngectomy: Alaryngeal Speech and Voice Restoration Rehabilitation

Unlike the consequences of surgery to the vocal tract, a total laryngectomy results in removal of the sound source itself: the true vocal folds. This obviously results in a significant problem for the resumption of verbal communication. The goal of voice restoration rehabilitation is to provide an alternative sound source in order to allow speech articulation, phoneme production, and meaningful verbal communication to occur. No one method for the alternative sound source is better than another. The goal is to match the method that is best for the patient at any particular time in the rehabilation process.

The first 10 to 14 postoperative days can be divided into two distinct periods: immediate (1 to 4 days) and transition (5 to 14 days) (2). The immediate postoperative period is characterized by a reduced ability of the patient to interact with the environment, the recovery from the effects of general anasthesia, nonambulation, connection to monitoring equipment, and a greater level of discomfort from surgery than will be evident in the transitional period. The transitional period usually includes ambulation; increased interaction with the environment as evidenced by writing, watching television, resumption of

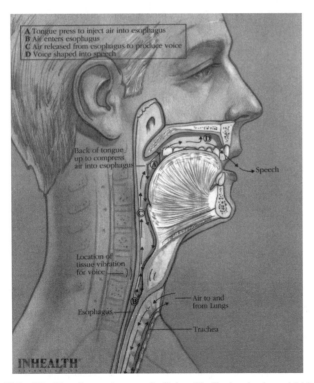

**FIG. 10.** Esophageal speech (Inhealth Technologies, 1110 Mark Ave., Carpinteria, CA 93013-2918).

oral feeding; and initiation of voice restoration rehabilitation with an electrolarynx.

Barring postoperative complications, the patient is usually discharged from the hospital after 10 to 14 days. Outpatient voice restoration rehabilitation continues the therapy begun during the transitional recovery period. Discussions with the speech-language pathologist regarding the use and timing of the various voice restoration techniques for verbal communication are carried out on a long-term basis so that an informed choice of optimal alaryngeal speech can be made.

Alaryngeal speech can be produced from four types of sources: (a) intrinsic (buccal, pharyngeal, and esophageal), (b) prosthetic (artificial or electrolarynx), (c) surgical (tracheoesophageal fistula or neoglottis), and (d) surgical-prosthetic (pharyngotomy with prosthesis or tracheoesophageal puncture with prosthesis) (28).

#### Intrinsic Voice Restoration

Intrinsic voice restoration does not rely on surgery or a prosthetic device. The sound source is produced by existing oral, pharyngeal, or esophageal structures. Buccal ("Donald Duck") and pharyngeal (high-frequency and squeaky) speech are not desirable and should be discouraged. Esophageal speech is a good goal is but not always obtainable.

Esophageal speech is produced by injecting or inhaling air into the upper esophagus at the C-4 to C-6 level, thereby vibrating the walls of the pharyngoesophageal segment as the air is returned to the mouth (Fig. 10). Several methods can be used to produce successful esophageal speech using air injection and air inhalation techniques (see references 2 and 29 for detailed discussions). This new sound source has greater mass than the true vocal folds, and therefore the voice produced has a lower fundamental frequency. In addition, less air is available with esophageal speech than from the lungs, resulting in fewer words per air charge (30,31). It should be mentioned that not all total laryngectomees can achieve fluent and intelligible esophageal speech; some estimates reporting that fewer than 10% of laryngectomees achieve acceptable fluency (28).

#### Prosthetic Voice Restoration with an Artificial Larynx and an Electrolarynx

An artificial larynx uses the laryngectomee's own lung air as the driving force for the new sound source. In order to do so, the artificial larynx connects the stoma with the oral cavity (Fig. 11). These devices are cumbersome to use, draw attention to the user, and are not generally used any more.

An electrolarynx provides the new sound source by vibrating the air in the remaining vocal tract, either direct-

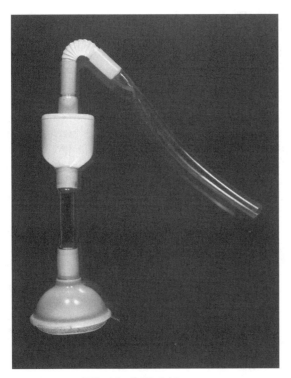

**FIG. 11.** Artificial larynx.

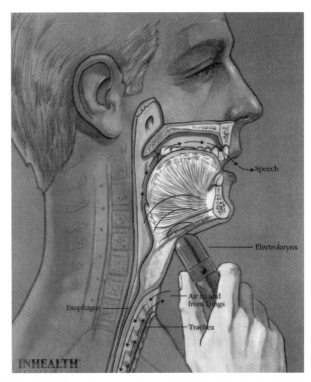

**FIG. 12.** Electrolaryngeal speech (Inhealth Technologies, 1110 Mark Ave., Carpinteria, CA 93013-2918).

ly, as with an intraoral device, or transcervically, as with a neck placement device (Fig. 12). The devices have built-in sound generators that are battery driven, and they have on/off, volume, and pitch controls that allow for some production of intonation and contrastive stress (32).

An electrolarynx should be provided to the new laryngectomee as soon as possible: 3 to 4 days postoperatively. Although optimal speech production and intelligibility will not be obtained, the positive psychological benefits of voice restoration rehabilitation provided by early introduction of an electrolarynx far outweigh any frustration due to early use of the device for speech production. An electrolarynx can also be used during all voice restoration rehabilitation techniques.

There are three types of electrolarynxes, those with (a) an extraoral sound source and intraoral connector only (b) an extraoral sound source with option of intraoral connector and transcervical (neck) placement, and (c) a totally intraoral sound source with extraoral control.

Figure 13 shows a typical device with an extraoral sound source and intraoral connector. Care must be taken so as not to block the end of the oral connector, and therefore the sound, with the tongue or with saliva. Optimal placement is usually 1.0 to 1.5 cm into the corner of the mouth between the buccal mucosa and tongue.

Figure 14 shows a typical device with an extraoral sound source but with two options for vibratory placement: intraoral and transcervical. The same technique as with the previous device (Fig. 13) is used with the optional intraoral tube. Approximately 1 month after

laryngectomy, when the neck has healed and if neck induration is not a confounding factor, neck placement can be attempted.

When neck placement is used, the vibrator head should be pressed comfortably but firmly on the neck to allow the sound source to travel through the skin and vibrate the air in the vocal tract (see Fig. 12). Experimentation with

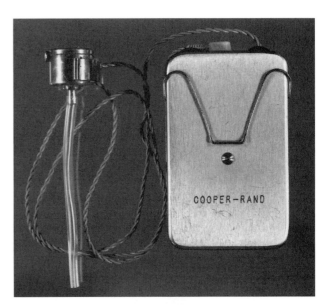

**FIG. 13.** Electrolarynx with extraoral sound source and only intraoral connector (Luminaud, Inc. [Cooper-Rand Electrolarynx], 8688 Tyler Blvd. Mentor, OH 44060).

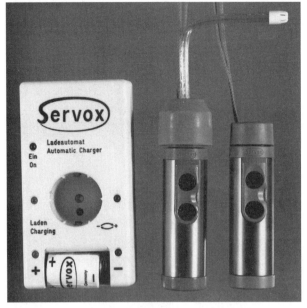

**FIG. 14.** Electrolarynx with extraoral sound source and both intraoral and transcervical vibratory placement options, with battery recharger (Siemens Hearing Instruments, Inc., 10 Constitution Ave., Piscataway, NJ 08855-1397).

different neck placement positions and pressures is usually necessary before the best vocal quality and speech intelligibility are produced. Precise articulation, as well as correct use of the on/off button and correct placement of the intraoral connector or neck placement, is stressed. Variable pitch control can be achieved if the device has two or more pitch controls, by neck tension, or by placement of the device. It is important to remember that lung air is not needed for speech; therefore, stoma noise from to exhaled air should be eliminated when an electrolarynx is used.

Figure 15 shows a device with a totally intraoral sound source with extraoral volume and pitch controls. The oral unit is custom-made to fit existing dentures or a new palatal retainer. The hand-held control unit houses the on/off, volume, and pitch controls and sends wireless radio commands to the oral unit, which houses the sound source and produces the desired pitch and loudness characteristics. The laryngectomee then uses the new vocal tract sound source for consonant and vowel articulation and phoneme production for intelligible verbal communication. The user holds the control unit out of sight in a pocket and does not have to use an intraoral or transcervical placement device.

### Surgical Voice Restoration

Surgical voice restoration attempts to use lung air for speech by utilizing various surgical techniques and the individual's own tissues, such as those of the esophageal mucosa, vein, skin tube, and tracheal tube (28). Unfortunately, unacceptable aspiration and tract stenosis leading to aphonia have occurred with most surgical procedure attempts. However, surgical voice restoration rehabilitation following total laryngectomy has not been abandoned completely (33), and innovative surgeons will surely continue to search for the optimal procedure.

### Surgical-Prosthetic Voice Restoration Rehabilation

Since the first reported successful total laryngectomy more than 100 years ago, many techniques, both surgical

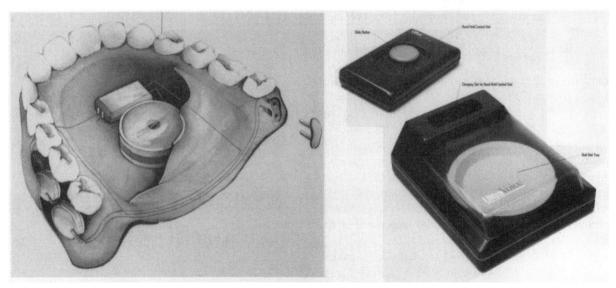

**FIG. 15.** Electrolarynx with totally intraoral sound source and extraoral volume and pitch controls, with battery recharger (Health Concepts Inc. [Ultra-Voice], Inc., 279-B Great Valley Pkwy., Malvern, PA 19355).

and mechanical, have been reported for speech restoration (34,35). Unfortunately, these early attempts were plagued by complication: aspiration, shunt stenosis, and fistula formation. Currently, the requisite essential for successful tracheoesophageal (TE) speech is a one-way prosthetic valve, placed in the tracheostoma by a surgically created TE puncture, which permits expired air to be directed into the esophagus during tracheostoma occlusion but is closed at all other times to prevent saliva and food from entering the trachea (Fig. 16).

The TE voice prosthesis is a hollow tube made of medical-grade silicone with a one-way valve at one end and retention collars on both ends (Fig. 17). Several different types are available, such as the Groningen button (36), the Provox (37), the Panje button (38), and the most widely used: the Blom-Singer TE prosthesis (39).

The TE voice prosthesis resides in the puncture tract at all times to prevent stenosis of the tract and aspiration through the puncture tract. When the stoma is covered and exhalation occurs, air travels from the lungs, into the trachea, through the voice prosthesis, and into the esophagus. The esophagus vibrates, creating a new sound source, which sets the column of air in the vocal tract into vibration, allowing for speech articulation, resonance, and verbal communication to occur.

A common frustration experienced by TE prosthesis users is the need to change the prosthesis every 3 to 4 days. In fact, early (40–42) as well as recent (43,44) studies reported the greatest disadvantage of a TE prosthesis to be that it must be inserted and changed frequently by the user. Users found changing to be bothersome to difficult to impossible.

Recent product development advances, specifically the "gel cap" insertion method (45) and the extended-wear "indwelling" TE voice prosthesis (46), have eliminated this problem (Fig. 18). The gel cap provides a smooth,

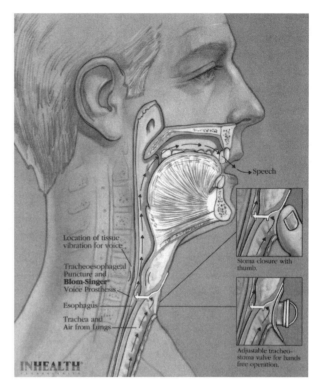

**FIG. 16.** Tracheoesophageal speech (Inhealth Technologies, 1110 Mark Ave., Carpinteria, CA 93013-2918).

rounded configuration that transiently eliminates the retention collar. The gel cap then dissolves in 2 to 3 minutes in the esophagus, releasing the retention collar for internal anchoring. The indwelling TE prosthesis has larger retention collars on the tracheal and esophageal ends, is inserted and changed only by the speech-language pathologist or otolaryngologist, and can stay in place for as long as 6 months. Daily in situ cleaning with

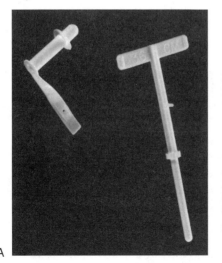
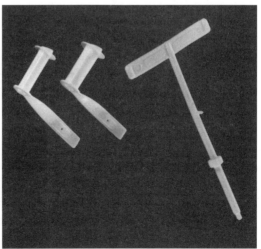

**FIG. 17.** Blom-Singer tracheoesophageal voice prosthesis (Inhealth Technologies, 1110 Mark Ave., Carpinteria, CA 93013-2918).

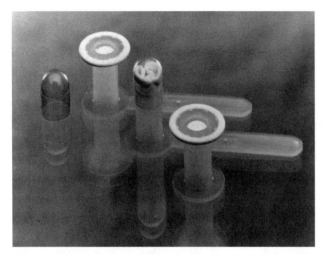

**FIG. 18.** Blom-Singer tracheoesophageal voice prosthesis with gel cap insertion in place and extended wear indwelling voice prosthesis (Inhealth Technologies, 1110 Mark Ave., Carpinteria, CA 93013-2918).

a flushing pipette is required of the user. Voice restoration rehabilitation is still required to achieve optimal speech intelligibility and pitch control by correct digital occlusion and pressure over the tracheostoma, and optimal use of a tracheostoma valve (45).

Tracheoesphageal speech has been a viable and proven alternative to esophageal and electrolaryngeal speech for patients with total laryngectomy since the introduction of the Blom-Singer TE puncture technique and prosthesis in 1980 (39). Subsequent studies evaluating the TE puncture procedure and TE prosthesis speech rehabilitation by its developers (35,47,48) and, more importantly, by independent investigators (40,42,49–52) have shown both the procedure and the prosthesis to be reliable for TE speech production following total laryngectomy.

As stated in their original paper, "Although this [TE puncture] method appears uncomplicated, it is not always 'easy' and a number of factors must be considered" (39:532). Some factors are surgically or medically related, e.g., tracheostoma size and position, cricopharyngeus spasm, and irradiated tissue. Other factors are patient related, e.g., motivation, capability to care for the stoma and prosthesis, visual disturbances, and arthritis. Still other factors are speech rehabilitation related, e.g., ability to follow directions, position and pressure for optimal digital stoma occlusion, TE valve use, and necessity of adequate followup (35,50,51). In all cases, the speech-language pathologist and otolaryngologist are a team that jointly selects, rehabilitates, and follows up the patient with a total laryngectomy and TE prosthesis (39,49,53,54).

The TE puncture procedure can be done primarily at the time of total laryngectomy (51,55) or secondarily, either following or in conjunction with esophageal and electrolarynx speech rehabilitation (39,52). A cricopharyngeal myotomy is done at the time of total laryngec-

tomy during a primary puncture procedure. When a secondary puncture is recommended, transnasal insufflation testing is performed to assess pharyngeal muscle response to esophageal distension (56). The insufflation test assesses cricopharyngeous spasm, and a cricopharyngeal myotomy (57) or pharyngeal plexus neurectomy (58) may be necessary to allow for the fluent production of TE prosthesis speech.

The new sound source does not necessarily have to be the esophagus. In patients with extensive disease, a pharyngolaryngoesophagectomy with gastric pull-up may be necessary. Reconstruction may also include microvascular free tissue grafts, myocutaneous flaps, cervical flaps, and visceral transposition. The standard TE puncture procedure has been shown to be successful in voice restoration rehabilitation with this population, although the resulting voice is characterized by lower pitch, reduced intensity, slower rate, and an overall "wet" or "gurgly" quality in comparison with TE prosthesis speakers (59).

*Tracheostema Valve.* The tracheostema valve was developed to eliminate the need for manual occlusion of the stoma to divert air into the voice prosthesis for speech production (60). The valve system has several parts. The circular valve housing is glued to the skin around the stoma every day. The adjustable valve fits into the housing, and its diaphragm remains open during normal respiration but closes with increased expiratory airflow, thereby diverting air into the voice prosthesis and esophagus for hands-free speech production (see Fig. 15; Fig. 19) The diaphragm opens automatically when the user stops talking to allow for resumption of normal inspiration.

### Hearing Loss

Hearing loss goes hand in hand with speech production in the communication cycle (61). If hearing is impaired, the potential is great for the communication process to fail. For the individual with cancer, participation in the care plan, family discussions, conferences with caregivers, and informed consent for therapeutic decisions all

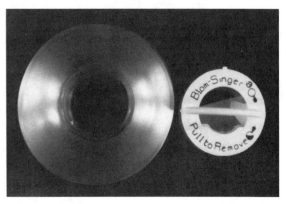

**FIG. 19.** Blom-Singer tracheostoma valve (Inhealth Technologies, 1110 Mark Ave., Carpinteria, CA 93013-2918).

rely on functional hearing. In addition, maintenance of orientation to the activities of daily living via the telephone, television, and radio are made much easier with the ability to hear at least as well as before treatment.

There are two types of hearing loss: conductive and sensorineural. Any impairment of the outer or middle ear with a normal inner ear results in a conductive hearing loss. The difficulty is not with the perception of sound but with the conduction of sound to the analyzing system. The severity of the conductive hearing impairment ranges from slight to moderate: 15 to 60 dB hearing level (HL) (62). When the loss of hearing is due to a pathologic condition of the inner ear or along the nerve pathway from the inner ear to the brain stem, the loss is called sensorineural. The severity of the sensorineural hearing impairment ranges from slight to profound, i.e., 15 to 91 dB HL (62). There also can be a mixed hearing loss, involving components of conductive and sensorineural loss, affecting both sound conduction and sound perception.

### Chemotherapy

Ototoxic chemotherapeutic drugs such as cisplatin have the potential to cause damage to the inner ear: the cochlea, vestibule, semicircular canals, and otoliths (63,64). The benefits of ototoxic therapy must be balanced with its potential for permanent damage to the inner ear and the resultant sensorineural hearing loss or balance disorders. Hearing and balance disturbances can have significant negative vocational, educational, and social ramifications. In an effort to minimize or even prevent ototoxic damage, audiologic testing before treatment and at regular intervals during and after treatment should be done. A comprehensive manual delineating guidelines for the audiologic management of individuals receiving ototoxic drug therapy is available (65).

### External Beam Radiation Therapy

Osteoradionecrosis of the temporal bone after external beam radiation therapy (EBRT) for malignant disease of the head and neck has been well described (66–69). Radiation can produce both early and late changes, ranging in time from 9 months to 20 years (70).

Hearing loss in 36% of irradiated ears has been reported to be caused by EBRT (71). Both types of hearing loss can occur. Osteoradionecrosis of the ossicular chain (72) and impaired eustachian tube functioning, which can lead to otitis media, can cause conductive hearing loss. Cochlea damage secondary to EBRT can lead to sensorineural hearing loss (71). Both conductive and sensorineural hearing loss can occur, depending on the extent of the radiated field.

### Aural Rehabilitation

Aural rehabilitation for patients with hearing loss secondary to cancer or its treatment may be different from aural rehabilitation for other adults with hearing loss (73). Cancer patients may be depressed or weak from the disease and its treatment. The hearing loss, if conductive, may be transient and will improve spontaneously, for instance, when EBRT has been completed. The hearing loss, if sensorineural, may or may not be amenable to improvement with hearing aids. If cost is an issue, low-cost alternatives—assistive listening devices such as pocket amplifiers and telephone receiver amplifiers—may provide the extra volume needed for hearing and successful participation in the communication dyad instead of hearing aids.

Appropriate communication strategies with the person who is newly hearing impaired should be stressed. Strategies include proper positioning of the speaker and listener for unobstructed vision, placement of the hearing-impaired listener in close proximity to the speaker, elimination of interfering background noise, and good lighting to take advantage of visual cues. In other words, conversation should not take place in a poorly illuminated and noisy environment, as is the case in most hospital rooms, and with the caregiver or listener performing tasks in the room that make optimal visual and auditory input impossible (73).

## CONCLUSION

The restoration of the best possible verbal communication is the goal of rehabilitation for people with impaired speech skills. Verbal communication, a uniquely human behavior, is critical to the patient's medical care, psychological functioning, and social interactions. Although cancer and its treatment may significantly alter the patient's ability to communicate verbally, many successful therapeutic interventions are available for the restoration of intelligible voice and speech production.

## REFERENCES

1. Denes PB, Pinson EN. The speech chain. New York: Bell Telephone Laboratories, 1969.
2. Doyle PC. Foundations of voice and speech rehabilitation following laryngeal cancer. San Diego: Singular Publishing Group, 1994.
3. Safar P, Grenvik A. Speaking cuffed tracheostomy tube. *Crit Care Med* 1975;3:23.
4. Levine SP, Koester DJ, Kett RL. Independently activated talking tracheostomy systems for quadriplegic patients. *Arch Phys Med Rehab* 1987;68:571.
5. Parker H. Communication breakdown: personal experience of being on ventilation. *Nurs Mirror* 1984;158:37.
6. Sparker AW, Robbins KT, Nevlud GN, Watkins CN, Jahrsdoerfer RA. A prospective evaluation of speaking tracheostomy tubes for ventilator dependent patients. *Laryngoscope* 1987;97:89.

7. Pickett JM. *The sounds of speech communication.* Baltimore: University Park Press, 1980.

8. Leder SB. Physiology of sound and speech perception. In: Kartush JM, Cass SP, Leder SB, Koch DB, eds. Cochlear implantation. Alexandria, Virginia: American Academy of Otolaryngology—Head and Neck Surgery Foundation, Inc., 1994:24.

9. Baken RJ. *Clinical measurement of speech and voice.* Boston: Little, Brown, 1987.

10. Baken RJ, Daniloff RG. *Readings in clinical spectrography of speech.* San Diego: Singular Publishing Group, 1991.

11. Halle M, Hughes GW, Radley J-PA. Acoustic properties of stop consonants. *J Acoust Soc Am* 1957;29:107.

12. Peterson GE, Barney HL. Control methods used in a study of the vowels. *J Acoust Soc Am* 1952;24:175.

13. Lisker L, Abramson AS. A cross-language study of voicing in initial stops: acoustical measurements. *Word* 1964;20:384.

14. Lisker L, Abramson AS. Some effects of context on voice onset time in English stops. *Lang Speech* 1967;10:1.

15. Kirchner JA. Growth and spread of laryngeal cancer as related to partial laryngectomy. *Laryngoscope* 1975;85:1516.

16. Kirchner JA. Treatment of laryngeal cancer. In: Chretien PB, Johns ME, Shedd DP, Strong EW, Ward PH, eds. *Head and neck cancer*, vol. 1. Philadelphia: BC Decker, 1985:199.

17. Sasaki CT. Horizontal supraglottic laryngectomy. In: Jafek BW, Sasaki CT, eds. *The atlas of head and neck surgery*. New York: Grune & Stratton, 1983:333.

18. Pearson BW, Woods RD, Hartman DE. Extended hemilaryngectomy for T3 glottic carcinoma with preservation of speech and swallowing. *Laryngoscope* 1980;90:1950.

19. Pearson BW. Subtotal laryngectomy. *Laryngoscope* 1981;91:1904.

20. Leeper HA, Heeneman H, Reynolds C. Vocal function following vertical hemilaryngectomy: a preliminary investigation. *J Otolaryngol* 1990;19:62.

21. Laccourreye O, Crevier-Buchmann LC, Weinstein G, Biacabe B, Laccourreye H, Brasnu D. Duration and frequency characteristics of speech and voice following supracricoid partial laryngectomy. *Ann Otol Rhinol Laryngol* 1995;104:516.

22. Leder SB. Importance of verbal communication for the ventilator dependent patient. *Chest* 1990;98:792.

23. Byrick RJ. Improved communication with the Passy–Muir valve: the aim of technology and the result of training. *Crit Care Med* 1993;21:483.

24. Manzano JL, Lubillo S, Henriquez D, et al. Verbal communication of ventilator-dependent patients. *Crit Care Med* 1993;21:512.

25. Leder SB, Traquina DN. Voice intensity of patients using a Communi-Trach I cuffed speaking tracheostomy tube. *Laryngoscope* 1989;99:744.

26. Leder SB. Verbal communication for the ventilator dependent patient: voice intensity with the Portex "Talk" tracheostomy tube. *Laryngoscope* 1990;100:1116.

27. Leder SB. Perceptual rankings of speech quality produced with one-way tracheostomy speaking valves. *J Speech Hear Res* 1994;37:1308.

28. Goldstein LP, Merwin GE. Speech rehabilitation after total laryngectomy. In: Million RR, Cassisi NJ, eds. *Management of head and neck cancer: a multidisciplinary approach*, 2nd ed. Philadelphia: JB Lippincott, 1994:499.

29. Lauder E. *Self-help for the laryngectomee*, 2nd ed. San Antonio: Lauder Publishing, 1995.

30. Snidecor JC, Curry ET. Temporal and pitch aspects of superior esophageal speech. *Ann Otol Rhinol Laryngol* 1959;68:1.

31. Snidecor JC, Curry ET. How effectively can the laryngectomee expect to speak? *Laryngoscope* 1960;70:62.

32. Gandour J, Weinberg B. Production of intonation and contrastive stress in electrolaryngeal speech. *J Speech Hear Res* 1984;27:605.

33. Brandenburg JH, Patil N, Swift EW. Modified neoglottis reconstruction following total laryngectomy: long-term follow-up and results. *Laryngoscope* 1995;105:714.

34. Schwartz AW, Devine KD. Some historical notes about the first laryngectomies. *Laryngoscope* 1959;69:194.

35. Singer MI. Tracheoesophageal speech: voice rehabilitation after total laryngectomy. *Laryngoscope* 1983;93:1454.

36. Manni JJ, van den Broek P. deGroot MA, Berends E. Voice rehabilitation after laryngectomy with the Groningen prosthesis. *J Otolaryngol* 1984;13:333.

37. Hilgers FJM, Schouwenburg PF. A new low-resistace self-retaining prosthesis (Provox) voice rehabilitation after total laryngectomy. *Laryngoscope* 1990;100:1202.

38. Panje WR. Prosthetic vocal rehabilitation following laryngectomy: the voice button. *Ann Otol Rhinol Laryngol* 1981;90:116.

39. Singer MI, Blom ED. An endoscopic technique for restoration of voice after laryngectomy. *Ann Otol Rhinol Laryngol* 1980;89:529.

40. Johns ME, Cantrell RW. Voice restoration of the total laryngectomy patient: the Singer–Blom technique. *Otolaryngol Head Neck Surg* 1981;89:82.

41. Donegan JO, Gluckman J, Singh J. Limitations of the Blom–Singer technique for voice restoration. *Ann Otol* 1981;90:495.

42. Wetmore SJ, Johns ME, Baker SR. The Singer-Blom voice restoration procedure. *Arch Otolaryngol* 1981;107:674.

43. Wang RC, Bui T, Sauris E, Ditkoff M, Anand V, Klatsky IA. *Arch Otolaryngol Head Neck Surg* 1991;117:1273.

44. Levine PA, Debo RF, Reibel JF. Pearson near-total laryngectomy: a reproducible speaking shunt. *Head Neck* 1994;16:323.

45. Blom ED, Hamaker RC, Freeman SB. Postlaryngectomy voice restoration. In: Lucente FE, ed. *Highlights of the instructional courses*. St. Louis: Mosby Year Book, 1994;7:3.

46. Leder SB, Erskine C. Voice restoration after laryngectomy: Experience with the Blom finger extended-wear indwelling, tracheoesophageal voice prothesis. *Head Neck* 1997;19:487.

47. Singer MI, Blom ED, Hamaker RC. Further experience with voice restoration after total laryngectomy. *Ann Otol Rhinol Laryngol* 1981;90:498.

48. Blom ED, Singer MI, Hamaker RC. A prospective study of tracheoesophageal speech. *Arch Otolaryngol Head Neck Surg* 1986;112:440.

49. Wood BG, Rusnov MG, Tucker HM, Levine HL. Tracheoesophageal punctue for alaryngeal voice restoration. *Ann Otol Rhinol Laryngol* 1981;90:492.

50. McConnell FMS, Duck SW. Indications for tracheoesophageal puncture speech rehabilitation. *Laryngoscope* 1986;96:1065.

51. Stiernberg CM, Bailey BJ, Calhoun KH, Perez DG. Primary tracheoesophageal fistula procedure for voice restoration: the University of Texas Medical Branch experience. *Laryngoscope* 1987;97:820.

52. Lavertu P, Scott SE, Finnegan EM, Levine HL, Tucker HM, Wood BG. Secondary tracheoesophageal puncture for voice rehabilitation after laryngectomy. *Arch Otolaryngol Head Neck Surg* 1989;115:350.

53. Kao WW, Mohr RM, Kimmel CA, Getch C, Silverman C. The outcome and techniques of primary and secondary tracheoesophageal puncture. *Arch Otolaryngol Head Neck Surg* 1994;120:301.

54. Leder SB, Sasaki CT. Incidence, timing, and importance of tracheoesophageal prosthesis resizing for successful tracheoesophageal speech production. *Laryngoscope* 1995;105:827.

55. Hamaker RC, Singer MI, Blom ED, Daniels HA. Primary voice restoration at laryngectomy. *Arch Otolaryngol* 1985;111:182.

56. Blom ED, Singer MI, Hamaker RC. An improved esophageal insufflation test. *Arch Otolaryngol* 1985;111:211.

57. Singer MI, Blom ED. Selective myotomy for voice restoration after total laryngectomy. *Arch Otolaryngol* 1981;107:670.

58. Singer MI, Blom ED, Hamaker RC. Pharyngeal plexus neurectomy for alaryngeal speech rehabilitation. *Laryngoscope* 1986;96:50.

59. Maniglia AJ, Leder SB, Goodwin WJ, Sawyer R, Sasaki CT. Tracheogastric puncture for vocal rehabilitation following total pharyngolaryngoesophagectomy. *Head Neck* 1989;11:524.

60. Blom ED, Singer MI, Hamaker RC. Tracheostoma valve for post-laryngectomy voice rehabilitation. *Ann Otol Rhinol Laryngol* 1982;91:576.

61. Leder SB, Spitzer JB. A perceptual evaluation of the speech of adventitiously deaf adult males. *Ear Hear* 1990;11:169.

62. Yantis PA. Puretone air-conduction testing. In: Katz J, Gabbay WL, Ungerleider DS, Wilde L. eds. *Handbook of clinical audiology*, 3rd ed. Baltimore: Williams & Wilkins, 1985:153.

63. Miller JJ. *Handbook of ototoxicity*. Boca Raton, CA: CRC Press, 1985.

64. Govaerts PJ, Claes J, van de Heyning PH, Jorens PG, Marquet J, de Broe ME. Aminoglycoside-induced ototoxicity. *Toxicol Lett* 1990;52:227.

65. American Speech-Language-Hearing Association. Guidelines for the audiologic management of individuals receiving cochleotoxic drug therapy. *Asha* 1994;36(Suppl 12):11.

66. Schuknecht HF, Karmody CS. Radionecrosis of the temporal bone. *Laryngoscope* 1966;76:1416.

67. Thornley GD, Gullane PJ, Ruby RRF. Heeneman H. Osteoradionecrosis of the temporal bone. *J Otolaryngol* 1979;8:396.

68. Ramsden RT, Bulman CH, Lorigan BP. Osteoradionecrosis of the temporal bone. *J Otolaryngol* 1975;89:941.

69. Wurster CF, Krespi YP, Curtis AW. Osteoradionecrosis of the temporal bone. *Otolaryngol Head Neck Surg* 1982;90:126.

70. Kveton JF. Surgical management of osteoradionecrosis of the temporal bone. *Otolaryngol Head Neck Surg* 1988;98:231.

71. Leach W. Irradiation of the ear. *J Otolaryngol Otol* 1965;79: 870.

72. Kveton JF, Sotelo-Avila C. Osteoradionecrosis of the ossicular chain. *Am J Otol* 1986;7:446.

73. Spitzer JB, Leder SB, Giolas TG. *Rehabilitation of late-deafened adults*. St. Louis: Mosby Year Book, 1993.

*Principles and Practice of Supportive Oncology,*
edited by Ann Berger et al.
Lippincott–Raven Publishers, Philadelphia ©1998

CHAPTER 50

# Home Care

Betty R. Ferrell

## THE INTENSIVE CARE OF HOME CARE

Since the mid-1980s there has been a major shift in home health care, caused originally by the prospective payment system and sustained by current trends toward managed care. Long hospital stays have been replaced by early discharges and the shifting of the burden of care to the home. The intensity of care for these home care patients has also changed because of the demographics of both patients and caregivers. Home care nurses and family caregivers have been charged with managing patients with complex and highly technical treatment plans. Home care is characterized by intensive management of symptoms and by needs for supportive care of both the patient and the family caregivers who assume the burdens of cancer and its treatment (1,2).

### Complexities of Home Care in the 1990s

Until recently, the study of symptom management has been largely confined to major symptoms such as cancer pain and to acute care settings. Recent studies have focused on the special needs of patients in other settings, including the nursing home (3), the hospice (4), and the home (2,5). Several factors can influence pain management in these settings. Heavy reliance on family members, access to diagnostic facilities, and often limited pharmacy services can influence the effectiveness of pain and symptom management at home.

It may be assumed that comfort is enhanced in home care, as the home environment has been considered preferable to institutional settings. Patients, families, and health care professionals often elect care at home, assuming that patients are more comfortable there. Research into pain management has served as a model case,

demonstrating that such treatment may not be substantially better at home (5,6). As researchers have extended studies into the home care setting, barriers have been described that actually hinder pain management in the home, including patient's and family's fears of addiction, failure of the patient to report pain, and limited access to needed services (7,8). These facts emphasize that fulfilling the patient's preference to be at home may not necessarily result in effective symptom management.

Symptom management is different at home than in the hospital or other institutional setting (5). Hospitals typically provide technical equipment and services for acutely ill patients. For patients with complex problems, inpatient care often includes a variety of aggressive or invasive strategies for diagnosis and definitive treatment of the underlying conditions. Home care, by contrast, relies heavily on low-tech strategies, concentrating mostly on symptom management. The overall effectiveness of these different strategies at home in comparison with hospitals remains difficult to analyze.

### Cancer As a Family Experience

Cancer and other life-threatening illnesses such as AIDS are generally recognized as affecting the entire family unit rather than a single individual. The recent shift in health care, with movement toward home care as the predominant setting, emphasizes the importance of family involvement in the total care needs of the patient. It is indeed remarkable that care which only a decade ago was reserved for intensive care units, by specially trained registered nurses, is now delegated to family caregivers in the home environment who have had little or no preparation to assume both the physical and emotional demands of illness (9–11). Recent literature has acknowledged the intense demands of family caregiving at home, largely in the areas of technical care, acquisition of skills, and provision of intense, 24-hour, physical caregiving. Less

B. R. Ferrell: Department of Nursing Research and Education, City of Hope National Medical Center, Duarte, CA 91010.

emphasis has been placed on the emotional burdens of assuming responsibilities for the patient's well-being or peaceful death in the home (12–14).

The home environment can be viewed as a delicate balance. At one end of the spectrum are the many demands that the home care environment offers that, if out of balance, can result in intense burdens for family caregivers and compromised care for patients. At the other end are the many benefits of home care. The home care environment often offers the patient improved physical comfort, the psychological comfort of familiar surroundings, an opportunity for healing of relationships, and the ability for patients and families to benefit from the compassion of giving and receiving comfort care and a shared transition from life to death (14).

Oncology and related specialties have moved into home care at excessive speed. Home care has advanced from low-tech care, focused on followup for patients discharged from hospitals, into its current status as the provision of active treatment in the form of chemotherapy, intravenous fluid administration, blood transfusion, complex wound care, and many other technical procedures.

Another significant trend has been the choice of home as the setting of care by patients and families. In the late 1970s and early 1980s, health care professionals generally made the decision whether to discharge a patient to the home or to offer an extended stay in an inpatient setting, based on patient or family preferences. The decade of the 1990s transformed home care as the primary setting of active treatment as well as palliative care. Very important, however, has been the diminished choice on the part of patients and families (16,17).

Patients and their family caregivers may reluctantly assume the burdens of home care. The benefits of home care are also threatened in recent years by the managed care movement. It is now common practice for patients to be discharged from acute care stays with a limited number or duration of home care visits, often limited to only a few nursing visits or a duration of care of only a few weeks, subsequent care is being provided only by the patient and family with no professional support.

The outcomes of home care may often be best evaluated by the effects on family caregivers following the death of the patient and during bereavement. Hospice providers have long recognized that positive experiences with caregiving in the home result in positive bereavement and adaptation by family members after the patient's death. Feelings of inadequacy in providing home care, patient complications, and deaths that are less optimal than anticipated can result not only in the patient's diminished quality of life or quality of death, but also in long-term consequences for the family. Home care, then, is best viewed as not merely care provided to a single individual in the home environment but rather as a family experience in which every aspect of care provided to the patient or the provision of care by the family caregiver will impact the others (18,19).

## Pain As a Metaphor for Death

Much literature has addressed the social need to deny death and the reluctance of individuals in society to accept death and dying amidst a health care focused on cure. Efforts by the hospice movement, the social influences of AIDs, the prevalence of cancer, and other factors have in many ways made our society confront the reality of death in recent years. These advances, however, have also been met with the new age of gene therapy, biomedical engineering, and advanced technologies. These trends afford us many opportunities to continue as a death-denying society. Health care providers should recognize that for many family caregivers and patients, the death that they are now witnessing is perhaps their first personal encounter with the termination of life. Family caregivers struggle with the sanctity of life and denial of death just as do health care professionals and society at large. However, the profound experience of dying, or of caring for a loved one who is dying, transcends all aspects of home care. This experience has been described as an all-encompassing aspect of the clinical care of the terminally ill patient at home (20–22).

## Other Physical and Psychosocial Issues

The needs of patients and family caregivers in home care span the domains of quality of life, as depicted in Figure 1. Home care needs most often involve physical needs, such as management of pain and other symptoms, and treatment of the side effects associated with treat-

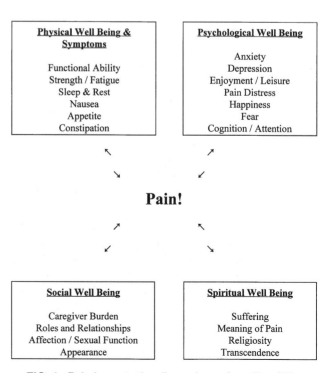

**FIG. 1.** Pain impacts the dimensions of quality of life.

ment of the disease. Nutritional needs, sleep disturbance, fatigue, incontinence, and other physical aspects of disease and treatment are common priorities of home care. In fact, the area of physical well-being and symptom management has been the focus of home care and also the area with the greatest scientific basis for the practice of care in the home (23).

Psychological well-being needs often include the pharmacologic management of symptoms such as anxiety and depression as well as counseling to address issues such as fears, loss of control, and the many other psychological demands of life-threatening illness (24–26). Similar to psychological needs are the patient's social needs, such as the ability to maintain appearance and normal roles and relationships, and family issues, such as financial concerns. The ability to meet psychological and social needs is more difficult outside palliative care programs, in which there is limited access to social workers, clinical psychologists, and other support personnel (27–31).

Spiritual well-being presents perhaps the greatest challenge in home care. In the institutional setting, such as the inpatient hospital, chaplaincy services are often more available. Yet, it is during the advanced stages of illness, when care takes place in the home, that psychological, social, and spiritual needs may become more prominent (32,33). This issue emphasizes the importance of psychosocial assessment to determine unmet needs. Innovative home care programs have begun to incorporate volunteer programs in order to meet the demands that simply will not be addressed in traditional home care services or those for which reimbursement is not possible. As a model example, the City of Hope National Medical Center has recently instituted a program in cooperation with the community Interfaith Council of churches to begin providing intensive volunteer support for respite care and other services in order to enhance the current services provided in home care.

## CHALLENGES TO SYMPTOM MANAGEMENT AT HOME

There are at present many uncertainties about the future of the health care system in the United States and in virtually all countries. A certainty, however, is that care continues to shift into the outpatient and home care environment; thus, it is patients and families who will assume the majority of care in the future. One of the greatest demands in this area will be social influences, such as the impact of a steadily aging population of patients with multiple chronic illnesses. Care of the cancer patient at home becomes far more difficult when the patient is 80 years old and also has concomitant illnesses such as cardiac disease, hypertension, and diabetes, with their associated medications and treatments, which greatly compound the already complex care of the patient (34–36).

An equal challenge rests in the demographics of family caregivers in the home. Research has revealed that approximately 70% of caregiving is provided by elderly spouses in the home and an additional 20% is provided by daughters or daughters-in-law, who are often balancing full-time employment as well as the demands of their own families while providing intensive care to their loved ones (37,38).

One of the most challenging aspects of home care will be the future impact of managed care and similar factors influencing the types and extent of care to be provided in the home. Factors such as limitations in the types of services available, the frequencies of visits, and the duration for which this care can continue will make home care extremely challenging. In essence, as the intensity of needs is increasing, the available resources in home care are diminishing.

## Involvement of Family Caregivers in Medications

A primary task of home care related to cancer and other terminal illness is management of medications. It is enlightening to realize that home care nurses and other professionals assume similar responsibilities in other settings only after formal courses in pharmacology and with support available from colleagues, pharmacists, and physicians reached by direct access. This is particularly true in oncology, where symptom management is often either accomplished on an as-needed basis for symptoms such as nausea or anxiety or with necessary titration of around-the-clock dosing of medication such as analgesics (22,39).

Management of medications is important not only to preserve the patient's comfort but also to diminish the burden on the family and avoid costly complications such as repeat hospitalizations when medications are not effectively used (40). Patients and family caregivers often do not have the necessary knowledge to judge indications for administration of medications or the delicate issues involved with titration or the side effects of medications. Health care providers can make a valuable contribution to the care of patients at home by insuring that medication schedules are made as simple as possible, using single agents rather than multiple drugs, and maintaining the simplest possible routes of administration and dosage schedules. Patients require assistance with important decisions regarding the use and titration of medications and practical techniques such as written dosage schedules, use of self-care logs, and provision of guidelines to help in medication choices. Table 1 includes examples of the types of decisions patients and families have reported in the use of pain medications at home. This illustrates the practical dosing decisions as well as the intense dilemmas patients and families may face in trying to seek relief of symptoms while avoiding the hazards of over-medication. Patients and families require information as

**TABLE 1.** *The caregiver's role in the administration of pain medications*

*Deciding what to give*
"I am the 'pill pusher.' I have to assess intensity, mix meds, and try to find the right combo."

*Deciding when to give*
"Totally, I regulate it. I can tell by the look on her face when she needs more pain medicine."
"I wonder about the time—whether to give it sooner or later."

*Night duty*
"I set my alarm to get up and get his meds."
"Dad gives Mom the medications she's taking. He sets the alarm during the night."

*Reminding/encouraging*
"She doesn't like to take them, so I encourage her."
"My mother has been reluctant to get involved in taking drugs for pain. I have tried to encourage her to take the drugs."
"My role has been more of an emotional support rather than one of dispensing any drugs."

*Keeping records*
"I write down what time it is and how many pills I give."

*Fear of addiction*
"I try to control pills. He's popping them before it's time. He's angry . . . was he liking them too much? The prescription said every four hours, but I would try to hold off if he was crying at 3 hours for 15 minutes. I kept them in my drawer after I found he was popping them."
"I know he needs the controlled drugs, but I hate to see him take them. So I don't remind him. He knows when he has pain. The only time I talk to him is when I think he has had too much medication."

*Doing everything*
"I do everything for her—give her the medications, et cetera."
"I administer the pills. I do every thing for him."

(Adapted from ref 21.)

## Other Concerns of Family Caregivers

An exploratory study investigated the experience of managing pain in the home from the perspectives of the patient, the primary family caregiver, and the home care nurse (39). In particular, the decisions and ethical conflicts encountered by members of 10 patient-caregiver-nurse triads were studied. The subjects reported that the use of medications prompted the majority of the decisions and provoked most of the conflicts; however, decisions related to assessment, the future, and how to live with pain were identified as well. The subjects also identified other areas that created conflict, such as spiritual and theological issues, determining when to tell the truth, and interpersonal relationships. Similar findings, emphasizing the importance of information and support for family caregivers, have been reported by other investigators (10–14, 17).

An additional burden of family caregiving, often neglected, is the costs assumed by patients and family caregivers themselves related to pain management and home care (40–42). Families incur significant expenses related to home care in advanced disease, much of which is not reimbursed. Costs include direct expenses, such as medications, as well as extensive indirect costs, such as loss of wages (42). Most of the cost savings to third-party payors have resulted in increased costs assumed by patients and families.

## Benefits of Care at Home

A primary benefit of home care, which has led to its growth, has been its cost. Care at home can significantly decrease the costs of care throughout the entire illness, from outpatient diagnostic procedures, to active treatments such as the administration of chemotherapy or blood products, to terminal care. Work at the City of Hope National Medical Center has demonstrated the significant cost reductions in comparing inpatient costs with those of home care (41). In this same setting, the potential cost savings of effective home care, which reduces unnecessary readmissions from controlled symptoms, have been demonstrated. Work by Grant and Ferrell initially documented a cost of $5.1 million for the years 1989 to 1990 related to admissions for uncontrolled pain by this institution. Followup analysis for the subsequent years of 1991 to 1993 has demonstrated initial cost savings to the institution of $2.7 million in reduced admissions costs because of efforts to improve the quality of pain management (40).

## Home Care of Children

Most literature regarding home care has focused on the care of adults. The care of children is often perceived to be less demanding or even normal, as families are usually expected to provide such pediatric home care. On the contrary, such care is quite demanding because of the characteristics of the ill child, the parents, the siblings, and the extended family. A recent study explored the experience of parents in caring for a child with pain. This study added a dimension to the previous research related to families and pain and also described the decisions and conflicts in pain management for children (43,44).

Parents of pediatric cancer patients in pain often reported that their health care team did not take their child's pain seriously and did not provide adequate analgesia to relieve the pain (43). This is consistent with recent literature describing the inadequate assessment and management of pediatric cancer pain. However, when specialized pain teams were involved, they were better able to relieve not only the child's pain but the parents' emotional suffering as well. The parents' role in decision making var-

well as support in their decisions regarding medications and treatments.

ied from allowing the child to have control whenever possible regarding his or her treatment to personally administering nondrug methods of pain relief that temporarily alleviated both the child's pain and the parents' feelings of helplessness.

## SUPPORTING FAMILY CAREGIVERS IN HOME CARE

The literature consistently supports the importance of family members during advanced illness. The caregiver's own health, attitudes, and knowledge have a profound effect on the successful management of the patient's symptoms. This is especially important in the care of terminal cancer patients at home (45).

The control of chronic pain remains a perplexing problem that may have important implications for stress experienced by the caregiver. Increased anxiety, depression, marital and family conflicts, embarrassment, guilt, resentment, low morale, and severe emotional and physical exhaustion are commonly reported by distressed caregivers (11–14,17). Indeed, pain management may present caregivers with unique kinds of stress. For example, pain management often requires drugs that must be monitored carefully to achieve maximum pain control safely with minimum side effects. Newer, high-tech pain strategies, such as morphine pumps and chronic spinal infusions, also require the caregivers to have special knowledge and skills. The areas of greatest burden for caregivers in the management of pain include demands on time, emotional adjustment, distressing symptoms, work adjustment, sleep adjustment, and family and relationship adjustments.

Studies of family factors influencing pain management among cancer patients at home, made by this author and colleagues, suggest that caregivers need education and support to cope with many of these issues (5,6). These unanswered questions may lead to increased anxiety, stress, and overall burden on the caregiver that, in turn, may translate into inadequate pain management. Education and support for caregivers cannot be overemphasized in the management of pain in the home.

An advocate of the ethical issues facing family caregivers, Callahan has been a champion of family caregivers and the struggles they face. Callahan has questioned the obligations of family caregivers when heroic, extraordinary care is needed. Improved social support from government agencies as well as a sensitive, responsive society that rewards the heroic efforts of family caregivers is required, given the current demands on families; yet, such social recognition and value is often not present (28).

Jennings and colleagues (10) discussed the ethical challenges the individual, family members, and society as a whole face as a result of the homebound chronically ill. Management of the chronically ill in the home results in

social withdrawal and isolation, transformation of family relationships and roles, and the placing of new burdens on both the patient and family caregivers.

### Assessment of Symptoms

Assessment of both acute and chronic symptoms can be difficult in the home. In the absence of diagnostic facilities and multidisciplinary specialists, care must be taken to avoid attributing symptoms to preexisting illness. Underreporting of symptoms may be common for a variety of reasons. Cancer patients may not report pain because they fear the social implications of opioid analgesics. Elderly patients are often stoic and dread additional diagnostic tests, hospitalization, and new medications (34,35). Although home care nurses and family caregivers may be extremely helpful, most patients require careful evaluation of significant new complaints as well as continued assessment for the management of chronic or persistent symptoms.

Patients with chronic pain should be evaluated for psychological problems. Functional assessment, including ambulation and a broad variety of activities, may represent important indicators of overall physical well-being. Most patients with chronic pain also have significant anxiety or depression at some time. The need to identify and manage anxiety and depression cannot be overemphasized in the adjunctive management of chronic pain. Formal assessment screening instruments for functional and psychological impairments are helpful in this evaluation and minimize the possibility that detectable problems will be missed (36).

### Nondrug Treatments

In addition to the extensive responsibilities related to the pharmacologic management of pain, patients and family caregivers use many nondrug strategies for pain relief at home. The home care environment offers the benefit of access to nondrug pain relief methods, and patients and families often feel more comfortable with these alternative methods at home. Previous research has demonstrated that patients and family caregivers infrequently receive formal information or guidance regarding nondrug strategies but rather rely on their own attempts to discover methods that may add to the patient's comfort (6,14,22). Our program of research at the City of Hope since 1991 has evaluated a structured program for introducing nondrug pain methods at home. These interventions include both physical and cognitive methods. Physical means of pain relief include such interventions as heat, cold, and massage, and cognitive strategies include relaxation, imagery, and a variety of distraction techniques (46,47).

Our experience has also demonstrated that patients and families are very eager to add nondrug interventions to their overall pain management (46,47). These provide great benefit to the patient by not only enhancing physical relief but also alleviating anxiety and giving the patient a better sense of control. We have also demonstrated that family caregivers have found nondrug comfort measures to be extremely valuable in reducing their sense of helplessness. Families are very eager to learn skills that will add to the patient's comfort. It is these family interventions that are often recalled during bereavement as positive memories of their ability to provide greater comfort during terminal illness.

Other more structured interventions can also be incorporated by referral to health care professionals such as clinical psychologists, psychiatrists, social workers, and others who can offer many other treatments that might assist in the patient's comfort at home.

## CONCLUSION

The home care environment can best be described as the intensive care unit of the future. Home care is indeed quite complex as a result of changing patient and family caregiver characteristics. The home environment is rich with benefits to enhance patient comfort but also provides challenges in providing optimum physical and psychosocial care. The literature has addressed many interventions that are helpful in assisting families in home care. Table 2 summarizes many of the suggestions derived from these reports. These interventions include a range of suggestions about physical care, and transferring information about physical caregiving back to families. Also important is offering validation and support to families for their efforts at home care, and including interventions to improve communication.

There is also a tremendous need for continuity of care, as patients are increasingly cared for across many settings. It is essential that issues of care in the home are communicated to those involved in ambulatory care, inpatient care, and other areas of care. Expert care for patients at home, similar to all aspects of palliative care, begins, however, with thorough assessment of the patient's needs. Organized care based on a comprehensive perspective, which recognizes the physical, psychological, social, and spiritual needs during advanced illness, is best accomplished by empowering families to provide excellent care for patients at home.

**TABLE 2.** *Interventions for assisting families in home care*

Acquisition of skills to perform treatments and procedures (e.g., care of decubitus ulcers, management of incontinence).

Knowledge regarding assessment of symptoms or disease status (e.g., signs of infection).

Scheduling of medical or laboratory appointments or coordination of home care services.

Information regarding the disease, treatments, and expected prognosis.

Emotional support in confronting the burdens of caregiving.

Counseling to promote communication within the family and with the health care providers.

Validation that the care they are providing is adequate to meet the patient's needs.

Assessment and guidance regarding the physical strains of caregiving (e.g., lifting, turning, personal care).

Spiritual support for changing belief systems as a result of life-threatening illness.

Assistance in maintaining a sense of normalcy in the household.

Skills in assessing cognitive changes in the loved one and in dealing with the emotional burden associated with cognitive changes.

Interventions to enhance the patient's and family's sense of control.

Information and assistance to access community resources.

Assistance in organizing the tasks of caregiving (e.g., teaching families to schedule assistance, establishing daily care schedules).

Coping skills to manage the uncertainty of illness.

Immediate access to health care services for emergencies.

Respite from emotional and physical exhaustion.

Care that preserves hope, with attention to preservation of hope even in advanced disease.

Respect for privacy in the home, and care that minimizes intrusions and preserves dignity.

## REFERENCES

1. Ferrell BR, Dean GE. Ethical issues in pain management at home. *J Palliat Care*, 1994;10:(3):67–72.
2. Ferrell BA, Ferrell BR. Pain management at home. *Clin Geriatr Med* 1991;7(4):765–776.
3. Ferrell BA, Ferrell BR, Osterweil D. Pain in the nursing home. *J Am Geriat Soc* 1990;38:409.
4. Morris JN, Mor V, Goldberg RJ, et al. The effect of treatment setting and patient characteristics on pain in terminal cancer patients: a report from the National Hospice Study. *J Chron Dis* 1968;39:27.
5. Ferrell BR, Schneider C. The experience and management of cancer pain at home. *Cancer Nurs* 1988;11(2):84.
6. Ferrell BR, Ferrell BA. Family factors influencing cancer pain management. *Postgrad Med J* 1991;67(Suppl 2):S64–S69.
7. Cook J, Rideout E, Brown G. The prevalence of pain complaints in a general population. *Pain* 1984;18:299.
8. Egbert AM, Parks LH, Short LM, et al. Randomized trial of postoperative patient controlled analgesia versus intramuscular narcotics in frail elderly men. *Arch Intern Med* 1990;150(9):1897–1903.
9. Ferrell BR, Taylor EJ, Sattler GR, Fowler M, Cheyney BL. Searching for the meaning of pain: cancer patients', caregivers', and nurses' perspectives. *Cancer Pract* 1993;1(3):185–194.
10. Jennings B, Callahan D, Caplan AL. Ethical challenges of chronic illness. *Hastings Center Rep* 1988;18(1):3–16.
11. Jones RVH, Hansford J, Fiske J. Death from cancer at home: the carers' perspective. *Br Med J* 1993;306:249–251.
12. Kristjanson LJ. Quality of terminal care: salient indicators identified by families. *J Palliat Care* 1989;5:21–30.
13. Kristjanson LJ. The family's cancer journey: a literature review. *Cancer Nurs* 1994;17:1–17.
14. Hull MM. Coping strategies of family caregivers in hospice home care. *Caring* 1993;February:78–88.
15. Leonard KM, Enzle SS, McTavish J, Cumming CE, Cumming DC. Prolonged cancer death. *Cancer Nurs* 1995;18:222–227.
16. Ferrell BA, Ferrell BR. Pain management at home. *Geriatr Home Care* 1991;7(4):765–776.
17. Hinds C. The needs of families who care for patients with cancer at home: are we meeting them? *J Adv Nurs* 1985;10:575–581.

18. Reimer JC, Daview B. Palliative care: the nurse's role in helping families through the transition of "fading away." *Cancer Nurs* 1991;14(6):321–327.

19. Musolf JM. Easing the impact of the family caregiver role. *Rehabil Nurs* 1991;16:82–84.

20. Faller H, Lang H, Schilling S. Emotional distress and hope in lung cancer patients, as perceived by patients, relatives, physicians, nurses and interviewers. *Psycho-Oncology* 1995;4:21–31.

21. Ferrell BR, Rhiner M, Cohen MZ, Grant M. Pain as a metaphor for illness. Part I: Impact of cancer pain on family caregivers. *Oncol Nurs Forum* 1991;18(8):1303–1309.

22. Ferrell BR, Rhiner M, Cohen MZ, Grant M. Pain as a metaphor for illness. Part II: Family Caregivers Management of Pain. *Oncol Nurs Forum* 1991;18(8):1315–1321.

23. Blank JJ, Clark L, Longman AJ, Atwood JR. Perceived home care needs of cancer patients and their caregivers. *Cancer Nurs* 1989;12:78–84.

24. Hull MM. Sources of stress for hospice caring families. *Hospice J* 1990;6/1990:29–53.

25. Schachter S. Quality of life for families in the management of home care patients with advanced cancer. *J Palliat Care* 1992;8(3):61–66.

26. Vachon LS, Kristjanson L, Higginson I. Psychosocial issues in palliative care: the patient, the family, and the process and outcome of care. *J Pain Symp Manag* 1995;10(2):142–150.

27. Beck-Friis B. The family in hospital-based home care with special reference to terminally ill cancer patients. *J Palliat Care*, 1993;9(1):5–13.

28. Callahan D. Families as caregivers: the limits of morality. *Arch Phys Med Rehabil* 1988;69:323–328.

29. Kristjanson LJ. Indicators of quality of care from a family perspective. *J Palliat Care* 1986;1:8–17.

30. Lewis FM. Strengthening family supports: cancer and the family. *Cancer* 1990;65:752–759.

31. Stetz KM. Caregiving demands during advanced cancer: the spouse's needs. *Cancer Nurs* 1989;10:260–268.

32. Ersek M, Ferrell BR. Providing relief from cancer pain by assisting in the search for meaning. *J Palliat Care* 1994;10(4):15–22.

33. Steele LL. The death surround: factors influencing the grief experience of survivors. *Oncol Nurs Forum* 1990;17:235–241.

34. Ferrell BA. Pain management in elderly people. *J Amer Geriatr Soc* 1991;39:64.

35. Ferrell BA, Ferrell BR. Assessment of chronic pain in the elderly. *Geriatr Med Today* 1989;8(5):123.

36. Rubenstein LZ, Campbell LJ, Kane RL, eds. Geriatric assessment. *Clin Geriatr Med* 1987;3.

37. Lubin S. Palliative care—could your patient have been managed at home? *J Palliat Care* 1992;8(2):18–22.

38. Bergen A. Nurses caring for the terminally ill in the community: a review of the literature. *Int J Nurs Stud* 1991;28(1):89–101.

39. Taylor EJ, Ferrell BR, Grant M, Cheyney L. Managing of cancer pain at home: the decisions and ethical conflicts of patients, family caregivers, and homecare nurses. *Oncol Nurs Forum* 1993;20(6):919–927.

40. Grant M, Ferrell B. Unscheduled readmissions. *Nurs Clin North Am* 1995;30(4):673–682.

41. Ferrell BR, Griffith H. Cost issues related to pain management: report from the Cancer Pain Panel of the Agency for Health Care Policy and Research. *J Pain Symp Manag* 1994;9(4):221–234.

42. Ferrell BR. Pain: how patients and families pay the price. In: Cohen MJM, Campbell JN, eds. *Pain treatment at the crossroads*, Vol. 7. Seattle: International Association for the Study of Pain (IASP), 1996.

43. Ferrell BR, Rhiner M, Shapiro B, Dierkes M. The experience of pediatric cancer pain. Part I: Impact of pain on the family. *J Pediatr Nurs* 1993;9(6):368–379.

44. Rhiner M, Ferrell BR, Shapiro B, Dierkes M. The experience of pediatric cancer pain. Part II: Management of pain. *J Pediatr Nurs* 1993;9(6):380–387.

45. Snelling J. The role of family in relation to chronic pain: review of the literature. *J Adv Nurs* 1990;15:771.

46. Rhiner M, Ferrell BR. A structured nondrug intervention program for cancer pain. *Cancer Pract* 1993;1(2):137–143.

47. Ferrell BR, Ferrell BA, Ahn C, Tran K. Pain management for elderly patients with cancer at home. *Cancer* 1994;74:2139–2146.

*Principles and Practice of Supportive Oncology,*
edited by Ann Berger et al.
Lippincott–Raven Publishers, Philadelphia ©1998

# CHAPTER 51

# Comprehensive Spiritual Care

Sally S. Bailey

Comprehensive spiritual care is an essential dimension of supportive care. This chapter is predicated on the assumption that each person has a spiritual dimension and on the principle that in the total care of a person, his or her spiritual nature must be considered along with the mental, emotional, and physical dimensions (1) (Fig. 1).

A second assumption is that spirituality has many facets; the corresponding principle is that a broad range of opportunities for experiencing and enhancing one's spirituality should be available and accessible (2) to persons who are being cared for in the health care setting.

The topic of spirituality is vast. Many books have been written on aspects of this subject, and articles increasingly appear in professional health care journals. Accordingly, I shall focus on the development and need for a concept of *comprehensive spiritual care* and address some of the components to support (a) patients who are confronting life-threatening illness, (b) their families, and (c) other caregivers.

In Fig. 2, the characters in the Chinese word *crisis*, which includes a character from the word *danger* and one from the word *opportunity*, reflect the ancient wisdom that inherent in every crisis is both danger and opportunity. The Chinese ideographs provide one of many images that may illumine and lift persons in the crisis of a life-threatening illness such as cancer. Competent and compassionate, comprehensive spiritual care can help patients and families discover opportunities for quality living at this special time in their lives.

Rather than hearing only a death knell, a cancer survivor had this to say: "Cancer is our 'wake-up call' and our awareness that our physical bodies are temporal. We are no longer anaesthetized from the fact of our mortality, and unconscious living for most survivors is no longer an option. With this awakening, we begin to acknowledge the human condition. We then strive to live well, pray to

live long, and bless ourselves for trying!" (2). Just as illness signals a crisis and an imbalance in one's body, so can it precipitate an imbalance in the intellect, emotions, and spirit as one begins to engage with the reality of one's mortality. That imbalance can be illustrated as a see-saw (Fig. 3):

One seeks to restore equipoise to one's life by searching for answers to such questions as these: Why me? What's happening to me? How can I live through this? Where is God in this? Spiritual caregivers help persons reexamine their lives to find the fulcrum now needed and relate it to the fulcrums that have given them equilibrium in the past. Fig. 4 shows one way to experience spiritual[1] homeostasis.

In order to maintain balance when confronting the crisis of a life-threatening illness, one needs to draw on every strength one has—physical, intellectual, emotional, and spiritual—to be free to make choices about the course of treatment as well as learn to live with the reality that the physical body is temporal—that there's no way out of a difficulty except by going through it. Competent and compassionate spiritual care can assist patients in finding the way through.

All persons in the health care team have the capacity and therefore the responsibility to extend spiritual care. The *special* task of chaplains is the general opportunity of all in the other disciplines. Therefore, to assist readers in reflecting on their own spirituality and the place of spiritual care in supporting patients and families and other members of the health care team, in this chapter the author shall present ideas drawn from 20 years of experience (18 of which were in the hospice setting) in ministering to the dying, their families, and caregivers, as well as selected readings. All of us can grow in our commitment and capacity in offering spiritual care. Our patients and their families are our best

---

S. S. Bailey: West Haven, CT 06515.

[1]Here spiritual is used in the broad sense to mean the human being's transphysical reality, as in the expressions "body and soul" and "spirit and body." This common speech should not be overread as metaphysical dualism.

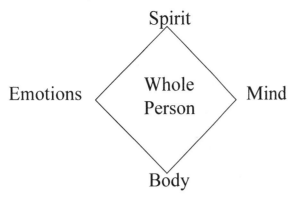

**FIG. 1.** The four dimensions of a human being.

¹Here this term includes the breadth and depth of the psyche: feelings, fantasies, day and night dreams, intuition.

teachers when we stop to listen to what they are saying and to what they are not saying. Further, spiritual care enables us to find and to stand on common ground with our fellow mortals in the presence of the Immortal.

## SPIRITUALITY AND SPIRITUAL CARE

Just as the concept of supportive oncology has grown out of the hospice movement, so has a concept of comprehensive spiritual care that addresses more than the religious issues. The first modern hospices, birthed in Eng-

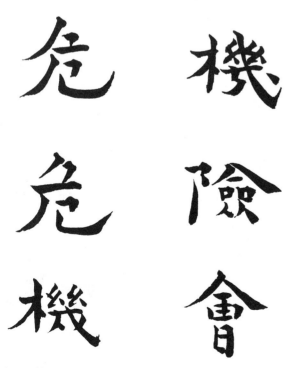

**FIG. 2.** Chinese ideographs for the word *crisis* (top), *danger* (middle), and *opportunity* (bottom). (Courtesy of Ching-ho Chang.)

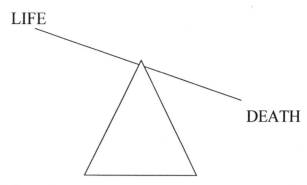

**FIG. 3.** The imbalance one feels when confronted by death.

land in the 1960s and early 1970s, had Christian roots: St. Joseph's, St. Christopher's, St. Columba's, St. Luke's. Du Boulay writes in her biography of Dame Cicely Saunders, the founder of the modern hospice movement and St. Christopher's Hospice: "Legally St. Christopher's is both a religious and medical foundation,... An agnostic St. Christopher's would be like bread without salt" (3). However, the hospices that were born in the United States in the mid-1970s and 1980s reflect our interfaith and diverse ethnic and racial culture. Early on we learned that some words used in health care institutional ministries, like chaplain, rabbi, or pastoral care, did not fit hospices developing in the Southwest and serving Native Americans. Furthermore, did only persons with an expressed religious faith have spiritual needs? What of the countless others who had never practiced any religion?

We began to see that we had to find a *language* as well as a *practice* that would reflect comprehensive and inclusive spiritual care. Recognizing the great diversity in our country, Florence Wald, former Dean of the Yale School of Nursing and a founder of the hospice movement in the United States, saw that a clearer articulation of the spiritual component of care needed to be made for spiritual care to be integral and available to the patient and family as well as supportive of the caregivers.

In 1986, the author was among the 12 first-generation hospice caregivers from different parts of the United

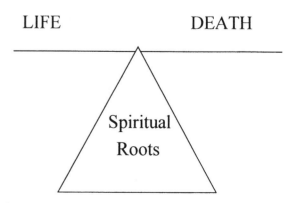

**FIG. 4.** The equipoise one feels when connected to spiritual roots.

States to be invited by Florence Wald to participate in a colloquy on this theme: In Quest of the Spiritual Component of Care for the Terminally Ill (4). Each person was from a different discipline and had a different spiritual base. Some were religious (Buddhist, Catholic, Jewish, Protestant) and others were based in the arts, humanism, social activism, and social science.

Among the questions explored by the participants were these:

1. How can we be perceptive of patient's spiritual beliefs and help put them to use?
2. Do caregivers have a spiritual foundation that is adequate to sustain their compassion and buoy their spirits in the hospice environment, where human suffering is so intense?
3. Who is responsible for providing spiritual support: the family, the institution, the chaplain, the interdisciplinary team, or all?

The basic assumption of the colloquium was that by articulating one's own spiritual foundation and discussing those of colleagues, one would become more sensitive to patients' needs and beliefs and more helpful in assisting them to express theirs.

From this initial gathering, the questions were further explored by participants at the Sixth World Congress on the Terminally Ill and by members of the International Work Group on Death, Dying and Bereavement (IWG) and finally developed by the Spiritual Care Work Group of the IWG into the document *Assumptions and Principles of Spiritual Care*, first published by Death Studies in 1990. All of the assumptions and principles grew out of everyone's respective clinical experience.

Because the document can serve as a lens through which to view and understand aspects of spirituality and spiritual care, helping people of diverse backgrounds to find common ground as they seek to provide comprehensive spiritual care, the document is being included in this chapter. Additional thoughts will be developed from it.

## Assumptions and Principles of Spiritual Care

In those areas of the world where medical care has been shaped by sophisticated technologies and complicated health care delivery systems, efforts to humanize patient care are essential if the integrity of the human being is not to be obscured by the system. This is especially needed by individuals with chronic maladies or those who are in the process of dying.

*Dying is more than a biological occurrence. It is a human, social, and spiritual event.* Often the spiritual dimensions of patients are neglected. The challenge to the health care provider is to recognize the spiritual dimension of patient care and to make resources available for those individuals who wish them and in the form desired.

Spirituality is concerned with the transcendental, inspirational, and existential way to live one's life as well as, in a fundamental and profound sense, with the person as a human being. The search for spirituality may be heightened as one confronts death. This uniquely human concern is expressed in a variety of ways, both formal and informal. Those who provide care for dying persons must respect each person's spiritual beliefs and preferences and develop the resources necessary to meet the spiritual needs of patients, family members, and staff. These resources and associated support should be offered as necessary throughout the bereavement period.

While the modern hospice movement has arisen within Western society with its particular cultural, social, and spiritual milieu, the principles may be applicable in and adapted to other countries and cultures. Ultimately, the Assumptions and Principles of Spiritual Care should influence other aspects of health care and be integrated into the larger system. Their need and manner of implementation, however, will be shaped by the spiritual life of a given individual and society (Table 1).

Let us turn our attention now to the document of *Assumptions and Principles of Spiritual Care*, to which a number of specific references will be made and illustrated by clinical experiences. The sections to be discussed will follow the order and item numbers of those in the document.

### Spirituality

Spirituality has become a buzz word in recent years. Its root is in the noun *spirit*, which derives from the Latin verb *spirare*, "to breathe." The breath is what gives life and vitality. Some have likened spirit also to a flame of fire or energy. One can't see the spirit when one dissects a corpse, but one can see manifestations of the spirit in one's devotions, decisions, actions, and creations—a spirit that theologian and poet Ted Loder describes as a power:

This power to speak
and have light burst upon a mind
or darkness descend upon a heart;
This power to make music
to which souls dance
or armies march;
This power to mold and paint and carve
and so spin out the stars
by which I plot my course to heaven or to hell;
This power to hear and touch and taste
the love and truth
by which life itself is birthed and built,
or the hate and lies
by which it shrivels and dies... (5)

We know that when the spirit flows out of the body, death occurs. (This is only one of many useful metaphors for describing dying as more than a merely physical process.) However, we also know that merely a body

**TABLE 1.** *Assumptions and principles of spiritual care*

| Assumptions | Principles |
|---|---|
| **General** | |
| 1. Each person has a spiritual dimension. | In the total care of a person, his or her spiritual nature must be considered along with the mental, emotional, and physical dimensions. |
| 2. A spiritual orientation influences mental, emotional, and physical responses to dying and bereavement. | Caregivers working with dying and bereaved persons should be sensitive to this interrelationship. |
| 3. Although difficult, facing terminal illness, death, and bereavement can be a stimulus for spiritual growth. | Persons involved in these circumstances may wish to give spiritual questions time and attention. |
| 4. In a multicultural society, a person's spiritual nature is expressed in religious and philosophical beliefs and practices that differ widely depending upon race, sex, class, religion, ethnic heritage, and experience. | No single approach to spiritual care is satisfactory for all in a multicultural society; many kinds of resources are needed. |
| 5. Spirituality has many facets. It is expressed and enhanced in a variety of ways both formal and informal, religious and secular. These expressons include, but are not limited to, symbols, rituals, practices, patterns and gestures, art forms, prayers, and meditation. | A broad range of opportunities for expressing and enhancing spirituality should be available and accessible. |
| 6. The environment shapes one's spirituality and can enhance or diminish it. | Care should be taken to offer settings that will accommodate individual preferences as well as communal experience. |
| 7. Spiritual concerns often have a low priority in health care systems. | Health care systems presuming to offer total care should plan for and include spiritual care as reflected in a written statement of philosophy and in resources of time, money, and staff. |
| 8. Spiritual needs can arise at any time of the day or night, any day of the week. | A caring environment should be in place to enhance and promote spiritual work at any time, not just at designated times. |
| 9. Joy is part of the human spirit. Humor is a leaven needed even, or especially, in times of adversity or despair. | Caregivers, patients, and family members should feel free to express humor and to laugh. |
| **Individual and family (natural and acquired)** | |
| 10. Human beings have diverse beliefs, understandings, and levels of development in spiritual matters. | Caregivers should be encouraged to understand various belief systems and their symbols as well as to attempt to understand an individual's particular interpretation of them. |
| 11. Individuals and their families may have divergent spiritual insights and beliefs. They may not be aware of these differences. | Caregivers should be aware of differences in spirituality within a family or a close relationship and should be alert to any difficulties which might ensue. |
| 12. The degree to which the patient and family wish to examine and share spiritual matters is highly individual. | Caregivers must be nonintrusive and sensitive to individual desires. |
| 13. Health care institutions and professionals may presume they understand, or may ignore, the spiritual needs of dying persons. | Spiritual needs can be determined only through a thoughtful review of spiritual assumptions, beliefs, practices, experiences, goals, and perceived needs with the patient or with family and friends. |
| 14. People are not always aware of, nor are able, nor wish to articulate spiritual issues. | Caregivers should be aware of individual desires and be sensitive to unexpressed spiritual issues. Individuals need access to resources and to people who are committed to deepened exploration of and communication about spiritual issues. |
| 15. Much healing and spiritual growth can occur in an individual without assistance. Many people do not desire or need professional assistance in their spiritual development. | Acknowledgment and support, listening to and affirming an individual's beliefs or spiritual concerns should be offered and may be all that is needed. |
| 16. Patients may have already provided for their spiritual needs in a manner satisfactory to themselves. | The patient's chosen way of meeting spiritual needs should be honored by caregivers. |
| 17. The spiritual needs of dying persons and their families may vary during the course of the illness and fluctuate with changes in the physical symptoms. | Caregivers need to be alert to the varying spiritual concerns that may be expressed directly or indirectly during different phases of illness. |
| 18. Patients and their families are particularly vulnerable at the time of impending death. | Caregivers should guard against proselytizing for particular types of beliefs and practices. |
| 19. As death approaches, spiritual concerns may arise that may be new or still unresolved. | Caregivers should be prepared to work with new concerns and insights as well as those of long standing. Caregivers must recognize that not all spiritual problems can be resolved. |

**TABLE 1.** *Continued.*

| Assumptions | Principles |
|---|---|
| 20. The spiritual care of the family may affect the dying person. | Spiritual care of family and friends is an essential component of total care for the dying. |
| 21. The family's need for spiritual care does not end with the death of the patient. | Spiritual care may include involvement by caregivers in the funeral and should be available throughout the bereavement period. |
| **Caregivers** | |
| 22. Caregivers, like patients, may have or represent different beliefs as well as different spiritual or religious backgrounds and insights. | Caregivers have the right to expect respect for their belief systems. |
| 23. Many health care workers may be unprepared or have limited personal development in spiritual matters. | Staff members should be offered skillfully designed opportunities for exploration of values and attitudes about life and death, their meaning and purpose. Caregivers need to recognize their limitations and make appropriate referrals when the demands for spiritual care exceed their abilities or resources. |
| 24. The clergy are usually seen as having primary responsibility for the spiritual care of the dying. | Caregivers should be aware that they each have the potential for providing spiritual care, as do all human beings, and should be encouraged to offer spiritual care to dying patients and their families as needed. |
| 25. Caregivers may set goals for the patient, the family, and themselves that are inflexible and unrealistic. This may inhibit spontaneity and impede the development of a sensitive spiritual relationship. | Caregivers and health care institutions should temper spiritual goals with realism. |
| 26. Ongoing involvement with dying and bereaved persons may cause a severe drain of energy and uncover old and new spiritual issues for the caregiver. | Ongoing spiritual education, growth, and renewal should be a part of a staff support program as well as a personal priority for each caregiver. |
| **Community Coordination** | |
| 27. Spiritual resources are available within the community and can make a valuable contribution to the care of the dying patient. | Spiritual counselors from the community should be integral members of the caregiving team. |
| 28. No one caregiver can be expected to understand or address all the spiritual concerns of patients and families. | Staff members addressing the needs of patients and families should utilize spiritual resources and caregivers available in the community. |
| **Education and Research** | |
| 29. Contemporary education for health care professionals often lacks reference to the spiritual dimension of care. | Health care curricula should foster an awareness of the spiritual dimension in the clinical setting. |
| 30. Education in spiritual care is impeded by a lack of fundamental research. | Research about spiritual care is needed to create a foundation of knowledge that will enhance education and enrich and increase the spiritual aspect of the provision of healthcare. |
| 31. Freedom from bias is a problem in the conduct of research into spiritual care. | Research should be carried out into the development and application of valid and reliable measures of evaluation. |

Developed by the Spiritual Care Work Group of the International Work Group on Death, Dying, and Bereavement: Inge Corless, R.N., Ph.D. (U.S.A.) *Chair*; Florence Wald, R.N., M.N., M.S. (U.S.A.) *Former Chair*; Rev. Canon Norman Autton (U.K.); Rev. Sally Bailey (U.S.A.); Marjory Cockburn, S.R.N., M.B.E. (U.K.); Rev. Roderick Cosh (U.K.); Barrie DeVeber, M.D. (Canada); Iola DeVeber, R.N. (Canada); Rev. David Head (U.K.); Dorothy C.H. Ley, M.D. (Canada); Rev. John Mauritzen (Norway); Jane Nichols (U.S.A.); Patrice O Connor, R.N., M.S. (U.S.A.); Rev. Takeshi Saito (Japan).

breathing does not make a life. To be fully alive, one seeks to find meaning, purpose, and a sense of direction for one's life.

Thus, the word *spirituality* points to the understanding that the human being has a spiritual core. Carmody and Carmody note this as "where he or she makes contact with God, ultimate reality, the holy, what gives life and creation their coherence, beauty, enduring significance...any comprehensive spirituality shapes political, economic, artistic and other realms of external, public culture" (6). One's spirituality will have interior as well as exterior expressions.

One lives one's spirituality. The German word *Weltanschauung*, world-view, expresses one way of speaking about spirituality. When persons confront the near prospect of death, their spirituality will be challenged as to the transcendental, inspirational, and existential ways they have been living their lives. Their understanding of what it means to be human with strengths, weaknesses, and limitations will be called into question. Caregivers need to be attuned to the spiritual questions that may arise as well as the kinds of spiritual care that may be needed and can be offered when a person has begun to confront the reality of death and its challenge to one's way of life, one's world-view, one's way of making sense, one's regrets, one's desire for forgiveness, one's urge to make amends, one's immortal yearning, one's longing for God.

### Spiritual Care

Just as *spirituality* has become a buzz word, so too has the word *care*, which Nouwen states is most often used in a negative way "'Do you want coffee or tea?' 'I don't care.' 'Do you want to stay home or go to a movie?' 'I don't care.' 'Do you want to walk or go by a car?' 'I don't care.' This expression of indifference toward choices in life has become commonplace. And often it seems that not to care has become more acceptable than to care, and a carefree lifestyle more attractive than a careful one. Real care is not ambiguous. Real care excludes indifference and is the opposite of apathy. The word *care* finds its roots in the Gothic *Kara*, which means 'lament.' The basic meaning of *care* is to grieve, to experience sorrow, to cry out with" (7).

One who cares has the capacity to enter into the suffering of another, to extend empathy. The absence of the recognition of spirituality, and a limited view of spiritual care in health care settings, have contributed to the dehumanizing of patient care. The presence of the recognition of spirituality and a broader understanding of the dimensions of spiritual care have contributed to the humanizing of patient care and the creating of environments that foster a sense of well-being.

In a broad sense, then, spiritual care is about enabling persons to find or reclaim spiritual roots, or to nurture their spirituality, which can bring vitality and meaning to their lives and empower them to engage with their realities to lead them forward to freedom as well as responsibility. Spiritual care helps persons to become open to truth, to be honest, to be real in relating to others. It helps them face their doubts as well as their faith, to live their questions as well as their answers. It helps them see hope through the darkness and so to gain while losing and to realize that love is stronger than death.

The spiritual caregiver brings light by helping the other to begin to see some of the possibilities for quality living that in fact remain in a situation otherwise hopeless. This theme, along with a clearer understanding of what hope is, is presented by Roy Fairchild: "Hope is not optimism. Optimism tends to minimize the tragic sense of life or foster belief that the remedy for life s ills is simple. According to Gabriel Marcel..., optimism is possible as a constant attitude only when people take a position that isolates them from the real evils and obstacles of the world... .

"The hoping person is fully aware of the harshness and losses of life. In order to hope, one must have experiences of fearing, doubting, or despairing. Hope is generated out of a tragic sense of life; it is painfully realistic about life and the obstacles to fulfillment, within and without. The Christian believer cannot simply focus attention on the positive in life, since there is a cross at the heart of Christian faith preceding any resurrection. For the devout Jew, there is the remembrance of the painful exile, out of which deliverance comes. Unless a person passes through meaninglessness, a 'valley of the shadow of death,' can genuine hope be born? With this understanding we can appreciate anew St. Paul's insistence that everyone lives by hope. Hope is the sense of possibility; in despair and trouble, it is the sense of a way out and a destiny that is going somewhere, even if not to the specific place one had in mind..." (8).

### General Statements

### Item 3

Confronting the reality of one's mortality in having a terminal illness has been the impetus for countless persons to grow spiritually when they enter their suffering. One who is in pain feels constricted and bound up, and can choose to endure by engaging the pain. The root of the word *suffer* is in the Middle English word *suff(e)ren*, which means "to undergo, endure, allow."[3] Spiritual growth can be seen in the strengths some suffering persons have been given. As they have struggled with their spiritual pain and inner turbulence that may have arisen from feelings of unresolved guilt, unmourned griefs, doubt, despair, anger, rage, or fear, many have found forgiveness, comfort, peace, renewed courage, deepened faith, hope, and love.

The role of the spiritual caregiver at these times is principally to stand by patients, to be present, and to listen as they wrestle with *their* questions. For the reality is that until persons live through the pain of their unanswered questions, they cannot be open to receive direct acts of solace or enter the final mystery of life. To stand by or to keep watch with another who is in pain of any kind is difficult for caregivers, because our natural response is to take away the pain, to fix it, or to make it better. But are not life's pains more friends than enemies? We live in a pain-killing culture. But a caregiver who expects good from pain may help others to do so.

Spiritual pain can be met by encouraging the person to "hang in there," to name the pain by identifying its root, if possible, rather than feeling that he or she is dealing with something amorphous. That is, naming one's fear can enable one to look at it realistically rather than expe-

---

[3]For further reading on the subject of suffering, see D. Soelle, Suffering (Philadelphia: Fortress Press, 1975).

riencing it as some vague dread. Anger, likewise, needs to be directed through healthful channels, otherwise it will become destructive and will not dissipate. Regretfully, feelings of anger are often denied, especially if one has been brought up to view anger as shameful or if the anger is rooted in anger against God.

Listening for the *images* a person uses in describing his or her experience and reflecting them back to the person also can serve as a mirror to enable the other to "keep on keeping on." Early one summer morning, a woman with metastatic breast cancer telephoned me when she was experiencing a crisis of faith. We later met, and I listened to her as we sat by the sea shore. A few days later, she returned to the cancer clinic bearing the following essay. It illustrates the water-related images that enabled her to move through a time of spiritual pain and regain deepened faith, hope, and courage.

## Swirling

### by Cheryl I. Carlson

Today, I feel at the mercy of a great river; a river, fast-flowing, strong, full of rushing water and rapids, tossing me helter-skelter against unforgiving rocks, up and down between waves, threatening, threatening to pull me within her wild folds. But, I don't get pulled under … I continue along, fighting without the use of paddles, in the middle of this boat. There is, I can sense, some protection in this boat despite being thrown about like a little cork.

Most days, I can handle much of what is tossed my way, some good, some bad. Yet, today, I awoke feeling horrifically vulnerable, devoid of inner peace, strength, and resilience. All components that I need to go on.

Perhaps this is a result of a week where the place that I am employed at, is trying to dissociate themselves from me. Having cancer can certainly be a blessing, opening one to all sorts of life's little wonders that heretofore went unappreciated. Yet, suddenly, one becomes persona non grata, a liability, an insurance nightmare. No one wants me because I have a disease that I did not ask for, yet have and will have. I am still the same person, though I feel more enriched from the cancer. I don't want sympathy or empathy from anyone. I just want to be normal. I can still think, talk, contribute to the American society, but now I must fight for the right to go on. Thank God, we don't have mass euthanasia. In this perfect society, I would face forced extinction. I am not perfect in man's eyes, only in the eyes of the Holy Spirit. I am the underdog. Ironically, my whole life, whether person or animal, whatever, I have always rooted for the underdog. My sympathies, love, and support have always been for those who the oddsmakers were against. Now, the oddsmakers are against me. Who will fight for me? ME. With the divine assistance that I need, I can beat the odds. Cancer is a tough enough adversary, but the immediate adversary is money. It costs money to fight this disease and Big Brother does not want to help. My coworkers are no longer supportive. Finding a new job at almost 44 years old, though educated, BUT with cancer, makes me about as desirable as a hurricane in June.

On the bright side, at the end of the rapids, there are smooth, calm waters that meander blissfully along. My tormented psyche must remember that those waters are there!! And, despite all the odds, I can reach safe, welcoming shores (9).

## Item 5

Living in a multicultural society, one has the opportunity to see as well as experience many facets of diverse spiritualities. This opportunity also presents many challenges for both the patient and the caregiver if they are of dissimilar backgrounds.

A variety of unique religious and secular practices can be seen in the United States, particularly during the December holidays observed as Hanukkah by Jews, Christmas by Christians, and Kwanzaa by some African Americans. Perhaps as a means to find unity in the midst of diversity, secular celebrations of the winter solstice, in which persons from many faith traditions participate, have been increasing. Every race, culture, and ethnic group in the United States, including the Native Americans, has its own set of belief systems and practices. The varieties of beliefs and practices become visible through the rituals, sacred writings, and sacred objects that people have chosen to support them when they confront life-threatening illnesses and/or death.

However, one must not assume that just because a person practices a particular ritual, or say that he or she comes from a particular tradition, that he or she has integrated what is espoused. In fact, the author's experience has been that very few persons, before the time of their dying, have an integrated faith. By this is meant that they have not used the resources of their traditions in their day-to-day living. Simply put, they have not practiced what they have said they believe.

But could this also reflect what it means to be human? That our human condition is such that until we are challenged we do not grow, we do not wake up? Have we not all heard cancer patients say: "I'm thankful for my cancer, otherwise I would never have known…" (positive life experience, or something good born out of the crisis)?

Thus, the spiritual caregiver can help the person rediscover what has had meaning in the other's life, and what has brought joy and strength in the past. One also listens to the person's regrets as well as wishes. However, all of this presumes that the other is open to such exploration. Again, the author's experience has been that when persons confront the reality of a life-threatening illness, their fear of the possibility of death often paralyzes them emotionally and their spiritual energies lie dormant. They have no energy to explore or engage with the issues before them. They become fragmented.

In a previous essay (10) this author stated that in the early days of chaplaincy training at Bellevue Hospital in New York City, she became acutely aware of the fragmentation in people's lives and pondered these questions: How does one become whole? How does one achieve balance? In facing the crises of aging, dying, and death, she saw people who had been cut off from their spiritual roots, who were detached from a strong religious faith—righteous people, paralyzed by fears with hearts that appeared "frozen." She pondered how the gospel could become real to them, how lives could become unlocked so the Creator might enter. She thought about how more persons could be set free to pray and praise, to mourn and celebrate life, to give thanks in every circumstance. She saw that traditional forms of ministry did not reach all people and was concerned that so many of the patients appeared to lack the spiritual energy to move through the crises before them.

From these initial experiences, she began to see that spirituality has many facets, for I also saw that the most alive patients were those in touch with their own creativity. Three patients—a poet and two painters—were pivotal in aiding her understanding that if one is in touch with one's creative center, the spirit is energized to move one forward on the journey of life. These three artists were pouring forth their rage, fear, and anger—some of it coming out on canvas, some through words. In the process, new creations came forth. With only one of the patients was the author able to follow through: the poet. In time she, who had raged against her lot and against those who cared for her, moved out into transcendence with a spirit of compassion for those about her—and then quietly died. Her spirit had been enlivened through her creativity. She lived as she was dying.

Since those days at Bellevue, the author's life's work has been to integrate the arts and creativity in spiritual care as a means of enabling persons to access spiritual roots. The reality is that one may have the intellectual acumen but not the spiritual strength to act on what one knows until the heart (emotions/spirit) is freed of its pain and the imagination liberated to explore or even to see the options before one. For this primary reason, it is imperative that the arts have a place in *all* health care settings, particularly where persons are confronting life-threatening illnesses, as well as in our personal lives as caregivers.

The arts help to keep our imaginations alive and maintain our connection to the earth and created order of the universe, for this is what the arts are all about. They are reflections and expressions of our engagement with our environment, with our surroundings, with our roots. The arts and creativity connect us to the energy and breath of life: the spirit. When we are cut off from the breath of life, we die, both literally and figuratively. When we stay in touch with our creativity, our imaginations are heightened to be alive to what confronts us, be it a life-threatening illness or the tremendous problems of injustice in our world.

In many ways it is difficult to write or speak about the arts because they are reflections of our spirituality and because one more fully understands the arts by experiencing them in every facet of one's being. However, for the purposes of this chapter it might be helpful to broadly and simply define the arts as the creative manifestations of a person's response to his or her surroundings through a variety of media: words, music, movement, film, paint, wood, stone, glass, metal, cloth, yarn, plants, and so on.

A creative artistic person works in a particular medium to make order out of what she or he may be experiencing. As Simone Weil has stated: "The first of the soul's needs, the one which touches most nearly its eternal destiny, is order" (11). Order is a conduit for truth. Therefore, one might say that the arts function to make truth more real to us, particularly the ineffable truths of life.

What do the arts do? The arts serve as regenerators of body, mind, emotions, and spirit. The whole person is touched when one engages with an art form. The arts enable people to find meaning for their lives, to become reconnected to their spiritual roots, to the source of life, to overcome the fragmentation in their lives. Engaging in the arts or the creative process can enable people to become more whole.

How is a person regenerated in body, mind, emotions, and spirit when engaging with the arts? One way to illustrate engagement with the environment and the act of creation is portrayed in Fig. 5.

We receive images and sounds from the environment through the senses of the body. The images are processed through our emotions, spirit, and mind and become inspirations and ideas that move through the body and are given form in other images and sounds. Thus, through the creative process, connections to each dimension of the self are made. All parts of our being are regenerated. We respond to the images and sounds in a variety of ways, depending on the meanings they may have for us (12).

Because engagement with the arts and creativity can enable all persons to survive and enhance their quality of life, artists need to be a part of the health care team. Perhaps it is the artist's own experience of constantly engaging with the negative and positive aspects of life—which is the foundation for all creation—that prepares the artist to be a special guide to those who are searching for meaning in their lives, particularly at a time of crisis. The artist in a health care team is a teacher who enables people to

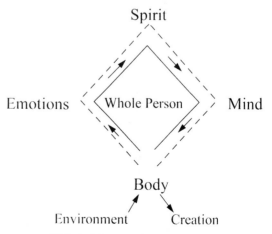

**FIG. 5.** The creative process.

enter the pain and suffering as well as the ecstasy of life and to create something new out of it. Through the creative process, persons are empowered to live out whatever days remain to them: the bad days as well as the good.

Hundreds of stories could be told about spiritual transformations in people's lives as they've entered their agonies of soul in confronting life-threatening illness by engaging in the arts and/or creative expression. This is manifest in the increasing number of published biographies, stories, collections of poetry, and works of art created by cancer survivors in particular. Regional and national touring art exhibits have reflected the painful as well as the beautiful and meaningful aspects of life the artists have discovered as they've journeyed with their illness—evidences of transcendence over chaos and despair.

A particularly heroic example of a contemporary artist's confrontation with her metastatic breast cancer is an exhibit of 14 paintings by Hollis Sigler: "Breast Cancer Journal: Walking with the Ghosts of My Grandmothers." The Chicago artist, whose mother and great-grandmother died of breast cancer, illustrates through her paintings her own spiritual and emotional journey.

Many cancer centers in the United States have seen the need to establish a department of spiritual care to support patients in their quality of life during cancer therapy, and some of them have been described in a published report (13). However, less than half of the centers reporting included opportunities for music or art support. A great opportunity to enrich the lives of patients, family members, and staff as well as a contribution to spiritual care is missed when the arts are not present in *all* supportive care programs. Arts may be absent from these programs for a variety of reasons, which could range from cost to finding well-trained artists, craftspersons, writers, and/or musicians who are comfortable in working with persons confronting life-threatening illness. It takes a particular kind of artist to work in supportive care.

Heretofore, when the arts have been present in health care settings, they have been seen generally as a therapeutic tool or as an add-on. Both views are too limited and need to be expanded when the arts are integrated into supportive care programs. When the arts are used as a therapeutic tool, the persons who offer them are generally trained principally from the psychological perspective to treat persons who are emotionally or mentally disturbed or physically deprived. The author's experience in working with people confronting a life-threatening illness is that they want to be seen as a whole person, not as fragmented or a diseased entity. Experience has shown that artists working as teachers enabling persons to create works of art or develop writing or other creative skills have been particularly helpful with populations in hos-

pices and in palliative care and oncology units in hospitals.[4] This has been substantiated throughout the years by countless patients with whom the author has personally worked and/or observed, and most clearly articulated by the members of the Spiritual Care and Arts Group, established at Yale Cancer Center, who have remarked: "We just want to be normal. We're tired of someone telling us what we should do. We just want to live."

In hospice care, most persons realize that they are nearing the end of their life's journey on earth, as do their caregivers—even though they may speak as if there will be a tomorrow. However, the major difference in working with persons through supportive care as opposed to hospice care is that persons who are treated with supportive care are fighting to live. Therefore, comprehensive spiritual care should be offered at the very beginning of a patient's care to provide the resources needed to empower them to access their spirituality, contribute to their quality of life, and enable them to live meaningfully and with vitality face-to-face with a life-threatening illness. As mentioned earlier, opportunities to engage with the arts and creativity may serve as an avenue to the spirit. Caregivers should be alert to what may be expressed by the patient, and careful not to impose their own interpretations or judgment.

A further contribution of the arts in spiritual care is that the arts can build bridges to persons of diverse backgrounds. A special bond arises among those who are experiencing the same crisis. The many walls that people erect to separate themselves from others, to be independent and self-sufficient, and to associate only with their own kind come tumbling down. In hospice care, we often see that the great leveler of imminent death bonds patients and families in supporting each other. In supportive care, the issues of dying and death are held at bay as persons fight to live. Persons bond through their common fight in having the same diagnosis or treatment. An esprit de corps evolves, expressed in such statements as these: "We're all in it together" and "It doesn't matter who you are or where you're from."

Thus, one of our roles as spiritual caregivers is to find ways to strengthen the support patients and families can give to each other and to offer that which can help connect persons of diverse backgrounds. Providing persons with opportunities to engage with the arts and creativity both individually and in groups can help establish common ground between people. Traditions and rituals can separate persons of different heritages, but the arts, with their language of images, symbols, and sounds expressing universal themes of life, death, and transcendence, can help unite persons of diverse backgrounds and build community.

This is not to say that tradition and ritual are not important in people's lives. On the contrary, traditions and rituals are what people have created and adhered to throughout the history of humankind to hold their lives together,

---

[4]For further reading on artists working in hospices and in oncology, see S Bailey, et al. Creativity and the close life (The Connecticut Hospice, 1990) and M Rockwood Lane M and J Graham-Pole, Development of an art program on a bone marrow transplant unit (Cancer Nurs 1994;17(3):185–192).

both interiorly and exteriorly. In all cultures, the traditions and rituals have arisen at all the major life moments: birth, coming of age, initiation ceremonies, marriage, anniversaries, death, remembering historical events. Traditions and rituals contribute to the rhythm and the seasons of life. However, they also reflect particular world views—how one sees and lives in the created world and in relation to others. Traditions and rituals reflect people's perspectives on what and whom they value and how they understand the world and their place in it.

All religious traditions have rituals that give external expression to an internal communal belief. Rituals can help people bond and enable a person to integrate his or her belief system. The spiritual caregiver needs to be attuned to the varieties of rituals that may be helpful to persons confronting life-threatening illness and provide opportunities for their expression. These could include sacraments, special prayers, or forms of meditation.

Through the interfaith and interracial Spiritual Care and Arts Group at Yale Cancer Center, we have seen how the arts and opportunities for creative expression can build a bridge between persons of dissimilar backgrounds and strengthen the support patients and families give each other. People have found common ground in doing creative arts projects together in a variety of media. They may also create together a work of art reflecting their shared experience. Other events have included listening to music and to each others' writings and songs. As a group, the patients have created their own rituals and prayers.

Since the group's inception, members have gone through the death of one of their members whom they supported during her dying. Following the death, several members participated in the interment and memorial services through writing, speaking, and singing. They found it especially important to have had the opportunity to accompany their friend's living, dying, and death in three settings: home, clinic and hospital. Comprehensive spiritual care provided the bridge that maintained the community and continuity of care. Bereavement support was extended to the patient's family, and attention was given to the group members' own bereavement needs, some of which were met as they participated in the memorial service.

We have seen that a multicultured society will reflect many facets of diverse spiritualities, many rooted in the varieties of religions with their particular traditions and rituals. Further opportunities to engage with the arts and creativity not only will contribute to persons' well-being but also can become avenues to spirituality that may enable persons of diverse backgrounds to find common ground and build community. The next issue that needs to be explored, therefore, is how an environment is created through supportive care to provide comprehensive spiritual care that will support persons facing life-threatening illness, their families, and their caregivers.

## Items 6 and 7

These two items are interrelated. The reality is that if there is not a written statement of philosophy about the need for spiritual care as well as resources of time, money, and staff appropriated for this component of supportive care, an environment will not be created that can enhance spirituality. The environment must be material as well as spiritual.

Hospitals were initially planned to accommodate primarily the persons who worked in them. Lo-Yi Chan, the architect of Connecticut Hospice, which opened in 1980 as the first free-standing hospice in the United States, helped to bring a new consciousness to the design of health care facilities: "I was taught that before you design a building you talk to the future users " (14). By this he meant the dying patients, and he took it upon himself to learn their needs and those of their families. When we look to the hospice movement, we see that much attention has been given to exploring and creating the kinds of materially comfortable and spiritually comforting spaces that can contribute to the well-being of patients, families, and staff. However, are the dying the only persons who need a comfortable and comforting environment? Since 1980 there has been a surge throughout the country in hospital renovation and construction, with serious attention being given to matters of comfort and aesthetics both inside and outside the buildings while hi-tech efficiency is maintained.

A manifestation of this growing consciousness since 1987 has been the annual Symposium on Healthcare Design. An increasing number of hospitals throughout the United States have established cultural affairs and/or arts departments that provide bedside opportunities in the arts for patients, curate permanent works of art, establish rotating art exhibits, and schedule musicians and other performing artists—all to support and enrich the quality of life of persons in the health care community.[5]

Also, both indoor atriums and outdoor gardens are contributing to the environments of health care settings. Of particular note is the healing garden designed by Topher Delaney, a distinguished landscape architect and a cancer survivor, for the Cancer Center of Marin General Hospital in California. It is adjacent to a waiting room and has one wall of floor-to-ceiling glass through which persons may look at the garden or walk out into it through sliding glass doors. There one sees and smells the refreshing green plants, or may sit quietly and be soothed by the sound of water flowing from a bamboo spout into a small Japanese well.

*Waiting* becomes one of the hardest realities for persons living with life-threatening illnesses. As caregivers,

---

[5]For further information on the integration of the arts in healthcare, see J Palmer and F Nash, The hospital arts handbook (Durham: Duke University Medical Center, 1991).

we need to look at all the spaces where patients have to wait and are treated, and ask whether those spaces contribute to the comfort of body and soul of those we serve. There are ways to transform any environment to serve and not to diminish, providing *we* see to it that the environment contributes to and/or will reflect the care we seek to give.

Too, when people are comfortable in the environment, communication between and among them is easier. The design of the material environment also contributes to the kinds of activities that may occur. Hospitals and hospices are being planned with attention to the need for both private and communal space. The same attention needs to be given to the design of clinics and treatment areas, in the spaces where patients become acutely aware of the criticalness of their illness. There should be a room or area where a patient can find solitude and/or be supported by a caregiver privately when the need arises. Examining and/or treatment rooms do not suffice, and a chapel may be too large unless it has been designed as an intimate or more personal space.

*Sounds* in the patient's environment should not be invasive but contribute to an atmosphere of peace and comfort. Earphones are necessary when there is a television and/or piped-in music. Many people find that listening to guided imagery, meditative, or music tapes is helpful. Again, individual differences and tastes should be taken into account when resources are provided for individual listening.

### Item 9

Because much of the spiritual care in the health care setting has focused on persons who are in crisis and confronting issues of life and death, caregivers need to remember that *joy* is one of the spiritual strengths that enable people to survive—including the capacity to see the funny side of life. In assessing spiritual needs, it's important to know what in the past has brought the person joy and what he or she has had fun doing.

When persons are encountering a life-threatening illness, many times they think "Life's over," or "I'll never be able to do *that* again." Here is another reason to integrate the arts into spiritual care. Given opportunities for creative expression, they take delight in doing and/or learning something new. They become empowered to *live* with a life-threatening illness. "Joy is part of the human spirit. Humor is a leaven which is needed even, or especially, in a time of adversity or despair."

The author remembers a dying man who loved the circus and had always wanted to be a clown. His wife thought he was ridiculous to think of something like that when he was dying. However, one of the arts staff in the hospice that day just happened to have her clown face paint and blue wig with her. Once informed of the patient's wish, she went to his bedside and made him into the clown he had always hoped to be. The joy and humor of a fulfilled wish helped carry him to his death two days later. Is there not more than one parable in this story for those of us who are caregivers?

### The Individual and Family (Natural and Acquired)

The hospice movement has brought into clearer focus that when persons are dying their family is affected also. That is why the family is the unit of care in hospice. I believe also that the family is affected and should be considered the unit of care when a patient is first diagnosed with cancer. The potential for a patient to survive well and/or thrive when living with a life-threatening illness will be enhanced or diminished by the family.

### *Item 11*

Rarely does one see uniform spiritual insights and beliefs among family members. Furthermore, because of such divergencies, there will not be unity among the family members unless there is a spirit of openness, respect, and tolerance.

Thomas Attig writes at length on the subject of respecting the other's spirituality, especially from the perspective of the caregiver. However, what if the patient or family member fails to thrive because of dysfunctional beliefs? Attig notes: "Perhaps the circumstances within which it is most difficult to define a respectful response are those where the dying or bereaved have firm convictions that are clearly dysfunctional.... In such cases respect requires extreme caution about judgement that the firmly held conviction is in fact dysfunctional." He continues: "Rather the judgement that the belief is dysfunctional must be based on caregiver perception that the belief is in fact contributing to the disorientation of the person or clearly undermining the person's own sense of meaningfulness in the experience."

He concludes: "It is good to remember that conviction, no matter how firm, neither changes the fundamental contours of reality and the human condition nor provides believers with immunity from suffering or death. At best it supplies a means of coping with or living in the face of death and suffering.... Where dysfunctional beliefs are present, respect for the believer requires recognition of the dysfunctional character of the belief and the courage to intervene caringly in the name of the person's own thriving ... imposition of the alternative beliefs is inappropriate. Yet, encouragement of exploration of (a) alternative interpretations of the beliefs in question or (b) alternative beliefs compatible with the person's values and life patterns is appropriate and respectful" (15).

What other ways might the caregiver intervene if he or she observes beliefs or attitudes that do not contribute to the patient's thriving? For example, a zealous family member may project his or her concern for the patient's well-being in the afterlife if the patient has not followed the same spiritual path that the family member has and thinks the patient should have, thereby causing high emotional stress for the patient. Caregivers need to be watchful about the kind of emotional and spiritual support the family is giving and should serve as advocate for the patient to help the patient articulate his or her own perception of needs.

At other times, when the patient has a stronger belief system than the family members, the caregiver can be an advocate for the patient to find the spiritual support he or she needs outside the family, as well as enable the patient to find ways to communicate his or her beliefs to the family members if that is desired.

### Items 14 and 19

People may not be aware of, nor able, nor wish to articulate spiritual matters. This does not mean that they have no spiritual concerns. A reality is that no one caregiver can be all things to all people nor expect to understand or address all spiritual concerns of patients and families. However, the clearer the caregiver is in his or her own spiritual grounding, the better can he or she enable others to explore their spiritual roots, if any. This points to the need for an interdisciplinary as well as an interfaith team of caregivers to provide supportive care, one of whom might have the resources or know how to find the resources to plumb the spiritual concerns of a particular patient.

Another reality, which is hard for caregivers to accept, is that not all spiritual problems can be resolved, just as not all cancers go into remission. Patients, family members, and caregivers alike have to learn to live with the unanswered questions and the mystery of life, which learning may be facilitated through a deepening spirituality.

### Item 20

Patients are deeply concerned about their families, especially those who have young children. The concerns range from who will take care of them physically as well as what kinds of persons they will grow to become if the parent dies. As competent and compassionate caregivers, we cannot *not* be concerned about what is happening to the family, so that we can help direct them to the individuals and resources that can assist them with the patient's concerns. One could look at this as prophylactic, a dimension of preventive medicine.

Another way the patient–family bond can be strengthened is by providing opportunities for them to do arts projects or share arts happenings together. Not only will lasting mementos be created from the gifts patients have made and left behind, but also life-affirming memories of shared experiences that were happy while family members lived through a crisis together. These experiences contribute greatly to empowering the bereaved to move through their mourning (16). Equally important to strengthening the patient–family bond are opportunities for them to participate in religious rituals or acts of worship together. These could include sharing sacraments, praying together, and reading passages from sacred texts.

### Caregivers

### Item 22

Our beauty and strength lie not only in unity but also in our *diversity*. Looking at the created world we live in, we can see the myriad variations in species and places—and yet they all fit together like the pieces in a beautiful puzzle. They support one another. Humankind has been slow to learn that we are interdependent and need to support one another without oppressing and destroying one another. Differences are real, and they occasion wars and separations. But another reality is that when people respond to others who are suffering, differences recede. One learns to view the other as a fellow human being. A spirituality of mutual respect and tolerance arises as each reaches across the divide once created by emphasis on differences, and common ground is found.

Teams of caregivers drawn to the common mission of supportive care will be strengthened as attention is given to respect for differences. However, the responsibility for creating and maintaining a climate of respect lies with the team facilitator. The team is made strong by each member's commitment to doing his or her part to reach the goals established in the mission.

### Item 23

To prepare health care workers to offer spiritual care, regular inservice educational opportunities should be scheduled to explore the concepts of spirituality and spiritual care, face-to-face with their own spirituality and their values and attitudes toward matters of life and death, meaning and purpose. Helpful here are some of the processes and learnings from clinical pastoral education.

To heighten consciousness as to the role of comprehensive spiritual care that integrates the arts, staff retreats for rest and renewal may be devoted to this exploration. Such retreats may be followed by workshops in a variety of media to allow participants to become familiar with the artists and kinds of materials being used with patients and families. It also gives caregivers opportunities to develop their own creativity. The arts can be integrated in inservice programs to help caregivers deal with issues of change and loss that affect both their personal and professional lives. Other ways to enhance awareness of the arts are to develop a library of related books, articles, video and music tapes; have art exhibits; include space for patients' work; and arrange for lectures, discussions, and grand rounds that integrate the themes of spirituality, the arts and medicine.

All these events and materials help foster an understanding of the breadth, or horizontal aspect, of spiritual care. But so. too, there is a need to understand the height and depth, or vertical aspect, of spiritual care, which includes a knowledge of particular faith systems with their respective beliefs and practices. Inservice programs should be regularly scheduled to familiarize health care workers with the belief systems of the people being served—particularly on issues of dying and death. Such information will help caregivers not only discuss the needs of particular patients but also make appropriate referrals. The wise caregiver knows his or her limits and when, where, and to whom to make necessary requests for spiritual support for the patient or family member.

### Item 24

The assumption has been that the religious leaders (ordained clergy, rabbis, imams, shamans, and practitioners) have the responsibility for spiritual care in health care settings. They are seen as persons specially trained and authorized to represent their religious traditions and assume the commensurate responsibilities of ministry. The reality is that not enough resources are allocated by the health care institution to implement spiritual care provided solely by the designated religious leaders. Because of limited resources, institutional spiritual care that is provided by designated religious leaders through departments of pastoral care or religious ministries has been directed principally to the following kinds of services: crisis intervention; counseling and comforting persons who have been identified to be in spiritual distress; giving support before and after surgery; offering sacraments, prayers, and spiritual related readings; coordinating care with community religious leaders when that is deemed helpful; establishing times for corporate worship services and leading them; participating in the ethical decision making of the institution; and supporting the staff. (We can expect an increased need for staff support as caregivers struggle to maintain high-quality patient care in the midst of the economic changes precipitated by managed care.)

A distinct support that a designated religious leader may offer is assurance that he or she is credible in representing the particular belief system. Accompanying this may be the expectation that the religious leader will help the other to find meaning amid the doubts of faith or fears that may have arisen at this time of crisis. Of particular

assistance will be the religious leader's capacity to enable the other to sort through matters of conscience or feelings of guilt from acts committed as well as regrets about what has been left undone. Each religious tradition has its practices, rituals, prayers, and/or sacraments to help restore a sense of at-one-ment with oneself, others, and the Other.

A unique role of the religious leader is to facilitate reconciliation by enabling one to make peace. Much spiritual work has been done and is done when persons have at last reached the place where they can say "thank you," like the patient quoted earlier: "If I hadn't had cancer, I would never have known..."(this gift, opportunity, beauty in life).

Fortunately, consciousness of the breadth of spiritual care has begun to intersect with the consciousness of its height and depth so that persons are more open to seeing the many facets of spirituality and spiritual care. Such an expanding consciousness not only provides more support for the patient and family but calls forth each person's responsibility and opportunity to be a spiritual caregiver one to another.

### Item 26

Caregivers who are constantly working with persons in crisis, particularly persons living with life-threatening illnesses and undergoing debilitating treatments, need to be in tune with their own physical, mental, emotional, and spiritual needs to be able to maintain the level of support required by patients and family members.

A natural human response when one has reached one's limits in any dimension is to withdraw. This is especially true when one is responsible for giving emotional and spiritual support. One becomes a "hardened" health care worker, and empathy ebbs. Both the one giving care and the one receiving it are diminished. To prevent this, the caregiver must tend to his or her needs. Sam Klagsbrun helped make it clear that it is the responsibility of caregivers to have their professional skills carefully honed and to be aware of their spiritual roots and be able to rely on them in the face of the high dosage of human suffering they receive when they care for the dying (17). However, given the high-stress nature of oncology, the institution should provide resources in time, money, and staff to establish ongoing educational and staff support programs (including days away and retreats) to nurture caregivers. It would be short-sighted not to recognize that this is required to maintain stability as well as enhance growth and efficacy.

### Community Coordination

Shrinking economic resources have an impact on all institutions. Increasingly, health care of patients and families will be given predominantly through clinics and at home. Staff giving spiritual care will need to be flexible, networking with others to assure that the spiritual needs of patients and families are being addressed by human and other institutional resources in the larger community.

To assure such collaboration, it is the responsibility of the health care institution to initiate and develop bridges to the larger community with its churches, synagogues, mosques, schools, and libraries to foster communication between professionals and lay persons. From opportunities to learn from each other, through educational forums and arts-related events reaching back and forth between the health care institution and the community, enhanced support may be provided to patients and families. This is preventive as well as applied medicine.

## Education and Research

The spiritual dimensions of care have received little attention in the education of health care professionals. Some believe that this is due to the scarcity of fundamental research in the areas of spirituality and spiritual care. Given the present scientific research methodology, how does one develop and apply valid reliable measures of evaluation to matters of the spirit? The same question is posed in the effort to evaluate the efficacy of arts experiences in people's lives. Have we not been pouring new wine into old wineskins in trying to use research methodologies inappropriate to matters of the spirit?

Our educational institutions have valued and fostered knowledge that is mechanistic and quantifiable and that cannot deal with the qualities of experience that include those from nature, color and sound, meaning, value, life, consciousness, self, and spirit. A cultural split has arisen from the undervaluing of the knowledge that comes from qualitative experience. On one side are the truths of knowledge given predominantly by science and discursive, empirical reason. On the other side are the truths of faith, religious experience, morality, meaning, and value. The latter are seen as grounded not in knowledge but variously in feeling, ethical action, communal convention, folk tradition, or unfathomable mystical experiences (18).

In order to overcome the faith–knowledge issue, Douglas Sloan gives at least four criteria that need to be met:

1. "There must be a fundamental transformation in our ways of knowing by developing qualitative ways of knowing on par with our quantitative....

2. "The positive potentials of modern consciousness must be preserved. The capacity for clear thinking consciousness, individual identity and selfhood, and the potential for freedom that individuality and clear-consciousness alone make possible...(This) transformation of knowing might best be thought of as the development of imagination in the fullest sense....

3. "A radical transformation of knowing will involve a transformation of ourselves. Knowledge of qualities in the world will depend on our being able to bring them to birth and recognize them within ourselves....

4. "The transformation of knowing will have consequences both for our knowledge of spirit and for our knowledge of nature (18)."

Can there be valid research of the spiritual dimension unless we indeed begin to value qualitative ways of knowing? The author believes that one of the mandates of our time is "to develop new capacities for valuing, knowing, and articulating the qualitative. This will begin to open new sources for the concrete and radical renewal of science, medicine, agriculture, economics, community, art, education, and religion [which] we so desperately need" (18).

## CONCLUSION

Just as it has been imperative for humankind to learn the benefits as well as the threats of the material world that scientific knowledge can teach us, so too, to maintain balance in our lives and help us to use our scientific knowledge wisely for human benefit, we need also to open ourselves to the other ways of knowing—the qualitative ways of experience that deepen our spirituality and empower us to offer spiritual care to others. This may be the hardest task of all, because it involves our becoming more vulnerable to the pain and suffering of others and also to the pain and suffering of our own lives in body, mind, emotions, and spirit.

However, we can be assured that those of us who practice our art in each discipline of supportive care will have also learned not to be afraid to be vulnerable. For haven't the most supportive spiritual caregivers always been the wounded healers?

May we remember this final message: Life is not our destination but rather a journey:

*The road
that stretches before our feet
is a challenge to our hearts
long before it tests the strength of our legs.
Our destiny
is to run to the edge of the world and beyond,
off into the darkness:
sure in spite of all our blindness,
secure in spite of all our helplessness,
strong in spite of all our weakness,
joyfully in love in spite of all
the pressures on our hearts.
In that darkness beyond the world
we can begin to know the world and ourselves—
and to understand
that we were not made to pace out our lives behind
    prison walls
but to walk into the arms of God (19).*

## REFERENCES

1. Spiritual Care Work Group. Assumptions and principles of spiritual care. In: Corr C, Morgan J, Wass H, eds. *Statements of death, dying and*

*bereavement*, Document No. 4. International Work Group on Death, Dying and Bereavement, through King's College, Ontario, 1993:33–41.

2. Suhadolc N. What does S.O.S. mean? *Coping* 1995;Nov/Dec:69.

3. Du Boulay S. *Cicely Saunders*. London: Hodder and Stoughton, 1984: 160.

4. Wald F, ed. *In Quest of the spiritual component of care for the terminally ill* [colloquium proceedings]. New Haven: Yale University School of Nursing, 1986.

5. Loder T. *Guerrillas of grace: prayers for the battle*. San Diego: Lura Media, 1985:104.

6. Carmody D, Carmody J. *In the path of the masters*. New York: Paragon House, 1994:8.

7. Nouwen H. *Out of solitude*. Notre Dame, IN: Ave Maria Press, 1974:33.

8. Fairchild RW. *Finding hope again*. San Francisco: Harper and Row, 1980:50.

9. Carlson C. Swirling. In: Bailey S, ed. The arts in spiritual care, *Sem Oncol Nurs* 1997;Vol. XIII, No. 4:242–247.

10. Bailey S. The arts as an avenue to the spirit. *New Catholic World Magazine* 1987;Nov/Dec:264–268.

11. Weil S. *The need for roots*. London: Routledge and Kegan Paul, 1952:9.

12. Bailey S. Creativity and the close of life. In: Corless I, Germino B, Pittman M, eds. *Dying, death and bereavement*. Boston: Jones and Bartlett, 1994:327.

13. Coluzzi P, Grant M, Doroshow J, Rhiner M, Ferrell B, Rivera L. Survey of the provision of supportive care services at National Cancer Institute—designated cancer centers. *J Clin Oncol* 1995;13:756–764.

14. Chan L. Hospice: a new building type to comfort the dying. *AIA J* 1976;Dec:42.

15. Attig T. Respecting the spirituality of the dying and bereaved. In Corless I, Germino B, Pittman M, eds. *A challenge for living*. Boston: Jones and Bartlett, 1995:117.

16. Bailey S. From mourning to morning. In: Morgan J. Dynamic caregiving with the dying and grieving. Amityville: Baywood, 1998 (in press).

17. Klagsbrun S. The ethics of hospice care. In: *Am Psychologist*. Nov 1982:1263.

18. Sloan D. *Faith and knowledge*. Louisville: Westminster John Knox Press, 1994:ix.

19. Elliott W. *Flow of flesh, reach of spirit*. Grand Rapids: Wm. B. Eerdmans, 1995:251. Adapted from the beginning of Farrell W and Healy M, eds, *My way of life: pocket edition of St. Thomas*. Brooklyn: Confraternity of the Precious Blood, 1952.

# SECTION III

# Terminal Care

*Principles and Practice of Supportive Oncology,*
edited by Ann Berger et al.
Lippincott–Raven Publishers, Philadelphia ©1998

CHAPTER 52

# The Evolution of Hospice and Palliative Medicine

Walter B. Forman

W. B. Forman: Department of Internal Medicine, University of New Mexico Health Sciences Center, Albuquerque, NM 87108.

Song Of A Man About To Die In A Strange Land
(Ojibwa poem, c. 1400)

> *If I die here in a strange land,*
> *If I die in a land not my own,*
> *Nevertheless, the thunder,*
> *The rolling thunder,*
> *Will take me home.*
> *If I die here, the wind,*
> *The wind rushing over the prairie,*
> *The wind will take me home.*
> *The wind and the thunder,*
> *They are the same everywhere,*
> *What does it matter, then,*
> *If I die in a strange land.*

## HISTORY OF THE HOSPICE MOVEMENT

### Before the 20th Century

The earliest hospice programs were not for the care of the dying but rather were developed to provided hospitality for pilgrims during their journeys. The first of these facilities appeared in the late 400s in Italy as a refuge for pilgrims from Africa. Over the next few centuries, hospice programs became disseminated throughout Europe. These hospices eventually became the earliest hospitals. Eventually, the term *hospice* became associated with a place to care for the dying, according to Dame Cicely Saunders. Madame J. Garnier founded several calvaries, or hospices, in the early 1840s in France, and the Sisters of Charity set up the first hospice in Ireland in 1879 (1). In the United States, Calvary Hospital in New York opened in 1899 with a mission to care for the incurable and dying. The foundation of the modern hospice move-

ment, the home care component, was not originally included. This concept was yet to be developed and unquestionably accounts for one of the most innovative changes in the care of the dying. It should be noted that not all cultures have taken the same approach to dying as those in the European tradition. The opening poem best exemplifies those differences. In this short passage, an American Indian, an Ojibwa from the Great Plains, is about to die in a strange land without benefit or in fact need of a hospice setting (2).

Why has the word *hospice*, which comes from the root word *hospes*, meaning "a host," come to connote a place—or, in the United States, a way—to pay for the care of the dying. There are at least two explanations. The founder of the Irish hospice in Dublin, Sister Mary Aikenhead, is thought to have used the word *hospice* because it was her view that death was part of an eternal journey, likened to that of pilgrims on their religious journeys (3). However, the first recorded injunction to attend to the dying person can be found in the *Shulhan Aruk*, the code of Jewish law compiled by Rabbi Joseph Karo in the 16th century. In chapter 194, verse 4, one finds the admonishment not "to leave a dying person in order that his soul may not depart when he is all alone because it is bewildered when departing from the body" (4). It is my contention that the coming together of these concepts—hospitality, a place to comfort the dying, and the postbiblical injunction not to leave the dying person alone—has led to the evolution of the modern hospice as well as to its current institutional adaptation in various countries throughout the world. Sloan (5) suggests that the diffusion of the hospice movement in the United States was a response to the perceived need for an alternative way to care for the dying. The hospice movement in the United States was a direct consequence of the death awareness movement, led by Dr. Elisabeth Kubler-Ross, seeking a change in the place of death from the hospital to that of the home (6–9).

## 1950 to the Present

### *World Wide Programs*

Three major programs are credited with firmly establishing the credibility of hospice care in the last quarter century. In 1967, after 19 years in planning, St. Christopher's Hospice opened under the medical direction of Dame Cicely Saunders. Dr. Saunders, who had shared with a survivor of the Warsaw ghetto her vision of a place to care for the dying with dignity, was bequeathed £500 by him to start the hospice program. Her vision was of an institution that would provide outstanding care but also where "there could be a place for scientific medicine and nursing" (10). Thus, one of Dr. Saunders' great achievements was to introduce and apply the scientific concept of research to the care of the dying, along with establishing many of our current clinical practices. At St. Christopher's she established the need to give pain medications by the clock rather than as needed or requested. She encouraged the person to determine the intensity of his or her own pain, and firmly incorporated the role of the family, particularly in the home care setting. Not only has this one individual and facility been responsible for many new concepts and changes in practice patterns, but she has also been the one primarily responsible for disseminating hospice care throughout the world. The second fellow at St. Christopher's was Dr. Robert Twycross. He subsequently established the World Health Organization's Collaborating Center for Hospice/Palliative Care at the Sir Michael Sobell House in Oxford. Dr. Twycross has written extensively on pain and symptom control. Dr. Balfour Mount, another trainee at St. Christopher's, opened the Palliative Care Service at the Royal Victorian Hospital in Montreal in 1975. Finally, Florence Wald, Dean of the Graduate School of Nursing at Yale University, who had also studied at St. Christopher's, opened the New Haven Connecticut Hospice in 1974. This was the first hospice home care program without an inpatient service in the United States; their inpatient service opened in 1979.

### *The United States*

The hospice in New Haven, Connecticut, opened in 1974, thereby ushering in the modern era of home care hospice in the United States. However, there were other hospital-based programs at the time: Calvary Hospital and St. Luke's–Roosevelt Hospital in New York. The New Haven program was responsible for bringing together North American advocates for hospice care in the late 1970's in order to establish guidelines for operational issues necessary to form hospice programs in this coun-

try. This meeting led to the development of the National Hospice Organization. Mor and colleagues (11) give five reasons why hospice was so quickly successful in the United States:

1. Consumerism. Societal changes in the 1960s and 1970s led to increased consumer demand for better products and services. As these changes were occurring the hospice movement appeared. What better way for people to express their distress with the health care industry's approach to dying than to take their loved ones home to die?

2. Naturalism. We have entered the era of "organic everything." Hospice, with its low-tech, high-touch approach to patient care, is a very acceptable alternative to traditional medical care.

3. Holism. The practice of medicine has become highly specialized. Patients are often viewed by their health care professionals as parts rather than as whole persons. Hospice has as its care model the whole person, including the family.

4. Discovering the total life span. The world population is aging. As a society, and as health care professionals, we can no longer avoid the fact that dying is a natural consequence of living. The concept of a good death has become a major theme in American culture. However, the U.S. Supreme Court has recently ruled that the individual states have the responsibility to determine the time and place of the terminally ill person's death.

5. Cost containment. Is it less expensive to die in a hospital or at home with a hospice program? We all hope that our medical decisions not only will be based on cost but, as our society looks at the cost of health care, also will consider quality of life. Cost savings were demonstrated by the study of Mor and colleagues. Nonetheless, Kane et al. (12) published results from a randomized controlled trial of hospice versus conventional care for the dying in 1984 and did not demonstrate that hospice care was a more cost-effective approach. It is important to continue to address these issues, since hospice and its concepts of care were originally driven by the need for social, rather than economic change.

In section 122 of the Tax Equity and Fiscal Responsibility Act (TEFRA) enacted on September 3, 1982, Congress authorized the Medicare Hospice benefit. This law, more than any other single factor, has defined hospice care in the United States (13). It is a landmark piece of legislation because it not only addresses the needs of the terminally ill but provides the framework for the first federally mandated managed care program in the United States. This benefit defines the type of services that are to be provided, the persons who are eligible to receive services, and a payment structure for services. For a hospice program to be certified to receive Medicare reimbursement, it must adhere to Federal guidelines and a defined set of patient eligibility criteria (Table 1).

**TABLE 1.** *The Medicare hospice benefit eligibility criteria*

1. Must be Medicare eligible.
2. Must have a terminal illness, i.e., physician-certified prognosis of less than 6 months to live.
3. The approach to care must be palliative.
4. Must give informed consent, i.e., understands the nature of the illness.

From its beginning in the 1970s, and enhanced by the TEFRA legislation in the early 1980s, hospice care in the United States has demonstrated tremendous growth. Its scope of care now includes home care as well as free-standing residential (inpatient) units and care in nursing homes. Currently, more than 2000 Medicare-approved hospices, including not-for-profit and for-profit agencies, serve over 300,000 patients and families each year. More than 80% of hospice patients have cancer as their major illness. The National Hospice Organization has recently published admission guidelines for patients with non-cancer diagnoses (13).

## THE EVOLUTION OF PALLIATIVE MEDICINE

### World Health Organization Activities

"[N]othing would have a greater impact on the quality of life of these patients than the dissemination and implementation of knowledge already available in relation to pain and symptom management" (14). This quotation is from a landmark 1990 World Health Organization (WHO) expert committee report, outlining guidelines for cancer pain and using palliative care (14). These guidelines were designed for patients living in developing countries and are based on the availability of a limited number of analgesic drugs, the lack of specialized health care professionals, and the remote locale of many people in the world. This type of planning was seen as the best type of care for all people with cancer. The WHO effort has been successful in improving pain management practices in many nations and helping others to consider development of progressive health policies that hopefully will lead to improved care.

### Palliative Medicine as a Medical Specialty

As hospice programs developed, and the need arose for physicians to have special knowledge and skills, the concept of palliative medicine as a distinct area of medical practice began to evolve. Why the name *palliative medicine*? There are several reasons. The root word *palliate* is derived from an article of clothing worn by Roman women to cover their undergarments. The modern usage of the word includes the concept of alleviating or relieving. Why the new word *palliative medicine* compared

with *hospice*, an already accepted term applied to care of the dying? Hospice, at least in the United States, defines a system that pays for the care of the dying. In other parts of the world, the term *hospice* means a place for care of the indigent. In some medical circles, the term *hospice* connotes a rather soft—i.e., without scientific credentials—area of patient care. *Hospice* has also come to be used as an exclusive term by those who are seeking alternative practice patterns. Finally, the term *hospice*, in regard to the physician, the patient, and the family, has come to mean the loss of hope—in other words, dying. In order to address these issues and to bring the role of the physician into greater focus, the term *palliative medicine* is rapidly being adopted. The term has been eloquently defined by Dr. Derek Doyle as "the study and management of patients with active, progressive, far-advanced disease for whom the prognosis is limited and the focus of care is quality of life" (15).

In the last decade, palliative medicine has grown as a medical specialty area. Numerous textbooks, peer reviewed journals, and curricula have been developed, and research efforts have been undertaken.

The first organized medical group to recognize palliative medicine as a new subspecialty of general internal medicine was The Royal College of Physicians in Great Britain, which in 1987 approved a training program for senior registrars. The Royal Australian Society of Physicians and Surgeons shortly followed this lead. No further developments outside the United States occurred until 1993, when the Canadian Society for Palliative Care Physicians was formed. It currently is attempting to gain medical specialty status. In 1988 the Academy of Hospice Physicians (n.k.a. The American Academy of Hospice and Palliative Medicine) formed in the United States under the guidance of Dr. Josephine Magno. It now numbers almost 1600 physicians, representing a wide variety of specialty areas. The first United States examination for added qualifications in palliative medicine was administered by the American Board of Hospice and Palliative Medicine in November 1996. There are now 125 physicians in the United States with credentials in palliative medicine.

## EDUCATIONAL OPPORTUNITIES IN PALLIATIVE MEDICINE

### Undergraduate Education

The need for curricula in death education was identified as early as the 1970s (16). In 1991, Mermann and colleagues noted that "personal involvement of students with patients in the process of learning about death and dying was minimal, despite the widely observed fact that students can hardly wait to go on the wards" (17). In the United States, one set of end-of-life education objectives has been published, and a growing number of medical schools are now incorporating the principles of palliative medicine in their curricula (18–22). As one example, Knight and colleagues (23) have published a curriculum for medical students and were able to show that it effected a major change in students' knowledge of pain and symptom management in the terminally ill.

In 1991, The Canadian Committee on Palliative Care Education published *The Canadian Palliative Care Curriculum*, a comprehensive set of curriculum objectives for Canadian medical schools (24). Great Britain has a Working Party of the Association for Palliative Medicine, which has issued a teaching syllabus, including guidelines for training medical students, generalists, and other physicians with a special interest in palliative medicine (25). A variety of other programs throughout the world now have curricula or clinical clerkships, designed to immerse medical students in the care of the dying. Many of these programs also offer experience in the home care setting.

When should palliative medicine be taught? Both Weissman (26) in the United States and MacDonald (27) in Canada have presented techniques to integrate palliative medicine education in the general hospital experience. Different approaches will no doubt emerge in the coming years, but no matter where palliative medicine is taught, it is essential that it be done at the bedside, within the context of an interdisciplinary team setting (28).

**Postgraduate Training**

Two general types of programs are available. In England, a special training program for senior registrars is available that can lead to a certificate in palliative medicine. In both Australia and England, diplomas can be obtained by completion of a rigorous course of study via the correspondence system (29,30). In the United States, several institutions now offer training in palliative medicine, including one-year palliative medicine fellowships or short preceptorship training experiences.

## PALLIATIVE MEDICINE: ONE ASPECT OF COMPREHENSIVE CANCER CARE

Our system of health care currently emphasizes the use of specialists in the care of particular diseases. Oncologists, whether of radiation or medical background, have had their training directed toward the cancer in the person, rather than the person with the cancer. All of these highly trained individuals are expected to also deliver excellent care at the end of life.

But while the medical establishment has aimed its care toward curing the disease, our patients and their payors are suggesting that times are changing. In particular, this applies to the care of the dying, or for that matter any person whose disease cannot be cured. How do we bring

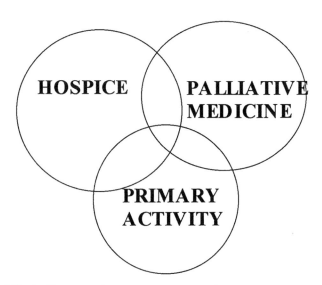

**FIG. 1.** The role of the primary care professional in regards to hospice and palliative medicine.

about this change in our professional culture? If a change is to be brought about, what will it be and to whom will it be directed: cancer patients, those with other incurable diseases, both? As members of a culture and as health care professionals, we must realize that there comes a time when medical intervention will no longer sustain the individual. It is at this point that palliative medicine can provide the person and the family unit with a different approach to their care.

The principles of palliative medicine need to be incorporated into our professional lives if total care is to be achieved. Is that not what we all wish—a time of peace and freedom from symptoms so that we can complete our life? This paradigm shift is essential if we are to provide whole-person care for our patients (Fig. 1).

Predicting the future of health care in this country is very difficult. As health care professionals, we need to address the concerns of whole persons and their families if we are to sustain our impact on their medical care. In order to accomplish this goal, palliative medicine must become part of our care plan early and throughout the course of treatment. It is no longer sufficient to say "there is nothing more I can do for you." Someone can and must assist the individual and the family. That person should be trained in those aspects of care that will provide relief from pain and other symptoms, assist the person and family to find meaning in their lives during and following the death of the individual, and assist individuals to live until they die.

## REFERENCES

1. Saunders C. Foreword. In: Doyle D, Hanks GWC, MacDonald N, eds. *Oxford Textbook of Palliative Medicine*. Oxford: Oxford University Press, 1993:vi.
2. Weir RF, ed. *Death in Literature*. New York: Columbia University Press, 1980:83.

3. Paradise LF. *Hospice handbook: a guide for managers and planners.* Rockville, MD: Aspen Systems Corporation, 1985.

4. Ganzfried S, ed. *Code of Jewish Law.* New York: Hebrew Publishing Co., 1961;89.

5. Sloan LS. The hospice movement: a study in the diffusion of innovative palliative care. *Am J Hospice Pall Care* 1992;May/June:24–31.

6. Stoddard S. Hospice in the United States: an overview. *J Pall Care* 1989;5:10–19.

7. Campbell L. History of the hospice movement. *Cancer Nurs* 1986;9: 333–338.

8. Rhymes J. Hospice care in America. *JAMA* 1990;264:369–372.

9. Amenta M. Hospice in the United States. *Nurs Clin North Am* 1985;20: 269–279.

10. Saunders C. The evolution of the modern hospices. In: Mann RD, ed. *The history of the management of pain.* Park Ridge, NJ: Parthenon Press, 1988:167–178.

11. Mor V, Greer DS, Kastenbaum R, eds. *The hospice experiment.* Baltimore, MD: John Hopkins University Press, 1988:13–15.

12. Kane RL, Wales J, Berstein L, et al. A randomized controlled trial of hospice care. *Lancet* 1984;1:890–894.

13. Federal Registry DHEW Health Care Financing Administration: Medicare program; hospice care; final rule. Part VII. December 16, 1983.

14. World Health Organization. *Cancer pain relief and palliative care: report of a WHO expert committee.* Technical Report Series 804. Geneva: World Health Organization, 1990:7.

15. Doyle D. Palliative medicine: a time for definition? *Pall Med* 1993;7: 253–255.

16. Dickinson GE. Death education in United States medical schools. *J Med Educ* 1976;51:34–36.

17. Mermann AC, Gunn DB, Dickinson GE. Learning to care for the dying: a survey of medical schools and a model course. *Acad Med* 1991;66: 35–38.

18. Schonwetter MD, Robinson BE. Educational objectives for medical training in the care of the terminally ill. *Acad Med* 1994;69(8):688–690.

19. Billings JA. Medical education for hospice care: a selected bibliography with brief annotations. *Hospice J* 1993;9(1):69–83.

20. Martin RW, Wylie N. Teaching third-year medical students how to care for terminally ill patients. *Acad Med* 1989;64:413–414.

21. Weissman DE. Pre-clinical palliative medicine education at the Medical College of Wisconsin. *J Cancer Ed* 1993;8(3):191–195.

22. Grauel RR, Eger R, Finley RC, et al. Educational program in palliative and hospice care at the University of Maryland School of Medicine. *J Cancer Educ* 11:144–147, 1996.

23. Knight CF, Knight PF, Gellula MH, Holman GH. Training our future physicians: a hospice rotation for medical students. *Am J Hospice Pall Care* 1992;Jan/Feb:23–28.

24. The Canadian Committee on Palliative Care Education. *The Canadian palliative care curriculum.* 1991.

25. The Working Party of the Association for Palliative Medicine. *Guidelines for teaching of palliative medicine.* Southhampton, UK:

26. Weissman D. Palliative medicine education: bridging the gap between acute care and hospice. *J Cancer Educ* 1991;6:67–8.

27. MacDonald N. Oncology and palliative care: the case for coordination. *Cancer Treat Rev* 1993;19(suppl. A):29–41.

28. Sheehan DC, Forman WB, eds. *Interdisciplinary hospice and palliative care: concepts and practice.* Boston: Jones and Bartlett, 1996.

29. Maddocks I, Donnell J. A master's degree and graduate diploma in palliative care. *Pall Med* 1992;6:317–320.

30. The course secretary, U.W.C.M. Diploma in palliative medicine, Marie Curie Centre, Holme Tower, Bridgeman Road, PENARTH, South Glamorgan, CF64 3YR, 1991.

*Principles and Practice of Supportive Oncology,*
edited by Ann Berger et al.
Lippincott–Raven Publishers, Philadelphia ©1998

# CHAPTER 53

# Symptom Control in Dying

## Porter Storey

Many people endure terrible suffering as they die of advanced cancer (1). The more we study and measure this distress, the broader and deeper we find this ocean of anguish to be (2). Not only does this suffering rob our patients of the opportunities for growth and enjoyment of their final days, but it tortures their loved ones (and health care providers) for years thereafter.

How can we help? In this chapter we will explore what many dying cancer patients have told us they need, and proven techniques for the alleviation of some of the more distressing and common syndromes of distress at the end of life. Our patients remind us that, particularly at this stage of life, they are more than failing organ systems and symptom complexes. Dying and suffering are deeply personal (3). They are central to one's life story. Suffering can sometimes be relieved by competent control of symptoms, but more often it will require more of us than prescribing the right dose of the best drug to bring effective relief.

## WHAT DO THE DYING NEED FROM US?

People have been dying without the help of oncologists and specialized treatments for many years. Dying is the inevitable result of being born; why medicalize this natural event? Our patients consistently tell us that they want to participate in decisions about their care and to exercise some control over their lives, and that they need honest, compassionately delivered information (4). They tell us they don't want to die in pain, gasping for breath, or suffer with other distressing symptoms. They tell us that they need to find meaning and hope in the midst of deterioration, distress, and despair.

P. Storey: The Hospice at the Texas Medical Center, Houston, TX 77030-4123.

## Honest Information

"Don't tell my mother that she's dying—she'll just give up!" We hear such statements often. A mere 30 years ago, few cancer patients in the United States were even told of their diagnosis, much less their prognosis. In 1985 Dame Cicely Saunders reported that despite their complete willingness to discuss the issues, 30% of St. Christopher's Hospice inpatients had not been informed of their diagnosis because they had not been specifically asked (5). Palliative medicine specialists in Poland and several Middle Eastern and Asian countries report that it is rarely acceptable to tell a patient of his or her short prognosis (6). Yet, how can patients make informed choices about their treatment options without some knowledge of their diagnosis and prognosis? Few physicians or oncology specialists in the United States would argue today that this information should be withheld from patients—but how do we avoid increasing our patients' suffering and despair?

Information about a lethal diagnosis or short prognosis must be delivered sensitively, in the context of a caring physician-patient relationship. There are no right words, particularly before we get to know our patient (7). Who is this person with cancer? What knowledge, experience, apprehensions, and expectations does he or she bring into the room? Physicians need to use the history and physical exam to find out not only the extent of the disease but who the person experiencing this illness is. Providing extra time, as scarce as it is, is essential at the beginning of the therapeutic relationship, at turning points, and near the end of life.

The preparation of the professional is also critical to a successful encounter. We must learn how to be fully present with the patient: to be centered, listening deeply to all levels of the interchange. At these times the patient will feel comfortable enough to tell us about his or her needs, fears, and hopes. We have to learn to trust this process, to breathe, to slow down, to really be there for the patient. There is a deep wisdom in all of us that we can cultivate, listen to, and trust. It knows what to say. When we speak, it should be the truth.

Delivering bad news and coping with conflicts and anger is difficult work. When family, significant others, colleagues, co-workers, and the patient dump strong emotions on us, they test our wisdom, centeredness, and endurance. Some days we can be the catalyst for great healing; other days we may be barely able to control a strong desire to retaliate. In some situations the best that can be hoped for is damage control. How well we care for ourselves—physically, emotionally, and spiritually—will strongly influence how much we have to give in these difficult situations (8). Another critical survival skill is the ability to let go of the need to control the outcome. Attachment to the fruits of our labors can drive us mad. Often all the right things are done and the family still goes away angry or the patient still dies "too soon." Do your best and then retreat in peace.

## Goal Setting

How much should be done to control hypercalcemia? Should every patient with bone metastases receive hemibody irradiation? When should a barbiturate coma be considered instead of neurosurgical ablation? How should psychosocial problems at the end of life be best managed?

After you have a sense of who the patient is and where this disease fits in his or her life story, you must determine the appropriate level of medical intensity for this patient's "big picture." For instance, a 10-year-old boy dying of leukemia is likely to receive more blood transfusions than a 65-year-old woman dying of colon cancer and dementia in a nursing home. A 75-year-old vibrant, active, retired professor dying of breast or prostate cancer might benefit from a transfusion early in the course of the illness but probably not at the end stage. Determining the appropriate levels of medical intensity is based on the patient's (and family's) wishes, the functional capabilities of the patient, the stage of disease progression, and the potential benefit/burden ratio of a given treatment compared with other available treatments. Oversimplifying these complex decisions—as in asking, "Do you want us to do everything to help your mother?"—is neither helpful nor responsible.

These decisions also involve the other physical, psychological, social, personal, and spiritual aspects of the patient—aspects best managed by an *interdisciplinary team*. For the 10-year-old with leukemia, for example, a well-trained palliative care nurse and social worker might be able to make it possible for the child to die at home instead of in the intensive care unit—a therapeutic maneuver that may be much more effective than dripping

**TABLE 1.** *To intervene effectively in advanced cancer*

Get to know *the person* with the disease.
Gauge the *medical intensity* appropriately.
Search for *treatable causes* when feasible.
*Treat specifically* whenever possible.
Use the *interdisciplinary team* to address the whole situation.

still more red blood cells into the child's overused veins. For the demented woman with colon cancer, a volunteer or music therapist might be able to alleviate the agitation and dyspnea with the singing of favorite melodies, or the nutritionist might point out that the six-cans-per-day gastric tube infusion is contributing as much to the dyspnea and secretions as is the anemia. For the retired professor, the chaplain might have noted that the patient is a Jehovah's Witness and thus would never want to be transfused with red blood cells, or the nurse might have noted the black tar-like stools, the high dosage of nonsteroidal antiinflammatory drugs, and the history of recurrent peptic ulcer disease. Thus, effective symptom management requires getting to know the person who has the disease, gauging the appropriate level of medical intensity, searching diligently for treatable causes (particularly in higher medical intensity situations), giving the appropriate level of specific therapy when possible, and using an interdisciplinary team effectively to address the multitude of physical, psychological, social, personal, and spiritual/existential aspects of the situation (Table 1).

## CRESCENDO PAIN SYMPTOM MANAGEMENT

Rapid escalation in the intensity of pain and anguish close to the end of life is well known. The incidence of this distress is uncertain, but estimates range from 5% to 50% (9). The first task is to recognize that this type of pain is occurring. Patients at home may require an urgent visit by a medical team member to identify the problem. Some common causes of severe distress are given in Table 2.

### Evaluation

Cicely Saunders has long taught the concept of *total pain*, that is, the multiple physical, psychological, social, and spiritual/existential components that together create the pain experience (10). As Table 2 points out, a call for help with pain in a terminal patient may require a great deal more than a prescription for a stronger analgesic. Often the situation is complicated by the patient's immobility at home. Someone must visit the patient at home, or the patient must travel (usually by ambulance) to an inpatient setting. With the help of a competent hospice/palliative care team, many such problems can be addressed at home. As has been noted in Great Britain and Australia,

**TABLE 2.** *Examples of possible causes of severe pain*

Physical
    Can't swallow/won't take medication (big pills, weak patient)
    New symptom (neuropathic pain, delirium, fracture, constipation)
    Medication ineffective (poor compliance or needs stronger medication)
    Unrealistic goals/excessive activity: (incident pain, falling)
Anxiety, anger
    Afraid to take medication (getting weak, drowsy, confused)
    Upset with family, friends, doctor ("If only...I'd be OK")
    Can't afford analgesics (financial stress, worry)
    Can't sleep (afraid of dying or losing control)
Interpersonal
    Stress from too many or too few visitors
    Righteous out-of-town relative arrives
    Caregiver exhausted, afraid, angry
    Fights over money or medication management
Nonacceptance
    "How could this be happening to me? NO!"
    "If I just have enough faith, God will heal me." (so no medications are needed)
    "How do I make sense of all this?"
    Hopelessness, despair ("What's the use?")

**TABLE 3.** *Evaluation of pain*

What disease is this? How far advanced?
What was working? How well?
What has changed? How fast?
What medications have been prescribed? Which taken? Why?
What are the separate components of the new situation?
Can we treat any of these complications specifically?
Are adjuvant medications indicated?
Is this problem likely to respond to opioids?
Who is caring for the patient? What does he or she see as the problem?
Can this be managed with oral medications? At home?
How can we best address the psychosocial and spiritual components?
What is the meaning of this pain to *this* patient and family?

when inpatient hospice care is available, 25% of cancer patients will want (or need) to spend their final week or two there (11). The most common reasons for transfer to an inpatient setting are uncontrolled pain and terminal restlessness or delirium. In whichever setting can be arranged, the clinician must do a thorough evaluation of the patient. A careful history and physical exam will reveal the answers to many of the questions in Table 3.

Special concerns arise as the patient approaches death. How severe is the pain? Few patients who are near death can complete extensive symptom control assessment tools. One hospital found it possible to reliably measure pain with simple yes/no questions (13). Some other available options are given in Table 4. The important point is that the severity of the pain must be assessed as a guide to therapy, and if at all possible, the patient should do the rating. Often in the final days, one must rely on facial expressions, grimacing on turning, and the number of boosts (rescue doses) given to judge the adequacy of pain control, but even this can be done in a valid manner, as

exemplified by assessment of discomfort in cognitively impaired patients (16).

## Treatment

How do you manage a patient who can't swallow tablets and wants to stay at home? Regular intramuscular (IM) injections are painful, require skilled nursing care, and are unsuitable for cachectic patients. Fortunately, new technologies together with old skills have made IM injections essentially obsolete in the care of the dying patient. Central venous catheters are also usually unnecessary. Transdermal fentanyl patches (Duragesic) are very useful but are expensive, are available in only four strengths, and have a slow onset of action (17). Sublingual soluble morphine or hydromorphone tablets or very concentrated liquid opioid preparations are simple to give and easy to titrate, and the bitter taste is a lessening problem as death approaches (18). Slow-release morphine tablets can be administered rectally as another means of delivering a wide range of morphine doses with readily available drugs (19). The slow-release morphine solutions and suppositories available in other countries should soon be available in the United States and will certainly help. Adjuvant analgesics such as indomethacin come in suppository form, and doxepin or carbamazepine can be given rectally in gelatin capsules for continued control of neuropathic pain (20).

**TABLE 4.** *Examples of pain scales*

| | Multiple dimensions of pain | Multiple symptoms | Single page | Reliable (correlate with patient rating) | Useful to guide therapy |
|---|---|---|---|---|---|
| Brief Pain Inventory (short form) (ref 15) | ✔ | | | ✔ | ✔ |
| Memorial Pain Assessment Card (ref 14) | ✔ | | ✔ | ✔ | ✔ |
| Edmonton Symptom Assessment Scale (ref 12) | | ✔ | ✔ | ✔ | ✔ |
| Liverpool Palliative Care Assessment Form (ref 13) | | ✔ | ✔ | ✔ | ✔ |
| Family ratings | | ✔ | ✔ | | ✔ |
| Staff ratings | | ✔ | ✔ | | ✔ |

Unfortunately, many patients and families find the rectal route unacceptable, especially for the rapid-dose titration so often necessary in crescendo pain. A visiting nurse can easily implant a subcutaneous needle and teach the family to give small (<1.5 ml) injections into the injection site cap (21).

The most ideal solution is often an infusion pump that can provide a continuous subcutaneous infusion and "booster" or rescue boluses as needed (22). Since the subcutaneous tissues will only absorb a few milliliters per hour (without hyaluronidase), hydromorphone concentrated solutions (10 mg/ml commercially available or custom mixed to 50–200 mg/ml) are very useful for the administration of high doses of opioid subcutaneously.

What if high-dose opioids (grams/day SC or IV) don't work? Certainly a reassessment is called for (see Tables 53-2 and 53-3). If the patient is completely alert and the pain unquestionably arises from progression of the disease, more invasive pain control techniques should be considered. An epidural or intrathecal infusion of an opioid, possibly with bupivacaine or clonidine, can bring welcome relief to some patients with severe cancer pain (23). Radiation therapy and nerve blocks such as a celiac plexus block or saddle block are sometimes helpful, but few actively dying patients can tolerate these procedures.

Other options include opioid rotation to decrease opioid tolerance (24). A few dramatic cases of pain relief by rotation to methadone have been described (25). Adjuvant drugs such as antidepressants or a continuous subcutaneous infusion of ketorolac (26) can also bring welcome relief in some patients (Table 5).

Most crescendo pain occurs not when patients are alert and can accurately describe their pain but mixed with restlessness or delirium. The situation is often a confusing mixture of fear, anguish, restlessness, pain, and family stress. If the pain seems to be incident in nature and exacerbated by agitation, then aggressive treatment of the agitation with haloperidol and/or midazolam can be effective. Rarely will the oral route be available, and if relief is not available quickly, the family will soon be unable to cope. A rapid evaluation for missed medication doses, urinary retention, or fecal impaction must be done immediately. Some patients can be calmed by gentle talking, familiar music, or helping the family to cope. Music thanatologists claim to be able to relieve this distress without medications by custom-composed skillfully performed harp music (27). However, most patients will require a potent sedative such as methotrimeprazine 30 mg IM or chlorpromazine (28). Families may need to be taught how to give analgesics and sedatives rectally or subcutaneously if no central venous catheter is available. In some instances, patients will need inpatient hospice or palliative care. A rapid titration of opioids and sedatives like midazolam can usually calm the crisis and may allow the return of some degree of responsiveness (29). Rapid response, careful evaluation, competent assertive use of medications, and family support are the keys to overcoming this crisis, allowing the patient to die peacefully and the family to recover in bereavement.

## TERMINAL RESTLESSNESS

### Identification

Anyone who has worked or lived with dying cancer patients knows about terminal restlessness: the terrible agitation, the calling out, the can't-get-comfortable distress often experienced in the final days of life.

Common features of this syndrome include a clouded sensorium coupled with discomfort or fear. It is often acute in onset and has a fluctuating course typical of agitated delirium (30). It is also common in patients with advanced dementia when they experience symptoms and cannot articulate the cause of distress (31). Terminal restlessness seems particularly common in anguished patients with "skeletons in the closet," who have not been able to resolve their guilt or conflicts before the approach of death. It is often drug induced or drug exacerbated (32) and may be simply brought about by misperceptions or the hypnagogic hallucinations common in people with normal mentation when they are drifting in and out of sleep (33).

### Evaluation

When the patient is close to death and the distress is severe, urgent evaluation and therapy are required. Table

**TABLE 5.** *Adjuvant drugs for pain*

| Pain type | Drug class | Oral example | If unable to swallow (example) |
|---|---|---|---|
| Bony/soft tissue | NSAID | naproxen 375 mg t.i.d. | indomethacin suppository 50 mg PR q 8 h OR ketorolac 60 mg/d by SC infusion (ref 26) |
| | Steroid | prednisone 20 mg b.i.d. | dexamethasone 4 mg SC q 8 H |
| Visceral/colic | Anticholinergic | oxybutynnin 10 mg q 8 h | glycopyrrolate 0.8 mg/d by SC infusion |
| Neuropathic | Antidepresant | nortriptyline 25–100 mg q h s | doxepin cap 50 mg PR b.i.d. |
| | Anticonvulsant | valproate 250 mg t.i.d. (may also give as liquid PR) | carbamazepine crushed in gel caps 600 mg PR b.i.d. |
| Anxiety-related | Phenothiazine | hydroxyzine 25–50 mg q 4 h | methotrimeprazine 50–200 mg/d by SC infusion (ref 28) |

**TABLE 6.** *Evaluation of terminal restlessness*

Was there a precipitating event? (drug overdose, new drug, fall)
Is there urinary retention (blocked Foley catheter) or severe constipation or fecal impaction?
Can you reorient the patient or help him or her reinterpret the delusion?
Is the patient taking medications that can cloud the sensorium (analgesics, psychotropics) and that he or she can reasonably do without?
Has the patient been missing (or doubling up on) medications?
Is there evidence for a metabolic ($\uparrow Ca^{++}$, $\downarrow Na^{+}$), infectious (pneumonia, urinary tract infection, sepsis), or neurologic (brain metastases, cerebral vascular accident) complication for which specific treatment would be reasonable and appropriate?
If the answer to the above 6 questions is *no*, then:
Will a sedative calm this crisis?
Can this patient be managed at home?

6 lists several questions that should be answered quickly in the evaluation of terminal restlessness. Families can often learn the meaning of the symbols some patients use to communicate (34).

## Management

Some patients with mild terminal restlessness can be helped by changing their medications or treating infections to clear their mentation. If pain or dyspnea is a prominent component of the distress, doubling the opioid dose should be tried first. If the risk of seizures is high, a benzodiazepine (lorazepam sublingually or rectally) may be the first choice. In most cases, a sedating phenothiazine like chlorpromazine (50–100 mg intramuscularly, intravenously, or rectally) will be most effective. Methotrimeprazine has the added benefit of potent analgesia

**TABLE 7.** *Examples of sedatives for terminal restlessness*

Mild
 pain-related: increase opioid
 family stress–related: calm family, or admit for respite care
 picking, hallucinations: haloperidol 0.5–2 mg/d PO or SC
 anxiety-related: lorazepam 1 mg q 2 h PRN
 nocturnal only: chloral hydrate 1–2 g qhs
Moderate
 chlorpromazine 25–50 mg PO or PR q 4–8 h
 OR
 haloperidol 2 mg PO or SC q 2 h PRN
Severe
 methotrimeprazine 30 mg IM q 30 min until calm,
  then haloperidol 10–20 mg/d + midazolam 5–100 mg/d
  by SC infusion
Extreme
 phenobarbital 130 mg SC q 30 min until calm (may take
  >1,000 mg/day)
 thiopental or methohexital IV titrated to unconsciousness
  (43,44)

(35) but is very expensive. A subcutaneous infusion of the required opioid with haloperidol and/or midazolam is another useful option (36) (Table 7).

## TERMINAL SEDATION

### Indications

Terminal sedation is the intentional use of pharmacologic agents to induce sleep (continuous if necessary) during the final days of life. The most common indications are distressing symptoms that cannot be controlled by other means: that further invasive or noninvasive interventions specifically directed toward the distressing symptom are either unlikely to be effective within a tolerable time frame or are associated with excessive or intolerable morbidity. The incidence of such refractory symptoms is controversial, but it probably falls somewhere between the 16% found in a Canadian inpatient palliative care ward (37) and the 52% found in an Italian home care hospice service (38). Pain, dyspnea, and agitation are the most common refractory symptoms. If they are truly refractory and the patient is rapidly nearing death, then aggressive symptom control measures, including sedation if necessary, should be used (39).

If the patient's distress is relational, psychological, spiritual, or existential, the evaluation process should be even more comprehensive. These types of suffering can be highly fluid, idiosyncratic, and persistent. Persistent distress is difficult for the patient, the family, and the health care providers. Repeated assessments and interventions by multiple, skilled, palliative care team members are essential. Patients can sometimes find meaning and hope in their present predicament by techniques such as biography therapy (40), image work (41), or religious rituals that may help them see their lives in a different context (42).

If no such innovative solution is effective or acceptable to the patient, the clinician should discuss the problem and review alternative approaches with the palliative care team, the patient, and the family. It is not unusual for the physician to misjudge the severity of the distress to the patient or the acceptability of alternative solutions. Prioritization of goals and informed decision making require a climate of trust and openness, a caring professional relationship, and enough time for all concerned to digest new information.

### Methods

If terminal sedation is required, agents should be chosen that will accomplish the patient's goals with the least morbidity. This means selecting an effective agent that can be administered in the location of the patient's choosing with adequate but not excessive potency (see Table 53-7). At home, the rectal route may be the most practical. Slow-release morphine tablets (19), chlorpromazine, diazepam, and pentobarbital can all be effectively administered rectally. Most patients will get faster relief as well as more accurate dose titration from continuous infusions of parenteral drugs. If a central venous catheter is in place, opioids and a benzodiazepine (e.g., lorazepam) and/or a phenothiazine (e.g., chlorpromazine) can be given in escalating doses until the desired amount of sedation is obtained. If no central venous catheter is available, morphine or hydromorphone can be combined with midazolam and/or methotrimeprazine and given by continuous subcutaneous infusion (22). Sometimes only a 50% increase in the opioid dose and 5 to 10 mg of midazolam per day are required. Other patients can be quite alert when receiving more than 100 mg/d of midazolam and grams of opioids.

If an opioid combined with benzodiazepine and/or a phenothiazine does not provide adequate sedation for symptom relief, barbiturates can be considered. Excellent results have been obtained with carefully titrated, short-acting barbiturates such as thiopental or methohexital by intravenous infusion or with subcutaneous boluses of phenobarbital (43,44).

Often the goal of symptom relief can be achieved and the patient can still be allowed occasional opportunities to interact with the family. Young children can often arouse a sedated patient enough for a smile and a kiss. Even when the patient shows no signs of response to the environment, the bedside vigil can be a time of remembrance and healing for all concerned.

### Ethics

Much has been written about the similarities (45) and important differences (46,47) between terminal sedation and assisted suicide or euthanasia. From our patients' point of view, the far more important ethical dilemma is that most dying patients do not get adequate palliative care. Hospital ethics committees are now beginning to address adequate symptom management as a moral imperative (48). The clinician's own conscience should press for the best possible answers to these questions:

1. Is there a way to relieve this suffering and keep the patient alert? Would consultation be helpful?
2. Are these symptoms troublesome enough to the patient and family to warrant sedation?
3. Is this what the patient wants (or would want in an optimal state of mind)?
4. Does everyone involved (including the staff) understand the palliative intent of these orders?

### DEHYDRATION

Cancer patients are commonly readmitted to the hospital at the end of their lives because of family concerns related to lack of oral intake. Intravenous fluids are often given and are often the excuse for keeping the patient hospitalized (49).

As with other troubling symptoms, a diligent search for a treatable cause is usually warranted. When the patient is relatively healthy, the underlying problem can usually be solved and the patient can be rehydrated at home with oral fluids. When the tumor burden is large and the patient is very ill, multiple problems often cause both increased loss and decreased intake. Is intravenous or nasogastric feeding justified at this point?

There is mounting evidence that these therapies can be more harmful than helpful in patients with advanced cancer. In 1957, force-fed cancer patients were found to have irreversible increases in their basal metabolic rates (50). Many tumors in cell culture and animal models demonstrate increased rates of growth when more nutrients are administered (51–55). In patients with colon cancer, sensitive measurements of tumor growth are increased when patients receive total parenteral nutrition (TPN) (56). In 1989, the American College of Physicians analyzed the 12 available controlled trials of TPN in cancer chemotherapy patients and concluded that TPN for cancer chemotherapy patients "resulted in *net harm* ... and no subgroup could be identified in which such treatment appeared to be of benefit" (57). Even if we discount this evidence of increased disease activity with intravenous or nasogastric feeding, many patients develop infections, bloating, dyspnea, diarrhea, or other severe symptoms from overfeeding in the final weeks of life (58). We should be certain that our therapy provides more benefits than burdens to the patient.

It is certainly possible to keep advanced cancer patients comfortable without intravenous or nasogastric fluids. The most troublesome symptom, a dry mouth, can be effectively relieved by dripping or swabbing a few drops of water or artificial saliva substitute into the mouth on a regular basis. An atomizer is another useful way of delivering moisture to the mouth. The eyes can be kept moist with saline drops, and the skin can be massaged with lotions. A humidifier for the room can also help. In the rare instance when patients complain of thirst, hypodermoclysis (59) or proctoclysis (60) can deliver 1 to 2 liters of fluid a day without the need for hospitalization.

### RATTLING SECRETIONS

Many cancer patients experience difficulty in clearing their pulmonary secretions. In an alert, semiambulatory patient, a careful history and physical exam may uncover correctable problems such as pneumonia, bronchitis, allergic rhinitis, aspiration, or volume overload. However, as with all rehabilitation efforts in advanced cancer patients, there comes a time when antibiotics, nebulizers, and physical therapy become more burdensome than

**TABLE 8.** *Anticholinergic medications for rattling secretions*

| Drug | Dosage | Route |
|------|--------|-------|
| oxybutynin (Ditropan) | 5–10 mg | t.i.d. PO or GT |
| hyoscyamine (Levsin SL) | 0.125 mg | t.i.d.–q.i.d. SL |
| transdermal scopalamine (Transderm Scop) | 1–3 patches | q 3 d topically |
| glycopyrrolate (Robinul) | 0.2 mg | q 4–8 h SC |
|  | 0.6–1.2 mg | q.d. by SC infusion |
| scopalamine | 0.8–2.4 mg | q.d. by SC infusion |

beneficial. If the patient is not overfed or overhydrated by the intravenous or nasogastric routes, there will be fewer secretions. for the patient to have to cope with. Frequent oral or nasotracheal suctioning is rarely effective enough to justify the discomfort that it causes to these very ill patients.

Anticholinergic drugs are the agents of choice for rattling secretions in patients too weak to cough (61). Low doses of oxybutynin (Ditropan) or hyoscyamine (Levsin) or transdermal scopalamine (Transderm Scop) are often effective and are reasonably well tolerated (Table 8). When secretions are more severe and the patient is unable to tolerate oral medications, glycopyrrolate (Robinul) or scopalamine can be given as an intravenous or subcutaneous bolus every 4 to 6 hours, or mixed with an opioid and given by subcutaneous infusion.

## HOPE

All of our patients, especially those with advanced cancer, need hope. This book is about supporting patients, and their sense of hope, through difficult times. Nothing destroys hope faster than untruthfulness, so we must be careful not to gloss over what is actually happening. Hope means different things to different people at different stages of the cancer experience, so the time we spend getting to know our patients and their families is often crucial.

Most people begin the cancer experience with a will to beat the disease, and hope may mean an aggressive chemotherapy or radiotherapy protocol. Severe symptoms rob the joy from hard-won extra days, so our skills at controlling symptoms must be well honed. Psychological pain, suffering, and depression are common in patients with advancing malignancy, and we must make sure our patients get the mental health services they need. Ironically, a referral to a well-trained hospice team can restore a great deal of hope by relieving the pain, anxiety, and family stress (62).

Some patients need us to lend strength to them during their times of great need. Eric Cassell describes this crucial role of the physician in the alleviation of suffering (3).

**TABLE 9.** *Burnout prevention*

| | |
|---|---|
| *Healthy body* | diet, exercise, adequate rest |
| *Healthy mind* | hobbies, reading, fun |
| *Healthy social life* | family, friends, sexuality |
| *Healthy spirit* | worship, meditation, prayer |

We lend our patients this strength by being vulnerable to them—by sharing our fallible human selves. Although this can be very difficult, it can be extremely rewarding.

With enough strength, with expert symptom management, with skillful psychological interventions, and with spiritual support, many patients find hope in their final weeks of life (62). They find that their life story has meaning and coherence. They find that they are part of an enduring social fabric. They find the light of the eternal shining through.

If we are there with them, our lives are made much richer. And even though the cost is high, we can find the strength to grieve their passing and to give ourselves again to the next patient (Table 9).

## REFERENCES

1. Ventafridda V, Ripamonti C, Tamburini M, Cassileth RB, De Conna F. Unendurable symptoms as prognostic indicators of impending death in terminal cancer patients. *Eur J Cancer* 1990;26(9):1000–1001.
2. Cleeland CS, Gonin R, Hatfield AK, et al. Pain and its treatment in outpatients with metastatic cancer. *N Engl J Med* 1994;330:592–596, 1994.
3. Cassel EJ. The nature of suffering and the goals of medicine. *N Engl J Med* 1982;306:639–645.
4. Mount B. Whole person care: beyond psychosocial and physical needs. *Am J Hosp Pall Care* 1993;10(1):28–37.
5. Saunders C. The moment of truth: care of the dying person. IIn: Pearson L, ed. *Death and dying: current issues in treatment of the dying person.* Case Western Reserve University Press, 1969:48–78.
6. Luczak J, Okupny M, Wieczorek-Cuske L. The program of palliative medicine and care in the curriculum of sixth-year medical students in Poland. *J Pall Care* 1992;8(2):39–43.
7. Fallowfield L. Giving sad and bad news. *Lancet* 1993;341;476–478.
8. Vachon MLS. Stress in oncologists. *Can J Oncol* 1993;3(1):166–172.
9. De Conno F, Saita L, Ripamonti C, Ventafridda V. In retrospect—on the last days of life. *J Pall Care* 1993;9(3):47–49.
10. Saunders C. Introduction—history and challenge. In: Saunders C, Sykes N, eds. *The management of malignant disease.* London: Edward Arnold, 1993:1–14.
11. Storey P. Hospice settings around the world. *Am J Hosp Pall Care* 1993; 10(4):4–5.
12. Bruera E, Kuehn N, Miller MJ, Selmser P, MacMillan K. The Edmonton symptom assessment system: a simple method for the assessment of palliative care patients. *J Pall Care* 1991;7(2):6–9.
13. Ellershaw JE, Peat SJ, Boys LC. Assessing the effectiveness of a hospital palliative care team. *Pall Med* 1995;9:145–152.
14. Portenoy RK, Thaler HT, Korblith AB, et al. The memorial symptom assessment scale: an instrument for the evaluation of symptom prevalence, characteristics and distress. *Eur J Cancer* 1994;30A(9): 1326–1336.
15. Daut RL, Cleeland CS, Flanery RC. Development of the Wisconsin Brief Plan Questionnaire to assess pain in cancer and other diseases. *Pain* 1983;17:197.
16. Cohen-Mansfield J, Marx MS, Rosenthal AS. A description of agitation in a nursing home. *J Gerontol* 1989;44:77–84.
17. Korte W, Morant R. Transdermal fentanyl in uncontrolled cancer pain: titration on a day-to-day basis as a procedure for safe and effective dose finding—a pilot study in 20 patients. *Support Care Cancer* 1994;2: 123–127.

18. Payne R. Novel routes of opioid administration: sublingual and buccal. *Primary Care & CA* 1989;1:55–56.
19. Wilkinson TJ, Robinson BA, Begg EJ, Duffull SB, Ravenscroft PJ, Schneider JJ. Pharmacokinetics and efficacy of rectal versus oral sustained release morphine in cancer patients. *Cancer Chemother Pharmacol* 1992;31:251–254.
20. Storey P, Trumble M. Rectal doxepin and carbamazepine therapy in patients with cancer. *N Engl J Med* 1992;327:1318–1319.
21. Crane RA. Intermittent subcutaneous infusion of opioids in hospice home care: an effective, economical, manageable option. *Am J Hosp Pall Care* 1994;1:8–12.
22. Storey P, Hill HH, St Louis RH, Tarver E. Subcutaneous infusions for control of cancer symptoms. *J Pain Symptom Manag* 1990;5:33–41.
23. Devulder J, Ghys L, Dhondt W, Rolly G. Spinal analgesia in terminal care: risk versus benefit. *J Pain Symptom Manag* 1994;9:75–81.
24. Stoutz ND, Bruera E, Suarez-Almazor M. Opioid rotation for toxicity reduction in terminal cancer patients. *J Pain Symptom Manag* 1995;10:378–384.
25. Thomas Z, Bruera E. Use of methadone in a highly tolerant patient receiving parenteral hydromorphone. *J Pain Symptom Manag* 1995;10:315–317.
26. Trotman IF, Myers KG. Use of ketorolac by continuous subcutaneous infusion for control of cancer-related pain. *Postgrad Med J* 1994;70:359–362.
27. Schroeder-Sheker T. Music for the dying: a personal account of the new field of music-thanatology—history, theories, and clinical narratives. *J Holistic Nurs* 1994;12(1):83–99.
28. Oliver DJ. The use of methotrimeprazine in terminal care. *Br J Clin Pract* 1985;22:339–340.
29. Burke AL, Diamond PL, Hubert J, Yeatman J, Farr EA. Terminal restlessness—its management and the role of midazolam. *Med J Austr* 1991;155:485–487.
30. Breitbart W, Bruera E, Chochinov H, Lynch M. Neuropsychiatric syndromes and psychological symptoms in patients with advanced cancer. *J Pain Symptom Manag* 1995;10:131–141.
31. Kunik ME, Yudofsky SC, Silver JM, Hales RE. Pharmacologic approach to management of agitation associated with dementia. *J Clin Psychiatry* 1994;55(2):13–17.
32. Dunlop RJ. Is terminal restlessness sometimes drug induced? *Pall Med* 1989;3:65–66.
33. Stedeford A. Confusion. In: Stedeford A. *Facing death: patients, families, professionals*. London: Wm Heinemann, 1984:122–136.
34. Callanan M, Kelly P. Final gifts: understanding the special awareness, needs, and communications of the dying. New York: Bantam, 1992.
35. Beaver WT, Wallenstein SL, Houde RW, Rogers A. A comparison of the analgesic effects of methotrimeprazine and morphine in patients with cancer. *Clin Pharmacol Ther* 1966;4:436–446.
36. Bottomley DM, Hanks GW. Subcutaneous midazolam infusion in palliat care. *J Pain Symptom Manag* 1990;5:259–261.
37. Fainsinger R, Miller MJ, Bruera E, Hanson J, Maceachem T. Symptom control during the last week on a palliative care unit. *J Palliat Care* 7(1):5–11, 1991.
38. Ventafridda V, Ripamonti C, DeConno F, Tamburini M, Cassileth BR. Symptom prevalence and control during cancer patients' last days of life. *J Palliat Care* 6(3):7–11, 1990.
39. Cherny NI, Portenoy RK. Sedation in the management of refractory symptoms: guidelines for evaluation and treatment. *J Palliat Care* 10(2)31–38, 1994.
40. Lichter I, Mooney J, Boyd M. Biography as therapy. *Palliat Med* 7:133–137
41. Kearney M. *Mortally wounded: stories of soul pain, death, and healing*. New York: Scribner, 1996.
42. Storey P, Knight C. *Unipac two:* psychological and spiritual aspects of dying and bereavement. American Academy of Hospice and Palliative Medicine, Gainesville, FL, 1997.
43. Truog RD, Berde CB, Mitchell C, Grier HE. Barbiturates in the care of the terminally ill. *N Engl J Med* 1992;327:1678–1682.
44. Greene WR, Davis WH. Titrated intravenous barbiturates in the control of symptoms in patients with terminal cancer. *South Med J* 1991;84:332–337.
45. Billings JA, Block SD. Slow euthanasia. *J Palliat Care* 12(4):21–30, 1996.
46. Portenoy RK. Morphine infusions at the end of life: the pitfalls of reasoning from anecdote. *J Palliat Care* 12(4):44–46, 1996.
47. Mount B. Morphine drips, terminal sedation, and slow euthanasia: definitions and facts not anecdotes. *J Palliative Care* 12:(4)31–37.
48. Editorial Medical Ethics Advisor, 86&89, July 1995.
49. Burge FI, King DB, Willison D. Intravenous fluids and the hospitalized dying: a medical last rite? *Can Fam Physician* 36:883–886, 1990.
50. Terepka AR, Waterhouse C. Metabolic observations during the forced feeding of patients with cancer. *Am J Med* 225–238, 1956.
51. Ota DM, Copeland EM, Strobel HW, Daly J, Gum ET, Guinn E, Dudrick SJ. The effect of protein nutrition on host and tumor metabolism. *J of Surg Res* 22:181–188, 1977.
52. Buzby GP Mullen, JL, Stein P, Miller EE, Hobbs CL, Rosato EF. Host-tumor interaction and nutrient supply. *Cancer* 45:2940–2948, 1980.
53. Popp MB, Morrison SD, Brennan MF. Total parenteral nutirion in a methycholanthrene-induced rat sarcoma model. *Cancer Treat Rep* 65(5):137–143, 1981.
54. Cameron IL. Effect of total parenteral nutrition on tumor-host responses in rats. *Cancer Treat Rep* 65(5):93–99, 1981.
55. Stragand JJ, Braunschweiger PG, Pollice AA, Schiffer LM. Cell kinetic alterations in murine mammary tumors following fasting and refeeding. *Eur J Cancer* 15:281–286, 1979.
56. Ota DM, Nishioka K, Grossie B, Dixon D. Erythrocyte polyamine levels during intravenous feeding of patients with colorectal carcinoma. *J Cancer Clin Oncol* 22(7):837–842, 1986.
57. American College of Physicians. Parenteral nutrition in patient receiving cancer chemotherapy. *Ann Int Med* 110(9):734–736, 1989.
58. Ciocon JO, Silverstone FA, Graver M, Foley CJ. Tube feedings in elderly patients—indications, benefits, and complications. *Arch Intern Med* 148:429–433, 1988.
59. Bruera E, Legris MA, Kuehn N, Miller MJ. Hypodermoclysis for the administration of fluids and narcotic analgesics in patients with advanced cancer. *J Pain Symptom Manag* 5:218–220, 1990.
60. Bruera E, Schoeller T, Pruvost M. Proctoclysis for hydration of terminal cancer patients. *Lancet* 344:1699, 1994.
61. Hughes AC, Wilcock A, Corcoran R. Management of "death rattle." *J Pain Symptom Manag* 12(5):271–272, 1996.
62. Herth K. Fostering hope in terminally-ill people. *J Adv Nursing* 15:1250–1259, 1990.

Principles and Practice of Supportive Oncology,
edited by Ann Berger et al.
Lippincott–Raven Publishers, Philadelphia ©1998

CHAPTER 54

# The Epidemiology of Cancer at the End of Life

Jane M. Ingham

Although many advances have occurred in the prevention and treatment of cancer, death from this condition remains a common occurrence. The end-of-life experience associated with cancer varies widely and may be influenced by the type and extent of the disease and by the palliative interventions that have been provided. Knowledge of the epidemiology of end-of-life concerns is essential for physicians who may be called upon to give advice to patients and families who are in, or approaching, the advanced phase of illness. Such knowledge is needed to facilitate optimal delivery of care and symptom management in addition to an informed public discussion about end-of-life care for cancer patients, the development of research initiatives aimed toward improving the quality of life at the end of life, and the further development of guidelines and treatment strategies for the care of the dying.

In oncology texts, the epidemiology of cancer is typically discussed in terms of the prevalence, incidence, and patterns of disease. Consequently, there is now a wealth of epidemiological data pertaining to the demographics of the dying population, including the causes of death and the likely site of death. Yet, there is a paucity of data describing the signs and symptoms of cancer and the other factors that contribute to the quality of life at the end of life. Given the absence of empirical data, anecdotal personal narratives, which provide only minimal insight into the nature of disease at the end of life, have frequently been given great credence (1–4). This chapter will review the data that relate to the epidemiology of cancer-related deaths, including causes, life expectancies, mortality rates, the pattern of institutionalization of medical care, and the nature of the dying process. While it must be acknowledged that there is a wide variability in the experience of cancer between countries, the predominant focus of this chapter will be on the experiences of cancer patients in the United States.

## MORTALITY STATISTICS

### Leading Causes of Death and Mortality Shifts

In 1990, there were nearly 50 million deaths worldwide, with 38.5 million occurring in developing countries and 11.7 million in developed countries (5). Cancer caused 10% of these deaths, infectious and parasitic diseases caused 34%, and circulatory diseases or chronic obstructive pulmonary disease together caused 26%. More specifically, 1995 statistics reveal that the three leading causes of death in the United States were diseases of the heart (32%), malignant neoplasms (23%), and cerebrovascular disease (7%) (6). Patterns of disease vary between developing and developed countries; a higher proportion of deaths from noncommunicable diseases occur in developed countries. Shifts in population demographics and patterns of disease are expected to alter the current patterns of mortality, and it is predicated that by the year 2015, noncommunicable diseases will become the main causes of death worldwide (7,8).

Given that death rates for specific diseases vary between countries and over time, a method for international comparison is required. The age-adjusted death rate is the figure generally used for this purpose and reflects the death rate established for each specific condition, applied to a standard population, and adjusted to eliminate the difference that would be accounted for by age differences in population composition. Table 54-1 shows recent age-adjusted death rates per hundred thousand population by select countries and causes of death (9). The wide variability in cancer and other disease mortality patterns among countries may be accounted for by many factors that affect both the incidence and treatment of disease. These include changes in life expectancy, decreasing infant mortality, availability of drugs, access to health care, altering patterns of smoking, and an increasing prevalence of infection with the human immunodeficiency virus (HIV). Some of these factors

J. M. Ingham: Lombardi Cancer Center, Georgetown University Medical Center, Washington, DC 20007.

**TABLE 1.** Death rates, by cause and country

| Country | Year | Ischemic heart disease | Cerebrovascular disease | Cancer of | | | Bronchitis,[1] emphysema, asthma | Chronic liver disease and cirrhosis | Motor vehicle traffic accidents | Suicide and self-inflicted injury |
|---|---|---|---|---|---|---|---|---|---|---|
| | | | | Lung trachea, bronchus | Stomach | Female breast | | | | |
| United States | 1991 | 169.9 | 48.3 | 57.5 | 5.4 | 31.6 | 9.2 | 10.8 | 16.3 | 12.1 |
| Australia | 1992 | 175.8 | 65.9 | 38.1 | 7.2 | 27.7 | 12.1 | 6.8 | 11.1 | 12.7 |
| Austria | 1993 | 152.3 | 86.4 | 35.6 | 16.6 | 31.4 | 15.5 | 25.9 | 14.0 | 19.5 |
| Belgium | 1989 | 90.5 | 72.3 | 52.7 | 11.3 | 37.9 | 12.8 | 11.3 | 17.4 | 17.9 |
| Bulgaria | 1993 | 237.8 | 241.8 | 32.8 | 19.9 | 20.6 | 10.3 | 17.8 | 11.8 | 16.0 |
| Canada | 1992 | 147.0 | 47.1 | 53.0 | 7.4 | 32.4 | 6.8 | 8.1 | 11.2 | 12.8 |
| Czech Republic | 1993 | 276.6 | 168.0 | 53.1 | 17.4 | 31.2 | 19.6 | 16.5 | 13.6 | 18.1 |
| Denmark | 1992 | 190.3 | 72.0 | 51.1 | 7.8 | 40.6 | 36.5 | 13.5 | 10.2 | 20.4 |
| Finland | 1993 | 224.4 | 97.0 | 32.5 | 12.0 | 23.6 | 16.5 | 9.9 | 8.4 | 26.6 |
| France | 1992 | 58.6 | 51.1 | 35.0 | 8.1 | 28.1 | 9.5 | 15.5 | 14.6 | 19.1 |
| Germany | 1993 | 157.7 | 84.9 | 36.2 | 14.8 | 32.1 | 18.5 | 21.5 | 11.4 | 13.8 |
| Hungary | 1993 | 260.5 | 169.9 | 65.7 | 22.9 | 35.0 | 41.0 | 78.8 | 16.9 | 34.2 |
| Italy | 1991 | 94.7 | 91.1 | 42.7 | 18.2 | 29.8 | 22.9 | 22.0 | 15.1 | 6.9 |
| Japan | 1993 | 34.0 | 77.9 | 27.6 | 31.8 | 9.2 | 10.3 | 11.8 | 10.3 | 15.0 |
| Netherlands | 1992 | 118.2 | 67.6 | 52.0 | 12.2 | 38.5 | 14.5 | 5.1 | 7.9 | 9.9 |
| New Zealand | 1992 | 206.3 | 76.4 | 42.9 | 9.4 | 34.1 | 11.9 | 3.6 | 18.0 | 14.6 |
| Norway | 1992 | 169.1 | 78.5 | 28.9 | 11.1 | 27.2 | 12.3 | 4.5 | 6.8 | 13.9 |
| Poland | 1993 | 118.2 | 81.3 | 52.3 | 19.0 | 22.1 | 20.7 | 12.6 | 17.8 | 15.3 |
| Portugal | 1993 | 85.0 | 204.8 | 23.1 | 24.1 | 24.9 | 11.0 | 26.4 | 23.2 | 7.4 |
| Spain | 1991 | 75.0 | 89.3 | 33.4 | 14.7 | 24.3 | 8.2 | 18.7 | 18.5 | 7.0 |
| Sweden | 1992 | 173.3 | 67.3 | 24.3 | 8.9 | 25.7 | 10.6 | 6.4 | 7.3 | 14.5 |
| Switzerland | 1993 | 104.1 | 50.0 | 34.9 | 8.4 | 34.7 | 17.4 | 8.3 | 9.2 | 18.8 |
| United Kingdom: | | | | | | | | | | |
| England and Wales | 1992 | 199.7 | 82.3 | 51.0 | 11.7 | 39.5 | 10.9 | 5.5 | 7.4 | 7.4 |
| Scotland | 1992 | 246.4 | 108.1 | 68.6 | 12.6 | 37.9 | 7.6 | 8.4 | 8.6 | 10.8 |

[1]Chronic and unspecified.

Age-standardized death rate per 100,000 population. The standard population for this table is the old European standard; see source for details. Deaths classified to ninth revision of *International Classification of Diseases.*

Source: World Health Organization, Geneva, Switzerland, *World Health Statistics Annual.*

Reproduced from Ref. 9.

will be discussed in detail below. As a consequence of these and other factors, and despite the development of new treatments for specific malignancies and the declining incidence of certain cancers, it is expected that there will be a proportionate increase in deaths of cancer worldwide (7,8,10–15).

A significant factor influencing patterns of cancer death is changing life expectancy. Life expectancy is rising, and it is expected to continue to rise at differing rates in each world region. In industrial market economies, the rise is expected to be from 76.2 years in 1985 to 77.9 years in 2015, whereas in sub-Saharan Africa, the change is expected to be from 51.3 to 61.3 years for the same period (7). These changes will increase the proportion of the elderly in the population. Between 1980 and 2020, it is expected that the total population of the developing world will increase by 95% and the elderly population will probably rise by almost 240% (16).

In the United States, overall life expectancy has increased from 70.8 years in 1970 to 75.8 years in 1995 (6,17). Although changes have been demonstrated widely, variability exists within certain subgroups. To date, the United States data, as they relate to race, have largely been

catigorized and reported in terms of the "black" and "white" populations, with some reference to the "other races." Although this broad classification may result in inaccuracies and may not be applicable in other settings, it nonetheless does provide some useful insights into some of the differences between subpopulations. In 1995, for example, the life expectancy for black men in the United States was 65.4 years, whereas for white men it was 73.4 years (6). In 1995, women were expected to outlive men by an average of 6.3 years, and white persons to outlive black persons by an average of 6.7 years (6). The increasing overall life expectancy is likely to affect the patterns of cancer diagnosis and also the need for society to provide care for the elderly, including those with cancer.

The 1995 mortality figures for the United States demonstrate that causes of death, mortality rates, and trends in cancer death are expected to be different for different age groups (18). Although malignant neoplasms were represented among the four major causes for death for every age group in the United States, the leading causes were "accidents and adverse effects" in the population under 25 years, HIV infection in those between 25 and 44 years, and heart disease in the age group 65 years

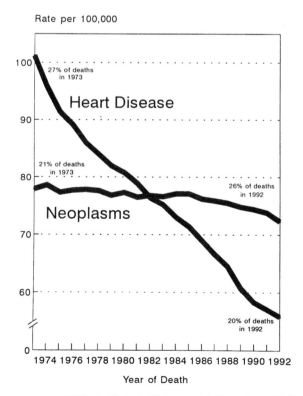

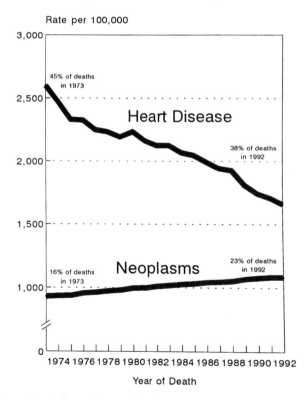

**FIG. 1.** United States mortality rates, 1973–1992. Reproduced from Kosary CL, GloecklerRies MS, Miller BA, Hankey BF, Harras A, Edwards BK. SEER Cancer Statistics Review, 1973–1992. Bethesda, MD: US Department of Health and Human Services, Public Health Services, National Institutes of Health, National Cancer Institute, 1996. Reproduced with permission from Ref. 19.

and over (6). Only in the age group 45 to 64 years were malignant neoplasms the leading cause of death. As with the life expectancy figures, there is also variability within subpopulations in the United States. For example, in 1993, the leading causes of death were the same for the white and black populations except for the age groups 15 to 24 and 25 to 44 years (18). In the white population, accidents and adverse effects were the most common cause of death for both of these age groups, whereas in the black population, "homicide and legal intervention" was listed as the leading cause of death for ages 15 to 24, and HIV infection led for those between the ages of 25 and 44 (18).

Age itself further affects mortality rates for specific illnesses. Figure 54-1 illustrates two examples of this by demonstrating the changes in mortality rates in the United States for heart disease and neoplasms over time in two different age groups (19). For both of these diseases, mortality is higher as age increases. Clearly, the influence of age on the prognosis in specific cancers is also likely to be relevant.

In addition to age, many social and disease-related factors are likely to affect the ranking of causes of death and the likelihood of death of specific conditions. For example, a major social factor affecting causes of death is smoking, which increases the prevalence of tobacco-related diseases. Some medical conditions may have an indirect effect on the incidence of malignant disease. One such condition is infection with the HIV virus. In the United States, HIV infection has continued to increase and has moved from being the tenth cause of death in 1990, to the ninth in 1991, and to the eighth in 1992 and 1993 (18,20,21). In 1995, HIV remained the eighth-ranked cause of death (6). As a consequence of this increasing prevalence, cancers associated with HIV infection may also increase.

Many of the data discussed above are derived from information obtained on death certificates. Although autopsy data would be more accurate, the rate of autopsies is low. For example, in 1993, 2,268,553 autopsies were performed in the United States, representing only 9.7% of the deaths that occurred in that year (18). Autopsy rates were particularly low when death was attributed to one of the leading causes of death. For example, the autopsy rate for death from malignant neoplasms was 2.5%. Less common causes of death, including those related to homicide and legal intervention, suicide, and accidents and adverse effects, were far more frequently investigated with autopsy. The autopsy rates in such cases were, respectively, 97.3%, 54.7%, and 48.4% (18). Although premortem investigations in patients with cancer often clarify the diagnosis, the very low autopsy rate for cancer-related deaths nonetheless hinders the evaluation of the dying process, both in individual cases and for the purpose of epidemiological research. This potential for inaccuracy, inherent in all data derived from death certificates, has important implications for the care of the dying. Specifi-

cally, the lack of detailed and accurate information impedes advancement in the medical understanding of the pathophysiology of symptoms and distress at the end of life, and may consequently slow the development of symptom-specific palliative interventions (22).

## Cancer Mortality

In 1990, there were 5 million deaths from cancer worldwide (5). As discussed above, cancer is proportionately more common as a cause of death in developed countries. In 1995, almost 538,000 (23.3%) of the 2.3 million deaths in the United States were attributed to cancer (6). During the same year, it was estimated that there were just over 1.25 million new cases of cancer (excluding basal and squamous cell skin cancer and in situ carcinomas except urinary bladder) (23). From 1990 to 1995, the overall age-adjusted cancer mortality rate in the United States declined by approximately 3.1%: the first sustained decline in cancer mortality since record-keeping began in the 1930s (15). Despite the latter encouraging statistic, death from cancer remains common.

Among the cancers in the United States, cancer of the lung is responsible for the largest number of deaths. In 1995, over 157,000 deaths were attributed to this condition, and it was estimated that almost 170,000 new cases would be diagnosed in that same year (Table 2). Also in 1995, the cancers that caused the next highest numbers of deaths were colon cancer, with 47,500 deaths (100,000 estimated new cases), and breast cancer, with 46,240 deaths (183,300 estimated new cases). For some cancers, including leukemia and cancers of the pancreas, brain, and esophagus, the estimated new case numbers approached the estimated number of deaths (23).

Mortality and 5-year survival figures vary for different cancers. These figures are influenced by many factors, including age, sex, race, and treatment strategies. Examples of trends from the United States cancer data base are included in Figure 2 and Tables 3 and 4 (9,19). Between 1988 and 1992, the median age at death for all cancers in the United States was 71 years (19), and for most cancers, the highest number of deaths occur between 64 and 74 years. In this population, the only common malignancies in which death commonly occurrs at an earlier age (less than 35 years) are testicular cancer, Hodgkin's disease, and acute lymphocytic leukemia (19). Variability in time from diagnosis to death is influenced by factors similar to those that influence survival. In the 1986 National Mortality Followback Survey, data on over 16,000 decedents in the United States was extrapolated to national mortality figures. The survey concluded that of the 511,114 deaths from cancer that occurred in that year, 140,944 (27.5%) occurred within 6 months of the cancer being noticed, 83,889 (16.4%) occurred from 6 to 12 months later, and 80,832 (15.8%) occurred from 1 to 2 years later (24).

**TABLE 2.** *Estimated new cancer cases and deaths for 1995 (all races, by sex)*

| Primary site | Estimated new cases | | | Estimated deaths | | |
|---|---|---|---|---|---|---|
| | Total | Males | Females | Total | Males | Females |
| All sites | 1,252,000 | 677,000 | 575,000 | 547,000 | 289,000 | 258,000 |
| Oral cavity and pharynx | 28,150 | 18,800 | 9,350 | 8,370 | 5,480 | 2,890 |
| Lip | 2,500 | 1,900 | 600 | 100 | 80 | 20 |
| Tongue | 5,550 | 3,600 | 1,950 | 1,870 | 1,200 | 670 |
| Mouth | 11,000 | 6,900 | 4,100 | 2,300 | 1,300 | 1,000 |
| Pharynx | 9,100 | 6,400 | 2,700 | 4,100 | 2,900 | 1,200 |
| Digestive system | 223,000 | 118,800 | 105,000 | 124,330 | 66,130 | 58,200 |
| Esophagus | 12,100 | 8,800 | 3,300 | 10,900 | 8,200 | 2,700 |
| Stomach | 22,800 | 14,000 | 8,800 | 14,700 | 8,800 | 5,900 |
| Small intestine | 4,600 | 2,400 | 2,200 | 1,120 | 590 | 530 |
| Colon | 100,000 | 49,000 | 51,000 | 47,500 | 23,000 | 24,500 |
| Rectum | 38,200 | 21,700 | 16,500 | 7,800 | 4,200 | 3,600 |
| Liver and intrahepatic Bile duct | 18,500 | 9,800 | 8,700 | 14,200 | 7,700 | 6,500 |
| Pancreas | 24,000 | 11,000 | 13,000 | 27,000 | 13,200 | 13,800 |
| Other digestive | 2,800 | 1,300 | 1,500 | 1,110 | 440 | 670 |
| Respiratory system | 186,300 | 108,400 | 77,900 | 162,950 | 99,470 | 63,480 |
| Larynx | 11,600 | 9,000 | 2,600 | 4,090 | 3,200 | 890 |
| Lung and bronchus | 169,900 | 96,000 | 73,900 | 157,400 | 95,400 | 62,000 |
| Other respiratory | 4,800 | 3,400 | 1,400 | 1,460 | 870 | 590 |
| Bones and joints | 2,070 | 1,100 | 970 | 1,280 | 750 | 530 |
| Soft tissues | 6,000 | 3,300 | 2,700 | 3,600 | 1,800 | 1,800 |
| Melanomas of skin | 34,100 | 18,700 | 15,400 | 7,200 | 4,500 | 2,700 |
| Breast | 183,400 | 1,400 | 182,000 | 46,240 | 240 | 46,000 |
| Genital organs | 333,100 | 252,200 | 80,900 | 67,380 | 40,980 | 26,400 |
| Cervix uteri | 15,800 | | 15,800 | 4,800 | | 4,800 |
| Corpus and uterus, NOS | 32,800 | | 32,800 | 5,900 | | 5,900 |
| Ovary | 26,600 | | 26,600 | 14,500 | | 14,500 |
| Other female genital | 5,700 | | 5,700 | 1,200 | | 1,200 |
| Prostate | 244,000 | 244,000 | | 40,400 | 40,400 | |
| Testis | 7,100 | 7,100 | | 370 | 370 | |
| Other male genital | 1,100 | 1,100 | | 210 | 210 | |
| Urinary system | 79,300 | 54,400 | 24,900 | 22,900 | 14,600 | 8,300 |
| Urinary bladder | 50,500 | 37,300 | 13,200 | 11,200 | 7,500 | 3,700 |
| Kidney and other Urinary | 28,800 | 17,100 | 11,700 | 11,700 | 7,100 | 4,600 |
| Eye and orbit | 1,870 | 1,000 | 870 | 240 | 130 | 110 |
| Brain and other nervous system | 17,200 | 9,700 | 7,500 | 13,300 | 7,300 | 6,000 |
| Endocrine glands | 15,380 | 3,900 | 11,480 | 1,780 | 760 | 1,020 |
| Thyroid | 13,900 | 3,200 | 10,700 | 1,120 | 440 | 680 |
| Other endocrine | 1,480 | 700 | 780 | 660 | 320 | 340 |
| Lymphomas and myelomas | 71,200 | 41,100 | 30,100 | 34,450 | 18,120 | 16,330 |
| Hodgkin's disease | 7,800 | 4,500 | 3,300 | 1,450 | 820 | 630 |
| Non-Hodgkin's lymphoma | 50,900 | 29,500 | 21,400 | 22,700 | 12,000 | 10,700 |
| Multiple myeloma | 12,500 | 7,100 | 5,400 | 10,300 | 5,300 | 5,000 |
| Leukemias | 25,700 | 14,700 | 11,000 | 20,400 | 11,100 | 9,300 |
| Lymphocytic leukemias | 11,000 | 6,700 | 4,300 | 6,400 | 3,500 | 2,900 |
| Myeloid leukemias | 11,100 | 5,900 | 5,200 | 8,400 | 4,600 | 3,800 |
| Other leukemias | 3,600 | 2,100 | 1,500 | 5,600 | 3,000 | 2,600 |
| All other sites | 45,230 | 30,300 | 14,930 | 32,580 | 17,640 | 14,940 |

Source: Reproduced with permission from ref. 19.

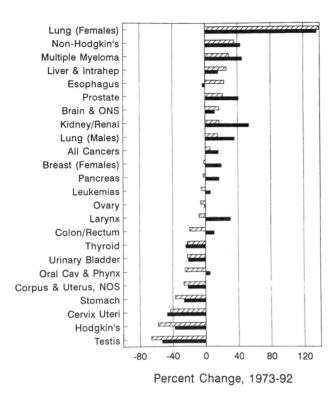

Percent Change, 1973-92

**FIG. 2.** Trends in United States cancer mortality rates, 1973–1992, whites (striped bars) and blacks (solid bars), all ages. Reproduced with permission from ref. 19.

## Place of Death

Although the epidemiological data above provide useful information about the demographics of cancer-related illness and death, they provide little insight into the nature of the illness. Place of death is one relevant concern. In a survey undertaken in the United Kingdom of 98 cancer patients, of whom 84 (86%) agreed to be interviewed, 58% expressed a preference to die at home, 20% preferred the hospital, and 20% preferred an inpatient hospice (25). Sixty-seven percent of these patients, given improved health-related and/or social circumstances, indicated that they would prefer to die at home.

Despite these preferences, most deaths in developed countries occur in medical institutions (26). For example, high rates of death in institutions are evident in Finland (75%), Sweden (79%), and Iceland (80%), while lower rates are recorded in some parts of Europe, in particular Bulgaria (25%), Spain (30%), and Italy (37%). Of the 2.2 million deaths occurring annually in the United States, 1990 death certificate data indicate that approximately 62% occurred in hospitals, 16% occurred in nursing homes, and 17% occurred in homes (National Center for Health Statistics: Unpublished data, general mortality, 1990, 1994). In comparison to deaths in the whole population, home death was more common for patients with malignant neoplasms. Of those dying from this condition, 25.8% died at home, 58.2% died in hospitals, and 13.3%

died in nursing homes. Although these death certificate records have been demonstrated to be highly consistent with the reports given by the next of kin, it has been suggested that the percentage of individuals dying in their homes may actually be slightly higher. This is considered likely because of those who were reported as dying in the hospital outpatient or emergency room or as dead on arrival, approximately one-third and just over one-half, respectively, actually died in their homes (24,27).

In the United States, the rate of in-hospital deaths varies with age and ranges from 48% to 91% (National Center for Health Statistics: Unpublished data, general mortality, 1990, 1994). The 1990 statistics indicate that the place of death for individuals dying before the age of 14 years is highly likely to be a hospital (69% to 91%). Between the ages of 15 and 24 years, deaths are often recorded as occurring in other places (29%). Twenty percent of those dying between 65 and 74 years die at home, and 38% of those over 85 years die in a nursing home. The diagnosis most commonly associated with a home death is malignant neoplasm (26%).

Although hospital deaths are reported to be most common (National Center for Health Statistics: Unpublished data, general mortality, 1990, 1994), this statistic does not clarify the site of treatment during the weeks prior to death. A recent survey of the deaths of elderly individuals found that 45% spent the night before their deaths in hospital and 25% were in a nursing home (28). Little has been reported about the number of moves between places of care that occur in the last weeks of life. Clinical experience suggests that moves between hospitals, homes, subacute care facilities, and hospices are not infrequent.

Social and disease-related factors also influence the place where death occurs. Marital status and cause of death, for example, have both been demonstrated to influence place of death (29,30). Patients with a recent cancer diagnosis and those with certain malignancies, for example leukemia and lymphoma, are more likely to die in the hospital setting than other groups with cancer (31). Although hospice participation has been associated with a higher likelihood of death at home (32), the availability of hospice-associated inpatient beds increases the likelihood of death in the inpatient setting (30). A cancer patient's symptom profile may also influence the site of death. For example, data from the 1981 National Hospice Study suggest that disorientation increases the likelihood that death will occur in the inpatient setting (30,33).

The economics of health care delivery clearly influence national differences in sites of death and the site of death within a specific country. In developing countries where access to heath care may be limited, death is less likely to occur in an institution. In the United States, the increase in deaths at home or in hospices during the last two decades, which has been particularly evident in patients with cancer, may reflect changes driven in part by the development of a Medicare hospice benefit (34).

**TABLE 3.** *Death rates from cancer, by sex and age: 1970 to 1993 (Deaths per 100,000 population in the specified age groups).*

| Age at death and selected type of cancer | Male | | | | | Female | | | | |
|---|---|---|---|---|---|---|---|---|---|---|
| | 1970 | 1980 | 1990 | 1992 | 1993 | 1970 | 1980 | 1990 | 1992 | 1993 |
| Total[1] | 182.1 | 205.3 | 221.3 | 220.8 | 222.1 | 144.4 | 163.6 | 186.0 | 188.2 | 189.8 |
| 25 to 34 years | 16.3 | 13.4 | 12.6 | 12.1 | 11.9 | 16.7 | 14.0 | 12.6 | 12.9 | 12.3 |
| 35 to 44 years | 53.0 | 44.0 | 38.5 | 38.1 | 38.0 | 65.6 | 53.1 | 48.1 | 46.5 | 44.1 |
| 45 to 54 years | 183.5 | 188.7 | 162.5 | 153.8 | 150.7 | 181.5 | 171.6 | 155.5 | 147.0 | 145.2 |
| 55 to 64 years | 511.8 | 520.8 | 532.9 | 513.4 | 507.4 | 343.2 | 361.7 | 375.2 | 369.7 | 366.7 |
| 65 to 74 years | 1,006.8 | 1,093.2 | 1,122.2 | 1,111.1 | 1,113.3 | 557.9 | 607.0 | 677.4 | 686.5 | 688.4 |
| 75 to 84 years | 1,588.3 | 1,790.5 | 1,914.4 | 1,882.7 | 1,885.4 | 891.9 | 903.1 | 1,010.3 | 1,025.6 | 1,046.1 |
| 85 years old and over | 1,720.8 | 2,369.5 | 2,739.9 | 2,802.3 | 2,830.7 | 1,095.7 | 1,255.7 | 1,372.1 | 1,393.9 | 1,415.3 |
| **Persons 35 to 44 years old** | | | | | | | | | | |
| Respiratory, intrathoracic | 17.0 | 12.6 | 9.1 | 8.6 | 8.3 | 6.5 | 6.8 | 5.4 | 5.6 | 5.0 |
| Digestive organs, peritoneum | 11.4 | 9.5 | 8.9 | 9.1 | 9.1 | 8.6 | 6.5 | 5.5 | 5.7 | 5.5 |
| Breast | 0.1 | — | (B) | 0.0 | (B) | 20.4 | 17.9 | 17.8 | 16.1 | 15.2 |
| Genital organs | 1.4 | 0.7 | 0.6 | 0.6 | 0.6 | 13.6 | 8.3 | 7.3 | 7.3 | 6.8 |
| Lymphatic and hematopoietic tissues, excl. leukemia | 5.6 | 4.3 | 4.5 | 4.9 | 4.7 | 3.2 | 2.4 | 2.1 | 2.2 | 2.0 |
| Urinary organs | 1.9 | 1.4 | 1.5 | 1.4 | 1.5 | 1.0 | 0.6 | 0.6 | 0.7 | 0.7 |
| Lip, oral cavity, and pharynx | 1.7 | 1.8 | 1.3 | 1.2 | 1.3 | 0.7 | 0.5 | 0.3 | 0.4 | 0.4 |
| Leukemia | 3.4 | 3.2 | 2.5 | 2.5 | 2.5 | 2.8 | 2.6 | 2.2 | 1.8 | 2.0 |
| **Persons 45 to 54 years** | | | | | | | | | | |
| Respiratory, intrathoracic | 72.1 | 79.8 | 63.0 | 57.7 | 54.6 | 22.2 | 34.8 | 35.3 | 32.5 | 31.6 |
| Digestive organs, peritoneum | 45.9 | 44.3 | 40.4 | 37.6 | 37.6 | 32.5 | 27.8 | 23.3 | 21.6 | 21.5 |
| Breast | 0.4 | 0.2 | 0.3 | 0.2 | 0.3 | 52.6 | 48.1 | 45.4 | 42.8 | 42.0 |
| Genital organs | 3.4 | 3.4 | 2.9 | 2.7 | 2.7 | 34.4 | 24.1 | 19.4 | 18.2 | 17.9 |
| Lymphatic and hematopoietic tissues, excl. leukemia | 12.8 | 10.2 | 10.9 | 10.8 | 10.3 | 8.3 | 6.6 | 6.0 | 6.1 | 6.0 |
| Urinary organs | 8.0 | 7.4 | 7.4 | 7.4 | 7.4 | 3.5 | 3.3 | 2.9 | 2.8 | 3.0 |
| Lip, oral cavity, and pharynx | 7.9 | 8.2 | 5.9 | 5.5 | 6.0 | 2.8 | 2.5 | 1.6 | 1.6 | 1.7 |
| Leukemia | 6.5 | 6.2 | 5.6 | 5.2 | 5.2 | 4.9 | 4.4 | 4.1 | 4.0 | 3.9 |
| **Persons 55 to 64 years old** | | | | | | | | | | |
| Respiratory intrathoracic | 202.3 | 223.8 | 232.6 | 217.0 | 216.0 | 38.9 | 74.5 | 107.6 | 108.4 | 107.3 |
| Digestive organs, peritoneum | 139.0 | 129.3 | 124.0 | 122.0 | 122.0 | 86.0 | 79.1 | 69.3 | 67.6 | 57.9 |
| Breast | 0.6 | 0.7 | 0.6 | 0.5 | 0.7 | 77.6 | 80.5 | 78.6 | 73.6 | 72.2 |
| Genital organs | 22.8 | 23.5 | 27.9 | 26.6 | 24.9 | 58.2 | 46.8 | 40.1 | 39.2 | 38.1 |
| Lymphatic and hematopoietic tissues excl. leukemia | 27.1 | 24.4 | 27.2 | 26.5 | 26.1 | 17.7 | 16.8 | 16.7 | 17.3 | 18.4 |
| Urinary organs | 26.4 | 22.9 | 23.5 | 23.1 | 22.3 | 9.4 | 8.9 | 8.8 | 9.1 | 8.4 |
| Lip, oral cavity, and pharynx | 20.1 | 17.9 | 15.2 | 14.8 | 14.2 | 6.2 | 6.0 | 4.7 | 4.4 | 4.3 |
| Leukemia | 15.4 | 14.7 | 14.7 | 14.9 | 14.7 | 9.0 | 9.3 | 8.8 | 9.0 | 8.7 |

**TABLE 3.** *Continued.*

| Age at death and selected type of cancer | Male | | | | | Female | | | | |
|---|---|---|---|---|---|---|---|---|---|---|
| | 1970 | 1980 | 1990 | 1992 | 1993 | 1970 | 1980 | 1990 | 1992 | 1993 |
| **Persons 65 to 74 years old** | | | | | | | | | | |
| Respiratory intrathoracic | 340.7 | 422.0 | 447.3 | 439.8 | 441.2 | 45.6 | 106.1 | 181.7 | 195.3 | 199.2 |
| Digestive organs, peritoneum | 293.3 | 284.1 | 267.4 | 263.6 | 259.6 | 185.8 | 173.6 | 153.0 | 148.4 | 151.8 |
| Breast | 1.4 | 1.1 | 1.1 | 1.1 | 1.2 | 93.8 | 101.1 | 111.7 | 109.3 | 105.7 |
| Genital organs | 103.7 | 107.6 | 123.5 | 122.0 | 117.9 | 85.6 | 73.6 | 71.0 | 70.5 | 67.0 |
| Lymphatic and hematopoietic tissues excl. leukemia | 50.3 | 48.1 | 56.8 | 58.7 | 59.0 | 34.6 | 34.4 | 39.5 | 41.0 | 42.5 |
| Urinary organs | 60.3 | 56.9 | 50.7 | 51.2 | 53.3 | 20.1 | 19.7 | 19.8 | 19.8 | 19.5 |
| Lip, oral cavity, and pharynx | 26.8 | 25.4 | 21.5 | 20.3 | 20.1 | 6.7 | 8.8 | 8.3 | 7.8 | 7.5 |
| Leukemia | 35.3 | 35.3 | 36.0 | 36.1 | 36.7 | 19.3 | 18.7 | 18.8 | 19.0 | 19.1 |
| **Persons 75 to 84 years old** | | | | | | | | | | |
| Respiratory, intrathoracic | 354.2 | 511.5 | 594.4 | 587.5 | 384.8 | 56.5 | 98.0 | 194.5 | 216.0 | 226.3 |
| Digestive organs, peritoneum | 507.5 | 496.6 | 468.0 | 444.0 | 441.7 | 353.3 | 326.3 | 293.3 | 288.7 | 287.7 |
| Breast | 2.7 | 2.1 | 1.6 | 2.0 | 2.3 | 127.4 | 126.4 | 146.3 | 140.8 | 146.4 |
| Genital organs | 299.4 | 315.4 | 358.5 | 355.7 | 356.6 | 104.9 | 95.7 | 95.3 | 97.2 | 97.4 |
| Lymphatic and hematopoietic tissues, excl leukemia | 74.0 | 80.0 | 104.5 | 106.5 | 107.8 | 49.4 | 57.8 | 71.2 | 74.6 | 78.4 |
| Urinary organs | 112.2 | 112.4 | 107.5 | 104.5 | 103.4 | 44.0 | 37.4 | 38.5 | 40.0 | 38.0 |
| Lip, oral cavity, and pharynx | 36.6 | 31.4 | 26.1 | 23.3 | 24.6 | 10.8 | 10.9 | 11.6 | 10.9 | 10.4 |
| Leukemia | 68.3 | 71.5 | 71.9 | 72.3 | 71.4 | 39.6 | 38.5 | 38.8 | 38.0 | 37.8 |
| **Persons 85 years old and over** | | | | | | | | | | |
| Respiratory, intrathoracic | 215.3 | 386.3 | 538.0 | 545.4 | 559.7 | 56.5 | 96.3 | 142.8 | 160.8 | 173.9 |
| Digestive organs, peritoneum | 583.7 | 705.8 | 699.5 | 683.8 | 668.5 | 465.0 | 504.3 | 497.6 | 495.7 | 487.0 |
| Breast | 2.9 | 2.6 | 2.4 | 4.4 | 5.1 | 157.1 | 169.3 | 196.8 | 195.5 | 206.0 |
| Genital organs | 434.2 | 612.3 | 750.0 | 808.3 | 842.2 | 107.3 | 115.9 | 115.5 | 115.8 | 114.4 |
| Lymphatic and hematopoietic tissues, excl. leukemia | 58.1 | 93.2 | 140.5 | 138.9 | 145.6 | 41.7 | 63.0 | 90.0 | 92.5 | 95.5 |
| Urinary organs | 140.5 | 177.0 | 186.3 | 192.9 | 190.3 | 59.9 | 63.8 | 68.5 | 69.6 | 64.5 |
| Lip, oral cavity, and pharynx | 47.0 | 40.2 | 37.4 | 32.8 | 31.1 | 19.2 | 16.0 | 17.5 | 16.9 | 16.8 |
| Leukemia | 83.3 | 117.1 | 116.0 | 116.8 | 115.6 | 50.9 | 61.1 | 65.0 | 67.7 | 68.2 |

—Represents zero. B Base figure too small to meet statistical standards for reliability of a derived figure.

[1] Includes persons under 25 years of age and malignant neoplasms of other and unspecified sites, not shown separately.

Source: U. S. National Center for Health Statistics. *Vital Statistics of the United States.* annual; and unpublished data.

**TABLE 4.** *Cancer—estimated new cases, 1996, and survival rates, 1974–77 to 1986–91*

| | Estimated new Cases.[1] 1996 (1,000) | | | 5-year relative survival rates (percent) | | | | | | | |
| | | | | White | | | | Black | | | |
| Site | Total | Male | Female | 1974– 77 | 1978– 81 | 1982– 85 | 1986– 91 | 1974– 77 | 1978– 81 | 1982– 85 | 1986– 91 |
|------|-------|------|--------|-------|-------|-------|-------|-------|-------|-------|-------|
| All sites[2] | 1,359 | 764 | 595 | 52.2 | 53.2 | 55.6 | 60.6 | 40.3 | 40.7 | 41.2 | 44.9 |
| Lung | 177 | 99 | 78 | 12.6 | 13.4 | 14.0 | 13.7 | 11.2 | 11.8 | 11.4 | 10.8 |
| Breast[3] | 186 | 1 | 184 | 75.1 | 75.8 | 79.2 | 84.3 | 62.9 | 64.0 | 64.2 | 69.0 |
| Colon and rectum | 134 | 68 | 66 | 50.2 | 53.4 | 57.7 | 61.7 | 44.8 | 45.9 | 47.3 | 52.4 |
| Prostate | 317 | 317 | (X) | 68.5 | 73.5 | 76.8 | 87.2 | 59.6 | 63.1 | 64.0 | 71.0 |
| Bladder | 53 | 38 | 15 | 73.8 | 77.9 | 79.1 | 82.1 | 49.4 | 57.2 | 58.5 | 58.6 |
| Corpus uteri | 34 | (X) | 34 | 88.8 | 84.9 | 85.1 | 85.7 | 61.4 | 55.4 | 55.7 | 57.3 |
| Non-Hodgkin's lymphoma[4] | 53 | 30 | 23 | 47.5 | 50.4 | 53.9 | 51.5 | 48.0 | 50.9 | 46.8 | 44.7 |
| Oral cavity and pharynx | 29 | 20 | 9 | 54.3 | 55.6 | 55.0 | 54.7 | 36.5 | 34.4 | 32.8 | 33.0 |
| Leukemia[4] | 28 | 15 | 12 | 35.8 | 38.1 | 40.5 | 41.2 | 31.9 | 30.8 | 32.9 | 32.4 |
| Melanoma of skin | 38 | 22 | 16 | 80.7 | 81.9 | 84.6 | 86.7 | 59.6 | 52.9 | 78.6 | 70.0 |
| Pancreas | 26 | 12 | 14 | 2.4 | 2.7 | 2.9 | 3.4 | 2.4 | 5.4 | 4.6 | 4.8 |
| Kidney | 31 | 19 | 12 | 50.1 | 52.2 | 54.8 | 58.7 | 49.5 | 55.8 | 52.5 | 53.5 |
| Stomach | 23 | 14 | 9 | 14.5 | 16.4 | 16.6 | 18.7 | 15.9 | 16.9 | 19.0 | 19.9 |
| Ovary | 27 | (X) | 27 | 36.8 | 38.2 | 39.7 | 44.0 | 40.1 | 39.0 | 40.7 | 38.0 |
| Cervix uteri[5] | 16 | (X) | 16 | 69.4 | 68.7 | 69.1 | 71.0 | 64.0 | 59.9 | 60.4 | 56.0 |

X Not applicable. [1]Estimates provided by American Cancer Society are based on rates from the National Cancer Institute's SEER program. [2]Includes other sites not shown separately. [3]Survival rates for female only. [4]All types combined. [5]Invasive cancer only.

The 5-year relative survival rate, which is derived by adjusting the observed survival rate for expected mortality, represents the likelihood that a person will not die from causes directly related to their cancer within 5 years. Survival data shown are based on those patients diagnosed while residents of an area listed below during the time periods shown. Data are based on information collected as part of the National Cancer Institute's Surveillance, Epidemiology and End Results (SEER) program, a collection of population-based registries in Connecticut, New Mexico, Utah, Iowa, Hawaii, Atlanta, Detroit, Seattle-Puget Sound, and San Francisco-Oakland.

Source: U. S. National Institutes of Health, National Cancer Institute, *Cancer Statistics Review,* annual.

The increase in the rate of nursing home death, particularly among the very elderly, may be related to changes in hospital reimbursement policies, such as prospective payment, utilization review, and preadmission screening (34,35). Some geographic trends also may relate, in part, to variations in the availability and reimbursability of hospice and home health care services. Differences may be compounded by variations in the availability of services in rural and urban areas. The dramatic impact of the utilization of services has been demonstrated in a survey of 12,343 cancer deaths in Italy (36). Although quality of life and quality of care were not explored in this study, home death was twice as frequent among the small number of patients who used the services of a palliative care team than among those who did not use such services (60.8% versus 29.3%).

Clinical experience suggests that many other ill-defined factors may influence place of death. Moreover, the choices that a patient or family make in the last days or hours of life may be different from their previously expressed preferences. Caring for a dying cancer patient in the home, although frequently a comforting and even rewarding experience for a patient and family, may also be burdensome. The availability of inpatient beds for the delivery of a hospice approach to care is imperative for the intensive management of certain symptoms and, in addition, provides an environment in which the family and patient may relax to some degree, spend time together, and be relieved of the responsibilities and burdens, both physical and psychological, of intensive home care.

Although much is speculated, there is very little information about the variation in the "quality" of either "care delivered" or "life of patients" among different sites. In 1981, the National Hospice Study assessed 1,754 terminal cancer patients in the United States and found that quality of life was similar for cancer patients in hospice and conventional care systems (37). While some indicators in this study suggested that control of pain and other symptoms may have been better in the inpatient hospice setting (30,33), the interpretation of the quality-of-life data is difficult owing to methodological difficulties. Most patients were unable to complete outcome measures in the weeks before death, and in these cases, data were provided by a caregiver, usually a family member. Although family perceptions are important and may in part reflect the patient's experience, retrospective third-party assessments have been demonstrated to correlate poorly with the patient's pain and other symptoms (38,39).

Little information is available to quantify the differences that exist within a particular site. In hospitals, the proportion of intensive care-related deaths, compared with ward deaths, is unknown, as is the proportion of patients who receive particular treatment interventions, such as palliative therapies, cardiopulmonary resuscitation (CPR), and mechanical ventilation. The recent SUPPORT study investigated the experiences of 4,301 seriously ill medical inpatients hospitalized in one of five teaching hospitals and found that a median of 8 days was spent in an intensive care unit (ICU), in a coma, or with ventilator support during the admission prior to death (40). The data from this study were combined with the information from another study of elderly patients to further explore the end-of-life experience associated with medical illness (41). The cancer patients in this population had either lung or colon cancer, and although the exact figures have not yet been reported in detail, the published data do give some indication of the cancer experience. For example, ICU involvement in the care of cancer patients was not as common as it was for other illnesses, 3% of colon cancer patients underwent a resuscitation attempt, and 2% received ventilator support.

Beyond the hospital, many patients die in nursing homes, and some hospices utilize nursing home beds for end-of-life care. Again, the care given at the end of life in nursing home environments has rarely been specifically explored. The nursing home environment presents particular challenges in the care of the dying, as the standard level of staffing in such facilities may be inadequate for the acute care of patients who may require frequent attention in response to symptomatic concerns. The evolution and increasing utilization of subacute care facilities presents yet another site wherein the care of the dying must also be specifically addressed.

In summary, the impact of the place of death on quality of life at the end of life remains largely unquantified. Although the proportion of patients dying in hospital and at home varies with age, diagnosis, and numerous sociodemographic factors, the reasons for this variability and its implications for patient morbidity and quality of life are unknown.

## Medical Involvement in Care During the Last Days of Life

In developed countries, those who are dying of chronic illness commonly have significant contact with health care professionals before death. The 1986 National Mortality Followback Survey collected data on over 16,000 decedents in the United States (24). This survey reported that 81% of decedents received some institutional care

during the last year of life, with 44% receiving between 1 week and 1 month of this care. Almost 9% of decedents received hospice care at home, and less than 0.5% received inpatient hospice care. In a retrospective study of cancer deaths in New York State, investigators found that although all of the patients surveyed had seen a doctor in the 6 months prior to death, a lack of face-to-face contact with the physicians was evident as death approached (42). More than half spent at least 1 of the last 2 weeks at home, 17% had no contact with their physician, and 31% had only telephone contact during this period.

These data demonstrate that most individuals seek and encounter physicians in the course of their medical care during the months before death. Physician involvement in the management of medical concerns as the end of life nears is most important and their involvement with patients with advanced disease places them in a position to play a pivotal role in the recognition of needs and the mobilization of resources to assist the patient and family. The possibility of deficiencies in involvement by physicians was suggested by the recent SUPPORT study, which demonstrated that despite contact with physicians during hospitalization, patient preferences regarding CPR were discussed in only 41% of cases, and physicians understood these patient preferences in only 47% of cases (40). The specific figures related to the cancer patients in this study have not been reported.

The system of care must be considered in the evaluation of medical involvement in the care of the dying. In the United States, *hospice* is defined broadly as a philosophy of care; however, practically it is most commonly a system of care distinct from the system that exists within the acute-care hospital system. Patients elect hospice and, for the most part, then seek to focus on comfort and quality of life without pursuing life-prolonging interventions. Hospice offers an array of services delivered through a team approach and aims to ensure quality of life for the patient and the family, most commonly in the home. In 1996, the National Hospice Organization estimated that 390,000 patients were treated in hospices in the United States (43). This represented approximately 17% of deaths nationally and a 15% increase from the previous year. It has been estimated that 58% of those in hospice care have cancer as their primary diagnosis and that almost 40% of those who die of cancer nationally receive hospice care (43,44). Survival data suggest that patients spent only short periods as hospice patients, despite eligibility that extends in the United States to those with a prognosis of less than 6 months' life expectancy. This statistic indicates a pattern of late referral to hospice. In a survey of 6,451 hospice patients, 80.2% of whom had cancer, Christakis and Escarce found that the median survival after enrollment was only 36 days, with 15.5% of the patients dying within 7 days (45). Survival varied substantially according to diagnosis even when this was adjusted for age and coexisting conditions. Table 54-5 contains these survival data

**TABLE 5.** *Survival according to cancer diagnosis among medicare beneficiaries enrolled in hospice programs*

| Diagnosis | Number of patients | Median survival (days) | Percentage who died within 7 days | Percentage who lived longer than 180 days |
|---|---|---|---|---|
| Leukemia or lymphoma | 291 | 23.0 | 20.6 | 14.1 |
| Urinary tract | 256 | 24.0 | 14.1 | 12.9 |
| Colon or rectum | 678 | 31.0 | 15.8 | 12.4 |
| Pancreas | 289 | 31.0 | 18.3 | 10.0 |
| Female genital tract | 223 | 34.0 | 17.5 | 14.8 |
| Upper gastrointestinal tract | 221 | 34.5 | 13.1 | 9.0 |
| Head or neck | 101 | 38.0 | 17.8 | 13.9 |
| Lung | 1378 | 38.0 | 14.2 | 11.8 |
| Breast | 364 | 43.5 | 13.5 | 9.0 |
| Central nervous system | 141 | 44.0 | 7.1 | 14.2 |
| Prostate | 480 | 46.0 | 14.0 | 13.7 |
| Liver or biliary tract | 205 | 50.0 | 22.4 | 8.8 |
| All other cancers | 548 | 32.5 | 15.1 | 12.0 |

Modified with permission from ref 45.

for the cancer patients in the study. For example, patients with breast, prostate, and central nervous system cancers tended to have a longer survivals after enrollment than did pancreas cancer patients.

## SYMPTOMS AND SIGNS IN THE LAST DAYS OF LIFE

Despite growing interest in quality-of-life outcomes, the oncological literature contains very little information about the nature of the dying process and the discomfort or distress associated with each different cancer. Optimal health care planning, on both an individual and a societal level, must be able to anticipate the problems that are likely to be encountered and plan accordingly. Without a clear understanding of the dying process, including recognition of the common sources of distress in patients and families, the medical care of this population will be suboptimal.

Only a few studies have described the experience of the last days or hours of patients with cancer. For the most part, these studies have been undertaken in the hospice or palliative care setting. Given that a large proportion of deaths in developed countries occur in the hospital setting, the absence of data on this group represents a significant gap in knowledge.

A survey of 486 dying patients by Dr. William Osler, performed between 1900 and 1904, represents the first important survey of the dying process. In this survey, a questionnaire was completed by the nurse who attended the patient at the hour of death (46,47). This survey was not confined to cancer patients. Osler described most patients as dying comfortably with "no sign of death one way or another, ... like their birth, death was a sleep and a forgetting." Despite this, many patients experienced distressing symptoms at least transiently. The distress was described as "bodily pain or distress" (*n*=90), "mental apprehension" (*n*=11), "positive terror" (*n*=2) and "bitter remorse" (*n*=1). The study did not go on to

describe the palliative interventions that were used to treat this distress, although it is known that Osler used opioid analgesia and held the view that uncontrolled symptoms should be adequately treated. Subsequent to this survey, several other investigators explored aspects of the dying process, including mental status and consciousness before death, individual awareness of impending death, and the distress experienced by the dying. Many of these studies were undertaken in patients with cancer, but very few were conducted in the United States. As a consequence, much of the following data originates from studies undertaken in the United Kingdom, Europe, and Canada.

### Mental Status and Consciousness Before Death

Epidemiological surveys have rarely focused on detailed descriptions of mental status at the end of life. The level of consciousness on the day of death is clearly influenced by a diverse range of factors, many of which are likely to be disease-specific. These factors include the rapidity of physical deterioration, coexisting organ failure, and use of medication. The 1986 National Mortality Followback Survey explored some issues relating to orientation during the last year of life (24). Among the 16,000 individuals who died of many diseases, 61% were described as "never or hardly ever ... having trouble understanding where he or she was during the last year of life." Fifteen percent were described as having this difficulty for the "last few hours or days," 13% for "some of the time," and 8% for "all or most of the time." In another large survey of the deaths of 1,227 United States elderly, 60% had no difficulty with orientation or with recognizing their family during the 3 days before death, and 51% had no difficulty on the day before death (28,48). This latter survey represented a mixed population, and data on the proportion of cancer patients have not been published. Recently, the data from the SUPPORT study population were combined with data from another group of elderly patients (total *N*=4,622) to evaluate, among other aspects of the dying experience, the level of consciousness before death (41). Eighty percent of the lung cancer patients and almost 70% of the colon cancer patients were reported to be conscious 3 days before death; 55% and 40% of these groups, respectively, were also reported to be able to communicate effectively at this time. A survey of 100 cancer patients who died at St. Christopher's Hospice in the United Kingdom described 10% as alert, 67% as drowsy or semiconscious, and 23% as unarousable or unconscious during the 24 hours before death (49). Finally, a recent survey of 154 inpatient and home-care cancer patients who died found one-third were able to interact 24 hours prior to death; this decreased to one-fifth at 12 hours before death and one-tenth in the hour before death (50).

The mental disturbances that occur before death have been specifically explored in several small studies. Massie et al., for example, found that eleven (85%) of 13 terminally ill cancer patients were delirious before death and noted that the early symptoms of delirium were frequently misdiagnosed as anxiety, anger, depression, or psychosis (51). Bruera et al. studied 66 episodes of cognitive failure in 39 patients admitted to a palliative care service and cited drugs, sepsis, and brain metastasis as the most frequently detected etiological factors (52). Of the episodes of cognitive failure that occurred in this population, 22 (33%) improved, 10 spontaneously and 12 as a result of treatment. This study demonstrated the benefits of an active approach to the diagnosis and treatment of cognitive decline (52).

In cancer patients, the potential causes of delirium and impaired cognition, particularly at the end of life, may be divided into direct effects related to tumor involvement and indirect effects (53). The latter category includes drugs, electrolyte imbalance, cranial irradiation, organ failure, nutritional deficiencies, vascular complications, paraneoplastic syndromes, and many other factors (53–59). Although no large prospective survey has assessed the relative contributions of these factors, a survey of cancer patients referred initially for a neurology consultation demonstrated a multifactorial etiology in most of the 94 patients with encephalopathy (60). In this survey, metabolic causes, drugs, and central nervous system metastases were the most common contributors to this state.

Although these studies reveal that a high proportion of cancer patients maintain alertness until they are close to death, it is apparent that impaired cognitive functioning is both prevalent and often reversible during the last weeks of life.

## Awareness of Impending Death

Several studies of medically ill patients, some involving patients with cancer, have attempted to explore the awareness of impending death. For example, Witzel eval-

uated 110 patients, 19% of whom had cancer, and found that 51% of the dying patients and only 5% of the control group felt that they were about to die (61). Interestingly, only 2.7% of the dying patients in this study expressed a fear of death, whereas almost 48% of the comparison group expressed such a fear. Moreover, it was observed that the dying patients expressed more fear during their last weeks of life than during their last days of life. Exton-Smith surveyed 220 dying geriatric patients and reported that 25% seemed to be aware of their approaching death (62). Of the 33 patients with cancer in this survey, 10 (30.3%) seemed to be aware that death was approaching. Hinton repeatedly interviewed 102 terminally ill patients (approximately 80% with cancer), all of whom subsequently died within 6 months. Seventy-five percent spoke of an awareness of a possible fatal outcome during one or more conversations (63). In a survey of 1,227 elderly decedents in the United States, 34% had some awareness of approaching death; 42% of these patients reported having had information about the imminence of death provided by a physician (28,48). Although cancer was documented as being present in 34% of this population it was listed as the first cause of death on the death certificate in only 10%.

## Symptom Distress Before Death

Several large surveys have evaluated symptom distress prior to death, and the experiences of those patients dying from cancer have been explored in numerous small studies undertaken in the hospice or palliative care setting. Unfortunately, there are still large gaps in our knowledge in this area, particularly regarding death from specific cancers in the hospital or home care setting.

Among the large surveys, Osler's report suggested that approximately one-fifth of dying patients experienced bodily pain or distress (46). This proportion is smaller than more recent studies have suggested. In the survey by Brock et al. of elderly decedents in the United States, caregivers reported that during the 24 hours before death, 44% were short of breath and 33% were in pain (28,48). Unfortunately, neither of these studies describe, in any detail, the medical and pharmacological interventions utilized for mangement of symptoms. It is therefore difficult to ascertain whether appropriate, state-of-the-art palliative medicine would have had any impact on these most significant levels of distress.

Many investigators have explored the spectrum of symptoms experienced by cancer patients at various points during the course of the disease, such as at admission to a hospice or to a palliative care unit (64–69). Several investigations, including those summarized in Table 54-6, have focused specifically on the dying process or the last weeks of life (28,37,48,49,61–63,70–78). Some studies have explored the prevalence and impact of particular symptoms in the setting of advanced malignant

**TABLE 6.** *Symptom prevalence in the last week of life in patients with cancer*

| Symptoms (%) | Bedard (76) n=952 (1,5) | Coyle (73) n=90 (3,5) | Fainsinger (77) n=100 (1,5,7) | Hinton (63) n=82 (2,4,10) | Lichter (74) n=200 (1,5) | Saunders (49) n=200 (1,5) | Ward (70) n=200 (2,7) |
|---|---|---|---|---|---|---|---|
| Pain | 12–30 | 34 | 99 | 71 | 51 | 23 | 62 |
| Dyspnea | 9 | 28 | 46 | 4–20 | 22 | 21 | 52 |
| Nausea | 16 | 13 | 71 | 12–17 | 14 | 3 | |
| Vomiting | 16 | | | 12–17 | 14 | 7 | 38 |
| Sleepiness | 5 | 57 | | | | 46 | |
| Congestion | | 6 | | | 56 | 53 | |
| Confusion | 4 | 28 | 39 | | 9 | 12 | 39 |
| Restlessness | | 7 | | | 42 | 31 | |
| Anorexia | 14 | 6 | | | | | 61 |
| Fatigue | | 52 | | | | | |
| Urinary incontinence | 4 | 6 | | | 32 | | 28 |

Symptoms are recorded if any 2 surveys demonstrated a prevalence of greater than 25% or if any one survey demonstrated a prevalence of 50% or more for specific symptom.
1. Hospice or palliative care inpatients only.
2. General patients, type of care not specified.
3. Cancer center inpatients and outpatients.
4. Data provided directly by patient.
5. Data provided by patient or primary caregiver.
6. Data provided by caregiver.
7. Indicators of overall distress included as well as prevalence.

disease (51,79–95), and others have highlighted other aspects of the dying process by characterizing the differences in the quality of care provided by inpatient and home care services (33,96–100).

Patients in the advanced stages of cancer commonly report fatigue, pain, anxiety, and anorexia, each with prevalence rates reported to be greater than 50% (65,68, 72,73,77,90,91,93,95,99). Moreover, most patients with advanced cancer experience multiple symptoms (68,73, 95). Although the most common symptoms are generally considered to be physical (e.g., pain, fatigue, or nausea), this finding can be ascribed to a survey methodology that often does not address psychological symptoms. When specific psychological measures are incorporated into survey methodologies, high prevalence rates for psychological symptoms have been reported (67,80,83,84,101). For example, depressed mood and anxiety have been found to be extremely common in ambulatory cancer patients when specific inquiries have been made (95).

Among the physical symptoms experienced by patients with advanced cancer, pain and dyspnea have been the focus of symptom-specific surveys in the cancer population. Large surveys have repeatedly documented that pain is experienced by 70% to 90% patients with advanced cancer (102–105). The National Hospice Study (N=1,754) documented that pain became more prevalent in cancer patients during the last weeks of life (86). Although a large proportion of patients in this study were not able to be interviewed directly, 25% of those who could provide self-report data indicated that persistent or severe pain was present within 2 days of death; this proportion increased from 17% in the previous 6 days.

Another survey demonstrated that 80% of cancer outpatients experienced pain as death approached (82), and yet another showed that only 35% of patients dying in the home care setting and 9% in hospital-based hospice care did not use analgesics during the last week of life (89). In the recent SUPPORT study, 50% of the 1,400 patients who had been conscious before death were reported by caregivers to have experienced moderate to severe pain for at least half of the time during their last three days of life (40). The data from this study were combined with data from another survey to clarify the perceptions of family members who observed the dying experiences of 3,357 patients, of whom approximately 12% had lung cancer and 5% had colon cancer (41). In the groups with cancer, 40% to 46% of patients with cancer were judged by their relatives to have moderate to severe pain for more than half of the time during the last 3 days of life.

It is difficult to draw conclusions concerning the factors that contribute to the severity of pain and distress before death, as most studies do not include detailed discussions of pain syndromes and treatments. Consequently, it is not possible to ascertain whether the high incidence of pain before death reflects worsening pathologic condition, undertreatment, or both. A large amount of data is available that confirms that pain and other distressing symptoms can be very effectively treated. Certainly, the undertreatment of pain, and perhaps of other symptoms, is likely to contribute to symptom distress. In the United States, many cancer patients continue to receive inadequate analgesia (106,107). In a survey of 1,308 oncology outpatients being treated by the physician members of the Eastern Cooperative Oncology Group,

67% reported recent pain and 36% described pain severe enough to impair function (107). Forty-two percent of the patients who reported pain were not given adequate analgesia. Eighty-six percent of the physicians believed that the majority of cancer patients with pain were undermedicated (106). Poor pain assessment was rated by 76% of physicians as the single most important barrier to adequate pain management, and 61% indicated that physicians' reluctance to prescribe opioids was also a barrier. In a similar survey undertaken in France, 69% of cancer patients rated their worst pain to be at a level that impaired their ability to function, and undertreatment was again a prominent factor (108).

Towards the end of life, cancer-related dyspnea has been reported to be in the range of 20% to 78% (71,88, 92,94). It is likely that this wide variation reflects variability in the definitions of dyspnea, the methods used for eliciting the symptom, and patient selection. In the National Hospice Study, dyspnea was seen in 70% of 1,754 patients during the final 6 weeks of life; the prevalence increased as death approached (88). Higginson and McCarthy studied a group of 86 cancer patients and noted that dyspnea was a severe and often uncontrollable symptom near death (92). In a survey of hospice inpatients with cancer, dyspnea was present in 55.5% of all patients on admission to the inpatient hospice and 78.6% of those who died within 1 day of admission (94). In the SUPPORT study, dyspnea was reported to be moderate to severe for the last few days of life in 30% of colon cancer patients and in almost 70% of those with lung cancer. As

with the data on pain, these studies contain no details of symptom management strategies.

Longitudinal studies provide further insight into the patient experience during the dying process (73). Coyle et al. reviewed the records of 90 cancer outpatients to describe the experiences of this population during the 4 weeks before death. These patients ranged in age from 23 to 82 years; and two-thirds cancers of the lung, colon, or breast. All patients were cared for at home during this 4-week period, and only 19% of patients were able to engage in some form of limited activity outside the home. Fifty-seven percent died at home, 41% in the hospital, and 2% in an emergency room. At various times within the last 4 weeks of life, patients spontaneously identified 44 different symptoms distressing enough to interfere with activity. The number of symptoms volunteered per person ranged from 1 to 9, with 71% describing 3 or more distinct symptoms at 4 weeks before death. Fatigue (58%), pain (54%), weakness (43%), sleepiness (24%), and cognitive impairment (24%) were the most prevalent symptoms (Table 54-7). Although the spectrum of symptoms reported were similar at 4 weeks and 1 week before death, there were changes in prevalence. The prevalence of sleepiness, for example, increased from 24% to 57%, whereas the prevalence of pain decreased from 54% to 34%. Although the population depicted in this survey had been referred because of difficult pain problems, the degree of distress remains informative. Eighteen of these patients acknowledged suicidal ideation, and an additional 4 patients were suicidal, each elaborating a specific plan.

**TABLE 7.** *Prevalence of symptoms volunteered by advanced cancer patients 4 weeks and 1 week before death (n=90)*

| Symptom | 4 weeks before death N (%) | 1 week before death N (%) |
|---|---|---|
| Fatigue | 52 (58) | 47 (52) |
| Pain | 49 (54) | 31 (34) |
| Generalized weakness | 39 (43) | 44 (49) |
| Sleepiness | 22 (24) | 51 (57) |
| Mental haziness, confusion | 22 (24) | 25 (28) |
| Anxiety | 19 (21) | 16 (18) |
| Weakness of legs | 16 (18) | 15 (17) |
| Shortness of breath | 15 (17) | 25 (28) |
| Nausea | 11 (12) | 12 (13) |
| Decreased hearing | 8 (9) | 5 (6) |
| Depression | 7 (8) | 4 (4) |
| Loss of appetite | 7 (8) | 5 (6) |
| Inability to sleep | 6 (7) | 5 (6) |
| Weakness of upper limb | 6 (7) | 5 (6) |
| Cough | 5 (6) | 6 (7) |
| Restlessness/irritability | 5 (6) | 6 (7) |
| Swollen limb | 4 (4) | 7 (8) |
| Constipation | 4 (4) | 6 (7) |
| Difficulty swallowing | 3 (3) | 6 (7) |
| Pulmonary congestion | 1 (1) | 5 (6) |
| Dizziness | 1 (1) | 5 (6) |
| Incontinence | 3 (3) | 5 (6) |
| Difficulty speaking | 5 (6) | 5 (6) |

Reproduced with permission from ref 73.

The latter patients were clinically depressed and required psychiatric intervention. Four patients requested euthanasia; in each case, the request was specific and spontaneous, without direct or indirect prompting from the clinician.

It is most important to note that a few studies specifically explore symptom distress. The mere prevalence of symptoms does not provide any information about the distress associated with the symptom, nor does it provide sufficient understanding of either their severity or their impact (90,95,109). Many studies from hospice literature provide data suggesting that most deaths can be comfortable. Further, there are minimal data that clarify the impact of far-advanced disease on function, physical or psychosocial needs, or the more global constructs of suffering and quality of life (110–112). Given the prevalence of impaired consciousness as the end of life approaches, exploration of many of these issues is likely to be challenging. It must be noted, however, that opportunities for further research abound in this population, as many patients do retain their ability to communicate until the very last days or hours of life. Despite the gaps in knowledge, the existing studies nonetheless highlight the spectrum of symptoms experienced by cancer patients who are nearing the end of life and provide some insights into the further studies that will be necessary for adequate characterization of the dying process.

### The Impact of Medications on Symptom Management at the End of Life

Specific strategies have evolved in the fields of pain management and palliative care to address common symptoms towards the end of life (113). For example, treatment approaches have been described for pain as very effective (105,114), dyspnea (115), confusion (116,117), and sleep disturbance (118). Notwithstanding, there is evidence that clinicians lack sufficient knowledge to implement these treatments optimally (106,107,119,120). Accurate assessment of the impact of drugs for symptom control, as well as assessment of the degree to which sedation is a necessary intervention for symptom management, has been hampered by the problems of underprescribing and poor methodology for symptom assessment.

The difficulties around this issue surfaced in a recent debate regarding the role of sedative medications in the management of unendurable symptoms at the end of life. Ventafridda et al. triggered a controversy in the palliative care literature by reporting that 52.5% of dying patients required sedation to obtain relief from symptoms (75). This finding contrasted starkly with data from hospice programs, which suggest that most deaths are peaceful (49,74), and by a subsequently published survey of 100 cancer patients that observed the majority of deaths were comfortable and only 18% of patients required sedating treatment for pain or delirium (although 57% of patients were unresponsive by the day of death) (77). Routine symptom assessment measures were used by Fainsinger

et al. in this latter study; however, in both of these studies, interpretation of the data was difficult, as symptoms were evaluated by observers and detailed data describing the palliative interventions were not included. The proportion of patients who have intolerable symptoms, therefore, remains unresolved.

Further studies of treatment strategies, which incorporate comprehensive symptom assessment measures, are needed to clarify the impact of therapy on symptoms in the dying. Although the role of sedative drugs for the management of refractory symptoms in the dying is controversial (77,121–124), the major concern continues to be the underutilization of palliative strategies for the management of distress. Research into these issues must be broadened to include individuals whose death occurs at home or outside of settings such as hospices, where palliation is the most common goal of care.

## CONCLUSION

Although many surveys have described the experience of patients who are in the advanced stages of cancer, many questions remain unanswered. These is a need to expand the epidemiological knowledge base particularly as it relates to specific cancers and specific sites of care. Information is needed about how patients are cared for and by whom; whether patients' goals for end of life care are being met; and which setting—home, hospital, or hospice—is most likely to meet these goals. Access to care, physicians' knowledge of palliative care, and patient-physician communication and patient-family-physician communication must be further explored. Special consideration also needs to be given to specific diseases and unique populations including the pediatric, the elderly, and the mentally handicapped. Much of the distress that may occur at the end of life is responsive to palliative interventions, but only with an understanding of many aspects of the end of life experience can health care strategies and standards for the care of the dying be developed so that the care of patient and families at this most difficult time becomes optimal.

## REFERENCES

1. Humphry D. *Final exit*. Secaucus, NJ: Carol Publishing, 1991.
2. Hill TP, Shirley D. *A good death: taking more control at the end of your life*. New York: Addison Wesley, 1992.
3. Quill TE. *Death and dignity: making choices and taking charge*. New York: WW Norton & Company, 1993.
4. Nuland SB. *How we die: reflections on life's final chapter*. New York: Alfred A. Knopf, 1994.
5. World Health Organization. Global health situation. *Weekly Epidemiol Record* 1993;68(6):33–6.
6. Rosenberg HM, Ventura SJ, Maurer JD, et al. Births and deaths: United States, 1995. In: National Center for Health Statistics. *Monthly Vital Statistics Report*. Hyattsville, MD: 1996;45(Suppl 21):1–40.
7. Bulatao RA. Mortality by cause, 1970–2015. In: *The epidemiological transition: policy and planning implications for developing countries*. Washington, DC: National Academy Press, 1993:42–68.
8. Bulatao RA, Stephens PW. *Global estimates and projections of mortality by cause, 1970–2015*. Washington, DC: World Bank, 1992.

9. United States Bureau of the Census. *Statistical abstract of the United States*, 116th ed. Washington, DC: National Technical Information Service, 1996.

10. Heligman L, Chen N, Babakol O. Shifts in the structure of population and deaths in less developed regions. In: Gribble JN and Preston SH, eds. *The epidemiological transition: policy and planning implications for developing countries*. Washington, DC: National Academy Press, 1993:9–41.

11. Lopez AD. Causes of death: an assessment of global patterns of mortality around 1985. *Wld Hlth Statist Q* 1990;43:91–104.

12. Lopez AD. Changes in tobacco consumption and cancer risk: evidence from national statistics. In: Hakama M, Beral V, Cullen JW, Parkin DM, eds. *Evaluating the effectiveness of primary prevention of cancer*, Vol 103. Lyon: International Agency for Research on Cancer, 1990:57–76.

13. Stjernsward J. Palliative medicine—a global perspective. In: Doyle D, Hanks GWC, MacDonald N, eds. *Oxford textbook of palliative medicine*, 1st ed. Oxford: Oxford University Press, 1993:805–816.

14. World Health Organization, Global Programme on AIDS. *The HIV pandemic: 1994 overview*. Geneva: World Health Organization, 1994.

15. Cole P, Rodu B. Declining cancer mortality in the United States. *Cancer* 1996;78(10):2045–2048.

16. World Health Organization. *Health of the elderly*. Technical Report Series. 1989;779:7–30.

17. Singh GK, Kochanek KD, MacDorman MF. Advance report of final mortality statistics, 1994. In: National Center for Health Statistics. *Monthly vital statistics report* 1996;45:19.

18. Gardner P, Hudson BL. Advance report of final mortality statistics, 1993. *Monthly vital statistics report* 1996;44(7 suppl).

19. Kosary CL, GloecklerRies MS, Miller BA, Hankey BF, Harras A, Edwards BK. *SEER cancer statistics review, 1973–1992*. Bethesda, MD: US Department of Health and Human Services, Public Health Services, National Institutes of Health, National Cancer Institute, 1996.

20. National Center for Health Statistics: Advance report of final mortality statistics, 1991. *Monthly vital statistics report* 1994;42(2 suppl).

21. Kochanek KD, Hudson BL. Advance report of final mortality statistics, 1992. *Monthly vital statistics report* 1995;43(6 suppl).

22. McGinnis JM, Foege WH. Real, true and genuine causes of death in the United States—what are they? *Mod Pathol* 1994;7(5):527–528.

23. Wingo PA, Tong T, Bolden S. Cancer statistics, 1995. *CA Cancer J Clin* 1995;45:8–30.

24. Seeman I. National mortality followback survey: 1986 summary. United States National Center for Health Statistics. *Vital Health Statistics* 1992;20(19).

25. Townsend J, Frank AO, Fermont D, et al. Terminal cancer care and patients' preference for place of death: a prospective study. *Br Med J* 1990;301(6749):415–417.

26. World Health Organization. *World health statistics annual*. Geneva: World Health Organization, xv–xvii.

27. Poe GS, Powell-Griner E, McLaughlin JK, et al. Compatibility of the death certificate and the 1986 National Mortality Followback Survey. National Center for Health Statistics. *Vital Health Statistics* 1993:2(118):5–14.

28. Foley DJ, Miles TP, Brock DB, Phillips C. Recounts of elderly deaths: endorsments for the patient self-determination act. *Gerontologist* 1995;35(1):119–121.

29. Polissar L, Severson RK, Brown NK. Factors affecting place of death in Washington State, 1968–1981. *J Comm Health* 1987;12(1):40–55.

30. Mor V, Hiris J. Determinants of site of death among hospice cancer patients. *J Health Soc Behav* 1983;24(12):375–385.

31. McCusker J. Where cancer patients die: an epidemiologic study. *Public Health Rep* 1983;98(2):170–177.

32. Moinpour CM, Polissar L. Factors affecting place of death of hospice and non-hospice cancer patients. *Am J Public Health* 1989;79(11):1549–1551.

33. Greer DS, Mor V, Morris JN, Sherwood S, Kidder D, Birnbaum H. An alternative in terminal care: results of the National Hospice Study. *J Chronic Dis* 1986;39(1):9–26.

34. McMillan A, Mentnech RM, Lubitz J, McBean AM, Russell D. Trends and patterns in place of death for Medicare enrollees. *Health Care Fin Rev* 1990;12(1):1–7.

35. Sager MA, Easterling DV, Kindig DA, Anderson OW. Changes in the location of death after passage of Medicare's prospective payment system. *N Engl J Med* 1989;320(7):433–439.

36. Costantini M, Camoirano E, Madeddu L, Bruzzi P, Verganelli E, Henriquet F. Palliative home care and place of death among cancer patients: a population-based study. *Pall Med* 1993;7(4):323–331.

37. Morris JN, Suissa S, Sherwood S, Wright SM, Greer D. Last days: a study of the quality of life of terminally ill cancer patients. *J Chron Dis* 1986;39(1):47–62.

38. Higginson I, Priest P, McCarthy M. Are bereaved family members a valid proxy for a patient's assessment of dying? *Soc Sci Med* 1994; 38(4):553–557.

39. Clipp EC, George LK. Patients with cancer and their spouse caregivers. Perceptions of the illness experience. *Cancer* 1992;69(4):1074–1079.

40. The SUPPORT study investigators: a controlled trial to improve care for seriously ill hospitalized patients: SUPPORT. *JAMA* 1995;274:1591–1598.

41. Lynn J, Teno JM, Phillips RS, et al: Perceptions by family members of the dying experience of older and seriously ill patients. *Ann Intern Med* 1997;126(2):97–106.

42. McCusker J. The terminal period of cancer: definition and descriptive epidemiology. *J Chronic Dis* 1984;37(5):377–385.

43. National Hospice Organization. *1995–1996 Hospice Statistics*. Arlington, VA: National Hospice Organization.

44. Haupt BJ. *Characteristics of patients receiving hospice care services: United States, 1994*. Advance data from Vital Health and Statistics, No. 282. Hyattsville, MD: National Center for Health Statistics, 1997.

45. Christakis NA, Escarce JJ. Survival of Medicare patients after enrollment in hospice programs. *N Engl J Med* 1996;335(3):172–178.

46. Osler W. The Ingersoll lecture. In: *Science and immortality*. New York: Houghton Mifflin, 1904:19.

47. Hinohara S. Sir William Osler's philosophy on death. *Ann Intern Med* 1993;118(8):638–642.

48. Brock DB, Holmes MB, Foley DJ, Holmes D. Methodological issues in a survey of the last days of life. In: Wallace RB, Woolson RF, eds. *The epidemiologic study of the elderly*. New York: Oxford University Press, 1992:315–332.

49. Saunders C. Pain and impending death. In: Wall P, Melzack R, eds. *Textbook of pain*. New York: Churchill Livingston, 1984:472–478.

50. Ingham JM, Layman-Goldstein M, Derby S, et al. The characteristics of the dying process in cancer patients in a hospice and a cancer center. *Proceedings of ASCO* 1994;13:172.

51. Massie MJ, Holland J, Glass E. Delirium in terminally ill cancer patients. *Am J Psychiatry* 1983;140(8):1048–1050.

52. Bruera E, Miller L, McCallion J, Macmillan K, Krefting L, Hanson J. Cognitive failure in patients with terminal cancer: a prospective study. *J Pain Symptom Manage* 1992;7(4):192–195.

53. Posner JB. Neurologic complications of systemic cancer. *Disease-a-Month* 1979;25:1–60.

54. Silberfarb PM, Philibert D, Levine PM. Psychosocial aspects of neoplastic disease: II. Affective and cognitive effects of chemotherapy in cancer patients. *Am J Psychiatry* 1980;137(5):597–601.

55. Oxman TE, Silberfarb PM. Serial cognitive testing in cancer patients receiving chemotherapy. *Am J Psychiatry* 1980;137(10):1263–1265.

56. Silberfarb PM. Chemotherapy and cognitive defects in cancer patients. *Ann Rev Med* 1983;34(35):35–46.

57. Patchell RA, Posner JB. Cancer and the nervous system. In: Holland JC, Rowland JH, eds. *Handbook of psychooncology*. New York: Oxford University Press, 1989:327–341.

58. Meyers CA, Abbruzzese JL. Cognitive functioning in cancer patient: effect of previous treatment. *Neurology* 1992;42:434–436.

59. Barbato M. Thiamine deficiency in patients admitted to a palliative care unit. *Pall Med* 1994;8:320–324.

60. Tuma R, DeAngelis L. Acute encephalopathy in patients with systemic cancer. *Ann Neurol* 1992;32:288.

61. Witzel L. Behavior of the dying patient. *Br Med J* 1975;2(April 12):81–82.

62. Exton-Smith A N. Terminal illness in the aged. *Lancet* 1961;2:305–308.

63. Hinton JM. The physical and mental distress of the dying. *Q J Med* 1963;32(125):1–21.

64. Wilkes E. Some problems in cancer management. *Proc Roy Soc Med* 1974;67:1001–1005.

65. Brescia FJ, Adler D, Gray G, Ryan MA, Cimino J, Mamtani R. Hospitalized advanced cancer patients: a profile. *J Pain Sympt Manag* 1990;5(4):221–227.

66. Brescia F. Approaches to palliative care: notes of a deathwatcher. In: Foley KM, Bonica JJ, and Ventafridda V, eds. *Advances in pain research and therapy*. Second International Congress on Cancer Pain. New York: Raven Press, 1990;16:393–397.

67. McCarthy M. Hospice patients: a pilot study in 12 services. *Pall Med* 1990;4:93–104.

68. Curtis EB, Krech R, Walsh TD. Common symptoms in patients with advanced cancer. *J Pall Care* 1991;7(2):25–29.

69. Donnelly S, Walsh D. The symptoms of advanced cancer. *Semin Oncol* 1995;22(2 Suppl 3):67–72.

70. Ward AWM. Terminal care in malignant disease. *Soc Sci Med* 1974;8: 413–420.

71. Hockley JM, Dunlop R, Davies RJ. Survey of distressing symptoms in dying patients and their families in hospital and the response to a symptom control team. *Br Med J (Clin Res Ed)* 1988;296:1715–1717.

72. Reuben DB, Mor V, Hiris J. Clinical symptoms and length of survival in patients with terminal cancer. *Arch Intern Med* 1988;148(7): 1586–1591.

73. Coyle N, Adelhardt J, Foley KM, Portenoy RK. Character of terminal illness in the advanced cancer patient: pain and other symptoms during the last four weeks of life. *J Pain Sympt Manag* 1990;5(2):83–93.

74. Lichter I, Hunt E. The last 48 hours of life. *J Pall Care* 1990;6(4):7–15.

75. Ventafridda V, Ripamonti C, De CF, Tamburini M, Cassileth BR. Symptom prevalence and control during cancer patients' last days of life. *J Pall Care* 1990;6(3):7–11.

76. Bedard J, Dionne L. The experience of La Maison Michel Sarrazin (1985–1990): profile analysis of 952 terminal cancer patients. *J Pall Care* 1991;7:48–53.

77. Fainsinger R, Miller MJ, Bruera E, Hanson J, MacEachern T. Symptom control during the last week of life on a palliative care unit. *J Pall Care* 1991;7(1):5–11.

78. Fakhoury WKH, McCarthy M, Addington-Hall J. The effects of the clinical characteristics of dying patients on informal caregivers' satisfaction with palliative care. *Pall Med* 1997;11:107–115.

79. Twycross RG. The use of narcotic analgesics in terminal illness. *J Med Ethics* 1975;1:10–17.

80. Plumb MM, Holland J. Comparative studies of psychological function in patients with advanced cancer—I. Self-reported depressive symptoms. *Psychosom Med* 1977;39(4):264–276.

81. Levine PM, Silberfarb PM, Lipowski ZJ. Mental disorders in cancer patients: a study of 100 psychiatric referrals. *Cancer* 1978;42(3): 1385–1391.

82. McKegney FP, Bailey LR, Yates JW. Prediction and management of pain in patients with advanced cancer. *Gen Hosp Psych* 1981;3:95–101.

83. Plumb M, Holland J. Comparative studies of psychological function in patients with advanced cancer. II. Interviewer-rated current and past psychological symptoms. *Psychosom Med* 1981;43(3):243–254.

84. Bukberg J, Penman D, Holland JC. Depression in hospitalized cancer patients. *Psychosom Med* 1984;46(3):199–212.

85. Heyse-Moore L, Baines MJ. Control of other symptoms. In: Saunders C, ed. *The management of terminal malignant disease.* London: Edward Arnold, 1984:100–132.

86. Morris JN, Mor V, Goldberg RJ, Sherwood S, Greer DS, Hiris J. The effect of treatment setting and patient characteristics on pain in terminal cancer patients: a report from the National Hospice Study. *J Chronic Dis* 1986;39(1):27–35.

87. Reuben DB, Mor V. Nausea and vomiting in terminal cancer patients. *Arch Intern Med* 1986;146(10):2021–2023.

88. Reuben DB, Mor V. Dyspnea in terminally ill cancer patients. *Chest* 1986;89(2):234–236.

89. Goldberg RJ, Mor V, Weimann M, Greer DS, Hiris J. Analgesic use in terminal cancer patients: report from the National Hospice Study. *J Chron Dis* 1986;39(1):37–45.

90. Dunlop GM. A study of the relative frequency and importance of gastrointestinal symptoms and weakness in patients with far advanced cancer. *Pall Med* 1989;4:37–43.

91. Grosvenor M, Bulcavage L, Chlebowski RT. Symptoms potentially influencing weight loss in a cancer population. Correlations with primary site, nutritional status, and chemotherapy administration. *Cancer* 1989;63(2):330–334.

92. Higginson I. McCarthy M. Measuring symptoms in terminal cancer: are pain and dyspnoea controlled? *J R Soc Med* 1989;82(5):264–267.

93. Ventafridda V, DeConno F, Ripamonti C, Gamba A, Tamburini M. Quality-of-life assessment during a palliative care programme. *Ann Oncol* 1990;1(6):415–420.

94. Heyse-Moore LH. How much of a problem is dyspnoea in advanced cancer? *Pall Med* 1991;5:20–26.

95. Portenoy RK, Thaler HT, Kornblith AB,; et al. Symptom prevalence, characteristics and distress in a cancer population. *Qual Life Res* 1994;3(3):183–189.

96. Kane RL, Wales J, Bernstein L, Leibowitz A, Kaplan S. A randomised controlled trial of hospice care. *Lancet* 1984;(April 21):890–894.

97. Vinciguerra V, Degnan TJ, Sciortino A, et al. A comparitive assessment of home versus hospital comprehensive treatment for advanced cancer patients. *J Clin Oncol* 1986;4(10):1521–1528.

98. Ventafridda V, De CF, Vigano A, Ripamonti C, Gallucci M, Gamba A. Comparison of home and hospital care of advanced cancer patients. *Tumori* 1989;75(6):619–625.

99. Dunphy KP, Amesbury BDW. A comparison of hospice and homecare patients: patterns of referral, patient characteristics and predictors on place of death. *Pall Med* 1990;4:105–111.

100. Searle C. A comparison of hospice and conventional care. *Soc Sci Med* 1991;32(2):147–152.

101. Holland JC, Rowland J, Plumb M. Psychological aspects of anorexia in cancer patients. *Cancer Res* 1977;37(7):2425–2428.

102. Portenoy RK. Cancer pain. Epidemiology and syndromes. *Cancer* 1989;63(11):2298–2307.

103. Bonica JJ. Treatment of cancer pain: current status and future needs. In: Fields HL, Dubner R, Cervero F, eds. *Advances in pain research and therapy.* New York: Raven Press, 1985:589–616.

104. Stjernsward J, Teoh N. The scope of the cancer pain problem. In: Foley KM, Bonica JJ, Ventafridda V, eds. *Advances in pain research and therapy,* Vol 16. Second International Congress on Cancer Pain. New York: Raven Press, 1990:7–12.

105. Foley KM. The treatment of cancer pain. *N Engl J Med* 1985;313(2): 84–95.

106. VonRoenn JH, Cleeland CS, Gonin R, Hatfield AK, Pandya KJ. Physician attitudes and practice in cancer pain management: a survey from the Eastern Cooperative Oncology Group. *Ann Intern Med* 1993;119: 121–126.

107. Cleeland CS, Gonin R, Hatfield AK, et al. Pain and its treatment in outpatients with metastatic cancer. *N Engl J Med* 1994;330:592–596.

108. Larue F, Colleau SM, Brasseur L, Cleeland CS. Multicentre study of cancer pain and its treatment. *Br Med J* 1995;310:1034–1037.

109. Portenoy RK, Thaler HT, Kornblith AB, et al. The Memorial Symptom Assessment Scale: an instrument for the evaluation of symptom prevalence, characteristics and distress. *Eur J Cancer* 1994;30A: 1326–1336.

110. Cherny NI, Coyle N, Foley KM. Suffering in the advanced cancer patient: a definition and taxonomy. *J Pall Care* 1994;10(2):57–70.

111. Cohen SR, Mount BM. Quality of life in terminal illness: defining and measuring subjective well-being in the dying. *J Pall Care* 1992;8(3): 40–45.

112. Higginson I. Palliative care: a review of past changes and future trends. *J Public Health Med* 1993;15(1):3–8.

113. Doyle D, Hanks G, Macdonald N, eds. *Oxford textbook of palliative medicine.* Oxford: Oxford University Press, 1993.

114. Cherny NI, Portenoy RK. Practical issues in the management of cancer pain. In: Wall PD, Melzack R, eds. *Textbook of pain,* 3rd ed. Edinburgh: Churchill Livingstone, 1994:1437–1467.

115. Ajemian I. Palliative management of dyspnea. *J Pall Care* 1991;7(3): 44–45.

116. Lipowski ZJ. Update on delirium. *Psychiatr Clin North Am* 1992; 15(2):335–346.

117. Fainsinger RL, Tapper M, Bruera E. A perspective on the management of delirium in terminally ill patients on a palliative care unit. *J Pall Care* 1993;9(3):4–8.

118. Sateia MJ, Silberfarb PM. Sleep in palliative care. In: Doyle D, Hanks G, MacDonald N, eds. *Oxford textbook of palliative medicine.* Oxford: Oxford University Press, 1993:472–486.

119. Vortherms R, Ryan P, Ward S. Knowledge of, attitudes toward, and barriers to pharmacologic management of cancer pain in a statewide random sample of nurses. *Res Nurs Health* 1992;15(6):459–466.

120. Cherny NI, Ho MN, Bookbinder M, Fahey TJ, Portenoy RK, Foley KM. Cancer pain: Knowledge and attitudes of physicians at a cancer center. *Proc Am Soc Clin Oncol* 1994;12:434.

121. Mount B. A final crescendo of pain. *J Pall Care* 1990;6(3):5–6.

122. Roy DJ. Need they sleep before they die? *J Pall Care* 1990;6(3): 3–4.

123. Bruera E. Issues of symptom control in patients with advanced cancer. *Am J Hospice Care* 1993(2):12–18.

124. Cherny NI, Portenoy RK. Sedation in the management of refractory symptoms: guidelines for evaluation and treatment. *J Pall Care* 1994; 10(2):31–38.

*Principles and Practice of Supportive Oncology,*
edited by Ann Berger et al.
Lippincott–Raven Publishers, Philadelphia ©1998

# CHAPTER 55

# Bereavement Care

## J. William Worden

## DEFINITIONS

*Bereavement*: the situation of losing to death a person to whom one is attached.

*Mourning*: the process that one goes through adapting to such a loss.

*Grief*: the thoughts, feelings, and behaviors one experiences after the loss.

Bereavement care should be a part of any comprehensive palliative care program. The well-being of the family and those close to a dying or recently deceased person is part of the health professionals' responsibility. Health care providers and the institutions they serve must understand the impact of grief and be sensitive to the needs of the bereaved by offering both support and information (1). Included in the understanding of bereavement must be an awareness of the negative consequences that can accrue to survivors after a death. Bereavement is not in and of itself a pathologic event. Quite the contrary, it is a normal human experience. However, for some the stress of bereavement may lead to pathologic consequences, either physical or mental.

Bereavement may place some at risk for morbidity and mortality following a loss. There have been several investigations into the morbidity and mortality effects of bereavement, especially conjugal bereavement. The findings are mixed. To date, the evidence suggests that there may be a higher risk for mortality among men, especially those over the age of 75, but not for women. Remarriage seems to reduce the risk for men, but the reasons for this are not clear. It may be that only the fittest of men remarry (2). The first year following the death of a spouse seems to be the time when men are most at risk. Also during the first year of bereavement, there is an increased risk of suicide, especially among older widowers and single men who lose their mothers.

The evidence for increased incidents of morbidity in the bereaved presents a mixed picture. Additional studies need to be done. It is clear, however, that there is a substantial increase in the use of alcohol, tobacco, tranquilizers, and hypnotics among the bereaved, both men and women. Recently, investigators have looked at the stress of bereavement on various immune functions in an attempt to find such a relationship (3–5). These studies may help clarify possible relationships between some bereavement and morbidity.

In addition to issues of morbidity and mortality, there is the problem of complicated bereavement. Although most people make an adequate adjustment to bereavement, the adjustment becomes complicated in some, and they develop abnormal patterns of grief (6). Among the types of complicated bereavement are those that follow.

1. *Chronic grief* does not seem to end, and several years later the mourner has the sense of being stuck in the process. Although there is no timetable for mourning, it is the subjective sense of stuckness for the mourner that helps identify this phenomenon.

2. *Delayed grief* appears at the time of a later loss but is clearly linked to an earlier loss that was insufficiently mourned. Frequently this mourning is interrupted because the loss is negated or seems overwhelming to the person, or the grieving behavior is not socially supported by others in the mourner's life.

3. *Exaggerated grief* is present when a normal grief response is exaggerated to the point where the person becomes dysfunctional. For example, it is normal to experience dysphoria after a loss, but if this affect is exaggerated to the level of clinical depression, it becomes a type of exaggerated grief. Likewise, it is normal to feel anxious after a loss. If the anxiety rises to a clinical level, such as panic attack, phobia, or major anxiety disorder, this would also qualify as an exaggerated grief reaction. Dysfunctional experiences that arise in the course of bereavement often receive a *DSM-IV* diagnosis. Fre-

J. W. Worden: Laguna Niguel, CA 92677.

quently, however, there has not been a previous episode of the disorder, the patient sees a relationship of his or her affect and behavior to the loss, and after treatment the patient may never again experience such a disorder.

4. *Masked grief* is the fourth type of complicated bereavement. Grief that was absent at the time of the loss appears later under the guise of a psychiatric or medical symptom. When the unmourned loss is grieved, then the symptoms usually abate. Unlike exaggerated grief, wherein the mourner sees a relationship of the symptom to the loss, in masked grief the mourner does not see such a relationship.

## THE TASKS OF MOURNING

The clinician who is interested in working with the bereaved needs to understand the process of mourning. Mourning does not involve clear-cut stages but rather involves certain tasks that need to be accomplished (6). Outlined in Table 1, these tasks do not require a specific ordering, but if they are not accomplished, the bereavement has not reached a satisfactory conclusion.

The first task of mourning is *to accept the reality of the loss*. Even in the case of an expected death from cancer, when the family may have observed the declining physical condition of the patient, there is a certain sense of unreality when the news comes that the person has died. This sense of unreality is heightened many times over when the death is sudden or violent. Following a death, many survivors experience searching behavior, looking for the lost loved one, or they may misidentify people on the street and have to remind themselves that the person is dead and will not return, at least in this life.

Disbelief that the person is dead can range from a simple hope that one will wake up from a bad dream and that this couldn't be happening to a full-blown delusion that the person is not dead. Illustrating the middle of this continuum of disbelief is the mother whose daughter was killed in a house fire. Although she visited the cemetery every day to put flowers on her daughter's grave, she went around the house saying, "I won't have you dead; I won't have you dead." This went on for 2 years until she was helped to acknowledge the reality of the loss, that her daughter was not coming back, and her own need to let her go and say goodbye to her.

Another form of thwarting this first task of mourning is efforts at "mummification" that keep the room, clothes,

and other belongings of the deceased undisturbed with the hope that one day the loved one may return. For most, the searching behavior and hope for reunion are short-lived, and people accept the reality that the person is gone and will never again return as they once were.

The second task of mourning is *to experience the pain of the loss*. Most people do not like pain and attempt to cut short the pain of grief. Others around the mourner who are not comfortable with the pain may try to thwart this process. Nevertheless, if the pain is not felt it may return later, associated with another loss, or it will manifest itself as some kind of physical symptom or some form of aberrant behavior.

The negation of this second task of working through the pain is not to feel. People can short-circuit this task in any number of ways. Some try to stop their feelings and deny that the pain is present through substance abuse, removing reminders of the deceased, or moving to a different location. Others idealize the dead and only allow themselves pleasant feelings. Still others cut the pain by minimizing the relationship to the deceased: "He was not very important to me." Moving after a death may be a way to cure the pain geographically. British psychiatrist John Bowlby has said, "Sooner or later, some of those who avoid all conscious grieving break down—usually with some form of depression." (7) One of the aims of grief counseling is to facilitate this difficult second task so people don't carry the pain with them throughout their life.

*Adjusting to an environment where the deceased is missing* is the third task of mourning. Adjusting to the loss means different things to different people, depending on their relationship with the deceased and the various roles the deceased played. Widows and widowers may take time to realize all that they have lost when a spouse dies: friend, lover, bill-payer, gardener, bed-warmer, etc. The awareness of all that one has lost takes time, and this contributes to bereavement being a lengthy process. One widow said 6 months after the death of her husband, "If you had asked me before he died who was the social director in our family, I would have said we both were. Now I realize that he was the one who planned the weekend events and made the arrangements." This was not the biggest loss she had sustained, but it illustrates how awareness of losses continue to come to the fore months after a death. Some survivors resent having to develop new skills after a death and thwart this third task by not adapting to the loss. They withdraw from the world, assume a helpless posture, and refuse to face up to environmental requirements. They are held in a state of suspended growth in which they are prisoners to a dilemma they cannot solve. (7)

Adjustments can be categorized as external, internal, or spiritual. External adjustments refer to the more obvious changes such as living in an empty house, taking on the role of a single parent, learning to drive, paying bills. Internal adjustments deal with changes in one's sense of

**TABLE 1.** *Tasks of mourning*

Accept the reality of the loss
Experience the pain of the loss
Adjust to the environment in which the deceased is missing
Find a way to remember the deceased while moving
  forward with life

self. Bereavement can lead to intense regression wherein the bereaved perceive themselves as inadequate, helpless, or otherwise incapable of functioning. Along with this may come the sense of being unlovable. Bereavement not only means the loss of a significant other but can also mean the loss of a sense of self, when one's self-esteem and self-efficacy are severely challenged. Lieberman found in a 7-year study of widowed persons that a third of widows experienced some growth after the death and that this often included a revision of their self-image. Such persons tended to be those who felt that their own self was submerged in the marriage and who found a sense of liberation after the death. (8)

Spiritual adjustment has to do with one's sense of the world and how the death has challenged one's fundamental life values and philosophical beliefs—beliefs that are influenced by families, peers, education, and religion as well as life experiences. Sudden and violent deaths frequently call for these adjustments as they challenge one's sense of God, the predictability of the universe, and why bad things often happen to good people.

The fourth task of mourning involves *finding a place in one's life for the deceased so that one can remember and appropriately memorialize the person, yet relocating that person so that one can move forward with one's life.* If a person tries to keep the relationship with the deceased just as it was before the death, the person may become stuck and not move forward with his or her life without the deceased and be open to new relationships and activities. A survivor's readiness to enter new relationships depends not on "giving up" the dead spouse but on finding a suitable place for the spouse in the psychological life of the bereaved—a place that is important but that leaves room for others (9). This task also applies to bereaved parents. A mother whose daughter was killed in a tragic accident was focused for months on that event and her loss. It was her first thought on awakening every day. Then one day she was surprised when her daughter did not occupy her first waking thought. She then realized that her daughter was dead and was never coming back, even though she wanted that desperately. She also realized that she was alive and needed to move forward with her life. Finding a way to remember the deceased while moving forward with life is the focus of this fourth task of mourning.

This task approach to mourning can be very useful to the clinician. First, it provides the clinician with an understanding of the process and supplies a focus for the types of intervention that may facilitate the process. Second, it offers a way to understand what is happening in the case of complicated bereavement: where and how a person is stuck and ways to develop grief therapy strategies. Third, it offers the caregiver something to do for the bereaved that can help reduce the feelings of helplessness stimulated when the mourner wants from us the one thing we cannot give—namely, the dead person back.

## DETERMINANTS OF THE GRIEF RESPONSE

Although all persons who have sustained a loss by death need to accomplish the tasks of mourning, a wide range of behavior can be classified as normal grief. Not all people grieve the same way any more than all people die the same way. For some, grief is strong and overpowering; for others, it is a very mild experience. For some, grief begins upon hearing of a death; for others, it takes longer to begin to grieve. For some, grief is a very brief experience; for others, it goes on and on and never seems to come to an end.

It is important for the clinician to understand that grief, the personal experience of loss, is a multidetermined phenomenon. No single factor such as type of death (sudden vs. expected) can explain the variations in experience. An understanding of these factors can be useful to the clinician who is trying to identify in advance how someone might grieve in order to offer preventive mental health intervention to those most likely to adapt poorly to the loss. Table 2 contains what seem to be the most important determinants of a grief response (6).

The first determinant of a grief response is the *nature of the attachment.* The most intense and often most difficult grief responses occur (a) when the attachment between the bereaved and the deceased was very strong, (b) when the deceased was needed to support the survivor's sense of self-worth and self-esteem, (c) when the survivor was highly dependent upon the deceased, and/or (d) when the relationship was a highly ambivalent one.

The *mode of death* can and does influence the grief response. A sudden death may be more difficult to grieve than one with advance warning. The natural death of an older person may be easier to grieve than the accidental death of a young child or the suicidal death of a teenager. Geographical distance at the time of death, multiple losses, and uncertain losses can all increase the probability of a poor outcome.

*Historical antecedents* are also important. How one handled previous losses and how well they were resolved can play a role in current loss. Also, a history of clinical depression may portend a more difficult mourning period.

*Personality variables*, such as age, gender, tolerance for pain and anxiety, personality structure, and ability to express feelings, also contribute to variations in grieving.

*Social factors* constitute another determinant of a grief response. Each person belongs to various social subcul-

**TABLE 2.** *Determinants of a grief response (6)*

Nature of attachment
Mode of death
Historical antecedents
Personality variables
Social factors
Changes and concurrent stressors

tures, such as ethnic and religious groups, which provide him or her with guidelines and rituals for grieving behavior. Social support is also an important factor in mourning. Those who feel supported by family and friends find it easier to grieve than those who do not or those whose social environment actively suppresses the expression of grief.

A final determinant is the *number of changes and concurrent stressors* experienced by the family as the result of the death. In the Harvard Child Bereavement Study of bereaved families who had lost a parent to death, the strongest predictor of both the depression of the surviving parent and the functioning of the school-age children was the number of changes that the family experienced as the result of the death (10). Families who experience fewer concurrent stressors as the result of the death do better than families for whom stressors are many. Closely related to these family stressors are the family coping styles. Families who could engage in more active coping and who could redefine and reframe problems were less affected by these concurrent stresses than families that could not do this.

## INTERVENTION PRINCIPLES

Given the tasks of mourning and the determinants of grief, there are certain implications for a comprehensive program of palliative care through which the bereaved can be helped (Table 3).

First, recognize that both the dying patient and the family can and do grieve before a death. Being aware of this and helping the patient and family to understand this can help them to cope with the alienation that can occur when someone is dying.

Second, encourage families of the dying to say those things to each other that need to be said before the death. This can leave the survivor with less unfinished business to be dealt with after the death. Family members often need permission from the caregiver to do this. A sentence or two can go a long way to help the family members do what they inwardly want to do but may feel awkward doing.

**TABLE 3.** *Intervention principles*

Facilitate anticipatory grieving
Before death, encourage communication between patient and family
At the time of death, encourage and provide for family presence
After death, encourage reminiscing
Help people deal with all of their feelings
Normalize grief behaviors
Identify complicated bereavement and make referrals to a professional for grief therapy
Be aware of the special features of the bereavement over the loss of a child

Third, allow the family to be with the person as he or she is dying, and allow them to be with the body after the death. This can be very salutary in facilitating the first task of mourning—making the death real. There is nothing like the confrontation with the loved one's body to bring home the reality of the loss. A program that encourages this and makes provision for it can make an important contribution to bereavement.

Fourth, after the death, encourage conversations about the deceased. Nothing works better to bring home the reality of the loss than verbalizing about the deceased. The problem is that many families cut short this process because they don't want to hear about something they already know. An enlightened caregiver can encourage those who want and need to talk to do so. The mourner must first believe that the death happened before he or she can deal with the feelings that go with such a loss.

Fifth, help people deal with their feelings. Most do not have difficulty with sadness but many have difficulty with the anger, guilt, and anxiety that may follow a loss. Helping them to understand that a wide range of these feelings is normal and to find appropriate outlets for these feelings is all part of a comprehensive program of bereavement care.

Sixth, know what is normal grief behavior, and offer reassurance if family members are having experiences they have never had before and feel that they are going crazy. In our research and clinical experience we find that people seldom decompensate and go insane following a loss, but they feel they are going crazy because of the unfamiliarity of the experiences. If the clinician knows that hallucinations, distractedness, nocturnal orgasms, sleep disturbance, appetite loss, and other anomalous experiences are normal, the appropriate reassurance can be given.

Seventh, the clinician should also know the signs of a complicated bereavement and, if these occur, make referral to a professional for grief therapy. This listing of these signs and symptoms is too long for this report but can be found in detail in other places (6, 11).

Eighth, know that pediatric oncology presents its own special features. Parents who lose children are among those with the most difficult grief to bear. To lose a child is not only to lose someone out of season but also to experience special strains on the whole family system. Much has been written on this subject, and support groups are available for bereaved parents, such as those sponsored by the Society of Compassionate Friends. The concerned oncologist should be familiar with these resources.

## BEREAVEMENT SERVICES

There are several considerations in the establishment of bereavement services as part of a palliative care service. They include such questions as these: Who should be served? Who should do the counseling? When should counseling begin and for how long should it be continued? Where should this counseling be done? Let's look at these questions one by one.

*Who should be served?* There are basically three philosophies of grief counseling. The first is to offer such services to everyone who is bereaved. This, however, is not a cost-effective approach, and not everyone needs grief counseling. Many, if not most, will do very well on their own without the need for special intervention. A second and very common philosophy is to wait and see which people get into difficulty in their mourning and to offer intervention at that point. There is nothing wrong with this approach except that it requires a person to experience a high level of distress or poor coping before intervention is offered. A third approach is to screen individuals around the time of death to predict who among them will not be doing well a year or two later. Preventive mental health counseling can be offered to those who are predicted to be at risk to preclude later negative sequelae. This type of approach makes sense when valid predictors and risk factors have been identified and there is a high level of reliability in a set of predictors. Parkes and others have identified such risk predictors for conjugal bereavement, and Worden and Silverman have developed a screening instrument for high-risk children who have lost a parent to death (12,13,10).

The question of who should be counseled raises the issue of unit of care. Who in a family should be given counseling?. When a spouse has died, the surviving spouse may prefer to be seen alone without other family members. When children die, the parents may prefer to be seen together. I prefer to have at least one session with the entire nuclear family, do an assessment of need, and make intervention referrals at that point.

*Who should do the counseling?* There are several possibilities. One involves a trained professional, such as a social worker, nurse clinician, psychologist, chaplain, or other mental health professional. The advantage here is the obvious training and experience of such personnel. Another possibility is the use of trained volunteers to intervene with or befriend the bereaved. Sometimes these volunteers have been bereaved themselves in the past and use their own experience to try and be helpful. Many hospice programs and groups like the Society of Compassionate Friends use this type of volunteer. A third possibility is the use of nonprofessional volunteers with professional backup. Decisions regarding personnel need to fit the particular organization that is offering counseling, but the emphasis clearly needs to be on trained individuals.

*When should counseling begin?* There is a general consensus that the best time to start is between 3 and 8 weeks after the event (12). Earlier than that, the bereaved may be very involved with family, and the reality of the loss may

not have set in. After 8 weeks, some will have sealed off their feelings and be hesitant to start the process all over again. For most bereaved individuals, 2 to 3 months after the death the reality of the loss and its consequences is setting in, pain is at a high point, and support that may have been there at the time of the funeral may be waning.

*How long should counseling for individuals and families continue?* There is no general agreement on this point. In the United States, hospice care programs usually follow up family members in one way or another for a year following the death. Such followup may be by phone, by letter, or by personal visit. This 1-year time frame was informally established and is not necessarily based on research. In fact, research shows that for some bereaved, the most difficult time and possibility for developing poor adjustment occurs in the second year of bereavement. This argues for the need of a good screening instrument to predict the individuals who are at most risk in the second year of bereavement.

*Where should counseling take place?* Some bereaved are hesitant to return for help to a hospital, a hospice, or the place where the loved one died. This is especially true in the early months after a loss. Many people feel most comfortable in their own homes, and this may be the best place to see them in the early weeks after a loss. Some bereaved prefer to talk to someone on the telephone because of the anonymity, but face-to-face contact is usually preferable so that nonverbal communication can be assessed and used in the intervention. Later on it can be useful for the bereaved person to return to the place of death as a point of reality for that loss.

Groups for bereaved individuals can be very effective in facilitating the grief process. In a well-run group, mourners can find others who have experienced similar losses and gain support from such individuals. Knowing that they are not alone in their loss, and knowing that others in the group will not be pushing them to finish their grieving, can be helpful to most people. However, not everyone wants to attend a bereavement group, and women are more frequent attenders than men. Men are more likely to attend a group whose aim is education about the grief experience or one whose aim is addressing specific problems such as how to be an effective single parent.

## CONCLUSION

Bereavement is one of life's greatest stresses and an experience from which none of us can escape. The clinician who learns from his or her own experience of loss can use this understanding to fashion interventions that can be helpful to the bereaved. Knowing what was and was not helpful to us in our time of need can direct us in making interventions, both verbal and programmatic, that will be healing to the families in our care.

# REFERENCES

1. Osterweis M, Solomon F, Green M, eds. *Bereavement*. Washington, DC: National Academy of Medicine, 1984.
2. Stroebe MS, Stroebe W, Gergen KJ. The broken heart: reality or myth? *Omega* 1982;87:12.
3. Irwin M, et al. Immune and neuroendricrine changes during bereavement. *Psychiatr Clin North Am* 1987;449:10.
4. Jacobs SC, et al. Urinary free cortisol and separation anxiety early in the course of bereavement and threatened loss. *Biol Psychiatry* 1987;448:22.
5. Schlifer SJ, Keller SE. Conjugal bereavement and immunity. *Israel J Psychiatry Relat Issues* 1987;111:24.
6. Worden JW. *Grief counseling and grief therapy*, 2nd ed. New York: Springer, 1991.
7. Bowlby J. *Attachment and loss*, vol 3. New York: Basic Books, 1980:158.
8. Lieberman M. *Doors close, doors open: widows, grieving and growing*. New York: Putnam, 1996.
9. Shuchter S, Zisook S. Treatment of spousal bereavement. *Psychiatr Ann* 1986;295:16.
10. Worden JW. *Children and grief: when a parent dies*. New York: Guilford, 1996.
11. Rando T. *Treatment of complicated mourning*. Champaign, IL: Research Press, 1993.
12. Parkes CM, Weiss RS. *Recovery from bereavement*. New York: Basic Books, 1983.
13. Raphael B. *The anatomy of bereavement*. New York: Basic Books, 1983.

*Principles and Practice of Supportive Oncology,*
edited by Ann Berger et al.
Lippincott–Raven Publishers, Philadelphia ©1998

CHAPTER 56

# Patient-Physician Communication in the Cancer Setting

Edward T. Creagan

## THE IMPORTANCE OF COMMUNICATION

Attitudes toward a malignant disease are largely shaped by social and cultural values (1,2). Although it is dangerous to generalize, the American culture is characterized by an emphasis on health, wealth, youth, and prominence. These characteristics evolved over several centuries and were typified by the pioneer-frontier spirit, which enable the early settlers to clearly change the face of North America and have an enormous impact on environmental, military, and economic forces. Physicians must recognize that when patients receive a diagnosis of cancer, these characteristics, among others, are clearly jeopardized and must become redefined and refocused by the patient. Another impact of a diagnosis of cancer is the difficulty in facing decisions. Retirement plans, vacation activities, the thought of building a new house, and so on are thrown into a chaotic state. Patients may become overwhelmed not only with the medical aspects of their predicament but also with far-reaching financial, insurance, and legal entanglements.

A primary responsibility of the physician in dealing with any patient is to impart factual, reasonable, and appropriate information so that the patient is appropriately informed and enabled to make reasonable decisions relative to lifestyle changes and treatment decisions. If the patient has a relatively mild and self-limited illness, such as a typical viral upper respiratory infection, communication between the patient and the physician will rarely have far-reaching implications. However, in dealing with a diagnosis of cancer, which may have fatal implications for the patient, communication becomes crucial. Only as a result of a thoughtful, thorough, and in-depth discussion can a patient be prepared to make lifestyle changes and to participate in decisions about treatment options.

Moreover, the diagnosis of cancer has far-reaching emotional implications for every patient. Most patients equate this diagnosis with death; disfigurement; a writhing, anguished terminal phase; loss of bodily functions; and loss of dignity and self-respect. It is fairly common in general oncology practice that once the term *cancer* is used, patients become psychologically overburdened and are unable to absorb the salient features of the discussion. Accordingly, physicians must be sensitive to this issue and recognize that small doses of information over a longer time impart information to patients much more effectively than a 1- or 2-hour discussion.

## PRACTICAL ISSUES

### Information

It is crucial, in discussing the implications of a malignant disease with a patient and family, to convey an atmosphere of professionalism and confidence. An important aspect of this phenomenon is to be absolutely certain about the technical, physiological, and anatomical details of the diagnosis. It is pointless to go into an in-depth discussion during the perioperative period when a patient is in pain and when the emotional atmosphere of the hospital room is psychically charged. When the patient is somewhat more comfortable, a review of the situation is then appropriate. In a case of breast cancer, for example, it is important that the clinician be aware of the size of the cancer, the number of involved lymph nodes, whether or not the disease extended beyond the nodes, and whether or not the disease was fully resected. Information about the estrogen and progesterone receptor

E. T. Creagan: Division of Medical Oncology, Mayo Medical School, Department of Medical Oncology, The Mayo Clinic, Rochester, MN 55905.

titers and morphologic characteristics of the cancer are important to appropriately impart to the patient (3,4).

Some individuals have a nearly insatiable need to have minute details of the problem reviewed with them. Other patients are somewhat less interested in the details, but the clinician should not be blindsided and must be aware that this is a perilous time. Likewise, many patients cannot be expected to understand the technical nuances of surgery. Surgeons may tell the patient and family that they "removed all the cancer that we could see." Some patients may interpret this as a gross total resection, whereas others may understand that there is a real possibility of either gross or microscopic residual disease. This issue is important in the approach to the bedside, and the clinician must know whether indeed there was residual disease. If the operative report and pathology review are unclear on this issue, a phone call to the surgeon is appropriate. It is sometimes helpful to physically read the operative report and pathology review as well as pertinent diagnostic studies at the bedside to reinforce the seriousness of the situation. Many patients are comforted in hearing the names of the radiologist, pathologist, and surgical team as an added reassurance that more than one individual has been involved in this difficult process.

If at all possible, friends or family members should be at the bedside during these informative discussions if this is the patient's wish. This approach can avoid much misinformation, since all concerned parties are hearing the same message. A delicate issue that sometimes arises is taping the physician's comments. If the physician is conscientious, thoughtful, and thorough, and is aware that he or she is being taped, this procedure should not cause undue distress. However, one must be especially discreet and recognize that the comments at the bedside may receive a completely different interpretation months or years later, once the acute emotional distress has subsided. The clinician must be especially mindful of flippant or uncomplimentary comments about other members of the health care team or other institutions, but not gloss over or minimize any egregious deviations in the standard of care. It is always important to emphasize that the initial signs and symptoms of a malignant process are vague, nondescript, and nonspecific, and only retrospectively would one make a diagnosis of cancer. One must be especially careful about "shooting from the hip" in these circumstances and recognize that some members of the family might have litigious inclinations. Previously estranged members of the family may be provoked into seeking legal redress, perhaps motivated by guilt or other nonaltruistic incentives.

## Location

If discussions relative to a serious cancer problem take place in the clinic, some guidelines are helpful. If the patient is new to the clinician, the use of a professional card helps the transition. It is very difficult for patients and family members to remember names, especially during a highly stressful situation. A firm handshake with the patient is most appropriate and sets that stage for a professional bonding between the physician and the patient. An awkward situation arises when there are multiple family members accompanying the patient—to shake the hands of every family member is similar to the ritual at the start of a football game. To shake the hand of the patient and acknowledge the other family members is a reasonable way of handling this situation.

Each physician has his or her own style in addressing patients at this time. To emphasize the importance of the patient, it is probably best that the patient sit near or closest to the physician, who is usually at a desk. If there are multiple family members between the physician and the patient, eye contact is clumsy and awkward. The answering of the telephone or the answering of pages or beepers during difficult discussions can completely erode the sacredness of the moment, especially since the physician may be called about a personal or relatively trivial issue. Turning off of the beeper or pager for a limited time signals to the patient that their time is important.

If it is apparent either in the hospital or in the clinic that the patient is in distress from pain, nausea, or other symptoms, it is pointless to launch into a detailed discussion about diagnosis, prognosis, and treatment options. In this situation, a few generic comments about the situation are most appropriate; they can then be expanded at a followup appointment. This obviously represents some administrative and scheduling issues. Likewise, if construction noises or other interruptions make meaningful dialogue impossible, scheduling a followup appointment is a humane and reasonable gesture.

## Physical Setting

The environment can have an enormous impact on the way patients absorb information about a diagnosis of a malignant disease. Some general guidelines are appropriate and sensible but are often overlooked.

In the hospital setting, if the physician does not know the patient or is being asked to consult with the patient for the first time, it is most appropriate that a professional card be given to the patient and the family. These are emotionally charged issues, and it is very difficult for patients to remember who the "cancer doctor" is, especially in an integrated multispecialty hospital practice, which is most typical in larger communities. If at all possible, the physician should sit down, since this is perceived by patients and families as showing more concern than when the physician stands. Obviously, this is not always physically possible. If there is another patient in the room, the curtain should be drawn to at least provide a semblance of privacy, in full recognition that this is clearly an artificial technique. The television, radio, CD player, and so on should be turned off so that attention is not diluted by other distractions. Patients should be asked whether there are other family members who are near by who should be participating in these discussions. It is most appropriate to close the door to the room and, if at all possible, avoid interruptions by custodial, culinary, security, and other support personnel. It is enormously distracting to be in the midst of a delicate discussion only to be interrupted by someone attempting to change a light bulb. The flushing of a toilet or the blaring of a "boom box" hardly provides a professional environment for dealing with some very difficult issues. The physician must be discreet and sensitive in these discussions and must recognize that his or her comments are being overheard by the other patient in the room and by family members of that patient. With the evolution of private rooms in most hospitals, these issues will become less crucial.

## SOCIAL AND CULTURAL ISSUES IN PATIENTS WITH ADVANCED MALIGNANT DISEASE

To a very real extent, physicians be sensitive to history, social issues, and anthropology in dealing with the patient with malignant disease. The typical American patient assumes a proactive posture and enters into a participatory relationship with the treating and responsible physician (5,6). This entails a complete disclosure about diagnosis, prognosis, and treatment options with particular attention to pros, cons, risks, options, expectations, and impact on quality of life. However, in other cultures, the situation is quite different. Some Latino, Chinese, African-American, and Native American communities view the family in a very generic and extended context. Illnesses affect not only the individual but also the clan or family as a group. Therefore, decisions relative to treatment must be filtered through family representatives. In the American judicial bioethical system, patients cannot make informed decisions relative to investigational programs or even conventional programs without this sort of background. However, health professionals must be sensitive that cultural issues have a profound impact in dealing with the patient with malignant disease. In many parts of the world—for example, Japan, some Mediterranean countries, and some South American countries—the diagnosis of cancer carries social implications similar to those of aquired immune deficiency disorder. Cancer is viewed as a death sentence, and patients interpret this diagnosis as the start of a downward spiral characterized by pain, disability, and total social isolation.

In many cultures, the terminology of cancer is anathema and must be avoided at all costs. This issue will become especially germane when the physician is dealing with the patient and family through interpreters and when using the word *cancer*. We must be respectful of the wishes of the patient and the family and avoid using terms that might strip the patients of hope. A difficult issue arises when potentially toxic treatments or surgical procedures with potentially high morbidity are recommended. There are few guidelines in this area, and one must proceed with tact and discretion. One approach is to carefully explain to a family representative the implications of the current situation and to stress to the patient that there are options and alternatives. If the word *cancer* is offensive in the patient's particular culture, it is certainly appropriate not to use that word but perhaps to substitute for it some other implication of a serious problem so as not to withdraw all hope from the patient (7).

Americans have typically focused on the family as the nuclear extension of society, and multigenerational families are increasingly rare. Grandparents and elderly aunts and uncles rarely live in the same home as their adult children, so decisions are typically made by the patients themselves, occasionally with a little input from other members of the family.

The disclosure of medical information to patients and families also must be approached in a delicate manner. Some individuals, especially upper–middle-class Americans from urban environments, demand an in-depth review of all pertinent aspects of their illness and potential treatments. In some cultures, this approach would have a devastating impact on the emotional well-being of the patient. It is the physician's responsibility to cooperate with the patient and the family within appropriate cultural guidelines while being sensitive to the patient's need to make informed decisions. Physicians will be far more effective in ministering to the patient and the family when they are sensitive to cultural issues.

### Practical Suggestions

A reasonable approach to ascertaining how much information the patient desires is to simply ask the patient, "What do you understand about the current situation?" This open-ended question provides an opportunity for the physician to develop an understanding of what the patient knows about the current oncologic situation. Most reasonable physicians can then sense whether the individual would like more information about diagnosis, treatment, and prognosis or whether he or she is comfortable with the current state of knowledge. An offer to share with the patient and family, if appropriate, the results of computed tomography, bone scans, magnetic resonance imaging, and other technical information is often helpful to clarify the extent of the disease process and the implications of the metastatic site. A magnetic resonance scan showing intracranial metastases can be shown to the patient and family, and this can be an effective technique to impress on them the seriousness of the problem. On the other hand, some patients become anxious when they see these images, so one obviously must be sensitive to the needs of patient and family.

Another challenging scenario is that of the patient from a non-American culture in which full disclosure of a serious oncologic situation is a cultural taboo. It is insensitive and inappropriate for the traditional health care provider to launch into an extensive discussion with the patient if this is inconsistent with cultural mores. In such situations, it is often helpful to discuss the situation with a responsible family member and determine from that person exactly how this type of situation should be handled. In some cultures, if patients are informed of a diagnosis of cancer, they may give up and have an accelerated downward clinical spiral. This most unfortunate situation can be avoided by ascertaining from responsible family members how these types of problems are traditionally handled. Admittedly, this is a time-consuming process, but great ill will is generated when one tries to circumvent cultural issues that have been firmly entrenched for centuries and generations.

## SPECIFIC COMMUNICATION TOPICS

### New Cancer Diagnosis

The physician must be mindful that the diagnosis of a malignant disease is one of the most significant events in the life of any individual (8–10). Patients must be allowed the time to verbalize their concerns, and physicians must be aware of their need to tell the story. Even though the clinician has the medical record at hand, patients need, in most circumstances, to recite the minute clinical details leading up to the diagnosis. Patients may be bewildered, and physicians must recognize that there are no shortcuts to outlining the diagnosis, prognosis, and treatment options. Scheduling should be flexible so that there is not a major professional or educational commitment that would interfere with the thoughtful and compassionate review of all pertinent details of the patient s case. Under these circumstances, it is most appropriate that some other responsible family member be with the patient, since the patient's ability to retrieve facts in this environment is marginal. It is the unusual patient who is able to grasp the enormity of the problem in one visit, and administrative channels should be available so that several consultations over a period of time are provided for the patient.

An often neglected dimension of this encounter is the issue of fatigue in the patient, the family, and the physician. An in-depth discussion of probabilities, percentages, and anticipated clinical course late on a Friday afternoon is hardly an ideal situation. In a perfect world, tests, consultations, and reviews are best organized early in the day, but obviously this is not always possible.

### Progressive Disease

From clinical experience, many patients have asserted that a recurrence is even more devastating than the initial diagnosis of a neoplasm. Even though most patients do understand the very high risk of recurrence, based on the clinical situation, when that event does occur, it can have dire implications for patient and family. Hopes are dashed, plans for the future are unraveled, and feelings of helplessness are common. The patient's situation is usually more complex if adjuvant chemotherapy has been recommended or if the patient has progressed through a first-line systemic therapy. This is a time for great tact and diplomacy on the part of the physician. Regardless of the circumstances, there are always symptomatic and supportive interventions, and patients must be aware that palliative care rather than aggressive, toxic, and unproven therapies is always a sensible option. Some family members may be uncomfortable with supportive care, whereas some patients are very much at peace with that recommendation.

Time has become the currency of contemporary clinical practice. If the physician suspects recurrence or metastasis, the patients so affected cannot be squeezed in at odd hours or between regularly scheduled patients. The time-consuming discussions likely to be necessary cannot be short-circuited. Another interesting dimension of this phenomenon is the sophistication of many patients with recurrent disease, in view of the proliferation of patient-centered computerized information via Web sites and Internet access. It is increasingly common that patients will come to the office with printouts of investigational programs, articles from newspapers and magazines, and well-meaning recommendations from friends and family members concerning complimentary therapies. These issues must be compassionately addressed, reviewed, and not dismissed. This is often a time of great desperation.

Many patients find comfort at the thought of referral to a cancer center or a tertiary care facility. Sometimes the input of the physician's colleague at the same clinic is reassuring to patients. It is sensible to tell patients that it is highly unlikely that a particular institution has a truly innovative therapy for their condition, because of the explosion in information technology. Should patients opt to go away for therapy, it is reasonable to explain to patients the implications of this, yet state the willingness of the physician to assume care when the patient returns home. Some patients are embarrassed about seeking complimentary or alternative therapies, and this issue should be openly addressed.

### Experimental Programs

Another dimension of the oncologist's responsibility to the cancer patient and family is the discussion of investigational therapies. These are situations where, by definition, there is no standard therapy for the patient's particular situation. Although several standard regimens may have been described in the literature, there is typically a consensus among oncologists that the current state of management is unsatisfactory and that one reasonable option is to enroll patients in prospective clinical trials.

A phase I trial involves an agent or a program for which there has been only limited clinical experience and most of the data relative to toxicity have been derived from animal tumor models. Although the goal of all therapeutic programs is to induce an objective tumor regression, patients must understand that this is not the goal of a phase I study. The focus of these programs is to obtain information relative to treatment toxicities. This point is sometimes glossed over when patients participate in these programs. The probability of an objective tumor response is vanishingly low, and this point—from a moral, ethical, and professional perspective—must be underscored with the patient and family. Many of these programs require elaborate pharmacologic testings and may require hospitalization, and these inconveniences may enhance the morbidity of the program.

A phase II study implies that there is a modicum of antitumor properties and the agent is being targeted for a specific tumor type. Patients must understand that in this setting there are always conventional alternatives and options, but these programs have not consistently been effective. A discussion of these programs by an overzealous oncologist can certainly sway the patient to either participate or decline participation. This raises the issue of the informed consent document. How should it be reviewed with the patient? One approach is to "walk through" the informed consent document with the patient and family. There may be an element of coercion in this approach, so an alternative is to allow the patient and family to review the document at their leisure. Since there is virtually never any emergency about a patient's participation, to allow the patient and family to review the document thoughtfully over a period of time is reasonable. Patients must understand that if they do decline to participate, conventional therapy and routine surveillance will still be offered to them.

A phase III trial implies a comparison of a relatively standard program with an investigational therapy. These trials may present a real conundrum to the patient and physician. The dilemma becomes even more difficult when a comparison is made between routine followup and potentially morbid intervention such as chemotherapy, surgery, or combinations thereof. It is very difficult to explain these trials to patients, especially when there is a tremendous divergence of therapeutic options. Cancer of the prostate is a case in point. Some trials may advocate observation in contrast to a treatment arm consisting of high-dose radiation therapy, which is obviously associated with some morbidity and inconvenience. The oncol-

ogist quite frequently is asked the question, "Doctor, what would you do if you were me?" This is a very difficult situation. One approach is to explain to the patient that each of us is different, and our willingness to participate reflects long-standing traditional values and methods of dealing with adversity. The oncologist cannot put himself or herself in the patient's position but is responsible for mapping out as objectively as possible the nuances of the program and assuring the patient that whatever the decision, the patient will be cared for and evaluated at periodic intervals.

### Acknowledging a Spiritual Dimension

Physicians must be aware of important historical developments in the way that illness is perceived (11). In the ancient cultures of Egypt and related peoples, all medical practitioners were priests. There was very little understanding about the biology of illness, so spiritual and magical forces were invoked to explain human illness.

With the emergence of Christianity, virtually all medical practitioners came from the ranks of the clergy; in fact, in the Middle Ages, ecclesiastical permission was required for individuals to practice medicine. The pendulum clearly shifted during the 1700s and 1800s, when medicine became more firmly based in sound biochemical and microbiological principles. These were used to explain virtually all human illnesses. However, the pendulum again shifted in the 1920s with the emergence of psychiatry and the writings of Sigmund Freud. These programs emphasized the impact of emotional issues on physical wellness.

The contemporary review of illness represents a composite, so that there is general acceptance of the biopsychosocial-spiritual model as a framework for human illness. It is becoming apparent that if each of these environments is not somehow addressed and reconciled, there will be major impediments to healing. The most technically superb anticancer program involving radiation therapy, infusional chemotherapy, and immune-related interventions has a very low likelihood of assisting the individual with a broken spirit or who has no form of psychosocial support. In this context, spirituality should be an integral aspect of communicating with the cancer patient.

Spirituality is a dimension, a capacity of our humanity by which we seek comfort, solace, and explanations for events that otherwise are without meaning or purpose. Spirituality can be viewed as a vehicle for providing order and reason out of chaotic and usually tragic events, such as a diagnosis of a malignant disease. A sensitivity and an understanding of this dimension can be of immeasurable help for the physician dealing with the cancer patient. Some aspects of this phenomenon may include the evaluation of the following:

1. The patient's sense of purpose and meaning in life.
2. Feelings of hope and views of the future.
3. The ability to believe in and draw strength from a higher power or from a transcendent process over and above the patient.

If physicians are not aware of these concepts, it may be very difficult, if not impossible, to meaningfully interpret patients' behaviors and to minister to them, not only from an emotional but from a physical perspective.

It is sometimes awkward and clumsy to specifically ask patients about their spirituality, but this issue can be addressed in a much more tactful manner. As part of a medical interview, it is important that the physician understand the patient's socioeconomic status and professional background. In the same context, an inquiry about the patient's church affiliation is a very nonconfrontational way to open up discussions on spirituality. Most patients are comforted in knowing that the physician is sensitive to these issues even though their belief systems may be quite different and unique.

### Uniquely Challenging Situations: The Doctor as Patient and the VIP

Although it is unlikely that one will be called upon to care for internationally prominent celebrities, it is certainly quite common that one may be responsible for high-profile individuals from the community (12). The well-connected patient, whether from the professional, political, or corporate world, presents some unique issues in communication, especially when the diagnosis is one of malignant disease. While it is certainly true that routine care is the best care, it would be professionally naive to ignore the stature of some patients whom we are called to see in consultation or as primary patients. These patients can be particularly challenging because, by virtue of their position, they have usually called the shots to attain their status and may be particularly demanding and inquisitive when asked to undergo diagnostic procedures that are sometimes unpleasant or frankly of high risk. These patients may require more of the physician's time, and schedules should be appropriately adjusted. Greater degrees of explanation may be required to assuage the anxiety of these patients and to enlist their cooperation or gain their confidence.

On one end of the spectrum in dealing with these patients is the attempt to alter diagnostic routines for the sake of convenience. Occasionally, the assessments of these individuals are streamlined so that usual and customary procedures are bypassed. This is a perilous approach and may, in the long run, subject the patient to more intrusions. The primary oncologist may be seduced into seeking "curbside consultations" from colleagues who do not actually see the patient. Obviously, this is not an ideal way to address complex situations. The other alternative, which sometimes occurs, is the pursuit of every trivial abnormality, either on x-rays or in laboratory studies, to provide the appearance of thoroughness and completeness. This approach may result in needless ancillary studies, the risks of morbidity, and a protracted clinical course in the hospital. The seeking of multiple consultations from subspecialists may open up a Pandora's box of diagnostic pursuits that may be completely unwarranted and needlessly heighten the angst of the patient and family.

An important dimension of dealing with the "celebrity" is to be certain that all appropriate individuals are aware of the patient's situation, if indeed this is the wish of the patient. These individuals often are accompanied by an entourage of physicians, and it is important to inform everyone about the patient's situation, if this is agreeable to the patient. It is quite customary that the high-profile individual will be bombarded with all sorts of medical recommendations and will be given the name of the medical guru for his or her particular problem. The responsible oncologist must be patient and sensitive, and allow time for these inquiries to be addressed. Although there is no biological distinction between a pope, a president, and a pipe-fitter, the physician needs to be sensitive and aware of the issues that each of these patients bring to the bedside.

A somewhat unique situation involves the doctor as patient. These individuals may be especially challenging, since it is virtually universal for physicians to tend to treat themselves, obtain informal consultations from colleagues, and not receive objective medical opinions. Many physicians will elicit the input from several colleagues until they hear the diagnosis and treatment that fits their biases. The interpretation of a physician's physical symptoms cannot ignore the high frequency of alcoholism, drug abuse, emotional issues, and cirrhosis that appear in some studies to be somewhat higher among physicians than in the general population.

Although it is difficult to present a cookbook or recipe for the handling the physician-patient, the following observations may be of help:

1. Do not assume that the patient-physician is conversant with the specific aspects of his or her illness. The cardiologist may have very little understanding of oncologic issues, and the gastroenterologist may have had no formal exposure to the nuances of chemotherapy and radiation therapy.
2. The responsible treating physicians must make every effort to ensure that the patient understands the situation and the implications of various diagnostic and therapeutic interventions.
3. The treating physician must accept that well-meaning colleagues will be most willing to share their advice and recommendations quite freely, often to the detriment and confusion of the patient. These suggestions must be

tactfully dealt with and accepted as genuine attempts to help. As with the VIP or the CEO, the requesting of consultations, when appropriate, may be a source of comfort to the patient, but there must be discretion so as to avoid an endless parade of specialist physicians who have a very narrow focus on the patient's problem.

4. The responsible treating physician must be wary of placing unnecessary burdens on patient-physicians by assuming that they are capable of outlining their own therapy.

5. The treating physician should clearly take the initiative in suggesting treatment options and also followup recommendations.

### Sharing a Dire Diagnosis or Prognosis over the Telephone

This awkward situation commonly arises in routine clinical practice. Several guidelines may make this difficult responsibility somewhat less burdensome.

1. Know to whom you are speaking. With complex and sometimes bewildering domestic arrangements in relationships, it is important for the physician to clearly identify with whom he or she is speaking and how that individual is related to the family.

2. A careful, deliberate, and slow introduction is most important. This is especially crucial if the phone call is late at night and the family is not expecting a dramatic downturn in the patient's condition. It is important to speak slowly so that all concerned parties are aware of who is "in the loop." It is also appropriate to offer a "warning shot" so that the caller is psychologically prepared for what may follow. An example might be as follows, "Good evening, my name is Dr. Smith; I am one of the cancer doctors who has been caring for Mr. Jones at the hospital. Although he had been doing well, there have been some complicated developments which have recently emerged, and I wanted to share some concerns with you." If the patient is still alive, it is important to say so and, if appropriate, to encourage the family to come to the clinic or the hospital. If the family member is alone, it is most sensible to offer to contact a friend, neighbor, clergyman, police officer, or some individual so that the individual does not remain alone. Under most circumstances that person should not attempt to drive to the hospital alone.

A delicate and awkward situation often arises when a patient has expired unexpectedly in the hospital and the family is at some distance away. It is sensible to inform the family if indeed the patient has died. It seems deceitful to have the family return to the hospital when the physician knows the individual has died. Offer to meet the family and explain the circumstances to them fully, recognizing that at this emotionally charged time, it is very difficult to have a meaningful dialogue.

## COMMUNICATING END-OF-LIFE ISSUES

### The "Big Questions" and How to Deal With Them

#### *"Doctor, how long do I have?"*

This question is implied in virtually all encounters with the medical oncologist or the practitioner in the first meetings with a patient newly diagnosed of malignant disease. This is a particularly perilous situation, since every comment of the physician will be carefully analyzed, dissected, and reinterpreted by the patient and the family. It is probably best to avoid making a specific estimate of time, since physicians are notoriously inaccurate in estimating survival. However, there is clearly a responsibility to provide some general guidelines. One approach is to inform the patient of some general parameters of survival. For example, among patients with metastatic nonsmall-cell lung cancer, the median survival is approximately 8 to 10 months. A small proportion of patients will succumb in a shorter time, whereas some will live longer. It would be reasonable to rephrase the patient's inquiry somewhat like this: "We do not have the technology to precisely estimate how long any one patient will live. However, among groups of patients in your particular situation, most will have significant problems and some may die within 8 to 10 months. However, let me clearly emphasize that this is a general and generic figure, and in any one patient we cannot estimate survival." This point should be carefully reemphasized so that there is no misinterpretation. It is typical that a patient will say, "my doctor gave me 3 months to live," and one has to be watchful for that problem.

As patients continue to deteriorate clinically, physicians can be somewhat more accurate in predicting ultimate survival. It is especially important not to mislead the family members. A declining performance score concomitant with apnea, unarousability, and worsening liver parameters usually portends a survival of days or weeks at the most. If this time frame is not made clear to family members, they may assume that survival is in terms of months and may defer or delay the appropriate work of closure. Physicians should take this opportunity to compassionately emphasize to the family that the end is near and that they should not wait to attend to issues of reconciliation, forgiveness, and reconnectedness. "If only we had known" is a very difficult burden for families to carry, and it is our responsibility, within reason, to inform them of the significance of clinical developments.

#### *"Doc, what will it be like?"*

This is obviously an open-ended question and an attempt by patients to express fears and concerns. The question may be rephrased by asking patients what specifically they are concerned about. Their issues and their fears may be quite different from what the physician believes. Perhaps a patient is fearful of not reconnecting with family members or of not completing some specific task, and not especially concerned about physical well-being.

### "Doc, am I terminal?"

The term *terminal* has dire and negative implications for the vast majority of individuals. It implies giving up, letting go, and a sense of isolation and abandonment. By asking patients what they mean by "terminal," physicians may become enlightened about the real issues.

### "Doctor, what exactly happens when I start to die?"

This question or a variant of it is very common in clinical practice. It is reasonable to explain to patients the anticipated natural history of a given condition, but with the clear understanding that each patient is unique and that there are techniques and programs available to control the vast majority of symptoms. Directly, many patients are concerned about pain, which is usually manageable in most circumstances.

### Advance Directives

Physicians and caregivers involved in the management of patients with advanced malignant disease must be cognizant of the medical-legal implications of this unique aspect of medical care. Some general guidelines will hopefully avoid unnecessary anxiety in dealing with complex and emotionally charged issues.

1. Each state has a variation of the patient self-determination act, which specifies the importance of advanced directives and the patient's assignment of durable power of attorney. As a general guideline, these issues should be addressed early in the patient's hospital stay, in writing, and with clear documentation of who was present and when these discussions were held.

2. Enlist a participatory relationship with several family members early during the patient's hospital stay. The 11th hour, the time of a crisis, or when family members are not physically present, is hardly the ideal time to embark upon a meaningful dialogue on issues of resuscitation and intubation.

3. Enlist the support and cooperation of each member of the medical team. Be certain that each health care provider, whether a physician, nurse, or allied health professional, has a voice in the patient's management. It is perilous to ignore the suggestions and comments of colleagues dealing with the terminally ill.

4. Be certain to have medical and legal procedures firmly in place before a crisis intervenes. If upon admission it is anticipated that the patient may have a complex or contentious relationship with some family members, it is important to be aware of these issues "up front" rather than at 3:00 in the morning.

5. Do not hesitate to obtain consultations with medical and legal services if it appears that the primary care team is not satisfying the needs of the patient and the family.

### Resuscitation: Practical Clinical Suggestions

There is now a clear legal mandate that patients be aware of resuscitative philosophy. If the patient's condition is clinically stable, this type of discussion can be reserved until after the history and physical examination have been performed and appropriate plans have been outlined to the patient and family. It is important to keep in mind the implications of resuscitation in the patient with advanced malignant disease. Many patients have a naive view of cardiac arrest from the media and do not recognize that the vast majority of patients who experience cardiac arrest in a hospital setting either do not leave the hospital or suffer significant neurologic impairment. By focusing on the concepts of comfort and quality of life and by explaining the implications of intubation, most patients can make an informed decision about resuscitation. A difficult decision always arises if a patient is admitted late at night or in the early morning hours. If the patient's condition is clinically stable and there is no anticipation of an untoward cardiopulmonary event, it would be most reasonable to reserve that discussion for a more sensible hour.

### Difficult Conflicts in the Management of the Dying Cancer Patient

Controversial areas in managing the patient with advanced malignant disease are the role of nasogastric or gastrostomy feeding tubes, the role of aggressive hydration and parenteral nutrition, and the pros and cons of intubation in the patient with advanced, progressive, and incurable malignant disease.

A fundamental concept, from legal, medical, and ethical perspectives, is respect for patient autonomy. If the patient is fully decisional and recognizes the futility of these interventions as a means of prolonging the dying process, the decision to forego these intrusions is relatively straightforward. It is clear that patients have the right to forego these measures even if, under unusual circumstances, they may prolong life. Anguish arises when a patient is unconscious or is not capable of making an informed decision. At these times, the patient's surrogate or legal representative must step forward to reflect the wishes of the patient. However, there is marked variation among states as to how specific the patient's wishes must have been shared with the surrogate. Some courts require clear and convincing evidence that the patient would not wish these procedures to be either introduced or maintained. In the absence of this evidence, some states have held that these measures cannot be withdrawn.

Hydration and nutrition have profound symbolism in the management of the cancer patient. However, most patients and families do not understand that aggressive hydration in the terminally ill cancer patient prolongs the dying process, increases pulmonary secretions, and typically provokes a worsening of edema, ascites, or dyspnea. Likewise, there is much confusion over the role of feeding gastrostomies, nasogastric tubes, and jejunostomy tubes. There are substantial risks of aspiration pneumonitis with these interventions, and there is no compelling evidence from any trial that parenteral nutrition in the advanced cancer patient enhances quality of life. One helpful technique in addressing this issue with patients and families is to explain that in the advanced cancer patient, aggressive hydration will prolong the dying process and aggressive nutrition will sustain the patient only to have him or her experience the clinical consequences of advanced malignant disease. When these discussions are conducted in a sensitive and caring manner with family members and with the patient present, there is generally a consensus not to proceed with these intrusions.

In some circumstances, the communications skills of the clinician will be tested. A case in point, which is all too common, involves a patient with progressive malignant disease who cannot make an informed decision and for whom some family members insist that "everything be done" including ventilatory support, whereas others are promoting a more rational course. If it becomes clear that the clinician cannot satisfactorily arbitrate diverse positions among family members, the input of an outside agency, individual, or committee can help resolve these sometimes bitter conflicts. These deliberations can be gut-wrenching and require the utmost skills in tact and diplomacy. The attending physician should meet with the patient and family with a clear recognition of the importance of the input of each family member. We cannot be naive in the era of blended families, stepfamilies, and mixed families. It may be that significant financial issues must be frankly addressed and brought into the open before there can be any resolution of the conflict. The clinician must be alert to the hidden agendas that may drive and support the position of a given family member.

Other individuals who should be included in these discussions include the entire care-giving team, a member of the pastoral care community, other clinical experts, and/or a patient representative. A representative from the ethics committee can be invited to review the details of the situation and participate in the discussion.

## Physician-Assisted Suicide and Euthanasia

By virtue of their training and moral orientation, physicians have a responsibility to care for their patients (13).

In the setting of malignant disease, there is a continuum of management that initially focuses on the cure of the disorder, but when that ceases to occur, there remains a fundamental responsibility to manage the symptoms of the illness. A natural corollary and extension of this responsibility is the conundrum of addressing the patient's request for information or assistance in taking his or her own life. This is a vexing issue for the patients, physicians, families, and also society as a whole. The scope of this discussion cannot encompass the far-reaching implications. Eloquent summaries of these issues have been published. However, it is this author's experience that requests for physician-assisted suicide are astonishingly infrequent. Nevertheless, if patients feel neglected, abandoned, and alienated from their culture and have their physiologic needs ignored, requests for assisted suicide are hardly surprising. The physician who is responsive and available to patients during their terminal days will infrequently be faced with this challenging dilemma (14). Clear and open communication between the caregiver, the patient, and the family may hopefully avoid these very difficult decisions.

## Financial and Estate-Planning Considerations

A will is a crucial document that allows for the orderly transfer of assets following the death of an individual. This document facilitates the wishes of the individual and allows for special bequests of assets to friends, employees, and distant relatives. It also is a vehicle for establishing trusts, providing direction for the care of minor children through guardians, and addressing other related issues. If a will is not prepared, there are state and legal guidelines, which may not be consistent with the wishes of the deceased.

It is appropriate that physicians remind patients and families about the importance of their ability to locate crucial financial documents, such as marriage and divorce decrees, birth certificates, and a whole spectrum of financial papers including insurance policies, deeds, and past income tax forms, and to identify family financial advisors, such as financial planners, attorneys, and accountants. It is always delicate for physicians to raise these issues, and it might be done in the following manner. A patient should be advised that when his or her health and stamina is perhaps at its optimum, that is the time to deal with financial issues. As the disease progresses, the patient's focus clearly becomes on nonfinancial issues, and that is not the optimum time to make far-reaching decisions that could affect survivors for generations.

## The Issue of Hope

The late Dr. Charles W. Mayo made this statement, "I never operate on a patient who thinks he is going to die." The sage clinician and surgeon recognized that this could become a self-fulfilling prophecy and underscored the importance of emotional issues relating to malignant disease. Hope is not the conviction that things will turn out well but the expectation that they will make sense, regardless of the outcome. Studies are emerging that show reasonably consistent results: hope, attitude, and disposition have something to do with the outcome of a malignant disease (15,16). Some studies have shown that appropriate psychological interventions can positively affect the quality of life of cancer patients, prolong survival, and positively affect the immune system. Most clinicians would agree that the socially, spiritually, and psychologically isolated individual, regardless of socioeconomic status, may have a very difficult time dealing with a malignant disease. A crucial dimension of hope in the cancer setting directly reflects the relationship between the patient and caregiver. Among 100 women with breast cancer who were surveyed 6 months after surgery, there was one unshakeable finding: their perception of the physicians' caring attitude was the most significant factor in psychological adjustment and decision making. Information-giving, though obviously important, was far less important in supporting patients during this difficult time.

Although there most clinicians generally agree about the value of optimism, fighting spirit, and hopefulness, there have been few hard data from patients that identify which techniques and procedures foster these phenomena. Studies among patients with advanced cancer have underscored that the following issues and topics are clearly important (8–10,15):

- Patients wish to receive the diagnosis in a face-to-face encounter that provides intimacy and privacy.
- The physician should be known to the patient if at all possible.
- A friend or family member should accompany the patient.
- A focus on the importance of alternative medical therapies and second-line treatments is important.
- Patients wish to know that some other individuals have done well in similar circumstances.
- Patients' participation in their own management is important.
- Patients want their physicians to emphasize the importance of exercise, diet, visualization, or psychotherapy,

recognizing that these techniques are not consistently endorsed by all clinicians.
- Fears of pain and the effects of treatment should be clearly addressed.
- Issues of abandonment are most important; appropriate physical expressions such as holding a hand, grasping the shoulder firmly, or a handshake are most important.
- Patients wish to have the hope that even if their disease is not curable, they may expect to have special times with families and friends, to have hope for personal growth and the achievement of a new awareness of priorities.

# REFERENCES

1. Holland JC, Geary N, Marchini A, Tross S. An international survey of physician attitudes and practice in regard to revealing the diagnosis of cancer. *Cancer Invest* 1987;5(2):151–154.
2. Trill MD, Holland J. Cross cultural difference in the care of patients with cancer. A review. *Gen Hosp Psychiatry* 1993;15:21–30.
3. Buckman R. *How to break bad news: a guide for health care professionals*. Baltimore: Johns Hopkins University Press, 1992.
4. Creagan ET. How to break bad news—and not devastate the patient. *Mayo Clin Proc* 1994;69:1015–1017.
5. Creagan ET. Psychosocial issues in oncologic practice. *Mayo Clin Proc* 1993;68:161–167.
6. Delbanco TL. Enriching the doctor-patient relationship by inviting the patient's perspective. *Ann Intern Med* 1992;116:414–418.
7. Broadhead WE, Kaplan BH. Social support and the cancer patient. *Cancer* 1991;67:794–799.
8. Sardell AN, Trierweiler SJ. Disclosing the cancer diagnosis. *Cancer* 1993;72:3355–3365.
9. Siminoff LA. Improving communications with cancer patients. *Oncology* 1992;6(10):83–89.
10. Spiro H. What is empathy and can it be taught? *Ann Intern Med* 1992;116:843–846.
11. Kuhn CC. A spiritual inventory of the medically ill patient. *Psychiatr Med* 1988;6(2):87–100.
12. Stoudemire A, Rhoads JM. When the doctor needs a doctor: special considerations for the physician-patient. Ann Intern Med 1983;98(Part 1):654–659.
13. Terry PB. Euthanasia and assisted suicide. *Mayo Clin Proc* 1995;70:189–192.
14. McCann RM, Hall WJ, Groth JA: Comfort care for terminally ill patients. The appropriate use of nutrition and hydration. *JAMA* 1994;272:1263–1266.
15. Roberts CS, Cox CE, Reintgen DS, Baile WF, Gibertini M. Influence of physician communication on newly diagnosed breast patients' psychologic adjustments and decision-making. *Cancer* 1994;74:336–341.
16. Ruckdeschel JC, Blanchard CG, Albrecht T. Psychosocial oncology research: where we have been, where we are going, and why we will not get there. *Cancer* 1994;74:1458–1463.

# SECTION IV

## Ethics

*Principles and Practice of Supportive Oncology,*
edited by Ann Berger et al.
Lippincott–Raven Publishers, Philadelphia ©1998

# CHAPTER 57

# Informed Consent

Robyn S. Shapiro

## INFORMED CONSENT IN CANCER TREATMENT

### History and Underlying Principles

The concept of informed consent in health care expresses the primacy of individualistic values in American society, and it facilitates good medical treatment decision-making by assuring the patient's receipt and understanding of information about alternative medical interventions. The historical roots of the informed consent doctrine lie in the tort of battery, under which liability is imposed for unpermitted touching. In *Schloendorff v. Society of New York Hospital* (1), to which most American informed consent court decisions cite, Judge Cardozo said: "Every human being of adult years and sound mind has a right to determine what shall be done with his own body; and a surgeon who performs an operation without his patient's consent commits an assault, for which he is liable in damages."

Consumer and civil rights developments in the succeeding decades broadened the foundation of the informed consent doctrine to include the concept that patients have significant power not only to authorize or veto a proposed procedure or treatment but also to participate in the medical decision-making process itself (2). As case law developed the informed consent doctrine during these years, courts increasingly recognized that even when consent is formally given and documented, it is legally ineffective unless patients *understand* information about the procedures they are authorizing (3).

### Required Elements of Disclosure

#### Elements of Disclosure

In 1957, the California appellate court's *Salgo* decision established that sufficient information must be communi-

R.S. Shapiro: Center for the Study of Bioethics, Medical College of Wisconsin, Milwaukee, WI 53226.

cated to the patient to render consent "informed," but that decision did not identify in detail the type and extent of information that must be disclosed. Later courts, which were left to transform the abstract *Salgo* principle into an operational rule, defined the following basic types of information as required under the informed consent doctrine:

1. Diagnosis
2. Nature, risks, and benefits of the proposed intervention
3. Alternative treatments
4. Likely results of no treatment
5. Likelihood of success

Of these disclosure elements, the two that have spawned the most litigation are risks and benefits of the proposed treatment, and alternative treatments.

### Risks and Benefits of Proposed Treatment

While courts have generally recognized that risks that are "too remote" need not be disclosed and that disclosure of "commonly known" risks is not required, specifically defining risks that are "too remote" or "commonly known" remains problematic. As a general rule, however, it can be said that the need for disclosure is a product of the probability that a particular risk will eventuate multiplied by the severity of the risk.

The obligation to disclose the likely *benefits* of proposed treatment was the issue in *Arato v. Avedon*, 5 Cal. 4th 1172, 23 Cal. Rptr. 2d 131, 858 P.2d 598 (1993), decided recently by the California Supreme Court. In that case, Mr. Arato, a 43-year-old electrical contractor, underwent an operation to remove a nonfunctioning kidney. In the course of surgery, physicians found a tumor in the tail of his pancreas, which was removed, along with surrounding tissue and lymph nodes. The surgeon told Mr. and Mrs. Arato that he thought he had removed all of the tumor but did not relate a prognosis or life expectancy estimate, and he referred Mr. Arato to an oncologist. The oncologist told the Aratos that there was a substantial chance of recurrence, although he was not asked for and did not give a prognosis, and he recommended chemotherapy and radiation treatment. During Mr. Arato's radiation treatment and chemotherapy, his cancer recurred. At that time, physicians believed that Mr. Arato would live no more than a few months, but they did not tell him so. Mr. Arato died 3 months after the recurrence was detected, approximately 1 year after his cancer first was diagnosed.

Mr. Arato's wife and children then sued the surgeons and the oncologist, alleging that they had an obligation under the informed consent doctrine to tell Mr. Arato, before recommending chemotherapy and radiation, that approximately 95% of people with pancreatic cancer die within 5 years. Mrs. Arato and her children alleged that had this statistical prognosis been disclosed, Mr. Arato would not have undergone the treatment, but rather would have lived out his final days with his family and made arrangements for his business affairs. At the trial, Mr. Arato's surgeon said that Mr. Arato had shown such great anxiety about his cancer that it was "medically inappropriate" to disclose specific mortality rates, and the chief oncologist said that reporting extremely high mortality rates was medically inadvisable because it could deprive patients of hope. The physicians also said that the statistical life expectancy of a group of patients does not have predictive value when applied to a particular patient.

On the basis of standard California jury instructions on informed consent, the jury ruled for the physicians. The California court of appeals reversed, holding that physicians do have to disclose life expectancy statistics so that patients can plan for their deaths. On appeal, the California Supreme Court upheld the jury. It is important to note, however, that the high court focused only on one question: whether California's standard jury instructions should be revised to require the disclosure of life expectancy statistics. While the court answered that question in the negative, it did not absolve physicians from their general obligation to inform patients about the success rates of proposed treatment in terms of the prospects for long-term survival and quality of life. The court concluded:

> Rather than mandate the disclosure of specific information as a matter of law, the better rule is to instruct the jury that a physician is under a legal duty to disclose to the patient all material information—that is, information which would be regarded as significant by a reasonable person in the patient's position when deciding to accept or reject a recommended medical procedure—needed to make an informed decision regarding a proposed treatment.

To facilitate the patient's thorough understanding, physicians should assure that he or she has enough time to assimilate and consider the risks and benefits of the proposed treatment and to ask questions. In addition, it may be beneficial for the patient to have an opportunity to speak with another patient who has undergone the recommended therapy. It is particularly important to facilitate thorough understanding when adjunctive therapy is recommended for women who have had surgical treatment for breast cancer and who are not known to have any cancer. While the theory is that such therapy maximizes the chance of complete cure because the level of tumor may be subclinical and not detectable, many of the therapies involved have a high level of toxicity. Because adjunctive therapy may cause significant side effects in an otherwise healthy woman, it is especially important for women to understand thoroughly the benefits and burdens of such treatment.

In all cancer treatment situations, the patient's thorough understanding of the potential risks and benefits allows her to control her medical course and also fosters a more realistic expectation of treatment outcomes—which can prevent future litigation. Moreover, data show marked clinical improvement in patients with advanced cancer who are able truly to collaborate with their physicians on account of their thorough understanding of the treatment (4).

### Alternative Treatments

Alternative medical intervention is another disclosure element that has been litigated extensively. According to case law and statutes in some states, all medically recognized approaches that are reasonably available under the circumstances should be discussed (5), even if they involve treatments that the treating physician cannot perform or provide.

At least 15 states have passed legislation imposing specific informed consent requirements with respect to breast cancer treatment alternatives. Many of these laws require physicians to disclose explicit alternative treatments to their breast cancer patients through the use of standardized written summaries or consent forms. Although these statutes were not necessarily enacted to encourage breast conservation treatment, studies have found higher rates of breast-conserving treatment in states with specific breast cancer treatment informed consent laws. In 1981, the national average of lumpectomies or wedge excisions of tumors under 1 centimeter was 4.8%. In Massachusetts, which had a 2-year-old informed consent law at the time, the incidence was 18%; in California, which had a 1-year-old law, the incidence was 10%; and in New York, which had no law, the incidence was 2% (6).

### Patients' Capacity to Give Consent

Adults are presumed to be capable of giving informed consent to treatment. However, a patient who lacks the mental capacity to understand the nature and consequences of authorizing treatment cannot give a valid consent.

In some cases, lack of decision-making capacity, as well as identification of the incapacitated patient's surrogate decision-maker, is clear. For example, if an individual is under guardianship or conservatorship of the person, it is the guardian or conservator from whom consent must be obtained. If the patient has previously executed a health care power of attorney appointing a health care agent to make treatment decisions on his or her behalf after incapacity and that document has been activated, consent must be obtained from the health care agent.

In other circumstances, however, determination of and response to decision-making incapacity are not as clear. Shock, trauma, alcohol or drug abuse, and several other factors can be responsible for a mental incapacity that temporarily or permanently impedes the patient's ability to consent to treatment. If the individual has periods of lucid and irrational thought, valid consent may be obtained while he or she is lucid and demonstrates the ability to understand the nature and consequences of consent. Likewise, the patient's withdrawal of consent during a lucid phase should be respected. On the other hand, consents, refusals, and withdrawals of consent made during a period when lucidity is absent should not be honored, because these decisions are not the products of deliberate, informed thinking. When a patient lacks decision-making capacity and has neither a guardian nor a health care agent, consent must be obtained from someone authorized to act on the patient's behalf.

### Suggested Informed Consent Process in Cancer Treatment

Decisions about various recommended cancer treatment regimens, including surgery, chemotherapy, and radiation, all raise important informed consent issues. In all cases, it is important for the physician and patient (or surrogate, if the patient is incapacitated) to have a thorough discussion about the treatment alternatives so that the patient (or surrogate) understands the choices and selects the treatment most consistent with the patient's values and preferences. For example, certain risks such as vomiting and hair loss, which commonly accompany many drugs used in cancer chemotherapy and may accompany radiation, are of much greater concern to some individuals than to others.

While it is advisable to document this conversation between physician and patient (or surrogate), consent must be viewed as a process, not a form. In this dialogue, both patient (or surrogate) and physician must exchange information and questions so that the patient (or surrogate) learns details about the proposed procedure, and the physician gains information about the patient's prefer-

ences and concerns in order to tailor appropriately the disclosure of risks and benefits.

## INFORMED CONSENT IN CANCER SCREENINGS

Many informed consent requirements in cancer treatment apply, as well, to cancer screening. For example, patient autonomy dictates that patients have the right to be fully informed before screenings as well as before treatment, and that they (or their surrogates, if they lack decision-making capacity) have the right to refuse screening as well as treatment. A unique issue in cancer screening, however, is determining for whom and when screening should be recommended.

Professional standards of care generally require screening tests to be offered whenever it is considered "reasonably prudent" to do so, often as determined by medical experts. The following have been suggested as important factors in determining which individuals should be screened:

1. The frequency and severity of the condition screened for
2. The availability of an efficacious therapy for the condition
3. The extent to which early detection improves the outcome
4. The validity and safety of the screening test
5. The costs in relation to the benefits of the screening test (7)

With respect to breast cancer screening, despite recent studies that demonstrate infrequent recommendations by physicians of these procedures for older women, (8) the role of age should be largely irrelevant to the application of the screening criteria described above. National health status surveys and longitudinal population studies have demonstrated that the physiologic health of older individuals is widely variable (9). For many women who are 85 or even 90, early detection and successful breast cancer treatment could allow them to live out their average life expectancy—a result comparable to the "5-year survival" considered an excellent outcome in many cancer protocols (10). These facts, along with application of the other generic screening criteria listed above, render difficult the argument that the older woman should not be screened for breast cancer—unless she herself rejects the screen on the basis of her own cost/benefit calculations.

Moreover, lack of decision-making capacity should not in and of itself preclude a screening procedure. Recommendations regarding the screen should be made to the patient's surrogate on the basis of the same generic screening criteria discussed above. Application of those criteria could be affected by the patient's incapacity if, for example, the test would greatly frighten or disturb the patient, so that the benefits would not outweigh the burdens. On the other hand, if the patient's life expectancy and quality of life would warrant treatment of a tumor found on a screening exam, and the costs (financial and otherwise) are not significant, consent should be sought from the surrogate.

## GENETIC RISK SCREENING AND NOTIFICATION

Advances in molecular oncology have resulted in enhanced capabilities to test for genetic cancer risks. Providing such cancer risk information, which may facilitate the patient's future participation in cancer prevention and surveillance programs, should be guided by principles applicable to informed consent to treatment. For example, a woman who is informed that she has a high risk of developing breast cancer on account of genetic predisposition should be given an opportunity to make an informed autonomous decision about the appropriate course of action in light of the medical facts and her own values. She may choose a prophylactic mastectomy if she is particularly anxious, or she may choose a more conservative approach.

Some issues raised by genetic cancer risk screening and notification raise new ethical and legal questions. Who should have access to such information? When should mass genetic cancer risk screening be advocated? When is mandatory genetic screening justified? If it is known that a patient's risk of cancer is increased because of genetic factors and there is no way to ameliorate the risk, how much should he or she be told? Must the physician inform family members of individuals who are identified as having a genetic cancer susceptibility? These questions demand that we refine strategies for communicating cancer risk information so as to minimize adverse psychologic or social consequences while maximizing prevention and surveillance regimens.

## INFORMED CONSENT IN THE TREATMENT OF ADOLESCENTS WITH CANCER

### Disclosure of Diagnosis

Regardless of determinations made later in the course of an adolescent's disease concerning responsibilities for treatment decision-making, the adolescent should be informed about the cancer and the contemplated treatment at the time of diagnosis—unless he or she has indicated a desire not to know. This conversation builds trust between the patient and the doctor, and it prevents the fear, isolation, and confusion that otherwise might occur.

### Informed Consent for Treatment

For the most part, consent for medical treatment of children younger than 18 years old is provided by their parents because these patients are statutorily defined as minors, unable to provide legal informed consent. However, a thorough understanding of the ethical principle of autonomy, of key concepts in child development, and of the legal doctrine of the "mature minor" suggests that determining the extent to which adolescents should be involved in treatment decisionmaking requires a case-by-case analysis.

Respect for autonomy protects the individual's opportunity to guide his or her own medical course, to the degree to which the individual is capable. Required capabilities for health care decision-making are (a) understanding and reasoning, which allow for thorough consideration of the salient medical aspects of the choice at hand, and (b) having and applying one's own set of values (11), which allow for personal evaluation of the treatment alternatives.

Some adolescents are sufficiently capable of understanding and reasoning to make their own medical decisions. Studies indicate that in adolescence, the individual begins to achieve full intellectual capacity, to be able to reason deductively, to hypothesize, and to deal with abstraction (12). With these abilities, the individual is capable of simultaneous consideration of alternative treatments and risks, as required in informed consent.

Moreover, psychological studies show that some adolescents have developed a consistent and stable set of values and that they can apply these values to medical decision-making. While children under 13 often have difficulty anticipating their future, some older children are able to give adequate weight to the effect of their medical decisions on their future interests (13).

In fact, on account of their illness, some adolescents with cancer may have decision-making capacities that exceed the expectations for patients their age. Some teenage cancer patients with advanced disease may have a more acute awareness and understanding of death because of their relationships with fellow patients who have died. Furthermore, the patient's own prior experience with cancer and its treatment may have given him or her a clearer idea about treatment benefits and burdens.

The legal doctrine of the "mature minor" supports the concept that some adolescents who are younger than 18 years old may be able to provide legal informed consent to treatment. Pursuant to this doctrine, a child under 18 may be judicially recognized as possessing sufficient understanding and appreciation of the nature and consequences of treatment—despite chronological age—to be able to give consent on his or her own.

For example, in one of the earliest "mature minor" cases, a 17-year-old underwent surgery for removal of a tumor in his ear (14). While the boy's father was aware of his condition, he did not know about the operation. Chloroform was administered just prior to surgery, and the boy suffered a fatal cardiopulmonary arrest. In a lawsuit by the father for wrongful death and unauthorized surgery, the Michigan Supreme Court sustained a directed verdict in favor of the defendants, noting the boy's independence concerning his illness. In fact, according to one commentator, a main feature in the case was the boy's apparent ability to make his own treatment decisions (15).

More recently, in *In re E.G.* (16), a 17-year-old Jehovah's Witness with leukemia refused blood transfusions. The Illinois Supreme Court affirmed the appellate court's finding that the patient was a mature minor, capable of refusing treatment, because she understood her disease and the consequences of her refusal.

## FUTURE INFORMED CONSENT ISSUES IN ONCOLOGY

The rapid changes in our health care delivery system are spawning changes and new challenges in informed consent. For example, recently there has been growing emphasis on outcomes data resulting from studies that identify treatments and procedures in a variety of efficacy categories. If such research is carried out with scientific integrity, and data are appropriately communicated to patients, treatment choices may be more informed and more tailored to patients' needs. In a study done by John Wennberg, for example, when severely symptomatic prostate cancer patients were fully informed of the risks and benefits of surgery, only one of five chose to undergo the procedure, despite the fact that it had been recommended by all of their physicians (17).

On the other hand, proliferating outcomes and cost data could lead to diminished patient choice. Managed care organizations and other health care payors increasingly are limiting or eliminating coverage for treatments and procedures determined to be cost ineffective. This practice, in turn, has given rise to new questions about the physician's disclosure obligations under informed consent. While the question of the managed care organization's liability exposure in some such situations may turn on the application of the ERISA preemption (18), the legal obligations of the physician remain essentially the same (19). Thus, doctors should adhere to recognized standards of practice in disclosing patient information to patients—including treatment alternatives not covered by a managed care entity.

## REFERENCES

1. 211 N.Y. 125, 105 N.E. 92 (1914).
2. See, eg., Katz J. *The Silent World of Doctor and Patient* (1984); and Andrews. Informed Consent Statutes and the Decisionmaking Process, *J Legal Med* 5:1163(1984).
3. See, eg., *Salgo v. Leland Stanford Jr. University Board of Trustees,* 154 Cal. App. 2d 560, 317 P 2d 170 (1957).
4. *Ethics and Alternative Medicine*. AHA Hospital Ethics, May/June 1993, 9;3:7.
5. See, eg., *Holt v. Nelson*, 11 Wash. App. 230, 523 P.2d 211(1974).
6. Dabice RL, Cordes, S. Informed consent heralds change in breast treatment. *Am Med News,* Nov. 11, 1985:1.
7. Annas G. Breast Cancer Screening in Older Women, Law and Patient Rights *Journal of Gerontology* 1992;47:121.
8. Weinberger M, Saunders AF, Samsa GP, et al. Breast Cancer Screening in Older Women: Practices and Barriers Reported by Primary Care Physicians. *J Am Geriatr Soc* 1991; 139:22–29.
9. Verbrugge LM. Comorbidity and its impact on disability. *Milbank Q* 1989;967: 450–484.
10. Yancik R, Ries LG, Yates JW. Breast Cancer in Aging Women: A population-based study of contrasts in stage, surgery, and survival. *Cancer* 1989;63:9676–9681.
11. Brock D. Children's Competence for Health Care Decisionmaking. In: Kopelman L, Moskop J. Eds, *Children and healthcare: Moral and social issues.* Boston: Kluwer Academic Publsihers, 1989:181–212.
12. Sussman E, Dorn L, Fletcher J. Reasoning about illness in ill and healthy children and adolescents: cognitive and emotional developmental aspects. *Develop Behav Pediatr* 1987;8:266–273.
13. Leikin S. The role of adolescents in decisions concerning their cancer therapy. *Cancer Suppl* 1993;71(10):3342–3346.
14. *Bakker v. Welsh*, 144 Mich. 632, 108 N.W. 94 (1906).
15. Wilkins, Children's rights: Removing the parental consent barrier to medical treatment of minors, 1975; *Ariz St L J*:31.
16. 133 Ill. 2d 98, 549 N.E. 2d 322 (Ill 1989).
17. Wennberg J. AHCPR and the strategy for healthcare reform. *Health Aff,* Winter 1992:69.
18. See, eg., *Corcoran v. United HealthCare Inc.* 965 F.2d 1321 (5th Cir.), *cert. denied*, 506 U.S. 1033 (1992).
19. See, eg, *Wickline v. California*, 192 Cal. App. 1630 (Ct. App. 1986), review dismissed, case remanded, 741 P.2d 613 (Cal 1987).

*Principles and Practice of Supportive Oncology,*
edited by Ann Berger et al.
Lippincott–Raven Publishers, Philadelphia ©1998

CHAPTER 58

# Advance Directives

Linda L. Emanuel

Many oncology patients would like to have some control over their medical care, not only when they are alert but also when they are too sick to participate in decisions. Similarly, those who have to make decisions for patients who are unable to participate would like to be guided by the patient's wishes. Advance care planning evolved in response to these needs.

## TERMS, HISTORY, AND LAW

There are two main modalities by which a person can make preparations in anticipation of future incapacity (1). One is to appoint a proxy to speak in the place of the principal person. The other is to write down wishes in a directive. These two modalities are usually complementary, since written statements cannot provide for all eventualities, and proxy decision-makers cannot speak as patients wished them to without guidance from the patients.

### Proxy Designation

Physicians should be aware of three key issues on which to advise patients and proxies. First, patients and proxies should understand the proxy's role. Speaking in place of the patient can take two distinctly different forms. In one form the patient asks the proxy to represent the patient's prior wishes. In this role, the proxy should not make decisions (a) based on what they would do for themselves (b) based on their assessment of the best interests of the patient, or (c) according to the interests of family, friends, or others. Instead, they should hold steadfast to the patient's known prior preferences, extrapolat-

ing them if necessary to the situation at hand. In the other form, the patient simply chooses the proxy and lets him or her speak according to the proxy's own judgment (2). In this alternative role, the proxy remains independent of the patient's prior wishes and tries instead to (a) imagine what the patient would have wanted in the circumstances (b) judge the best interests of the patient, and (c) balance other issues as he or she sees fit. These two modalities can be merged. For instance, a patient may tell a proxy to apply his or her prior wishes, albeit with latitude and taking particular types of unpredictable family issues into consideration (3).

Second, patients and proxies should know that studies have found that proxies often guess the prior wishes of patients inaccurately and furthermore that proxies often imagine that the patients' prior wishes are for more intervention than patients actually select (4). Even a proxy who has had a close relationship with the patient may not be able to make accurate judgments. It is possible that close relationships do not often include discussions about medical aspects of dying, or that patients do not even know their own preferences until they have discussed or faced a relevant matter. It is also possible that proxies face significant emotional issues that may hinder their ability to imagine the patients' wishes. Regardless, physicians must counsel patients to discuss relevant perspectives explicitly and well in advance of a deteriorating medical situation that may result in incompetence.

Third, patients should be aware that friends and family members have their own interests and issues, which may conflict with their role as proxy. Common examples include the difficulty of letting go of the loved patient, the great emotional burden of making life-and-death decisions, the difficulty of finding the extensive time it takes to perform the proxy role well, and the difficulty of choosing how to allocate limited family resources (e.g., to the patient's medical care versus the children's education) (4). Conflicting motivations are inevitable and need not prohibit the proxy role. Nonetheless, the proxy may

L.L. Emanuel: Ethics Standards Division, American Medical Association, Chicago, IL 60610.

This chapter has been modified from *Geriatric Medicine* (C Cassel, ed). New York: Springer-Verlag, 1997.

need help distinguishing different motivations and abiding by those that are most suited to the proxy role.

### Instructional Directives

The history of the development of instructional directives reflects the search for the most valid form of expressing prior wishes. The earliest commonly used instructional directive was the Do Not Resuscitate (DNR) order, written by the physician after discussion with the patient and family (5). After its proposal in 1976, a set of studies and a culture evolved around the DNR discussion. It is still relevant and can be included in comprehensive advance planning discussions (6). A hazard of isolated DNR discussions is that they occur too late, either missing the patients who need them or occurring in such "out of the blue" conversations that patients get unintended messages, perhaps feeling that they are being abandoned (7).

An earlier modality for making instructional directives, which never achieved widespread use in the medical system, was the living will. This was introduced in 1968 by a lawyer, Louis Kutner. The living will attempted to express the widespread view that heroic levels of technological intervention should be avoided if the patient's prognosis was hopeless. The statements made in living wills were true enough to the sentiment, but in practice they were insufficient to guide the specific decision-making needed in real clinical circumstances. Different interpretations of what constitutes a heroic intervention and what constitutes a hopeless prognosis meant that this early type of living will was liable to bring as much confusion as clarity to the decisions.

Efforts to increase the specificity of living wills began, starting most notably with Sissela Bok's and Michigan's living will (8,9). Thereafter, developments began along two lines: one to better describe the general health-related values of the patient (values histories) and one to formulate ways in which patients could make very specific treatment preference statements (treatment-specific directives) (10,11). Empirical evidence that general statements cannot predict specific wishes has supported the more balanced view that these two modalities work best together (12–14). Some patients are inclined to write a free-prose letter encapsulating their wishes. Such letters can be worthwhile, but many patients do not have the writing skills or the specialized knowledge that ensures coverage of relevant decisions. In such cases, concurrent use of predrafted documents is to be encouraged.

More recently, efforts have been focused on the need to validate predrafted instructional directives, just as any other instrument that seeks to record subjective matters needs to be validated (15). Specific forms that have been extensively validated are still few, and validated forms tailored to oncology patients are even fewer; one of the more studied forms, which is generic and adaptable, is reproduced in Appendix 1. Physicians should advise patients to use validated forms, since using nonvalidated forms risk misrepresentation of patients' true wishes and can confuse decision-making. Validated forms also provide a succinct method of ensuring that patients have considered the major areas that most people need to cover. The use of a validated form as a worksheet for thought and discussion can be as important as its use as a recorded document.

### Statutory versus Advisory Documents

All states and the District of Columbia have statutes that endorse advance directives in one way or another. Some endorse the use of proxies, others endorse the use of instructional directives, and most now endorse both (16). Most state statutes have a corresponding document, which is often available from local health care facilities or state medical organizations. The fundamental purpose of state statutes is to allow physicians to follow the patient's wishes without fear of liability. The interests of the patient are served indirectly by protecting physicians who follow patients' wishes and rendering physicians vulnerable if they do not. Many states specifically honor the statutory documents of other states, although some differences exist, and frequent travelers may wish to have documents from their frequented state bound together with those from their home state.

It is part of common law that competent patients have the right to accept or refuse medical intervention, even life-sustaining intervention. Even casual statements have been honored as sufficient evidence, although written statements have been explicitly identified as desirable evidence of patients' preferences (17,18). Physicians can therefore be assured that patients' statements recorded in a fashion not specifically designed for local state statutes—they can be considered advisory documents—still carry legal authority. Distinctions between legal and "nonlegal" or "illegal" forms in this context are erroneous. A statutory form is legally binding, and a nonstatutory advisory document is also binding if it provides clear evidence of the patient's wishes. Since statutory forms are written to comply with legal criteria, they are often far less informative than advisory documents, which can address personal values and clinical issues.

### The Patient Self-Determination Act, and Recommendations of the Joint Commission on Accreditation of Health Care Organizations

In 1990, the United States Congress passed the Patient Self-Determination Act, which requires that patients be asked about the existence of an advance directive at the time of enrollment or admission to a health care facility. The intent of the law was to increase awareness and documentation of advance directives. In addition, the Joint

Commission on Accreditation of Health Care Organizations recommends that facilities have arrangements for counseling patients who wish to complete advance directives. Completion of advance directives is best done in the more stable setting of continuing outpatient care, but occasionally their completion in the inpatient setting is unavoidable. Thus, although minimal compliance with the Patient Self-Determination Act and the recommendations of the Joint Commission require relatively little from physicians, the spirit of both requirements involves thoughtful, longitudinal involvement of the physician in discussion with the patient.

## CONCEPTUAL FOUNDATIONS

### Honoring Patients' Wishes

The basic precept on which advance directives depend is somewhat confusing. The notion that autonomy can be extended into times of incompetence by recording wishes ahead of time is problematic. How can anyone know whether the wishes of an incompetent person are represented by previously recorded wishes? What about patients who are incompetent for decision-making but are awake and appear to be capable of feelings and wishes, and these apparent wishes differ from the prior wishes? Responding to these two questions, which motivated considerable criticism of the advance directive movement, depends on understanding two things. First, the justifying principle for advance directives is surviving interests, rather than the broader principle of autonomy. Second, the patient condition in which advance directives pertain is actually wishlessness, not the more general condition of incompetence (19).

### Surviving Interests

Ordinarily, autonomy involves application of real-time wishes. But since it is impossible to create real-time wishes when there are none, autonomy can be extended only by applying prior wishes. A surviving interest constitutes a distinct form of autonomy and should not be confused with the more general autonomy. *Surviving interest*, ordinarily a legal term, refers to the right of the individual to determine decisions on matters in which he or she has an overriding interest even after losing the direct ability to act on these matters. The most common example is the estate will, in which individuals exercise their right to determine disposal of their property after death. A related arrangement that relies on a surviving interest concerns the funeral directions by the principal planning for his or her own death. Another example is the organ donor card. The important point is that arrangements predicated on surviving interests do not rely on real-time wishes; they rely on prior wishes. Advance directives rely on prior wishes in just the same

way as these more traditional applications of surviving interests. Even when a proxy is instructed to make decisions without reference to the patient's prior wishes, the proxy's authority relies on the patient's prior wishes to designate him or her, and while proxies may make use of their own real-time judgments, there is no application of the patients' (nonexistent) real-time wishes. The question: How can anyone know if the wishes of the incompetent patient are represented by the recorded wishes? can now be answered: When there are no real-time wishes, it is prior wishes that must be represented.

### The Zone Between Incompetence and Wishlessness

Patients who are in a state in which it is not possible to have wishes, such as occurs when there is complete absence of neocortical function, clearly meet the criteria by which advance directives can be activated. A problem arises when a patient is not wishless but is decisionally incapacitated, as is commonly the case after a stroke or in many types of dementia or debilitated states. Many such circumstances involve such a significant change in patients' personality or states of being that they are very different from the former selves who made out the directive. There is limited ethical imperative to apply the wishes of the former person to the current person if the latter is a significantly altered or truncated version of the former (20). Many patients fall into this "twilight zone," and advance directives should be used as no more than one factor (the representation of prior wishes of the former person) in the assessment of what the current person's wishes and needs may be. Under these circumstances, advance directives may be said to represent a weak version of the surviving interests of the patients, and other factors must therefore be considered. Technical and legal statements as to when advance directives can be activated often fail to make this distinction. Nonetheless, physicians should be particularly careful to meet ethical standards as well as legal ones under these circumstances. The question: How should one represent decisionally incapacitated patients who seem to have wishes that differ from the recorded wishes? can now be answered: A combination of guidance by the advance directive and substituted or best interests judgment should determine the physicians' and proxies' decisions for patients in this circumstance.

### Substituted Judgment and Best Interests Judgment

Whenever patients' surviving interests are unknown, decisions must be made by using standards of substituted judgment or best interests judgment. The application of prior wishes is not the same thing as using substituted judgment. Even when prior wishes are inferred from stated wishes to fit unpredicted decisions, this is a form of prior-preference–guided judgment that is justified by surviving interests.

Substituted judgment usually refers to attempts to judge as the patient would have if he or she could have. In the words of Justice Hughes, who wrote the opinion for Karen Quinlan's case, "if Karen were herself miraculously lucid for an interval (not altering the existing prognosis of the condition to which she would soon return) and perceptive of her . . . condition, she [would] decide upon . . . [the decision of the court offered on her behalf]" (21). Substituted judgment is an intrinsically difficult concept and is just as difficult to implement in reality. Understanding what a person would want is hard enough in ordinary circumstances. Understanding what a person would want when the person is in a state that the proxy has never been in is even harder. When that state is such that the individual is incapable of having wishes, it is impossible. This last key difficulty centers on the fact that real-time wishes are being created when there are none. Commentators have noted that substituted judgment usually ends up being a version of best interest judgment. It may also end up being a version of prior-preference–guided judgment in that attempts are made to guess what the prior healthy person would have wanted if he or she could have anticipated the eventual condition.

Best interests judgment is somewhat easier conceptually, but still difficult to implement. The idea is to judge according to the best interests of the patient. It has this advantage: not only is real time used, but also there need be no reliance on notions of the patient's wishes. The difficulty for this concept is determining what the best interests of the patient are, since this involves highly subjective value assessments. It may also be the case that the patient is so debilitated and "absent" that ordinary real-time interests do not exist. Despite these difficulties, it is the best guiding standard available when prior preferences cannot be used.

## AUTHENTICITY OF WISHES

### Informed Consent and Competence Standards for Advance Directives

Patients' prior wishes are articulated in real time and must be held to the same standards as any other real-time decisions, namely, to ordinary standards of informed consent. Informed consent has received considerable attention, and its standards can be read about elsewhere (22–24). Although standards may evolve, for the present physicians should ensure that patients understand the nature of the decision, understand the alternatives, and understand the risks (common or serious) and benefits. Patients should be over 18 years of age, have decision-making capacity in the relevant areas, and give evidence of having made actual active decisions.

Informed consent specifically for advance directives can be considered in two parts. First, patients must consent to making out an advance directive. Patients must know what the basic procedures are (to discuss the issues and record preferences) and understand that traditional decision-making (having physicians and legal next of kin use their best judgment) is the alternative. They must know that there are risks either way (e.g., careless advance directives can lead to unintended actions, but traditional decision-making is known to correspond poorly to patients' wishes). To be competent in the use of instructional directives, patients have to be competent in the use of imagined scenarios. Otherwise, they will not be able to understand the intervention choices they are making for future potential situations. This is not as dissimilar as it may initially seem from real-time decisions, since real-time decisions are also based on how people think they will feel in the future while living with the consequences of the immediate decision.

Second, discussions of advance directives need to ensure adequate informed consent for any specific treatment decisions made. This can be difficult because of the large number of decisions included in some instructional directives and because of the sketchy nature of delineated scenarios in the advance directive. Many instructional directives specifically state that they are to be used as a guide to the patient's wishes rather than as a series of treatment decisions. For this reason, standards of informed consent can be relaxed to some degree. Nonetheless, the standards must be sufficient to provide an accurate picture of the patient's wishes. The use of well-designed brochures or other information packets that describe key interventions can help ensure informed consent standards. The key interventions should include resuscitation, mechanical respiration, chemotherapy or radiation therapy, dialysis, simple diagnostic tests, and pain control (including the potential side effect of respiratory depression). Whether or not information aids are used, physicians must ensure evidence of patients' comprehension.

### Valid Expressions

The validity of prior preferences can be judged in essentially the same way that the validity of real-time wishes is judged. Validation of predrafted instruments for the articulation of subjective matters is a well-developed discipline in itself. Generally speaking, instruments must meet standards of content validity, construct validity, criterion-related validity, and test-retest reliability. The first requires that the instrument cover the relevant content matter, the second that items in the instrument be constructed to fit the concepts of the subject matter, the third that the items bear sensible relationships to existing relevant scales and to one another, and the fourth that if the same items were used over again at a different time a reasonably similar set of responses would be obtained (15). Predrafted advance directives should meet these standards, as adapted to the needs of advance directives (19).

An efficient way for physicians to assist patients in valid expressions and recordings of prior preferences is to provide them with a validated predrafted instructional directive and go through it. If patients have been able to complete such a directive, meeting standards of informed consent for the wishes they express, then the statements recorded must be considered valid.

## HOW TO DO IT

### Five Steps in a Continuing Process

The creation of recorded advance directives is one step in a longitudinal process that should be integrated into the totality of clinical care. Although five steps can be identified, they will rarely be so distinct in actual practice. First is raising the topic. Second, and most important, is structuring a core discussion to cover the main issues and start the patient thinking about his or her views. Third is reviewing the final document and putting it in the medical record. Fourth is updating the directive from time to time. Fifth is ensuring its availability and use, applying it to decisions that arise after the patient has become wishless (25).

### *Raising the Topic, Providing Background Information, and Advising on Proxy Choice*

First, the topic must be raised. This may be the hardest part, although among physician groups, oncologists may be the best at it. Both providers and patients need to be comfortable with the idea that advance planning should be a routine part of good practice, and providers need skill and experience in conducting the requisite conversations. Once expected and routinized, it is a surprisingly easy matter.

With whom should the topic be raised? Among oncology patients, everyone should have the opportunity for advance care planning, whether the prognosis for cure is excellent or poor. Occasionally, patients will have discussed advance care planning with their primary care or other physician. The oncologist can build on this foundation. The topic should not be avoided on the assumption that it has been dealt with. Patients who have completed advance care planning before receiving their oncologic diagnosis may have since changed their perspective. The extent and structure of the planning may not have been as good as that the oncologist can offer. Most important of all, the oncologist needs to know the substance of the patient's current health advance care planning.

In an oncology or a palliative care practice, the topic can be raised by the fourth or fifth visit, depending on the emotional and medical circumstances. Time should be allowed before advance care planning for confirmation of the diagnosis, exploration of treatment options, establishment of a solid therapeutic relationship, and some adjustment by the patient to his or her diagnosis. Earlier mention, say at the second or third visit, that advance planning will be a component of routine care (as should occur for all patients with or without cancer) can facilitate the process. In a long-term care facility, an analogous process is possible, with early mention that the discussion will occur, within the first 3 months of a patient's residency.

One fashion in which the topic can be raised is as follows:

"Ms/r. X, I want to talk with you about planning for future medical care. Many now recommend that people make plans whether or not they have an illness, and that doctors discuss these issues routinely with patients. There is even a federal law that aims to let people know that advance planning is available to all people. We should go through these issues together. It is part of getting to know your values and helping to ensure that you are cared for the way you would want to be even in times of life-threatening illness when communication may be impossible. There is nothing new about your health, and I am not hiding bad news that we have not already discussed; planning for the future simply is prudent. Is this something you have explored before?"

It is helpful to be able to add, as is true for many oncologists:

"I myself have done this as a routine matter, despite being in good health."

Some issues for the patient to consider in selecting a proxy can be included at this point, in particular that being a proxy is a complex and burdensome task, and that family members and close friends may have interests that conflict with the patient's. Most people prefer to select someone close to them as a proxy nonetheless, and usually for good reason, but the possibilities of appointing a more distant friend or a professional such as a social worker or lawyer are worth considering. Some patients suggest appointing the physician as proxy. Since the idea of a proxy is to have someone to talk with the physician, this is not usually the best idea. The patient should be reassured that the physician will in any case be working to make the best decision for the patient and additional proxy powers are usually unnecessary; participation by the physician in creating a written directive, perhaps without a designated proxy, assists the aspiration.

Nonphysician health care providers can assist in the first step of raising the topic and providing background information. Brochures and predrafted forms and videos or closed-circuit television programs can also be made available in patient information libraries and patient rooms.

### *Structured Discussion*

Second, the topic must be discussed. The proxy should be present at this discussion whenever possible. He or she can be advised to listen and limit participation to needed clarification, in preparation for the potential role of speaking for the patient, and may even act as scribe, penciling down the patient's statements.

The most efficient way of structuring a discussion is simply to go through a validated blank directive, using it as a worksheet (19). The sections can be gone through systematically. Using a pencil rather than a pen to fill in the patient's wishes, and having the pencil in the patient's or proxy's hand, can help to emphasize explicitly that in this discussion the directive is being used as a worksheet and not a final document. When scenario-based documents are used, it is possible to start the discussion in something like the following fashion:

"Let's look at these standardized circumstances. We will go through three and then perhaps another one or two more.

"Imagine this first case in the worksheet. You are in a coma with no awareness. Assume there is a chance that you might wake up, but it isn't likely, and recovery may involve serious disability.

Some people would want us to withdraw treatment and let them die, others would want us to attempt everything possible, and yet others would want us to try to restore quality of life but stop treatment if it was not working. What do you think your goals for medical care would be?"

Useful scenarios to go through include (a) a coma with a small chance of recovery (as above), (b) a persistent vegetative state, and (c) a moribund state with waxing and waning consciousness. In each scenario the patient's goals for care are illustrated with some selected intervention preferences. The commonly considered intervention preferences are (a) resuscitation (b) mechanical respiration (c) chemo- or radiation therapy (d) renal dialysis (e) major surgery, and (f) artificial nutrition/hydration. In addition, preferences regarding (g) simple diagnostic tests and (h) antibiotics provide useful information. Finally, preferences should be elicited on (i) comfort measures such as pain medications when they may hasten death by causing respiratory depression. Most people can also say whether pain control or being alert and unconfused to the last possible moment is more important to them. Although not a great deal of time need be spent on informed consent for each intervention, it is wise to provide brochures on the interventions for patients to review on their own time.

The first three or so scenarios should be standard scenarios designed to cover the major situations commonly encountered when advance directives pertain. Then two or three additional scenarios can be used that are tailored to the patient. One may be created by the physician, based on the patient's illness and expectable circumstances (26). Another may be created by the patient if he or she wishes, based on what the patient considers to be a state worse than death that has not already been covered in previous scenarios (27). It can also be important to consider a scenario in which the patient is in his or her current health

and acquires a new life-threatening illness involving incompetence.

After these scenarios, patients can be asked what, if anything, they would consider to be "good dying." Most can say, for instance, that they want enough time to settle things with people they are involved with, that they want to have done one particular thing, or that they want to be in a particular place. Elicitation of these images of a good dying should not be construed as promises to fulfill them; rather, the physician should tell the patient that the images may help in orchestrating care that frees the patient as much as possible to do as he or she wishes with the last stages of life, before unconsciousness or death occur.

There are certain key positions that patients should be encouraged to articulate during or after their consideration of the scenarios. One is their position on withholding versus withdrawing life-sustaining therapy, since some people have strong positions on the distinction or lack thereof between the two, and it is well to have a specific indication whether or not an unwanted intervention, if in place already, should be withdrawn. Another topic that can be included in the scenarios is the place of pain control. Use of pain medications intended to control pain but with a known side effect of hastening death is generally considered morally acceptable. Physician-assisted suicide, while not generally accepted, is receiving wide attention, and it may be helpful to clearly articulate preferences and positions on this matter. Physicians who have patients requesting actions they cannot condone should advise the patients of the fact at this early stage. Similarly, the proxy should raise objections at this stage if necessary.

This entire process need take no more than 15 minutes once the physician has gained experience with it. The intent is not to reach final resolution or to elicit extended narratives. Rather, it is to identify the key issues that patients should think about and to provide them with a good method for recording their preferences. Nonetheless, during these steps patients commonly communicate deeply held values. Witnessing such expressions can give physicians a strong sense of the privilege of caring for patients, and the knowledge that ensues about how health issues fit with the individual patient's sense of meaning in life can be of great practical importance. Reciprocally, patients can feel clearer, more understood, and confident.

Patients should be encouraged to absorb the informational materials and talk over all the issues with their family, friends, pastor, lawyer, counselor, or whomever they consider to be relevant. The patient should then prepare a final statement, preferably in a fashion that includes a validated advisory form and a statutory form that can then be stapled together if they are not already combined.

### Finalizing and Recording the Document

Once the patient has completed the essential personal discussions outside the physician's office, he or she can bring the document in for final review by the physician. At this point, the physician can check for medical misconceptions and major changes that may need inquiry. This should take only a few moments in most cases. It is useful to have a space where the physician can cosign the document (28). This signature should not be a requirement, but its presence fosters the physician's involvement and carries an important implicit message of partnership between patient and physician.

### Updating the Document

Documents should be reviewed at routine intervals. For a patient who has undergone a cure or for whom the prognosis is good, this review should occur every 1 to 5 years and after major life changes such as childbirth, marriage, divorce, significant health status changes, bereavement, and important experiences of others' ill health. Most reviews will be rapid. Specific treatment decisions are about as durable as other major life decisions, such as marriage (29–32). When a patient shows a particularly high level of instability, this may indicate incompetence for advance decision-making, and the physician should review the matter, perhaps advising simple designation of a proxy instead of instructional directives.

### Applying the Document to Real Decisions

Certain patterns of decisions have high degrees of predictability. If a patient's prior directives do not cover the decision at hand, it may well be possible to extrapolate from the preferences that are provided in the directive. Such predictions can be far more accurate than unguided judgments. Decline of less invasive interventions predicts decline of more invasive interventions, and acceptance of more invasive interventions predicts acceptance of less invasive interventions. Acceptance of intervention in poor-prognosis scenarios predicts acceptance in better-prognosis scenarios, and decline in better-prognosis scenarios predicts decline in poorer prognoses. The use of simple calculations can even provide probability estimates of specific decisions, which, when very high or very low, can be a comforting guide to proxy decision-makers (33). This approach is illustrated and necessary reference statistics are provided in Appendix 1 and Tables 58-1 and 58-2.

### Pitfalls and Preventive Measures

As advance directives gradually come into more general use, common pitfalls are emerging (34). Assessment of a patient's competence to undertake advance care planning can be difficult if profound psychological issues or psychiatric diagnoses are involved. Occasionally, for instance, a patient will show major inconsistency in treatment plans or will ask for extremes of no treatment or undue intervention. These may be indications of ineffective emotional adjustment to medical circumstance. Although perhaps not strictly incompetent for completing advance directives, these patients may do better using proxy designation rather than instructional directives to preserve flexible decision-making. Alternatively, advance care planning can be deferred or updated frequently until psychotherapy or other assistance has secured better emotional adjustment.

A further problem is noninclusion of relevant parties at early stages of planning. Noninclusion of the proxy or of family members or close friends who have divergent opinions can lead to fractured decision-making. Noninclusion of the physician can lead to inadequate sensitization of the physician to the patient's thinking. For instance, a recent major study showed that when a nurse is the main communicator in advance planning, the physician's understanding of the patient's wishes is not improved (35).

Poor informed consent and documentation constitute another pair of pitfalls. For example, a patient may express a strong desire to avoid perpetual dependence on a respirator, but the wording of the advance directive may indicate that a respirator should never be used. In the event of reversible pneumonia, the patient may well want temporary use of a respirator. A properly validated directive should require this kind of distinction, and physicians should ensure this minimum level of patients' understanding. Physicians should check the document for improbable statements and ask patients to briefly state their wishes in free words, checking for correspondence with medical possibilities.

Perhaps the most common pitfall of all is activation of advance directives before patients have reached a wishless state, and sometimes even before they have reached an incompetent state for the decision(s) at hand. A widespread tendency to avoid direct communication with patients appears to exacerbate this problem. Advance directives, as distinct from their predecessor, the Do Not Resuscitate order, have no authority when they are first written and must not be activated until the patient is decisionally incapacitated and wishless.

A final crucial pitfall is poor application of wishes to eventual decisions. Some studies have indicated that physicians rather commonly override advance directives (36). Whether this is because patients are decisionally incapacitated but not wishless, or because proxy opinions persuade physicians more than the patient's advance directives, or for other reasons is not well studied. Nonetheless, if a patient has a validated advance directive that uses scenarios and specific intervention choices, extrapolation to unstated decisions can be accomplished with considerable accuracy in many cases.

## BROADER USES

### Structured Deliberation

An unforeseen benefit brought about by the idea of advance directives was a general increase in attention to the questions of how patients' health care values can be elicited, understood, documented, and used as the driving force behind therapeutic decision-making. In a sense, the field emerged from a desire to move the medical question from "What is the right decision?" to "Who should make the decision?" with the intended answer being "the patient." However, as the desirability of multilateral decision-making became more accepted, the question has become "What is the right kind of deliberative process for the decision?" This latter question is potentially relevant to a wide range of decisions and circumstances. In delineating a set of validated worksheets and structured deliberations for advance directives, the concept of structured deliberation for a wide range of medical decisions and approaches has emerged (37,38).

### Structuring Other Care Plans

The use of care plans need not be limited to scenarios involving incompetence and wishlessness. Plans can usefully be made for situations involving no loss of competence as well. Nursing home and hospice facilities often make use of such plans. A common example is prior decision-making regarding transfer to a hospital facility in case of medical deterioration. Those who decline may have a written "Do Not Hospitalize" order. Similar decisions about levels of medical care within the facility can also be made. For instance, some patients may elect comfort care only, whereas others may elect simple diagnostic maneuvers but no invasive ones, and others may elect full aggressive care. Corresponding orders and/or notes can be written in patients' records. Such decisions must always be subject to change if the patient wishes, just as advance directives are adjustable while the patient is competent. Nonetheless, such planning provides important communication and often streamlines decision-making in the event of otherwise difficult decisions.

### Intervention for Turbulent Thought Processes

Patients in difficult medical circumstances often face existential decisions. Turbulent emotions and turbulent thinking are common. For instance, a patient may understand that he or she has incurable cancer and therefore decline chemotherapy, but when faced with the need to make a decision about resuscitation may be precipitated into an emotional crisis by the sense of imminent death or impending abandonment and may decline a "Do Not Resuscitate" order. Such decisions are often perplexing to providers, and discord between parties readily ensues. Discord over goals or treatment decisions should alert physicians to the likelihood that patients are facing emotional and moral turbulence. A structured dialogue can be very helpful. The preset scenarios in a validated generic advance directive provide an excellent structure. By going back over preset scenarios that the patient knows were designed independently and that cover questions likely to be relevant (because the document is validated), the physician may be able to discern the structure of the patient's nonturbulent moral thought. With the more stable structure returned, it is possible to reapproach a scenario that is tailored to the patient and, finally, the patient's current situation. Often, the patient no longer feels threatened by the sense of imminent mortality, and coherent thought processes and decisions can occur again. If these discussions are conducted in the presence of the proxy and other relevant care providers, there can be a refocusing of the entire group of providers on the retrieved coherent plan. Difficult personal interactions and time-consuming confusions can be put aside, allowing people to get on with the business of preparing for departure on a personally meaningful level.

Structured deliberations such as these can also provide an approach to patients who request euthanasia or physician-assisted suicide. Some patients may have firm and persuasive reasons for requesting such actions, but many patients are in fact seeking something else. Some seek control, some attempt to avoid pain, and some try to address concerns about being a burden or being abandoned. A structured path through scenarios allows patients to assert control and gain assurances that pain can be controlled in the great majority of cases, that there are ways of planning for burden and nonabandonment, and that there are ways to exit this world without active euthanasia or assisted suicide. Some physicians find active euthanasia morally defensible in some instances, and others do not. But all must agree that patients who request it erroneously, actually seeking care, should be identified and guided toward the actions they really desire. Structured deliberations can provide a sensitive, professional, and efficient method to help patients understand their own desires. Importantly, they also provide the physician with a chance to communicate explicitly what their moral position is; physicians who do not find active euthanasia or physician-assisted suicide acceptable can make this clear in the supportive setting while simultaneously making clear what comfort care they can offer.

## LIMITATIONS AND FUTURE DIRECTIONS

As important as advance directives may be, they have clear limitations and should not be construed as a panacea for decision-making about life-sustaining interventions. Especially in the case of moderately demented patients or otherwise decisionally incapacitated but not wishless patients, advance directives offer no more than tangible evidence of one among other perspectives to be weighed in the decision. Even for wishless patients, advance directives provide a way to augment the honoring of surviving interests, but they do not offer perfect evidence of all relevant wishes.

## No Evidence for Cost Savings

Some advocates have suggested that the use of advance directives can effect considerable cost savings. This perspective has been motivated by the assumption that their use would help avoid unwanted and costly interventions and therefore help reduce the costs of medical care. While end-of-life care is very costly, there is evidence that patients tend to opt for more treatment than physicians and nurses, and that proxies opt for even more intervention (39,40). In addition, although hospice and palliative care have traditionally been less costly than hospital care for dying patients, these populations are self-selecting. A randomized controlled trial found no cost savings, perhaps indicating that patients, taken in the aggregate, may be getting more or less the degree of intervention that they want (41,42). Individual matches with patients' wishes are, however, found to be poor in many studies, and advance planning should continue with the goal of closing this gap. These motivations for advance planning have overwhelming independent merit and should not be confused with false economic incentives.

## When Patients Have No Advance Directive

About half of all patients have an estate will. If even this form of well-accepted planning for death is not used by more patients, it is likely that advance directives will also have a similar "ceiling." To meet the objective of attempting to match decisions with patients' prior preferences, it can be helpful to have supplementary approaches (43). In circumstances when the patient comes from a population of patients whose preferences have been studied and documented, it is possible refer to those data to help guide decisions for them. Thus, if it is known that the patients registered at the hospital in question declined resuscitation for the situation at hand in 85% of instances, the proxy may find this useful guiding information. In cases when the proxy has no idea how to speak on behalf of the patient, the physician may indicate that the greatest likelihood of matching the patient's prior wishes, if only the patient had had a chance to articulate them, will be by following the majority preferences of others. Naturally, these default guidelines should not be coercive or replace valid personal directives.

## APPENDIX 1

### The Medical Directive

*Introduction.* As a part of person's right to self-determination, every adult may accept or refuse any recommended medical treatment. This is relatively easy when people are well and can speak. Unfortunately, during serious illness they are often unconscious or otherwise unable to communicate their wishes—at the very time when many critical decisions need to be made.

The Medical Directive allows you to record your wishes regarding various types of medical treatments in several representative situations so that your desires can be respected. It also lets you appoint a proxy, someone to make medical decision in your place if you should become unable to make them on your own.

The Medical Directive comes into effect only if you become incompetent (unable to make decisions and too sick to have wishes). You can change it at any time until then. As long as you are competent, you should discuss your care directly with your physician.

*Completing the form.* You should, if possible complete the form in the context of a discussion with your physician. ideally, this should occur in the presence of your proxy. This lets your physician and your proxy know how to think about these decisions, and it provides you and your physician with the opportunity to give or clarify relevant personal or medical information. You may also wish to discuss the issues with your family, friends, or religious mentor.

The Medical Directive contains six illness situations that include incompetence. For each one, you consider possible interventions and goals of medical care. Situation A is permanent coma; B is near death; C is with weeks to live in and out of consciousness; D, is extreme dementia; E is a situation you describe; and F is temporary inability to make decisions.

For each scenario you identify your general goals for care and specific intervention choices. The interventions are divided into six groups: 1) cardiopulmonary resuscitation or major surgery; 2) mechanical breathing or dialysis; 3) blood transfusions or blood products; 4) artificial nutrition and hydration; 5) simple diagnostic tests or antibiotics; and 6) pain medications, even if they dull consciousness and indirectly shorten life. Most of these treatments are described briefly. if you further questions, consult your physician.

Your wishes for treatment options (I want this treatment; I want this treatment tried, but stopped if there is no clear improvement, I am undecided; I do not want this treatment) should be indicated. If you choose a trail of treatment, you should understand that this indicates you want the treatment *withdrawn* if your physician and proxy believe that it has become futile.

The Personal Statement section allows you to explain your choices, and say anything you wish to those who may make decisions for your concerning the limits of your life and the goals of intervention. For example, in situation B, if you wish to define "uncertain chance" with numerical probability, you may do so here.

Next you may express your preferences concerning organ donation. Do you wish to donate your body or some or all of your organs after your death? If so, for what purpose(s) and to which physician or institution? If not, this should also be indicated in the appropriate box.

In the final section you may designate one or more proxies, who would be asked to make choices under circumstances in which your wishes are unclear. You can indicae whether or not the decisions of the proxy should override your wishes if there are differences. And, should you name more than one proxy, you can state who is to have the final say if there is disagreement. Your proxy must understand that this role usually involves making judgments that you would have made for yourself, had you been able—and making them by

the criteria you have outlined. Proxy decisions should ideally be made in discussion with your family, friends, and physician.

*What to do with the form.* Once you have completed the form, you and two adult witnesses (other than your proxy) who have no interest in your estate need to sign and date it.

Many states have legislation covering documents of this sort. To determine the laws in your state, you should call the state attorney general's office or consult a lawyer. If your stat has a statutory document, you may wish to use the Medical Directive and append it to this form.

You should give a copy of the completed document to your physician. His or her signature is desirable but not mandatory. The Directive should be placed in your medical records and flagged so that anyone who might be involved in your care can be aware of its presence. Your proxy, a family member, and/or a friend should also have a copy. In addition, you may want to carry a wallet card noting that you have such a document and where it can be found.

---

## MY MEDICAL DIRECTIVE

This Medical Directive shall stand as a guide to my wishes regarding medical treatments in the event that illness should make me unable to communicate them directly. I make this Directive, being 18 years or more of age, of sound mind, and appreciating the consequences of my decisions.

## SITUATION A

If I am in a coma or a persistent vegetative state and, in the opinion of my physician and two consultants, have no known hope of regaining awareness and higher mental functions no matter what is done, then my goals and specific wishes—if medically reasonable—for this and may additional illness would be:

☐ prolong life; treat everything
☐ attempt to cure, but reevaluate often
☐ limit to less invasive and less burdensome interventions
☐ provide comfort care only
☐ other *(please specify):* _____

*Please check appropriate boxes:*

1. **Cardiopulmonary resuscitation** (chest compressions, drugs, electric shocks, and artificial breathing aimed at reviving a person who is on the point of dying). _____
2. **Major surgery** (for example, removing the gallbladder or part of the colon). _____
3. **Mechanical breathing** (respiration by machine, through a tube in the throat). _____
4. **Dialysis** (cleaning the blood by machine or by fluid passed through the belly). _____
5. **Blood transfusions or blood products.**

   _____
6. **Artificial nutrition and hydration** (given through a tube in a vein or in the stomach). _____
7. **Simple diagnostic tests** (for example, blood tests or x-rays).

   _____
8. **Antibiotics** (drugs used to fight infection).

   _____
9. **Pain medication, even if they dull consciousness and indirectly shorten my life.**

| I want | I want treatment tried. If no clear improvement, stop | I am undecided | I do not want |
|---|---|---|---|
|  | Not applicable |  |  |
|  | Not applicable |  |  |
|  |  |  |  |
|  |  |  |  |
|  | Not applicable |  |  |
|  |  |  |  |
|  | Not applicable |  |  |
|  | Not applicable |  |  |
|  | Not applicable |  |  |

## SITUATION B

If I am near death and in a coma and, in the opinion of my physician and two consultants, have a small but uncertain chance of regaining higher mental functions, a somewhat greater chance of surviving with permanent mental and physical disability, and a much greater chance of not recovering at all, then my goals and specific wishes—if medically reasonable—for this and any additional illness would be:

☐ prolong life; treat everything
☐ attempt to cure, but reevaluate often
☐ limit to less invasive and less burdensome interventions
☐ provide comfort care only
☐ other *(please specify):* _____

*Please check appropriate boxes:*

1. **Cardiopulmonary resuscitation** (chest compressions, drugs, electric shocks, and artificial breathing aimed at reviving a person who is on the point of dying). _____
2. **Major surgery** (for example, removing the gallbladder or part of the colon). _____
3. **Mechanical breathing** (respiration by machine, through a tube in the throat). _____
4. **Dialysis** (cleaning the blood by machine or by fluid passed through the belly). _____
5. **Blood transfusions or blood products.**

   _____
6. **Artificial nutrition and hydration** (given through a tube in a vein or in the stomach). _____
7. **Simple diagnostic tests** (for example, blood tests or x-rays).

   _____
8. **Antibiotics** (drugs used to fight infection).

   _____
9. **Pain medication, even if they dull consciousness and indirectly shorten my life.**

| I want | I want treatment tried. If no clear improvement, stop | I am undecided | I do not want |
|---|---|---|---|
|  | Not applicable |  |  |
|  | Not applicable |  |  |
|  |  |  |  |
|  |  |  |  |
|  | Not applicable |  |  |
|  |  |  |  |
|  | Not applicable |  |  |
|  | Not applicable |  |  |
|  | Not applicable |  |  |

## SITUATION C

If I have a terminal illness with weeks to live, and my mind is not working well enough to make decisions for myself, but I am sometimes awake and seem to have feelings, then my goals and specific wishes—if medically reasonable—for this and any additional illness would be:

☐ prolong life; treat everything
☐ attempt to cure, but reevaluate often
☐ limit to less invasive and less burdensome interventions
☐ provide comfort care only
☐ other *(please specify):* _____

*In this state, prior wishes need to be balanced with a best guess about your current feelings. The proxy and physician have to make this judgment for you.

*Please check appropriate boxes:*

| | I want | I want treatment tried. If no clear improvement, stop | I am undecided | I do not want |
|---|---|---|---|---|
| 1. **Cardiopulmonary resuscitation** (chest compressions, drugs, electric shocks, and artificial breathing aimed at reviving a person who is on the point of dying). ___ | | Not applicable | | |
| 2. **Major surgery** (for example, removing the gallbladder or part of the colon). ___ | | Not applicable | | |
| 3. **Mechanical breathing** (respiration by machine, through a tube in the throat). ___ | | | | |
| 4. **Dialysis** (cleaning the blood by machine or by fluid passed through the belly). ___ | | | | |
| 5. **Blood transfusions or blood products.** ___ | | Not applicable | | |
| 6. **Artificial nutrition and hydration** (given through a tube in a vein or in the stomach). ___ | | | | |
| 7. **Simple diagnostic tests** (for example, blood tests or x-rays). ___ | | Not applicable | | |
| 8. **Antibiotics** (drugs used to fight infection). ___ | | Not applicable | | |
| 9. **Pain medication, even if they dull consciousness and indirectly shorten my life.** | | Not applicable | | |

## SITUATION D

If I have brain damage or some brain disease that in the opinion of my physician and two consultants cannot be reversed and that makes me unable to think or have feelings, *but I have no terminal illness,* then my goals and specific wishes—if medically reasonable—for this and any additional illness would be:

☐ prolong life; treat everything
☐ attempt to cure, but reevaluate often
☐ limit to less invasive and less burdensome interventions
☐ provide comfort care only
☐ other *(please specify):* _____

*Please check appropriate boxes:*

| | I want | I want treatment tried. If no clear improvement, stop | I am undecided | I do not want |
|---|---|---|---|---|
| 1. **Cardiopulmonary resuscitation** (chest compressions, drugs, electric shocks, and artificial breathing aimed at reviving a person who is on the point of dying). ___ | | Not applicable | | |
| 2. **Major surgery** (for example, removing the gallbladder or part of the colon). ___ | | Not applicable | | |
| 3. **Mechanical breathing** (respiration by machine, through a tube in the throat). ___ | | | | |
| 4. **Dialysis** (cleaning the blood by machine or by fluid passed through the belly). ___ | | | | |
| 5. **Blood transfusions or blood products.** ___ | | Not applicable | | |
| 6. **Artificial nutrition and hydration** (given through a tube in a vein or in the stomach). ___ | | | | |
| 7. **Simple diagnostic tests** (for example, blood tests or x-rays). ___ | | Not applicable | | |
| 8. **Antibiotics** (drugs used to fight infection). ___ | | Not applicable | | |
| 9. **Pain medication, even if they dull consciousness and indirectly shorten my life.** | | Not applicable | | |

## SITUATION E

If I . . .
(describe a situation that is important to you and/or your doctor believes you should consider in view of your current medical situation):

- ☐ prolong life; treat everything
- ☐ attempt to cure, but reevaluate often
- ☐ limit to less invasive and less burdensome interventions
- ☐ provide comfort care only
- ☐ other (please specify): _____

*Please check appropriate boxes:*

1. **Cardiopulmonary resuscitation** (chest compressions, drugs, electric shocks, and artificial breathing aimed at reviving a person who is on the point of dying). _____
2. **Major surgery** (for example, removing the gallbladder or part of the colon). _____
3. **Mechanical breathing** (respiration by machine, through a tube in the throat). _____
4. **Dialysis** (cleaning the blood by machine or by fluid passed through the belly). _____
5. **Blood transfusions or blood products.** _____
6. **Artificial nutrition and hydration** (given through a tube in a vein or in the stomach). _____
7. **Simple diagnostic tests** (for example, blood tests or x-rays). _____
8. **Antibiotics** (drugs used to fight infection). _____
9. **Pain medication, even if they dull consciousness and indirectly shorten my life.**

| I want | I want treatment tried. If no clear improvement, stop | I am undecided | I do not want |
|---|---|---|---|
| | Not applicable | | |
| | Not applicable | | |
| | | | |
| | | | |
| | Not applicable | | |
| | | | |
| | Not applicable | | |
| | Not applicable | | |
| | Not applicable | | |

---

## SITUATION F

If I am in my current state of health (describe briefly): _____ and then have an illness that, in the opinion of my physician and two consultants, is life threatening but reversible, and I am temporarily unable to make decisions, then my goals and specific wishes—if medically reasonable—would be:

- ☐ prolong life; treat everything
- ☐ attempt to cure, but reevaluate often
- ☐ limit to less invasive and less burdensome interventions
- ☐ provide comfort care only
- ☐ other (please specify): _____

*Please check appropriate boxes:*

1. **Cardiopulmonary resuscitation** (chest compressions, drugs, electric shocks, and artificial breathing aimed at reviving a person who is on the point of dying). _____
2. **Major surgery** (for example, removing the gallbladder or part of the colon). _____
3. **Mechanical breathing** (respiration by machine, through a tube in the throat). _____
4. **Dialysis** (cleaning the blood by machine or by fluid passed through the belly). _____
5. **Blood transfusions or blood products.** _____
6. **Artificial nutrition and hydration** (given through a tube in a vein or in the stomach). _____
7. **Simple diagnostic tests** (for example, blood tests or x-rays). _____
8. **Antibiotics** (drugs used to fight infection). _____
9. **Pain medication, even if they dull consciousness and indirectly shorten my life.**

| I want | I want treatment tried. If no clear improvement, stop | I am undecided | I do not want |
|---|---|---|---|
| | Not applicable | | |
| | Not applicable | | |
| | | | |
| | | | |
| | Not applicable | | |
| | | | |
| | Not applicable | | |
| | Not applicable | | |
| | Not applicable | | |

## HEALTH CARE PROXY

I appoint as my proxy decision-maker(s):

_____ and _____
Name and Address   *(optional)*   Name and Address

I direct my proxy to make health-care decisions based on his/her assessment of my personal wishes. If my personal desires are unknown, my proxy is to make health-care decisions based on his/her best guess as to my wishes. My proxy shall have the authority to make all health-care decisions for me, including decisions about life-sustaining treatment, if I am unable to make them myself. My proxy's authority becomes effective if my attending physician determines in writing that I lack the capacity to make or to communicate health-care decisions. My proxy is then to have the same authority to make health-care decisions as I would if I had the capacity to make them, EXCEPT *(list the limitations, if any, you wish to place on your proxy's authority):*

*I wish my written preference to be applied as exactly as possible/with flexibility according to my proxy's judgment.* (Delete as appropriate)

Should there be any disagreement between the wishes I have indicated in this document and the decisions favored by my above-named proxy, I wish my proxy to have authority over my written statements/I wish my written statements to bind my proxy. *(Delete as appropriate)*

If I have appointed more than one proxy and there is disagreement between their wishes, _____ shall have final authority.

Signed:
Signature _____   Printed Name _____
Address _____   Date _____
Witness:
Signature _____   Printed Name _____
Address _____   Date _____
Witness:
Signature _____   Printed Name _____
Address _____   Date _____

Physician *(optional):*
*I am _____'s physician. I have seen this advance care document and have had an opportunity to discuss his/her preferences regarding medical interventions at the end of life. If _____becomes incompetent, I understand that it is my duty to interpret and implement the preferences contained in this document in order to fulfill his/her wishes.*

An earlier version of this form was originally published as part of an article by Linda L. Emmanuel and Ezekiel J. Emanuel. "The Medical Directive: A New Comprehensive Advance Care Document," *Journal of the American Medical Association* 261:3288–3293, June 9, 1989. It does not reflect the official policy of the American Medical Association.

*Signed:*
Signature _____   *Printed Name* _____
Address _____   Date _____

## ORGAN DONATION

—I hereby make this anatomical gift, to take effect after my death:

I give
☐ my body
☐ any needed organs or parts
☐ the following parts _____

to

☐ the following person or institution _____
☐ the physician in attendance at my death
☐ the hospital in which I die
☐ the following physician, hospital storage bank, or other medical institution: _____

for

☐ any purpose authorized by law
☐ therapy of another person
☐ medical education
☐ transplantation
☐ research

—I do not wish to make any anatomical gift from my body.

## MY PERSONAL STATEMENT

*(Use additional page if necessary)*
Please mention anything that would be important for your physician and your proxy to know. In particular, try to answer the following questions: 1) What medical conditions, if any, would make living so unpleasant that you would want life-sustaining treatment *withheld?* (Intractable pain? Irreversible mental damage? Inability to share love? Dependence on others? Another condition you would regard as intolerable?) 2) Under what medical circumstances would you want to stop interventions that might already have been started? 3) Why do you choose what you choose?

If there is any difference between my preferences detailed in the illness situations and those understood from my goals or from my personal statement, I wish my treatment selections/my goals/my personal statement *(please delete as appropriate)* to be given greater weight.

When I am dying, I would like—if my proxy and my health-care team think it is reasonable—to be cared for:

☐ at home or in a hospice
☐ in a nursing home
☐ in a hospital
☐ other *(please specify):* _____

## APPENDIX 2

### Extrapolating Stated Preferences

It is often necessary to infer a prior preference, since advance directives cannot foresee all possible decisions. In addition to using the general rules noted in the text of the chapter, it may be possible to use what a patient did state along with population preference data to calculate the probability that a particular prior preference would have been made if the patient had considered it. For many physicians and proxies, these calculations are very reassuring.

Survey preference data from patients completing the Medical Directive provide prior odds for treatment preferences (see Table 58-1). The same data allow particular preferences to be used as a "test" for other particular preferences. Each decision pair has a likelihood ratio that has been calculated from this data set. So if the patient stated a prior preference that fits the test preference, the likelihood for all other decisions on the Medical Directive can

be found (see Table 58-2 and its accompanying explanatory footnotes). Together, the prior odds of a preference and the likelihood ratio of the relevant preference pair can be used to calculated the posterior odds that a patient would have had a particular preference.[32]

Take the following example:

A patient who is unconscious and has a small chance of recovery has an advance directive stating that (s)he does not want artificial feeding in such a situation, but the question is whether to write a "Do Not Resuscitate" order. The family have no idea what the patient would have wanted. From Table 1 we see that the prior odds of declining resuscitation in this circumstance is 1.2 (55% of the population declined it). We also know from Table 2 that the likelihood ratio for this decision is 12.6. Therefore, the posterior odds are $1.2 \times 12.6 = 15.1$ that (s)he would have declined resuscitation. Therefore, the posterior probability that (s)he would have stated a wish to decline CPR in an advance directive is $15.1/(1 - 15.1) = 94\%$.

**TABLE 1.** *Prior odds for treatment choices*

| Rx | Coma/Chance | | PVS | | Dementia | | Dementia/Terminal | |
|---|---|---|---|---|---|---|---|---|
| | Decline | Accept | Decline | Accept | Decline | Accept | Decline | Accept |
| abx | 0.9 | 1.1 | 3.1 | 0.3 | 1.9 | 0.5 | 3.3 | 0.3 |
| blood | 1.2 | 0.9 | 4.2 | 0.2 | 2.5 | 0.4 | 4.6 | 0.2 |
| cpr | 1.3 | 0.8 | 4.8 | 0.2 | 2.4 | 0.4 | 4.7 | 0.2 |
| dxc | 0.8 | 1.2 | 3.7 | 0.3 | 2.4 | 0.4 | 4.2 | 0.2 |
| dxs | 0.9 | 1.1 | 2.3 | 0.4 | 1.6 | 0.6 | 2.7 | 0.4 |
| feed | 1.2 | 0.8 | 4.0 | 0.3 | 2.7 | 0.4 | 4.2 | 0.2 |
| iv | 1.1 | 0.9 | 3.3 | 0.3 | 2.4 | 0.4 | 4.0 | 0.3 |
| ormaj | 1.6 | 0.6 | 5.1 | 0.2 | 3.0 | 0.3 | 5.3 | 0.2 |
| ormin | 1.3 | 0.8 | 4.1 | 0.2 | 2.2 | 0.5 | 3.9 | 0.3 |
| dialysis | 1.3 | 0.8 | 4.1 | 0.2 | 2.6 | 0.4 | 4.6 | 0.2 |
| resp | 1.2 | 0.8 | 4.0 | 0.3 | 2.7 | 0.4 | 4.8 | 0.2 |

Letter abbreviations: abx, antibiotics; blood, blood transfusions; cpr, cardiopulmonary resuscitation; dxc, invasive diagnostics; dxs, noninvasive diagnostics; feed, artificial tube feeding; iv, intravenous fluids; ormaj, major operations; ormin, minor operations; dialysis, peritoneal or hemodialysis; resp, mechanical respiration; coma/chance, coma with a chance of recovery; PVS, persistent vegetative state; dementia/terminal, dementia with terminal illness.

The prior odds for preferences are derived from population data that have been published elsewhere (44). The assumption is that prior odds of a given choice = (proportion of population with that choice)/(1 − proportion of population with that choice).

Some proxies or physicians will have reason to understand that the patient was not well represented by the population data. In these cases, if a calculation is still desired, a numerical estimate of the prior odds will have to be derived from whatever information is available.

**TABLE 2.** *Defining and using likelihood ratios for preference pairs*

Likelihood ratio of declines- all scenarios and treatments.

| | abx1 | abx2 | abx3 | abx4 | blood1 | blood2 | blood3 | blood4 | cpr1 | cpr2 | cpr3 | cpr4 | dxc1 | dxc2 | dxc3 | dxc4 | dxs1 | dxs2 | dxs3 | dxs4 | feed1 | feed2 |
|---|---|---|---|---|---|---|---|---|---|---|---|---|---|---|---|---|---|---|---|---|---|---|
| abx1 | . | 1.6 | 1.9 | 1.6 | 8.7 | 1.4 | 1.6 | 1.4 | 5.7 | 1.4 | 1.6 | 1.3 | 6.7 | 1.4 | 1.6 | 1.4 | 18.1 | 1.7 | 2.0 | 1.6 | 7.0 | 1.5 |
| abx2 | 4.9 | . | 2.7 | 2.4 | 2.7 | 3.9 | 2.0 | 1.9 | 2.6 | 2.6 | 2.2 | 1.9 | 3.0 | 4.6 | 2.3 | 1.9 | 3.7 | 12.2 | 2.7 | 2.4 | 2.5 | 3.8 |
| abx3 | 3.4 | 1.8 | . | 2.6 | 2.3 | 1.6 | 5.5 | 1.9 | 2.4 | 1.6 | 5.8 | 1.7 | 2.2 | 1.7 | 5.4 | 1.9 | 3.4 | 2.0 | 52.5 | 2.7 | 2.5 | 1.7 |
| abx4 | 5.7 | 2.7 | 11.9 | . | 3.0 | 2.2 | 3.8 | 4.2 | 3.0 | 2.0 | 4.0 | 3.4 | 2.6 | 2.4 | 4.4 | 4.3 | 5.5 | 2.9 | 8.8 | 26.6 | 3.8 | 2.4 |
| blood1 | 68.0 | 1.5 | 1.7 | 1.5 | . | 1.4 | 1.7 | 1.4 | 7.0 | 1.3 | 1.6 | 1.3 | 8.0 | 1.4 | 1.6 | 1.4 | 32.7 | 1.5 | 1.9 | 1.5 | 9.0 | 1.4 |
| blood2 | 4.1 | 21.9 | 3.0 | 2.9 | 3.3 | . | 3.0 | 2.4 | 2.7 | 3.6 | 2.8 | 2.3 | 2.7 | 7.5 | 2.8 | 2.2 | 3.7 | 27.0 | 3.2 | 2.8 | 2.9 | 5.3 |
| blood3 | 3.4 | 1.8 | 64.3 | 2.5 | 3.3 | 1.8 | . | 2.3 | 2.5 | 1.6 | 10.3 | 1.9 | 2.4 | 1.8 | 8.3 | 2.0 | 3.5 | 2.0 | 120.7 | 2.5 | 2.8 | 1.7 |
| blood4 | 5.0 | 2.8 | 11.5 | 82.2 | 5.0 | 2.7 | 9.4 | . | 3.1 | 2.4 | 5.6 | 7.1 | 2.8 | 2.7 | 6.1 | 8.4 | 4.4 | 3.2 | 8.0 | 77.6 | 4.3 | 2.7 |
| cpr1 | 23.2 | 1.5 | 1.8 | 1.5 | 9.3 | 1.4 | 1.6 | 1.4 | . | 1.4 | 1.7 | 1.4 | 7.8 | 1.4 | 1.7 | 1.4 | 20.0 | 1.6 | 1.9 | 1.6 | 7.3 | 1.4 |
| cpr2 | 4.4 | 7.6 | 3.4 | 2.9 | 2.9 | 5.0 | 2.7 | 2.5 | 3.9 | . | 3.1 | 2.7 | 2.8 | 6.1 | 3.3 | 2.4 | 4.3 | 17.9 | 3.8 | 3.2 | 3.0 | 5.3 |
| cpr3 | 2.7 | 1.8 | 22.5 | 2.4 | 2.3 | 1.7 | 7.4 | 2.0 | 2.7 | 1.7 | . | 2.1 | 2.5 | 1.8 | 6.9 | 2.0 | 3.1 | 2.1 | 31.7 | 2.6 | 2.4 | 1.7 |
| cpr4 | 4.1 | 3.0 | 6.1 | 13.3 | 3.1 | 2.6 | 4.2 | 7.7 | 3.7 | 2.7 | 9.1 | . | 3.2 | 3.0 | 5.5 | 6.3 | 4.8 | 3.5 | 7.0 | 25.4 | 3.2 | 2.8 |
| dxc1 | 5.2 | 1.4 | 1.5 | 1.4 | 3.9 | 1.3 | 1.4 | 1.3 | 3.5 | 1.3 | 1.5 | 1.3 | . | 1.4 | 1.6 | 1.4 | 5.1 | 1.5 | 1.6 | 1.4 | 3.8 | 1.3 |
| dxc2 | 3.8 | 9.9 | 3.1 | 2.7 | 2.4 | 4.5 | 2.3 | 2.1 | 2.4 | 3.1 | 2.5 | 2.2 | 3.0 | . | 3.0 | 2.3 | 4.0 | . | 3.5 | 2.9 | 2.5 | 4.2 |
| dxc3 | 3.2 | 1.9 | 19.0 | 2.5 | 2.4 | 1.7 | 6.6 | 2.0 | 2.5 | 1.7 | 7.2 | 2.0 | 3.0 | 1.9 | . | 2.4 | 3.3 | 2.1 | 63.2 | 2.9 | 2.8 | 1.8 |
| dxc4 | 4.1 | 2.5 | 6.2 | 12.7 | 3.1 | 2.2 | 3.8 | 5.4 | 3.2 | 2.1 | 4.1 | 4.4 | 4.2 | 2.7 | 9.0 | . | 5.3 | 2.9 | 8.8 | 85.3 | 3.6 | 2.4 |
| dxs1 | 13.0 | 1.5 | 1.9 | 1.6 | 6.7 | 1.4 | 1.6 | 1.4 | 5.0 | 1.3 | 1.6 | 1.4 | 5.9 | 1.4 | 1.6 | 1.4 | . | 1.8 | 2.1 | 1.7 | 5.3 | 1.4 |
| dxs2 | 3.1 | 3.9 | 2.4 | 2.0 | 2.2 | 2.5 | 1.9 | 1.7 | 2.1 | 2.2 | 2.0 | 1.7 | 2.2 | 3.4 | 2.0 | 1.7 | 4.0 | . | 3.1 | 2.5 | 2.0 | 2.5 |
| dxs3 | 3.0 | 1.7 | 7.9 | 2.1 | 2.3 | 1.5 | 3.7 | 1.7 | 2.2 | 1.5 | 3.9 | 1.6 | 2.1 | 1.7 | 4.0 | 1.8 | 3.6 | 2.1 | . | 2.9 | 2.1 | 1.5 |
| dxs4 | 3.5 | 2.1 | 4.7 | 5.3 | 2.5 | 1.8 | 2.7 | 2.8 | 2.6 | 1.8 | 3.1 | 2.6 | 2.4 | 2.1 | 3.5 | 3.3 | 5.1 | 3.1 | 13.9 | . | 2.7 | 1.9 |
| feed1 | 96.0 | 1.5 | 1.8 | 1.6 | 12.6 | 1.4 | 1.7 | 1.4 | 7.1 | 1.3 | 1.6 | 1.4 | 9.3 | 1.4 | 1.7 | 1.4 | 22.8 | 1.5 | 1.9 | 1.6 | . | 1.6 |
| feed2 | 5.3 | 10.2 | 3.0 | 3.0 | 3.1 | 4.3 | 2.5 | 2.3 | 2.6 | 3.3 | 2.6 | 2.3 | 3.1 | 5.2 | 2.9 | 2.3 | 4.0 | 10.6 | 3.1 | 2.9 | 6.1 | . |
| feed3 | 3.3 | 1.8 | 59.9 | 2.6 | 2.4 | 1.7 | 9.7 | 2.1 | 2.5 | 1.6 | 10.4 | 2.0 | 2.4 | 1.8 | 12.6 | 2.1 | 3.0 | 2.0 | 56.0 | 2.7 | 3.4 | 2.0 |
| feed4 | 4.9 | 2.9 | 9.4 | 45.0 | 2.6 | 2.5 | 4.0 | 6.2 | 3.0 | 2.3 | 4.9 | 5.1 | 2.9 | 2.9 | 5.3 | 7.1 | 4.4 | 3.5 | 7.0 | 28.3 | 4.4 | 3.2 |
| iv1 | 43.2 | 1.5 | 1.8 | 1.6 | 11.3 | 1.4 | 1.7 | 1.4 | 6.5 | 1.4 | 1.6 | 1.4 | 7.4 | 1.4 | 1.7 | 1.4 | 18.6 | 1.6 | 1.9 | 1.6 | 14.8 | 1.5 |
| iv2 | 5.8 | 7.2 | 3.1 | 2.7 | 3.1 | 3.9 | 2.5 | 2.1 | 2.8 | 3.0 | 2.5 | 2.0 | 2.5 | 4.1 | 2.6 | 2.0 | 3.9 | 9.2 | 3.2 | 2.7 | 3.8 | 7.2 |
| iv3 | 3.6 | 1.8 | 44.5 | 2.6 | 2.4 | 1.7 | 9.4 | 2.1 | 2.5 | 1.7 | 9.9 | 1.9 | 2.3 | 1.8 | 8.1 | 2.0 | 3.0 | 2.1 | 62.6 | 2.8 | 3.0 | 1.9 |
| iv4 | 5.2 | 2.8 | 9.9 | 31.5 | 2.8 | 2.3 | 4.2 | 5.7 | 3.0 | 2.4 | 5.2 | 5.1 | 2.7 | 2.6 | 4.9 | 5.3 | 4.6 | 3.5 | 8.2 | 44.8 | 4.3 | 2.9 |
| ormaj1 | 76.7 | 1.6 | 1.8 | 1.6 | 16.5 | 1.4 | 1.7 | 1.5 | 9.8 | 1.4 | 1.7 | 1.4 | 20.2 | 1.4 | 1.9 | 1.6 | 49.6 | 1.6 | 1.9 | 1.7 | 14.1 | 1.5 |
| ormaj2 | 4.5 | 72.8 | 3.3 | 3.2 | 2.7 | 8.5 | 2.8 | 2.6 | 3.0 | 5.5 | 2.9 | 2.6 | 2.8 | 25.2 | 3.4 | 2.8 | 3.6 | . | 3.5 | 3.0 | 3.0 | 7.5 |
| ormaj3 | 3.3 | 1.9 | 108.3 | 2.6 | 2.7 | 1.8 | 16.6 | 2.3 | 2.5 | 1.7 | 16.3 | 2.1 | 2.6 | 1.9 | 38.5 | 2.4 | 3.4 | 2.1 | . | 2.8 | 2.9 | 1.9 |
| ormaj4 | 3.6 | 2.9 | 10.1 | 36.0 | 3.0 | 2.5 | 5.0 | 10.9 | 2.9 | 2.5 | 6.4 | 9.5 | 3.1 | 3.0 | 8.1 | 18.8 | 4.3 | 3.2 | 9.4 | 34.0 | 3.5 | 2.8 |
| ormin1 | 62.7 | 1.5 | 1.8 | 1.6 | 13.3 | 1.4 | 1.6 | 1.4 | 7.9 | 1.3 | 1.6 | 1.4 | 11.2 | 1.4 | 1.7 | 1.4 | 25.7 | 1.5 | 1.8 | 1.6 | 12.0 | 1.5 |
| ormin2 | 4.3 | 17.9 | 3.2 | 2.8 | 2.5 | 5.2 | 2.4 | 2.0 | 2.5 | 3.6 | 2.7 | 2.1 | 2.7 | 7.7 | 3.0 | 2.1 | 3.3 | 27.7 | 3.1 | 2.8 | 3.7 | 9.4 |
| ormin3 | 3.0 | 1.7 | 20.9 | 2.4 | 2.3 | 1.6 | 6.1 | 1.9 | 2.3 | 1.6 | 6.5 | 1.8 | 2.3 | 1.7 | 6.5 | 1.9 | 2.9 | 2.0 | 27.5 | 2.4 | 2.5 | 1.7 |
| ormin4 | 3.9 | 2.6 | 7.4 | 12.1 | 2.7 | 2.2 | 3.4 | 4.5 | 3.0 | 2.2 | 4.0 | 4.2 | 2.8 | 2.6 | 5.1 | 5.8 | 4.1 | 3.2 | 8.5 | 23.1 | 3.5 | 2.6 |
| pd1 | 182.0 | 1.5 | 1.8 | 1.6 | 17.7 | 1.4 | 1.7 | 1.4 | 14.2 | 1.4 | 1.7 | 1.4 | 12.5 | 1.4 | 1.7 | 1.5 | 88.3 | 1.6 | 1.9 | 1.7 | 16.6 | 1.5 |
| pd2 | 5.1 | 22.5 | 2.9 | 2.9 | 2.7 | 5.8 | 2.5 | 2.1 | 2.7 | 3.7 | 2.5 | 2.1 | 2.5 | 7.7 | 2.8 | 2.2 | 3.6 | 83.6 | 2.8 | 2.6 | 3.5 | 7.8 |
| pd3 | 3.4 | 1.8 | . | 2.7 | 2.6 | 1.8 | 14.5 | 2.1 | 3.0 | 1.7 | 16.1 | 2.0 | 2.8 | 1.9 | 10.6 | 2.2 | 3.7 | 2.2 | 114.8 | 3.0 | 3.1 | 1.9 |
| pd4 | 5.0 | 2.9 | 11.5 | . | 3.2 | 2.8 | 5.3 | 8.6 | 3.7 | 2.5 | 5.6 | 7.1 | 3.3 | 3.1 | 6.6 | 10.6 | 5.4 | 3.5 | 9.2 | . | 4.7 | 3.1 |
| resp1 | 28.0 | 1.5 | 1.7 | 1.5 | 13.1 | 1.4 | 1.7 | 1.4 | 7.7 | 1.4 | 1.6 | 1.4 | 8.7 | 1.4 | 1.7 | 1.4 | 18.8 | 1.5 | 1.8 | 1.6 | 11.9 | 1.5 |
| resp2 | 5.8 | 11.4 | 3.1 | 2.9 | 3.4 | 5.3 | 2.8 | 2.3 | 3.0 | 4.2 | 2.8 | 2.2 | 2.7 | 5.2 | 2.8 | 2.1 | 4.3 | 21.3 | 3.2 | 2.9 | 3.8 | 7.3 |
| resp3 | 3.1 | 1.8 | 39.8 | 2.5 | 2.6 | 1.8 | 14.2 | 2.1 | 2.5 | 1.6 | 25.5 | 2.0 | 2.3 | 1.7 | 9.6 | 2.0 | 3.2 | 2.0 | 112.5 | 2.6 | 2.8 | 1.8 |
| resp4 | 5.3 | 3.0 | 9.4 | 78.8 | 3.5 | 2.9 | 5.0 | 10.3 | 3.1 | 2.7 | 7.0 | 13.9 | 3.1 | 3.0 | 6.4 | 9.0 | 5.9 | 3.8 | 8.8 | 74.4 | 3.9 | 3.2 |

Likelihood ratio of accepts- all scenarios and treatments.

| | abx1 | abx2 | abx3 | abx4 | blood1 | blood2 | blood3 | blood4 | cpr1 | cpr2 | cpr3 | cpr4 | dxc1 | dxc2 | dxc3 | dxc4 | dxs1 | dxs2 | dxs3 | dxs4 | feed1 | feed2 |
|---|---|---|---|---|---|---|---|---|---|---|---|---|---|---|---|---|---|---|---|---|---|---|
| abx1 | . | 6.7 | 4.1 | 8.0 | 70.9 | 5.9 | 4.4 | 7.3 | 24.9 | 6.4 | 3.4 | 5.9 | 4.7 | 5.3 | 4.0 | 5.9 | 12.0 | 3.8 | 3.3 | 4.6 | 103.1 | 7.6 |
| abx2 | 2.2 | . | 3.2 | 6.4 | 2.1 | 69.6 | 3.3 | 6.9 | 2.2 | 23.2 | 3.4 | 7.6 | 1.8 | 29.4 | 3.5 | 6.0 | 2.0 | 9.1 | 2.7 | 4.3 | 2.1 | 30.9 |
| abx3 | 2.3 | 4.8 | . | 25.3 | 2.1 | 5.7 | 132.9 | 26.1 | 2.3 | 6.7 | 44.9 | 13.2 | 1.7 | 5.9 | 38.0 | 13.2 | 2.2 | 3.7 | 13.3 | 8.8 | 2.4 | 5.7 |
| abx4 | 2.2 | 5.7 | 5.5 | . | 2.2 | 7.6 | 5.5 | 290.8 | 2.3 | 7.7 | 5.3 | 45.1 | 1.7 | 6.8 | 5.7 | 42.0 | 2.1 | 4.0 | 4.0 | 14.7 | 2.5 | 7.8 |
| blood1 | 9.1 | 3.7 | 2.9 | 4.4 | . | 5.0 | 4.5 | 8.1 | 11.0 | 4.4 | 2.9 | 4.8 | 3.9 | 3.4 | 3.2 | 4.6 | 6.8 | 2.7 | 2.7 | 3.3 | 14.9 | 4.6 |
| blood2 | 2.0 | 12.4 | 3.0 | 5.8 | 2.1 | . | 4.0 | 8.1 | 2.1 | 48.4 | 3.6 | 8.0 | 1.7 | 15.2 | 3.7 | 6.0 | 1.9 | 6.6 | 2.7 | 4.1 | 2.1 | 14.9 |
| blood3 | 2.1 | 3.7 | 11.3 | 8.5 | 2.4 | 6.7 | . | 25.1 | 2.2 | 5.8 | 16.9 | 10.3 | 1.7 | 4.7 | 14.9 | 8.8 | 2.0 | 3.1 | 6.9 | 5.4 | 2.4 | 5.1 |
| blood4 | 2.0 | 4.6 | 4.3 | 14.9 | 2.3 | 7.3 | 6.1 | . | 2.2 | 7.8 | 4.8 | 32.0 | 1.7 | 5.8 | 5.0 | 21.2 | 1.9 | 3.6 | 3.3 | 8.4 | 2.4 | 6.7 |
| cpr1 | 6.2 | 3.7 | 3.0 | 4.5 | 8.3 | 4.1 | 3.4 | 4.9 | . | 6.4 | 3.7 | 6.0 | 3.6 | 3.5 | 3.4 | 5.0 | 5.3 | 2.8 | 2.7 | 3.6 | 8.6 | 4.0 |
| cpr2 | 2.0 | 7.9 | 3.1 | 5.3 | 2.0 | 13.3 | 3.5 | 7.6 | 2.3 | . | 3.7 | 9.0 | 1.7 | 10.5 | 3.8 | 6.3 | 1.9 | 5.7 | 2.8 | 4.3 | 2.1 | 11.6 |
| cpr3 | 1.9 | 4.1 | 11.5 | 8.9 | 2.0 | 6.0 | 23.3 | 13.7 | 2.4 | 6.9 | . | 23.4 | 1.7 | 5.0 | 15.8 | 9.5 | 2.0 | 3.4 | 7.1 | 6.0 | 2.2 | 5.3 |
| cpr4 | 2.0 | 4.8 | 3.8 | 11.5 | 2.1 | 7.0 | 4.6 | 29.7 | 2.3 | 9.2 | 5.4 | . | 1.7 | 6.4 | 4.8 | 16.5 | 2.0 | 3.7 | 3.2 | 7.7 | 2.2 | 6.7 |
| dxc1 | 6.1 | 3.8 | 2.5 | 3.3 | 7.9 | 3.6 | 2.9 | 3.8 | 8.0 | 3.7 | 2.9 | 4.4 | . | 3.8 | 3.5 | 5.8 | 5.3 | 2.6 | 2.2 | 2.8 | 9.5 | 4.1 |
| dxc2 | 2.0 | 13.6 | 3.3 | 6.1 | 1.9 | 25.4 | 3.5 | 7.5 | 2.0 | 20.6 | 3.5 | 8.6 | 1.8 | . | 4.1 | 7.6 | 2.0 | 8.6 | 2.9 | 4.6 | 2.0 | 16.7 |
| dxc3 | 2.1 | 4.2 | 10.7 | 10.0 | 2.1 | 6.0 | 18.7 | 15.1 | 2.3 | 7.4 | 15.2 | 13.6 | 1.9 | 6.3 | . | 22.8 | 2.0 | 3.4 | 7.3 | 7.1 | 2.4 | 6.1 |
| dxc4 | 2.0 | 4.5 | 4.0 | 14.3 | 2.1 | 6.0 | 4.7 | 32.8 | 2.2 | 7.1 | 4.5 | 24.0 | 1.9 | 6.4 | 6.0 | . | 2.0 | 3.5 | 3.5 | 9.7 | 2.3 | 6.3 |
| dxs1 | 16.7 | 4.9 | 4.0 | 7.6 | 33.3 | 5.2 | 4.4 | 6.3 | 21.0 | 6.1 | 3.8 | 6.9 | 4.6 | 5.4 | 4.1 | 7.6 | . | 5.0 | 4.0 | 6.7 | 23.9 | 5.5 |
| dxs2 | 2.1 | 28.6 | 3.3 | 5.8 | 2.0 | 69.9 | 3.4 | 6.8 | 2.0 | 46.7 | 3.5 | 7.6 | 1.7 | . | 3.6 | 6.0 | 2.2 | . | 3.3 | 6.0 | 1.9 | 26.2 |
| dxs3 | 2.2 | 4.3 | 88.6 | 16.6 | 2.2 | 5.6 | 222.8 | 15.9 | 2.3 | 7.0 | 56.9 | 13.8 | 1.7 | 6.1 | 114.6 | 17.3 | 2.4 | 4.7 | . | 25.3 | 2.2 | 5.3 |
| dxs4 | 2.1 | 4.9 | 5.0 | 73.3 | 2.1 | 6.4 | 5.0 | 232.0 | 2.2 | 7.8 | 5.2 | 74.7 | 1.7 | 6.5 | 6.0 | 250.7 | 2.2 | 4.9 | 5.3 | . | 2.3 | 6.5 |
| feed1 | 7.5 | 3.5 | 3.2 | 5.8 | 10.6 | 4.4 | 3.9 | 7.2 | 8.9 | 4.7 | 3.2 | 5.1 | 3.8 | 3.6 | 3.8 | 5.7 | 5.5 | 2.5 | 2.6 | 3.8 | . | 10.0 |
| feed2 | 2.1 | 11.6 | 3.1 | 6.3 | 2.1 | 18.1 | 3.6 | 8.0 | 2.1 | 18.7 | 3.5 | 8.3 | 1.8 | 13.5 | 3.8 | 6.8 | 1.9 | 6.2 | 2.7 | 4.4 | 2.7 | . |
| feed3 | 2.0 | 3.6 | 9.4 | 8.7 | 2.0 | 5.3 | 16.3 | 14.2 | 2.2 | 5.6 | 13.1 | 11.1 | 1.7 | 4.6 | 15.2 | 10.1 | 1.9 | 3.0 | 6.0 | 5.6 | 2.5 | 6.9 |
| feed4 | 2.1 | 5.1 | 4.4 | 18.6 | 2.0 | 7.2 | 4.8 | 42.1 | 2.2 | 8.3 | 4.9 | 32.4 | 1.7 | 6.9 | 5.1 | 26.6 | 2.0 | 3.9 | 3.4 | 9.0 | 2.4 | 8.9 |
| iv1 | 11.0 | 4.2 | 3.3 | 6.2 | 19.7 | 5.4 | 4.4 | 7.6 | 13.0 | 6.1 | 3.2 | 5.2 | 4.0 | 3.5 | 3.9 | 5.4 | 7.0 | 2.9 | 2.8 | 4.0 | . | 8.8 |
| iv2 | 2.2 | 15.0 | 3.4 | 6.9 | 2.2 | 31.6 | 4.0 | 8.3 | 2.2 | 32.2 | 3.6 | 8.2 | 1.7 | 16.2 | 3.9 | 6.2 | 2.0 | 7.3 | 2.9 | 4.7 | 2.5 | 327.1 |
| iv3 | 2.1 | 4.0 | 12.2 | 10.7 | 2.1 | 6.1 | 28.5 | 18.8 | 2.2 | 7.0 | 19.8 | 12.6 | 1.7 | 4.9 | 17.2 | 9.7 | 2.0 | 3.5 | 7.2 | 6.6 | 2.5 | 6.5 |
| iv4 | 2.1 | 5.0 | 4.6 | 21.3 | 2.0 | 6.9 | 5.1 | 54.7 | 2.2 | 9.2 | 5.2 | 45.7 | 1.7 | 6.3 | 5.1 | 23.1 | 2.0 | 4.1 | 3.6 | 10.2 | 2.5 | 8.5 |
| ormaj1 | 4.7 | 3.7 | 2.8 | 4.8 | 6.3 | 4.3 | 3.5 | 6.0 | 6.4 | 4.8 | 3.3 | 5.6 | 3.5 | 3.6 | 3.8 | 6.6 | 4.2 | 2.6 | 2.4 | 3.4 | 7.2 | 5.2 |
| ormaj2 | 2.0 | 9.7 | 3.0 | 5.5 | 1.9 | 16.0 | 3.6 | 7.4 | 2.1 | 18.0 | 3.4 | 7.6 | 1.7 | 14.2 | 3.8 | 7.0 | 1.8 | 5.9 | 2.6 | 4.0 | 2.1 | 12.5 |
| ormaj3 | 2.0 | 3.8 | 7.8 | 7.3 | 2.1 | 5.1 | 14.6 | 14.6 | 2.2 | 5.9 | 11.7 | 11.5 | 1.7 | 4.9 | 14.5 | 11.2 | 2.0 | 3.1 | 5.5 | 5.1 | 2.3 | 5.8 |
| ormaj4 | 1.9 | 4.5 | 4.0 | 11.0 | 2.0 | 6.1 | 4.6 | 23.7 | 2.1 | 7.3 | 4.7 | 23.4 | 1.7 | 5.9 | 5.0 | 19.7 | 1.9 | 3.5 | 3.3 | 7.0 | 2.2 | 6.2 |
| ormin1 | 7.0 | 3.4 | 3.0 | 4.7 | 10.3 | 3.7 | 3.4 | 5.3 | 9.4 | 4.2 | 3.0 | 4.8 | 4.0 | 3.3 | 3.5 | 5.0 | 5.5 | 2.6 | 2.4 | 3.3 | 13.4 | 5.0 |
| ormin2 | 2.0 | 12.6 | 3.2 | 5.6 | 1.9 | 20.3 | 3.4 | 6.2 | 2.0 | 19.4 | 3.5 | 7.1 | 1.7 | 16.6 | 3.9 | 5.9 | 1.8 | 6.8 | 2.7 | 4.2 | 2.3 | 27.5 |
| ormin3 | 2.1 | 3.9 | 15.4 | 10.2 | 2.1 | 5.5 | 28.5 | 15.2 | 2.2 | 6.3 | 20.6 | 11.3 | 1.7 | 4.8 | 22.2 | 9.3 | 2.0 | 3.3 | 8.2 | 5.8 | 2.3 | 5.3 |
| ormin4 | 2.0 | 4.9 | 4.4 | 10.1 | 2.0 | 6.6 | 4.6 | 38.5 | 2.2 | 8.4 | 4.7 | 33.4 | 1.7 | 6.6 | 5.4 | 32.8 | 2.0 | 3.9 | 3.7 | 10.2 | 2.3 | 7.5 |
| pd1 | 6.7 | 3.9 | 3.1 | 5.5 | 10.3 | 5.3 | 4.0 | 6.4 | 13.1 | 6.2 | 3.6 | 5.8 | 3.9 | 3.7 | 3.6 | 5.6 | 5.7 | 2.9 | 2.7 | 4.1 | 14.0 | 6.0 |
| pd2 | 2.1 | 13.2 | 3.0 | 5.8 | 2.0 | 23.7 | 3.5 | 6.8 | 2.1 | 21.1 | 3.3 | 6.7 | 1.6 | 16.6 | 3.7 | 6.2 | 1.9 | 7.2 | 2.5 | 3.9 | 2.3 | 23.3 |
| pd3 | 2.1 | 3.7 | 10.6 | 9.4 | 2.1 | 6.0 | 23.9 | 15.2 | 2.4 | 7.2 | 17.8 | 11.7 | 1.8 | 5.1 | 14.9 | 11.3 | 2.0 | 3.4 | 6.4 | 6.5 | 2.4 | 5.9 |
| pd4 | 2.0 | 4.8 | 4.3 | 15.7 | 2.1 | 7.6 | 5.1 | 36.1 | 2.3 | 8.2 | 4.8 | 32.0 | 1.8 | 6.8 | 5.2 | 24.7 | 2.0 | 3.8 | 3.4 | 8.7 | 2.4 | 7.5 |
| resp1 | 7.2 | 3.8 | 2.9 | 4.7 | 13.2 | 5.1 | 3.9 | 6.9 | 11.3 | 5.6 | 3.1 | 4.9 | 3.9 | 3.3 | 3.5 | 5.1 | 5.7 | 2.7 | 2.4 | 3.4 | 19.0 | 6.2 |
| resp2 | 2.1 | 11.7 | 3.2 | 6.1 | 2.2 | 23.1 | 3.9 | 8.1 | 2.2 | 30.4 | 3.6 | 8.0 | 1.7 | 13.0 | 3.7 | 6.0 | 2.0 | 6.8 | 2.7 | 4.3 | 2.4 | 24.6 |
| resp3 | 2.0 | 3.6 | 9.0 | 7.9 | 2.1 | 6.4 | 21.0 | 13.1 | 2.2 | 5.3 | 19.3 | 12.0 | 1.7 | 4.3 | 13.0 | 8.4 | 2.0 | 3.1 | 6.2 | 5.2 | 2.3 | 5.5 |
| resp4 | 2.0 | 4.8 | 4.1 | 13.5 | 2.1 | 7.6 | 4.9 | 33.8 | 2.2 | 9.0 | 5.0 | 47.6 | 1.7 | 6.3 | 5.0 | 19.3 | 2.0 | 3.8 | 3.3 | 7.9 | 2.3 | 7.5 |

**TABLE 2.** *Continued*

| feed3 | feed4 | iv1 | iv2 | iv3 | iv4 | ormaj1 | ormaj2 | ormaj3 | ormaj4 | ormin1 | ormin2 | ormin3 | ormin4 | pd1 | pd2 | pd3 | pd4 | resp1 | resp2 | resp3 | resp4 |
|---|---|---|---|---|---|---|---|---|---|---|---|---|---|---|---|---|---|---|---|---|---|
| 1.6 | 1.4 | 10.9 | 1.6 | 1.7 | 1.5 | 4.0 | 1.3 | 1.5 | 1.3 | 6.5 | 1.4 | 1.7 | 1.4 | 6.0 | 1.4 | 1.6 | 1.4 | 6.9 | 1.5 | 1.5 | 1.4 |
| 1.9 | 2.1 | 3.0 | 5.3 | 2.2 | 2.1 | 2.4 | 2.9 | 1.9 | 1.7 | 2.4 | 4.0 | 2.2 | 2.1 | 2.6 | 4.2 | 2.0 | 1.9 | 2.7 | 3.9 | 1.9 | 1.9 |
| 4.4 | 2.0 | 2.7 | 1.8 | 6.0 | 2.1 | 2.1 | 1.5 | 3.6 | 1.7 | 2.4 | 1.6 | 7.9 | 2.1 | 2.4 | 1.6 | 5.0 | 1.9 | 2.3 | 1.7 | 4.3 | 1.8 |
| 3.7 | 5.4 | 4.2 | 2.8 | 4.7 | 6.3 | 2.9 | 2.0 | 3.1 | 3.1 | 3.1 | 2.2 | 4.8 | 5.6 | 3.5 | 2.2 | 4.0 | 4.4 | 3.2 | 2.3 | 3.4 | 3.8 |
| 1.5 | 1.3 | 17.6 | 1.5 | 1.6 | 1.4 | 4.9 | 1.3 | 1.5 | 1.3 | 8.6 | 1.3 | 1.6 | 1.4 | 8.4 | 1.4 | 1.6 | 1.4 | 11.3 | 1.4 | 1.6 | 1.4 |
| 2.4 | 2.5 | 3.6 | 9.8 | 2.8 | 2.4 | 2.6 | 4.0 | 2.3 | 2.0 | 2.5 | 5.7 | 2.7 | 2.4 | 3.3 | 6.5 | 2.7 | 2.4 | 3.3 | 6.5 | 2.8 | 2.4 |
| 6.8 | 2.0 | 3.3 | 2.0 | 12.3 | 2.1 | 2.4 | 1.6 | 5.8 | 1.8 | 2.5 | 1.7 | 13.1 | 2.0 | 2.8 | 1.7 | 9.8 | 2.0 | 2.8 | 1.8 | 8.6 | 1.9 |
| 5.4 | 10.6 | 4.9 | 3.1 | 7.4 | 14.1 | 3.4 | 2.3 | 5.1 | 5.4 | 3.3 | 2.2 | 6.4 | 10.4 | 3.8 | 2.4 | 5.8 | 8.6 | 4.3 | 2.7 | 5.0 | 7.8 |
| 1.6 | 1.4 | 11.3 | 1.5 | 1.7 | 1.4 | 4.8 | 1.3 | 1.5 | 1.3 | 7.7 | 1.4 | 1.7 | 1.4 | 10.4 | 1.4 | 1.7 | 1.4 | 9.4 | 1.4 | 1.6 | 1.4 |
| 2.5 | 2.7 | 4.0 | 9.8 | 3.1 | 3.0 | 2.8 | 4.4 | 2.5 | 2.2 | 2.7 | 5.4 | 3.0 | 2.9 | 3.7 | 5.8 | 3.1 | 2.6 | 3.6 | 8.1 | 2.4 | 2.7 |
| 5.7 | 2.1 | 2.5 | 1.9 | 8.8 | 2.2 | 2.3 | 1.6 | 4.8 | 1.8 | 2.3 | 1.7 | 9.8 | 2.1 | 2.6 | 1.7 | 7.6 | 2.0 | 2.3 | 1.8 | 8.0 | 2.0 |
| 4.3 | 8.3 | 3.5 | 3.0 | 5.1 | 11.8 | 3.2 | 2.3 | 4.2 | 5.3 | 3.1 | 2.4 | 5.0 | 9.1 | 3.5 | 2.4 | 4.6 | 7.7 | 3.2 | 2.7 | 4.6 | 10.7 |
| 1.4 | 1.3 | 4.2 | 1.4 | 1.4 | 1.3 | 3.2 | 1.2 | 1.4 | 1.2 | 3.9 | 1.3 | 1.5 | 1.3 | 3.7 | 1.3 | 1.5 | 1.3 | 3.9 | 1.3 | 1.4 | 1.3 |
| 2.2 | 2.5 | 2.5 | 5.5 | 2.5 | 2.4 | 2.3 | 3.8 | 2.3 | 2.0 | 2.3 | 4.9 | 2.5 | 2.5 | 2.5 | 4.9 | 2.4 | 2.3 | 2.3 | 4.0 | 2.1 | 2.2 |
| 6.4 | 2.1 | 3.0 | 2.0 | 7.7 | 2.2 | 2.6 | 1.6 | 5.8 | 1.9 | 2.5 | 1.8 | 10.5 | 2.3 | 2.6 | 1.7 | 6.4 | 2.0 | 2.6 | 1.8 | 5.6 | 2.0 |
| 4.0 | 7.1 | 3.6 | 2.5 | 4.1 | 6.5 | 3.7 | 2.2 | 4.2 | 4.7 | 3.2 | 2.2 | 4.2 | 9.1 | 3.5 | 2.3 | 4.5 | 6.2 | 3.3 | 2.2 | 3.5 | 4.9 |
| 1.5 | 1.4 | 7.1 | 1.5 | 1.6 | 1.4 | 3.7 | 1.3 | 1.5 | 1.3 | 5.2 | 1.4 | 1.6 | 1.4 | 5.3 | 1.4 | 1.6 | 1.4 | 5.6 | 1.4 | 1.6 | 1.4 |
| 1.8 | 1.8 | 2.3 | 3.1 | 2.0 | 1.9 | 1.9 | 2.2 | 1.8 | 1.6 | 2.0 | 2.6 | 2.0 | 1.9 | 2.2 | 2.7 | 1.9 | 1.7 | 2.1 | 2.7 | 1.8 | 1.7 |
| 3.2 | 1.7 | 2.4 | 1.7 | 4.0 | 1.8 | 1.9 | 1.4 | 2.9 | 1.6 | 2.0 | 1.5 | 4.7 | 1.9 | 2.2 | 1.5 | 3.4 | 1.7 | 2.1 | 1.6 | 3.3 | 1.7 |
| 2.7 | 3.1 | 3.0 | 2.2 | 3.3 | 3.5 | 2.3 | 1.7 | 2.4 | 2.3 | 2.4 | 1.9 | 3.1 | 3.6 | 2.8 | 1.8 | 3.1 | 2.9 | 2.5 | 1.9 | 2.6 | 2.6 |
| 1.7 | 1.5 | . | 1.6 | 1.8 | 1.5 | 5.4 | 1.3 | 1.6 | 1.3 | 10.9 | 1.5 | 1.7 | 1.5 | 11.1 | 1.5 | 1.7 | 1.5 | 15.9 | 1.5 | 1.6 | 1.4 |
| 3.0 | 2.9 | 5.7 | 95.9 | 3.0 | 2.9 | 3.1 | 3.4 | 2.5 | 2.0 | 3.2 | 7.5 | 2.7 | 2.7 | 3.7 | 6.5 | 2.7 | 2.5 | 4.0 | 6.9 | 2.5 | 2.4 |
| . | 2.5 | 3.3 | 2.1 | 42.9 | 2.5 | 2.4 | 1.6 | 6.2 | 1.9 | 2.6 | 1.8 | 31.1 | 2.3 | 2.7 | 1.8 | 10.7 | 2.2 | 2.6 | 1.8 | 9.2 | 2.0 |
| 6.9 | . | 4.5 | 3.7 | 6.7 | 31.1 | 2.9 | 2.2 | 3.8 | 4.7 | 3.2 | 2.7 | 5.5 | 10.1 | 3.5 | 2.7 | 5.1 | 8.6 | 3.1 | 2.7 | 3.8 | 6.3 |
| 1.7 | 1.5 | . | 1.6 | 1.8 | 1.5 | 4.7 | 1.3 | 1.5 | 1.3 | 8.1 | 1.4 | 1.7 | 1.5 | 8.6 | 1.5 | 1.7 | 1.4 | 11.4 | 1.5 | 1.6 | 1.4 |
| 2.5 | 2.5 | 5.3 | . | 3.1 | 2.8 | 2.5 | 2.9 | 2.3 | 1.8 | 2.9 | 4.5 | 2.6 | 2.3 | 3.4 | 4.9 | 2.5 | 2.2 | 3.6 | 6.0 | 2.4 | 2.1 |
| 10.3 | 2.3 | 3.5 | 2.2 | . | 2.5 | 2.3 | 1.6 | 5.3 | 1.9 | 2.5 | 1.8 | 12.4 | 2.2 | 2.8 | 1.7 | 8.9 | 2.1 | 2.6 | 1.8 | 7.9 | 1.9 |
| 5.4 | 14.0 | 4.7 | 3.9 | 8.5 | . | 3.0 | 2.1 | 3.8 | 4.3 | 3.4 | 2.6 | 5.4 | 7.9 | 3.4 | 2.5 | 5.0 | 7.0 | 3.3 | 2.7 | 4.0 | 5.4 |
| 1.7 | 1.5 | 27.1 | 1.6 | 1.7 | 1.5 | . | 1.5 | 1.7 | 1.5 | 17.1 | 1.5 | 1.8 | 1.5 | 14.4 | 1.5 | 1.7 | 1.5 | 13.8 | 1.5 | 1.7 | 1.4 |
| 2.5 | 2.8 | 3.2 | 14.7 | 2.9 | 2.8 | 4.0 | . | 3.3 | 2.6 | 2.4 | 12.8 | 3.0 | 2.8 | 3.2 | 19.3 | 2.9 | 2.8 | 3.1 | 10.9 | 2.7 | 2.8 |
| 10.6 | 2.3 | 3.0 | 2.1 | 19.2 | 2.4 | 3.0 | 1.8 | . | 2.2 | 2.5 | 1.8 | 28.0 | 2.4 | 2.9 | 1.8 | 14.7 | 2.2 | 2.8 | 1.8 | 10.6 | 2.2 |
| 5.5 | 18.8 | 3.6 | 2.9 | 6.5 | 24.9 | 4.2 | 2.7 | 6.9 | . | 3.3 | 2.5 | 7.0 | 18.5 | 3.4 | 2.6 | 6.0 | 19.1 | 3.2 | 2.7 | 5.1 | 9.5 |
| 1.6 | 1.4 | 19.7 | 1.5 | 1.7 | 1.5 | 6.0 | 1.3 | 1.5 | 1.3 | . | 1.4 | 1.7 | 1.5 | 10.4 | 1.4 | 1.7 | 1.4 | 11.8 | 1.4 | 1.5 | 1.4 |
| 2.6 | 2.6 | 3.9 | 13.0 | 2.8 | 2.7 | 2.9 | 4.3 | 2.3 | 2.0 | 3.1 | . | 3.1 | 2.6 | 3.0 | 9.5 | 2.6 | 2.3 | 2.9 | 6.2 | 2.2 | 2.2 |
| 5.9 | 2.0 | 2.7 | 1.8 | 6.9 | 2.1 | 2.2 | 1.5 | 4.3 | 1.8 | 2.5 | 1.7 | . | 2.3 | 2.4 | 1.6 | 5.4 | 1.9 | 2.3 | 1.7 | 4.6 | 1.8 |
| 4.0 | 6.2 | 3.7 | 2.8 | 4.3 | 6.6 | 2.9 | 2.0 | 3.4 | 3.7 | 3.3 | 2.4 | 7.1 | . | 3.2 | 2.3 | 4.4 | 5.3 | 3.1 | 2.4 | 3.2 | 4.4 |
| 1.7 | 1.5 | 48.4 | 1.6 | 1.8 | 1.5 | 6.4 | 1.4 | 1.6 | 1.4 | 13.3 | 1.4 | 1.7 | 1.5 | . | 1.5 | 1.8 | 1.5 | 19.7 | 1.5 | 1.7 | 1.4 |
| 2.5 | 2.6 | 4.2 | 18.3 | 2.7 | 2.6 | 2.8 | 4.8 | 2.3 | 2.0 | 2.8 | 9.5 | 2.6 | 2.5 | 3.4 | . | 2.7 | 2.4 | 3.4 | 10.5 | 2.5 | 2.3 |
| 9.4 | 2.3 | 3.2 | 2.0 | 18.6 | 2.4 | 2.5 | 1.6 | 6.6 | 1.9 | 2.8 | 1.8 | 15.7 | 2.4 | 3.6 | 1.8 | . | 2.4 | 3.0 | 1.8 | 9.4 | 2.0 |
| 5.8 | 21.4 | 4.9 | 3.4 | 6.7 | 28.3 | 3.6 | 2.4 | 4.5 | 6.7 | 3.5 | 2.7 | 6.4 | 16.8 | 4.8 | 2.9 | 10.9 | . | 4.3 | 2.7 | 5.0 | 7.8 |
| 1.6 | 1.4 | 23.2 | 1.6 | 1.7 | 1.4 | 4.9 | 1.3 | 1.5 | 1.3 | 8.8 | 1.4 | 1.6 | 1.4 | 9.9 | 1.4 | 1.7 | 1.4 | . | 1.5 | 1.6 | 1.4 |
| 2.6 | 2.5 | 4.7 | 31.4 | 3.0 | 2.7 | 3.0 | 3.9 | 2.3 | 2.0 | 3.0 | 5.6 | 2.8 | 2.5 | 3.9 | 8.8 | 2.6 | 2.3 | 4.6 | . | 2.9 | 2.5 |
| 9.2 | 2.1 | 3.0 | 2.0 | 18.2 | 2.3 | 2.4 | 1.6 | 6.2 | 1.9 | 2.3 | 1.7 | 11.1 | 2.1 | 2.8 | 1.8 | 10.7 | 2.1 | 3.0 | 1.9 | . | 2.1 |
| 4.8 | 16.4 | 4.3 | 3.5 | 5.4 | 20.3 | 3.3 | 2.6 | 4.6 | 6.0 | 3.4 | 2.6 | 6.2 | 13.4 | 4.0 | 2.8 | 5.5 | 10.3 | 4.1 | 3.4 | 5.5 | . |
| | | | | | | | | | | | | | | | | | | | | | |
| 4.3 | 7.2 | 43.7 | 8.1 | 4.5 | 7.5 | 90.4 | 6.7 | 4.4 | 5.3 | 67.8 | 6.1 | 3.6 | 5.5 | 200.5 | 7.4 | 4.4 | 7.3 | 29.4 | 8.4 | 3.9 | 7.9 |
| 3.3 | 7.3 | 2.1 | 20.4 | 3.4 | 6.7 | 2.4 | 244.6 | 3.7 | 7.4 | 2.1 | 56.3 | 3.1 | 6.1 | 2.3 | 71.1 | 3.3 | 7.3 | 2.1 | 34.8 | 3.3 | 7.8 |
| 126.2 | 20.8 | 2.2 | 5.7 | 90.5 | 21.7 | 2.5 | 6.7 | 235.1 | 23.3 | 2.3 | 6.2 | 40.7 | 15.8 | 2.4 | 5.5 | . | 26.1 | 2.2 | 6.0 | 83.5 | 21.3 |
| 6.2 | 155.4 | 2.3 | 6.8 | 6.0 | 106.9 | 2.7 | 9.0 | 6.3 | 128.7 | 2.3 | 7.1 | 5.1 | 39.3 | 2.5 | 7.5 | 6.3 | . | 2.3 | 7.7 | 5.8 | 280.7 |
| 3.2 | 3.9 | 12.6 | 4.4 | 3.2 | 4.1 | 21.4 | 4.1 | 3.8 | 4.6 | 15.8 | 3.5 | 3.0 | 4.0 | 21.4 | 4.0 | 3.5 | 4.9 | 15.2 | 5.2 | 3.6 | 5.4 |
| 3.7 | 7.2 | 2.1 | 12.5 | 3.7 | 6.5 | 2.4 | 33.7 | 3.9 | 7.7 | 2.0 | 18.5 | 3.3 | 6.0 | 2.3 | 21.3 | 4.0 | 8.6 | 2.2 | 18.9 | 4.2 | 9.0 |
| 23.4 | 9.4 | 2.3 | 5.1 | 21.8 | 9.9 | 2.6 | 6.3 | 42.0 | 12.7 | 2.2 | 4.9 | 13.2 | 7.7 | 2.5 | 5.1 | 35.4 | 13.3 | 2.3 | 6.1 | 34.9 | 12.7 |
| 5.7 | 24.7 | 2.2 | 5.6 | 5.4 | 22.3 | 2.6 | 8.3 | 6.6 | 47.6 | 2.2 | 5.6 | 4.5 | 16.8 | 2.4 | 6.1 | 5.7 | 36.1 | 2.3 | 6.8 | 5.5 | 44.5 |
| 3.4 | 4.7 | 7.5 | 4.1 | 3.4 | 4.6 | 13.0 | 4.7 | 3.6 | 4.6 | 9.7 | 3.8 | 3.0 | 4.5 | 17.9 | 4.0 | 4.2 | 6.1 | 9.2 | 4.6 | 3.5 | 5.0 |
| 3.6 | 7.1 | 2.1 | 10.0 | 3.8 | 7.3 | 2.4 | 22.8 | 4.0 | 8.2 | 2.1 | 13.0 | 3.3 | 6.5 | 2.4 | 13.7 | 4.1 | 7.9 | 2.2 | 15.7 | 3.5 | 9.2 |
| 24.1 | 11.7 | 2.1 | 4.8 | 22.2 | 12.3 | 2.5 | 6.3 | 39.6 | 16.3 | 2.1 | 5.6 | 13.7 | 9.1 | 2.4 | 5.0 | 37.9 | 13.7 | 2.1 | 5.7 | 61.1 | 17.8 |
| 5.1 | 20.1 | 2.0 | 5.5 | 4.8 | 19.7 | 2.5 | 8.4 | 5.9 | 41.6 | 2.2 | 6.1 | 4.1 | 15.2 | 2.3 | 5.9 | 5.1 | 29.7 | 2.1 | 6.6 | 5.3 | 61.7 |
| 2.9 | 3.9 | 7.1 | 3.2 | 2.7 | 3.5 | 22.4 | 3.7 | 3.2 | 4.3 | 11.4 | 3.4 | 2.6 | 3.7 | 13.0 | 3.2 | 3.4 | 4.4 | 8.7 | 3.5 | 2.8 | 4.3 |
| 3.7 | 8.4 | 1.9 | 12.0 | 3.5 | 7.0 | 2.3 | 95.4 | 4.2 | 8.9 | 2.0 | 26.0 | 3.2 | 7.0 | 2.1 | 26.0 | 3.9 | 9.2 | 1.9 | 16.5 | 3.5 | 8.8 |
| 29.6 | 12.7 | 2.2 | 5.2 | 18.0 | 11.5 | 2.8 | 7.8 | 96.4 | 21.2 | 2.3 | 6.5 | 13.8 | 12.0 | 2.4 | 5.9 | 24.7 | 16.7 | 2.2 | 5.8 | 22.2 | 16.1 |
| 5.4 | 26.6 | 2.1 | 4.9 | 4.6 | 18.9 | 2.8 | 8.9 | 6.4 | 78.9 | 2.2 | 5.8 | 4.1 | 21.1 | 2.4 | 6.0 | 5.5 | 42.1 | 2.2 | 5.7 | 4.9 | 35.6 |
| 3.7 | 6.2 | 18.4 | 5.2 | 3.7 | 6.5 | 57.1 | 5.2 | 4.4 | 6.2 | 27.2 | 4.5 | 3.5 | 5.6 | 95.0 | 4.9 | 4.6 | 7.9 | 19.4 | 5.9 | 4.1 | 8.6 |
| 3.4 | 7.6 | 2.0 | 21.5 | 3.6 | 7.5 | 2.2 | . | 3.7 | 7.2 | 2.0 | 71.4 | 3.2 | 6.7 | 2.2 | 218.7 | 3.8 | 7.7 | 2.0 | 54.1 | 3.5 | 8.5 |
| 105.0 | 13.5 | 2.2 | 5.4 | 113.8 | 15.9 | 2.4 | 6.5 | . | 19.4 | 2.1 | 5.4 | 48.1 | 16.4 | 2.4 | 4.8 | 214.9 | 18.4 | 2.1 | 5.6 | 211.7 | 17.7 |
| 5.6 | 81.8 | 2.2 | 5.9 | 5.7 | 129.3 | 2.5 | 7.2 | 5.8 | 102.7 | 2.2 | 6.3 | 4.5 | 65.3 | 2.4 | 5.7 | 6.4 | . | 2.1 | 6.4 | 5.3 | 224.0 |
| 4.9 | 7.2 | 17.1 | 5.9 | 4.2 | 6.9 | 18.8 | 4.7 | 4.3 | 5.8 | 14.7 | 5.8 | 3.3 | 5.4 | 20.9 | 5.4 | 4.4 | 7.9 | 14.3 | 6.0 | 4.0 | 6.3 |
| 4.6 | 9.9 | 2.4 | 24.4 | 4.0 | 8.7 | 2.6 | 28.0 | 4.5 | 8.5 | 2.3 | 34.4 | 3.3 | 7.2 | 2.5 | 28.0 | 4.1 | 9.4 | 2.3 | 26.1 | 4.0 | 10.0 |
| . | 18.6 | 2.3 | 5.2 | 25.2 | 14.0 | 2.5 | 5.7 | 27.7 | 15.0 | 2.2 | 5.7 | 13.5 | 9.8 | 2.4 | 5.5 | 23.5 | 15.5 | 2.1 | 5.6 | 23.1 | 12.6 |
| 6.9 | . | 2.2 | 7.1 | 5.6 | 55.3 | 2.5 | 8.9 | 6.0 | 78.9 | 2.2 | 7.8 | 4.5 | 22.6 | 2.4 | 7.8 | 5.8 | 88.4 | 2.1 | 7.4 | 5.2 | 67.4 |
| 4.5 | 6.9 | . | 7.9 | 4.8 | 7.2 | 34.1 | 4.8 | 4.1 | 5.5 | 22.8 | 6.0 | 3.4 | 5.4 | 57.2 | 6.5 | 4.4 | 7.6 | 26.2 | 7.2 | 4.1 | 6.6 |
| 4.3 | 10.3 | 2.5 | . | 4.6 | 10.9 | 2.5 | 50.2 | 4.6 | 8.0 | 2.3 | 42.5 | 3.5 | 7.2 | 2.5 | 60.8 | 4.2 | 9.3 | 2.4 | 105.7 | 4.2 | 10.1 |
| 105.4 | 16.7 | 2.4 | 6.5 | . | 21.5 | 2.5 | 6.5 | 47.5 | 16.7 | 2.3 | 5.9 | 14.7 | 9.9 | 2.5 | 5.7 | 44.5 | 16.9 | 2.2 | 6.4 | 43.8 | 13.4 |
| 6.5 | 122.7 | 2.3 | 7.8 | 6.4 | . | 2.6 | 8.5 | 6.3 | 101.3 | 2.3 | 7.8 | 4.7 | 23.2 | 2.4 | 7.4 | 6.1 | 113.3 | 2.2 | 7.6 | 5.6 | 81.0 |
| 3.5 | 4.9 | 6.0 | 4.0 | 3.3 | 5.1 | . | 7.4 | 4.9 | 7.9 | 8.2 | 5.0 | 3.1 | 4.8 | 8.8 | 4.7 | 3.7 | 6.5 | 6.4 | 5.1 | 3.5 | 5.8 |
| 3.6 | 7.0 | 2.0 | 10.0 | 3.5 | 6.4 | 2.7 | . | 4.8 | 9.8 | 1.9 | 17.4 | 3.2 | 6.0 | 2.2 | 19.7 | 3.8 | 8.1 | 2.1 | 15.1 | 3.8 | 8.9 |
| 16.1 | 9.9 | 2.1 | 5.0 | 13.1 | 9.9 | 2.8 | 8.5 | . | 20.6 | 2.1 | 5.3 | 10.0 | 8.7 | 2.4 | 5.3 | 17.4 | 12.5 | 2.2 | 5.2 | 16.1 | 12.9 |
| 5.3 | 19.7 | 2.0 | 5.0 | 4.8 | 17.4 | 2.7 | 9.4 | 6.6 | . | 2.2 | 5.8 | 4.3 | 14.6 | 2.2 | 6.1 | 5.3 | 30.4 | 2.1 | 6.1 | 5.1 | 26.7 |
| 3.6 | 5.0 | 9.4 | 4.3 | 3.4 | 5.3 | 23.2 | 3.6 | 3.5 | 5.4 | . | 4.9 | 3.3 | 5.2 | 16.7 | 4.3 | 3.9 | 5.7 | 10.6 | 4.7 | 3.1 | 5.4 |
| 4.0 | 8.1 | 2.2 | 14.8 | 3.7 | 7.5 | 2.5 | 51.3 | 4.1 | 7.5 | 2.2 | . | 3.5 | 6.6 | 2.3 | 35.7 | 3.9 | 7.9 | 2.1 | 19.8 | 3.4 | 7.9 |
| 70.6 | 12.6 | 2.2 | 5.0 | 26.5 | 12.2 | 2.5 | 6.2 | 65.2 | 16.9 | 2.3 | 6.3 | . | 16.3 | 2.3 | 5.1 | 34.8 | 15.2 | 2.1 | 5.5 | 24.3 | 14.6 |
| 5.7 | 36.8 | 2.2 | 6.0 | 5.0 | 27.9 | 2.5 | 8.2 | 6.1 | 72.2 | 2.3 | 7.1 | 5.3 | . | 2.3 | 6.8 | 5.9 | 64.0 | 2.2 | 6.7 | 4.9 | 50.7 |
| 3.9 | 5.6 | 10.2 | 5.3 | 4.0 | 5.5 | 19.9 | 5.3 | 4.3 | 5.6 | 13.1 | 4.8 | 3.2 | 5.1 | . | 5.4 | 5.3 | 8.3 | 12.2 | 6.3 | 4.0 | 6.7 |
| 3.9 | 8.1 | 2.2 | 16.4 | 3.6 | 7.2 | 2.5 | 79.0 | 4.1 | 7.9 | 2.1 | 35.7 | 3.2 | 6.4 | 2.4 | . | 4.0 | 8.8 | 2.2 | 32.8 | 3.9 | 8.8 |
| 26.8 | 13.0 | 2.2 | 5.1 | 21.3 | 12.7 | 2.6 | 6.7 | 38.3 | 16.3 | 2.3 | 5.6 | 12.1 | 10.8 | 2.7 | 5.9 | . | 30.5 | 2.3 | 5.8 | 26.8 | 14.6 |
| 5.9 | 35.3 | 2.2 | 6.0 | 5.2 | 28.1 | 2.7 | 9.3 | 6.2 | 86.7 | 2.3 | 6.9 | 4.5 | 20.2 | 2.5 | 7.5 | 6.8 | . | 2.3 | 6.8 | 5.5 | 44.5 |
| 3.5 | 4.8 | 12.9 | 5.3 | 3.5 | 5.0 | 18.1 | 4.8 | 3.9 | 5.1 | 14.1 | 4.3 | 2.9 | 4.6 | 24.3 | 5.2 | 4.2 | 6.9 | . | 7.2 | 4.1 | 6.6 |
| 4.0 | 7.9 | 2.3 | 20.2 | 3.9 | 7.6 | 2.6 | 42.3 | 4.1 | 8.2 | 2.2 | 21.9 | 3.3 | 6.5 | 2.5 | 39.1 | 4.0 | 8.1 | 2.4 | . | 4.4 | 10.8 |
| 23.1 | 9.5 | 2.2 | 5.1 | 19.0 | 10.0 | 2.5 | 6.4 | 27.7 | 13.7 | 2.1 | 4.6 | 10.0 | 7.5 | 2.4 | 5.5 | 23.5 | 13.1 | 2.3 | 6.5 | . | 14.9 |
| 5.3 | 25.7 | 2.1 | 6.1 | 4.8 | 21.7 | 2.5 | 9.6 | 6.1 | 42.8 | 2.2 | 6.6 | 4.4 | 16.6 | 2.4 | 7.2 | 5.4 | 33.8 | 2.3 | 8.1 | 5.6 | . |

## Footnotes to Table 2

Within each pair, one preference (regarding treatment A) is considered a test for the other preference (regarding treatment B) which is considered an outcome. For each test preference it is possible to define the test sensitivity and specificity from the population data, as for any other clinical test. The likelihood ratio provides a measure of the likelihood that decision A will predict decision B. The likelihood ratio is defined as (sensitivity)/(1-specificity).

For likelihood ratios for declining treatment, sensitivity = (correctly predicted treatment B declines)/(total treatment B declines), and specificity = (correctly predicted treatment B accepts)/(total treatment B accepts). For likelihood ratios for accepting treatment, sensitivity = (correctly predicted treatment B accepts)/(total treatment B accepts), and specificity = (correctly predicted treatment B declines)/(total treatment B declines).

Likelihood ratios are related to the prior odds (odds before the predictor test) and posterior odds (odds after the predictor test by the following formula: posterior odds = likelihood ratio x prior odds. A likelihood ratio of 1 indicates that the test choice has no ability to predict the other choice. A value greater than 1 indicates predictive power; for instance, a likelihood ratio of 10 for decision A predicting for decision B multiplies the odds that decision B will be the same as decision A tenfold.

Letter abbreviations: abx, antibiotics; blood, blood transfusions; cpr, cardiopulmonary resuscitation; dxc, invasive diagnostics; dxs, noninvasive diagnostics; feed, artificial tube feeding; iv, intravenous fluids; ormaj, major operations; ormin, minor operations; dialysis, peritoneal or hemodialysis; resp, mechanical respiration; coma/chance, coma with a chance of recovery; PVS, persistent vegetative state; dementia/terminal, dementia with terminal illness; pd = peritoneal or hemo dialysis. Numerical digits refer to scenarios: 1 = coma/chance; 2 = PVS; 3 = dementia; 4 = dementia/terminal.

# REFERENCES

1. President's Commission for the Study of Ethical Problems in Medicine and Biomedical Research. *Deciding to forego life-sustaining treatment: a report on the ethical, medical, and legal issues in treatment decisions.* Washington, DC: Government Printing Office, 1983.
2. Lynn J. Why I don t have a living will. *Law Med Health Care* 1991;19: 101–104.
3. Seghal A, Galbraith A, Chesney M, Schoenfeld P, Charles G, Lo B. How strictly do dialysis patients want their advance directives followed? *JAMA* 1992;267:59–63.
4. Emanuel EJ, Emanuel LL. Proxy decision making. *JAMA* 1992;267: 2221–2226.
5. Rabkin MT, Gillerman G, Rice NR. Orders not to resuscitate. *N Engl J Med* 1976;295:364–366.
6. Emanuel LL. Does the do-not-resuscitate order need life sustaining intervention? Time for advance care directives. *Am J Med* 1989;86:87–90.
7. Bedell SE, Delbanco TL. Choices about cardiopulmonary resuscitation in the hospital: when do physicians talk with patients? *N Engl J Med* 1984;310:1089–1093.
8. Bok S. Personal directions for care at the end of life. *N Engl J Med* 1976; 295:367–369.
9. Relman AS. Michigan's sensible living will. *N Engl J Med* 1979;300: 1270–1272.
10. Doukas DJ, McCullough LB. The values history: the evaluation of the patient's values and advance directives. *J Fam Pract* 1991;32:145–153.
11. Emanuel LL, Emanuel EJ. The medical directive: a new comprehensive advance care document. *JAMA* 1989;261:3288–3293.
12. Schneiderman LJ, Pearlman RA, Kaplan RM, Anderson JP, Rosenberg EM. Relationship of general advance directive instructions to specific life-sustaining treatment preferences in patients with serious illness. *Arch Intern Med* 1992;152:2114–2122.
13. Fischer G, Alpert H, Stoeckle JD, Emanuel LL. Relationship between goals and treatment preferences in advance directives. *J Gen Intern Med* 1994;9:93.
14. Doukas DJ, Gorenflo DW. Analyzing the values history: an evaluation of patient medical values and advance directives. *J Clin Ethics* 1993;4: 41–45.
15. Nunally JC. *Psychometric theory*, 2nd ed. New York: McGraw-Hill, 1978:265–270.
16. *Right to die legislation.* New York: Choice in Dying, 1994.
17. Weir RF, Gostin L. Decisions to abate life-sustaining treatment for non-autonomous patients: ethical standards and legal liability for physicians after Cruzan. *JAMA* 1990;264:1846–1853.
18. Emanuel EJ. A review of the ethical and legal aspects of terminating medical care. *Am J Med* 1988;84:291–301.
19. Emanuel LL. What makes a directive valid? *Hastings Cent Rep* 1994; 24(Suppl):S27–S29.
20. Dresser RS. Advance directives, self-determination, and personal identity. In: Hackler C, Moseley R, Vawter DE, eds. *Advance directives in medicine.* New York: Praeger Publishers, 1989:155–170.
21. *In re Karen Ann Quinlan* 70 N.J. 10, 355 A.2d 647 (1976).
22. Appelbaum PS, Lidz CW, Meisel A. *Informed consent: legal theory and clinical practice.* New York: Oxford University Press, 1987.
23. Faden RR, Beauchamp TL. Decision-making and informed consent: a study of the impact of disclosed information. *Soc Indicators Res* 1980; (7):313–336.
24. Shapiro R. Informed consent. In: Berger A, Levy MH, Portenoy RK, Weissman DE, eds. *Principles and practice of supportive oncology.* Philadelphia: JB Lippincott, 1996.
25. Emanuel LL, Danis M, Pearlman RA, Singer PA. Advance care planning as a process. *Am Geriatr Soc* 1995;43:440–446.
26. Singer PA. Disease-specific advance directives. *Lancet* 1994;344: 594–596.
27. Patrick DO, Starks HE, Cain KC, Uhlmann RF, Pearlman RA. *Measuring preferences for health states worse than death. Medical decision making.* 1994;14:9–18.
28. Orentlicher D. Advance medical directives. *JAMA* 1990;263:2365–2367.
29. Silverstein MD, Stocking CB, Antel JP, Beckwith J, Roos RP, Siegler M. Amyotrophic lateral sclerosis and life-sustaining therapy: patient s desires for information, participation in decision making, and life-sustaining therapy. *Mayo Clin Proc* 1991;66:906–913.
30. Everhart MA, Pearlman RA. Stability of patient preferences regarding life-sustaining treatments. *Chest* 1990;97:159–164.
31. Emanuel LL, Emanuel EJ, Stoeckle JD, Hummel LR, Barry MJ. Advance directives: stability of patients treatment choices. *Arch Intern Med* 1994;154:209–217.
32. Danis, Patrick DL, Garrett J, Harris R, Patrick DL. Stability of choices about life- sustaining treatments. *Ann Intern Med* 1994;120: 567–573.
33. Emanuel LL, Barry MJ, Emanuel EJ, Stoeckle JD. Advance directive: can patients stated treatment choices be used to infer unstated choices? *Med Care* 1994;32:95–105.
34. Emanuel LL. Appropriate and inappropriate use of advance directives. *Clin Ethics* 1994;5(4):357–359.
35. The SUPPORT investigators. A controlled trial to improve decision-making for seriously ill hospitalized patients: The struggle to understand prognoses and preferences for outcomes and risks of treatments (SUPPORT). *JAMA* 1995;274(20):1591–1598.
36. Danis M, Southerland LI, Garrett JM, et al. A prospective study of advance directives for life-sustaining care. *N Engl J Med* 1991;324: 882–888.
37. Emanuel LL. Structured deliberation for medical decision making for the seriously ill. *Hastings Center Rep* 1995;25(6):514–518.
38. Kasper JF, Mulley AG Jr, Wennberg JE. Developing shared decision-making programs to improve the quality of health care. *Qual Rev Bull* 1992;18(6):183–190.
39. Steiber SR. Right to die: public balks at deciding for others. *Hospitals* 1987;61:72.
40. Gillick MR, Hesse K, Massapica N. Medical technology at the end of life. What would physicians and nurses want for themselves? *Arch Intern Med* 1993;153:2542–2547.
41. Kane RL, Wales J, Bernstein L, Leibowitz A, Kaplan S. A randomized controlled trial of hospice care. *Lancet* 1984;1:890–894.
42. Emanuel EJ, Emauel LL. The economics of dying–the illusion of cost savings at the end of life. *N Engl J Med* 1994;330:540–544.
43. Emanuel LL, Emanuel EJ. When patients have no advance directives: institutional default guidelines defined by communities of patients. *Hastings Cent Rep* 1993;23:6–14.
44. Emanuel LL, Barry MJ, Stoeckle JD, Ettelson LM, Emanuel EJ. Advance care directives: a case for greater use. *N Engl J Med* 1991; 324:889–895.

*Principles and Practice of Supportive Oncology,*
edited by Ann Berger et al.
Lippincott–Raven Publishers, Philadelphia ©1998

CHAPTER 59

# Withholding and Withdrawing Treatment

## The Doctor-Patient Relationship and the Changing Goals of Care

David Barnard

This chapter will review the ethical considerations involved in withholding or withdrawing treatment of cancer patients. It will have two major objectives. The first will be to explore ethical aspects of decisions beginning with the transition from active treatment to palliative care, and subsequent decisions concerning life-sustaining treatments and care in the terminal phase. The second objective will be to explore the impact of these decisions on the doctor-patient relationship, when cure of the patient's disease is no longer a realistic goal.

Two quotations suggest important starting points:

1. "The kinds of decisions that have to be taken with, and often on behalf of, the seriously ill are not purely technical. These decisions become an intrinsic component of the dying process. Depending on which decisions are taken, and on how they are reached, some people will have the chance to die well, as masters of their dying, not alone and not lonely. Others may die before their time, without a chance to live through their dying. Others may die too late, reduced to impersonal biological systems that have to be tended. Some may be uninformed and unenlightened, caught in the act of playing scene two when the drama is about to close. Still others may die, who could have lived" (1).

2. "To the dying person his doctor, however much he is trusted and regarded as a source of treatment, is no longer one with the power to cure; to the doctor, the patient becomes one whose death, despite every possible effort, he is impotent to prevent. This gives rise to problems in the special relationship which often develops between a patient and his doctor, and besides that they have the difficulties that face any two people trying to adjust to the fact that one of them is shortly going to die" (2).

Quotation 1 suggests these points:

- In the context of modern scientific medicine, death is timed and shaped to a great extent by human choice and decision.
- It is possible for patients to die either "too soon" or "too late."
- There is a need to respect the choices made by competent patients while not abandoning patients with seriously impaired decision-making capacity to the harmful results of their incompetent decisions.
- Decision-making near the end of life often takes place under conditions of medical uncertainty.

Quotation 2 suggests these points:

- Regardless of the scientific and technical issues at stake, end-of-life decision-making occurs in the context of human relationships.
- Doctor and patient face the patient's death together, with an impact on both.
- End-of-life decisions raise important issues of meaning, hope, and communication.

In keeping with these starting points, the present chapter will be divided into two parts. The first part will focus on the ethics of decision-making, the second will focus on the doctor-patient relationship.

D. Barnard: Department of Humanities, The Pennsylvania State University College of Medicine, Hershey, PA 17033-0850.

## ETHICS OF DECISION-MAKING

Three frameworks are useful for approaching the ethical aspects of decisions to withdraw or withhold medical treatment for cancer patients: the goals of medical care, the current ethical and legal consensus regarding withdrawal or withholding of life-sustaining treatment, and the ideal decision-making process and reasons for departures from the ideal.

### The Goals of Medical Care

In the context of cancer there are three major goals of care. The first is *cure or long-lasting remission of the disease.* In pursuit of this goal, which when completely achieved results in the total eradication of the disease, major side effects of treatment are usually acceptable. The second goal is *prolongation of survival.* Although a complete cure may be unlikely, moderate to major side effects are acceptable in the attempt to arrest the progression of the disease. The third goal is *comfort and optimum quality of life.* The primary emphasis is to palliate the symptoms of advanced disease and to help the patient maintain the highest possible quality of life. No significant side effects are acceptable that are inconsistent with the patient's comfort (3).

In practice these goals often overlap. The patient's comfort and quality of life, for example, ought to be of concern from the very beginning, despite the rigors of aggressive treatment. Moreover, the points of transition from one goal to another are rarely clear-cut. Because of the combination of clinical uncertainty, the sometimes erratic or surprising behavior of a particular patient's tumor, and the patient's and the doctor's ambivalence, these transitions are often gradual and subtle.

Nevertheless, over the course of any patient's treatment the two key questions are these:

1. Which goal should be pursued as the *primary* goal at any given time?
2. When is it appropriate to *change* goals and begin the process of withholding or withdrawing treatments?

In the majority of cases these questions are answered in ways that are acceptable to both patient and doctor, even though decisions to withhold or withdraw treatment are typically accompanied by feelings of disappointment and sadness. Conflicts arise when the patient and the physician differ on the desirability of continuing active treatment of the patient's disease. In one common scenario, the physician sees the potential benefits of continued treatment, either in pursuit of cure or an improved quality of life, but the patient expresses the desire to stop. Another troubling scenario is the reverse: the physician believes that further active treatment is likely to do more harm than good, but the patient or the patient's family insists on continuing the fight.

## The Ethical and Legal Consensus

A strong ethical and legal consensus has emerged over the past two decades regarding patients' preferences to withhold or withdraw medical treatment. No similar consensus yet exists with respect to the physician's responsibilities when a patient insists on treatments that the physician believes to be contrary to the patient's best interests, though such a consensus may well be forming.

The following points are well established in the statements of professional medical societies, bioethics groups, judicial opinions, and actions by state legislatures (4–10):

1. Competent adults may refuse medical treatment.
2. Treatment refusals may include all forms of life-sustaining treatment, including artificial nutrition and hydration.
3. From an ethical and legal point of view, there is no difference between withholding a treatment (not starting it) and withdrawing a treatment (stopping it after it has been started), as long as either action is in accord with the patient's preferences.
4. Complying with a competent adult's wishes to refuse or discontinue life-sustaining treatment is considered to be neither homicide nor assisted suicide.
5. Treatments intended primarily to maintain comfort near the end of life that have as a side effect the hastening of death are morally permissible and are not the moral equivalent of active euthanasia.
6. Incompetent or otherwise nonautonomous people have the same rights as do people with decision-making capacity, though their rights must be exercised either through a written advance directive or by a person who is authorized to make decisions on their behalf.

Central to the development of this consensus has been the increasing recognition of the value of patients' self-determination in medical decision-making, and decreasing deference either to the authority and judgment of health professionals or to an abstract state interest in the preservation of life. There has been greater acceptance of judgments about the quality of life as determined by the patient's own preferences and values, instead of an unquestioned commitment to the extension of biological existence. Patients' desires for comfort, companionship, and control near the end of life, and not only the prolongation of life, have come to the forefront of the health professional's responsibilities. The emergence of palliative care as a field of special expertise within medicine is itself a manifestation of this trend.

In principle, then, according to this consensus any and all treatments may be withheld or withdrawn. The important factor is whether or not the treatment in question, and the goal it serves, are in accord with the patient's informed and considered preferences. These preferences set the limit to the authority for medical intervention.

Respect for patients' self-determination means that competent patients have the right to say "no" to the physician's recommendations. The physician who strongly believes that the patient will benefit from continued treatment may attempt to educate and persuade the patient but may not impose treatment on a competent patient who has refused it (11).

In the reverse situation, when the physician believes that a patient's insistence on continuing active treatment is contrary to the patient's best interests, the ethical and legal consensus is less clear, though the outlines of consensus are beginning to emerge. There is general agreement on two points: patients' self-determination, which underlies patients' rights to *refuse* medical treatments, does not entail a right to *demand* medical treatments that are contrary to medical judgment, and the integrity of the medical profession requires that physicians not be obligated to provide nonbeneficial treatment (12). What makes this consensus problematic is unavoidable ambiguity in deciding when a treatment is nonbeneficial.

Current debates on this issue are usually framed in terms of the concept of futility (13–15). Like *nonbeneficial*, the term *futility* is an objective-sounding word that masks two sorts of value judgments. A treatment is futile only with respect to a given goal. Therefore, in addition to a probability judgment (the statistical likelihood of achieving a particular goal) there is a judgment whether that goal is worth pursuing at all. An example is cardiopulmonary resuscitation (CPR) of the elderly, chronically ill patient. Studies suggest that only a small percentage of such patients who receive CPR will survive to be discharged from the hospital. The first value judgment in labeling CPR futile in this situation is that the given percentage of patients likely to survive is too low for the treatment to be regarded as effective. The second value judgment is that short-term survival after CPR is not a worthwhile goal of the intervention.

Patients differ in their willingness to undergo burdensome or painful side effects; in their judgment as to the length of life, quality of life, or other nonmedical values that would justify those side effects; and in their willingness to pursue long odds. In the face of this variability, and the inescapably value-laden nature of futility judgments, ethical and legal consensus has been slower to form than in the previous context of the patient's right to refuse treatment. Courts, for example, have ruled in opposite directions. A district court in Minnesota refused to allow a hospital to discontinue mechanical ventilation for an 86-year-old woman in a persistent vegetative state over the objections of the patient's husband, who asserted that his wife would want every chance for a miracle to restore her to health (16). A superior court in Massachusetts, on the other hand, upheld the decision of Massachusetts General Hospital to refuse CPR to a comatose, irreversibly brain-damaged patient on the grounds that such treatment would be futile, even though the patient's

family insisted that she be given every possible treatment to maintain her life (17).

Social policy is still evolving on the question of physicians' legal ability to withhold nonbeneficial treatments that are demanded by patients or their families, though there is reason to expect that broad agreement will emerge, at least in certain areas. Cases involving persistent vegetative state, for example, constitute an area where professional groups and bioethics organizations have begun to articulate limits to the obligations to provide intensive care (14). Even in the absence of clear legal consensus, however, certain guidelines for clinical behavior are relatively clear. Patients or families who insist on continuing treatment that appears contrary to medical judgment should be given clear, sensitive explanations of the physician's rationale for advising against the treatment or for changing the goals of care (13). Education and emotional support, often over an extended time, will usually lead to agreement about the proper course to pursue. Unresolved conflicts can be moved to the setting of an institutional ethics committee or, in extreme cases of disagreement, arrangements can be made to transfer the patient to the care of another physician. Fortunately, it is the exceptional case in which disagreement persists to that extent, or to the point where recourse to the courts is required.

## The Ideal Decision-Making Process

Regardless of whose initiative prompts consideration of a change in the goals of care, a crucial first step is to establish a therapeutic dialogue that facilitates optimal decision making. The clinician's goal should be to promote an accommodation between reasonably expected outcomes of treatment (or nontreatment) and the preferences and values of the patient. An ideal decision-making process includes at least the following elements:

1. Joint participation of doctor and patient, with the additional participation of significant others of the patient's choice
2. Clear and truthful communication by the physician
3. Clear and thoughtful deliberation by the patient
4. Consideration of both medical and nonmedical factors, including

- The reasonable probability that a particular goal of medical treatment can be achieved
- The reasonably expected proportion of benefits to harmful side effects of treatment or nontreatment, including the nature and availability of palliative care services
- The patient's values and life goals
- The patient's tolerance for risks and harms
- The patient's assessment of his or her quality of life in terms of his or her personal values and sources of meaning

5. A reasonable accommodation of the resulting decision to the medical facts, and consistency of the decision with the patient's values and the physician's conscience

## Departures From the Ideal

In the real world, of course, things are rarely so simple and neat. We may look in three directions for the main factors that tend to complicate physician-patient deliberation about withholding or withdrawing treatment: medical uncertainty, physicians' attitudes and values, and patients' attitudes and values.

### Medical Uncertainty

There is little dispute that it is inappropriate to apply maximum life-prolonging medical treatment to a patient who is irreversibly dying. The problem is to determine when the dying process has begun. In the setting of contemporary medical technology and intensive care, the line between life and death is almost always blurred. Something can usually be done to stave off death for an additional time, during which additional treatments are often proposed. Even if the chance that these treatments will benefit the patient is small, it is rarely possible to demonstrate that the chance is zero. In this context, and given the inherent uncertainties in medical prognosis (especially regarding the future time of death except when death is expected within a few days or hours), many physicians are reluctant to pronounce a definitive judgment that the patient is dying, or that it is time to consider a change in the goals of care.

### Physicians' Attitudes and Values

A cluster of physicians' attitudes and values—some which reflect attitudes toward death in the culture at large, some which seem peculiar to the medical profession—add to the difficulty of carrying out a clear and forthright dialogue with patients with advanced disease. There is, first, denial that the patient has deteriorated—something often easier to recognize in the patients of one's colleagues! There is also the belief, particularly in the field of oncology, that the role of the physician is to push back the frontiers of medical knowledge and power, so that the oncologist's most pressing and legitimate goals are to offer new treatments to fight the disease and to encourage patients to try them. To recommend anything less, it is frequently asserted, is tantamount to annihilating the patient's hope.

The blurred line between life and death and the ability to postpone death technologically have given rise to an attitude that every patient's death is the result of the physician's act or omission. The notion that death (in the abstract) may be inevitable, but that every particular cause of death is or should be curable or preventable, places an enormous psychological and moral burden on the physician, who has come to believe that he or she is responsible for every patient's death (18). To say that this patient died because I failed to do X or Y is very different from saying that the patient died because he or she was too sick to live anymore. The latter formulation has come to seem hopelessly out of date, yet it conveys an important truth about the naturalness of dying that medical advances (and human resistance) have tended to obscure (19).

### Patients' Attitudes and Values

Although physicians most often become concerned about patients' ability to make treatment decisions when they refuse recommended therapy, in the case of advanced cancer there may also be reasons for concern when patients accept or demand continuing treatment. The patient's denial of his or her deterioration or closeness to death can be an adaptive, protective response, enabling the patient to pursue tasks of living free from debilitating fear or worry. Yet, denial can also seriously impair the patient's ability to assess realistically the benefits and harms of continuing active treatment (20). (When both patient and physician are in a state of denial, the chances of inappropriately continuing active treatment are high.) Other patients may accept or demand continuing treatment, not because they genuinely desire it but because they believe that they owe it to their family to keep up the fight.

On the other hand, patients' refusals of treatment may be a language for indirectly expressing other things. When explored further, many patients' initial requests to stop active treatment (or more drastic requests for assisted suicide or active euthanasia) turn out to be indirect communications of—for example—uncontrolled symptoms, fear of being a burden, anger, mistrust of doctors or family members, loneliness, or helplessness (21–24). Common symptoms include unrelieved pain, nausea, anxiety, and sleep disturbances accompanied by exhaustion or fatigue (25). Some patients who refuse treatment, or express the desire to die, may be suffering from a clinical depression or other psychiatric disorder (21,26).

In summary, to insure optimal decision-making when considering withdrawal or withholding of medical treatment, the physician must undertake a thorough assessment of these facts:

- His or her own biases, motivations, emotional reactions to the patient and the patient's illness, and the factual bases for his or her prognostic judgment
- The personal meaning to the patient of the illness, symptoms, and treatment

- The patient's perceptions of the health care system, especially the communication of information and the functioning of the health care team
- The dynamics of the patient's family as they affect the patient's experience of being ill
- The presence of inadequately treated physical symptoms, clinical depression, or other psychiatric disorder
- The patient's current goals and values as they influence the patient's weighing of the benefits and burdens of continued treatment

In making this assessment, it is important to distinguish disagreement between physician and patient that is due to some severe impairment of the patient's ability to deliberate and choose, from the diversity of values that people can bring to bear on matters of life and death (21). The current consensus is that for the mentally competent patient, his or her self-determination is the primary value that we must respect.

## Competence

The concept of competence obviously bears very great weight in these decisions. In assessing competence, the aim must be to avoid two sorts of harm: (a) refusing to respect the wishes of a competent patient or (b) abandoning an incompetent patient to the harmful consequences of his or her incompetently chosen course of action.

A clinically useful definition of competence is the ability of the patient to understand the facts of his or her situation, appreciate their significance in terms of the likely consequences of choosing among the available alternatives of treatment or nontreatment, and give reasons for his or her choice that relate the choice to the patient's values and life goals.

Competence is decision-specific. It is not a global state. Thus, the important determination is whether the patient is competent to make this particular decision, not whether he or she is competent to make any and all decisions. The higher the stakes, the more stringent ought to be the test for competence. But in deciding what the stakes of a patient's decision actually are, it must be remembered that the balance of goods and harms that may follow a particular choice is always relative to the alternatives that are actually available. Moreover, competence refers to the *process* of the patient's decision, not to its *outcome*. As noted previously, people differ widely in their weighing of the benefits and harms of medical treatment, the acceptability of side effects, or an acceptable quality of life (11,27).

Respect for patients' self-determination is most likely to be upheld when we presume that the patient is competent and test for incompetence, rather than the reverse. Four potential indicators of incompetence, however, should be grounds for concern:

- The patient gives evidence of a psychiatric disorder.

- The patient's stated preference appears to depart radically from previous patterns and preferences.
- The patient appears to hold inconsistent or contradictory preferences.
- The patient's choice appears irrational, and not simply evidence of a profound difference in values.

Even in cases when these suspicions lead to an assessment that the patient is incompetent, efforts should be made to restore the patient's competence, if that is possible, before identifying a surrogate decision-maker.

## Withholding and Withdrawing Treatment, Assisted Suicide, and Euthanasia

Can the withholding or withdrawing of life-sustaining treatment be reliably differentiated from assisting in the patient's suicide or from active euthanasia? Judges, legislatures, and position statements of professional societies have consistently answered "yes." Nevertheless, certain decisions at the very end of life provoke unease in many clinicians. Most provocative are the withdrawal of artificial nutrition and hydration, and continuous sedation in response to otherwise intractable physical, psychological, or existential suffering. In both cases it appears as if the physician has introduced a specific cause of death, independent of the fatal outcome that will ultimately result from the patient's disease. Withholding nutrition and hydration deprives the patient of the basic necessities that all people need, while continuous sedation brings about a state of unconsciousness that prevents the patient from taking in these necessities. In either case, the patient dies sooner than he or she would have if these actions had not been taken.

Some have argued that these situations demonstrate that the distinction between withholding and withdrawing treatment and assisted suicide or euthanasia does not, in fact, hold. It would be inconsistent, in this view, to permit withholding or withdrawing while legally prohibiting physician-assisted suicide or active voluntary euthanasia. Conversely, if assisted suicide and euthanasia are impermissible, then the withholding of artificial nutrition and hydration, and continuous sedation, should be impermissible as well (28,29).

Though the distinction is admittedly very fine in certain cases, I would claim that it is *generally* tenable. Moreover, besides being firmly established in the law, the distinction is useful not only clinically but socially. Should it be abandoned, this should be done only with great care and in full awareness of the possible consequences (30). There are, in any event, three main points of difference that support maintaining the distinction between withholding and withdrawing, on one hand, and assisted suicide or active euthanasia, on the other: intention, the right to be left alone, and the possibility for continuing care (31).

## Intention

Withholding or withdrawing treatment is usually undertaken in order to spare the patient from treatments that can no longer accomplish their goal, or that impose greater burdens than can be justified by the benefit to be gained. Euthanasia, by contrast, is an act intended to end the patient's life. In this context, artificial nutrition and hydration, for example, are properly regarded as medical treatments whose benefits must be weighed against the potential burdens. There are situations in which continuing hydration of the moribund patient may well serve valuable goals of the patient's comfort (32). But that—and not the foreseeable hastening of the patient's death or the particular nature of the treatment itself—is the important question that must be evaluated in the specific case. If no benefit to the patient can be demonstrated, then the treatment may be withdrawn—assuming this action is in accord with the preferences of the patient to avoid further medical intervention (33). In the case of continuous sedation, the primary intention is to alleviate symptoms and the patient's suffering. The foreseeable but unintended side effect of the patient's earlier death is not, in and of itself, sufficient reason to classify continuous sedation as an act of euthanasia (34).

## The Right to Be Left Alone

The patient's choice to refuse further life-sustaining treatment is an expression of a *negative* right. It expresses our right to say "no": to set limits on the power of others to enter our bodies or direct our lives. This right to be left alone is the meaning of self-determination and personal autonomy, as these concepts have been employed and interpreted in the common law and in bioethics for the past century. As noted in the previous discussion of futility, the notion of self-determination does not extend to the right to demand medical treatment that is contrary to medical judgment or the physician's conscience. Yet, a request for assisted suicide or euthanasia is just such a positive request for an active intervention.

## The Possibility for Continuing Care

The decision to withhold or withdraw treatment can usually be reconsidered and sometimes reversed. Euthanasia, by contrast, is immediate and irreversible. Moreover, for patients who have refused further life-prolonging treatments there are almost always opportunities to continue acts of comfort and supportive care. Even when a patient is under continuous sedation, caregivers and loved ones may still attempt to communicate their tenderness, presence, and love.

Public pressures for the legalization of physician-assisted suicide or euthanasia are mounting. As this chapter is written the legislature of the Northern Territory of Australia has passed a law—since repealed—permitting active voluntary euthanasia by physicians, and voters in the state of Oregon have approved a referendum permitting physicians to prescribe lethal doses of medication to terminally ill patients who request help in committing suicide. (Implementation of the Oregon measure has been delayed pending judicial review.) Although in 1997 the Supreme Court (in *Vacco v. Quill* and *Washington v. Glucksberg*) found no constitutional right to physician-assisted suicide, similar initiatives in other states are likely in the future. A major stimulus for this activity is the public's lack of trust in physicians and hospitals to provide care that assures patients comfort and dignity at the end of life.

People on both sides of the divisive euthanasia debate agree on the importance of making excellent palliative care available as a realistic option for the dying. This will be possible only with adequate financing of these services, and excellence in health professionals' education in palliative care. The current mismatch between funding for curative cancer treatments and for palliative care will have to be redressed if withholding or withdrawing treatment is to be a genuinely humane alternative for the advanced cancer patient (35).

## THE DOCTOR-PATIENT RELATIONSHIP

As was suggested by Hinton at the beginning of this chapter, decisions to withhold or withdraw treatment take place in the context of human relationships. Both doctor and patient face the patient's inevitable death together, and there is a personal impact on both. The physician has the opportunity and responsibility to maintain strong ties to the patient during this period and to support the patient's hope even though cure of the disease is no longer a realistic goal. In Oratz's words:

> In choosing palliative rather than curative treatment, the patient is not abandoning all hope of life, but is choosing one kind of life over another. She should be assured that she will not be deserted by her physician or any other member of the health care team as she leads that life. All health care providers have an obligation to continue to provide symptomatic relief of pain and suffering, emotional reassurance, physical contact, and social support to the patient who chooses palliative, rather than curative therapy (36).

### Maintaining Hope

The desire to maintain hope is frequently cited by physicians as the reason for withholding bad news from patients, or for continuing to offer curative treatments even when they are likely to be of little benefit. It is a nearly universal belief among health professionals that hope is important to the patient, though there is no unanimous opinion as to exactly why. There are suggestive but by no means conclusive data on the correlations between hope and longevity, survival, and other physiological parameters. There are better correlations to subjective factors such as the patient's assessment of quality of life, the quality of interpersonal relationships, and the ability to make the most of the time that is left (37–41). In the face of a grave prognosis and the changing goals of care, the important questions for the clinician are these: what is the basis for the patient's hope, and what is the role of the physician in maintaining that hope?

### The Changing Focus of Hope

Though both patient and physician undertake cancer therapy with the hope of a cure, the patient's hopefulness need not be focused exclusively on the expectation of cure or prolonged survival. Other important objects of hope include comfort and freedom from pain, companionship, completion of tasks, and security for those who will be left behind.

In a survey undertaken as part of a national study of hospice care, Kastenbaum and his colleagues asked a group of dying patients to describe the last three days of their life as they would like them to be, including whatever aspects of the situation seemed to be of greatest importance. Among the most frequent responses were these:

- "I want certain people to be here with me."
- "I want to be physically able to do things."
- "I want to feel at peace."
- "I want to be free from pain."
- "I want the last three days of my life to be like any other days" (42).

In interviews with 30 terminally ill patients, Herth (41) found several categories of experience or interaction that patients found to be supportive of hope:

- Connection to others
- Lightheartedness or playfulness
- Determination, courage, serenity
- Attainable aims (which would shift according to time horizon and medical condition)
- A spiritual base
- Review of uplifting memories
- Having one's worth affirmed and one's individuality accepted

By contrast, three categories were associated with the loss of hope:

- Abandonment and isolation
- Uncontrollable pain and discomfort
- Depersonalization

It is important to note that none of the hope-inducing categories is related to length of survival. All of them relate to the experience of continuing relationship with others, the quality of those relationships, and the patient's inner spiritual resources.

In a more personal narrative form, a cancer patient expressed her hopes this way:

> As patients we want to be able to trust our doctors. Most of us do not want legislation for active euthanasia. We want informed clinical judgment about when to stop treatment. We want to remain clear-headed to be able to attend to our affairs and relate to family and friends. We don't want to pretend pain is controlled if it is not—in order not to offend. We want to use our gifts and talents to the end. We want to be treated lovingly, knowing we may become unlovable. Most of us would like to die at home in our own surroundings, and hope we will still have friends there when we do (43).

Two additional perspectives on hope provide useful guidance to the physician:

1. *Hope is not the physician's to dispense or to remove.* Hope originates from within the patient, and the patient's resources for maintaining hope will likely be very different from what the physician expects.

2. *To support a patient's hope requires, first, that we know the patient's fears and despair.* Only when we have allowed the patient to express himself or herself about his or her deepest fears can we offer anything more than vague, placating generalities that the patient will not trust. Taking time for honest, empathic dialogue is a prerequisite for supporting the patient's hope.

### Maintaining Connection

The patient's feeling of hopefulness is sustained primarily by his or her experience of continuing to be in relationships. For many patients, especially those who are actively religious, the sense of ongoing relatedness may well include their relationship to God. But for all patients the sense of relatedness will depend in important ways on human relationships of comfort, respect, empathy, and love (44).

The physician's willingness to maintain connection and not withdraw from the patient is crucial. This is so not only because of the value of continuity in the doctor-patient relationship itself. At times the physician's steadiness in relationship with the patient will serve as an important example to the patient's family and friends. Some family members and friends may, for their own reasons, be tempted to withdraw and distance themselves from the patient. They may need the physician's example, support, and encouragement to stay close.

The inspiriting, hope-inducing power of relationship is something of a mystery, and it is not easily reduced to biological or psychological explanations. A psychologist working on a palliative care unit in France has written (my translation from the French):

> If I insist so much on this aspect of emotional connection, of touch, of presence, it is because in the face of our utter pow-

erlessness at the hands of this terrible disease [AIDS], often not knowing what to do, how to comfort, how to soothe the pain, the only possible way out is to offer the patient our very being in all its genuineness and authenticity. For it is there, in the depth of our own being, that we find our reserves of love and faith. This quality of presence that we are trying to achieve in the midst of the other's despair requires us at one and the same time to be in contact with our own deepest selves but also to be able to forget ourselves in order to be truly with the other, and in giving comfort to him to soothe our own pain...It is with love and solidarity that we must try to bear with the other through suffering and death (45).

## Dying, Death, and the Doctor

There is an undeniable price to pay for trying to maintain deep bonds of solidarity and connection with the dying. One enters into direct confrontation with his or her own feelings about death and loss. One is brought face to face with one's own vulnerability, helplessness, and mortality. This sets another challenge for the clinician: to identify the people and the settings in his or her life that help with this encounter. The physician's tasks are to place inevitable losses in perspective, to grieve, and to move on.

In changing the goals of care it is not only the patient but also the doctor who is challenged to shift the focus of his or her hope and meaning. The power to cure or to prolong life need not be the only source of validation of one's personal and professional effort. There are also profound rewards in maintaining relationships, and helping people in significant ways during the final passages of their lives. In the words of an oncologist:

In the long run, particularly if one is engaged in treating patients with far advanced illness, a large number of one's patients die. If keeping patients alive is one of the goals, a large part of one's life can be sheer misery when most patients die. If the physician is able to change his goal, his life may be more tolerable. When the physician's goal can change from that of curing patients to that of trying his best to help and to care for the patient, then success is much less related to whether the patient lives or dies. The physician can succeed when success means that he has tried, that he has done his very best, and that his patient has not died alone, has not died unloved, has not died in any more discomfort than necessary...With this new set of values, success can be an internal thing, measured by one's feeling that he has tried, with all his skill and technique and love, to help a patient through a trying time. If the patient improves and may live longer, this is in part a success and in part a bonus; if the patient has worsened or died, this may still be a success, although a sad one. Under these new values, death becomes reality and not defeat (46).

## REFERENCES

1. Roy DJ, Williams JR, Dickens, BM. *Bioethics in Canada.* Scarborough, Ontario: Prentice Hall Canada, 1994:381.
2. Hinton J. The dying and the doctor. In: Toynbee A, ed. *Man's concern with death.* St. Louis: McGraw-Hill, 1969:36.
3. Miller RJ. The role of chemotherapy in the hospice patient: a problem of definition. *Am J Hospice Care* 1989;6(3):19.
4. ACCP/SCCM Consensus Panel. Ehtical and moral guidelines for the initiation, continuation, and withdrawal of intensive care. *Chest.* 1990; 97:949.
5. American College of Physicians. Ethics manual; part2: the physician and society; research; life-sustaining treatment; other issues. *Ann Intern Med* 1991;111:327
6. American Thoracic Society. Withholding and withdrawing life sustaining therapy. *Ann Intern Med* 1991;115:478.
7. Council on Ethical and Judicial Affairs, American Medical Association. Decisions near the end of life. *JAMA* 1992;267:2229.
8. Gostin L, Weir RF. Life and death choices after Cruzan: case law and standards of professional conduct. *Milbank Q* 1991;69:143.
9. The Hastings Center. *Guidelines on the terminaton of life-sustaining treatment and the care of the dying.* Briarcliff Manor, NY: The Hastings Center, 1987.
10. Meisel A. The legal consensus about forgoing life-sustaining treatment: its status and prospects. *Kennedy Inst Ethics J* 1993;2:309.
11. President's Commission for the Study of Ethical Problems in Medicine and Biomedical and Behavioral Research. *Making health care decisions: the ethical and legal implications of informed consent in the patient-practitioner relationship.* Washington, DC: US Government Printing Office, 1982.
12. Brett AS, McCullough LB. When patients request specific interventions: defining the limits of the physician's obligation. *N Engl J Med* 1986;315:1347.
13. Tomlinson T, Brody H. Futility and the ethics of resuscitation. *JAMA* 1990;264:1276.
14. Truog RD, Brett AS, Frader J. The problem with futility. *N Engl J Med* 1992;326:1276.
15. Youngner SJ. Who defines futility? *JAMA* 1988;260:2094.
16. Capron AM. In re Helga Wanglie. *Hastings Cent Rep* 1991;21(5):26.
17. Capron AM. Abandoning a waning life. *Hastings Cent Rep* 1995;25(4): 24.
18. Callahan D. *The troubled dream of life: living with mortality.* New York: Simon and Schuster, 1993.
19. McCue JD. The naturalness of dying. *JAMA* 1995;273:1039.
20. Wool MS. Understanding denial in cancer patients. *Adv Psychosom Med* 1988;18:37.
21. Goldberg RJ. Systematic understanding of cancer patients who refuse treatment. *Psychother Psychosom* 1983;39:180.
22. Jackson DL, Youngner S. Patient autonomy and death with dignity : some clinical caveats. *N Engl J Med* 1979;301:404.
23. Quill TE. Doctor, I want to die. Will you help me? *JAMA* 1993;270:870.
24. Block SD, Billings JA. Patient requests to hasten death: evaluation and management in terminal care. *Arch Intern Med* 1994;154:2039.
25. Foley KM. The relationship of pain and symptom management to patient requests for physician-assisted suicide. *J Pain Sympt Manag* 1991;6:289.
26. Lynch ME. The assessment and prevalence of affective disorders in advanced cancer. *J Palliat Care* 1995;11(1):10.
27. Buchanan A, Brock DW. Deciding for others. *Milbank Q* 1986;64 (Suppl)2:17.
28. Brody H. Causing, intending, and assisting death. *J Clin Ethics* 1993;4: 112.
29. Brock DW. Voluntary active euthanasia. *Hastings Cent Rep* 1992;22(2): 10.
30. Wolf SM. Holding the line on euthanasia. *Hastings Cent Rep* 1989;19 (1,Suppl):13.
31. Weir RF. *Abating treatment with critically ill patients: Ethical and legal limits to the medical prolongation of life.* New York: Oxford University Press, 1989.
32. Fainsinger R, Bruera E. The management of dehydration in terminally ill patients. *J Palliat Care* 1994;10(3):55.
33. Lynn J, Childress JF. Must patients always be given food and water? *Hastings Cent Rep* 1983;13(5):17.
34. Cherny NI, Portenoy RK. Sedation in the management of refractory symptoms: guidelines for evaluation and treatment. *J Palliat Care* 1994;10(2):31.
35. *Cancer pain relief and palliative care.* Geneva: World Health Organization, 1990.
36. Oratz R. Commentary. In: Cohen CB, ed. *Casebook on the termination of life-sustaining treatment and the care of the dying.* Bloomington: Indiana University Press, 1988:77.

37. Good MD, Good BJ, Schaffer C, Lind E. American oncology and the discourse on hope. *Cult Med Psychiatry* 1990;14:59.

38. Cassileth BR, Lusk EJ, Miller DS, et al. Psychosocial correlates of survival in advanced malignant disease? *N Engl J Med* 1985;312:1551.

39. Optimism plays no definitive role in survival of patients with advanced prognostically poor cancers. *Clin Cancer Lett* 1987;10:1.

40. Levy SM, Wise BD. Psychosocial risk factors, natural immunity, and cancer progression: implications for intervention. In: Johnston M, Mareau T, eds. *Applications in health psychology.* New Brunswick, NJ: Transaction, 1989:141.

41. Herth K. Fostering hope in terminally ill people. *J Adv Nurs* 1990;15: 1250.

42. Kastenbaum R. *Death, society, and human experience,* 3rd ed. Columbus: Merrill, 1986.

43. Jolley MG. Ethics of cancer management from the patient's perspective. *J Med Ethics* 1988;14:188.

44. Barnard D. Chronic illness and the dynamics of hoping. In: Toombs SK, Barnard D, Carson RA, eds. *Chronic illness: from experience to policy.* Bloomington: Indiana University Press, 1995:38.

45. De Hennezel M. Le mythe de la mort parfaite: le nouveau sens de la mort dans le contexte du sida. In: de Montigny J, de Hennezel M. *L'amour ultime.* Montreal: Les editions internationales Stanke, 1990: 130.

46. White LP. The self-image of the physician and the care of dying patients. *Ann NY Acad Sci* 1969;164:822.

*Principles and Practice of Supportive Oncology,*
edited by Ann Berger et al.
Lippincott–Raven Publishers, Philadelphia ©1998

# CHAPTER 60

# Palliative Care and Physician-Assisted Death

Barbara A. Supanich, Howard Brody, and Karen S. Ogle

Physician-assisted death is a very challenging ethical issue for all citizens and health care professionals, but it poses special concerns for those involved in hospice and palliative care. In this chapter we will review some of the major ethical arguments, look more specifically at the challenges posed for palliative care, and, finally, propose clinical strategies for responding to a patient's request for death assistance.

## DEFINITIONS

A cogent ethical analysis of the concerns about assisted death must start with clear definitions.

*Withdrawing or withholding life-sustaining treatment* refers to decisions to stop or not begin certain medical therapies, with the anticipated outcome that the patient will die from the underlying disease. Common examples include withdrawing a ventilator from a patient in end-stage emphysema; foregoing the use of antibiotics in a patient with terminal cancer and suspected pneumonia; and refusal of tube feeding by a patient with an end-stage neuromuscular disease.

*Active euthanasia* refers to the direct administration of a lethal agent to the patient by another party, with a merciful intent. As commonly practiced today in the Netherlands, this might involve the physician injecting intravenously a quick-acting sedative followed by a paralytic agent to halt respiration. Active euthanasia may be voluntary, involuntary, or nonvoluntary, depending on whether the patient has freely chosen it, has freely rejected it, or has offered no opinion. In the remainder of this chapter, we will only consider *voluntary active euthanasia* because that is the only form being seriously advocated in the United States today.

*Assisted suicide* refers to the patient intentionally and willfully ending his or her own life, with the assistance of another party. This assistance may include different levels of involvement —merely providing information about how to commit suicide; providing the means to commit suicide, such as a lethal quantity of pills; or actively participating in the suicide, such as being present at the scene and inserting an intravenous line through which the patient may then administer a lethal dose (1). The widely publicized actions of Drs. Timothy Quill (2) and Jack Kevorkian (3,4) provide examples of the second and third levels of involvement, respectively.

*Assisted death* is the term we will use in the remainder of this chapter to refer jointly to the practices of voluntary active euthanasia and assisted suicide. Most of the ethics literature has focused on the special problems of the physician's role; and so we will most commonly refer to *physician-assisted death*. However, in a hospice context the roles of the other health care professionals and the family are extremely important, and in some cases the patient may request assistance in dying from one or more of them as well as (or instead of) from the physician.

It is also important to be clear about what is *not* assisted death. As noted, it is *not* an assisted death if a competent person decides not to initiate a specific therapy (e.g., further chemotherapy, antibiotics for a pneumonia or another septic process, or artificial nutrition or hydration); nor is it assisted death to withdraw any of these options from the terminal patient. The use of high doses of opioids, where the intent is to relieve pain and not to hasten death, is *not* physician-assisted death. Although many still believe that high-dose opioids pose a serious risk of fatal respiratory depression, palliative specialists know that this very seldom occurs with proper titration of analgesic doses, even when very large doses of opioids are administered in terminal illness (5). Even in the rare case where respiratory depression is a foreseen (but unintended) consequence of adequate analgesia, administering the analgesics is not considered to be physician-assisted death.

B. A. Supanich, H. Brody, and K.S. Ogle: Department of Family Practice, Michigan State University College of Human Medicine, East Lansing, MI 48824.

Withholding and withdrawing life-sustaining treatment is widely accepted today, both in ethics and law, as appropriate and compassionate care, so long as the competent patient is fully informed and freely chooses that management option. Some, notably Rachels (6), have argued that there is no morally relevant difference between this practice and the practice of assisted death. In this chapter, without giving detailed arguments, we will dissent from this view. That is, we will leave open the question of whether assisted death is morally justifiable, offering a review of arguments on both sides of that question. But we will assume that if assisted death can be justified, it must be justified on its own merits and not merely because it shares some moral features with the relatively uncontroversial practice of withdrawing or withholding life-sustaining treatment (7–10).

## ETHICAL ARGUMENTS

### Patient Integrity

Most patients with terminal illnesses want to maintain their personal integrity and autonomy. From the patient's perspective, this means that one's belief system and life goals will be valued and respected, and will play a vital role in decisions about the treatment plan. Most patients have the expectation that their suffering will be moderated, their pain will be controlled, and they will have the opportunity to have rational discussions with their physicians about the type and extent of their treatments (11–13).

Proponents of assisted death would argue that they are honoring the personal integrity and personal autonomy of the patient by being willing to discuss and assist the patient with *all* treatment/care choices for the patient, including assisted death. Proponents also claim that physician-assisted death minimizes harm to the patient and others. They argue that the patient should determine what counts as a harm and may legitimately decide that ongoing life with severe suffering is a greater harm than a painless death (14,15).

Opponents claim that however important the moral value of patient autonomy, it is insufficient to justify the practice of assisted death (7,16–18). Autonomy may justify withdrawing or withholding treatment because that constitutes a negative right of noninterference, which is strongly grounded in the concept of respecting personal bodily integrity. But it cannot justify a positive right to demand that others take specific actions to promote one's own idea of one's welfare—especially when those actions cause death. Moreover, opponents insist that death be considered one of the greatest harms that a health care professional could inflict on a patient. The basic principle of "Do no harm" should be understood as requiring a healing relationship between the physi-

cian and the patient and, thus, in direct conflict with respect for patient autonomy when assistance in dying is requested.

### Compassionate Response to Suffering

For some physicians, a request by a patient for death assistance is viewed as a plea to release the patient from intolerable suffering, and so assistance is an act of compassion. Quill and others (19–21) have argued that a willingness to discuss this option with the patient may often act as a suicide preventive because once the patient's concerns and fears have been fully discussed, the physician may be able to propose alternative means of relieving suffering short of death (22). By contrast, if physicians refuse to offer assistance, suffering patients may avoid these searching conversations and instead commit suicide in a manner that actually increases their own and their family's suffering.

It is a serious mistake to equate suffering narrowly with pain and other unpleasant physical symptoms. Suffering is defined through the experiences of the individual, which includes a personal sense of impaired quality of life, and is understood as a fundamental threat to one's wholeness as a person. Suffering is ultimately tied to one's personal belief system and how those beliefs define the reality of the human person, and how one experiences an illness in the overall context of one's life journey and personal expectations for the future. Two patients may report similar symptoms but have vastly different experiences of suffering (23,24).

Proponents of assisted death point to the multifaceted and complex nature of suffering as a defense for the individual's right to choose a quicker death because no one can really comprehend the severity of anyone else's suffering. Palliative care may be able to relieve unpleasant symptoms very well; but it may be much less capable of restoring meaning and function to a life that has irreversibly lost both. Thus, while excellent palliative care and hospice care should greatly reduce the number of patients who may request death assistance, it would not negate the need for this option in other cases.

By contrast, opponents claim that proponents have a short-sighted and simplistic approach to the relief of suffering. Precisely because suffering is multifaceted and intimately tied to personal meaning, one has numerous ways to work with the suffering individual to restore a sense of meaning in life even with severely reduced function and increased physical distress. To relieve suffering by eliminating the sufferer must always be viewed as an inadequate response. Attending adequately to loneliness, fear of death, depression, unresolved conflicts, lack of forgiveness, anger, and hopelessness is harder work but ultimately will allow a better personal resolution. This is especially important because physicians and families may tend to project their own suffering onto the patient

**TABLE 1.** *Safeguards and guidelines for the discussion of assisted death (19,26)*

The patient must have a condition that is incurable (not necessarily terminal) and is associated with severe suffering without hope of relief.

All reasonable comfort-oriented measures must have been considered or tried.

The patient must express a clear and repeated request to die that is not coerced (e.g., emotionally or financially).

The physician must ensure that the patient's judgment is not distorted, i.e., the patient is competent to make a rational treatment choice.

Physician-assisted death must be carried out only in the context of a meaningful physician–patient relationship.

Consultation must be obtained from another physician to ensure that the patient's request is rational and voluntary.

There must be clear documentation that the previous six steps have been taken and a system of reporting, reviewing, and studying such deaths must be established.

and, therefore, conclude that a premature death is actually the merciful choice from the patient's perspective (25).

## Safeguards

Both proponents and opponents of physician-assisted death agree that safeguards are needed to protect the patient's safety and integrity and to protect society from physicians who might abuse this end-of-life choice (14,19,26,27). Table 1 lists some commonly proposed safeguards and guidelines for discussing the choice of assisted death (19,26).

As previously discussed, proponents believe that patients are the best judge of their own suffering and should have the option of discussing their situation with their personal physicians and developing a mutually agreeable plan for control of their pain and suffering. Proponents also believe that repeated and compassionate conversations between the patient and the primary physician over time will build the trust and rapport necessary for honest and uncoerced conversations among the patient, family members, and the physician. Many proponents also believe that consultation with at least one other physician is a vital safeguard. A parallel safeguard is the assurance of accurate and clear documentation that all of the guidelines have been followed.

Most opponents would agree that patients are the best judge of their own suffering and that all reasonable comfort-oriented measures should be considered and tried. They would argue that more open and frank discussions between the physician and the patient should occur on topics such as pain control and the patient's perception and experience of suffering. In their opinion, these types of discussions and the subsequent individualized plan of treatment for the patient would negate the need for the option of assisted death. Opponents see the potential for

coercion as very real and often quite difficult to ascertain, so that the proposed guidelines would be inadequate in practice. Opponents are also concerned about erosion of the physician–patient relationship occurring when physicians start providing the means of death for their patients. They see flaws in the consultation and documentation guidelines; they think that a physician could and would choose another physician of like mind to serve as consultant, and are skeptical that any documentation system could assure consistency and compassion among physicians and guarantee safety and sensitivity for patients.

## Professional Integrity

Opponents of physician-assisted death often argue that causing death is inconsistent with the moral integrity of the physician, who should always strive to be a healer and never a killer. In this view, even if society deemed it appropriate to permit assistance in dying, ethical physicians would be obligated to refuse to provide such assistance; and some other group of professionals or technicians would have to be appointed by society for that role (28,29). Similar arguments of integrity have been made on behalf of nurses, pharmacists, and other health care professionals (18,30–33).

But some proponents of physician-assisted death claim that the opponents rely on too narrow a conception of the moral goals of medicine. Healing in the usual sense, they claim, is but one of the goals that define the content of the physician's professional integrity; relief of suffering, respect for the patient's voluntary choices, and aiding patients to achieve the most peaceful and dignified death possible are also worthy aims. Therefore, suffering that has been unrelieved by excellent palliative care in a patient who has made repeated voluntary requests for death assistance would constitute an exception to the general prohibition. In such narrowly defined cases, a physician could assist death while maintaining ethical integrity (so long as assisting death did not violate any of that physician's personal moral or religious commitments) (34).

## Slippery Slope

This is one of the main arguments raised by opponents. They contend that once the legal barriers to physician-assisted death are broken there will be little justification for limiting this practice to only the terminally ill. What is today an *option* to choose assisted death might become an *obligation* to choose it, especially under pressures of cost containment and biases toward vulnerable populations such as the aged, the HIV-positive, minorities, and the disabled (35).

In particular, Steven Miles (25) discusses a concern that vulnerable populations will be subtly pressured into choosing death by messages that they are not worth saving. Many family members and physicians who care for persons with chronic illnesses may become exhausted and exasperated and, therefore, might be driven to go along with or even encourage a suicide request.

Proponents respond that proper attention to safeguards will prevent many problems and concerns raised by the slippery slope argument. Typical of the dispute between proponents and opponents of assisted death are sharply divergent interpretations of the euthanasia debate in the Netherlands (26,27). One side views the Dutch experience as having confirmed our worst fears of the slippery slope (38,39). The other side uses the same data to maintain that the Dutch policy of assisted death has generally worked well and that the occasional abuses have been successfully detected and contained (14,40).

### Substituted Judgment

Opponents worry that society will extend physician-assisted death to incompetent patients. Most proposals for physician-assisted death in the United States today specifically exclude the option of choosing physician-assisted death by an advance directive. The slippery slope argument, however, claims that this barrier will become impossible to maintain once physician-assisted death is legally permitted (9,41). In 1996, a U.S. Court of Appeals ruled both that patients have a constitutional right to physician-assisted death, and also that such a right might be exercised by a surrogate on behalf of an incompetent patient. Whether this is an accurate statement of constitutional law is, however, debatable (42–44).

### IMPLICATIONS FOR PALLIATIVE CARE AND HOSPICE

### Official Policies

Both the National Hospice Organization (NHO) and the Academy of Hospice Physicians (AHP) have position statements opposing the legalization of assisted death (45,46). The AHP statement is brief and states that competent palliative care usually relieves the pain and suffering of terminally ill persons and their families. This statement calls for policy reforms to ensure comprehensive hospice services for all. The NHO position paper (Table 2) is considerably more detailed and reviews all of the major points we have discussed in this chapter. In summary, the NHO statement maintains that allowing unpreventable death to occur with dignity and comfort is quite different from accepting death as an expeditious way out of difficult situations for individuals or society.

Both organizations see hospice as an ethically sound model of compassionate, cost-effective, patient- and family-oriented care. They also would argue that hospice care should be available to all and affordable for all who

**TABLE 2.** *Major points of the National Hospice Organization's position statement on assisted death*

In November 1990, a resolution was adopted rejecting the practice of voluntary euthanasia and assisted suicide.

These practices are counter to the NHO's core principles of relief of suffering, coordination of palliative and support services for the patient and family, a focus on maintaining the quality of remaining life, and a commitment to affirm life and neither hasten nor postpone death.

Hospice offers competent, appropriate, and compassionate palliative care to patients and their families as an effective choice for the care of dying patients and their families.

Aggressive palliative care can improve the quality and quantity of remaining life, as defined by the patient's life goals and choices.

Patients and their families need to be given the opportunity to discuss the accuracy, prognosis, and range of palliative treatment options appropriate for their personal situation and lifestyle.

The administrative and financial requirements of developing and maintaining assisted death as a component of the health care delivery system could competitively diminish the support needed to increase access to appropriate health care and palliative care.

would opt for supportive palliative care, and that all health care professionals should possess basic knowledge of palliative care and hospice management principles.

### Attitudes

As one might expect from official policy statements, there is a marked difference in attitudes toward physician-assisted death among hospice workers compared to U.S. health care workers in general. A slight majority of physicians in the states of Washington and Michigan favor a policy that would permit the option of physician-assisted death; and other surveys have shown from 33% to 40% of physicians in favor of such a policy (47–49). By contrast, surveys of hospice physicians, nurses, and volunteers show only a small minority in favor of allowing physician-assisted death, and about two thirds strongly opposed (18,50). Still, during the 1994 debate over assisted suicide in Oregon, a considerable split emerged within the hospice community in that state (18).

It is natural for those who devote so much of their energy to relief of symptoms, and who see the vast majority of their patients relishing the period of life that remains to them, to view the occasional patient who chooses physician-assisted death as either a failure or a threat. Some of those patients had prior exposure to hospice care, and the later choice of assisted death seems therefore to count as a rejection of the hospice philosophy. Even patients who had never experienced organized palliative care may seem to be saying, by choosing assisted death, that they do not value what is offered by palliative care. So there are understandable philosophical and emotional reasons for hospice workers reacting negatively to physician-assisted death.

If the underlying philosophy of hospice is that all patients with appropriate help and support can enjoy a high-quality existence until such time as death occurs naturally, then physician-assisted death would appear to be inappropriate, unnecessary, or both in every case (41). But another strand of hospice philosophy in the United States seems at first glance to be much more consistent with the views of proponents of assisted death. Both have in common a rejection of the dominant mode of dying that seems to characterize the American hospital setting—a death prolonged by excessive use of technology, inadequately attended by concern for amelioration of symptoms, and above all a depersonalized and deindividualized death, as patients' true choices are routinely ignored and human relationships and human caring are given short shrift in a world of machines. Both hospice workers and assisted death advocates agree that there are much better ways to die, and that the direction lies in more appreciation of human needs and of individual choices and values.

**Success of Palliative Care**

Advocates of physician-assisted death assume that palliative care modalities, while normally highly successful, cannot work in 100% of patients. There will of necessity be a few patients whose unpleasant symptoms or inability to function in basic ways cannot be ameliorated by even the most highly skilled palliative interventions. Many advocates of physician-assisted death would favor restricting the option of death to that small percentage of patients who cannot be helped effectively by palliative means. This suggestion angers some palliative care specialists who contend that their treatment modalities are much more effective than physician-assisted death advocates appreciate. Knowing full well how often the average U.S. practitioner underestimates the effectiveness of quality patient-centered palliative technology—and how often a so-called failure of palliative care is the result of an untrained practitioner either undertreating or choosing suboptimal treatment strategies—palliative care specialists may confidently predict that if they could only offer all needy patients in the United States the best quality hospice care, then the demand for physician-assisted death would soon be nil (51,52).

But both well-designed studies and common sense would lead to the conclusion that no medical therapy, however marvelous, can always succeed (21,53). Thus challenged, palliative specialists sometimes suggest that they can indeed effectively treat all terminal patients with distressing symptoms. Even the 3–5% or so of patients whose physical suffering does not respond well to either pharmacologic management or more invasive approaches can be offered heavy sedation (to the point of coma, if necessary) (54). Since the intent is to relieve symptoms and not to shorten life, even though shortening of life can be confidently predicted in most such cases, pharmacologically induced coma does not constitute physician-assisted death but instead is an acceptable, if extreme, use of palliative technology (55).

Defenders of physician-assisted death have offered two rebuttals to this argument. First, they have argued that in many instances in which pharmacologically induced coma might be used, death follows so surely and within so short a span of time that it is a semantic quibble not to view this as physician-assisted death *from a moral point of view* (while recognizing of course that from a *legal* point of view, sedation to the point of coma is quite acceptable even in jurisdictions where physician-assisted death would be a crime). In order to understand these moral and legal nuances, it is important to discuss the application of the ethical principle of double effect to high-dose opiates for analgesia and to pharmacologically induced coma. To opponents of physician-assisted death, the two instances are quite analogous. In both cases, one intends relief of symptoms, not death. One foresees the risk that the means used to relieve symptoms could cause a hastened death, but hastening death is not one's true intent (as is shown by the fact that if one had an alternative agent that effectively relieved symptoms but carried no risk of death, one would unhesitatingly use that agent instead). Thus, death is a foreseen but unintended consequence of an action that is itself morally defensible, and so the use of that means is morally justified despite the risk.

To proponents of physician-assisted death, however, the two cases are quite different. Very few patients actually suffer respiratory depression from properly administered narcotics in terminal illness. By contrast, in most instances where pharmacologically induced coma is employed (most commonly with barbiturates), death follows with near certainty and within a much shorter time frame. Moreover, if one sees respirations being depressed, one would not lower the dose because the patient's awakening would mean the cruel reinfliction of the intolerable suffering that one sought to avoid by inducing the coma in the first place. More to the point, the question of intent is more clouded in the case of induced coma. The fact that one elects to use this extreme measure, which often results in death within days or even hours, means that one has decided that any prolongation of conscious life is incompatible with this patient's true interests. If, by chance, the coma persists for many days or for weeks, the palliative care professional will seldom regard this as a good outcome. Indeed, this may make the death an even more poignant tragedy for the family as well as for the caregivers.

A second rebuttal is that some terminally ill patients who have demanded the right to physician-assisted death have claimed that a drug-induced coma typifies the loss of control and dignity that it is their overriding goal to avoid. For at least this small group of patients, palliative care experts might relieve unpleasant physical symptoms, but only at the cost of violating the patient's own deeply held values regarding quality of life.

## Pain Versus Suffering

We have already mentioned that suffering is a much broader concept than is pain or any set of unpleasant physical symptoms. The best available study of patient attitudes in a setting where physician-assisted death is openly practiced and legally tolerated reveals that only about 10% of patients requesting euthanasia suffer principally from pain and only about 50% suffer from any physical symptoms of the sort that can easily be relieved by palliative medical intervention. A significant number of requests to die arise from those who state that they are merely tired of life or whose general level of functioning has deteriorated below their personally acceptable minimum (36). Anecdotal evidence in the United States would tend to support these statistics (2,22). Possibly many or even most patients could be aided by emotional and/or spiritual counseling to the point where they would no longer request assisted death. A more sensitive and patient-centered approach requires understanding the meaning the patient attaches to the individual circumstances and not merely the assumption that palliative care technology has been underutilized (11,13,17,56).

Requests for physician-assisted death by patients with severe degenerative neuromuscular disease are usually made out of a concern by these patients that they do not want to experience the later stages of their illness, despite strong reassurances that they will receive compassionate and competent care. This subgroup of patients often identifies maintenance of their personal autonomy and integrity as important personal values, which they want health care professionals to respect and honor.

## Funding for Palliative Care

One recurring argument against allowing physician-assisted death is that hospice and palliative care have historically been under-funded in the United States. According to this argument, as soon as physician-assisted death is a legal option, patients will be steered toward a quick, painless, cheap death, and will be discouraged from seeking potentially expensive hospice care. The net result will be the serious underfunding of all types of palliative care programs, and the option to choose palliative care will be an option on paper only for most U.S. patients. Many U.S. hospice workers charge that palliative care has been very slow to develop in the Netherlands and that country's euthanasia policy is directly to blame. To hospice workers

this argument is self-evident. They have experienced the problems of chronic underfunding and of working with physicians and administrators who were often ill informed about hospice care. Understandably, they are skeptical of any proposal that assumes that palliative care has arrived and that adequate funding is on the horizon (50).

Defenders of the assisted death option have argued in reply that a properly regulated and legalized option for physician-assisted death could actually support the expansion of hospice. Many such proposals include the stipulation that no patient will be granted the request to die until palliative care experts have concluded that the patient cannot be effectively helped by appropriate treatments. In effect, the proposals would require that every patient requesting physician-assisted death undergo a trial of palliative care (19,26). The proponents further assume that in the vast majority of cases, the patients would be so impressed with the success of the treatment that they would elect to remain in the hospice program rather than be put to death. The result, they argue, will be additional political support for hospice programs and for palliative care training and research.

It is possible, of course, that health care professionals might merely rubber-stamp requests for assisted death rather than engaging in detailed conversations with their patients. Ironically, this outcome would be more likely if the nation moves toward legalizing physician-assisted death and if (as opinion polls now suggest) the best trained palliative care specialists refuse as a matter of conscience to have anything to do with the assisted death program, even to the extent of screening patients and consulting on available palliative alternatives (18,50).

## CLINICAL MANAGEMENT OF REQUESTS FOR ASSISTED DEATH

While we have shown that the debate between opponents and proponents of assisted death is complex and apparently intractable, many aspects of the practical management of patients who request direct assistance in dying will be the same, regardless of the provider's moral stance. We will suggest approaches that should fit both moral positions comfortably and highlight those few areas of practice where approaches must differ to remain consistent with one's own moral commitments (Table 3).

## Reactions to Patient Request

As noted above, a hospice patient who requests physician-assisted death may well trigger intensely negative emotional reactions among members of the care team. It is very important that those emotional reactions be validated by other team members but not be allowed to derail the necessary conversations with the patient that will support the patient's values and choices, as well as assess

**TABLE 3.** *Suggested steps for the clinical management of a request for assisted death*

The provider should listen to the request for assisted death in an open and sympathetic manner and evaluate the issues underlying the request.

The provider should share her personal stance with the patient in an open and professional manner, always assuring the patient that he will be supported throughout the process of his personal decision making process.

All providers should take appropriate steps to process their personal emotional reactions to the patient's request, e.g., hospice team meetings.

The provider should have a continuing dialogue with the patient and appropriate family members or support persons concerning the development and implementation of the therapeutic treatment plans, including a request for assisted death, in a manner consistent with the provider's moral values and belief system.

future care needs. Ideally, the patient's request will be received sympathetically but matter of factly. The patient may be told that she is hardly alone among patients facing death in making such a request and that the provider very much appreciates the trust shown by the patient in stating the request openly.

A patient may confide this request, or the fact that she is seriously considering suicide, to only one member of the palliative care team with whom she may experience a deeper personal trust. In that event, the team member ought initially to respect the confidence but state clearly that she feels a very strong obligation to share that information with all other team members, so that as a team they can discuss how best to offer future assistance to the patient. The provider should persist in seeking the patient's permission to share the disclosure with the rest of the team members. If the selective disclosure indicates that there are unresolved issues of distrust between the patient and other team members, the most therapeutic approach may be to address those issues head-on as part of the negotiations about disclosure. If the patient continues to refuse permission to share this information, then the provider is faced with the very difficult ethical conflict about when it is justifiable to violate a patient's confidence (57). One must balance the goal of preventing harm to the patient against the possibility that violating a confidence (or threatening to do so) may lead to even less disclosure of key information and, therefore, a lessened opportunity to help the patient in the future. If the provider, on balance, thinks that the secret ought to be revealed to co-workers, the justification would be that the provider is at the patient's bedside not as a solo practitioner but as a representative of the team; and not to allow the team to function cohesively is in a sense to reject that provider's care. This justification will be most plausible when the team aspects of care, and the sharing of information in the team, have been fully disclosed to

the patient as a part of the admission process. Also, in order to minimize further loss of trust, the provider who feels obligated to reveal secret information should frankly inform the patient of this and the reasons for the disclosure.

Some requests for death assistance are transparently a result of a temporary stress or mood change and are very unlikely to represent the considered, enduring posture of the patient. The provider may deal with such requests by validating the emotional state of the patient and responding with appropriate brief counseling.

All patients should be informed at this stage that it is the practice of the team to take all requests for death assistance very seriously. The patient should be informed that it is the experience of the team that the concerns and problems that prompt such requests can usually be ameliorated once the team has carefully assessed the patient's situation and further care options. The provider should promise speedy attention to the concerns that the patient raises and full communication of the team's planning processes.

At this point in the inquiry, the provider or the organization will take different approaches depending on their moral position on physician-assisted death. A provider (or team) who is morally opposed to this practice in all cases should share this information with the patient, lest the patient entertain unrealistic hopes of later assistance. The statement of refusal to consider the option of assisted death should in our view be coupled with the promise to stand by the patient until the moment of death and to continue to search exhaustively for any means other than death assistance to ameliorate the patient's suffering. The provider should then request that the patient continue to be open about his own suffering and what he plans to do about it, so that patient and provider can continue to engage in dialogue and seek mutually acceptable solutions. The provider may wish to add that a moral distaste for the action of assisting death does not equate with a moral condemnation of the suffering individual who feels driven to make the request.

The provider (or team) who is morally willing to consider the permissibility of assisting a patient's death in carefully selected cases may at this point share that stance with the patient. The provider should next point out the procedure the team has agreed to follow in order to be sure that the patient is making a voluntary, considered choice and is suffering in ways that cannot be relieved by any other means. The estimated amount of time needed for this determination, and to consider and suggest alternatives, should be shared with the patient. In any event, the patient needs to be told that no quick and easy acquiescence is contemplated. The provider may wish to inform the patient of the statistical chances that the patient will select an alternative means of addressing his suffering and will, in that event, no longer request a quick death.

## Possible Scenarios

After this initial discussion around the patient's first request for assisted death, the palliative care team should engage in a careful inquiry to determine the nature and origin of the patient's suffering, taking at face value that if the patient was prompted to ask to die the suffering must be more severe than the team had previously appreciated. The inquiry will be aided by understanding some common scenarios observed among patients making such requests (58). We have found very useful the categories suggested by Quill (22). The following six categories illustrate scenarios in which all observers should agree that the best option lies not in assisting death but in providing some other type of care.

### Inadequately Treated Physical Symptoms

The easiest category to deal with is the patient who seeks death because of suffering caused by inadequately treated physical symptoms. The palliative care team may have missed the onset, duration, or severity of the symptom. The patient may have felt compelled for a variety of emotional reasons to deny or to minimize the symptom. Or the previously prescribed treatment may be producing unpleasant or intolerable side effects that the patient similarly feels obligated to deny or minimize, possibly to avoid hurting the feelings of the providers. In any case, a searching discussion in which physical symptoms and treatment side effects are explicitly asked about should reveal the source of the problem, or other family members may be able to enlighten the hospice team on the nature of the complaint. A trial of improved treatment, to show the patient that the troublesome symptom can indeed be relieved without dying, may have to accommodate any fear of side effects or of lack of duration of relief that the patient may be entertaining.

### Depression

Untreated depression can cause a patient uncharacteristically to wish to die and to consider the future hopeless. A team member skilled in the differential diagnosis of depression should interview the patient with this possibility in mind. In an elderly patient, special expertise in geropsychiatry may be required both to distinguish the signs of depression from the effects of aging or chronic illness, and to determine a type and dose of antidepressant medication that can be successfully and safely be administered to the patient (59,60).

The diagnosis of depression does not necessarily lead to the successful treatment of depression soon enough to preserve the terminal patient's quality of life, and thus it is of no benefit to label her as depressed. As always in palliative care, the treatment of depression in the terminal patient should be aimed at the actual relief of troublesome symptoms rather than the cure of a disease. This may require flexibility and creativity in combining medication with emotional support.

### Family Dysfunction or Conflict

A patient's wish to die may grow out of conflict within a troubled family relationship. A patient may wish to die because of a fear that painful and dissatisfying family relationships are not going to improve; or in other cases a request may be a manipulative counteroffensive aimed at punishing other family members. Most hospice teams have social workers and chaplains, as well as family practice physicians and nurses who are capable of evaluating family dysfunction and developing an appropriate management plan.

### Spiritual Crisis

A request for assisted death may signal the fact that whatever belief system that previously provided the patient with a sense of meaning in his life is no longer experienced as supportive or meaningful, and the patient now feels that further existence would be without meaning for him. It may also suggest that this patient had been able to cope with previous life stressors without invoking any spiritual belief system and is now belatedly confronting the fact that he has no such resource to draw upon in looking at his own impending death.

Spiritual counseling may help to resolve the crisis and to restore a sense of meaning to the patient's life in the context of his illness and impending death. To be effective, the counseling will have to be tailored to the patient's beliefs and current needs. A careful assessment of the patient's sense of the nature of the current conflict and of why previously helpful spiritual or emotional supports no longer seem to be working is essential for identifying the type of counselor who would be most helpful. Human beings often assign meaning to events through the construction of narratives; and so engaging the patient in telling or writing stories about his past life or his present illness, or about his hopes for his survivors, may facilitate the process of restoring meaning (11,17, 23,52,56,61,62).

### Unremitting Suffering Despite Adequate Support

This category, which with high-quality palliative care will include relatively few patients, presents the starkest contrast between those morally opposed to and morally accepting of physician-assisted death. If the patient has failed to achieve adequate relief of suffering through appropriate trials of palliative treatments, with proper attention to emotional, social, and spiritual factors, and the patient has been shown to be competent and persists in requesting death, then those providers who accept the permissibility of physician-assisted death would regard this patient as a candidate for that assistance (58). We have elected not to address in this chapter the actual medical means that might be employed in such a case because this information is available elsewhere (63,64).

A problem will arise for providers opposing physician-assisted death if the patient has refused to try an offered mode of therapy or has ceased treatment before full therapeutic benefit occurred because of unpleasant side effects or fear of them. In some such cases the provider will judge that the side effects were truly severe and debilitating, or that their likelihood of occurring was exactly as the patient predicted. In such cases the provider might in good conscience proceed to assist death. But in other cases the provider may judge, fairly or unfairly, that the patient's reasons for refusing the offered therapy were inadequate or insubstantial; and that, in effect, the patient was so intent on receiving assistance with death that he was not really trying to achieve relief of suffering by any other route. This presents a serious dilemma for supporters of physician-assisted death. On the other hand, it is evident that only the patient can truly know how much he is suffering; and judgments by third parties that his reasons for refusing an offered therapy are inadequate seem to undermine the respect for free choice that motivated support for assisted death policies in the first place. On the other hand, if patients may receive assistance in dying after refusing all offered therapies for any reason whatsoever, then we have in fact created a policy of death on demand in which all so-called medical safeguards are spurious.

In our view, it is important for providers to recall in such cases that it is much harder to make the case that assistance in dying is a *right* of a terminally ill patient than that such death assistance is *permissible* in rare, selected instances. If patients have no moral right to death assistance, then physicians can refuse to assist death in all dubious cases. This effectively places the burden of proof on the patient rather than on the physician—a negative situation if one adopts a strongly libertarian posture but a positive one if one is concerned about the ease with which any policy of assisted death may be abused to the detriment of vulnerable persons.

Those morally opposed to assisted death who are facing a patient with unremitting suffering will again wish to affirm their commitment not to abandon the patient and to always stand by her in her suffering, while continuing to try new approaches and new combinations of treatments despite the waning likelihood of success. Spiritual counseling becomes critically important at this juncture because even patients who may continue to have some suffering before death may be helped to attach new and profound meanings to that suffering, so that the suffering becomes personally more bearable. If heavy sedation or barbiturate coma has not previously been considered, they should be reviewed with the patient and the family at this point. Knowing that these modalities are available may help the patient find the strength to endure.

## Hastening Death by Withdrawing Nutrition and Hydration

A policy proposal (65) and a case report (66) have recently awakened interest in a legally permissible strategy allowing patients to hasten death, even in jurisdictions proscribing physician-assisted suicide. The patient refuses to eat and drink and the physician provides palliative support to prevent any discomfort of dying by dehydration. Providers may legitimately differ over the moral assessment of this practice. For some, it will seem a clear-cut case of providing compassionate symptom relief while a patient exercises the legal and moral right to refuse medical interventions, including artificial nutrition and hydration. For others, it will seem an obvious subterfuge in which one stays on the right side of the law while engaging in an act which is morally indistinguishable from physician-assisted suicide. After all, the patient refuses artificial nutrition and hydration not because of an inability to drink or eat in the regular manner, and not because artificial administration is excessively painful or burdensome, but because the patient has determined that future life is not worth living and that an early death is preferable. Thus, such cases are easily distinguishable from the more usual hospice case in which symptom relief is offered and artificial hydration and nutrition are seldom used because they would add no comfort and merely prolong the dying process. We anticipate that palliative care providers and organizations may be divided on this strategy. Some who favor physician-assisted death will regard a prolonged death from dehydration, even if symptoms are well controlled, as an undignified travesty of what could otherwise have been a quick and painless death had more direct means been used. However, we imagine that some physicians who are morally opposed to physician-assisted death might find this strategy to be an acceptable compromise for patients who are suffering and who have repeatedly requested aid in dying. And some physicians who advocate physician-assisted death but fear the legal repercussions may find this an acceptable temporary solution. In that event, they could mention it as an option to patients who repeatedly request assistance in dying and whose suffering has not been adequately relieved by other means.

Considerable patient and family education is helpful and necessary because few health care providers and lay persons are aware that such a death can be relatively painless and comfortable (11,65,66). Some patients or families may still find the prospect unacceptable even after several conversations. For those patients who might elect to use this method, it will be important to allow for changes of heart along the way as well as to provide the promised symptom relief promptly and adequately throughout the process.

## CONCLUSIONS

We have discussed the ethical issues, the professional implications for hospice caregivers, and the clinical management of requests for assisted death from hospice patients. We would agree with Campbell et al. (18) that hospice caregivers and proponents of physician-assisted death have consensus on the following issues: the right of a terminally ill patient to control end-of-life decisions; medical assistance to keep the terminally ill person as pain-free as possible (and we would add proper management of suffering as well); a supportive network of caregivers; and a death that expresses personal dignity (18).

Physician-assisted death is a very controversial topic of concern to palliative care professionals. We hope that our discussion in this chapter will assist our readers in their reflections and management discussions with their peers, patients, and family members as they compassionately attend to the needs of persons with terminal illnesses.

### Acknowledgments

The authors acknowledge the valuable assistance of Pat Bayer and Debbie Richardson in the preparation of this manuscript.

## REFERENCES

1. Watts DT, Howell T. Assisted suicide is not voluntary active euthanasia. *J Am Geriatr Soc* 1992;40:1043.
2. Quill T. Death and dignity: A case of individualized decision making. *N Engl J Med* 1991;324:691.
3. Kevorkian J. *Prescription: medicide—the goodness of planned death.* Buffalo: Prometheus Books, 1991.
4. Annas G. Physician-assisted suicide-Michigan's temporary solution. *N Engl J Med* 1993;328:1573.
5. Wilson WC, Smedira NG, Fink C, et al. Ordering and administration of sedatives and analgesics during the withholding and withdrawal of life support from critically ill patients. *JAMA* 1992;267:949.
6. Rachels J. *The end of life: euthanasia and morality.* New York: Oxford University Press, 1986.
7. Annas G. Death by prescription—the Oregon Initiative. *N Engl J Med* 1994;331:1240.
8. Callahan D. Pursuing a peaceful death. *Hastings Center Rep* 1993 Jul/Aug;33.
9. Euthanasia: California Proposition 161. Commonweal supplement 1992 Sept.
10. Emanuel EJ. The history of euthanasia debates in the United States and Britain. *Ann Intern Med* 1994 November;121(10):793.
11. Peteet J. Treating patients who request assisted suicide. *Arch Fam Med* 1994;3:723.
12. Ferrel B, Rhiner M. High-tech comfort: Ethical issues in cancer pain management for the 1990's. *J Clin Ethics* 1991(Summer):108.
13. Steinmetz D, Walsh M, Gabel LL, William PT. Family physician's involvement with dying patients and their families. *Arch Fam Med* 1993;2:753.
14. Battin M. Voluntary euthanasia and the risks of abuse: Can we learn anything from the Netherlands? *Law Med Health Care* 1992;20(1–2, Spring–Summer):133.
15. Davies J. Altruism towards the end of life. *J Med Ethics* 1993 Jun;19(2):111.
16. Pain management—theological and ethical principles governing the use of pain relief for dying patients. *Health Progr* 1993 Jan/Feb:30.
17. Derezinski K. Moving beyond the pain. *Perspectives* 1994 Fall:4.
18. Campbell CS, Hare J, Mathews P. Conflicts of conscience: Hospice and assisted suicide. *Hastings Center Rep* 1995;25(3):36.
19. Quill T, Cassel C, Meier D. Care of the hopelessly ill—proposed clinical criteria for physician-assisted suicide. (Sounding Board). *N Engl J Med* 1992;327:1380.
20. Brody H. Assisted death—A compassionate response to a medical failure. *N Engl J Med* 1992;327:1384.
21. Quill TE. *Death and dignity: Making choices and taking charge.* New York: WW Norton, 1993.
22. Quill T. Doctor, I want to die, will you help me? *JAMA* 1993;270:870.
23. Cassell EJ. The nature of suffering and the goals of medicine. *N Engl J Med* 1982;306:639.
24. Cassell EJ. *The nature of suffering and the goals of medicine.* New York: Oxford University Press, 1991.
25. Miles S. Physicians and their patient's suicides. *JAMA* 1994;271:1786.
26. Miller F, Quill T, Brody H, et al. Regulating physician-assisted death. *N Engl J Med* 1994;31:119.
27. Weir RF. The morality of physician-assisted suicide. *Law Med Health Care* 1992 Spring–Summer;20(1–2):116.
28. Gaylin W, Kass LR, Pellegrino ED, et al. Doctors must not kill. *JAMA* 1988;259:2139.
29. Kass LR. Neither for love nor money: Why doctors must not kill. *The Public Interest* 1989;94 Winter: 25.
30. Haddad A. Physician-assisted suicide: The impact on nursing and pharmacy. *Of Value (SHHV Newslett)* 1994 Dec.
31. Rupp MT, Isenhower HL. Pharmacists attitudes toward physician-assisted suicide. *Am J Hosp Pharm* 1994 Jan;51(1):69.
32. Young A, Volker D. Oncology nurses attitudes regarding voluntary, physician-assisted dying for competent, terminally ill patients. *Oncol Nurse Forum* 1993 Apr;20(3):445.
33. Kowalski S. Assisted suicide: Where do nurses draw the line? *Nurse Health Care* 1993 Feb;14(2):70.
34. Miller FG, Brody H. Professional integrity and physician-assisted death. *Hastings Center Rep* 1995;25(3):8.
35. Campbell CS. Aid-in-dying and the taking of human life. *J Med Ethics* 1992 Sep;18(3):128.
36. Van der Maas PJ, Van Delden JJM, Pijnenborg L, Looman CWN. Euthanasia and other medical decisions concerning the end of life. *Lancet* 1991;338:669.
37. Pijnenborg L, van der Maas PJ, van Delden JJM., Looman CWN. Life-terminating acts without explicit request of patient. *Lancet* 1993;341:1196.
38. Gomez CP. *Regulating death: the case of the Netherlands.* New York: Free Press, 1991.
39. Report of the Board of Trustees of the American Medical Association. Euthansia/physician-assisted suicide: Lessons in the Dutch experience. *Issues Law Med* 1994 Summer;10(1):81.
40. VanderWal G, Dillmann RJ. Euthanasia in the Netherlands. *Br Med J* 1994 May;308(6940):1346.
41. Callahan D. Aid in dying: the social dimensions. *Commonweal* 1991 (Suppl 9 Aug):12.
42. Anonymous. Physician-assisted suicide and the right to die with assistance. *Harvard Law Rev* 1992;105:2021.
43. Kamisar Y. Are laws against assisted suicide constitutional? *Hastings Center Rep* 1993;23(3):32.
44. Sedler RA. The constitution and hastening inevitable death. *Hastings Center Rep* 1993 Sept/Oct;23(5):20.
45. Position statement. Gainesville, FL: Academy of Hospice Physicians, 1988.
46. Statement opposing the legalization of euthanasia and assisted suicide. Arlington, VA: National Hospice Organization.
47. Cohen J, Fihn S, Boyko EJ, et al. Attitudes toward assisted suicide and euthanasia among physicians in Washington state. *N Engl J Med* 1994;331:89.
48. Bachman JG, Alcser KH, Doukas D, et al. Attitudes of Michigan physicians and public toward legalizing assisted suicide and voluntary active euthanasia. *N Engl J Med.* 1997;334(5):303–309.
49. Doukas DJ, Waterhouse D, Gorenflo DW, Seid J. Attitudes and behaviors on physician-assisted death: a study of Michigan oncologists. *J Clin Oncol* 1995;13:1055.

50. Miller RJ. Hospice care as an alternative to euthanasia. *Law Med Health Care* 1992 Spring–Summer;20(1–2):127.

51. Cundiff D. *Euthanasia is not the answer: a hospice physician's view.* Totowa, NJ: Humana Press, 1992.

52. Foley KM. The relationship of pain and symptom management to patient requests for physician-assisted suicide. *J Pain Sympt Manag* 1991;6:289.

53. Management of Cancer Pain Guideline Panel. *Management of cancer pain (Clinical practice guideline no. 9).* Rockville, MD: Agency for Health Care Policy and Research, 1994.

54. Truog R, Berde C, Mitchell C, Grier HE. Barbiturates in the care of the terminally ill. (Sounding Board). *N Engl J Med* 1992;327:1678.

55. Byock IR. The euthanasia/assisted suicide debate matures. *Am J Hospice Palliat Care* 1993(March–April):8.

56. Freeman J, Pelligrino E. Management at the end of life. *Arch Fam Med* 1993;2:1078.

57. Jonsen A, Siegler M, Winslade W. *Clinical ethics,* 3rd ed, New York: McGraw-Hill, 1992.

58. Block SD, Billings JA. Patient requests to hasten death: Evaluation and management in terminal care. *Arch Intern Med* 1994 September;154(18):2039.

59. Conwell Y, Caine ED. Rational suicide and the right to die: reality and myth. *N Engl J Med* 1991;325:1100.

60. Baile WF, DiMaggio JR, Schapira DV, Janofsky JS. The request for assistance in dying: the need for psychiatric consultation. *Cancer* 1993 Nov;72(9):2786.

61. Frank AW. *The wounded storyteller: body, illness and ethics.* Chicago: University of Chicago Press 1995.

62. Billings JA, Block SD. Patient request to hasten death: Evaluation and management in terminal care. *Arch Intern Med* 1994;154:2039.

63. Humphry D. *Final exit: the practicalities of self-deliverance and assisted suicide for the dying.* Oregon: Hemlock Society, 1991.

64. Admiraal PV. *Justified euthanasia: a manual for the medical profession.* Amsterdam: Dutch Society for Voluntary Euthanasia, 1984.

65. Bernat JL, Gert B, Mogielnicki, et al. Patient refusal of hydration and nutrition: an alternative to physician-assisted suicide or voluntary active euthanasia. *Arch Intern Med* 1993;153:2723.

66. Eddy DM. A conversation with my mother. *JAMA* 1994;172:179.

# SECTION V

## Special Topics

*Principles and Practice of Supportive Oncology,*
edited by Ann Berger et al.
Lippincott–Raven Publishers, Philadelphia ©1998

CHAPTER 61

# Stress and Burnout in Oncology

Mary L. S. Vachon

The stress of caregivers in oncology is different from that of caregivers working in the hospice/palliative care field. The long-term, often collaborative, nature of the relationships established in oncology involves staff in assisting patients to deal with an initial diagnosis; helping them through their treatment; rejoicing with them when they go into remission; supporting them when and if they develop a recurrence; being present as they deal with the realization that there will be no cure and that the intent of treatment is palliative; and grieving with them as they prepare to die. Oncology caregivers must also deal with fiscal constraints and managed care limiting the resources and care they can provide to patients and families. Economic forces may require the transfer of patients from one system of care to another at a time when both patients and caregivers might have preferred to maintain their relationship. These variables, added to the aggressive treatments and high technology that are a part of the daily life of oncology professionals and the role strain that results from trying to juggle the multiple roles of clinician, teacher, and researcher, can combine to make work in oncology potentially both very stressful and very rewarding.

This chapter will provide a historical overview of the literature on occupational stress and burnout; highlight the personal and occupational variables that may lead to stress and burnout in oncology; and discuss the literature on stress, burnout, and coping in oncology.

## INTRODUCTION AND HISTORICAL OVERVIEW

### Caregiver Stress

Interest in the issue of professional caregiver stress can be seen to date from the late 1950s. The psychologist

M. L. S. Vachon: Department of Psychiatry and Behavioural Science, University of Toronto, Toronto Sunnybrook Regional Cancer Centre/Sunnybrook Health Science Centre, Toronto, Ontario M4N 3M5, Canada .

Herman Feifel (1) noted that physicians were found to have a greater fear of death than laypersons. In the same year, the sociologist Renée Fox (2) studied the stress experienced by physicians conducting pioneering work on the artificial kidney and kidney transplantation. Intervention to assist with the management of stress began with nurses (3,4), moving on to teams (5) and then to physicians (6). Most of the early work was anecdotal in nature and made no attempt to define or measure the stress experienced by staff, much less to document ways of managing such stress.

The hospice/palliative care movement began in England in 1967 and in North America in 1974 and interest in the area of caregiver stress burgeoned (7). Gradually, work emerged that focused on measuring and managing staff stress in both hospice and oncology settings (8,9).

### The Concept of Burnout

As interest in caregiver stress increased, the concept of burnout developed. The term is generally credited to Freudenberger (10,11) who used the analogy of a building that has been burned out. Where once there was a throbbing vital structure, pulsating with energy, now there are only crumbling reminders of energy and life. While the outer shell may seem to be intact, if you go inside you will be struck by the force of desolation (11,12).

Burnout has been characterized as "the progressive loss of idealism, energy and purpose experienced by people in the helping professions as a result of the conditions of their work" (13, p. 14). Burnout has also been described as a syndrome of responses involving increased feelings of emotional exhaustion, negative attitudes toward the recipients of one's service (depersonalization), a tendency to evaluate oneself negatively with regard to one's work, and a feeling of dissatisfaction with accomplishments on the job (14,15) (Table 1).

**TABLE 1.** *Burnout and work environment*

| |
|---|
| Burnout is associated with: |
| Work overload |
| Role ambiguity |
| Role conflict |
| Time and staffing limitations |
| Lack of advancement opportunities |
| Poor working relationships |
| Lack of chairperson and peer support |
| Poor head nurse leadership style |
| Increased demands by patients and families |
| Frequent exposure to death and dying |

Modified from ref 15.

Burnout is generally seen to result from the interaction between the needs of a person to sacrifice himself or herself for a job and a job situation that places inordinate demands on an individual. The person prone to burnout is apt to have unrealistically high personal expectations for satisfaction in a given area of life. The phenomenon can occur not only in an individual but also within a system (13,16).

Pines (17) proposed a social-psychological model of burnout positing certain characteristics of the work environment as contributing to burnout. According to her model, professionals with a high level of motivation can either achieve peak performance if working within a positive environment or develop burnout symptoms if the individual continues to confront a stressful, discouraging environment. Individual differences determine how soon an individual develops burnout and how extreme the experience might be.

The most commonly used instrument to measure burnout is the Maslach Burnout Inventory (MBI) (18), which measures emotional exhaustion, depersonalization, and a lack of personal accomplishment on two dimensions—*frequency* (how often a feeling occurs) and *intensity* (the strength of that feeling). The MBI was studied on 169 nurses, 43 physicians, and 1025 helping professionals as a normative group. The levels of emotional exhaustion were similar for nurses and physicians but they differed significantly in depersonalization. For physicians, the greater the amount of time they spent with patients, the higher was their score on the MBI. Emotional exhaustion was linked to feelings of lack of control and was higher for nurses than for physicians (19,20).

## THE INDIVIDUAL AND THE WORK ENVIRONMENT IN ONCOLOGY

### Personality Variables

In looking at the stress of those in oncology the personal characteristics that professionals bring to their profession is relevant as is the impact of professional training programs. Those who choose medicine have been found to have strong obsessive-compulsive personality traits that lead them to "choose a career in which long hours of study, heavy responsibility and devotion to work are required. In fact, the more these traits are exaggerated the more outstanding a student may be" (21, p. 647, references in original). This personality trait added to the fact that physicians have been shown to have a greater fear of death than laypersons (1) may lead to increased distress as a physician agonizes over a decision that he or she may see as a personal failure to save a life. "This compulsiveness, when present in conjunction with other characteristics of overly controlled emotions and low need for relaxation and pleasure, makes the medical student, and later the physician more vulnerable than others to depression, alcoholism, psychiatric disorders, and suicide" (21, p. 647). Such problems have been found to be more associated with adjustment before medical school than to occupational hazards (22). Physicians with the least stable childhoods and adolescent adjustment have been identified as being most vulnerable to occupational hazards (22).

Research on the personality of oncology nurses using the Personal Style Inventory (23) based on the 1923 work of Jung (24) showed that the most common personality type for oncology nurses was ISFJ, where feeling is introverted and perception is practical so that helping others is both a responsibility and a pleasure. Caregivers with these personality characteristics value interpersonal interactions and have great empathy. The strengths of this personality type include independence, ability to work alone, diligence, and attention to detail. Traits that could be a hindrance include the proclivity to work alone and the tendency to act on internal reasoning without consulting others. The latter personality trait could be a problem because oncology nurses play a pivotal role in collaborative groups in today's health care environment. The introvert prefers quiet time to concentrate and time to think before making decisions. This personality type also dislikes interruptions, which can be a problem in the busy oncology clinic or unit (25).

Theories that emphasize the role of the individual in the development of burnout assert that the degree of burnout depends on personal characteristics such as the individual's cognitive appraisal and coping strategies under stressful circumstances, motivation for entering the health field, expectations of self and others, and a failure to live up to one's ideals (15). The personality characteristic of hardiness (26,27) has been found to be associated with decreased rates of burnout in ICU nurses and was associated with improved coping in house officers at Memorial Sloan-Kettering Cancer Center (MSKCC) (21). Hardiness consists of three characteristics: commitment, control, and challenge. "The combination of a sense of commitment to one-self and the various areas in life including work, an attitude that one has influence over what occurs, and a sense of being challenged in the face of a changing environment has been shown, when present, to be associated with fewer mental and physical symptoms of stress. Hardiness is said to lead to a perception, interpretation, and handing of stressful events that prevents excessive activation of arousal and therefore results in fewer symptoms of stress" (21, p. 652).

## Stressors in Oncology

Work in oncology can be described as being emotional labor, which is "the labor involved in dealing with other people's feelings, a core component of which is the regulation of emotions" (28, p. 15). This work is often performed by women. "Emotional labor is hard work and can be sorrowful and difficult. It demands that the laborer give personal attention which means that they must give something of themselves, not just a formulaic response" (28, p. 19). Such work also involves the regulation of emotion between the carer and the person being cared for, which is one of the sometimes tremendous but rewarding challenges of work in oncology.

Mount (29) delineated the stressors of oncologists as including exposure to death as an existential fact, emphasizing the finite nature of life; the cumulative grief associated with repeated unresolved losses; the pressures of a medical care system fueled by the medical information system; the inability to achieve the idealistic goals embraced by holistic medical care; the stressors inherent in working as a team; and the issues involved in treatment failure.

It has been suggested that oncology nurses may be particularly susceptible to the more chronic situational stressors associated with the nature of their responsibilities and patient/family needs associated with deteriorating illness (30). The stressors in oncology nursing have changed in the past decade (31); they are now work overload, lack of resources, and staff shortages. Conflicts with other health care workers (doctors in particular) seem to have decreased, possibly due to changes in pain and symptom control management. Nurses continue to be concerned about patient deterioration and death.

In a Bavarian study (32) comparing 57 physicians and 91 nurses on cancer wards in 13 settings, nurses were found to report greater stress and to have a vulnerability to stress in areas involving the empathic component of their relationship with patients. Physicians had stress associated with decision making and communicating diagnoses. In this study the stress–complaints relationship for physicians and nurses was quite different. For nurses, it was primarily interpersonal stress that related to physical distress. Nurses were more likely to have physical symptoms if their outside life failed to relieve the stress generated on their job. Physicians had much less stress associated with interpersonal difficulties. Their symptoms were much more strongly correlated with

space, dealing with patients, and the events of the workday. Having to work with trainees was seen as a stressor in both nurses and physicians. Small hospitals engendered less job critique among nurses but more stress through identification with patients. Doctors found such hospitals to be cramped. The variables in this study were not linked to gender with the exception that females of both professions had a greater tendency to cry. With age, stress reduced for most stress areas as was found previously (33).

Kunkel and Shmuely (34) reported on the stress of ancillary staff working in radiation oncology. Stress was found to be related to "difficult to manage" patients who were defined as having characteristics that "interfered with patient compliance with either radiation treatments or the clinic routine. Such patients typically asked many questions, were often anxious, angry or psychotic, had bad prior experiences with medical care, had cognitive deficits or were actively using drugs or alcohol. Most difficult patients were identified as having some emotional or behavioral disturbance" (34, p. 242).

### Is Stress Greater in Oncology?

Cohen et al. (35) reviewed the literature and suggested that when comparisons were performed, oncology nurses differed little from or fared better than other nurses in terms of stress levels and stressors identified. Van Servellen and Leake (36) compared 237 nurses from AIDS special care units, oncology special care units, medical intensive care units, and general medical care units and found no significant differences in scores on the Maslach Burnout Inventory. They found that greater job influence had a significant protective effect on emotional exhaustion and enhanced personal accomplishment and job tension was a significant predictor of exhaustion.

In a British study, Wilkinson (37) measured the anxiety of 65 nurses working on six units in two cancer hospitals. The Spielberger State-Trait Anxiety Inventory (38) was used. Oncology nurses were found to be no more anxious than other working women. Newly qualified nurses were more anxious than sisters and enrolled nurses. Nurses who never went to church had a higher state anxiety score than those who went to church weekly or occasionally. There was some difference in the level of state anxiety on different wards and the authors noted that the ward on which nurses worked appeared to influence the levels of stress and job satisfaction experienced. This was thought to be due in part to managerial style affecting ward climate.

When the team in a hospital-based home care unit (HBHC) working with severely ill cancer patients was compared with the staff working with a similar population of patients on three inpatient units, both groups showed a limited degree of continuous stress and a high degree of job satisfaction (39). However, there were differences between the two work environments. The HBHC group reported more freedom to make their own decisions, better cooperation between day and night shifts, a more reasonable workload, fewer problems in communication with patients, and fewer problems with tension and sleeping. These findings were felt to be due to the fact that the HBHC team was older, more often married, had worked longer in health care, and thus were more experienced.

When 581 professionals from all major disciplines and specialty areas working with the critically ill and dying were compared, the stressors of those in oncology differed from those in other settings in that they reported equal numbers of stressors in the areas of *patients and families* (patients and families with coping or personality problems, patients and families with whom they had communication problems, and identification with patient and family); *occupational role* (role overload, role ambiguity, role conflict, lack of control); and *environmental stressors* (team communication problems, inadequate resources, communication problems with others in the system, and unrealistic expectations of the organization) (33,40). The other specialty areas were far more likely to report the major stressors as coming from their work environment.

A more recent German study compared 299 physicians and 592 nurses from 54 different hospitals and clinics (41). The staff worked in oncology, cardiac, intensive care, or surgical units. Although the groups experienced the same overall degree of work-related stress and physical complaints, the oncology group suffered more from feelings of emotional involvement and self-doubt. However, the oncology group suffered less from stress connected with institutional factors than did the comparison group despite few objective differences in their situations. The author hypothesized that the stress accompanying the care of people with cancer is no greater than that which accompanies the care of other medically ill people but it is of a different quality. For oncology staff, institutional stressors move into the background when compared with the personal emotional involvement of working with patients.

While the stress of those in oncology may not differ significantly from that of their colleagues in other medical specialties, it is generally greater than that of colleagues in palliative care. A comparison of hospice and oncology nurses showed that the latter experienced more burnout that was directly related to role overload, patient/staff ratio, less opportunity to express work-related feelings and problems, and a greater dissonance between their ideal and real work situation (42).

In a British survey sent to all consultant nonsurgical oncologists in the United Kingdom, the stressors of medical oncologists ($N = 69$), clinical oncologists (formerly known as radiotherapists) [$N = 253$], and palliative care specialists were assessed ($N = 126$). Sources of stress were segregated into four factors: feeling overloaded and its effect on home life, having organizational responsibil-

ities/conflicts, dealing with the patient's suffering, and being involved with treatment toxicity and errors. Clinical oncologists reported significantly higher stress from treatment toxicity and errors and dealing with patients suffering than medical oncologists who reported more stress from organizational responsibilities/conflicts. Palliative care specialists generally reported the lowest mean percentage of items rated as contributing "quite a bit" or "a lot' to overall job stress (43).

### Stressors Versus Rewards

Although oncology can be stressful, some authors have also tried to measure the rewards of the specialty. Papadatou et al. (15) suggest that the challenge of working with cancer patients may serve as a reward that counterbalances the stressful aspects of practice. Bean and Holcombe (25) point out the way in which the personality types of oncology nurses may be complementary to the stressors identified in the work setting (25,44), leading presumably to increased job satisfaction. There is some evidence, however, that job satisfaction in oncology nurses is declining (37).

Cohen et al. (35) found that the three most important sources of rewards for oncology nurses were, in the order of importance, patients, co-workers, and new skills, but that each source of rewards could also be a source of difficulty (e.g., relationships with patients were rewarding but emotions could be evoked as nurses watched patients suffer). Oncology nurses experience difficulty with "excessive demands, negative expectations from patients/families, unexpected crises, poor staffing/overwork/inadequate time, patient deaths, and balancing work and personal life" (25, p. 484, quoting 44). Critical incidents that showed the essence of oncology nursing consisted of handling emergencies, preventing serious errors, helping with emotional distress, and empathizing with patients. The rewards of oncology nursing were identified as patients getting well and patients' expressions of gratitude for emotional support (44).

In the British study of oncologists and palliative care specialists (43), 20 sources of satisfaction items were aggregated into four factors. The four satisfaction items were dealing well with patients and relatives, which contributed most to overall job satisfaction, followed by having professional status and esteem, deriving intellectual stimulation, and having adequate resources to perform one's role. The overall pattern was for clinical oncologists to report the lowest levels of satisfaction for all the factors. Medical oncologists reported higher levels of satisfaction from deriving intellectual stimulation than either of the other two groups. Palliative care specialists reported the highest levels of satisfaction from dealing well with patients and relatives and having adequate resources.

In a study of 147 physician American Society of Clinical Oncologists (ASCO) members, 80% reported that they were somewhat or very satisfied with working in oncology whereas 61.9% found that working in oncology was stressful (45). Physicians reported the satisfactions of oncology as being effective treatment (44.8%), challenge of oncology, positive relations with patients and families, personal satisfactions, symptom management, positive professional interactions, and emotional support to patients and families (11.2%). Dissatisfactions included the pressures of practice (40%), negative relationships with patients/families, dealing with dying patients, ineffective treatments, emotional support to patients and families, negative relations with other professionals, and impact on personal life (20.8%).

The stressors and rewards in an oncology hospital were identified (46). All professional disciplines received their greatest rewards from helping patients but physicians more often described satisfaction from curing cancer and learning and advancing research whereas nurses emphasized the rewards of meeting personal goals for patient care. The major source of discomfort for physicians was being unable to help patients and not being able to provide optimal medical care. For nurses, it was dealing with ethical issues such as truth telling, interference with patient comfort and dying in the context of medical experimentation, and the determination of "do not resuscitate" status.

## MANIFESTATIONS

### Physical

A strong association was found between specific, situational stressors and reported psychosomatic complaints (32). For nurses, interpersonal difficulties, whether on or off the job, related to physical distress, whereas for physicians dissatisfaction with the job and working conditions, including space problems involving the work environment and dealing with patients, related to a general malaise. Irregular working hours related to stress in both groups.

Nurses were more apt to report problems with headaches/pressure in head, tiredness, tendency to cry, loss of appetite, irritability, and neck/shoulder pain if their life outside the work situation did not relieve their stress generated on the job. For nurses there were three distinct phenomena associated with the stress of dealing with patients: interpersonal conflict (leading to irritability and headaches), physical distaste for certain tasks (leading to visceral pain and nausea), and physical strain, causing back pain, heaviness in legs, and neck/shoulder pain. Identification with the patient correlated most markedly with tiredness in its various forms. If the reported symptom level, rather than the reported stress level, was taken as an indicator of objective stress, then neither lack of satisfaction with the job and the surroundings nor proximity to the dying was linked to health-

related concerns. Identification with the patient's suffering was itself principally tiring. However, the effects of interpersonal difficulties (*private life* and *dealing with patients*) were most worrisome (32).

The authors observe that for physicians "the findings can be summarized in one over-simple phrase: stressed doctors are tired" (32, p. 1017). For the physician group, the authors described a subpattern of symptoms that "linked stress to loss of control, in the form of irregular heartbeat, diarrhea, discomfort in the throat, dizziness, and breathlessness. The doctors' stress may derive in part from lack of confidence when faced with their limited ability to alter the course of illness [references in original]. Identification with the patients' suffering, which was linked to tiredness among nurses, had effects among doctors that suggest an almost physical rejection of the patient" (32, p. 1021).

### Psychological

### *Burnout*

In the largest study of the stress of oncologists to date (47), 56% of oncologist subscribers to the *Journal of Clinical Oncology* reported experiencing burnout in their professional lives. Burnout was measured using an author-constructed questionnaire, as opposed to one of the more usual instruments used to measure burnout (18). When asked to define the specific nature of their burnout, 56% mentioned frustration or a sense of failure, 34% depression, 20% disinterest in practice, and 18% boredom. Almost half felt that burnout was inherent to the practice of oncology. Institution or university-based oncologists on salary reported a lower incidence of burnout (47%) than those in private adult oncology practice (63%).

In the Ramirez et al. study of UK oncologists and palliative care specialists (43), the Maslach Burnout Inventory was used (18). The percentage of cancer clinicians reporting high levels of exhaustion was similar to that of the normative sample (31% versus 33%) (19). Thirty-three percent of both the cancer clinicians and the normative sample reported low personal accomplishment. Significantly fewer of the UK cancer clinicians reported high levels of depersonalization compared to the U.S. sample (23% versus 33%, $p < 0.0001$). *Demographic factors* associated with burnout included being age 55 or younger and being a clinical oncologist rather than a medical oncologist or palliative care specialist. *Job characteristics* associated with burnout included emotional exhaustion associated with high levels of stress from "being overloaded and its effect on home life," "dealing with patients suffering," and low levels of satisfaction from "not having adequate resources to perform one's role." Depersonalization was associated with "being overloaded" and "dealing with patients' suffering" as well as low levels of satisfaction from "dealing well with patients and relatives." Being a clinical oncologist and working part-time were independent risk factors for depersonalization. "Low personal accomplishment was associated with stress from 'being involved with treatment toxicity and errors' and low levels of satisfaction from 'dealing well with patients and relatives' and from 'having professional status and esteem' " (43, p. 1268).

A large Finnish study of 2671 physicians (48) found that male oncologists were among those physicians most likely to report burnout; the same finding was not reported for female oncologists. The authors speculated that higher burnout was associated with the specialties associated with dealing with chronically ill, uncurable, or dying patients. They hypothesized that hope and the lack of it in medical work have important influences on feelings of burnout. As with the U.S. study (47), they found that those with a university position were less likely to report burnout.

A comparison of hospice and oncology nurses (42) showed that the latter experienced more burnout that was directly related to role overload, patient/staff ratio, less opportunity to express work-related feelings and problems, and a greater dissonance between their ideal and real work situations. Descriptive data in that study indicated that hospice nurses experienced slightly less dissonance between their ideal and real work situations.

A study of burnout in oncology clinical nurse specialists showed that while the oncology group had lower burnout scores than other nursing groups previously studied, the best predictors of burnout were dissatisfaction with one's role, high levels of job stress, feelings of apathy and withdrawal, and inadequate psychological support at work (49). Jenkins and Ostchega (50) replicated the previous study (49) with oncology nurses and found similar results, suggesting that oncology nurses experienced moderate amounts of burnout. Those nurses with relatively higher scores indicating burnout reported greater levels of job stress, a greater degree of job dissatisfaction, and lower levels of available perceived support in their work environment. Papadatou et al. (15) warn that both of the previous studies must be viewed with some caution because no control groups were used.

At MSKCC studies showed that oncology nurses were high on emotional exhaustion but lower than house staff members on the dimensions of diminished empathy. The author hypothesized that this finding might have a particularly adverse effect on sensitivity and compassion in patient care for the house staff (30).

In a Greek study using a control group, Papadatou et al. (15) found no statistically significant difference in burnout scores comparing oncology nurses with nurses in general hospitals. Personal characteristics were found to predict a greater percentage of variability in the burnout experience than either occupational or demographic variables. Among the personality dimensions, the existence

of the hardy personality—especially the perceived control aspect of this personality type—seemed to be significant (cf. 21). This sense of control over things that happen in life and in the work environment was found to protect nurses from emotional exhaustion, depersonalization, and a lack of personal accomplishment. Nurses who experienced higher degrees of burnout reported a lack of a sense of control over external events. Among all the job stressors studied, only the stress of a heavy workload was found to be associated positively with burnout (and emotional exhaustion in particular). This finding is similar to that reported by oncologists (47), although the self-controlled aspects of workload (e.g., involvement in research and teaching) may be negatively related to burnout (15). Among house staff hardiness was found to be negatively related to burnout and physical illness; negative work stressors were positively related to burnout as was supervisor support (21).

The finding that self-controlled workload may be negatively related to burnout is interesting in view of the fact that in a large study of professionals from a variety of settings, those in oncology were most apt to mention developing the multiple roles of clinician, researcher, and teacher as one of their major coping mechanisms (33). In the same study, only 4% of the psychological manifestations of stress mentioned by caregivers involved burnout.

### Depression and Burnout: Do They Differ?

Feelings of depression must be distinguished from those of burnout. Maslach states that one phase of the burnout syndrome involves a sense of reduced accomplishment and a loss of self-esteem, which is a central characteristic of depression. The loss may be that of early ideals or of "good people" to work with. A professional's sense of self-worth and self-esteem may be threatened by the inevitable outcome of patients' deaths and the physical, psychological, and social pain of terminal illness (51). Caregivers may also feel that they have failed at their work or have failed to live up to their original standards (14). Burnout is generally regarded as being associated with overinvolvement in any one area of life to the exclusion of all others. Usually this is the occupational role (12).

Although the burned-out person may be depressed, his symptoms are not primarily intrapsychic but are at least partially situationally induced. An appropriate evaluation of burnout requires that the possibility of a clinical depression be ruled out. A clinical depression might be suspected if the person has had a recent loss, has the vegetative symptoms of depression, has had a previous history of depression, or has a family history of depression (12). If the symptoms are worse in the work situation, associated with conflict or feeling misunderstood by colleagues in a person who tends to work long hours and/or always takes work home and has no time for outside interests or support from others, then the problem may well be burnout.

Ramirez et al. (43) attempted to distinguish between the phenomenon of burnout and psychiatric disturbance. They used the 12-item General Health Questionnaire (GHQ) (52). The GHQ has been used in a variety of studies of occupational stress (see 7 for a review of its use in palliative care studies). The estimated prevalence of psychiatric disorder from the GHQ was 28% and was not significantly different among the three oncology specialty groups, nor did their findings differ from other studies (43). They therefore concluded that although clinical oncologists experienced the greatest amount of work-related stress and lowest satisfaction from work-related sources, they are not at any greater risk of psychiatric disorder that their colleagues.

No demographic or job characteristics predicted psychiatric disorder as measured by the GHQ. However, high GHQ scores indicative of psychiatric disorder were associated with high levels of stress from feeling overloaded, from being involved with treatment toxicity and errors, and from deriving low levels of satisfaction from having professional status and esteem.

## COPING WITH STRESS AND BURNOUT IN ONCOLOGY

The research on coping with job stress is still limited. There have been few long-term longitudinal studies of coping. The effectiveness of strategies for handling stress and burnout have not been studied with reference to impact on performance, productivity, or client outcome (20,35). In a multidisciplinary, multispecialty study, caregivers were twice as likely to report personal coping strategies, rather than environmental strategies, as being helpful in dealing with and preventing occupational stress (33).

### Personal Coping Strategies

On the basis of the findings of the subsample of 110 professionals in oncology, the most helpful personal coping strategies included developing a sense of competence, control, and pleasure from one's work; having control over aspects of one's practice; having a personal philosophy of illness, death, and one's professional role; managing one's lifestyle; and leaving the work situation.

#### A Sense of Competence, Control, and Pleasure in One's Work

A sense of competence, control, and pleasure in work was often associated with a sense of belonging to a team "that knew what it was doing." Through team affiliation

one may derive an ongoing sense of personal worth that survives even though individual patients die (33).

A sense of competence is very similar to the sense of personal hardiness found to be helpful in other studies (15,21). Hardiness protected oncology nurses from emotional exhaustion on the MBI. The personality factors that best predicted personal accomplishment on the MBI included a sense of mastery and control over the difficulties of life and a problem-focused coping style when faced with adversity. The role-related variables that predicted high personal accomplishment included a tendency to assume at the beginning of one's career somewhat neutral expectations (neither high nor low) regarding job satisfaction (15).

A sense of competence can also be associated with having a good person–environment fit between one's personal characteristics and the work environment (33). Bean and Holcombe (25) note the ways in which the personality types of the oncology nurses they studied were complementary to the essence of oncology nursing identified by the nurses in the Cohen and Sarter study (44). The introvert's attention to detail could prevent serious errors, which was viewed as a part of the essence of oncology nursing. The critical incidences of "empathizing with patients and helping with emotional distress were consistent with feeling as the preferred way of making judgments" (36, p. 484).

A sense of control included redefining particular situations as being a challenge instead of a threat, redefining one's role and involvement with people (e.g.,"It is not my role to save people from their illness; rather it is my role to help people to lift the burden which is theirs"), developing more complex skills, and sharing decision making and control with patients (33).

A sense of pleasure in one's work evolved "from one's work with individual patients, from pleasure in the utilization of professional skills, or satisfaction with the indirect impact that one's work can have on groups of patients and families that one might influence indirectly through teaching or administrative roles" (33, p. 188). Caregivers reported allowing themselves to feel pleasure at a job well done. This approach requires a certain maturity as well as an ability to distance oneself from the pain of others and to derive satisfaction objectively from one's role in helping to alleviate at least some of this suffering. Some caregivers have difficulty in distancing in this way and feel guilty if they experience a sense of satisfaction that is associated with the suffering of others.

#### Control Over Aspects of One's Practice

This problem-focused coping strategy entailed setting limits on some aspect of one's practice and organizing work to give one a sense of personal satisfaction. In a study of 289 nurses, those with a high workload and little control suffered significantly more from negative stress consequences such as a lack of job satisfaction or health impairment when compared with others (53). An attempt to gain control over one's practice can lead to difficulty for the clinician who is convinced that he or she knows what is best for the patient, which may or may not be congruent with the patient's needs (54,55).

### A Personal Philosophy

The caregiver who is going to stay in oncology for an extended period often feels the need for something "beyond" the present role. A personal philosophy of illness, death, and one's professional role is an important coping mechanism for many (33).

For some, a religious philosophy centered around a commitment to serve others may be both helpful and key to deriving a sense of meaning in difficult times. Heim (56) found that religion could be a helpful coping mechanism for a certain group of nurses. The religious beliefs of house staff were also found to be associated with lower burnout levels (21). However, when caregivers use their own personal religious beliefs to reach out to patients, this may or may not be helpful to patients (54).

It may also be useful to assume the philosophical perspective that "it's not my fault that this person has the disease, but my responsibility is to do what I can to help lift the burden." Consistent with this view, decision making is a shared responsibility. By participating in a collaborative relationship, caregivers can enable patients to heighten their sense of control through increased self-awareness and understanding of the disease process and treatment.

Inherent in a philosophy of practice is the right, and indeed obligation, to mourn for those who have died. Although not all patients will touch caregivers equally, in many situations patient deaths and the ensuing staff grief deserve recognition. Acknowledging the deaths of individual patients can enable practitioners to avoid the accumulation of grief that comes from repeated, unresolved losses (29). However, at times multiple losses can lead to a sense of grief overload that may need to be dealt with in a variety of ways, including memorial services, journaling, staff "wakes," or attending a funeral. In addition, participating in a grief process can enable caregivers to assess gains that have been made and what one has gained from this relationship, in a manner that may be helpful to future clinical practice.

### Lifestyle Management

Although lifestyle management is certainly not a panacea for dealing with work stress, it enables one to have the energy to cope with stressors. It reflects acknowledgment of an individual's need to learn his or her own body's response to stress in order to detect signals of significant overload. When one finds oneself experiencing symptoms of stress, such as headaches, gastric disturbances, increased infections, a lack of pleasure in one's professional roles and responsibilities, or feeling overwhelmed by responsibilities, it is often time to take a break before one develops more serious symptoms. This break may be a few hours away from one's desk to pursue another interest or a longer break of a few days or weeks. Oncologists suggested decreasing burnout through time away from the clinical setting including more vacation or personal time and sabbaticals (47).

Effective lifestyle management involves developing a balance between one's personal and professional lives. Job home interaction has been found to be a significant source of stress in several studies (32,33,43). Controlling job–home interaction can be very difficult, particularly for those who have developed multiple professional roles, such as clinician, researcher, and writer, while trying to maintain a healthy personal life. Certainly, there are times when career demands must take precedence, but if one always bows to career demands at personal sacrifice, one may need to do some looking at one's sense of self-esteem.

Although lifestyle management and good health habits, including diet, exercise, and rest, are all helpful in stress reduction (Table 2), those in oncology often do not mention using these coping strategies (35).

### Organizational Coping Mechanisms

### Team Philosophy, Team Support and Team Building

Although personal coping mechanisms are important, the work environment does have a role to play in helping caregivers provide effective care to those with cancer. A sense of team philosophy, support, and team building has been identified as the most important organizational coping mechanism for oncology professionals (33). Improving interprofessional cooperation and team processes and group support in nursing was found to provide the best protective or buffering approach to many health stressors, especially burnout (56). The perception of social support

**TABLE 2.** *Lifestyle management techniques*

Other lifestyle management techniques that have been shown to be effective include:
Recognize and monitor symptoms
Change pace and balance diet
Decrease overtime work
Exercise
Maintain sense of humor
Seek consultation if symptoms are severe
Discuss work-related stresses with others who share the same problems
Visit counterparts in other institutions; look for new solutions to problems (21).

at work was also correlated with lower burnout in a study comparing hospice and oncology nurses (42).

Nason (57) notes that team development always involves tension and conflict. This may be viewed as the result of competition, lack of role definition, or poor leadership, but it can also be viewed as a reflection of contradictory institutional goals. Team members may become entrapped in conflicting relationships through the interaction of limited resources, competing demands, and unrealistic institutional priorities and, as a consequence, come to represent differing value systems within the organization. For example, team members of different disciplines may become involved in rivalry and "turf wars" in the current tight economic climate in which the roles of many professional groups are being challenged.

An effective team must have clarity of objectives, mission, and priorities that are shared by all team members. Role expectations should be realistic and well defined when they overlap. Effective decision making and problem solving processes should be in place to arrive at the "best" possible solution; environmental norms should exist that support the tasks of problem solving. There should be a concern for each other's needs and an opportunity for individuals to enlarge their roles and optimize their chances for personal growth (58).

### Support Groups

While support groups are recommended almost as a panacea for either team stress or problems with patients, they were found in one study to be the least commonly mentioned organizational coping strategy (33). Horowitz et al. (59) reported on interdisciplinary "pizza rounds" held weekly on the Neurooncology Service at MSKCC. The purpose of the rounds is to "enhance patient care by improving interdisciplinary functioning and by providing staff with the opportunity to exchange ideas, solve problems involving difficult patients and families, develop consistent plans for patient management, and ventilate their emotional responses to job-related stress. Food is served as a means of increasing attendance and reducing hierarchical barriers between staff members" (p. 330). The group is led by a social worker and psychiatrist. Although no formal evaluation of the meetings have been conducted, the authors feel that the fact that the group has endured for a period of years attests to its effectiveness.

### Administrative Policies

Effective administrators and administrative policies can be extremely important in maximizing productivity and job satisfaction. Oncology nurses valued administrators who were able and willing to change the work environment for staff. "Competent, caring administrators provided leadership, were flexible and available, communicated with staff, fostered development, and allowed opportunities for growth and input into decisions...Nurses spoke about how important it was to 'have a voice in fixing' a problem at work" (35, p. 13). In view of the stress experienced by those in oncology because of work overload, it will be important to develop realistic workloads that recognize the needs of both caregivers and organizations.

Effective administrative policies need to recognize the importance of the emotional labor of oncology and to recognize that this activity will sometimes take time away from other activities (28).

An environment should be provided in which the feelings generated in oncology care can be recognized and expressed. James (28) warns that although the repression of emotion at work may appear to lead to greater efficiency in production, it does not mean that emotions disappear, merely that they are concealed but will eventually be expressed elsewhere, i.e., at home or possibly in leisure pursuits. It takes time to work through frightening or worrying feelings, helping ill people and their families to work out a strategy that they can live with. Time needs to be worked in to provide job flexibility to deal with emotional labor in a highly technological environment (28). By making the expression of feelings in the workplace unacceptable, labor processes may affect not only how feelings are expressed in the workplace but also the emotional labor that is likely to be necessary at home. In a Swedish study, a home-based care program was able to provide very satisfactory work conditions, despite demanding work with cancer patients, by ensuring a continuous education program and providing an environment that stimulated the staff's own initiative but was also capable of supporting staff when necessary (39).

Recognizing the economic constraints of the current work environment, all professional groups will need to work with administration to develop new roles. In addition, opportunities abound for the development of roles in a variety of settings (60).

### Educational Interventions

Training in management skills appears to reduce the stress of overload and increase professional esteem. Equiping clinicians with these skills should increase personal competence in meeting the demands of the job and reduce levels of burnout and psychiatric disorder (43). Developing programs that target specific identified areas might also be helpful. For example, the research of Ulrich and FitzGerald (32) suggests that intervention into particular problem areas—interpersonal difficulties for nurses and job dissatisfaction for doctors—might be effective.

Dealing with patients and families was generally seen as being the most important source of work satisfaction. Communication skills training has been suggested to reduce stress and enhance the satisfaction of dealing with patients as well as reducing the stress of dealing with treatment toxicity and errors and enhancing professional self-esteem (43). Strategies to improve communication between caregivers and patients have been suggested (61,62).

An educational and supportive intervention program showed that it was possible to reduce burnout in medical oncology house staff at MSKCC (21,63). Furthermore, the patients on the intervention unit perceived the house staff as being more empathic, sensitive, and compassionate.

## CONCLUSIONS

The evidence shows that the stress and burnout caregivers in oncology experience may be no greater than that of colleagues in other medical specialties but is greater than that reported in palliative care. Clearly there is stress associated with the empathic relationship with patients and families, particularly those approaching death. However, the major difference in stress and burnout in oncology, as compared to palliative care, appears to be related to the greater workload experienced by those in oncology. In addition, there is not the same recognition that exists in palliative care settings that personal and organizational support systems are required in order to enable caregivers to care effectively for patients and their families without totally depleting themselves.

There is some evidence that caregivers in oncology are feeling increasing stress from work overload and limited resources and that job satisfaction is decreasing as a result. In today's restricted economic climate it will be important to determine realistic workloads for caregivers in oncology and to develop educational and organizational structures that will provide appropriate support. Evidence from the United Kingdom has shown the greater risk of burnout in clinical oncologists whose workloads are on average two and one half times that of their colleagues in major European countries and the United States (43). To date most studies have dealt with the perception of work overload that caregivers report without attempting to document the actual work being performed. Future research will need to determine at what point increasing workloads jeopardize patient care, caregiver health, and home life. The evidence has shown that younger caregivers may be at particular risk of burnout. Programs to target this group have been shown to be effective (63), but more evaluation studies are needed. Further work on personality hardiness as a buffer in the work environment is also indicated. Perhaps those with hardy personalities and the ability to exert control in the work environment will have a role to play in helping to determine realistic expectations in the work setting.

With the current economic climate necessitating significant changes in models of care delivery, it will be important to continue to assess the stress of oncology practitioners over the coming years in order to assure that optimal patient/family care is provided by practitioners who recognize the need to care for themselves in order to be able to care for patients within organizations that provide the necessary administrative support needed for a healthy organization with realistic workloads.

## REFERENCES

1. Feifel H. *The meaning of death.* New York: Blakiston/McGraw-Hill, 1959.
2. Fox RC. *Experiment perilous.* Glencoe, IL: Free Press, 1959.
3. Wodinsky A. Psychiatric consultation with nurses on a leukemia service. *Ment Hygiene* 1964;48:282–287.
4. Klagsbrun SC. Cancer, emotions and nurses. *Am J Psychiatry* 1964; 126:71–81.
5. Jones RG, Weisz AE. Psychiatric liason with a cancer research center. *Comp Psych* 1970;111:336–345.
6. Arliss KL, Levine AS. Doctor–patient relationship in severe illness. *N Engl J Med* 1973; 288:1210–1213.
7. Vachon MLS. Staff stress in hospice/palliative care: a review. *Palliat Med* 1995;9:91–122.
8. Lyall WAL, Rogers J, Vachon MLS. Report to palliative care unit of Royal Victoria Hospital regarding professional stress in the care of the dying. In: Ajemian I, Mount B, eds. *Palliative care service report.* Montreal: Royal Victoria Hospital, 1976;457–468.
9. Vachon MLS, Lyall WAL, Freeman SJJ. Measurement and management of stress in health professionals working with advanced cancer patients. *Death Educ* 1978;1:365–375.
10. Freudenberger HJ. Staff burnout. *J Soc Issues* 1974;30:159–165.
11. Freudenberger HJ, Richelson G. *Burn out: the high cost of high achievement.* New York: Anchor Press, 1980.
12. Vachon MLS. Are your patients burning Out? *Can Fam Phys* 1982;28: 1570–1574.
13. Edelwich J, Brodsky A. *Burn-out: stages of disillusionment in the helping professions.* New York: Springer, 1980.
14. Maslach M. Burnout: the cost of caring. New York: Prentice-Hall, 1982.
15. Papadatou D, Anagnostopoulos F & Monos D. Factors contributing to the development of burnout in oncology nursing. *Br J Med Psychol* 1994;67:187–199.
16. Vachon MLS. Battle fatigue in hospice/palliative care. In: Gilmore A, Gilmore S, eds. *A safer death.* New York: Plenum Press, 1988;149–160.
17. Pines AM. Who is to blame for helper's burnout? Environmental impact. In: Scott CD, Hawk J, eds. *Heal thyself: the health of health care professionals.* New York: Brunner/Mazel, 1986.
18. Maslach C, Jackson SE. *The Maslach burnout inventory (Manual),* 2nd ed. Palo Alto, CA: Consulting Psychologists Press, 1986.
19. Maslach C, Jackson SE. Burnout in health professions: a social psychological analysis. In: Sanders GS, Suls J, eds. *Social psychology of health and illness.* London: Erlbaum, 1982.
20. Delvaux N, Razavi D, Farvacques C. Cancer care: a stress for health professionals. *Soc Sci Med* 1988;27:159–166.
21. Kash KM, Holland JC. Special problems of physicians and house staff in oncology. In: Holland JC, Rowland JH, eds. *Handbook of psychooncology.* New York: Oxford University Press, 1989;647–657.
22. Vaillant GE, Sobowale NC, McArthur C. Some psychologic vulnerabilities of physicians. *N Engl J Med* 1972;287:372–375.
23. Hogan C, Champagne D. Hogan-Champagne reference survey. In: Champagne D, Hogan C, eds. *Supervisory and management skills: a competency-based training program for middle managers of educational systems.* Pittsburgh: University of Pittsburgh Press, 1979.
24. Jung C. *Psychological types.* Princeton, NJ: Princeton University Press, 1980.
25. Bean CA, Holcombe JK. Personality types of oncology nurses. *Cancer Nursing* 1993;16:479–485.
26. Kobasa SC. Stressful life events, personality and health: an inquiry into hardiness. *J Pers Soc Psychol* 1979;37:1–11.

27. Kobasa SC, Maddi SR, Kahn S. Hardiness and Health: a prospective inquiry. *J Pers Soc Psychol* 1982;42:168–177.
28. James N. Emotional labour: skill and work in the social regulation of feelings. *Sociol Rev* 1989; 37:15–42.
29. Mount BM.. Dealing with our losses. *J Clin Oncol* 1986; 4:1127–1134.
30. Hansell PS. Stress on nurses in oncology. In: Holland JC, and Rowland JH, eds. *Handbook of psychooncology.* New York: Oxford University Press, 1989;658–663.
31. Wilkinson SM. The changing pressures for oncology nurses 1986–93. *Eur J Cancer Care* 1995;4(2):69–74.
32. Ulrich A, FitzGerald P. Stress experienced by physicians and nurses in the cancer ward. *Soc Sci Med* 1990; 31:1013–1022.
33. Vachon MLS. *Occupational stress in the care of the critically ill, dying and bereaved.* Washington, DC: Hemisphere, 1987.
34. Kunkel EJS, Shmuely Y. Sources of ancillary oncology staff stress in radiation oncology. *Psycho-oncology* 1994 3:241–243.
35. Cohen MZ, Haberman MR, Steeves R, Deatrick JA. Rewards and difficulties of oncology nursing. *Oncol Nursing Forum,* 1994;21(8), Supplement, 9–17.
36. Van Servellen G, Leake B. Burn-out in hospital nurses: a comparison of acquired immunodeficiency syndrome, oncology, general medical, and intensive care unit nurse samples. *J Prof Nursing* 1993;9:169–177.
37. Wilkinson SM. Stress in cancer nursing: does it really exist? *J Adv Nursing* 1994;20:1079–1084.
38. Spielberger CD, Gorsch RL, Lushene RE, Vagg PR, Jacobs GA. *Manual for the state-trait anxiety inventory.* Palo Alto, CA: Counselling Psychologists Press, 1983.
39. Beck-Friis B, Strang P, Sjödén P-O. Caring for severely ill cancer patients: a comparison of working conditions in hospital-based home care and in hospital. *Support Care Cancer* 1993;1:145–151.
40. Vachon MLS. Stress in oncologists. *Can J Oncol* 1993;3:166–172.
41. Herschbach P. Work-related stress specific to physicians and nurses working with cancer patients. *J Psychosoc Oncol* 1992; 10(2);79–99.
42. Bram PJ, Katz LF. A study of burnout in nurses working in hospice and hospital oncology settings. *Oncol Nursing Forum* 1989;16:555–560.
43. Ramirez AJ, Graham J, Richards MA, Cull A, Gregory WM, Leaning MS, Snashall DC, Timothy AR. Burnout and psychiatric disorder among cancer clinicians. *Br J Cancer* 1995;71:1263–1269.
44. Cohen M, Sarter B. Love and work: oncology nurses' view of the meaning of their work. *Oncol Nursing Forum* 1992;19:1481–1486.
45. Schmale J, Weinberg N, Pieper S. Satisfactions, stresses and coping mechanisms of oncologists in clinical practice. *Am Soc Clin Oncol* 1987;6:A1003.
46. Peteet JR, Murray-Ross D, Medeiros C, Walsh-Burke K, Rieker P, Finkelstein D. Job stress and satisfaction among the staff members at a cancer center. *Cancer* 1989;64:975–982.
47. Whippen DA, Canellos GP. Burnout syndrome in the practice of oncology. *J Clin Oncol* 1991;9:1916–1921.
48. Olkinuora M, Asp S, Juntunen J, Kauttu K, Strid L, Aarimaa M. Stress symptoms, burnout and suicidal thoughts in Finnish physicians. *Soc Psychiatry Psychiatr Epidemiol* 1990;25:81–86.
49. Yasko JM. Variables which predict burnout experienced by oncology clinical nurse specialists. *Cancer Nursing* 1983;6:109–116.
50. Jenkins JF, Ostchega Y. Evaluation of burnout in oncology nurses. *Cancer Nursing* 1986;9:108–116.
51. McWilliam CL, Burdock J, Wamsley J. The challenging experience of palliative care support-team nursing. *Oncol Nursing Forum* 1993;20: 770–785.
52. Goldberg D, Williams P. *A users guide to the general health questionnaire.* Windsor, Berkshire: NFER-Nelson, 1988.
53. Landsbergis PA. Occupational stress among health care workers: a test of the job demands-control-model. *J Org Behav* 1988;217–239.
54. Steeves R, Cohen MZ, Wise CT. An analysis of critical incidents describing the essence of oncology nursing. *Oncol Nursing Forum* 1994;21(8)(Suppl):19–26.
55. Grossman SA, Sheidler VR, Swedeen K, Mucenski J, Piantadosi S. Correlation of patient and caregiver ratings of cancer pain. *J Pain Sympt Manag* 1991;6(2),53–57.
56. Heim E. Job stressors and coping in health professions. *Psychother Psychsom* 1991;55:90–99.
57. Nason F. Team tension as a vital sign. *Gen Hosp Psychiatry* 1981;3: 32–36.
58. Beckhard R. Organizational implications of team building. In: Wise H, Beckhard R, Rubin I, Kyte AL, eds. *Making health teams work.* Cambridge, UK: Ballinger, 1974;69–94.
59. Horowitz SA, Passik SD, Brish M, Breitbart WS. *Psycho-Oncology* 1994;3:329–332.
60. Boyle DM, Engelking C, Harvey C. Making a difference in the 21st century: are oncology nurses ready? *Oncol Nursing Forum* 1994;21: 53–55.
61. Cowan DH, Laidlaw JC. A strategy to improve communication between health care professionals and people living with cancer. *J Cancer Educ* 1993;8:109–117.
62. Faulkner A, Maguire P. *Talking to cancer patients and their relatives.* Oxford: Oxford University Press, 1994.
63. Kash K, Breitbart W, Holland Jr, Berenson S, Marks E, Lesko L, Ouellette-Kobasa S. A stress-reducing intervention for medical oncology housestaff. *Am Soc Clin Oncol* 1989;8:A1214.

*Principles and Practice of Supportive Oncology,*
edited by Ann Berger et al.
Lippincott–Raven Publishers, Philadelphia ©1998

# CHAPTER 62

# Supportive Care in Children with Cancer

Steven J. Weisman

## THE CONCEPT OF SUPPORTIVE CARE

The field of supportive care in children has evolved as a direct outgrowth of the care of children with cancer. Initially, the focus of supportive care was on the terminally ill child with cancer. Improved treatment protocols, involving progressively more intensive therapy, have now led to more prolonged survival and cure. This has created a population of children with a wide variety of supportive care problems, in addition to the smaller group of children who need terminal palliative care. Supportive/palliative care in children differs from that in adults because of differences in diseases, differences in the intensity of treatment, and because of the developmental and cognitive differences present in children. The importance of supportive care in the management of children with cancer is highlighted by a recent monograph on the subject by the Children's Cancer Study Group (1), as well as an extensive discussion in the recent text of Pizzo and Poplack (2).

This chapter provides an overview of the clinical issues that are important for providing effective supportive and palliative care in children. Most of the principles and therapies already presented in this volume apply to the care of children as well as adult patients. Rather than attempt to rehash the vast majority of the topics already presented, this chapter will focus on the aspects of supportive and palliative care in children that might require special techniques or approaches based on the nature of the diseases involved or based on the specific stage of development the child has achieved.

Palliative care has been defined by the World Health Organization (WHO) as the active total care of patients whose disease is not responsive to curative treatment. Control of pain, of other symptoms, and of psychological, social, and spiritual problems is paramount. The goal of palliative care is achievement of the best quality of life for patients and their families (3). Throughout much of the following discussion, concepts can be applied virtually synonymously to both palliative and supportive care. In fact, it should be stated that palliative care must begin when children are diagnosed with cancer. There should be continued and meticulous attention directed to alleviating all aspects of the child's distress including his or her physical, psychological, and spiritual needs. In this way, supportive care, or symptom relief, and palliative care ultimately both work toward the same goal.

## THE SUPPORTIVE/PALLIATIVE CARE TEAM: HOSPITAL, HOSPICE, HOME

There are three common settings in which supportive/palliative care must be provided for chronically ill children: home, hospice, and hospital. It should be obvious that during all hospitalizations children should be afforded the highest level of care to treat disease symptoms or complications of diagnostic or therapeutic interventions. In addition, aggressive management of disease- or treatment-related events must be incorporated into the care plan for the child at home. Child-specific hospice units remain uncommon in the United States.

It is unusual for most pediatric facilities to provide the resources for a specific supportive/palliative care team. Indeed, however, a few such programs exist in North America such as at the IWK Children's Hospital in Halifax, Nova Scotia. In contrast, most pediatric specialty treatment centers have a variety of general and specialized pediatric providers who have the potential to provide all of the elements ideally present in a supportive/palliative care team. Many pediatric specialty facilities have formally or informally organized pain management teams that serve as a tangible resource for providing pain treatment. Often these teams are led by pediatric anesthesiol-

S. J. Weisman: Departments of Anesthesiology and Pediatrics, Yale University School of Medicine, New Haven, CT 06520-8051.

ogists who can provide sound pharmacologic advice for analgesic use as well as providing rare interventional pain management techniques for difficult-to-manage patients. Child life programs, including in-hospital teachers, should also be involved in the care of children who require supportive/palliative care. Their programs help to establish a more normal daily schedule for hospitalized children, as well as providing behaviorally therapeutic distractive activities. Pediatric rehabilitation departments can also play a pivotal role in providing supportive/palliative care services.

The supportive care/palliative care team for children with cancer should be organized by the physician who is primarily responsible for the care of the child. In most circumstances in the United States, this responsibility falls to a subspecialty-trained pediatrician, such as the pediatric oncologist. It is less common for this professional to be the primary pediatrician who may have provided most of the child's care before the diagnosis of malignancy was made. However, one physician must be identified who can assume coordinating responsibilities for a youngster's supportive care.

Because children who require supportive/palliative care may be in various states of acute or chronic distress, and because virtually every one of these patients suffers from a potentially overwhelming disease, it is critical for any supportive/palliative care team to have very active and visible psychological providers available. These individuals may be social workers and psychiatric social workers or they may be child psychiatrists or psychologists. Unfortunately, these providers often cannot successfully recover reimbursement for their services and hence this aspect of a supportive/palliative care program may be one of the most difficult to support. Ideally, every child who will be cared for by the supportive/palliative care team should undergo psychological assessment so that the entire team can appreciate the child's temperament and the psychological resources that will be available to the child and family to help cope with their disease or treatment side effects.

Nurses can participate in the supportive/palliative care team in many different roles. Some may be fortunate enough to serve as clinical nurse specialists directly assigned to such a team, whereas others may participate as clinical nurse specialists for the primary pediatric subspecialty caring for the child. Clinical nurse specialists for pediatric pain services may be able to provide important clinical care, especially for those youngsters who require palliative care in the terminal phases of their illness. Yet the staff nurse, assigned to the care of the child in the hospital or at home, may be the most pivotal of the nursing providers on the supportive/palliative care team. These caretakers are able to spend the most consistent time with the patient and have the most direct contact with the child's immediate family. This permits the nurse to develop a close personal relationship with the child, which may then foster recognition of that child's emotional and physical needs.

## DRUG ADMINISTRATION: ROUTES FOR CHILDREN, CENTRAL LINES

Symptom control in many children is confounded by the challenge of medication administration. In most circumstances, one might argue that the oral route should be chosen over parenteral administration of medications. However, young children cannot swallow tablets. Certain sustained release medications cannot be crushed or chewed to permit use in younger patients. Many medications are not formulated in elixirs or suspensions, and it is quite uncommon to find palatable chewable tablets. In addition, medication administration can be one of the more challenging aspects of overall care of children with cancer. In fact, it is often the source of considerable distress and psychological struggling between the child and the caregivers.

Many medications, including preoperative sedatives, analgesics, and anxiolytics, can be administered rectally (4–6). Acetaminophen or aspirin has been given safely by this route for many years. The non steroidal antiinflammatory drug ibuprofen has been employed for the management of postoperative pain via the rectal route (7). The obvious drawback to this route for routine use is that it can be invasive for some children. For the child who is toilet-trained, the rectal route may not only be uncomfortable, but it also invades their personal privacy. Thus, although it might prove useful in the younger school-aged child, it rarely is chosen as the preferred route of medication administration. In infants and toddlers, it can be a very helpful delivery route.

It is quite reasonable to maximize the use of parenteral drug administration routes in children with cancer. The intramuscular route is the least preferred method for use in children. Most importantly, this route is painful and when PRN drugs are offered to children via this route, they will refuse them. Children also have reduced muscle mass when compared to adults, which makes the intramuscular site choice more difficult to effect. Subcutaneous drugs, particularly opioids, have been used for end-of-life care in children (8).

The intravenous route, especially with the popularization of central venous access catheters, is clearly the route of choice for most pharmacologic interventions for children (9,10). These catheters permit administration of chemotherapeutic agents, blood products, parenteral nutrition, antibiotics, and pain medications as needed (11). In addition, the catheters allow minimally traumatic blood sampling, which otherwise has been a source of considerable distress in children with cancer.

The single major problem with their use has been the associated increased risk of infection (12–15). Much of this risk has been reduced by the acceptance of the use of implantable ports (16–18).

The intravenous route, as in adults, can be employed to deliver analgesics using patient-controlled analgesia (PCA) (19,20). It can be employed with or without a background basal infusion and many commercially available pumps permit application both in hospital and at home in children (21,22). It has been employed with excellent success and patient satisfaction for the management of mucositis in bone marrow transplant patients (23,24).

Other alternative routes of administration of opioids and other drugs have been described. Considerable experience with fentanyl administered via the transdermal route in adults has led to it being used in children (25,26). Its use in children may be limited by the slow onset of action and the difficulty in achieving rapid titration of the system for changing levels of pain. In addition, often the lowest dosage form delivers too much opioid for use in many children. On the other hand, transdermal administration of local anesthetics using EMLA cream (eutectic mixture of local anesthetic) stands out as a major advance in cancer treatment and palliative care (27). It has been successfully employed in children with cancer for the management of lumbar puncture as well as for reducing the discomfort of central venous access port puncture (28,29). The nasal route has been described for administration of sedatives in children. Unfortunately, medications given via this route can be quite uncomfortable (30–32). Midazolam, for example, because of its low pH, can cause intense burning. The buccal mucosa can serve as another readily available delivery site for some drugs. When midazolam is administered via this route, it is better tolerated than via the nasal mucosa (32). Transmucosal fentanyl has been used for the management of painful procedures in children (33,34). It can also be used for the treatment of cancer breakthrough pain and postoperative pain (35–37). However, it has not been formally studied in children in these latter applications.

Epidural and subarachnoid drug delivery, although not often necessary in the management of cancer pain in children, has certainly gained wide acceptance and application in the management of postoperative pain. Regional anesthetic techniques do have application in children with terminal malignancy (38). In general, children unresponsive to extremely high-dose opioid infusions or children with unacceptable opioid toxicity benefited from this invasive approach to drug delivery.

## SYMPTOM CONTROL

### Pain Control

Pain management has become a priority in the management of symptoms in children with cancer. An extensive volume on the subject of pain management in children has recently been published (39). In addition, another specific discussion of cancer pain management in children can be found in Pizzo and Poplack (2).

Tables 1–3 contain general guidelines for pain management in the child receiving supportive or palliative care.

**TABLE 1.** Nonopioid analgesics

| Drug | Dose (mg/kg) | Route | Formulation | Comments |
|---|---|---|---|---|
| Acetaminophen | 10–30 q3–4h | PO, PR | Liquid, tablet (chewable), suppository | Maximum 60 mg/kg/day<br>Limited antiinflammatory effect |
| Ibuprofen | 5–10 q6–8h | PO | Tablet, suspension | Antiplatelet effect<br>Gastritis<br>Interstitial nephritis<br>Hepatic toxicity (chronic use) |
| Ketorolac | 0.5 q6h | IV, IM | Parenteral | Limit to 48–72 hr<br>Only NSAID approved for parenteral analgesia |
|  | 10 mg (total dose) q6h | PO | Tablet | See ibuprofen |
| Choline magnesium trisalicylate | 25 q8–12h | PO | Liquid, tablet | Less gastritis<br>?? less antiplatelet effect |
| Acetyl salicylic acid | 10–15 q4h | PO | Tablet (chewable) | Associated with Reye Syndrome<br>Gastritis<br>Antiplatelet effect |
| Indomethacin | 1 q6h | PO, IV, PR | Liquid, tablet, suppository | Used in premature infants to close patent ductus arteriosus |
| Naproxen | 5–10 q6–8h | PO | Liquid, tablet | See ibuprofen |
| Tolmetin | 5–10 q6–8h | PO | Tablet | See ibuprofen |

**TABLE 2.** *Opioid analgesics*

| Drug | Equianalgesic initial dose (mg/kg) | Interval and route | Comments |
| --- | --- | --- | --- |
| Codeine | 1 | q4–6h PO | Dose limited by constipation, nausea, vomiting; ceiling effect |
| Oxycodone | 0.15 | q4h PO | Opioid in Percocet, Roxicet |
| Morphine sulfate | 0.1 | q2–3h IV | Histamine release (pruritis), |
| Continuous | 0.03–0.05 | per hr IV, SC | nausea, vomiting, |
| PCA | 0.01–0.02 | per hr basal | urinary retention |
| | 0.01–0.02 | q6–10 min per dose | |
| Oral | 0.3 | q3–4h PO | |
| MS-Contin (slow-release morphine) | 0.3 | q8–12h PO | Chronic pain Smallest tablet is 15 mg; cannot divide |
| Hydromorphone (Dilaudid) | 0.015–0.02 0.075–0.1 q3h IV | q3h IV q3–4h PO | Less itching, nausea, dysphoria than morphine; can be used for PCA; infusions |
| Methadone | 0.1–0.2 | q4h (initial (ts) 2–3) IV then q 8–12h | Long acting |
| | 0.2–0.4 | q8–12h PO | |
| Fentanyl | 0.001 | q1–2h IV | Rapid onset and short duration (single doses); useful for procedure pain |
| | 0.005–0.015 | x 1 transmucosal | Preop sedation or procedure pain |
| Meperidine (Demerol) | 1.0 2.0–3.0 | q3–4h IV q3–4h PO | Avoid chronic use. Metabolite normeperidine accumulates and causes CNS stimulation/seizures |

**TABLE 3.** *Adjuvant drugs useful in pediatric pain management*

| Drug class | Uses | Drug and dosages | Comments |
| --- | --- | --- | --- |
| Tricyclic antidepressants | Neuropathic pain Decrease pain by central action on pain inhibitory systems Improve sleep cycles Improve mood | Amitriptyline (Elavil): 0.1 mg/kg qhs PO advanced as tolerated to 0.5–2 mg/kg Doxepine: As for amitriptyline (liquid) Imipramine (Tofranil): 1.5 mg/kg/day t.i.d. PO | Anticholinergic effect (morning somnolence and dry mouth) diminished by starting with small doses Use with caution in patients with cardiac conduction defects Imipramine causes photosensitization, lowers seizure threshold, and has lower metabolism in the presence of methylphenidate (Ritalin) |
| Anticonvulsants | Used for neuropathic pain (trigeminal neuralgia) and migraine Appear to alter neuronal excitability | Phenytoin (Dilantin): 5 mg/kg/day Carbamazepine (Tegretol): 100–200 bid Clonazepam (Klonopin): 0.01–0.2 mg/kg/day, increased to 0.1–0.2 mg/kg/day | Side effects include sedation, ataxia, dysphoria, GI symptoms, and hepatotoxicity Drug level must be monitored Hematologic/hepatic side effects |
| Stimulants | Increase analgesia and decrease sedation by chronic use of opioids Provide some euphoria | Methylphenidate: 0.1–0.2 mg/kg/dose b.i.d. PO Dextroamphetamine: 0.1–0.2 mg/kg/dose b.i.d. PO | Given in early morning and midday to avoid nighttime insomnia |
| Corticosteroids | Used for neuropathic pain (trigeminal neuralgia) and migraine Appear to alter neuronal excitability Headache from increased intracranial pressure | Dexamethasone/prednisone/ prednisolone: variable, as per patient requirements | Dosage and route determined by patient's medical condition |
| Sedatives/ anxiolytics | Decrease anxiety when given as premedication Provide amnesia Most useful for very short term use or for single procedures muscle spasms | Diazepam (Valium): 0.02–0.1 mg/kg q6–8h Midazolam (Versed): 0.05–0.1 mg/kg q2–4h Lorazepam (Ativan): 0.02–0.05 mg/kg q8–12h | Increased respiratory depression when given with opioids Do not provide analgesia Midazolam is short acting Lorazepam has antiemetic qualities and causes hallucinations in children under 6 years of age |

**TABLE 4.** Antiemetics

| Class/Agent | Dose | Comments |
|---|---|---|
| Phenothiazines | | Extrapyramidal side effects |
|   Chlorpromazine (Thorazine) | 0.5 mg/kg IV q6–8h | Orthostatic hypotension, sedation |
|   Prochlorperazine (Compazine) | 0.1 mg/kg IV q4h | Modest antiemetic effect |
|   Promethazine (Phenergan) | 0.25–0.5 mg/kg IV q4–6h | |
|   Perphenazine (Trilafon) | 0.02–0.05 mg/kg IV q6h | |
|   Methotrimeprazine (Levoprome) | 0.05 mg/kg IV q6h | Analgesic 3:2 ratio to morphine sulfate |
| Serotonin antagonists | | Headache and diarrhea |
|   Ondansetron (Zofran) (51) | 0.1–0.15 mg/kg q2–6h | |
|   Granisetron (Kytril)(52,53) | 0.01 mg/kg q6h | |
| Metaclopramide (Reglan) | 0.5–1.0 mg/kg IV q2–4h | Central (antidopaminergic) and peripheral (increases gastric emptying) effects |
| | | Extrapyramidal side effects |
| Butyrophenones | | |
|   Droperidol (Inapsine) | 0.01–0.02 mg/kg IV q6h | Sedation, hypotension, extrapyramidal side effects |
| Antihistamines | | |
|   Diphenhydramine (Benadryl) | 0.5–1.0 mg/kg IV q4–6h | Can be used to treat/prevent extrapyramidal side effects |
| Steroids | | |
|   Dexamethasone (Decadron) | 0.1–0.2 mg/kg q6h | |
| Cannabinoids | | |
|   Tetrahydrocannabinol (Marinol) | 2.5–7.5 mg/m2 | Dysphoria |

## Nausea/Vomiting

Many options are available for successful management of nausea and vomiting in children with cancer. Prophylactic approaches are usually the most successful. Behavioral interventions, as well as more traditionally accepted pharmacologic interventions, have been used for prevention and treatment of nausea and vomiting (40) (Table 4). An excellent review of this topic is included in a recent text of pediatric oncology (2).

## Pruritis

Pruritis is a common problem seen with opioid administration in children. It is common for them to not complain of this symptom; rather, caretakers will notice incessant rubbing of the eyes and face or trunk and abdomen. It can be annoying and cause distress in children and one should aggressively attempt to control it.

It is less commonly a direct manifestation of the malignancy, such as Hodgkin's or non-Hodgkin's lymphoma. In these latter examples, antipruritic therapy may be less effective than the primary treatment of the disease. See Table 5 for a listing of antipruritics.

## Mouth Care

Maintenance of adequate oral hygiene is an essential component of supportive care. The mouth is the site of therapy-related complications such as mucositis, cellulitis, dental abscesses, and bleeding (41). Dental evaluation and maintenance treatments should be continued during all phases of cancer therapy. Patients should be taught a daily hygiene regimen that includes brushing, flossing, and using an oral rinse. Often 0.1% chlorhexidine gluconate (Peridex) is used to reduce oral bacterial flora.

Mucositis/gingivitis can be managed with continuation of the daily oral hygiene regimen. Sucralfate suspension

**TABLE 5.** Antipruritics

| Class/Agent | Dose | Comments |
|---|---|---|
| Antihistamines | | |
|   Diphenhydramine (Benadryl) | 0.5–1.0 mg/kg IV/PO q4–6h | |
|   Hydroxyzine (Atarax) | 0.5–1.0 mg/kg IV/POq 6 h | |
| Opioid antagonists | | |
|   Naloxone infusion | 0.5–1.0 µg/kg IV | Titrate slowly for opioid pruritis |
| | 0.5–1.0 µg/kg/h IV | |
|   Nalmefene | 0.25 µg/kg IV q8–12h | Long half-life |
| Opioid agonist/antagonist | | |
|   Nalbuphine (Nubain) | 0.1 mg/kg IV q6h | |

swishes several times a day has been shown to have some salutary effect on the oral mucosa (42). In addition, oral capsaicin, administered as candied lozenges, can be employed to reduce the pain in cancer patients (43). However, the hallmark of good management of mucositis involves a combination of systemic analgesia and local analgesic care. Dyclonine (0.5%) is a topical local anesthetic that can be applied directly to injured mucosa. Its major advantage is that it has not been reported to cause system toxicity due to absorption through the mucosa. Viscous lidocaine (2%) can also be used for topical local anesthesia; however, with repeated use or use of large volumes, lidocaine neurotoxicity can occur (seizures). One part viscous lidocaine (2%) can be combined with 1 part diphenhydramine elixir, 2 parts antacid (Maalox or Mylanta), plus 2 parts water and used plain or with flavoring as "magic mouthwash." This concoction can be used as a swish and *spit* gargle or mouthwash with excellent pain relief.

Mucosal or gingival bleeding, which is usually related to thrombocytopenia, can be managed with adopting a more gentle oral hygiene regimen and, most commonly, with platelet replacement. Topical thrombin and/or antifibrinolytic agents can also be used. Aminocaproic acid can be administered at 100 mg/kg IV followed by 30 mg/kg every 2–6 hours to help control bleeding. Alternatively, tranexamic acid (25 mg/kg PO t.i.d. or 10 mg/kg IV t.i.d.) can be started.

## Constipation

Constipation in children receiving supportive care will usually be the result of chemotherapeutic interventions (vinca alkaloids) or opioid therapy. In either case, expectant therapy should be the norm. Mineral oil–based stool softeners, such as Kondremul (1–2 tsp once to twice a day), offer a pleasant-tasting alternative for treatment. Senekot tablets can be quite effective for children capable of swallowing tablets. In addition, Pericolace syrup or tablets (docusate and casanthranol) can be used. Addition of dietary fiber to a child's diet can be difficult and therefore psyllium-containing laxatives are often not employed. Although oral naloxone therapy has been reported for management of constipation in adults (1–3 mg q6h), its use has not been formally reported in children (44).

## Convulsions

Convulsions in the child receiving supportive care can be quite distressing to the caretakers. Certainly all children with known convulsive disorders must be maintained on therapeutic levels of their normal anticonvulsants. For those on oral therapy, adjustments may need to take place if oral intake is not possible. Seizures in children without underlying histories of such are apt to be caused by primary or metastatic lesions in the central nervous system.

Particularly in children on home therapy, plans for management of convulsions should be in place. This might include instruction in the use of home benzodiazepines (midazolam, diazepam) for the acute onset of seizures.

## Anxiety/Agitation

A caring, loving supportive care environment may be the most effective intervention for the management of anxiety and agitation. If agitation and anxiety result in distress, especially in the terminal phases of therapy, cautious use of anxiolytics may be indicated. Benzodiazepines, butyrophenones (haloperidol), or phenothiazines may all be helpful. Occasionally, agitation/delirium may result from progressive hepatic or renal impairment and reduction in any of a variety of supportive care measures may be quite helpful in treating these symptoms. Also, children may experience paradoxical reactions to the benzodiazepines, manifested by hyperactivity, irritability, and restlessness. In these cases, alternative sedative agents should be chosen.

## Urinary Incontinence/Retention

Urinary retention is often seen as a side effect of either chemotherapy or opioid treatment. Conservative management with warm compresses applied to the bladder, ambulation, and gentle massage/pressure (in the young infant) may all facilitate the passage of urine. When these simple maneuvers fail, single-time straight catheterization or placement of an indwelling urine catheter may be needed.

## Cardiorespiratory: Dyspnea

Shortness of breath or air hunger can be extremely distressing to children and their parents. Causes for new-onset dyspnea should be sought and, if possible, treatment directed at any discovered etiologies. Treatment will clearly be determined by the stage of treatment. Initially, symptoms from space-occupying lesions, such as mediastinal masses, will require aggressive and very prompt interventions. However, in end-of-life situations, dyspnea must be treated as aggressively as pain. The popular notion that because opioids may lead to respiratory depression, they should not be employed in patients with dyspnea may be quite inappropriate. Certainly a combination of judicious doses of opioids and anxiolytics with supplemental oxygen should be the foundation of therapy (45).

## Nutrition

Nutritional support for children with cancer has become one of the cornerstones of effective care. The major impact that malnutrition had on children with malignancies was clearly recognized in the early 1980s, especially as therapeutic regimens intensified (46–48). Aggressive nutritional assessment must be part of the overall care plan for any child with malignancy. Because children have ongoing developmental and growth caloric requirements in addition to the metabolic stress of malignancy, they will have enormous nutritional needs. Children who may be expected to be in negative nitrogen balance during the initial phases of therapy are at extremely high risk and are unlikely to be able to maintain their weight. Serum albumin and serum transferrin levels should be monitored along with weight and other anthropomorphic parameters. Early intervention with enteral or parenteral treatment regimens can prevent and even reverse protein-energy malnutrition (49).

The convenience of central venous catheters in children with malignancy has facilitated the use of aggressive parenteral nutritional supplementation techniques. Specific recommendations for such therapy are beyond the scope of this brief section, although several reviews are available (50).

## REFERENCES

1. Ablin AR. Supportive care of children with cancer. In: Spivak JL, Abeloff MD, eds. *The Johns Hopkins series in hematology/oncology.* Baltimore: The Johns Hopkins University Press, 1993;170.
2. Pizzo PA, Poplack DG. *Principles and practice of pediatric oncology.* Philadelphia: Lippincott–Raven, 1997.
3. World Health Organization. *Cancer pain relief: With a guide to opioid availability.* Geneva, 1996;63.
4. Lindahl S, Olsson AK. Rectal premedication in children. *Anaesthesia* 1981;36:376–379.
5. Cole L, Hanning CD. Review of the rectal use of opioids. *J Pain Sympt Manag* 1990;5:118–126.
6. Shane SA, Fuchs SM, Khine H. Efficacy of rectal midazolam for the sedation of preschool children undergoing laceration repair. *Ann Emerg Med* 1994;24:1065–1073.
7. Maunuksela EL, Ryhanen P, Janhunen L. Efficacy of rectal ibuprofen in controlling postoperative pain in children. *Can J Anaesth* 1992; 39:226.
8. Miser AW, Davis DM, Hughes CS, et al. Continuous subcutaneous infusion of morphine in children with cancer. *Am J Dis Child* 1983; 137:383–385.
9. Dawson S, Pai MKR, Smith S, Rothney M, Ahmed K, Barr RD. Right atrial catheters in children with cancer: a decade in the use of tunnelled, exteriorized devices at a single institution. *Am J Pediatr Hematol Oncol* 1991;13:126–129.
10. Weiner ES, McGuire P, Stolar CJ, et al. The CCG prospective study of venous access devices: an analysis of insertions and causes for removal. *J Pediatr Surg* 1992;27:155–164.
11. Kingston JE, Fowler PC, Jackson DB, Potter V, Malpas JS. Experience with central intravenous catheters in a peditric oncology unit. *Eur Pediatr Hematol Oncol* 1985;2:29–34.
12. Hiemenez J, Skelton J, Pizzo P. Perspective on the management of catheter-related infections in cancer patients. *Pediatr Inf Dis* 1986;5: 20–24.
13. Prince A, Heller B, Levy J, Heird W. Management of fever in patients with central vein catheters. *Pediatr Infect Dis* 1986;5:20–24.
14. Ingram J, Weitzman S, Greenberg ML, Parkin P, Filler R. Complications of indwelling venous access lines in the pediatric hematology patient: a prospective comparison of external venous catheters and subcutaneous ports. *Am J Pediatr Hematol Oncol* 1991;13:130–136.
15. Johnson PR, Decker MD, Edwards KM, Schaffner W, Wright PF. Frequency of Broviac catheter infections in pediatric oncology patients. *J Inf Dis* 1986;154:570–578.
16. Hockenberry M, Schultz W, Bennett B, Bryant R, Falletta J. Experience with minimal complications in implanted catheters in children. *Am J Pediatr Hematol Oncol* 1989;11:295–299.
17. Mirro J, Rao B, Stokes D, et al. A prospective study of Hickman/Briviac catheters and implantable ports in pediatric oncology patients. *J Clin Oncol* 1989;7:214–222.
18. Mirro J, Jr, Rao BN, Kumar M, et al. A comparison of placement techniques and complications of externalized catheters and implantable port use in children with cancer. *J Pediatr Surg* 1990;25:120–124.
19. Berde CB, Lehn BM, Yee JD, Sethna NF, Russo D. Patient-controlled analgesia in children and adolescents: a randomized, prospective comparison with intramuscular morphine for postoperative analgesia. *J Pediatrics* 1991;118:460–446.
20. Gaukroger PB, Omkins DP, Van Der Walt JH. Patient-controlled analgesia with low dose background infusions after lower abdominal surgery in children. *Anaesth Intensive Care* 1989;17:264.
21. Doyle E, Robinson D, Morton NS. Patient-controlled analgesia with low dose background infusions after lower abdominal surgery in children. *Br J Anaesth* 1993;71:818–822.
22. Skues MA, Watson DM, O'Meara M, Goddard JM. Patient-controlled analgesia in children: a comparison of two infusion techniques. *Paediatr Anaesth* 1993;3:223–228.
23. Mackie AM, Coda BC, Hill HF. Adolescents use patient-controlled analgesia effectively for relief from prolonged oropharyngeal mucositis pain. *Pain* 1991;46:265–269.
24. Dunbar PJ, Buckley P, Gavrin JR, Sanders JE, Chapman CR. Use of patient-controlled analgesia for pain control for children receiving bone marrow transplant. *J Pain Sympt Manag* 1995;10:604–611.
25. Miser AW, Narang PK, Dothage JA, Young RC, Sindelar W, Miser JS. Transdermal fentanyl for pain control in patients with cancer. *Pain* 1989;37:15–21.
26. Patt RB, Lustik S, Litman RS. The use of transdermal fentanyl in a six-year-old patient with neuroblastoma and diffuse abdominal pain. *J Pain Sympt Manage* 1993;8:317–319.
27. Maunuksela E, Korpela R. Double-blind evaluation of lignocaine-prilocaine cream (EMLA) in children. *Br J Anaesth* 1986;58:1242–1245.
28. Kapelushnik J, Koren G, Solh H,Greenberg M, DeVeber L. Evaluating the efficacy of EMLA in alleviating pain associated with lumbar puncture; comparison of open and double-blinded protocols in children. *Pain* 1994;42:31–34.
29. Miser Aw, Goh S, Dose AM, et al. Trial of a topically administered local anaesthetic (EMLA cream) for pain relief during central venous port access in children with cancer. *J Pain Sympt Manag* 1994;9:259–264.
30. Theroux MC, West DW, Corddry DH, et al. Efficacy of intranasal midazolam in facilitating suturing of lacerations in preschool children in the emergency department. *Pediatrics* 1993;91:624–627.
31. Connors K, Terndrup TE. Nasal versus oral midazolam for sedation of anxious children undergoing laceration repair. *Ann Emerg Med* 1994;24:1074–1079.
32. Karl HW, Rosenberger JL, Larach MG, Ruffle JM. Transmucosal administration of midazolam for premedication of pediatric patients. *Anesthesiology* 1993;78:885–891.
33. Schutzman SA, Burg J, Liebelt E, et al. Oral transmucosal fentanyl citrate for premedication of children undergoing laceration repair. *Ann Emerg Med* 1994;24:1059–1064.
34. Schechter NL, Weisman SJ, Rosenblum M, Bernstein B, Conrad PL. The use of oral transmucosal fentanyl citrate for painful procedures in children. *Pediatrics* 1995;95:335–339.
35. Ashburn MA, Lind GH, Gillie MH, de Boer AJ, Pace NL, Stanley TH. Oral transmucosal fentanyl citrate (OTFC) for the treatment of postoperative pain. *Anaesth Analg* 1993;76:377–381.
36. Fine PG, Marcus M, de Boer AJ, Van der Oord B. An open label study of oral transmucosal fentanyl citrate (OTFC) for the treatment of breakthrough cancer pain. *Pain* 1991;45:149–153.
37. Ashburn MA, Fine PG, Stanley TH. Oral transmucosal fentanyl citrate for the treatment of breakthrough cancer pain: a case report. *Anesthesiology* 1989;71:615–617.
38. Collins JJ, Grier HE, Sethna NF, et al. Regional anesthesia for pain associated with terminal malignancy. *Pain* 1996;65:63–69.
39. Schechter NL, Berde CB, Yaster M. *Pain in infants, children, and adolescents.* Baltimore: Williams and Wilkins, 1993.

40. Zeltzer L, LeBaron S, Zeltzer PM. The effectiveness of behavioral interventions for reduction of nausea and vomiting in children and adolescents receiving chemotherapy. *J Clin Oncol* 1984;2:683–690.

41. Simon AR, Roberts MW. Management of oral complications associated with cancer therapy in pediatric patients. *ASDC J Dent Children* 1991;58:384–389.

42. Shenep JL, Kalwinsky DK, Hutson PR, et al. Efficacy of oral sucralfate suspension in prevention and treatment of chemotherapy-induced mucositis. *J Pediatrics* 1988;113:758–763.

43. Berger A, Henderson M, Nadoolman W, et al. Oral capsaicin provides temporary relief for oral mucositis pain secondary to chemotherapy/radiation therapy. *J Pain Sympt Manag* 1995;10:243–248.

44. Culpepper-Morgan JA, Inturrisi CE, Portenoy RK, et al. Treatment of opioid-induced constipation with oral naloxone: a pilot study. *Clin Pharmacol Ther* 1992;52:90–95.

45. Davis CL. The therapeutics of dyspnea. *Cancer Surv* 1994;21:85–98.

46. Van Eys J. Nutritional therapy in children with cancer. *Cancer Res* 1977;37:2457–2461.

47. Rickard KA, Baehner RL, Coates TD, et al. Supportive nutritional intervention in pediatric cancer. *Cancer Res* 1982;42:766–773.

48. Donaldson SS. Effects of therapy on nutritional status of the pediatric cancer patient. *Cancer Res* 1982;42:729–736.

49. Rickard KA, Loghmani ES, Grosfeld JL, et al. Short- and long-term effectiveness of enteral and parenteral nutrition in reversing or preventing protein-energy malnutrition in advanced neuroblastoma. *Cancer* 1985;56:2881–2897.

50. Mauer Am, Burgess JB, Donaldson SS, et al. Special nutritional needs of children with malignancies: a review. *J Parenter Enter Nutr* 1990;14:315–324.

51. Jurgens H, McQuade B. Ondansetron as prophylaxis for chemotherapy and radiotherapy-induced emesis in children. *Oncology* 1992;49:279–285.

52. Hahlen K, Quintana E, Pinkerton R, Cedar E. A randomized comparison of intravenously administered granisetron versus chlorpromazine plus dexamethasone in the prevention of ifosfamide-induced emesis in children. *J Pediatrics* 1995;126:309.

53. Jacobson SJ, Shore RW, Greenberg M, Speilberg SP. The efficacy and safety of granisetron in pediatric cancer patients who had failed standard antiemetic therapy during anticancer therapy. *Am J Pediatr Hematol Oncol* 1994;16:213.

*Principles and Practice of Supportive Oncology,*
edited by Ann Berger et al.
Lippincott–Raven Publishers, Philadelphia ©1998

CHAPTER 63

# Supportive Care in Elderly People

Bruce A. Ferrell

Elderly people have traditionally been defined by demographers, insurers, and employers as those over 65 years of age. In regions where geriatric medicine has emerged as a distinct specialty, the elderly are more commonly regarded as those over age 75. Often the elderly are identified by individual patient characteristics, the presence of disease and disability that often characterize the elderly, and by the capacity of existing health care systems to meet specific needs. Younger patients who are chronically ill and disabled are often cared for by geriatric practitioners in long-term care facilities that are designed largely to meet the needs of geriatric patients. By the age of 75, almost all people are frail, with diminished reserve, and are particularly vulnerable to illness associated with aging. In the latter half of the twentieth century, the need for understanding this rapidly growing population has caused substantial growth in the fields of gerontology and geriatric medicine. Gerontology is the study of aging, whereas geriatric medicine is a subdiscipline specifically devoted to the medical care of elderly people (1). In general, practitioners in geriatric medicine care for the oldest, sickest, most frail, and most complicated patients with multiple medical problems (1).

## BIOLOGY OF AGING

Aging is a poorly understood process (2). In general, aging converts healthy adults to frail ones, with diminished reserves in most physiologic systems and an exponentially increasing vulnerability to most diseases and to death. The impact of aging on health and well-being eclipses that of any single disease category. Although even laypersons can identify observable differences between young and old people, the fundamental

processes that control the rate at which people age remains essentially unknown. Likewise, despite hundreds of research papers generated every year describing the effects of age at increasingly more sophisticated levels of cellular and molecular detail, an explanation of how the passage of time leads to diseases of aging remains a mystery.

It is beyond the scope of this chapter to review the various theories of aging. Several excellent references are provided for those who wish to explore these issues more deeply (2–5). Suffice it to say that aging is a ubiquitous biological process characterized by a progressive, predictable, inevitable evolution of an organism until death. Aging does not appear to represent the accumulation of disease, even though aging and disease may be related in subtle and complex ways. Although aging is conveniently quantified in chronologic terms, aging appears to occur at different rates among individuals and at different rates among biological process and organ systems within individuals (3). Despite the lack of a unified theory of aging, in the last 20 years at least several fundamental findings have emerged. First, the general pattern of aging is similar across nearly all mammalian species. Second, the rate of aging appears to be determined by genes that vary across species. Third, the rate of aging can be decreased by caloric restriction, at least in rodents (2). Current aging research appears to be focusing on the molecular mechanisms that might account for the synchrony of structural and functional change in different cells and tissues of individual members of a given species. Interest continues to expand about genes and processes that control the rate of aging in different species and how caloric restriction might slow this rate (2).

Normal aging in the absence of disease is a remarkably benign process. Normal aging entails the steady erosion of organ system reserves and homeostatic controls. Decline in organ function is often evident only during periods of maximum stress. Organ systems eventually reach a critical point where minimum insults cannot be overcome, eventually resulting in death. Consequently in

B. A. Ferrell: Department of Geriatric Medicine, UCLA School of Medicine and Sepulveda VA Medical Center, Sepulveda, CA 91343.

normal aging, morbidity is often compressed into the last period of life (6). In reality, it is extremely difficult to separate the effects of aging alone from those of disease, environmental, and other factors that may contribute to functional decline over time.

At the cellular level, cells from older persons are often altered in function and appearance compared to those from younger persons. One example is the well-known Hayflick phenomenon, in which the number of in vitro fibroblast cell doubling has been observed to decrease in cells taken from older persons (7). The cells of older persons also accumulate lipofuscin pigment, and have lower rates of oxidative phosphorylation and RNA and protein synthesis. Older cells generally have lower numbers of cell surface receptors. These biochemical and morphologic changes in cells tend to be most marked in the postmitotic organs such as the central nervous system and cardiac and skeletal muscle (8).

A fundamental process of aging has been observed in connective tissue. Collagen undergoes progressively greater crosslinking with age, resulting in greater stability and increased resistance to movement. Elastin demonstrates greater fragmentation and decreased elasticity with aging. These changes are seen in internal structures such as arterial walls as well as in skin, although the processes are accelerated in the skin from exposure to ultraviolet light (9).

Substantial changes also occur in body composition with aging. Between the ages of 25 and 75, the lipid compartment may double as a percentage of body weight. In general, there is a reduction in lean body mass. Shrinkage of the bone and viscera contributes less to this change in fat-to-lean body mass ratio. Hypothetically, hormonal changes with aging are key factors in these phenomenon (10). This change in composition has important implications for nutrition, metabolic activity, and pharmacokinetic activity of drugs. However, variability among individuals in considerable. Thus estimates such as volume of distribution for drugs and other measurements are highly variable and more problematic in older individuals.

Total body metabolism also varies with age. The basal metabolic rate declines slightly with age. The maximum oxygen consumption with exercise ($VO_2$ max) declines more dramatically with age largely due to the age-related fall in maximum hear rate. The $VO_2$ max remains higher in those who exercise regularly compared to sedentary elderly people and still higher in elderly athletes (11).

A large number of age-associated changes are observed in various organ systems. Readers interested in specific organ system changes with aging should consult other reviews and recent texts on the subject (1,2,8,11,12). The following will focus on age-associated changes that directly impact symptom management and specifically pharmacology among elderly people.

The brain and central nervous system remains relatively stable from maturity and then slowly atrophies with aging. In general, differentiated neurons do not proliferate and are not replaced when they die, but glial cells may. Most evidence indicates with normal aging there is neuronal loss as well as loss of dendritic arborization, and some loss of enzymes and receptors in neurotransmission. The extent of neuronal loss associated with normal aging remains controversial, and it clearly varies by region of the brain. Compensatory dendrite proliferation with aging, which has been observed in several laboratories, has been proposed as a means by which selected neuronal pathways are able to maintain contact with their target despite neuronal loss (neuroplasticity) (13). Age-associated changes in nerve conduction as well as changes in sensory, integrative, and motor functions have been observed in elderly patients. However, the extent to which many of these observations can be isolated from those due to occult disease or environmental injuries remains to be shown.

Age-associated changes in pain perception have been a topic of interest for many years. Elderly people are often observed to present with unusual presentation of illness, e.g., painless myocardial infarction or painless intraabdominal catastrophes. Whether these clinical observations represent distinct age-related changes remains controversial (14). Studies using a variety of methods to induce pain in experimental subjects have resulted in mixed results. The most recent study suggested that aging may result in a different effect on pain perception mediated by C fibers compared to A-delta fibers (15). In an elegant review of this subject, Harkins concluded that clinically significant age-related changes in pain perception probably do not occur (16). Moreover, the generalizability of these studies are questionable because induced pain may not be analogous to pain caused by disease.

Renal changes with aging indicate the number of functioning nephrons declines with age in many species. Cross-sectional and longitudinal studies of large human populations usually have shown a decline in creatinine clearance with age. Recent evidence suggests that this relationship is not linear and falls more steeply at very advanced ages. However, in some older persons studied for as long as 18 years, there was absolutely no fall in creatinine clearance over time and even a slight rise in some individuals. Other renal functions that have been observed with aging include decreased renal plasma flow, tubular secretion, tubular reabsorption, hydrogen ion secretion, and water absorption and excretion. As in other organ systems the relative contributions of aging and disease on the kidney in not known with certainty, but they are clearly additive (17).

The importance of declining renal function with aging is relevant to the large number of drugs that either rely on renal excretion or are directly toxic to the kidney. Drugs that have active metabolites that rely on renal excretion are particularly prone to accumulate and cause side effects. For example, delayed renal excretion of meperidine's metabolite, normeperidine, may result in delirium, central nervous system excitement, and seizure activity. Other drugs, including aminoglycoside antibiotics, non-steroidal antiinflammatory drugs (NSAIDs), contrast media, and many other drugs are also much more likely to cause direct renal toxicity in elderly patients with base-line renal impairment (18).

In general, the gastrointestinal tract shows less change in function with age than many other systems. The esophagus commonly, but not universally, shows delayed transit time and altered lower esophageal sphincter func-tion. The stomach maintains relatively normal motility but undergo age-related atrophy of the gastric glands and decreased acid secretion. Total achlorhydria, however, is not normal and usually signifies disease. Small intestinal transit speed does not appear to change with aging but colonic transit is significantly slowed. Absorption is not grossly altered with age but decreases in metabolism and absorption of sugars (especially lactose and d-xylose), iron, and calcium have been observed. There is a decrease in the lymphoid tissue in the intestinal wall and the ade-quacy of IgA has been examined, but no solid evidence of impaired function has been proven (19).

The solid organs of the gastrointestinal tract appear to maintain adequate function throughout the life span. Rarely does hepatic or pancreatic failure become clini-cally relevant in extreme old age. Pancreatic function is well maintained. Trypsin secretion may be decreased but the other enzymes and bicarbonate production are unchanged.

By detailed testing, cytochrome P-450 microsomal oxidase systems of the liver have been shown to decline in efficiency with age and liver enzyme systems of older individuals may be less inducible. However, nonmicroso-mal oxidation, e.g., alcohol dehydrogenase, does not appear to decline with aging. Demethylation, the process by which benzodiazepines, clordiazepine, and diazepam are metabolized in the liver, has been shown to markedly decrease. This altered mechanism is directly linked to the need for dosage adjustments in older patients. Hepatic conjugation reactions such as acetylation in the case of isoniazid or glucuronidation, the primary metabolism of oxazepam or lorazepam, are not altered by age. Drugs that undergo high hepatic first-pass metabolism by extraction from the blood may have altered clearance with age due to reduced hepatic blood flow. This effect has been demon-strated most clearly with propranolol (19).

## AGING AND DISABILITY

The most challenging issue in medical care of elderly people is the decline in functional status and resultant dependency on others. In 1985 it was estimated that about 20% of those over 65 in the United States were disabled or were limited in their capacity to preform normal activ-ities of daily living (20). In 1987, the National Medical Expenditure Survey described the number and character-istics of functionally impaired elderly persons living in the community (21). Of 5.6 million functionally impaired elderly, about 20% required formal home care services. Of these, 41% required homemakers and 25% required home health aids. Approximately 23% were receiving skilled nursing visits at home. These patients were mostly female (2:1 female-to-male ratio) and almost 50% lived alone. Forty-seven percent needed help with more than three activities of daily living (bathing, dressing, toilet-ing, feeding, and transfers to bed or chair) (22).

In the United States, the 1982 National Long Term Care Survey estimated that approximately 2.2 million people were acting as informal caregivers to disabled elderly persons (23). Of these, 35.5% were spouses and 37.4% were children of the patient, and about 75% resided with the patient (29). Caregivers were predomi-nantly female (72%) and their mean age was 57 years (25% were age 65–74 and 10% were age 75 and over). Approximately one in three caregivers was poor or near-poor in income, and a similar proportion rated their own health as fair or poor. Spouses were more likely to be the single source of care (63%), whereas children were more likely to be the primary caregivers when other informal or formal caregivers and services were being utilized. Per-sons with other relationships (siblings, grandchildren, other relatives, and nonrelatives) were likely to play sec-ondary roles. Most informal caregiver responsibilities lasted more than 4 years (67%) and almost all spouse caregivers, and approximately 75% of children, provided assistance on a daily basis. Over 86% of caregivers assisted with shopping, transportation, and household tasks such as cleaning, meal preparation, and laundry. Approximately half administered medication and assisted with finances. Almost three fourths assisted with hygiene and two thirds assisted with activities of daily living (23).

The health, psychological, social, and economic issues related to informal caregivers is described extensively in the literature (20–24). Although it is beyond the scope of this chapter to review this expansive literature, it is clear that care of frail elderly people can place a significant strain on family and informal caregivers and can have substantial negative impacts on their medical and mental health as well as their economic resources. For example, caregiver responsibilities often result in major time and work constraints for those who are employed. Although support networks can often be highly effective in sustain-ing care in the home, many families eventually become completely "burned out." In this situation, and because many elderly people do not have family, adequate resources, or support at home, nursing homes remain the last safety net for a large number of elderly people (25).

In the United States there are almost two million elderly persons residing in almost 20,000 nursing homes (26). This is almost triple the number of acute care hos-pitals and double the number of hospital beds. It is estimated that about 5% of elderly people reside in nursing homes at this time. However this figure is somewhat misleading. Among those 65–74 years of age, <2% live in nursing homes. The figure rises to about 7% for those 75–84, whereas for those over age 85, almost 20% live in nursing homes. Longitudinal studies in the United States suggest that persons 65 years of age and older have better than a 40% chance of spending some time in a nursing home before they die. Of those who enter nursing homes, 55% will spend at least 1 year there and >20% will spend more than 5 years there. The need for nursing homes is not simply the result of the presence of disease and functional disabilities. It is also a result of lack of social support. Many nursing home patients have outlived close family; also, often the family becomes exhausted after caring for a patient for a long period of time. Among the most disturbing symptoms that result in early family fatigue involve incontinence and behavioral problems such as wandering or disruptive behavior often associated with dementia and Alzheimer's disease (25,26).

Patients in alternate care settings such as nursing homes and those confined to their homes present substantial challenges to medical care (27,28). In these settings logistic barriers, such as the lack of availability to laboratory, radiographic, and pharmaceutical services with the capability of rapid response, make evaluation and treatment more difficult. Many physicians do not see patients at home or in nursing homes and those who do often provide substandard care. These patients are often sent to distant clinics or the emergency room where they are evaluated by personnel who are generally not familiar with their baseline status, goals of care, and who lack training or interest in the care of frail and dependent elderly patients (28).

## PAIN IN ELDERLY PEOPLE

Although pain is common among elderly people, the epidemiology of pain in elderly populations has not been widely studied. Small population-based studies have estimated between 25% and 50% of community-dwelling elderly people suffer important pain problems (29). In a Canadian survey by Crook et al. of 500 randomly selected households in Burlington, Ontario, the incidence of "significant" pain in the proceeding 2 weeks was twofold higher in those age 60 and older compared to those <60 years of age (25% versus 12.5%) (29). Among nursing home patients the prevalence of pain may be even higher and estimates range from 45% to almost 80% (28).

The most predominant causes of pain in elderly people appear to be musculoskeletal factors, especially osteoarthritis. Indeed, arthritis may affect as many as 80% of people over age 65, and most suffer significant pain (30). Cancer of almost every type is more common among elderly people, and as many as 80% will have substantial pain (31). A number of other specific pain syndromes are known to disproportionately affect elderly populations, including herpes zoster, temporal arteritis, polymyalgia rheumatica, and atherosclerotic peripheral vascular disease (32). The consequences of pain are also widespread in the elderly population. Depression, decreased socialization, sleep disturbance, impaired ambulation, and increased health care utilization and costs have each been associated with the presence of pain in elderly people. Though less thoroughly explored, deconditioning, gait disturbances, falls, slow rehabilitation, polypharmacy, cognitive dysfunction, and malnutrition are among the common geriatric conditions that are potentially worsened by poorly managed pain (14).

## Pain Assessment

Elderly people often present substantial problems in pain assessment. Failures in memory, depression, and sensory impairments may often hinder history taking. More importantly, elderly people may underreport symptoms because they expect pain with aging and their disease. Cancer patients may not report pain because they fear the meaning of the pain. To them pain may be a metaphor for advancing illness and approaching death (33), a natural basis for denial in most people. Dependent elderly people may not report pain because of the distress they see it causes in others. Often, family and caregivers become the most important source of information, which presents another set of problems in the validity and reliability of pain assessment by proxy.

Because elderly patients often suffer multiple medical problems, care must be taken to avoid attributing new pain to preexisting conditions. Making this problem worse is the fact that the character and intensity of chronic pain fluctuates with time. Injuries due to trauma as well as other acute arthritides, such as gout, and calcium pyrophosphate arthritis are easily overlooked in this setting. Only astute questioning and comprehensive evaluation can possibly avoid these potential pitfalls (34).

Evaluation of function is important so that mobility and independence can be maximized for elderly patients in pain. Scales frequently used in routine geriatric assessment include basic activities of daily living and instrumental activities, and gait and balance evaluation. However, at least several investigators have suggested that advanced activities or elective activities may be more sensitive to changes in pain (35). It is important to remember that most available quantitative functional assessment scales have not been well established in typical nursing home or home care populations.

Cognitive impairment may be a substantial barrier to pain assessment in some elderly patients (36). Both qualitative and quantitative pain assessment scales established in younger populations have not be extensively studied in those with significant cognitive impairment, delirium, or dementia. It has been estimated that as many as 15% of elderly patients may have some cognitive impairment. Among nursing home residents, >50% may have substantial dementia or psychological illness. These patients typically have deficits in memory, attention, visual spatial skills, and language (aphasia). Behavioral problems are also not uncommon.

Despite these potential barriers, Parmelee et al. found no evidence of "masking" of pain complaints by cognitive patients in a study of 758 nursing home residents from a single long-term care facility in Philadelphia (37). The authors of this study concluded that despite the fact that elderly patients were observed to under-report pain slightly, their reports were no less valid than those of cognitively intact patients. Findings from our studies suggest that most cognitively impaired elderly patients in pain can respond to available pain intensity scales if they are administered in a manner sensitive to the patients disabilities (36). Such patients often require time to assimilate questions about pain and respond appropriately. They have limited attention spans and are easily distracted. It is helpful to provide visual cues in large print and prepare these patients by providing adequate ambient light and hearing devices when necessary. With these issues in mind, most cognitively impaired patients appear capable of reliably reporting pain at the moment. On the other hand, the extent to which they are able to accurately report pain in the last week or in the last month remains to be studied. These early investigations suggest that assessment in cognitively impaired patients will likely require frequent and constant assessment of pain at the moment in order that management strategies can be maximized. It is also clear that much additional work is needed to establish methods for pain evaluation among those who are mute or who have more profound impairment.

**Pain Control in Elderly People**

The most common treatment for pain in elderly people is the use of oral or parenteral analgesic medications. The analgesic drugs of choice for elderly people are those with the lowest side effect profiles. Adverse effects of drugs are more common in the elderly including drug–drug, drug–disease, and untoward drug reactions. Therefore several considerations should be made when prescribing analgesic drugs in the elderly.

Acetaminophen is the most often prescribed analgesic in the nursing home (36,38). It appears to be reasonably safe and effective for mild and moderate pain complaints in this frail population. Alternatives to acetaminophen, most commonly NSAIDs, must be weighed against their known side effect profiles.

NSAIDs often work well for elderly people whether given alone or in combination with opioid analgesics for inflammatory conditions and metastatic bone pain. However, these drugs have been associated with increased risk of side effects in elderly people including an increased risk of peptic ulcer disease, renal injury, and bleeding diathesis compared to younger persons. Among frail elderly persons, these drugs have occasionally been reported to also cause constipation, cognitive impairment, and headaches (14).

A recent review pointed out that older persons have generally been omitted from clinical trials of NSAIDs (39). Between 1987 and 1990, 83 randomized trials involving almost 10,000 patients included only 203 patients over age 65 and none were over 85 years of age. This is particularly disturbing in light of the high incidence of gastric bleeding associated with NSAIDs in elderly people. Griffin and colleagues estimated that the relative risk of peptic ulcer disease associated with NSAIDs in the elderly was more than fourfold higher (relative risk ratio = 4.1; 95% confidence interval 3.5–4.7) compared to elderly persons who did not use them (40). Moreover, the relative risk increases with dose from 2.8 among the lowest dosage to 8.0 for the highest dosage.

Although opioid analgesic drugs will be discussed in more detail elsewhere in this book, some opioids require special considerations. Propoxyphene is a controversial drug that is probably overprescribed in elderly people. Reports suggest efficacy no better than aspirin or acetaminophen and it has a potential for dependency and renal injury. Pentacozine is an opioid that should be avoided because it frequently causes delirium and agitation in elderly persons. Meperidine is also particularly hazardous in the elderly, especially those with underlying renal impairment. The active metabolite normeperidine is particularly prone to accumulate and cause delirium and seizure activity. Methadone should be used with caution because of its long half-life and propensity to accumulate. Finally, transdermal fentanyl is an extremely potent drug that because of its unique transdermal delivery system and prolonged half-life is particularly dangerous, especially in opiate-naive persons (14,41).

Adjuvant analgesic drugs, such as antidepressants, neuroleptics, and some systemically administered local anesthetic drugs, may be helpful in some patients with recalcitrant pain syndromes. Of concern is the high side effect profiles these drugs often have in the elderly. Elderly patients are particularly sensitive to the anticholinergic effects of amitriptyline and other antidepressants. Movement disorders, bowel and bladder dysfunction, and dry mucus membranes are particularly common in the elderly. Elderly patients are also particularly sensitive to the central nervous system side effects of neuroleptic drugs including local anesthetic agents. Delirium, agitation, and seizure activity are particularly problematic with these drugs. In general, most adjuvant analgesic drugs should probably be reserved for patients with severe pain and disability in whom safer and more traditional treatments have failed (42).

Many nonpharmacologic pain management strategies are effective in elderly people, especially when combined with drug strategies. Most nondrug strategies commonly used for elderly people are discussed elsewhere in this book; however, the importance of physical therapy, activities, exercise, and recreation cannot be overemphasized. Deconditioning alone is an important cause of disability among elderly people. Inactivity and immobility often contribute extensively to depression and worsening pain among elderly people. Many recent studies of exercise in elderly people have clearly shown that programs aimed at improving strength, endurance, and overall fitness are successful in preserving independence and quality of life among most disabled elderly people (43–45). Our studies of frail elderly with chronic low back pain have shown that a simple program of self-limited fitness walking may significantly improve overall pain management (45). Likewise, others have shown that walking may significantly improves chronic knee pain due to osteoarthritis (44).

Finally, recent developments in pain management have focused on highly technical and sometimes invasive strategies for pain management including new drug delivery systems. Many of these systems are being used among selected elderly patients with postoperative pain, cancer pain, and some recalcitrant other chronic pain syndromes. A randomized trial found that patient-controlled analgesia using morphine infusions is safe and effective for the postoperative management of nondemented frail elderly (46). However, parenteral morphine infusions for chronic pain are expensive and may cost several thousands of dollars a month to maintain (47).

Although these procedures have been effective in selected cases, more work is needed to define expanded roles for these technologies among frail elderly. Because of potential side effects and costs, it is usual to consider these strategies only after other treatments have been tried. Further study is needed to determine the risk–benefit and cost-effectiveness ratios to justify their routine use for nonmalignant or less intense pain syndromes. Although most of these strategies are expensive, they are often at least partially reimbursed by Medicare and other health insurers. These issues have raised ethical questions about the application of high-tech treatment strategies in patients who might be equally managed with oral medications that are not much less expensive but are not reimbursable (48).

## REFERENCES

1. Hazzard WR. Introduction: The practice of geriatric medicine. In: Hazzard WR, Bierman EL, Blass JP, Ettinger WHJr, Halter JB, eds. *Principles of geriatric medicine and gerontology*. New York: McGraw-Hill, 1994;xxiii–xxiv.
2. Miller RA, The biology of aging and longevity. In: Hazzard WR, Bierman EL, Blass JP, Ettinger WH Jr, Halter JB, eds. *Principles of geriatric medicine and gerontology*. New York: McGraw-Hill, 1994;3–18.
3. Finch CE. *Longevity, senescence and the genome*. Chicago: University of Chicago Press, 1990.
4. Schneider EL, Rowe RW. *Handbook of the biology of aging*, 3rd ed. San Diego: Academic Press, 1990.
5. Comfort A. *The biology of senescence*, 3rd ed. New York: Elsevier, 1979.
6. Fries JF. Aging, natural death and the compression of morbidity. *N Engl J Med* 1990;303:130.
7. Hayflick L, Moorehead PS. The serial cultivation of human diploid cell strains. *Exp Cell Res* 1961;25:585.
8. Abrass IB. Biology of aging. in Wilson JD, Braunwald E, Isselbacher KJ, et al, eds. *Principles of internal medicine* 12th ed. New York: McGraw-Hill, 1991.
9. Uitto J. Connective tissue biochemistry of the aging dermis. Age associated alterations in collagen and elastin. *Clin Geriatr Med* 1989; 5(1)127–147.
10. Fulop T, Worum I, Csongor J, Foris G, Leavey A. Body composition in elderly people. *Gerontology* 1985;31.6–14.
11. Lakatta EG. Changes in cardiovascular function with aging. *Eur Heart J (Suppl C)* 1990;11.22–28.
12. Gilchrest BA (Ed.) Geriatric dermatology. *Clin Geriatr Med* 1989;5(1).
13. Coleman PD, Flood DG. Neuron numbers and dendritic extent in normal aging and Alzheimer's disease. *Neurobiol Aging* 1987;8;521.
14. Ferrell BA. Pain management in elderly people. *J Am Geriatr Soc* 1991; 39:64–73.
15. Cakour MC, Gibson SJ, Bradbeer M, Helme RD. The effect of age on Aδ- and C-fiber thermal pain perception. *Pain* 1996;64:143–152.
16. Harkins SA. Pain perceptions in the old. *Clin Geriatr Med* 1996;12(3): 435–459.
17. Lindeman RD, Tobin J, Shock NW. Longitudinal studies of the rate of decline in renal function with age. *J Am Geriatr Soc* 1985;33:278–285.
18. Perneger TV, Whelton PK, Klag MJ. Risk of kidney failure associated with use of acetaminophen, aspirin, and nonsteroidal antiinflammatory drugs. *N Engl J Med* 1994;331:1675–1679.
19. Baime MJ, Nelson JB, Castell DO. Aging of the gastrointestinal system. In: Hazzard WR, Bierman EL, Blass JP, Ettinger WH Jr, Halter JB, eds. *Principles of geriatric medicine and gerontology*. New York: McGraw-Hill, 1994;665–681.
20. Manton KG. Epidemiological, demographic and social correlates of disability among the elderly. *Milbank Q* 1989;67:13.
21. Short P, Leon J. Use of home and community services by persons aged 65 and older with functional disabilities. National Medical Expenditure Survey Findings 5, Agency for Health Care Policy and Research. DHHS Publ. No. (PHS) 90-4366. Rockville, MD: US Public Health Service, 1990.
22. Ferrell BA. Home care. In: Cassel CK, Cohen HJ, Larson EB, Meier DE, Resnick NM, Rubenstein LZ, eds. *Geriatric medicine*, 3rd ed. New York: Springer-Verlag, 1997.
23. Stone R, Cafferata GL, Sangl J. Caregivers of frail elderly: A national profile. *Gerontologist* 1987;27:616.
24. Ferrell BA, Rubenstein LZ, eds. Home care. *Clin Geriatr Med* 1991; 7(7):645–847.
25. Ouslander JG. Medical care in the nursing home. *JAMA* 1989;262; 2582–2590.
26. Ouslander GJ, Osterweil D, Morley J. *Medical care in the nursing home*. New York: McGraw-Hill, 1991;3–19.
27. Ferrell BA. Pain evaluation and management. In: Katz P, Kane RL, eds. *Adv Long Term Care* 1994;195–209.
28. Ferrell BA. Pain evaluation and management in the nursing home. *Ann Intern Med* 1995;123(9):681–687.
29. Crook J, Rideout E, Brown G. The prevalence of pain complaints among a general population. *Pain* 1984;18:299–314.
30. Davis MA. Epidemiology of osteoarthritis. *Clin Geriatr Med* 1988; 4(2):241–255.
31. Foley K. Pain in the elderly. In: Hazzard WR, Bierman EL, Blass JP, Ettinger WHJr, Halter JB, eds. *Principles of geriatric medicine and gerontology*. New York: McGraw-Hill, 1994.
32. Gordon, RS. Pain in the elderly. *JAMA* 1979;241(23):2191–2192.
33. Ferrell BR, Rhiner M, Cohen MZ, Grant M. Pain as a metaphor for illness. Part 1: Impact of cancer pain on family caregivers. *Oncol Nursing Forum* 1991;18:1303–1309.
34. Nishikawa ST, Ferrell BA. Pain assessment in the elderly. *Clinical geriatrics and issues in long term care* 1993;1:15–28.
35. Turk DC, Melzack R, eds. *Handbook of pain assessment*. New York: Guilford Press, 1992.
36. Ferrell BA, Ferrell BR, Rivera L. Pain in cognitively impaired nursing home patients. *J Pain Sympt Manag* 1995;10(8):591–595.
37. Parmelee PA, Smith B, Katz IR. Pain complaints and cognitive status

among elderly institution residents. *J Am Geriatr Soc* 1993;41:
517–522.

38. Ferrell BA, Ferrell BR, Osterweil D. Pain in the nursing home. *J Am
Geriatr Soc* 1990;38:409–414.

39. Rochon PA, Fortin PR, Dear KB, Minaker KL, Chalmers TC. Reporting of age in data in clinical trials of arthritis. *Arch Intern Med* 1993;
153:243–248.

40. Griffin MR, Piper JM, Doughtery JR, Snowden M, Ray WA. Nonsteroidal antiinflammatory drug use and increased risk for peptic ulcer
disease in elderly persons. *Ann Intern Med* 1991;114:257–263.

41. Ferrell BA. Pain. In: Yoshikawa TT, Cobbs EL, Brummel-Smith K, eds.
*Ambulatory geriatric care*. St. Louis: CV Mosby, 1993;382–390.

42. Lipman AG. Analgesic drugs for neuropathic and sympathetically
maintained pain. *Clin Geriatr Med* 1996;12(3):501–515.

43. Province MA, Hadley EC, Hornbrook MC, et al. The effects of exercise
on falls in elderly patients. A preplanned meta-analysis of the FICSIT
Trials. Frailty and injuries: cooperative studies of intervention techniques. *JAMA* 1995;273(17):1381–1383.

44. Ettinger WH, Burns R, Messier SP, Applegate W, Rejeeski WJ, Morgan T, Sumaker S, Berry MJ, O'Toole M, Monu J, Craven T. A randomized trial comparing aerobic exercise and resistance exercise with
a health education program in older adults with knee osteoarthritis:
the Fitness Arthritis and Seniors Trial (FAST) *JAMA* 1997;227(1):
25–31.

45. Ferrell BA, Josephson KR, Pollan AM, Loy S, Ferrell BR. A randomized trial of walking versus physical methods for chronic pain management. *Aging Clin Exp Res* 1997;9(1):99–105.

46. Egbert AM, Parks LH, Short LM, Burnett ML. Randomized trial of
postoperative patient controlled analgesia vs intramuscular narcotics in
frail elderly men. *Arch Intern Med* 1990;150:1897–1903.

47. Ferrell BR, Griffith H. Cost issues related to pain management. Report
from the Cancer Pain Panel of the Agency for Health Care Policy and
Research. *J Pain Sympt Manag* 1994;9:221–234.

48. Wedon M, Ferrell BR. Professional and ethical considerations in the
use of high tech pain management. *Oncol Nursing Forum* 1991;18:
1135–1143.

*Principles and Practice of Supportive Oncology,*
edited by Ann Berger et al.
Lippincott–Raven Publishers, Philadelphia ©1998

# CHAPTER 64

# Supportive Care of Patients with AIDS

Charles F. von Gunten and Jamie H. Von Roenn

One of the challenges in caring for patients with human immunodeficiency virus (HIV) is to appropriately balance medical treatment between the sometimes opposing poles of disease control and quality of life. The goals of medical care for an individual patient evolve over the course of the illness. With the exception of an aggressive malignancy, there is rarely a point in the spectrum of HIV illness where one can determine with certainty where "curative" therapy ends and "palliative" therapy begins. While this turning point may be clearly evident in the care of patients with cancer (i.e., when the cancer is no longer responsive to anticancer therapy), it is usually more appropriate to gradually shift the emphasis from prolongation of life toward quality of life as acquired immune deficiency syndrome (AIDS) progresses. Clinical scenarios that suggest that the illness is reaching its end stages include an accelerating tempo of the disease, an increasing number of opportunistic infections over short periods of time, the incomplete recovery from one problem before the advent of another, or relentless refractory wasting.

The conceptual approach to the supportive care of patients with AIDS does not differ fundamentally from that of patients with cancer. Attention to control of symptoms and the relief of suffering should be appropriately integrated with therapy directed at cure.

The purpose of this chapter is to discuss some of the common clinical situations that may arise in the care of a patient with AIDS and a malignancy aside from the treatment of specific AIDS-defining illnesses or malignancies. We will emphasize useful approaches for patients with advanced AIDS when palliative care strategies are particularly appropriate.

This chapter is written with the full knowledge that treatment of HIV infection and its associated opportunis-

tic infections and conditions is changing rapidly. With new drugs and approaches being introduced every few months, no book chapter can hope to be as up to date as we would like. Therefore, this chapter is meant to be a general introduction. Clinicians are advised to check with HIV specialists for the latest developments when questions arise.

This chapter is also written in the knowledge that clinical practice, especially in regard to palliative and supportive care issues, often progresses in advance of carefully performed studies in patients with AIDS. At the risk of confusing anecdote with science, some of our assertions are based on collective clinical experience or extrapolation from other patient populations rather than from rigorous clinical trials in patients with AIDS.

AIDS was first described in 1981 (1,2). As experience has grown, the management of the illness has improved with earlier diagnosis, better treatment, and prophylaxis of the associated opportunistic infections. For example, the death rate from *Pneumocystis carinii* pneumonia in patients with AIDS has dropped from 40% to 3% over the course of a decade (3). As a result of longer survival, up to 40% of patients will develop a malignancy at some point in the course of the illness: 20% Kaposi's sarcoma, 10% non-Hodgkin's lymphoma, and 10% other cancers, including squamous cell carcinoma of the cervix or anus.

## DISEASE TRAJECTORY OF AIDS

Although AIDS is a result of the slow destruction of the host's immune response by HIV, the disease trajectory, or the course of the illness in an individual, is highly variable. The helper T cell (CD4) count is the most widely used surrogate marker of host immunity; it declines over many years and correlates with survival (4). However, it alone is clearly not an adequate predictor of the disease course or degree of illness for an individual patient. It appears that the viral load, a measure of the

C. F. von Gunten and J. H. Von Roenn: Division of Hematology/Oncology, Department of Medicine, Northwestern University Medical School, Chicago, IL 60611.

number of copies of the HIV RNA in the blood, increases in advanced HIV infection and may be a more direct marker of activity of the virus (5). Together, the CD4 count and viral load may be more predictive of the disease course than either one alone. However, neither CD4 count nor viral load replaces the clinical assessment of the "tempo" of illness as judged by the number and frequency of opportunistic infections, performance status, refractory weight loss, etc. (6). In this regard, it is important to note that the case definition of AIDS by the U.S. Centers for Disease Control is, in large part, a public health definition for the purpose of keeping statistical records. Many patients with a CD4 count under 50 cells/mm$^3$ are otherwise clinically well. In contrast, there are patients with a CD4 count over 100 cells/mm$^3$ who are quite ill.

For the clinician, it is important to understand that infection with HIV causes a spectrum of illness. Most of the course of HIV infection may be completely asymptomatic. However, as immunosuppression progresses, patients are increasingly likely to develop symptoms associated with opportunistic infections, malignancies, and progressive HIV infection itself. The causes of clinical complaints are often difficult to sort out.

## PROPHYLAXIS

While it is beyond the scope of this chapter to discuss specific therapies of opportunistic infections associated with AIDS, the treatment and prophylaxis of opportunistic infections has been an area of rapid progress in the management of patients with AIDS (7). Not only does treatment cure or control these infections, but it relieves and prevents symptoms such as dyspnea, cough, fever, and odynophagia. Because these treatments may simultaneously improve quality of life as well as survival, their continuation even in the end stages of AIDS may be justified.

## ANEMIA, LEUKOPENIA, AND THROMBOCYTOPENIA

Cytopenia is a frequent complication of HIV infection and may be a result of drugs used to treat HIV and its associated conditions, the HIV-associated opportunistic diseases, or HIV infection itself. Common causes of cytopenia in the setting of HIV infection are listed in Table 1.

### Assessment

The assessment of any HIV-infected patient with any cytopenia begins with a review of the patient's medications. A few deserve special mention. Zidovudine (AZT), an anti-HIV reverse transcriptase inhibitor, may cause

**TABLE 1.** *Common causes of cytopenia in HIV-infected patients*

| Cause | Disorder |
|---|---|
| *Drugs* | |
| Zidovudine (AZT) | anemia, granulocytopenia |
| Trimethoprim/sulfamethoxazole | anemia, granulocytopenia |
| Ganciclovir | granulocytopenia |
| Dapsone | anemia, granulocytopenia |
| Pyrimethamine | anemia, granulocytopenia |
| Interferon (esp. with AZT) | anemia, granulocytopenia |
| Antineoplastic therapy | pancytopenia |
| *Infections* | |
| HIV | pancytopenia |
| *Mycobacterium avium* | pancytopenia |
| Cytomegalovirus | pancytopenia |
| *Malignancy* | |
| Lymphoma | pancytopenia |
| Gastrointestinal Kaposi's sarcoma | anemia (blood loss) |
| *Immunological* | |
| Autoimmune | pancytopenia |
| Immune thrombocytopenic purpura (ITP) | thrombocytopenia |

anemia and, less frequently, leukopenia or pancytopenia. In the ACTG 019 clinical trial, zidovudine at 1500 mg/day was compared with 500 mg/day and placebo. There was no difference in the incidence of anemia between the 500-mg dose and placebo. Those patients at greatest risk for anemia were those receiving the higher dose of zidovudine, with prior anemia, a low CD4 count, and/or a low leukocyte count before zidovudine was begun. For patients receiving cytotoxic chemotherapy for a malignancy, alternative nonmyelosuppressive antiviral agents may be substituted for zidovudine. Ganciclovir, a drug commonly used to treat cytomegalovirus infection, may cause severe leukopenia, which can usually be ameliorated with a myeloid colony-stimulating factor. Foscarnet, a relatively nonmyelosuppressive anti-CMV agent, may be used if blood counts cannot otherwise be maintained. The combination of trimethoprim and sulfamethoxazole (Bactrim, Septra, and others) is the regimen of choice for prophylaxis against *Pneumocystis carinii* pneumonia. This drug combination may cause anemia and leukopenia. Some have advocated the addition of folinic acid (vitamin B$_6$) to counter this effect, but in our experience, this is often not helpful. Other problems associated with the sulfa drugs include a high rate of intolerance that may present clinically with fever and leukopenia, with or without a skin rash.

Several opportunistic infections commonly cause cytopenia. In advanced HIV infection, *Mycobacterium avium* complex (MAC) and cytomegalovirus (CMV) are particularly common causes. HIV infection itself may cause any of the cytopenias. Immune thrombocytopenic purpura (ITP) may also occur; it may be the most common HIV-related cytopenia.

## Diagnosis

The anemia of HIV infection occurs in the setting of moderately advanced immune suppression (CD4 count <500 cells/ml). The anemia is typically normochromic and normocytic. It is an anemia of chronic disease characterized by a slightly shortened erythrocyte life span, impaired iron reutilization, and an inappropriately low reticulocyte count. The erythropoietin level may be elevated. Macrocytosis is rare in the absence of zidovudine. A bone marrow biopsy commonly shows dyserythropoiesis, megaloblastoid changes, an increased number of plasma cells, an increase in reticulin, and an overall increase in cellularity. Late in the course of the disease, the bone marrow may show a myelophthisic picture. Cobalamin (vitamin $B_{12}$) and folate (vitamin $B_6$) levels are usually normal unless there is an associated malabsorption syndrome. If iron deficiency is detected, it is important to test for occult bleeding. Vitamin supplementation in the absence of deficiencies is not indicated.

The leukopenia associated with AIDS is often most prominent in the granulocytic series. Lymphocyte counts are usually normal but may appear atypical. Lymphopenia implies the presence of a separate pathologic process. Patients may often be neutropenic according to standard oncology criteria (absolute neutrophil count <500 cells/ml). Clinicians may be faced with patients who are neutropenic and febrile without having been exposed to any antineoplastic chemotherapeutic agents. One clinical approach is to support patients with myeloid colony-stimulating factors administered as infrequently as once weekly on a long-term basis.

The thrombocytopenia associated with AIDS generally falls into one of two categories: decreased production, or increased destruction. As with other cytopenias, the incidence increases as immunosuppression progresses. The peripheral smear may be helpful in making the distinction between the two, and a bone marrow aspiration and biopsy is definitive. With decreased production (often due to HIV itself or to drugs) the platelets are small. The bone marrow shows decreased numbers of megakaryocytes. With increased destruction—usually due to immune mechanisms, as in immune thrombocytopenic purpura (ITP)—the platelets often appear large and may be reported as giant platelets. The marrow shows normal or increased numbers of megakaryocytes. This HIV-associated ITP is clinically indistinguishable from classic ITP and may be the presenting manifestation of HIV infection. It does not imply rapid progression to AIDS.

A common question is whether or not to perform a bone marrow biopsy. The biopsy itself is technically easy, can be performed in the outpatient setting, and is associated with minimal risk. It is often the most expeditious way to assess a fever of unknown origin, diagnose a disseminated malignancy, or determine the cause of an observed cytopenia. In a retrospective review of bone marrow aspiration biopsies performed to diagnose the cause of a fever of unknown origin, the positive yield for AIDS patients was 45.8% (8). While the results of such a biopsy may provide a definitive diagnosis, it may not change the management of the patient. Review the etiologic possibilities and therapeutic implications with patients and families *before* the bone marrow biopsy is done.

**TABLE 2.** *Currently available HIV antiviral drugs*

*Nucleoside reverse transcriptase inhibitors*
Zidovudine (AZT Retrovir)
Zalcitabine (DDC, Hivid)
Didanosine (DDI, Videx)
Stavudine (D4T, Zerit)
Lamivudine (3TC, Epivir)
*Nonnucleoside reverse transcriptase inhibitors*
Nevirapine (Viramune)
*Protease inhibitors*
Saquinavir (Invirase)
Ritonavir (Norvir)
Indinavir (Crixivan)
Nelfinavir (Viracept)

## Management

Although it may seem paradoxical, the addition of an anti-HIV agent may reverse the cytopenias due to HIV (9). Combinations of antiviral agents may be more efficacious than single agent-therapy in some patients. Currently approved drugs are listed in Table 2.

### Anemia

The reversible causes of anemia should be treated. When the anemia cannot be reversed, red blood cell transfusion should be considered. The evaluation of transfusion requirements requires the distinction between laboratory abnormalities and illness. Many patients with a stable hemoglobin of 8 mg/dl are otherwise asymptomatic.

In general, blood transfusions may relieve fatigue, headache, and dyspnea on exertion. In the absence of symptoms or coronary artery disease, there is no a priori reason to give a transfusion to a patient who is otherwise stable. Bed-bound patients rarely achieve any benefit from transfusion. The fatigue of end-stage AIDS in a bed-bound patient is not responsive to transfusion. If dyspnea is a problem in a bed-bound patient, there are better ways to relieve it than transfusion.

In making a decision about transfusions in a patient with AIDS, a clinical trial is often helpful. Transfuse 2 to 4 units, then reassess symptom relief over a 1-week period. If symptoms are improved, then it may be useful to continue transfusions as required. Relief of symptoms after an hour is more likely related to the placebo effect than to the transfusion. If there is no improvement in symptoms, or if the benefit is lost, then stop transfusions and stop blood sampling.

Erythropoietin may be an effective alternative to transfusions for some patients. Determination of the serum erythropoietin level is helpful in predicting who will benefit. If the endogenous erythropoietin level is over 500 units/mL, then erythropoietin is less likely to be effective. Initiate erythropoietin at 10,000 IU subcutaneously three times weekly, and give supplemental iron. Vitamin $B_{12}$ and folate may require supplementation if deficiencies are demonstrated. Clinical response is usually seen in 4 to 6 weeks. If zidovudine is implicated, it may be prudent to consider alternative antiviral agents.

### Leukopenia

Leukopenia in the setting of HIV infection is often responsive to the colony-stimulating factors sargramostim (GM-CSF) or filgrastim (G-CSF). Their use may permit the administration of curative antineoplastic chemotherapy on schedule, reduce the incidence of neutropenic fever, or permit the continued administration of a vital antibiotic, such as ganciclovir. The administration of these growth factors may also be associated with fever, myalgia, arthralgia, and the burden of frequent injections. These symptoms are usually controlled with antiinflammatory analgesics. As with transfusion, it is important to determine how these colony-stimulating factors will affect the overall care of the patient, not just the absolute neutrophil count.

### Thrombocytopenia

The distinction between the decreased production and increased destruction thrombocytopenias is critical because of the implications for treatment. For patients with thrombocytopenia due to decreased production unresponsive to anti-HIV drugs, transfusion of platelets may prevent hemorrhage. However, as in patients with myelodysplastic syndromes, repeated transfusions may induce antithrombocyte antibodies and render platelet transfusion useless. Reserve platelet transfusions for patients who have demonstrated bleeding diathesis as a result of the thrombocytopenia.

For patients with thrombocytopenia due to increased destruction from immune mechanisms, platelet transfusion is never indicated. Several treatment options exist; they are summarized in Table 3. A few clinical points are worth noting. Failure of one anti-HIV drug does not imply that this strategy should be abandoned. A serial trial of agents, or combinations, may prove to be effective. Interferon-alpha may also be useful. Although

**TABLE 3.** *Treatment of HIV-related ITP*

| |
|---|
| Antiviral therapy |
|   Zidovudine (AZT) |
|   Interferon |
| Anti Rh (D) |
| Intravenous immune globulin |
| Splenectomy |
| Protein A sepharose column apheresis |
| Prednisone |
| Vincristine |

platelet counts often increase in response to corticosteroids, because of their immunosuppressive effects and the often long-term requirement for them, they should be reserved for patients who are otherwise refractory or who have advanced HIV disease and are in the hospice or palliative care setting. Immune globulin administration or Sepharose-A column adsorption should be considered after zidovudine or interferon has been tried. Splenectomy should be considered for patients who have relapsed or are refractory to other treatments.

## WEIGHT LOSS AND FATIGUE

Independently of malignancy or its treatment, advanced HIV infection is associated with weight loss in excess of 5% of the usual body weight. While this ultimately affects the majority of patients with AIDS, it may also be an early finding (i.e., 17% of patients will have wasting as their AIDS-defining illness, and 24% will have it as a component of their presentation). There is no clear relationship between weight loss and the level of immunosuppression.

### Assessment

A careful assessment is critical. Anorexia and decreased oral intake are components of weight loss in the majority of patients (10). Symptoms of nausea, dysgeusia, dysphagia, odynophagia, early satiety, constipation, or diarrhea should be elicited. Many commonly prescribed drugs may cause these symptoms, which iatrogenically interfere with caloric intake and lead to weight loss.

Weight loss may be associated with significant generalized fatigue or asthenia. It is associated with an increased likelihood of hospitalization and portends a poor prognosis (11). Although weight loss is associated with decreased performance status and decreased activity level, it is not yet clear that it affects the likelihood of opportunistic infections. The patient's anxiety about the meaning of the weight loss, as well as the loss of pleasure associated with eating, may have a profound impact on quality of life.

**TABLE 4.** *Conditions and symptoms that interfere with oral intake*

*Oral/esophageal*
Aphthous ulcers
Dysgeusia
Candidiasis
Herpes simplex/zoster
Xerostomia
Cytomegalovirus
Dysphagia
Odynophagia
*Gastrointestinal tract*
Nausea/vomiting
Gastric dysmotility
Early satiety
Pain
Gas
Constipation
Diarrhea
*Macrobiotic diet*
*Depression*
*Infection*
*Malignancy*
*Fever*
*Anorexia*
*Neuropsychiatric disease*

## Diagnosis

Many factors contribute to the development of HIV-associated weight loss. They include decreased caloric intake; hormone, cytokine, and/or metabolic effects; malabsorption; and alterations in energy expenditure. Significant weight loss may be prevented or delayed by identification and treatment of reversible causes of decreased dietary intake such as mucositis, nausea, pain, diarrhea, depression, malignancy, or infection. The diagnostic evaluation should include measurement of the serum testosterone level in male patients, as this is the most common endocrine abnormality; testosterone is essential for maintenance of lean body mass in men. Patients should also be evaluated for occult opportunistic infections.

Unfortunately, the causes of weight loss in many patients are neither readily identifiable nor reversible. It is rarely due to isolated causes such as hypogonadism or simple starvation. Table 4 lists the common symptoms associated with weight loss and decreased oral intake.

## Management

General measures should be pursued first. They may include a physical therapy evaluation and regimen to build endurance. Many patients report that dysgeusia responds to an increase in food seasoning. A nutrition evaluation may be helpful in identifying foods that are likely to be appetizing as well as high in calories. Some patients may have been pursuing alternative diet therapies that may be counterproductive. To be effective, however, dietary counseling, nutritional supplements, and exercise often require the patient to be truly motivated. In the absence of a remediable cause, the clinician and patient may feel that therapy directed at increasing appetite might be useful, as decreased caloric intake is a primary predictor of overall outcome. Careful exploration and clarification of treatment goals is important before specific therapy is undertaken. Megestrol acetate (Megace) is an oral progestational agent widely used to treat advanced hormone-responsive neoplasms. It has been demonstrated to improve appetite, increase weight, and improve the overall sense of well-being in patients with AIDS. As a dose response with respect to weight gain has been demonstrated, begin therapy with 800 mg/day. More than 60% of patients will respond at this dose level (12). The dose can be titrated downward to maintain the desired weight. The drug is associated with minimal side effects, but it is expensive.

Hypogonadism should be treated with testosterone. Growth hormone, oxandrolone, and other anabolic steroids for patients with weight loss may be effective, and clinical trials are currently underway.

Dronabinol (Marinol) has been demonstrated to improve appetite in patients with AIDS without significant increase in weight (13). Begin with 2.5 mg twice a day before meals, and gradually increase the dose until the desired effect is achieved. It is associated with clinically significant euphoria or dysphoria in some patients, particularly the elderly. Patients with a history of marijuana use are more likely to tolerate the drug well.

Corticosteroids (prednisone, dexamethasone, and others) are associated with a short-term increase in appetite (approximately 4 weeks) without significant weight gain. Several randomized placebo controlled trials have failed to show a beneficial effect in the cachexia of cancer. Some clinicians fear the use of these drugs in patients with HIV in view of the underlying immune deficiency. However, in patients with advanced HIV infection in whom a generalized improvement in well-being and stamina is desired, and for whom long-term therapy is not contemplated, corticosteroid therapy may be useful. Dexamethasone in a single morning dose of 2 to 6 mg may be effective, although a higher dose may be required.

The use of total parenteral nutrition (TPN) in patients with HIV infection, as well as in patients with cancer, is often controversial. It is recommended for HIV-seropositive patients who have one of four conditions and are otherwise well: (a) severe refractory diarrhea associated with progressive weight loss and malnutrition, (b) persistent intolerance to enteral feeding in the absence of any acute remediable AIDS-related condition, (c) persistent severe gastrointestinal malabsorption (e.g. cryptosporidiosis, microsporidiosis, or HIV enteropathy), or (d) intraabdominal pathologic condition resulting in indefinite continuous mechanical bowel obstruction (14). For patients with such unremediable gastrointestinal syndromes, long-term TPN may be crucial to the maintenance of normal activity and quality of life. However, in advanced HIV disease, in the absence of one of the four conditions just named, it rarely helps the symptoms of fatigue and anorexia for which it is given. Although weight gain may be accomplished, fatigue may persist, and anorexia generally worsens.

Significant risks and burdens are associated with TPN. Infection, pancreatitis, hepatitis, symptomatic hypoglycemia or hyperglycemia, other electrolyte abnormalities, and edema are common. The therapy requires semipermanent intravenous access and significant time (8 to 12 hours) spent while the patient receives the therapy each day.

For patients with advanced HIV disease for whom palliation is the predominant goal of care, clinicians should educate families and patients about what to expect and about the emotional meaning of weight loss and feeding. It is usually best to stop weighing the patient, thus removing another focus on a numerical value.

## PAIN

### Assessment

Pain may be as prevalent in patients with HIV as it is in patients with cancer (15). The approach to pain in the patient with HIV is not fundamentally different from that in the patient with cancer (16). Good pain management relies on good pain assessment, including an adequate pain history and an ongoing evaluation of the response to analgesics as part of routine medical care. Patients with HIV and AIDS often require strong narcotics to relieve the pain that may be associated with the disease itself or its treatment. The WHO three-step ladder can be very useful way to approach the medical management of pain in these patients.

The most significant clinical difference between cancer pain and AIDS pain is the marked prevalence of neuropathic pain in AIDS patients, particularly associated with peripheral neuropathy, which occurs in 30% to 40% of patients. Patients commonly describe a severe burning pain in their hands and/or feet, which may be so severe that they are unable to walk. Although some of the drugs that are commonly used in the management of HIV disease may cause peripheral neuropathy, it may be due to HIV itself.

A significant clinical question when pain occurs in a patient with HIV is how far to pursue a specific diagnosis as opposed to focusing on analgesic control of symptoms. Headache is a good example. Patients with HIV commonly have headaches. Although they may be associated with medications, stress, or migraine, they may be

the first indication of a life-threatening intracranial infection (such as toxoplasmosis) or malignancy (such as lymphoma). A careful consideration of the overall condition of the patient and the assessment of the patient's and family's goals should be made before specific diagnostic studies are undertaken.

### Diagnosis

Pain may be due to HIV infection, to one of the opportunistic infections or malignancies, to aspects of the treatment of the patient, or to some cause not related to the disease or treatment. In all instances, pain should be managed to the patient's satisfaction.

Patients describe the pain of peripheral neuropathy as burning, shooting, numbness, or like pins and needles. On physical examination, the impression of neuropathic pain may be supported by finding allodynia (a nonpainful stimulus such as light touch provoking the pain), hyperesthesia, numbness, or color changes in the affected area. Incipient CMV infection may exacerbate neuropathic pain. Extensive diagnostic tests, such as electromyography (EMG), are not necessary to confirm the diagnosis of neuropathic pain. Although these tests may be required for other reasons, pain management may begin after an adequate history and physical examination have been completed.

When headache is the complaint, evaluate the patient for evidence of increased intracranial pressure. The patient may experience the headaches as being worst upon waking in the morning, stiff neck, or blurred vision. The presence or absence of papilledema on physical examination is not of sufficient sensitivity or specificity to rule out an intracerebral process. Most patients with a new headache, and for whom a diagnosis will result in specific treatment, will require a contrast-enhanced MRI scan of the head. The most common cause of contrast-enhancing intracerebral lesions in AIDS is toxoplasmosis (90%). As these frequently respond to therapy, a biopsy may safely await a clinical trial of antitoxoplasmosis antibiotics for a 2-week period. However, if serum antibody titers to toxoplasmosis are low, or if there is evidence of clinical deterioration, a needle biopsy should be performed immediately. Cryptococcal meningitis may present clinically without meningeal signs or fever, just fatigue or headache. Determination of the serum cryptococcal antigen is helpful in making this diagnosis.

### Management

As with the management of cancer pain, management of the pain associated with HIV should be incorporated into the entire spectrum of HIV care, not just reserved for the end stages of illness. While reversible causes of the pain should be searched for, medical management should begin even while diagnostic studies are being carried out.

Medical pain management should generally follow the guidelines described for cancer pain management (16). The WHO three-step analgesic ladder is useful in guiding the choice of therapy for those who are learning how to use these analgesics.

Neuropathic pain is one of the most difficult pain syndromes to manage. It is important to tell this to the patient, so that expectations of a quick fix are not generated. Several medication changes may be required before pain control is satisfactory.

Tricyclic antidepressants are the most widely used adjuvant or coanalgesic drugs for neuropathic pain. As a group, these drugs are thought to improve pain management in part through enhanced negative modulation of pain stimuli at the level of the dorsal horn in the spinal cord. These drugs do not promote analgesia merely though their antidepressant properties. Amitriptyline (Elavil) is the most widely described drug for analgesia in this class, but desipramine and nortriptyline are commonly used because they have fewer side effects. Any tricyclic antidepressant may work. The choice of drug is usually based on the side effect profile of the drug. For example, if sedation at bedtime would be helpful because of insomnia, amitriptyline may be very useful because of its sedating effects. A low dose of these drugs, such as amitriptyline 25 mg orally, at bedtime, is the usual starting dose. Analgesia usually begins within 4 and 7 days after the drug is begun. The dose may then be elevated over the course of several weeks until analgesia is achieved or side effects intervene. If no benefit is achieved, serum levels may be checked to ascertain whether therapeutic levels have been achieved.

The anticonvulsants may be useful for neuropathic pain that has a lancinating quality (such as postherpetic neuralgia) or is unrelieved with a tricyclic analgesic alone. Carbamazepine (Tegretol) is the most commonly used, although valproic acid (Depakote) and phenytoin (Dilantin) may also be useful. There are anecdotal reports of the effectiveness of the newer anticonvulsants such as gabapentin (Neurontin) for this indication as well. The anticonvulsants may safely be added to tricyclic and opioid analgesics.

The class I oral antiarrhythmic class of drugs may significantly benefit patients with neuropathic pain. Developed as oral agents to mimic the effects of lidocaine on cardiac conduction abnormalities, these drugs were also noted to ease peripheral neuropathic pain. Although definitive clinical studies are scant, there is widespread clinical use of the drug mexiletine (Mexitil) for refractory neuropathic pain. Patients with a history of cardiac disease or evidence of conduction abnormalities should not receive these drugs. The gastrointestinal intolerance (particularly nausea and vomiting) limits the utility of mexiletine in some patients with advanced AIDS. Similar drugs with fewer side effects (such as flecainide) may be more useful in these patients (17).

The relief of abdominal pain merits a few additional comments. It is common and often is diffuse and crampy. An antispasmodic agent may be required in addition to an opioid drug. While prudence regarding opioids and new abdominal pain is warranted, excessive anxiety about "masking" symptoms of pain in the abdomen is unwarranted and should not prevent the use of opioid analgesics for this problem. The time-honored tradition of withholding analgesics during the evaluation of acute abdominal pain is unsupported scientifically and is particularly inappropriate in the management of chronic abdominal pain.

### History of Drug Substance Use

A past or present history of recreational drug use raises an additional concern in the treatment of pain in patients with AIDS. While this is treated as a general topic elsewhere in this text, a few remarks are in order. Most importantly, nonopioids should *not* be substituted for opioids in the management of pain merely because of a history of substance use (16). When treating patients with HIV infection and a history of opioid abuse, the clinician should anticipate using much larger doses of the opioid analgesics than usual because of the incipient tolerance that may be present. Concerns regarding drug diversion or abuse need to be openly discussed with the patient.

### NAUSEA AND VOMITING

Nausea and/or vomiting are common in patients with advanced HIV disease. The possible causes are legion.

### Assessment

Begin the assessment with a careful history. The relationship of nausea to vomiting and the timing of associated symptoms are often important clues to the underlying cause. Besides the usual considerations discussed elsewhere in this text, a few notes about common clinical situations associated with nausea and vomiting in patients with AIDS is in order.

Because of the polypharmacy that almost always accompanies the treatment of a patient with advanced HIV infection, drug-induced nausea and vomiting are exceedingly common. The history should include the relationship of the nausea and vomiting to newly instituted drugs or to the time of day that drugs are administered.

Patients who describe early satiety, or who report persistent nausea and vomitiing only after eating, may be suffering from a HIV-associated diffuse gastroenteric neuropathy with consequent dysmotility.

## Diagnosis

Although an extensive workup to discover specific causes may be undertaken, empirical therapy is often effective. It is helpful to remember that there are five major pharmacologic targets for the treatment of nausea and vomiting:

- Serotonin receptors—principally located in the gut and chemoreceptor trigger zone
- Dopamine receptors—principally located in the chemoreceptor trigger zone
- Cholinergic receptors—principally located in the vestibular and chemoreceptor trigger zone areas
- Histamine receptors—principally located in the chemoreceptor trigger zone
- Cerebral cortex—where emotions, learned responses, and intracerebral pressure affect nausea and vomiting

Remember that poor gastric motility due to opiates, HIV neuropathy, infection, or an infiltrative tumor (such as Kaposi's sarcoma or lymphoma) may cause persistent nausea and vomiting. When constipation is relieved or gastric motility improved, nausea and vomiting may disappear. Hyperacidity with or without gastroesophageal reflux and gastric, esophageal, or duodenal erosions or ulcers due to infection, stress, or medications may also be implicated.

## Management

As with most symptoms, the first step in the management of nausea and vomiting is to identify any reversible causes. In patients with AIDS, the most common causes are drug related. Therefore, try to eliminate or substitute alternatives for those drugs that may be responsible.

Often the proximate cause cannot be identified or removed. The five targets for nausea and vomiting are important to remember in the choice of empiric antiemetics. Begin with an antidopaminergic drug (such as prochlorperazine). Use metoclopramide instead if dysmotility is suspected. If there are side effects (excessive sedation or dystonia), then change to an alternate antidopaminergic drug (such as haloperidol). If there is partial relief, increase the dose of the drug before changing drugs or adding a new agent. If there is no relief, then combine a second agent from a different class with the antidopaminergic drug. Continue this process until the symptoms have been brought under control. Ignorance of the actions of these drugs results in the sequential trial of multiple medications with the same mechanism of action, and results in the persistence of unrelieved symptoms. Table 5 lists common drugs from each class.

The serotonin antagonists, including ondansetron (Zofran) and granisetron (Kytril), merit special mention. These drugs are highly specific for the Ht-3 serotonin receptor, which is particularly implicated in chemother-

**TABLE 5.** *Antiemetics*

| |
|---|
| *Serotonin antagonists* |
| Ondansetron |
| Granisetron |
| *Dopamine antagonists* |
| Prochlorperazine |
| Haloperidol |
| Metoclopramide |
| *Anticholinergics* |
| Scopolamine |
| Hyoscyamine |
| *Antihistamines* |
| Diphenhydramine |
| *Cerebral cortex* |
| Corticosteroids |
| Benzodiazepines |
| Tetrahydrocannabinol |

apy-associated nausea and vomiting. Although controlled trials in HIV-infected patients are lacking, anecdotal reports support their effectiveness in selected patients. It makes intuitive sense that this class may be useful for drug-induced nausea and vomiting that is not controlled by antidopaminergic antiemetics. However, these drugs are expensive; may be given by the oral route, which is equivalent or superior to the intravenous route in many patients; and may be effective at far lower doses than the doses that were initially advocated. Therefore, until adequate studies are available, it makes sense to use the lowest oral dose of the antiserotonergic drug that is effective. If the drug class is tried and fails to control the target symptom, then discontinue the drug and use other classes of agents as described above.

## DIARRHEA

### Assessment

Diarrhea is usually a result of one of the following:

- HIV infection
- Malabsorption
- Lactose intolerance
- Tumor invasion
- Treatable infection
- Untreatable infection

In the supportive care setting, it is important to both identify the cause and control the symptom. There is a time-honored tradition in medicine of not treating diarrhea until after infectious causes have been excluded and/or completely treated. The fear has been that if the natural cleansing action of the diarrhea is stopped pharmacologically, an invasive toxigenic infection could be worsened. While this is a consideration, it should not preclude a measured approach to the relief of the symptom at the same time a diagnostic workup is pursued.

## Diagnosis

There has been some controversy over what constitutes a judicious evaluation of diarrhea in patients with HIV. Although some have suggested that a clear cause can be identified in 95% of cases given a thorough evaluation, the treatment for many of the causes remains symptomatic only. The workup should be extensive enough to identify treatable, reversible causes without subjecting the patient to unnecessary and burdensome procedures that will not change management (18). If the diarrhea is not bloody, prudent evaluation begins with a stool culture, examination for ova and parasites, and administration of antidiarrheal medication. If the diarrhea is unresponsive to modest symptomatic therapy (such as diphenoxylate), the workup should then proceed to a search for protozoa, esophagogastroduodenoscopy with biopsy, and colonoscopy with biopsy.

## Management

During the search for and treatment of the proximate cause (if possible), an antidiarrheal agent should be administered and a lactose-free diet instituted. In general, a graduated approach using the following ladder of treatments is effective. The ladder goes from least to most potent in much the same way that the WHO three-step ladder goes from least potent to most potent analgesic. As with the three-step ladder, if diarrhea is severe, there is no need to begin at the bottom of the ladder. Routine dosing may be more effective than intermittent or as-needed dosing.

- Bismuth subsalicylate (Pepto-Bismol): This over-the-counter product contains aspirin and is useful for mild diarrhea, especially if there are abdominal cramps.
- Attapulgite (Kaopectate): This over-the-counter product helps solidify liquid stools without really modifying the cause of the diarrhea and is useful in mild watery diarrhea.
- Loperamide (Imodium): This poorly absorbed opiate analog slows intestinal motility and is now available without prescription in the United States.
- Diphenoxylate with atropine (Lomotil): This combination medicine includes an opiate to decrease motility and an anticholinergic to decrease abdominal cramping.
- Tincture of opium: An alcohol-solubilized opium, this high-potency opiate may be very effective in diarrhea that is refractory to the other antidiarrheal drugs. Seven drops every 4 hours is a reasonable starting dose, but the dosage can be escalated until symptoms are relieved, or side effects intervene, in the same manner as with opioid analgesics.
- Octreotide (Sandostatin): This injectable analog of somatostatin inhibits the secretion of fluids in the intestinal tract. It may be highly effective in the secretory diarrhea associated with AIDS that is refractory to other management. Start with 100 µg subcutaneously, two or three times daily, or 10 µg subcutaneously every hour by infusion, and titrate until a good effect is obtained.

## DELIRIUM AND DEMENTIA

### Assessment

Infection with HIV is associated with a progressive dementia characterized by a loss of short-term memory, mental slowing, decreased concentration, and poor judgment not unlike the dementias seen in geriatric populations. It is often a late manifestation of AIDS. For this reason, it is imperative that advance directives and surrogate decision makers are identified early in the course of HIV illness. Many patients will have strong views about their overall medical care if HIV dementia occurs. It behooves the clinician to ascertain these views far in advance of any clinical symptoms.

For appropriate patients with a new onset of a change in personality or orientation, it is important to distinguish dementia from delirium. As for patients with cancer, many causes of delirium in a patient with HIV are highly treatable and lead to vastly improved quality of life, as well as length of life.

### Diagnosis

For a patient in whom it is appropriate to pursue diagnostic testing, a contrast-enhanced MRI of the head is an important first step. Computed tomography is rarely definitive. The HIV infection alone is often associated with diffuse atrophy, which is a nonspecific finding. This may be the only abnormality found in patients with HIV-associated dementia. Enhancing lesions are most commonly toxoplasmosis (90%), although primary central nervous system lymphoma and other fungal infections are possible. Demyelination associated with progressive multifocal leukoencephalopathy (PML) may be seen. If the MRI scan is not diagnostic, a lumbar puncture should be performed. Cryptococcal meningitis, CMV encephalitis, neurosyphilis, and tuberculous meningitis may present with no more than subtle changes in personality, mood, or progressive fatigue. Meningeal signs may be absent on physical examination.

### Management

Specific causes of delirium should be treated in patients for whom it is agreed that relief is of value and the burden of treatment will not exceed benefit. Although a diagnosis of exclusion, HIV-associated dementia may improve or stabilize with zidovudine.

Nevertheless, one of the most difficult management issues concerns the patient who was previously independent and is now demented and unable to care for himself or herself. Social work intervention is invariably required. The patient's safety must be ensured. Often this means that 24-hour monitoring is needed. Help the patient maintain orientation by providing a calendar, a clock, and night lights. If behavior requires control, pharmacological restraints may be more helpful than physical restraints. Haloperidol in doses ranging from 2 to 20 mg per day, chlorpromazine (Thorazine) in doses from 25 to 200 mg/day, or lorazepam 2 to 8 mg/day may be particularly useful. New neuroleptic medications such as risperidone (Risperdal) have fewer anticholinergic side effects than do standard agents and may be better choices for patients with advanced HIV infection.

## DEHYDRATION

### Assessment

Dehydration may be due to excessive vomiting, diarrhea, or progressive inability to imbibe adequate fluids because of dysphagia, odynophagia, dementia, or generalized fatigue. In the care of patients who do not have an obviously remediable cause of the dehydration, a significant question often arises as to whether parenteral or enteral hydration should be administered. Exertional fatigue and orthostatic hypotension due to dehydration may be reversed with parenteral or enteral fluids. Some have suggested that delirium may be reversed with fluids if it is due primarily to dehydration or secondarily to decreased renal clearance of medications.

Exogenous fluids may also be associated with several adverse effects that are not commonly considered, particularly when the patient has hypoalbuminemia. They can increase secretions and worsen bronchospasm, cough, peripheral edema, ascites, diarrhea, and incontinence. If fluids are given intravenously, there may be local complications of phlebitis and ecchymosis. If they are given via a percutaneous gastrostomy, the risk of aspiration increases. Excess fluids can provoke congestive heart failure and dyspnea and can increase the risk of skin breakdown.

### Diagnosis

Diarrhea, vomiting, sweating, and fever as the cause of dehydration can be readily evaluated and controlled. Hypoalbuminemia, hyperglycemia, and hypercalcemia should be excluded. For a patient who has refractory orthostatic blood pressure changes despite adequate provision of intravenous fluids, it is important to consider the diagnosis of dysautonomia. The same neuropathic process that results in the pain or gastric dysmotility syndromes associated with AIDS may selectively result in the dysregulation of vessel tone.

### Management

In a patient for whom intravenous or subcutaneous fluids may be beneficial, a clinical trial of parenteral fluids should be performed. For example, administer 2 liters of normal saline intravenously and assess the change in symptoms. If the patient experiences a clear benefit, then continue to monitor orthostatic blood pressures and treat as needed. If dysautonomia is suspected, a trial of fludrocortisone acetate (Florinef) may be helpful.

If the symptoms do not improve, then discontinue the hydration and assure the patient's safety. Stop checking the blood pressure. Keep mucous membranes moist (oral mucosa, lips, nares, and eyes). It is important to note that attention to oral hygiene may often relieve the dry mouth of a patient who is predominantly bed-bound. Oral candidiasis (thrush) should be searched for and treated.

## CONSTITUTIONAL SYMPTOMS

### Assessment

Besides weight loss, the most common constitutional symptoms in patients with HIV infection are fevers, sweats, and fatigue. These symptoms can be debilitating, and their treatment can result in significant improvement in quality of life. Their causes can be legion, and a judicious search for the cause is often justified.

### Diagnosis

Bacterial infections in AIDS patients are usually straightforward in their diagnosis. For a patient with persistent fevers, sweats and/or fatigue in the absence of other localizing findings, the occult causes are more likely to be mycobacterial [*Mycobacterium avium* complex (MAC) or *Mycobacterium tuberculosis*, (MTb)] fungal, viral (cytomegalovirus in particular), or malignancy (lymphoma). Evaluation includes blood cultures for MAC, a retinal examination for CMV, and determination of serum lactate dehydrogenase, which is commonly elevated in lymphoma.

### Management

The nonsteroidal antiinflammatory drugs are often useful in the management of persistent fevers and sweats. As with constant pain, these drugs should be administered on a schedule, not as needed. The goal is to keep the symptoms under control. The fear that a significant fever will be obscured is overrated. Significant fevers are only blunted by antiinflammatory drug treatment; they are not completely suppressed.

*Mycobacterium avium* complex (MAC) infection is the most common disseminated bacterial opportunistic disease in patients with AIDS (19). Its seroprevalence reaches 41% at 2 years from the diagnosis of AIDS (20). Blood cultures may take several weeks to turn positive for this organism. Therefore, patients with advanced HIV infection (CD4 <75 cells/ml) and clinical signs and symptoms suggestive of MAC infection (weight loss, persistent fever, diarrhea, night sweats, anemia, fatigue, generalized wasting) should be empirically treated with clarithromycin or azithromycin plus ethambutol until culture results are available.

## DYSPNEA

### Assessment

Dyspnea is the sensation of shortness of breath. It is caused by both central and peripheral mechanisms. Centrally, a lowered $pO_2$ or increased $pCO_2$ may stimulate a sensation of shortness of breath. Anxiety may cause identical symptoms. Inflammatory or infiltrative processes in the lungs may also cause a sense of dyspnea through poorly described stretch receptors.

### Diagnosis

The most common cause of dyspnea is an inflammatory process in the lungs such as pneumonia (bacterial, protozoal, fungal). Infiltrative processes such as Kaposi's sarcoma or lymphoma may also be responsible. Other common conditions such as congestive heart failure, bronchospasm, pulmonary embolism, pleural effusions, pneumonia, and drug reactions should also be considered. Although a chest radiograph, oxygen saturation determination, and blood gas determination may be helpful in diagnosing the cause of dyspnea, the values obtained should not be confused with the symptom itself. Dyspnea is what the patient says it is.

### Management

As with other symptoms, the physician may begin symptom management and therapy directed against the cause at the same time. This is true even if the cause is likely to be infectious. There are four common symptomatic treatments: oxygen, bronchodilators, opiates, and anxiolytics.

### Oxygen

Many patients describe relief of dyspnea when oxygen is supplied, either by nasal prongs or by face mask.

Patients may describe relief even when their hemoglobin oxygen saturation is normal without additional oxygen. This has been ascribed to the reassurance that the oxygen brings as well as to the effect of cool air moving against the face. Hospice workers have noted that the same effect can be achieved by directing a gentle breeze against the face from a fan or an open window.

### Bronchodilators

There may be bronchoconstriction without a previous history of asthma. A clinical trial of a bronchodilator such as salbutamol may bring significant relief of dyspnea.

### Opiates

The opiates act both centrally and at the peripheral receptors in the lung to decrease the sensation of dyspnea. Physicians may be reticent to use opiates at the same time they are trying to treat a lung infection, owing to exaggerated fears of respiratory depression. Dyspnea is a more potent stimulus to breathe than pain. In addition, in the studies performed in patients with cancer and dyspnea, the dyspnea was relieved before there was any change in the respiratory rate. This highlights a critical aspect of dyspnea management: the patient's self-report is to be used as the clinical outcome. It is wrong to titrate the opiates to respiratory rate.

### Anxiolytics

Dyspnea is one of the most frightening sensations that a patient can experience. For some, the application of reassurance, oxygen, and an opiate are sufficient to relieve the sensation. In others, however, anxiety plays a disproportionate part in the symptom complex. The addition of a benzodiazepine (such as lorazepam 0.5 to 1 mg orally every 6 to 8 hours) may help.

## ORAL SYMPTOMS

### Assessment

Dry or sore mouth is common in patients with AIDS. Hairy leukoplakia is commonly seen on the lateral borders of the tongue and correlates with advanced HIV disease but is usually not symptomatic. Aphthous ulcers and candidiasis may be very painful. Drugs may cause mucositis. Poor dentition may be a result of decreased saliva production, the immune suppression associated with HIV infection, and low-grade bacterial superinfection and may be painful. Kaposi's sarcoma or lymphoma may be cosmetically distressing, disfiguring, and painful if ulcerated. Thrush, herpes simplex virus, and cytomegalovirus may cause painful oral lesions.

## Diagnosis

If visual inspection is not diagnostic, culture and biopsy may yield definitive diagnoses. Oral candidiasis may be atypical in appearance. The oral mucosa may only be reddened rather than demonstrating the more familiar white plaques. A swab of oral lesions for herpes simplex virus is a simple way to make that diagnosis. Isolated aphthous lesions may require a biopsy to eliminate CMV as a cause. If the patient experiences jaw pain or fever, dental evaluation and a panoramic radiograph of the mouth may be helpful to rule out an abscess.

## Management

Specific causes may be treated with specific therapy. However, for the common complaint of aphthous ulcers, the usual mucositis cocktails common in oncology may be relatively useless. A cocktail developed by the otorhinolaryngologists may be more helpful. Combine:

Hydrocortisone 200 mg,
Nystatin 2 million units,
Tetracycline 1500 mg, and
Diphenhydramine (Benadryl) elixir to bring the total volume to 250 ml.

Swish and spit 5 to 10 ml every 4 hours.
Systemic steroids may also be helpful. There are anecdotal reports of thalidomide being helpful. Clinical trial results are pending.

## DERMATOLOGIC COMPLAINTS

### Assessment

For reasons that are not entirely clear, patients with AIDS are commonly afflicted by various dermatologic complaints (Table 6). Seborrheic dermatitis occurs in up

**TABLE 6.** *Common oral/dermatologic conditions*

| |
| --- |
| Candidiasis (thrush) |
| Hairy leukoplakia |
| Periodontal disease |
| Seborrheic dermatitis |
| Xerosis (dry skin) |
| Herpes simplex |
| Herpes zoster |
| Molluscum contagiosum |
| Staphylococcal folliculitis |
| Secondary syphilis |
| Kaposi's sarcoma |
| Scabies |
| *Mycobacterium avium* |
| *Mycobacterium tuberculosis* |
| Tinea corporis/cruris |

to 80% of patients (21). Seborrheic patches may involve the face, scalp, back, axillae, and groin. Dry skin of such severity that it approaches that of ichthyosis may be accompanied by disabling pruritus. Patients are also prone to boils and carbuncles that may develop into skin abscesses or cellulitis. Rashes are common and may be related to drug sensitivity. Disseminated herpes simplex or herpes zoster may be seen. Molluscum contagiosum, which is due to papillomavirus infection, is common on the face and may be extensive.

## Diagnosis

If a rash has pustules, a Tzanck preparation and viral culture to rule out herpesvirus may be often useful. A potassium hydroxide preparation of a scraping from an angry red patch may easily exclude a fungal infection. Any new maculopapular rash that appears up to 7 to 10 days after the addition of a new medicine should be considered a drug eruption. For skin conditions that persist, or that do not yield to specific therapy, the help of a dermatologist may be required.

## Management

In addition to the treatment of specific conditions, liberal amounts of skin moisturizers should be recommended to counteract dry skin and pruritus. Since many of the nonprescription drugstore preparations are water-based and of minimal utility, choose products that are oil-based. Seborrheic dermatitis will often respond to 1% hydrocortisone. A topical antifungal such as clotrimazole (Lotrimin) may provide added benefit.

## REFERENCES

1. Gottlieb MS, Schroff R, Schanker HM, et al. *Pneumocystis carinii* pneumonia and mucosal candidiasis in previously healthy homosexual men. *N Engl J Med* 1981;305:1425–31.
2. Masu H. Michelis MA, Greene JB, et al. Outbreak of community-acquired *Pneumocystis carinii* pneumonia. *N Engl J Med* 1981;305:1431–8.
3. Peters BS, Beck EF, Coleman DG, et al. Changing disease patterns in patients with AIDS in a referral center in the United Kingdom: the changing face of AIDS. *Br Med J* 1991;302:203–7.
4. Yarchoan R. Venzon DJ, Plue JM, et al. CD4 counts and the risk for death in patients infected with HIV receiving antiretroviral therapy. *Ann Intern Med* 1991;115:184–98.
5. Mellors JW, Kingsley LA, Rinaldo CR, et al. Quantitation of HIV-1 RNA in plasma predicts outcome after seroconversion. *Ann Intern Med* 1995;122:573–9.
6. Apolonio EG, Hoover DR, He Y, et al. Prognostic factors in human immunodeficiency virus-positive patients with a CD4-lymphocyte count <50/µl. *J Infect Dis* 1995;171:829–36.
7. CDC USPHS/DISA guidelines for the prevention of opportunistic infections in persons infected with HIF: a summary. *MMWR* 1995;44(RRR-8):1–34.
8. Shah P, Mullai N, Hussain MA, Kocka FE, Allen S. Bone marrow culture in fever of unknown origin (FUO): a retrospective analysis. *Proc ASCO* 1995;14:288.

9. Oksenhendler E, Bierling P, Ferchal F, Clauvel J, Seligmann M. Zidovudine for thrombocytopenic purpura related to Human Immunodeficiency virus (HIV) infection. *Ann Intern Med* 1989:110:365–8.

10. O'Sullivan P, Linke RA, Dalton S. Evaluation of body weight and nutritional status among AIDS patients. *J Am Diet Assoc* 1985;85:1483–4.

11. Hickey MS, Weaver KE. Nutritional management of patients with ARC or AIDS. *Gastroenterol Clin North Am* 1988:17:545–61.

12. Von Roenn JH, Armstrong D, Dickmeyer, MS, et al. Megestrol acetate in patients with AIDS-related cachexia. *Ann Intern Med* 1994;121(6):393–9.

13. Gorter R, Seefried M, Volberding P. Dronabinol effects on weight in patients with HIV infection. *AIDS* 1992:6(1)127.

14. Kotler DP, Tierney AR, Culpepper-Morgon JA, et al. Effect of home total parenteral nutrition on body composition in patients with acquired immunodeficiency syndrome. *J Parenter Enteral Nutr* 1990;14:454–8.

15. Breibart W, Rosenfeld BO, Passik SD, McDonald MV, Thaler H, Portenoy RK. The undertreatment of pain in ambulatory AIDS patients. *Pain* 1996;65:243–9.

16. US Department of Health and Human Services, Public Health Service, Agency for Health Care Policy and Research. *Clinical Practice Guideline No. 9: Management of Cancer Pain.* 1994;139–41.

17. Ferris FD, Flannery JS, McNeal HB, et al. *A comprehensive guide for the care of persons with HIV disease. Module 4: Palliative care.* Toronto: Kirkpatrick & Associates Printing, 1995.

18. Johanson JF, Sonnenberg A. Efficient management of diarrhea in the acquired immunodeficiency syndrome (AIDS): a medical decision analysis. *Ann Intern Med* 1990;112:942–8.

19. Zakowski P, Gligiel S, Berlin OBW, Johnson Jr, BL. Disseminated *Mycobacterium avium* intracellulare infection in homosexual men dying of acquired immunodeficiency. *JAMA* 1982;248:2980–2.

20. Nightingale SB, Byrd LT, Souther PM, et al. Incidence of *Mycobacterium avium* intracellulare complex bacteremia in human immunodeficiency virus-positive patients. *J Infect Dis* 1992;165:1082–5.

21. Gerber TG, Obuch ML, Goldschmidt RH. Dermatologic manifestations of HIV infection. *Am Fam Pract* 1990;41(6): 1729–42.

*Principles and Practice of Supportive Oncology,*
edited by Ann Berger et al.
Lippincott–Raven Publishers, Philadelphia ©1998

CHAPTER 65

# Measurement of Outcomes in Supportive Oncology

## Quality of Life

Roland T. Skeel

## QUALITY OF LIFE OUTCOMES

### Importance of Quality of Life Outcomes in Supportive Oncology

Patients regularly ask physicians and nurses for quality of life information about their cancer and its treatment: "How much pain will I have? How much nausea and vomiting will the chemotherapy cause? How long will it last? Will I have enough energy to work? Is it safe for me to have sex? Will all my hair fall out? Will it come back? How much time will I have to spend in the hospital? How much is this all going to cost? When is my appetite going to come back? Why am I feeling so depressed? Will I ever stop being so nervous?" And they often ask the ultimate question that requires the physician to integrate knowledge of the anticancer treatment, the supportive care efforts, and the quality of life effect of the disease and the treatment: "Will I be better off because of this treatment?" Too often the answers given are limited to anecdotal, incomplete, or misinformed replies, because quality of life evaluations in cancer clinical trials and in supportive care have been either uncommon or limited in scope.

The goal of supportive care in oncology is to make patients feel and function better than they would have without that supportive care. This goal is explicitly different from that of curative or life-extending therapy, in which there is regularly a moderate to high tolerance for side effects and temporary functional impairments (1,2). Even with these curative or life-extending therapies, sup-

portive care measures are necessary, and the success of these measures may determine whether or not the patient is willing to tolerate repeated cycles of the treatment, as is usually necessary with chemotherapy. Whether the supportive oncology care is given in conjunction with other cancer treatment or is used exclusively to palliate the effects of the cancer, the criteria of success for the supportive care are that the patient feels and functions better. When patients are less pleased with how they are feeling or functioning—that is, when they believe their quality of life is not better—then the supportive care has not been successful. The patients' personal, subjective perception of how they are feeling and how they are functioning thus becomes a critical outcome measure of this aspect of cancer care. As stated by Roy, "Quality of life studies and measurements are a systematic way of paying attention to the details in which effective compassion will be found or found wanting"(3).

### Health-Related Quality of Life: Subjectivity of Assessments and Multidimensionality of Dimensions

Quality of life measurement is neither a concept nor a procedure with which nurses and physicians caring for patients with cancer are really comfortable, because it seems so difficult to define the meaning of the phrase "quality of life." This is not to say that there is disagreement over the importance of quality of life. In a 1987 survey of physicians in the Eastern Cooperative Oncology Group, 89% of ECOG physicians said that they felt more satisfied when they could improve the quality of their

R. T. Skeel: Division of Hematology/Oncology, Department of Medicine, Medical College of Ohio, Toledo, OH 43614-5809.

patients' lives rather than simply prolong survival. Thus, even clinicians who have been self-selected to perform clinical research to find more effective cancer therapies value the notion of quality of life, despite lack of agreement on a precise meaning of the concept or on our ability to measure what is meant (4).

"Quality of life" is a phrase and a concept that also has crept into common parlance. When used in everyday language, it is assumed to cover many aspects of life, including the availability of food and shelter, climate, occupation, and other aspects of economic well-being as well as social, psychological, and physical health. An article about the Federal Emergency Management Agency's report on "Nuclear Attack Planning Base—1900" discussed optimistic and pessimistic predictions about "the quality of life after World War III" (5). When measured in general populations by social scientists, "quality of life" usually refers to these broader terms. Domains that national surveys have identified as important to quality of life include the following:

- Physical and material well-being (which includes health and personal safety)
- Relations with other people
- Social, community, and civic activities
- Personal development and fulfillment
- Recreation (6)

Specific instruments used to measure quality of life determine the precise meaning for an individual study more definitively, and it is important to recognize that a single definition does not apply equally to all quality of life measurements. It is of interest that health and personal safety were ranked as important or very important by 95% to 98% of a sample of 3,000 30- to 70-year-old subjects from the general United States population, higher than any other of the 15 different components that were ranked for importance to their quality of life. Fifteen percent to 20% reported that this component was moderately, only slightly, or not at all well met in their lives (6).

When limited to the narrower realm of illness and health, "quality of life" takes on more specific meanings, though it remains multidimensional and is clearly affected by factors that may be included in the more broadly designated quality of life. For the remainder of this chapter we will use the term *health-related quality of life* (HQL) to designate a more focused concept related to the impact of a medical condition or its treatment on a person's expected physical, psychological, and social well-being (2). Calman has posited that quality of life evaluations measure the difference between the "hopes and expectations of the individual and that individual's present experiences" (7). This postulate carries the implication that the perceived quality of life could be improved either by reducing expectations or by improving the actual symptoms, functional status, and psychological well-being that the patient compares with his or her expectations.

Implicit in these definitions of HQL is that the designation of the extent of variation from that expected by the patient must be determined by the individual in order to have greatest validity. Perceptions are by their very nature subjective. Therefore, reliance on family members or health professionals may produce misleading information on what the patient's quality of life is (8–10). In contrast to this general caveat, when treatment-related symptoms are focused on, others have found that at least with some instruments, there are minor differences in HQL (11).

While it is possible—and logical—to draw some conclusions about the relative HQL impairment from certain symptoms or objective functional impairments, what appears logical may not in fact obtain. Two studies in patients with advanced cancer demonstrate this (12,13). In these studies, despite increased side effects from a more aggressive regimen (colon cancer) or a more prolonged regimen of chemotherapy versus shorter radiotherapy (lung cancer), patients did not report greater impairment of quality of life. It has been suggested that the overall improvement in quality of life in such active therapy may be related to "optimism and support provided by close medical supervision" (14). It becomes even more hazardous to try to extrapolate the effect on psychological or social components of perceptions of HQL from objectively measured impairments. The subjectivity of HQL comes about in part because a person's designation of perceived HQL is psychologically derived from both his or her current (momentary) self-observed quality and the current quality that the person expects. The current quality expected is not static, but varies with many factors, including psychological adjustment to disease (e.g., the long-term paraplegic who is quite satisfied with his or her quality of life), culture, and personality. The momentary self-observed quality of life is itself derived from a complex integration of factors that constitute the multidimensionality that is commonly assessed in quality of life measures (15–17):

1. Physical symptoms of the disease or its treatment or concurrent illness
2. Functional capacity (ability and energy) for daily routine, social interactions, intellectual activity, emotional reactions and adjustments, economic independence
3. Self-perceptions of wellness or its absence

The physical symptoms of disease and side effects of treatment include such elements as pain, nausea and vomiting, hair loss, anorexia, and fatigue. While these are discrete elements that contribute to global HQL, they also have an impact on functional capacity. The latter is usually separated into three distinct domains: psychological functioning, social functioning, and physical functioning. Psychological functioning includes anxiety, depression, adjustment to the disease and its treatment, and satisfaction with care. Physical functioning includes mobility, ability for self care, and ability to carry on daily routine (such as child care or work activities). Social functioning includes family interactions, relationships with friends, and ability to function on the job beyond the physical level. Additional considerations in HQL may relate to spiritual concerns, sexual functioning, and body image (18). Variability among respondents may also occur because of the assessment environment and the manner and form of evaluation (19). Thus, subjectivity and multidimensionality are two critical factors in understanding and measuring HQL and in interpreting data from HQL assessments.

## Quality of Life Outcomes Important to Cancer Patients

Somatic and physiologic symptoms and complaints are generally the most immediate concerns of patients with cancer. Dame Cicely Saunders, the founding director of St. Christopher's Hospice, London, England, stated it a lecture at Yale in the early 1970s that when a patient is in pain or lying in a bed of feces, it is difficult to converse with family and friends and to reminisce about the good times. The simple physical problems must be addressed first. "Successful symptomatic treatment should enable a patient to be so relieved of physical distress that he is freed to concentrate on other matters" (20).

Physicians and nurses are usually attuned to the physical, symptomatic distress expressed by patients. How likely it is that the range of HQL effects of this distress will be addressed depends on a willingness to take time with the patient and to ask appropriate questions that are relevant to the patient's disease. Asking the appropriate questions requires a knowledge of how specific factors about the disease and its treatment are likely to affect the patient's HQL.

### Influence of Cancer Characteristics on HQL

The types of symptoms and physical distress experienced by patients are greatly influenced not only by the type of cancer but also by the stage of the disease, the specific organs and tissues involved, and the current or most recent treatment. For example, in early breast cancer, paresthesia on the chest wall consequent to surgery, nausea and vomiting, hair loss, or weight gain from chemotherapy may be important quality of life concerns. In advanced breast cancer, bone pain, loss of appetite and cachexia, or shortness of breath may be predominant physical quality of life concerns. For any patient who has completed active therapy, primary physical concerns may be persistent lack of energy with its resultant functional deficits, loss of organ function (e.g., of speech or swallowing), or the potential for second malignancies. As with other dimensions of HQL, patients' expectations

about how they should feel play an important role in the degree to which their physical problems affect their HQL.

The influence of the cancer, its stage, and the treatment employed on the social and psychological domains of HQL are not as evident as with the physical domains. In contrast to somatic and physiologic symptoms and complaints, social and emotional issues get inadequate attention from physicians and are underemphasized in many HQL measures (21). Physicians often feel that emotional support is better relegated to other health professionals, though many patients prefer to get their support from their primary oncology physician (14). The emotional benefit of psychological interventions for patients with cancer in reducing emotional distress, enhancing coping, and improving "adjustment" have been well demonstrated (22). There is even some suggestion that there is a physical, life-prolonging benefit as well (23), though this is far from being established (24).

### Influence of Age and Other Factors on HQL

Any discussion of HQL measurement must also recognize that HQL is influenced by considerations other than the disease in question and its therapy. Because the measured quality of life is dependent upon expectations as well on as the patient's current situation, anything that can affect expectations will have an influence on the measured quality. Younger people have different expectations regarding life expectancy than do older persons; they may also have different expectations about functional ability, pain, or other symptoms that could affect their perceived HQL. Age has been found to affect decision making by patients with cancer when they are presented with options of willingness to trade survival for quality of life: younger patients are more likely to accept a treatment with more severe side effects to gain an increment in survival than are older patients who have a greater interest in maintaining their current quality of life (25). In addition, patients with higher scores on the social well-being subscale of the Functional Assessment of Cancer Therapy (FACT) assessment, and those with children living at home, were more willing to have aggressive cancer treatment (26). Debilities from the disease or comorbid conditions may be greater in older patients and result in a worse baseline quality of life.

It has been found that older patients with cancer do have lower HQL scores when uncorrected data are used. However. once complicating comorbidities or performance status were controlled for, the older patients have a quality of life similar to that younger patients, according to various physical and psychosocial scales (27). Because the results obviously reflect how the analysis is designed and what measure is used, it is not possible to generalize from these data that age was not a factor in HQL measurement or perception. In fact, the opposite might be true, since only after "correction" for performance status or comorbidities or functional status were the HQL scores similar. Age is clearly a potentially important patient variable to be taken into consideration and controlled for when possible.

Similar arguments can be made for socioeconomic status, which has a significant effect on overall health (28). Because the cultural context in which the HQL is being evaluated is important, a determination of cross-cultural validity of HQL assessments is essential (29). Finally, personality factors, such as ability to adjust to and cope with stressful situations, can also have an impact on the patient's perceived quality of life, since they will impinge on the patient's expectations.

### Evolution of HQL Measurements from Curiosity to Commonplace

When Spitzer reviewed the state of the science of quality of life, he found only four papers in the medical literature (by physicians and surgeons) with "quality of life" in their titles between 1966 and 1970 (30). In the next 5 years there were 34, and since then the rise has been seemingly exponential: In 1993 alone, 165 articles met the specific criteria of focusing on HQL and were believed to be significant contributions to the HQL literature (31). It was reported that in 1992, more than 1,000 titles indexed in MEDLINE (National Library of Medicine, Bethesda, Maryland) contained the phrase "quality of life" (32). The growth of the area is further attested to by the fact that there is now a dedicated journal (*Quality of Life Research*) to deal with this topic. With the growth in the research has been a concomitant growth in the instruments to measure quality of life. In an update of a quality of life bibliography and measurement instruments, over 170 different HQL instruments were reported as being used in 1993 (31).

Many of these are measures designed for use either in the general population to assess health status or in patients with disease states, but they are not directed specifically at any one health problem (33,34). Other measures are much more specific and are designed with a limited population in mind, such as patients with systemic lupus erythematosus, chronic lung disease, or cancer. Even within disease groups there are specific measures that aim to address the particular problems posed by a unique group of patients. Thus, for example, within cardiovascular diseases, there is a questionnaire for patients with chronic heart failure. Whether the approach is broad and general or narrow and specific, the aim is to gain information that will enhance understanding of the disease process, the illness that people experience from their diseases, the consequences of the therapy for the diseases, and the predictive value of the information about groups or individuals with disease.

Just as there is often a gap between a patients' expectation about their HQL and current reality, there is also a gap between the health profession's affirmation of the importance of quality of life in medical care and how the outcomes from measurements of HQL using standardized instruments are used to inform patients, shape clinical decisions, and establish health policy. As a consequence, physicians continue to use unsystematic approaches to learn about their patients' perceived quality of life and to apply this knowledge to clinical decisions (2).

Although HQL evaluations in oncology, particularly in clinical trials (35–37), became prevalent somewhat later than HQL evaluations in cardiovascular (38) or chronic lung disease (39), there has been a flurry of activity in the past 5 to 10 years that has resulted in HQL evaluations being companion studies or an integral component of many clinical trials in oncology (36,37,40).

### Use of HQL as a Clinical Endpoint

The most prevailing use of HQL assessment in oncology is as an endpoint in clinical trials (18,21,29,35,36, 40–47). Gotay and colleagues (42) suggested that for HQL to serve as a study endpoint, two conditions must be met:

1. The predicted survival differences between treatment arms are expected to be small.
2. Moderate to large differences are expected on at least one quality of life dimension.

This set of conditions describes one important situation where HQL should be an endpoint, but if applied strictly, may be unduly restrictive to investigators who may have valid reasons to study HQL effects in other situations. For example, significant differences in HQL could be important to some patients despite substantial (or at least statistically significant) differences in survival. A determination of what is a "small" difference in survival, after all, requires a value judgment: a judgment of the relative importance of survival and quality of life to the patient. Importantly, a significant change in survival or HQL as seen through the eyes of the statistician may not be viewed as clinically important by the patient or physician. As pointed out by Edlund and Tancredi (48), to understand quality of life measures, we need to know "who is talking about quality of life? what sort of quality is being specified? defined by whom, for whom? decided by whom? One must consider the different social and economic (or bureaucratic) groups who use the phrase, when they use it, how they use it, and finally, why they use it." Predictability about preferences is treacherous, and contrary to some expectations, patients with cancer may forgo a better quality of life and choose a more radical treatment with minimal chance of benefit than those without cancer, including medical professionals (49).

### Use of HQL to Inform and to Develop Health Care Policy

Once HQL data have been derived from clinical trials that are deemed valid and generalizable, several uses can be made of the information. One obvious and direct use is to enable health care professionals to better inform patients about the risks and benefits of a proposed treatment, particularly if the alternatives being considered are the same as those that were compared in a clinical trial. Because HQL data may be a useful prognostic variable (50–53), they can be of further benefit to clinicians and patients in helping them to make informed treatment decisions.

Thus far, most HQL evaluations have been used in attempts to learn about the impact of cancer and the treatments on groups of patients. This has led to a focus on disease rather than on individual patient outcome. As familiarity with HQL assessments increases and their value and limitations become clearer, it is anticipated that they will become an aid in patient management, because they (a) have prognostic value, (b) can be used as independent outcome measures that will help determine the benefit or harm of current antineoplastic or supportive therapy, and (c) can be used as clinical tools to direct earlier initiation of psychological, social, or physical support or rehabilitative measures.

Quality of life data can also be used to determine health policy (54). The information might be used to select alternatives for additional clinical trials or to make decisions about approval of new drugs for marketing. The United States Food and Drug Administration has declared that "a favorable effect [of an anticancer drug] on survival or quality of life is generally required for approval" (55). Assessments of HQL have the potential to enhance decision making about the utilization of health care resources, but because of the pervasive issues of value that are associated with various HQL outcomes (or lack thereof), the information thus gained is open to misuse. As pointed out by Ganz, it will "be imperative that the QL data incorporated into policy decisions be of high quality and that both patient advocates and clinicians play an important role in their interpretation" (18).

## MEASUREMENT OF HQL

### Clinical Assessment

Physicians have placed a premium on the quality of life of their patients throughout the history of medicine. Hippocrates wrote: "I will define what I conceive medicine to be. In general terms, it is to do away with the sufferings of the sick, to lessen the violence of their diseases, and to refuse to treat those who are overmastered by their disease, realizing that in such cases medicine is powerless"

(56). In most clinical oncology offices, physicians regularly obtain HQL information from their patients when they ask "How are you?" or "How's it going?" (57). This question is equivalent to the global HQL evaluation that asks "How would you rate your quality of life today?" or "How satisfied are you at present with your life?" (58). The physician then follows up this question with further questions that probe the ways in which quality of life has been affected by the cancer and its treatment. This assessment is usually qualitative rather than quantitative, but it explores those domains that patients believe have an impact on their quality of life. For example, one patient may have a low satisfaction with his or her current quality of life because of persistent nausea, another because of pain, and another because of a disinterest in talking with friends. These clinical assessments are essential in dealing with individual patient concerns, but they are of little value in collating information about the general and particular effects of cancer and its treatment on the "average" patient. For these purposes, standardized evaluation instruments are needed.

### Standardized Instruments

In order to obtain useful information from groups of patients about HQL, standardized instruments are necessary (21,29,35,36,58–61). Questions that are asked of patients can fall into two major categories: they can be *open questions* to which the respondent may make any response, or *closed questions*, in which the respondent is supplied with a list of responses or a fixed scale on which to indicate a response. Open questions are less likely to restrict possible responses, but they are more difficult to categorize and analyze than responses to open questions and may not cover all important areas because of the patient's reluctance, memory lapses or impairments, or lack of understanding of the scope of acceptable responses (60,62).

### Psychometric and Utility Approaches to HQL Evaluation

Cella has emphasized that there have been two different approaches to measuring quality of life: psychometric and utility (2).

With the *psychometric approach*, instruments are used to measure the impact of the disease, condition, or treatment on the physical, psychological, social, and functional domains of HQL and on overall perceived well-being. This approach does not quantify the weight or importance that patients place on these HQL domains or individual components when it comes to making decisions about alternative treatments, nor does it assess the impact of each component on their overall quality of life.

For example, nausea and vomiting or anxiety may be rated by the patient as severe, but that alone does not tell the investigator how important that is to the patient's feeling of or absence of well-being and further, how that will affect choices of therapeutic alternatives.

The *utility approach* is concerned with decision making and a comparison of two different conditions or treatment approaches in which an assessment is made by the investigator or the patient of the cost-to-benefit ratio of therapy. When utility measurements are made, there is always an explicit or implied evaluation of relative importance. The psychometric approach assesses intensity of symptoms, ability to function, and the psychological state of the patient; the utility approach tries to assess the importance of these factors, relative to each other or other factors, and the impact that they have on practical decisions (63). Utility assessments may involve

1. Offering theoretical choices between the patient's current state of health and various probabilities of cure or death
2. Asking the patient how much time he or she would be willing to give up in order to live the rest of life in perfect health
3. Having the patient subjectively assign the effect of specific HQL impairments on overall quality of life (21)

One current area of development in standardized instruments is to blend the psychometric data with utility estimates in the anticipation that the results will facilitate more informed decision making by individual patients, physicians, and policy makers. This kind of extension of HQL data permits formal assessments of various derived cost-utility parameters. In one type of analysis, total survival is adjusted for quality of that survival to obtain a measure called quality of life years (QALY). One can than compare treatments and calculate the cost for the gain in QALYs. What is done with that information is then a broad societal question that requires the imposition of value of incremental years lived in comparison with cost for the intervention under consideration relative to other health care or societal costs. One criterion states that treatments are reasonably cost effective up to $50,000 per QALY gained (54). When patients themselves are asked about preferences for therapy, there is a reluctance to trade off survival for quality of life (64). This is consistent with the results of Slevin (49), who found that patients were more likely than doctors and nurses to accept radical treatment for minimal benefit.

The majority of HQL instruments in use today are primarily based on the psychometric approach. Examples of 17 generic, cancer-specific, and cancer-site–specific instruments are reviewed elsewhere (65). Their application to cancer clinical trials has been reviewed by Moinpour (36) and Maguire (66).

## Development and Testing of Instruments

The design of a valid, reliable, and useful instrument is not as simple or straightforward as picking some questions that are thought to be important to quality of life, applying a scale, and administering the instrument to patients. In the best-tested instruments there is a systematic process of item generation, item review and reduction, scale construction and piloting, and initial evaluation. Included in the initial evaluation are item analysis, factor analysis, creation of subscales (if there are to be any), and validity testing. Additional evaluation includes test-retest reliability and measurement of sensitivity to change. Validity testing tries to answer this question: Does the instrument measure what it is intended to measure? Measures of validity (21,29,35,60,61) include

1. Content validity—does the measure cover all of the issues of interest and appear to be applicable for the stated purpose?
2. Construct validity—does the measure correlate with other similar measures completed at the same time, and do the results diverge from dissimilar measures completed at the same time?
3. Clinical validity or interpretability—are there correlations with other measures of health status, is there a responsiveness to a change in health status over time, and do the results have clinical relevance?

Once the instrument has undergone development and initial assessment, repeated evaluations over time in different populations are required to determine its specificity for unique populations and generalizability to broader categories of patients or healthy people.

## Generic versus Specialized Instruments

In the search for a gold standard, it was once believed that the choice was between either a broad generic instrument that gave information about general health status and HQL but was not specific enough to detail information relevant to a disease or treatment, or a specific instrument designed for each disease or stage or treatment. Aaronson (67) suggested an alternative modular approach whereby one could design an instrument with a number of general questions that would apply to many situations (e.g., to all patients with cancer) and append to this a module of disease-specific or even trial-specific measures of disease symptoms and treatment side effects. This approach has been carried out by Cella and colleagues (21) and Aaronson and colleagues (29). A related approach uses an established general health measure, such as the Short-Form Health Survey: Medical Outcomes Study (33) and combines this with a global measure of quality of life and specific measures for antici-

**TABLE 1.** *The functional assessment of cancer therapy-lung (FACT-L) HQL instrument*

FACT-L (Version 3)   Below is a list of statements that other people with your illness have said are important. By circling one number per line, please indicate how true each statement has been for you *during the past 7 days.*

| During the past 7 days: | not at all | a little bit | somewhat | quite a bit | very much |
|---|---|---|---|---|---|
| **Physical well-being** | | | | | |
| 1. I have a lack of energy | 0 | 1 | 2 | 3 | 4 |
| 2. I have nausea | 0 | 1 | 2 | 3 | 4 |
| 3. Because of my physical condition, I have trouble meeting the needs of my family | 0 | 1 | 2 | 3 | 4 |
| 4. I have pain | 0 | 1 | 2 | 3 | 4 |
| 5. I am bothered by side effects of treatment | 0 | 1 | 2 | 3 | 4 |
| 6. I feel sick | 0 | 1 | 2 | 3 | 4 |
| 7. I am forced to spend time in bed | 0 | 1 | 2 | 3 | 4 |

8. Looking at the above 7 questions, how much would you say your PHYSICAL WELL BEING affects your quality of life? (Circle one number)

   0  1  2  3  4  5  6  7  8  9  10
*Not at all*                             *Very Much so*

| During the past 7 days: | not at all | a little bit | somewhat | quite a bit | very much |
|---|---|---|---|---|---|
| **Social/Family well-being** | | | | | |
| 9. I feel distant from my friends | 0 | 1 | 2 | 3 | 4 |
| 10. I get emotional support from my family | 0 | 1 | 2 | 3 | 4 |
| 11. I get support from my friends and neighbors | 0 | 1 | 2 | 3 | 4 |
| 12. My family has accepted my illness | 0 | 1 | 2 | 3 | 4 |
| 13. Family communication about my illness is poor | 0 | 1 | 2 | 3 | 4 |
| 14. I feel close to my partner (or the person who is my main support) | 0 | 1 | 2 | 3 | 4 |
| 15. Have you been sexually active during the past year? No___ Yes___ If yes: I am satisfied with my sex life | 0 | 1 | 2 | 3 | 4 |

16. Looking at the above 7 questions, how much would you say your SOCIAL/FAMILY WELL-BEING affects your quality of life? (circle one number)

   0  1  2  3  4  5  6  7  8  9  10
*Not at all*                             *Very Much so*

| During the past 7 days: | not at all | a little bit | somewhat | quite a bit | very much |
|---|---|---|---|---|---|
| **Relationship with doctor** | | | | | |
| 17. I have confidence in my doctor(s) | 0 | 1 | 2 | 3 | 4 |
| 18. My doctor is available to answer my questions | 0 | 1 | 2 | 3 | 4 |

19. Looking at the above 2 questions, how much would you say your RELATIONSHIP WITH THE DOCTOR affects your quality of life? (circle one number)

   0  1  2  3  4  5  6  7  8  9  10
*Not at all*                             *Very Much so*

| During the past 7 days: | not at all | a little bit | somewhat | quite a bit | very much |
|---|---|---|---|---|---|
| **Emotional well-being** | | | | | |
| 20. I feel sad | 0 | 1 | 2 | 3 | 4 |
| 21. I am proud of how I'm coping with my illness | 0 | 1 | 2 | 3 | 4 |
| 22. I am losing hope in the fight against my illness | 0 | 1 | 2 | 3 | 4 |
| 23. I feel nervous | 0 | 1 | 2 | 3 | 4 |
| 24. I worry about dying | 0 | 1 | 2 | 3 | 4 |
| 25. I worry that my condition will get worse | 0 | 1 | 2 | 3 | 4 |

26. Looking at the above 6 questions, how much would you say your EMOTIONAL WELL-BEING affects your quality of life? (circle one number)

   0  1  2  3  4  5  6  7  8  9  10
*Not at all*                             *Very Much so*

| During the past 7 days: | not at all | a little bit | somewhat | quite a bit | very much |
|---|---|---|---|---|---|
| **Functional well-being** | | | | | |
| 27. I am able to work (include work in home) | 0 | 1 | 2 | 3 | 4 |
| 28. My work (include work in home) is fulfilling | 0 | 1 | 2 | 3 | 4 |
| 29. I am able to enjoy life | 0 | 1 | 2 | 3 | 4 |
| 30. I have accepted my illness | 0 | 1 | 2 | 3 | 4 |
| 31. I am sleeping well | 0 | 1 | 2 | 3 | 4 |
| 32. I am enjoying the things I usually do for fun | 0 | 1 | 2 | 3 | 4 |
| 33. I am content with the quality of my life right now | 0 | 1 | 2 | 3 | 4 |

34. Looking at the above 7 questions, how much would you say your FUNCTIONAL WELL-BEING affects your quality of life? (circle one number)

   0  1  2  3  4  5  6  7  8  9  10
*Not at all*                             *Very Much so*

**TABLE 1.** *Continued*

| During the past 7 days: | not at all | a little bit | somewhat | quite a bit | very much |
|---|---|---|---|---|---|
| Additional concerns | | | | | |
| 35. I have been short of breath | 0 | 1 | 2 | 3 | 4 |
| 36. I am losing weight | 0 | 1 | 2 | 3 | 4 |
| 37. My thinking is clear | 0 | 1 | 2 | 3 | 4 |
| 38. I have been coughing | 0 | 1 | 2 | 3 | 4 |
| 39. I have been bothered by hair loss | 0 | 1 | 2 | 3 | 4 |
| 40. I have a good appetite | 0 | 1 | 2 | 3 | 4 |
| 41. I feel tightness in my chest | 0 | 1 | 2 | 3 | 4 |
| 42. Breathing is easy for me | 0 | 1 | 2 | 3 | 4 |
| 43. Have you ever smoked? | | | | | |
|     No___ Yes___ If yes: I regret my smoking | 0 | 1 | 2 | 3 | 4 |
| 44. Looking at the above 9 questions, how much would you say your ADDITIONAL CONCERNS affect your quality of life? (circle one number) | *0  1  2  3  4  5  6  7  8  9  10*<br>*Not at all*                                            *Very Much so* | | | | |

pated disease and treatment-specific HQL outcomes, such as unique symptoms.

### Example of HQL Instruments in Cancer

The Functional Assessment of Cancer Therapy (FACT) measurement system is an example of a psychometric instrument with a utility component (21). The FACT measurement is a 34- to 50-item compilation of a generic core of 34 items and specific subscales that can be appended for specific diseases. These subscales reflect symptoms and other problems that may be associated with disease sites, such as lung, breast, bladder, cervix, colon/rectum, head and neck, ovary, or prostate, or with human immunodeficiency virus (HIV) infection. Table 1 provides an example of one of these instruments, the FACT-L (Lung). Items 1 through 34 constitute the FACT-G (General), which can be given to any patient with cancer. Items 35 through 44 are administered only to patients with lung cancer. The FACT is broken into six components from which subscales can be derived: (a) physical well-being, (b) social/family well-being, (c) relationship with doctor, (d) emotional well-being, (e) functional well-being, and (f) additional concerns (disease specific, treatment specific, or both).

Questionnaires such as the FACT are usually completed by the patients themselves, with instructions by a research assistant or nurse but without assistance in completing the questions. The importance of patient-assessed HQL has been confirmed in cardiovascular disease (9) and cancer (10,68). Following the completion of the questionnaire, the nurse or research assistant reviews the responses to help ensure that all questions are completed (if possible) so as to minimize the number of unanswered questions. For patients who have difficulty in completing the questionnaire by themselves, it is preferable to have a nurse or research assistant help with the questions, since family members are more likely to insert their own biases about patients' responses than a person who has been trained to be neutral. Results are then analyzed by use of a manual provided by the developer of the instrument.

While instruments such as the FACT are not widely used in the clinic to inform health care professionals about their patients' ongoing quality of life concerns or to make individual decisions about patients, these self-administered instruments can be easily adapted to such a purpose, particularly as the health care professional becomes more familiar with the instrument and with the interpretation of individual responses.

The European Organization for Research and Treatment (EORTC) QLQ-C30 (29,69) is a similar core questionnaire developed by the EORTC. It has an additional virtue of having consistent reliability and validity across three language-cultural groups: patients from English-speaking countries, those from northern Europe, and those from southern Europe. In contrast to the FACT, it does not ask patients to render a judgment regarding how much each of the domains (e.g., social well-being) affects their quality of life, though it does ask global questions about how patients rate their overall physical condition during the past week and how they rate their overall quality of life during the past week. The selection of the question time frame is influenced by the disease and treatment under study: if one is looking at a relatively short duration of side effects, then there must be a clearly defined time of interest in the questions. This will also relate to the timing of administration of the instrument relative to the treatment. As pointed out by Aaronson, even in the case of long-term effects, the use of a relatively short time frame, such as a week, will minimize problems associated with memory loss or a tendency over time to minimize or exaggerate symptoms or functional impairment (67).

A different type of instrument used in patients with cancer is the Cancer Rehabilitation Evaluation System (CARES), developed by Schag, Ganz, and others (70,71).

This is a comprehensive list of 139 problems encountered by patients with cancer. Patients rate each problem on a five-point scale. The first 88 items apply to all patients. The remaining questions apply to subgroups of patients. For instance, if a person does not have children, that section is skipped; if the person has not been employed, that section is skipped. A short form with 59 items has also been developed. It is intended particularly for use in research protocols where repeated measures may be needed and too long a time taken completing an instrument would be undesirable.

A third example of a quality of life instrument is a newly developed Hospice Quality of Life Index (72). This is a 25-item satisfaction questionnaire that has visual analog scales with adjectival anchors on each end of a 100-mm line on which the patient must make a single mark. Each item is then weighted by the patient relative to its importance for his or her quality of life. This instrument has been much less rigorously tested and validated than the first two, but it may have broader validity for patients who are only receiving supportive care.

## QUALITY OF LIFE OUTCOMES IN CANCER PATIENTS

Quality of life outcomes in patients with cancer that have been assessed by well-validated instruments have become much more common in the past several years, though their interpretation and usefulness to the oncology community has not yet been fully realized (73,74). Most studies have been in breast cancer, with fewer studies in other types of cancer, and fewer yet in the supportive care or palliative care setting. Some have addressed palliative care offered by cancer treatment. Because HQL evaluations have been most developed for patients with specific cancers, some examples of what has been done and the types of results will be discussed in this section, followed by a description of the development of HQL in supportive care and the potential for future directions both in research and in clinical care.

### HQL in Breast, Lung, and Other Cancers

#### Breast Cancer

An earlier study of HQL was an evaluation of patients receiving treatment for advanced breast cancer using a linear analogue self-assessment (LASA) by Priestman and Baum (75). In one group of women with breast cancer they evaluated HQL with this technique before and after 3 months of endocrine therapy. In another group, they compared subjective toxicity with two different cytotoxic regimens. While the analysis was not highly sophisticated, they reached the following conclusions:

1. Patient age does not greatly influence the degree of subjective disturbance.
2. A smaller fall in the LASA score during the second cycle of chemotherapy suggested that patients tend to adjust to their side effects with time.

The National Institutes of Health Consensus Development Conference Statement, "Adjuvant chemotherapy for breast cancer," stated that "The goal of adjuvant therapy is to significantly prolong survival while maintaining an acceptable quality of life" (76). Many HQL studies that addressed primarily "psychosocial" problems have been done in patients receiving adjuvant therapy for breast cancer. For example, Meyerowitz (77) studied 50 women receiving adjuvant chemotherapy and found that 88% reported a decrease in activities from the adjuvant chemotherapy, 54% reported an increased financial burden, and 41% said their treatment had an adverse effect on their family or sexual life. Interestingly, 74% said they would definitely recommend the treatment to their friends. This disparity demonstrates that the psychometric analysis (how much of a problem they have experienced) without the utility analysis (the relative importance of the symptoms versus possible benefit from treatment) gives incomplete information. A 2-year followup of 35 of these patients 21 months after treatment ended found that there were significant improvements in quality of life in most areas, though there were continuing problems in the physical area (78). Anxiety levels were found by Cassileth to be similar in patients randomized to adjuvant chemotherapy versus observation in women on two Eastern Cooperative Oncology Group studies (79). While the sample was small, the data were sufficient to rule out major differences in anxiety levels among women randomized to each arm.

The effectiveness of supportive care, such as for nausea and vomiting, clearly can make a difference in HQL outcome. The investigators in one early study of adjuvant chemotherapy in breast cancer and its effects on quality of life believed that the side effects from multiple drug regimens were so severe that they decided to stop a study of doxorubicin, vincristine, fluorouracil, methotrexate, and chlorambucil. Major side effects were nausea and vomiting, alopecia, and feeling "off color." Nearly 30% of the patients said the treatment was unbearable or that they would "never again" undertake it (80).

Kemeny and associates looked at psychosocial outcome in 52 (62%) of 83 patients randomized to mastectomy versus segmentectomy (81). They found that women with segmentectomies felt less anxious, less sad, and more in control of their lives. Even the fear of recurrence was less in the segmentectomy group. Offering a choice of surgery in early breast cancer has been shown to reduce anxiety in both patients and their husbands (82).

Coates and others (43) looked at the HQL effect of intermittent versus continuous treatment strategies for advanced breast cancer and concluded that continuous chemotherapy was better than intermittent chemotherapy. In other words, it does not help to take a break and wait for the disease to progress. The implication is that cancer (or the concern about doing nothing for the cancer) has a greater adverse effect on HQL than does chemotherapy.

A different approach that tried to put some relative value on health states regarding adjuvant therapy of breast cancer was pioneered by Gelber and associates, who coined the concept "time without symptoms or toxicity" (TWiST) and a modification of it, the quality-adjusted TWiST (Q-TWiST) (44,83,84). Their studies supported adjuvant therapy as providing more quality time to patients, even when the toxic periods were subtracted from the total survival.

### Lung Cancer

In lung cancer, Cella found that the psychological distress was correlated with worsening performance status and that when the performance status was poor, the extent of disease was also a determinant of distress (85). An early study in lung cancer using the Functional Living Index–Cancer (FLIC) found that when patients did not complete the instrument, not enough information was obtained for rigorous analysis (86), but correlations were found, as might be expected, between HQL and performance status. Compliance problems are not trivial, but there appear to be methods that minimize their occurrence (87). Psychological response has been compared in patients with lung cancer receiving either intravenous methotrexate, doxorubicin, cyclophosphamide, and oral lomustine (repeated in 21 days) or intravenous cyclophosphamide, doxorubicin, vincristine, and oral lomustine, (with the doxorubicin and vincristine repeated in 21 days) (88). This study showed a "strong trend" to more fatigue and depression in the second group, which was hypothesized to be due to the vincristine, despite no differences in clinical response. It demonstrated the value of HQL studies in lung cancer or other cancers, though the conclusions themselves have no importance for current lung cancer therapy. Other studies, as mentioned previously, have shown that assessment of HQL can be a predictor of survival in lung cancer. Assessment of HQL by the Functional Living Index—Cancer (FLIC) is superior to performance status for predicting survival in patients with lung cancer (50,51).

Systematic evaluation of symptoms at presentation in patients with lung cancer has shown that the chest symptoms commonly inquired about are not the only issues of concern to patients. Tiredness, lack of appetite, worry, and anxiety as well as cough and shortness of breath are most common and are equally present in patients with both small-cell and non–small-cell carcinomas of the lung (89). The authors suggest that all symptoms at the outset of disease must be taken into account when the benefit of palliative therapy is assessed.

Other cancers have been studied less regularly, though each common cancer, modality of therapy, and age group has probably had some HQL or psychosocial evaluation (46,90–95).

### HQL in Symptomatic Care

In contrast to the burgeoning development of HQL assessments in clinical trials of cancer therapy, there has been relatively little systematic advancement in the design of specific instruments or the use of standardized instruments for patients receiving supportive, palliative, or posttreatment followup care (96–98). In their literature review of the psychologic and psychosocial implications of survivorship of cancer in adults, Welch-McCaffrey and associates (99) point to significant psychosocial concerns of patients who have had cancer and are no longer undergoing active treatment. They include fear of recurrence and death, relationships with the health care team, adjustment to physical compromise, alterations in customary social support, isolationism, psychosocial reorientation, and employment and insurance problems. For many patients who are no longer undergoing active therapy, psychological and social support are necessary for optimal rehabilitation. Survivors of various cancers have been studied in a systematic fashion by use of validated instruments (100). One conclusion has been that patients who survive cancer do not return to a state of normal health, which emphasizes the need for continuing supportive care after active cancer treatment has ended. The relative absence of good prospective studies, however, has meant that retrospective studies, case reports, and legal overviews have been the primary source of information about such effects (99).

Farncombe (101) has suggested that the model for palliative care has shifted in recent years from one in which there was a sharp break between active aggressive therapy and palliative therapy to one in which there is a gradual shift in the balance between the approaches. This means that the HQL evaluations of supportive oncology care must not be relegated only to patients who will no longer be offered active antineoplastic therapy, but can, in fact, take place throughout the course of management of the cancer (97,98,102). The need for supportive care as a key ingredient of total cancer care is being recognized by many National Cancer Institute—designated cancer centers that have ongoing research programs in supportive care (103). The prevalence of symptoms has been shown to be highly associated with psychological distress and poorer quality of life (104). This association highlights the need for regular assessment of HQL in the evaluation of symptom management during all phases of cancer care.

Occasional chemotherapy studies have been done in which palliation was the primary endpoint of therapy. Moore and co-workers (105) treated hormone-resistant prostate cancer with mitoxantrone and prednisone and used HQL as the endpoint. Evaluation tools included a pain intensity score and a modification of the EORTC core questionnaire. By these criteria, 9 of 25 patients achieved a palliative response for 6 or more weeks of therapy, despite the fact that only 1 patient had a measurable objective partial response.

HQL has been compared in patients with terminal cancer who were dying in palliative care units or in the hospital. Using a variety of psychological scales, Viney and associates (106) looked at uncertainty, anxiety, depression, anger, helplessness, competence, sociability, and good feelings through content analysis of interview material. They found that patients in specialized palliative care units showed less indirectly expressed anger and more positive feelings. Interestingly, they also reported more anxiety about death but less anxiety about isolation.

HQL has been found to deteriorate in most patients during the last weeks of life, though a substantial group (20%) of patients cared for in hospices felt that they had a good quality of life even toward the end of life (107). This suggested that attention to patients' concerns could play a role in the maintenance of HQL as perceived by the patients and that factors other than physical function are contributors to HQL in terminal cancer. When patients with varying prognoses were compared by use of the EORTC QLQ-C30, the main effect of prognosis was on the general QOL scale and the physical aspects of HQL, with little effect on social or psychological functioning (102).

Because of the weak physical state of most patients who are terminally ill, Cohen and Mount (97) have suggested that the ideal palliative care HQL instrument is one that can be administered verbally (orally) in 10 to 15 minutes. They believe that the measure should determine how satisfied the patients are with the various aspects of their lives that are evaluated, and that they should be asked how important that aspect is to them (utility weight).

Single-problem issues can be important and legitimate foci for HQL evaluations in supportive care. In such circumstances, the HQL instrument may be limited to various facets of the single problem, such as the response of anorexia to megestrol acetate, which was reported to improve appetite, increase weight, food intake (108). Pain relief has been a common single-problem focus in the HQL arena. An example of this is a study of palliative pamidronate in the treatment of patients with bone metastasis from breast cancer (109). As an alternative to the study of only one symptom, broader instruments may be used to determine the impact of one problem on overall HQL.

Issues of feeding, nutrition, and hydration are among those that will benefit from more systematic evaluation of HQL. Patients who have been monitored during terminal illness to determine the frequency of hunger and thirst reveal that hunger is infrequent and can be usually be palliated by small amounts of food (110). Thirst can be relieved by careful mouth care and sips of water—less than would be ordered to prevent hydration. It is concluded that attention to what the patient requests is probably of greatest benefit to most patients. If patients have stopped eating, the production of ketones may lead to suppression of hunger and mild euphoria. Administration of carbohydrates (as in 5% dextrose and water) could serve to reverse this and reawaken hunger (111). If artificial feeding is deemed appropriate, the enteral approach should be used if possible. Padilla (112) reported that even in those who had lost the normal ability to eat, enteral tube feedings gave patients more perceived control, were less stressful, and produced fewer psychosocial problems than parenteral feeding. Finally, vigorous attempts at hydration in patients whose heart and kidneys are failing may inadvertently lead to fluid overload, pulmonary congestion, and a more uncomfortable death than had the natural processes been allowed to take place.

An additional area of supportive care that is as least as difficult to study is that of the use of drugs for symptoms control during the last days of life (113). Issues that must be addressed not only include the quality of the living and dying by the patient and the predominance of the patient's own wishes for the relief of suffering, but also the perceptions of the family about the patient's suffering and their own suffering. Consideration must also be given to ethical, social and religious issues surrounding suffering and its relief by allowing death to occur in the process of relieving the suffering (114,115).

While there obviously is a limit to when and under what circumstances HQL testing can be done, it may be possible to formally ask alert patients in the terminal stages of disease how much relief or discomfort they experience from those things we do to try to help. Indeed, it has been suggested that many palliative care patients welcome the opportunity to participate in clinical research, because they recognize that they will receive state-of-the-art care and also that hey will continue to provide meaning for their lives by contributing to society as they and their families deal with their life-wrenching illness.

One such study has been done by the Methylprednisolone Preterminal Cancer Study Group, which studied the effect of an 8-week course of methylprednisolone, 125 mg daily, in a double-blind, placebo-controlled trial (116). Assessment of HQL was made by use of the Nurses' Observational Scale for Inpatient Evaluation (NOISIE), the Linear Analog Self-assessment Scale (LASA), and the Physicians' Global Evaluation. In all scales, treatment was more effective in improving HQL but was associated with a higher mortality rate in females. The reason for the latter result was not established.

One problem in the evaluation of HQL in patients receiving cancer treatment is a high attrition rate (86). This is a particular problem in patients receiving palliative chemotherapy who may die during therapy or become too ill to be able to or wish to continue reporting on their HQL (117). This does not mean that HQL evaluations should not be done but that the limitations of the population must be considered when studies are designed.

The Staunton Harold Sue Ryder Hospice used a method of assessing HQL at the time of patients' admission to their program that deliberately avoided standardized instruments. This was based upon their opinion that standardized measures in the later stages of terminal illness were inappropriate because of poor patient acceptance, the "danger" of missing an aspect of suffering that was of most immediate concern to the patient, and the unreliability of observers' assessments of of these patients' needs (118). They found this technique helpful in identification of previously unrecognized or underrated problems, particularly those that were psychosocial. They found that the use of the Patient Evaluated Problem Score (PEPS) was also helpful in evaluating progress and that it was acceptable to patients, even those who were within a week of dying. The authors recognized that this type of questionnaire cannot easily be used as a research tool, nor is it appropriate for interpatient comparison.

Another approach to the evaluation of palliation is the "audit." Such an approach can determine the perspective of health care providers on symptom relief, objective response, and improved activity status. This approach can be used to assess the cost-effectiveness of palliative therapy (119). While this use of predetermined criteria for effectiveness is valuable and is one component of the determination of effectiveness of symptom management, it is necessarily incomplete without the patients' perspective obtained from HQL evaluations (120).

## CONCLUSION

As society becomes more concerned about the cost of high-technology care, legitimate questions can be raised about how to integrate the patient's subjectively determined quality of life into the formulation of total medical benefits and costs incurred with supportive oncology care. The costs of care will be most problematic if the care given is seen as "futile" or "marginal" (121). Without a doubt, HQL measurements will be factored into clinical practice guidelines and policies by professional societies, insurance carriers, states, and perhaps the federal government.

It has been proposed that HQL tools will be more widely used in the future, so that oncologists will become as familiar with them as they now are with performance status, and find them as useful (18). If standardized HQL scores are found to be reliable and clinically meaningful

endpoints for groups of patients in clinical trials, they may become integral to the process of making individual patient treatment recommendations and decisions. The degree to which this happens will depend on the results of current clinical trials and the ease with which these results and their meanings are translated to individual patient scenarios by clinicians. Such a development will be contingent on the maturation of HQL evaluations in clinical trials now under way, dissemination of the findings, and a demonstration of their discriminatory value for prognosis and for understanding the benefits and burdens of cancer therapy in cancer. If this comes about, such HQL evaluations may be able to identify problems that can be addressed immediately by the physicians or other members of the health care team. As Till points out, it is not just those who are directly involved in HQL research who have legitimate priorities, nor even the health care providers, but especially patients and their advocates (73).

## REFERENCES

1. Cella DF. Measuring quality of life in palliative care. *Semin Oncol* 1995;22(2 Suppl 3):73.
2. Cella DF. Using quality of life and cost-utility assessments in cancer treatment decisions. In: Skeel RT, Lachant NA, eds. *Handbook of cancer chemotherapy*, 4th ed. Boston: Little, Brown, 1995:80.
3. Roy DJ. Measurement in the service of compassion [editorial]. *J Palliat Care* 1992;8:3.
4. Taylor KM, Feldstein ML, Skeel RT, Pandya KJ, Ng P, Carbone P. Fundamental dilemmas of the randomized clinical trial process: results of a survey of the 1737 Eastern Cooperative Oncology Group Investigators. *J Clin Oncol* 1994;12:1796.
5. Marshall E. Armageddon revisited. *Science* 1987;236:1421.
6. Flanagan JC. Measurement of quality of life: current state of the art. *Arch Phys Med Rehabil* 1982;63:56
7. Calman KC. Quality of life in cancer patients—an hypothesis. *J Med Ethics* 1984;10:124
8. Clipp EC, George LK. Patients with cancer and their spouse caregivers: perceptions of the illness experience. *Cancer* 1992;69:1074.
9. Jachuck SJ, Brierley H, Jachuck S, Willcox PM. The effect of hypotensive drugs on the quality of life. *J R Coll Gen Pract* 1982; 32:103.
10. Jennings BM, Muhlenkamp AF. Systematic misperceptions: oncology patients' self-reported affective states and their caregivers' perceptions. *Cancer Nurs* 1981;4:485
11. Bell DR, Tannock IF, Boyd NF. Quality of life measurement in breast cancer patients. *Br J Cancer* 1985;51:577.
12. Glimelius B, Hoffman K, Olafsdottir,M, Pahlman L, Sjoden P, Wennberg A. Quality of life during cytostatic therapy for advanced symptomatic colorectal carcinoma: a randomized comparison of two regimens. *Eur J Cancer Clin Oncol* 1989;25:829.
13. Kaasa S, Mastekassa A Naess S. Quality of life of lung cancer patients in a randomized clinical trial evaluated by a psychosocial well-being questionnaire. *Acta Oncol* 1988;27:335.
14. Slevin ML. Quality of life: philosophical question or clinical reality? *Br Med J* 1992;305:466.
15. Wenger NK, Mattson, AME, Furgerg CD, Elinson J. Assessment of quality of life in clinical trials of cardiovascular therapies. *Am J Cardiol* 1984;54:908.
16. Moinpour C. Assessment of quality of life in clinical trials. In: Nayfield SG, Hailey BJ, McCabe M, eds. *Quality of life assessment in cancer clinical trials*. Report of the Workshop on Quality of Research in Cancer Clinical Trials. July 16–17, 1990. Bethesda, MD: US Department of Health and Human Services, 1991:21
17. Nayfield SG, Ganz PA, Moinpour CM, Cella DF, Hailey BJ. Report

from a National Cancer Institute (USA) workshop on quality of life assessment in cancer clinical trials. *Qual Life Res* 1992;1:203.

18. Ganz PA. Quality of life and the patient with cancer. Individual and policy implications [Review]. *Cancer* 1994;74(4 Suppl):1445.

19. Testa MA, Nackley JF. Methods for quality-of-life studies. *Ann Rev Public Health* 1994;15:535.

20. Saunders CM. Appropriate treatment, appropriate death. In: Saunders CV, ed. *The management of terminal disease*. London: Edward Arnold, 1978:3.

21. Cella DF, Tulsky DS, Gray G, et al. The functional assessment of cancer therapy scale: development and validation of the general measure. *J Clin Oncol* 1993;11:570.

22. Andersen BL. Psychological interventions for cancer patients to enhance the quality of life. *J Consult Clin Psychol* 1992;60:552.

23. Spiegel D, Bloom JR, Kraemer HC, Gottheil E. Effect of psychosocial treatment on survival of patients with metastatic breast cancer. *Lancet* 1989;2:888.

24. Fox BH. The role of psychological factors in cancer incidence and prognosis. *Oncology* 1995;9:245.

25. Yellen SB, Cella DF, Leslie WT. Age and clinical decision making in oncology patients. *J Natl Cancer Inst* 1994;86:1766.

26. Yellen SB, Cella DF. Someone to live for: social well-being, parenthood status, and decision-making in oncology. *J Clin Oncol* 1995; 13:1255.

27. Mor V. QOL measurement scales for cancer patients: differentiating effects of age from effects of illness. *Oncology* 1992;6(Suppl):146.

28. Adler NE, Boyce T, Chesney MA, et al. Socioeconomic status and health: the challenge of the gradient. *Am Psychologist* 1994;49:15.

29. Aaronson NK, Amedzai S, Bergman B, et al. The European Organization for Research and Treatment of Cancer QLC-C30: a quality-of-life instrument for use in international clinical trials in oncology. *J Natl Cancer Inst* 1993;85:365.

30. Spitzer WO. State of science 1986: Quality of life and functional status as target variables for research. *J Chronic Dis* 1987;40:465.

31. Berzon RA, Simeon GP, Simpson RL, Donnelly MA, Tilson HH. Quality of life bibliography and indexes: 1993 update. *Qual Life Res* 1995;4:53.

32. Osoba D. Lessons learned from measuring health-related quality of life in oncology [Review]. *J Clin Oncol* 1994;12:608.

33. Stewart AL, Hays RD, Ware JE. The MOS Short-form General Heath Survey. Reliability and validity in a patient population. *Med Care* 1988;26:724.

34. Hunt SM, McKenna SP, McEwen J, et al. The Nottingham Health Profile: subjective health status and medical consultations. *Soc Sci Med* 1981;15A:221.

35. Donovan K, Sanson-Fisher RW, Redman S. Measuring quality of life in cancer patients. *J Clin Oncol* 1989;7:959.

36. Moinpour CM, Feigel P, Metch B, Hayden KA, Meyskens FL, Crowley J. Quality of life end points in cancer clinical trials: review and recommendations. *J Natl Cancer Inst* 1989;81:485.

37. Skeel RT. Quality of life assessment in cancer clinical trials—it's time to catch up. *J Natl Cancer Inst* 1989;81:472.

38. Wenger NK, Mattson ME, Furberg CD, Elinson J, eds. *Assessment of quality of life in clinical trials of cardiovascular therapies*. New York: LeJacq Publishing, 1984.

39. Grant I, Heaton RK, McSweeny AJ, et al. Neuropsychologic findings in hypoxemic chronic obstructive pulmonary disease. *Arch Intern Med* 1982;143:1941.

40. Ganz PA, Moinpour CM, Cella DF, Fetting JH. Quality-of-life assessment in cancer clinical trials: a status report [Editorial; Comment]. *J Natl Cancer Inst* 1992;84:994.

41. Gotay CC, Korn EL, McCabe MS, Moore TD, Cheson BD. Building quality of life assessment into cancer treatment studies. *Oncology* 1992;6:25.

42. Gotay CC, Korn EL, McCabe MS, Moore TD, Cheson BD. Quality-of-life assessment in cancer treatment protocols: research issues in protocol development [Review]. *J Natl Cancer Inst* 1992;84:575.

43. Coates A, Gebski V, Bishop JF, et al. Improving the quality of life during chemotherapy for advanced breast cancer. A comparison of intermittent and continuous treatment strategies. *N Engl J Med* 1987; 317:1490.

44. Gelber RD, Goldhirsch A. A new endpoint for the assessment of adjuvant therapy in postmenopausal women with operable breast cancer. *J Clin Oncol* 1986;4:1772.

45. Kornblith AB, Anderson J, Cella DF, et al. Comparison of psychosocial adaptation and sexual function of survivors of advanced Hodgkin disease treated by MOPP, ABVD, or MOPP alternating with ABVD. *Cancer* 1992;70:2508.

46. Chang AE. Functional and psychosocial effects of multimodality limb-sparing therapy in patients with soft tissue sarcoma. *J Clin Oncol* 1989;7:1217.

47. Silverfarb PM, Holland, JCB, Anbar D, et al. Psychological response of patients receiving two drug regimens for lung carcinoma. *Am J Psychiatry* 1983; 140:110.

48. Edlund M, Tancredi LR. Quality of life: an ideological critique. *Perspect Biol Med* 1985;28:591.

49. Slevin ML, Stubbs L, Plant HJ, Wilson P, Gregory WM. Attitudes to chemotherapy: comparing views of patients with cancer with those of doctors, nurses, and general public. *Br Med J* 1990;300:1458.

50. Ganz PA, Lee JJ, Siau J. Quality of life assessment. An independent prognostic variable for survival in lung cancer. *Cancer* 1991;67:3131.

51. Ruckdeschel JC, Piantadosi S, and the Lung Cancer Study Group. Quality of life assessment in lung surgery for bronchogenic carcinoma. *J Thorac Surg* 1991;6:201.

52. Coates A, Gebski V, Signorini D, et al. Prognostic value of quality of life scores during chemotherapy for advanced breast cancer. *J Clin Oncol* 1992; 10:1833.

53. Seidman AD, Portnoy R, Yao T-J, et al. Quality of life in phase II trials: a study of methodology and predictive value in patients with advanced breast cancer treated with paclitaxel plus granulocyte colony stimulating factor. *J Natl Cancer Inst* 1995;87:1316.

54. Porzsolt F, Tannock I. Goals of palliative cancer therapy. *J Clin Oncol* 1993;11:378.

55. Johnson JR, Temple R. Food and Drug Administration requirements for approval of new anticancer drugs. *Cancer Treat Rep* 1985;69:1155.

56. Jones WHS, ed. *Hippocrates, "the art,"* vol II. Cambridge, Harvard University Press. The Loeb Classical Library. 1923:193.

57. Szalai A. In: Salazi A, Andrews FM, eds. *The quality of life: comparative studies*, 7–21. Beverly Hills: Sage, 1980. Cited in Barofsky I: Quality of life assessment: evolution of the concept. In: Ventafridda V, Van Dam FSAM, Yancik R, Tamburini M, eds. *Assessment of quality of life and cancer treatment*. Amsterdam: Excerpta Medica International Congress Series 702. Elsevier Science Publishers, 1986:11.

58. Olschewski M, Schumacher M. Statistical analysis of quality of life data in cancer clinical trials. *Statist Med* 1990;9:749.

59. Cella DF, Tulsky DS. Quality of life in cancer: definition, purpose, and method of measurement [Review]. *Cancer Invest* 1993;11:327.

60. Fayers PM, Jones DR. Measuring and analyzing quality of life in cancer clinical trials: a review. *Statist Med* 1983;2:429.

61. Guyatt GH, Feeny DH, Patrick DL. Measuring health-related quality of life. *Ann Intern Med* 1993;118:622.

62. Schuman H, Scott J. Problems in the use of survey questions to measure public opinion. *Science* 1987;236:957.

63. Kaplan RM. Quality of life assessment for cost/utility studies in cancer [Review]. *Cancer Treat Rev* 1993;19(Suppl A):85.

64. O'Connor AMC, Boyd NF, Warde P, Stolbach L, Till JE. Eliciting preferences for alternative drug therapies in oncology: influence of treatment outcome description, elicitation technique and treatment experience on preferences. *J Chronic Dis* 1987;40:811.

65. Tchekmedyian NS, Cella DF, eds. Quality of life in current oncology practice and research. *Oncology* 1990;4:21.

66. Maguire P, Selby P. Assessing quality of life in cancer patients. *Br J Cancer.* 1989;60:437.

67. Aaronson NK. Methodologic issues in psychosocial oncology with special reference to clinical trials. In: Ventafridda V, Van Dam FSAM, Yancik R, Tamburini M, eds. *Assessment of quality of life and cancer treatment*. Excerpta Medica International Congress Series 702. Amsterdam: Elsevier Science Publishers, 1986:29.

68. Kahn SB, Houts PS, Harding SP. Quality of life in patients with cancer: a comparative study of patient versus physician perceptions and its implications for cancer education. *J Cancer Educ* 1992;7:241.

69. Osoba D, Zee B, Pater J, Warr D, Kaizer L, Latreille J. Psychometric properties and responsiveness of the EORTC Quality of Life Questionnaire (QLQ-C-30) in patients with breast, ovarian, and lung cancer. *Qual Life Res* 1994;3:353.

70. Schag CC, Heinrich RL, Aadland R, Ganz PA. Assessing problems of cancer patients: psychometric properties of the Cancer Inventory of Problem Situations. *Health Psychol* 1990;9:83.

71. Ganz PA, Schag CAC, Lee JJ, Sims MS. The CARES: a generic measure of health related quality of life for patients with cancer. *Qual Life Res* 1992; 1:19.

72. McMillan SC, Mahon M. Measuring quality of life in hospice patients using a newly developed hospice quality of life index. *Qual Life Res* 1994;3:437.

73. Till JE, Osoba D, Pater JL, Young JR. Research on health-related quality of life: dissemination into practical applications. *Qual Life Res* 1994;3:279.

74. Hopwood P, Stephens RJ, Machin D. Approaches to the analysis of quality of life data: experiences gained from a medical research council lung cancer working party palliative chemotherapy trial. *Qual Life Res* 1994;3:339.

75. Priestman TJ, Baum M. Evaluation of quality of life in patients receiving treatment for advanced breast cancer. *Lancet* 1976;1:899.

76. Adjuvant chemotherapy for breast cancer. *NIH Consensus Statement Outline* 1985 Sep 9–11;5(12):1–19.

77. Meyerowitz BE, Sparks FC, Spears IK. Adjuvant chemotherapy for breast carcinoma. Psychosocial implications. *Cancer* 1979;43:1613.

78. Meyerowitz BE, Watkins IK, Sparks FC. Psychosocial implications of adjuvant chemotherapy. A two-year followup. *Cancer* 1983;52:1541.

79. Cassileth BR, Lusk EJ, Walsh WP. Anxiety levels in patients with malignant disease. *Hospice J* 1986;2:56.

80. Palmer BV, Walsh GA, McKinna JA, Greening WP. Adjuvant chemotherapy for breast cancer: side effects and quality of life. *Br Med J* 1980;281:1594.

81. Kemeny MM, Wellisch DK, Schain WS. Psychosocial outcome in a randomized surgical trial for treatment of breast cancer. *Cancer* 1988; 62:1231.

82. Morris J, Royle GT. Offering patients a choice of surgery for early breast cancer: a reduction in anxiety and depression in patients and their husbands. *Soc Sci Med* 1988;26:583.

83. Gelber RD, Goldhirsch A, Cole BF. Evaluation of effectiveness: Q-TWiST. The International Breast Cancer Study Group. *Cancer Treat Rev* 1993;19 Suppl A:73.

84. Goldhirsch A, Gelber RD, Simes RJ, Glasziou P, Coates AS. Costs and benefits of adjuvant therapy in breast cancer: a quality adjusted survival analysis. *J Clin Oncol* 1989;7:36.

85. Cella D, Orofiamma B, Holland JC, et al. The relationship of psychological distress, extent of disease, and performance status in patients with lung cancer. *Cancer* 1987;60:1661.

86. Finkelstein DM, Cassileth BR, Bonomi PD, Ruckdeschel JC, Ezdinli EZ, Wolter JM. A pilot study of the functional living index—Cancer (FLIC) scale for the assessment of quality of life for metastatic lung cancer patients. *Am J Clin Oncol* 1988;11:630.

87. Sadura A, Pater J, Osoba D, Levine M, Palmer M, Bennett K. Quality-of-life assessment: patient compliance with questionnaire completion [see comments]. *J Natl Cancer Inst* 1992;84:1023.

88. Silverfarb PM, Holland JCB, Anbar D, Bahna G, Maurer H, Chahinian AP, Comis R. Psychological response of patients receiving two drug regimens for lung carcinoma. *Am J Psychiatry* 1983;140:110.

89. Hopwood P, Stephens RJ. Symptoms at presentation for treatment in patients with lung cancer: implications for the evaluation of palliative treatment. The Medical Research Council (MRC) Lung Cancer Working Party. *Br J Cancer* 1995;71:633.

90. Danoff B, Kramer S, Irwin P, Gottlieb A. Assessment of the quality of life in long-term survivors after definitive radiotherapy. *J Clin Oncol* 1983;6:339.

91. Herr HH Quality of life measurement in testicular cancer patients. *Cancer* 1987;60:1412.

92. Mulhern RK, Ochs J, Armstrong FD, Horowitz ME, Friedman AG, Copeland K, Kun L. Assessment of quality of life among pediatric patients with cancer. *Psychol Assess J Consult Clin Psychol* 1989;1:130.

93. Scheithauer W, Rosen H, Kornek GV, Sebesta C, Depisch D. Randomized comparison of combination chemotherapy plus supportive care with supportive care alone in patients with metastatic colorectal cancer. *Br Med J* 1993;306:752.

94. Fossa SD, Aass N, Opjordsmoen S. Assessment of quality of life in patients with prostate cancer [Review]. *Semin Oncol* 1994;21:657.

95. Poon MA. Biochemical modulation of fluorouracil: evidence of significant improvement of survival and quality of life in patients with advanced colorectal cancer. *J Clin Oncol* 1989;7:1407.

96. Bullinger M. Quality of life assessment in palliative care. *J Palliat Care* 1992;8:34.

97. Cohen SR, Mount BM. Quality of life in terminal illness: defining and measuring subjective well-being in the dying. *J Palliat Care* 1992; 8:40.

98. Finlay IG, Dunlop R. Quality of life assessment in palliative care [Review]. *Ann Oncol* 1994;5:13.

99. Welsh-McCaffrey D, Hoffman B, Leigh SA, Loescher LJ, Meyskens FL. Surviving adult cancers. Part 2: Psychologic implications. *Ann Intern Med* 1989;111:517.

100. Schag CAC, Gans PA, Wing DS, Sim M.-S, Lee JJ. Quality of life in adult survivors of lung, colon and prostate cancer. *Qual Life Res* 1994; 3:127.

101. Farncombe ML. Ambulatory supportive care for the cancer patient [Review]. *Curr Opin Oncol* 1994;6:335.

102. Ringdal GI, Ringdal K, Kvinnsland S, Gotestam KG. Quality of life of cancer patients with different prognoses. *Qual Life Res* 1994;3:143.

103. Coluzzi PH, Grant M, Doroshow JH, Rhiner M, Ferrell B, Rivera L. Survey of the provision of supportive care services at National Cancer Institute—designated cancer centers. *J Clin Oncol* 1995;13:756.

104. Portenoy RK, Thaler HT, Kornblith AB, et al. Symptom prevalence, characteristics and distress in a cancer population. *Qual Life Res* 1994;3:183.

105. Moore MJ, Osoba D, Murphy K, et al. Use of palliative end points to evaluate the effects of mitoxantrone and low-dose prednisone in patients with hormonally resistant prostate cancer. *J Clin Oncol* 1994; 12:689.

106. Viney LL, Walker BM, Robertson T, Lilley B, Ewan C. Dying in palliative care units and in hospital: a comparison of the quality of life of terminal cancer patients. *J Consult Clin Psychol* 1994;62:157.

107. Morris JN, Suissa S, Sherwood S, Wright SM, Greer D. Last days: a study of the quality of life of terminally ill cancer patients. *J Chronic Dis* 1986;39:47.

108. Tchekmedyian NS, Hickman M, Siau J, Greco FA, Keller J, Browder H, et al. Megestrol acetate in cancer anorexia and weight loss. *Cancer* 1992;69:1268.

109. van Holten-Verzantvoort AT, Kroon HM, Bijvoet OL, Cleton FJ, Beex LV, Blijham G, et al. Palliative pamidronate treatment in patients with bone metastases from breast cancer. *J Clin Oncol* 1993;11:491.

110. McCann RM, Hall WJ, Groth-Juncker A. Comfort care for terminally ill patients. The appropriate use of nutrition and hydration. *JAMA* 1994;272:1263.

111. Sullivan RJ. Accepting death without artificial nutrition or hydration. *J Gen Intern Med* 1993;8:220.

112. Padilla GV, Grant MM. Psychosocial aspects of artificial feeding. *Cancer* 1985;55:301.

113. Enck RE. Drug-induced terminal sedation for symptom control. *Am J Hospice Palliat Care* 1991;8:3.

114. Latimer E. Caring for seriously ill and dying patients: the philosophy and ethics. *Can Med Assoc J* 1991;144:859.

115. Cain JM, Hammes BJ. Ethics and pain management: respecting patient wishes. *J Pain Sympt Manag* 1994;9:160.

116. Della Cuna GR, Pellegrini A, Piazzi M. Effect of methylprednisolone sodium succinate on quality of life in preterminal cancer patients: a plecebo-controlled, multicenter trial. *Eur J Clin Oncol* 1989;25: 1817.

117. Payne SA. A study of quality of life in cancer patients receiving palliative chemotherapy. *Soc Sci Med* 1992;35:1505.

118. Rathbone GV, Horsley S, Goacher J. A self-evaluated assessment suitable for seriously ill hospice patients. *Palliat Med* 1994;8:29.

119. Towlson K, Rubens R. Quality of life: outcome evaluation. *J Palliat Care* 1992;8:22.

120. Rubens RD. Approaches to palliation and its evaluation. *Cancer Treat Rev* 1993;19(Suppl A):67.

121. Lundberg GD. American health care system management objectives: the aura of inevitability becomes incarnate. *JAMA* 1993;269:2554.

*Principles and Practice of Supportive Oncology,*
edited by Ann Berger et al.
Lippincott–Raven Publishers, Philadelphia ©1998

# CHAPTER 66

# Long-Term Survivorship

## Late Effects

Wendy S. Harpham

Long-term cancer survivorship is a modern phenomenon, thanks to progress in diagnosis and treatment. This success has been won at some cost: ongoing and/or new medical problems are common after treatments have been completed. Late effects are those physiological changes or complications that first appear months or years following treatment and are due to the cancer or its treatment. They are of increasing concern because advancements in supportive therapies made dose escalation possible before the advent of methods to prevent the unintended late effects of toxic antineoplastic treatments, and survivors now live long enough to express late effects.

The comprehensive care of cancer survivors demands maximum efforts to prevent, minimize, and effectively treat long-term medical sequelae throughout the survivorship trajectory. An understanding of the spectrum of posttreatment problems will enable researchers and clinicians to develop treatment modifications that will decrease their incidence and severity without compromising disease control. When it can be better determined at the time of diagnosis which patients need aggressive therapy for cure and which will do better with less, physicians will be able to prevent more of the long-term medical consequences by individualizing the type and intensity of therapy. We can hope that basic research will facilitate the trend toward more targeted therapies, so that fewer normal cells are damaged as innocent bystanders. In addition, research will yield insights into the biology of late effects, promoting clinical trials of measures that prevent or minimize their development.

Physicians today are caught in a paradox when they grapple with late effects: as methods of treatment progress, information obtained from long-term survivors of now obsolete therapies becomes meaningless regarding the newer therapies, and information about these newer therapies remains unavailable until adequate time has elapsed to enable assessment of the associated late effects. The literature reflects a lack of consensus regarding how long-term survivors of adult cancers should be screened for recurrent cancer, a new second primary cancer, or nonmalignant late effects. Consequently, the responsibility for choosing specific methods of followup for long-term survivors rests in the hands of individual doctors.

Until definitive data and recommendations are available, primary care physicians and specialists are faced with the challenge of integrating a patient's cancer history into a comprehensive wellness program. Late effects clinics for survivors of childhood malignancies offer a useful model for long-term followup of survivors of adult cancers (1). This chapter presents information and suggestions from the perspective of an internist who is a survivor. The goal is to help health care professionals tailor their current practices to facilitate comprehensive care of their patients who have a history of cancer.

## BIOLOGY OF LATE EFFECTS

An individual's course throughout life reflects the dynamic interaction between insults (infection, toxin exposure, surgery, injury, genetically programmed pathologic conditions, medications, psychosocial stresses) and the body's responses to maintain homeostasis. In the normal aging process, progressive loss of homeostatic reserves occurs gradually over years, the rate of decline of each organ system being influenced by diet, personal habits, environment, and genetic factors. In the long-term

W. S. Harpham: Department of Internal Medicine, Presbyterian Hospital of Dallas, Dallas, TX 75231.

survivor, this loss of reserves may be accelerated depending on the type of cancer and its treatment. Late effects are the end result of physiologic insults, many of which are unique to cancer survivors, and the long-term survivors' decreased ability to respond in a manner that minimizes the clinical expression of pathologic conditions.

Cancer treatments can be responsible for causing late effects (Table 1). Surgery performed to diagnose or treat cancer can cause late effects because of the physiologic changes due to altered or removed body part(s), or subsequent scarring. Chemotherapy and radiation therapy are responsible for most late effects. The therapeutic benefits of chemotherapy and radiation therapy depend on the selective cytotoxicity of malignant cells over normal cells. When injury to normal tissues is not repaired completely, late effects may develop: stem cell depletion in the bone marrow can lead to changes in the blood that persist indefinitely or develop at a later time; repair processes such as fibrosis may distort normal tissue architecture in a functionally significant way; arteriocapillary fibrosis challenges circulatory reserve; radiation and many chemotherapeutic agents are themselves mutagenic or carcinogenic.

Radiation therapy is a local treatment modality, causing changes in the organs in the radiated field and, to a lesser degree, in tissues receiving scatter radiation. The techniques of administering radiation therapy have improved over the past 30 years, offering greater protection of normal tissues. Rapidly dividing normal cells, such as the lining of the intestines, the bone marrow, and the skin, are most at risk of acute radiation injury. Once treatment ends, repair processes proceed over a finite period of time, either restoring the tissue to its pretreatment state or resulting in residual abnormalities. In contrast to acute radiation reactions, chronic damage from radiation also occurs in tissues that normally have little cell turnover, is less easily identified or treatable, and tends to be progressive rather than self-limited (2). Patients who experience skin induration, ulceration, and fibrosis in the radiated field months or years later may require biopsy to differentiate benign postradiation changes from malignancy (3).

Chemotherapy is a systemic treatment modality; late effects can occur in organ systems far removed from the tumor being treated. Immunotherapy such as interferons,

interleukins, colony-stimulating factors, T-cell preparations, tumor vaccines, tumor necrosis factors, and monoclonal antibodies may be responsible for late effects that are hard to distinguish from those that are due to chemotherapy and/or radiation therapy that was delivered before, during, or after biologic agents. Although one of the theoretical advantages of these agents relates to better target-cell selectivity, even a minor perturbation of the highly complex immune system may lead to clinical sequelae. Treatment with antibodies that are conjugated to toxins or radioactive isotopes may carry the long-term risks of these active agents.

The clinical expression of late effects is influenced by many factors related to the treatment course in addition to the type of drugs or radiation used: the dose per treatment, total dose, dose frequency, duration of treatment, and local circumstances due to infection, postoperative state, injury, or prior or concurrent therapies (Table 2). The age and developmental stage of the patient at the time of treatment, and the age at the time of presentation, also play a role. Although the risk of most late effects increases with increased exposure to antineoplastic therapy, some late effects can occur at any dose (e.g., interstitial fibrosis following bleomycin) (4). Exposure to both chemotherapy and radiation therapy, even when they are given at different times, can have additive or synergistic effects on the risk or severity of certain late sequelae. The development of acute or delayed problems does not always predict the development or severity of subsequent late effects, nor does their absence always result in a sparing of late complications.

The risk of radiation-induced late effects other than second malignant neoplasm appears to be influenced by preexisting damage to end-organ arterioles (3). In addition, radiation may sensitize blood vessels to hypertensive changes (3,5). After the completion of treatment, hypertension from any cause may be associated with significant vascular damage in irradiated blood vessels (3). Thus, irradiation to vital tissues (brain, spinal cord, bowel, heart, or lung) may predispose the patient to the increased risk of devastating late sequelae of organ ischemia or infarction in the setting of subsequent hypertension.

When looked at from a comprehensive care point of view, cancer or treatment-related physiologic changes

**TABLE 1.** *Causes of late effects*

Surgery
  Altered or removed body parts
  Scarring (fibrosis)
Immunotherapy
  Permanent changes in the immune system
  Injury due to the attached toxin (drug or isotope)
Chemotherapy and radiation therapy
  Depletion of stem cells (blood changes)
  Scarring (fibrosis)
  DNA damage (benign and malignant tumors)

**TABLE 2.** *Factors affecting clinical expression of late effects*

Treatment course
  Type of drugs or radiation
  Dose per treatment
  Total dose
  Dose frequency
  Duration of treatment
Local tissue factors
Prior or concurrent therapies
Age at time of treatment
Other medical conditions (e.g., metabolic, circulatory)

**TABLE 3.** *Clinical disease expression in long-term survivors*

Premature development of a normal, age-related change
Atypical presentation of a common medical problem
Increased risk of developing a common problem
Increased risk of developing an unusual problem
Poor response to treatment that is usually effective

may affect the clinical expression of disease (Table 3). Patients may demonstrate (a) premature development of normal, age-related changes, (b) atypical presentations of common medical problems, (c) an increased risk of developing a common medical problem, (d) an increased risk of developing an unusual medical problem, and (e) a poor response to medical or surgical treatment that is usually effective. In long-term survival, the risk-benefit ratio for many of the methods of disease prevention, screening, and treatment is shifted and must be reflected in survivor-specific recommendations.

## MEDICAL EVALUATION OF LONG-TERM SURVIVORS

Throughout the history-taking, physical examination, diagnostic evaluation, assessment, and treatment, the potential impact of the patient's cancer history on normal aging and nonmalignant pathologic processes must be kept in mind. The medical history needs to include the precise cancer diagnosis (histology, extent of disease) and details of antineoplastic treatments received (Table 4). Medical problems experienced by the long-term survivor during and after treatment should be included, as well as all supportive care therapies used, such as reconstructive surgery, chemoprophylactic and replacement hormonal agents, all other medications, and psychosocial support. Survivors' fear of recurrence, and their greater awareness of their own mortality, help shape their perception of symptoms that develop during remission. The effect can vary widely between survivors, or for one survivor at different times, from downplaying or denying serious symptoms to amplifying minor ones.

The patient's family history should be updated annually because new diagnoses may occur and prior diagnoses may come to light that may affect the cost-benefit

**TABLE 4.** *Medical evaluation of long-term survivors*

Medical history
    Cancer diagnosis (histology, extent of disease)
    Antineoplastics received
    Medical problems experienced during and after treatment
    Medications, surgical procedures, psychosocial support
Family history (update annually)
Social history
    Nonprescription medications/therapies
    Alternative therapies

ratio of preventive or screening measures. When eliciting a social history, the health care team must encourage patients to report all nonprescription medicines and therapies they have used or are using. Alternative therapies are frequently pursued by cancer survivors, but information about these measures often is not volunteered unless the patient is asked about them specifically. Even then, patients may be reluctant to admit to their use for fear of reprisal or abandonment. Judgment-free acknowledgment of patients' normal and appropriate desire to do everything possible to regain and maintain good health helps maintain open communication. Patients need to understand why the health care team's complete knowledge of all the patient's therapies is vital to high-quality care. In this setting, physicians have the opportunity to teach patients the facts about alternative therapies.

Routine followup for the lifetime of the long-term survivor offers repeated opportunities to reestablish a baseline, pursue primary prevention of late effects, provide counsel regarding the signs and symptoms of late effects, encourage health-promoting lifestyle changes, offer genetic counseling when appropriate, and pursue disease monitoring and early detection for second malignancies and other late effects.

How should the long-term survivor be educated about his or her role in the prevention, early detection, and treatment of late effects, and encouraged to act on sound knowledge in a health-promoting way? The concept of late sequelae is emotionally charged, both for the patient who has survived a brush with death and for the health care team that made the decisions and administered the treatments that enabled that survival. The health care team should focus on the modifiable risk factors that influence the survivor's overall risk of developing specific late effects.

The health care team can help survivors overcome the fear, anxiety, anger, depression, and maladaptive denial that often accompany discussions of late effects by providing the information that most serious late effects occur in only a minority of long-term survivors. Reminding survivors that continuing research will provide a narrowing of the spectrum of late effects, and an expansion and enhanced efficacy of preventive and treatment options, helps survivors find and nourish hope. Comprehensive care of the cancer patient demands that the same expertise, energy, empathy, and support that were provided during the crises of diagnosis and treatment are provided throughout survivorship, which is "from the time of discovery and for the balance of life" (6).

## SECOND MALIGNANT NEOPLASMS

The feared late effect of a second malignant neoplasm is becoming more common. The exact contribution of treatments to patients' increased risk of a second malignant neoplasm is difficult to determine because the increased risk over age-matched controls may be due to a combination of (a) genetic vulnerability to a series of malignancies, (b) ongoing risk-carrying lifestyle behavior(s), (c) the carcinogenetic effect of chemotherapy, (d) the carcinogenetic effect of radiation, (e) treatment-induced hormonal changes, or (f) immunosuppression due to a preexisting immunodeficiency; permanent, treatment-induced immunologic changes; or the need for exogenous immunosuppressive therapy (Table 5).

Surgery can be associated with an altered risk of second malignant neoplasm. Ureterosigmoidostomy, as in the treatment of bladder cancer, increases the risk of subsequent adenocarcinoma of the colon (7). Postsurgical chronic lymphedema has been associated with a small but increased risk of angiosarcoma (8,9). Adenocarcinoma of the gastric stump is a recognized complication of gastrectomy and gastroenterostomy (10). Splenectomy may be a risk factor for the subsequent development of a hematologic malignancy following successful treatment for Hodgkin's disease (11–14). Surgical menopause has been associated with a decreased risk of subsequent breast cancer (15,16).

Hormone manipulation can play a role in oncogenesis. Survivors of prostate cancer who take exogenous estrogens have an increased risk of developing breast cancer, hepatoma, and desmoid tumors (17). Unopposed estrogen use has been associated with an increased risk of endometrial cancer. Combination birth control pills with an adequate progesterone component have been associated with temporary protection from ovarian cancer (18,19).

Radiation therapy can initiate and promote tumorigenesis. The risk of radiation-associated leukemia appears greatest after low-dose irradiation to a large volume of bone marrow, attributed to sublethal genetic alterations, in contrast to cell death after high-dose irradiation (18–21). Lymphomas and solid tumors (carcinomas of breast, thyroid, salivary glands, skin, gastrointestinal tract, bone, and soft tissues; sarcomas; meningiomas; and astrocytomas) have been associated with direct radiation to tissue or, less often, indirect radiation scatter (18–32). Studies suggest that high-dose irradiation >50 Gy is more likely to induce a solid second malignant neoplasm than low-dose radiation (33). Regarding radiation-associated breast cancer, an increased incidence has been reported among long-term survivors, especially those who received irradiation to the breast at a relatively young age (34–42). Although

many factors affect an individual's risk of developing breast cancer, exposure to radiotherapy (the field, dose, patient's age at time of treatment, posttreatment interval) must be considered in the assignment of risk for a second malignant neoplasm of the breast.

The incidence pattern over time differs for postradiation leukemia versus solid tumors, and it differs among the various solid malignancies. Most excess incidence of leukemia occurs in the 2 to 12 years following treatment; most studies indicate that the increased incidence gradually disappears by 15 years after treatment. In contrast, the increased incidence of solid tumors tends to appear 10 or more years after radiotherapy and continues indefinitely (43). Latency intervals of 2 to 45 years for various solid second malignant neoplasms have been reported. This wide range is consistent with the observation that some radiation-induced solid tumors seem to occur at the same age at which spontaneous tumors of the same type are most prevalent, and may reflect differences in growth rates of neoplasms originating in various organ sites, or the influence of age-dependent factors (26). However, some secondary cancers, such as breast cancer following mantle radiation therapy, are evident at an earlier age than when they are commonly encountered as a primary neoplasm (41).

Chemotherapy can be tumorigenic, although secondary solid tumors are infrequently associated with antineoplastic drugs and are associated with a shorter latency than those that are radiation-induced (44). Long-term cyclophosphamide administration is associated with an increased risk of urothelial carcinomas as well as transitional cell and, occasionally, squamous cell carcinomas of the bladder (45). Various chemotherapeutic agents, but especially alkylating agents, have been associated with the development of myelodysplastic syndromes, acute myelocytic leukemia, and non-Hodgkin's lymphoma, the three most common second malignant neoplasms following chemotherapy.

Alkylating agents are notorious leukemogens, the risk of myelodysplastic syndrome/acute myelocytic leukemia being increased with increased age, exposure to increased cumulative dose or increased number of alkylating agents, or cotreatment with 4-epidoxorubicin, an Adriamycin congener that affects DNA-topoisomerase II (46,47). Standard-dose cyclophosphamide-containing adjuvant chemotherapy for breast cancer has not been associated with an increased risk of leukemia (48). The median latency from the beginning of treatment with an alkylating agent to the onset of detectable myelodysplastic syndromes is 4 to 5 years (range <1 year to >25 years). The peak incidence occurs at 4 years, with a continued increased incidence until a plateau is reached at 10 years, when the risk becomes the same as in the general population.

Other chemotherapeutic agents have been found to be leukemogens. The epipodophyllotoxins etoposide and

**TABLE 5.** *Factors predisposing to second malignant neoplasms*

Genetic vulnerability
Ongoing risk-carrying lifestyle behaviors
Carcinogenetic effect of chemotherapy
Carcinogenetic effect of radiation
Hormonal changes
Immunosuppression

teniposide have been found to be leukemogenic through their effect on DNA-topoisomerase II. Other drugs that act on this enzyme include doxorubicin, 4-epi-doxorubicin, dactinomycin, and mitoxantrone. Risk is increased with increased cumulative dose and increased frequency of administration of epipodophyllotoxins, and it appears to be independent of patient age. In contrast to alkylating agent-induced myelodysplastic syndrome/acute myelocytic leukemia, epipodophyllotoxins are associated with acute myelocytic leukemia without a detectable preceding myelodysplastic syndrome phase, and usually have a shorter latency period (21,46). The cytogenetic changes are different from those seen with alkylating agent-related myelodysplastic syndrome/acute myelocytic leukemia, and the response to intensive chemotherapy is better.

Cisplatin is probably leukemogenic, but there are far fewer cases of myelodysplastic syndrome or acute myelocytic leukemia following cisplatin-containing regimens that do not include either alkylating agents or epipodophyllotoxins (49). Leukemogenic effects may be synergistic or additive between drugs that act on topoisomerase II and those that act on DNA directly (cisplatin and alkylators) (46,50,51). Studies in breast cancer survivors suggest that anthracycline exposure in combination with cisplatin or alkylating agents may be leukemogenic (48). The risk of myelodysplastic syndrome is increased in patients exposed to antilymphocyte globulin for the treatment of aplastic anemia.

A constellation of findings in peripheral blood and in bone marrow is necessary to diagnose myelodysplastic syndrome and classify it into one of the five myelodysplastic syndrome subtypes. Although the incidence of leukemic progression and average length of survival differs among the types of myelodysplastic syndrome, the prognosis is also affected by the degree of cytopenia and the presence of certain genetic abnormalities. The risk of infection and bleeding is disproportionate to the degree of cytopenia because of associated cell dysfunction. The majority of patients with myelodysplastic syndrome have symptoms at the time of diagnosis: fatigue, weakness, fever, or signs and symptoms of cytopenia. Fewer than 10% have hepatomegaly, splenomegaly, lymphadenopathy, gingival hypertrophy, skin infiltration, or neurological abnormalities secondary to central nervous system involvement (21).

Bone marrow transplantation is associated with an increased risk of second malignant neoplasm. Data are beginning to accrue regarding the risk of myelodysplastic syndrome/leukemia or a new solid cancer following transplantation (52–56). More studies are needed to assess the degree of risk over a lifetime of specific second malignant neoplasms in relation to specific conditioning regimens, patient factors, primary malignancies, and posttreatment factors such as graft-versus-host disease. A recent study of solid second malignant neoplasms following bone marrow transplantation revealed an ele-

vated risk for melanoma and cancers of the buccal cavity, liver, brain, thyroid, bone, and connective tissue. The risk increased over time and rose significantly in survivors who were under 10 years of age at the time of transplantation. Longer followup was needed before conclusions could be drawn about the risk of other solid cancers, such as those of the breast or lung (56).

Lifelong cancer prevention and screening for a second malignant neoplasm must be part of the routine followup care of long-term survivors for the rest of their lives, especially survivors of carcinogenic treatments. The specific studies pursued in each long-term survivor are determined by an assessment of risk, keeping in mind both the general incidence patterns of the various malignancies and the wide range of latency periods reported for almost all types of second malignant neoplasm. Notation should be made of all potentially carcinogenic treatments received for benign or malignant disease, any personal or family history of disease associated with later development of malignancy, and any past or current lifestyle behaviors that affect risk. The results of a thorough physical examination and appropriate preliminary screening studies will then dictate which additional studies are indicated, if any. Although treatment-induced leukemias respond poorly to available treatments, many of the solid second malignant neoplasms are potentially curable. One would expect prognosis of the latter to be improved with earlier diagnosis.

A history of radiation to an organ must be considered one risk factor for the development of cancer of that organ and nearby structures. Meticulous examination of organs in previously radiated fields, and compliance with available cancer screening (e.g., urinalysis, Papanicolaou smear, stool test for occult blood, sigmoidoscopy, mammography) must be continued for the life of the long-term survivor in order to increase the likelihood of early detection of a second malignant neoplasm. Any signs and symptoms of possible malignancy, such as a mass, must prompt an immediate evaluation. Plain x-rays with a minimum of two views should be taken of any painful area or mass in a previously irradiated field. Sonography, computed tomography, or magnetic resonance imaging may be indicated in some cases where plain x-ray films are inconclusive.

A history of chest irradiation in the long-term survivor of Hodgkin's disease is an important factor when the methods of breast cancer screening, evaluation, and treatment are being determined. Studies in women with a history of Hodgkin's disease treated with mantle irradiation indicate a markedly increased risk of breast cancer, the risk increasing dramatically after a latency of 15 years, and with an increased relative risk in the first 15 years in those woman who also received chemotherapy with methotrexate, oncovin, prednisone, and procarbazine (40). Careful clinical breast examinations should be done routinely (39,40,44); some authors cite 6 months as a minimum interval between evaluations (39). There is variability in authors' recommendations for the timing of screening mammography. The recommendations for patients treated with mantle irradiation before age 30 include baseline films 5 or 10 years later, or at age 30 or 35 if that comes sooner (41,44), and annual mammography begun 8 or 10 years after irradiation, or at age 30 if that comes sooner (39,41,44). The evaluation of a breast mass should reflect the rising evidence of increased risk of malignancy, significant numbers of false-negative mammograms in the presence of a mass (39,40,42), and the prevalence of synchronous bilateral disease (39,42) in this population.

After ureterosigmoidostomy, annual intravenous pyelogram and barium enema are recommended by some authors. Symptoms referable to the urinary tract or the large bowel should prompt immediate evaluation (7). The followup routine care of a long-term survivor after long-term cyclophosphamide or ifosfamide, or irradiation to the abdomen or pelvis should include a urology-directed history and urinalysis. Counseling about modifiable risk factors for urinary system malignancies such as tobacco smoking, excessive use of phenacetin, and exposure to aromatic amines takes on heightened importance. When abnormalities are detected, or when the patient develops urinary symptoms, workup should be immediate with urine cytology and flow cytometry, and intravenous pyelography followed by cystoscopy (24).

Increased risk for skin cancers is found in some long-term survivors, such as Hodgkin's disease survivors with their increased risk of melanoma, or patients who have received radiation to the skin. Counseling regarding protection from exposure to ultraviolet light, and aggressive surveillance for and removal of dysplastic nevi and non-melanoma skin cancers, can decrease the risk and impact of developing these malignancies (57). The development of a meningioma in a patient who has received brain irradiation should be approached with an awareness of the tendency of these tumors to behave atypically (23).

Long-term survivors who have received nitrosamine-containing treatments or radiation to the mediastinum should be questioned about esophageal symptoms. There is evidence from animal models for a risk of esophageal cancers, both squamous cell and adenocarcinoma—a risk affected by dietary factors and esophageal reflux (58,59). Since these putative risk factors may be additive or synergistic for squamous cell carcinoma of the esophagus in humans, (60) efforts should be made to control reflux, maintain adequate nutrition, and limit exposure to tobacco, alcohol, and dietary nitrosamines (tobacco, barbecued meats, pickled vegetables, nitrite-containing foods).

Regarding myelodysplastic syndrome/acute myelocytic leukemia, environmental and occupational exposure to agents associated with acute myelocytic leukemia such as benzene, ethylene oxide, and petrol and diesel fumes or liquids should be avoided. As diagnostic radiation may carry a small but real risk, judicious use of these studies is indicated; alternative imaging that provides similar information is preferred. The potential small risk should not sway physicians from using diagnostic irradiation that enables appropriate followup of long-term survivors.

Routine hemograms may reveal anemia and/or neutropenia and/or thrombocytopenia in a long-term survivor exposed to an alkylating agent, procarbazine, or a topoisomerase II inhibitor. Since monocytosis or macrocytosis, or abnormal cell structure without cytopenia, occasionally indicates the presence of myelodysplastic syndrome, a new onset of hematologic changes suggests the possibility of myelodysplastic syndrome even if the changes are subtle. Cytopenia that persists indefinitely following the completion of cytotoxic therapy may be due to the development of myelodysplastic syndrome. Bone marrow aspirate and biopsy will be needed to enable a diagnosis (17). When hematologic changes are noted, care must be taken to exclude deficiency of vitamin $B_{12}$ or folate, heavy metal poisoning, alcohol injury, chronic liver disease, and chronic inflammation, all of which can be accompanied by dysplastic changes. Myelodysplastic syndrome also can occur in the setting of lymphoma or malignant neoplasms, suggesting its presence as a paraneoplastic phenomenon.

When myelodysplastic syndrome is diagnosed, treatment options must be discussed, including those available through clinical trials. The approach to treatment for myelodysplastic syndrome will depend on the patient's age and life expectancy, the degree of cytopenia, the subtype of myelodysplastic syndrome, and comorbid disease. Survival after combination chemotherapy is poor. The best survival results are seen after allogenic bone marrow transplant, the only treatment to date that offers patients the possibility of cure.

Physicians cannot overemphasize to a long-term survivor the importance of making lifestyle changes that minimize additional physiologic or genetic insults. The excessive incidence of many second cancers, such as lung cancer or melanoma in long-term survivors of Hodgkin's lymphoma, may reflect a cofactor role of smoking or ultraviolet light, respectively. Counseling regarding smoking cessation, moderation of alcohol consumption, compliance with a low-fat diet, use of a carcinogen-free diet, participation in doctor-approved exercise programs, and so on should be an integral part of the routine followup care of a long-term survivor.

## LATE EFFECTS ON THE CARDIOVASCULAR SYSTEM

Cardiovascular late effects may be related to treatment-induced changes in the blood vessels, myocardium, endocardium, pericardium, heart valves, aorta, or coronary arteries.

## Systemic and Coronary Vascular Disease

Radiation damages blood vessels of all sizes. Weakening of the walls of large vessels may lead to aneurysm or rupture, two postirradiation risks that are influenced by the extent of any surgery in the area and the amount of supportive structures. Acute and chronic radiation injury of small blood vessels leads to reactive and reparative processes that can be associated with progressive decreased capillary permeability; increased extracapillary fibrosis; occlusion of small vessels; and luminal narrowing due to concentric fibrosis, loss of vascular elasticity, thrombosis, and intimal proliferation. Radiation may sensitize blood vessels to subsequent hypertensive injury (3,5). Hypertension that develops decades after high-dose irradiation may lead to localized vascular insufficiency, and even necrosis of the irradiated volume. Since vascular compromise may remain silent in the setting of adequate collateral flow, one would intuit the potential value of minimizing vasculopathy from any cause in patients who have received radiation.

Control of blood pressure may offer an important means of decreasing the overall risk of some potentially serious late effects of radiation, not only by preserving collateral circulation in nonirradiated vessels but by slowing the rate of radiation-induced vasculopathy. When a long-term survivor develops new-onset hypertension, especially if he or she has received radiation to critical tissues such as the brain, workup must proceed and treatment be instituted as soon as possible. The likelihood of a secondary cause of new-onset hypertension is increased in certain long-term survivors. Renovascular hypertension has been noted in up to 24% of men after cisplatin-based chemotherapy for germ cell tumors (17). Chemotherapy-associated dysautonomia may play a role in some cases of systemic hypertension. Mitomycin and cisplatin have been associated with a thrombotic microangiopathy several months after the end of treatment (61,62). In patients who have received upper abdominal irradiation, radiation nephropathy of one kidney must be considered as a possible cause of malignant hypertension (3).

Radiation has been associated with epicardial coronary artery disease (63–68). The pathophysiology includes endothelial cell damage leading to accelerated atherosclerosis and, more commonly, severe medial and adventitial fibrosis without atherosclerotic changes of the intima. The risk of coronary artery disease increases as the radiation dose increases. It begins 5 years after irradiation, is usually progressive, and is probably due, at least in part, to age-associated changes. Animal and retrospective human studies suggest that radiation may be synergistic with hyperlipidemia in causing accelerated atherogenesis (64,65). The incidence of myocardial infarction attributable to prior radiation is low; it is expected to be even lower in the cohort of long-term survivors treated with modern techniques of radiation therapy. The presentation and course are affected by any radiation-induced changes in the lung, thyroid, pulmonary vasculature, or heart, such as cardiomyopathy or endocardial fibrosis.

Regarding the care of a long-term survivor at risk of radiation-induced coronary artery disease, many advise evaluation and followup of coronary artery disease risk factors (such as hypertension, hyperlipidemia, diabetes, and hypothyroidism) and counseling about behavioral modification (diet, smoking, exercise, stress management) (66). In particular, the results of animal studies suggest that vigilant screening for and treatment of hypertension would help protect against the development of clinically significant coronary atherosclerotic disease. As the recommendations regarding screening for silent ischemia in various populations continue to evolve, and the increased risk of pericardial disease in long-term survivors who have received chest irradiation is high, periodic studies might include a chest x-ray (to measure cardiac silhouette,) electrocardiogram, and/or echocardiography. Periodic image-enhanced stress testing may be considered in asymptomatic long-term survivors who have other risk factors for coronary artery disease or who have received irradiation to the mediastinum prior to the implementation of multiple radiation portals and use of subcarinal blocks.

In male and female long-term survivors with symptoms suggestive of myocardial ischemia several months to decades after mediastinal radiation, early evaluation should be pursued even in the absence of other cardiac risk factors (66). The measurement of left ventricular function at rest can identify adverse effects of irradiation on that function, but exercise imaging studies are more sensitive. The absence of regional wall motion abnormalities makes coronary artery disease as the cause of left ventricular dysfunction less likely (68). Most postirradiation patients are candidates for angioplasty and coronary artery bypass graft. When heart surgery is being considered as primary treatment or as a backup to angioplasty, the possibility of radiation-induced mediastinal and pericardial fibrosis, sclerosis of the proximal aorta, and poor wound healing in previously irradiated tissues must be considered (63).

Raynaud's phenomenon, common in the general population, may be uncovered or exacerbated in the long-term survivor who develops vascular disease. Raynaud's phenomenon is seen during and after treatment with bleomycin, which is often given in combination with vinblastine or cisplatin. Numerous potential mechanisms have been proposed, including hyperreactivity of the central sympathetic nervous system, damage to the vascular endothelium and/or musculature, and impaired nonneurogenic autoregulation of the arteriolar smooth muscle cells (17,61,69). The vasculopathy is usually chronic, improving slowly over the years after completion of chemotherapy in half of patients (17).

## Congestive Heart Failure

Anthracyclines are responsible for the majority of therapy-related cardiotoxicity in long-term survivors. The risk of anthracycline-induced cardiomyopathy-related congestive heart failure is correlated to total cumulative dose, each specific drug having a unique dose-risk curve. An increased risk of clinically significant left ventricular dysfunction is seen when the total cumulative dose of doxorubicin is equal to or greater than 450–500 mg/m$^2$, but toxicity can occur at lower doses (71). The risk of cardiomyopathy is related to the schedule of drug administration: low-dose continuous infusions have less toxicity than high-dose intermittent infusions. Higher risk is also related to age <15 years or >70 years, concurrent or subsequent mediastinal irradiation, prior anthracycline exposure, and preexisting heart disease or cardiac risk factors such as hypertension, hyperlipidemia, or diabetes. Mild cardiomyopathy may be asymptomatic despite evidence of left ventricular dysfunction as revealed by exercise radionuclide angiography (72). The natural history of anthracycline-related cardiomyopathy is highly variable: some patients show gradual improvement in symptoms and objective measures of left ventricular ejection fraction (LVEF), others remain stable, and still others experience progressive—and ultimately lethal—congestive heart failure despite maximal medical therapy (73).

Mitoxantrone is an anthracycline-related anthracene associated with a significantly decreased incidence of cardiotoxicity at equi-myelotoxic doses as doxorubicin (72,74). Prior therapy with anthracyclines increases the risk of mitoxantrone cardiotoxicity. Cardiac irradiation is associated with cardiomyopathy characterized by interstitial myocardial fibrosis (75). The risk is escalated with increased dosage (a dose-response curve with a steep rise above 40 Gy, and especially above 60 cGy), increased percent volume of cardiac muscle irradiated, increased fraction size, prior irradiation, or concomitant or sequential cardiotoxic chemotherapy (76). As cardiac and pulmonary function are highly interdependent, the threshold for the clinical expression of radiation-induced cardiac injury is lowered by the presence of lung disease, radiation induced or otherwise. In patients who received mediastinal irradiation through a single anteroposterior portal or without subcarinal blocks, the possibility of asymptomatic biventricular dysfunction should be kept in mind in light of studies of Hodgkin's disease survivors that showed abnormal results of exercise imaging studies as a common finding 5 to 20 years following radiation therapy (68). Constrictive changes of the pericardium may cause or contribute to decreased diastolic compliance following irradiation.

When a long-term survivor has risk factors for chronic cardiomyopathy, the physician should inquire about dyspnea and symptoms of decreased exercise tolerance, and examine the patient for signs of pulmonary and circulatory congestion. Sinus tachycardia in a patient whose condition is otherwise stable can be the earliest sign of myocardial toxicity (17). Although routine noninvasive cardiac evaluation in asymptomatic long-term survivors has not yet been justified by an ability to predict or intervene in the development of late treatment-induced cardiomyopathy, measures used for evaluating and following other types of cardiomyopathy can be considered, such as obtaining chest x-ray, electrocardiogram, echocardiography, or periodic radionuclide angiography. Assessing for subclinical myocardial disease allows for appropriate cardiac monitoring when patients are likely to be subjected to fluid overload states (as with transfusion), high-output states (such as anemia), or other physiologic stresses that may unmask decreased myocardial contractility (such as pregnancy or major surgery).

When symptoms develop, evaluation of LVEF can be accomplished using multiple gated image acquisition radionuclide scanning or Doppler echocardiography. The advantages of the latter are that the valves, pericardium, and myocardial systolic and diastolic function can be evaluated while the use of radioisotopes is avoided. When the cause of a long-term survivor's decreased LVEF remains unclear and needs to be determined, endomyocardial biopsy can be considered if the special expertise necessary for obtaining and interpreting the specimen is available.

In counseling the long-term survivor with risk factors for the development of chronic cardiomyopathy, it makes sense to discourage the use of excessive alcohol because of the risk of myocardial toxicity. Until information becomes available for this population, drugs with a potential for causing cardiotoxicity, such as lithium, catecholamines, or phenothiazines, should be prescribed with caution (77). Treatment for drug- or radiation-induced cardiomyopathy is similar to that for any cardiomyopathy.

## Arrhythmias and Valvular Disease

Arrhythmias as a late effect are uncommon but may occur in the setting of significant drug-induced cardiomyopathy. In contrast, sinus tachycardia is common in patients with otherwise asymptomatic drug-induced cardiomyopathy. Pulmonary venous hypertension can precipitate supraventricular arrhythmias. Although left ventricular failure is associated with ventricular arrhythmias, sudden death attributable to anthracycline-related heart disease is rare (17). Radiation to the chest can result in damage to the conduction system of the heart, pericardium, coronary arteries, and thyroid, all of which may manifest as rhythm disturbances. Radiation-induced valvular defects can be associated with signs and symptoms of valve stenosis and/or regurgitation, subvalvular stenosis, or outflow tract obstruction (78).

## Pericardial Disease

Pericarditis with effusion is the most common cardiac manifestation of radiation injury and is related to the administered dose and percent volume of heart irradiated (76). Acute pericarditis can appear weeks to several years after irradiation, although the peak incidence is between 5 and 9 months following treatment (17,79). The clinical picture may be similar to that of common idiopathic pericarditis (fever, substernal pain, and dyspnea), although many patients are asymptomatic. Examination may reveal tachycardia and a pericardial friction rub. Effusion is nearly always present and usually resolves spontaneously (17). Signs and symptoms of tamponade may develop if the fluid develops rapidly and/or if there is a large volume of fluid. Chest x-ray may reveal a widened cardiac silhouette. The electrocardiogram may show inversion and flattening of the T waves, elevation of the ST segment, and decrease of the QRS segment. The differential diagnosis for acute pericarditis or effusion includes malignancy (primary or metastatic, involving the pericardium or obstruction of venous/lymphatic vessels) and more treatable causes such as drugs (e.g., hydralazine, procainamide), or collagen vascular disease. Thyroid function must be evaluated, especially in long-term survivors at risk for radiation-induced hypothyroidism.

Radiation-induced acute pericarditis and pericardial effusion is usually self-limited (80). Patients will need followup care that includes clinical assessment and echocardiography or magnetic resonance imaging (68). If the patient is symptomatic, treatment with antipyretics for fever, and nonsteroidal anti-inflammatory agents should be considered (75). The acute syndrome may recur or progress to chronic constrictive pericarditis caused by fibrosis and calcification of the pericardial exudate. Pericardiocentesis or pericardiectomy may be indicated in the treatment of chronic, symptomatic pericardial effusion or tamponade (17,79).

Chronic constrictive changes of the pericardium with varying degrees of effusion characterize chronic pericarditis, a late effect that can first become manifest from 6 months to many years following treatment. Patients may have fatigue, dyspnea, chest pain, pericardial knock, Kussmaul's sign, venous distension, peripheral edema, pleural effusion, and evidence of bowel or hepatic congestion. Paradoxical pulse, fever, and a history of acute pericarditis may or may not be present. The electrocardiogram may show decreased QRS voltage, flat or inverted T waves, and elevation of the ST segment. The chest x-ray may reveal a normal or an enlarged cardiac silhouette. Computed tomography or magnetic resonance imaging may be useful in assessing the degree of pericardial thickening and calcification. Doppler echocardiography, although not as helpful in studying the pericardium, helps to define cardiac hemodynamics. Treatment is geared to the severity of hemodynamic compromise with

pericardiocentesis for tamponade, and pericardiectomy for severe constrictive symptoms (17). The higher complication rate of pericardiectomy in irradiated patients is at least partly due to concomitant radiation-induced restrictive cardiomyopathy (78).

## LATE EFFECTS INVOLVING THE PULMONARY SYSTEM

Cytotoxic therapy can cause late pulmonary effects that compromise quality of life and even lead to premature death. Two major issues are second malignant neoplasms and, more commonly, the early manifestations of chronic, progressive diseases like chronic obstructive pulmonary disease in the setting of loss of lung reserve. Late lung injury due to radiation is a toxic effect characterized by progressive fibrosis and thickening of alveolar septa with alveolar collapse. Some chemotherapeutic agents cause a similar toxic effect (e.g., bleomycin, chlorambucil, nitrosoureas). In addition, an allergic reaction (e.g., to cyclosphosphamide, methotrexate, procarbazine, or bleomycin) or an idiosyncratic reaction such as that seen after low-dose bleomycin may lead to pulmonary fibrosis as a result of interstitial or eosinophilic pneumonitis, alveolar proteinosis, or pulmonary veno-occlusive disease (81,82). Agents that cause pulmonary toxicity may act synergistically (82,83).

Pleural effusions can occur months to years following mediastinal radiation and may be due to pleural changes, constrictive pericarditis, or mediastinal fibrosis causing obstruction of the superior vena cava or lymphatic drainage (84,85). Spontaneous pneumothorax is an unusual late effect that is often small and asymptomatic (86,87). Rarely, radiation-induced bronchial vasculopathy presents as hemoptysis (88). Endobronchial high-dose radiation therapy (brachytherapy) has been associated with the late development of bronchial stenosis, the risk being increased in those who have also received external beam irradiation to the area (89).

Late-onset pulmonary fibrosis has been reported months to decades following radiation or discontinuation of drugs such as cyclophosphamide or BCNU (82,90). Following acute radiation pneumonitis, permanent fibrosis is an expected sequela over the subsequent 6 to 24 months (17). Importantly, significant pulmonary fibrosis can develop as a late effect in the absence of a history of acute radiation pneumonitis. The risk of radiation-associated late pulmonary problems depends on the volume of lung irradiated, dose per fraction, and total dose. The clinical expression of late effects is influenced by preexisting or subsequent pulmonary disease from other causes such as asthma, infection, smoking, chemotherapy associated with pulmonary toxicity, and steroid withdrawal.

Most patients who receive radiation to any part of the lung develop asymptomatic radiographic abnormalities.

Radiographic evidence of scarring often reflects the treatment portal but can show regional contraction, pleural thickening, tenting of the diaphragm, and linear streaking radiating beyond the field of irradiation. Significant lung contraction can be associated with a compensatory hyperinflation of the remaining lung, which accentuates the changes. With time, the radiograph can reveal benign fibrotic pulmonary nodules, which are difficult to distinguish from malignant neoplasms. Computed tomography, Gallium-67 citrate imaging, and single photon emission computerized tomography (SPECT) ventilation-perfusion scans are more sensitive tools than plain radiographs for detecting and following lung fibrosis. Magnetic resonance imaging may find a place in the noninvasive evaluation of pulmonary abnormalities (91).

Scar represents an area of decreased or absent gas exchange. Pulmonary function tests may reveal persistent defects following large lung volume irradiation: a reduction in maximum breathing capacity and tidal volume, and an increase in minute ventilation. Diffusion capacity is the most sensitive indicator of reduced whole lung function.

Radiation-induced fibrosis can be associated with chronic cough, dyspnea on exertion, decreased exercise tolerance, orthopnea, chest pain, cyanosis, and clubbing. Cor pulmonale can lead to failure of the right side of the heart. The clinical expression of treatment-induced pulmonary changes usually occurs only when more than half of the lung volume is involved, but it may be accelerated or exacerbated by coexisting cardiac disease, infection, or certain drugs. The differential diagnosis of respiratory symptoms in long-term survivors includes malignancy, infection, embolic or allergic disease, and other pulmonary disease. Without effective measures to prevent or reverse fibrosis, the treatment remains supportive with bronchodilators, expectorants, antibiotics, rest, and oxygen (17).

Routine chest x-rays and pulmonary function tests that assess lung volumes, compliance, and diffusion capacity should be obtained every 2 to 5 years in asymptomatic survivors who have undergone whole-lung irradiation or exposure to agents that cause pulmonary toxicity (98). The role of prophylactic pneumococcal and influenza vaccines should be discussed. Vigorous counseling about smoking cessation by the health care team is a followup task that cannot be overemphasized. Long-term survivors with pulmonary compromise must be informed of the risks of general anesthesia and evaluated with spirometry, $DL_{co}$, and arterial blood gas analysis before they undergo major surgery (92). Long-term survivors who have been treated with bleomycin should inform all subsequent physicians of this history. When supplemental oxygen is necessary, the lowest fraction of inspired oxygen possible to maintain adequate oxygen saturation should be used (92).

## LATE EFFECTS ON THE URINARY SYSTEM

Late effects of the urinary system include decreased renal function, impairment or obstruction of ureteral or urethral flow, diminished or altered bladder capacity and function, increased risk of infection, vesicovaginal fistula formation, and second malignant neoplasms. Cisplatin-based chemotherapy can be associated with mild persistent compromise of renal function (93,94). Most radiation-associated bladder problems are dose dependent and are due to vasculopathy. They usually occur within 3 years of treatment, although the latency period may last for decades (95,96). Ureteral stricture may first appear years after irradiation.

Determination of serum creatinine level and evaluation of a clean urine specimen for cells and bacteria, as well as examination of the external genitalia, abdomen, flanks, and suprapubic regions, are part of routine followup care. In long-term survivors previously exposed to nephrotoxic drugs such as cisplatin, serum creatinine may remain within normal limits despite substantially impaired creatinine clearance, an abnormality that should be quantitated before potential nephrotoxins are prescribed. Hematuria, flank pain, or a rising serum creatinine level should prompt evaluation with ultrasonography of the kidneys and ureters (96). Long-term survivors should be asked about irritative or obstructive urinary symptoms or incontinence. When urinary tract symptoms are attributed to infection, their resolution should be recorded after treatment. When symptoms persist in the uninfected patient, cytologic study of the urine and ultrasonography of the kidneys and ureters are indicated (96). Large-volume or continuous incontinence in a woman may indicate a urinary tract fistula. Urodynamic studies and fluoroscopy of the lower urinary tract will help define urinary dysfunction. In comparison with similar symptoms in the patient who has not received irradiation, surgical intervention in bladder, ureter, or urethral dysfunction may be more difficult, and the results may be less complete or durable, because of concomitant late effects of the small bowel and vasculature in the irradiated field.

## LATE EFFECTS INVOLVING THE GASTROINTESTINAL TRACT

Most late gastrointestinal sequelae in long-term survivors are due to postoperative changes (e.g., stricture, adhesions, shortened bowel) or postradiation changes. Radiation injury to any part of the gastrointestinal tract can lead to late effects. Radiation to the esophagus may result in fibrosis, leading to dysmotility or benign stricture-related dysphagia. The patient's age, the use of intraluminal brachytherapy, the length of esophagus irradiated, and chemotherapy administered concurrently or soon after radiation may affect the risk and severity of late stricture. Long-term survivors who have undergone high-dose irradiation to the esophagus should be questioned periodically about dysphagia. If dysphagia is present, esophagography or endoscopy can be performed. After malignancy has been ruled out, symptomatic stricture may be managed with dietary modifications, antireflux measures, and dilatation. Reflux esophagitis is usually treated pharmacologically with $H^2$ antagonists, proton pump inhibitors, or prokinetic drugs. Symptomatic spasm can be approached with trials of nitrates, calcium channel blockers, and anticholinergic agents (97).

Radiation to the stomach can cause decreased gastric motility and decreased secretions that may persist for years despite apparent histologic recovery of the mucosa. Dyspepsia has been reported to first develop 6 months to years following gastric irradiation (97). In the light of altered digestion due to changes in gastric motility and secretions, periodic nutritional assessments of serum protein, albumin, iron, and vitamin $B_{12}$ levels seem prudent. Gastric ulceration, or even rupture, is the major significant postirradiation late effect—a risk that appears to be increased after high dose per fraction or high total dose radiation, and previous abdominal surgery (98).

The intestinal epithelium is one of the tissues most sensitive to radiation damage, thus making enteropathy a significant complication of radiation therapy to the abdomen and/or pelvis in terms of both frequency and morbidity. Chronic radiation enteropathy is due to obliterative vascular injury, fibrosis, and mucosal ulcers. Progressive vascular damage and ischemic fibrosis can remain silent for months or years following radiation but become clinically evident in the setting of vasculopathy, such as that due to hypertension, diabetes mellitus, generalized atherosclerosis, or hypoperfusion related to volume depletion or heart failure. Even in the absence of any other conditions, radiation-induced vasculopathy and fibrosis can progress and cause significant morbidity. Factors that increase the risk for late complications of radiation include treatment volume, fraction size, thin body build, and postoperative or postpelvic-inflammatory adhesions before radiation therapy is given. Doxorubicin, 5FU, and mitomycin-C may potentiate the effects of radiation therapy on normal tissues (97).

The symptoms of this potentially debilitating and life-threatening late effect include diarrhea, abdominal cramping, nausea, vomiting, weight loss, obstruction, perforation, fistula formation, or chronic blood loss. Symptoms may first occur 6 months to many decades after treatment; a differential diagnosis for gastrointestinal symptoms must include radiation enteropathy for the rest of the long-term survivor's life, even in the absence of a history of acute radiation injury (99).

In the followup care of long-term survivors at risk of enteritis, physicians should be alert to signs, symptoms, or laboratory results that suggest nutritional deficiency. The evaluation of suspected radiation enteropathy should include the determination of levels of intestinal absorption markers such as vitamin $B_{12}$, carotene, protime, and folate. Seventy-two-hour fecal fat collection and a differential Schilling test may also be useful. In particular, vitamin $B_{12}$ absorption may be impaired by intrinsic factor deficiency, ileal enteropathy, and/or bacterial overgrowth secondary to strictures, fistulas, or defunctionalized areas of intestine. Malabsorption of bile salts caused by ileal damage can lead to significant diarrhea and steatorrhea. Imaging studies can be helpful in the evaluation of these conditions. A small bowel series may show a malabsorption pattern consisting of mucosal edema, separation of small bowel loops, and increased secretions in the bowel lumen. Progressive fibrosis may lead to narrowed, tubular intestinal segments and strictures. Endoscopic examination of involved mucosa may show granularity, multiple telangiectasias, ulcerations, or necrotic areas.

Often, evaluation is nonspecific and the diagnosis is made on clinical grounds (100). The treatment approach should begin with nonsurgical measures: a low-fiber lactose-free or elemental diet, antidiarrheal medication, antispasmodics, and cholestyramine (to bind bile salts that are not absorbed in the ileum) (97,100,101). If partial obstruction does not respond to dietary manipulation, it may respond to temporary bowel rest and total parenteral nutrition at home for several weeks to months. Bacterial overgrowth should be treated with antibiotics. When medical measures fail, surgical resection or bypass is indicated. Optimal surgical technique and timing of this high-risk surgery is controversial and is subject to factors such as the length of intestine involved and the presence of fistulas, occult perforation, or closed loop obstruction. Total parenteral nutrition and broad-spectrum antibiotics should be given before and after definitive surgery (105). Conditions that predispose to intestinal ischemia or vascular compromise, such as hypertension, diabetes, or hypovolemia, should be prevented or treated perioperatively.

At times, the radiographic appearance of radiation-induced enteropathy is indistinguishable from that of chronic ulcerative colitis, granulomatous disease, or neoplasm. Biopsy may be the only way to make a definitive diagnosis, but it must be done with caution because of the additional risk of bleeding or progressive ischemic necrosis due to the compromised vasculature of irradiated tissue.

Radiation enteritis can lead to intestinal lymphangeiectasia, a syndrome of dilated telangiectatic lymphatic vessels of the submucosa of the small intestine; severe peripheral edema; hypoproteinemia; lymphocytopenia; impaired cellular immunity; and mild or absent gastrointestinal symptoms, which when present may include nausea, vomiting, diarrhea, and edema. Other possible causes of lymphangiectasia in long-term survivors include retroperitoneal fibrosis or tumor, mesenteric or diffuse lymphoma, and constrictive pericarditis. Serum protein and immunoelectrophoretic studies, diagnostic paracentesis or thoracentesis, and lymphangiogram may help make the diagnosis. Medical treatment begins with a very-low-fat diet or a diet in which fat is provided only by medium-chain triglycerides. When symptoms are not controlled, elective resection of isolated or severely affected areas of lymphangiectasia can be considered, with the caveat that healing of radiation-injured tissues is impaired.

Chronic radiation injury to the rectum can lead to ulceration, hemorrhage, strictures, fistulization, abscess, or decreased rectal capacity and compliance. Blood-streaked stools or gross rectal bleeding, excessive mucus, colicky abdominal pain, decreasing stool caliber, tenesmus, or progressive obstipation may indicate the development of colonic or rectal stricture. Steroid retention enemas may help proctitis; steroids and oral sulfasalazine have been used for colitis (100,101). In one study, sodium pentosanpolysulfate showed promise (102). Mild symptoms of partial sigmoid or rectal obstruction may be alleviated with mineral oil. Rectal strictures can be dilated manually. Significant obstruction due to stricture requires endoscopic dilatation or surgical intervention. Often, when the colon is seriously injured the small intestine is also involved, and the extent and severity of small bowel involvement will determine the patient's prognosis and overall approach to treatment.

Radiation to the pancreas can lead to pancreatic enzyme deficiency, but rarely to islet cell dysfunction. Radiation-induced hepatopathy has become more common since high-dose irradiation to primary and metastatic hepatic tumors has been added to the range of antineoplastic therapies.

Few chemotherapeutic agents cause long-lasting gastrointestinal problems. Vincristine and vinblastine can cause an autonomic neuropathy that can persist after a prolonged course of treatment, or when administered to elderly patients. The colicky abdominal pain, constipation, and adynamic ileus often respond to conservative treatment.

## LATE EFFECTS INVOLVING THE ENDOCRINE SYSTEM

Endocrine dysfunction may be a consequence of cancer therapy, either as an intended component of antineoplastic therapy or as an undesired complication. Clinically apparent radiation-induced endocrine dysfunction usually has a latency measured in months to years. Surgical or pharmacological alteration of endocrine function usually is evident postoperatively or during chemotherapy; however, endocrinopathies may remain subclinical until unmasked by age-related or other changes. Nonspecific symptoms such as fatigue and anxiety should

prompt assessment of endocrine status. Long-term followup care must include periodic reevaluation and titration of replacement therapies.

Thyroid dysfunction can be a late effect after irradiation or immunotherapy. Irradiation of the pituitary in the course of treating tumors of the pituitary, brain, or head and neck can lead to hypothalamic, pituitary, or primary hypothyroidism many years later (109). Irradiation of the thyroid with mantle or neck irradiation is associated with the development of hypothyroidism and, rarely, hyperthyroidism. Hypothyroidism is common after mantle irradiation, evident clinically or subclinically as defined by elevated serum thyroid-stimulating hormone levels and abnormal thyroid-stimulating hormone response to thyrotropin-releasing hormone (103,104). Cases of hyperthyroidism with low radioiodine uptake, presumably due to radiation-induced thyroiditis, have been reported (105). Exophthalmos can be seen by itself, with hyperthyroidism, or following treatment of hyperthyroidism. Interleukin-2 and/or interferon therapy has been associated with hypothyroidism, initially or following a period of hyperthyroidism, and is probably due to an immune thyroiditis (106). Long-term survivors at risk of treatment-related thyroid dysfunction require lifelong annual evaluation of thyroid anatomy and function. Screening for subclinical hypothyroidism with ultrasensitive determination of serum thyroid-stimulating hormone may be justified by experimental evidence suggesting a role for thyroid-stimulating hormone stimulation in the development of thyroid neoplasms (104,107–110). Signs and symptoms of hypothyroidism, including pleural or pericardial effusions, bradycardias, and hypercholesterolemia, should prompt reevaluation of thyroid status. Overt hypothyroidism should be treated with the goal of keeping the patient euthyroid with a normal level of thyroid-stimulating hormone.

Thyroid neoplasms may also occur in long-term survivors who received neck radiation. Postirradiation thyroid malignancies are usually well differentiated and slow-growing; multicentric lesions are common. They need annual followup of the thyroid with careful palpation of the gland and the cervical lymph nodes. The detection of a single nodule should prompt evaluation with scintiscan and fine needle aspiration. Unless the workup reveals a definitive diagnosis of thyroiditis or Graves' disease, surgery is usually recommended, although some physicians offer patients a trial of exogenous suppression and meticulous followup of a small benign nodule (17,111). A decrease in nodule size while the patient is receiving exogenous thyroid does not rule out malignancy. In light of the higher risk that an irradiated thyroid will develop carcinoma, when surgery is recommended the usual approach is total or near-total thyroidectomy followed by lifelong suppressive therapy (111,112).

Hypothalamic-pituitary dysfunction is a potential complication of irradiation to the face, brain, or neck. The clinical sequelae for irradiated children can be obvious and devastating, whereas the same hormonal perturbations can be associated with more subtle clinical abnormalities in the adult. Growth hormone deficiency may be associated with a decrease in muscle mass and an increase in adipose tissue—changes of import not so much for the cosmetic outcome as for the possible impact on exercise tolerance and lipid metabolism (113). Impaired gonadotropin function can be associated with infertility, sexual dysfunction, and decreased libido; adrenocorticotropic hormone deficiency with poor stamina, lethargy, fasting hypoglycemia, and dilutional hyponatremia (114). Hyperprolactinemia in women is signaled by galactorrhea and/or amenorrhea, and in men by impotence and decreased libido. When symptoms suggest impairment of the hypothalamic-pituitary axis, hyperprolactinemia or evaluation for deficiency of adrenocorticotropic hormone, thyroid-stimulating hormone, growth hormone, or gonadotropins may reveal a treatable late effect. Long-term survivors of endocrine neoplasias that can be part of a syndrome of multiple endocrine neoplasias must be screened serially for the development of the associated second neoplasm(s) (17).

Antineoplastic hormonal therapy can have long-term effects. Tamoxifen is used in the treatment of breast cancer and is being evaluated for its role in the prevention of breast cancer in high-risk women. During the time of use, Tamoxifen appears to exert a beneficial effect on bone density (115) and cholesterol profile (116)—changes that have the potential of translating into a lowered risk of clinically significant osteoporosis and cardiovascular disease. These benefits must be balanced against the increased risk of endometrial cancer (117–119). Any endocrine treatment that results in premature menopause, such as ovarian ablation, increases the risk of premature cardiovascular disease and osteoporosis.

Long-term corticosteroid use may cause or exacerbate medical problems in long-term survivors: secondary and opportunistic infection, myopathy, diabetes, hypertension, coagulopathy, thrombosis, embolization, osteoporosis, osteonecrosis, cataracts, and various types of cancer. Glucocorticoid-induced osteoporosis is related to the dose used and the duration of therapy, as well as many other factors such as hormone status and physical activity. Although daily doses of as little as 7.5 mg of prednisone are believed to cause significant loss of trabecular bone in most patients, bone loss can occur with lower-dose therapy in men and postmenopausal women. Preventive and treatment measures include maintaining physical activity whenever possible, maintaining good nutrition, and restriction of sodium to 2 to 3 grams per day (120). Treatment with calcitonin or bisphosphonate should be strongly considered; however, decisions about these and other treatments, such as calcium supplementation, estrogen or testosterone replacement therapy, diuretics for hypercalciuria, vitamin D for low serum 25-OHD,

sodium fluoride, or anabolic hormones, must weigh the potential risks related to the long-term survivor's history of malignancy and current hormonal and metabolic milieu (17,121–123).

Long-term survivors exposed to corticosteroids may have an increased risk of osteonecrosis, one form of which is aseptic vascular necrosis, a potentially debilitating late effect that usually involves the femoral or humeral head. The risk depends on the administered dose, the duration of therapy, and the cumulative dose, as well as many other factors such as activity level, coexistent vascular disease, and alcohol use. Radiation can also lead to osteonecrosis, in particular aseptic vascular necrosis of the femoral or humeral head following radiation to that area.

Long-term survivors at risk for osteoporosis or osteonecrosis should be counseled about the possible benefits of exercise, and control of blood pressure and lipid levels (16,124). When a patient experiences pain or weakness of the back or a joint, evaluation with x-ray and T-1 and T-2 weighted magnetic resonance imaging on frontal and transversal planes may help rule out other pathologic processes and reveal the characteristic changes of precollapse aseptic vascular necrosis or ischemic vertebral collapse (124). Early detection is important for intervention with protective weight bearing and for optimal timing of core decompression (17,124).

## LATE EFFECTS ON THE NERVOUS SYSTEM

Improved techniques have decreased therapeutic irradiation as a cause of late neurotoxicities. However, supportive therapies that allow dose escalation of chemotherapeutic agents, together with new antineoplastic treatments, have resulted in an increase in certain neurological sequelae. Most signs and symptoms of neurotoxicity appear acutely during cancer treatment, but some therapies cause late effects that first appear months or years later.

### Peripheral, Autonomic, and Cranial Nerve Neuropathies

Chemotherapy-induced peripheral neuropathies, autonomic neuropathies, and cranial nerve palsies usually appear during the treatment course (for example, with vinca alkaloids, cisplatin, or taxol). When potentially neurotoxic chemotherapeutic agents are given when peripheral nerves have already been irradiated (125), or to patients with an underlying neuropathy (e.g., diabetes or Charcot-Marie-Tooth disease), severe neuropathy can develop even with relatively low doses of chemotherapy. Most acute peripheral neuropathies are reversible and do not present prominent long-term problems (126–128). However, the resolution of severe deficits may be slow and incomplete. Cisplatin has been associated with acute and delayed onset of peripheral neuropathy as well as an autonomic neuropathy, which may present as isolated impotence caused by parasympathetic dysfunction (68).

Peripheral nerves are relatively radioresistant; however, cranial nerve and/or cervical sympathetic nerve palsies have been reported in a few patients with nasopharyngeal carcinoma treated with irradiation (129). Sacral plexopathy is a possible complication of pelvic irradiation (130). A late complication of radiation to the axilla can be brachial plexoplathy, the incidence and severity of which appears related to the dose per fraction and total dose (131). Latent periods of 12 to 20 months are common; 20-year latent intervals have been reported. Severe pain usually precedes the development of paresthesias and sensory loss (132).

Long-term survivors with new peripheral neuropathies should be evaluated for all the usual causes seen in the general population. When there is an increased risk of malignancy (e.g., in a middle-aged or elderly patient with weight loss) or if the evaluation does not reveal the cause, a more aggressive search for occult malignancy may be indicated, since polyneuropathy can occur as a remote complication of carcinoma, in up to one-half of patients with osteosclerotic myeloma, and in a small percentage of patients with lymphoma (133,134).

Efforts should be made to minimize trauma to affected nerves and to avoid medications that can cause or exacerbate existing neuropathy. When symptoms of peripheral neuropathy are troublesome, pain relief, supportive measures (e.g., orthosis for foot drop), and physiotherapy may provide relief. Definitive treatment is aimed at the underlying disorder. Analgesic pharmacotherapy with amitriptyline has the potential for unmasking an underlying dysautonomia (e.g., constipation, bladder dysfunction, orthostatic hypotension). Bladder and bowel dysfunction may be less of a problem when desipramine is given. Anticonvulsants such as carbemazepine or phenytoin can also be used as analgesics (17,134).

## Myelopathy, Ototoxicity, Encephalopathy

The differential diagnosis for spinal cord dysfunction in long-term survivors includes recurrent cancer causing spinal cord compression, a paraneoplastic myelopathy, carcinomatous meningitis, or intramedullary metastases. Noncancer causes of myelopathy include postradiation changes, abscess, and hematoma. Postradiation myelopathy is a devastating late effect that can appear as progressive unilateral spastic paralysis and loss of proprioception, and contralateral loss of pain and temperature below a single cord level (Brown-Sequard syndrome,) Lhermitte's sign, and incontinence. The initial symptoms,

which can begin 6 months to years after treatment and may be subtle, may include clumsiness, gait changes, or pain. The symptoms usually progress, but they may stabilize at any degree of severity (135). Magnetic resonance imaging may show cord edema, but radiation-induced myelopathy is a diagnosis of exclusion and is difficult to distinguish from other demyelinating myelopathies. Cases have been reported of myelopathy due to late-occurring radiation vasculopathy precipitating a hemorrhage in the radiation field but at a site distant from the original tumor (136).

Permanent hearing loss is a dose-related late effect of cisplatin. The risk is significantly increased in those who receive >200 mg/m$^2$ (137), are older than 46 at the time of cisplatin administration, or are treated with cranial irradiation involving the ears or temporal lobes before or after cisplatin. Hearing impairment and recurrent otitis media can occur following irradiation to the nasopharyngeal region. Periodic audiograms can be used to identify and monitor hearing loss in long-term survivors. As with any patient with hearing deficit, ototoxins should be avoided when possible.

Methotrexate and high-dose ara-C are drugs that when given intravenously or intrathecally can cause leukoencephalopathy, a chronic neurotoxicity that can first appear months to years following treatment. The risk is increased in younger patients, when methotrexate levels in the central nervous system are elevated, and when methotrexate is administered following cranial radiation therapy. Intrathecal thioTEPA and intraarterial BCNU or cisplatin also have been reported to be associated with leukoencephalopathy (17). Clinically significant chemotherapy-related leukoencephalopathy usually becomes evident 6 to 24 months after the completion of treatment. It appears with insidious, progressive, irreversible focal neurologic signs and loss of cognitive function, sometimes with seizures or ataxia, and may progress to dementia, coma, and death. In addition, postirradiation diffuse injury to the white matter, a form of chronic leukoencephalopathy, is one end of a spectrum of late sequelae that can develop in adult survivors treated with whole-brain cranial irradiation. This demyelinating necrotizing reaction usually appears with dementia and dysarthria and may progress to seizures, ataxia, focal long-tract signs, encephalopathy, or death. The initial symptoms can be subtle, with mild fatigue, headache, personality changes, or loss of recent memory. Evidence of atrophy, calcifications, diffuse white matter degeneration, or focal necrosis can be seen on brain imaging. Current techniques of radiation therapy have all but eliminated radiation as a cause of severe diffuse leukoencephalopathy. At the other end of the spectrum of late effects are varying degrees of cognitive impairment, which appear to correlate with the severity of white matter changes seen on magnetic resonance imaging (150). More studies are needed regarding the incidence, pattern, and relationship to radiation exposure, because current studies have drawn divergent conclusions.

Evaluation of encephalopathy in the long-term survivor must rule out treatable causes, as the diagnosis of chemotherapy or radiation-induced leukoencephalopathy is one of exclusion. A thorough diet and medication history should include inquiry about prescription and over-the-counter medications, as well as alternative therapies. Studies should evaluate the status of the patient's serum electrolyte and glucose levels, liver and renal function, oxygenation, calcium and magnesium, ammonia, and thyroid hormone. Other studies to consider include tests of adrenal function, a urine toxicology screen, and an electroencephalogram. Brain imaging with computed tomography or magnetic resonance imaging should be done to assess for a mass lesion or large-area abnormalities of the white matter suggestive of leukoencephalopathy (16). If the cause remains unclear, and after an imaging scan has ruled out a mass lesion, lumbar puncture can be done to rule out infectious or neoplastic meningitis and to evaluate the cerebrospinal fluid with a protein screen (IgG, oligoclonal bands) (139). Without preventive or therapeutic measures available to reverse or halt the progression, care of the long-term survivor with this complication is solely supportive.

Focal radiation necrosis, which occurs most often after high-dose exposure of a localized area, can present a diagnostic dilemma to physicians who care for patients in remission. Clinical signs and symptoms reflecting the site of focal lesion(s) usually begin 3 months to 4 years following radiation therapy, and the findings on computed tomography and magnetic resonance imaging (mass effect, enhancement, and/or cyst formation) can mimic residual or recurrent tumor. Positron emission tomography, although expensive and not universally available, may be helpful in differentiating radiation-induced necrosis from recurrent malignancy. Temporal lobe necrosis following irradiation of nasopharyngeal carcinoma is infrequent but is potentially disabling or lethal, with a median latency of 5 years (129). High-dose stereotactic radiosurgery and interstitial brain implants have been associated with a delayed (beginning 6 months or more following treatment) subacute reaction that resembles late-occurring radionecrosis but is self-limited. Treatment options for focal radionecrosis include long-term high-dose steroids or resection (135).

## Seizures

Long-term survivors who present with new-onset seizures need evaluation to rule out brain metastases, meningeal carcinomatosis, or one of the many nonmalignant precipitants to seizures that can occur more commonly following treatment for certain types of cancer. An ischemic or hemorrhagic event can occur in the setting of a cancer-related hypercoaguable state or vasculopathy. A CNS infection (bacterial, fungal, viral), brain abscess or infective endocarditis can be related to a persistent immunocompromised state. Seizures can also occur as part of a chronic leukoencephalopathy.

## Carotid Artery Disease/Central Nervous System Hemorrhage

Radiation therapy to the carotid arteries has been associated with premature atherosclerosis, especially when the patient is hyperlipidemic at the time of radiation treatments (140). Narrowing occurs in atypical locations as well as in areas commonly involved in the general population. The clinical presentation is the same as that seen with similarly located lesions in people who have never received radiation. Prevention, early detection, and life-long treatment of hypertension play important roles in preventing and minimizing carotid artery disease after neck irradiation. Patient followup care should include inquiry about symptoms due to possible carotid disease, and screening evaluation with physical examinations and, when indicated, serial ultrasonic vascular imaging. Counseling about modifiable risk factors for carotid disease, in particular hypertension, hyperlipidemia, and smoking, would be expected to decrease the development of clinically significant extracranial arterial occlusive disease, since radiation-induced lesions can remain silent when there is adequate collateral flow. The role of noninvasive imaging in long-term followup is being evaluated; some authors recommend periodic imaging of the carotid arteries following higher-dose (>150 Gy) radiotherapy for head and neck cancer (141).

The surgical approach to carotid disease in the patient who has previously received irradiation should be the same as for the general population, although periarterial fibrous connective tissue around the radiated carotids, and more involvement of the arterial wall by plaque, may make surgery more technically difficult (3).

Long-term survivors with a cerebrovascular accident may have suffered an intraparenchymal central nervous system hemorrhage caused by recurrent cancer. However, survivors of brain tumors have been reported to develop small arteriovenous malformation-like vascular abnormalities. These are associated with microhemorrhages and parenchymal necrosis in the radiation field, distant from the original tumor, which can bleed years after the completion of radiation. Symptoms can develop insidiously or dramatically many years after radiation therapy has ended (136,142,143). Surgical resection of a symptomatic hematoma may be the only way to make the diagnosis (136). Recurrent hemorrhages are not uncommon in this setting because the radiation-induced vasculopathy can be difficult to identify radiographically or pathologically.

## LATE EFFECTS INVOLVING THE HEAD AND NECK

Most late effects from treatment of head and neck cancer are radiation induced. Premature cataracts or glaucoma may develop after local radiation. Problems with the nervous system, endocrine glands, and upper gastrointestinal tract and second malignant neoplasms are discussed elsewhere. Soft-tissue necrosis of the oral cavity mucosa and osteonecrosis of the mandible are late complications caused by progressive vasculopathy that compromises circulation. The risk of tissue necrosis and osteonecrosis is increased after radiation by high doses, large fraction size or treatment volume, interstitial implantation, continued smoking or drinking, and local trauma or dental extraction. Edentulous status lowers the overall risk, but not to the level of that in the general population. Long-term survivors at risk of osteonecrosis should be instructed on the importance of excellent dental hygiene, self-examination of the oral cavity, and regular professional dental evaluation and hygiene. Osteoporosis may be an important factor in postmenopausal tooth loss; estrogen replacement therapy may be beneficial in decreasing oral bone loss, and, consequently, tooth loss (144). Signs and symptoms of dental caries and soft tissue necrosis or infection should be reported immediately. Long-term survivors need to understand that infection can occur spontaneously in an area of compromised blood supply, that tissue injury and infection are often painless, and that early intervention decreases the risk of a chronic or life-threatening problem. The development of a mucosal ulcer can present a diagnostic challenge: differentiating recurrent or new malignancy from benign pathology may be difficult, and biopsy may worsen a benign process caused by radiation-induced small vessel damage. When biopsy or dental extraction is indicated, the risk of complications from the procedure is minimized by taking special precautions such as the use of prophylactic antibiotics, techniques that minimize tissue trauma, specially formulated toothpaste, and possibly pretreatment hyperbaric oxygen (17,145). Radiation-induced laryngeal edema can persist for years (146), causing respiratory obstruction or repeated aspiration, as well as providing a diagnostic dilemma regarding recurrent malignancy. Followup care of head and neck primary sites in long-term survivors must include aggressive counseling and support regarding the increased risk of malignancy associated with continued exposure to tobacco and alcohol.

## MISCELLANEOUS

Sseveral physical and medical issues will be mentioned that deserve attention by health care workers. Various degrees of immunodeficiency, compromised blood supply, and/or barrier defects (anatomic or functional abnormalities of skin or epithelial lining of the gastrointestinal or genitourinary tracts) may be associated with an increased risk of clinically significant viral, bacterial, or fungal infections. Immunodeficiency may be related to prior splenectomy or antineoplastic treatments, current medications, or an underlying genetic defect. Long-term survivors should be encouraged to report signs or symptoms of possible infection and should be reminded about preventive measures such as good hygiene and nutrition. Many are candidates for prophylactic antibiotics and vaccinations and for postexposure immunoglobulin therapy. One must not be lulled into a false sense of security after vaccinations, as the immunocompromised long-term survivor may have an attenuated immune response.

Attention to survivor-specific issues such as recurrent cancer should supplement, not replace, attention to comprehensive wellness issues: cardiovascular screening, screening for other cancers when the long-term survivor has no increased risk for second malignancy, weight control, emotional well-being, etc. Medications and their metabolism may be an ongoing issue for a long-term survivor. The effects of medications taken over a long period must be kept in mind when problems are being evaluated, as must the possibility of altered metabolism related to renal or hepatic dysfunction when therapy is prescribed. Many sequelae that affect quality of life for long-term survivors are not life-threatening or even health-threatening, and are difficult to quantitate. Physical deformity can shape self-esteem and ability to function in certain social, professional, and private settings. This is true of obvious changes such as a facial deformity or aphonia, hidden changes such as a missing breast or testicle, and subtle changes such as fatigue or decreased ability to concentrate. Progress in the field of psychoneuroimmunology will clarify the relationship between health and the chronic stresses of survivorship. The heightened awareness of one's own mortality, and the psychosocial and economic consequences of one's survivorship, can be associated with heightened anxiety or depression which persists for years. These psychological states may have an impact on physical well-being and may be responsive to intervention.

## REFERENCES

1. Schwartz CL, Hobbie WL, et al., eds. *Survivors of childhood cancer: assessment and management.* St. Louis: CV Mosby, 1994.
2. Pavy JJ, Denekamp J, Letschert J, et al. Late effects toxicity scoring: the Soma scale. *Int J Radiat Oncol Biol Phys* 1995;31(5):1044.
3. Cox JD: *Moss's radiation oncology: rationale, technique, results.* St. Louis: CV Mosby, 1994:100,311,501,315.
4. Jules-Elysee K, White DA. Bleomycin-induced pulmonary toxicity. Clin Chest Med 1990;11(1):2.
5. Asscher AW. The delayed effects of renal irradiation. *Clin Radiol* 1064;15:320–325.
6. National Coalition of Cancer Survivorship Charter, Albuquerque, NM 1986.
7. Recht KA, Belis JA, Kandzari SJ, Milan DF. Ureterosigmoidostomy followed by carcinoma of the colon. *Cancer* 1979;44:1538.

8. Stewart FW, Treves N. Lymphangiosarcoma in postmastectomy lymphedema: a report of three cases. *Cancer* 1948;1:64.

9. Edeiken S, Russo DP, Knecht J, et al. Angiosarcoma after tylectomy and radiation therapy for carcinoma of the breast. *Cancer* 1992; 70:644.

10. Sleisenger MH, Fordtran JS. *Gastrointestinal disease*. Philadelphia: WB Saunders, 1993:769.

11. Meadows A, Obringer A, et al. Second malignant neoplasms following childhood Hodgkin's disease: treatment and splenectomy as risk factors. *Med Pediatr Oncol* 1989;17:477–484.

12. Van Leeuwen FE, Somers R, Hart AAM. Splenectomy in Hodgkin's disease and second leukaemias. *Lancet* 1987;2:210–211.

13. Boivin JF, Hutchison GB, et al. Incidence of second cancers in patients treated for Hodgkin's disease. *J Natl Cancer Inst* 1995;87(10): 732–741.

14. Rosenberg SA. Exploratory laparotomy and splenectomy for Hodgkin's disease: a commentary. *J Clin Oncol* 1988;6:574.

15. Trichopoulos D, MacMahon B, Cole P. Menopause and breast cancer risk. *J Natl Cancer Inst* 1972;48:605–613.

16. Feinleib M. Breast cancer and artificial menopause: a cohort study. *J Natl Cancer Inst* 1968;41:315–339

17. Abeloff MD, Armitage JO, et al. *Clinical oncology*. New York: Churchill Livingstone, 1995:844,1986,1521,810,812,16,796,816, 805, 1052,1064,2204,778,779,749.

18. The WHO collaborative study of neoplasia and steroid contraceptives: epithelial ovarian cancer and combined oral contraceptives. *Int J Epidemiol* 1989;18:538.

19. Greene MH, Clark JW, Blaynew DW. The epidemiology of ovarian cancer. *Semin Oncol* 1984;11:3,209.

20. Boice JD. Cancer following medical irradiation. *Cancer* 1981;47 (Suppl):1081–1090.

21. Levine EG, Booomfield CD. Leukemias and myelodysplastic syndromes secondary to drug, radiation, and environmental exposure. *Semin Oncol* 1992;19(1):47–84.

22. Robinson E, Neugut AI, Wylie P. Clinical aspects of postirradiation sarcomas. *J Natl Cancer Inst* 1988;80(4):233–240.

23. Laitt RD, Chambers EJ, et al. Magnetic resonance imaging and magnetic resonance angiography in long term survivors of acute lymphoblastic leukemia treated with cranial irradiation. *Cancer* 1995;76(10): 1846–1852.

24. Marks LB, Carroll PR, Dugan TC, Anscher MS. The response of the urinary bladder, urethra, and ureter to radiation and chemotherapy. *Int J Radiat Oncol Biol Phys* 1995;31(5)1270–1271.

25. Sherrill DJ, Grishkin BA, Galal FS, et al. Radiation associated malignancies of the esophagus. *Cancer* 1984;54:726.

26. Moller H, Mellemgaard, et al. Incidence of second primary cancer following testicular cancer. *Eur J Cancer* 1993;29A(5):672–676.

27. Soffer D, Gomori JM, Siegl T, Shalit MN. Intracranial meningiomas after high-dose irradiation. *Cancer* 1989;63:1514.

28. Enghold G, Kleinerman RA, et al. Radiation dose and second cancer risk in patients treated for cancer of the cervix. *Radiat Res* 1988; 116:3–55.

29. Arai T. et al. Second cancer after radiation therapy for cancer of the uterine cervix. *Cancer* 1991;398–405.

30. Mark, RJ, Poen J, et al. Postirradiation sarcomas. *Cancer* 1994;73(10): 887–893.

31. Kumar PP, Good RR, et al. Radiation-induced neoplasms of the brain. *Cancer* 1987;59:1274–1282.

32. Harrison MJ, Wolfe DE, et al. Radiation induced meningiomas: experience at Mount Sinai Hospital and review ofthe literature. *J Neurosurg* 1991;75:564–566.

33. Boice JD, Day NE, Andersen A, et al. Second cancer following radiation treatment for cervix cancer: an international collaboration among cancer registries. *J Natl Cancer Inst* 1985;74:955–975.

34. Basco VE, Coldman AJ, Elwood JM, Young MEF. Radiation dose and second breast cancer. *Br J Cancer* 1985;52:319.

35. Horn PL, Thompson WD. Risk of contralateral breast cancer: associations with histologic, clinical, and therapeutic factors. *Cancer* 1988; 62:412.

36. Boice JD Jr, Harvey EB, Blettner M, et al. Cancer in the contralateral breast after radiotherapy for breast cancer. *N Engl J Med* 1992; 326:781.

37. Yahalom J, Petrek JA, Biddinger PW, et al. Breast cancer in patients irradiated for Hodgkin's disease: a clinical and pathologic analysis of 45 events in 37 patients. *J Clin Oncol* 1992;10:1674.

38. Boice JD Jr, Monson RR. Breast cancer in women after repeated fluoroscopic examinations of the chest. *J Natl Cancer Inst* 1977;59: 823–832.

39. O'Brien PC, Barton MB, et al. Breast cancer following treatment for Hodgkin's disease: the need for screening in a young population. *Aust Radiol* 1995;39:271–276.

40. Hancock SL, Tucker MA, Hoppe RT. Breast cancer after treatment of Hodgkin's disease. *J Natl Cancer Inst* 1993;85:25–31.

41. Peters MH, Indukumar MS, et al. Breast cancer in women following mantle irradiation for Hodgkin's disease. *Am Surg* 1995;61(9) 763–766.

42. Dershaw DD, et al. Breast carcinoma in women previously treated for Hodgkin's disease: mammographic evaluation. *Radiology* 1992;184: 421–423.

43. Blayney DW, Longo DL, Young RC, et al. Decreasing risk of leukemia with prolonged follow-up after chemotherapy and radiotherapy for Hodgkin's disease. *N Engl J Med* 1987;316:710–714.

44. Colvett KT. Bilateral breast carcinoma after radiation therapy for Hodgkin's disease. *South Med J* 1995;88(2):239–242.

45. Pedersen-Bjergaard J, Ersboll J, et al. Carcinoma of the urinary bladder after treatment with cyclophosphamide For non-Hodgkin's lymphoma. *N Engl J Med* 1988;318:1028.

46. Whitlock JA, Greer JP, Lukens JN. Epipodophyllotoxin-related leukemia: identification of a new subset of secondary leukemia. *Cancer* 1991;68:600.

47. Pedersen-Bjergaard J, Daugaard G, Hansen SW, Philip P, et al. Increased risk of myelodysplasia and leukaemia after etoposide, cisplatin, and bleomycin for germ-cell tumours. *Lancet* 1991;338: 359–363.

48. Tallman MS, Gray R, Bennett JM, et al. Leukemogenic potential of adjuvant chemotherapy for early-stage breast cancer: the Eastern Cooperative Oncology Group experience. *J Clin Oncol* 1995;13(7): 1557–1563.

49. Pedersen-Bjergaard J, Sigsgaard TC, Neilsen D, et al. Acute monocytic or myelomonocytic leukemia with balanced chromosome translocations to band 11q23 after therapy with 4-epi-doxorubicin and cisplatin or cyclophosphamide for breast cancer. *J Clin Oncol* 1992;10: 1444–1451.

50. Boice JD Jr, Greene MH, Killen JY Jr, et al. Leukemia and preleukemia after adjuvant treatment of gastrointestinal cancer with semustine (methyl CCNU.) *N Engl J Med* 1983;309:1079.

51. Green MH, Boice JD Jr, Strike TA. Carmustine as a cause of acute nonlymphocytic leukemia. *N Engl J Med* 1985;313:579.

52. Bhatia S, Ramsay NDC, Steinbuch M et al. Malignant neoplasms following bone marrow transplantation. *Blood* 1996;87(9):3633–3639.

53. Lowsky R, Lipton J, Fyles G, et al. Secondary malignancies after bone marrow transplantation in adults. *J Clin Oncol* 1994;12(10):2187–2192.

54. Witherspoon RP, Fisher LD, et al. Secondary cancers after bone marrow tranplantation for leukemia or aplastic anemia. *N Engl J Med* 1989;321(12):784–789.

55. Kolb HJ, Bender-Gotze CH. Late complications after allogenic bone marrow transplantation for leukemia. *Bone Marrow Transplant* 1990; 6:61–72.

56. Curtis RE, Rowlings PA, et al. Solid cancers after bone marrow transplantation. *N Engl J Med* 1997;326(13):897–904.

57. Tucker MA, Coleman CN, Cox RS, Varghese A, Rosenberg SA. Risk of second cancers after treatment for Hodgkin's disease. *N Engl J Med* 1988;318(2):76–80.

58. Mervish S. Nitrosamine action and metabolism in the rat and human esophagus in relation to the etiology of squamous and adenocarcinoma of the esophagus. International Congress on Cancer of the Esophagus, St. Margherita Ligure, Italy, 1992.

59. Attwood SE, Smyrk TC, DeMeester TR, et al. Esophageal reflux and the development of esophageal carcinoma in rats. *Surgery* 1992;111: 503–510.

60. Haubrich WS, et al. *Gastroenterology*, 5th ed. Philadelphia: WB Saunders 1995:537.

61. Doll DC, Ringenberg QS, Yarbro JW. Vascular toxicity associated with antineoplastic agents. *J Clin Oncol* 1086;4(9):1405–1417.

62. Jackson AM, Rose BD, Graff LG, et al. Thrombotic microangiopathy and renal failure associated with antineoplastic chemotherapy. *Ann Intern Med* 1984;101:41–44.

63. McEniery PT, Dorosti K, Schiavone WA, et al. Clinical and angiographic features of coronary artery disease after chest irradiation. *Am J Cardiol* 1987;60:1020.

64. Simon EB, Ling J, Mendiazabal RC, Midawell J. Radiation-induced coronary artery disease. *Am Heart J* 1984;108:1032.

65. Amromin GD, Gidldenhorn HL, Solomaon RD, et al. The synergism of x-irradiation and cholesterol-fat feeding on the development of coronary artery lesions. *J Atherosclerosis Res* 1964;4:325–334.

66. DeVita VT, et al. *Cancer: principles and practice of oncology*, 4th ed. Philadelphia: JB Lippincott:1993.

67. Gustavsson A, Eskilsson J, et al. Late cardiac effects after mantle radiotherapy in patients with Hodgkin's disease. *Ann Oncol* 1990;1:361.

68. Gottdiener JS, Michael JK, et al. Late cardiac effects of therapeutic mediastinal irradiation. *N Engl J Med* 1983;308(10):371.

69. Hansen SW. Late effects after treatment for germ-cell cancer with cisplatin, vinblastine, and bleomycin. *Dan Med Bull* 1992;39(5):395.

70. Von Hoff DD. Risk factors for doxorubicin-induced congestive heart failure. *Ann Intern Med* 1979;91:710–717.

71. Braunwald E. *Heart disease: a textbook of cardiovascular medicine*, 4th ed. Philadelphia: WB Saunders, 1992.

72. Henderson IG, Allegra JC, Woodcock T, et al. Randomized clinical trial comparing mitoxantrone with doxorubicin in previously treated patients with metastatic breast cancer. *J Clin Oncol* 1989;7:560–571.

73. Schlant RC. et al. *The heart, arteries, and veins*. New York: McGraw-Hill, 1993:1992.

74. Posner LE, Kukart G, Goldberg J, et al. Mitoxantrone: an overview of safety and toxicity. *Invest New Drugs* 1985;3:123–132.

75. Stewart JR, Fajardo LF. Radiation-induced heart disease: an update. *Prog Cardiovasc Dis* 1984;27:173.

76. Stewart JR, Fajardo LF, et al. Radiation injury to the heart. *Int J Radiat Oncol Biol Phys* 1995;31(5):1205–1211.

77. *Physician's desk reference*, 49th ed. Montvale, NJ: Medical Economics Data Production Company, 1995.

78. Pohjola-Sintonen S, Totterman KJ, et al. Late cardiac effects of mediastinal radiotherapy in patients with Hodgkin's disease. *Cancer* 1987;60:31–37.

79. Martin RG, Ruckdeschel JC, Chang P, et al. Radiation-related pericarditis. *Am J Cardiol* 1975;35:216.

80. DeVita VT, et al. *Cancer: principles and practice of oncology*, 4th ed. Philadelphia: JB Lippincott, 1993.

81. Lombard CM, Churg A, Winokur S. Pulmonary veno-occlusive disease following therapy for malignant neoplasms. *Chest* 1987;92(5).

82. McDonald S, Rubin P, et al. Injury to the lung from cancer therapy: clinical syndromes, measurable endpoints, and potential scoring systems. *Int J Radiat Oncol Biol Phys* 1995;31(5):1187–1203.

83. Lehne G, Lote K. Pulmonary toxicity of cytotoxic and immunosuppressive agents. *Acta Oncol* 1990;29(2):118.

84. Rodriquez-Garcia JL, Fraile G, et al. Recurrent massive pleural effusion as a late complication of radiotherapy in Hodgkin's disease. *Chest* 1992;100:4.

85. Cwikiel M, Albertsson M, Hambraeus G. Acute and delayed effects of radiotherapy in patients with oesophageal squamous cell carcinoma treated with chemotherapy, surgery and pre-and postoperative radiotherapy. *Acta Oncol* 1994;33(1):49–53.

86. Shapiro SJ, Shapiro SD, et al. Prospective study of long-term pulmonary manifestations of mantle irradiation. *Int J Radiat Oncol Biol Phys* 1990;19(3):707–714.

87. Libshitz HI, Banner MP. Spontaneous pneumothorax as a complication of radiation therapy to the thorax. *Radiology* 1974;112:199–201.

88. Isaacs RD, Wattie WJ, et al. Massive hemoptysis as a late consequence of pulmonary irradiation. *Thorax* 1987;42:77–78.

89. Speiser BL, Spratiling L. Radiation bronchitis and stenosis secondary to high dose rate endobronchial irradiation. *Int J Radiat Oncol Biol Phys* 1992;25:589–597.

90. O'Driscoll BR, Hasleton PS, et al. Active lung fibrosis up to 17 years after chemotherapy With carmustine (BCNU) in childhood. *N Engl J Med* 1990;323(6).

91. Glazer HS, Lee JKT, Levitt RG, et al. Radiation fibrosis: differentiation from recurrent tumor by MR imaging. *Radiology* 1985;156:721–726.

92. Hubbard SM, Longo DL. Treatment-related morbidity in patients with lymphoma. *Curr Opin Oncol* 1992;3:857.

93. Markman M, Rothman R, et al. Late effects of cisplatin-based chemotherapy on renal function in patients with ovarian carcinoma. *Gynecol Oncol* 1991;41:217–219.

94. Osanto S, Bukman A, et al. Long-term effects of chemotherapy in patients with testicular cancer. *J Clin Oncol* 1992;10(4):574–579.

95. Marks LB, Carroll PR, et al. The response of the urinary bladder, urethra, and ureter to radiation and chemotherapy. *Int J Radiat Oncol Biol Phys* 1995;31(5):1257–1280.

96. Soubek J, McGuire EJ, et al. The late occurrence of urinary tract damage in patients successfully treated by radiotherapy plus cervical carcinoma. *J Urol* 1989l;141:1347–1349.

97. Coia LR, Myerson RJ, Tepper JE. Late effects of radiation therapy on the gastrointestinal tract. *Int J Radiat Oncol Biol Phys* 1995;31(5):1213–1236.

98. Cosset J, Henry-Amar M, et al. Late radiation injuries of the gastrointestinal tract in the H2 and H5 EORTC Hodgkin's disease trials: emphasis on the role of exploratory laparotomy and fractionation. *Radiother Oncol* 1988;13:61–68.

99. Lucarotti ME, Mountford RA, Bartolo CC. Surgical management of intestinal radiation injury. *Dis Colon Rectum* 1991;34(10):865–869.

100. Yeoh EK, Horowitz M. Radiation enteritis. *Surg Gynecol Obstet* 1987;165:373–379.

101. Sleisenger MH, Fordtran JS. *Gastrointestinal disease: pathophysiology/diagnosis/management*, vol 2. Philadelphia: WB Saunders, 1993;1267.

102. Grigsby PW, Pilepich MV, Parsons CL. Preliminary results of a Phase I/II study of sodium pentosanpolysulfate in the treatment of chronic radiation-induced proctitis. *Am J Clin Oncol* 1990;13:28–31.

103. Hancock SL, McDougall IR, Constine LS. Thyroid abnormalities after therapeutic external radiation. *Int J Radiat Oncol Biol Phys* 1995;31(5):1165–1170.

104. Smith RE, Adler RA, Clark P, et al. Thyroid function after mantle irradiation in Hodgkin's disease. *JAMA* 1981;245:46.

105. Petersen M, Keeling CA, McDougall RM. Hyperthyroidism with low radioiodine uptake after head and neck irradiation for Hodgkin's disease. *J Nucl Med* 1989;30(2):255–257.

106. Schwartzentruber DJ, White DE, et al. Thyroid dysfunction associated with immunotherapy for patients with cancer. *Cancer* 1991;68:2384–2390.

107. Doniach I. Experimental induction of tumours of the thyroid by radiation. *Br Med Bull* 1958;14:181–183.

108. Lindsay S, Michols CW Jr, Chaikoff IL. Induction of benign and malignant thyroid neoplasms in the rat. *Arch Pathol* 1966;81:308–316.

109. Morgan GW, Freeman AP, et al. Late cardiac, thyroid, and pulmonary sequelae of mantle radiotherapy for Hodgkin's disease. *Radiat Oncol Biol Phys* 1985;11(11).

110. Moroff SV, FLuks JZ. Thyroid cancer following radiotherapy for Hodgkin's fisease: a vase report and review of the literature. *Med Pediatr Oncol* 1986;14:216–220.

111. DeGroot LJ. *Endocrinology*, 3rd ed. Philadelphia: WB Saunders, 1995, 839.

112. Schneider AB, Recant W, Pinsky SM, et al. Radiation-induced thyroid cancer. *Ann Intern Med* 1986;105:405.

113. Salomon F, Cuneo RC, et al. The effects of treatment with recombinant human growth hormone on body composition and metabolism in adults with growth hormone deficiency. *N Engl J Med* 1989;321:1797–1803.

114. Sklar CA, Constine LS. Chronic neuroendocrinological sequelae of radiation therapy. *Int J Radiat Oncol Biol Phys* 1995;31(5):1113–1121.

115. Powles TJ, Tillyer CR, Jones AL, et al. Prevention of breast cancer with tamoxifen: an update on the Royal Marsden Hospital pilot program. *Eur J Cancer* 1990;26:680.

116. Cuzick J, Allen D, et al. Long-term effects of tamoxifen. Biological effects of Ttamoxifen working party. *Eur J Cancer* 1993;29A(1):15–21.

117. Killackey MA, Hakes TB, et al. Endometrial adenocarcinoma in breast cancer patients receiving antiestrogens. *Cancer Treat Rep* 1985;69:237.

118. Malfetano JH. Tamoxifen-associated endometrial carcinoma in postmenopausal breast cancer patients. *Gynecol Oncol* 1990;39:82.

119. Fisher B, Costantino J, Redmond C, et al. Endometrial cancer in tamoxifen-treated breast cancer patients: findings from the National Surgical Adjuvant Breast and Bowel Project (NSABP) B-14. *J Natl Cancer Inst* 1994;86:527–537.

120. Lukert BP, Paisz LG. Glucocorticoid-induced osteoporosis: pathogenesis and management. *Ann Intern Med* 1990;112(5):352–364.

121. Lukert BP. Etidronate in the management of glucocorticoid-induced osteoporosis. *Am J Med* 1995;99:233–234.

122. Sambrook P, Birmingham J, et al. Prevention of corticosteroid osteoporosis. *N Engl J Med* 1993;328(24)1747–1752.

123. Struys A, Snelder AA, Mulder H. Cyclical etidronate reverses bone loss of the spine and proximal femur in patients with established corticosteroid-induced osteoporosis. *Am J Med* 1995;99:235–242.

124. Arlet J. Nontraumatic avascular necrosis of the femoral head. Past, present, and future. *Clin Orthop Rel Res* 1992;12–22.

125. Cassady JR, Tonnesen GL, Wolfe LC, Sallan SE. Augmentation of vincristine neurotoxicity by irradiation of peripheral nerves. *Cancer Treat Rep* 1980;64:963.

126. Rosenthal S, Kaufman S. Vincristine neurotoxicity. *Ann Intern Med* 1974;80:733.

127. Cavaletti G, Marzorati L, Bogliun G, et al. Cisplatin-induced peripheral neurotoxicity is dependent on total-dose intensity and single-dose intensity. *Cancer* 1992;69:203.

128. Postma TJ, Benard BA, et al. Long-term effects of vincristine on the peripheral nervous system. *J Neuro Oncol* 1993;15:23–27.

129. Lee AWM, Law SCK, et al. Retrospective analysis of nasopharyngeal carcinoma treated during 1976–1985: late complications following megavoltage irradiation. *Br J Radiol* 1992;65:918–928.

130. Stryker JA, Sommerville K, Perez R, Velkley D. Sacral plexus injury after radiotherapy for carcinoma of cervix. *Cancer* 1990; 1488–1492.

131. Fulton DS. Brachial plexopathy in patients with breast cancer. *Dev Oncol* 1987;51:249–257.

132. Rowland LP. *Merritt's textbook of neurology*, 9th ed. Baltimore: Williams & Wilkins, 1995:661,662,672.

133. Wiederholt W. *Neurology for non-neurologists*. New York: Academic Press, 1982:280.

134. Rakel RE. *1996 Conn's current therapy*. Philadelphia: WB Saunders, 1996:920,923.

135. Schuyltheiss TE, Kun LE, et al. Radiation response of the central nervous system. *Int J Radiat Oncol Biol Phys* 1995;31(5):1093–1112.

136. Allen JC, Miller DC, et al. Brain and spinal cord hemorrhage in long-term survivors of malignant pediatric brain tumors: a possible late effect of therapy. *Neurology* 1991;41(1):148–150.

137. Schaefer SD, Post JD, Close LG, Wright CG. Ototoxicity of low- and moderate dose cisplatin. *Cancer* 1985;56:1934.

138. Constine LS, Konski A, Ekholm S. Adverse effects of brain irradiation correlated with MR and CT imaging. *Int J Radiat Oncol Biol Phys* 1988;15:319–330.

139. Haerer AF. *DeJong's the neurologic examination*, 5th ed. Philadelphia: JB Lippincott, 1992:781–783.

140. Silverberg GD, Britt RH, Goffinet DR. Radiation-induced carotid artery disease. *Cancer* 1978;41:130–137.

141. Moritz MW, Higgins RF, Jacobs JR. Duplex imaging and incidence of carotid radiation injury after high-dose radiotherapy for tumors of the head and neck. *Arch Surg* 1990;125:1181–1183.

142. Chung E, Bodensteiner J, Hogg JP. Spontaneous intracerebral hemorrhage: a very late delayed effect of radiation therapy. *J Child Neurol* 1992;7:259–263.

143. Woo E, Chan YF, et al. Apoplectic intracerebral hemorrhage: an unusual complication of cerebral radiation necrosis. *Pathology* 1987;19:95–98.

144. Paganini-Hill A. The benefits of estrogen replacement therapy on oral health. *Arch Intern Med* 1995;155:2325–2329.

145. Larson DL. Long-term effects of radiation therapy in the head and neck. *Clin Plast Surg* 1993;20(3):485–490.

146. Deore SM, et al. Late radiation-induced laryngeal oedema in the treatment of vocal cord cancer: analysis using the linear quadratic model. *Ind J Cancer* 1993;30:113–119.

*Principles and Practice of Supportive Oncology,*
edited by Ann Berger et al.
Lippincott–Raven Publishers, Philadelphia ©1998

# CHAPTER 67

# Psychosocial Aspects of Cancer Survivorship

Susan A. Leigh and Elizabeth J. Clark

---

What happens when my body breaks down happens not just to that body but also to my life, which is lived in that body. When the body breaks down, so does the life. Even when medicine can fix the body, that doesn't always put the life back together again (1).

Survivorship is not just about long-term survival but about quality of life from the moment of diagnosis onward. In order to better understand this issue from the consumer's perspective, it is helpful to understand the difference between curing and healing. The concept of cure has become a medical reality for many types of cancer; yet, the concept of healing after cancer and its treatment is a completely different story. While curing resides within a disease-repair system and is defined biomedically, healing focuses on health and wellness and can be explained both physically and psychosocially. Disease is what is seen, treated, and measured and is the tangible focus for cure. Illness is what is felt and experienced and is a more intangible focus for healing. Lerner notes that "Although the capacity to heal physically is necessary to any successful cure, healing can also take place on deeper levels whether or not physical recovery occurs" (2). By understanding the differences between the treatment of an external disease and the personal, lived experience of illness, physicians can more readily acknowledge and appreciate the psychosocial sequelae that often accompany or follow a diagnosis of cancer. This chapter will attempt to redefine the cancer experience, especially from the consumer's perspective; review psychosocial aspects of survival along an expanded continuum; and offer strategies to enhance survivorship.

## CANCER MYTHS

At the beginning of fall semester, 1995, the question "What does cancer mean to you?" was posed to a class of second-year medical students at the University of Arizona. Their responses reflect current feelings within Western society as a whole and include descriptives such as *death, terminal, sadness, fear, chemotherapy, mutilation, pain, financial loss,* and, last but not least, *cure.* Their attitudes about cancer echo the generally negative sentiments that would have been expected decades ago. The only positive word was *cure,* and it was at the bottom of the list.

Cancer continues to instill dread and to masquerade as a ruthless, secretive assailant. Early in this century it was believed that "if it was not fatal, it was not cancer" (3). In *Illness as Metaphor,* Sontag (3) writes that a diagnosis of cancer will remain an automatic death sentence until its causes are known and effective treatments are discovered. Even though recent advances in science and medical technology have increased the chances for survival, the often paralyzing fear of eventual death of the disease still lingers today.

Along with the myth of imminent death, cancer evokes other misunderstandings, especially concerning causation. Decades ago, many people theorized that cancer was caused by emotional resignation and hopelessness (3). While attempts to identify "cancer personalities" became a popular trend in the 1970s, there were suggestions that patients unfortunate enough to be diagnosed with cancer must have done, thought, or repressed something to allow this disease to happen. Current pop psychology, which often oversimplifies causation and blames the sick individual for having done something wrong, may be rooted in this myth. Although the paranoia surrounding cancer is gradually diminishing, the disease continues to harbor

S. A. Leigh: Tucson, AZ 85739.

E.J. Clark: National Coalition for Cancer Survivorship, Silver Spring, MD 20910.

elements of fear, stigma, shunning, discrimination, and withdrawal of support (4).

When the biology of a disease is not understood, mythologic speculation and oversimplification are apt to define the sickness. Of major importance in defining cancer is that it continues to be identified as a homogeneous disease. Cancer is less often seen as many diseases with multiple causes and treatments and more frequently seen as a single entity with simple causation. The prevalent idea that stress causes cancer often overrules other causative factors, such as genetic predisposition, decreased or damaged immune competence, dangerous health habits, and environmental carcinogens. But not all myths are rooted in the individual. The health care system itself is also full of myths and misunderstandings.

## HEALTH CARE MYTHS

As medical researchers and clinicians focus on extending and saving lives, patients become acutely aware of issues affecting the quality of their lives. Two current myths involved with quality of life concerns are (a) the all-powerful role of the physician and (b) the healing environment within our hospitals (4).

The power and control in the management of patients was historically held by doctors. In this current age of increased bureaucracy, expensive delivery of care, and cost containment, decision-making powers are now shifting to financing and regulatory agencies (5). Physicians are required to spend increasing amounts of time on administrative matters, which decreases the amount of time available for patient care. Patients have longer waits for appointments, and the choice of doctors is more limited. Meanwhile, out of necessity a new prototype of health care consumer is emerging. Consumers who are more assertive in asking questions and requesting information are more inclined toward partnership *with* rather than paternalism *from* their providers of care. As the decision-making powers shift, this attitude can either enhance or strain the already challenged physician-patient relationship.

The second area of misunderstanding is the type of environment in which healing is fostered. The delivery of care is now complicated by diagnosis-related groups, cost containment, utilization reviews, managed care, and mountains of paperwork. While the old system allowed unlimited stays in the hospital and actually encouraged passivity and invalidism, the new system has gone to the other extreme. Since discharging patients from the hospital as soon as possible has become fiscally prudent, patients return home sooner and sicker. The healing environment, then, becomes the home rather than the hospital, and greater responsibility is placed on the patient and family members or other caregivers. These changing social trends are actually

forcing a shift from passive patienthood to a more proactive survivorship.

## SEMANTICS OF SURVIVORSHIP

The concept of survivorship was initially introduced to the field of oncology in 1986 with the founding of the National Coalition for Cancer Survivorship (NCCS). The events preceding this organizational meeting included medical advances and social trends that provoked exploration of new issues related to cancer.

As new therapies became available to treat cancer, the hopes and expectations of surviving this disease were elevated. Access to information about scientific breakthroughs became readily available to the general public; awareness about cancer prevention, early detection, second opinions, and treatment options increased; many types of cancers shifted from acute to chronic diseases; and some patients were actually cured. Oncologists were finally able to rejoice, along with their patients, that not everyone would die of this feared disease. Yet, as patients and family members savored the sweetness of survival they also realized that life would never be the same and that it would always be full of uncertainty. In *Of Dragons and Garden Peas*, wherein a patient talks to doctors, Trillin sums up this dilemma: "So, once we have recognized the limitations of the magic of doctors and medicine, where are we? We have to turn to our own magic, to our ability to 'control' our bodies" (6).

Control comes in many forms. Before this decade, the cancer patient's agenda was more often than not set by health care providers, especially physicians. Eventually, patients decided to take more control, either directly or indirectly, over all aspects of cancer care that affected their lives. Thus, support groups, hotlines, resource materials, and patient networks proliferated. As the shift to recognize the consumer voice began, the concept of *survivorship* emerged.

Mullan describes survivorship as "the act of living on...a dynamic concept with no artificial boundaries" (7). Carter further describes this theme as a process of *going through*, suggesting movement through phases (8). From these models, the concept of survivorship is viewed as a continual, ongoing process rather than a stage or outcome of survival (9). It is not just about long-term survival, which is how the medical profession generally defines it. Rather, it is the experience of living with, through, or beyond cancer (10,11). From this point of view, survivorship begins at the moment of diagnosis and continues for the remainder of life (7).

Other discrepancies in semantics revolve around who is or is not a cancer survivor. When cancer was considered incurable, the term *survivor* applied to the family members whose loved one had died of the disease. This terminology was used for years by the medical profession and insurance companies. But when potentially curative therapy became a reality, physicians selected a 5-year parameter to measure survival. Freedom from disease and biomedical longevity became the standards of success where the outcome was measurable and quantifiable.

As treatment successes improved over the years, this limited definition failed to consider patients who are not cured of their disease, require maintenance therapy, or periodically change treatment modalities, yet remain alive for more than 5 years. Others experience late recurrences, are diagnosed with second malignancies, or develop delayed effects of treatment. Even as the 5-year landmark has been modified as a parameter for describing survival, medical professionals seem inclined to categorize anyone receiving therapy or not completely free of disease as a "patient" and everyone who is not under treatment or with no evidence of disease as a "survivor."

Many people who have histories of cancer feel that survivorship extends far beyond the restrictions of time and treatment. As the empowered consumer encourages the shift from paternalism to partnership, survivors are describing themselves as victors, graduates, triumphers, veterans, thrivers, activists, and, of course, survivors. All these labels can confuse providers and consumers alike, but as Gray (12) notes in *Persons With Cancer Speak Out*, "The act of defining is an act of power." This is all about the people—the survivors—identifying their own issues and defining themselves rather than relying on the agendas and descriptives of the health care community (9). Any or all of these labels can be considered correct, both quantitatively and qualitatively; they simply need to be defined within the context in which they are used. Thus, the term *survivor* in this chapter reflects the NCCS definition: "from the time of its discovery and for the balance of life, an individual diagnosed with cancer is a survivor" (7).

## STAGES OF SURVIVAL

Obviously, cancer survivors have different issues depending on their circumstances along the survival continuum. In the classic article "Seasons of survival: reflections of a physician with cancer," Mullan (13) was the first to propose a model of survival that includes acute, extended, and permanent stages.

### Acute Stage

The acute (or immediate) stage begins at the time of the diagnostic workup and continues through the initial courses of medical treatment. The survivor is commonly called a patient during this stage, and the primary focus is on physical survival. Usually, without any prior training, those who are ill are required to make sophisticated medical decisions at a time of intense vulnerability, fear, and pressure. Inexperienced in navigating the complicated culture of medicine, many patients continue to rely solely on their physicians to make treatment-related decisions for them. Others, though, ask for information, explanations, and more effective communication in an attempt to understand their choices.

Supportive services are most available at this time. Access to the medical team, counselors, patient support networks, resource libraries, hotlines, and family support systems helps patients navigate this stage. But the picture changes, sometimes dramatically, once treatment ends.

### Extended Stage

If the disease responds during the initial course of therapy, the survivor moves into the extended (or intermediate) stage of survival. This stage is often described as one of watchful waiting, limbo, or remission as survivors monitor their bodies for symptoms of disease recurrence. Uncertainty about the future prevails, as medical-based support systems are no longer readily available. Recovery entails dealing with the physical and emotional effects of treatment, and reentry into social roles is often challenged by ignorance and discrimination.

While no longer a patient, the person may not feel entirely healthy and may have difficulty feeling like a survivor. Ambiguity defines this stage, as survivors find themselves afloat in a mixture of joy and fear, happy to be alive and finished with treatments, yet afraid of what the future may hold.

The need for continued supportive care during this transitional stage has recently received attention (7–11). Community and peer networks often replace institutional support, and recovery entails regaining both physical and psychological stamina.

### Permanent Stage

A certain level of trust and comfort gradually returns, and survivors enter the permanent (or long-term) stage of survival. This is roughly equivalent to cure or sustained remission. While most survivors experience a gradual evolution from a state of "surviving to thriving," as described by Hassey-Dow (14), others must deal with the chronic, debilitating, or delayed effects of therapy. Although many of these long-term survivors have no physical evidence of disease and appear to have fully recovered, the life-threatening experience of having survived cancer is never forgotten. The metaphor of the Damocles syndrome illustrates the apprehension or fear of living under the sword, never knowing whether or when it might drop (15,16).

For many cancer survivors, long-term followup tends to be as unpredictable as today's health care system. Generally, there are scant, if any, guidelines for specific followup, nor are there wellness-focused programs tailored to the altered health care needs of this population. One exception is pediatric oncology, which is far beyond adult oncology in the systematic followup of long-term survivors. Standardized assessments in specialized clinics help identify problems such as disease recurrence, second malignancies, or late effects of treatment, and interventions can be initiated as soon as possible.

Adults, on the other hand, often feel burdened by a "glorification of recovery" (17) whereby they are praised for overcoming adversity and encouraged to minimize their complaints. The appearance of health can actually hamper the identification of real problems, as no one wants to believe that something might still be wrong (17,18). But symptoms of distress, both biomedical and psychosocial, must be taken seriously. And in this age of cost containment and managed care, survivors need continued access to appropriate specialists who understand the consequences of survival and can treat accordingly.

As the population of cancer survivors increases, attention to survival issues needs to be encouraged. Even if the disease is eradicated, the psychosocial sequelae of surviving a life-threatening experience must be recognized as barriers to a full recovery.

## PSYCHOSOCIAL ASPECTS

How well an individual adapts psychologically and socially to living with cancer depends on a wide variety of factors. First are the physical factors, including the age and sex of the individual, the type and stage of disease, the kinds and duration of recommended treatments, the outcomes of treatment, disease progression, and residual side effects. Added to these are permanent disabilities, physical limitations, and possible disfigurement and altered body image. Next are the psychological variables. Where is the individual in life-stage development? What previous experiences has the person had with illness in general and with cancer in particular? What individual psychological strengths and weaknesses are brought to the cancer experience? What kinds of coping mechanisms usually are employed by the individual in crisis situations? Does the individual have a prior history of emotional problems such as depression, anxiety, or other mental health concerns? Self-esteem, independence and motivation, as well as interactional skills, also play a part.

When aspects of social functioning are added to the equation, many other variables need to be considered. These include the sociodemographic factors such as marital status, race, ethnicity, religious orientation, educational level, employment history, and financial stability. Next are the social roles ascribed to the individual, such as spouse, parent, employee, and friend. In addition to the sociodemographic variables, other social factors include the type of social support available to the individual.

What kinds of changes will a history of cancer bring for the individual and the family? Will the individual be able to fulfill existing job requirements, or will joblessness or employment discrimination become a factor? Despite this wide range of individual variability, there are numerous shared experiences that occur along the continuum of cancer survivorship. Also shared are the most common problems and needs faced by persons with cancer.

### Needs of Cancer Survivors

Houts and his colleagues (19) conducted one of the most comprehensive studies to date on the needs of cancer survivors. They interviewed a random sample of 629 persons who had been diagnosed with cancer within the past 2 years and also interviewed 397 persons involved in their care. Four major categories of unmet needs were identified: (a) emotional/social needs (including family issues) (b) economic needs (financial, insurance, and employment issues) (c) medical staff needs (the need for information and increased availability) and (d) community needs (including home care and transportation) (19).

In 1988, the Canadian Cancer Society conducted a needs assessment with over 2,000 persons who had been diagnosed with cancer or had had a cancer recurrence between 1982 and 1989 (20). Subjects were selected to represent a cross-section of types and stages of cancer and of various geographic locations. The greatest needs identified were for prompt medical attention, emotional support, pain management, practical assistance, attention to employment and financial problems, and information.

Loescher and her colleagues (21) evaluated the needs of long-term survivors of adult cancer using the Cancer Survivor Questionnaire. They interviewed a small sample of individuals more than 2 years after cancer therapy. Deduction content analysis revealed several themes. The needs identified were for reassurance, control, information, insurance coverage, and money as well as the need to talk about the cancer experience.

In one of the most recent quality of life studies in long-term cancer survivors, Ferrell and colleagues (22) used a mailed survey approach to assess the quality of life of 687 cancer survivors. Of the four domains of well-being (physical, social, psychological, and spiritual) that were evaluated using a Quality of Life–Cancer Survivors Tool, the psychological well-being subscale had the lowest score. The authors conclude that while distress related to the cancer experience abates over time, the psychological impact of the distress lingers.

Addressing the wide variety of psychosocial needs and concerns of cancer patients mentioned above is beyond the scope of this chapter. However, several salient themes have been selected to receive expanded coverage and to indicate some psychosocial sequelae that perhaps are specific to the cancer experience.

## Normlessness (Lack of Societal Norms) of the Cancer Experience

Many of the psychological problems associated with cancer are related to a lack of knowledge and requisite skills needed for negotiating the cancer experience. Cancer survivors experience a sequence of crises for which habitual problem-solving activities are not adequate and that do not lead to the previously achieved balanced state (23). Therefore, cancer may be a normless or anomic situation for a significant number of persons.

Anomia can be defined as "a temporary state of mind occasioned by a sudden alteration in one's life situation, and characterized by confusion and anxiety, uncertainty, loss of purpose, and a sense of separateness from one's usual social support system" (24). Persons newly diagnosed with cancer may not know how to think or talk about their situation. They need information, but because of the shock and unfamiliarity of the situation, they may be unable to understand the broad significance or assimilate what information they do receive.

Added to this is the stigma that accompanies a cancer diagnosis. Despite treatment advances and extended survival rates for various cancers, cancer remains a stigmatized disease, and persons with cancer must contend with the consequent societal attitudes, prejudices, and discrimination (1,3).

Eventually, most persons with cancer become expert about their own illness and treatment. They know more or less what to expect medically, and they learn how best to navigate the health care system. They develop the requisite language and needed coping skills to manage the crisis periods. They often interact with other cancer patients, and perhaps by attending support groups or with the help of their medical team and counselors, they find that while the disease of cancer is a personal experience, there are numerous commonalities among individuals regarding the illness process and its consequences. In short, they learn how to live with cancer. There may be recurrent crisis situations, both physical and psychosocial, but gradually the normlessness first experienced after the cancer diagnosis subsides, and life takes on a somewhat normal, albeit a "new normal," cadence that incorporates the physical, emotional, and spiritual changes catalyzed by the cancer experience (25).

## Problems with Reentry

For many patients, active cancer therapy eventually ends, but the successful end of cancer treatment does not necessarily signal an end to the difficulties and stresses faced by persons with cancer and their family members. The period of waiting to see whether the treatment abated the disease process, and worry about not receiving any active intervention, may create new anxiety and fear (26). The survivor enters what Hurt and her colleagues (27) refer to as "neutral time": a period of remission characterized by uncertainty and lacking in "safety signals" indicating that the disease will not return. At this time, some individuals face an illness-related identity crisis. They may no longer be perceived as cancer "patients" because they are not in active treatment, yet they may have difficulty thinking about themselves as cancer "survivors" or achieving reentry into a "well-role" (11). Another anomic situation, what Maher (24) refers to as "the anomia of good fortune," may occur.

When the concept of anomia is applied to cancer recovery, the positive experience of doing well, perhaps even of being cured, may be mixed with negative elements, including (a) the withdrawal of the intensified social support that accompanied diagnosis and treatment, (b) ambivalence about the discontinuation of treatment, (c) anxiety about recurrence of disease, (d) adjustment to permanent disabilities resulting from the disease or its treatment, (e) the need to resume life-oriented modes of thought after a successful adjustment to the idea of death, (f) anger at perceived inadequacies, or (g) confusion about feelings of depression when the objective situation has improved (24).

Reentry also entails problems with assuming previous roles and responsibilities, and with readjustment and readaptation to daily life (28). The stress of a diagnosis of cancer and its subsequent treatment disrupts the patterns of a lifetime and requires adaptation to personal and interpersonal changes. While active treatment is ongoing, family members frequently assume some of the instrumental, and even emotional, duties of the person with cancer. This redistribution of tasks can have a marked impact on the family unit. When cancer treatment ends, interpersonal relationships may be further strained because the new patterns of interaction and functionality need to be negotiated once again. Another area of reentry that may be of concern for some cancer survivors is rejoining the workforce. The majority of persons with cancer remain actively employed during the treatment phase, but some experience brief or extended absences from work. Returning to work can entail various psychological stresses. There may be a difference in the way the employee is treated by others. Some co-workers may still believe that cancer carries an automatic death sentence and may stigmatize and isolate the returning employee. There may be changes in physical appearance, such as permanent disfigurement from cancer surgery, or temporary changes in appearance, such as hair loss, that initially make the cancer survivor feel insecure and awkward. An added concern may be reduced physical stamina, which makes it difficult to meet the previous work demands and can have an impact on relationships with co-workers.

## Employment Discrimination

Of paramount importance to most survivors is financial stability and the opportunity to retain their jobs during or after therapy. Yet, many who are able and willing to work encounter discrimination by being dismissed or demoted, by having benefits reduced or eliminated, or by experiencing conflict with co-workers because of a lack of understanding, ignorance, or fear about cancer (11,29, 30). Hoffman (30) estimates that approximately 25% of individuals with a history of cancer experience some form of employment discrimination solely on the basis of their medical histories. Health care professionals, as well as cancer survivors, must take action on three levels to combat cancer-based discrimination: individual and group advocacy, public and professional education, and appropriate use of legal remedies (31).

Legal protection against employment discrimination is more readily available for qualified survivors with the recent passage of the Americans With Disabilities Act (ADA). Also, the Federal Rehabilitation Act of 1973 affords limited protection to those survivors whose employers receive federal funds. Most states have laws against discrimination in general, while a few states protect cancer survivors specifically. A major challenge is to test the system and file suit when discrimination is suspected.

## Living with Uncertainty

Reentry may require some compromises on both the personal and the interpersonal levels. The cancer survivor may have to learn to live with physical compromises related to the disease or to the effects of the cancer therapy. Adverse late effects of treatment may not appear for years after the completion of therapy, and the person with a history of cancer has to live with an awareness of the vulnerability associated with delayed treatment effects, recurrence of disease, or susceptibility to a second cancer. Family members also must live with these fears, and overprotectiveness by family members may be an issue after the completion of treatment. Schmale and his colleagues (32) found that 1 year after diagnosis, both survivors and family members were careful about the survivors' activity level, even when there were no obvious physical limitations.

## Maintaining a Positive Future Orientation

For a while after a cancer diagnosis, the future is foreshortened, reduced to the span of time between treatments or between episodes of active disease (24), and frustration and disappointment may occur as a result of

the nonlinear quality of healing (7). Cancer in the family can have a profound negative impact, and yet hopefulness and a positive future orientation are important components for quality of life in cancer survivorship. Hope is a complex concept and often is misunderstood by health care professionals. Much of the reason for this confusion is that health care professionals generally think only in terms of therapeutic hope, i.e., hope that refers to a cure or remission of disease (33). Many other kinds of hope, generalized and particular, are described in the literature.

Farran et al. (34) maintain that hope is a critical clinical construct and provide the following working definition of hope (34):

> Hope constitutes an essential experience of the human condition. It functions as a way of feeling, a way of thinking, a way of behaving, and a way of relating to oneself and one's world. Hope has the ability to be fluid in its expectations, and in the event that the desired object or outcome does not occur, hope can still be present (34).

Staats and Stassen (35) define hope as a cognitive-affective resource that is a psychological asset. The purpose of hope is to guard against despair, and as a coping strategy it can reduce ongoing stress and discomfort quickly and for prolonged periods of time.

Hope is individualistic, and persons have various capacities for hoping and different approaches for maintaining hope. Individual hope is generally influenced by the patterns of hoping within the family (36).

There is a temporal aspect to hope that involves a consideration of the future, and hope changes as situations and circumstances change. Even when hope for survival is dim, individuals will find other things to hope for: pain control, mending strained relationships, or even a dignified death. Disconfirmation of one's hope usually leads to a reformulation of hope, not to its destruction (37).

Cancer survivors need and desire accurate and honest information about their disease, its treatment, and the potential side effects. They need to be aware of problems that they may have to face in the future. If these issues and concerns are presented with compassion and with assurance for continuing support, they can accept even bad news, and new, more realistic goals can be assimilated into the hoping process.

Cancer survivors are challenged to find ways to cope with uncertainty and with maintaining a positive future orientation. The fear of recurrence of cancer and heightened vulnerability may diminish over time, but the consensus is that it never completely goes away (38).

## Survivor Guilt

One additional related aspect of long-term cancer survival deserves special mention. Numerous long-term survivors express guilt over the fact that they have survived when many others have not (39). This may be a particularly salient issue for persons who have been well integrated into a support group and who have watched other members of that group succumb to their disease.

Arthur Frank, in his book *At the Will of the Body*, gives an excellent example of the concept of survivor guilt: "At the same time I was diagnosed as having cancer, a good friend my age also was diagnosed, and my mother-in-law came out of remission again. They both have died. I can make no sense of their deaths and my survival" (1).

Many survivors search for meaning and purpose in their survival and make a renewed commitment to life (40). They also may decide to try to "give something back" in practical and tangible ways. This often includes advocacy efforts on behalf of other survivors.

## Living with Loss

Nothing ever prepares us for the really bad things in life, and loss is an encompassing life theme. Losses are a part of life—we lose loved ones, we lose jobs, we lose chances, and we lose dreams. There are many necessary losses when one has cancer. Some of these losses, like hair loss and loss of fertility, are physical, but emotional losses are associated with cancer as well. For example, cancer survivors may have to learn to live with some limitations, and they may have to alter goals, expectations, and hopes to fit the current after-cancer reality.

Every loss requires a concomitant grief response or some type of mourning, but American society is uncomfortable with grief. Therefore, persons tend to hide their feelings and emotions. A secondary factor is that the person who appears to be coping well relieves others of the burden of support, so hidden grief is reinforced.

Grief, however, cannot be postponed indefinitely. It must reach expression in some way, and hidden grief may be transformed into a variey of emotional responses such as anger, guilt, anxiety, helplessness, or sadness.

The literature on the tasks of mourning is well developed (41,42). These tasks can be summarized as (a) accepting the reality of the loss, (b) experiencing the pain of the grief, (c) adjusting to a changed environment, and (d) emotionally relocating the loss in one's life and moving on.

Perhaps the most important way of helping persons experiencing loss is to "enfranchise" their grief (43). This includes recognizing their right to express emotions and encouraging them to verbalize their feelings and sadness (44). A basic step in helping people live with loss is educating them about the grief process and encouraging them to openly discuss loss issues. Through expression can come emotional healing.

## REDEFINING THE CANCER EXPERIENCE

With an increasing sense of empowerment, survivors are redefining the cancer experience for themselves. For example, the Cancer Survivors' Bill of Rights (see Appendix 67-1) was published in 1988 by the American Cancer Society but was written by a survivor for survivors. It addresses quality of life issues and identifies individual, interpersonal, and social rights to greater care and satisfaction throughout the cancer experience. Also, survivors are requesting—and sometimes demanding—that nonmedical supportive services be an integral part of cancer care and recovery. Many are working on their own to provide support, resources, and education for fellow survivors, while others are working in conjunction with health care institutions to provide these services. Survivors are joining support groups, producing publications, manning telephone hotlines, and sharing information through online services. Others are developing community-based mutual aid networks, are testifying before Congress, and are forming national organizations and coalitions. Advocacy—on personal, community, national, and political levels—has become a major component of the cancer care equation.

## FINDING MEANING

Weil (45) suggests that there is no meaning to cancer—it is simply cancer. The meaning attached to the experience is different for everyone and reflects individual interpretations of the disease, treatments, and circumstances. Formulas or recipes are not enough in the assessment and care of people who are distressed and suffering. Ferrell fears that the concept of quality of life is an endangered species in today's medical and political climate and "may be lost during healthcare reform and amidst what [she has] termed the 'dehumanization' of cancer" (46). In response to this growing concern, the Texas Cancer Council outlined ten Ethical Principles for Cancer Care (see Appendix 67-2) as the moral basis for delivering comprehensive care to people with cancer. Guidelines for action are also delineated in the complete work so that these principles can be put into practice.

The increasing needs, both biomedical and psychosocial, of this expanding population of survivors call for cooperative efforts among the recipients and providers of care, the payors who finance care, the scientists who develop better methods of care, and the politicians who set public policy as to what kind of care will be available to whom. To insure the integrity of our health care system, the mythology of cancer must be dispelled, caring must expand into long-term survival, and attention must be paid to the psychosocial aspects of living with, through, and beyond cancer.

The American Cancer Society presents this Survivors' Bill of Rights to call public attention to survivor needs, to enhance cancer care, and to bring greater satisfaction to cancer survivors, as well as to their physicians, employers, families and friends:

1. Survivors have the right to assurance of lifelong medical care, as needed. The physicians and other professionals involved in their care should continue their constant efforts to be:
   — sensitive to the cancer survivors' lifestyle choices and their need for self-esteem and dignity;
   — careful, no matter how long they have survived, to have symptoms taken seriously, and not have aches and pains dismissed, for fear of recurrence is a normal part of survivorship;
   — informative and open, providing survivors with as much or as little candid medical information as they wish, and encouraging their informed participation in their own care;
   — knowledgeable about counseling resources, and willing to refer survivors and their families as appropriate for emotional support and therapy which will improve the quality of individual lives.
2. In their personal lives, survivors, like other Americans, have the right to the pursuit of happiness. This means they have the right:
   — to talk with their families and friends about their cancer experience if they wish, but to refuse to discuss it, if that is their choice and not to be expected to be more upbeat or less blue than anyone else;
   — to be free of the stigma of cancer as a "dread disease" in all social relations;
   — to be free of blame for having gotten the disease and of guilt for having survived it.
3. In the workplace, survivors have the right to equal job opportunities. This means they have the right:
   — to aspire to jobs worthy of their skills, and for which they are trained and experienced, and thus not to have to accept jobs they would not have considered before the cancer experience;
   — to be hired, promoted, and accepted on return to work, according to their individual abilities and qualifications, and not according to "cancer" or "disability" stereotypes;
   — to privacy about their medical histories.
4. Since health insurance coverage is an overriding survivorship concern, every effort should be made to assure all survivors adequate health insurance, whether public or private. This means:
   — for employers, that survivors have the right to be included in group health coverage, which is usually less expensive, provides better benefits, and covers the employee regardless of health history;
   — for physicians, counselors, and other professionals concerned, that they keep themselves and their survivor-clients informed and up-to-date on available group or individual health policy options, noting, for example, what major expenses like hospital costs and medical tests outside the hospital are covered and what amount must be paid before coverage (deductibles);
   — for social policy makers, both in government and in the private sector, that they seek to broaden insurance programs like Medicare to include diagnostic procedures and treatment which help prevent recurrence and ease survivor anxiety and pain.

Adapted from Spingarn ND. *The cancer survivors' bill of rights.* Atlanta: American Cancer Society, 1988.

**APPENDIX 67-2.** *Ethical principles for cancer care*

I. Since cancer affects a person's entire sense of well- being, cancer care cannot be equated with or limited to prevention, early detection, and treatent of bodily disease. To deal with the effects of cancer, this care should address humans as whole persons with biological, emotional, social, economic, informational, moral, and spiritual needs.
II. Benefiting persons with cancer is the highest priority of health care professionals. Individuals fully benefit when they receive personalized, comprehensive, coordinated, and culturally sensitive care.
III. Patients are to be respected as autonomous, self-governing persons with the right to express their needs and emotions and make informed decisions in their own best interests.
IV. To make informed decisions, patients must be provided with information that is understandable, sufficient, and applicable to their circumstances.
V. Effective communication is essential in order to benefit persons with cancer and respect their autonomy. This communication rests on trust, concern, mutual respect, honesty, and self-awareness.
VI. Terminally ill patients are to receive continued health care, support, respect, and assurance.
VII. Collegial teamwork is essential for attending to the total human dimensions of cancer care.
VIII. Teamwork is sustained by caregiver collegiality, which is based on a mutual understanding of and respect for the individual and professional contributions of colleagues.
IX. The ability of health care professionals to care for patients and those close to the patient depends on caregivers attending to their own personal, psychological, social, moral, and spiritual needs.
X. Basic, clinical, and psychosocial research is integral to improving cancer prevention, early detection, diagnosis, treatment, long-term followup, and the personal dimensions of cancer care. All research should contribute to, not detract from, beneficial and respectful care of individuals with cancer.

From Vanderpool HY, ed. *The human dimensions of cancer care: principles and guidelines for action.* Galveston: The Texas Cancer Council and Institute for the Medical Humanities, The University of Texas Medical Branch at Galveston, 1994. Copyright 1994, Texas Cancer Council.

## REFERENCES

1. Frank AW. *At the will of the body*. Boston: Houghton Mifflin, 1991:8, 137.
2. Lerner M. *Choices in healing*. Cambridge: MIT Press, 1994:14.
3. Sontag S. *Illness as metaphor and AIDS and its metaphors*. New York: Anchor, 1988:19.
4. Leigh S. Myths, monsters, and magic: personal perspectives and professional challenges of survival. *Oncol Nurs Forum* 1992;19:1475.
5. Anderson JG. The deprofessionalization of American medicine. In: Miller G, ed. *Current research on occupations and professions*. Vol 7. Greenwich, CT: JAI Press, 1992:241.
6. Trillin AS. Of dragons and garden peas. *N Engl J Med* 1981;304: 699–700.
7. Mullan F. Survivorship: an idea for everyone. In: Mullan F, Hoffman B, eds. *Charting the journey: an almanac of practical resources for cancer survivors*. Mount Vernon, NY: Consumers Union, 1990:1.
8. Carter B. Going through: a critical theme in surviving breast cancer. *Innov Oncol Nurs* 1989;5:2.
9. Leigh S. Cancer survivorship: a consumer movement. *Semin Oncol* 1994;21:783.
10. Leigh S, Logan C. The cancer survivorship movment. *Cancer Invest* 1991;9:571.
11. Welch-McCaffrey D, Loescher LJ, Leigh SA, Hoffman B, Meyskens F. Surviving adult cancer. Part 2: Psychosocial implications. *Ann Intern Med* 1989;3:517.
12. Gray RE. Persons with cancer speak out: reflections on an important trend in Canadian health care. *J Palliat Care* 1992;8:30.
13. Mullan F. Seasons of survival: reflections of a physician with cancer. *N Engl J Med* 1985;313:270.
14. Hassey-Dow K. The enduring seasons in survival. *Oncol Nurs Forum* 1990;17:511.
15. Koocher G, O'Malley J, eds. *The Damocles syndrome: psychosocial consequences of surviving childhood cancer*. New York: McGraw Hill, 1981.
16. Smith D, Lesko LM. Psychosocial problems in cancer survivors. *Oncology* 1988;2:33.
17. Siegal K, Christ GH. Hodgkins disease survivorship: psychosocial consequences. In: Lacher MJ, Redman JR, eds. *Hodgkins disease: consequences of survival*. Philadelphia: Lea & Febiger, 1990:383.
18. Smith DW. *Survival of illness*. New York: Springer, 1981.
19. Houts PS, Yasko JM, Kahn SB, Schelzel GW, Marconi KM. Unmet psychological, social, and economic needs of persons with cancer in Pennsylvania. *Cancer* 1986;58:2355.
20. Canadian Cancer Society. *Final report on the needs of people living with cancer across Canada*. Toronto: Canadian Cancer Society, 1992.
21. Loescher LJ, Welch-McCaffrey D, Leigh SA, Hoffman B, Meyskens, F. Surviving adult cancer. Part 1: Physiologic effects. *Ann Intern Med* 1989;3:411.
22. Ferrell BR, Dow KH, Leigh S. Quality of life in long-term cancer survivors. *Oncol Nurs Forum* 1995;22:915.
23. Clark E. The role of the social environment in adaptation to cancer. *Soc Work Res Abstr* 1983;19:32.
24. Maher EL. Anomic aspects of recovery from cancer. *Soc Sci Med* 1982; 16:907–911.
25. Harpham WS. *After cancer: a guide to your new life*. New York: WW Norton, 1994.
26. Tross S, Holland JC. Psychological sequelae in cancer survivors. In: Holland JC, Rowland JH, eds. *Handbook of psychooncology*. New York: Oxford University Press, 1990:101.
27. Hurt GJ, McQuellon RP, Darrett RJ. After treatment ends. *Cancer Pract* 1994;2:417.
28. Mullan F. Re-entry: the educational needs of the cancer survivor. *Health Educ Q* 1984;10(suppl):88.
29. Leigh S, Welch-McCaffrey D, Loescher LJ, Hoffman B. Psychosocial issues of long-term survival from adult cancer. In: Groenwald SL, Frogge MH, Goodman M, Yarbro CH, eds. *Cancer nursing: principles and practice*, 3rd ed. Boston: Jones & Bartlett, 1993:484.
30. Hoffman B. Employment discrimination: another hurdle for cancer survivors. *Cancer Invest* 1989;9:589.
31. Hoffman B. *Working it out: your employment rights as a cancer survivor* (booklet). Silver Spring, MD: National Coalition for Cancer Survivorship, 1993.
32. Schmale A, Morrow G, Schmitt M, et al. Well-being of cancer survivors. *Psychosom Med* 1983;45:163.
33. Nuland SB. *How we die*. New York: Alfred A. Knopf, 1993.
34. Farran CJ, Herth KA, Popovich JM. *Hope and hopelesness*. Thousand Oaks, CA: Sage, 1995:6.
35. Staats S, Stassen M. Hope: an affective cognition. *Soc Indicat Res* 1985;17:235.
36. Murphy JB. Managing hope. *Illness, crises and loss* 1991;1(3):46.
37. Callan DB. Hope as a clinical issue in oncology social work. *J Psychosoc Oncol* 1989;7(3):31.
38. Christ G. Psychosocial tasks throughout the cancer experience. In: Stearns NM, Lauria MM, Hermann JF, Fogelberg PR. *Oncology social work: a clinician's guide*. Atlanta: American Cancer Society Inc., 1993:79.
39. Shanfield SB. On surviving cancer: psychological considerations. *Comprehen Psychol* 1980;21(2):128.
40. Maxwell T, Aldredge-Clanton J. Survivor guilt in cancer patients: a pastoral perspective. *J Pastoral Care* 1994;48(1):25.
41. Lindemann E. Symptomatology and management of acute grief. *Am J Psychiatry* 1944;101:141.
42. Worden JW. *Grief counseling and grief therapy: a handbook for the mental health practitioner*. New York: Springer Publishing Co., 1991.
43. Doka KJ. *Disenfranchised grief: recognizing hidden sorrow*. New York: Lexington Books, 1989.
44. Clark E. The rights of the bereaved. In: Kutscher A, Carr AC, Kutscher LG, eds. *Principles of thanatology*. New York: Columbia University Press, 1987:186.
45. Weil A. *Health and healing*. Boston: Houghton Mifflin, 1988.
46. Ferrell BR. To know suffering. *Oncol Nurs Forum* 1993;20:1471.

# Subject Index

# Subject Index